NURSE'S REFERENCE LIBRARY®

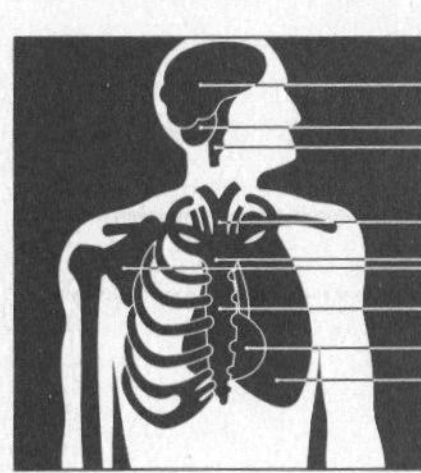

Diseases

Second Edition

Nursing88 Books™
Springhouse Corporation
Springhouse, Pennsylvania

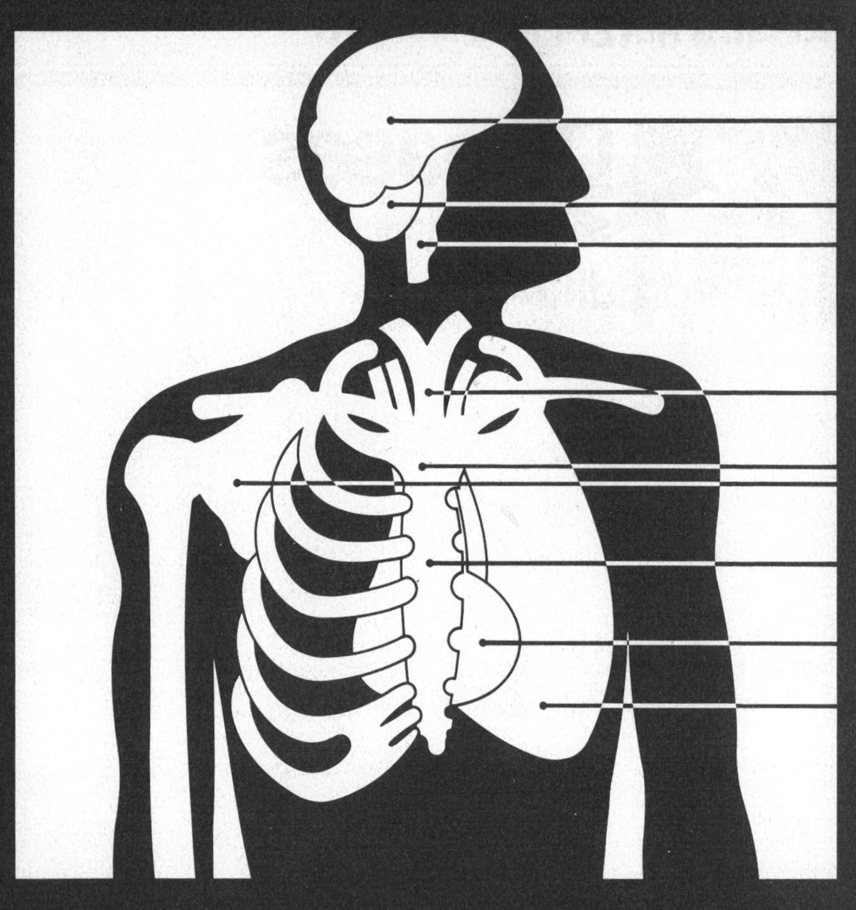

CAUSE	RATE
Leukemia	7.0
Cerebral and other intracranial hemorrhage	6.7
Emphysema	5.7
Congenital anomalies	5.4
Birth trauma, hypoxia, and respiratory distress	2.7
Hypertension	2.5
Peptic and duodenal ulcer	2.2
Hernia and intestinal obstruction	2.2
Rheumatic fever and chronic rheumatic heart disease	2.1
Asthma	1.6
Anemia	1.5
Bronchitis	1.4
Hypertensive heart and renal disease	1.3
Cholelithiasis, cholecystitis, and cholangitis	1.2
Infections of kidney	0.8
Meningitis	0.6
Tuberculosis	0.5
Cerebral embolism	0.4
Appendicitis	0.2
Angina pectoris	0.2
Complications of pregnancy, childbirth	0.1

From the National Center for Health Statistics, *Vital Statistics Report*, Vol. 34, No. 11, February 20, 1986.

Diseases

Second Edition

Nursing88 Books™
Springhouse Corporation
Springhouse, Pennsylvania

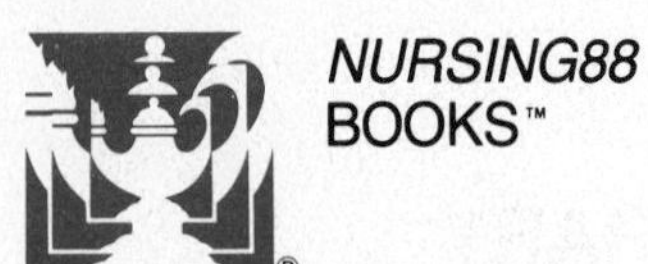

The clinical procedures described and recommended in this publication are based on research and consultation with medical and nursing authorities. To the best of our knowledge, these procedures reflect currently accepted clinical practice; nevertheless, they can't be considered absolute and universal recommendations. For individual application, recommendations must be considered in light of the patient's clinical condition and, before administration of new or infrequently used drugs, in light of latest package-insert information. The authors and the publisher disclaim responsibility for any adverse effects resulting directly or indirectly from the suggested procedures, from any undetected errors, or from the reader's misunderstanding of the text.

First edition published 1981; second edition, 1987

NRL1-020188

Library of Congress Cataloging-in-Publication Data
Diseases.
(Nurse's reference library)
"Nursing87 books."
Includes bibliographies and index.
1. Medicine. 2. Nursing. I. Series. [DNLM: 1. Medicine—nurses' instruction. WB 100 D6112]
RT65.D55 1987 616 86-14396
ISBN 0-916730-95-6

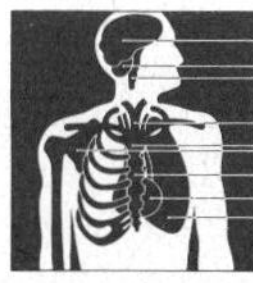

NURSE'S REFERENCE LIBRARY®

Staff for this edition

EDITORIAL DIRECTOR
Helen Klusek Hamilton

CLINICAL DIRECTOR
Barbara F. McVan, RN

ART DIRECTOR
Sonja E. Douglas

Clinical Editor: Joanne Patzek DaCunha, RN, BS

Contributing Clinical Editors: Linda Buschiazzo, RN, CEN; Mary Chapman Gyetvan, RN, BSEd; Robin Castle White, RN, BSN

Acquisitions: Margaret L. Belcher, RN, BSN

Drug Information Manager: Larry Neil Gever, PharmD

Editors: Kevin J. Law, Elizabeth L. Mauro, Nancy J. Priff, Patricia Shinehouse

Editorial Services Manager: David R. Moreau

Copy Editors: Jaclyn A. Bootel, Traci A. Deraco, Mary Teresa Durkin, Nancy K. Gibson, Diane M. Labus, Doris Weinstock

Production Coordinator: Sally Johnson

Designers: Carol Cameron-Sears, Ann Croft, Jacalyn Bove Facciolo, Christopher Laird, Matie Anne Patterson

Art Production: Robert Perry (manager), Donald Knauss, Mark Marcin, Lisa Rich, Louise Stamper, Bob Wieder

Typography: David C. Kosten (manager), Elizabeth DiCicco, Amanda C. Erb, Ethel Halle, Diane Paluba, Nancy Wirs

Production: Deborah C. Meiris (manager), T. A. Landis

Editorial Assistants: Maree DeRosa, Marlene Rosensweig

Indexer: Barbara Hodgson

Researcher: Nancy H. Lange

Special thanks to Marie Connor, Rose Foltz, and Peter Johnson, who assisted in preparation of this volume.

Staff for the preceding edition

EDITORIAL DIRECTOR
Helen Klusek Hamilton

CLINICAL DIRECTOR
Minnie Bowen Rose, RN, BSN, MEd

Senior Editor: Thomas Leibrandt

Associate Editors: Lisa Z. Cohen, Martin DiCarlantonio

Assistant Editors: Laura Albert, William Kelly, Brenda Moyer

Clinical Editors: Joanne Patzek DaCunha, RN; Susan M. Glover, RN, BSN; Lenora Haston, RN, MSN; Patrice Nasielski, RN

Clinical Pharmacy Editor: Larry Gever, PharmD

Production Coordinator: Patricia A. Hamilton

Copy Editors: Linda S. Hewlings, Barbara Hodgson, Jo Lennon

Associate Designer: Kathaleen Motak Singel

Assistant Designer: Christopher Laird

Art Production Manager: Wilbur D. Davidson

Art Assistants: Diane Fox, Sandra Simms, Bob Walsh, Joan Walsh, Ron Yablon

Illustrators: Jean Gardner, Robert Jackson, Thomas Lewis, Cynthia Mason, Kim Milnazik, Richard Oden, Bud Yingling

Typography Manager: David C. Kosten

Typography Assistants: Nancy Merz Ballner, Ethel Halle, Diane Paluba

Production Manager: Robert L. Dean

Editorial Assistants: Maree DeRosa, Helen O'Connor Smith

Indexer: Grinstead/Feik Indexers

Researcher: Vonda Heller

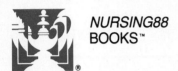

NURSING88 BOOKS™

NURSE'S REFERENCE LIBRARY®

This volume is part of a series conceived by the publishers of *Nursing88®* magazine and written by hundreds of nursing and medical specialists. This series, the NURSE'S REFERENCE LIBRARY, is the most comprehensive reference set ever created exclusively for the nursing profession. Each volume brings together the most up-to-date clinical information and related nursing practice. Each volume informs, explains, alerts, guides, educates. Taken together, the NURSE'S REFERENCE LIBRARY provides today's nurse with the knowledge and the skills that she needs to be effective in her daily practice and to advance in her career.

Other volumes in the series:

Assessment
Diagnostics
Drugs
Procedures
Definitions
Practices
Emergencies
Signs & Symptoms
Patient Teaching
Treatments

Other publications:

NEW NURSING SKILLBOOK™ SERIES

Giving Emergency Care Competently
Monitoring Fluid and Electrolytes Precisely
Assessing Vital Functions Accurately
Coping with Neurologic Problems Proficiently
Reading EKGs Correctly
Combatting Cardiovascular Diseases Skillfully
Nursing Critically Ill Patients Confidently
Dealing with Death and Dying
Managing Diabetes Properly
Giving Cardiovascular Drugs Safely

NURSING PHOTOBOOK™ SERIES

Providing Respiratory Care
Managing I.V. Therapy
Dealing with Emergencies
Giving Medications
Assessing Your Patients
Using Monitors
Providing Early Mobility
Giving Cardiac Care
Performing GI Procedures
Implementing Urologic Procedures
Controlling Infection
Ensuring Intensive Care
Coping with Neurologic Disorders
Caring for Surgical Patients
Working with Orthopedic Patients
Nursing Pediatric Patients
Helping Geriatric Patients
Attending Ob/Gyn Patients
Aiding Ambulatory Patients
Carrying Out Special Procedures
1987 Nursing Photobook Annual

***Nursing88* DRUG HANDBOOK™**

Nursing Yearbook88

NURSE REVIEW™ SERIES

Cardiac Problems
Respiratory Problems
Gastrointestinal Problems
Neurologic Problems
Vascular Problems
Genitourinary Problems
Endocrine Problems
Musculoskeletal Problems
Metabolic Problems
Hematologic Problems

CLINICAL POCKET MANUAL™ SERIES

Diagnostic Tests
Emergency Care
Fluids and Electrolytes
Signs and Symptoms
Cardiovascular Care
Respiratory Care
Critical Care
Neurologic Care
Surgical Care
Medications and I.V.s
Ob/Gyn Care
Pediatric Care
Assessment
Drug Interactions
Documentation

Contents

4 Trauma

5 Immune Disorders

6 Mental and Emotional Disorders

7 Respiratory Disorders

8 Musculoskeletal Disorders

19 Eye Disorders

20 Ear, Nose, and Throat Disorders

21 Skin Disorders

Appendices and Index

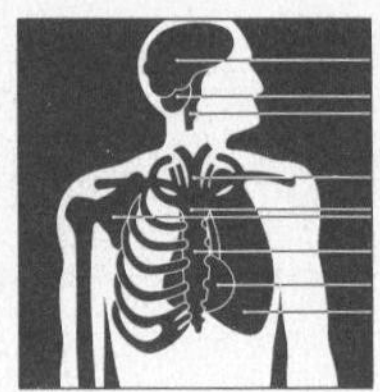

Advisory Board

At the time of publication, the advisors, clinical consultants, and contributors held the following positions.

Lillian S. Brunner, MSN, ScD, Litt D, FAAN, Nurse/Author, Brunner Associates, Inc., Berwyn, Pa.

Donald Charles Cannon, MD, PhD, Resident in Internal Medicine, University of Kansas School of Medicine, Wichita

Luther P. Christman, RN, PhD, Vice-President, Nursing Affairs, and Dean, College of Nursing, Rush–Presbyterian–St. Luke's Medical Center, Chicago

Kathleen Dracup, RN, DNSc, CCRN, FAAN, Associate Professor, UCLA School of Nursing

Stanley J. Dudrick, MD, FACS, Clinical Professor of Surgery, The University of Texas Medical School at Houston/St. Luke's Episcopal Hospital

Halbert E. Fillinger, MD, Forensic Pathologist and Assistant Medical Examiner, Philadelphia

M. Josephine Flaherty, RN, PhD, Principal Nursing Officer, Department of National Health and Welfare, Ottawa

Joyce LeFever Kee, RN, MSN, Associate Professor, College of Nursing, University of Delaware, Newark

Dennis E. Leavelle, MD, Associate Professor and Consultant, Mayo Medical Laboratories, Mayo Clinic, Rochester, Minn.

Roger M. Morrell, MD, PhD, FACP, Diplomate, American Board of Psychiatry and Neurology; Professor, Neurology and Immunology, Wayne State University, Detroit; Chief, Neurology, Veterans Administration Medical Center, Allen Park, Mich.

Ara G. Paul, PhD, Dean, College of Pharmacy, and Professor of Pharmacognosy, University of Michigan, Ann Arbor

Rose Pinneo, RN, MS, Associate Professor of Nursing and Clinician II, University of Rochester (N.Y.)

Thomas E. Rubbert, BSL, LLB, JD, Attorney-at-Law, Pasadena, Calif.

Maryanne Schreiber, RN, BA, Product Manager, Patient Monitoring, Hewlett-Packard Co., Waltham (Mass.) Division

Frances J. Storlie, RN, PhD, CANP, Director, Personal Health Services, Southwest Washington Health District, Vancouver

Claire L. Watson, RN, Clinical Documentation Associate, IVAC Corporation, San Diego

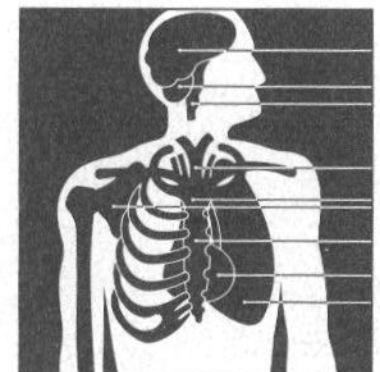

Clinical Consultants

Victoria J. Allen, RN, BSN, Clinical Nurse, National Institutes of Health, Clinical Center, Bethesda, Md.

John P. Atkinson, MD, Head, Division of Rheumatology, and Investigator, Howard Hughes Medical Institute, St. Louis; Professor of Microbiology and Immunology, Washington University School of Medicine, St. Louis

Edmund Martin Barbour, MD, Assistant Clinical Professor of Medicine, Wayne State University, Detroit

Garrett E. Bergman, MD, FAAP, Associate Professor of Pediatrics, Medical College of Pennsylvania, Philadelphia

Barbara Gross Braverman, RN, MSN, CS, Psychiatric Clinical Nurse Specialist, Medical College of Pennsylvania, Philadelphia

Lawrence W. Brown, MD, FAAP, FAAN, Associate Professor of Pediatrics and Neurology, Medical College of Pennsylvania, Philadelphia

A. Bruce Campbell, MD, PhD, Hematologist and Oncologist, Scripps Memorial Hospital, La Jolla, Calif.

G. Carpenter, MD, Associate Professor of Pediatrics, Thomas Jefferson University, Philadelphia

Maribel J. Clements, RN, MA, Clinical Associate, Puget Sound Blood Center, Seattle

Jerome M. Cotler, MD, Professor, Orthopaedic Surgery, Jefferson Medical College of Thomas Jefferson University, Philadelphia

Robert L. Cox, MD, Clinical Consultant, Infectious Diseases, Porter Memorial Hospital, Rose Medical Center, Rocky Mountain Hospital, Denver; Swedish Medical Center, Craig Hospital, Englewood, Colo.

Janie Daddario, RN, MSN, Instructor, Maternal-Child Nursing, Vanderbilt University School of Nursing, Nashville, Tenn.

Patricia I. Dolan, RNC, BSN, Clinical Instructor of Obstetrics and Director of Childbirth Education, Pennsylvania Hospital, Philadelphia

Richard M. Donner, MD, Pediatric Cardiologist and Director, Echo Laboratory, St. Christopher's Hospital for Children, Department of Pediatrics, Temple University School of Medicine, Philadelphia

Brian B. Doyle, MD, Clinical Professor of Psychiatry and of Family and Community Medicine, Georgetown University School of Medicine, Washington, D.C.

Jeanne E. Doyle, RN, BS, Nurse Consultant, Peripheral Vascular Surgery, University Hospital at Boston University Medical Center

Stephen C. Duck, MD, Director, Endocrinology and Metabolism, Medical College of Wisconsin, Milwaukee; Associate Professor of Pediatrics, Milwaukee Children's Hospital

Roland D. Eavey, MD, FAAP, Director, ENT Pediatric Services, and Director, Emergency and Ambulatory Services, Massachusetts Eye and Ear Infirmary, Boston

Diane Erlandson, RN, MS, Clinical Specialist in Rheumatology, Brigham and Women's Hospital, Boston

Richard K. Gibson, RN, MN, JD, Critical Care Nurse, Kaiser Foundation Hospital, San Diego

Sheila Glennon, RN, MA, CCRN, Chief of Critical Care Nursing, Norwalk (Conn.) Hospital

Donald P. Goldsmith, MD, Associate Professor of Pediatrics, Temple University School of Medicine, Philadelphia; Director, Rheumatic Diseases Center, St. Christopher's Hospital for Children, Philadelphia

Marcia Goldstein, RN, BSN, CHN, Nephrology Clinical Nurse Specialist, Albert Einstein Medical Center, Northern Division, Philadelphia

Kathleen D. Groves, RN, MS, Clinical Nursing Instructor, The Johns Hopkins Hospital, Baltimore

Mitchell M. Jacobson, MD, Clinical Professor of Medicine, University of Wisconsin Medical School, Madison; Associate Clinical Professor of Medicine, Medical College of Wisconsin, Milwaukee

Elizabeth Johnstone, RNC, BS, Home Health Nurse, Department of Continuing Care, Dartmouth-Hitchcock Medical Center, Hanover, N.H.

Sande Jones, RN, MS, Inservice Education Coordinator, Mount Sinai Medical Center, Miami Beach, Fla.

William M. Keane, MD, Surgeon, Pennsylvania Hospital, Philadelphia; Assistant Clinical Professor, University of Pennsylvania School of Medicine, Philadelphia

Paul M. Kirschenfeld, MD, Assistant Attending Physician and Co-Director, Medical-Surgical Intensive Care Unit, Atlantic City (N.J.) Medical Center; Private Practice in Pulmonary Diseases and Critical Care Medicine, Absecon, N.J.

Mary Ann Lafferty-Della Valle, PhD, Research Associate, Department of Human Genetics, School of Medicine, and Lecturer, School of Nursing, University of Pennsylvania, Philadelphia

Katherine Lambros, RN, BSN, Clinical Nurse, National Institutes of Health, Clinical Center, Bethesda, Md.

Peter G. Lavine, MD, Director, Coronary Care Unit, Crozer-Chester Medical Center, Chester, Pa.

Harold I. Lief, MD, Professor of Psychiatry, University of Pennsylvania School of Medicine, Philadelphia; Psychiatrist, Pennsylvania Hospital, Philadelphia

Herbert A. Luscombe, MD, Professor and Chairman, Department of Dermatology, Jefferson Medical College of Thomas Jefferson University, Philadelphia

Neil MacIntyre, MD, Assistant Professor of Medicine, Duke University Medical Center, Durham, N.C.

Kenneth J. Mamot, RN, BS, Infection Control Consultant, The Genesee Hospital, Rochester, N.Y.

Linda L. Martin, RN, MSN, Pulmonary Clinical Nurse Specialist, University of Virginia Medical Center, Charlottesville

Margaret E. Miller, RN, MSN, Head and Neck Nurse Coordinator, Illinois Masonic Medical Center, Chicago

Terri Murrell, RN, MSN, Cardiovascular Clinical Nurse Specialist, Scripps Clinic, La Jolla, Calif.

John J. O'Shea, Jr., MD, Chief Medical Staff Fellow, Clinical Immunology Section, Laboratory of Clinical Investigation, National Institute of Allergy and Infectious Diseases, National Institutes of Health, Bethesda, Md.

Linda C. Pachucki, RN, MS, Diabetes Educator, Mount Sinai Medical Center, Milwaukee

Teresa A. Pellino, RN, MS, Director, Division of Education, National Association of Orthopaedic Nurses, Pitman, N.J.; Lecturer, University of Wisconsin, Madison

Frances W. Quinless, RN, PhD, Assistant Professor, Rutgers University College of Nursing, Newark, N.J.

Daniel W. Rahn, MD, Clinical Assistant Professor of Medicine, Yale University School of Medicine, New Haven, Conn.

Barbara Riegel, RN, MN, CS, Cardiovascular Clinical Nurse Specialist, Scripps Clinic and Research Foundation, San Diego

Janice R.J. Salyers, BS, RRT, Assistant Director, Respiratory Care, Duke University Medical Center, Durham, N.C.

Grannum R. Sant, MD, Assistant Professor of Urology, Tufts University School of Medicine, Boston

Joseph A. Scarola, MD, Staff Rheumatologist, Abington (Pa.) Memorial Hospital

Eric Z. Silfen, MD, Staff Physician, Emergency Department, and Clinical Instructor, Departments of Medicine and Emergency Medicine, Georgetown University Hospital, Washington, D.C.

Bryan P. Simmons, MD, Medical Director, Infection Control, Methodist Hospitals of Memphis

Janis B. Smith, RN, MSN, Nurse Consultant in Parent-Child Nursing, Pediatric Intensive Care, and Pediatric Cardiology and Cardiac Surgery, Wilmington, Del.

Brenda M. Splitz, RN, MSN, ANP, Adult Clinical Specialist; Clinical Coordinator, Nurse Practitioner Program; and Adjunct Faculty for Health Care Sciences, George Washington University Hospital, Washington, D.C.

Paul C. Summerell, RN, BSN, Assistant Head Nurse, Medical Intensive Care Unit, Duke University Medical Center, Durham, N.C.

Basia Belza Tack, RN, MSN, ANP, Nursing Consultant, Mountain View, Calif.

Richard W. Tureck, MD, Assistant Professor of Obstetrics and Gynecology, and Coordinator, In Vitro Fertilization/Embryro Transfer Program, University of Pennsylvania School of Medicine, Philadelphia

A. Eugene Washington, MD, MSc, Assistant to the Director, Division of Sexually Transmitted Diseases, Centers for Disease Control, Atlanta

John K. Wiley, MD, FACS, Associate Clinical Professor of Neurosurgery, Wright State University School of Medicine, Dayton, Ohio

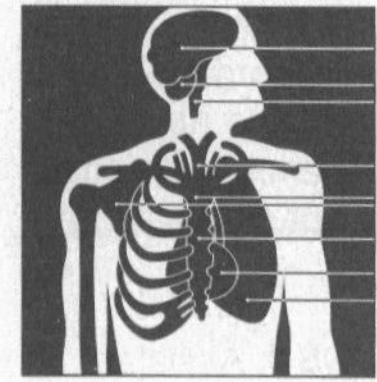

Contributors

Virginia P. Arcangelo, RN, MSN, Instructor, Helene Fuld School of Nursing, Camden, N.J.

Charold L. Baer, RN, PhD, Professor, Department of Adult Health and Illness, The Oregon Health Sciences University School of Nursing, Portland

Katherine G. Baker, RN, MN, Clinical Specialist, UCLA Center for Health Sciences

Ardelina Albano Baldonado, RN, PhD, Assistant Dean and Director, Undergraduate Program, The Marcella Niehoff School of Nursing, Loyola University of Chicago

Cynthia Ashe Beebe, RN, Clinical Gynecologic Oncology Nurse, University of Virginia Medical Center, Charlottesville

Judy Beniak, RN, MPH, Program Director, Continuing Nursing Education, University of Minnesota, Minneapolis

Jo Anne Bennett, RN, MA, CNA, Adjunct Instructor, Lienhard School of Nursing, Pace University, Pleasantville, N.Y.

Patricia M. Bennett, RN, BSN, Unit Teacher, Urology Service, Massachusetts General Hospital, Boston

Margaret Hamilton Birney, RN, MSN, Lecturer, College of Nursing, Wayne State University, Detroit

Nora Lynn Bollinger, RN, MSN, Oncology Clinical Nurse Specialist, Walter Reed Army Medical Center, Washington, D.C.

Heather Boyd-Monk, RN, BSN, Assistant Director for Nursing Education Programs, Wills Eye Hospital, Philadelphia

Hirotaka Katsumata Bralley, RN, BSN, CRNA, Certified Registered Nurse Anesthetist, Cookeville (Tenn.) General Hospital

Barbara Gross Braverman, RN, MSN, CS, Psychiatric Clinical Nurse Specialist, Medical College of Pennsylvania, Philadelphia

Phyllis Bitner Brehm, RN, Medical Oncology Coordinator, Medical College of Pennsylvania, Philadelphia

Christine S. Breu, RN, MN, Research Associate, University of California, Los Angeles

Lillian S. Brunner, MSN, ScD, LittD, FAAN, Nurse/Author, Brunner Associates, Inc., Berwyn, Pa.

Joanne D'Agostino Bryanos, RN, MSN, Former Clinical Nurse Leader, Massachusetts General Hospital, Boston

Lizabeth A. Burke, RN, BSN, CPNP, Nurse Clinician, Children's Hospital of Philadelphia

Judith Suter Burkholder, RN, MSN, Clinical Director, Ambulatory Services, Yale–New Haven (Conn.) Hospital

Barbara J. Burns, RN, BSN, Medical Surgical Instructor, St. Elizabeth Hospital School of Nursing, Utica, N.Y.

Barbara R. Burroughs, RN, MSN, Home Infusion Clinical Nurse Specialist, nmc Homecare, Theranutrix, Delran, N.J.

Priscilla A. Butts, RN, MSN, Lecturer, School of Nursing, University of Pennsylvania, Philadelphia

Mary P. Cadogan, RN, MN, Former Instructor, Community Health Nursing, Yale University School of Nursing, New Haven, Conn.; Former Family Nurse Practitioner, Hill Health Center, New Haven

Linda Pelczynski Cagle, RN, MSN, Vice-President, Dynamedics Inc., St. Louis

G. Carpenter, MD, Associate Professor, Pediatrics, Thomas Jefferson University, Philadelphia

Barbara Walsh Clark, RN, MSN, Former Associate Professor of Nursing, Bucks County Community College, Newtown, Pa.

Constance C. Cooper, RN, Supervisor, Gastroenterology Services, Allegheny General Hospital, Pittsburgh

Susan Corbett, RN, Dermatology Nurse, Skin and Cancer Hospital and Mycosis Fungoides Center of Temple University Hospital, Philadelphia

Pam Cross, BSN, MS, Major, Army Nurse Corps; Clinical Head Nurse; Acute Care Psychiatric Ward, Eisenhower Army Medical Center, Fort Gordon, Ga.

Joanne Patzek DaCunha, RN, BS, Clinical Editor, Springhouse Corp., Springhouse, Pa.

T. Forcht Dagi, MD, FACS, Assistant Professor, Surgery and Anatomy, Georgetown University Hospital, Washington, D.C.

Mary Lou Damiano, RN, BA, ADN, Program Coordinator, Mountain States Regional Hemophilia Center, University of Arizona Health Sciences Center, Tucson

Helen Kline Davis, RN, MSN, Staff Nurse, Labor and Delivery, Thomas Jefferson University Hospital, Philadelphia

Fleda Dean, RN, BSN, AB, Staff Nurse, Yale–New Haven (Conn.) Hospital

Andrea L. Devoti, RN, MSN, CNRN, Nursing Supervisor, The Bryn Mawr (Pa.) Hospital

Stella R. Doherty, RN, MSN, Nursing Services Consultant for Tuberculosis, Commonwealth of Pennsylvania, Pennsylvania Department of Health, Division of Acute Infectious Disease Control, Harrisburg

Judy Donlen, RNC, MSN, Assistant Director of Nursing, Children's Hospital of Philadelphia

Gail D'Onofrio, RN, MS, Critical Care Specialist, Boston

Kathleen Dracup, RN, DNSc, CCRN, FAAN, Associate Professor, UCLA School of Nursing

Diane Dressler, RN, MSN, CCRN, Clinical Nurse Specialist, Midwest Heart Surgery Institute, Milwaukee

Colleen Jane Dunwoody, RN, BA, Clinical Instructor, Nursing Inservice Education, Presbyterian–University Hospital, Pittsburgh

Jeanne Dupont, RN, Staff Nurse, Laconia (N.H.) State School and Training Center

Susan Lynn Earl, RN, BA, Staffing Coordinator, Health Sciences Centre, Winnipeg, Manitoba, Canada

Joan Edmiston-Davis, RN, Critical Care Specialist, Alvarado Medical Center, San Diego

Marjorie M. Eichler, RN, MPH, Health Program Assistant, State of Connecticut Department of Health Services, Hartford

Mary Ellen Florence, RN, PhD, Assistant Professor of Nursing, Stockton State College, Pomona, N.J.

Dawn Flowers, RN, BSN, Staff Nurse (Clinical), National Institutes of Health, Bethesda, Md.

Kathleen T. Flynn, RN, MS, Associate Professor/Clinical Specialists General Surgery, Yale University School of Nursing, Yale–New Haven (Conn.) Hospital

Bernadette M. Forget, RN, MSN, BS, Head Nurse, Dermatology, Yale–New Haven (Conn.) Hospital

Carolyn P. Fritz, RN, BSN, Nurse Consultant—ER, Critical Care Registered Nursing Inc., Holmes, Pa.

Sally S. Gammon, RN, BSN, MS, PCNS, Medical Clinical Nurse Specialist, St. Mary's Hospital, Richmond, Va.

Cathy Garofano, RN, BS, Nurse Specialist in Endocrinology and Diabetes, Senior Instructor in Medicine, Hahneman University Hospital, Philadelphia

Carolyn L. Garson, RN, MSN, PNP/O, Doctoral Student, University of Pennsylvania School of Nursing, Philadelphia

Anna Gawlinski, RN, MSN, CCRN, Cardiovascular Clinical Nurse Specialist, UCLA Medical Center

Mary Lillian "Lillee" Gelinas, RNC, MSN, Director of Nursing, Memorial Hospital of Burlington County, Mount Holly, N.J.

Susan M. Glover, RN, MSN, Educational Services Coordinator, Anne Arundel General Hospital, Annapolis, Md.

Marcia Goldstein, RN, BSN, CHN, Nephrology Clinical Nurse Specialist, Albert Einstein Medical Center, Northern Division, Philadelphia

Christine Grady, RN, MSN, CNS, Clinical Specialist, Immunology, Allergy, and Infectious Disease, National Institutes of Health, Clinical Center, Bethesda, Md.

Carol Ann Gramse, RN, PhD, CNA, Assistant Professor of Nursing, Hunter College–Bellevue School of Nursing, New York

Sherry Pawlak Greifzu, RN, Head Nurse, Acute Medical Oncology Unit, St. Raphael's Hospital–Verdi North, New Haven, Conn.

Donna H. Groh, RN, MSN, Assistant Director of Nursing, Children's Hospital of Los Angeles

Irma Guerra-Ellis, RN, BSN, FNP, PHN Coordinator, National Hansen's Disease Contract Health Services Program, National Hansen's Disease Center, Carville, La.

Mary Lou L. Hamilton, RN, MS, Assistant Professor, University of Delaware, Newark

Rebecca G. Hathaway, RN, MSN, Assistant Director of Nursing, Assistant Clinical Professor, UCLA Medical Center, UCLA School of Nursing

Laura Lucia Hayman, RN, PhD, Chair and Program Director, Nursing of Children, University of Pennsylvania School of Nursing, Philadelphia

Eddie R. Hedrick, BS, MT(ASCP), Manager, Infection Control Department, University of Missouri–Columbia Hospital and Clinics

Constance Ann Henderson, RN, MA, Certified Psychiatric and Mental Health Nurse, Director of Psychiatric Nursing, North Charles General Hospital, Baltimore

Nancy M. Holloway, RN, MSN, CCRN, Critical Care and Emergency Consultant, Nancy Holloway & Associates, Oakland, Calif.

Patricia Turk Horvath, RN, MSN, Corporate Health Programs Coordinator, The Standard Oil Company (Ohio), Cleveland

Mary Kay Hull, RN, BSN, Former Clinical Research Associate, Medical Service Consultants, Inc., Arlington, Va.

Elizabeth Johnstone, RNC, BS, Home Health Nurse, Department of Continuing Care, Dartmouth-Hitchcock Medical Center, Hanover, N.H.

Mary Louise H. Jones, RN, MSN, Nursing Coordinator, Perinatal Center, Florida Hospital Medical Center, Orlando

Karen Joseph, RN, AD, Staff Nurse, Dermatology Unit, Yale–New Haven (Conn.) Hospital

Kathleen Joyce, MSN, Supervisory Clinical Nurse, Nephrology, National Institutes of Health, Clinical Center, Bethesda, Md.

Joyce LeFever Kee, RN, MSN, Associate Professor, College of Nursing, University of Delaware, Newark

Margaret A. Keen, RN, MSN, CNM, Associate Director/Midwifery Service, Kennedy Memorial Hospital–University Medical Center, Turnersville, N.J.

Karen Mabry Kennedy, RN, BSN, Formerly on Staff, Emergency Room, Winter Park (Fla.) Memorial Hospital

Ruth S. Kitson, RN, BAA(N), MBA, Director of Nursing, Critical Care, Toronto Western Hospital

Deborah J. LaCamera, RN, BSN, Nurse Epidemiologist, National Institutes of Health, Clinical Center, Bethesda, Md.

Mary Ann Lafferty-Della Valle, PhD, Research Associate, Department of Human Genetics, School of Medicine, and Lecturer, School of Nursing, University of Pennsylvania, Philadelphia

Cheryl Ann Gross Lane, RN, Former Oncology Nurse Specialist, Bowman Gray School of Medicine of Wake Forest University, Winston-Salem, N.C.

Linda Lass-Schuhmacher, RN, MEd, Adjunct Faculty, Department of Sociology, Suffolk University, Boston

Deborah J. Leisifer, RN, CCRN, Head Nurse, Medical/Surgical Intensive Care, Saint Francis Medical Center, Pittsburgh

Blanche M. Lenard, RN, Nurse Epidemiologist, Crozer-Chester Medical Center, Chester, Pa.

Dorrett N. Linton, RN, AD, Occupational Health Nurse, Rohm and Haas Company, Philadelphia

Patricia A. Lockhart-Pretti, RN, MS, Clinical Nurse Specialist in Neurology/Neurosurgery/Neuro-Rehabilitation, University Hospital, Boston

Pamela Peters Long, RN, BSN, Oncology Program Administrator and Clinical Coordinator, South Fulton Hospital, East Point, Ga.

Kenneth J. Mamot, RN, BS, Infection Control Consultant, The Genesee Hospital, Rochester, N.Y.

Joan Kern Manny, RN, Clinical Nurse, National Institutes of Health, Bethesda, Md.

Shirley Heaton Marshburn, RN, BSN, Assistant Director of Nursing, Hamad General Hospital Corporation, Doha Qatar, Arabian Gulf

Linda L. Martin, RN, MSN, Pulmonary Clinical Nurse Specialist, University of Virginia Medical Center, Charlottesville

Celestine B. Mason, RN, BSN, MA, Associate Professor, Pacific Lutheran University, Tacoma, Wash.

Donna McCarthy, RN, PhD, Post Doctoral Fellow, School of Nursing, University of Rochester (N.Y.)

Mary R. McCole, RN, BSN, Nurse Manager–Critical Care, Albert Einstein, Northern Division, Philadelphia

Edwina A. McConnell, RN, MS, Independent Nurse Consultant; Staff Nurse, Madison (Wis.) General Hospital

Joan P. McNamara, RN, I.V. Nurse Therapist, Abington (Pa.) Memorial Hospital

Vivian Meehan, RN, BA, Nurse Clinician for Eating Disorders Program, Highland Park (Ill.) Hospital; President and Founder, National Association for Anorexia Nervosa and Associated Disorders, Highland Park

Rita V. Miller, RN, BA, Former Nurse Manager, Presbyterian–University of Pennsylvania Medical Center, Philadelphia

M. Leslie Mitman, RN, BSN, Formerly on Staff, Thomas Jefferson University Hospital, Philadelphia

Marilee Warner Mohr, RN, MSN, Supervisor, Women and Children Division, The Bryn Mawr (Pa.) Hospital

Anna P. Moore, RN, BSN, MS, Assistant Professor, Coordinator of Psychiatric Mental Health Nursing, Petersburg (Va.) General Hospital School of Nursing

Brenda M. Nevidjon, RN, MSN Cancer Program Manager, Providence Medical Center, Seattle

Elaine H. Niggemann, RN, MD, Fellow, Division of Cardiology, Southwestern Medical School, Dallas

John J. O'Shea, Jr., MD, Chief Medical Staff Fellow, Clinical Immunology Section, Laboratory of Clinical Investigation, National Institute of Allergy and Infectious Diseases, National Institutes of Health, Bethesda, Md.

Mary Beth Lyman Pais, RN, BSN, MNEd, Head Nurse, Orthopaedics and Arthritis Rehabilitation, Presbyterian–University Hospital, Pittsburgh

A. June Partyka, RN, ET, Rehabilitation Nurse Coordinator, St. Francis Medical Center, Trenton, N.J.

Christene Perkins, RN, MN, Chairperson, Department of Nursing, Kettering (Ohio) College of Medical Arts

Adele W. Pike, RN, MSN, Clinical Nurse, National Institutes of Health, Clinical Center, Bethesda, Md.

Patricia Hogan Pincus, RN, MS, Technical Associate, University of Rochester (N.Y.) Medical Center; Infection Control Consultant, Hill Haven Nursing Home and Health Related Facility, Webster, N.Y.

Rosemary Carol Polomano, RN, MSN, CS, Oncology Clinical Specialist, Hospital of the University of Pennsylvania, Philadelphia

Katherine S. Puls, RN, MS, CNM, Nurse Midwife in Private Practice, Women's Alternative Health Care of Barrington (Ill.), Ltd.

Jo-Ellen Quinlan, RN, MSN, Gastrointestinal Nurse Clinician, Children's Hospital, Boston

Roger L. Ready, RN, CNA, Nurse Endoscopist, Mayo Clinic, Rochester, Minn.

Hazel V. Rice, RN, MS, EdS, Associate Chairman, Southern College of SDA, Orlando, Fla.

Marilyn A. Roderick, RN, BSN, MD, Physician, General Practice, Redwood City, Calif.

Lisa Sehrt Rodriguez, RN, BSN, Staff Development Coordinator, Alton Ochsner Medical Foundation Hospital, New Orleans

Mary E. Ropka, RN, MS, Doctoral Student, University of Virginia, Charlottesville

Pamela M. Rowe, RN, BSN, MEd, Assistant Director of Nursing Education, Dartmouth-Hitchcock Medical Center, Hanover, N.H.

Sherrill Jantzi Rudy, RN, BSN, Pediatric Dermatology, Children's Hospital of Pittsburgh

Sarah A. Ryan, RN, Nurse Epidemiologist, Crozer-Chester Medical Center, Chester, Pa.

Linda Patti Sarna, RN, MN, Assistant Clinical Professor, UCLA School of Nursing

Karen Moore Schaefer, RN, MSN, Assistant Professor in Nursing, Cedar Crest College, Allentown, Pa.

Sandra Schuler, RN, MSN, Assistant Professor of Nursing, Montgomery College, Takoma Park, Md.

Marilyn R. Shahan, RN, MS, Nurse Epidemiologist, Denver Department of Health and Hospitals, Disease Control Service

Susan Budassi Sheehy, RN, MSN, CEN, Assistant Director/Trauma Service, St. Joseph Hospital, Tacoma, Wash.; Associate Clinical Professor, University of Washington School of Nursing, Seattle

Charlotte Shields, RN, BSN, Outreach Nurse Coordinator, Comprehensive Pediatric Rheumatology Center, Children's Hospital National Medical Center, Washington, D.C.

Jean A. Shook, RN, MS, CS, Psychiatric Clinical Nurse Specialist, Medical College of Pennsylvania, Philadelphia

Frances "Billie" Sills, RN, MSN, ARNP, Assistant Administrator, Nursing, The Institute for Rehabilitation and Research, Houston

Christine McNamee Smith, RN, BSN, Nurse Clinician, Thomas Jefferson University Hospital, Philadelphia

Janis B. Smith, RN, MSN, Nurse Consultant in Parent-Child Nursing, Pediatric Intensive Care, and Pediatric Cardiology and Cardiac Surgery, Wilmington, Del.

Sandra J. Somma, RN, BSN, Head Nurse. Department of Dermatology, Yale–New Haven (Conn.) Hospital

Brenda M. Splitz, RN, MSN, ANP, Adult Clinical Specialist; Clinical Coordinator, Nurse Practitioner Program; and Adjunct Faculty for Health Care Sciences, George Washington University Hospital, Washington, D.C.

Charlene Wandel Stanich, RN, MN, Associate Vice-President, Medical Nursing, Presbyterian–University Hospital, Pittsburgh

June L. Stark, RN, BSN, CCRN, Critical Care Instructor, Renal Nurse Consultant, New England Medical Center, Boston

Janice G. Stewart, RN, MSN, Manager of Nursing Support Resources, Thomas Jefferson University Hospital, Philadelphia

Frances J. Storlie, RN, PhD, CANP, Director, Personal Health Services, Southwest Washington Health District, Vancouver

Nancy S. Storz, RD, EdD, Adjunct Assistant Professor, University of Pennsylvania School of Nursing, Philadelphia

Mona R. Sutnick, RD, EdD, Nutrition Consultant, Sutnick Associates, Philadelphia; Lecturer in Community and Preventive Medicine, Medical College of Pennsylvania, Philadelphia

Basia Belza Tack, RN, MSN, ANP, Nursing Consultant, Mountain View, Calif.

Janet D'Agostino Taylor, RN, MSN, Program Director, Comprehensive Pulmonary Care Program, St. Elizabeth's Hospital, Brighton, Mass.

Maureen K. Toal, RN, BSN, Staff Nurse, Critical Care Unit, Sacred Heart Medical Center, Chester, Pa.

Sharon McBride Valente, RN, MN, CS, FAAN, Adjunct Assistant Professor, University of Southern California, Department of Nursing, Los Angeles; Clinical Specialist in Mental Health in Private Practice, Los Angeles

Susan VanDeVelde-Coke, RN, MA, MBA, Director of Nursing, Health Sciences Centre, Winnipeg, Manitoba, Canada

Mary Mishler Vogal, RN, MSN, CHN, Course Coordinator and Instructor, Helene Fuld School of Nursing, Camden, N.J.

Peggy L. Wagner, RN, MSN, CCRN, Cardiovascular Clinical Nurse Specialist, St. Michael Hospital, Milwaukee

Madeline Wake, RN, MSN, Administrator, Continuing Education in Nursing, Marquette University, Milwaukee

Connie A. Walleck, RN, MS, CNRN, Clinical Nurse Supervisor/Clinical Nurse Specialist, Neuro Trauma Center, Maryland Institute of Emergency Medical Services Systems, Baltimore

Joanne Schlosser Ware, RN, CCRN, Head Nurse, Progressive Care Unit, Martin Memorial Hospital, Stuart, Fla.

Joseph B. Warren, RN, BSN, Territory Manager/Neurosurgical Nurse Consultant, Kinetic Concepts, San Antonio, Tex.

Juanita Watson, RN, MSN, Director, Department of Continuing Education, Saint Agnes Medical Center, Philadelphia

Rosalyn Jones Watts, RN, EdD, Associate Professor of Nursing, University of Pennsylvania, Philadelphia

Terri E. Weaver, RN, MSN, CS, Pulmonary Clinical Nurse Specialist, Hospital of the University of Pennsylvania, Philadelphia; Clinical Instructor, University of Pennsylvania School of Nursing, Philadelphia

Erma L. Webb, RN, MS, Assistant Professor, Southern College of SDA, Orlando, Fla.

Joanne F. White, RN, MNEd, Associate Dean, School of Nursing, Duquesne University, Pittsburgh

Barbara A. Wojtklewicz, RNC, BSN, Former Adult Nurse Practitioner, Martha Eliot Health Center/Children's Hospital Medical Center, Jamaica Plain, Mass.

Hilary A. Wood, RN, SCM, Director, Cancer Treatment Center, Bethesda Hospital, Inc., Cincinnati

Gayle L. Ziegler, RN, MSN, Senior Research Assistant, University of Pittsburgh School of Medicine

Mary R. Zimmerman, RN, BSN, MS, Director of Nursing, Madison (Wis.) General Hospital

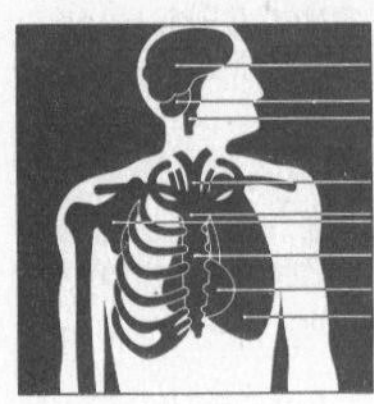

Foreword

Two dramatic changes in patient care have taken place this past year that directly affect nurses and nursing care: hospitalized patients are more acutely ill, requiring more concentrated and intensive nursing in a shorter time; and hospital patients are being discharged earlier and are therefore sicker than they used to be when moved to a step-down-care facility, a nursing home, or their own homes.

And our clients/patients are increasingly knowledgeable about health care: more consumers are maintaining good body care, recognizing early symptoms, and changing undesirable life-styles; and, when illness occurs, they are seeking second, even third, opinions before consenting to treatment. They want to know the latest technological diagnostic and treatment methods; after hospitalization, they expect concise and complete instructions on what to do to facilitate recovery, to recognize untoward signs and symptoms, and to achieve and maintain optimum well-being.

Over and above these changes, the continual stream of expanded technologies, better laboratory analyses, new drugs, and the latest research findings are adding to the volume of medical and nursing information.

To deal with these changes, nurses must have an expanding knowledge base that is current and available. You will need to sharpen your assessment skills, such as making an accurate observation, taking an informative nursing history, performing a useful physical examination, and even developing a nursing diagnosis. You will need to know what is generally accepted in treating a particular disease. What complications are likely and how can they be prevented, minimized, or managed? What are the essential elements of a good nursing care plan to facilitate the patient's recovery? What does the patient need to know to promote his recovery and prevent recurrence of his medical problem? Have the initial goals developed into expected outcomes?

DISEASES, the first volume in the Nurse's Reference Library, provides you with this information. An invaluable reference source for the practicing nurse, DISEASES includes over 600 entries—each complete in itself—on virtually every major disease and an appendix that summarizes characteristics, causes, and treatments of more than 160 rare disorders. Written by a nurse or another health care specialist, each entry presents current clinical information about a disease and emphasizes relevant nursing aspects.

The book divides the discussion of diseases into two major sections. Section I (chapters 1 through 6) deals with disorders that affect the whole body, such as immune disorders and neoplasms. Section II (chapters 7 through 21) covers diseases that primarily affect a specific body system, such as cardiovascular, gastrointestinal, renal, and dermatologic disorders. Each chapter begins with an *Introduction* that summarizes general considerations and normal anatomy and physiology, enabling you to review normal function before considering the abnormal. The introduction also summarizes relevant assessment procedures.

Each entry that follows the introduction begins with a concise definition of the disease, often including incidence and prognosis. The entry continues with a brief summary of *Causes* and, when appropriate, pathophysiology. Next, a section called *Signs and symptoms* details the disease's expected clinical effects. *Diagnosis* follows, summarizing the clinical findings and special tests that confirm, suggest, or support the presence of the disease. Tests that unequivocally confirm a diagnosis are graphically highlighted.

The next section, *Treatment,* covers therapy, including surgery, and summarizes complications. Ominous clinical changes that signal the onset of life-threatening deterioration in the patient's condition are also graphically highlighted. Finally, the section on *Special considerations,* another distinctive feature, lists relevant nursing actions to help you formulate a comprehensive care plan.

When appropriate, each entry includes information on patient teaching, rehabilitation, and prevention. Charts, anatomic drawings, and illustrations clarify and amplify the text; carefully selected marginalia emphasize useful supplementary information. For example, in the chapter on neoplastic diseases, most entries offer guidelines for recognizing the clinical stages of a specific neoplasm.

I am convinced you will find DISEASES an invaluable resource and a worthwhile addition to your library. Properly used, it can help you untangle the complexities of the disease process and can enable you to plan patient care more skillfully, confidently, and effectively.

—LILLIAN S. BRUNNER, MSN, SCD, LITT D, FAAN
Coauthor of the *Textbook of Medical-Surgical Nursing* and *The Lippincott Manual of Nursing Practice*

Overview

Disease: The twilight process

Definitions of health and disease are easy to come by, but hard to live with. In most cases, they're concrete statements drawn from highly fluid abstractions—private beliefs and prejudices, religion and folklore—and only occasionally from rational thought and scientific evidence.

Not too long ago, health was understood to be simply the absence of disease—a definition we now realize is unrealistic. Even more utopian is the concept that health is a state of absolute physical, mental, and social well-being. Recent proof of the long-term gestation of chronic disease renders one part of this notion obsolete, and if health depended on perfect mental and social equanimity, it would be an even rarer commodity than it already is.

The fact is that health and disease are parallel dimensions in the life of every human being, overlapping and intermingling in such a way as to defy precise definition.

Consider the individual who's fully recovered from a myocardial infarction. He takes no medication, observes only minimal restrictions in his diet and daily activities, appears perfectly healthy in every respect—yet he does have heart disease. Do you interrupt this man in the middle of a red-hot tennis game to tell him he's sick? Or is he again healthy?

A hemophiliac may strike most of us as being far from healthy. But what it means to be healthy and what it means to be sick are concepts so colored by one's personal perceptions that many who are physically or mentally impaired—if they're able to function in what, for them, is a normal manner—may consider themselves in perfect health. And who can argue with them?

Disease, in other words, is often a twilight process—capable of flagrant and awful destruction, but just as likely to lapse into remission—during which the individual is neither totally healthy nor totally sick. As nurses, we must take this less starry-eyed view of the disease process into account, recognize the myriad factors that can cause the process to begin, and above all, strive to prevent it from getting started in the first place.

Environment: The inescapable factor

A thoroughly pragmatic examination of health and disease begins by considering human beings in relation to environment. Human interaction with environment starts at conception and continues throughout life until the very moment of death, clearly influencing health and disease in many ways. To simplify matters, we'll distinguish between internal and external environmental factors, noting, however, that no part of a person's environment can be strictly divorced from any other aspect.

Genetic endowment, familial tendency, and personal predisposition appear to be the primary determinants of *internal environment*. The line between genetic endowment and familial tendency is fine but real. Scientific proof firmly supports the existence of genetic defects, such as muscular dystrophy, Down's syndrome, and many forms of mental retardation, while theories of familial tendency stand on less solid ground. Nevertheless, familial tendency can be defined as the apparent inclination of family members to acquire the same disease.

By personal predisposition, we mean certain physical and psychological traits that seem to characterize the majority of persons with a particular disease. Men with Type A behavior patterns (success-oriented, hard-driving), for example, are said to run a greater risk of having myocardial infarctions than those with Type B patterns (placid, easy-going). A link may also exist between personality and somatic disorders such as ulcers and colitis.

Only recently have the destructive effects of *external environment* on health become clear. Pure food, clean water, and fresh air are treasures to be cherished in our highly mobile, heavily industrialized society. At one time the burning environmental issue of the day was sewage treatment versus septic tanks. Now we must find safer ways to dispose of all sorts of deadly environmental debris—gases, chemicals, and nuclear waste.

Today, entire populations may develop eye problems, hearing disorders, lung diseases, or cancer simply because of where they live or work. Occupational diseases caused by handling or breathing coal, asbestos, or wheat dust and various chemical sprays are becoming commonplace. Unfortunately, not all of us can escape such hazards by altering our life-styles or moving to healthier environments. The well-to-do may find it feasible, but poverty traps countless others—coal-mining families, migrant workers and their children—forcing them to live under perilous conditions.

Food poisoning could once be traced rather easily to bacterial contamination during preparation or storage. Today, the widespread use of preservatives in commercially prepared foods raises more complex health questions. How much of a chemical preservative is it safe to use? How can we monitor the long-term effects of preservatives?

The scarcity of scientific data from human populations hampers researchers and restricts our role in this area. Many of us feel unqualified to evaluate the available information; we hesitate to suggest limits to those seeking advice. All too often we ourselves are trying to decide whether to stop using hair dryers, to start buying bread with no preservatives, or to give up sugar.

Knowledge of genetic aberrations, family history, personal inclination, and the impact of external environment on health allows us to screen patients more effectively for disease. Our role can only broaden as we perfect our skills in history-taking and physical assessment, as we become more sensitive to the need for providing emotional support, and as we learn more about cue syndromes—unique clusters of signs and symptoms indicative of specific disease states—and the disease process in general.

Pathogenesis: The imperfect science

Pathogenesis—the process of tracing the history of a disease from its inception—is hardly a simple matter. Many intermediate factors that contribute to disease never come to light. Elevated blood cholesterol, hypertension, and cigarette smoking, for example, are the primary risk factors in heart disease, according to the American Heart Association. Yet these same factors don't figure at all in more than half the cases of coronary artery disease.

In short, pathogenesis is an imperfect science, which makes our role in screening and referral all the more important.

Disease usually begins in one of two ways: either a pathogen invades a person whose resistance to that particular pathogen has decreased, as a result of a breakdown in the body's homeostatic mechanisms, the integrity of the skin or other body organs, or the entire reticuloendothelial system; or a person, perhaps in perfect health, comes in contact with an unusually toxic pathogen (rabies virus or heavy smoke, for example).

Multisystem diseases occur, of course, but most illnesses are limited in scope and time. Renal disease, treated early, can be controlled; the cardiovascular, pulmonary, and endocrine systems may remain unimpaired for years. Pneumonia, appendicitis, and acute infectious diseases last only so long. In most cases, the disease runs its course; signs and symptoms eventually abate.

During our initial contact with patients, we should define the scope and expected duration of their illnesses, since for most people these factors indicate the gravity of a disease. Our patients will be anxious and troubled until we answer their questions in terms they can understand.

Pathogens such as viruses and bacteria represent readily identifiable *physiologic stressors*, directly linked to disease. However, other kinds of stressors—loud noise, for example—affect physiologic functions as well as attitudes and feelings. Noise above 70 decibels triggers a predictable response from the sympathetic nervous system. Cardiac rate changes, respirations increase, and blood pressure may rise, but the point at which loud noise can consistently raise blood pressure and sustain hypertension until symptoms of heart disease appear is not clear. Research has linked noise exposure to elevated blood cholesterol in animals, but we can't say for certain that the same thing happens in humans. We can only say that noise may contribute to the development of cardiac disease in some people.

The same is true of *psychological stress* and its concomitant emotions of anger, worry, bitterness, and anxiety. While health-care professionals find it hard to define stress precisely, most people have no trouble recognizing it in their daily lives. So many things can cause it—loss of a job, disaffection for a spouse, death of a loved one, financial problems. We say that people in the Western civilization live under greater stress than their more contemplative Eastern counterparts, that city folks pursue a more stressful existence than their country cousins. We often evaluate one another by our ability to "handle" stress, naively prizing the appearance of being at harmony with the world and oneself despite adversity.

The energy needed to maintain such outward calm, to create the illusion of coping successfully with life in the eyes of others, may exact a heavy toll. We know that stressful physical, psychologic, and symbolic stimuli can—separately or in concert—elicit a physiologic response from the body.

Such a response, however, cannot be elicited indefinitely; at some point, disease begins.

In most cases, we can identify physiologic stressors and weaken their effect by altering the patient's environment or by attenuating his reaction to the stressor. We may advise a patient with cardiac disease, for example, to find a new house or apartment so he won't have to climb flights of stairs. In addition, we may instruct him to take medication, such as digitalis, to strengthen his heart's contractions. Both approaches represent viable nursing interventions.

But how can we help patients cope with psychological stress? Providing sound health information, taking the time to teach the facts about this more subtle form of stress, is perhaps the most important contribution we can make.

Moreover, we must learn to emphasize the positive aspects of dealing with stress. Don't tell your patient what he stands to *lose* if he doesn't learn to cope with stress intelligently and maturely; tell him what he stands to *gain*—a fuller and more bountiful life—if he does learn to cope.

Health expectations: The new emphasis

As Diagnosis-Related Groups (DRGs) gain in popularity, more patients will feel the effects of restricted hospital stays and medical cost reductions. The result? Patients will wait to seek medical attention. They'll be more acutely ill when they enter the hospital—and when they leave. Many of them will choose alternatives to prolonged hospital stays, such as ambulatory care, extended care, home health care, or treatment in hospices or self-care units. Clearly, the DRGs will change the health care system dramatically, as well as the public's view of it.

Because of these changes, which have already begun, prevention and health education have become as important as treatment, if not more so. Today, people don't want a good doctor—or a good nurse—so much as they want to avoid getting sick in the first place.

This change in the public's perception of health and disease has created disturbing repercussions throughout the health care system in the United States. Interest has shifted so dramatically from sickness to "wellness," from medical cure to healthful living, that we can no longer ignore a corresponding shift in society's expectations of its members entrusted with health care. This provocative new emphasis underlies the philosophy behind health maintenance organizations (HMOs), proliferating group cooperatives which hold that health and well-being are better served through education and prevention than through attempts to treat disease.

Because these organizations are regulated by the Department of Health and Human Services, the extent of our participation is subject to guidelines. But as a matter of practice, we enjoy great flexibility in their day-to-day functioning. If the stated goal of HMOs—to provide quality health care at the lowest possible cost—is to be realized, we must play a more active role in the future.

The hard fact is that socioeconomic status, a measure of affluence, often determines the amount and quality of health care that people seek for themselves and their families in the United States. The poor visit a doctor only when symptoms become acute. A migrant worker explained his reason for not seeing a doctor: "I wasn't bleeding anywhere and I didn't even have a temperature." This man was experiencing constant but subdued pain, which was later attributed to cancer.

Our responsibility to the public has never been greater, nor has it ever been under more intense scrutiny. DRGs require us to give quality care in less time for less money. Our expanded role in the health care system calls for advanced knowledge of health and disease. We can no longer rely on "basic training" to see us through because, in most cases, that training did not cover the in-depth anatomy, physiology, and pharmacology required for today's responsibilities. Nor did it offer sufficient understanding of cue syndromes or vital skills, such as auscultation, palpation, percussion, and inspection.

Fortunately, most of us want to acquire the knowledge and skills necessary to serve our patients in the most effective way. Understanding health and disease in the context of both internal and external environments is one step toward this goal. Shifting the focus of our professional care from merely treating disease to advocating healthful living is another direction in which we must begin to move.

With these goals firmly in mind, and with proper dedication and discipline, we can act as indispensable catalysts to far-reaching change.

—FRANCES J. STORLIE, RN, PhD, CANP

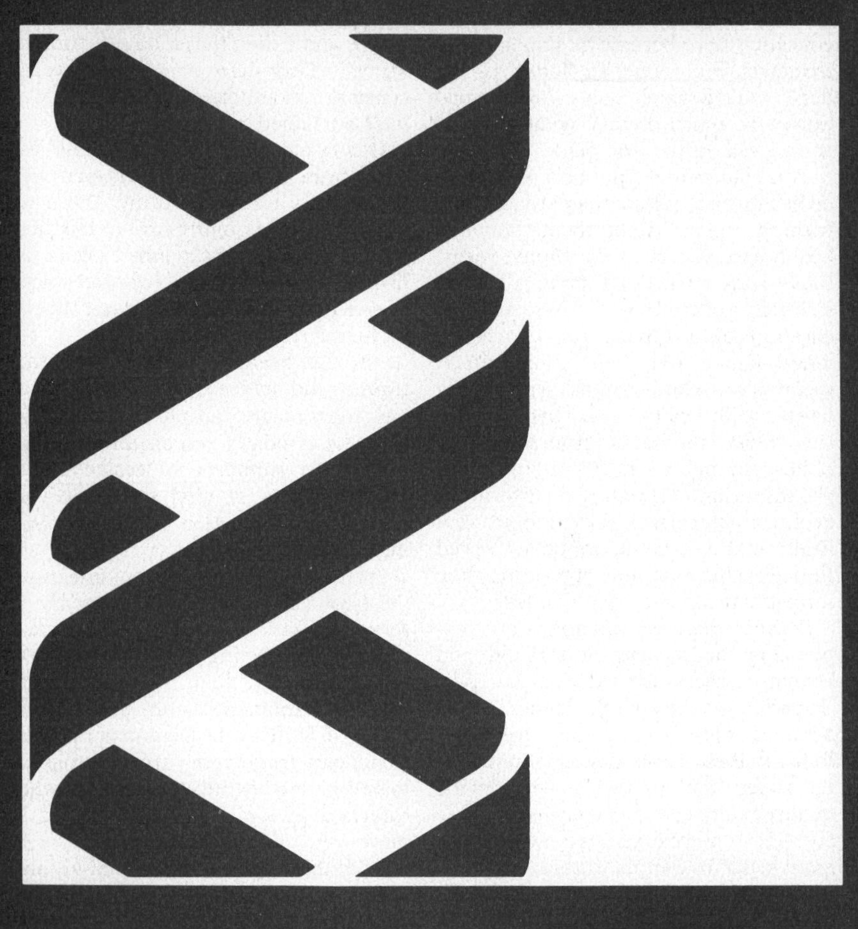

1 Genetic Disorders

Genetic Disorders

Introduction

Genetic diseases result from single gene (mendelian) substitutions, chromosome abnormalities, or multifactorial (polygenic) errors. Well over 2,000 such abnormalities have been identified in humans, ranging from mild differences (as in certain hemoglobin abnormalities) to fatal or overwhelmingly disabling conditions, such as Down's syndrome (trisomy 21). In the United States alone approximately 200,000 infants are born each year with an overt genetic abnormality. Such abnormalities account for up to 20% of all pediatric hospital admissions and at least 10% to 20% of all stillbirths and neonatal deaths.

Although genetic disorders are determined entirely by a person's genetic makeup and, as such, are unchangeable throughout life, they can and do interact with environmental factors. For example, albinism (an inherited inability to generate the protective pigment melanin) greatly increases susceptibility to skin cancer after excessive exposure to sunlight.

Pedigree analysis

Genetics, the study of heredity, uses pedigree (family tree) analysis, karyotypic (chromosomal) analysis, and biochemical analysis of blood, urine, or body tissues to unravel the effects and patterns of inheritance. With the resulting increased understanding of heredity, genetic influences are likely to assume greater importance in health care delivery as time goes by.

The essential ingredient of heredity is *DNA* (deoxyribonucleic acid), which makes up *genes* (basic units of hereditary material) that are arranged into threadlike organelles called *chromosomes* in the cell nucleus. Together, these contribute to a person's genotype and phenotype (genetic and physical makeup). In humans, each body cell (except ova and sperm) has 46 chromosomes arranged in 23 pairs. One such pair is the sex chromosomes: females have a matched (homologous) pair of X chromosomes; males, an unmatched (heterologous) pair, an X and a Y. Thus, the normal human chromosome complement is 46,XX in females and 46,XY in males. The remaining 22 chromosome pairs (autosomes) are all homologous.

The position that the gene for a given trait occupies on a chromosome is called a *locus*. Different loci exist for hair color, blood group, and so on. The number and arrangement of the locus on homologous chromosomes are the same. A different form of the same gene that occupies a corresponding locus on a homologous chromosome is called an *allele* and determines alternative (and inheritable) forms of the same characteristic. Some alleles control normal trait variation, such as hair color; other defective alleles may cause a congenital defect or even induce abortion. Both heterologous (co-dominant) alleles may express their own effects, or one (the dominant allele) may be expressed and the other (the recessive) suppressed.

A mutation—a permanent, inheritable change in a gene—may cause serious,

PATTERNS OF TRANSMISSION IN GENETIC DISORDERS

- **Autosomal recessive**
  Hartnup disease
  Xeroderma pigmentosum
  Congenital afibrinogenemia
  Congenital virilizing adrenal hyperplasia
  Fabry's disease
  Galactosemia
  Niemann Pick disease
  Retinitis pigmentosa
  Thalassemia
  Cystic fibrosis
  Tay-Sachs disease
  Cystinuria
  Cretinism
  Phenylketonuria
  Albinism
  Fanconi's syndrome
  Sickle cell anemia

- **Chromosomal**
  Turner's syndrome
  Trisomy 13
  Trisomy 18
  Down's syndrome (trisomy 21)
  Klinefelter's syndrome
  Hermaphroditism
  Cri du chat syndrome

- **Autosomal dominant**
  Achondroplastic dwarfism
  Colorectal polyposis
  Familial nonhemolytic jaundice
  Renal glycosuria
  Spherocytosis
  Pituitary diabetes insipidus
  Hyperlipidemias
  Neurofibromatosis
  Huntington's chorea
  Osteogenesis imperfecta
  Retinoblastoma
  Marfan's syndrome
  Hereditary hemorrhagic telangiectasia

- **X-linked**
  Some immunodeficiencies
  Pseudohypoparathyroidism
  G 6-PD deficiency
  Hemophilia
  Duchenne-type muscular dystrophy

- **Multifactorial**
  Rheumatoid arthritis
  Diabetes mellitus (some cases)
  Congenital heart anomalies
  Neural tube anomalies
  Mental retardation (some cases)
  Cleft lip/palate

DNA AND HOW IT WORKS

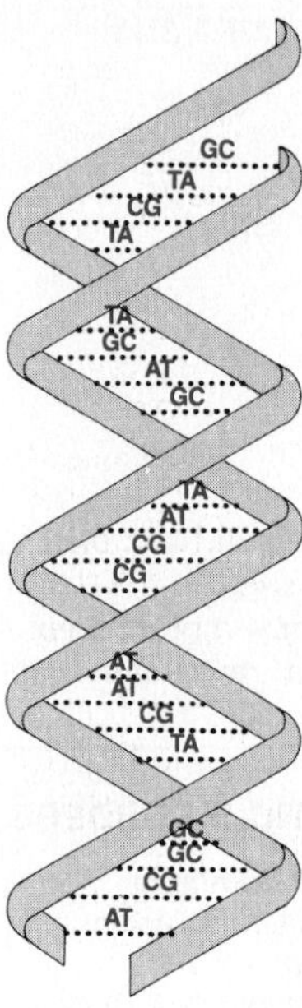

Deoxyribonucleic acid (DNA) is a polymer (macromolecule) made up of individual units called *nucleotides*. Each nucleotide is composed of the pentose (5-carbon) sugar deoxyribose and phosphate, plus two nitrogen-containing bases—a purine and a pyrimidine. These bases are paired by hydrogen bonds to form two coiled chains, known as a double helix. In DNA, the purines are adenine (A) and guanine (G); the pyrimidines, thymine (T) and cytosine (C) (see illustration).

DNA transmits its genetic code by acting as a template (pattern) for the synthesis of messenger ribonucleic acid (RNA). Messenger RNA, in turn, arranges amino acids in the correct sequence to build polypeptide chains, the basis for enzymes that control the cell's essential biochemical processes and other proteins.

even lethal defects, or it may be relatively benign. Teratogenic agents such as radiation, drugs, viruses, and synthetic chemicals may produce mutations (gene changes), but such changes may also occur spontaneously. Mutations can occur anywhere in the DNA chain of bases that transmit the genetic code.

Types of genetic defects

Genetic disorders occur in three different forms:

- *Mendelian* or *single-gene disorders* are inherited in clearly identifiable patterns.
- *Chromosomal aberrations or abnormalities* include structural defects within a chromosome, such as deletion and translocation, plus absence or addition of complete chromosomes.
- *Multifactorial (polygenic) disorders* reflect the interaction of at least two abnormal genes and environmental factors to produce a defect.

Single-gene disorders

Single-gene disorders are inherited through a single allelic gene form and, except for new mutations, usually follow mendelian rules of inheritance. They may be autosomal (result from defective genes on one of the 22 pairs of autosomes) or X-linked (result from a defective gene on the X chromosome). Autosomal defects are by far the most common genetic disorders; in fact, about 90% of *all* genetic defects result from this type of inheritance. In addition, single-gene disorders may be further classified as dominant or recessive, depending on whether the defective gene is a dominant or a recessive allele.

Single-gene inheritance patterns

A dominant gene produces its effect even in heterozygotes (persons who also carry a normal gene for the same trait), since the dominant gene masks the effects of the normal paired gene. Because a person with an autosomal dominant disease is usually a heterozygote and carries a normal gene, his children have a 50% chance of inheriting the defective dominant gene and the disease (see page 7).

This probability remains the same for each and every pregnancy, since each pregnancy is a separate event. Unaffected persons (normal homozygotes) don't carry the gene and therefore can't transmit it to their children (except as a new mutation). Gender doesn't influence transmission of the abnormal autosomal dominant trait. Unless the defective dominant gene has arisen as a new mutation, every affected person has an affected parent, so autosomal dominant traits don't tend to skip generations.

Since a defective recessive gene can only produce a disorder in homozygotes *(autosomal recessive inheritance),* to inherit the recessive trait, offspring must receive one copy of the same defective gene from each parent. Since both parents must be heterozygous carriers, such autosomal recessive disorders are more common in children of consanguineous parents (blood relatives). Autosomal recessive disorders affect males and females equally.

In *X-linked recessive inheritance,* nearly all affected persons are male, since females inherit a dominant normal allelic gene that doesn't permit expression of the recessive trait. Females do, however, act as carriers for such traits. X-linked recessive disorders are never transmitted directly from father to son, since the father gives the son a Y chromosome, which can't carry the trait.

In *X-linked dominant inheritance,* which is rare, an affected male transmits the defective trait to all his daughters but none of his sons. His daughters, in turn, may pass on the trait (and the disorder) to their sons. Such inheritance also affects heterozygous females but to a lesser extent than males.

Genetic accidents

During germ cell formation by meiosis, failure of chromosomes to divide (*nondisjunction*) results in a germ cell that contains less or more than the normal 23 chromosomes. Usually, such abnormal germ cells fail to unite at conception; or if fertilization does take place, the embryo is aborted early. Experts believe

MITOSIS AND MEIOSIS

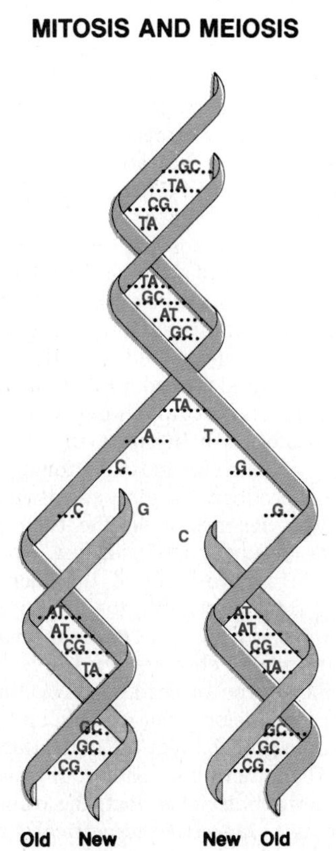

The body grows and replaces all dividing cells other than germ cells (sperm and ova) by *mitosis.* In mitosis, the cell's DNA exactly replicates itself and leads to the creation of a new daughter cell with the identical genetic makeup as the parent cell. Each new cell has a diploid number of chromosomes (in humans, 46).

Germ cells, however, form by *meiosis.* In meiosis, DNA first replicates. Then, through a complicated process, two cell divisions create four daughter cells (a sperm or ovum) from each parent cell, each of which has a haploid number of chromosomes (in humans, 23).

that up to 60% of spontaneous abortions at less than 90 days' gestation result from abnormal fetal chromosome number; offspring with grosser abnormalities are probably never even implanted. Absence of an autosomal chromosome is incompatible with life; but absence of a sex chromosome, as in Turner's syndrome (in which a female offspring receives only one X chromosome) is better tolerated. Presence of an extra chromosome (a trisomy), as in Down's syndrome, produces some combination of physical malformation and mental retardation.

Chromosomal disorders may also result from structural changes within chromosomes. For instance, in *deletion*, loss of part of a chromosome during cell division produces varying effects in the offspring, depending on the type and amount of genetic material lost. An example of a chromosomal disorder resulting from deletion is the cri du chat syndrome, in which part of the short arm of the number 5 chromosome is missing.

Another type of chromosome abnormality is *translocation*, in which part of a chromosome breaks off and attaches itself to another chromosome. If little or no genetic material is lost, the translocation is balanced (symmetrical), and the person is normal.

Another abnormality, *ring chromosomes*, results when a chromosome loses a section of genetic material from each end and the remaining stumps join together to form a ring. The effect of such a structural abnormality varies with the type of genetic material lost.

In *mosaicism*, a rare condition, abnormal chromosomal division in the *zygote* (the cell formed at conception by the union of the sperm and ova) results in two or more cell lines with different chromosomes. One cell line may be normal, the other abnormal, such as trisomy 21. The patient's phenotype depends on the percentage of normal cells, but usually he shows the effect of the abnormal cell line.

Multifactorial (polygenic) disorders are inherited abnormalities that result from the interaction of at least two inherited abnormal genes and environmental factors. They include common malformations such as neural tube abnormalities, cleft lip, and cleft palate, as well as disorders that might not become apparent until later in life. Such disorders don't follow the mendelian patterns of inheritance, but a study of the frequency of specific birth defects within families suggests familial transmission. So far, however, exactly *how* multifactorial disorders result remains unclear.

Detecting genetic disorders

Although genetic disorders can't be cured, genetic testing and counseling can help prevent them and can help patients and their families deal with such disorders when they do develop. Genetic testing relies primarily on pedigree (family tree) analysis, karyotype (chromosomal) analysis, biochemical analysis of blood, urine, or body tissues (including amniocentesis), and chorionic villus biopsy, to detect abnormal gene products. Newborn screening for inherited metabolic disorders such as phenylketonuria (PKU) has become standard, and prompt treatment of such disorders can avoid or minimize their results. Simple blood tests can detect carriers of recessive genes such as Tay-Sachs and sickle cell anemia. This gives a couple at risk the option of prenatal diagnosis (amniocentesis) to detect affected offspring. Recent developments, such as chromosomal banding and identifying areas on chromosomes responsible for specific abnormalities, have further helped unravel genetic mysteries. But even with such developments, certain genetic disorders remain undetectable until they produce irreversible clinical features. Unfortunately, we still have no way to look at a specific gene directly.

A *pedigree*, the study of a trait or a disease in the patient's family, helps determine its inheritance pattern, including the probability of occurrence. The pedigree chart begins with the patient (index) and traces all living and remembered blood relatives in order of their birth, listing the following data:

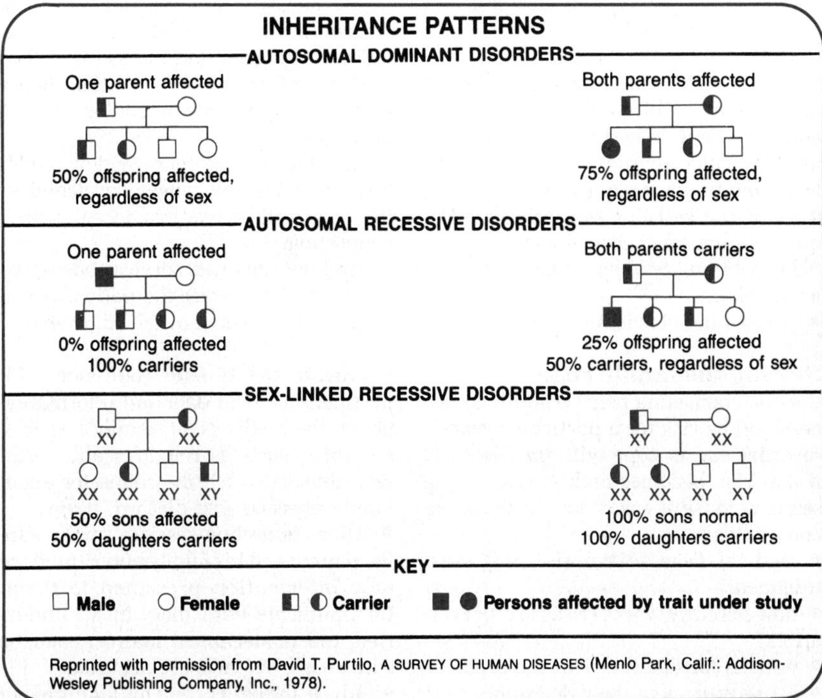

Reprinted with permission from David T. Purtilo, A SURVEY OF HUMAN DISEASES (Menlo Park, Calif.: Addison-Wesley Publishing Company, Inc., 1978).

- current age or age at death
- health status (including abortions, miscarriages, stillbirths, and their reasons; the site and nature of congenital anomalies; acquired heart lesions; primary site malignancies; and types of arthritis)
- relationships (if he's a twin or involved in a consanguineous marriage).

This information can be culled from the patient's memory, autopsy and pathology reports, and photographs. After gathering such information, the pedigree chart is viewed in relation to the clinical features of the suspected genetic disorder and appropriate laboratory tests. One such test is the *karyotype.* In a karyotype, blood cells drawn from the patient's vein are grown in a special culture until the stage of mitosis, when chromosomes are most easily seen with a microscope. Then the cells are broken open and stained to show specific bands on the chromosomes. Staining techniques can be varied to help identify each chromosome and the bands it contains.

Amniocentesis, needle aspiration of amniotic fluid following transabdominal puncture of the uterus under local anesthetic, can now detect over a hundred genetic disorders before birth by:

- karyotyping fetal chromosomes.
- culturing fetal cells in amniotic fluid to measure fetal enzymes or identify cell characteristics.
- analyzing alpha-fetoprotein (AFP). Usually, this procedure is done at 15 to 16 weeks' gestation.

Amniocentesis allows parents to choose elective abortion or prepare themselves during pregnancy for the birth of a child with a genetic disorder. It's recommended in:

- maternal age over 35 years.
- familial history of chromosomal abnormalities or translocations.
- history of previous children or a primary relative with a neural tube defect.
- parents who are known carriers for

an autosomal recessive disease that can be detected prenatally, such as Tay-Sachs disease.

In most other situations, the risks of amniocentesis (bleeding, fluid leakage, abortion, and infection) outweigh the benefits. Safer alternatives to amniocentesis now under study include:

- culturing fetal chorionic cells that desquamate into the cervical canal.
- karyotyping fetal lymphocytes in maternal blood.
- performing chorionic villus biopsy.

Helping the family cope

Genetic counseling helps a family to understand its risk for a particular genetic disorder and to cope with the disorder, if that risk becomes reality. Counseling sessions make it easier for the family to comprehend:

- medical facts (diagnosis, prognosis, treatment)
- how heredity works (risks to other relatives)
- options for dealing with the problem
- consequences of their decision.

Psychological support to relieve stress and improve the patient's or parents' self-concept is as important as the correct information. Birth of a child with a genetic defect may provoke parental feelings of isolation, insecurity, and helplessness; strain marital relations; and initiate a period of shock and denial, followed by grief and mourning. When testing confirms a genetic disease, here's how you can provide psychological support:

- Help the persons concerned deal with their initial shock, anger, or denial so that they will be ready to accept genetic counseling.
- Find out the exact services offered by the counseling center the patient's been referred to so you can tell him what to expect.
- Provide the genetic counselor with pertinent medical data and information about the patient's or family's special concerns, such as religious and social restraints. Also tell the counselor about family pressure and discord, if any.
- After counseling sessions, make sure the patient and his family understand the new information presented to them. Communicate with them in an unhurried and nontechnical manner, and be sure your own facts are accurate.
- Advise the patient and his family about community resources and agencies that are available to help them deal with genetic disorders. If they're interested, help them get in touch with the families of other patients with the same disorder.
- Coordinate the assistance needed from other members of the health care team, such as doctors, psychologists, and social workers.
- Recognize the parents' stresses in caring for their child and allow them to vent their feelings.

AMNIOCENTESIS

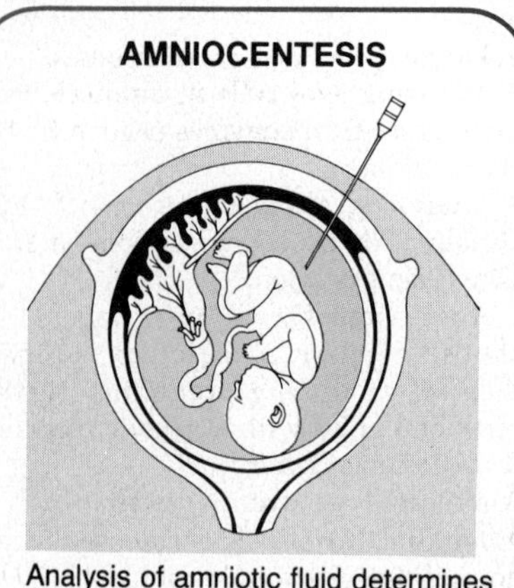

Analysis of amniotic fluid determines fetal maturity and detects genetic abnormalities.

List of genetic counseling units

The National Foundation of the March of Dimes publishes a list of genetic counseling units located throughout the United States. To obtain this list, write to the Professional Education Department, The National Foundation of the March of Dimes.

Local March of Dimes chapters can also provide information about local genetic counseling services and educational material about birth defects.

AUTOSOMAL DOMINANT INHERITANCE

Neurofibromatosis

(Von Recklinghausen's disease)

Neurofibromatosis is an inherited developmental disorder of the nervous system, muscles, bones, and skin that causes formation of multiple, pedunculated, soft tumors (neurofibromas), and café-au-lait spots. About 80,000 Americans are known to have neurofibromatosis; in many others, this disorder is overlooked because symptoms are mild. The disease occurs in about 1 in 3,000 births; prognosis varies, though spinal or intracranial tumors can shorten life span.

Causes and incidence

Neurofibromatosis is present at birth, but symptoms generally appear during childhood or adolescence. Sometimes progression stops as the patient matures, but it may accelerate at puberty, during pregnancy or after menopause. It's often associated with meningiomas, suprarenal medullary secreting tumors, kyphoscoliosis, vascular and lymphatic nevi, and ocular and renal anomalies. In some patients, the disease is transmitted as an autosomal dominant trait; in others, it occurs as a new mutation. Persons with neurofibromatosis have a 50% risk that their offspring will have this disease.

Signs and symptoms

Symptoms result from an overgrowth of mesodermal and ectodermal elements in the skin, central nervous system, and other organs. Such overgrowth produces multiple pedunculated nodules (neurofibromas) of varying sizes on the nerve trunks of extremities and on the nerves of head, neck, and body. Symptoms generally worsen during puberty and pregnancy. Effects vary with the location and size of the tumors and include:

- neurologic impairment from intracranial, spinal, and orbital tumors—and in 10% of patients, seizures, blindness, deafness, developmental delay, and mental deficiency
- cutaneous lesions—six or more flat-pigmented or hyperpigmented skin areas
- skeletal involvement—scoliosis, severe kyphoscoliosis, macrocephaly, and short stature
- endocrine abnormalities
- renal damage—hypertension.

Complications include congenital tibial pseudoarthrosis; cancer of the nerve sheath, or neurofibrosarcoma, which occurs in up to 8% of patients; and malignant changes in tumors themselves.

Diagnosis

Diagnosis rests on typical clinical findings, especially neurofibromas and café-

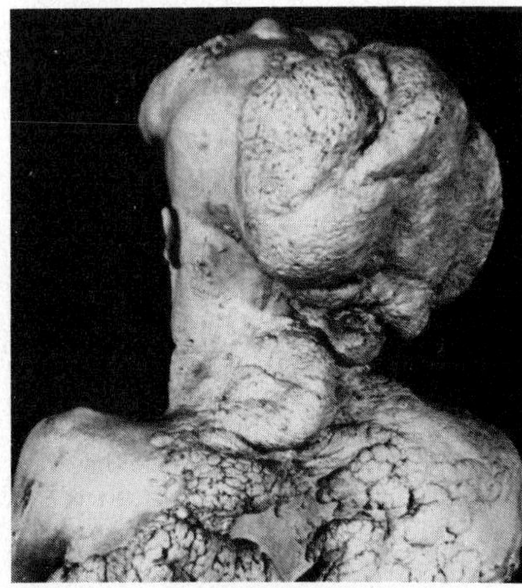

Severe neurofibromatosis—postmortem cast of the back of the head of John Merrick, "the Elephant Man."

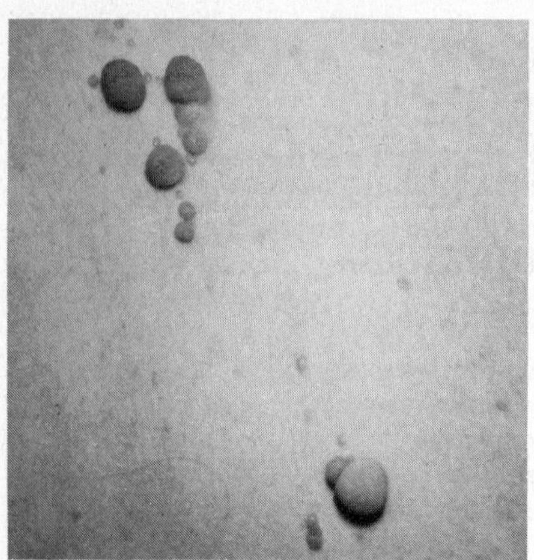

Multiple pedunculated nodules (neurofibromas) of varying sizes

au-lait spots. X-rays showing a widening internal auditory meatus and intervertebral foramen support this diagnosis, which rarely requires a tumor biopsy.

Treatment

Treatment consists of surgical removal of intracerebral or intraspinal tumors, when possible; correction of kyphoscoliosis; and, if necessary, cosmetic surgery for disfiguring or disabling growths.

Special considerations

- Disfigurement may cause overwhelming social embarrassment and regression. By showing your own acceptance, you can help the patient adjust to his condition.
- Advise the patient to choose attractive clothing that covers unsightly nodules; suggest special cosmetics to cover skin lesions.
- Refer the patient for genetic counseling to discuss the 50% risk of transmitting this disorder to offspring. Refer for more information to the National Neurofibromatosis Foundation.

Osteogenesis Imperfecta

Osteogenesis imperfecta (brittle bones) is a hereditary disease of bones and connective tissue that causes skeletal fragility, thin skin, blue sclera, poor teeth, hypermobility of joints, and progressive deafness. This disease occurs in two forms. In the rare congenital form, fractures are present at birth. This form is usually fatal within the first few days or weeks of life. In the late-appearing form (osteogenesis imperfecta tarda)*, the child appears normal at birth but develops recurring fractures (mostly of the extremities) after the first year of life.*

Causes

Osteogenesis imperfecta can result from autosomal dominant or recessive inheritance. Clinical signs may result from defective osteoblastic activity and a defect of mesenchymal collagen (embryonic connective tissue) and its derivatives (scleras, bones, and ligaments). The reticulum fails to differentiate into mature collagen or causes abnormal collagen development, leading to immature and coarse bone formation. Cortical bone thinning also occurs.

Signs and symptoms

Both congenital and delayed osteogenesis imperfecta produce bilaterally bulging skull, triangular-shaped head and face, prominent eyes, and blue sclera. One third of patients become deaf by ages 30 to 40 because of osteosclerosis, pressure on the auditory nerve, and neurogenic deafness. These disorders also cause thin, translucent skin; possible subcutaneous hemorrhages; and discolored (blue-gray or yellow-brown) teeth, which break easily and are cavity-prone. Other findings are poorly developed skeletal muscles (atrophy) and hypermobility of joints.

The hallmark of this disease, though, is fractures that occur with even slight trauma. In the congenital form, hundreds of fractures may be present before birth and birth itself may cause fractures; other skeletal deformities reflect intrauterine fractures that healed in abnormal positions. In both forms, incomplete and relatively painless fractures after birth that receive no treatment can produce deformities from bones healing in poor alignment. The incidence of such fractures decreases after puberty.

Osteogenesis imperfecta tarda may also cause stunted growth from epiphyseal fractures, or short stature from deformities following fractures.

Diagnosis

Family history and characteristic features, such as blue sclera or deafness, establish this diagnosis. X-rays showing evidence of multiple old fractures and skeletal deformities and skull X-ray showing wide sutures with small, irregularly shaped islands of bone (wormian bones) between them support the diagnosis. Serum calcium and serum phosphorus levels are normal.

Treatment

Treatment aims to prevent deformities by traction, immobilization, or both, and to aid normal development and rehabilitation. Support includes:

- checking the patient's circulatory, motor, and sensory abilities
- encouraging him to walk when possible (these children develop a fear of walking)
- teaching preventive measures. For example, the child must avoid contact sports or strenuous activity or must wear knee pads, helmets, or other protective devices when he engages in them
- assessing for and treating scoliosis, a common complication
- promoting preventive dental care and repair of dental caries.

Special considerations

- Educate the family. Teach the parents and child how to recognize fractures and how to correctly splint a fracture.
- Advise parents to encourage their child to develop interests that don't require strenuous physical activity, and to develop his fine motor skills. These will promote the child's self-esteem.
- Help parents make arrangements for tutoring.
- Teach the child to assume some responsibility for precautions during physical activity to help foster his independence.
- Stress good nutrition to heal bones.
- Refer the parents and child for genetic counseling.
- Administer analgesics, as ordered.
- Monitor dental and hearing needs. Stress nutrition, dental care, and immunizations in well-child visits.

Marfan's Syndrome

(Arachnodactyly)

Marfan's syndrome is a rare inherited, degenerative, generalized disease of the connective tissue that causes ocular, skeletal, and cardiovascular anomalies. It probably results from elastin and collagen abnormalities.

Death is usually attributed to cardiovascular complications and may occur anytime from early infancy to adulthood, depending on the severity of the symptoms. Marfan's syndrome affects males and females equally. Probably its most famous victim was Abraham Lincoln.

Causes

Marfan's syndrome is inherited as an autosomal dominant trait. In 85% of patients with this disease, family history confirms Marfan's syndrome in one parent as well. In the remaining 15%, a negative family history suggests fresh mutation, possibly because of advanced paternal age.

Signs and symptoms

Characteristically, the clinical effects of Marfan's syndrome may show linear disparity at birth and develop slowly over a period of years. These effects vary even among siblings.

The most common signs and symptoms of this disorder are skeletal abnormalities, particularly excessively long tubular bones and an arm span exceeding the patient's height. Usually, the patient is taller than average for his family, with the upper half of his body shorter than average and the lower half, longer. His fingers are long and slender (spider fingers). Weakness of ligaments, tendons, and joint capsules results in joints that are loose, hyperextensible, and habitually dislocated. Excessive growth of the rib bones gives rise to chest deformities, such as funnel breast and pigeon breast.

Eye problems are also common: 75% of patients have crystalline lens displacement (ectopia lentis), the ocular hallmark of Marfan's syndrome. Frequently, quivering of the iris with eye movement (iridodonesis) suggests this disorder. Most patients are severely myopic, many have retinal detachment, and some have glaucoma.

The most serious complications occur in the cardiovascular system and include weakness of the aortic media that leads to progressive dilation or dissecting aneurysm of the ascending aorta. Such dilation appears first in the coronary sinuses and is often preceded by aortic regurgitation. Less common cardiovascular complications include mitral regurgitation and endocarditis.

Other general symptoms and associated problems include sparsity of subcutaneous fat, frequent hernia, cystic lung disease, recurrent spontaneous pneumothorax, and scoliosis.

Diagnosis

Because no specific test confirms Marfan's syndrome, diagnosis rests on typical clinical features (particularly skeletal deformities *and* ectopia lentis) and a history of the disease in close relatives. Useful supplementary procedures, though not definitive for diagnosis, include X-rays for skeletal abnormalities and auscultation for abnormal heart sounds.

Treatment

Attempts to stop the degenerative process have met with little success. Therefore, treatment of Marfan's syndrome is basically symptomatic, such as surgical repair of aneurysms and of ocular deformities. In young patients with early dilation of the aorta, prompt treatment with propranolol can often decrease ventricular ejection and protect the aorta; extreme dilation requires surgical replacement of the aorta and the aortic valve. Steroids and sex hormones have been successful (especially in girls) in inducing precocious puberty and early epiphyseal closure to prevent abnormal adult height. Genetic counseling is important, particularly since pregnancy and resultant increased cardiovascular work load can produce aortic rupture.

Special considerations

- The patient needs supportive care, as appropriate for his clinical status.
- Also provide information for the patient and his family about the course of this disease and its potential complications, such as lung disease and pneumothorax.
- Stress the need for frequent checkups so the degenerative changes can be discovered and treated early.
- Emphasize the importance of taking prescribed medication as ordered.
- If recommended by the doctor, encourage hormonal therapy to induce early epiphyseal closure, thus preventing abnormal adult height.
- Encourage normal adolescent development by telling the parents not to have unrealistic expectations for the child just because he is tall and looks older than his years.

Epidermolysis Bullosa

Epidermolysis bullosa (EB) is a heterogeneous group of disorders that affect the skin and mucous membranes, producing blisters in response to normally harmless heat and frictional trauma. As many as 16 scarring and nonscarring forms may exist, including an acquired form (epidermolysis acquisita bullosa) that develops after childhood and is not genetically inherited.

Prognosis depends on the severity of the disease. In the nonscarring forms of EB, blisters eventually become less severe and less frequent as the patient matures. But the severe scarring forms commonly cause disability or disfigurement and may be fatal during infancy or childhood.

Causes and incidence

The nonscarring forms of EB result from autosomal dominant inheritance—except for junctional EB (EB Herlitz or EB letalis), which is recessively inherited. All nonscarring forms produce a split *above* the basement membrane, the layer between the epidermis and dermis.

Except for dominant dystrophic EB, the scarring forms result from autosomal recessive inheritance and produce a split *below* the basement membrane in the upper part of the dermis. Sometimes, EB occurs as a mutation in families with no history of blistering disorders.

Although the cause of EB is unknown, children with dystrophic EB have been found to have fewer—and abnormal—anchoring fibrils securing the epidermis to the dermis. These children also have more—and abnormal—collagenase, an enzyme that may destroy the anchoring fibrils. Some patients with EB simplex also have deficiencies of other enzymes involved in collagen synthesis.

The Dystrophic Epidermolysis Bullosa Research Association of America estimates 25,000 to 50,000 Americans have EB. EB occurs in 1 per 50,000 births; the more severe scarring forms, in 1 per 500,000 births.

Signs and symptoms

Blisters may be generalized or develop only on hands, feet, knees, or elbows. In some forms of EB, they can develop in areas that haven't been exposed to trauma or heat.

In all scarring forms and some nonscarring forms, parturition causes widespread blistering and occasional sloughing of large areas of newborn skin.

Newborns with the severe scarring forms, affecting mucous membranes can develop sucking blisters as well as blistering in the gastrointestinal, respiratory, or genitourinary tracts that may lead to strictures or adhesions.

Ocular complications may include eyelid blisters, conjunctivitis, blepharitis, adhesions, and corneal opacities. Other findings may be fusion of fingers and toes, delayed tooth eruption, malformed or carious teeth, alopecia, abnormal nails, retarded growth, anemia, constipation, malnutrition, infection, squamous cell carcinoma, and pyloric atresia.

Diagnosis

Skin biopsy of a freshly induced blister using immunofluorescence and electron microscopy confirms which type of EB is present. Prenatal diagnosis of the severe scarring forms can be confirmed at 20 weeks' gestation by fetoscopy and biopsy. Diagnosis cannot be confirmed by amniocentesis alone.

Differential diagnosis of EB should rule out other chronic, nonhereditary bullous diseases, such as juvenile bullous pemphigus, chronic bullous disease of childhood, and congenital herpes.

Treatment

Phenytoin (Dilantin) may help in reces-

WHEN CARING FOR PATIENTS WITH E.B.

For neonates:
- Use DeLiss catheter or bulb syringe. Avoid wall suction.
- Use sheepskin or soft blanket, not harsh linen.
- Keep skin scrupulously clean, but avoid alcohol or iodine preparations and harsh antibacterial soaps.
- Use Isolette, not overhead warmer, to maintain normal temperature. Check temperature with axillary thermometer.
- Cover large areas of denuded skin with petrolatum gauze and place strips of it between fingers and toes to delay fusion. Avoid tape; elastic bandages; or adherent, dry dressings.
- Release fluid in blisters by puncturing both sides with a sterile needle or small scissors. Press gently with a gauze pad. Apply wet soaks or antibiotic cream. DO NOT remove blister roof.
- Secure dressings with soft fleece or gauze bandages; remove them by soaking in warm water. Never use adhesive tape or pull clothing from skin.
- Encourage breast feeding. For formula feeding, use unheated formula and a preemie nipple or rubber-tipped syringe.
- Bathe infant in foam-cushioned plastic tub. Avoid stainless steel basins and washcloths.
- Encourage parents to use infant stimulation techniques, such as music, talking, and mobiles. Encourage them to hold their newborn.

For infants and children:
- Keep child's environment safe by using skin lubricants, padded walkers and swings, and air conditioning. Dress child in soft clothing.
- Lift child from under the buttocks—never from under the arms.
- Provide sheepskin, air, or water mattress for sleeping and don't place wool, sharp objects, or toys near child.
- Observe for signs of infection but don't treat without a doctor's order.
- Feed the child small portions of a high-protein, complex-carbohydrate diet at frequent intervals, giving him cool fluids, sherbet, or ice pops to soothe his throat before and after each feeding. Use medium-chain triglycerides oil or Polycose, an enteral nutritional supplement. Provide lactose-free products for children who can't tolerate lactose. Avoid simple sugars, megadoses of vitamins or minerals, and hot, spicy, acidic, or hard-crusted foods.
- Promote good bowel habits with fresh fruits and vegetables, bran, and plenty of fluids. Avoid laxatives.
- Clean teeth with a soft toothbrush, gauze, or sponge.
- Encourage an exercise program of stretching or swimming. Avoid jogging or contact sports.

sive dystrophic forms of EB and corticosteroids and retinoids in other forms.

Supportive treatment consists of preventing infection and guarding the skin from trauma and friction through application of protective dressings and skin lubricants. A high-calorie diet containing vitamin and mineral supplements helps combat chronic malnutrition. Iron supplements or transfusions help counteract anemia. Occupational and physical therapy help prevent contractures and deformities.

Special considerations

Because EB is a visible skin disorder, it tends to disrupt the patient's body image as well as his family's dynamics: In many such families, parents and siblings become overprotective, fostering overdependence in the patient. Such parents must also deal with the burden of providing time-consuming personal care, as well as continual advocacy in their child's behalf. Sadly, these parents are sometimes unjustly accused of child abuse by strangers who assume the child's distressing appearance resulted from being burned or beaten.

To help the patient and his family deal with this disease, encourage parents to seek family counseling and join a support group.

AUTOSOMAL RECESSIVE INHERITANCE

Cystic Fibrosis

(Mucoviscidosis)

Cystic fibrosis is a generalized dysfunction of the exocrine glands, affecting multiple organ systems in varying degrees of severity. It's transmitted as an autosomal recessive trait and is the most common fatal genetic disease of white children. Cystic fibrosis is a chronic disease that severely shortens the patient's life span. About 50% of affected children die by age 16; of the rest, some survive to age 30.

Causes and incidence

Incidence of cystic fibrosis is highest (approximately 1 in 2,000 live births) in persons of northern European ancestry. Incidence is lower in American blacks (1 in 17,000 live births), American Indians, and persons of Asian ancestry. Frequency is equal in both sexes.

The underlying biochemical defect probably reflects an alteration in a protein or enzyme. In fact, cystic fibrosis accounts for almost all cases of pancreatic enzyme deficiency in children.

The immediate causes of symptoms in cystic fibrosis are increased viscosity of bronchial, pancreatic, and other mucous gland secretions and consequent obstruction of glandular ducts.

Signs and symptoms

The clinical effects of cystic fibrosis may become apparent soon after birth or may take years to develop. They include major aberrations in sweat gland, respiratory, and gastrointestinal functions. Sweat gland dysfunction is the most consistent abnormality. Increased concentrations of sodium and chloride in the sweat lead to hyponatremia and hypochloremia and can eventually induce fatal shock and arrhythmias, especially in hot weather, when sweating is profuse.

Respiratory symptoms reflect disabling obstructive changes in the lungs: wheezy respirations; a dry, nonproductive paroxysmal cough; dyspnea; and tachypnea. These changes stem from the accumulation of thick, tenacious secretions in the bronchioles and the alveoli, and eventually lead to severe atelectasis and emphysema. Consequently, children with cystic fibrosis typically display a barrel chest, cyanosis, and clubbing of the fingers and toes. They suffer recurring bronchitis and pneumonia, and may have associated nasal polyps and sinusitis. Pneumonia, emphysema, or atelectasis usually causes death.

The gastrointestinal effects of cystic fibrosis occur mainly in the intestines, pancreas, and liver. One of the earliest such symptoms is meconium ileus; the newborn with cystic fibrosis doesn't excrete meconium, a dark green mucilaginous material found in the intestine at birth. Therefore, he develops symptoms of intestinal obstruction, such as abdominal distention, vomiting, constipation, dehydration, and electrolyte imbalance. Eventually, obstruction of the pancreatic ducts and resulting deficiency of trypsin, amylase, and lipase prevent the conversion and absorption of fat and protein in the intestinal tract. The undigested food is then excreted in characteristically frequent, bulky, foul-smelling, and pale stools with a high fat content. This malabsorption induces other abnormalities: poor weight gain, poor growth, ravenous appetite, distended abdomen, thin extremities, and sallow skin with poor turgor. The inability to absorb fats produces deficiency of fat-soluble vitamins (A, D, E, and K), leading to clotting problems, retarded bone growth and delayed sexual development. Males may experience azoospermia; females may experience secondary amenorrhea. A common complication in infants and children with these signs and symptoms is rectal prolapse, secondary to malnutrition and wasting of perirectal supporting tissues.

In the pancreas, fibrotic tissue, multiple cysts, thick mucus, and eventually fat replace the acini (small, saclike swellings normally found in this gland), producing symptoms of pancreatic insufficiency: insufficient insulin production, abnormal glucose tolerance, and glycosuria. Biliary obstruction and fibrosis may prolong neonatal jaundice. In some patients, cirrhosis and portal hypertension may lead to esophageal varices, episodes of hematemesis and, occasionally, hepatomegaly.

Diagnosis

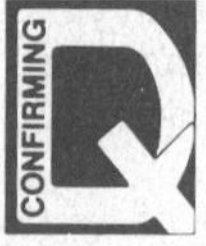

The presence of elevated electrolyte (sodium and chloride) concentration in sweat in a patient with pulmonary disease or pancreatic insufficiency confirms cystic fibrosis. The sweat test (stimulation of sweat glands, collection of samples, and laboratory analysis) shows that the volume of sweat is normal, but that its weight is increased because of increased chloride and sodium concentration. (Normal sodium concentration of sweat is less than 40 mEq/liter; in cystic fibrosis, it rises to more than 60 mEq/liter.) The sodium and chloride concentration of sweat normally rises with age, but any value greater than 50, even in adults, strongly suggests cystic fibrosis and calls for repeated testing.

Examination of duodenal contents for pancreatic enzymes and stools for trypsin can confirm pancreatic insufficiency; trypsin is absent in over 80% of children with cystic fibrosis. Chest X-rays, pulmonary function tests, and arterial blood gas determination assess the patient's pulmonary status. Sputum culture can detect concurrent infectious diseases. Family history may show siblings or other relatives with cystic fibrosis.

Treatment and special considerations

Since cystic fibrosis has no cure, the aim of treatment is to help the child lead as normal a life as possible. The child's family needs instruction about the disease and its complications; referral for genetic counseling will also be helpful. The emphasis of treatment depends on the organ systems involved.

- To combat sweat electrolyte losses, treatment includes generous salting of foods and, during hot weather, administration of salt supplements.
- To offset pancreatic enzyme deficiencies, treatment includes oral pancreatic enzymes with meals and snacks. Such supplements improve absorption and digestion and satisfy hunger on a reasonable calorie intake. The child's diet should be low in fat, but high in protein and calories, and should include supplements of water-miscible, fat-soluble vitamins (A, D, E, and K).
- Pulmonary dysfunction management includes physical therapy, postural drainage, and breathing exercises several times daily, to aid removal of secretions from lungs. Patients with cystic fibrosis shouldn't receive antihistamines, since they have a drying effect on mucous membranes, making expectoration of mucus difficult or impossible. Aerosol therapy includes intermittent nebulizer treatments before postural drainage, to loosen secretions.

Treatment of pulmonary infection requires:

- loosening and removal of mucopurulent secretions, using an intermittent nebulizer and postural drainage to relieve obstruction. Use of a mist tent is controversial, since mist particles may become trapped in the esophagus and stomach and never even reach the lungs.
- aggressive use of broad-spectrum antimicrobials (usually with acute pulmonary infections, since prophylactic use causes resistant bacterial strains)
- oxygen therapy as needed.

Hot, dry air increases vulnerability to respiratory infections, so cystic fibrosis patients benefit from such things as air conditioners and humidifiers.

Throughout this illness:

- Thoroughly explain all treatment measures and teach the patient and his family about his disease.
- Provide much needed emotional support. Be flexible with care and visiting hours during hospitalization to allow continuation of schooling and friendships.

For further information and support, refer the patient and his family to the Cystic Fibrosis Foundation.

Tay-Sachs Disease

(Amaurotic familial idiocy)

The most common of the lipid storage diseases, Tay-Sachs disease results from a congenital enzyme deficiency. It's characterized by progressive mental and motor deterioration and is always fatal, usually before age 5.

Causes and incidence

Tay-Sachs disease is an autosomal recessive disorder in which the enzyme hexosaminidase A is deficient. This enzyme is necessary for metabolism of gangliosides, water-soluble glycolipids found primarily in CNS tissues. Without hexosaminidase A, accumulating lipid pigments distend and progressively destroy and demyelinate CNS cells. Tay-Sachs disease is quite rare and appears in fewer than 100 infants born each year in the United States. However, it strikes persons of Ashkenazic Jewish ancestry about 100 times more often than the general population, occurring in about l in 3,600 live births in this ethnic group. About 1 in 30 such persons are heterozygous carriers of this defective gene. If two such carriers have children, each of their offspring has a 25% chance of having Tay-Sachs disease.

Signs and symptoms

A newborn with Tay-Sachs disease appears normal at birth, although he may have an exaggerated Moro reflex. By age 3 to 6 months, he becomes apathetic and responds to loud sounds only. Increasing physical and mental deterioration follows. His neck, trunk, arm, and leg muscles grow weaker, so that soon he can't sit up or lift his head. He has difficulty turning over, can't grasp objects, and has progressive vision loss.

By 18 months, such an infant is usually deaf, and has seizures and generalized paralysis and spasticity. Although he's blind, he may hold his eyes wide open and roll his eyeballs. His pupils are always dilated and don't react to light.

Decerebrate rigidity and a complete vegetative state follow. After age 2, the child suffers recurrent bronchopneumonia and usually dies before age 5.

Diagnosis

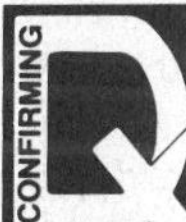

Typical clinical features point to Tay-Sachs disease, but serum analysis showing deficient hexosaminidase A is the key to diagnosis. An ophthalmic examination showing optic nerve atrophy and a distinctive cherry-red spot on the retina further supports diagnosis.

Diagnostic screening is essential for all couples of Ashkenazic Jewish ancestry and for others with a familial history of the disease. A simple blood test evaluating hexosaminidase A levels can identify carriers. If carriers wish to have children, amniocentesis at 15 to 16 weeks of gestation is recommended to detect hexosaminidase A deficiency and, consequently, Tay-Sachs disease in the fetus.

Treatment

Tay-Sachs disease has no known cure. Supportive treatment includes tube feedings using nutritional supplements, suctioning and postural drainage to remove pharyngeal secretions, skin care to prevent decubiti in such children once they're bedridden, and mild laxatives to relieve neurogenic constipation. Unfortunately, anticonvulsants usually fail to prevent seizures. Because these children need round-the-clock physical care, their parents often place them in long-term special care facilities.

Special considerations

Your most important job is to help the family deal with inevitably progressive illness and death.

- Refer parents for genetic counseling, and stress the importance of amniocentesis in future pregnancies. Refer siblings for screening to determine if they're carriers. If they are carriers and are adults, refer them for genetic counseling, but stress that there's no danger of transmitting the disease to offspring if they don't marry another carrier.
- Because parents may feel excessive stress or guilt due to their child's illness and the emotional and financial burden it places on them, refer them for psychological counseling if indicated.
- If parents care for their child at home, teach them how to do suctioning, postural drainage, and tube feeding. Also teach them how to give good skin care to prevent decubiti.

For more information on this disease, refer parents to National Tay-Sachs and Allied Diseases Association, Inc.

Phenylketonuria

(Phenylalaninemia, phenylpyruvic oligophrenia)

Phenylketonuria (PKU) is an inborn error in phenylalanine metabolism, resulting in high serum levels of phenylalanine, cerebral damage, and mental retardation.

Causes and incidence

In the United States, this disorder occurs once in approximately 14,000 births. (About one person in 60 is an asymptomatic carrier.) It has a low incidence in Finland, in Japan, and among Ashkenazic Jews and American blacks.

PKU is transmitted by an autosomal recessive gene. Patients with this disorder have insufficient phenylalanine hydroxylase, an enzyme that acts as a catalyst in the conversion of phenylalanine to tyrosine. As a result, phenylalanine and its metabolites accumulate in the blood, causing mental retardation. The exact biochemical mechanism that causes this retardation isn't clearly understood.

Signs and symptoms

An infant with PKU appears normal at birth but by 4 months of age begins to show signs of arrested brain development, including mental retardation and, later, personality disturbances (schizoid and antisocial personality patterns and uncontrollable temper). Such a child may have a lighter complexion than unaffected siblings and often has blue eyes. He may also have macrocephaly; eczematous skin lesions or dry, rough skin; and a musty (mousy) odor due to skin and urinary excretion of phenylacetic acid. Approximately 80% of these children have abnormal EEG patterns, and about one third have seizures, which usually begin when they are 6 to 12 months old.

Children with this disorder show a precipitous decrease in IQ in their first year, are usually hyperactive and irritable, and show purposeless, repetitive motions. They have increased muscle tone and an awkward gait.

Although blood phenylalanine levels approach normal at birth, they begin to rise within a few days. By the time they reach significant levels (roughly 30 mg/dl), cerebral damage has begun. Such irreversible damage probably is complete by age 2 to 3. However, early detection and treatment can minimize this cerebral damage.

Diagnosis

Most states require screening for PKU at birth; the Guthrie screening test on a capillary blood sample (bacterial inhibition assay) reliably detects PKU. However, since phenylalanine levels may be normal at birth, the infant should be reevaluated after he has received dietary protein for 24 to 48 hours. Adding a few drops of 10% ferric chloride solution to a wet diaper is another method of detecting PKU. If the area turns a deep, bluish-green color, phenylpyruvic acid is present in the urine.

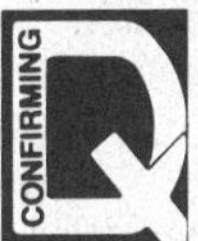

Detection of elevated blood levels of phenylalanine and the presence of phenylpyruvic acid in the infant's urine confirm the diagnosis. (Urine should also be tested 4 to 6 weeks after birth, since urinary levels of phenylpyruvic acid vary with the amount of protein ingested.)

Treatment

Treatment consists of restricting dietary intake of the amino acid phenylalanine to keep phenylalanine blood levels between 3 and 9 mg/dl. Since most natural proteins contain 5% phenylalanine, they must be limited in the child's diet. An enzymatic hydrolysate of casein, such as Lofenalac powder or Progestimil powder, is substituted for milk in the diets of affected infants. This milk substitute contains a minimal amount of phenylalanine, normal amounts of other amino acids, and added amounts of carbohydrate and fat. When blood and urine tests are acceptable, phenylalanine restrictions may be relaxed.

Such a diet calls for careful monitoring. Since the body doesn't make phenylalanine, overzealous dietary restriction can induce phenylalanine deficiency, producing lethargy, anorexia, anemia, skin rashes, and diarrhea.

Special considerations

In caring for a phenylketonuric child, it's especially important to teach both the parents and child about this disease and to provide emotional support and counseling. (Psychological and emotional problems may result from the difficult dietary restrictions.) Teach the child and his parents about the critical importance of adhering to his diet. The child must avoid breads, cheese, eggs, flour, meat, poultry, fish, nuts, milk, legumes, and Nutrasweet. He'll need frequent tests for urine phenylpyruvic and blood phenylalanine levels to evaluate the diet's effectiveness. As the child grows older and is supervised less closely, his parents have less control over what he eats. As a result, deviation from the restricted diet becomes more likely, and so does the risk of further brain damage. Encourage parents to allow the child some choices in the kinds of low-protein foods he wants to eat; this will help make him feel trusted and more responsible. Teach parents about normal physical and mental growth and development, so they

PHENYLALANINE, PROTEIN, AND CALORIE RECOMMENDATIONS IN PHENYLKETONURIA

AGE	PHENYLALANINE (MG PER POUND)	PROTEIN (G PER POUND)	CALORIES (PER POUND)
0 to 3 months	20-22	1.75-2.0	60-65
4 to 12 months	18-20	1.5	55-60
1 to 3 years	16-18	32 g total	50-55
4 to 7 years	10-16	40 g total	40-50

From Corinne H. Robinson, *Normal and Therapeutic Nutrition*. Copyright © 1972 by Macmillan Publishing Co., Inc. Used by permission.

can recognize any developmental delay that may point to excessive phenylalanine intake.

To prevent this disorder:

• Infants should be routinely screened for PKU, since detection and control of phenylalanine intake soon after birth can prevent severe mental retardation.

• Refer phenylketonuric females who reach reproductive age for genetic counseling, since recent research indicates that their offspring may have a higher than normal incidence of brain damage; microcephaly; and major congenital malformations, especially of the heart and central nervous system. Such damage may be prevented with a low-phenylalanine diet during pregnancy.

Albinism

Albinism is a rare inherited defect in melanin metabolism of the skin and eyes (oculocutaneous albinism) or just the eyes (ocular albinism). Ocular albinism impairs visual acuity. Oculocutaneous albinism also causes severe intolerance to sunlight and increases susceptibility to skin cancer in exposed skin areas.

Causes and incidence

Oculocutaneous albinism results from autosomal recessive inheritance; ocular albinism from an X-linked recessive trait that causes hypopigmentation only in the iris and the ocular fundus.

Normally, melanocytes synthesize melanin. Melanosomes, melanin-containing granules within melanocytes, diffuse and absorb the sun's ultraviolet light, thus protecting the skin and eyes from its dangerous effects. In tyrosinase-negative albinism (most common), melanosomes don't contain melanin since they lack tyrosinase, the enzyme that stimulates melanin production. In tyrosinase-positive albinism, melanosomes contain tyrosine, a tyrosinase substrate, but a defect in the tyrosine transport system impairs melanin production. In tyrosinase-variable albinism (rare), an unidentified enzyme defect probably impairs synthesis of a melanin precursor. Other rare forms of albinism are Hermansky-Pudlak syndrome (tyrosinase-positive albinism with platelet dysfunction, bleeding abnormalities and ceroidlike inclusions in many organs); Chédiak-Higashi syndrome (tyrosine-negative albinism with hematologic and neurologic manifestations); and Cross-McKusick-Breen syndrome (tyrosinase-positive albinism with neurologic involvement).

Tyrosinase-negative albinism affects 1 in every 34,000 persons in the United States and is equally common in whites and blacks. Tyrosinase-positive albinism affects more blacks than whites. American Indians have a high incidence of both forms.

Signs and symptoms

Light-skinned whites with tyrosinase-negative albinism have pale skin and hair color ranging from white to yellow; their pupils appear red because of translucent irides. Blacks with the same disorder have hair that may be white, faintly tinged with yellow, or yellow-brown. Both whites and blacks with tyrosinase-positive albinism grow darker as they age. For instance, their hair may become straw-colored or light brown and their skin cream-colored or pink. People with tyrosinase-positive albinism may also have freckles and pigmented nevi that may require excision.

In tyrosinase-variable albinism, at birth the child's hair is white, his skin is pink, and his eyes are gray. As he grows older, though, his hair becomes yellow, his irides may become darker, and his skin may even tan slightly.

The skin of a person with albinism is

easily damaged by the sun. It may look weather-beaten and is highly susceptible to precancerous and cancerous growths. The patient may also have photophobia, myopia, strabismus, and congenital horizontal nystagmus.

Diagnosis

Diagnosis is based on clinical observation and the patient's family history. Microscopic examination of the skin and of hair follicles determines the amount of pigment present. Testing plucked hair roots for pigmentation when incubated in tyrosine distinguishes tyrosinase-negative albinism from tyrosinase-positive albinism. Tyrosinase-positive hair bulbs will develop color.

Treatment and special considerations

Teach the child and his parents what measures best protect him from solar radiation, and inform them of its danger signals (excessive drying of skin, crusty lesions on exposed skin, changes in skin color). Advise the patient to wear full-spectrum sunblocks, dark glasses, and appropriate protective clothing.

If the patient's appearance causes him social and emotional problems, he may need psychiatric counseling. Such counseling may also be in order for his family, if they too find it difficult to accept his disorder. To help parents work through any feelings of guilt and depression, encourage early infant/parent bonding. Also inform parents of cosmetic measures (glasses with tinted lenses, makeup foundation) that can lessen disfigurement when their child gets older. Stress the need for frequent refractions and eye examinations to correct visual defects. As needed, suggest genetic counseling.

Sickle Cell Anemia

A congenital hemolytic anemia that occurs primarily but not exclusively in blacks, sickle cell anemia results from a defective hemoglobin molecule (hemoglobin S) that causes red blood cells (RBCs) to roughen and become sickle-shaped. Such cells impair circulation, resulting in chronic ill health (fatigue, dyspnea on exertion, swollen joints), periodic crises, long-term complications, and premature death.

At present, only symptomatic treatment is available. Half of such patients die by their early twenties; few live to middle age.

Causes and incidence

Sickle cell anemia results from homozygous inheritance of the hemoglobin S–producing gene, which causes substitution of the amino acid valine for glutamic acid in the B hemoglobin chain. Heterozygous inheritance of this gene results in sickle cell trait, generally an asymptomatic condition. Sickle cell anemia is most common in tropical Africans and in persons of African descent; about 1 in 10 Afro-Americans carries the abnormal gene. If two such carriers have offspring, there is a 1 in 4 chance that each child will have the disease. Overall, 1 in every 400 to 600 black children has sickle cell anemia. This disease also occurs in Puerto Rico, Turkey, India, the Middle East, and the Mediterranean area. Possibly, the defective hemoglobin S–producing gene has persisted because in areas where malaria is endemic, the heterozygous sickle cell trait provides resistance to malaria and is actually beneficial.

The abnormal hemoglobin S found in such patients' RBCs becomes insoluble whenever hypoxia occurs. As a result, these RBCs become rigid, rough, and elongated, forming a crescent or sickle shape. Such sickling can produce hemolysis (cell destruction). In addition, these

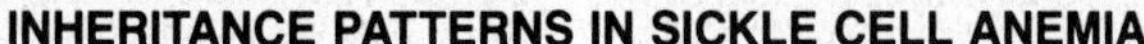

INHERITANCE PATTERNS IN SICKLE CELL ANEMIA

As this chart shows, in only two situations can you predict the outcome with certainty.

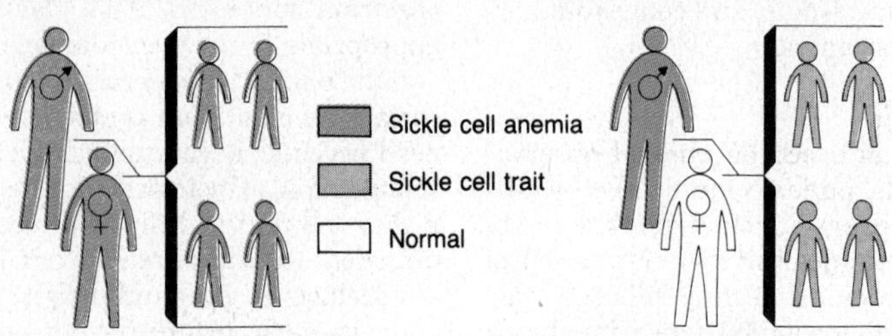

The first and most serious risk occurs when both parents have sickle cell anemia; childbearing—if possible at all—is dangerous for the mother, and all offspring will have sickle cell anemia.

When one parent has sickle cell anemia and one is normal; all offspring will be carriers of sickle cell anemia.

altered cells tend to pile up in capillaries and smaller blood vessels, making the blood more viscous. Normal circulation is impaired, causing pain, tissue infarctions, and swelling. Such blockage causes anoxic changes that lead to further sickling and obstruction.

Signs and symptoms

Characteristically, sickle cell anemia produces tachycardia, cardiomegaly, systolic and diastolic murmurs, pulmonary infarctions (which may result in cor pulmonale), chronic fatigue, unexplained dyspnea or dyspnea on exertion, hepatomegaly, jaundice, pallor, joint swelling, aching bones, chest pains, ischemic leg ulcers (especially around the ankles), and increased susceptibility to infection. Such symptoms usually don't develop until after 6 months of age, since large amounts of fetal hemoglobin protect infants for the first few months after birth. Low socioeconomic status and related problems, such as poor nutrition and education, may delay diagnosis and supportive treatment.

Infection, stress, dehydration, and conditions that provoke hypoxia—strenuous exercise, high altitude, unpressurized aircraft, cold, and vasoconstrictive drugs—may all provoke periodic crisis. A *painful crisis* (vasoocclusive crisis, infarctive crisis), the most common crisis and the hallmark of this disease, usually appears periodically after age 5. It results from blood vessel obstruction by rigid, tangled sickle cells, which causes tissue anoxia and possible necrosis. It's characterized by severe abdominal, thoracic, muscular, or bone pain and possibly increased jaundice, dark urine, or a low-grade fever. Autosplenectomy, in which splenic damage and scarring is so extensive that the spleen shrinks and becomes impalpable, occurs in patients with long-term disease. This can lead to increased susceptibility to *Streptococcus pneumoniae* sepsis, which can be fatal without prompt treatment. After the crisis subsides (in 4 days to several weeks), infection may develop, so watch for lethargy, sleepiness, fever, or apathy.

An *aplastic crisis* (megaloblastic crisis) results from bone marrow depression and is associated with infection, usually viral. It's characterized by pallor, lethargy, sleepiness, dyspnea, possible coma, markedly decreased bone marrow activity, and RBC hemolysis.

In infants between 8 months and 2 years old, an *acute sequestration crisis* may cause sudden massive entrapment of red cells in the spleen and liver. This rare crisis causes lethargy and pallor and, if untreated, commonly progresses to hypovolemic shock and death.

A *hemolytic crisis* is quite rare and usually occurs in patients who have glucose 6-phosphate dehydrogenase (G6PD) deficiency with sickle cell anemia. It probably results from complications of sickle cell anemia, such as infection, rather than from the disorder itself. Hemolytic crisis causes liver congestion and hepatomegaly as a result of degenerative changes. It worsens chronic jaundice, although increased jaundice doesn't always point to a hemolytic crisis.

Suspect any of these crises in a sickle cell anemia patient with pale lips, tongue, palms, or nail beds; lethargy; listlessness; sleepiness, with difficulty awakening; irritability; severe pain; temperature over 104° F. (40° C.) or a fever of 100° F. (37.8° C.) that persists for 2 days.

Sickle cell anemia also causes long-term complications. Typically, such a child is small for his age, and puberty is delayed. (However, fertility isn't impaired.) If he reaches adulthood, his body build tends to be spiderlike—narrow shoulders and hips, long extremities, curved spine, barrel chest, and elongated skull. An adult usually has complications from organ infarction, such as retinopathy and nephropathy. Premature death commonly results from infection or repeated occlusion of small blood vessels and consequent infarction or necrosis of major organs. For example, cerebral blood vessel occlusion causes cerebrovascular accident.

Diagnosis

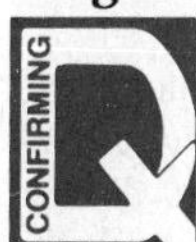

A positive family history and typical clinical features suggest sickle cell anemia; a stained blood smear showing sickle cells and hemoglobin electrophoresis showing hemoglobin S confirm it. Ideally, electrophoresis should be done on umbilical cord blood samples at birth, especially if the parents are known to carry the sickle cell trait. Additional lab studies show low RBC, elevated white blood cell (WBC) and platelet counts, decreased erythrocyte sedimentation rate, increased serum iron, decreased RBC survival, and reticulocytosis. Hemoglobin may be low or normal. During early childhood, palpation may reveal splenomegaly, but as the child grows older, the spleen shrinks.

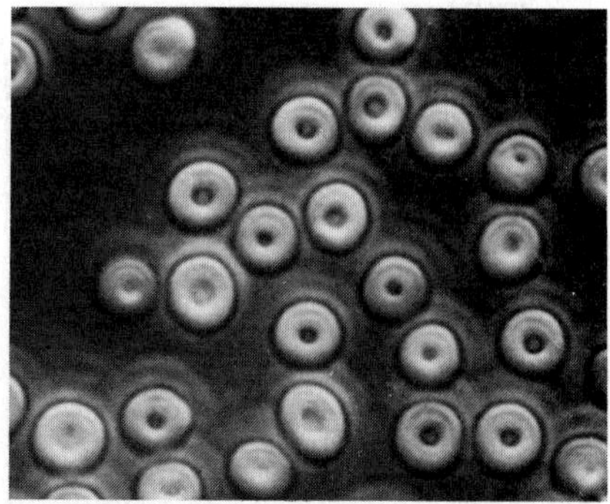

Normal red blood cells

Treatment

Treatment is primarily symptomatic and can usually take place at home. If the patient's hemoglobin drops suddenly or if his condition deteriorates rapidly, hospitalization is needed for transfusion of packed red cells. In a sequestration crisis, treatment may include sedation and administration of analgesics, blood transfusion, oxygen administration, and large amounts of oral or I.V. fluids. A good antisickling agent isn't yet available; the most commonly used drug, sodium cyanate, has many adverse effects.

Special considerations

Supportive measures during crises and precautions to avoid them are important.

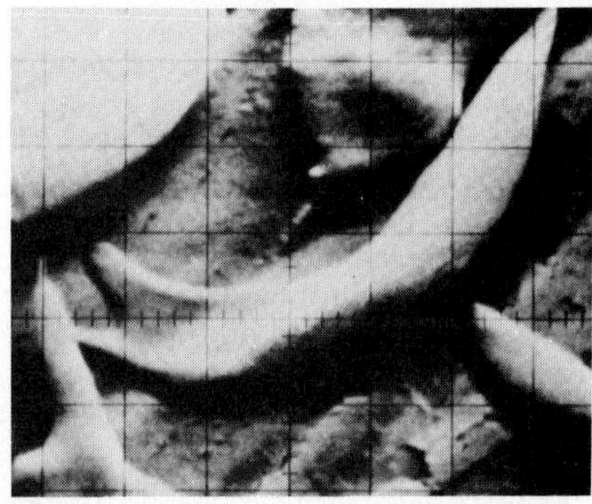

Sickle cells

SICKLE CELL TRAIT

This relatively benign condition results from heterozygous inheritance of the abnormal hemoglobin S–producing gene. Like sickle cell anemia, this condition is most common in Blacks. Sickle cell trait *never* progresses to sickle cell anemia.

In persons with sickle cell trait (also called carriers), 20% to 40% of their total hemoglobin is hemoglobin S; the rest is normal.

Such persons usually have no symptoms. They have normal hemoglobin and hematocrit values and can expect a normal life span. Nevertheless, they must avoid situations that provoke hypoxia, since these occasionally cause a sickling crisis similar to that in sickle cell anemia.

Genetic counseling is essential for sickle cell carriers. If two sickle cell carriers marry, each of their children has a 25% chance of inheriting sickle cell anemia.

Here are some actions you can take during a painful crisis:

- Apply warm compresses to painful areas, and cover the child with a blanket. (Never use cold compresses, since this aggravates the condition.)
- Administer an analgesic-antipyretic, such as aspirin or acetaminophen.
- Encourage bed rest, and place the patient in a sitting position. If dehydration or severe pain occurs, hospitalization may be necessary.
- When cultures indicate, give antibiotics as ordered.

During remission, help the patient prevent exacerbation by:

- advising him to avoid tight clothing that restricts circulation
- warning against strenuous exercise, vasoconstricting medications, cold temperatures (including drinking large amounts of ice water and swimming), unpressurized aircraft, high altitude, and other conditions that provoke hypoxia
- stressing the importance of normal childhood immunizations, meticulous wound care, good oral hygiene, regular dental checkups, and a balanced diet as safeguards against infection
- emphasizing the need for prompt treatment of infection
- making him aware of the need to increase fluid intake to prevent dehydration that results from impaired ability to concentrate urine properly. Tell parents to encourage such a child to drink more fluids, especially in the summer, by offering such fluids as milkshakes, ice pops, and eggnog.

To encourage normal mental and social development, warn parents against being overprotective. Although the child must avoid strenuous exercise, he can enjoy most everyday activities.

Refer parents of children with sickle cell anemia for genetic counseling to answer their questions about the risk to future offspring. Recommend screening of other family members to determine if they're heterozygote carriers. These parents may also need psychological counseling to cope with guilt feelings. In addition, suggest they join an appropriate community support group.

Sickle cell anemia calls for special precautions during pregnancy or surgery:

- Warn women with sickle cell anemia that they're poor obstetrical risks. However, their use of oral contraceptives is also risky; refer them for birth control counseling by a gynecologist. If such women *do* become pregnant, they should maintain a balanced diet during pregnancy and may benefit from a folic acid supplement.
- During general anesthesia, a sickle cell anemia patient requires adequate ventilation, to prevent hypoxic crisis. Therefore, make sure the surgeon and the anesthesiologist are aware that the patient has sickle cell anemia, and provide a preoperative transfusion of packed red cells, as needed.

Men with sickle cell anemia may develop sudden, painful episodes of priapism. Reassure them that these episodes are common and have no permanent harmful effects.

X-LINKED INHERITANCE

Hemophilia

Hemophilia is a hereditary bleeding disorder resulting from deficiency of specific clotting factors. Hemophilia A (classic hemophilia), which affects over 80% of all hemophiliacs, results from deficiency of Factor VIII; hemophilia B (Christmas disease), which affects 15% of hemophiliacs, from deficiency of Factor IX. However, recent evidence suggests that hemophilia may actually result from nonfunctioning Factors VIII and IX, rather than from their deficiency.

Severity and prognosis of bleeding disorders vary with the degree of deficiency and the site of bleeding. The overall prognosis is best in mild hemophilia, which doesn't cause spontaneous bleeding and joint deformities. Advances in treatment have greatly improved prognosis, and many hemophiliacs live normal life spans. Surgical procedures can be done safely at special treatment centers for hemophiliacs under the guidance of a hematologist.

Causes and incidence

Hemophilia A and B are inherited as X-linked recessive traits. This means that female carriers have a 50% chance of transmitting the gene to each daughter, who would then be a carrier, and a 50% chance of transmitting the gene to each son, who would be born with hemophilia. Hemophilia is the most common X-linked genetic disease and occurs in approximately 1.25 in 10,000 live male births. Hemophilia A is five times more common than hemophilia B. Hemophilia causes abnormal bleeding because of a specific clotting factor malfunction. After a person with hemophilia forms a platelet plug at a bleeding site, clotting factor deficiency impairs capacity to form a stable fibrin clot.

Signs and symptoms

Hemophilia produces abnormal bleeding, which may be mild, moderate, or severe, depending on the degree of factor deficiency. Mild hemophilia frequently goes undiagnosed until adulthood, because the patient with a mild deficiency does not bleed spontaneously or after minor trauma but has prolonged bleeding if challenged by major trauma or surgery. Postoperative bleeding continues as a slow ooze or ceases and starts again, up to 8 days after surgery.

Severe hemophilia causes spontaneous bleeding. Often, the first sign of severe hemophilia is excessive bleeding after circumcision. Later, spontaneous bleeding or severe bleeding after minor trauma may produce large subcutaneous and deep intramuscular hematomas. Bleeding into joints and muscles causes pain, swelling, extreme tenderness, and, possibly, permanent deformity.

Moderate hemophilia causes symptoms similar to severe hemophilia but produces only occasional spontaneous bleeding episodes.

Bleeding near peripheral nerves may cause peripheral neuropathies, pain, paresthesias, and muscle atrophy. If bleeding impairs blood flow through a major vessel, it can cause ischemia and gangrene. Pharyngeal, lingual, intracardial, intracerebral, and intracranial bleeding may all lead to shock and death.

Diagnosis

A history of prolonged bleeding after surgery (including dental extractions) or trauma or of episodes of spontaneous bleeding into muscles or joints usually indicates some defect in the hemostatic mechanism. Specific coagulation factor assays can diagnose the type and severity of hemophilia. A positive family history can also help diagnose hemophilia, but 20% of all cases have no family history. Characteristic findings in hemophilia A are:

- Factor VIII assay 0% to 30% of normal
- prolonged activated partial thromboplastin time (PTT)
- normal platelet count and function, bleeding time, and prothrombin time.

Characteristics of hemophilia B:

- deficient Factor IX assay
- baseline coagulation results similar to hemophilia A, with normal Factor VIII.

In hemophilia A or B, the degree of factor deficiency determines severity:

- mild hemophilia—factor levels 5% to 40% of normal
- moderate hemophilia—factor levels 1% to 5% of normal
- severe hemophilia—factor levels less than 1% of normal.

PARENT-TEACHING AID

Managing Hemophilia

Dear Parents:
Your child has hemophilia, a lifelong condition that requires special care.

- Notify your doctor immediately after even minor injury, but especially after injury to the head, neck, or abdomen. Such injuries may require special blood factor replacement. Also, check with your doctor before you allow dental extractions or any other surgery. Get the names of other doctors you can contact in case your regular doctor isn't available.
- Teach your child the importance of regular, careful toothbrushing to prevent any need for dental surgery. Have him use a soft toothbrush to avoid gum injury.
- Always watch for signs of severe internal bleeding, such as severe pain or swelling in a joint or muscle, stiffness, decreased joint movement, severe abdominal pain, blood in urine, black tarry stools, and severe headache.
- Because your child receives blood components, he risks hepatitis. Watch for early signs of this disease, which may appear 3 weeks to 6 months after treatment with blood components: headache, fever, decreased appetite, nausea, vomiting, abdominal tenderness, and pain over the liver.
- Make sure your child wears a medical identification bracelet at all times.
- *Never give him aspirin!* It can aggravate his tendency to bleed. Give acetaminophen instead.
- Protect your child from injury, but avoid unnecessary restrictions that impair his normal development. For example, for a toddler, sew padded patches into the knees and elbows of clothing to protect these joints during frequent falls. You must forbid an older child to participate in contact sports such as football, but you can encourage him to swim or to play golf.
- After injury, apply cold compresses or ice bags and elevate the injured part, or apply light pressure to the bleeding site. To prevent recurrence of bleeding after treatment, restrict activity for 48 hours after bleeding is under control.
- If you've been trained to administer blood factor components at home to avoid frequent hospitalization, know proper venipuncture and infusion techniques, and don't delay treatment during bleeding episodes. Keep blood factor concentrate and infusion equipment with you at all times, even when you're on vacation. Don't let your child miss routine follow-up examinations at your local hemophilia center. To answer your questions about the vulnerability of future offspring, get genetic counseling. Your daughters should have genetic screening to determine if they're hemophilia carriers.

For more information, contact the National Hemophilia Foundation.

Treatment

Hemophilia is not curable, but treatment can prevent crippling deformities and prolong life expectancy. Correct treatment quickly stops bleeding by increasing plasma levels of deficient clotting factors to help prevent disabling deformities that result from repeated bleeding into muscles and joints.

In hemophilia A, cryoprecipitated antihemophilic factor (AHF), lyophilized AHF, or both given in doses large enough to raise clotting factor levels above 25% of normal can permit normal hemostasis. Before surgery, AHF is administered to raise clotting factors to hemostatic levels. Levels are then kept within a normal range until the wound has completely healed.

In hemophilia B, administration of Factor IX concentrate during bleeding episodes increases Factor IX levels.

A person with hemophilia who undergoes surgery needs careful management by a hematologist with expertise in hemophilia care. The patient will require deficient factor replacement before and after surgery. Such replacement may be necessary even for minor surgery, such as a dental extraction. In addition, epsilon-aminocaproic acid is frequently used for oral bleeding to inhibit the active fibrinolytic system present in the oral mucosa. Preventive treatment teaches the patient how to avoid trauma, manage minor bleeding, and recognize bleeding that requires immediate medical intervention. Genetic counseling helps those who are carriers understand how this disease is transmitted.

FACTOR REPLACEMENT PRODUCTS

Cryoprecipitate
- Contains Factor VIII (70 to 100 units/bag). Does not contain Factor IX.
- Can be stored frozen up to 12 months but must be used within 6 hours after it thaws.
- Given through a blood filter. Compatible with normal saline solution only.

Lyophilized Factor VIII or IX
- Freeze-dried.
- Can be stored up to 2 years at about 36° to 46° F. (2° to 8° C.); up to 6 months at room temperature not exceeding 88° F. (31° C.)
- Labeled with exact units of Factor VIII or IX contained in vial.
- Vials range from 200 to 1,500 units of Factor VIII or IX each and contain 20 to 40 ml after reconstitution with diluent.
- Collected from large donor pools, so may cause hepatitis.
- No blood filter needed. Usually given slow I.V. push through a butterfly infusion set.

Fresh frozen plasma
- Contains Factor VIII (approximately .75 unit/ml) and Factor IX (approximately 1 unit/ml). Not practical to use for most hemophiliacs because a large volume is needed to raise factors to hemostatic levels.
- Can be stored frozen up to 12 months but must be used within 2 hours after it thaws.
- Given through a blood filter. Compatible with normal saline solution only.

Special considerations

During bleeding episodes:
- Give deficient clotting factor or plasma, as ordered. The body uses up AHF in 48 to 72 hours, so repeat infusions, as ordered, until bleeding stops.
- Apply cold compresses or ice bags and raise the injured part.
- To prevent recurrence of bleeding, restrict activity for 48 hours after bleeding is under control.
- Control pain with an analgesic, such as acetaminophen, propoxyphene, codeine, or meperidine, as ordered. Avoid I.M. injections because of possible hematoma formation at the injection site. Aspirin and aspirin-containing medications are contraindicated, since they decrease platelet adherence and may increase the bleeding.

If the patient has bled into a joint:
- Immediately elevate the joint.
- To restore joint mobility, if ordered, begin range-of-motion exercises at least 48 hours after the bleeding is controlled. Tell

patient to avoid weight bearing until bleeding stops and swelling subsides.

After bleeding episodes and surgery:

• Watch closely for signs of further bleeding, such as increased pain and swelling, fever, or symptoms of shock.
• Closely monitor PTT.
• Teach parents special precautions to prevent bleeding episodes. Reassure them that with proper management, their child can lead a productive life.
• Refer new or suspected patients to a hemophilia treatment center for evaluation. The center will devise a treatment and management plan for the patient's primary care physician and is a resource for medical personnel, dentists, school personnel, or anyone else involved in such a patient's care.

CHROMOSOMAL ABNORMALITIES

Down's Syndrome

(Mongolism, trisomy 21)

The first disorder attributed to a chromosome aberration, Down's syndrome characteristically produces mental retardation, abnormal facial features, and other distinctive physical abnormalities. It's often associated with congenital heart defects and other congenital disorders.

Life expectancy for patients with Down's syndrome has increased significantly because of improved treatment for related complications (heart defects, tendency toward respiratory and other infections, acute leukemia). Nevertheless, up to one third die before they're 10 years old. Mortality is highest in patients with congenital heart disease.

Causes and incidence

Down's syndrome usually results from trisomy 21, an aberration in which chromosome 21 has three copies instead of the normal two because of faulty meiosis (nondisjunction) of the ovum or, sometimes, the sperm. This results in a karyotype of 47 chromosomes instead of the normal 46. About 4% of the time, though, Down's syndrome results from an unbalanced translocation in which the long arm of chromosome 21 breaks and attaches to another chromosome.

One of the parents of a child with such an unbalanced translocation is a "balanced translocation carrier" with no physical or mental abnormalities. A mother who is a balanced translocation carrier has a 10% chance of having a Down's child; a carrier father has a less than 5% chance.

Overall, Down's syndrome occurs in 1 per 650 live births, but the incidence increases with maternal age, especially after age 35. For instance, at age 20, a mother has about one chance in 2,000 of having a child with Down's syndrome; by age 49, she has one chance in 12. Although women over age 35 account for fewer than 5% of all births, they bear 20% of all children with Down's syndrome. The role of paternal age is not yet known. This suggests that sometimes the chromosome abnormality responsible for Down's syndrome results from deterioration of the oocyte because of age alone or because of the accumulated effects of environmental factors, such as radiation and viruses. However, if a mother has had one child with Down's syndrome, the risk of recurrence remains 0.5% to 2%, unless trisomy results from translocation.

Signs and symptoms

The physical signs of Down's syndrome

(especially hypotonia) are readily apparent at birth; mental retardation is obvious as such infants grow older. Typically, these persons have craniofacial anomalies, such as slanting, almond-shaped eyes (epicanthic folds); protruding tongue; small open mouth; a single transverse palmar crease (simian crease); small white spots (Brushfield's spots) on the iris; strabismus; small skull; flat bridge across the nose; slow dental development, with abnormal or absent teeth; flattened face; small external ears; short neck; and occasionally cataracts.

Other physical effects include dry, sensitive skin with decreased elasticity, umbilical hernia, short stature, and short extremities, with broad, flat, and squarish hands and feet. These patients have clinodactyly (small little finger that curves inward), a wide space between the first and second toe, and abnormal fingerprints and footprints. Hypotonic limb muscles impair reflex development, posture, coordination, and balance.

Such patients have an IQ between 30 and 50. So, as infants, they're slow to sit up, walk, and talk, but they're usually docile and easily managed. Their intellectual development slows with age. Commonly, they have congenital heart disease (septal defects or pulmonary or aortic stenosis), duodenal atresia, megacolon, and pelvic bone abnormalities. Their genitalia are poorly developed, and puberty is delayed. Females may menstruate and be fertile. Males are infertile with low serum testosterone levels; in many, the testicles fail to descend. These patients are especially susceptible to leukemia and to acute and chronic infections. Thyroid disorders are common.

Diagnosis

Physical findings at birth, especially hypotonia, suggest this diagnosis, but no physical feature is diagnostic in itself.

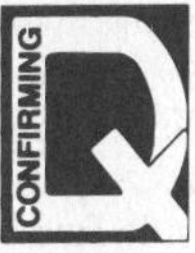

A karyotype showing the chromosome abnormality can confirm it. Amniocentesis allows prenatal diagnosis; 80% of all amniocenteses are done for this purpose and are recommended for pregnant women past age 35. Amniocentesis is indicated for a pregnant woman of any age when either she or the father carries a translocated chromosome.

Treatment

Down's syndrome has no known cure. Surgery to correct heart defects and other related congenital abnormalities and antibiotic therapy for recurrent infections have improved life expectancy considerably. Plastic surgery may be done to correct the characteristic facial traits, especially the protruding tongue. Benefits beyond improved appearance include improved speech, reduced susceptibility to dental caries, and fewer orthodontic problems later. Down's syndrome patients may be cared for at home and attend special education classes or, if profoundly retarded, may be institutionalized. As adults, some may work in a sheltered workshop.

Special considerations

Support for the parents of a child with Down's syndrome is vital. By following the guidelines listed below, you can help them meet their child's physical and emotional needs:

- Establish a trusting relationship with parents, and encourage communication during the difficult period soon after diagnosis and when parents face the difficult decision of whether or not to care for their child at home.
- Teach parents the importance of a balanced diet. Stress the need for patience while feeding their child, since he may have difficulty sucking, and may be less demanding and seem less eager to eat than normal babies.
- Encourage parents to hold and nurture their child, even though their first reaction may be to reject him because he isn't normal.
- Emphasize the importance of adequate exercise and maximal environmental stimulation, and refer them for infant stimulation classes, which may begin at age 3 months.

• Assist parents in setting realistic goals for their child. His mental development may seem normal at first, but warn parents not to view this early development as a sign of future progress. By the time he's 1 year old, his development will clearly lag behind that of normal children. Help them view their child's successful achievements positively, even though he's slow. The Denver Developmental Screening Test for noninstitutionalized Down's children can help chart progress.
• Refer parents and older siblings for genetic counseling and, if necessary, for psychological counseling, to help them evaluate future risks and adopt a positive outlook.
• Warn parents not to overlook the emotional needs of other children in the family.

Klinefelter's Syndrome

This relatively common genetic abnormality results from one or more extra X chromosomes, and it affects only males. It usually becomes apparent at puberty, when the secondary sex characteristics develop; although the penis is normal, the testicles fail to mature, and degenerative testicular changes begin that eventually result in irreversible infertility. Klinefelter's syndrome often causes gynecomastia and is also associated with a tendency toward mental deficiency.

Causes and incidence

Klinefelter's syndrome, probably the most common cause of hypogonadism, appears in approximately 1 in every 600 males. (For information on another common cause of hypogonadism, see *Turner's syndrome.*) Also, it accounts for roughly 10 in every 1,000 institutionalized mentally retarded males.

This disorder usually results from one extra X chromosome, giving such patients a 47,XXY complement instead of the normal 46,XY. Sometimes additional X chromosomes are present (XXXY, XXXXY). Usually, the larger the number of extra chromosomes, the more severe the disorder. In the rare, mosaic form of this syndrome, only some cells contain the extra X chromosomes, while others contain the normal XY complement.

The extra chromosome or chromosomes responsible for Klinefelter's syndrome probably result from either meiotic nondisjunction during parental gametogenesis or from meiotic nondisjunction in the zygote. The incidence of meiotic nondisjunction increases with maternal age.

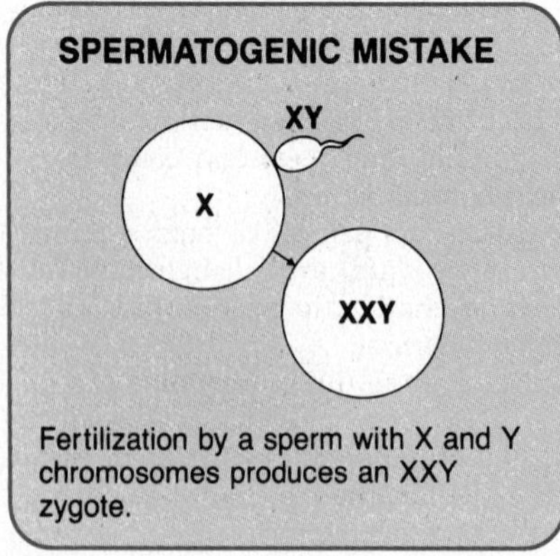

Fertilization by a sperm with X and Y chromosomes produces an XXY zygote.

Signs and symptoms

Klinefelter's syndrome usually isn't apparent until puberty or later and many cases probably go undetected—especially mild ones, with no abnormalities except infertility. Its characteristic features include a small penis and prostate; small, firm testicles; sparse facial and abdominal hair; feminine distribution of pubic hair; sexual dysfunction (impotence, lack of libido); and, in less than 50% of patients, gynecomastia. Aspermatogenesis and infertility result from

TURNER'S SYNDROME

In Turner's syndrome, the missing X chromosome (or missing part of the second X chromosome), may be lost from either ovum or sperm through nondisjunction or chromosome lag. Mixed aneuploidy may result from mitotic nondisjunction.

Incidence of Turner's syndrome is 1 per 2,500 to 1 per 7,000 births; 95% to 98% of fetuses with this syndrome are spontaneously aborted.

Turner's syndrome produces certain characteristic signs. At birth, 50% of infants with this syndrome measure below the third percentile in length. Commonly, they have swollen hands and feet, a wide chest with laterally displaced nipples, and a low hairline that becomes more obvious as they grow. They may have severe webbing of the neck; some have coarse, enlarged, prominent ears. Gonadal dysgenesis is seen at birth and typically causes sterility in adults.

Cardiovascular malformations occur in 10% to 40% of patients, but renal abnormalities are even more common. Short stature (usually under 59″ [150 cm]) is the most common adult sign.

Most patients have average or slightly below average intelligence; they commonly show space-form blindness, right-left disorientation for extrapersonal space, and defective figure drawing. They're typically immature, socially naive, and conforming.

Turner's syndrome can be diagnosed by chromosome analysis. Differential should rule out mixed gonadal dysgenesis, Noonan-Ehmke's syndrome, and other similar disorders. Treatment should begin in early childhood and include hormonal therapy: androgens, human growth hormone, and, possibly, small doses of estrogen. Later, progesterone and estrogen can induce sexual maturation.

progressive sclerosis and hyalinization of the seminiferous tubules in the testicles and from testicular fibrosis during and after puberty. In the mosaic form, such changes and resulting infertility may be delayed.

Klinefelter's syndrome is also associated with mental retardation, osteoporosis, abnormal body build (long legs with short, obese trunk), tall stature, and a tendency toward alcoholism, antisocial behavior, and other personality disorders. In addition, it's associated with increased incidence of pulmonary disease, varicose veins, and breast cancer.

Diagnosis

Typical clinical features suggest Klinefelter's syndrome, but only a karyotype (chromosome analysis) determined by culturing lymphocytes from peripheral blood can clearly confirm it.

Characteristically, Klinefelter's syndrome decreases urinary 17-ketosteroids, increases follicle-stimulating hormone (FSH) excretion, and decreases plasma testosterone levels after puberty.

Treatment and special considerations

Depending on severity, treatment may include mastectomy in persistent gynecomastia, and supplemental testosterone in sexual dysfunction. However, not all patients need hormonal treatment. The testicular changes that lead to infertility can't be prevented. But earlier treatment may be more effective.

Psychotherapy with sexual counseling is indicated when sexual dysfunction causes emotional maladjustment. If patients with the mosaic form of the syndrome are fertile, genetic counseling is essential, since they may transmit this chromosomal abnormality.

Encourage such patients to discuss feelings of confusion and rejection that may arise, and reinforce their male identity. Improve compliance with hormone therapy by making sure they understand testosterone's benefits and side effects.

Cri du Chat Syndrome

(Cat's cry syndrome, 5p-syndrome)

Cri du chat syndrome is a rare congenital disorder characterized by a catlike cry in infancy, and severe mental and physical retardation. Many cri du chat infants do not live past their first year, but of those who do survive, some may live to adulthood.

Causes and incidence

Cri du chat syndrome results from abnormal deletion of the short arm of chromosome 5 (5*p*–). About 10% of infants with this disorder have a parent who is a balanced carrier for a translocation of the short arm of chromosome 5. The risk of cri du chat does not increase with parental age. Incidence is probably about 1 in every 20,000 live births and is more common in females than in males.

Signs and symptoms

An infant with this disorder usually has a normal prenatal history and birth. At birth he is abnormally small and shows microencephaly, wide-set eyes, receding chin, high-arched palate, round face, and decreased muscle tone, which makes feeding difficult. The high-pitched catlike cry appears soon after birth and later disappears. Other symptoms include low-set ears, simian crease, epicanthal folds, severe mental retardation (IQ is less than 50), and associated defects, such as congenital heart disease, joint and bone deformities, and inguinal hernia.

Diagnosis

These typical clinical features (cat cry, facial disproportions, microencephaly, small birth size, poor physical and mental development) strongly suggest cri du chat syndrome.

A karyotype showing deleted short arms of chromosome 5 confirms it.

Treatment

No specific treatment exists for cri du chat. Individualized treatment includes evaluation and treatment of congenital heart and eye defects. When these infants survive past their first year, management is primarily nonmedical and emphasizes education, training in self-care and socialization, recreational and social services, vocational training, and custodial arrangements. Ideally, such management requires the cooperation of a team of specialists to develop a personalized and realistic care plan. Whenever possible, such a plan should emphasize home care, early education (which may use behavior modification), and parent teaching to maximize stimulation.

Special considerations

- Because an affected infant is usually a poor eater, closely monitor fluid intake and output, caloric intake, and weight. To help him meet caloric requirements, offer small feedings frequently. Large meals are apt to tire him because of his decreased muscle tone.
- Amniocentesis can detect cri du chat syndrome prenatally. Encourage parents of such a child to receive genetic counseling. If the male is the translocation carrier, artificial insemination may be a viable alternative.
- Explain the child's potential so his family can understand and accept long-term plans (including whether or not to institutionalize the child). Refer the parents to an infant stimulation program, which will help their child reach his potential. To avoid rejection or overprotection of such a child, help the parents set realistic goals.
- If parents have trouble coping, refer them for psychologic counseling.

MULTIFACTORIAL ABNORMALITIES

Cleft Lip and Palate

Cleft lip and cleft palate deformities occur in 1 in every 800 births. They originate in the second month of pregnancy, when the front and sides of the face and the palatine shelves fuse imperfectly. Cleft deformities fall into four categories: clefts of the lip (unilateral or bilateral); clefts of the palate (along the midline); unilateral clefts of the lip, alveolus (gum pad), and palate, which are twice as common on the left side as on the right; and bilateral clefts of the lip, alveolus, and palate. Cleft lip with or without cleft palate is more common in males, while cleft palate alone is more common in females.

Causes and incidence

Although cleft lips and palates occur in infants with chromosomal abnormalities, they are also found in infants who are otherwise normal. Incidence of cleft deformities is higher in children with a positive family history. If normal parents have a baby with a cleft, the risk that subsequent offspring will have the defect is 5%; if they have two children with this disorder, the risk in subsequent offspring climbs to 12%.

Signs and symptoms

Congenital clefts of the face occur most often in the upper lip. They range from a simple notch to a complete cleft, extending from the lip edge through the floor of the nostril, on either side of the midline. A cleft lip rarely runs along the midline itself, unless accompanied by other congenital anomalies.

A cleft palate may be partial or complete. A complete cleft includes the soft palate, the bones of the maxilla, and the alveolus on one or both sides of the premaxilla. A double cleft—the severest of all cleft deformities—runs from the soft palate forward to either side of the nose, separating the maxilla and premaxilla into free-moving segments. The tongue and other muscles can displace these bony segments, enlarging the cleft. In Pierre Robin syndrome, micrognathia and glossoptosis coexist with cleft palate.

Diagnosis

Typical clinical picture confirms diagnosis. Cleft lips, with or without cleft palates, are obvious at birth. Cleft palates without cleft lips may not be detected until a thorough mouth examination is done, or until feeding difficulties develop.

Treatment

Treatment consists of surgical correction, but the timing of surgery varies. Some plastic surgeons repair cleft lips within the first few days of life. This makes it easier to feed the baby and makes him more acceptable to his parents. However, many surgeons delay lip repairs for 8 to 10 weeks and sometimes as long as 6 to 8 months, to allow time for maternal bonding, and most important, to rule out associated congenital anomalies. Cleft palate repair is usually completed by the 12th to 18th month. Still other surgeons repair cleft palates in two steps, repairing the soft palate between 6 and 18 months and the hard palate as late as 5 years old. In any case, surgery is performed only after the infant is gaining weight satisfactorily and is free of any respiratory, oral, or systemic infections.

When a wide horseshoe defect makes surgery impossible, a contoured speech bulb is attached to the posterior of a denture to occlude the nasopharynx and help the child develop intelligible speech. Surgery must be coupled with speech therapy. Because the palate is essential to speech formation, structural changes, even in a repaired cleft, can permanently affect speech patterns. To compound the problem, children with cleft palates often have hearing difficulties because of middle ear damage or infections.

Special considerations

- Never place a child with Pierre Robin syndrome (micrognathia, glossoptosis) on his back, since his tongue can fall back and obstruct his airway. Therefore, train such a baby to sleep on his side. All other cleft palate babies can sleep on their backs without difficulty.
- Maintain adequate nutrition for normal growth and development. Experiment with feeding devices. A baby with a cleft palate has an excellent appetite but often has trouble feeding because of air leaks around the cleft and nasal regurgitation. He often feeds better from a nipple with a flange that occludes the cleft, a lamb's nipple (a big soft nipple with large holes), or just a regular nipple with enlarged holes.

Teach the mother to hold the infant in a near-sitting position, with the flow directed to the side or back of the baby's tongue. Tell her to burp the baby frequently, since he tends to swallow a lot of air. If the underside of the nasal septum becomes ulcerated and the child refuses to suck because of the pain, instruct the mother to direct the nipple to the side of his mouth, to give the mucosa time to heal. Tell her to gently clean the palatal cleft with a cotton-tipped applicator dipped in half-strength hydrogen peroxide or water after each feeding.

- Encourage the mother of a baby with cleft lip to breast-feed if the cleft doesn't prevent effective sucking. Breast-feeding an infant with a cleft palate or one who has just had corrective surgery is impossible. (Postoperatively, the infant can't suck for up to 6 weeks.) However, if the mother desires, suggest that she use a breast pump to express breast milk and then feed it to her baby from a bottle.
- Following surgery, record intake and output, and maintain good nutrition. To prevent atelectasis and pneumonia, the doctor may gently suction the nasopharynx (this may be necessary before surgery, too). Restrain the infant to stop him from hurting himself. Elbow restraints allow the baby to move his hands while keeping them away from his mouth. When necessary, use an infant seat to keep the child in a comfortable sitting position. Hang toys within reach of restrained hands.
- Surgeons sometimes place a curved metal Logan bow over a repaired cleft lip to minimize tension on the suture line. Remove the gauze before feedings, and replace it often. Moisten it with normal saline solution until the sutures are removed. Check your hospital policy to confirm this procedure.
- Help the parents deal with their feelings about the child's deformity. Start by telling them about it immediately and showing them their baby as soon as possible. Because society places undue importance on physical appearance, parents often feel shock, disappointment,

CLEFT LIP AND PALATE

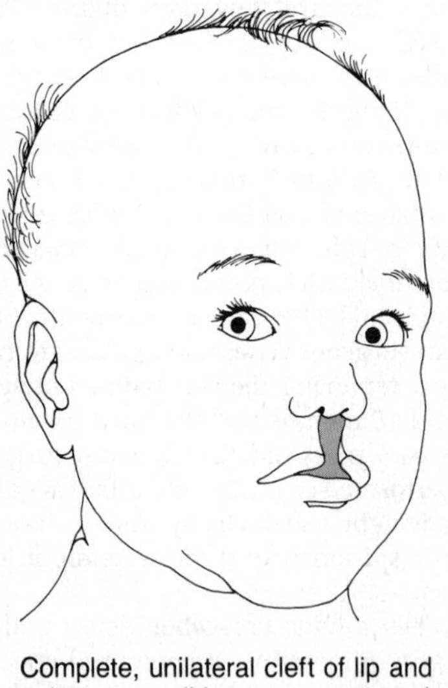

Complete, unilateral cleft of lip and palate, a condition more common in males than in females

and guilt when they see the child. Help them by being calm and providing positive information. Direct parents' attention to their child's assets; show them what is "right" about their baby. Stress the fact that surgical repairs can be made. Include the parents in the care and feeding of the child right from the start to encourage normal bonding. Provide the necessary instructions, emotional support, and reassurance the parents will need to take proper care of the child at home. Refer them to a social worker who can guide them to community resources.

Selected References

Aumonier, M.E., and Cunningham, C.C. "Health and Medical Problems in Infants with Down's Syndrome," *Health Visitor* 57(5):137-40, May 1984.

Cohen, Felissa L. *Clinical Genetics in Nursing Practice*. Philadelphia: J.B. Lippincott Co., 1984.

Guerrein, Ann Therese. "Osteogenesis Imperfecta: A Disorder That Breaks More Than Our Hearts," *Maternal Child Nursing* 7:315-18, September/October 1982.

Knudson, A.G. "A Geneticist's View of Neurofibromatosis," *Advances in Neurology* 29:237-43, 1981.

McKusick, Victor. *Mendelian Inheritance in Man: Catalogs of Autosomal Dominant, Autosomal Recessive, and X-linked Phenotypes,* 6th ed. Baltimore: Johns Hopkins Press, 1983.

Polloch, R.A., et al. "Malignant Hyperthermia in Head and Neck Surgery Patients: An Update and Review," *Laryngoscope* 93(3):318-25, March 1983.

Sutton, Eldon H. *An Introduction to Human Genetics.* New York: Holt, Rinehart & Winston, 1975.

Thompson, James S., and Thompson, Margaret W. *Genetics in Medicine,* 3rd ed. Philadelphia: W.B. Saunders Co., 1980.

Vaughan, V., and McKay, R. J., eds. *Nelson Textbook of Pediatrics,* 12th ed. Philadelphia: W.B. Saunders Co., 1983.

Whaley, L., and Wong, D. *Nursing Care of Infants and Children,* 2nd ed. St. Louis: C.V. Mosby Co., 1983.

Williams, J.K. "Reproductive Decisions: Adolescents with Down's Syndrome," *Pediatric Nursing* 9(1):43-44, January/February 1983.

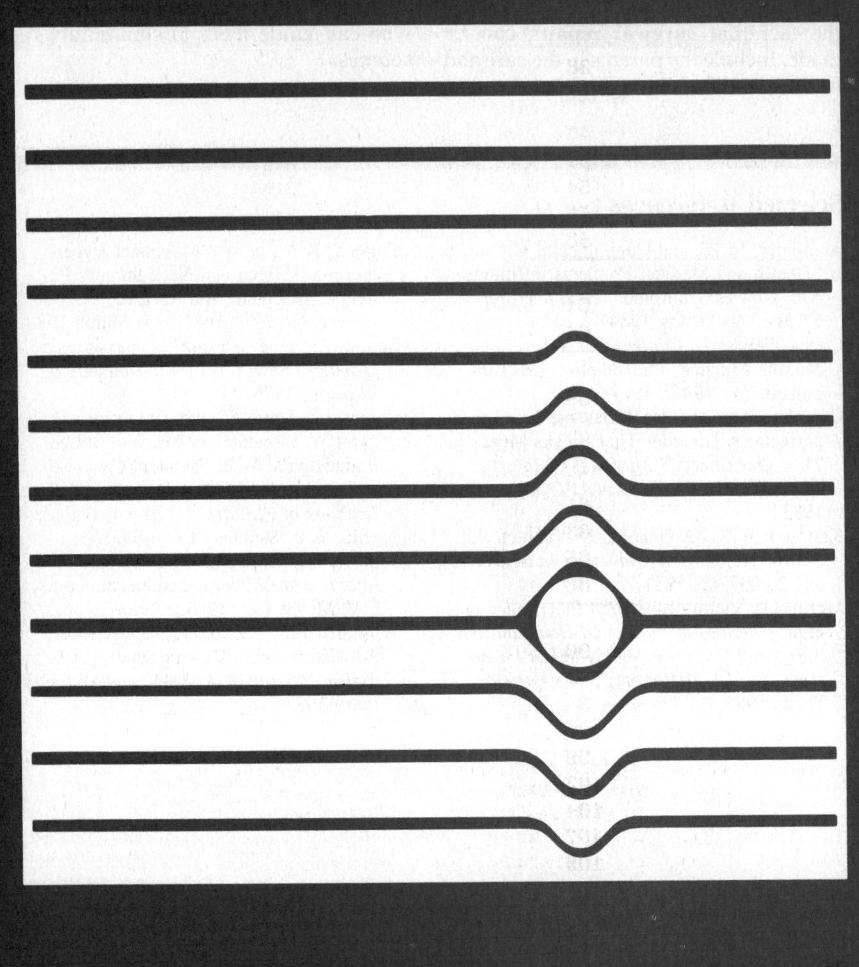

2 Neoplasms

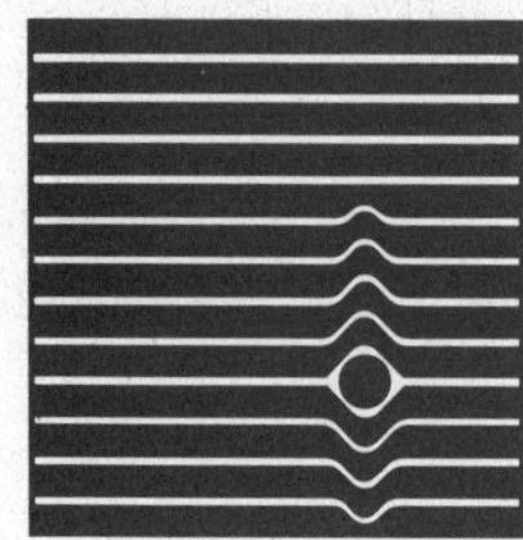

Neoplasms

Introduction

Cancer is second only to cardiovascular disease as the leading cause of death in the United States (over 400,000 deaths annually). Predominantly a disease of older adults (incidence increases geometrically with age), it's generally more common in men. Although cancer isn't very common in children, only accidental death exceeds it as the leading cause of death in this age-group.

Abnormal cell growth

Conveniently classified according to their histologic origin, malignant tumors derived from epithelial tissues are known as carcinomas, while those arising from connective, muscle, and osseous tissues are known as sarcomas.

Neoplastic cells differ from normal cells in size—they are larger and divide more quickly—and in function, as they serve no useful purpose. The most characteristic difference, however, is the malignant cells' ability to grow and spread throughout the body rapidly, uncontrollably, and independently from the primary site to other tissues, and to establish secondary foci called metastases. Malignant cells can metastasize by way of blood or lymphatics, by accidental transplantation from one site to another during surgery, and by local extension.

What causes cancer?

All available evidence indicates that malignant transformation of cells (carcinogenesis) results from complex interactions of viruses, physical and chemical carcinogens, genetic predisposition, immunologic factors, and diet. Through studies on animals that monitor the ability of viruses to transform cells, some human viruses have been shown to have carcinogenic potential. For example, the Epstein-Barr virus (EBV), the cause of infectious mononucleosis, has been linked to lymphomas. Other DNA viruses (such as herpes simplex, type 2) have been associated with cancer of the nasopharynx and of the cervix; RNA viruses, with breast cancer.

Of all known carcinogens, radiation is perhaps the most dangerous and unpredictable because it damages DNA, possibly inducing genetically transferable abnormalities. Although radiation can induce many different types of tumors, other factors, such as tissue type, age, and the patient's hormonal state, also interact to promote its carcinogenic effect. Even the sun's ultraviolet rays can cause skin cancer on exposed body areas.

Many substances commonly found in the environment may induce carcinogenesis by damaging the DNA. Some of these substances have been proven carcinogenic in humans:

- asbestos—mesothelioma of the lung
- vinyl chloride—angiosarcoma of the liver

- aromatic hydrocarbons and benzopyrene (from polluted air)—lung cancer
- alkylating agents—leukemia
- tobacco—cancer of the lung, oral cavity and upper airways, esophagus, pancreas, kidneys, and bladder.

Diet has also been implicated, especially in the development of gastrointestinal cancer as a result of a high-protein and high-fat diet. Additives composed of nitrates and certain methods of food preparation—particularly charbroiling—are also recognized factors.

The role of hormones in carcinogenesis is still controversial, but it seems that excessive use of some hormones, especially estrogen, produces cancer in animals. Also, the synthetic estrogen diethylstilbestrol (DES) causes vaginal cancer in some daughters of women who were treated with it. It's unclear, however, whether changes in human hormonal balance retard or stimulate cancer development.

Some forms of cancer and precancerous lesions result from genetic predisposition either directly (as in Wilms' tumor and retinoblastoma) or indirectly (in association with inherited conditions such as Down's syndrome or immunodeficiency diseases). Expressed as autosomal recessive, X-linked, or autosomal dominant disorders, their common characteristics include:

- early onset of malignant disease
- increased incidence of bilateral cancer in paired organs (breasts, adrenal glands, kidneys, and eighth cranial nerves [acoustic neuroma])
- increased incidence of multiple primary malignancies in nonpaired organs
- abnormal chromosome complement in tumor cells.

Immune tumor response

Other factors that interact to increase susceptibility to carcinogenesis are immunologic competence, age, nutritional status, hormonal balance, and response to stress. Theoretically, the body develops cancer cells continuously, but the immune system recognizes them as foreign cells and destroys them. This defense mechanism, known as *immunosurveillance*, has two major components: humoral immune response and cell-mediated immune response; their interaction promotes antibody production, cellular immunity, and immunologic memory. Presumably, the intact human immune system is responsible for spontaneous regression of tumors.

Theoretically, the *cell-mediated immune response* begins when T lymphocytes become sensitized by contact with a specific antigen. After repeated contacts, sensitized T cells release chemical factors called *lymphokines*, some of which begin to destroy the antigen. This reaction triggers the transformation of an additional population of T lymphocytes into "killers" of antigen-specific cells—in this case, cancer cells.

Similarly, the *humoral immune response* reacts to an antigen by triggering the release of antibodies from plasma cells and activating the serum-complement system, which destroys the antigen-bearing cell. However, an opposing immune factor, a "blocking antibody," enhances tumor growth by protecting malignant cells from immune destruction.

Theoretically, cancer arises when any one of several factors disrupts the immune system:

- *Aging cells,* when copying their genetic material, may begin to err, giving rise to mutations; the aging immune system may not recognize these mutations as foreign and thus may allow them to proliferate and form a malignant tumor.
- *Cytotoxic drugs* or *steroids* decrease antibody production and destroy circulating lymphocytes.
- *Extreme stress* or *certain viral infections* can depress the immune system.
- *Increased susceptibility to infection* often results from radiation, cytotoxic drug therapy, and lymphoproliferative and myeloproliferative diseases, such as lymphatic and myelocytic leukemia. These cause bone marrow depression, which can impair leukocyte function.
- *Acquired immunodeficiency syndrome* (AIDS) weakens cell-mediated immunity.
- *Cancer* itself is immunosuppressive; advanced cancer exhausts the immune response. (The absence of immune reactivity is known as *anergy.*)

Diagnostic methods

A thorough medical history and physical examination should precede sophisticated diagnostic procedures. Useful tests for the early detection and staging of tumors include X-ray, isotope scan, computed tomography scan, and magnetic resonance imaging, but the single most important diagnostic tool is a biopsy for direct histologic study of tumor tissue. Biopsy tissue samples can be taken by curettage, fluid aspiration (pleural effusion), needle aspiration biopsy (breast), dermal punch (skin or mouth), endoscopy (rectal polyps), and surgical excision (visceral tumors and nodes).

An important tumor marker, carcinoembryonic antigen (CEA), although not diagnostic by itself, can signal malignancies of the large bowel, the stomach, the pancreas, lungs, breasts, and sometimes sarcomas, leukemias, and lymphomas. CEA titers range from normal (less than 5 ng) to suspicious (5 to 10 ng) to very suspect (over 10 ng). CEA provides a valuable baseline during chemotherapy to evaluate the extent of tumor spread, regulate drug dosage, prognosticate after surgery or radiation, and detect tumor recurrence.

Although no more specific than CEA, alpha-fetoprotein (AFP), a fetal antigen uncommon in adults, can suggest testicular, ovarian, gastric, pancreatic, and primary lung cancers. Beta human chorionic gonadotropin (beta HCG) may point to testicular cancer or choriocarcinoma.

Staging and grading

Choosing effective therapeutic options depends on correct *staging* of malignant disease, often with the internationally known TNM staging system (*t*umor size, *n*odal involvement, *m*etastatic progress). This classification allows an accurate tumor description that's adjustable as the disease progresses. TNM staging allows reliable comparison of treatment and survival among large population groups; it also identifies nodal involvement and metastasis to other areas. TNM staging is applicable to most cancers (but not to Hodgkin's disease and other lymphomas).

Grading is another objective way to define a tumor. Grading takes into account resemblance of tumor tissue to normal cells (differentiation) and its estimated growth rate (for example, a well-differentiated tumor with a slow growth rate would be termed "low grade"). Grading also names the lesion according to corresponding normal cells, such as lymphoid or mucinous lesions.

READER'S DIGEST
GIFT SERVICE DEPT.
PLEASANTVILLE, N.Y. 10570

Use this Stamp to receive your FREE GIFT

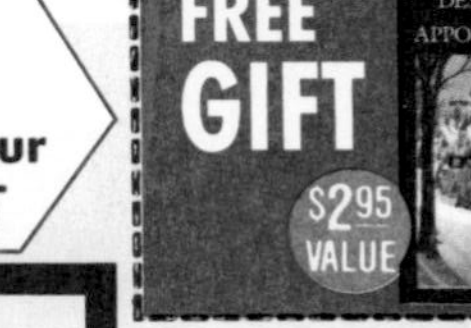

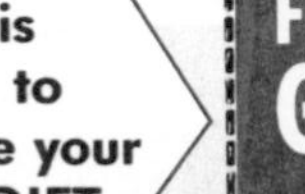

CONFIRMATION OF $11.59 SAVING

This attached Confirmation Card is an *Important Document* which is valid for an $11.59 Saving plus a Free Gift for your personal use. PLEASE REPLY before *November 15th* so we can rush your Free Gift to you.

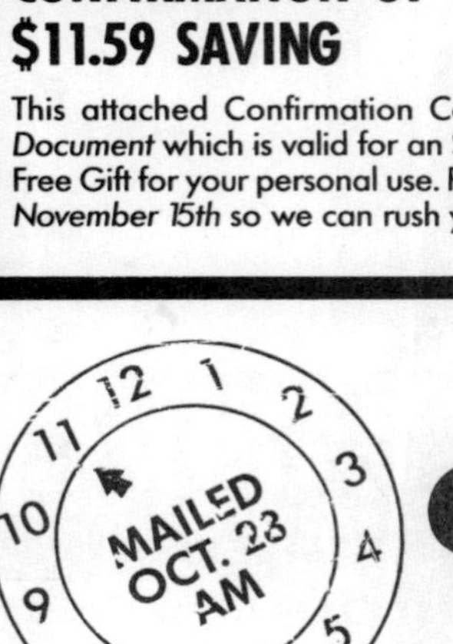

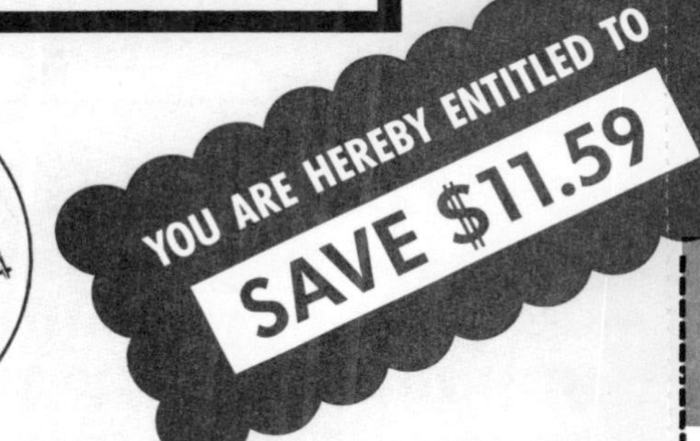

▼ KEEP THIS RECEIPT FOR YOUR RECORDS ▼

Mail Your Official Confirmation Card above to give a 12-month new gift subscription to Reader's Digest for only $7.97 plus $1.44 postage.

Give a gift subscription and we'll send a **FREE** copy of the **1987 DESK CALENDAR** to:

DAVID
ELLISON

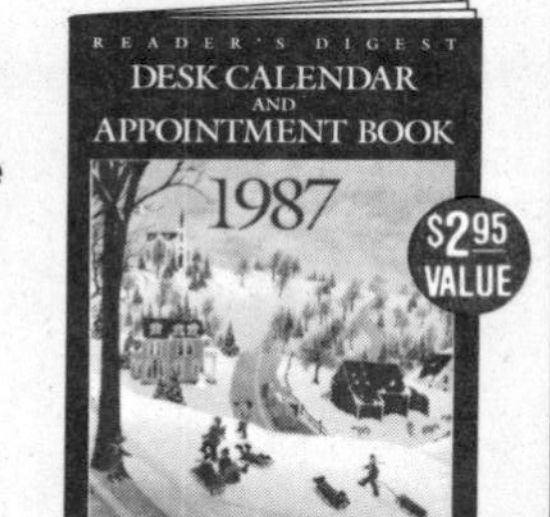

YOU SAVE:

$6.00

off the regular subscription price.

$11.59

off the yearly single-copy price.

SAVE MORE THAN HALF OFF!

TERMS: Send no money now. We won't bill you for your gift until after January 6, 1987.

THIS SPECIAL DISCOUNT VALID FOR ONE NEW GIFT SUBSCRIPTION ONLY.

Prices shown good only in U.S. Price for foreign delivery of U.S. Edition and foreign editions is $21.41.

ESSENTIAL DIFFERENCES BETWEEN BENIGN AND MALIGNANT TUMORS

	BENIGN	MALIGNANT
Growth	Slow expansion; push aside surrounding tissue but do not infiltrate	Usually infiltrate surrounding tissues rapidly, expanding in all directions
Limitation	Frequently encapsulated	Seldom encapsulated; often poorly delineated
Recurrence	Rare after surgical removal	When removed surgically, frequently recur due to infiltration into surrounding tissues
Morphology	Cells closely resemble cells of tissue of origin	Cells may differ considerably from those of tissue of origin
Differentiation	Well differentiated	Variable
Mitotic activity	Variable	Extensive
Tissue destruction	Usually slight	Extensive due to infiltration and metastatic lesion
Spread	No metastasis	Spread via blood and/or lymph systems; establish secondary tumors
Effect on body	Cachexia rare; usually not fatal but may obstruct vital organs, exert pressure, produce excess hormones; can become malignant	Cachexia typical—anemia, loss of weight, weakness, etc.; fatal if untreated

Three major therapies

The major therapies used to treat cancer are surgery, radiation, and chemotherapy, employed independently or in combination. (Immunotherapy to bolster the patient's immune response to cancer is still an unproven form of therapy.) In every case, treatment depends on the type, stage, localization, and responsiveness of the tumor.

Surgery, once the mainstay of cancer treatment, is now more often combined with radiation and chemotherapy (surgery to remove the bulk of the tumor, then chemotherapy and radiation to discourage proliferation of residual cells). Surgery can also relieve pain, correct obstruction, and alleviate pressure. Today's less radical surgery (for example, a lumpectomy instead of a radical mastectomy) is more acceptable to patients.

Radiation therapy aims to destroy the rapidly dividing cancer cells, while damaging normal cells as little as possible. Radiation consists of two types: ionizing radiation and particle radiation. Both types have the cellular DNA as their target; however, particle radiation produces less skin damage.

Radiation treatment approaches include external beam radiation and intracavitary and interstitial implants. The latter therapy requires personal radiation protection for all staff members who come in contact with the patient.

Normal and malignant cells respond to radiation differently, depending on blood supply, oxygen saturation, previous irradiation, and immune status. Generally, normal cells recover from radiation faster than malignant cells. The success of the treatment and damage to normal tissue also vary with the intensity of the radiation. Although a large single

RADIATION SIDE EFFECTS

AREA RADIATED	EFFECT	MANAGEMENT
Abdomen/ pelvis	Cramps, diarrhea, cystitis	Administer camphorated opium tincture and diphenoxylate with atropine; provide low-residue diet; maintain fluid and electrolyte balance.
Head	Alopecia	Encourage patient to wear wig or head covering.
	Mucositis	Provide mouthwash with viscous lidocaine, cool carbonated drinks, ice pops, and a soft, nonirritating diet.
	Monilia	Provide medicated mouthwash—avoid commercial mouthwash.
	Dental caries	Apply fluoride to teeth prophylactically; provide gingival care.
Chest	Lung tissue irritation	Tell the patient to stop smoking and to avoid people with upper respiratory infections; provide steroid therapy, as ordered; provide humidifier, if necessary.
	Pericarditis, myocarditis	Control dysrhythmias with appropriate agents (procainamide, disopyramide phosphate); monitor for heart failure.
	Esophagitis	Provide I.V. hyperalimentation; maintain fluid balance.
Kidneys	Nephritis, lassitude, headache, edema, dyspnea on exertion, hypertensive nephropathy, azotemia, secondary anemia	Maintain fluid and electrolyte balance; watch for signs of renal failure.

dose of radiation has greater cellular effects than fractions of the same amount delivered sequentially, a protracted schedule allows time for normal tissue to recover in the intervals between individual sublethal doses.

Radiation is often used palliatively to relieve pain, obstruction, malignant effusions, cough, dyspnea, ulcerative lesions, and hemorrhage; it can also promote the repair of pathologic fractures and delay tumor spread. Radiation can give a cancer patient an important psychologic lift just by shrinking a visible tumor.

Combining radiation and surgery can minimize radical surgery, prolong survival, and preserve anatomical function. For example, small preoperative doses of radiation shrink a tumor, making it operable, while preventing further spread of the disease during surgery. After the wound has healed, larger postoperative doses prevent residual neoplastic cells from multiplying or metastasizing.

Systemic side effects of radiation include weakness, fatigue, and possibly anorexia, nausea, vomiting, anemia, and diarrhea. (For localized side effects, see the chart above.) These side effects may respond to treatment with antiemetics, sedatives, steroids, frequent small meals, fluid maintenance, medications to control diarrhea (diphenoxylate with atropine or camphorated opium tincture), and bed rest. Systemic effects are seldom severe enough to require discontinuation of treatment, but they often necessitate careful adjustment of radiation dosage. Radiation therapy also requires frequent blood counts (with particular attention to WBCs and platelets).

Chemotherapy includes a wide array of drugs and may induce regression of a tumor and its metastasis. It's particularly useful in controlling residual disease or as an adjunct to surgery or radiotherapy and can induce long remissions and possibly effect cures, especially in patients with childhood leukemia, Hodgkin's disease, choriocarcinoma, and testicular cancer. As palliative treatment, chemotherapy aims to improve the patient's quality of life by temporarily relieving pain or other symptoms. The major cancer chemotherapeutic agents are as follows:

- *Alkylating agents* inhibit cell growth and division by reacting with DNA (antineoplastic agents of the nitrosurea group act in the same way).
- *Antimetabolites* prevent cell growth by competing with metabolites in the production of nucleic acid.
- *Anticancer antibiotics* block cell growth by binding with DNA and interfering with DNA-dependent RNA synthesis.
- *Plant alkaloids* prevent cellular reproduction by disrupting cell mitosis.
- *Steroid hormones* inhibit the growth of hormone-susceptible tumors by changing their chemical environment.

Chemotherapy side effects

Although antineoplastic agents are toxic to cancer cells, they can also cause transient changes in normal tissues, especially among rapidly proliferating body cells. For example, antineoplastic agents often depress bone marrow, causing anemia, leukopenia, and thrombocytopenia; irritate gastrointestinal epithelial cells, causing ulceration, bleeding, and vomiting; and destroy the cells of the hair follicles and skin, causing alopecia and dermatitis. Many I.V. drugs cause pain on administration and venous sclerosis and, if extravasated, can produce deep cutaneous necrosis requiring debridement and skin grafting.

Therefore, all patients undergoing chemotherapy need special care:

- Watch for any signs of infection, especially if the patient is receiving simultaneous radiation treatment. Be especially alert for fever when the granulocyte count falls below 500/mm^3; take the patient's temperature frequently.
- Increase the patient's fluid intake before and throughout chemotherapy.
- Inform the patient of the possibility of temporary hair loss (if he's receiving drugs that cause this condition), and reassure him that his hair should grow back after therapy ends (although it may then be a different color and texture). Suggest that he obtain a hairpiece or other head covering.
- Check skin for petechiae, ecchymoses, and chemical cellulitis and for secondary infection during treatment with sclerosing drugs.
- Minimize the possibility of venous sclerosis by frequently checking for blood return during I.V. push administration and by maintaining a properly running I.V. In case of extravasation, notify the doctor immediately (he should order local infiltration with a rapid-acting steroid for vesicant agents). Apply an ice pack to the site, and repeat at regular intervals for the next 24 hours; afterward, apply a warm, moist soak.

Chemotherapy can be administered orally, subcutaneously, I.M., I.V., intracavitarily, intrathecally, and by arterial infusion, depending on the drug and its pharmacologic action; usually, administration is intermittent to allow for bone marrow recovery between doses. Dosage is calculated according to the patient's body surface area, with adjustments for general condition and degree of myelosuppression. When calculating dosage, make sure your information is current, since chemotherapy dosages may change due to constant research.

Because many patients approach chemotherapy with apprehension, be sure to emphasize its beneficial results when teaching the patient about possible side effects. Explain that not all patients who undergo chemotherapy experience nausea and vomiting and, for those who do, antiemetic drugs, relaxation therapy, and diet can minimize these problems. Your support and encouragement throughout the course of chemotherapy will also help the patient.

Immunotherapy

Generally, immunotherapeutic agents are used in combination with chemotherapy or radiation therapy and are most effective in the early stages of cancer. Because much of the work done on immunotherapy is still experimental, the availability of treatment may be limited, and side effects are often unpredictable. Several promising approaches are currently under investigation:

• *Nonspecific immunostimulation* uses biological agents such as BCG (bacille Calmette-Guérin) vaccine or *C. parvum* (*Corynebacterium parvulum*) to stimulate the body's reticuloendothelial system, augmenting the patient's own immunosurveillance and combating the immunosuppressive effects of cancer and its treatment.

• *Intralesional stimulation* involves injection of a biological agent directly into the tumor; this initiates specific and nonspecific responses that lead to local destruction of cancer cells.

• *Active specific immunostimulation* uses specific tumor antigen vaccines to stimulate the patient's own immune mechanism to control or reject malignant cells by producing antibodies plus lymphocytes.

• *Adoptive transfer of immunity* involves the transfer of immunologically active cells from a donor with established immunity to stimulate active immunity in the patient.

Exciting advances have occurred in three other areas of immunotherapy. *Interferons,* once confined to antiviral applications, are now used to stimulate antibody production and cell-mediated immunity as well. *Bone marrow transplantation* restores hematologic and immunologic function in patients with immunodeficiencies and acute leukemia who don't respond to conventional immunotherapy. When tagged with radioisotopes and injected into the body, biochemicals known as *monoclonal antibodies* help detect cancer by attaching to tumor cells. In the future, these antibodies may be linked with toxins to destroy specific cancer cells without disturbing surrounding healthy cells.

Maintaining nutrition and fluid balance

Tumors grow at the expense of normal tissue by competing for nutrients and vitamins; consequently, the cancer patient often suffers protein deficiency and may also be hypermetabolic from the large number of dividing cells. Moreover, cancer treatments themselves produce fluid and electrolyte disturbances, such as vomiting, diarrhea, draining fistulae, and anorexia. Understandably, maintaining adequate nutrition, fluid intake, and electrolyte balance should be a major focus of your care.

• Obtain a comprehensive dietary history to pinpoint nutritional problems and their past causes, such as diabetes; help plan the diet accordingly.

• Ask the dietitian to provide a liquid, high-protein, high-carbohydrate, high-calorie diet if the patient can't tolerate solid foods. If the patient has stomatitis, provide soft, bland, nonirritating foods.

• Encourage the patient's family to bring his favorite foods from home.

• Make mealtime as relaxed and pleasant as possible. Encourage visitors to eat with the patient or, if possible, encourage him to dine with other patients. Let him choose from a varied menu.

• With the doctor's approval, suggest a glass of wine or a cocktail before dinner to help the patient relax and to stimulate his appetite.

• Urge him to drink juice or other caloric beverages instead of water.

If the patient can't eat

An alternate method of providing nourishment for the patient who has had recent head, neck, or GI surgery or who has dysphagia or pain when swallowing is through a nasogastric tube. If the patient still needs to use the tube after he's discharged, teach him how to insert it, how to test its position in his stomach by aspirating stomach contents, and how to use it to feed himself.

If a nasogastric tube isn't appropriate, other alternatives are gastrostomy, je-

HOW TO PREPARE THE PATIENT FOR EXTERNAL RADIATION THERAPY

- Show the patient where radiation therapy takes place, and introduce him to the radiation therapist.
- Tell him to remove all metal objects (pens, buttons, jewelry) that may interfere with therapy. Explain that the areas to be treated will be marked with water-soluble ink, and that *he must not scrub these areas,* because it's important to radiate the same areas each time.
- Reinforce the doctor's explanation of the procedure, and answer any questions as honestly as you can. If you don't know the answer to a question, refer the patient to the doctor.
- Teach the patient to watch for and report possibility of side effects. Since radiation therapy may increase susceptibility to infection, warn him to avoid persons with colds or other infections during therapy. However, emphasize the benefits (such as the outpatient treatment) instead of the side effects.
- Reassure the patient that treatment is painless and won't make him radioactive. Stress that he'll be under constant surveillance during radiation administration and need only call out if he needs anything.

junostomy, and, occasionally, esophagostomy. These make it possible for you to feed prescribed protein formulas and semiliquids, such as cream soups and eggnog, and also make it easier for the patient to feed himself. Remember to warn the patient that if spilled gastric or intestinal juices come in contact with the skin, they will cause abdominal excoriation if they're not washed off immediately. Some patients may prefer to chew their food before it's placed with the liquid in the tube and, while you may find this distasteful, allow them this option. Always flush the tube well with water after each feeding. Also, to provide adequate hydration, instill 4 to 6 ounces (118 to 177 ml) water or other clear liquid between meals. After jejunostomy, begin with very small feedings, slowly and carefully increasing the amounts and variety of food. Provide additional fluids and calories during these days of limited food intake by supplementing jejunostomy feedings with I.V. fat emulsions or alcohol.

Hyperalimentation is often an important part of cancer care, since patients who receive it during aggressive chemotherapy or radiotherapy experience less nausea, vomiting, diarrhea, and weight loss than patients who don't. Because of their improved nutritional status, these patients may respond better to the therapeutic effects of treatment. Hyperalimentation can also bring a severely debilitated patient into positive protein balance so he can better tolerate surgery. It can cause a slight weight gain in the patient receiving radiation therapy, provide optimum nutrition for wound healing, and help the patient combat infection after radical surgery.

Pain control critical

Cancer patients have a great fear of overwhelming pain. Therefore, controlling pain is a major consideration at every stage of cancer—from localized cancer to advanced metastasis. Cancer pain may result from inflammation of or pressure on pain-sensitive structures, tumor infiltration of nerves or blood vessels, or metastatic extension to bone. Chronic and unrelenting pain can wear down the patient's tolerance, interfere with eating and sleeping, and color his life with anger, despair, and anxiety.

Narcotic analgesics, either alone or in combination with nonnarcotic analgesics or antianxiety agents, are the mainstay of pain relief in advanced cancer. In terminal illness, narcotic dosages may be quite high, since drug tolerance invariably develops and the danger of addiction is unimportant. Provide such analgesics generously. Anticipate the need for pain relief, and provide it on a schedule that doesn't allow pain to break through. Don't wait to relieve pain until it becomes severe. Reassure the patient that you'll provide pain medication whenever he needs it.

Noninvasive pain relief techniques can be used alone or in combination with drug therapy. Popular noninvasive techniques include cutaneous stimulation, relaxation, distraction, and guided imagery.

Surgery or treatment with antibiotics can relieve the pressure and pain caused by inflamed necrotic tissue; radiation therapy can shrink metastatic tissue and control bone pain. When a tumor invades nervous tissue, pain control requires anesthetics, destructive nerve blocks, electronic nerve stimulation with a dorsal column or transcutaneous electrical nerve stimulator, rhizotomy, or chordotomy.

PATIENT-CONTROLLED ANALGESIA SYSTEM

A new method of pain relief, the patient-controlled analgesia system (PCA), is now being used in some cancer care centers with encouraging results. This system permits the patient to self-administer a premeasured dosage of analgesic by pressing a button at the bedside that activates a pump fitted with a prefilled syringe containing the analgesic. Small intermittent doses of the analgesic administered I.V. maintain blood levels that ensure comfort and minimize the risk of oversedation. Dosages and time intervals (usually 8 to 10 minutes) that allow for the patient to determine his comfort level are preset by the doctor or the nursing staff. The syringe is locked inside the pump as a safety feature. The system will only dispense the analgesic until the correct (preset) time interval has elapsed.

Clinical studies report that patients on PCA tend to titrate analgesic drugs effectively and maintain comfort without oversedation. They tend to use less of the drug than the amount normally given by I.M. injection.

PCA provides other significant advantages:

- Patients are alert and active during daytime hours.
- Patients no longer need to suffer pain while awaiting their injections.
- Patients are free from pain caused by injections.
- The nursing staff is free for other clinical duties.

The hospice approach

A holistic approach to patient care modeled after St. Christopher's Hospice in London, hospice care provides comprehensive physical, psychologic, social, and spiritual care for terminally ill patients. Many hospices are associated with hospitals, but some are independent or use home care programs. (As a variation of the hospice approach for non-terminal patients, several large cities in the United States have facilities that offer children with leukemia and their families a homelike environment during outpatient treatment at a nearby hospital.) The goal of the hospice is to maintain the patient's quality of life by providing treatment in as homelike an atmosphere as possible. Pain control, using morphine or methadone, is considered the first priority. Hospice care also emphasizes a coordinated team effort to overcome the anxiety, fear, and depression that often affect the terminally ill patient. Hospice staffs encourage family members to assume an active role in the patient's care, provide warmth and security, and help them begin to work out their grief before the patient dies.

Everyone involved in this method of care must be committed to high quality patient care, unafraid of emotional involvement, and comfortable with personal feelings about death and dying. Good hospice care also requires open communication among team members, not just for the evaluation of patient care, but also to help the staff cope with their own feelings.

Psychological aspects

No illness evokes as profound an emotional response as the diagnosis of cancer. Patients express this response in several ways. A few face this difficult reality immediately from the outset of diagnosis and treatment. Many use denial as a coping mechanism and simply refuse to accept the truth, but this stance is increasingly difficult for them to maintain. As evidence of the tumor becomes inescapable, the patient may plunge into deep depression. Family members may express denial in attempts to cope by encouraging unproven methods of cancer treatment, which often delay effective care. Some patients cope by intellectualizing about their disease, enabling them to obscure the reality of the cancer and regard it as unrelated to themselves. Generally, intellectualization is a more productive coping behavior than denial because the patient is receiving treatment. Be aware of the possible behavioral responses so you can identify them and then interact supportively with the patient and his family. For many malignancies, you can offer realistic hope for long-term survival or remission; even in advanced disease, you can offer short-term achievable goals. To help a patient cope with cancer, make sure you understand your own feelings about it. Then listen sensitively to the patient so you can offer genuine understanding and support. When caring for a patient with terminal cancer, increase your effectiveness by seeking out someone to help you through your own grieving.

HEAD, NECK, AND SPINE

Malignant Brain Tumors

Malignant brain tumors (gliomas, meningiomas, and schwannomas) are common (slightly more so in men than in women), with an incidence of 4.5 per 100,000.

Tumors may occur at any age. In adults, incidence is generally highest between ages 40 and 60. The most common tumor types in adults are gliomas and meningiomas; these tumors are usually supratentorial (above the covering of the cerebellum). In children, incidence is generally highest before age 1 and then again between ages 2 and 12. The most common tumors in children are astrocytomas, medulloblastomas, ependymomas, and brain stem gliomas. In children, brain tumors are one of the most common causes of death from cancer.

Causes

The cause of brain tumors is unknown.

Signs and symptoms

Brain tumors cause central nervous system changes by invading and destroying tissues and by secondary effect—mainly compression of the brain, cranial nerves, and cerebral vessels; cerebral edema; and increased intracranial pressure (ICP). Generally, clinical features result from increased ICP; these features vary with the type of tumor, its location, and the degree of invasion. Onset of symptoms is usually insidious, and brain tumors are commonly misdiagnosed.

Diagnosis

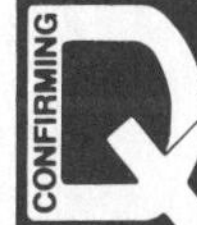

Definitive diagnosis is made from biopsy of the lesion to identify the histologic type. Patient history, neurologic assessment, and the following tests can locate the tumor: skull X-rays, brain scan, computed tomography scan, magnetic resonance imaging, and cerebral angiography. Lumbar puncture shows increased pressure and

MALIGNANT BRAIN TUMORS

TUMOR	CLINICAL FEATURES
Glioblastoma multiforme *(spongioblastoma multiforme)* • Peak incidence at 50 to 60 years; twice as common in males; most common glioma • Unencapsulated, highly malignant; grows rapidly and infiltrates the brain extensively; may become enormous before diagnosed • Occurs most often in cerebral hemispheres, especially frontal and temporal lobes (rarely in brain stem and cerebellum) • Occupies more than one lobe of affected hemisphere; may spread to opposite hemisphere by corpus callosum; may metastasize into CSF, producing tumors in distant parts of the nervous system	*General:* • Increased ICP (nausea, vomiting, headache, papilledema) • Mental and behavioral changes • Altered vital signs (increased systolic pressure; widened pulse pressure, respiratory changes) • Speech and sensory disturbances • In children, irritability, projectile vomiting *Localizing:* • Midline: headache (bifrontal or bioccipital); worse in A.M.; intensified by coughing, straining, or sudden head movements • Temporal lobe: psychomotor seizures • Central region: focal seizures • Optic and oculomotor nerves: visual defects • Frontal lobe: abnormal reflexes, motor responses
Astrocytoma • Second most common malignant glioma (approximately 30% of all gliomas) • Occurs at any age; incidence higher in males • Occurs most often in white matter of cerebral hemispheres; may originate in any part of the CNS • Cerebellar astrocytomas usually confined to one hemisphere	*General:* • Headache; mental activity changes • Decreased motor strength and coordination • Seizures; scanning speech • Altered vital signs *Localizing:* • Third ventricle: changes in mental activity and level of consciousness, nausea, pupillary dilation and sluggish light reflex; later—paresis or ataxia • Brain stem and pons: early—ipsilateral trigeminal, abducens, and facial nerve palsies; later—cerebellar ataxia, tremors, other cranial nerve deficits • Third or fourth ventricle or aqueduct of Sylvius: secondary hydrocephalus • Thalamus or hypothalamus: variety of endocrine, metabolic, autonomic, and behavioral changes
Oligodendroglioma • Third most common glioma • Occurs in middle adult years; more common in women • Slow-growing	*General:* • Mental and behavioral changes • Decreased visual acuity and other visual disturbances • Increased ICP *Localizing:* • Temporal lobe: hallucinations, psychomotor seizures • Central region: seizures (confined to one muscle group or unilateral) • Midbrain or third ventricle: pyramidal tract symptoms (dizziness, ataxia, paresthesias of the face) • Brain stem and cerebrum: nystagmus, hearing loss, dizziness, ataxia, paresthesias of face, cranial nerve palsies, hemiparesis, suboccipital tenderness, loss of balance

TUMOR	CLINICAL FEATURES
Ependymoma • Rare glioma • Most common in children and young adults • Locates most often in fourth and lateral ventricles	*General:* • Similar to oligodendroglioma • Increased ICP and obstructive hydrocephalus, depending on tumor size
Medulloblastoma • Rare glioma • Incidence highest in children age 4 to 6 • Affects males more than females • Frequently metastasizes via CSF	*General:* • Increased ICP *Localizing:* • Brain stem and cerebrum: papilledema, nystagmus, hearing loss, flashing lights, dizziness, ataxia, paresthesias of face, cranial nerve palsies (V, VI, VII, IX, X, primarily sensory), hemiparesis, suboccipital tenderness; compression of supratentorial area produces other general and focal symptoms
Meningioma • Most common nongliomatous brain tumor (15% of primary brain tumors) • Peak incidence among 50-year-olds; rare in children; more common in females (ratio 3:2) • Arises from the meninges • Common locations include parasagittal area, sphenoidal ridge, anterior part of the base of the skull, cerebellopontile angle, spinal canal • Benign, well-circumscribed, highly vascular tumors that compress underlying brain tissue by invading overlying skull	*General:* • Headache • Seizures (in two thirds of patients) • Vomiting • Changes in mental activity • Similar to schwannomas *Localizing:* • Skull changes (bony bulge) over tumor • Sphenoidal ridge, indenting optic nerve: unilateral visual changes and papilledema • Prefrontal parasagittal: personality and behavioral changes • Motor cortex: contralateral motor changes • Anterior fossa compressing both optic nerves and frontal lobes: headaches and bilateral vision loss • Pressure on cranial nerves causes varying symptoms
Schwannoma *(acoustic neurinoma, neurilemoma, cerebellopontile angle tumor)* • Accounts for approximately 10% of all intracranial tumors • Higher incidence in women • Onset of symptoms between ages 30 and 60 • Affects the craniospinal nerve sheath, usually cranial nerve VIII; also, V and VII, and to a lesser extent, VI and X on the same side as the tumor • Benign, but often classified as malignant because of its growth patterns; slow-growing—may be present for years before symptoms occur	*General:* • Unilateral hearing loss with or without tinnitus • Stiff neck and suboccipital discomfort • Secondary hydrocephalus • Ataxia and uncoordinated movements of one or both arms due to pressure on brain stem and cerebellum *Localizing:* • V: early—facial hypoesthesia/paresthesia on side of hearing loss; unilateral loss of corneal reflex • VI: diplopia or double vision • VII: paresis progressing to paralysis (Bell's palsy) • X: weakness of palate, tongue, and nerve muscles on same side as tumor

Adapted with permission from CANCER NURSING—A HOLISTIC MULTIDISCIPLINARY APPROACH, 2nd ed., by Ardelina A. Baldonado and Dulcelina A. Stahl. (Garden City, N.Y.: Medical Examination Publishing Co., Inc., 1980)

protein, decreased glucose, and occasionally, tumor cells in cerebrospinal fluid (CSF).

Treatment

Treatment includes removing a resectable tumor, reducing the size of a nonresectable tumor, relieving cerebral edema or ICP, relieving symptoms, and preventing further neurologic damage.

Mode of therapy depends on the tumor's histologic type, radiosensitivity, and anatomic location and may include surgery, radiation, chemotherapy, or decompression of increased ICP with diuretics, corticosteroids, or possibly ventriculoatrial or ventriculoperitoneal shunting of CSF.

A glioma usually requires resection by craniotomy, followed by radiation therapy. A combination of carmustine (BCNU), lomustine (CCNU), or procarbazine combined with postoperative radiation may prove to be more effective than radiation alone.

For low-grade cystic cerebellar astrocytomas, surgical resection brings long-term survival. For other astrocytomas, treatment consists of repeated surgery, radiation therapy, and shunting of fluid from obstructed CSF pathways. Some astrocytomas are highly radiosensitive, but others are radioresistant.

Treatment for oligodendrogliomas and ependymomas includes surgical resection and radiation therapy; for medulloblastomas, surgical resection and possibly intrathecal infusion of methotrexate or another antineoplastic drug. Meningiomas require surgical resection, including dura mater and bone (operative mortality may reach 10% because of large tumor size).

For schwannomas, microsurgical technique allows complete dissection of tumor and preservation of facial nerves. Although schwannomas are moderately radioresistant, postoperative radiation therapy is necessary.

Chemotherapy for malignant brain tumors includes methotrexate, nitrogen mustard, cyclophosphamide, vincristine, hydroxyurea, thiotepa, and doxorubicin. Intrathecal administration of such drugs is still under investigation.

Palliative measures for gliomas, astrocytomas, oligodendrogliomas, and ependymomas include dexamethasone for cerebral edema, and antacids and histamine receptor antagonists (such as cimetidine) for stress ulcers. These tumors and schwannomas may also require anticonvulsants.

Special considerations

A patient with a brain tumor requires comprehensive neurologic assessment, teaching, and supportive care. During your first contact with the patient, perform a comprehensive assessment (including a complete neurologic evaluation) to provide baseline data and to help develop your care plan. Obtain a thorough health history concerning onset of symptoms. Assist the patient and his family in coping with the treatment, potential disabilities, and changes in lifestyle resulting from his tumor.

Throughout hospitalization:

- Carefully document seizure activity (occurrence, nature, and duration).
- Maintain airway patency.
- Monitor patient safety.
- Administer anticonvulsive drugs, as ordered.
- Check continuously for changes in neurologic status, and watch for increase in ICP.

- Watch for and immediately report sudden unilateral pupillary dilation with loss of light reflex; this ominous change indicates imminent transtentorial herniation.
- Monitor respiratory changes carefully (abnormal respiratory rate and depth may point to rising ICP or herniation of the cerebellar tonsils from expanding infratentorial mass).
- Monitor temperature carefully. Fever commonly follows hypothalamic anoxia but might also indicate meningitis. Use hypothermia blankets preoperatively and postoperatively to keep the patient's temperature down and minimize cerebral metabolic demands.

• Administer steroids and antacids, as ordered. Observe and report signs of stress ulcer: abdominal distention, pain, vomiting, and tarry stools.
• Restrict fluids to 1,500 ml/24 hours. Administer osmotic diuretics, such as mannitol or urea, as ordered. Carefully monitor fluid and electrolyte balance.
• Radiation therapy is usually delayed until after the surgical wound heals, but it can induce wound breakdown even then. Therefore, observe the wound carefully for infection and sinus formation. Because radiation may cause brain inflammation, monitor closely for signs of rising ICP.
• Since the nitrosoureas—carmustine (BCNU), lomustine (CCNU), and procarbazine—used as adjuncts to radiotherapy and surgery can possibly cause delayed bone marrow depression, tell the patient to watch for and immediately report any signs of infection or bleeding that appear within 4 weeks after the start of chemotherapy. Before chemotherapy, give prochlorperazine or another antiemetic, as ordered, to minimize nausea and vomiting.
• Teach the patient and his family early signs of recurrence; urge compliance with therapy.
• Since brain tumors may cause residual neurologic deficits that handicap the patient physically or mentally, begin rehabilitation early. Encourage independence in daily activities. As necessary, provide aids for self-care and mobilization, such as bathroom rails for wheelchair patients. If the patient is aphasic, arrange for consultation with a speech pathologist.

Surgery requires additional nursing care. After craniotomy, continue to monitor general neurologic status and watch for signs of increased ICP, such as an elevated bone flap and typical neurologic changes. To reduce the risk of increased ICP, restrict fluids to 1,500 ml/24 hours. To promote venous drainage and reduce cerebral edema after supratentorial craniotomy, elevate the head of the patient's bed about 30°. Position him on his side to allow drainage of secretions and prevent aspiration. As appropriate, instruct the patient to avoid Valsalva's maneuver or isometric muscle contractions when moving or sitting up in bed; these can increase intrathoracic pressure and thereby increase ICP. Withhold oral fluids, which may provoke vomiting and consequently raise ICP.

After infratentorial craniotomy, keep the patient flat for 48 hours, but logroll him every 2 hours to minimize complications of immobilization. Prevent other complications by paying careful attention to ventilatory status and to cardiovascular, gastrointestinal, and musculoskeletal functions.

Pituitary Tumors

Pituitary tumors, which constitute 10% of intracranial neoplasms, originate most often in the anterior pituitary (adenohypophysis). They occur in adults of both sexes, usually during the third and fourth decades of life. The three tissue types of pituitary tumors include chromophobe adenoma (90%), basophil adenoma, and eosinophil adenoma.

Prognosis is fair to good, depending on the extent to which the tumor spreads beyond the sella turcica.

Causes

Although the exact cause is unknown, a predisposition to pituitary tumors may be inherited through an autosomal dominant trait. Pituitary tumors aren't malignant in the strict sense, but because their growth is invasive, they're considered a neoplastic disease.

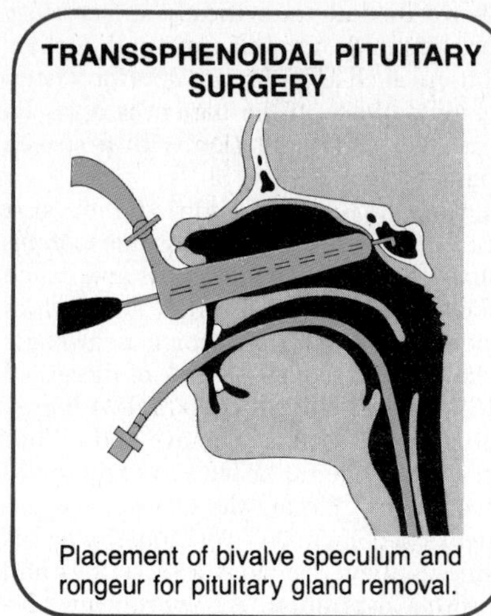

Placement of bivalve speculum and rongeur for pituitary gland removal.

Chromophobe adenoma may be associated with production of adrenocorticotropic hormone (ACTH), melanocyte-stimulating hormone, growth hormone, and prolactin; basophil adenoma, with evidence of excess ACTH production and, consequently, with signs of Cushing's syndrome; eosinophil adenoma, with excessive growth hormone.

Signs and symptoms

As pituitary adenomas grow, they replace normal glandular tissue and enlarge the sella turcica, which houses the pituitary gland. The resulting pressure on adjacent intracranial structures produces these typical clinical manifestations:

Neurologic:

- frontal headache
- visual symptoms, beginning with blurring and progressing to field cuts (hemianopias) and then unilateral blindness
- cranial nerve involvement (III, IV, VI) from lateral extension of the tumor, resulting in strabismus; double vision, with compensating head tilting and dizziness; conjugate deviation of gaze; nystagmus; lid ptosis; and limited eye movements
- increased intracranial pressure (secondary hydrocephalus)
- personality changes or dementia, if the tumor breaks through to the frontal lobes
- seizures
- rhinorrhea, if the tumor erodes the base of the skull
- pituitary apoplexy secondary to hemorrhagic infarction of the adenoma. Such hemorrhage may lead to both cardiovascular and adrenocortical collapse.

Endocrine:

- hypopituitarism, to some degree, in all patients with adenoma, becoming more obvious as the tumor replaces normal gland tissue. Symptoms include amenorrhea, decreased libido and impotence in men, skin changes (waxy appearance, decreased wrinkles, and pigmentation), loss of axillary and pubic hair, lethargy, weakness, increased fatigability, intolerance to cold, and constipation (because of decreased ACTH and thyroid-stimulating hormone production).
- addisonian crisis, precipitated by stress and resulting in nausea, vomiting, hypoglycemia, hypotension, and circulatory collapse
- diabetes insipidus, resulting from extension to the hypothalamus
- prolactin-secreting adenomas (in 70% to 75%), with amenorrhea and galactorrhea; growth hormone-secreting adenomas, with acromegaly; and ACTH-secreting adenomas, with Cushing's syndrome.

Diagnosis

- *Skull X-rays* with tomography show enlargement of the sella turcica or erosion of its floor; if growth hormone secretion predominates, X-rays show enlarged paranasal sinuses and mandible, thickened cranial bones, and separated teeth.
- *Carotid angiogram* shows displacement of the anterior cerebral and internal carotid arteries if the tumor mass is enlarging; it also rules out intracerebral aneurysm.
- *Computed tomography scan* may confirm the existence of the adenoma and accurately depict its size.
- *Cerebrospinal fluid* analysis may

show increased protein levels.

• *Endocrine function tests* may contribute helpful information, but results are often ambiguous and inconclusive.

Treatment

Surgical options include transfrontal removal of large tumors impinging on the optic apparatus and transsphenoidal resection for smaller tumors confined to the pituitary fossa. Radiation is the primary treatment for small, nonsecretory tumors that don't extend beyond the sella turcica or for patients who may be poor postoperative risks; otherwise, it's an adjunct to surgery.

Postoperative treatment includes hormone replacement with cortisone, thyroid, and sex hormones; correction of electrolyte imbalance; and, as necessary, insulin therapy.

Drug therapy may include bromocriptine, an ergot derivative that shrinks prolactin-secreting and growth hormone-secreting tumors. Cyproheptadine, an antiserotonin drug, can reduce increased corticosteroid levels in the patient with Cushing's syndrome.

Adjuvant radiotherapy is used when only partial removal of the tumor is possible. Cryohypophysectomy (freezing the area with a probe inserted by transsphenoidal route) is a promising alternative to surgical dissection of the tumor.

Special considerations

• Conduct a comprehensive health history and physical assessment to establish the onset of neurologic and endocrine dysfunction and provide baseline data for later comparison.

• Establish a supportive, trusting relationship with the patient and family to assist them in coping with the diagnosis, treatment, and potential long-term changes. Make sure they understand that the patient needs lifelong evaluations and, possibly, hormone replacement.

• Reassure the patient that some of the distressing physical and behavioral signs and symptoms caused by pituitary dysfunction (for example, altered sexual drive, impotence, infertility, loss of hair, and emotional lability) will disappear with treatment.

• Maintain a safe, clutter-free environment for the visually impaired or acromegalic patient. Reassure him that he'll probably recover his sight.

• Position patients who have undergone supratentorial or transsphenoidal hypophysectomy with the head of the bed elevated about 30°, to promote venous drainage from the head and reduce cerebral edema. Place the patient on his side to allow drainage of secretions and prevent aspiration.

• Withhold oral fluids, which can cause vomiting and subsequent increased intracranial pressure. Don't allow a patient who's had transsphenoidal surgery to blow his nose. Watch for cerebrospinal fluid drainage from the nose. Monitor for signs of infection from the contaminated upper respiratory tract. Make sure the patient understands that he'll lose his sense of smell.

• Regularly compare the patient's postoperative neurologic status with your baseline assessment.

• Monitor intake and output to detect fluid and electrolyte imbalances.

• Before discharge, encourage the patient to purchase and wear a Medic Alert bracelet or necklace that identifies his hormone deficiencies and their proper treatment.

POSTCRANIOTOMY CARE

• Monitor vital signs (especially level of consciousness), and perform a baseline neurologic assessment from which to plan further care and assess progress.
• Maintain the patient's airway; suction as necessary.
• Monitor intake and output carefully.
• Give the patient nothing by mouth for 24 to 48 hours, to prevent aspiration and vomiting, which increases intracranial pressure.
• Observe for cerebral edema, bleeding, and CSF leakage.
• Provide a restful, quiet environment.

Laryngeal Cancer

The most common form of laryngeal cancer is squamous cell carcinoma (95%); rare forms include adenocarcinoma, sarcoma, and others. Such cancer may be intrinsic or extrinsic. An intrinsic *tumor is on the true vocal cord and does not have a tendency to spread, because underlying connective tissues lack lymph nodes. An* extrinsic *tumor is on some other part of the larynx and tends to spread early. Laryngeal cancer is nine times more common in males than in females; most victims are between ages 50 and 65.*

Causes and incidence

In laryngeal cancer, major predisposing factors include smoking (it's especially common in heavy smokers and rare in nonsmokers) and alcoholism; minor factors include chronic inhalation of noxious fumes, familial tendency, and, less commonly, a history of frequent laryngitis and vocal straining.

Laryngeal cancer is classified according to its location:

- supraglottis (posterior surface of the epiglottis, aryepiglottic folds, false vocal cords)
- glottis (true vocal cords)
- subglottis (downward extension from vocal cords [rare]).

Signs and symptoms

In intrinsic laryngeal cancer, the dominant and earliest symptom is hoarseness that persists longer than 3 weeks; in extrinsic cancer, it's a lump in the throat or pain or burning in the throat when drinking citrus juice or hot liquid. Later clinical effects of metastases include dysphagia, dyspnea, cough, enlarged cervical lymph nodes, and pain radiating to the ear.

Diagnosis

Any hoarseness that lasts longer than 2 weeks requires visualization of the larynx by indirect laryngoscopy (mirror visualization) or direct laryngoscopy.

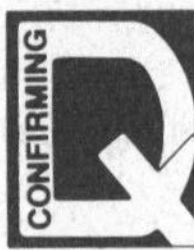

Firm diagnosis also requires xeroradiography, laryngoscopy, biopsy, laryngeal tomography, computed tomography scan, or laryngography to define the borders of the lesion, and chest X-ray to detect metastases.

Treatment

In laryngeal cancer, the goal of treatment is to eliminate the cancer through surgery, radiation, or both, and to preserve speech. If speech preservation isn't possible, speech rehabilitation may include esophageal speech or prosthetic devices; surgical techniques to construct a new voice box are still experimental. Surgical procedures vary with tumor size and can include cordectomy, partial or total laryngectomy, supraglottic laryngectomy, or total laryngectomy with laryngoplasty.

Special considerations

Psychologic support and good preoperative and postoperative care can minimize complications and speed recovery.

Before partial or total laryngectomy:

- Instruct the patient to maintain good oral hygiene; if appropriate, instruct a male patient to shave off his beard to facilitate postoperative care.
- Encourage the patient to verbalize his concerns before surgery temporarily cuts off effective verbal communication. Prepare him for this by helping him choose an alternate method of communication that he finds comfortable (such as pencil and paper, sign language, or alphabet board).
- If you are preparing the patient for total laryngectomy, arrange for a laryngectomee to visit him. Explain postoperative procedures (suctioning, nasogastric feeding, care of laryngec-

tomy tube) and their results (breathing through neck, speech alteration). Also prepare him for other functional losses; he won't be able to smell, blow his nose, whistle, gargle, sip, or suck on a straw.

After partial laryngectomy:

• Give I.V. fluids and, usually, tube feedings for the first 2 days postoperatively; then resume oral fluids. Keep the tracheostomy tube (inserted during surgery) in place until tissue edema subsides.

• Make sure the patient doesn't use his voice until the doctor gives permission (usually 2 to 3 days postoperatively). Then caution the patient to whisper until healing is complete.

After total laryngectomy:

• As soon as he returns to his bed, position the patient on his side and elevate his head 30° to 45°. When you move him, remember to support the back of his neck to prevent tension on sutures and possible wound dehiscence.

• The patient will probably have a laryngectomy tube in place until his stoma heals (about 7 to 10 days). This tube is shorter and thicker than a tracheostomy tube but requires the same care. Watch for crusting and secretions around the stoma, which can cause skin breakdown. To prevent crust formation, provide adequate room humidification. Remove crusting with petrolatum, an-

PATIENT TEACHING AID

Neck Stoma Care

Dear Patient:
After you're discharged, you'll have to do your own neck stoma care.

• To prevent infection, wash your hands before touching your stoma.

• Then, wet a washcloth with warm water (don't use wet cotton or soap); wring it out, and place it over the stoma.

• To keep the stoma moist, apply petrolatum thinly around its edges. Wipe off any excess.

• Use a stoma bib (crocheted cover or cotton cloth) over the stoma to filter and warm air before it enters the stoma. Fasten the bib with a tie around your neck. You can wear an ascot, a turtleneck sweater, or a regular shirt (sew the second button from the top over the buttonhole as though it were fastened, to leave access for a handkerchief when coughing); you can also wear jewelry or scarves.

• If you're a man, be careful when shaving, as some of your sensory nerve endings may have been cut in surgery. These endings will regenerate in about 6 months.

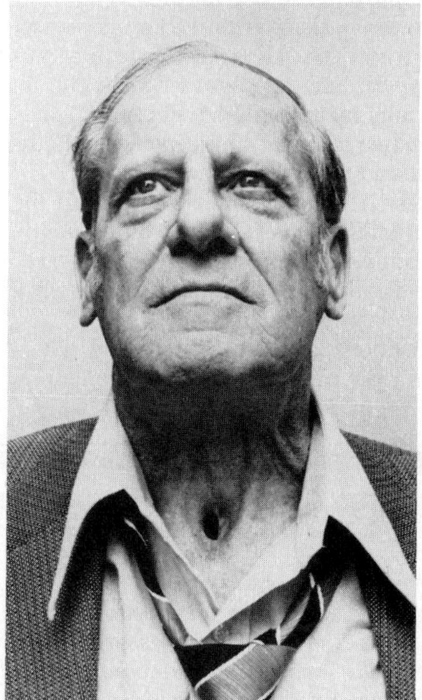

Patient shows well-healed neck stoma.

timicrobial ointment, and moist gauze.

• Watch for and report complications: fistula formation (redness, swelling, secretions on suture line), carotid artery rupture (bleeding), and tracheostomy stenosis (constant shortness of breath). A fistula may form between reconstructed hypopharynx and the skin. This eventually heals spontaneously but may take weeks or months. Carotid artery rupture usually occurs in patients who have had preoperative radiation, particularly those with a fistula that constantly bathes the carotid artery with oral secretions. If carotid rupture occurs, apply pressure to the site; call for help immediately and take patient to the operating room for carotid ligation. Tracheostomy stenosis occurs weeks to months after laryngectomy; treatment includes fitting the patient with successively larger tracheostomy tubes until he can tolerate insertion of a large one. If the patient has a fistula, feed him through a nasogastric tube; otherwise, food will leak through the fistula and delay healing. Monitor vital signs (be especially alert for fever, which indicates infection). Record fluid intake and output, and watch for dehydration.

• Give frequent mouth care. Scrub the patient's tongue and the sides of his mouth with a soft toothbrush or a terry washcloth, and rinse his mouth with a deodorizing mouthwash.

• Suction gently; unless ordered otherwise, do not attempt deep suctioning, which could possibly penetrate the suture line. Suction through both the tube and the patient's nose, since the patient can no longer blow air through his nose; suction his mouth gently.

• After insertion of drainage catheter (usually connected to a blood drainage system or a gastrointestinal drainage system), don't stop suction without the doctor's consent. After catheter removal, check dressings for drainage.

• Give analgesics, as ordered. Keep in mind that narcotics depress respiration and inhibit coughing.

• If the doctor orders nasogastric tube feeding, check tube placement, and elevate the patient's head to prevent aspiration. Be ready to suction after nasogastric tube removal or oral fluid intake, since the patient may have difficulty swallowing.

• Reassure the patient that speech rehabilitation (laryngeal speech, esophageal speech [air bolus techniques], artificial larynx, various mechanical aids) can help him speak again. Encourage him to contact the American Speech and Hearing Association, the International Association of Laryngectomees, the American Cancer Society, or the local chapter of the Lost Chord Club or the New Voice Club.

• Support the patient through some inevitable grieving. If the depression seems severe, consider psychiatric referral.

Thyroid Cancer

Thyroid carcinoma occurs in all age-groups, especially in persons who have had radiation treatment to the neck area. Papillary and follicular carcinomas are most common and are usually associated with prolonged survival.

Papillary carcinoma accounts for half of all thyroid cancers in adults; it can occur at any age, but is most common in adult females during childbearing years. It is usually multifocal and bilateral, and metastasizes slowly into regional nodes of the neck, mediastinum, lungs, and other distant organs. It is the least virulent form of thyroid cancer. Follicular carcinoma is less common (30% of all cases), but is more likely to recur and metastasize to the regional nodes and through blood vessels into the bones, liver, and lungs. Medullary (solid) carcinoma originates in *the parafollicular cells derived from the last branchial pouch and contains amyloid and calcium deposits. It can produce calcitonin, histaminase, ACTH (producing Cushing's syndrome), and prostaglandin E_2 and F_3 (producing diarrhea). This form of thyroid cancer is familial, possibly inherited as an autosomal dominant trait, and is often associated with pheochromocytoma. This rare (5%) form of thyroid cancer usually occurs in women over age 40. It is completely curable when detected before it causes symptoms. Untreated, it grows rapidly, frequently metastasizing to bones, liver, and kidneys.*

Giant and spindle cell cancer (anaplastic tumor) resists radiation and is almost never curable by resection. It metastasizes rapidly and causes death by tracheal invasion and compression of adjacent structures.

Causes and incidence

Predisposing factors include radiation exposure, prolonged thyroid-stimulating hormone (TSH) stimulation (through radiation or heredity), familial predisposition, or chronic goiter.

Radiation therapy in childhood was common in the 1950s to shrink enlarged thymus gland, tonsils, or adenoids, and to treat acne and other skin disorders. Twenty-five percent of those so treated later developed thyroid nodules; 25% of those nodules became malignant. Risk of malignancy after radiation correlates with dose (a threshold dose has not been defined) and age (malignancy is rare in patients who begin radiation treatment after age 21).

Signs and symptoms

The dominant signs of thyroid cancer are a painless nodule, a hard nodule in an enlarged thyroid gland, or palpable lymph nodes with thyroid enlargement. Eventually, the pressure of such a nodule or enlargement causes hoarseness, dysphagia, dyspnea, and pain on palpation. If the tumor is large enough to destroy the gland, hypothyroidism follows, with its typical signs of low metabolism (mental apathy, cold sensitivity). However, if the tumor stimulates excess thyroid hormone production, it induces signs of hyperthyroidism (heat sensitivity, restlessness, overactivity). Other clinical features include diarrhea, anorexia, irritability, vocal cord paralysis, and symptoms of distant metastases.

Diagnosis

The first clue to thyroid cancer is usually an enlarged, palpable node in the thyroid gland, neck, lymph nodes of the neck, or vocal cords. Patient history of radiation therapy or a family history of thyroid cancer supports diagnosis. However, tests must rule out nonmalignant thyroid enlargements, which are much more common. Thyroid scan differentiates between functional nodes (rarely malignant) and hypofunctional nodes (commonly malignant) by measuring

GIANT CELL THYROID CANCER

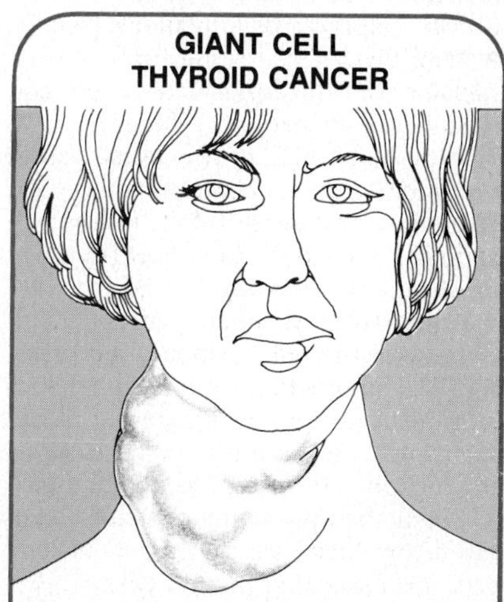

The most disfiguring, destructive, and deadly form of thyroid carcinoma, giant (or spindle) cell cancer has the poorest prognosis. Although this tumor rarely metastasizes to distant organs, its size produces severe anatomical distortion of nearby structures. Treatment usually consists of a total thyroidectomy but is rarely successful.

how readily nodules trap isotopes compared with the rest of the thyroid gland. In thyroid cancer, the scintiscan shows a "cold," nonfunctioning nodule. Other tests include needle biopsy, ultrasonic scan, and serum calcitonin assay to diagnose medullary cancer. Calcitonin assay is a reliable clue to silent medullary carcinoma. Calcitonin level is measured during a resting state and during an infusion of calcium (15 mg/kg) over a 4-hour period. An elevated fasting calcitonin and an abnormal response to calcium stimulation (high release of calcitonin from the node in comparison with the rest of the gland) are indicative of medullary cancer.

Treatment

Treatment varies and may include one or any combination of the following:

• Total or subtotal thyroidectomy, with modified node dissection (bilateral or homolateral) on the side of the primary cancer (papillary or follicular cancer)

• Total thyroidectomy and radical neck excision (for medullary, or giant and spindle cell cancer)

• Radiation (^{131}I), with external radiation (for large inoperable cancer and sometimes postoperatively in lieu of radical neck excision) or by itself (for local or distant metastases)

• Adjunctive thyroid suppression, with exogenous thyroid hormones suppressing TSH production, and simultaneous administration of an adrenergic blocking agent, such as propranolol, increasing tolerance to surgery and radiation

• Chemotherapy, which is experimental; doxorubicin is sometimes beneficial with metastasizing thyroid cancer.

Special considerations

Before surgery, tell the patient to expect temporary voice loss or hoarseness lasting several days after surgery. Also, explain the operation and postoperative procedures and teach proper postoperative positioning.

Ideally, the patient should be euthyroid before surgery, as demonstrated by a normal electrocardiogram, thyroid function tests, and pulse rate.

Plan meticulous postoperative care:

• When the patient regains consciousness, keep him in semi-Fowler's position, with his head neither hyperextended nor flexed, to avoid pressure on the suture line. Support his head and neck with sandbags and pillows; when you move him, continue this support with your hands.

• After monitoring vital signs, check the patient's dressing, neck, and back for bleeding. If he complains that the dressing feels tight, loosen the dressing and call the doctor immediately. Check serum calcium levels daily, and watch for and report other complications: hemorrhage and shock (elevated pulse and hypotension), tetany (carpopedal spasm, twitching, convulsions), thyroid storm (high fever, severe tachycardia, delirium, dehydration, and extreme irritability), and respiratory obstruction (dyspnea, crowing respirations, retraction of neck tissues). Keep a tracheotomy set and oxygen equipment handy in case of respiratory obstruction. Use continuous steam inhalation in the patient's room until his chest is clear.

• The patient may need I.V. fluids or a soft diet, but many patients can tolerate a regular diet within 24 hours of surgery.

Care of the patient after extensive tumor and node excision is identical to other radical neck postoperative care.

Spinal Neoplasms

Spinal neoplasms may be any one of many tumor types similar to intracranial tumors; they involve the cord or its roots and, if untreated, can eventually cause paralysis. As primary tumors, they originate in the meningeal coverings, the parenchyma of the cord or its roots, the intraspinal vasculature, or the vertebrae. They can also occur as metastatic foci from primary tumors.

Causes and incidence

Primary tumors of the spinal cord may be extramedullary (occurring outside the spinal cord) or intramedullary (occurring within the cord itself). Extramedullary tumors may be intradural (meningiomas and schwannomas), which account for 60% of all primary spinal cord neoplasms; or extradural (metastatic tumors from breasts, lungs, prostate, leukemia, or lymphomas), which account for 25% of these neoplasms.

Intramedullary tumors, or gliomas (astrocytomas or ependymomas), are comparatively rare, accounting for only about 10%; in children, they're low-grade astrocytomas.

Spinal cord tumors are rare compared with intracranial tumors (ratio of 1:4). They occur with equal frequency in both men and women, with the exception of meningiomas, which occur most often in women. Spinal cord tumors can occur anywhere along the length of the cord or its roots.

Signs and symptoms

Extramedullary tumors produce symptoms by pressing on nerve roots, the spinal cord, and spinal vessels; intramedullary tumors, by destroying the parenchyma and compressing adjacent areas. Because intramedullary tumors may extend over several spinal cord segments, their symptoms are more variable than those of extramedullary tumors.

The following clinical effects are likely with all spinal cord neoplasms:

- *Pain*—Most severe directly over the tumor, radiates around the trunk or down the limb on the affected side, and is unrelieved by bed rest
- *Motor symptoms*—Asymmetric spastic muscle weakness, decreased muscle tone, exaggerated reflexes, and a positive Babinski's sign. If the tumor is at the level of the cauda equina, muscle flaccidity, muscle wasting, weakness, and progressive diminution in tendon reflexes are characteristic.
- *Sensory deficits*—Contralateral loss of pain, temperature, and touch sensation (Brown-Séquard syndrome). These losses are less obvious to the patient than functional motor changes. Caudal lesions invariably produce paresthesias in the nerve distribution pathway of the involved roots.
- *Bladder symptoms*—Urinary retention is an inevitable late sign with cord compression. Early signs include incomplete emptying or difficulty with the urinary stream, which is usually unnoticed or ignored. Cauda equina tumors cause bladder and bowel incontinence due to flaccid paralysis.
- *Constipation.*

Diagnosis

- A *spinal tap* shows clear yellow cerebrospinal fluid (CSF) as a result of increased protein levels if the flow is completely blocked. If the flow is partially blocked, protein levels rise, but the fluid is only slightly yellow in proportion to the CSF protein level. A Pap smear of the CSF may show malignant cells of metastatic carcinoma.
- *X-rays* show distortions of the intervertebral foramina; changes in the vertebrae or collapsed areas in the vertebral body; and localized enlargement of the spinal canal, indicating an adjacent block.
- *Myelography* identifies the level of the lesion by outlining it if the tumor is causing partial obstruction; it shows anatomic relationship to the cord and the dura. If obstruction is complete, the injected dye can't flow past the tumor. (This study is dangerous if cord compression is nearly complete, since withdrawal or escape of CSF will actually allow the tumor to exert greater pressure against the cord.)
- A *radioisotope bone scan* demonstrates metastatic invasion of the verte-

brae by showing a characteristic increase in osteoblastic activity.
• *Computed tomography scan* shows cord compression and tumor location.
• *Frozen section biopsy* at surgery identifies the tissue type.

Treatment

Treatment of spinal cord tumors generally includes decompression or radiation. Laminectomy is indicated for primary tumors that produce spinal cord or cauda equina compression; it's *not* usually indicated for metastatic tumors. If the tumor is slowly progressive, or if it's treated before the cord degenerates from compression, symptoms are likely to disappear, and complete restoration of function is possible. In a patient with metastatic carcinoma or lymphoma who suddenly experiences complete transverse myelitis with spinal shock, functional improvement is unlikely, even with treatment, and his outlook is ominous. If the patient has incomplete paraplegia of rapid onset, emergency surgical decompression may save cord function. Steroid therapy minimizes cord edema until surgery can be performed. Partial removal of intramedullary gliomas, followed by radiation, may alleviate symptoms for a short time. Metastatic extradural tumors can be controlled with radiation, analgesics, and, in the case of hormone-mediated tumors (breast and prostate), appropriate hormone therapy. Transcutaneous electrical nerve stimulation (TENS) may control radicular pain from spinal cord tumors and is a useful alternative to narcotic analgesics. In TENS, an electrical charge is applied to the skin to stimulate large-diameter nerve fibers and thereby inhibit transmission of pain impulses through small-diameter nerve fibers.

Special considerations

The care plan for patients with spinal cord tumors should emphasize emotional support and skilled intervention during acute and chronic phases, early recognition of recurrence, prevention and treatment of complications, and maintenance of quality of life.
• On your first contact with the patient, perform a complete neurologic evaluation to obtain baseline data for planning future care and evaluating changes in his clinical status.
• Care for the patient with a spinal cord tumor is basically the same as that for the patient with spinal cord injury and requires psychologic support, rehabilitation (including bowel and bladder retraining), and prevention of infection and skin breakdown. After laminectomy, care includes checking neurologic status frequently, changing position by logrolling, administering analgesics, monitoring frequently for infection, and aiding in early walking.
• Help the patient and his family to understand and cope with the diagnosis, treatment, potential disabilities, and necessary changes in life-style.
• Take safety precautions for the patient with impaired sensation and motor deficits. Use side rails if the patient is bedridden; if he's not, encourage him to wear flat shoes, and remove scatter rugs and clutter to prevent falls.
• Encourage the patient to be independent in performing daily activities. Avoid aggravating pain by moving the patient slowly and by making sure his body is well aligned when giving personal care. Advise him to use TENS to block radicular pain.
• Administer steroids and antacids, as ordered, for cord edema after radiation therapy. Monitor for sensory or motor dysfunction, which indicates the need for more steroids.
• Enforce bed rest for the patient with vertebral body involvement until the doctor says he can safely walk, because body weight alone can cause cord collapse and cord laceration from bone fragments.
• Logroll and position the patient on his side every 2 hours to prevent decubitus ulcers and other complications of immobility.
• If the patient is to wear a back brace, make sure he does wear it whenever he gets out of bed.

THORAX

Lung Cancer

Lung cancer usually develops within the wall or epithelium of the bronchial tree. Its most common types are epidermoid (squamous cell) carcinoma, small-cell (oat cell) carcinoma, adenocarcinoma, and large-cell (anaplastic) carcinoma. Although, generally, prognosis is poor, it varies with the extent of spread at the time of diagnosis and cell type growth rate. Only 13% of patients with lung cancer survive 5 years after diagnosis. Lung cancer is the most common cause of cancer death in men and is fast becoming the most common cause in women, even though it's largely preventable.

Causes and incidence

Most experts agree that lung cancer is attributable to inhalation of carcinogenic pollutants by a susceptible host. Who is most susceptible? Any smoker over age 40, especially if he began to smoke before age 15, has smoked a whole pack or more per day for 20 years, or works with or near asbestos.

Pollutants in tobacco smoke cause progressive lung cell degeneration. Lung cancer is 10 times more common in smokers than in nonsmokers; indeed, 80% of lung cancer patients are smokers. Cancer risk is determined by the number of cigarettes smoked daily, the depth of inhalation, how early in life smoking began, and the nicotine content of cigarettes. Two other factors also increase susceptibility: exposure to carcinogenic industrial and air pollutants (asbestos, uranium, arsenic, nickel, iron oxides, chromium, radioactive dust, and coal dust), and familial susceptibility.

Signs and symptoms

Because early-stage lung cancer usually produces no symptoms, this disease is often in an advanced state at diagnosis. The following late-stage symptoms often lead to diagnosis:

- With epidermoid and small-cell carcinomas—smoker's cough, hoarseness, wheezing, dyspnea, hemoptysis, and chest pain
- With adenocarcinoma and large-cell carcinoma—fever, weakness, weight loss, anorexia, and shoulder pain.

In addition to their obvious interference with respiratory function, lung tumors may also alter the production of hormones that regulate body function or homeostasis. Clinical conditions that result from such changes are known as hormonal paraneoplastic syndromes:

- *Gynecomastia* may result from large-cell carcinoma.
- *Hypertrophic pulmonary osteoarthropathy* (bone and joint pain from cartilage erosion due to abnormal production of growth hormone) may result from large-cell carcinoma and adenocarcinoma.
- *Cushing's* and *carcinoid syndromes* may result from small-cell carcinoma.
- *Hypercalcemia* may result from epidermoid tumors.

Metastatic symptoms vary greatly, depending on the effect of tumors on intrathoracic and distant structures:

- *bronchial obstruction*: hemoptysis, atelectasis, pneumonitis, dyspnea
- *recurrent nerve invasion*: hoarseness, vocal cord paralysis
- *chest wall invasion*: piercing chest pain; increasing dyspnea; severe shoulder pain, radiating down arm
- *local lymphatic spread*: cough, hemoptysis, stridor, pleural effusion
- *phrenic nerve involvement*: dyspnea; shoulder pain; unilateral paralyzed diaphragm, with paradoxical motion

• *esophageal compression*: dysphagia
• *vena caval obstruction*: venous distention and edema of face, neck, chest, and back
• *pericardial involvement*: pericardial effusion, tamponade, dysrhythmias
• *cervical thoracic sympathetic nerve involvement*: miosis, ptosis, exophthalmos, reduced sweating.

Distant metastases may involve any part of the body, most commonly the central nervous system, liver, and bone.

Diagnosis

Typical clinical findings may strongly suggest lung cancer, but firm diagnosis requires further evidence.

• *Chest X-ray* usually shows an advanced lesion, but it can detect a lesion up to 2 years before symptoms appear. It also indicates tumor size and location.
• *Sputum cytology*, which is 75% reliable, requires specimen coughed up from lungs and tracheobronchial tree, *not* postnasal secretions or saliva.
• *Bronchoscopy* can locate the tumor site. Bronchoscopic washings provide material for cytologic and histologic examination. The flexible fiberoptic bronchoscope increases test effectiveness.
• *Needle biopsy* of the lungs employs biplane fluoroscopic visual control to detect peripherally located tumors. This allows firm diagnosis in 80% of patients.
• *Tissue biopsy* of accessible metastatic sites includes supraclavicular and mediastinal node and pleural biopsy.
• *Thoracentesis* allows chemical and cytologic examination of pleural fluid.

Additional studies include chest tomography, bronchography, esophagography, angiocardiography (contrast studies of bronchial tree, esophagus, and cardiovascular tissues). Tests to detect metastasis include bone scan (positive scan may lead to bone marrow biopsy; bone marrow biopsy is also recommended in small-cell carcinoma), computed tomography scan of the brain, liver function studies, and gallium scan (noninvasive nuclear scan) of liver, spleen, and bone.

After histologic confirmation, staging determines the extent of the disease and helps in planning treatment and understanding prognosis.

Treatment

Recent treatment—which consists of combinations of surgery, radiation, and chemotherapy—may improve prognosis and prolong survival. Nevertheless, because treatment usually begins at an advanced stage, it is largely palliative.

Surgery is the primary treatment for Stage I, Stage II, or selected Stage III squamous cell carcinoma; adenocarcinoma; and large-cell carcinoma, unless the tumor is nonresectable or other conditions (such as cardiac disease) rule out surgery. Surgery may include partial removal of a lung (wedge resection, segmental resection, lobectomy, radical lobectomy) or total removal (pneumonectomy, radical pneumonectomy).

Preoperative radiation therapy may reduce tumor bulk to allow for surgical resection, but this is of questionable value. Radiation therapy is ordinarily recommended for Stage I and Stage II lesions if surgery is contraindicated, and for Stage III when the disease is confined to the involved hemithorax and the ipsilateral supraclavicular lymph nodes. Generally, radiation therapy is delayed until 1 month after surgery, to allow the wound to heal, and is then directed to the part of the chest most likely to develop metastasis.

Several new chemotherapy combinations show promise. The combination of fluorouracil, vincristine, and mitomycin induces remission in 40% of patients with adenocarcinomas. Promising combinations for treating small-cell carcinomas include cyclophosphamide, doxorubicin, and vincristine (CAV); cyclophosphamide, doxorubicin, vincristine, and etoposide (CAVE); and etoposide and cisplatin (VP16).

Immunotherapy is still experimental. Nonspecific immunotherapy using bacille Calmette-Guérin (BCG) vaccine or, possibly, *Corynebacterium parvulum* appears the most promising.

In laser therapy, also largely experi-

STAGING LUNG CANCER

TO: No evidence of primary tumor

TX: Tumor proven by the presence of malignant cells in bronchopulmonary secretions but not visualized roentgenographically or bronchoscopically, or any tumor that cannot be assessed

TIS: Carcinoma in situ

T1: A tumor that is 3 cm or less in greatest diameter, surrounded by lung or visceral pleura, and without evidence of invasion proximal to a lobar bronchus at bronchoscopy.

T2: A tumor more than 3 cm in greatest diameter, or a tumor of any size that invades the visceral pleura or has associated atelectasis or obstructive pneumonitis extending to the hilar region. At bronchoscopy, the proximal extent of demonstrable tumor must be within a lobar bronchus or at least 2 cm distal to the carina. Any associated atelectasis or obstructive pneumonitis must involve less than an entire lung, and there must be no pleural effusion.

T3: A tumor of any size with direct extension into an adjacent structure such as the parietal pleura, the chest wall, the diaphragm, or the mediastinum and its contents; or a tumor demonstrable bronchoscopically to involve a main bronchus less than 2 cm distal to the carina; or any tumor associated with atelectasis, obstructive pneumonitis of an entire lung, or pleural effusion.

N0: No demonstrable metastasis to regional lymph nodes

N1: Metastasis to lymph nodes in the peribronchial or the ipsilateral hilar region, or both, including direct extension

N2: Metastasis to lymph nodes in the mediastinum

M0: No distant metastasis

M1: Distant metastasis such as in scalene, cervical, or contralateral hilar lymph nodes, brain, bones, liver, or contralateral lung.

Occult Carcinoma	Stage I	Stage II	Stage III
TX N0 M0	TIS N0 M0	T2 N1 M0	T3 any N or M
	T1 N0 M0		N2 any T or M
	T1 N1 M0		M1 any T or N
	T2 N0 M0		

From David T. Carr and Edward C. Rosenow, "Bronchogenic Carcinoma," *Basics of Respiratory Disease,* Vol. 5, No. 5, 1977, p. 5. Used by permission of the authors and the American Lung Association.

mental, laser energy is directed through a bronchoscope to destroy local tumors.

Special considerations

Comprehensive supportive care and patient teaching can minimize complications and speed recovery from surgery, radiation, and chemotherapy.

Before surgery:

- Supplement and reinforce what the doctor has told the patient about the disease and the surgical procedure itself.
- Explain expected postoperative procedures, such as insertion of a Foley catheter, endotracheal tube, dressing changes, and I.V. therapy. Instruct the patient in coughing, deep diaphragmatic breathing, and range-of-motion exercises. Reassure him that analgesics and proper positioning will control postoperative pain.
- Inform the patient that he may take

DISTRIBUTION OF THE SIX MOST COMMON CANCER SITES

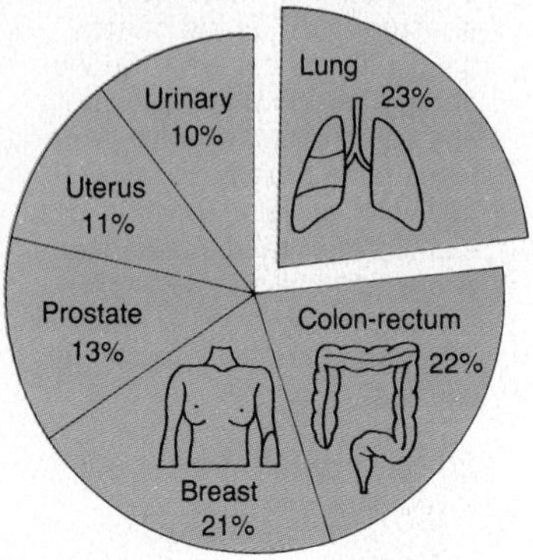

nothing by mouth (NPO) after midnight the night before surgery; that a povidone-iodine shower the night or morning before surgery is required; and that he'll be given preop medications, such as a sedative, and an anticholinergic to dry secretions.

After thoracic surgery:

- Maintain a patent airway, and monitor chest tubes to reestablish normal intrathoracic pressure and prevent postoperative and pulmonary complications.
- Check vital signs every 15 minutes during the first hour after surgery, every 30 minutes during the next 4 hours, and then every 2 hours. Watch for and report abnormal respiration and other changes.
- Suction patient often, and encourage him to begin deep breathing and coughing as soon as possible. Check secretions often. Initially, sputum will be thick and dark with blood, but it should become thinner and grayish-yellow within a day.
- Monitor and record closed chest drainage. Keep chest tubes patent and draining effectively. Fluctuation in the water seal chamber on inspiration and expiration indicates that the chest tube is patent. Watch for air leaks, and report them immediately. Position the patient on the surgical side to promote drainage and lung reexpansion.
- Watch for and report foul-smelling discharge and excessive drainage on dressing. Usually, the dressing is removed after 24 hours, unless the wound appears infected.
- Monitor intake and output. Maintain adequate hydration.
- Watch for and treat infection, shock, hemorrhage, atelectasis, dyspnea, mediastinal shift, and pulmonary embolus.
- To prevent pulmonary embolus, apply antiembolism stockings and encourage range-of-motion exercises.

If the patient is receiving chemotherapy and radiation:

- Explain possible side effects of radiation and chemotherapy. Watch for, treat, and, when possible, try to prevent them.
- Ask the dietary department to provide soft, nonirritating foods that are high in protein, and encourage the patient to eat high-calorie between-meal snacks.
- Give antiemetics and antidiarrheals, as needed.
- Schedule patient care to help the patient conserve his energy.
- Impose reverse isolation if patient develops bone marrow suppression.
- During radiation therapy, give good skin care to minimize skin breakdown. If the patient receives radiation therapy as an outpatient, warn him to avoid tight clothing, sunburn, and harsh ointments on his chest. Teach exercises to prevent shoulder stiffness.

Educate high-risk patients in ways to reduce their chances of developing lung cancer:

- Refer smokers who want to quit to local branches of the American Cancer Society, Smoke Enders, I Quit Smoking Clinics, or I'm Not Smoking Clubs; or suggest group therapy, individual counseling, or hypnosis.
- Recommend that all heavy smokers over age 40 have a chest X-ray annually and sputum cytology every 6 months. Also encourage patients with recurring or chronic respiratory infections and those with chronic lung disease who detect any change in the character of a cough to see their doctor promptly for evaluation.

Breast Cancer

Breast cancer is the second most common malignancy affecting women and is the number two killer (after lung cancer) of women age 35 to 54. It occurs in men, but rarely. The 5-year survival rate has improved from 53% in the 1940s to 65% in the 1970s. This is because of earlier diagnosis and the variety of treatment modes now available. The death rate, however, has not changed in the past 50 years.

Although breast cancer may develop any time after puberty, it's uncommon before age 35.

Causes and incidence

The cause of breast cancer isn't known, but its high incidence in women implicates estrogen. Certain predisposing factors are clear; women at *high risk* include those who:

- have a family history of breast cancer.
- have long menstrual cycles; began menses early or menopause late.
- were first pregnant after age 35.
- have had unilateral breast cancer.
- have endometrial or ovarian cancer.
- are whites of middle or upper socioeconomic class.
- are under constant stress or undergo unusual disturbances in their home or work lives.

Many other predisposing factors have been researched, such as radiation, hair dyes, estrogen therapy, antihypertensives, diet, and fibrocystic disease of the breasts. However, none of these has been demonstrated conclusively.

Women at *lower risk* include those who:

- were pregnant before age 20.
- had multiple pregnancies.
- are Indian or Asian.
- are of lower socioeconomic class.

Pathophysiology

Breast cancer occurs more often in the left breast than the right, and more often in the upper outer quadrant. Growth rates vary. Theoretically, slow-growing breast cancer may take up to 8 years to become palpable at ⅜″ (1 cm) in size. It spreads by way of the lymphatic system and the bloodstream, through the right heart to the lungs, and to the other breast, chest wall, liver, bone, and brain.

Many refer to the estimated growth rate of breast cancer as "doubling time," or the time it takes the malignant cells to double in number. Survival time for breast cancer is based on tumor size; the number of involved nodes is the single most important factor in predicting survival time.

Classified by histologic appearance and location of the lesion, breast cancer may be:

- *adenocarcinoma*—arising from the epithelium
- *intraductal*—developing within the ducts (includes Paget's disease)
- *infiltrating*—occurring in parenchymal tissue of the breast
- *inflammatory (rare)*—rapid tumor growth, in which the overlying skin becomes edematous, inflamed, and indurated
- *lobular carcinoma in situ*—tumor growth involving lobes of glandular tissue
- *medullary or circumscribed*—large tumor with rapid growth rate.

These classifications should be coupled with a staging or nodal status classification system for a clearer understanding of the extent of the cancer. The most common system for staging, both before and after surgery, is the tumor-nodes-metastasis (TNM) system.

Signs and symptoms

Warning signals of possible breast cancer include:

- a lump or mass in the breast (a hard, stony mass is usually malignant).

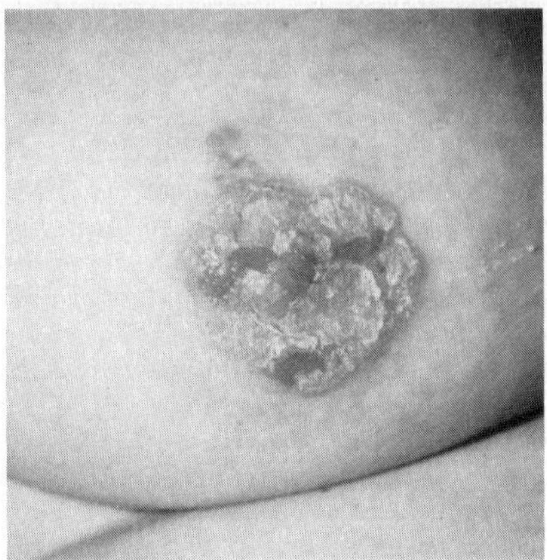

Paget's disease (cancer of the nipple), in which erosion and bleeding of the nipple occur

• change in breast symmetry or size.
• change in breast skin, such as thickening, dimpling, edema (peau d'orange), or ulceration.
• change in skin temperature (a warm, hot, or pink area; suspect cancer in a nonlactating woman past childbearing age until proven otherwise).
• unusual drainage or discharge (a spontaneous discharge of any kind in a nonnursing, nonlactating woman warrants investigation; so does any discharge produced by breast manipulation [greenish black, white, creamy, serous, or bloody]). If a nursing infant rejects one breast, this may suggest possible breast cancer.
• change in the nipple, such as itching, burning, erosion, or retraction.
• pain (not usually a symptom of breast cancer unless the tumor is advanced, but it should be investigated).
• bone metastasis, pathologic bone fractures, and hypercalcemia.

Diagnosis

The most reliable method of detecting breast cancer is the regular breast exam (breast self-examination), followed by immediate evaluation of any abnormality. Other dependable diagnostic measures include mammography, ultrasonography, thermography, and surgical biopsy. Mammography is indicated for any woman whose physical exam might suggest breast cancer. It should be done as a baseline on women between ages 35 and 40 (some say all women over 50), and annually on women who've had unilateral breast cancer, to check for new disease. However, the value of mammography is questionable for women under 35 (because of the density of the breasts), except those who are strongly suspected of having breast cancer. Consequently, in the presence of a suspicious mass, a negative mammogram should be disregarded and surgical biopsy done.

Bone scan, computed tomography scan, measurement of alkaline phosphatase levels, liver function studies, and liver biopsy can detect distant metastases. A hormonal reception assay done on the tumor can determine if the tumor is estrogen- or progesterone-dependent. (This test is important in making therapy decisions. Such therapy then aims to block the action of the estrogen hormone that supports tumor growth.)

Treatment

Much controversy exists over treatment of breast cancer; therapy should take into consideration the stage of the disease, the woman's age and menopausal status, and the disfiguring effects of the surgery. Treatment may include one or any combination of the following:

• Surgery

Lumpectomy (excision of the tumor) is the initial surgery; this procedure also aids in determining tumor cell type. It is often done on an outpatient basis and is the only surgery some patients require, especially those with a small tumor and no evidence of axillary node involvement. Radiation therapy is often combined with this surgery.

A two-stage procedure, in which the surgeon removes the lump, confirms that it's malignant, and discusses treatment options with the patient, is desirable because it allows the patient to participate in her treatment plan. Sometimes, if the tumor is diagnosed as clinically malignant, such planning can be done before surgery. In lumpectomy and dissection of the axillary lymph nodes, the tumor and the axillary lymph nodes are removed, leaving the breast intact. A simple mastectomy removes the breast but not the lymph nodes or pectoral muscles. Modified radical mastectomy removes the breast and the axillary lymph nodes. Radical mastectomy, the performance of which has declined, removes the breast, pectoralis major and minor, and the axillary lymph nodes.

Postmastectomy, reconstructive surgery can create a breast mound if the patient desires it and if she doesn't demonstrate evidence of advanced disease. Additional surgery to modify hormone production may include oophorectomy, adrenalectomy, and hypophysectomy. (With adrenalectomy or hypophysectomy, the patient is required to take daily cortisone supplements for the rest of her life.)

- Chemotherapy

Various cytotoxic drug combinations are being used, either as adjuvant therapy (in patients with axillary lymph node involvement but no evidence of distant metastasis) or as primary therapy (when metastasis has occurred), based on a number of factors, including the patient's premenopausal or postmenopausal status. The most commonly used drugs are cyclophosphamide, 5-fluorouracil, methotrexate, doxorubicin, vincristine, and prednisone. A common combination of such drugs, for example, is cyclophosphamide, methotrexate, and 5-fluorouracil (CMF); it's used in both premenopausal and postmenopausal women.

- Radiation therapy

Primary radiation therapy *after* tumor removal is effective for small tumors in early stages with no evidence of distant metastasis; it's also used to prevent or treat local recurrence.

- Other methods

Breast cancer patients may also re-

PATIENT TEACHING AID

Preventing Infection After Axillary Node Dissection or Radiation Therapy

Dear Patient:
Because edema makes tissue especially vulnerable to injury, take special care of the arm and hand on the surgical side.

Some don'ts

- Don't hold a cigarette in the affected hand.
- Don't use it to carry your purse or anything heavy.
- Don't wear a wristwatch or other jewelry on it.
- Don't cut or pick at cuticles or hangnails.
- Don't work near thorny plants or dig in the garden without heavy gloves.
- Don't reach into a hot oven with it.
- Don't permit injection into it.
- Don't permit blood to be drawn from it.
- Don't allow your blood pressure to be taken on it.

Some do's

- Do wear a loose rubber glove on this hand when washing dishes.
- Do wear a thimble when sewing.
- Do apply lanolin hand cream daily if your skin is dry.
- Do wear your Life Guard Medical Aid tag engraved with CAUTION OR PREVENT—LYMPHEDEMA ARM—NO TESTS—NO HYPOS.
- Do contact your doctor immediately if your arm gets red, feels warm, or is unusually hard or swollen.
- Do elevate your arm if it feels heavy.
- Do show this hand care sheet to your surgeon.

Information courtesy of the Cleveland Clinic, Department of Physical Medicine and Rehabilitation.

POSTOPERATIVE ARM AND HAND CARE

Hand exercises for the patient who is prone to lymphedema can begin on the day of surgery. Plan arm exercises with the doctor, because he can anticipate potential problems with the suture line.

- Have the patient open her hand and close it tightly six to eight times every 3 hours while she's awake.
- Elevate the arm on the affected side on a pillow above the heart level.
- Encourage the patient to wash her face and comb her hair—an effective exercise.
- Measure and record the circumference of the patient's arm 2¼" (6 cm) from her elbow. Indicate the exact place you measured. By remeasuring a month after surgery, and at intervals during and following radiation therapy, you will be able to determine whether lymphedema is present. The patient may complain that her arm is heavy—an early sign of lymphedema.
- When the patient is home, she can elevate her arm and hand by supporting it on the back of a chair or a couch.

ceive estrogen, progesterone, or androgen therapy; anti-androgen therapy with aminoglutethimide; or anti-estrogen therapy, specifically tamoxifen—a new drug with few side effects that inhibits DNA synthesis. Tamoxifen is used in postmenopausal women and is most effective against estrogen-receptor positive tumors. The success of these newer drug therapies along with growing evidence that breast cancer is a systemic, not local, disease, has led to a decline in ablative surgery.

Special considerations

To provide good care for a breast cancer patient, begin with a history; assess the patient's feelings about her illness, and determine what she knows about it and what she expects. Preoperatively, be sure you know what kind of surgery the patient is going to have, so you can prepare her properly. If a mastectomy is scheduled, in addition to the usual preoperative preparation (skin preparations, not allowing the patient anything by mouth), provide the following information for your patient:

- Teach her how to deep breathe and cough, to prevent pulmonary problems.
- Instruct her to rotate her ankles to help prevent thromboembolism.
- Tell her she can ease her pain by lying on the affected side, or by placing a hand or pillow on the incision. Preoperatively, show her where the incision will be. Inform her that she'll receive pain medication and that she needn't fear addiction. Remember, adequate pain relief encourages coughing and turning and promotes general well-being. A small pillow under the arm anteriorly provides comfort.
- Tell her that she may move about and get out of bed as soon as possible (even as soon as the anesthesia wears off or the first evening after surgery).
- Explain to her that after mastectomy, an incisional drain or some type of suction (Hemovac) is used to remove accumulated serous or sanguineous fluid and to keep the tension off the suture line, promoting healing.

Postoperative care:

- Inspect the dressing anteriorly and posteriorly, and report excessive bleeding promptly.
- Measure and record the amount and color of drainage. It's bloody during the first 4 hours and then becomes serous.
- Monitor circulatory status (blood pressure, pulse, respirations, and bleeding).
- Monitor intake and output for at least 48 hours after general anesthesia.
- Prevent lymphedema of the arm, which may be an early complication of any breast cancer treatment that involves lymph node dissection. Help the patient prevent lymphedema by instructing her to exercise her hand and arm regularly and to avoid activities that might cause infection in this hand or arm (infection increases the chance of developing lymphedema). Such prevention is very important, because lymphedema can't be

treated effectively.

• Inspect the incision. Encourage the patient and her partner to look at her incision as soon as feasible, perhaps when the first dressing is removed.

• Advise the patient to ask her doctor about reconstructive surgery or to call the local or state medical society for the names of plastic reconstructive surgeons who regularly perform surgery to create breast mounds. Such reconstruction may be planned prior to the mastectomy.

• Instruct the patient about breast prostheses. The American Cancer Society's Reach to Recovery group can provide instruction, emotional support, and a list of area stores that sell prostheses.

• Give psychological and emotional support. Many patients react to the fear of cancer and to disfigurement, and worry about loss of sexual function. Explain that breast surgery doesn't interfere with sexual function and that the patient may resume sexual activity as soon as she desires after surgery. She may experience "phantom breast syndrome" (a phenomenon in which a tingling or a pins-and-needles sensation is felt in the area of the amputated breast tissue) or depression following mastectomy. Listen to the patient's concerns, offer support, and refer her to an appropriate organization, such as the American Cancer Society's Reach to Recovery—which offers caring and sharing groups to help breast cancer patients in the hospital and at home.

ABDOMEN AND PELVIS

Gastric Carcinoma

Gastric carcinoma is common throughout the world and affects all races; however, unexplained geographic and cultural differences in incidence occur; for example, mortality is high in Japan, Iceland, Chile, and Austria. In the United States, during the past 25 years, incidence has decreased 50%, with the resulting death rate from gastric carcinoma one third that of 30 years ago. Incidence is higher in males over 40. Prognosis depends on the stage of the disease at the time of diagnosis; however, overall, the 5-year survival rate is approximately 15%.

Causes

The cause of gastric carcinoma is unknown, but predisposing factors include gastritis with gastric atrophy, achlorhydria, hypochlorhydria, and pernicious anemia. Polyps and chronic ulcers are occasionally associated with carcinoma of the stomach, but the data linking them are insubstantial. (Apparently, no correlation exists between duodenal ulcers and carcinoma of the stomach.) Genetic factors have also been implicated, since this disease occurs more frequently among people with type A blood than among those with type O; similarly, it occurs more frequently in people with a family history of such carcinoma. Dietary factors also seem related, including types of food preparation, physical properties of some foods, and certain methods of food preservation (especially smoking, pickling, or salting).

The parts of the stomach affected by gastric carcinoma, listed in order of decreasing frequency, are the pylorus and antrum, the lesser curvature, the cardia, the body of the stomach, and the greater curvature.

Gastric carcinoma infiltrates rapidly to regional lymph nodes, omentum, liver, and lungs by the following routes: walls of the stomach, duodenum, and esophagus; lymphatic system; adjacent organs; bloodstream; and peritoneal cavity.

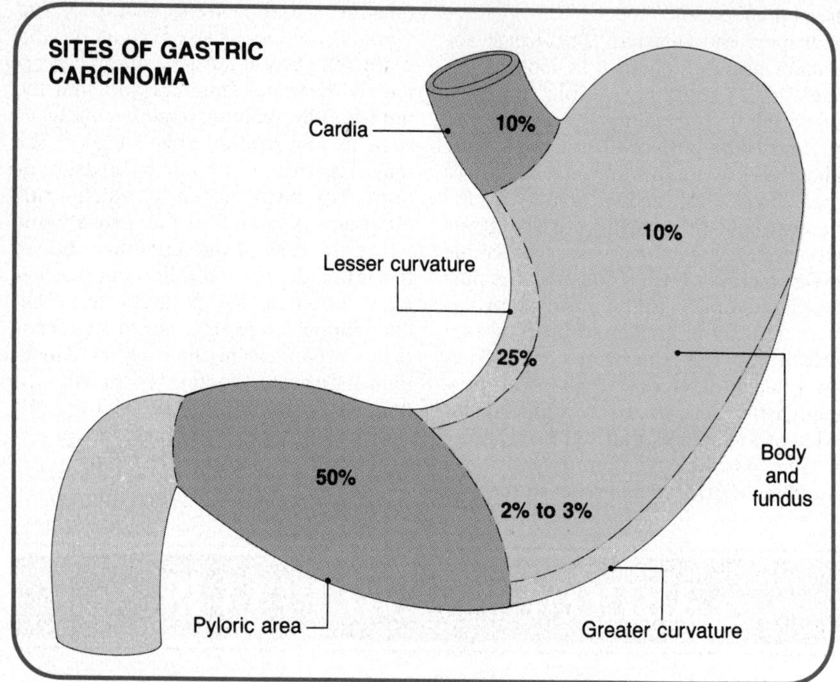

The decrease in the frequency of gastric carcinoma during the past 25 years in the United States has been attributed, without proof, to the improved and well-balanced diets most Americans enjoy.

Signs and symptoms

Early clues to gastric cancer are chronic dyspepsia and epigastric discomfort, followed in later stages by weight loss, anorexia, feeling of fullness after eating, anemia, and fatigue. If the carcinoma is in the cardia, the first symptom may be dysphagia and, later, vomiting (often coffee grounds vomitus). Affected patients may also have blood in their stools.

The course of gastric cancer may be insidious or fulminating. Unfortunately, the patient typically treats himself with antacids until the symptoms of advanced stages appear.

Diagnosis

Diagnosis depends primarily on reinvestigations of any persistent or recurring gastrointestinal changes and complaints. To rule out other conditions producing similar symptoms, diagnostic evaluation must include the testing of blood, stool, and stomach fluid samples.

Diagnosis of carcinoma of the stomach often requires these studies:

- *Barium X-rays of the GI tract, with fluoroscopy* show changes (tumor or filling defect in the outline of the stomach; loss of flexibility and distensibility; and abnormal gastric mucosa with or without ulceration).
- *Gastroscopy with fiberoptic endoscopy* helps rule out other diffuse gastric mucosal abnormalities by allowing direct visualization and gastroscopic biopsy to evaluate gastric mucosal lesions.
- *Photography with fiberoptic endoscope* provides a permanent record of gastric lesions that can later be used to determine disease progression and effect of treatment.

Certain other studies may rule out specific organ metastases: computed tomography scans, chest X-rays, liver and bone scans, and liver biopsy.

Treatment

Surgery is often the treatment of choice. Excision of the lesion with appropriate margins is possible in over one third of patients. Even in patients whose disease isn't considered surgically curable, resection offers palliation and improves potential benefits from chemotherapy and radiation.

The nature and extent of the lesion determine what kind of surgery is most appropriate. Common surgical procedures include subtotal gastric resection (subtotal gastrectomy) and total gastric resection (total gastrectomy). When carcinoma involves the pylorus and antrum, gastric resection removes the lower stomach and duodenum (gastrojejunostomy or Billroth II). If metastasis has occurred, the omentum and spleen may also have to be removed.

If gastric cancer has spread to the liver, peritoneum, or lymph glands, palliative surgery may include gastrostomy, jejunostomy, or a gastric or partial gastric resection. Such surgery may temporarily relieve vomiting, nausea, pain, and dysphagia, while allowing enteral nutrition to continue.

Chemotherapy for gastrointestinal malignancies may help to control symptoms and prolong survival. Adenocarcinoma of the stomach has responded to several agents including 5-fluorouracil, BCNU, and doxorubicin. Antiemetics can control nausea, which increases as the malignancy grows. In later stages, sedatives and tranquilizers may be necessary to control overwhelming anxiety. Narcotics are often necessary to relieve pain. However, morphine itself may produce nausea, so a synthetic derivative has been used more often recently.

Radiation has not been highly effective against carcinoma of the stomach but is still used occasionally. It should be given on an empty stomach, and shouldn't be used preoperatively, since it may damage viscera and impede healing.

Patients for whom extensive spread of malignancy rules out surgery may benefit from a medical regimen. Antispasmodics and antacids may relieve distress.

Special considerations

Before surgery, prepare the patient for its effects and for postsurgical procedures such as a nasogastric tube for drainage and I.V.s.

- Reassure the patient who is having a partial gastric resection that he may eventually be able to eat normally. Prepare the patient who is having a total gastrectomy for slow recovery and only partial return to a normal diet.
- Include the family in all phases of the patient's care.
- Emphasize the importance of changing position every 2 hours and of deep breathing.

After surgery, give meticulous supportive care to promote recovery and prevent complications.

Following any type of gastrectomy, pulmonary complications may result. Oxygen may be needed postoperatively. Regularly assist the patient with coughing, deep breathing, and turning. Hourly turning and judicious use of analgesic narcotics (these depress respiration) may prevent pulmonary problems. Intermittent positive pressure breathing (IPPB) or incentive spirometry breathing may be necessary for complete expansion of the lungs if the patient isn't able to breathe effectively on his own. Proper positioning is important; the semi-Fowler's position facilitates breathing and drainage.

After gastrectomy, little (if any) drainage comes from the nasogastric tube,

BILLROTH II PROCEDURE

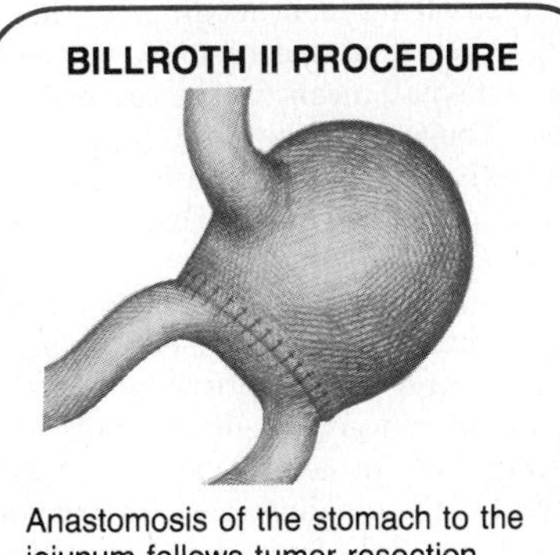

Anastomosis of the stomach to the jejunum follows tumor resection.

DUMPING SYNDROME

After gastric resection, rapid emptying of gastric contents into the small intestine produces the following:

- *Early dumping syndrome,* which may be mild or severe, occurs a few minutes after eating and lasts up to 45 minutes. Onset is sudden, with nausea, weakness, sweating, palpitations, dizziness, flushing, borborygmi, explosive diarrhea, and increased blood pressure and pulse rate.
- *Late dumping syndrome,* which is less serious, occurs 2 to 3 hours after eating. Similar symptoms include profuse sweating, anxiety, fine tremor of the hands and legs accompanied by vertigo, exhaustion, lassitude, palpitations, throbbing headache, faintness, sensation of hunger, glycosuria, and marked decrease in blood pressure and blood sugar.

These symptoms may persist for 1 year after surgery or for the rest of the patient's life.

because no secretions form after the stomach is removed. Since the stomach's storage function has been eliminated, the patient often suffers from a dumping syndrome. Intrinsic factor is absent from gastric secretions, which leads to malabsorption of vitamin B_{12}. To prevent vitamin B_{12} deficiency, the patient needs to replace this vitamin the rest of his life, as well as take an iron supplement.

During radiation treatment, encourage the patient to eat high-calorie, well-balanced meals. Offer fluids, such as orange juice, grapefruit juice, or ginger ale, to minimize nausea and vomiting. Watch for radiation side effects (nausea, vomiting, hair loss, malaise, and diarrhea).

Watch for complications of surgery:

- Patients who experience poor digestion and absorption after gastrectomy need a special diet: frequent feedings of small amounts of clear liquids, increasing to small frequent feedings of bland food. After total gastrectomy, patients must eat small meals for the rest of their lives. (Some patients need pancreatin and sodium bicarbonate after meals to prevent or control steatorrhea and dyspepsia.)
- Wound dehiscence and delayed healing, stemming from decreased protein, anemia, and avitaminosis, occur frequently in cancer patients. Preoperative vitamin and protein replacement can prevent such complications. Observe the wound regularly for redness, swelling, failure to heal, or warmth. Parenteral administration of vitamin C may improve wound healing.
- Vitamin deficiency that results from obstruction, diarrhea, or an inadequate diet. Ascorbic acid, thiamine, riboflavin, nicotinic acid, and vitamin K supplements may be beneficial. Good nutrition promotes weight gain, strength, independence, and positive emotional outlook, and promotes tolerance for surgery, radiotherapy, or chemotherapy. Aside from meeting caloric needs, good nutrition must provide adequate protein, fluid, and potassium intake to facilitate glycogen and protein synthesis. Anabolic agents, such as methandrostenolone, may induce nitrogen retention. Steroids, antidepressants, wine, or brandy may stimulate the appetite.

When all treatment has failed, concentrate on keeping the patient comfortable and free of unnecessary pain, and provide as much psychologic support as possible. Talk with him and encourage him to verbalize his feelings and fears. When he asks questions about his illness, answer them honestly. Evasive answers will make him retreat and feel isolated. Talk with family members, and answer any questions they may have. Tell them to let the patient talk about his future, but encourage them to maintain a realistic outlook. If the patient is going home, arrange for a visiting nurse or homemaker, if needed, as well as for his sickroom needs (for example, a bedside commode or a walker).

Esophageal Cancer

Esophageal cancer usually develops in men over 60 years of age and is nearly always fatal. This disease occurs worldwide, but incidence varies geographically. It's most common in Japan, Russia, China, the Middle East, and in the Transkei region of South Africa, where esophageal cancer has reached almost epidemic proportions. More than 8,000 cases of esophageal cancer are reported annually in the United States alone.

Causes

The cause of esophageal cancer is unknown, but predisposing factors have been identified: chronic irritation, as in heavy smoking and excessive use of alcohol; stasis-induced inflammation, as in achalasia or stricture; previous head and neck tumors; and nutritional deficiency, as in untreated sprue and Plummer-Vinson syndrome. Esophageal tumors are usually fungating and infiltrating. Most arise in squamous cell epithelium; a few are adenocarcinomas; fewer still, melanomas and sarcomas.

About half the squamous cell cancers occur in the lower portion of the esophagus, about 40% in the midportion, and the remaining 10% in the upper or cervical esophagus. Regardless of cell type, prognosis for esophageal cancer is grim. Five-year survival rates don't exceed 10%.

In most cases, the tumor partially constricts the lumen of the esophagus. Regional metastasis occurs early, by way of submucosal lymphatics, and often fatally invades adjacent vital intrathoracic organs. Direct invasion of adjoining structures may lead to dramatic complications: mediastinitis, tracheo- or bronchioesophageal fistulas (causing an overwhelming cough induced by swallowing liquids); or aortic perforation with sudden exsanguination. If the patient survives primary extension, the liver and lungs are the usual sites of distant metastasis. Rarer sites of metastasis include bone, kidneys, and adrenals.

Signs and symptoms

Dysphagia and weight loss are the most common presenting symptoms. At first, dysphagia is usually mild and intermittent, occurring only after ingestion of solid food (especially meat). Before long, however, dysphagia becomes constant, with pain on swallowing, hoarseness, coughing, and glossopharyngeal neuralgia. In later stages, signs of esophageal obstruction appear—sialorrhea, nocturnal aspiration, regurgitation, and inability to swallow even liquids. Cachexia usually develops.

Diagnosis

X-rays of the esophagus, with barium swallow and motility studies, reveal structural and filling defects and reduced peristalsis.

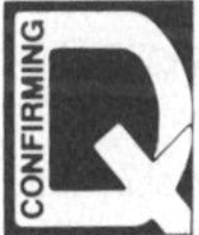

Endoscopic examination of the esophagus, punch and brush biopsies, and exfoliative cytologic tests confirm esophageal tumors.

Treatment

Whenever possible, treatment includes resection to maintain a passageway for food. This often involves radical surgery, such as esophagogastrectomy with jejunal or colonic bypass grafts. Palliative surgery may include a feeding gastrostomy. Treatment also consists of radiation; chemotherapy with, for example, bleomycin; or installation of prosthetic tubes (such as the Mousseau Barbin or Celestin tubes), to bridge the tumor and alleviate dysphagia. Unfortunately, none of these methods is completely successful. Surgery can cause its own complications (anastomotic leak, fistula formation, pneumonia, empyema, malnutrition); radiation can cause esophageal perforation, pneumonitis and fibrosis of the lungs, or myelitis of the spinal cord; and prosthetic tubes can become blocked or dislodged, causing a perforation of the mediastinum, or can precipitate tumor erosion.

Special considerations

- Before surgery, answer the patient's questions, and offer reassurance by letting him know what to expect. Explain the procedures he'll experience after surgery—closed chest drainage, nasogastric suctioning, and gastrostomy tubes.
- After surgery, monitor vital signs. Report any unexpected changes to the doctor immediately. If surgery has included an anastomosis to the esophagus, position the patient flat on his back to prevent tension on the suture line.
- Your primary goal is to promote adequate nutrition—a difficult task in such patients. Assess the patient's nutritional and hydrational status for possible supplementary parenteral feedings.
- Prevent aspiration of food by placing the patient in Fowler's position for meals and allowing plenty of time to eat. Provide high-calorie, high-protein, "blenderized" food, as needed. Since the patient will probably regurgitate some food, clean his mouth carefully after each meal. Keep mouthwash handy.
- If the patient has a gastrostomy tube, give food slowly—by gravity—in prescribed amounts (usually 200 to 500 ml). Offer something to chew before each feeding. This promotes gastric secretions and provides some semblance of normal eating.
- Instruct the family in gastrostomy tube care (checking tube patency before each feeding, providing skin care around the tube, keeping the patient upright during and after feedings).
- Provide emotional support for the patient and family; refer them to appropriate organizations such as the American Cancer Society.

Pancreatic Cancer

Second only to cancer of the colon as the deadliest GI cancer, pancreatic cancer now ranks fourth among all fatal carcinomas. Prognosis is poor, and most patients die within a year after diagnosis.

Tumors of the pancreas are almost always adenocarcinomas and arise most frequently (67% of the time) in the head of the pancreas. Rarer tumors are those of the body and tail of the pancreas and islet cell tumor. The two main tissue types of pancreatic cancer, both of which form fibrotic nodes, are cylinder cell (which arises in ducts and degenerates into cysts) and large, fatty, granular cell (which arises in parenchyma).

Causes and incidence

Pancreatic adenocarcinoma occurs most often among blacks, particularly in men between ages 35 and 70. Geographically, incidence of pancreatic cancer is highest in Israel, the United States, Sweden, and Canada; lowest in Switzerland, Belgium, and Italy.

Evidence suggests that pancreatic cancer is linked to inhalation or absorption of carcinogens which are then excreted by the pancreas:

- cigarette smoking—pancreatic cancer is three to four times more common among smokers
- diets high in fat and protein—induce chronic hyperplasia of the pancreas with increased turnover of cells
- food additives
- exposure to industrial chemicals, such as beta-naphthalene, benzidine, and urea.

TYPES OF PANCREATIC CANCER

PATHOLOGY	CLINICAL FEATURES
Head of pancreas • Often obstructs ampulla of Vater and common bile duct • Directly metastasizes to duodenum • Adhesions anchor tumor to spine, stomach, and intestines.	• Jaundice (predominant symptom)—slowly progressive, unremitting; may cause skin (especially of the face and genitals) to turn olive green or black • Pruritus—often severe • Weight loss—rapid and severe (as great as 30 lbs [13.6 kg]); may lead to emaciation, weakness, and muscle atrophy • Slowed digestion, gastric distention, nausea, diarrhea, and steatorrhea with clay-colored stools • Liver and gallbladder enlargement from lymph node metastasis to biliary tract and duct wall results in compression and obstruction; gallbladder may be palpable (Courvoisier's sign). • Dull, nondescript, continuous abdominal pain radiating to upper right quadrant; relieved by bending forward • GI hemorrhage and biliary infection common
Body and tail of pancreas • Large nodular masses become fixed to retropancreatic tissues and spine. • Direct invasion of spleen, left kidney, suprarenal gland, diaphragm • Involvement of celiac plexus results in thrombosis of splenic vein and spleen infarction.	**Body** • Pain (predominant symptom)—usually epigastric, develops slowly and radiates to back; relieved by bending forward or sitting up; intensified by lying supine; most intense 3 to 4 hours after eating; when celiac plexus is involved, pain is more intense and lasts longer • Venous thrombosis and thrombophlebitis—frequent; may precede other symptoms by months • Splenomegaly (from infarction), hepatomegaly (occasionally), and jaundice (rarely) **Tail** Symptoms result from metastasis: • Abdominal tumor (most common finding) produces a palpable abdominal mass; abdominal pain radiates to left hypochondrium and left chest. • Anorexia leads to weight loss, emaciation, and weakness. • Splenomegaly and upper GI bleeding

Other possible predisposing factors are chronic pancreatitis, diabetes mellitus, and chronic alcohol abuse.

Signs and symptoms

The most common features of pancreatic carcinoma are weight loss, abdominal or low back pain, jaundice, and diarrhea. Other generalized effects include fever, skin lesions (usually on the legs), and emotional disturbances, such as depression, anxiety, and premonition of fatal illness.

Diagnosis

Definitive diagnosis requires a laparotomy with a biopsy. However, a biopsy may miss relatively small or deep-seated cancerous tissue or create a pancreatic fistula. Other tests used to detect pancreatic cancer include:

- *X-rays*—retroperitoneal insufflation, cholangiography, scintigraphy, and, particularly, barium swallow (to locate neoplasm and detect changes in the duodenum or stomach relating to carcinoma of the head of the pancreas)
- *ultrasound*—can identify a mass but not its histology
- *computed tomography scan*—similar to ultrasound but shows greater detail
- *angiography*—shows vascular supply of tumor
- *endoscopic retrograde cannulization of the pancreas* or *endoscopic pancreatography*—allows visualization, instillation of contrast medium, and possible specimen
- *secretin test*—shows absence of pancreatic enzymes; suggests pancreatic

ISLET CELL TUMORS

Relatively uncommon, islet cell tumors (insulinomas) may be benign or malignant and produce symptoms in three stages:

1. *Slight hypoglycemia*—fatigue, restlessness, malaise, and excessive weight gain.
2. *Compensatory secretion of epinephrine*—pallor, clamminess, perspiration, palpitations, finger tremors, hunger, decreased temperature, increased pulse and blood pressure.
3. *Severe hypoglycemia*—ataxia, clouded sensorium, diplopia, episodes of violence and hysteria.

Usually, insulinomas metastasize to the liver alone but may metastasize to bone, brain, and lungs. Death results from a combination of hypoglycemic reactions and widespread metastasis. Treatment consists of enucleation of tumor (if benign) and chemotherapy with streptozocin or resection to include pancreatic tissue (if malignant).

duct obstruction and tumors of body and tail.

Laboratory values supporting this diagnosis include increased serum bilirubin, serum amylase-lipase (occasionally elevated); prolonged prothrombin time; serum glutamic-oxaloacetic transaminase and serum glutamic-pyruvic transaminase (elevation of enzymes indicates necrosis of liver cells); alkaline phosphatase (marked elevation occurs with biliary obstruction); plasma insulin immunoassay (shows measurable serum insulin in the presence of islet cell tumors); hemoglobin/hematocrit (may show mild anemia); fasting blood sugar (may indicate hypoglycemia or hyperglycemia); and stools (occult blood may point to ulceration in GI tract or ampulla of Vater).

Treatment

Treatment of pancreatic cancer is rarely successful, because this disease is often widely metastasized at diagnosis. Therapy consists of surgery and, possibly, radiation and chemotherapy.

Small advances have been made in the survival rate with surgery:

- Total pancreatectomy has perhaps increased survival time by resecting a localized tumor or by controlling postoperative gastric ulceration.
- Cholecystojejunostomy, choledochoduodenostomy, and choledochojejunostomy have partially replaced radical resection to bypass obstructing common bile duct extensions, and thereby ease jaundice and pruritus.
- Whipple's operation, or pancreatoduodenectomy, has a high mortality but can obtain wide lymphatic clearance, except with tumors located near the portal vein, superior mesenteric vein and artery, and celiac axis. This rarely used procedure removes the head of the pancreas, duodenum, and portions of the body and tail of pancreas, stomach, jejunum, pancreatic duct, and distal portion of the bile duct.
- Gastrojejunostomy is performed if radical resection isn't indicated and duodenal obstruction is expected to develop later.

Although pancreatic carcinoma generally responds poorly to chemotherapy, recent studies using combinations of carmustine (BCNU), 5-fluorouracil, and doxorubicin show a trend toward longer survival time. Other medications used in pancreatic cancer include:

- antibiotics (oral, I.V., or I.M.)—prevent infection and relieve symptoms
- anticholinergics—particularly propantheline, decrease GI tract spasm and motility and reduce pain and secretions
- antacids (oral or by nasogastric tube)—decrease secretion of pancreatic enzymes; they also suppress peptic activity and thereby reduce stress-induced damage to gastric mucosa
- diuretics—mobilize extracellular fluid from ascites
- insulin—provides adequate exoge-

nous insulin supply after pancreatic resection

- narcotics—relieve pain; but since morphine, meperidine, and codeine can lead to biliary tract spasm and increase common bile duct pressure, they're used only after other analgesics fail
- pancreatic enzymes—(average dose 0.5 to 1 mg with meals) assist digestion of proteins, carbohydrates, and fats when pancreatic juices are insufficient due to surgery or obstruction.

Radiation therapy is usually ineffective except when used as an adjunct to 5-fluorouracil chemotherapy; then it may prolong survival time from 4 to 9 months. It can also ease the pain associated with nonresectable tumors.

Special considerations

Comprehensive supportive care can prevent surgical complications, increase patient comfort, and help the patient and his family cope with inevitable death.

Before surgery:

- Ensure that the patient is medically stable, particularly regarding nutrition (this may take 4 to 5 days). If the patient can't tolerate oral feedings, provide total parenteral nutrition and I.V. fat emulsions to correct deficiencies and maintain positive nitrogen balance.
- Give blood transfusions (to combat anemia), vitamin K (to overcome prothrombin deficiency), antibiotics (to prevent postoperative complications), and gastric lavage (to maintain gastric decompression), as ordered.
- Tell the patient about expected postoperative procedure and expected side effects of radiation and chemotherapy.

After surgery:

- Watch for and report complications, such as fistula, pancreatitis, fluid and electrolyte imbalance, infection, hemorrhage, skin breakdown, nutritional deficiency, hepatic failure, renal insufficiency, and diabetes.
- If patient is receiving chemotherapy, watch for and symptomatically treat its toxic effects.

Throughout this illness, provide meticulous supportive care:

- Monitor fluid balance, abdominal girth, metabolic state, and weight daily. In weight loss, replace nutrients I.V., P.O., or with a nasogastric tube; with weight gain (due to ascites), impose dietary restrictions, such as a low-sodium or fluid retention diet, as ordered. Maintain a 2,500-calorie diet.
- Serve small, frequent meals. Consult the dietitian in planning meals to ensure proper nutrition, and make mealtimes as pleasant as possible. Administer an oral pancreatic enzyme at mealtimes, if needed. As ordered, give an antacid to prevent stress ulcers.
- To prevent constipation, administer laxatives, stool softeners, and cathartics, as ordered; modify diet; and increase fluid intake. To increase GI motility, position the patient properly during and after meals, and assist him with walking when he's able.
- Ensure adequate rest and sleep (with a sedative, if warranted). Assist with range-of-motion exercises and isometrics, as appropriate.
- Administer analgesics for pain, and antibiotics and antipyretics for fever, as ordered. Note time, site (if injected), and response.
- Observe closely for signs of hypoglycemia or hyperglycemia; administer glucose or a hypoglycemic agent, such as tolbutamide, as ordered. Monitor blood glucose concentration, urine sugar, acetone, and response to treatment. Document progression of jaundice.
- Provide scrupulous skin care to avoid pruritus and necrosis. Keep skin clean and dry. If the patient has overwhelming pruritus, prevent excoriation by clipping his nails and persuading him to wear light cotton gloves.
- Watch for signs of upper GI bleeding; Hematest stools and emesis, and maintain a flow sheet of frequent hemoglobin/hematocrit determinations. To control active bleeding, promote gastric vasoconstriction with medication and iced saline lavage through a nasogastric or duodenal tube. Replace any fluid loss. Ease discomfort from pyloric obstruction with a nasogastric tube.

• To prevent thrombosis, apply antiembolism stockings and assist in range-of-motion exercises. If thrombosis occurs, elevate legs, apply moist heat to thrombus site and give an anticoagulant or aspirin, as ordered, to prevent further clot formation and pulmonary embolus.
• Encourage the patient to verbalize his fears, which are valid. Promote family involvement, and offer the assistance of a chaplain or psychologist. Help the patient and his family deal with the impending reality of death. Examine and work out your own feelings about death to provide maximum support.

Colorectal Cancer

Colorectal cancer is the second most common visceral neoplasm in the United States and in Europe. Incidence is equally distributed between men and women.

Colorectal malignant tumors are almost always adenocarcinomas. About half of these are sessile lesions of the rectosigmoid area; the rest are polypoid lesions.

Colorectal cancer tends to progress slowly and remains localized for a long time. Consequently, it's potentially curable in 75% of patients if early diagnosis allows resection before nodal involvement. With improved diagnosis, the overall 5-year survival rate is nearing 50%.

Causes

The exact cause of colorectal cancer is unknown, but studies showing concentration in areas of higher economic development suggest a relationship to diet (excess animal fat, particularly beef, and low fiber). Other factors that magnify the risk of developing colorectal cancer include:
• other diseases of the digestive tract.
• age (over 40).
• history of ulcerative colitis (average interval before onset of cancer is 11 to 17 years).
• familial polyposis (cancer almost always develops by age 50).

Signs and symptoms

Signs and symptoms of colorectal cancer result from local obstruction and, in later stages, from direct extension to adjacent organs (bladder, prostate, ureters, vagina, sacrum) and distant metastasis (usually liver). In the early stages, signs and symptoms are typically vague and depend on the anatomical location and function of the bowel segment containing the tumor. Later, they generally include pallor, cachexia, ascites, hepatomegaly, or lymphangiectasis.

On the right side of the colon (which absorbs water and electrolytes), early tumor growth causes no signs of obstruction, since the tumor tends to grow along the bowel rather than surround the lumen, and the fecal content in this area is normally liquid. It may, however, cause black, tarry stools; anemia; and abdominal aching, pressure, or dull cramps. As the disease progresses, the patient develops weakness, fatigue, exertional dyspnea, vertigo, and, eventually, diarrhea, obstipation, anorexia, weight loss, vomiting, and other signs of intestinal obstruction. In addition, a tumor on the right side may be palpable.

On the left side, a tumor causes signs of an obstruction even in early stages, since in this area stools are of a formed consistency. It commonly causes rectal bleeding (often ascribed to hemorrhoids), intermittent abdominal fullness or cramping, and rectal pressure. As the disease progresses, the patient develops obstipation, diarrhea, or "ribbon" or pencil-shaped stools. Typically, he notices that passage of a stool or flatus relieves the pain. At this stage, bleeding from the colon becomes obvious, with dark or bright red blood in the feces and mucus in or on the stools.

With a rectal tumor, the first symptom is a change in bowel habits, often beginning with an urgent need to defecate on arising ("morning diarrhea") or obstipation alternating with diarrhea. Other signs are blood or mucus in stool and a sense of incomplete evacuation. Late in the disease, pain begins as a feeling of rectal fullness that later becomes a dull, and sometimes constant, ache confined to the rectum or sacral region.

Diagnosis

Only tumor biopsy can verify colorectal cancer, but other tests help detect it:

- *Digital examination* can detect almost 15% of colorectal cancers.
- *Hemoccult test* (guaiac) can detect blood in stools.
- *Proctoscopy* or *sigmoidoscopy* can detect up to 66% of colorectal cancers.
- *Colonoscopy* permits visual inspection (and photographs) of the colon up to the ileocecal valve, and gives access for polypectomies and biopsies of suspected lesions.
- *Intravenous pyelography* verifies bilateral renal function and checks for any displacement of the kidneys, ureters, or bladder.
- *Barium X-ray,* utilizing a dual contrast with air, can locate lesions that are undetectable manually or visually. Barium examination should *follow* endoscopy or intravenous pyelography, because the barium sulfate interferes with these tests.
- *Carcinoembryonic antigen (CEA),* though not specific or sensitive enough for early diagnosis, is helpful in monitoring patients before and after treatment to detect metastasis or recurrence.

Treatment

The most effective treatment for colorectal cancer is surgery to remove the malignant tumor and adjacent tissues, and any lymph nodes that may contain cancer cells. The type of surgery depends on the location of the tumor:

- *Cecum and ascending colon*—right hemicolectomy (for advanced disease) may include resection of the terminal segment of the ileum, cecum, ascending colon, and right half of the transverse colon with corresponding mesentery
- *Proximal and middle transverse colon*—right colectomy to include transverse colon and mesentery corresponding to midcolic vessels, or segmental resection of transverse colon and associated midcolic vessels
- *Sigmoid colon*—surgery is usually limited to sigmoid colon and mesentery
- *Upper rectum*—anterior or low anterior resection (newer method, using a stapler, allows for resections much lower than were previously possible)
- *Lower rectum*—abdominoperineal resection and permanent sigmoid colostomy.

Chemotherapy is indicated for patients with metastasis, residual disease, or a recurrent inoperable tumor. Drugs used in such treatment commonly include 5-fluorouracil, lomustine, mitomycin, methotrexate, and vincristine.

Radiation therapy induces tumor regression and may be used before or after surgery. Immunotherapy using BCG (bacille Calmette-Guérin) vaccine is still experimental.

Special considerations

Before colorectal surgery, monitor patient's diet modifications, laxatives, enemas, and antibiotics—all used to cleanse the bowel and to decrease abdominal and perineal cavity contamination during surgery. If the patient is to have a colostomy, teach him and his family what he needs to know about the procedure:

- Emphasize that the stoma will be red, moist, and swollen, and that postoperative swelling will eventually subside.
- Show a diagram of the intestine before and after surgery, stressing how much of the bowel remains intact. Supplement your teaching with instruction booklets (available for a fee from the United Ostomy Association and free from various companies that manufacture ostomy

PATIENT TEACHING AID

How to Care for a Stoma

Dear Patient:

- Keep the skin around the stoma clean after removing the pouch, by washing with mild soap and water, rinsing well with clear water, and drying. Coat the skin with a silicone skin protector and cover with a collection pouch.
- Keep the skin around the stoma unirritated. For irritation and breakdown, apply a layer of antacid precipitate to the clean and dry skin, dust with karaya gum powder, allow to dry, and coat with a silicone skin protector.
- Measure the stoma, and prepare the face plate of the pouch to clear the stoma, with a ⅛″ (3.2 mm) margin.
- Protect the skin from the effluent and abrasiveness of the adhesive.
- Cut the opening in the barrier the same size as the stoma to prevent skin irritation.
- Check the pouch frequently to make sure the skin seal is still intact.
- Control odor within the pouch with any of the commercial products available.

This patient teaching aid may be reproduced by office copier for distribution to patients.

supplies). Arrange a postsurgical visit from a recovered ostomate.

- Prepare the patient for postoperative I.V.s, nasogastric tube, and Foley catheter.
- Discuss importance of cooperation during coughing and deep breathing exercises.

After surgery, explain to the patient's family the importance of their positive reactions to the patient's adjustment. Consult with an enterostomal therapist, if available, for questions on setting up a regimen for the patient.

Encourage the patient to look at the stoma and participate in its care as soon as possible. Teach good hygiene and skin care. Allow him to shower or bathe as soon as the incision heals. If appropriate, instruct the patient with a sigmoid colostomy to do his own irrigation as soon as he's able after surgery. Advise him to schedule irrigation for the time of the day when he normally evacuated before surgery. Many patients find that irrigating every 1 to 3 days is necessary for regulation. If flatus, diarrhea, or constipation occurs, eliminate suspected causative foods from the patient's diet. He may reintroduce them later.

After several months, many ostomates establish control with irrigation and no longer need to wear a pouch. A stoma cap or gauze sponge placed over the stoma protects it and absorbs mucoid secretions.

Before achieving such control, the patient can resume physical activities, including sports, providing there is no threat of injury to the stoma or surrounding abdominal muscles. He can place a pouch or stoma cap (if regulated) over the stoma when swimming. However, he should avoid heavy lifting, as herniation or prolapse may occur through weakened muscles in the abdominal wall. A structural, gradually progressive exercise program to strengthen abdominal muscles may be instituted under the doctor's supervision.

Schedule a visiting nurse to call on the patient at home to check on his physical care. Suggest sexual counseling for male patients; most are impotent after an abdominoperineal resection and suffer fear of rejection.

Anyone who has had colorectal cancer runs an increased risk of developing another primary cancer and should have yearly screening and follow-up testing, as well as a diet high in fiber (bulk).

Kidney Cancer

(Nephrocarcinoma, renal cell carcinoma, hypernephroma, Grawitz's tumor)

Kidney cancer usually occurs in older adults. About 85% of kidney cancers originate in the kidneys; other kidney cancers include metastases from other primary-site carcinomas. Renal pelvic tumors and Wilms' tumor occur primarily in children.

Usually, kidney tumors—which may affect either kidney—are large, firm, nodular, encapsulated, unilateral, and solitary. Occasionally, they're bilateral or multifocal. Kidney cancer can be separated histologically into clear cell, granular, and spindle cell types. Prognosis is sometimes considered better for the clear cell type than it is for the other two types; in general, however, prognosis seems more dependent on the stage of the disease than on the type.

Overall, prognosis for kidney cancer has improved considerably, with the 5-year survival rate now at approximately 50% of patients and the 10-year survival rate at 18% to 23% of patients.

Causes and incidence

The causes of kidney cancer aren't known. However, the incidence of this malignancy is rising, possibly as a result of exposure to environmental carcinogens as well as increased longevity. Even so, such cancer accounts for only about 2% of all adult cancers. Kidney cancer is twice as common in men as in women, and usually strikes after age 40, with peak incidence between ages 50 and 60.

Signs and symptoms

Kidney cancer produces a classic clinical triad: hematuria, pain, and a palpable mass. Any one of these may occur as the first sign of cancer. Microscopic or gross hematuria (which may be intermittent) often indicates that the cancer has spread to the renal pelvis. Constant abdominal or flank pain may be dull or, if the cancer causes bleeding or clot formation, acute and colicky. The palpable mass is generally smooth, firm, and nontender. All three major signs coexist in only about 10% of patients.

Other symptoms include fever (perhaps a result of hemorrhage or tumor necrosis); hypertension (a result of compression of the renal artery with renal parenchymal ischemia); rapidly progressing, and occasionally fatal, hypercalcemia (possibly due to ectopic parathyroid hormone production by the tumor); and urinary retention, from an obstructing blood clot. Weight loss, edema in the legs, nausea, and vomiting point to advanced disease.

Diagnosis

Studies to identify kidney cancer usually include computed tomography scans, intravenous pyelography, retrograde pyelography, ultrasound studies, cystoscopy (to rule out associated bladder cancer), and nephrotomography or renal angiography to distinguish a kidney cyst from a tumor.

Other relevant tests include liver func-

STAGING KIDNEY CANCER

Stage I: Tumor confined to kidney

Stage II: Perirenal spread confined to Gerota's space (fascia around the kidney)

Stage III: Spread to renal vein or inferior vena cava, with or without lymphatic involvement

Stage IV: Advanced disease, with spread to adjacent organs (except for adrenal glands) or metastases, usually to distant lymph nodes, lungs, liver, and bone

NEPHROCARCINOMA

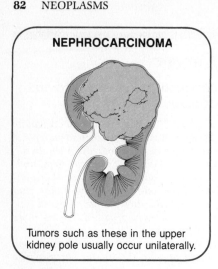

Tumors such as these in the upper kidney pole usually occur unilaterally.

tion studies, showing increased alkaline phosphatase, bilirubin, transaminase, and prolonged prothrombin time. Such results may point to liver metastasis, but if the tumor hasn't metastasized, these abnormalities reverse after tumor resection.

Routine lab studies that show hematuria, anemia (unrelated to blood loss), polycythemia, hypercalcemia, and increased erythrocyte sedimentation rate call for further testing to rule out kidney cancer.

Treatment

Radical nephrectomy, with or without regional lymph node dissection, offers the only chance of being cured for a patient with kidney cancer. Since this disease is radiation resistant, radiation is used only when the cancer has spread into the perinephric region or the lymph nodes, or when the primary tumor or metastatic sites can't be completely excised. Then, high radiation doses are usually necessary.

Drug therapy has been only erratically effective against kidney cancer. Chlorambucil, 5-fluorouracil, cyclophosphamide, vinblastine, lomustine, vincristine, cisplatin, tamoxifen, interferons, and hormones, such as medroxyprogesterone and testosterone, have been used with varying success.

Special considerations

Meticulous postoperative care, supportive treatment (including relief from associated symptoms and side effects) during radiation and chemotherapy, and psychological support can hasten recovery and minimize complications.

Before surgery:

- Encourage the patient to express his anxieties and fears. Assure him that his body will adequately adapt to the loss of a kidney.
- Explain the possible side effects of radiation and chemotherapy.
- Teach the patient about the expected postoperative procedures, as well as diaphragmatic breathing, how to cough properly, and how to splint his incision while coughing.

After surgery:

- Encourage diaphragmatic breathing and coughing.
- Assist the patient with leg exercises to reduce the risk of phlebitis, and turn him every 2 hours.
- Check dressings often for excessive bleeding. Watch for signs of internal bleeding, such as restlessness, sweating, and increased pulse rate.
- Position the patient on the operative side to allow the pressure of adjacent organs to fill the dead space at the operative site and thus improve dependent drainage. If possible, assist the patient with walking within 24 hours after surgery.
- Maintain adequate fluid intake, and monitor intake and output. Monitor lab results for anemia, polycythemia, or abnormal blood chemistries that may point to bone or hepatic involvement or may result from radiation or chemotherapy.
- Symptomatically treat all drug side effects.

When preparing a patient for discharge, stress the importance of compliance with any prescribed outpatient treatment. This includes an annual follow-up chest X-ray to rule out lung metastasis and intravenous pyelography every 6 to 12 months to check for contralateral tumors.

Liver Cancer

(Primary hepatic carcinoma)

Liver cancer is a rare form of cancer with a high mortality. It's responsible for roughly 2% of all malignancies in the United States and for 10% to 50% in Africa and parts of Asia. Liver cancer is most prevalent in men (particularly over age 60); incidence increases with age. It is rapidly fatal, usually within 6 months from gastrointestinal hemorrhage, progressive cachexia, hepatic failure, or metastatic spread.

Most primary liver tumors (90%) originate in the parenchymal cells and are hepatomas (hepatocellular carcinoma, primary lower-cell carcinoma). Some primary tumors originate in the intrahepatic bile ducts and are known as cholangiomas (cholangiocarcinoma, cholangiocellular carcinoma). Rarer tumors include a mixed-cell type, Kupffer cell sarcoma, and hepatoblastomas (which occur almost exclusively in children and are usually resectable and curable). The liver is one of the most common sites of metastasis from other primary cancers, particularly colon, rectum, stomach, pancreas, esophagus, lung, breast, or melanoma. In the United States, metastatic carcinoma occurs over 20 times more often than primary carcinoma and, after cirrhosis, is the leading cause of fatal hepatic disease. At times, liver metastasis may appear as a solitary lesion, the first sign of recurrence after a remission.

Causes

The immediate cause of liver cancer is unknown, but many consider it a congenital disease in children. Adult liver cancer may result from environmental exposure to carcinogens, such as the chemical compound aflatoxin (a mold that grows on rice and peanuts), thorium dioxide (a contrast dye medium used in liver radiography in the past), Senecio alkaloids, and possibly androgens and oral estrogens.

Roughly 30% to 70% of patients with hepatomas also have cirrhosis, and it is estimated that a person with cirrhosis is 40 times more likely to develop hepatomas than someone with a normal liver. Whether cirrhosis is a premalignant state, or alcohol and malnutrition predispose the liver to develop hepatomas, is still unclear. Another high-risk factor is exposure to the hepatitis B virus.

Signs and symptoms

Clinical effects of liver cancer include:

- a mass in the right upper quadrant
- tender, nodular liver on palpation
- severe pain in the epigastrium or the right upper quadrant
- bruit, hum, or rubbing sound if tumor involves a large part of the liver
- weight loss, weakness, anorexia, fever
- occasional jaundice or ascites
- occasional evidence of metastatsis through venous system to lungs, from lymphatics to regional lymph nodes, or by direct invasion of portal veins
- dependent edema.

Diagnosis

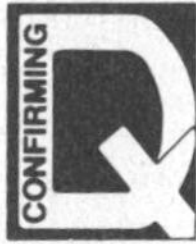

The confirming test for liver cancer is liver biopsy by needle or open biopsy. Liver cancer is difficult to diagnose in the presence of cirrhosis, but several tests can help identify it:

- Serum glutamic-oxaloacetic transaminase, serum glutamic-pyruvic transaminase, alkaline phosphatase, lactic dehydrogenase, and bilirubin all show abnormal liver function.
- Alpha-fetoprotein rises to a level above 500 mcg/ml.
- Chest X-ray may rule out metastasis.
- Liver scan may show filling defects.
- Arteriography may define large tumors.

• Electrolyte studies may indicate an increased retention of sodium (resulting in functional renal failure) and hypoglycemia, leukocytosis, hypercalcemia, or hypocholesterolemia.

Treatment

Because liver cancer is often in an advanced stage at diagnosis, few hepatic tumors are resectable. A resectable tumor must be a single tumor in one lobe, without cirrhosis, jaundice, or ascites. Resection is done by lobectomy or partial hepatectomy.

Radiation therapy for unresectable tumors is usually palliative. But because of the liver's low tolerance for radiation, this therapy has not increased survival.

Another method of treatment is chemotherapy with I.V. 5-fluorouracil, methotrexate, or doxorubicin or with regional infusion of 5-fluorouracil or floxuridine (catheters are placed directly into the hepatic artery or left brachial artery for continuous infusion for 7 to 21 days, or permanent implantable pumps are used on an outpatient basis for long-term infusion).

Appropriate treatment for liver metastasis may include resection by lobectomy or chemotherapy (with results similar to those in hepatoma). Liver transplantation is now a possible alternative for some patients.

Special considerations

The patient care plan should emphasize comprehensive supportive care and emotional support.

• Control edema and ascites. Monitor the patient's diet throughout. Most patients need a special diet that restricts sodium, fluids (no alcohol allowed), and protein. Weigh the patient daily, and note intake and output accurately. Watch for signs of ascites—peripheral edema, orthopnea, or dyspnea on exertion. If ascites is present, measure and record abdominal girth daily. To increase venous return and prevent edema, elevate the patient's legs whenever possible.

• Monitor respiratory function. Note any increase in respiratory rate or shortness of breath. Bilateral pleural effusion (noted on chest X-ray) is common, as is metastasis to the lungs. Watch carefully for signs of hypoxemia from intrapulmonary arteriovenous shunting.

• Relieve fever. Administer sponge baths and aspirin suppositories if there are no signs of GI bleeding. Avoid acetaminophen, since the diseased liver can't metabolize it. High fever indicates infection and requires antibiotics.

• Give meticulous skin care. Turn the patient frequently and keep his skin clean to prevent decubitus ulcers. Apply lotion to prevent chafing, and administer an antipruritic, such as diphenhydramine, for severe itching.

Watch for encephalopathy. Many patients develop end-stage symptoms of ammonia intoxication, including confusion, restlessness, irritability, agitation, delirium, asterixis, lethargy, and, finally, coma. Monitor the patient's serum ammonia level, vital signs, and neurologic status. Be prepared to control ammonia accumulation with sorbitol (to induce osmotic diarrhea), neomycin (to reduce bacterial flora in the GI tract), lactulose (to control bacterial elaboration of ammonia), and sodium polystyrene sulfonate (to lower potassium level).

• If a transhepatic catheter is used to relieve obstructive jaundice, irrigate it frequently with prescribed solution (normal saline or, sometimes, 5,000 units of heparin in 500 ml 5% dextrose in water). Monitor vital signs frequently for any indication of bleeding or infection.

• After surgery, give standard postoperative care. Watch for intraperitoneal bleeding and sepsis, which may precipitate coma. Monitor for renal failure by checking urine output, blood urea nitrogen, and creatinine levels hourly. Remember that throughout the course of this intractable illness, your primary concern is to keep the patient as comfortable as possible.

Bladder Cancer

Bladder tumors can develop on the surface of the bladder wall (papillomas, benign or malignant) or grow within the bladder wall (generally more virulent) and quickly invade underlying muscles. Almost all bladder tumors (90%) are transitional cell carcinomas, arising from the transitional epithelium of mucous membranes. They may result from malignant transformation of benign papillomas. Less common bladder tumors include adenocarcinomas, epidermoid carcinomas, squamous cell carcinomas, sarcomas, tumors in bladder diverticula, and carcinoma in situ.

Bladder tumors are most prevalent in people over age 50 and are more common in men than in women. The incidence of bladder tumors rises in densely populated industrial areas. Bladder cancer accounts for about 2% to 4% of all cancers.

Causes

Certain environmental carcinogens, such as 2-naphthylamine, benzidine, tobacco, nitrates, and coffee, are known to predispose to transitional cell tumors. Thus, certain industrial groups are at high risk for developing such tumors: rubber workers, cable workers, weavers, aniline dye workers, hairdressers, petroleum workers, spray painters, and leather finishers. The latent period between exposure to the carcinogen and development of symptoms is approximately 18 years.

Squamous cell carcinoma of the bladder also occurs with great frequency in geographic areas where schistosomiasis is endemic (such as Egypt). It's also associated with chronic bladder irritation and infection in people with kidney stones, Foley catheters, and chemical cystitis caused by cyclophosphamide.

Signs and symptoms

In early stages, approximately one fourth of patients with bladder tumors have no symptoms. Commonly, the first sign is gross, painless, intermittent hematuria (often with clots in the urine). Patients with invasive lesions often have suprapubic pain after voiding. Other clinical effects include bladder irritability, urinary frequency, nocturia, and dribbling.

Diagnosis

Only cystoscopy and biopsy confirm bladder cancer. Cystoscopy should be performed when hematuria first appears. When it is performed under anesthesia, a bimanual examination is usually done to determine if the bladder is fixed to the pelvic wall. A careful history and thorough physical examination may help determine whether the tumor has invaded the prostate or the lymph nodes.

The following tests can provide essential information about the size and location of the tumor:

- *Intravenous pyelography* can identify a large, early-stage tumor or an infiltrating tumor; can delineate functional problems in the upper urinary tract; and can assess the degree of hydronephrosis.
- *Urinalysis* can detect blood in the urine and malignant cytology.
- *Excretory urography* can detect ureteral obstruction or rigid deformity of the bladder wall.
- *Pelvic arteriography* can reveal tumor invasion into the bladder wall.
- *CAT scan* demonstrates the thickness of the involved bladder wall and detects enlarged retroperitoneal lymph nodes.

Treatment

Superficial bladder tumors are removed through transurethral (cystoscope) resection and fulguration (electrical destruction). This procedure is adequate when the tumor has not invaded the muscle. However, additional tumors may develop, and the fulguration may have to be repeated every 3 months for years.

TWO TYPES OF URINARY DIVERSION

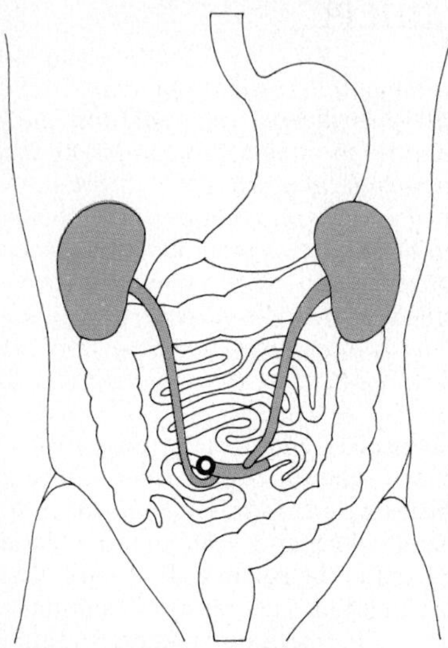

Ileal conduit (preferred method)—diversion of urine through a loop in the ileum to a stoma on the abdomen.

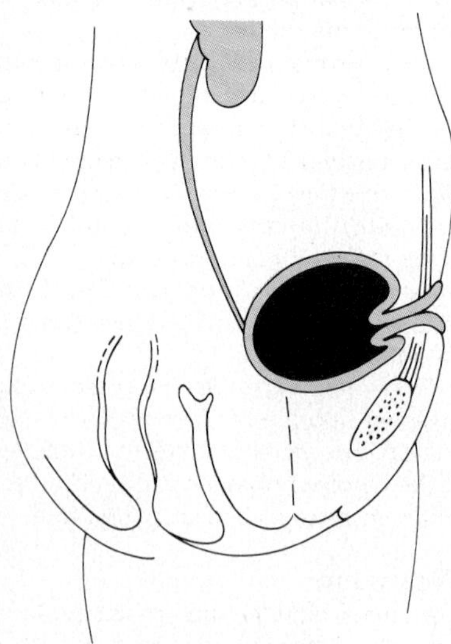

Continent vesicostomy (alternative method)—diversion of urine to a stoma on the abdomen formed from part of the bladder wall; urine is drained through catheterization.

Once the tumors penetrate the muscle layer or recur frequently, cystoscopy with fulguration is no longer appropriate.

Tumors too large to be treated through a cystoscope require segmental bladder resection to remove a full-thickness section of the bladder. This procedure is feasible only if the tumor isn't near the bladder neck or ureteral orifices. Bladder instillations of thiotepa after transurethral resections may also help control such tumors.

For infiltrating bladder tumor, radical cystectomy is the treatment of choice. The week before cystectomy, treatment may include 2,000 rads of external beam therapy to the bladder. Then, resection removes the bladder with perivesical fat, lymph nodes, urethra, and, in males, the prostate and seminal vesicles; in females, the uterus and adnexa. The surgeon forms a urinary diversion, usually an ileal conduit. The patient must then wear an external pouch continuously. Other diversions include ureterostomy, nephrostomy, vesicostomy, ileal bladder, ileal loop, and sigmoid conduit.

Males are impotent following radical cystectomy and urethrectomy, because such resection damages the sympathetic and the parasympathetic nerves that control erection and ejaculation. At a later date, the patient may desire a penile implant, to make sexual intercourse (without ejaculation) possible.

Treatment for patients with advanced bladder cancer includes cystectomy to remove the tumor, radiation therapy, and systemic chemotherapy, such as cyclophosphamide, 5-fluorouracil, doxorubicin, and cisplatin. This combined treatment has sometimes been successful in arresting this disease.

Special considerations

- Provide psychological support; encourage the patient to have a positive outlook about the stoma.
- Before surgery, assist in selection of the stoma site by assessing the patient's abdomen in varying positions; the usual site is in the rectus muscle, to minimize the risk of subsequent herniation. Make

sure that the selected stoma site is visible to the patient.

• After surgery, encourage the patient to look at the stoma. If he has difficulty doing this, leave the room for a few minutes while the stoma is exposed. Offer the patient a mirror to make viewing easier.

• To obtain a specimen for culture and sensitivity, catheterize the patient, using sterile technique. Insert the lubricated tip of the catheter into the stoma about 2″ (5 cm). (In many hospitals, a double telescope-type catheter is available for ileal conduit catheterization.)

• If the patient with surgically induced impotence was sexually active before surgery, elicit psychologic support and understanding for the patient from the patient's partner. Also, suggest alternate methods of sexual expression.

• Except for heavy lifting and contact sports, the patient with a urinary stoma may participate in various athletics and physical activities.

• When a patient with a urinary diversion is discharged, arrange for follow-up home care from a visiting nurse.

• Make a referral to the enterostomal therapist, if one is available, who will then work with you to coordinate the patient's care.

• Teach the patient about his urinary stoma. Instruction usually begins 4 to 6 days after surgery. Encourage the patient's spouse or a friend or relative to attend the teaching session, and advise this person beforehand that a negative reaction to the stoma can impede the patient's adjustment.

First, teach the patient how to prepare and apply the pouch. The pouch may be either reusable or disposable. If he chooses the reusable type, at least two are needed.

Selecting the right sized pouch is important; measure the stoma and order a pouch with an opening that clears the stoma with a ⅛″ margin. Instruct the patient to remeasure the stoma after he goes home, in case the size changes. The pouch should have a push-button or twist-type valve at the bottom that will allow for drainage. Tell the patient to empty the pouch when it is one third full, or every 2 to 3 hours.

Assuring a good skin seal is crucial. Since urine tends to destroy skin barriers that contain a lot of karaya, select a skin barrier that contains synthetics and little or no karaya. Check the pouch frequently to ascertain that the skin seal is still intact. A good skin seal with a skin barrier may last for 3 to 6 days, so only change the pouch that often. Tell the patient he can wear a loose-fitting elastic belt to help secure the pouch.

The ileal conduit stoma reaches its permanent size about 2 to 4 months after surgery. Since the intestine is normally mucus-producing, mucus will appear in the draining urine. Assure the patient that this is normal.

Keep the skin around the stoma clean and free of irritation. After removing the pouch, wash the skin with water and mild soap. Rinse well with clear water to remove soap residue, and then gently pat the skin dry; don't rub. Place a gauze sponge soaked with vinegar-water (1 part:3 parts) over the stoma for a few minutes to prevent uric acid crystal buildup. While preparing the skin, place a rolled-up dry sponge over the stoma to collect draining urine. Coat the skin with a silicone skin protector, and cover with the collection pouch. If skin irritation or breakdown occurs, apply a layer of antacid precipitate to the clean, dry skin before coating with the silicone skin protector.

The patient can level uneven surfaces on his abdomen, such as gullies, scars, or wedges, with a variety of specially prepared products or skin barriers.

• All high-risk people—for example, aniline dye or chemical workers, those in areas where schistosomiasis is endemic, and those with histories of benign bladder tumors or persistent unexplained cystitis—should have periodic cytologic examinations and should know about the danger of significant exposure to irritants, toxins, and carcinogens. Many industries have taken measures to protect workers from possible exposure to aromatic amines, such as 2-naphthylamine and benzidine, and have reduced incidence of bladder cancer among their workers. For added information, refer ostomates to the American Cancer Society or to the United Ostomy Association.

Gallbladder and Bile Duct Carcinoma

Gallbladder carcinoma is rare, comprising less than 1% of all malignancies. It's normally found coincidentally in patients with cholecystitis; 1 in 400 cholecystectomies reveals malignancy. This disease is most prevalent in females over age 60. It's rapidly progressive and usually fatal; patients seldom live a year after diagnosis. Poor prognosis is due to late diagnosis; gallbladder cancer is usually not diagnosed until after cholecystectomy, when it is often in an advanced, metastatic stage.

Extrahepatic bile duct carcinoma is the cause of approximately 3% of all cancer deaths in the United States. It occurs in both males and females (incidence is slightly higher in males) between ages 60 and 70. The usual site is at the bifurcation in the common duct. Carcinoma at the distal end of the common duct is often confused with carcinoma of the pancreas. Characteristically, metastatic spread occurs to local lymph nodes, the liver, lungs, and the peritoneum.

Causes

Many consider gallbladder carcinoma a complication of gallstones. However, this inference rests on circumstantial evidence from postmortem examinations: from 60% to 90% of gallbladder carcinoma patients also have gallstones; but postmortem data from patients with gallstones show gallbladder carcinoma in only 0.5%.

The predominant tissue type in gallbladder cancer is adenocarcinoma, 85% to 95%; squamous cell, 5% to 15%. Mixed-tissue types are rare.

Lymph node metastasis is present in 25% to 70% of patients at diagnosis. Direct extension to the liver is common (in 46% to 89%); direct extension to both the cystic and the common bile ducts, stomach, colon, duodenum, and jejunum also occurs, and produces obstructions. Metastasis also spreads by portal or hepatic veins to the peritoneum, ovaries, and lower lung lobes.

The cause of extrahepatic bile duct carcinoma isn't known; however, statistics report an unexplained increased incidence of this carcinoma in patients with ulcerative colitis. This association may be due to a common cause—perhaps an immune mechanism, or chronic use of certain drugs by the colitis patient.

Signs and symptoms

Clinically, gallbladder cancer is almost indistinguishable from cholecystitis: pain in the epigastrium or right upper quadrant, weight loss, anorexia, nausea, vomiting, and jaundice. However, chronic, progressively severe pain in an afebrile patient suggests malignancy. In patients with simple gallstones, pain is sporadic. Another telling clue to malignancy is palpable gallbladder (right upper quadrant), with obstructive jaundice. Some patients may also have hepatosplenomegaly.

Progressive profound jaundice is commonly the first sign of obstruction due to extrahepatic bile duct cancer. The jaundice is usually accompanied by chronic pain in the epigastrium or the right upper quadrant, radiating to the back. Other common symptoms, if associated with active cholecystitis, include pruritus, skin excoriations, anorexia, weight loss, chills, and fever.

Diagnosis

No test or procedure is, in itself, diagnostic of gallbladder carcinoma. However, the following laboratory tests support this diagnosis when they suggest hepatic dysfunction and extrahepatic biliary obstruction:

- *baseline studies* (complete blood count, routine urinalysis, electrolyte studies, enzymes)
- *liver function tests* (bilirubin, urine bile and bilirubin, and urobilinogen are elevated in more than 50% of patients; serum alkaline phosphatase levels are consistently elevated)
- *sulfur colloid liver-spleen scan*
- *upper GI series* (shows abnormality of pylorus or duodenum)
- *occult blood in stools* (linked to the associated anemia)
- *cholecystography* (may show stones or calcification—a "porcelain" gallbladder)
- *cholangiography* (may locate the site of common duct obstruction)
- *chest X-ray* (may show elevation [displacement by the tumor] of right side of diaphragm).

The following tests help confirm extrahepatic bile duct carcinoma:

- *liver function studies* indicate biliary obstruction; elevated bilirubin (5 to 30 mg/100 ml), alkaline phosphatase, and blood cholesterol; prolonged prothrombin time; response to vitamin K.
- *barium studies, cholangiography, and endoscopic retrograde cannulization of the pancreas* (may help locate the obstruction but are not diagnostic).

Treatment

Surgical treatment of gallbladder cancer is essentially palliative, and includes cholecystectomy, common bile duct exploration, T-tube drainage, and wedge excision of hepatic tissue. If the cancer invades gallbladder musculature, the survival rate is less than 5%, even with massive resection. Although some long-term survivals (4 to 5 years) have been reported, few patients survive longer than 6 months after surgery.

Surgery is normally indicated to relieve obstruction and jaundice that result from extrahepatic bile duct carcinoma. The procedure depends on the site of the carcinoma and may include cholecystoduodenostomy or T tube drainage of the common duct.

Other palliative measures for both kinds of carcinomas include radiation (mostly used for local and incisional recurrences) and chemotherapy (especially with 5-fluorouracil), both of which have limited effects.

Special considerations

After biliary resection:

- Monitor vital signs.
- Use strict aseptic technique when caring for the incision and the surrounding area.
- Place the patient in low Fowler's position.
- Prevent respiratory problems by encouraging deep breathing and coughing. The high incision makes the patient want to take shallow breaths; using analgesics and splinting his abdomen with a pillow or an abdominal binder may aid in greater respiratory efforts.
- Monitor bowel sounds and bowel movements. Observe patient's tolerance to diet.
- Provide pain control.
- Check intake and output carefully. Watch for electrolyte imbalance; monitor I.V. solutions to avoid overloading the cardiovascular system.
- Monitor the nasogastric tube, which will be in place for 24 to 72 hours postoperatively to relieve distention, and the T tube. Record amount and color of drainage each shift. Secure the T tube to minimize tension on it and prevent its being pulled out.
- Help the patient and his family cope with their initial fears and reactions to the diagnosis by offering information and support.
- Advise the patient of the side effects of both chemotherapy and radiation therapy. Monitor the patient on radiation therapy closely for side effects, and observe the patient receiving chemotherapy for side effects of cytotoxic drugs.

MALE AND FEMALE GENITALIA

Prostatic Cancer

Prostatic cancer is the second most common neoplasm found in men over age 50 and the third leading cause of male cancer death. Adenocarcinoma is its most common form; only rarely does it occur as a sarcoma. About 85% of prostatic carcinomas originate in the posterior part of the prostate gland; the rest originate near the urethra. Malignant prostatic tumors are seldom a result of the benign hyperplastic enlargement that commonly develops around the prostatic urethra in elderly men.

Prostatic carcinoma seldom produces symptoms until it's well advanced. When treated in its localized form, the 5-year survival rate is 70%; after metastasis, it's under 35%. When prostatic cancer is fatal, it's usually the result of widespread bone metastases.

Causes and incidence

Although androgens regulate prostatic growth and function and may also speed tumor growth, a definite link between increased androgen levels and prostatic cancer hasn't been found. Typically, when primary prostatic lesions spread beyond the prostate gland, they invade the prostatic capsule and then spread along the ejaculatory ducts in the space between the seminal vesicles or perivesicular fascia.

Prostatic cancer accounts for 17% of all cancers. Incidence is highest among blacks and in men with blood type A; it is lowest in Orientals. Its occurrence is unaffected by socioeconomic status or fertility.

Signs and symptoms

Signs and symptoms of prostatic cancer appear only in the advanced stages of the disease. Clinical effects include difficulty initiating a urinary stream, dribbling, urine retention, unexplained cystitis, and, rarely, hematuria.

Diagnosis

A rectal examination that reveals a small, hard nodule may help diagnose prostatic cancer before symptoms develop (except in Stage A of the disease, when the cancer is still occult). Therefore, a routine physical examination of men over age 40 should *always* include a rectal examination to check for prostatic cancer.

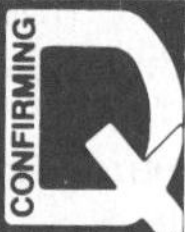

Biopsy confirms this diagnosis. Serum acid phosphatase is elevated in two-thirds of patients with metastasized prostatic cancer. Successful therapy returns the serum acid phosphatase level to normal; a subsequent rise points to recurrence.

Elevated alkaline phosphatase levels and a positive bone scan point to bone metastasis; routine bone X-rays don't always show evidence of such metastasis.

Treatment

Correct management of prostatic cancer depends on clinical assessment, tolerance to therapy, expected life span, and the stage of the disease. Treatment must be chosen carefully, since prostatic cancer usually affects older men, who frequently have serious coexisting disorders such as hypertension, diabetes, or cardiac disease.

Therapy varies with each stage of the disease and generally includes radiation, prostatectomy, orchiectomy (removal of the testes) to reduce androgen production, and hormone therapy with synthetic estrogen (diethylstilbestrol [DES]). Radical prostatectomy is usually effective for localized lesions with no evidence of metastasis.

Radiation therapy is used for Stage B and C prostatic cancer and locally invasive lesions in Stage A, and also to relieve bone pain from metastatic skeletal involvement.

If hormone therapy, surgery, or radiation therapy aren't feasible or successful, chemotherapy may be tried. Chemotherapy for prostatic cancer employs various combinations of cyclophosphamide, vinblastine, doxorubicin, bleomycin, cisplatin, and vindesine; research is continuing on the most effective chemotherapeutic regimens.

Special considerations

The patient care plan should emphasize psychologic support of patients facing prostatectomy, good postoperative care, and symptomatic treatment of radiation side effects.

Before prostatectomy:

- Explain the expected effects of surgery (such as impotence and possible incontinence), as well as the side effects of radiation.
- Encourage the patient to express his fears.
- Instruct the patient about postoperative procedures, such as placement of tubes and dressing changes.
- Teach the patient perineal exercises (done either sitting or standing) to minimize incontinence. (To develop his perineal muscles, the patient should squeeze his buttocks together and hold this position for a few seconds; then relax. He should do this exercise one to ten times an hour.)

After prostatectomy:

- Regularly check dressing, incision, and drainage systems for excessive bleeding; watch for signs of bleeding (cold clammy skin, pallor, restlessness, falling blood pressure, and rising pulse rate).
- Watch for signs of infection (fever, chills, inflamed incisional area). Maintain adequate fluid intake (at least 2,000 ml daily).
- Give antispasmodics, as ordered, to control postoperative bladder spasms. Give analgesics, as needed.
- Since urinary incontinence is a frequent problem after prostatectomy, keep the patient's skin clean and dry.

After a suprapubic prostatectomy:

- Keep the skin around the suprapubic drain dry, and free from drainage and urine leakage. Encourage the patient to begin perineal exercises within 24 to 48 hours after surgery.
- Allow the patient's family to assist in his care, and encourage their psychologic support.
- Give meticulous catheter care. After

STAGING PROSTATIC CANCER

Staging procedures for prostatic cancer include X-rays and laboratory and radioisotopic studies for clinical diagnosis; laparotomy, bone marrow aspiration, open or needle biopsy; and surgical resection and histologic examination of the prostate gland and possibly the regional lymph nodes.

Stage A: Incidental finding without symptoms
- Stage A1: Three or fewer well-differentiated foci
- Stage A2: More than three foci, poorly differentiated and more extensive than in Stage A1

Stage B: Palpable prostatic lesion
- Stage B1: Lesion less than 2 cm in diameter involving one lobe
- Stage B2: Lesion greater than 2 cm in diameter with diffuse involvement

Stage C: Extension of lesion beyond the prostatic capsule, but with no signs of metastasis

Stage D: Metastatic carcinoma
- Stage D1: Involvement of pelvic lymph nodes below the aortic bifurcation
- Stage D2: Lymph node involvement above the aortic bifurcation or metastasis to other distant sites.

prostatectomy, a patient often has a three-way catheter with a continuous irrigation system. Check the tubing for kinks, mucus plugs, and clots, especially if the patient complains of pain. Warn the patient not to pull on the tubes or the catheter.

After transurethral resection:
• Watch for signs of urethral stricture (dysuria, decreased force and caliber of urinary stream, and straining to urinate) and for abdominal distention (a result of urethral stricture or catheter blockage by a blood clot). Irrigate the catheter, as ordered.

After a perineal prostatectomy:
• Avoid taking rectal temperature or inserting enema tubes or other rectal tubes. Provide pads to absorb urinary drainage and a rubber ring for the patient to sit on. Frequent sitz baths relieve pain and inflammation.

After perineal and retropubic prostatectomy:
• Give reassurance that urine leakage after catheter removal is normal and will disappear in time.
• When a patient receives radiation or hormonal therapy, watch for and treat nausea, vomiting, dry skin, and alopecia. Also watch for side effects of DES, (gynecomastia, fluid retention, nausea, and vomiting). Keep alert for thrombophlebitis (pain, tenderness, swelling, warmth, and redness in calf), which is always a possibility in patients receiving DES.

Testicular Cancer

Malignant testicular tumors primarily affect young to middle-aged adults and are the leading cause of death from solid tumors in men between the ages of 15 and 34. In testicular tumors occurring in children (which are rare), 50% are detectable before age 5.

With few exceptions, testicular tumors are of gonadal cell origin. Such tumors may be seminomas *(about 40%), in which uniform, undifferentiated cells resemble primitive gonadal cells, or* nonseminomas, *in which tumor cells show various degrees of differentiation.*

Prognosis varies with the cancer cell type and staging. When treated with surgery and radiation, 100% of patients with Stage I or II seminomas and 90% of those with Stage I nonseminomas survive beyond 5 years. Prognosis is poor if this disease is advanced beyond Stage II at diagnosis.

Causes and incidence

The cause of testicular cancer isn't known, but incidence is higher in men with cryptorchidism (even when this condition has been surgically corrected). Testicular cancer rarely occurs in nonwhite males and accounts for less than 1% of all male cancer deaths. Peak incidence of the disease is at age 32. Typically, when testicular cancer extends beyond the testes, it spreads through the lymphatic system to the iliac, para-aortic, and mediastinal nodes, with metastases to the lungs, liver, viscera, and bone.

Signs and symptoms

Characteristically, testicular cancer becomes apparent with the development of a firm, painless, and smooth testicular mass, which may be as small as a pea or as large as a grapefruit. Often there is also a feeling of testicular heaviness. When such a tumor produces chorionic gonadotropin or estrogens, it may also cause gynecomastia and nipple tenderness. In late stages, lymph node involvement and distant metastases lead to ureteral obstruction, abdominal mass, cough, hemoptysis, shortness of breath, weight loss, fatigue, pallor, and lethargy.

Diagnosis

The most effective means for early detection of testicular cancer are regular self-examination and palpation of the testes as part of a routine physical examination. When such examination reveals a testicular mass, transillumination can distinguish between a tumor (which will *not* transilluminate) and a hydrocele or spermatocele (which will). Further diagnostic measures should include a breast examination for gynecomastia and abdominal palpation to detect abdominal masses.

Confirming lab tests include intravenous pyelography to search for ureteral deviation resulting from para-aortic node involvement, determination of urinary or serum-luteinizing hormone levels, lymphangiography followed by ultrasound examination, and a hematologic workup, including a complete blood count. Serum alpha-fetoprotein and beta-human chorionic gonadotropin are important indicators of testicular tumor activity and can provide a baseline to measure response to therapy and to help determine prognosis.

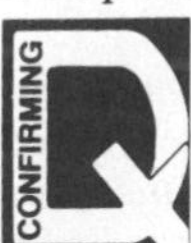

When a tumor is present, surgical removal of the entire testis for biopsy permits histologic verification of tumor cell type—essential for effective treatment. Inguinal exploration determines nodal involvement.

Treatment

Treatment includes surgery, radiation, and chemotherapy; the intensity of such therapy varies with tumor cell type and staging. Surgery includes orchiectomy and retroperitoneal node dissection to prevent extension of the disease and to aid in staging. Most surgeons remove just the testis, not the scrotum, which allows for a prosthetic testicular implant at a later date. Hormone replacement may be necessary to supplement depleted hormonal levels, especially after bilateral orchiectomy.

Treatment of seminomas involves postoperative radiation to the retroperitoneal and homolateral iliac nodes and, in patients with retroperitoneal extension, prophylactic radiation to the mediastinal and supraclavicular nodes. In nonseminomas, treatment includes radiation to all positive nodes.

Chemotherapy is essential in patients with large abdominal or mediastinal nodes and frank distant metastases or in others at high risk of developing metastases. Cyclophosphamide produces excellent results in seminomas; and combinations of vinblastine, doxorubicin, bleomycin, cisplatin, and vindesine are effective in nonseminomas.

Special considerations

Begin to develop a care plan as soon as the diagnosis is made. Care should emphasize dealing with the patient's psychological response to the disease, preventing postoperative complications, and minimizing and controlling the side effects of radiation and chemotherapy. The young patient with testicular cancer faces difficult treatment, and fears sexual impairment and disfigurement.

Before orchiectomy:

- Encourage the patient to talk about his fears. Try to establish a trusting relationship so that he feels comfortable asking questions.
- Give reassurance that sterility and impotence do not follow unilateral orchiectomy. Explain that synthetic hormones

STAGING TESTICULAR CANCER

Staging work-up in testicular cancer combines surgical evaluation with pathologic staging. Usually, it includes testicular and tumor resection with lymph node dissection (especially inguinal exploration) to determine nodal involvement.

Stage I: Tumor confined to one testis, with no clinical or radiographic evidence of extratesticular spread

Stage II: Cancer metastasized to regional lymph nodes but not beyond

Stage III: Metastasis beyond regional nodes, usually to abdominal, mediastinal, supraclavicular, or pulmonary nodes

can supplement depleted hormonal levels. Inform the patient that most surgeons don't remove the scrotum, and that implant of a testicular prosthesis can correct disfigurement.

After orchiectomy:

• For the first day after surgery, apply an ice pack to the scrotum and provide analgesics, as ordered.
• Check for excessive bleeding, swelling, and signs of infection.
• Provide a scrotal athletic supporter to minimize pain during ambulation.
• During chemotherapy, know what side effects to expect and how to prevent or ease them. Give antiemetics, as needed, to prevent severe nausea and vomiting, and small, frequent feedings to maintain oral intake despite anorexia. Develop a good mouth care regimen, and check for stomatitis. Watch for signs of myelosuppression. If the patient receives vinblastine, assess for neurotoxicity (manifested by such symptoms as peripheral paresthesias, jaw pain, muscle cramps). If he receives cisplatin, check for ototoxicity. To prevent renal damage, increase fluid intake, give I.V. hydration, as ordered, with a potassium supplement, and provide diuresis, as ordered, with furosemide or mannitol.

Penile Cancer

Penile carcinoma rarely affects circumcised men in modern cultures; when it does occur, it's usually in men who are over age 50. The most common form, epidermoid squamous cell carcinoma, is usually found in the glans but may also occur on the corona glandis, and, rarely, in the preputial cavity. This malignancy produces ulcerative or papillary (wartlike, nodular) lesions, which may become quite large before spreading beyond the penis; such lesions may destroy the glans prepuce and invade the corpora.

Prognosis varies according to staging at time of diagnosis. If begun early enough, radiation therapy increases the 5-year survival rate to over 60%; surgery only, to over 55%. Unfortunately, many men delay treatment of penile cancer, because they fear disfigurement and loss of sexual function.

Causes

The exact cause of penile cancer is unknown; however, it's generally associated with poor personal hygiene, and phimosis in uncircumcised men. This may account for the low incidence among Jews, Muslims, and people of other cultures that practice circumcision at birth or shortly thereafter. (Incidence isn't decreased in cultures that practice circumcision at a later date.) Early circumcision seems to prevent penile cancer by allowing for better personal hygiene and minimizing inflammatory (and often premalignant) lesions of the glans and prepuce. Such lesions include:

• *leukoplakia*—inflammation, with thickened patches that may fissure
• *balanitis*—inflammation of the penis associated with phimosis
• *erythroplasia of Queyrat*—squamous cell carcinoma in situ; velvety, erythematous lesion that becomes scaly and ulcerative
• *penile horn*—scaly, horn-shaped growth.

Signs and symptoms

In a circumcised man, early signs of penile cancer include a small circumscribed lesion, a pimple, or a sore on the penis. In an uncircumcised man, however, such early symptoms may go unnoticed, so penile cancer first becomes apparent when it causes late-stage symptoms, such as pain, hemorrhage, dysuria, purulent discharge, and obstruction of the urinary meatus. Rarely are metastases the first signs of penile cancer.

Diagnosis

Diagnosis of penile cancer requires tissue biopsy. Preoperative baseline studies include complete blood count, urinalysis, electrocardiogram, and a chest X-ray. Enlargement of inguinal lymph nodes because of infection from the primary lesion makes lymphangiographic preoperative evaluation of lymph node metastasis difficult.

Treatment

Depending on the stage of progression, treatment includes surgical resection of the primary tumor and, possibly, chemotherapy and radiation. Local tumors of the prepuce only require circumcision. Invasive tumors, however, require partial penectomy (unless contraindicated because of the patient's young age); tumors of the base of the penile shaft require total penectomy and inguinal node dissection (done less often in the United States than in other countries where incidence is higher). Radiation therapy may improve treatment effectiveness after resection of localized lesions without metastasis; it may also reduce the size of lymph nodes before nodal resection. It's not adequate primary treatment for groin metastasis, however. Bleomycin and methotrexate are generally used in chemotherapy but are not very effective.

Special considerations

Penile cancer calls for good patient teaching, psychological support, and comprehensive postoperative care. The patient with penile cancer fears disfigurement, pain, and loss of sexual function.

Before penile surgery:

- Spend time with the patient, and encourage him to talk about his fears.
- Supplement and reinforce what the doctor has told the patient about the surgery and other treatment measures, and explain expected postoperative procedures, such as dressing changes and catheterization. Show him diagrams of the surgical procedure and pictures of the results of similar surgery to help him adapt to an altered body image.
- If the patient needs urinary diversion, refer him to the enterostomal therapist.

Although postpenectomy care varies with the procedure used and the doctor's protocol, certain procedures are always applicable:

- Constantly monitor the patient's vital signs and record his intake and output accurately.
- Provide comprehensive skin care to prevent skin breakdown from urinary diversion or suprapubic catheterization. Keep the skin dry and free from urine. If the patient has a suprapubic catheter, make sure the catheter is patent at all times.
- Administer analgesics, as ordered. Elevate the penile stump with a small towel or pillow to minimize edema.
- Check the surgical site often for signs of infection, such as foul odor or excessive drainage on dressing.
- If the patient has had inguinal node dissection, watch for and immediately report signs of lymphedema, such as decreased circulation or disproportionate swelling of a leg.
- After partial penectomy, reassure the patient that the penile stump should be

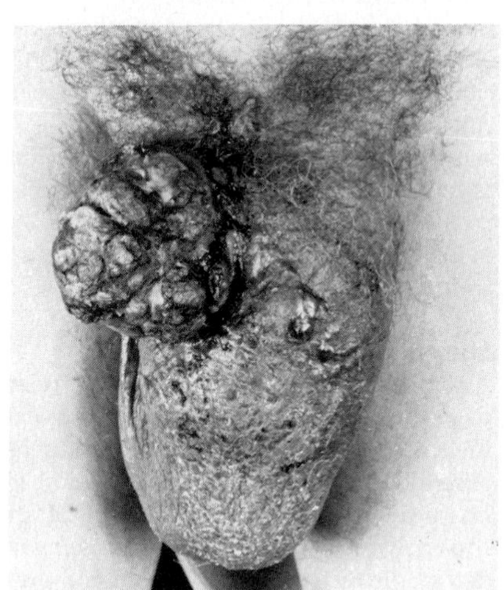

Penile carcinoma

sufficient for urination and sexual function. Refer him for psychological or sexual counseling if necessary.

Cervical Cancer

The third most common cancer of the female reproductive system, cervical cancer is classified as either preinvasive or invasive.

Preinvasive carcinoma ranges from minimal cervical dysplasia, in which the lower third of the epithelium contains abnormal cells, to carcinoma in situ, in which the full thickness of epithelium contains abnormally proliferating cells (also known as cervical intraepithelial neoplasia [CIN]). Preinvasive cancer is curable 75% to 90% of the time with early detection and proper treatment. If untreated (and depending on the form in which it appears), it may progress to invasive cervical cancer.

In invasive carcinoma, cancer cells penetrate the basement membrane and can spread directly to contiguous pelvic structures or disseminate to distant sites by lymphatic routes. Invasive carcinoma of the uterine cervix is responsible for 8,000 deaths annually in the United States alone. In almost all cases (95%), the histologic type is squamous cell carcinoma, which varies from well-differentiated cells to highly anaplastic spindle cells. Only 5% are adenocarcinomas. Usually, invasive carcinoma occurs between ages 30 and 50; rarely, under age 20.

Causes

While the cause is unknown, several predisposing factors have been related to the development of cervical cancer: intercourse at a young age, multiple sexual partners, multiple pregnancies, and herpesvirus II and other bacterial or viral venereal infections.

Signs and symptoms

Preinvasive cervical cancer produces no symptoms or other clinically apparent changes. Early invasive cervical cancer causes abnormal vaginal bleeding, persistent vaginal discharge, and postcoital pain and bleeding. In advanced stages, it causes pelvic pain, vaginal leakage of urine and feces from a fistula, anorexia, weight loss, and anemia.

Diagnosis

A cytologic examination (Pap smear) can detect cervical cancer before clinical evidence appears. (Systems of Pap smear classification may vary from hospital to hospital.) Abnormal cervical cytology routinely calls for colposcopy, which can detect the presence and extent of preclinical lesions requiring biopsy and histologic examination. Staining with Lugol's solution (strong iodine) or Schiller's solution (iodine, potassium iodide, and purified water) may identify areas for biopsy when the smear shows abnormal cells but there's no obvious lesion. While the tests are nonspecific, they do distinguish between normal and abnormal tissues: normal tissues absorb the iodine and turn brown; abnormal tissues are devoid of glycogen and won't change color. Additional studies, such as lymphangiography, cystography, and scans, can detect metastasis.

Treatment

Appropriate treatment depends on accurate clinical staging. Preinvasive lesions may be treated with total excisional biopsy, cryosurgery, laser destruction, conization (and frequent Pap smear follow-up), or, rarely, hysterectomy. Therapy for invasive squamous cell carcinoma may include radical hysterectomy and radiation therapy (internal, external, or both).

Special considerations

Management of cervical cancer requires

skilled preoperative and postoperative care, comprehensive patient teaching, and emotional and psychological support.

- If you assist with a biopsy, drape and prepare the patient as for routine Pap smear and pelvic examination. Have a container of formaldehyde ready to preserve the specimen during transfer to the pathology lab. Explain to the patient that she may feel pressure, minor abdominal cramps, or a pinch from the punch forceps. Reassure her that pain will be minimal, because the cervix has few nerve endings.
- If you assist with cryosurgery, drape and prepare the patient as if for a routine Pap smear and pelvic examination. Explain that the procedure takes approximately 15 minutes, during which time the doctor will use refrigerant to freeze the cervix. Warn the patient that she may experience abdominal cramps, headache, and sweating, but reassure her that she'll feel little, if any, pain.
- If you assist with laser therapy, drape and prepare the patient as if for a routine Pap smear and pelvic examination. Explain that the procedure takes approximately 30 minutes and may cause abdominal cramps.
- After excisional biopsy, cryosurgery, and laser therapy, tell the patient to expect a discharge or spotting for about 1 week after these procedures, and advise her not to douche, use tampons, or engage in sexual intercourse during this time. Tell her to watch for and report signs of infection. Stress the need for a follow-up Pap smear and a pelvic ex-

INTERNAL RADIATION SAFETY PRECAUTIONS

There are three cardinal safety rules in internal radiation therapy:

- *Time.* Wear a radiosensitive badge. Remember, your exposure increases with time, and the effects are cumulative. Therefore, carefully plan the time you spend with the patient to prevent overexposure. (However, don't rush procedures, ignore the patient's psychologic needs, or give the impression you can't get out of the room fast enough.)
- *Distance.* Radiation loses its intensity with distance. Avoid standing at the foot of the patient's bed, where you're in line with the radiation.
- *Shield.* Lead shields reduce radiation exposure. Use them whenever possible.

In internal radiation therapy, remember that the patient is radioactive while the radiation source is in place, usually 48 to 72 hours.

- Pregnant women should not be assigned to care for these patients.
- Check the position of the source applicator every 4 hours. If it appears dislodged, notify the doctor immediately. If it's completely dislodged, remove the patient from the bed; pick up the applicator with long forceps, place it on a lead-shielded transport cart, and notify the doctor immediately.
- *Never* pick up the source with your bare hands. Notify the doctor and radiation safety officer whenever there's an accident, and keep a lead-shielded transport cart on the unit as long as the patient has a source in place.

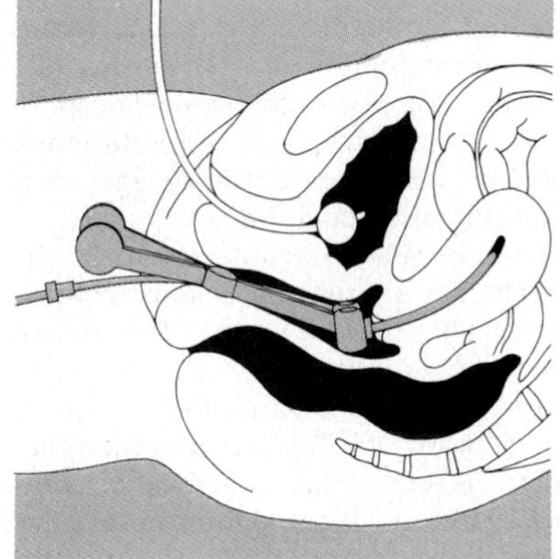

Positioning of internal radiation applicator for uterine cancer

STAGING CERVICAL CANCER

Stage 0: Carcinoma in situ, intraepithelial carcinoma
Stage I: Carcinoma is strictly confined to the cervix (extension to the corpus should be disregarded)
Stage Ia: Microinvasive carcinoma (early stromal invasion)
Stage Ib: All other cases of Stage I. Occult cancer should be marked "occ."
Stage II: Carcinoma extends beyond the cervix but has not extended to the pelvic wall. The carcinoma involves the vagina, but not as far as the lower third.
Stage IIa: No obvious parametrial involvement
Stage IIb: Obvious parametrial involvement
Stage III: Carcinoma has extended to the pelvic wall. On rectal examination, there is no cancerfree space between the tumor and the pelvic wall. The tumor involves the lower third of the vagina. All cases with a hydronephrosis or nonfunctioning kidney are included, unless they are known to be due to other cause.
Stage IIIa: No extension to the pelvic wall
Stage IIIb: Extension to the pelvic wall and/or hydronephrosis or nonfunctioning kidney
Stage IV: Carcinoma has extended beyond the true pelvis or has clinically involved the mucosa of the bladder or rectum. A bullous edema as such does not permit a case to be allotted to Stage IV.
Stage IVa: Spread of the growth to adjacent organs
Stage IVb: Spread to distant organs

amination within 3 to 4 months after these procedures and periodically thereafter. Also, inform the patient what to expect postoperatively if a hysterectomy is necessary.

• After surgery, monitor vital signs every 4 hours. Watch for and immediately report signs of complications, such as bleeding, abdominal distention, severe pain, wheezing, or other breathing difficulties. Administer analgesics, prophylactic antibiotics, and subcutaneous heparin, as ordered. Encourage deep breathing and coughing.

• Explain that external outpatient radiation therapy, when necessary, continues for about 4 to 6 weeks. The patient may be hospitalized for a 2- to 3-day course of internal radiation treatment (an intracavitary implant of radium, cesium, or some other radioactive material). Find out if the patient is to have internal or external therapy, or both. Usually, internal radiation therapy is the first procedure.

• Check to see if the radioactive source will be inserted while the patient is in the operating room (preloaded) or at bedside (afterloaded). If the source is preloaded, the patient returns to her room "hot," and safety precautions begin immediately.

• *Remember* that safety precautions—time, distance, and shielding—begin as soon as the radioactive source is in place. Inform the patient that she'll require a private room.

• Explain the *preloaded* internal radiation procedure, and answer the patient's questions. Internal radiation requires a 2- to 3-day hospital stay, a bowel preparation, a povidone-iodine vaginal douche, a clear liquid diet, and nothing by mouth the night before the implantation; it also requires a Foley catheter. Tell the patient that the procedure is performed in the operating room under general anesthetic, during which time she is placed in lithotomy position, and a radium applicator is inserted. The radioactive source is implanted in the applicator by the doctor.

• If the patient is to have *afterloaded* radiation therapy, explain that a member of the radiation team will implant the source after she is returned to her room from surgery.

• Encourage the patient to lie flat and limit movement while the source is in place. If she prefers, elevate the head of the bed slightly.

• Check vital signs every 4 hours; watch for skin reaction, vaginal bleeding, abdominal discomfort, or evidence of dehydration. Make sure the patient can reach everything she needs without stretching or straining. Assist her in range-of-motion *arm* exercises (leg exercises and other body movements could dislodge the source). If ordered, administer a tranquilizer to help the patient relax and remain still. Organize the time you spend with the patient to minimize your exposure to radiation.

• Inform visitors of safety precautions, and hang a sign listing these precautions on the patient's door.

• Teach the patient to watch for and report uncomfortable side effects. Since radiation therapy may increase susceptibility to infection by lowering WBCs, warn the patient during therapy to avoid persons with obvious infections.

• Reassure the patient that this disease and its treatment shouldn't radically alter her life-style or prohibit sexual intimacy.

Uterine Cancer

Uterine cancer (cancer of the endometrium) is the most common gynecologic cancer. Usually, it affects postmenopausal women between ages 50 and 60; it's uncommon between ages 30 and 40, and extremely rare before age 30. Most premenopausal women who develop uterine cancer have a history of anovulatory menstrual cycles or other hormonal imbalance. An average of 37,000 new cases of uterine cancer are reported annually; of these, 3,300 are eventually fatal.

Causes

Uterine cancer seems linked to several predisposing factors:

- low fertility index and anovulation
- abnormal uterine bleeding
- obesity, hypertension, or diabetes
- familial tendency
- history of uterine polyps or endometrial hyperplasia
- estrogen therapy (still controversial).

Generally, uterine cancer is an adenocarcinoma that metastasizes late, usually from the endometrium to the cervix, ovaries, fallopian tubes, and other peritoneal structures. It may spread to distant organs, such as the lungs and the brain, through the blood or the lymphatic system. Lymph node involvement can also occur. Less common uterine tumors include adenoacanthoma, endometrial stromal sarcoma, lymphosarcoma, mixed mesodermal tumors (including carcinosarcoma), and leiomyosarcoma.

Signs and symptoms

Uterine enlargement, and persistent and unusual premenopausal bleeding, or any postmenopausal bleeding, are the most common indications of uterine cancer. The discharge may at first be watery and blood-streaked but gradually becomes more bloody. Other symptoms, such as pain and weight loss, don't appear until the cancer is well advanced.

Diagnosis

Unfortunately, a Pap smear, so useful for detecting cervical cancer, doesn't dependably predict early-stage uterine cancer. Diagnosis of uterine cancer requires endometrial, cervical, and endocervical biopsies. Negative biopsies call for a fractional dilatation and curettage (D & C) to determine diagnosis. Positive diagnosis requires the following tests to provide baseline data and permit staging:

- multiple cervical biopsies and endocervical curettage to pinpoint cervical involvement
- Schiller's test, staining the cervix and vagina with an iodine solution that turns healthy tissues brown; cancerous tissues resist the stain.
- complete physical examination
- chest X-ray or computed tomography scan
- intravenous pyelography and, possibly, cystoscopy
- complete blood studies
- electrocardiogram
- proctoscopy or barium enema studies (rarely used).

Treatment

Treatment varies, depending on the extent of the disease:

- *Surgery* generally involves total abdominal hysterectomy, bilateral salpingo-oophorectomy, or possibly omentectomy with or without pelvic or paraaortic lymphadenectomy. Total exenteration removes all pelvic organs, including the vagina, and is only done when the disease is sufficiently contained to allow surgical removal of diseased parts. Partial exenteration may retain an unaffected colorectum or bladder.
- *Radiation therapy.* When the tumor isn't well differentiated, intracavitary or external radiation, or both, given 6 weeks before surgery, may inhibit recurrence and lengthen survival time.
- *Hormonal therapy* using progesterone or chemotherapy with doxorubicin. Other combinations are useful for recurrence, especially vincristine, cyclophosphamide, and actinomycin D.

Special considerations

The care plan for patients with uterine cancer should emphasize comprehensive patient teaching to help them cope with surgery, radiation, and chemotherapy. Provide good postoperative care and psychological support.

Before surgery:

- Reinforce what the doctor told the patient about the surgery, and explain the routine tests (e.g., repeated blood tests the morning after surgery) and postoperative care. If the patient is to have a lymphadenectomy *and* a total hysterectomy, explain that she'll probably have a blood drainage system for about 5 days

STAGING UTERINE CANCER

Stage 0: Carcinoma in situ. Histologic findings are suspicious of malignancy; cases of Stage 0 should not be included in any therapeutic statistics.

Stage I: Carcinoma confined to the corpus

Stage Ia: Length of the uterine cavity 8 cm or less

Stage Ib: Length of the uterine cavity more than 8 cm

Stage I cases should be subgrouped by histologic type of the adenocarcinoma as follows:

- G1: Highly differentiated adenomatous carcinoma
- G2: Moderately differentiated adenomatous carcinoma with partly solid areas
- G3: Predominantly solid or entirely undifferentiated carcinoma

Stage II: Carcinoma has involved the corpus and the cervix but has not extended outside the uterus.

Stage III: Carcinoma has extended outside the uterus but not outside the true pelvis.

Stage IV: Carcinoma has extended outside the true pelvis or has obviously involved the mucosa of the bladder or rectum. A bullous edema as such does not permit a case to be allotted to Stage IV.

Stage IVa: Spread of the growth to adjacent organs

Stage IVb: Spread of the growth to distant organs

MANAGING PELVIC EXENTERATION

Before pelvic exenteration

- Teach the patient about ileal conduit and possible colostomy, and make sure the patient understands that her vagina will be removed.
- To minimize the risk of infection, supervise a rigorous bowel and skin preparation procedure. Decrease the residue in the patient's diet for 48 to 72 hours, then maintain a diet ranging from clear liquids to nothing by mouth. Administer oral or I.V. antibiotics, as ordered, and prep skin daily with antibacterial soap.
- Instruct the patient about postop procedures: I.V. therapy, central venous pressure (CVP) catheter, blood drainage system, and an unsutured perineal wound with gauze packing.

After pelvic exenteration:

- Check the stoma, incision, and perineal wound for drainage. Be especially careful to check the perineal wound for bleeding after the packing is removed. Expect red or serosanguineous drainage, but notify the doctor immediately if drainage is excessive, continuously bright red, foul-smelling, or purulent, or if there's bleeding from the conduit.
- Provide excellent skin care because of draining urine and feces. Use warm water and saline solution to clean the skin, because soap may be too drying and may increase skin breakdown.

after surgery. Also explain Foley catheter care. Fit the patient with antiembolism stockings for use during and after surgery. Make sure the patient's blood has been typed and cross-matched. If the patient is premenopausal, inform her that removal of her ovaries will induce menopause.

After surgery:

- Measure fluid contents of the blood drainage system every shift. Notify the doctor immediately if drainage exceeds 400 ml.
- If the patient has received subcutaneous heparin, continue administration, as ordered, until the patient is fully ambulatory again. Give prophylactic antibiotics, as ordered, and provide good Foley catheter care.
- Check vital signs every 4 hours. Watch for and immediately report any sign of complications, such as bleeding, abdominal distention, severe pain, wheezing, or other breathing difficulties. Provide analgesics, as ordered.
- Regularly encourage the patient to breathe deeply and cough to help prevent complications. Promote the use of an incentive spirometer once every waking hour to help keep lungs expanded.
- Find out if the patient is to have internal or external radiation or both. Usually, internal radiation therapy is done first. Check to see if the radioactive source will be inserted while the patient is in the operating room (preloaded) or at bedside (afterloaded). If the source is preloaded, the patient returns to her room "hot," and safety precautions begin immediately.
- Explain the *preloaded* internal radiation procedure, and answer the patient's questions. Explain that internal radiation requires a 2- to 3-day hospital stay, bowel prep, povidone-iodine vaginal douche, clear liquid diet, and nothing taken by mouth the night before the implantation; it also requires a Foley catheter. Tell the patient that the procedure is performed in the operating room under general anesthetic. She will be placed in a dorsal position, with knees and hips flexed, heels resting in footrests. The source is implanted in the vagina by the doctor. If the patient is to have *afterloaded* radiation therapy, explain that a member of the radiation team will implant the source while she is in her room.
- *Remember* that safety precautions—**time, distance, and shielding—must be imposed as soon as the patient's radioactive source is in place.**

Tell the patient that she'll require a private room.

• Encourage the patient to limit movement while the source is in place. If she prefers, elevate the head of the bed slightly. Make sure the patient can reach everything she needs (call bell, telephone, water) without stretching or straining. Assist her in range-of-motion *arm* exercises (leg exercises and other body movements could dislodge the source). If ordered, administer a tranquilizer to help the patient relax and remain still. Organize the time you spend with the patient to minimize your exposure to radiation.

• Check the patient's vital signs every 4 hours; watch for skin reaction, vaginal bleeding, abdominal discomfort, or evidence of dehydration.

• Inform visitors of safety precautions and hang a sign listing these precautions on the patient's door.

If the patient receives external radiation:

• **Teach the patient and her family about** the therapy before it begins. Tell the patient that treatment is usually given 5 days a week for 6 weeks. Warn her not to scrub body areas marked with indelible ink for treatment, because it's important to direct treatment to exactly the same area each time.

• Instruct the patient to maintain a high-protein, high-carbohydrate, low-residue diet to reduce bulk and yet maintain calories. Administer diphenoxylate with atropine, as ordered, to minimize diarrhea, a possible side effect of pelvic radiation.

• To minimize skin breakdown and reduce the risk of skin infection, tell the patient to keep the treatment area dry, to avoid wearing clothes that rub against the area, and to avoid using heating pads, alcohol rubs, or irritating skin creams. Since radiation therapy increases susceptibility to infection (possibly by lowering WBC), tell the patient to avoid people with colds or other infections.

Remember, a uterine cancer patient needs special counseling and psychologic support to help her cope with this disease and the necessary treatment measures. Fearful about her survival, she may also be concerned that treatment will alter her life-style and prevent sexual intimacy. Explain that except in total pelvic exenteration, the vagina remains intact and that once she recovers, sexual intercourse is possible. Your presence and interest alone will help the patient, even if you can't answer every question she may ask.

Vaginal Cancer

Vaginal cancer accounts for approximately 2% of all gynecologic malignancies. It usually appears as squamous cell carcinoma, but occasionally as melanoma, or sarcoma, or adenocarcinoma (clear cell adenocarcinoma has an increaced incidence in young women whose mothers took diethylstilbestrol). Vaginal cancer generally occurs in women in their early to mid-50s, but some of the rarer types do occur in younger women, and rhabdomyosarcoma appears in children.

Pathophysiology

Vaginal cancer varies in severity according to its location and effect on lymphatic drainage. (The vagina is a thin-walled structure with a rich lymphatic drainage.) Vaginal cancer is similar to cervical cancer in that it may progress from an intraepithelial tumor to an invasive cancer. However, it spreads more slowly than cervical cancer.

A lesion in the upper third of the vagina (the most common site) usually metastasizes to the groin nodes; a lesion in the lower third (the second most common site) usually metastasizes to the hypogastric and iliac nodes; but a lesion in the middle third metastasizes erratically. A posterior lesion displaces and distends the vaginal posterior wall before spreading to deep layers. By contrast, an anterior lesion spreads more rapidly into other structures and deep layers, because unlike the posterior wall, the anterior vaginal wall is not flexible.

Signs and symptoms

Commonly, the patient with vaginal cancer has experienced abnormal bleeding and discharge. Also, she may have a small or large, often firm, ulcerated lesion in any part of the vagina. As the cancer progresses, it commonly spreads to the bladder (producing frequent voiding and bladder pain), the rectum (bleeding), vulva (lesion), pubic bone (pain), or other surrounding tissues.

Diagnosis

The diagnosis of vaginal cancer is based on the presence of abnormal cells on a vaginal Pap smear. Careful examination and biopsy rule out the cervix and vulva as the primary sites of the lesion. In many cases, however, the cervix contains the primary lesion that has metastasized to the vagina. Then, any visible lesion is biopsied and evaluated histologically. It is sometimes difficult to visualize the entire vagina because the speculum blades may hide a lesion, or the patient may be uncooperative because of discomfort. When lesions are not visible, colposcopy is used to search out abnormalities. Painting the suspected vaginal area with Lugol's solution (strong iodine solution) also helps identify malignant areas by staining glycogen-containing normal tissue, while leaving abnormal tissue unstained.

Treatment

Early-stage treatment aims to treat the malignant area, while preserving the normal parts of the vagina. Radiation or surgery varies with the size, depth, and location of the lesion, and the patient's desire to maintain a functional vagina.

STAGING VAGINAL CANCER

Stage 0: Carcinoma in situ; intraepithelial carcinoma

Stage I: Carcinoma limited to vaginal wall

Stage II: Carcinoma involves subvaginal tissue but not the pelvic wall.

Stage III: Carcinoma has extended to the pelvic wall.

Stage IV: Carcinoma has extended beyond the true pelvis or has involved the mucosa of the bladder or rectum. Bullous edema as such does not permit assignment to Stage IV.

Stage IVa: Spread to adjacent organs

Stage IVb: Spread to distant organs.

Reprinted from *Manual for Staging of Cancer* (Chicago: American Joint Committee for Cancer Staging and End Results Reporting, 1983). Used with permission.

Preservation of a functional vagina is generally possible only in the early stages. Survival rates are the same for patients treated with radiation as for those with surgery.

Surgery is usually recommended only when the tumor is so extensive that exenteration is needed, because close proximity to the bladder and rectum permits only minimal tissue margins around resected vaginal tissue.

Radiation therapy is the preferred treatment for advanced vaginal cancer. Most patients need preliminary external

SAFE TIME FOR RADIATION IMPLANT

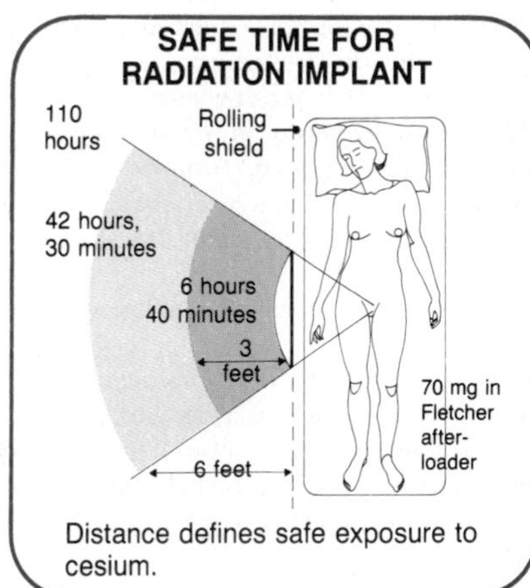

Distance defines safe exposure to cesium.

radiation treatment to shrink the tumor before internal radiation can begin. Then, if the tumor is localized to the vault and the cervix is present, radiation (radium or cesium) can be given with an intrauterine tandem or ovoids; if the cervix is absent, then a specially designed vaginal applicator is used instead. To minimize complications, radioactive sources and filters are carefully placed away from radiosensitive tissues, such as the bladder and the rectum. Such treatment lasts 48 to 72 hours, depending on dosage.

Special considerations

The patient receiving internal radiation needs special care:

- Before treatment begins, find out if the radiation source will be preloaded in the operating room or afterloaded while the patient is in her bed, so that you know how to plan patient care to minimize your exposure to radiation.
- Since the effects of radiation are cumulative, wear a radiosensitive badge and a lead shield (if available), when you enter the patient's room. Check with the radiation therapist concerning the maximum recommended time that you can safely spend with the patient when giving direct care.
- While the radiation source is in place, the patient must lie flat on her back. Insert a Foley catheter (usually done in the operating room), and do not change the patient's linens unless they are soiled. Give only partial bed baths, and make sure the patient has a call bell, phone, water, or anything else she needs within easy reach. The doctor will order a clear liquid or low-residue diet and an antidiarrheal drug to prevent bowel movements.
- To compensate for immobility, encourage the patient to do active range-of-motion exercises with both arms.
- Before radiation treatment, explain the necessity of immobilization, and tell the patient what it entails (such as no linen changes and the use of a Foley catheter). Throughout therapy, encourage her to express her anxieties and fears.
- Instruct the patient to use a stent or prescribed candle exercises to prevent vaginal stenosis. Coitus is also helpful in preventing such stenosis.

Ovarian Cancer

After cancer of the breast, the colon, or the lung, primary ovarian cancer ranks as the most common cause of cancer deaths among American women. In women with previously treated breast cancer, metastatic ovarian cancer is more common than cancer at any other site.

Prognosis varies with the histologic type and staging of the disease but is generally poor because ovarian tumors tend to progress rapidly. Although about 25% of women with ovarian cancer survive for 5 years, prognosis may be improving because of recent advances in chemotherapy.

Three main types of ovarian cancer exist:

- *Primary epithelial tumors* account for 90% of all ovarian cancers and include serous cystoadenocarcinoma, mucinous cystoadenocarcinoma, and endometrioid and mesonephric (clear-cell) malignancies.
- *Germ cell tumors* include endodermal sinus malignancies, embryonal carcinoma (a rare ovarian cancer that appears in children), immature teratomas, and dysgerminoma.
- *Sex cord (stromal) tumors* include granulosa cell tumors (which produce estrogen and may have feminizing effects), thecomas, and the rare arrhenoblastomas (which produce androgen

STAGING OVARIAN CANCER

Stage I: Growth limited to the ovaries
Stage Ia: Growth limited to one ovary; no ascites*
Stage Iai: No tumor on the external surface; capsule intact
Stage Iaii: Tumor on the external surface, or capsule(s) ruptured, or both
Stage Ib: Growth limited to both ovaries; no ascites
Stage Ibi: No tumor on the external surface; capsule intact
Stage Ibii: Tumor on the external surface, or capsule(s) ruptured, or both
Stage Ic: Tumor either Stage 1a or 1b, but with ascites present or with positive peritoneal washings
Stage II: Growth involving one or both ovaries with pelvic extension
Stage IIa: Extension and/or metastases to the uterus and/or tubes
Stage IIb: Extension to other pelvic tissues
Stage IIc: Tumor either stage IIa or Stage IIb, but with ascites present or with positive peritoneal washings
Stage III: Growth involving one or both ovaries with intraperitoneal metastases outside the pelvis, or positive retroperitoneal nodes, or both. Tumor limited to the true pelvis with histologically proven malignant extension to small bowel or omentum.
Stage IV: Growth involving one or both ovaries with distant metastasis. If pleural effusion is present, there must be positive cytology to allot a case to Stage IV. Parenchymal liver metastasis signifies Stage IV.
Special Category: Unexplored cases thought to be ovarian carcinoma

*Ascites is peritoneal effusion that, in the opinion of the surgeon, is pathologic, clearly exceeds normal amounts, or both.

Reprinted from *Manual for Staging of Cancer* (Chicago: American Joint Committee for Cancer Staging and End Results Reporting, 1983). Used with permission.

and have virilizing effects).

Causes and incidence

Exactly what causes ovarian cancer isn't known, but its incidence is noticeably higher in women of upper socioeconomic level between ages 40 and 65, and in single women (although the disease may occur anytime, including childhood or during pregnancy). In a study involving a limited number of patients, a history of endometrial carcinoma seemed linked with ovarian cancer.

Primary epithelial tumors arise in the müllerian epithelium; germ cell tumors, in the ovum itself; and sex cord tumors, in the ovarian stroma (the ovary's supporting framework). Ovarian tumors spread rapidly intraperitoneally by local extension or surface seeding and, occasionally, through the lymphatics and the bloodstream. Generally, extraperitoneal spread is through the diaphragm into the chest cavity, which may cause pleural effusions. Other metastasis is rare.

Signs and symptoms

Typically, symptoms vary with the size of the tumor. Occasionally, in the early stages, ovarian cancer causes vague abdominal discomfort, dyspepsia, and other mild gastrointestinal disturbances. As it progresses, it causes urinary frequency, constipation, pelvic discomfort, distention, and weight loss. Tumor rupture, torsion, or infection may cause pain, which, in young patients, may mimic appendicitis. Granulosa cell tumors have feminizing effects (such as bleeding between periods in premenopausal women); conversely, arrhenoblastomas have virilizing effects. Advanced ovarian cancer causes ascites, rarely postmenopausal bleeding and pain, and symptoms relating to metastatic sites (most often pleural effusions).

Diagnosis

Diagnosis of ovarian cancer requires clinical evaluation, complete patient history, surgical exploration, and histologic studies. Preoperative evaluation in-

cludes a complete physical examination, including pelvic examination with Pap smear (an inconclusive test, as it is positive in only a small number of women with ovarian cancer)
• abdominal ultrasonography, computed tomography scan, or X-ray (may delineate tumor size)
• complete blood count, blood chemistries, and electrocardiogram
• intravenous pyelography for information on renal function and possible urinary tract anomalies or obstruction
• chest X-ray for distant metastasis and pleural effusions
• barium enema (especially in patients with gastrointestinal symptoms) to reveal obstruction and size of tumor
• lymphangiography to show lymph node involvement
• mammography to rule out primary breast cancer
• liver function studies or a liver scan in patients with ascites
• ascites fluid aspiration for identification of typical cells by cytology.

Despite extensive testing, accurate diagnosis and staging are impossible without exploratory laparotomy, including lymph node evaluation and tumor resection.

Treatment

According to the staging of the disease and the patient's age, treatment of ovarian cancer requires varying combinations of surgery, chemotherapy, and, in some cases, radiation.

Occasionally, in girls or young women with a unilateral encapsulated tumor who wish to maintain fertility, a conservative approach may be appropriate:
• resection of the involved ovary
• biopsies of the omentum and the uninvolved ovary
• peritoneal washings for cytologic examination of pelvic fluid
• careful follow-up, including periodic chest X-rays to rule out lung metastasis.

Ovarian cancer usually requires more aggressive treatment, including total abdominal hysterectomy and bilateral salpingo-oophorectomy with tumor resection, omentectomy, appendectomy, lymph node palpation with probable lymphadenectomy, tissue biopsies, and peritoneal washings. Complete tumor resection is impossible if the tumor has matted around other organs or if it involves organs that can't be resected. Bilateral salpingo-oophorectomy in a girl who hasn't reached puberty necessitates hormone replacement therapy, beginning at the age of puberty, to induce the development of secondary sex characteristics.

Chemotherapy extends the length of survival time in most ovarian cancer patients but is largely palliative in advanced disease. However, prolonged remissions are being achieved in some patients. Chemotherapeutic drugs useful in ovarian cancer include melphalan, chlorambucil, thiotepa, methotrexate, cyclophosphamide, doxorubicin, vincristine, vinblastine, actinomycin D, bleomycin, and cisplatin. These drugs are usually given in combination.

In early-stage ovarian cancer, instillation of a radioisotope, such as ^{32}P, is occasionally useful when peritoneal washings are positive. Radiation treatment is likely to be more than merely palliative only if residual tumor size is ¾" (2 cm) or less; if there's no evidence of ascites or no metastatic deposits on the peritoneum, the liver, or kidneys; and if no distant metastases and no prior history of abdominal radiation exist. Immunotherapy is controversial and consists of I.V. or, in chronic ascites, intraperitoneal injection of *Corynebacterium parvulum* or bacille Calmette-Guérin (BCG) vaccine.

Special considerations

Because treatment for ovarian cancer varies widely, so must the patient care plan.

Before surgery:
• Thoroughly explain all preoperative tests, the expected course of treatment, and surgical and postoperative procedures.
• Reinforce what the surgeon has told the patient about the surgical procedures

listed in the surgical consent form. Explain that this form lists multiple procedures because the extent of the surgery can only be determined after the surgery itself has begun.

• In premenopausal women, explain that bilateral oophorectomy artificially induces early menopause, so they may experience hot flashes, headaches, palpitations, insomnia, depression, and excessive perspiration.

After surgery:

• Monitor vital signs frequently, and check I.V. fluids often. Monitor intake and output, while maintaining good catheter care. Check the dressing regularly for excessive drainage or bleeding, and watch for signs of infection.

• Provide abdominal support, and watch for abdominal distention. Encourage coughing and deep breathing. Reposition the patient often, and encourage her to walk shortly after surgery.

• Monitor and treat side effects of radiation and chemotherapy.

• If the patient is receiving immunotherapy, watch for flulike symptoms that may last 12 to 24 hours after drug administration. Give aspirin or acetaminophen for fever. Keep the patient well covered with blankets, and provide warm liquids to relieve chills. Administer an antiemetic, as needed.

• Provide psychological support for the patient and her family. Encourage open communication, while discouraging overcompensation or "smothering" of the patient by her family. If the patient is a young woman who grieves for her lost ability to bear children, help her (and her family) overcome feelings that "there's nothing else to live for." If the patient is a child, find out whether or not her parents have told her she has cancer, and deal with her questions accordingly. Also, enlist the help of a social worker, chaplain, and other members of the health-care team for additional supportive care.

Cancer of the Vulva

Cancer of the vulva accounts for approximately 5% of all gynecologic malignancies. It can occur at any age, even in infants, but its peak incidence is in the mid-60s. The most common vulval cancer is squamous cell carcinoma. Early diagnosis increases the chance of effective treatment and survival. Lymph node dissection allows 5-year survival in 85% of patients if it reveals no positive nodes; otherwise, the survival rate falls to less than 75%.

Causes

Although the cause of cancer of the vulva is unknown, several factors seem to predispose women to this disease:

• leukoplakia (white epithelial hyperplasia)—reported in about 25% of patients
• chronic vulvar granulomatous disease, including venereal disease
• chronic pruritus of the vulva, with friction, swelling, and dryness
• pigmented moles that are constantly irritated by clothing or perineal pads
• irradiation of the skin, such as nonspecific treatment for pelvic cancer
• obesity
• hypertension
• diabetes
• nulliparity.

Signs and symptoms

Cancer of the vulva usually begins with vulval pruritus, bleeding, or a small vulval mass (which may start as a small ulcer on the surface; eventually, it becomes infected and painful), so such symptoms call for immediate diagnostic evaluation. Less common indications include a mass in the groin, abnormal urination or defecation, or cachexia.

STAGING VULVAR CANCER

Stage 0: Carcinoma in situ
Stage I: Tumor confined to vulva—2 cm or less in diameter. Nodes are not palpable or are palpable in either groin, not enlarged, mobile (not clinically suspicious of neoplasm).
Stage II: Tumor confined to the vulva—more than 2 cm in diameter. Nodes are not palpable or are palpable in either groin, not enlarged, mobile (not clinically suspicious of neoplasm).
Stage III: Tumor of any size with (1) adjacent spread to the urethra and any or all of the vagina, the perineum, and the anus, and/or (2) nodes palpable in either or both groins (enlarged, firm, and mobile, not fixed but clinically suspicious of neoplasm).
Stage IV: Tumor of any size (1) infiltrating the bladder mucosa or the rectal mucosa or both, including the upper part of the urethral mucosa, and/or (2) fixed to the bone or other distant metastases. Fixed or ulcerated nodes in either or both groins.

Diagnosis

A Pap smear that reveals abnormal cells or the typical clinical picture (pruritus, bleeding, or small vulvar mass) strongly suggests vulvar cancer.

Firm diagnosis requires histologic examination. Abnormal tissues for biopsy are identified by colposcopic examination to pinpoint vulvar lesions or abnormal skin changes and by staining with toluidine blue dye, which, after rinsing with dilute acetic acid, is retained by diseased tissues.

Other diagnostic measures include complete blood count, X-ray, electrocardiogram, and thorough physical (including pelvic) examination. Occasionally, lymphangiography may pinpoint lymph node involvement.

Treatment

Depending on the stage of the disease, cancer of the vulva usually calls for radical or simple vulvectomy (or laser therapy, for some small lesions). Radical vulvectomy requires bilateral dissection of superficial and deep inguinal lymph nodes. Depending on the extent of metastasis, resection may include the urethra, vagina, and bowel, leaving an open perineal wound until healing—about 2 to 3 months. Plastic surgery, including mucocutaneous graft to reconstruct pelvic structures, may be done later.

Small, confined lesions with no lymph node involvement may require a simple vulvectomy or hemivulvectomy (without pelvic node dissection). Personal considerations (young age of patient, active sexual life) may also mandate such conservative management. However, a simple vulvectomy requires careful postoperative surveillance, since it leaves the patient at higher risk of developing a new lesion.

If extensive metastasis, advanced age, or fragile health rules out surgery, irradiation of the primary lesion offers palliative treatment.

Special considerations

Patient teaching, preoperative and postoperative care, and psychologic support can help prevent complications and speed recovery.

Before surgery:

- Supplement and reinforce what the doctor has told the patient about the surgery and postoperative procedures, such as the use of a Foley catheter, preventive respiratory care, and exercises to prevent venous stasis.
- Encourage the patient to ask questions, and answer them honestly.

After surgery:

- Provide scrupulous routine gynecologic care and special care to reduce pressure at the operative site, reduce tension on suture lines, and promote healing through better air circulation.
- Place the patient on an air mattress or egg crate mattress, and use a cradle to support the top covers.

• Periodically reposition the patient with pillows. Make sure her bed has a half-frame trapeze bar to help her move.
• For several days after surgery, the patient will be maintained on I.V. fluids or a clear liquid diet. As ordered, give her an antidiarrheal drug three times daily to reduce the discomfort and possible infection caused by defecation. Later, as ordered, give stool softeners and a low-residue diet to combat constipation.
• Teach the patient how to thoroughly cleanse the surgical site.
• Check the operative site regularly for bleeding, foul-smelling discharge, or other signs of infection. The wound area will look lumpy, bruised, and battered, making it difficult to detect occult bleeding. This situation calls for a doctor or a primary nurse, who can more easily detect subtle changes in appearance.
• Within 5 to 10 days after surgery, as ordered, help the patient to walk. Encourage and assist her in coughing and range-of-motion exercises.
• To prevent urine contamination, the patient will have a Foley catheter in place for 2 weeks. Record fluid intake and output, and provide standard catheter care.
• Counsel the patient and her partner. Explain that sensation in the vulva will eventually return after the nerve endings heal, and they will probably be able to have sexual intercourse 6 to 8 weeks following surgery. Explain that they may want to try different sexual techniques, especially if surgery has removed the clitoris. Help the patient adjust to the drastic change in her body image.

Fallopian Tube Cancer

Primary fallopian tube cancer is extremely rare and accounts for fewer than 0.5% of all gynecologic malignancies. It usually occurs in postmenopausal women in their 50s and 60s but occasionally is found in younger women. Because this disease is generally well advanced before diagnosis (up to 30% of such cancers are bilateral with extratubal spread), prognosis is poor.

Causes
The causes of fallopian tube cancer aren't clear, but this disease appears to be linked with nulliparity. In fact, over half the women with this disease have never had children.

Signs and symptoms
Generally, early-stage fallopian tube cancer produces no symptoms. Late-stage disease is characterized by an enlarged abdomen with a palpable mass, amber-colored vaginal discharge, excessive bleeding during menstruation, or, at other times, abdominal cramps, frequent urination, bladder pressure, persistent constipation, weight loss, and unilateral colicky pain produced by hydrops tubae profluens. (This last symptom occurs when the abdominal end of the fallopian tube closes, causing the tube to become greatly distended until its accumulated secretions suddenly overflow into the uterus.) Metastases develop by local extension or by lymphatic spread to the abdominal organs or to the pelvic, aortic, and inguinal lymph nodes. Extraabdominal metastases are rare.

Diagnosis
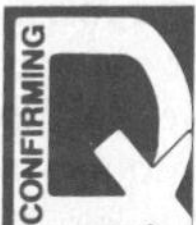

Unexplained postmenopausal bleeding and an abnormal Pap smear (suspicious or positive in up to 50% of all cases) suggest this diagnosis, but laparotomy is usually necessary to confirm fallopian tube cancer. When such cancer involves both the ovary and fallopian tube, the primary site is very difficult to identify.

Preoperative workup includes:
• an ultrasound or plain film of the ab-

domen to help delineate tumor mass
- intravenous pyelography to assess renal function, and show urinary tract anomalies and ureteral obstruction
- chest X-ray to rule out metastases
- barium enema to rule out intestinal obstruction
- routine blood studies
- electrocardiogram.

Treatment

Treatment of fallopian tube cancer consists of total abdominal hysterectomy, bilateral salpingo-oophorectomy, and omentectomy; chemotherapy with progestogens, 5-fluorouracil, melphalan, cyclophosphamide, and cisplatin; and external radiation for 5 to 6 weeks. All patients should receive some form of adjunctive therapy (radiation or chemotherapy), even when surgery has removed all evidence of the disease.

Special considerations

Good preoperative patient preparation and postoperative care, patient instruction, psychologic support, and symptomatic measures to relieve radiation and chemotherapy side effects can promote a successful recovery and minimize complications.

For example, reinforce the doctor's explanation of the diagnostic and treatment procedures. Explain the need for preoperative studies, and tell the patient what to expect: fasting from the evening before surgery; an enema to clear the bowel, using a Foley catheter attached to a drainage bag; an abdominal and possibly a pelvic preparation; an I.V. line; and, possibly, a sedative. Describe the tubes and dressings the patient can expect to have in place when she returns from surgery. Teach the patient deep breathing and coughing techniques to prepare for postoperative exercises.

After surgery:

- Check vital signs every 4 hours. Report fever, tachycardia, and hypotension to the doctor.
- Monitor I.V. fluids.
- Change dressings regularly, and check for excessive drainage and bleeding and signs of infection.
- Provide antiembolism stockings, as ordered.
- Encourage regular deep breathing and coughing. If necessary, institute intermittent positive pressure breathing, as ordered.
- Turn the patient often, and help her reposition herself, using pillows for support.
- Auscultate for bowel sounds. When the patient's bowel function returns, ask the dietitian to provide a clear liquid diet; then, when it can be tolerated, a regular diet.
- Encourage the patient to walk within 24 hours after surgery. Reassure her that she won't harm herself or cause wound dehiscence by sitting up or walking.
- Provide psychologic support. Encourage the patient to express anxieties and fears. If she seems worried about the effect of surgery on her sexual life, reassure her that this surgery will not inhibit sexual intimacy.
- Before radiation therapy begins, explain that the area to be irradiated is marked with water-soluble ink to precisely locate the treatment field. Explain that radiation may cause a skin reaction, bladder irritation, myelosuppression and other systemic reactions, or a drop in blood pressure. During and after treatment, watch for and treat side effects of radiation and chemotherapy.
- Before discharge, to minimize side effects during outpatient radiation and chemotherapy, advise the patient to maintain a high-carbohydrate, high-protein, low-fat, low-bulk diet to maintain caloric intake but reduce bulk. Suggest that she eat several small meals a day instead of three large ones.
- Include the patient's husband or other close relatives in patient care and teaching as much as possible.

To help detect fallopian tube and other gynecologic cancers early, stress the importance of a regular pelvic examination to *all* patients. Tell them to contact a doctor promptly about any gynecologic symptom.

BONE, SKIN, AND SOFT TISSUE

Primary Malignant Bone Tumors

(Sarcomas of the bone, bone cancer)

Primary malignant bone tumors are rare, constituting less than 1% of all malignant tumors. Most bone tumors are secondary, caused by seeding from a primary site. Primary malignant bone tumors are more common in males, especially in children and adolescents, although some types do occur in persons between ages 35 and 60. They may originate in osseous or nonosseous tissue. Osseous bone tumors arise from the bony structure itself and include osteogenic sarcoma (the most common), parosteal osteogenic sarcoma, chondrosarcoma, and malignant giant cell tumor. Together they make up 60% of all malignant bone tumors. Nonosseous tumors arise from hematopoietic, vascular, and neural tissues and include Ewing's sarcoma, fibrosarcoma, and chordoma. Osteogenic and Ewing's sarcomas are the most common bone tumors in childhood.

Causes

Causes of primary malignant bone tumors remain unknown. Some suggest that primary malignant bone tumors arise in areas of rapid growth, since children and young adults with such tumors seem to be much taller than average. Additional theories point to heredity, trauma, and excessive radiotherapy.

Signs and symptoms

Bone pain is the most common indication of primary malignant bone tumors. It's often more intense at night and is not usually associated with mobility. The pain is dull and is usually localized, although it may be referred from the hip or spine and result in weakness or a limp. Another common sign is the presence of a mass or tumor. The tumor site may be tender and may swell; the tumor itself is often palpable. Pathologic fractures are common. In late stages, the patient may be cachectic, with fever and impaired mobility.

Diagnosis

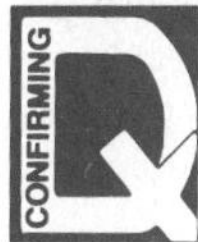

A biopsy (by incision or by aspiration) is essential for confirming primary malignant bone tumors. Bone X-rays and radioisotope bone and computed tomography scans show tumor size. Serum alkaline phosphatase is usually elevated in patients with sarcoma.

Treatment

Surgery (usually amputation) and radiation are the treatments of choice, sometimes combined with chemotherapy and immunotherapy. Sometimes radical surgery (such as hemipelvectomy or interscapulothoracic amputation) is necessary. However, surgical resection of the tumor (often with preoperative radiation *and* postoperative chemotherapy) has saved limbs from amputation. Chemotherapeutic drugs include doxorubicin, high-dose methotrexate with leucovorin rescue, vincristine, cyclophosphamide, cisplatin, bleomycin, dactinomycin, and melphalan. Adjuvant immunotherapy uses interferon or the transfer factor (a dialyzable extract of immune lymphocytes that transfers cell-mediated immunity).

Special considerations

• Be sensitive to the enormous emotional strain caused by the threat of amputation. Encourage communication, and help the patient set realistic goals. If amputation is inevitable, teach him how to readjust his body weight so he'll be able to get in and out of bed and wheelchair. Teach exercises that will help him do this even before surgery.

- Before surgery, start I.V. infusions to maintain fluid and electrolyte balance, and to have an open vein if blood or plasma is needed during surgery.
- After surgery, check vital signs every hour for the first 4 hours; then every 2 hours for the next 4 hours; and then every 4 hours if the patient is stable. Tape a tourniquet to the bed in case of hemorrhage. Check dressing periodically for oozing. Elevate the foot of the bed or the stump on a pillow for the first 24 hours. (Be careful not to leave the stump elevated for more than 48 hours, as this may lead to contractures.)
- To ease the patient's anxiety, administer analgesics for pain before morning care. If necessary, brace the patient with pillows, keeping the affected part at rest.
- Urge the patient to eat foods high in protein, vitamins, and folic acid, and to get plenty of rest and sleep to promote recovery. Encourage some physical exercise. Administer laxatives, if necessary, to maintain proper elimination.
- Since the patient may have thrombocytopenia, make sure he uses a soft toothbrush and an electric razor to avoid bleeding. Don't give I.M. injections or take rectal temperatures. Be careful not to bump the patient's arms or legs; his low platelet count causes bruising.
- Encourage fluids to prevent dehydration. Record intake and output accurately. After a hemipelvectomy, insert nasogastric tube to prevent abdominal distention. Continue low gastric suction for 2 days after surgery or until the patient can tolerate a soft diet. Administer antibiotics to prevent infection of the rectum. Give transfusions, if necessary, and administer medication to control pain. Keep drains in place to facilitate wound drainage and prevent infection. Use a Foley catheter until the patient can void voluntarily.
- Watch for adverse reactions to radiation treatment: nausea, vomiting, and dryness of skin with excoriation.

Encourage early rehabilitation:

- Start physical therapy 24 hours postop. Pain is usually not severe after amputation. If it is, watch for a wound complication, such as hematoma, excessive stump edema, or infection.
- Be aware of the "phantom limb" syndrome. The patient may "feel" an itch or tingling in an amputated extremity. This can last for several hours or persist for years. Tell the patient this sensation is normal after amputation and usually subsides.
- To avoid contractures and assure the best conditions for wound healing, warn the patient not to hang the stump over the edge of the bed; sit in a wheelchair with the stump flexed; place a pillow under his hip, knee, or back, or between his thighs; lie with knees flexed; rest an above the knee (AK) stump on the crutch handle; or abduct an AK stump.
- Wash the stump, massage it gently, and keep it dry until it heals. Make sure the bandage is firm and is worn day and night. Know how to reapply the bandage to shape the stump for a prosthesis.
- Help the patient select a prosthesis by informing him of the needs to be considered and the types of prostheses available. The rehabilitation staff will make the final decision, but since most patients are totally uninformed about choosing a prosthesis, give some guidelines. Keep in mind the patient's age and possible vision problems. Generally, children need relatively simple devices, while elderly patients may require prostheses that provide more stability. Consider personal and family finances too. Children outgrow prostheses, so advise parents to select inexpensive ones.
- The same points are applicable for an interscapulothoracic amputee, but losing an arm causes a greater cosmetic problem.
- Try to instill a positive attitude toward recovery. Urge the patient to resume an independent life-style. Refer elderly patients to community health services, if necessary. Suggest tutoring for children to help them keep up with schoolwork.

PRIMARY MALIGNANT BONE TUMORS

TYPE	CLINICAL FEATURES	TREATMENT
OSSEOUS ORIGIN		
Osteogenic sarcoma	• Osteoid tumor present in specimen • Tumor arises from bone-forming osteoblast and bone-digesting osteoclast • Occurs most often in femur, but also tibia and humerus; occasionally, in fibula, ileum, vertebra, or mandible • Usually in males aged 10 to 30 years	• Surgery (tumor resection, high thigh amputation, hemipelvectomy, interscapulothoracic surgery) • Radiation • Chemotherapy • Combination of above
Parosteal osteogenic sarcoma	• Develops on surface of bone instead of interior • Progresses slowly • Occurs most often in distal femur, but also in tibia, humerus, and ulna • Usually in females aged 30 to 40 years	• Surgery (tumor resection, possible amputation, interscapulothoracic surgery, hemipelvectomy) • Chemotherapy • Combination of above
Chondrosarcoma	• Develops from cartilage • Painless; grows slowly, but is locally recurrent and invasive • Occurs most often in pelvis, proximal femur, ribs, and shoulder girdle • Usually in males aged 30 to 50 years	• Hemipelvectomy, surgical resection (ribs) • Radiation (palliative) • Chemotherapy
Malignant giant cell tumor	• Arises from benign giant cell tumor • Found most often in long bones, especially in knee area • Usually in females aged 18 to 50 years	• Curettage • Total excision • Radiation
NONOSSEOUS ORIGIN		
Ewing's sarcoma	• Originates in bone marrow and invades shafts of long and flat bones • Usually affects lower extremities, most often femur, innominate bones, ribs, tibia, humerus, vertebra, and fibula; may metastasize to lungs • Pain increasingly severe and persistent • Usually in males aged 10 to 20 years • Prognosis poor	• High-voltage radiation (tumor is very radiosensitive) • Chemotherapy to slow growth • Amputation only if there's no evidence of metastases
Fibrosarcoma	• Relatively rare • Originates in fibrous tissue of bone • Invades long or flat bones (femur, tibia, mandible) but also involves periosteum and overlying muscle • Usually in males aged 30 to 40 years	• Amputation • Radiation • Chemotherapy • Bone grafts (with low-grade fibrosarcoma)
Chordoma	• Derived from embryonic remnants of notochord • Progresses slowly • Usually found at end of spinal column and in spheno-occipital, sacrococcygeal, and vertebral areas • Characterized by constipation and visual disturbances • Usually in males aged 50 to 60 years	• Surgical resection (often resulting in neural defects) • Radiation (palliative, or when surgery not applicable, as in occipital area)

Multiple Myeloma

(Malignant plasmacytoma, plasma cell myeloma, myelomatosis)

Multiple myeloma is a disseminated neoplasm of marrow plasma cells that infiltrates bone to produce osteolytic lesions throughout the skeleton (flat bones, vertebrae, skull, pelvis, ribs); in late stages, it infiltrates the body organs (liver, spleen, lymph nodes, lungs, adrenal glands, kidneys, skin, and gastrointestinal tract). Multiple myeloma strikes about 9,600 people yearly—mostly men over age 40. Prognosis is usually poor, because diagnosis is often made after the disease has already infiltrated the vertebrae, pelvis, skull, ribs, clavicles, and sternum. By then, skeletal destruction is widespread and, without treatment, leads to vertebral collapse; 52% of patients die within 3 months of diagnosis, 90% within 2 years. Early diagnosis and treatment prolong the lives of many patients by 3 to 5 years. Finally, death usually follows complications, such as infection, renal failure, hematologic imbalance, fractures, hypercalcemia, hyperuricemia, or dehydration.

Signs and symptoms

The earliest indication of multiple myeloma is severe, constant back pain that increases with exercise. Arthritic symptoms may also occur: achiness, joint swelling, and tenderness, possibly from vertebral compression. Other effects include fever, malaise, slight evidence of peripheral neuropathy (such as peripheral paresthesias), and pathologic fractures. As multiple myeloma progresses, symptoms of vertebral compression may become acute, accompanied by anemia, weight loss, thoracic deformities (ballooning), and loss of body height—5″ (12.7 cm) or more due to vertebral collapse. Renal complications such as pyelonephritis (caused by tubular damage from large amounts of Bence Jones protein, hypercalcemia, and hyperuricemia) may occur. Severe, recurrent infection, such as pneumonia, may follow damage to nerves associated with respiratory function.

Diagnosis

After a physical examination and a careful medical history, the following diagnostic tests and nonspecific laboratory abnormalities confirm the presence of multiple myeloma:

- *Complete blood count* shows moderate or severe anemia. The differential may show 40% to 50% lymphocytes but seldom more than 3% plasma cells. Rouleaux formation (often the first clue) seen on differential smear results from elevation of the red cell sedimentation rate.
- *Urine studies* may show Bence Jones protein and hypercalciuria. Absence of Bence Jones protein doesn't rule out multiple myeloma; however, its presence almost invariably confirms the disease.
- *Bone marrow aspiration* detects myelomatous cells (abnormal number of immature plasma cells).
- *Serum electrophoresis* shows elevated globulin spike that is electrophoretically and immunologically abnormal.
- *X-rays* during early stages may show only diffuse osteoporosis. Eventually, they show multiple, sharply circumscribed osteolytic (punched out) lesions, particularly on the skull, pelvis, and spine—the characteristic lesions of multiple myeloma.
- *Intravenous pyelography* can assess renal involvement. To avoid precipitation of Bence Jones protein, iothalamate or diatrizoate is used instead of the usual contrast medium. And although oral fluid restriction is usually the standard procedure before an intravenous pyelogram (IVP), patients with multiple myeloma receive large quantities of fluid, generally orally but sometimes intrave-

nously, before an IVP is done.

Treatment

Long-term treatment of multiple myeloma consists mainly of chemotherapy to suppress plasma cell growth and control pain. Combinations of melphalan and prednisone or of cyclophosphamide and prednisone are used. Also, adjuvant local radiation reduces acute lesions, such as collapsed vertebrae, and relieves localized pain. Other treatment usually includes a melphalan-prednisone combination in high intermittent doses or low continuous daily doses, and analgesics for pain. If the patient develops spinal cord compression, he may require a laminectomy; if he has renal complications, he may need dialysis.

Because the patient may have bone demineralization and may lose large amounts of calcium into blood and urine, he is a prime candidate for renal stones, nephrocalcinosis, and, eventually, renal failure due to the hypercalcemia. Hypercalcemia is managed with hydration, diuretics, corticosteroids, oral phosphate, and mithramycin I.V. to decrease serum calcium levels.

Special considerations

- Push fluids; encourage the patient to drink 3,000 to 4,000 ml fluids daily, particularly before his IVP. Monitor fluid intake and output (daily output should not be less than 1,500 ml).
- Encourage the patient to walk (immobilization increases bone demineralization and vulnerability to pneumonia), and give analgesics, as ordered, to lessen pain. Never allow the patient to walk unaccompanied; be sure that he uses a walker or other supportive aid to prevent falls. Since the patient is particularly vulnerable to pathologic fractures, he may be fearful. Give reassurance, and allow him to move at his own pace.
- Prevent complications by watching for fever or malaise, which may signal the onset of infection, and for signs of other problems, such as severe anemia and fractures. If the patient is bedridden, change his position every 2 hours. Give passive range-of-motion and deep breathing exercises. When he can tolerate them, promote active exercises.
- If the patient is taking melphalan (a phenylalanine derivative of nitrogen mustard that depresses bone marrow), make sure his blood count (platelet and white blood cell) is taken before each treatment. If he is taking prednisone, watch closely for infection, since this drug often masks it.
- Whenever possible, get the patient out of bed within 24 hours after laminectomy. Check for hemorrhage, motor or sensory deficits, and loss of bowel or bladder function. Position the patient as ordered, maintain alignment, and logroll when turning.
- Provide much-needed emotional support for the patient and his family, as they are likely to be very anxious. Help relieve their anxiety by truthfully informing them about diagnostic tests (including painful procedures, such as bone marrow aspiration and biopsy), treatment, and prognosis. If needed, refer them to an appropriate community resource for additional support.

ALL ABOUT BENCE JONES PROTEIN

The hallmark of multiple myeloma, this protein (a light chain of gamma globulin) was named for Henry Bence Jones, an English doctor who in 1848 noticed that patients with a curious bone disease excreted a unique protein—unique in that it coagulated at 113° to 131° F. (45° to 55° C.), then redissolved when heated to boiling. It remained for Otto Kahler, an Austrian, to demonstrate in 1889 that Bence Jones protein was related to myeloma. Bence Jones protein is not found in the urine of *all* multiple myeloma patients, but it is almost never found in patients without this disease.

Basal Cell Epithelioma

(Basal cell carcinoma)

Basal cell epithelioma is a slow-growing destructive skin tumor. This carcinoma usually occurs in persons over age 40; it's more prevalent in blond, fair-skinned males and is the most common malignant tumor affecting whites.

Causes

Prolonged sun exposure is the most common cause of basal cell epithelioma, but arsenic ingestion, radiation exposure, burns, and, rarely, vaccinations are other possible causes. Most of these tumors (94%) occur on parts of the body with abundant pilosebaceous follicles, especially on the face.

Although the pathogenesis of basal cell epithelioma is uncertain, some experts now hypothesize that it originates when, under certain conditions, undifferentiated basal cells become carcinomatous instead of differentiating into sweat glands, sebum, and hair.

Signs and symptoms

Three types of basal cell epithelioma occur:

- *Noduloulcerative* lesions occur most often on the face, particularly the forehead, eyelid margins, and nasolabial folds. In early stages, these lesions are small, smooth, pinkish, and translucent papules. Telangiectatic vessels cross the surface, and the lesions are occasionally pigmented. As the lesions enlarge, their centers become depressed and their borders become firm and elevated. Ulceration and local invasion eventually occur. These ulcerated tumors, known as "rodent ulcers," rarely metastasize; however, if untreated, they can spread to vital areas and become infected, or cause massive hemorrhage if they invade large blood vessels.
- *Superficial basal cell epitheliomas* are often multiple and commonly occur on the chest and back. They're oval or irregularly shaped, lightly pigmented plaques, with sharply defined, slightly elevated threadlike borders. Due to superficial erosion, these lesions appear scaly and have small, atrophic areas in the center that resemble psoriasis or eczema. They're usually chronic and don't tend to invade other areas. Superficial basal cell epitheliomas are related to ingestion of or exposure to arsenic-containing compounds.
- *Sclerosing basal cell epitheliomas (morphealike epitheliomas)* are waxy, sclerotic, yellow to white plaques without distinct borders. Occurring on the head and neck, sclerosing basal cell epitheliomas often look like small patches of scleroderma.

Diagnosis

All types of basal cell epitheliomas are diagnosed by clinical appearance, incisional or excisional biopsy, and histologic study.

Treatment

Depending on the size, location, and depth of the lesion, treatment may include curettage and electrodesiccation, chemotherapy, surgical excision, irradiation, or chemosurgery.

- Curettage and electrodesiccation offer good cosmetic results for small lesions.
- Topical 5-fluorouracil is often used for superficial lesions. This medication produces marked local irritation or inflammation in the involved tissue but no systemic effects.
- Microscopically controlled surgical excision carefully removes recurrent lesions until a tumor-free plane is achieved. After removal of large lesions, skin grafting may be required.
- Irradiation is used for elderly or debilitated patients who might not withstand surgery.

• Chemosurgery is often necessary for persistent or recurrent lesions. Chemosurgery consists of periodic applications of a fixative paste (such as zinc chloride) and subsequent removal of fixed pathologic tissue. Treatment continues until tumor removal is complete.

Special considerations

• Instruct the patient to eat frequent small meals that are high in protein. Suggest egg nogs, "blenderized" foods, or liquid protein supplements if the lesion has invaded the oral cavity and caused eating problems.
• Tell the patient that to prevent disease recurrence, he needs to avoid excessive sun exposure and use a strong sunscreen or sunshade to protect his skin from damage by ultraviolet rays.
• Advise the patient to relieve local inflammation from topical 5-fluorouracil with cool compresses or with corticosteroid ointment.
• Instruct the patient with noduloulcerative basal cell epithelioma to wash his face gently when ulcerations and crusting occur; scrubbing too vigorously may cause bleeding.

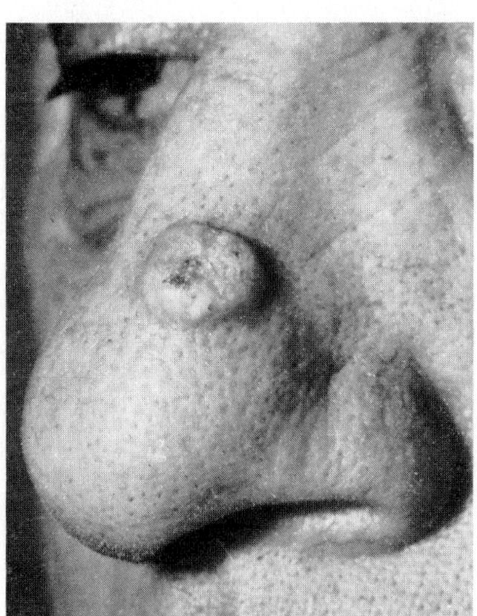

The photograph above shows an enlarged nasal nodule in basal cell carcinoma.

Squamous Cell Carcinoma

Squamous cell carcinoma of the skin is an invasive tumor with metastatic potential that arises from the keratinizing epidermal cells. It occurs most often in fair-skinned white males over age 60. Outdoor employment and residence in a sunny, warm climate (southwestern United States and Australia, for example) greatly increase the risk of developing squamous cell carcinoma.

Causes

Predisposing factors associated with squamous cell carcinoma include overexposure to the sun's ultraviolet rays, the presence of premalignant lesions (such as actinic keratosis or Bowen's disease), X-ray therapy, ingestion of herbicides containing arsenic, chronic skin irritation and inflammation, exposure to local carcinogens (such as tar and oil), and hereditary diseases (such as xeroderma pigmentosum and albinism). Rarely, squamous cell carcinoma may develop on the site of smallpox vaccination, psoriasis, or chronic discoid lupus erythematosus.

Signs and symptoms

Squamous cell carcinoma commonly develops on the skin of the face, the ears, the dorsa of the hands and forearms, and other sun-damaged areas. Lesions on sun-damaged skin tend not to be as invasive, with less tendency to metastasize than lesions on unexposed skin. Notable exceptions to this tendency are squamous cell lesions on the lower lip and the ears. These are almost invariably

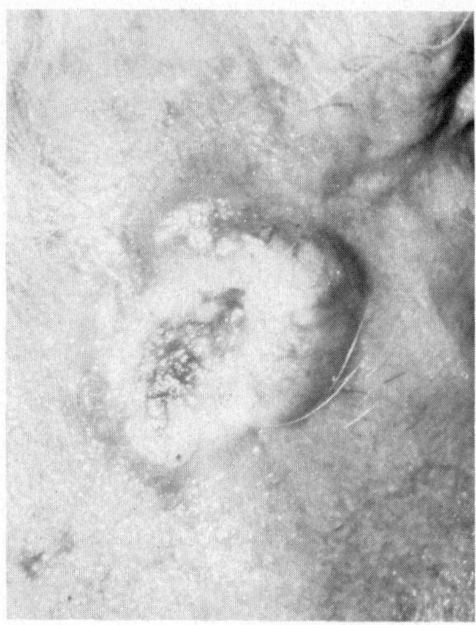

Ulcerated nodule with indurated base in squamous cell carcinoma

TREATING ACTINIC KERATOSES WITH TOPICAL 5-FLUOROURACIL

5-fluorouracil is available in different strengths (1%, 2%, and 5%) as a cream or solution. Local application causes immediate stinging and burning, followed later by erythema, vesiculation, erosion, superficial ulceration, necrosis, and re-epithelialization. The 5% solution induces the most severe inflammatory response, but provides complete involution of the lesions with little recurrence. Be careful to keep 5-fluorouracil away from eyes, scrotum, or mucous membranes. Warn the patient to avoid excessive exposure to the sun during the course of treatment because it intensifies the inflammatory reaction.

Continue application of 5-fluorouracil until the lesions reach the ulcerative and necrotic stages (usually 2 to 4 weeks); then consider application of a corticosteroid preparation as an anti-inflammatory agent. Possible side effects of treatment include postinflammatory hyperpigmentation. Complete healing occurs within 1 to 2 months, with excellent results.

markedly invasive metastastic lesions, with a generally poor prognosis.

Transformation from a premalignant lesion to squamous cell carcinoma may begin with induration and inflammation of the preexisting lesion. When squamous cell carcinoma arises from normal skin, the nodule grows slowly on a firm, indurated base. If untreated, this nodule eventually ulcerates and invades underlying tissues. Metastasis can occur to the regional lymph nodes, producing characteristic systemic symptoms of pain, malaise, fatigue, weakness, and anorexia.

Diagnosis

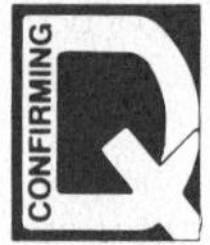

An excisional biopsy provides definitive diagnosis of squamous cell carcinoma. Other appropriate laboratory tests depend on systemic symptoms.

Treatment

The size, shape, location, and invasiveness of a squamous cell tumor and the condition of the underlying tissue determine the treatment method used; a deeply invasive tumor may require a combination of techniques. All the major treatment methods have excellent rates of cure; generally, prognosis is better with a well-differentiated lesion than with a poorly differentiated one in an unusual location. Depending on the lesion, treatment may consist of:

- wide surgical excision
- electrodesiccation and curettage (offer good cosmetic results for smaller lesions)
- radiation therapy (generally for older or debilitated patients)
- chemosurgery (reserved for resistant or recurrent lesions).

Special considerations

The care plan for patients with squamous cell carcinoma should emphasize meticulous wound care, emotional support, and thorough patient instruction.

- Coordinate a consistent care plan for changing the patient's dressings. Estab-

PREMALIGNANT SKIN LESIONS

DISEASE	CAUSE	PATIENT	LESION	TREATMENT
Actinic keratosis	Solar radiation	Caucasian men with fair skin (middle-aged to elderly)	Reddish-brown lesions 1 mm to 1 cm in size (may enlarge if untreated) on face, ears, lower lip, bald scalp, dorsa of hands and forearms	Topical 5-fluorouracil, cryosurgery using liquid nitrogen, or curettage by electrodesiccation
Bowen's disease	Unknown	Caucasian men with fair skin (middle-aged to elderly)	Brown to reddish-brown lesions, with scaly surface on exposed and unexposed areas	Surgical excision, topical 5-fluorouracil
Erythroplasia of Queyrat	Bowen's disease of the mucous membranes	Men (middle-aged to elderly)	Red lesions, with a glistening or granular appearance on mucous membranes, particularly the glans penis in uncircumcised males	Surgical excision
Leukoplakia	Smoking, alcohol, chronic cheek-biting, ill-fitting dentures, misaligned teeth	Men (middle-aged to elderly)	Lesions on oral, anal, and genital mucous membranes vary in appearance from smooth and white to rough and gray	Elimination of irritating factors, surgical excision, or curettage by electrodesiccation (if lesion is still premalignant)

lishing a standard routine helps the patient and family learn how to care for the wound.

- Keep the wound dry and clean.
- Try to control odor with balsam of Peru, yogurt flakes, oil of cloves, or other odor-masking substances, even though they are often ineffective for long-term use. Topical or systemic antibiotics also temporarily control odor and eventually alter the lesion's bacterial flora.
- Be prepared for other problems that accompany a metastatic disease (pain, fatigue, weakness, anorexia).
- Help the patient and family set realistic goals and expectations.
- Disfiguring lesions are distressing to both the patient and you. Try to accept the patient as he is and to increase his self-esteem and strengthen a caring relationship.

To prevent squamous cell carcinoma, tell patients to:

- avoid excessive sun exposure.
- wear protective clothing (hats, long sleeves).
- periodically examine the skin for precancerous lesions; have any removed promptly.
- use strong sunscreening agents containing para-aminobenzoic acid (PABA), benzophenone, and zinc oxide. Apply these agents 30 to 60 minutes before sun exposure.
- use lipscreens to protect the lips from sun damage.

Malignant Melanoma

A neoplasm that arises from melanocytes, malignant melanoma is relatively rare and accounts for only 1% to 2% of all malignancies. The three types of melanomas are superficial spreading melanoma, nodular malignant melanoma, and lentigo maligna melanoma. Melanoma is slightly more common in women than in men, and is rare in children. Peak incidence occurs between ages 50 and 70, although the incidence in younger age-groups is increasing.

Melanoma spreads through the lymphatic and vascular systems and metastasizes to the regional lymph nodes, skin, liver, lungs, and central nervous system. Its course is unpredictable, however, and recurrence and metastases may not appear for more than 5 years after resection of the primary lesion. Prognosis varies with tumor thickness. Generally, superficial lesions are curable, while deeper lesions tend to metastasize. The Breslow level method measures tumor depth from the granular level of the epidermis to the deepest melanoma cell. Melanoma lesions less than 0.76 mm deep have an excellent prognosis, while deeper lesions (more than 0.76 mm) are at risk for metastasis. Prognosis is better for a tumor on an extremity (which is drained by one lymphatic network) than for one on the head, neck, or trunk (drained by several networks).

Causes

Several factors seem to influence the development of melanoma:

• *Excessive exposure to sunlight.* Melanoma is most common in sunny, warm areas and often develops on parts of the body that are exposed to the sun.

• *Skin type.* Most persons who develop melanoma have blond or red hair, fair skin, and blue eyes; are prone to sunburn; and are of Celtic or Scandinavian ancestry. Melanoma is rare among blacks; when it does develop, it usually arises in lightly pigmented areas (the palms, plantar surface of the feet, or mucous membranes).

• *Hormonal factors.* Pregnancy may increase risk and exacerbate growth.

• *Family history.* Melanoma occurs slightly more often within families.

• *Past history of melanoma.* A person who has had one melanoma is at greater risk of developing a second.

Signs and symptoms

Common sites for melanoma are on the head and neck in men, on the legs in women, and on the backs of persons exposed to excessive sunlight. Up to 70% arise from a preexisting nevus. It rarely appears in the conjunctiva, choroid, pharynx, mouth, vagina, or anus.

Suspect melanoma when any skin lesion or nevus enlarges, changes color, becomes inflamed or sore, itches, ulcerates, bleeds, undergoes textural changes, or shows signs of surrounding pigment regression (halo nevus or vitiligo).

Each type of melanoma has special characteristics:

• *Superficial spreading melanoma* (SSM), the most common, usually develops between ages 40 and 50. Such a lesion arises on an area of chronic irritation. In women, it's most common between the knees and ankles; in blacks and Orientals, on the toe webs and soles (lightly pigmented areas subject to trauma). Characteristically, this melanoma has a red, white, and blue color over a brown or black background and an irregular, notched margin. Its surface is irregular, with small elevated tumor nodules that may ulcerate and bleed. Horizontal growth may continue for many years; when vertical growth begins, prognosis worsens.

• *Nodular malignant melanoma* (NMM) usually develops between ages 40 and 50, grows vertically, invades the dermis, and metastasizes early. Such a lesion is usually a polypoidal nodule, with uniformly dark discoloration (it may be grayish), and looks like a blackberry. Occasionally, this melanoma is flesh-colored, with flecks of pigment around its base (which may be inflamed).

- *Lentigo maligna melanoma* (LMM) is relatively rare. It arises from a lentigo maligna on an exposed skin surface and usually occurs between ages 60 and 70. Such a lesion looks like a large (3 to 6 cm) flat freckle of tan, brown, black, whitish, or slate color, and has irregularly scattered black nodules on the surface. It develops slowly, usually over many years, and eventually may ulcerate. This melanoma commonly develops under the fingernails, on the face, and on the back of the hands.

Diagnosis

A skin biopsy with histologic examination can distinguish malignant melanoma from a benign nevus, seborrheic keratosis, and pigmented basal cell epithelioma, and can also determine tumor thickness. Physical examination, paying particular attention to lymph nodes, can point to metastatic involvement.

Baseline lab studies include complete blood count with differential, erythrocyte sedimentation rate, platelet count, liver function studies, and urinalysis. Depending on the depth of tumor invasion and metastatic spread, baseline diagnostic studies may also include chest X-ray, lung tomography, a computed tomography (CT) scan of the chest and abdomen, and a gallium scan. Signs of bone metastasis may call for a bone scan; CNS metastasis, a CT scan of the brain.

Treatment

A patient with malignant melanoma always requires surgical resection to remove the tumor. The extent of resection depends on the size and location of the primary lesion. Closure of a wide resection may necessitate a skin graft. If so, new plastic surgery techniques provide excellent cosmetic repair. Surgical treatment may also include regional lymphadenectomy.

Deep primary lesions may merit adjuvant chemotherapy and immunotherapy to eliminate or reduce the number of tumor cells. Although new drug therapies for primary and metastatic lesions are constantly being developed, their effectiveness awaits further clinical eval-

STAGING MELANOMA

Primary tumor (T)

T_0 Tumor confined to epidermis (Clark level I)
T_1 Tumor invades papillary dermis (level II), or tumor $\leq$ 0.75 mm thickness
T_2 Tumor extends to interface between papillary and reticular dermis (level III), or tumor of 0.76 to 1.5 mm thickness
T_3 Tumor extends into reticular dermis (level IV), or tumor of 1.51 to 4 mm thickness
T_4 Tumor invades subcutaneous tissue (level V), or tumor $\geq$ 4.1 mm thickness, or satellite within 2 cm of a primary melanoma

Nodal involvement (N)

N_0 No evidence of regional lymph node involvement
N_1 Movable nodes ($\leq$ 5 cm diameter), involving one regional lymph node station, or no regional lymph node involvement with less than five in-transit (between primary tumor and primary lymph node drainage site) metastases beyond 2 cm from primary site
N_2 Involvement of more than one regional lymph node station, or regional nodes more than 5 cm in diameter or fixed, or five or more in-transit metastases or any in-transit metastases beyond 2 cm from primary site with regional lymph node involvement

Distant metastasis (M)

M_0 No evidence of metastasis
M_1 Metastasis to skin or subcutaneous tissues beyond the site of primary lymph node drainage
M_2 Metastasis to any distant site other than skin or subcutaneous tissues

uation.

Radiation therapy is usually reserved for metastatic disease. It doesn't prolong survival but may reduce tumor size and relieve pain. Regardless of treatment, melanomas require close long-term follow-up to detect metastases and recurrences. Statistics show that 13% of recurrences develop more than 5 years after primary surgery.

RECOGNIZING POTENTIALLY MALIGNANT NEVI

Nevi (moles) are skin lesions that are often pigmented and may be hereditary. They begin to grow in childhood (occasionally they're congenital) and become more numerous in young adults. Up to 70% of patients with melanoma have a history of a preexisting nevus at the tumor site. Of these, approximately one third are reported to be congenital; the remainder develop later in life.

Changes in nevi (color, size, shape, texture, ulceration, bleeding, or itching) suggest possible malignant transformation. The presence or absence of hair within a nevus has no significance.

Types of Nevi:

- *Junctional nevi* are flat or slightly raised and light to dark brown, with melanocytes confined to the epidermis. Usually, they appear before age 40. These nevi may change into compound nevi if junctional nevus cells proliferate and penetrate into the dermis.
- *Compound nevi* are usually tan to dark brown and slightly raised, although size and color vary. They contain melanocytes in both the dermis and epidermis, and they rarely undergo malignant transformation. Excision is necessary only to rule out malignant transformation or for cosmetic reasons.
- *Dermal nevi* are elevated lesions from 2 to 10 mm in diameter, and vary in color from flesh to brown. They usually develop in older adults and generally arise on the upper part of the body. Excision is necessary only to rule out malignant transformation.
- *Blue nevi* are flat or slightly elevated lesions from 0.5 to 1 cm in diameter. They appear on the head, neck, arms, and dorsa of the hands and are twice as common in women as in men. Their blue color results from pigment and collagen in the dermis, which reflect blue light but absorb other wavelengths. Excision is necessary to rule out pigmented basal cell epithelioma or melanoma, or for cosmetic reasons.
- *Dysplastic nevi* are generally greater than 5 mm in diameter, with irregularly notched or indistinct borders. Coloration is usually a variable mixture of tan and brown, sometimes with red, pink, and black pigmentation. No two lesions are exactly alike. They occur in great numbers (typically over 100 at a time), never singly, usually appearing on the back, scalp, chest, and buttocks. Dysplastic nevi are potentially malignant, especially in patients with a personal or familial history of melanoma. Skin biopsy confirms diagnosis; treatment is by surgical excision, followed by regular physical examinations (every 6 months) to detect any new lesions or changes in existing lesions.
- *Lentigo maligna* (melanotic freckles, Hutchinson freckles) is a precursor to malignant melanoma. (In fact, about one third of them eventually give rise to malignant melanoma.) Usually, they occur in persons over age 40, especially on exposed skin areas such as the face. At first, these lesions are flat, tan spots, but they gradually enlarge and darken and develop black speckled areas against their tan or brown background. Each lesion may simultaneously enlarge in one area and regress in another. Histologic examination shows typical and atypical melanocytes along the epidermal basement membrane. Removal by simple excision (not electrodesiccation and curettage) is recommended.

Special considerations

Management of the melanoma patient requires careful physical, psychological, and social assessment. Preoperative teaching, meticulous postoperative care, and psychological support can make the patient more comfortable, speed recovery, and prevent complications.

- After diagnosis, review the doctor's explanation of treatment alternatives. Tell the patient what to expect before and after surgery, what the wound will look like, and what type of dressing he'll have. Warn him that the donor site for a skin graft may be as painful, if not more painful, than the tumor excision site itself. Honestly answer any questions he may have regarding surgery, chemotherapy, and radiation.
- After surgery, be careful to prevent infection. Check dressings often for excessive drainage, foul odor, redness, or swelling. If surgery included lymphadenectomy, minimize lymphedema by applying a compression stocking, and instruct the patient to keep the extremity elevated.
- During chemotherapy, know what side effects to expect and do what you can to minimize them. For instance, give an antiemetic, as ordered, to reduce nausea and vomiting.

To prepare the patient for discharge:

- Emphasize the need for close follow-up to detect recurrences early. Explain that recurrences and metastases, if they occur, are often delayed, so follow-up must continue for years. Tell him how to recognize signs of recurrence.
- Provide psychological support to help the patient cope with anxiety. Encourage him to verbalize his fears. Answer his questions honestly without destroying hope.

In advanced metastatic disease:

- Control and prevent pain with consistent, regularly scheduled administration of analgesics. *Don't* wait to relieve pain until after it occurs.
- Make referrals for home care, social services, and spiritual and financial assistance, as needed.
- If the patient is dying, identify the needs of patient, family, and friends, and provide appropriate support and care.

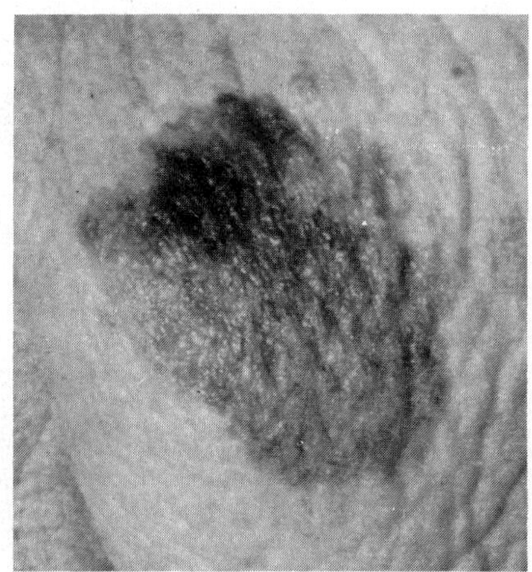

Lentigo maligna melanoma (LMM) of the cheek

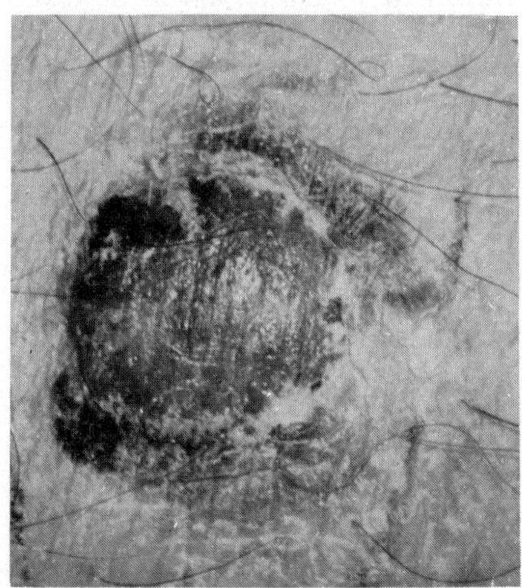

Superficial spreading melanoma (SSM) of the ankle

To help prevent malignant melanoma, stress the detrimental effects of overexposure to solar radiation, especially to fair-skinned, blue-eyed patients. Recommend that they use a sunblock or sunscreen. In all physical examinations, especially in fair-skinned persons, look for unusual nevi or other skin lesions.

BLOOD AND LYMPH

Hodgkin's Disease

Hodgkin's disease is a neoplastic disease characterized by painless, progressive enlargement of lymph nodes, spleen, and other lymphoid tissue resulting from proliferation of lymphocytes, histiocytes, eosinophils, and Reed-Sternberg giant cells. The latter cells are its special histologic feature. Untreated, Hodgkin's disease follows a variable but relentlessly progressive and ultimately fatal course. However, recent advances in therapy make Hodgkin's disease potentially curable, even in advanced stages, and appropriate treatment yields a 5-year survival rate of approximately 90% of patients.

Causes and incidence

The cause of Hodgkin's disease is unknown. It is most common in young adults, with a higher incidence in males than in females. It occurs in all races but is slightly more common in whites. Its incidence peaks in two age-groups: 15 to 38 and after age 50—except in Japan, where it occurs exclusively among people over 50.

Signs and symptoms

The first sign of Hodgkin's disease is usually a painless swelling of one of the cervical lymph nodes (but sometimes the axillary, mediastinal, or inguinal lymph nodes), occasionally in a patient who gives a history of recent upper respiratory infection. In older patients, the first symptoms may be nonspecific—persistent fever, night sweats, fatigue, weight loss, and malaise. Rarely, if the mediastinum is initially involved, Hodgkin's may produce respiratory symptoms.

Another early and characteristic indication of Hodgkin's disease is pruritus, which, while mild at first, becomes acute as the disease progresses. A rare symptom is the presence of the Pel-Ebstein fever pattern (intermittent fever of several days duration, alternating with afebrile periods). Other symptoms depend on the degree and location of systemic involvement.

Lymph nodes may enlarge rapidly, producing pain and obstruction, or enlarge slowly and painlessly for months or years. It's not unusual to see the lymph nodes "wax and wane," but they usually don't return to normal. Sooner or later, most patients develop systemic manifestations, including enlargement of retroperitoneal nodes and nodular infiltrations of the spleen, the liver, and bones. At this late stage other symptoms include edema of the face and neck, progressive anemia, possible jaundice, nerve pain, and increased susceptibility to infection.

Diagnosis

Diagnostic measures for confirming Hodgkin's disease include a thorough medical history and a complete physical examination, followed by a lymph node biopsy checking for Reed-Sternberg's abnormal histiocyte proliferation and nodular fibrosis and necrosis. Other appropriate diagnostic tests include bone marrow, liver, and spleen biopsies; and routine chest X-ray, abdominal computed tomography scan, lung scan, bone scan, and lymphangiography, to detect lymph node or organ involvement.

Hematologic tests show mild to severe normocytic anemia; normochromic anemia (in 50%); elevated, normal, or reduced white blood cell count and differential showing any combination of neutrophilia, lymphocytopenia, monocytosis, and eosinophilia. Elevated serum alkaline phosphatase indicates liver or bone involvement.

THE STAGES OF HODGKIN'S DISEASE

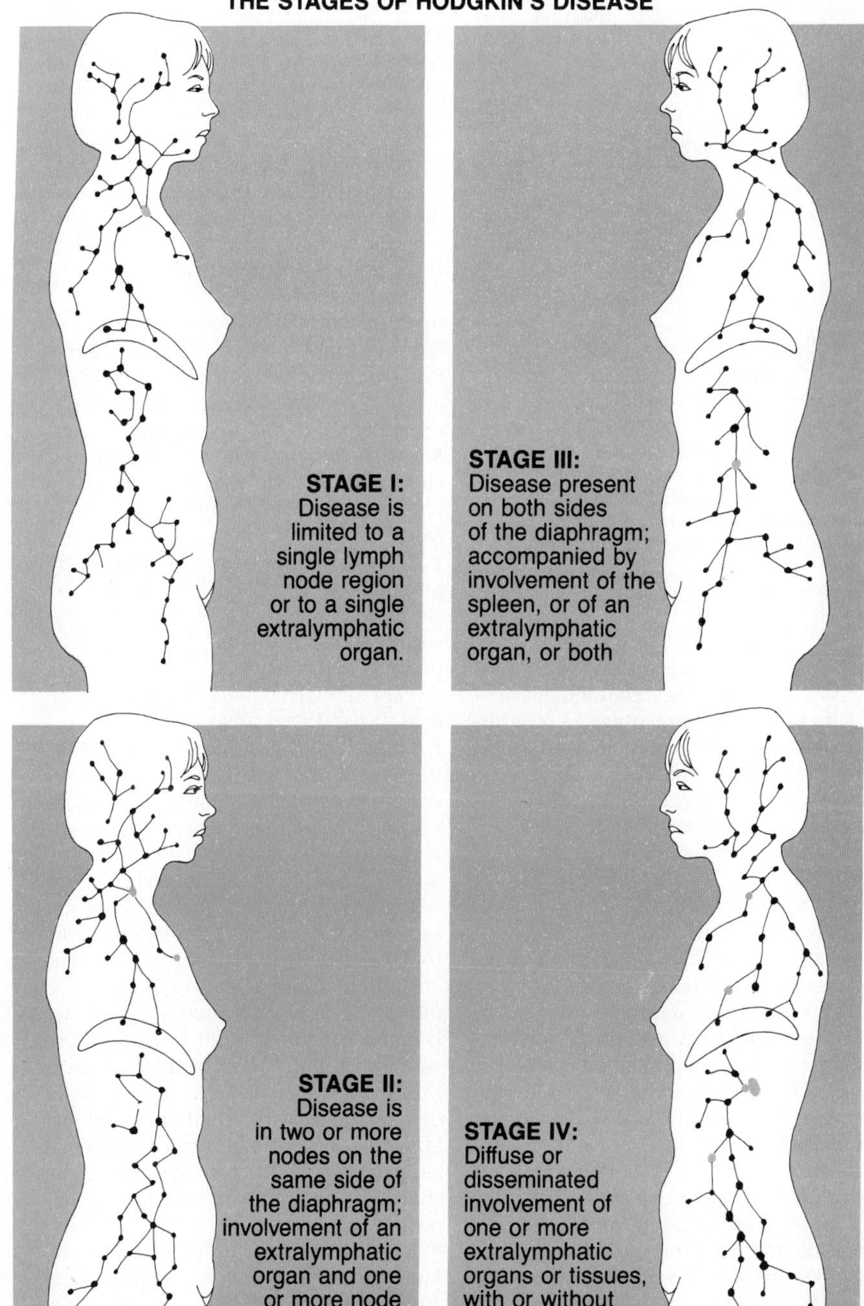

STAGE I:
Disease is limited to a single lymph node region or to a single extralymphatic organ.
STAGE III:
Disease present on both sides of the diaphragm; accompanied by involvement of the spleen, or of an extralymphatic organ, or both
STAGE II:
Disease is in two or more nodes on the same side of the diaphragm; involvement of an extralymphatic organ and one or more node regions, or of the spleen.
STAGE IV:
Diffuse or disseminated involvement of one or more extralymphatic organs or tissues, with or without associated lymph node involvement

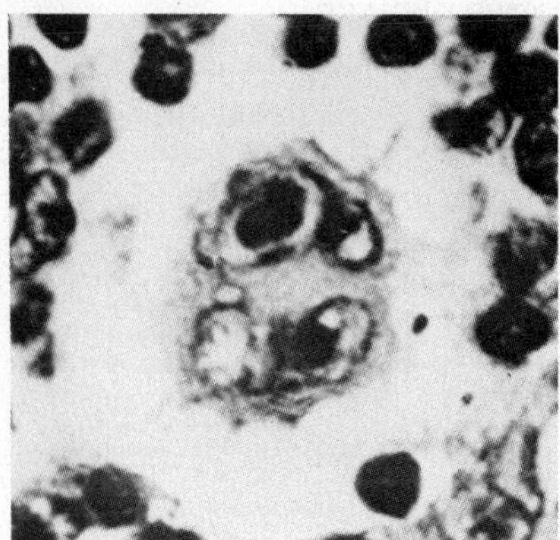

These enlarged, abnormal histocytes (Reed-Sternberg cells) from an excised lymph node suggest Hodgkin's disease. Note the large, distinct nucleoli. Reed-Sternberg cells indicate Hodgkin's disease when they coexist with one of these four histologic patterns: lymphocyte predominance, mixed cellularity, lymphocyte depletion, and nodular sclerosis.

The same diagostic tests are also used for staging. A staging laparotomy is necessary for patients under age 55 or without obvious Stage III or Stage IV disease, lymphocyte predominance subtype histology, or medical contraindications. Diagnosis must rule out other disorders that also enlarge the lymph nodes.

Treatment

Appropriate therapy (chemotherapy or radiation, or both, varying with the stage of the disease) depends on careful physical examination with accurate histologic interpretation and proper clinical staging. Correct treatment allows longer survival and even induces an apparent cure in many patients. Radiation therapy is used alone for Stage I and Stage II, and in combination with chemotherapy for Stage III. Chemotherapy is used for Stage IV, sometimes inducing a complete remission. Chemotherapy includes various combinations of mechlorethamine (nitrogen mustard), vincristine, procarbazine, prednisone, cyclophosphamide, vinblastine, carmustine, bleomycin, doxorubicin, and dacarbazine. The well-known MOPP protocol (mechlorethamine, vincristine [Oncovin], procarbazine, and prednisone) was the first to provide significant cures to patients with generalized Hodgkin's; another useful combination is ABVD (doxorubicin [Adriamycin], bleomycin, vinblastine, and dacarbazine). Treatment with these drugs may require concomitant antiemetics, sedatives, or antidiarrheals to combat gastrointestinal side effects.

Special considerations

Because many patients with Hodgkin's disease receive radiation or chemotherapy as outpatients, tell the patient to observe the following precautions:

- Watch for and report radiation and chemotherapy side effects (particularly anorexia, nausea, vomiting, and diarrhea).
- Minimize radiation side effects by maintaining good nutrition (aided by eating small, frequent meals of his favorite foods); drinking plenty of fluids; pacing his activities to counteract therapy-induced fatigue; and keeping the skin in irradiated areas dry.
- Control pain and bleeding of stomatitis by using a soft toothbrush, cotton swab, or anesthetic mouthwash such as viscous lidocaine (as prescribed); by applying petrolatum to his lips; and by avoiding astringent mouthwashes.
- If a woman patient is of childbearing age, advise her to delay pregnancy until prolonged remission, because radiation and chemotherapy can cause genetic mutations and spontaneous abortions. Because the patient with Hodgkin's disease has usually been healthy up until this point, he is likely to be especially distressed. Provide emotional support and offer appropriate counseling and reassurance. Ease the patient's anxiety by sharing your optimism about his prognosis.
- Make sure both the patient and his family know that the local chapter of the American Cancer Society is available for information, financial assistance, and supportive counseling.

Malignant Lymphomas

(Non-Hodgkin's lymphomas, lymphosarcomas)

Malignant lymphomas are a heterogeneous group of malignant diseases originating in lymph glands and other lymphoid tissue. Lymphomas are categorized by Rappaport histologic classification according to the degree of cellular differentiation and the presence or absence of nodularity. Nodular lymphomas yield a better prognosis than the diffuse form of the disease, but in both, prognosis is less hopeful than in Hodgkin's disease.

Causes and incidence

The cause of malignant lymphomas is unknown, although some theories suggest a viral source. Up to 8,000 new cases of malignant lymphomas appear annually in the United States alone. They're two to three times more common in males than in females, and occur in all age-groups. Although rare in children, they occur about one to three times more often and cause twice as many deaths as Hodgkin's disease in children under age 15. Incidence rises with increasing age (median age is 50). These lymphomas seem linked to racial or ethnic status, with increased incidence in whites and people of Jewish ancestry.

Signs and symptoms

Usually, the first indication of malignant lymphoma is swelling of the lymph glands, enlarged tonsils and adenoids, and painless, rubbery nodes in the cervical supraclavicular areas. In children, these nodes are usually in the cervical region, and the disease causes dyspnea and coughing. As the lymphoma progresses, the patient develops symptoms specific to the area involved and systemic complaints of fatigue, malaise, weight loss, fever, and night sweats.

Diagnosis

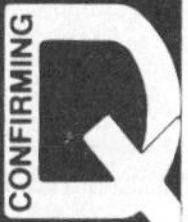

Diagnosis requires histologic evaluation of biopsied lymph nodes; of tonsils, bone marrow, liver, bowel, or skin; or, as needed, of tissue removed during exploratory laparotomy. (Biopsy differentiates malignant lymphoma from Hodgkin's disease.) Other relevant tests include bone and chest X-rays, lymphangiography, liver and spleen scan, computed tomography scan of the abdomen, and intravenous pyelography. Lab tests include complete blood count (may show anemia), uric acid (elevated or normal), serum calcium (elevated if bone lesions

STAGING MALIGNANT LYMPHOMA

Stage I: Involvement of a single lymph node region or of a single extralymphatic organ or site

Stage II: Involvement of two or more lymph node regions on the same side of the diaphragm, or localized involvement of an extralymphatic organ or site of one or more lymph node regions on the same side of the diaphragm

Stage III: Involvement of lymph node regions on both sides of the diaphragm, which may also be accompanied by localized involvement of extralymphatic organ or site or by involvement of the spleen or both

Stage IV: Diffuse or disseminated involvement of one or more extralymphatic organs or tissues with or without associated lymph node enlargement.

Reprinted from *Manual for Staging of Cancer* (Chicago: American Joint Committee for Cancer Staging and End Results Reporting, 1983). Used with permission.

are present), serum protein (normal), and liver function studies.

Treatment

Treatment for malignant lymphomas may include radiotherapy or chemotherapy. Radiotherapy is used mainly in the early localized stage of the disease. Total body irradiation is often effective for both nodular and diffuse histologies.

Chemotherapy is most effective with multiple combinations of antineoplastic agents. For example, cyclophosphamide, vincristine, and prednisone can induce a complete remission in 70% to 80% of patients with nodular histology and in 20% to 55% of patients with diffuse histology. Other combinations—such as bleomycin, Adriamycin, Cytoxan, vincristine (Oncovin), and prednisone (BACOP)—induce prolonged remission and possible cure in patients with diffuse histology.

Special considerations

- Observe the patient who's receiving radiation or chemotherapy for side effects (anorexia, nausea, vomiting, diarrhea). Consult with the dietitian, and plan small, frequent meals scheduled around the patient's treatment and including his favorite foods.
- If the patient can't tolerate oral feedings, administer I.V. fluids and, if necessary, give antiemetics and sedatives, as ordered.
- Instruct the patient to keep irradiated skin dry.
- Provide emotional support by informing the patient and family about the prognosis and diagnosis and by listening to their concerns. If needed, refer them to the local chapter of the American Cancer Society for information and counseling. Stress the need for continued treatment and follow-up care.

Mycosis Fungoides

(Malignant cutaneous reticulosis, granuloma fungoides)

Mycosis fungoides (MF) is a rare, chronic malignant T-cell lymphoma of unknown cause that originates in the reticuloendothelial system of the skin, eventually affecting lymph nodes and internal organs. In the United States, it strikes over 1,000 patients of all races annually; most are between ages 40 and 60. Unlike other lymphomas, MF allows an average life expectancy of 7 to 10 years after diagnosis. If correctly treated, particularly before it has spread past the skin, MF may go into remission for many years. However, after MF has reached the tumor stage, progression to severe disability or death is rapid.

Signs and symptoms

The first sign of MF may be generalized erythroderma, possibly associated with itching. Eventually, MF evolves into varied combinations of infiltrated, thickened, or scaly patches, tumors, or ulcerations.

Diagnosis

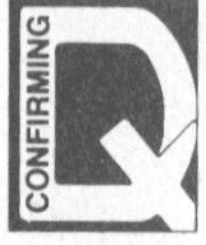

A clear diagnosis of mycosis fungoides depends on a history of multiple, varied, and progressively severe skin lesions associated with characteristic histologic evidence of lymphoma cell infiltration of the skin, with or without involvement of lymph nodes or visceral organs. Consequently, this diagnosis is often missed during the early stages until lymphoma cells are sufficiently numerous in the skin to show up in biopsy.

Other diagnostic tests help confirm mycosis fungoides: complete blood count and differential; a finger stick smear for Sézary cells (abnormal circulating lymphocytes), which may be present in the erythrodermic variants of MF (Sézary syndrome); blood chemistries to screen for visceral dysfunction; chest X-ray; liver-spleen isotopic scanning; lymphangiography; and lymph node biopsy to assess histologic involvement. These tests also help to stage the disease—a necessary prerequisite to treatment.

STAGING MYCOSIS FUNGOIDES

Magnitude of skin involvement (T):
T_0 Clinically or histopathologically suspicious lesions
T_1 Premycotic lesions, papules, or plaques involving less than 10% of the skin surface
T_2 Premycotic lesions, papules, or plaques involving more than 10% of the skin surface
T_3 One or more tumors of the skin
T_4 Extensive, often generalized erythroderma

Status of peripheral lymph nodes (N):
N_0 Clinically normal; no pathologic involvement
N_1 Clinically abnormal; no pathologic involvement
N_2 Clinically normal; pathologic involvement
N_3 Clinically abnormal; pathologic involvement

Status of visceral organs (M):
M_0 No pathologic involvement
M_1 Pathologic involvement

Treatment

Depending on the stage of the disease and its rate of progression, past treatment and results, the patient's age and overall health, treatment facilities available, and other factors, treatment of MF may include topical, intralesional, or systemic corticosteroid therapy; phototherapy; methoxsalen photochemotherapy; radiation; topical, intralesional, or systemic mechlorethamine hydrochloride; and other systemic chemotherapy.

Application of topical mechlorethamine hydrochloride (nitrogen mustard) is the preferred treatment for inducing remission in pretumorous stages. Preliminary I.V. infusions of small amounts of mechlorethamine hydrochloride are given before beginning this treatment to reduce the risk of allergic sensitization. However, the value of this practice hasn't been definitely established.

Total body electron beam radiation, which is less toxic to internal organs than standard photon beam radiation, has induced remission in some patients with early-stage MF.

Chemotherapy is employed primarily for patients with advanced-stage MF; chemotherapeutic agents used include cyclophosphamide, chlorambucil, methotrexate (with or without folinic acid rescue), doxorubicin, vincristine, and bleomycin.

Special considerations

- If the patient applying nitrogen mustard has difficulty reaching all skin surfaces, give assistance. But wear gloves to prevent contact sensitization.
- If the patient is receiving drug treatment, report side effects, particularly infection, immediately.
- If the patient is receiving radiation, he'll probably develop alopecia and erythema. Suggest that he wear a wig to boost his self-image until hair regrowth begins, and suggest or give medicated oil baths to ease erythema.
- Since pruritus is often worse at night, the patient may need larger bedtime doses of antipruritics or sedatives, as ordered, to ensure a good night's sleep. When the patient has had a difficult night's sleep, postpone early morning care to allow him more sleep.
- The patient with pruritus has an overwhelming need to scratch—often to the point of removing epidermis and replacing pruritus with pain, which some patients find easier to endure. Realize that you can't keep such a patient from scratching; the best you can do is help minimize the damage. Advise the patient to keep fingernails short and clean and to wear a pair of white gloves when itching is unbearable.
- The malignant skin lesions are likely

to make the patient depressed, fearful, and self-conscious. Fully explain the disease and its stages to help the patient and family understand and accept the disease. Provide reassurance and support by demonstrating a positive but realistic attitude. Reinforce your verbal support by touching the patient without any hint of anxiety or distaste.

Acute Leukemia

Acute leukemia is a malignant proliferation of white blood cell precursors (blasts) in bone marrow or lymph tissue and their accumulation in peripheral blood, bone marrow, and body tissues. Its most common forms are acute lymphoblastic (lymphocytic) leukemia (ALL), abnormal growth of lymphocyte precursors (lymphoblasts); acute myeloblastic (myelogenous) leukemia (AML), rapid accumulation of myeloid precursors (myeloblasts); and acute monoblastic (monocytic) leukemia, or Schilling's type, marked increase in monocyte precursors (monoblasts). Other variants include acute myelomonocytic leukemia and acute erythroleukemia.

Untreated, acute leukemia is invariably fatal, usually because of complications that result from leukemic cell infiltration of bone marrow or vital organs. With treatment, prognosis varies. In ALL, treatment induces remissions in 90% of children (average survival time: 5 years) and in 65% of adults (average survival time: 1 to 2 years). Children between ages 2 and 8 have the best survival rate—about 50%—with intensive therapy. In AML, the average survival time is only 1 year after diagnosis, even with aggressive treatment. In acute monoblastic leukemia, treatment induces remissions lasting 2 to 10 months in 50% of children; adults survive only about 1 year after diagnosis, even with treatment.

Causes and incidence

Research on predisposing factors isn't conclusive but points to some combination of viruses (viral remnants have been found in leukemic cells), genetic and immunologic factors, and exposure to radiation and certain chemicals.

Pathogenesis isn't clearly understood, but immature, nonfunctioning white blood cells (WBCs) appear to accumulate first in the tissue where they originate (lymphocytes in lymph tissue, granulocytes in bone marrow). These immature WBCs then spill into the bloodstream and from there infiltrate other tissues, eventually causing organ malfunction because of encroachment or hemorrhage.

Acute leukemia is more common in males than in females, in whites (especially people of Jewish descent), in children (between ages 2 and 5; 80% of all leukemias in this age-group are ALL), and in persons who live in urban and industrialized areas. Acute leukemia ranks 20th in causes of cancer-related deaths among people of all age-groups. Among children, however, it's the most common form of cancer. In the United States, an estimated 11,000 persons develop acute leukemia annually.

Signs and symptoms

Signs of acute leukemia are sudden onset of high fever accompanied by thrombocytopenia and abnormal bleeding, such as nosebleeds, gingival bleeding, purpura, ecchymoses, petechiae, easy bruising after minor trauma, and prolonged menses. Nonspecific symptoms, such as low-grade fever, weakness, and lassitude, may persist for days or months before visible symptoms appear. Other insidious signs include pallor, chills, and recurrent infections. In addition, ALL, AML, and acute monoblastic leukemia may cause dyspnea, anemia, fatigue, malaise, tachycardia, palpitations, systolic ejection murmur, and abdominal or bone pain. When leukemic cells cross the blood-brain barrier and escape the effects of systemic chemotherapy, the patient may develop meningeal leukemia (confusion, lethargy, headache).

Diagnosis

Typical clinical findings and bone marrow aspirate showing a proliferation of immature WBCs confirm acute leukemia. An aspirate that's dry or free of leukemic cells in a patient with typical clinical findings requires bone marrow biopsy, usually of the posterior superior iliac spine. Blood counts show thrombocytopenia and neutropenia. Differential leukocyte count determines cell type. Lumbar puncture detects meningeal involvement.

Treatment

Systemic chemotherapy aims to eradicate leukemic cells and induce remission (restore normal bone marrow function). Chemotherapy varies:

- Meningeal leukemia—intrathecal instillation of methotrexate or cytarabine with cranial radiation
- ALL—vincristine and/or prednisone with intrathecal methotrexate or cytarabine; I.V. asparaginase, daunorubicin, and doxorubicin. Maintenance is with mercaptopurine and methotrexate.
- AML—a combination of I.V. daunorubicin or doxorubicin, cytarabine, and oral thioguanine; or, if these fail to induce remission, a combination of cyclophosphamide, vincristine, prednisone, or methotrexate; high-dose cytarabine alone or with other drugs; amsacrine; and 5-azacytidine and mitoxantrone (both investigational). Maintenance treatment is with additional chemotherapy.
- Acute monoblastic leukemia—cytarabine and thioguanine with daunorubicin or doxorubicin.

Bone marrow transplant is now possible in some cases. Treatment also may include antibiotic, antifungal, and antiviral drugs and granulocyte injections to control infection, platelet transfusions to prevent bleeding, and red blood cell transfusions to prevent anemia.

Special considerations

The care plan for the leukemic patient should emphasize patient comfort, minimize the side effects of chemotherapy, promote preservation of veins, manage complications, and provide psychological support and patient education. Because so many of these patients are children, be especially sensitive to their emotional needs and those of their families. Before treatment begins:

- Explain the disease course, treatment and side effects.

PREDISPOSING FACTORS IN ACUTE LEUKEMIA

Although the exact causes of most leukemias remain unknown, increasing evidence suggests a combination of contributing factors:

Acute lymphoblastic leukemia
- familial tendency
- monozygotic twins
- congenital disorders, such as Down's syndrome, Bloom's syndrome, Fanconi's anemia, ataxia-telangiectasia, and congenital agammaglobulinemia
- viruses

Acute myeloblastic leukemia
- familial tendency
- monozygotic twins
- congenital disorders, such as Down's syndrome, Bloom's syndrome, Fanconi's anemia, ataxia-telangiectasia, and congenital agammaglobulinemia
- ionizing radiation
- exposure to the chemical benzene and cytotoxins, such as alkylating agents
- viruses

Acute monoblastic leukemia
- unknown (irradiation, exposure to chemicals, heredity, and infections show little correlation to this disease)

• Teach the patient and his family how to recognize infection (fever, chills, cough, sore throat) and abnormal bleeding (bruising, petechiae), and how to stop such bleeding (pressure, ice to area).
• Promote good nutrition. Explain that chemotherapy may cause weight loss and anorexia, so encourage the patient to eat and drink high-calorie, high-protein foods and beverages. However, chemotherapy and adjunctive prednisone may cause weight gain, so dietary counseling and teaching are helpful.
• Help establish an appropriate rehabilitation program for the patient during remission.

Plan meticulous supportive care:
• Watch for signs of meningeal leukemia (confusion, lethargy, headache). If these occur, know how to manage care after intrathecal chemotherapy. After such instillation, place the patient in the Trendelenburg position for 30 minutes. Force fluids, and keep the patient supine for 4 to 6 hours. Check the lumbar puncture site often for bleeding. If the patient receives cranial radiation, teach him about potential side effects, and do what you can to minimize them.
• Prevent hyperuricemia, a possible result of rapid chemotherapy-induced leukemic cell lysis. Force fluids to about 2 liters daily, and give acetazolamide, $NaHCO_3$ tablets, and allopurinol. Check urine pH often—it should be above 7.5. Watch for rash or other hypersensitivity reaction to allopurinol.
• Watch for early signs of cardiotoxicity, such as dysrhythmias, and signs of heart failure if the patient receives daunorubicin or doxorubicin.
• Control infection by placing the patient in a private room and imposing re-

TYPES OF LEUKEMIA

GENERAL CLASS	SUBCLASS AND CELL TYPE	HISTOCHEMISTRY OR OTHER FEATURES	PROGNOSIS
Acute leukemias	• Subclass: acute lymphatic (ALL) • Cell: lymphoblasts	• Sudan black and PAS +	• Children (2 to 8 years): 50% cured, 90% show response to therapy • Adults: average survival 2 years
	• Subclass: acute myeloblastic (AML) • Cell: myeloblasts	• Peroxidase +	• Adults (15 to 75 years): response to therapy 65% • Average survival 1 year
	• Subclass: acute monoblastic (monocytic) (AMOL) • Cell: monoblasts	• Muramidase +	• Children: response to therapy 50% • Adults: average survival 1 year
Chronic leukemias	• Subclass: chronic granulocytic (CGL) • Cell: granulocytic precursors	• Ph^1 chromosome • Low LAP	• After chronic phase: 3 to 4 years • After acute phase: 3 to 6 months
	• Subclass: lymphocytic • Cell: B type	• Immunoglobulin or surface markers	• Average survival 5 years

verse isolation, if necessary. (The benefits of reverse isolation are controversial.) Coordinate patient care so the leukemic patient doesn't come in contact with staff who also care for patients with infections or infectious diseases. Avoid using Foley catheters and giving I.M. injections, since they provide an avenue for infection. Screen staff and visitors for contagious diseases, and watch for and report any signs of infection.

- Provide thorough skin care by keeping the patient's skin and perianal area clean, applying mild lotions or creams to keep skin from drying and cracking, and thoroughly cleaning skin before all invasive skin procedures. Change I.V. tubing according to your hospital's policy. Use strict aseptic technique and a metal scalp vein needle (metal butterfly needle) when starting I.V.s. If the patient receives total parenteral nutrition, give scrupulous subclavian catheter care.
- Monitor temperature every 4 hours; patients with fever over 101° F and decreased WBC counts should receive prompt antibiotic therapy.
- Watch for bleeding; if it occurs, apply ice compresses and pressure, and elevate the extremity. Avoid giving I.M. injections, aspirin, and aspirin-containing drugs. Also avoid taking rectal temperatures, giving rectal suppositories, and doing digital examinations.
- Prevent constipation by providing adequate hydration, a high-residue diet, stool softeners, and mild laxatives, and by encouraging walking.
- Control mouth ulceration by checking often for obvious ulcers and gum swelling and by providing frequent mouth care and saline rinses. Tell the patient to use a soft toothbrush and to avoid hot, spicy foods and overuse of commercial mouthwashes. Also check the rectal area daily for induration, swelling, erythema, skin discoloration, or drainage.
- Provide psychological support by establishing a trusting relationship to promote communication. Allow the patient and his family to verbalize their anger and depression. Let the family participate in his care as much as possible.
- Minimize stress by providing a calm, quiet atmosphere that's conducive to rest and relaxation. For children particularly, be flexible with patient care and visiting hours to promote maximum interaction with family and friends and to allow time for schoolwork and play.
- For those patients who are refractory to chemotherapy and in the terminal phase of the disease, supportive nursing care is directed to comfort; management of pain, fever, and bleeding; and patient and family support. Provide the opportunity for religious counseling. Discuss the option of home or hospice care.

Chronic Granulocytic Leukemia

(Chronic myelogenous [or myelocytic] leukemia [CML])

Chronic granulocytic leukemia (CGL) is characterized by the abnormal overgrowth of granulocytic precursors (myeloblasts, promyelocytes, metamyelocytes, and myelocytes) in bone marrow, peripheral blood, and body tissues. CGL is most common in young and middle-aged adults and is slightly more common in men than in women; it is rare in children. In the United States, approximately 3,000 to 4,000 cases of CGL develop annually, accounting for roughly 20% of all leukemias.

CGL's clinical course proceeds in two distinct phases: the insidious chronic phase, *with anemia and bleeding abnormalities and, eventually, the* acute phase (blastic crisis), *in which myeloblasts, the most primitive granulocytic precursors, proliferate rapidly. This disease is invariably fatal. Average survival time is 3 to 4 years after onset of the chronic phase and 3 to 6 months after onset of the acute phase.*

Causes

Almost 90% of patients with CGL have the Philadelphia (Ph^1) chromosome, an abnormality discovered in 1960 in which the long arm of chromosome 22 is translocated, usually to chromosome 9. Radiation and carcinogenic chemicals may induce this chromosome abnormality. Myeloproliferative diseases also seem to increase the incidence of CGL, and some clinicians suspect that an unidentified virus causes this disease.

Signs and symptoms

Typically, CGL induces the following clinical effects:

- anemia (fatigue, weakness, decreased exercise tolerance, pallor, dyspnea, tachycardia, and headache)
- thrombocytopenia, with resulting bleeding and clotting disorders (retinal hemorrhage, ecchymoses, hematuria, melena, bleeding gums, nosebleeds, and easy bruising)
- hepatosplenomegaly, with abdominal discomfort and pain in splenic infarction from leukemic cell infiltration.

Other symptoms include sternal and rib tenderness from leukemic infiltrations of the periosteum; low-grade fever; weight loss; anorexia; renal calculi or gouty arthritis from increased uric acid excretion; occasionally, prolonged infection and ankle edema; and, rarely, priapism and vascular insufficiency.

Diagnosis

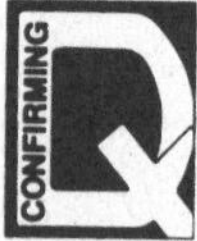

In patients with typical clinical changes, chromosomal analysis of peripheral blood or bone marrow showing the Philadelphia chromosome and low leukocyte alkaline phosphatase levels confirm CGL. Other relevant lab results show:

- white blood cell abnormalities: leukocytosis (leukocytes more than 50,000/mm^3, ranging as high as 250,000/mm^3), occasional leukopenia (leukocytes less than 5,000/mm^3), neutropenia (neutrophils less than 1,500/mm^3) despite high leukocyte count, and increased circulating myeloblasts
- hemoglobin: often below 10 g
- hematocrit: low (less than 30%)
- platelets: thrombocytopenia common (less than 50,000/mm^3), but platelet levels may be normal or elevated
- serum uric acid: possibly more than 8 mg
- bone marrow aspirate or biopsy: hypercellular, shows bone marrow infiltration by increased number of myeloid elements (biopsy is done only if aspirate is dry); in the acute phase, myeloblasts predominate.

Treatment

Control of abnormal myeloid proliferation requires rigorous chemotherapy. During the chronic phase, outpatient chemotherapy induces excellent remissions; it is often continued at lower doses during remissions. Such chemotherapy usually includes busulfan and, occasionally, melphalan, other nitrogen mustards, thioguanine, and hydroxyurea.

Ancillary treatments may include:

- local splenic radiation to reduce peripheral blood counts and splenic size, or splenectomy (controversial)
- leukapheresis (selective leukocyte removal) to reduce leukocyte count
- bone marrow transplant
- allopurinol to prevent hyperuricemia or colchicine to relieve gouty attacks caused by elevated serum uric acid
- prompt treatment of infections that may result from chemotherapy-induced bone marrow suppression.

During the acute phase, treatment is the same as for acute myeloblastic leukemia (although it is less likely to induce remission) and emphasizes supportive measures and chemotherapy with doxorubicin or daunorubicin, thioguanine, cyclophosphamide, vincristine, methotrexate, cytarabine, or daunorubicin with prednisone. Despite vigorous treatment, CGL is rapidly fatal after onset of the acute phase.

Special considerations

In patients with CGL, meticulous supportive care, psychological support, and careful patient teaching help make the most of remissions and minimize complications. When the disease is diagnosed, be prepared to repeat and reinforce the doctor's explanation of the disease and its treatment to the patient and his family.

Throughout the chronic phase of CGL when the patient is hospitalized:

- If the patient has persistent anemia, plan your care to help avoid exhaustion. Schedule lab tests and physical care with frequent rest periods in between, and assist the patient with walking, if necessary. Regularly check the patient's skin and mucous membranes for pallor, petechiae, and bruising.
- To minimize bleeding, suggest a soft-bristle toothbrush, an electric razor, and other safety precautions.
- To minimize the abdominal discomfort of splenomegaly, provide small, frequent meals. For the same reason, prevent constipation with a stool softener or laxative, as needed. Ask the dietary department to provide a high-bulk diet, and maintain adequate fluid intake.
- To prevent atelectasis, stress the need for coughing and deep breathing exercises.

Because the patient with CGL often receives outpatient chemotherapy throughout the chronic phase, sound patient teaching is essential:

- Explain expected side effects of chemotherapy; pay particular attention to dangerous side effects, such as bone marrow suppression.
- Tell the patient to watch for and immediately report signs and symptoms of infection: any fever over 100° F. (37.7° C.), chills, redness or swelling, sore throat, and cough.
- Instruct the patient to watch for signs of thrombocytopenia, to immediately apply ice and pressure to any external bleeding site, and to avoid aspirin and aspirin-containing compounds because of the risk of increased bleeding.
- Emphasize the importance of adequate rest to minimize the fatigue of anemia. To minimize the toxic effects of chemotherapy, stress the importance of a high-calorie, high-protein diet.

For more information on treatment during the acute phase, see ACUTE LEUKEMIA, pages 130 to 133.

Chronic Lymphocytic Leukemia

A generalized, progressive disease that is common in the elderly, chronic lymphocytic leukemia is marked by an uncontrollable spread of abnormal, small lymphocytes in lymphoid tissue, blood, and bone marrow. Nearly all patients with chronic lymphocytic leukemia are men over age 50. According to the American Cancer Society, chronic lymphocytic leukemia accounts for almost one third of new leukemia cases annually.

Causes

Although the cause of chronic lymphocytic leukemia is unknown, researchers suspect hereditary factors (higher incidence has been recorded within families), still-undefined chromosome abnormalities, and certain immunologic defects (such as ataxia-telangiectasia or acquired agammaglobulinemia). The disease does not seem to be associated with radiation exposure.

Signs and symptoms

Chronic lymphocytic leukemia is the most benign and the most slowly progressive form of leukemia. Clinical signs derive from the infiltration of leukemic cells in bone marrow, lymphoid tissue, and organ systems.

In early stages, patients usually complain of fatigue, malaise, fever, and nodal enlargement. They're particularly susceptible to infection.

In advanced stages, patients may experience severe fatigue and weight loss, with liver or spleen enlargement, bone tenderness, and edema from lymph node obstruction. Pulmonary infiltrates may appear when lung parenchyma is involved. Skin infiltrations, manifested by macular to nodular eruptions, occur in about half the cases of chronic lymphocytic leukemia.

As the disease progresses, bone marrow involvement may lead to anemia, pallor, weakness, dyspnea, tachycardia, palpitations, bleeding, and infection. Opportunistic fungal, viral, and bacterial infections commonly occur in late stages.

Diagnosis

Typically, chronic lymphocytic leukemia is an incidental finding during a routine blood test that reveals numerous abnormal lymphocytes. In early stages, white blood cell (WBC) count is mildly but persistently elevated. Granulocytopenia is the rule, but the WBC count climbs as the disease progresses. Blood studies also show hemoglobin count under 11 g, hypogammaglobulinemia, and depressed serum globulins. Other common developments include neutropenia (under 1,500/mm^3), lymphocytosis (over 10,000/mm^3), and thrombocytopenia (under 150,000/mm^3). Bone marrow aspiration and biopsy show lymphocytic invasion.

Treatment

Systemic chemotherapy includes alkylating agents, usually chlorambucil or cyclophosphamide, and sometimes steroids (prednisone) when autoimmune hemolytic anemia or thrombocytopenia occurs.

When chronic lymphocytic leukemia causes obstruction or organ impairment or enlargement, local radiation treatment can be used to reduce organ size. Allopurinol can be given to prevent hyperuricemia, a relatively uncommon finding.

Prognosis is poor if anemia, thrombocytopenia, neutropenia, bulky lymphadenopathy, and severe lymphocytosis are present. Gross bone marrow replacement by abnormal lymphocytes is the most common cause of death, usually within 4 to 5 years after diagnosis.

Special considerations

- Plan patient care to relieve symptoms and prevent infection. Clean the patient's skin daily with mild soap and water. Frequent soaks may be ordered. Watch for signs of infection: temperature over 100° F. (37.7° C.), chills, redness, or swelling of any body part.
- Watch for signs of thrombocytopenia (black tarry stools, easy bruising, nosebleeds, bleeding gums) and anemia (pale skin, weakness, fatigue, dizziness, palpitations). Advise the patient to avoid aspirin and products containing aspirin. Explain that many medications contain aspirin, even though their names don't make this clear. Teach him how to recognize aspirin variants on medication labels.
- Explain chemotherapy and its possible side effects. If the patient is to be discharged, tell him to avoid coming in contact with obviously ill persons, especially children with common contagious childhood diseases. Urge him to eat high-protein food and drink high-calorie beverages.
- Stress the importance of follow-up care, frequent blood tests, and taking all medications exactly as prescribed. Teach the patient the signs of recurrence (swollen lymph nodes in the neck, axilla, and groin; increased abdominal size or discomfort), and tell him to notify his doctor immediately if he detects any of these signs.
- Provide emotional support and be a good listener. Most patients with chronic lymphocytic leukemia are elderly; some are frightened. Try to keep their spirits up by concentrating on little things like improving their personal appearance, providing pleasant environment, asking questions about their families. If possible, provide opportunities for their favorite activities.

Selected References

Bouchard, Rosemary, and Owens, Norma F. *Nursing Care of the Cancer Patient,* 3rd ed. St. Louis: C.V. Mosby Co., 1976.

Casciato, Dennis A., and Bennett, B.B. Lowitz. *Manual of Bedside Oncology.* Boston: Little, Brown & Co., 1983.

Cooper, J. *Concepts in Cancer Care.* Philadelphia: Lea & Febiger, 1980.

Cooper, Richard G., et al. "Adjuvant Chemotherapy of Breast Cancer," *Journal of Cancer* 44:793-98, September 1979.

Coppleson, Malcolm. *Gynecologic Oncology: Fundamental Principles and Clinical Practice.* New York: Churchill Livingstone, 1981.

Doubilet, P., et al. "Treatment Choice in Gastric Carcinoma. A Decision-Analytic Approach," *Medical Decision Making* 2(3):261-74, 1982.

DeVita, V. T., Jr., and Hellman, S. *Cancer: Principles and Practices of Oncology.* Philadelphia: J.B. Lippincott Co., 1982.

DiSaia, Philip J., and Creasman, William T. *Clinical Gynecologic Oncology.* St. Louis: C.V. Mosby Co., 1981.

Donovan, M., and Pierce, S. *Cancer Care Nursing.* East Norwalk, Conn.: Appleton-Century-Crofts, 1984.

Dorr, R. and Fritz, W. *Cancer Chemotherapy Handbook.* New York: Elsevier Science Publishing Co., 1980.

Douglass, H.O. "Gastric Cancer: How We Can Improve Survival," *Consultant* (10):177-93, October 23, 1983.

Green, P.H.R., et al. "Early Gastric Cancer," *Gastroenterology* 81(2):247-56, August 1981.

Henderson, I. Craig, and Canellos, George P. "Cancer of the Breast," *New England Journal of Medicine* 302:17-30, January 3, 1980.

Holland, J., and Frei, E. *Cancer Medicine.* Philadelphia: Lea & Febiger, 1982.

Kurtz, R. and Owens, N. *The Cancer Patient.* St. Louis: C.V. Mosby Co., 1981.

Lynch, H., et al. "Hereditary Cancer: Ascertainment and Management," *CA-A Cancer Journal for Clinicians* 29:216-32, July/August 1979.

Marino, Lisa Begg. *Cancer Nursing.* St. Louis: C.V. Mosby Co., 1981.

Plum, Fred, and Posner, Jerome. *The Diagnosis of Stupor and Coma,* 3rd ed. Philadelphia: F.A. Davis, 1983.

Rudy, Ellen B., *Advanced Neurologic and Neurosurgical Nursing.* St. Louis: C.V. Mosby Co., 1984.

Vogt, G., et al. *Manual of Neurosurgical Care.* St. Louis: C.V. Mosby Co., 1985.

Williams, W., et al. *Hematology,* 2nd ed. New York: McGraw-Hill Book Co., 1977.

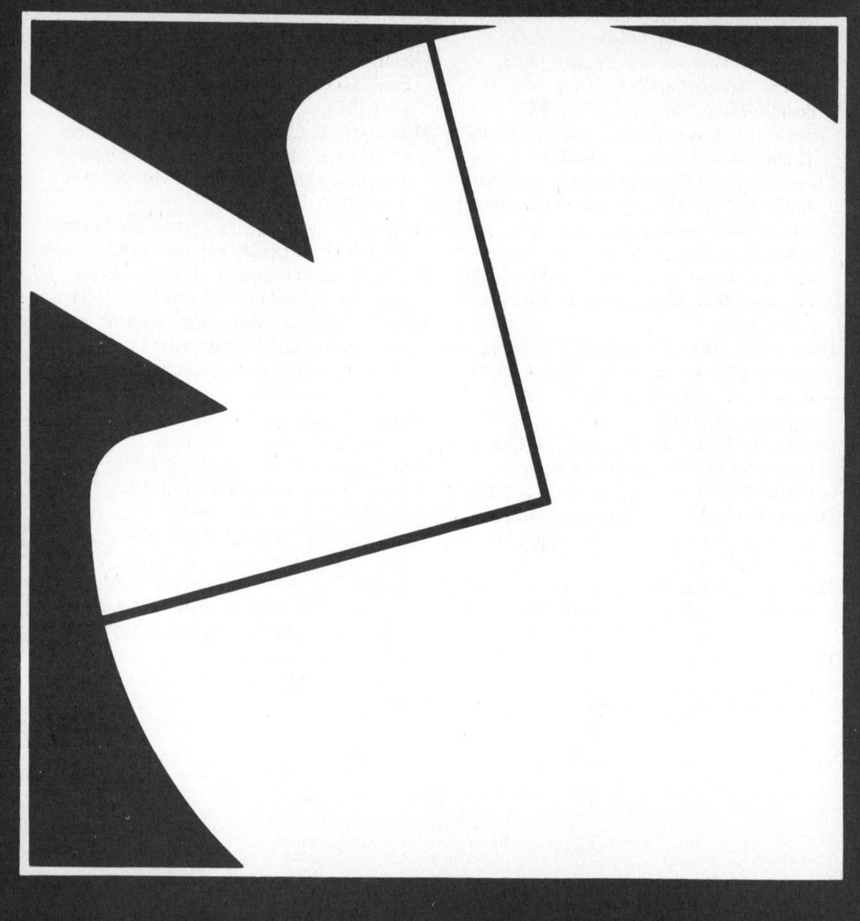

3 Infection

Infection

Introduction

Despite improved methods of treating and preventing infection—potent antibiotics, complex immunizations, and modern sanitation—infection still accounts for much serious illness, even in highly industrialized countries. In developing countries, infection is one of the most critical health problems.

What is infection?

Infection is the invasion and multiplication of microorganisms in or on body tissue that produce signs and symptoms as well as an immunologic response. Such reproduction injures the host by causing cellular damage from microorganism-produced toxins or intracellular multiplication, or by competing with host metabolism. The host's own immune response may compound the tissue damage; such damage may be localized (as in infected decubitus ulcers) or systemic. The severity of the infection varies with the pathogenicity and number of the invading microorganisms, and the strength of host defenses.

Why are the microorganisms that cause infectious diseases so hard to overcome? There are many complex reasons:

- Some bacteria—especially gram-negative bacilli—develop resistance to antibiotics.
- Some microorganisms—such as the influenza virus—include so many different strains that a single vaccine can't provide protection against them all.
- Most viruses resist antiviral drugs.
- Some microorganisms localize in areas that make treatment difficult, such as the central nervous system and bone.

Moreover, certain factors that contribute to improved health—such as the affluence that allows good nutrition and living conditions, and advances in medical science—can increase the risk of infection. For example, travel can expose persons to diseases for which they have little natural immunity. The expanded use of immunosuppressives, surgery, and other invasive procedures increases the risk of infection.

Kinds of infections

A laboratory-verified infection that causes no signs and symptoms is called a *subclinical*, *silent*, or *asymptomatic* infection. A multiplication of microbes that produces no signs, symptoms, or immune responses is called a *colonization*. A person with a subclinical infection or colonization may be a carrier and transmit infection to others. A *latent* infection occurs after a microorganism has been dormant in the host, sometimes for years. An *exogenous* infection results from environmental pathogens; an *endogenous* infection, from the host's normal flora (for instance, *Escherichia coli* displaced from the colon, which causes urinary tract infection).

The varied forms of microorganisms responsible for infectious diseases include bacteria, viruses, rickettsiae, chlamydiae, spirochetes, fungi (yeasts and molds), and protozoa; larger organisms, such as helminths (worms), may also cause disease.

Bacteria are single-cell microorganisms with well-defined cell walls, that can grow independently on artificial media without the need for other cells. In developing countries, where poor sanitation potentiates infection, bacterial diseases are prevalent sources of death and disability. In industrialized countries, bacterial infections are the most common fatal infectious diseases.

Bacteria can be classified according to shape. Spherical bacterial cells are called *cocci*; rod-shaped bacteria, *bacilli*; and spiral-shaped bacteria, *spirilla*. They can also be classified according to their response to staining (gram-positive, gram-negative, or acid-fast bacteria), their motility (motile or nonmotile bacteria), tendency to capsulation (encapsulated or nonencapsulated bacteria), and their capacity to form spores (sporulating or nonsporulating bacteria).

EPIDEMIOLOGY DEFINED

Epidemiology is the dynamic study of various factors as they relate to the occurrence, frequency, and distribution of disease in a given population. This includes the origin of the disease, how it's transmitted, and host and environmental factors that influence the development of the disease. Several terms describe the occurrence or frequency of a disease. In an *epidemic*, a disease occurs at a level that is higher than normal. An *outbreak*, however, is a sudden appearance of the disease, often in a small portion of the population. An *endemic* disease is persistently present in a given locale; a *hyperendemic* disease is persistent and has a high incidence. *Reservoir* refers to the natural habitat of the organism responsible for the disease; *source*, to the site (or milieu) from which the host (victim) directly acquires the disease. Infectious organisms can multiply within the source. A source includes a *vector*, which is usually an arthropod (for example, a mosquito) that transmits the disease indirectly from person to person, but it may be a person who has the disease, was recently exposed to it, or is a carrier. Transmission may also occur through a *vehicle*, like contaminated food or water. Infectious organisms can multiply within a vehicle.

HOW TO COLLECT CULTURE SPECIMENS

CULTURE SITE	SPECIMEN SOURCE	SPECIAL CONSIDERATIONS
Infected wound	• Aspiration of exudate with syringe (preferred technique)	• Use only sterile syringe. Pungent odor suggests the presence of anaerobes. Use oxygen free collection tubes, if available.
	• Applicator swab	• Firmly but gently saturate swab with exudate from infected site. If surface is dry, moisten swab with sterile saline solution before taking culture.
Skin lesions	• Excision or puncture	• Thoroughly cleanse skin before excision or puncture and follow procedure for infected wound.
Upper respiratory tract	• Nasopharyngeal swab (generally used to detect carriers of *Staphylococcus aureus* and viral infections)	• Gently pass swab through nose into nasopharynx. Immediately send specimen to lab for culture.
	• Throat swab	• Under adequate light, swab the area of inflammation or exudation.
Lower respiratory tract	• Expectorated sputum	• Instruct patient to cough deeply and to expectorate into cup. Culture requires expectorated sputum, not just saliva from mouth.
	• Induced sputum (used when patient can't expectorate sputum)	• Use aerosol mist spray of saline solution or water to induce sputum production. Apply cupping and postural drainage, if needed.
	• Nasotracheal suction	• Measure approximate distance from patient's nose to his ear. Note the distance; then, insert a sterile suction catheter this length, with a collection vial attached, into his nose. Maintain suction during catheter withdrawal.
	• Pleural tap	• Advise patient that he may feel discomfort even though skin is anesthetized before this procedure. After tap, check site often for local swelling, and report dyspnea and other adverse reactions.
Lower intestinal tract	• Rectal swab	• Lesion on colon or on rectal wall may require colonoscopy or sigmoidoscopy to obtain specimen. If so, explain the procedure. Help patient to assume a left lateral decubitus or a knee-chest position.
	• Stool specimen	• Specimen should contain any pus or blood present in feces and a sampling of the first, middle, and last portion of stool. Urine with stool can invalidate results. Immediately send specimen to lab in a clean, tightly covered container, especially stools being examined for ova and parasites.

Viruses are subcellular organisms made up only of an RNA or a DNA nucleus covered with proteins. They are the smallest known organisms (so tiny they're visible only through an electron microscope). Independent of host cells, viruses can't replicate. Rather, they invade a host cell and stimulate it to participate in the

Proper identification of the causative organism requires proper culture collection. Label culture specimen with date, time, patient's name, suspected diagnosis, and source of culture

CULTURE SITE	SPECIMEN SOURCE	SPECIAL CONSIDERATIONS
Eye	• Cotton swab	• Carefully retract lower lid, and gently swab the conjunctiva.
	• Corneal scrapings	• Doctor uses swab loop to scrape specimen from site of corneal infection. Reassure patient that procedure is short and discomfort minimal.
Genital tract	• Swab specimen	• In males, specimen should contain urethral discharge or prostatic fluid; in females, urethral or cervical specimens. Always collect specimens on two swabs simultaneously.
Urinary tract	• Midstream clean catch urine (avoids specimen contamination with microorganisms commonly found in the lower urethra and perineum)	• In an uninfected person, midstream clean catch should contain less than 10,000 bacteria/ml. • Instruct patient how to collect specimen or supervise collection. In males, retract foreskin and cleanse glans penis; in females, cleanse and separate labia so urinary meatus is clearly visible; then, cleanse meatus. Tell patient to void 25 to 30 ml and, without stopping urine stream, to collect specimen. • In infants, apply the collection bag carefully and check it frequently to avoid mechanical urethral obstruction. • Immediately send urine to lab, or refrigerate it to retard growth.
	• Foley catheter specimen	• Cleanse specimen port of catheter with alcohol, and aspirate urine with a sterile needle, or from a latex catheter, at a point distal to the "Y" branch.
Body fluids	• Needle aspiration	• Immediately send peritoneal and synovial fluid and cerebrospinal fluid (CSF) to lab. *Don't* retard growth of CSF organisms by refrigerating specimen. After pericardial and pleural fluid aspiration, observe patient carefully, and check vital signs often. Watch for signs of pneumothorax or cardiac tamponade.
Blood	• Venous or arterial aspiration	• Prep skin according to your hospital's policy. • Using a sterile syringe, collect 12 to 15 ml blood, changing needles before injecting blood into the aerobic and anaerobic collection bottles. Continue the procedure according to your hospital's policy. • If patient is receiving penicillin, note this on lab slip, since lab may add penicillinase to culture to inactivate drug.

formation of additional virus particles. The estimated 400 viruses that infect humans are classified according to their size, shape (spherical, rod-shaped, or cubic), or means of transmission (respirational, fecal, oral, or sexual).

Rickettsiae are relatively uncommon in the United States. They're small, gram-negative, bacterialike organisms that frequently induce life-threatening infections. Like viruses, they require a host cell for replication. Three genera of rickettsiae include *Rickettsia*, *Coxiella*, and *Rochalimaea*.

Chlamydiae are smaller than rickettsiae and bacteria but larger than viruses. They too depend on host cells for replication, but unlike viruses, they are susceptible to antibiotics.

IMMUNIZATION SCHEDULE

Usually, childhood immunizations are given on a fixed schedule, as follows:

AGE	IMMUNIZATION
2 months	First dose: diphtheria/ pertussis/tetanus (DPT) vaccine; polio vaccine (OPV)
4 months	Second dose: DPT and OPV
6 months	Third dose: DPT and OPV (optional)
12 months	Tuberculin test
15 months	Rubella vaccine; measles; mumps
18 months	DPT and OPV (third)
4-6 years	DPT; polio booster
14-16 years	Tetanus and diphtheria toxoids only

Before immunization:
- Ask the parents if the child receives corticosteroids or other drugs that depress immune response, or if he's had a recent febrile illness.
- Obtain a history of allergies, especially to antibiotics, eggs, or feathers, and past reaction to immunization.

After immunization:
- Tell parents to report a severe reaction, especially to first dose of pertussis vaccine.
- Give them an immunization record.

Spirochetes are flexible, slender, undulating spiral rods that have cell walls. Most are anaerobic. The three forms pathogenic in humans include *Treponema*, *Leptospira*, and *Borrelia*.

Fungi are single-cell organisms, with nuclei enveloped by nuclear membranes. They have rigid cell walls like plant cells but lack chlorophyll, the green matter necessary for photosynthesis; they also show relatively little cellular specialization. Fungi occur as yeasts (single-cell oval-shaped organisms) or molds (organisms with hyphae, or branching filaments). Depending on the environment, some fungi may occur in both forms. Fungal diseases in humans are called mycoses.

Protozoa are the simplest single-cell organisms of the animal kingdom but show a high level of cellular specialization. Like other animal cells, they have cell membranes rather than cell walls, and their nuclei are surrounded by nuclear membranes.

In addition to these microorganisms, infectious diseases may also result from larger parasites, such as roundworms or flatworms.

Modes of transmission

Most infectious diseases are transmitted in one of four ways.

1. In *contact transmission*, the susceptible host comes into direct contact (as in venereal disease) or indirect contact (contaminated inanimate objects or the close-range spread of respiratory droplets) with the source.

2. *Airborne transmission* results from inhalation of contaminated evaporated saliva droplets (as in pulmonary tuberculosis), which are sometimes suspended in airborne dust particles.

3. In *enteric* (oral-fecal) *transmission*, the organisms are found in feces and are ingested by susceptible victims, often through fecally contaminated food (as in salmonella infections).

4. *Vectorborne transmission* occurs when an intermediate carrier (vector), such as a flea or a mosquito, transfers an organism.

ISOLATION PRECAUTIONS

DISEASES THAT REQUIRE ISOLATION	Private room	Mask	Gown	Gloves	Special handling of waste or contaminated articles
Strict isolation (may require room with special ventilation) Pharyngeal diphtheria, viral hemorrhagic fevers, pneumonic plague, smallpox, varicella (chicken pox), zoster (localized in immunocompromised patient or disseminated)	X with door closed	X	X	X	X
Contact isolation Group A *Streptococcus* endometritis; impetigo; pediculosis; *Staphylococcus aureus* or pneumonia; rabies; rubella; scabies; scalded skin syndrome; major skin, wound, or burn infection; vaccinia; primary disseminated herpes simplex; and infection or colonization with multiply-resistant bacteria. In infants and young children: acute respiratory infections; influenza; infectious pharyngitis; viral pneumonia. In newborns: gonococcal conjunctivitis; staphylococcal furunculosis; neonatal disseminated herpes simplex	X	O	⊗	⊗	X
Respiratory isolation *Hemophilus influenzae* epiglottitis; erythema infectiosum; measles; *H. influenzae* or meningococcal meningitis; meningococcal pneumonia; meningococcemia; mumps; pertussis; *H. influenzae* pneumonia in children	X with door closed	O	—	—	X
Acid-fast bacillus isolation (requires room with special ventilation) Tuberculosis	X with door closed	O	⊗	—	X
Enteric precautions Amebic dysentery; cholera; coxsackievirus disease; acute diarrhea with suspected infection; echovirus disease; encephalitis caused by enteroviruses; *Clostridium difficile* or *Staphylococcus* enterocolitis; enteroviral infection; gastroenteritis caused by *Campylobacter* species, *Cryptosporidum* species, *Dientamoeba fragilis, Escherichia coli, Giardia lamblia, Salmonella* species, *Shigella* species, *Vibrio parahaemolyticus*, viruses, *Yersinia enterocolitica;* hand, foot and mouth disease; hepatitis A; herpangina; viral meningitis caused by enteroviruses; necrotizing enterocolitis; pleurodynia; poliomyelitis; typhoid fever; viral pericarditis, myocarditis, or enteroviral meningitis	D	—	⊗	⊗	X
Drainage/secretion precautions Conjunctivitis; minor or limited abscess; minor or limited burn, skin, wound, or decubitus ulcer infection	—	—	⊗	⊗	X
Blood/body fluid precautions AIDS; arthropodborne viral fevers, such as dengue and yellow fever; babesiasis; Creutzfeldt-Jakob disease; hepatitis B; hepatitis non-A, non-B; leptospirosis; malaria; rat-bite fever; relapsing fever; primary and secondary syphilis with lesions	D	—	⊗	⊗	X

Key
X = Always necessary
⊗ = Necessary if soiling of hands or clothing is likely
O = Necessary for close contact or if patient is coughing and does not reliably cover mouth
D = Desirable but optional; necessary only if patient has poor hygiene
— = Unnecessary

REPORTABLE INFECTIOUS DISEASES

Most states require that certain diseases be reported to local public health authorities by mail, telephone, or telegraph. Such reports should include the patient's name, address, age, race, and sex, along with the disease or suspected disease and the means of exposure, if known.

Reportable diseases vary from state to state but usually include acute respiratory viral diseases, AIDS, anthrax, botulism, chancroid, cholera, neonatal inclusion conjunctivitis, keratoconjunctivitis, epidemic neonatal diarrhea, diphtheria, infectious encephalitis, gonorrhea, hepatitis A and B as well as non-A and non-B, histoplasmosis, influenza, leprosy, leptospirosis, listeriosis, malaria, rubeola, meningococcal meningitis, meningococcemia, mumps, paratyphoid fever, pertussis, plague, poliomyelitis, psittacosis, Q fever, rabies, rat-bite fever, relapsing fever, rubella, shigellosis, smallpox, syphilis, tetanus, pulmonary and extrapulmonary tuberculosis, typhoid fever, typhus, and yersiniosis.

Some states also require the reporting of: actinomycosis, amebiasis, lymphocytic choriomeningitis, coccidioidomycosis, acute bacterial conjunctivitis and epidemic hemorrhagic conjunctivitis, granuloma inguinale, hemorrhagic jaundice, impetigo contagiosa, lymphogranuloma venereum, pediculosis, bacterial and mycoplasmal pneumonia, ringworm, Rocky Mountain spotted fever, scabies, staphylococcal infections, streptococcal infections, trachoma, and tularemia.

Adapted from information provided by the American Public Health Association, 1015 18th St., N.W., Washington, D.C. 20036

Much can be done to prevent transmission of infectious diseases:
- comprehensive immunization (including the required immunization of travelers to or emigrants from endemic areas)
- drug prophylaxis
- improved nutrition, living conditions, and sanitation
- correction of environmental factors.

Immunization can now control many diseases, including diphtheria, tetanus, pertussis, measles, rubella, some forms of meningitis, poliovirus, hepatitis B, pneumococcal pneumonia, influenza, rabies, and tetanus. Smallpox (variola)—which killed and disfigured millions—is believed to have been successfully eradicated by a comprehensive World Health Organization program of surveillance and immunization.

Vaccines—which contain live but attenuated (weakened) or killed microorganisms—and toxoids—which contain bacterial exotoxins—induce active immunity against bacterial and viral diseases by stimulating antibody formation. Immune serums contain previously formed antibodies from hyperimmunized donors or pooled plasma, and provide temporary passive immunity. Antitoxins provide passive immunity to various toxins. Generally, passive immunization is used only when active immunization is perilous or impossible, or when complete protection requires both active and passive immunization.

While prophylactic antibiotic therapy may prevent certain diseases, the risks of superinfection and emergence of drug-resistant strains may outweigh the benefits. So prophylactic antibiotics are usually reserved for patients at high risk of exposure to dangerous infection.

Nosocomial infections

A *nosocomial* infection is one that develops after a patient is admitted to a hospital or other institution. Most infections of this type are caused by group A *Streptococcus pyogenes*, *Staphylococcus*, *Escherichia coli*, *Klebsiella*, *Proteus*, *Pseudomonas*, *Hemophilus influenzae*, hepatitis viruses, and *Candida albicans*.

Transmission of nosocomial infection usually occurs by direct contact. Less often, transmission occurs by inhalation of or wound invasion by airborne organisms, or by contaminated equipment and solutions.

Despite hospital programs of infection control that include surveillance, prevention, and education, about 5% of patients who enter hospitals contract a nosocomial infection. Since the 1960s, staphylococcal infection has been declining, but gram-negative bacilli and fungal infections have been steadily increasing.

Nosocomial infections continue as a difficult problem, because most hospital patients are older and more debilitated than in the past. The very advances in treatment that increase longevity in many diseases that alter immune defenses also create a high-risk population. Moreover, the increased use of invasive and surgical procedures, immunosuppressives, and antibiotics predisposes patients to infection and superinfection. At the same time, the growing number of personnel that can come in contact with each patient makes the risk of exposure greater.

Here's how you can prevent nosocomial infections:

- Follow strict infection control procedures.
- Document hospital infections as they occur.
- Identify outbreaks early, and take steps to prevent their spread.
- Eliminate unnecessary procedures that contribute to infection.
- Strictly follow necessary isolation techniques.
- Observe *all* patients for signs of infection, especially those at high risk.
- Follow good handwashing techniques, and encourage other staff members to do the same.
- Keep staff and visitors with obvious infection, as well as known carriers, away from susceptible patients.
- Take special precautions with vulnerable patients—those with Foley catheters, mechanical ventilators, or I.V.s, and those recuperating from surgery.

Accurate assessment vital

Accurate assessment helps identify infectious diseases and prevents avoidable complications. Complete assessment consists of patient history, physical examination, and laboratory data. History should include the patient's sex, age, address, occupation, and place of work; known exposure to illness; and date of disease onset. It should also detail information about recent hospitalization, blood transfusions, blood donation denial by Red Cross or other agencies, vaccination, travel or camping trips, and exposure to animals. If applicable, ask about possible exposure to sexually transmitted diseases or about drug abuse. Also, try to determine the patient's resistance to infectious disease. Ask about usual dietary patterns, unusual fatigue, and any conditions, such as neoplastic disease or alcoholism, that may predispose him to infection. Notice if the patient is listless or uneasy, lacks concentration, or has any obvious abnormality of mood or affect.

In suspected infection, a physical examination must assess the skin, mucous membranes, liver, spleen, and lymph nodes. Check for and note the location of and type of drainage from skin lesions. Record skin color, temperature, and turgor; ask if the patient has pruritus. Take his temperature, using the same route consistently, and watch for a fever (the best indicator of many infections). Note and record the pattern of temperature change and the effect of antipyretics. Be aware that certain analgesics may contain antipyretics. In high fever, especially in children, watch for convulsions.

Check the pulse rate. Infection often increases pulse rate, but some infections, notably typhoid fever and psittacosis, may decrease it. In severe infection or when complications are possible, watch for hypotension, hematuria, oliguria, hepatomegaly, jaundice, bleeding from gums or into joints, and altered level of consciousness. Obtain laboratory studies and appropriate cultures, as ordered.

GRAM-POSITIVE COCCI

Staphylococcal Infections

PREDISPOSING FACTORS	SIGNS AND SYMPTOMS	DIAGNOSIS
Bacteremia • Infected surgical wounds • Abscesses • Infected I.V. or intraarterial catheter sites or catheter tips • Infected vascular grafts or prostheses • Infected decubitus ulcers • Osteomyelitis • Parenteral drug abuse • Source unknown (primary bacteremia) • Cellulitis • Burns • Immunosuppression • Debilitating diseases, such as chronic renal insufficiency, diabetes, and leukemia • Infective endocarditis, which may be caused by coagulase-positive staphylococci, and subacute bacterial endocarditis, which is usually caused by coagulase-negative staphylococci	• Fever (high fever with no obvious source in children under age 1), shaking chills, tachycardia • Cyanosis or pallor • Confusion, agitation, stupor • Skin microabscesses from emboli-containing bacteria • Joint pain • Complications: shock (likely in gram-negative bacteremia); acute bacterial endocarditis (in prolonged infection; indicated by new or changing systolic murmur); retinal hemorrhages (Roth's spots); splinter hemorrhages under nails and small, tender red nodes on pads of fingers and toes (Osler's nodes); metastatic abscess formation in skin, bones, lungs, brain, and kidneys; pulmonary emboli if tricuspid valve is infected • Prognosis poor in patients over age 60 or with advanced malignancy	• Blood cultures (two to four samples from different sites at different times): growing staphylococci and leukocytosis (usually 12,000 WBCs/mm^3), with shift to the left of polymorphonuclear leukocytes (70% to 90% neutrophils) • Urinalysis shows microscopic hematuria. • ESR elevated, especially in chronic or subacute bacterial endocarditis • Severe anemia or thrombocytopenia (possible) • Prolonged PTT and PT, low fibrinogen and platelet counts, and low factor assays; possible DIC • Cultures of urine, sputum, and draining skin lesions may identify primary infection site. So may chest X-rays and scans of lungs, liver, abdomen, and brain. • Echocardiogram may show heart valve vegetation.
Pneumonia • Immune deficiencies, especially in elderly and children under age 2 • Chronic lung diseases and cystic fibrosis • Malignancies • Antibiotics that kill normal respiratory flora but spare *S. aureus* • Viral respiratory infections, especially influenza • Hematogenous (bloodborne) bacteria spread to the lungs from primary sites of infections (such as heart valves, abscesses, and pulmonary emboli)	• High temperature: adults, 103° to 105° F. (39.4° to 40.6° C.); children, 101° F. (38.3° C.) • Cough, with purulent, yellow or bloody sputum • Dyspnea, rales, and decreased breath sounds • Pleural pain • In infants: mild respiratory infection that suddenly worsens: irritability, anxiety, dyspnea, anorexia, vomiting, diarrhea, spasms of dry coughing, marked tachypnea, expiratory grunting, sternal retractions, and cyanosis • Complications: necrosis, lung abscess, pyopneumothorax; empyema; pneumatocele; shock, hypotension, oliguria or anuria, cyanosis, loss of consciousness	• WBC elevated (15,000 to 40,000/mm^3; 15,000 to 20,000/mm^3 in children), with predominance of polymorphonuclear leukocytes • Sputum Gram stain: mostly gram-positive cocci in clusters, with many polymorphonuclear leukocytes • Sputum culture: mostly coagulase-positive staphylococci • Chest X-rays: usually patchy infiltrates • Arterial blood gas analysis (in shock): hypoxia and respiratory acidosis

Staphylococci are coagulase-negative (S. epidermidis) *or coagulase-positive* (S. aureus) *gram-positive bacteria. Coagulase-negative staphylococci, which grow abundantly as normal flora on skin and in the upper respiratory tract, are usually nonpathogenic but can cause serious infections. Pathogenic strains of staphylococci are found in many adults—"carriers"—usually on the nasal mucosa, axilla, or groin. Sometimes, carriers shed staphylococci, infecting themselves or other susceptible people. Coagulase-positive staphylococci tend to form pus; they cause many types of infections.*

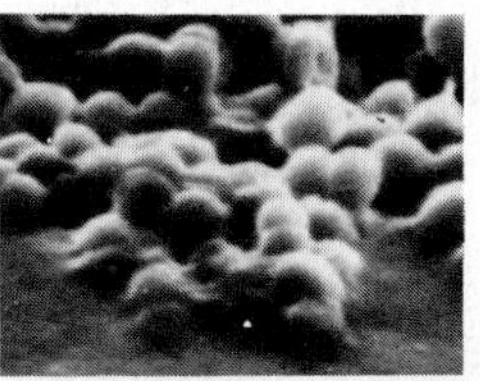

TREATMENT	SPECIAL CONSIDERATIONS
• Semisynthetic penicillins (methicillin, nafcillin) or cephalosporins (cefazolin) given I.V. • Vancomycin I.V. for those with penicillin allergy or methicillin-resistant organism • Probenecid may be given to partially prevent urinary excretion of penicillin and to prolong blood levels. • I.V. fluids to reverse shock • Removal of infected catheter or foreign body • Surgery	• *S. aureus* bacteremia can be fatal within 12 hours. Be especially alert for it in debilitated patients with intravenous catheters or in those with a history of drug abuse. • Administer antibiotics on time to maintain adequate blood levels, but give them slowly, using the prescribed amount of diluent, to prevent thrombophlebitis. • Watch for signs of penicillin allergy, especially pruritic rash (possible anaphylaxis). Keep epinephrine 1:1,000 and resuscitation equipment handy. Monitor vital signs, urine output, and mental state for signs of shock. • Obtain cultures carefully, and observe for clues to the primary site of infection. Never refrigerate blood cultures; it delays identification of organisms by slowing their growth. • Impose appropriate isolation if the primary site of infection is draining. Special blood precautions are not necessary, since the number of organisms present, even in fulminant bacteremia, is minimal. • Obtain peak and trough levels to determine the adequacy of treatment.
• Semisynthetic penicillins (methicillin, nafcillin) or cephalosporins given I.V. • Vancomycin I.V. for those with penicillin allergy or methicillin-resistant organisms • Isolation until sputum shows minimal numbers of *S. aureus* (about 24 to 72 hours after starting antibiotics)	• Use masks with isolated patient because staphylococci from lungs spread by air as well as direct contact. Use gown and gloves only when handling contaminated respiratory secretions. • Keep the door to the patient's room closed. Don't store extra supplies in his room. Empty suction bottles carefully. Place any articles containing sputum (tissues, clothing, etc.) in a sealed plastic bag. Mark them "contaminated," and dispose of them promptly by incineration. • When obtaining sputum specimens, make sure you're collecting thick sputum, not saliva. The presence of epithelial cells (found in the mouth, not lungs) indicates a poor specimen. • Administer antibiotics strictly on time, but slowly. Watch for signs of penicillin allergy and for signs of infection at I.V. sites. Change the I.V. site at least every third day. • Perform frequent chest physical therapy. Do chest percussion and postural drainage after intermittent positive pressure breathing treatments. Concentrate on consolidated areas (revealed by X-rays or auscultation).

(continued)

PREDISPOSING FACTORS	SIGNS AND SYMPTOMS	DIAGNOSIS
Enterocolitis • Broad-spectrum antibiotics (tetracycline, chloramphenicol, or neomycin) as prophylaxis for bowel surgery or treatment of hepatic coma • Usually occurs in elderly, but also in newborn infants (associated with staphylococcal skin lesions)	• Sudden onset of profuse, watery diarrhea usually 2 days to several weeks after start of antibiotic therapy, I.V. or P.O. • Nausea, vomiting, abdominal pain and distention • Hypovolemia and dehydration (decreased skin turgor, hypotension, fever)	• Stool Gram stain: many gram-positive cocci and polymorphonuclear leukocytes, with few gram-negative rods • Stool culture: *S. aureus* • Sigmoidoscopy: mucosal ulcerations • Blood studies: leukocytosis, moderately increased blood urea nitrogen level, and decreased serum albumin level
Osteomyelitis • Hematogenous organisms • Skin trauma • Infection spreading from adjacent joint or other infected tissues • *S. aureus* bacteremia • Orthopedic surgery or trauma • Cardiothoracic surgery • Usually occurs in growing bones, especially femur and tibia, of children under age 12 • More common in males	• Abrupt onset of fever—usually 101° F. (38.3° C.) or lower; shaking chills; pain and swelling over infected area; restlessness; headache • About 20% of children develop a chronic infection if not properly treated.	• Possible history of prior trauma to involved area • Positive bone and pus cultures (and blood cultures in about 50% of patients) • X-ray changes apparent after second or third week. • ESR elevated with leukocyte shift to the left.
Food poisoning • Enterotoxin produced by toxogenic strains of *S. aureus* in contaminated food (second most common cause of food poisoning in U.S.)	• Anorexia, nausea, vomiting, diarrhea, and abdominal cramps 1 to 6 hours after ingestion of contaminated food • Symptoms usually subside within 18 hours, with complete recovery in 1 to 3 days.	• Clinical findings sufficient. • Stool cultures usually negative for *S. aureus.*
Skin infections • Decreased resistance • Burns or decubitus ulcers • Decreased blood flow • Possibly skin contamination from nasal discharge • Foreign bodies • Underlying skin diseases, such as eczema and acne • Common in persons with poor hygiene living in crowded quarters	• Cellulitis—diffuse, acute inflammation of soft tissue (no drainage) • Pus-producing lesions in and around hair follicles (folliculitis) • Boil-like lesions (furuncles and carbuncles) extend from hair follicles to subcutaneous tissues. These painful, red, indurated lesions are 1 to 2 cm and have a purulent yellow discharge. • Small macule or skin bleb that may develop into vesicle containing pus (bullous impetigo); common in school-age children • Mild or spiking fever • Malaise	• Clinical findings and analysis of pus cultures if sites are draining • Cultures of nondraining cellulitis taken from the margin of the reddened area by infiltration with 1 ml sterile saline solution and immediate fluid aspiration

TREATMENT	SPECIAL CONSIDERATIONS
• Broad-spectrum antibiotics should be discontinued. • Antistaphylococcal agents, such as vancomycin P.O., may be given.	• Monitor vital signs frequently to prevent shock. Force fluids to correct dehydration. • Know serum electrolyte levels. Measure and record bowel movements when possible. Check serum chloride level for alkalosis (hypochloremia). • Collect serial stool specimens for Gram stain, and culture for diagnosis and for evaluating effectiveness of treatment.
• Surgical debridement • Prolonged antibiotic therapy (4 to 8 weeks) • Vancomycin I.V. for those with penicillin allergy or methicillin-resistant organisms	• Identify the infected area, and mark it on the care plan. • Check the penetration wound from which the organism originated for evidence of present infection. • Severe pain may render the patient immobile. If so, perform passive range-of-motion exercises. Apply heat, as needed, and elevate the affected part. (Extensive involvement may require casting until the infection subsides.) • Before such procedures as surgical debridement, warn the patient to expect some pain. Explain that drainage is essential for healing, and that he will continue to receive analgesics and antibiotics after surgery.
• No treatment necessary unless dehydration becomes a problem (usually in infants and elderly); then, I.V. therapy may be necessary to replace fluids	• Obtain a complete history of symptoms, recent meals, and other known cases of food poisoning. • Monitor vital signs, fluid balance, and serum electrolyte levels. • Check for dehydration if vomiting is severe or prolonged, and for decreased blood pressure. • Observe and report the number and color of stools.
• Topical ointments; bacitracin-neomycin-polymyxin or gentamicin • P.O. cloxacillin, dicloxacillin, or erythromycin; I.V. oxacillin, nafcillin, or methicillin for severe infection; I.V. vancomycin for methicillin-resistant organisms • Application of heat to reduce pain • Surgical drainage • Identification and treatment of sources of reinfection (nostrils, perineum) • Cleansing and covering the area with moist, sterile dressings	• Identify the site and extent of infection. • Keep lesions clean with saline solution and peroxide irrigations, as ordered. Cover infections near wounds or genitourinary tract with gauze pads. Keep pressure off the site to facilitate healing. • Be alert for the extension of skin infections. • Severe infection or abscess may require surgical drainage. Explain the procedure to the patient. Determine if cultures will be taken, and be ready to collect a specimen. • Impetigo is contagious. Isolate the patient and alert his family. Use secretion precautions for all draining lesions.

Streptococcal Infections

CAUSES AND INCIDENCE	SIGNS AND SYMPTOMS
***STREPTOCOCCUS PYOGENES* (group A streptococcus)**	
Streptococcal pharyngitis (strep throat) • Accounts for 95% of all cases of bacterial pharyngitis • Most common in children aged 5 to 10, and during October to April • Spread by direct person-to-person contact via droplets of saliva or nasal secretions • Organism frequently colonizes throats of persons with no symptoms; up to 20% of school children may be carriers	• After 1- to 5-day incubation period: temperature of 101° to 104° F. (38.3° to 40° C.), sore throat with severe pain on swallowing, beefy red pharynx, tonsillar exudate, edematous tonsils and uvula, swollen glands along the jaw line, generalized malaise and weakness, anorexia, occasional abdominal discomfort • Up to 40% of small children have symptoms too mild for diagnosis. • Fever abates in 3 to 5 days; nearly all symptoms subside within a week.
Scarlet fever (scarlatina) • Usually follows streptococcal pharyngitis; may follow wound infections or puerperal sepsis • Caused by streptococcal strain that releases an erythrogenic toxin • Most common in children age 2 to 10 • Spread by inhalation or direct contact	• Streptococcal sore throat, fever, strawberry tongue, fine erythematous rash that blanches on pressure and resembles sunburn with goosebumps • Rash usually appears first on upper chest, then spreads to neck, abdomen, legs, and arms, sparing soles and palms; flushed cheeks, pallor around mouth • Skin sheds during convalescence.
Erysipelas • Occurs primarily in infants and adults over age 30 • Usually follows strep throat • Exact mode of spread to skin unknown	• Sudden onset, with reddened, swollen, raised lesions (skin looks like an orange peel), usually on face and scalp, bordered by areas that often contain easily ruptured blebs filled with yellow-tinged fluid. Lesions sting and itch. Lesions on the trunk, arms, or legs usually affect incision or wound sites. • Other symptoms: vomiting, fever, headache, cervical lymphadenopathy, sore throat
Impetigo (streptococcal pyoderma) • Common in poor children aged 2 to 5 in hot, humid weather; high rate of familial spread • Predisposing factors: close contact in schools, overcrowded living quarters, poor skin hygiene, minor skin trauma • May spread by direct contact, environmental contamination, or arthropod vector	• Small macules rapidly develop into vesicles, then become pustular and encrusted, causing pain, surrounding erythema, regional adenitis, cellulitis, and itching. Scratching spreads infection. • Lesions frequently affect the face, heal slowly, and leave depigmented areas.
Streptococcal gangrene (necrotizing fasciitis) • More common in elderly with arteriosclerotic vascular disease or diabetes • Predisposing factors: surgery, wounds, skin ulcers • Spread by direct contact	• Mimics gas gangrene; within 72 hours of onset, patient shows red-streaked, painful skin lesion with dusky red surrounding tissue. Bullae with yellow or reddish black fluid develop and rupture. • Other symptoms: fever, tachycardia, lethargy, prostration, disorientation, hypotension, jaundice, hypovolemia, severe pain followed by anesthesia (due to nerve destruction)

Streptococci are small gram-positive bacteria linked together in pairs of chains. Although researchers have identified 21 species of streptococci, three classes—groups A, B, and D—cause most of the infections. When streptococci cause infection, drainage tends to be thin and serous.

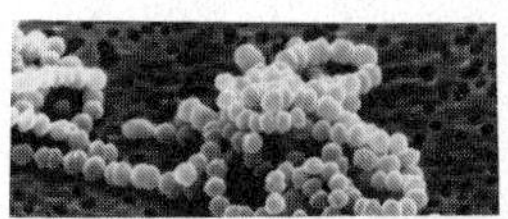

DIAGNOSIS	COMPLICATIONS	TREATMENT AND SPECIAL CONSIDERATIONS
• Clinically indistinguishable from viral pharyngitis • Throat culture shows group A beta-hemolytic streptococci (carriers have positive throat culture). • Elevated white blood cell (WBC) count • Serology shows a four-fold rise in streptozyme titers during convalescence.	• Acute otitis media or acute sinusitis occurs most frequently. • Rarely, bacteremic spread may cause arthritis, endocarditis, meningitis, osteomyelitis, or liver abscess. • Post-streptococcal sequelae: acute rheumatic fever or acute glomerulonephritis	• Penicillin or erythromycin • Stress the need for bed rest and isolation from other children for 24 hours after antibiotic therapy begins. Patient should finish prescription; even if symptoms subside; abscess, glomerulonephritis, and rheumatic fever can occur. • Tell the patient not to skip doses and to properly dispose of soiled tissues.
• Characteristic rash and strawberry tongue • Culture and Gram stain show *S. pyogenes* from nasopharynx • Granulocytosis	• Although rare, complications may include high fever, arthritis, and jaundice.	• Penicillin or erythromycin • Isolation for first 24 hours • Carefully dispose of purulent discharge. • Stress the need for prompt and complete antibiotic treatment.
• Typical reddened lesions • Culture taken from edge of lesions shows group A beta-hemolytic streptococci • Throat culture is almost always positive for group A beta-hemolytic streptococci	• Untreated lesions on trunk, arms, or legs may involve large body areas and lead to death.	• Penicillin I.V. or P.O. • Cold packs, analgesics (aspirin and codeine for local discomfort) • Prevention: prompt treatment of streptococcal infections and drainage/secretion precautions
• Characteristic lesions with honey-colored crust • Culture and Gram stain of swabbed lesions show *S. pyogenes*	• Septicemia (rare) • Ecthyma, a form of impetigo with deep ulcers	• Penicillin I.V. or P.O., or erythromycin, or antibiotic ointments • Frequent washing of lesions with soap and water followed by thorough drying • Isolation of patient with draining wounds • Prevention: good hygiene and proper wound care
• Culture and Gram stain usually show *S. pyogenes* from early bullous lesions and frequently from blood	• Extensive necrotic sloughing • Bacteremia, metastatic abscesses, and death • Thrombophlebitis, when lower extremities are involved	• Immediate, wide, deep surgery of all necrotic tissues • High-dose penicillin I.V. • Good preoperative skin preparation; aseptic surgical and suturing technique

(continued)

CAUSES AND INCIDENCE	SIGNS AND SYMPTOMS
***STREPTOCOCCUS AGALACTIAE* (group B streptococcus)**	
Neonatal streptococcal infections • Incidence of early-onset infection (age 5 days or less): 2/1,000 live births • Incidence of late-onset infection (age 7 days to 3 months): 1/1,000 live births • Spread by vaginal delivery or hands of nursery staff • Predisposing factors: maternal genital tract colonization, membrane rupture over 24 hours before delivery, crowded nursery.	• Early onset: bacteremia, pneumonia, and meningitis; mortality from 14% for infants over 1,500 g at birth to 61% for infants under 1,500 g at birth • Late onset: bacteremia with meningitis, fever, and bone and joint involvement; mortality 15% to 20% • Other symptoms, such as skin lesions, depend on the site affected.
Adult group B streptococcal infection • Most adult infections occur in postpartum women, usually in the form of endometritis or wound infection following Caesarian section. • Incidence of group B streptococcal endometritis: 1.3/1,000 live births	• Fever, malaise, uterine tenderness
***STREPTOCOCCUS PNEUMONIAE* (group D streptococcus)**	
Pneumococcal pneumonia • Accounts for 70% of all cases of bacterial pneumonia • More common in men, elderly, blacks, and American Indians, in winter and early spring • Spread by air and contact with infective secretions • Predisposing factors: trauma, viral infection, underlying pulmonary disease, overcrowded living quarters, chronic diseases, immunodeficiency • Among the 10 leading causes of death in the United States	• Sudden onset with severe shaking chills, temperature of 102° to 105° F. (38.9° to 40.6° C.), bacteremia, cough (with thick, scanty, blood-tinged sputum) accompanied by pleuritic pain • Malaise, weakness, and prostration common • Tachypnea, anorexia, nausea, and vomiting less common • Severity of pneumonia usually due to host's cellular defenses, not bacterial virulence
Otitis media • About 76% to 95% of all children have otitis media at least once. *S. pneumoniae* causes half of these cases.	• Ear pain, ear drainage, hearing loss, fever, lethargy, irritability • Other possible symptoms: vertigo, nystagmus, tinnitus
Meningitis • Can follow bacteremic pneumonia, mastoiditis, sinusitis, skull fracture, or endocarditis • Mortality (30% to 60%) highest in infants and in the elderly	• Fever, headache, nuchal rigidity, vomiting, photophobia, lethargy, coma
Endocarditis • Group D streptococcus (enterococcus) causes 10% to 20% of all bacterial endocarditis. • Most common in elderly patients and in those who abuse I.V. substances • Often follows bacteremia from an obvious source, such as a wound infection • Most cases are subacute.	• Weakness, fatigability, weight loss, fever, night sweats, anorexia, arthralgia, splenomegaly

DIAGNOSIS	COMPLICATIONS	TREATMENT AND SPECIAL CONSIDERATIONS
• Isolation of group B streptococcus from blood, cerebrospinal fluid (CSF), or skin • Chest X-ray shows massive infiltrate similar to that of respiratory distress syndrome or pneumonia	• Overwhelming pneumonia, sepsis, and death	• Penicillin or ampicillin I.V. • Patient isolation is unnecessary unless open draining lesion is present, but careful handwashing is essential. If draining lesion is present, take drainage/secretion precautions. • Vaccine is in developmental stages.
• Isolation of group B streptococcus from blood or infection site	• Bacteremia followed by meningitis or endocarditis	• Ampicillin or penicillin I.V. • Careful observation for symptoms of infection following delivery • Drainage/secretion precautions
• Gram stain of sputum shows gram-positive diplococci; culture shows *S. pneumoniae* • Chest X-ray shows lobular consolidation in adults; bronchopneumonia in children and elderly • Elevated WBC count • Blood cultures often positive for *S. pneumoniae*	• Pleural effusion occurs in 25% of patients. • Pericarditis (rare) • Lung abscess (rare) • Death possible if bacteremia is present	• Penicillin or erythromycin I.V. or I.M. • Monitor and support respirations, as needed. Record sputum color and amount. • Prevent dehydration. • Avoid sedatives and narcotics to preserve cough reflex. • Carefully dispose of all purulent drainage. (Respiratory isolation is unnecessary.) Advise high-risk patients to receive vaccine and to avoid infected persons.
• Fluid in middle ear • Isolation of *S. pneumoniae* from aspirated fluid, if necessary	• Recurrent attacks may cause hearing loss.	• Amoxicillin or ampicillin • Tell patient to report lack of response to therapy after 72 hours.
• Isolation of *S. pneumoniae* from CSF or blood culture • Increased CSF cell count and protein level; decreased CSF glucose level	• Persistent hearing deficits, convulsions, hemiparesis, or other nerve deficits	• Penicillin I.V. or chloramphenicol • Monitor closely for neurologic changes. • Watch for symptoms of septic shock, such as acidosis and tissue hypoxia.
• Anemia, increased ESR and serum immunoglobulin, and positive blood culture for Group D Streptococcus.	• Embolization • Pulmonary infarction • Osteomyelitis	• Penicillin for *S. bovis* (nonenterococcal group D strep) • Penicillin or ampicillin *and* an aminoglycoside for enterococcal group D strep

GRAM-NEGATIVE COCCI

Meningococcal Infections

Two major meningococcal infections (meningitis and meningococcemia) are caused by the gram-negative bacteria Neisseria meningitidis, *which also causes primary pneumonia, purulent conjunctivitis, endocarditis, sinusitis, and genital infection. Meningococcemia occurs as simple bacteremia, fulminant meningococcemia, and rarely, chronic meningococcemia. It often accompanies meningitis. (For more information on meningitis, see* MENINGITIS *in Chapter 9. Meningococcal infections may occur sporadically or in epidemics; virulent infections may be fatal within a matter of hours.*

Causes and incidence

Meningococcal infections occur most often among children (ages 6 months to 1 year) and men, usually military recruits, because of overcrowding.

N. meningitidis has seven serogroups (A, B, C, D, X, Y, Z); group A causes most epidemics. These bacteria are often present in upper respiratory flora. Transmission takes place through inhalation of an infected droplet from a carrier (an estimated 2% to 38% of the population). The bacteria then localize in the nasopharynx. Following an incubation period of approximately 3 or 4 days, they spread through the bloodstream to joints, skin, adrenal glands, lungs, and the central nervous system. The tissue damage that results (possibly due to the effects of bacterial endotoxins) produces symptoms and, in fulminant meningococcemia and meningococcal bacteremia, progresses to hemorrhage, thrombosis, and necrosis.

Signs and symptoms

Clinical features of meningococcal infection vary. Symptoms of *meningococcal bacteremia* include sudden spiking fever, headache, sore throat, cough, chills, myalgia (in back and legs), arthralgia, tachycardia, tachypnea, mild hypotension, and a petechial, nodular, or maculopapular rash.

In about 10% to 20% of patients, this progresses to *fulminant meningococcemia*, with extreme prostration, enlargement of skin lesions, disseminated intravascular coagulation (DIC), and shock. Unless it is treated promptly, fulminant meningococcemia results in death from respiratory or heart failure in 6 to 24 hours.

Characteristics of the rare *chronic meningococcemia* include intermittent fever, maculopapular rash, joint pain, and enlarged spleen.

Diagnosis

Isolation of *N. meningitidis* through a positive blood culture, CSF culture, or lesion scraping confirms the diagnosis except in nasopharyngeal infections, since *N. meningitidis* exists as part of the normal nasopharyngeal flora.

Tests that support the diagnosis include counterimmunoelectrophoresis of CSF or blood, low WBC, and, in patients with skin or adrenal hemorrhages, decreased platelet and clotting levels. Diagnostic evaluation must rule out Rocky Mountain spotted fever and vascular purpuras.

Treatment

As soon as meningococcal infection is suspected, treatment begins with large doses of aqueous penicillin G, ampicillin, or some cephalosporins, such as cefoxitin and moxalactam; or, for the patient who is allergic to penicillin, chloramphenicol I.V. Therapy may also include mannitol for cerebral edema, heparin I.V. for DIC, dopamine for shock, and digoxin and a diuretic if congestive heart failure develops. Supportive measures include fluid and electrolyte maintenance, proper ventilation (patent airway and oxygen, if necessary), insertion of an arterial or central venous pressure (CVP) line to monitor cardiovascular status, and bed rest.

Chemoprophylaxis with rifampin or minocycline is useful for hospital workers in close contact with the patient; minocycline can also temporarily eradicate the infection in carriers.

Special considerations

- Give I.V. antibiotics, as ordered, to maintain blood and CSF drug levels.
- Enforce bed rest in early stages. Provide a dark, quiet, restful environment.
- Maintain adequate ventilation with oxygen or a ventilator, if necessary. Suction and turn the patient frequently.
- Keep accurate intake and output records to maintain proper fluid and electrolyte levels. Monitor blood pressure, pulse, arterial blood gases, and CVP.
- Watch for complications, such as DIC, arthritis, endocarditis, and pneumonia.
- If the patient is receiving chloramphenicol, monitor CBC.
- Check the patient's drug history for allergies before giving antibiotics.

To prevent the spread of meningococcal infection:

- Isolate the patient until he has received antibiotic therapy for 24 hours.
- Label all meningococcal specimens. Deliver them to the laboratory quickly because meningococci are very sensitive to changes in humidity and temperature.
- Report all meningococcol infections to public health department officials.

GRAM-POSITIVE BACILLI

Diphtheria

Diphtheria is an acute, highly contagious toxin-mediated infection caused by Corynebacterium diphtheriae, *a gram-positive rod that usually infects the respiratory tract, primarily involving the tonsils, nasopharynx, and larynx. Currently, both cutaneous and wound diphtheria are seen more frequently in the United States and are often caused by nontoxigenic strains. The gastrointestinal and urinary tracts, conjunctivae, and ears are rarely involved.*

Causes

Transmission usually occurs through intimate contact or by airborne respiratory droplets from apparently healthy carriers or convalescing patients, since many more people carry this disease than contract active infection. Diphtheria is more prevalent during the colder months because of closer person-to-person contact indoors. But it may be contracted at any time during the year.

Thanks to effective immunization, diphtheria is rare in many parts of the world, including the United States. Since 1972, there has been an increase in cutaneous diphtheria, especially in the Pacific Northwest and the Southwest, particularly in areas where crowding and poor hygienic conditions prevail. Most victims are children under age 15. Diphtheria's mortality is up to 10%.

Signs and symptoms

Most infections go unrecognized, especially in partially immunized individuals. After an incubation period of less than a week, clinical cases of diphtheria characteristically show a thick, patchy, grayish green membrane over the mucous membranes of the pharynx, larynx, tonsils, soft palate, and nose; fever; sore throat; a rasping cough, hoarseness, and other symptoms similar to croup. Attempts to remove the membrane usually cause bleeding, which is highly characteristic of diphtheria. If this membrane causes airway obstruction (particularly likely in laryngeal diphtheria), symptoms include tachypnea, stridor, possibly cyanosis, suprasternal retractions, and suffocation, if untreated. In cutaneous diphtheria, skin lesions resemble impetigo.

Complications include myocarditis, neurologic involvement (primarily affecting motor fibers but possibly also sensory neurons), renal involvement, and pulmonary involvement (bronchopneumonia) due to *C. diphtheriae* or other superinfecting organisms.

Diagnosis

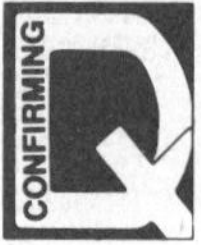

Examination showing the characteristic membrane and throat culture, or culture of other suspect lesions growing *C. diphtheriae,* confirm this diagnosis. Treatment must begin based on clinical findings and not wait for confirmation by culture.

Treatment

Standard treatment includes diphtheria antitoxin administered I.M. or I.V.; antibiotics, such as penicillin or erythromycin, to eliminate the organisms from the upper respiratory tract and other sites, to terminate the carrier state; and measures to prevent complications.

Special considerations

Diphtheria requires comprehensive supportive care with psychological support.

- To prevent spread of this disease, stress the need for strict isolation. Teach proper disposal of nasopharyngeal secretions. Maintain infection precautions until after two consecutive negative nasopharyngeal cultures—at least 1 week after drug therapy stops. Treatment of exposed individuals with antitoxin remains controversial. Suggest that family members later receive diphtheria toxoid (usually given as combined diphtheria and tetanus toxoids [DT] or a combination including pertussis vaccine [DPT] for children under age 6) if they haven't been immunized.

Administer drugs, as ordered. Although it is time-consuming and hazardous, desensitization should be attempted if tests are positive, since diphtheria antitoxin is the only *specific* treatment available. Since mortality increases directly with delay in antitoxin administration, the antitoxin is given before laboratory confirmation of diagnosis if sensitivity tests are negative. Before giving diphtheria antitoxin, which is made from horse serum, obtain eye and skin tests to determine sensitivity. After giving antitoxin and/or penicillin, be alert for anaphylaxis, and keep epinephrine 1:1,000 and resuscitative equipment handy. In patients who receive erythromycin, watch for thrombophlebitis.

- Monitor respirations carefully, especially in laryngeal diphtheria (usually, such patients are in a high-humidity or croup tent). Watch for signs of airway obstruction, and be ready to give immediate life support, including intubation and tracheotomy.
- Watch for signs of shock, which can develop suddenly.
- Obtain cultures, as ordered.
- If neuritis develops, tell the patient it's usually transient. Be aware that peripheral neuritis may not develop until 2 to 3 months after onset of illness.

Be alert for signs of myocarditis, such as development of heart murmurs or EKG changes. Ventricular fibrillation is a common cause of sudden death in diphtheria patients.

- Assign a primary nurse to increase the effectiveness of isolation. Give reassurance that isolation is temporary.
- Stress the need for childhood immunizations to all parents. Report all cases to local public health authorities.

Listeriosis

Listeriosis is an infection caused by the weakly hemolytic, gram-positive bacillus Listeria monocytogenes. *It occurs most often in fetuses, in neonates (during the first 3 weeks of life), and in older or immunosuppressed adults. The infected fetus is usually stillborn or is born prematurely, almost always with lethal listeriosis. This infection produces milder illness in pregnant women and varying degrees of illness in older and immunosuppressed patients; their prognoses depend on the severity of underlying illness.*

Causes

The primary method of person-to-person transmission is neonatal infection *in utero* (through the placenta) or during passage through an infected birth canal. Other modes of transmission may include inhaling contaminated dust; drinking contaminated, unpasteurized milk; coming in contact with infected animals, contaminated sewage or mud, or soil contaminated with feces containing *L. monocytogenes*; and, possibly, person-to-person transmission.

Signs and symptoms

Contact with *L. monocytogenes* commonly causes a transient asymptomatic carrier state. But sometimes it produces bacteremia and a febrile, generalized illness. In a pregnant woman, especially during the third trimester, listeriosis causes a mild illness with malaise, chills, fever, and back pain. However, her fetus may suffer severe uterine infection, abortion, premature delivery, or stillbirth. Transplacental infection may also cause early neonatal death or granulomatosis infantiseptica, which produces organ abscesses in infants.

Infection with *L. monocytogenes* commonly causes meningitis, resulting in tense fontanelles, irritability, lethargy, convulsions, and coma in neonates; and low-grade fever and personality changes in adults. Fulminant manifestations with coma are rare.

Diagnosis

L. monocytogenes is identified by its diagnostic tumbling motility on a wet mount of the culture. Other supportive diagnostic results include positive culture of blood, spinal fluid, drainage from cervical or vaginal lesions, or lochia from a mother with an infected infant, but isolation of the organism from these specimens is often difficult. Listeriosis also causes monocytosis.

Treatment

The treatment of choice is ampicillin or penicillin I.V. for 3 to 6 weeks, possibly with gentamicin to increase its effectiveness. Alternate treatments include erythromycin, chloramphenicol, or tetracycline.

Ampicillin and penicillin G are best for treating meningitis due to *L. monocytogenes*, since they more easily cross the blood-brain barrier. Pregnant women require prompt, vigorous treatment to combat fetal infection.

Special considerations

- Deliver specimens to the laboratory promptly. Because very few organisms may be present, take at least 10 cc of spinal fluid for culture.
- Use secretion precautions until a series of cultures of bodily discharges are negative. Be especially careful when handling lochia from an infected mother and secretions from her infant's eyes, nose, mouth, and rectum, including meconium.
- Evaluate neurologic status at least every 2 hours. In an infant, check fontanelles for bulging. Maintain adequate I.V. fluid intake; measure intake and output accurately.

- If the patient has CNS depression and becomes apneic, provide respiratory assistance, monitor respirations, and obtain frequent ABG measurements.
- Provide adequate nutrition by total parenteral nutrition, nasogastric tube feedings, or a soft diet, as ordered.
- Allow parents to see and, if possible, hold their infant in the ICU. Be flexible about visiting privileges. Keep parents informed of the infant's status and prognosis at all times.
- Reassure parents of an infected newborn who may feel guilty about the infant's illness.
- Educate pregnant women to avoid infective materials on farms where listeriosis is endemic among livestock.

Tetanus

(Lockjaw)

Tetanus is an acute exotoxin-mediated infection caused by the anaerobic, spore-forming, gram-positive bacillus Clostridium tetani. *Usually, such infection is systemic; less often, localized. Tetanus is fatal in up to 60% of unimmunized persons, usually within 10 days of onset. When symptoms develop within 3 days after exposure, the prognosis is poor.*

Causes and incidence

Normally, transmission is through a puncture wound that is contaminated by soil, dust, or animal excreta containing *C. tetani*, or by way of burns and minor wounds. After *C. tetani* enters the body, it causes local infection and tissue necrosis. It also produces toxins that then enter the bloodstream and lymphatics and eventually spread to CNS tissue.

Tetanus occurs worldwide, but it's more prevalent in agricultural regions and developing countries that lack mass immunization programs. It's one of the most common causes of neonatal deaths in developing countries, where infants of unimmunized mothers are delivered under unsterile conditions. In such infants, the unhealed umbilical cord is the portal of entry.

In America, about 75% of all cases occur between April and September.

Signs and symptoms

The incubation period varies from 3 to 4 weeks in mild tetanus to under 2 days in severe tetanus. When symptoms occur within 3 days after injury, death is more likely. If tetanus remains localized, signs of onset are spasm and increased muscle tone near the wound.

If tetanus is generalized (systemic), indications include marked muscle hypertonicity; hyperactive deep tendon reflexes; tachycardia; profuse sweating; low-grade fever; and painful, involuntary muscle contractions:

- neck and facial muscles, especially cheek muscles—locked jaw (trismus) and a grotesque, grinning expression called *risus sardonicus*
- somatic muscles—arched-back rigidity (opisthotonos); boardlike abdominal rigidity
- intermittent tonic convulsions lasting several minutes, which may result in cyanosis and sudden death by asphyxiation.

Despite such pronounced neuromuscular symptoms, cerebral and sensory functions remain normal. Complications include atelectasis, pneumonia, pulmonary emboli, acute gastric ulcers, flexion contractures, and cardiac dysrhythmias.

Neonatal tetanus is always generalized. The first clinical sign is difficulty in sucking, which usually appears 3 to 10 days after birth. It progresses to total inability to suck with excessive crying, irritability, and nuchal rigidity.

Diagnosis

Frequently, diagnosis must rest on clinical features, and a history of trauma and no previous tetanus immunization. Blood cultures and tetanus antibody tests are often negative; only a third of patients have a positive wound culture. CSF pressure may rise above normal. Diagnosis also must rule out meningitis, rabies, phenothiazine or strychnine toxicity, and other conditions that mimic tetanus.

Treatment

Within 72 hours after a puncture wound, a patient with no previous history of tetanus immunization first requires tetanus immune globulin (TIG) or tetanus antitoxin to confer temporary protection. Next, he needs active immunization with tetanus toxoid. A patient who has not received tetanus immunization within 5 years needs a booster injection of tetanus toxoid. If tetanus develops despite immediate postinjury treatment, the patient will require airway maintenance and a muscle relaxant, such as diazepam, to decrease muscle rigidity and spasm. If muscle contractions aren't relieved by muscle relaxants, a neuromuscular blocker may be needed. The patient with tetanus needs high-dose antibiotics (penicillin administered I.V., if he's not allergic to it).

Special considerations

When caring for the tetanus victim:

- Thoroughly debride and cleanse the injury site with 3% hydrogen peroxide, and check the patient's immunization history. Record the cause of injury. If it's a dog bite, report the case to local public health authorities.
- Before giving penicillin and TIG, antitoxin, or toxoid, obtain an accurate history of allergies to immunizations or penicillin. If the patient has a history of any allergies, keep epinephrine 1:1,000 and resuscitative equipment available.
- Stress the importance of maintaining active immunization with a booster dose of tetanus toxoid every 10 years.

After tetanus develops:

- Maintain an adequate airway and ventilation to prevent pneumonia and atelectasis. Suction often and watch for signs of respiratory distress. Keep emergency airway equipment on hand, since the patient may require artificial ventilation or oxygen administration.
- Maintain an I.V. line for medications and emergency care, if necessary.
- Monitor EKG frequently for dysrhythmias. Accurately record intake and output, and check vital signs often.
- Turn the patient frequently to prevent bedsores and pulmonary stasis.
- Since even minimal external stimulation provokes muscle spasms, keep the patient's room dark and quiet. Warn visitors not to upset or overly stimulate the patient.
- If urinary retention develops, insert a Foley catheter.
- Give muscle relaxants and sedatives, as ordered, and schedule patient care to coincide with heaviest sedation.
- Insert an artificial airway, if necessary, to prevent tongue injury and maintain airway during spasms.
- Provide adequate nutrition to meet the patient's increased metabolic needs. The patient may need nasogastric feedings or hyperalimentation.

Botulism

Botulism, a life-threatening paralytic illness, results from an exotoxin produced by the gram-positive, anaerobic bacillus Clostridium botulinum. *It occurs with botulism food poisoning, wound botulism, and infant botulism. The mortality from botulism is about 25%, with death most often caused by respiratory failure during the first week of illness.*

Causes and incidence

Botulism is usually the result of ingesting inadequately cooked contaminated foods, especially those with low acid content, such as home-canned fruits and vegetables, sausages, and smoked or preserved fish or meat. Rarely, it is a result of wound infection with *C. botulinum.*

Botulism occurs worldwide and affects adults more often than children. Recently, findings have shown that an infant's GI tract can become colonized with *C. botulinum* from some unknown source, and then the exotoxin is produced within the infant's intestine. Incidence had been declining, but the current trend toward home canning has resulted in an upswing (approximately 250 cases per year in the United States) in recent years.

Signs and symptoms

Symptoms usually appear within 12 to 36 hours (range is 6 hours to 8 days) after the ingestion of contaminated food. Severity varies with the amount of toxin ingested and the patient's degree of immunocompetence. Generally, early onset (within 24 hours) signals critical and potentially fatal illness. Initial symptoms include dry mouth, sore throat, weakness, vomiting, and diarrhea. The cardinal sign of botulism, though, is acute symmetrical cranial nerve impairment (ptosis, diplopia, dysarthria), followed by descending weakness or paralysis of muscles in the extremities or trunk, and dyspnea from respiratory muscle paralysis. Such impairment doesn't affect mental or sensory processes and isn't associated with fever.

Infant botulism usually afflicts infants between 3 and 20 weeks of age and can produce hypotonic (floppy) infant syndrome. Symptoms are constipation, feeble cry, depressed gag reflex, and inability to suck. Cranial nerve deficits also occur in infants and are manifested by a flaccid facial expression, ptosis, and ophthalmoplegia. Infants also develop generalized muscle weakness, hypotonia, and areflexia. Loss of head control may be striking. Respiratory arrest is likely.

Diagnosis

Identification of the offending toxin in the patient's serum, stool, gastric content, or the suspected food confirms the diagnosis. An electromyogram (EMG) showing diminished muscle action potential after a single supramaximal nerve stimulus is also diagnostic.

Diagnosis also must rule out other diseases often confused with botulism, such as Guillain-Barré syndrome, myasthenia gravis, cerebrovascular accident (CVA), staphylococcal food poisoning, tick paralysis, chemical intoxications, carbon monoxide poisoning, fish poisoning, trichinosis, and diphtheria.

Treatment and special considerations

Treatment consists of I.V. or I.M. administration of botulinum antitoxin (available through the Center for Disease Control).

If you suspect ingestion of contaminated food:

- Obtain a careful history of the patient's food intake for the past several days. Check to see if other family members exhibit similar symptoms and share a common food history.
- Observe carefully for abnormal neurologic signs. If the patient returns home, tell his family to watch for signs of weakness, blurred vision, and slurred speech, and to return the patient to the hospital immediately if such signs appear.
- If ingestion has occurred within several hours, induce vomiting, begin gastric lavage, and give a high enema to purge any unabsorbed toxin from the bowel.

If clinical signs of botulism appear:

- Admit the patient to the ICU, and monitor cardiac and respiratory functions carefully.
- Administer botulinum antitoxin, as ordered, to neutralize any circulating toxin. Before giving antitoxin, obtain an accurate patient history of allergies, especially to horses, and perform a skin test. Afterward, watch for anaphylaxis

or other hypersensitivity, and serum sickness. Keep epinephrine 1:1,000 (for subcutaneous administration) and emergency airway equipment available.

• Closely assess and accurately record neurologic function, including bilateral motor status (reflexes, ability to move arms and legs).

• Give I.V. fluids, as ordered. Turn the patient often, and encourage deep-breathing exercises. Isolation is not required.

• As botulism is sometimes fatal, keep the patient and family informed regarding the course of the disease.

• Immediately report all cases of botulism to local public health authorities.

To help prevent botulism, encourage patients to observe proper techniques in processing and preserving foods. Warn them to avoid even *tasting* food from a bulging can or one with a peculiar odor, and to sterilize by boiling any utensil that comes in contact with suspected food; ingestion of even a small amount of food contaminated with botulism toxin can prove fatal.

Gas Gangrene

Gas gangrene results from local infection with the anaerobic, spore-forming, gram-positive rod Clostridium perfringens *(or another clostridial species). It occurs in devitalized tissues and results from compromised arterial circulation following trauma or surgery. This rare infection carries a high mortality unless therapy begins immediately. However, with prompt treatment, 80% of patients with gas gangrene of the extremities survive; prognosis is poorer for gas gangrene in other sites, such as the abdominal wall or the bowel. The usual incubation period is 1 to 4 days but can vary from 3 hours to 6 weeks or longer.*

Causes

C. perfringens is a normal inhabitant of the gastrointestinal and the female genital tracts; it's also prevalent in soil. Transmission occurs by entry of organisms during trauma or surgery. Since *C. perfringens* is anaerobic, gas gangrene is most often found in deep wounds, especially those in which tissue necrosis further reduces oxygen supply. When *C. perfringens* invades soft tissues, it produces thrombosis of regional blood vessels, tissue necrosis, and localized edema. Such necrosis releases both carbon dioxide and hydrogen subcutaneously, producing interstitial gas bubbles. Gas gangrene most commonly occurs in the extremities and in abdominal wounds, and less frequently in the uterus.

Signs and symptoms

True gas gangrene produces myositis and another form of this disease, involving only soft tissue, called anaerobic cellulitis. Most signs of infection develop within 72 hours of trauma or surgery. The hallmark of gas gangrene is crepitation, a result of carbon dioxide and hydrogen accumulation as a metabolic by-product in necrotic tissues. Other typical indications are severe localized pain, swelling, and discoloration (often dusky brown or reddish), with formation of bullae and necrosis within 36 hours from onset of symptoms. Soon the skin over the wound may rupture, revealing dark red or black necrotic muscle, a foul-smelling watery or frothy discharge, intravascular hemolysis, thrombosis of blood vessels, and evidence of infection spread. In addition to these local symptoms, gas gangrene produces early signs of toxemia and hypovolemia (tachycardia, tachypnea, and hypotension), with moderate fever usually not above 101° F. (38.3° C.). Although pale, prostrate, and motionless, most patients remain alert and oriented

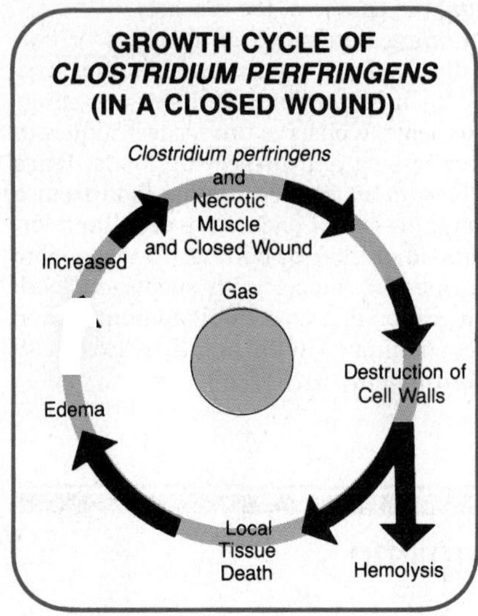

and are extremely apprehensive. Usually death occurs suddenly, often during surgery for removal of necrotic tissue. Less often, death is preceded by delirium and coma, and is sometimes accompanied by vomiting, profuse diarrhea, and circulatory collapse.

Diagnosis

A history of recent surgery or a deep puncture wound and the rapid onset of pain and crepitation around the wound

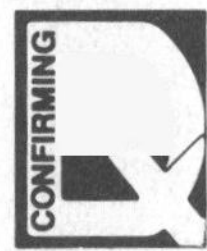

suggest this diagnosis. It is confirmed by anaerobic cultures of wound drainage showing *C. perfringens*; a Gram stain of wound drainage showing large, gram-positive, rod-shaped bacteria; X-rays showing gas in tissues; and blood studies showing leukocytosis and, later, hemolysis. Diagnosis must rule out synergistic gangrene and necrotizing fasciitis; unlike gas gangrene, both these disorders anesthetize the skin around the wound.

Treatment

Treatment includes careful observation for signs of myositis and cellulitis and *immediate treatment* if these signs appear; *immediate* wide surgical excision of all affected tissues and necrotic muscle in myositis (delayed or inadequate surgical excision is a fatal mistake!); intravenous administration of high-dose penicillin; and, after adequate debridement, hyperbaric oxygenation, if available. For 1 to 3 hours every 6 to 8 hours, the patient is placed in a hyperbaric chamber and is exposed to pressures designed to increase oxygen tension and prevent multiplication of the anaerobic clostridia. Surgery may be done within the hyperbaric chamber if the chamber is large enough.

Special considerations

Careful observation may result in *early* diagnosis. Look for signs of ischemia (cool skin; pallor or cyanosis; sudden, severe pain; sudden edema; and loss of pulses in involved limb).

After diagnosis, provide meticulous supportive care:

- Throughout this illness, provide adequate fluid replacement, and assess pulmonary and cardiac functions often. Maintain airway and ventilation.
- To prevent skin breakdown and further infection, give good skin care. After surgery, provide meticulous wound care.
- Before penicillin administration, obtain a patient history of allergies; afterward, watch closely for signs of hypersensitivity.
- Psychological support is critical, since these patients can remain alert until death, knowing that death is imminent and unavoidable.
- Deodorize the room to control foul odor from wound. Prepare the patient emotionally for a large wound after surgical excision, and refer him for physical rehabilitation, as necessary.
- Institute wound precautions. Dispose of drainage material properly (double-bag dressings in plastic bags for incineration), wear sterile gloves when changing dressings, and, after the patient is discharged, have the room cleaned with a germicidal solution.

To prevent gas gangrene, routinely take precautions to render all wound sites unsuitable for growth of clostridia by attempting to keep granulation tissue viable; adequate debridement is imperative to reduce anaerobic growth conditions. Be alert for devitalized tissues, and notify the surgeon promptly. Position the patient to facilitate drainage, and eliminate all dead spaces in closed wounds.

Actinomycosis

Actinomycosis is an infection primarily caused by the gram-positive anaerobic bacillus Actinomyces israelii, *which produces granulomatous, suppurative lesions with abscesses. Common infection sites are the head, neck, thorax, and abdomen, but it can spread to contiguous tissues, causing multiple draining sinuses.*

Sporadic and infrequent, actinomycosis affects twice as many males—especially those aged 15 to 35—as females. It is likely to infect people with dental disease.

Causes

A. israelii occurs as part of the normal flora of the throat, tonsillar crypts, and mouth (particularly around carious teeth); infection results from its traumatic introduction into body tissues.

Signs and symptoms

Symptoms appear from days to months after injury and may vary, depending on the site of infection.

In *cervicofacial actinomycosis* (lumpy jaw), painful, indurated swellings appear in the mouth or neck up to several weeks following dental extraction or trauma. They gradually enlarge and form fistulas that open onto the skin. Sulfur granules (yellowish gray masses that are actually colonies of *A. israelii*) appear in the exudate.

In *pulmonary actinomycosis*, aspiration of bacteria from the mouth into areas of the lungs already anaerobic from infection or atelectasis produces a fever and a cough that becomes productive and occasionally causes hemoptysis. Eventually, empyema follows, a sinus forms through the chest wall, and septicemia may occur.

In *gastrointestinal actinomycosis*, ileocecal lesions are caused by swallowed bacteria, which produce abdominal discomfort, fever, sometimes a palpable mass, and an external sinus. This follows intestinal mucosa disruption, usually by surgery or an inflammatory bowel condition, such as appendicitis.

Rare sites of actinomycotic infection are the bones, brain, liver, kidneys, and female reproductive organs. Symptoms reflect the organ involved.

Diagnosis

Isolation of *A. israelii* in exudate or tissue confirms actinomycosis. Other tests that help identify it are:

- *microscopic examination* of sulfur granules.
- *Gram staining* of excised tissue or exudate to reveal branching gram-positive rods.
- *chest X-ray* to show lesions in unusual locations, such as the shaft of a rib.

Treatment

High-dose I.V. penicillin or tetracycline therapy precedes surgical excision and drainage of abscesses in all forms of the disease and continues for 3 to 6 weeks. Following parenteral therapy, treatment with oral penicillin or tetracycline may continue for 1 to 6 months.

Special considerations

- Dispose of all dressings in a sealed plastic bag.
- After surgery, provide proper aseptic wound management.
- Administer antibiotics, as ordered. Before giving the first dose, obtain an accurate patient history of allergies. Watch for hypersensitivity reactions,

such as rash, fever, itching, and signs of anaphylaxis. If the patient has a history of any allergies, keep epinephrine 1:1,000 and resuscitative equipment available.

- Stress the importance of good oral hygiene and proper dental care.

Nocardiosis

Nocardiosis is an acute, subacute, or chronic bacterial infection caused by a weakly gram-positive species of the genus Nocardia*—usually* Nocardia asteroides. *It is most common in men, especially those with compromised immune defense mechanisms. Its mortality in brain infection exceeds 80%; in other forms, mortality is 50%, even with appropriate therapy.*

Causes

Nocardia are aerobic gram-positive bacteria with branching filaments similar in appearance to fungi. Normally found in soil, these organisms cause occasional sporadic disease in humans and animals throughout the world. Their incubation period is unknown but is probably several weeks. The usual mode of transmission is inhalation of organisms suspended in dust. Less often it's transmitted by direct inoculation through puncture wounds or abrasions.

Signs and symptoms

Nocardiosis originates as a pulmonary infection and causes a cough that produces thick, tenacious, purulent, mucopurulent, and possibly blood-tinged sputum. It may also cause a fever as high as 105° F. (40.6° C.), chills, night sweats, anorexia, malaise, and weight loss. This infection may lead to pleurisy, intrapleural effusions, and empyema. Other effects include tracheitis, bronchitis, pericarditis, endocarditis, peritonitis, mediastinitis, septic arthritis, and keratoconjunctivitis.

If the infection spreads through the blood to the brain, abscesses form, causing confusion, disorientation, dizziness, headache, nausea, and seizures. Rupture of a brain abscess can cause purulent meningitis. Extrapulmonary, hematogenous spread may cause endocarditis and lesions of kidneys, liver, subcutaneous tissue, and bone.

Diagnosis

Identification of *Nocardia* by culture of sputum or discharge is difficult. Special staining techniques often must be relied upon to make the diagnosis, in conjunction with a typical clinical picture (usually progressive pneumonia, despite antibiotic therapy). Occasionally, diagnosis requires biopsy of lung or other tissue. Chest X-rays vary and may show fluffy or interstitial infiltrates, nodules, or abscesses. Unfortunately, up to 40% of nocardial infections elude diagnosis until postmortem examination.

In brain infection with meningitis, lumbar puncture shows nonspecific changes, such as increased opening pressure; CSF shows increased WBC and protein levels, and decreased glucose levels compared to serum glucose.

Treatment

Nocardiosis requires 12 to 18 months of treatment, preferably with trimethoprim-sulfamethoxazole or high doses of sulfonamides. In patients who do not respond to sulfonamide treatment, other drugs, such as ampicillin or erythromycin, may be added. Treatment also includes surgical drainage of abscesses and excision of necrotic tissue. The acute phase requires complete bed rest; as the patient improves, activity can increase.

Special considerations

Nocardiosis requires no isolation: it's not transmitted from person to person.

• Provide adequate nourishment through total parenteral nutrition, nasogastric tube feedings, or a balanced diet.
• Give tepid sponge baths and antipyretics, as ordered, to reduce fever.
• Monitor for allergic reactions to antibiotics.
• High-dose sulfonamide therapy (especially sulfadiazine) predisposes to crystalluria and oliguria. So assess frequently, force fluids, and alkalinize the urine with sodium bicarbonate, as ordered, to prevent these complications.
• In patients with pulmonary infection, administer intermittent positive-pressure breathing (IPPB), as ordered, with chest physiotherapy. Auscultate the lungs daily, checking for increased rales or consolidation. Note and record amount, color, and thickness of sputum.
• In brain infection, regularly assess neurologic function. Watch for signs of increased intracranial pressure, such as decreased level of consciousness, and respiratory abnormalities.
• In long-term hospitalization, turn the patient often, and assist with range-of-motion exercises.

Before the patient is discharged, stress the need for a regular medication schedule to maintain therapeutic blood levels and continuation of drugs even after symptoms subside. Explain the importance of frequent follow-up examinations. Provide support and encouragement to help the patient and his family cope with this long-term illness.

GRAM-NEGATIVE BACILLI

Salmonellosis

One of the most common infections in the United States (over 2 million new cases appear annually), salmonellosis is caused by gram-negative bacilli of the genus Salmonella, *a member of the Enterobacteriaceae family. It occurs as enterocolitis, bacteremia, localized infection, typhoid, or paratyphoid fever. Nontyphoidal forms of salmonellosis usually produce mild to moderate illness, with low mortality.*

Typhoid, the most severe form of salmonellosis, usually lasts from 1 to 4 weeks. Mortality is about 3% of persons who are treated and 10% of those untreated, usually as a result of intestinal perforation or hemorrhage, cerebral thrombosis, toxemia, pneumonia, or acute circulatory failure. An attack of typhoid confers lifelong immunity, although the patient may become a carrier.

Causes and incidence

The most common species of *Salmonella* include *Salmonella typhi*, *Salmonella enteritidis*, and *Salmonella choleraesuis*. Of an estimated 1,700 serotypes of *Salmonella*, 10 cause the diseases most common in the United States; all 10 can survive for weeks in water, ice, sewage, or food. Nontyphoidal salmonellosis generally follows the ingestion of contaminated or inadequately processed foods, especially eggs, chicken, turkey, and duck. Proper cooking reduces the risk of contracting salmonellosis but doesn't eliminate it. Other causes include contact with infected persons or animals, or ingestion of contaminated dry milk, chocolate bars, or pharmaceuticals of animal origin. Salmonellosis may occur in children under age 5 from fecal-oral spread. Enterocolitis and bacteremia are especially common (and more virulent) among infants, the elderly, and people already weakened by other infections; paratyphoid fever is rare in the United States.

Typhoid results most frequently from drinking water contaminated by excre-

CLINICAL VARIANTS OF SALMONELLOSIS

VARIANT	CAUSE	CLINICAL FEATURES
Enterocolitis	Any species of nontyphoidal *Salmonella,* but usually *S. enteritidis*. Incubation period, 6 to 48 hours.	Mild to severe abdominal pain, diarrhea, sudden fever to 102° F. (38.8° C.), nausea, vomiting; usually self-limiting, but may progress to enteric fever (resembling typhoid), local abscesses (usually abdominal), dehydration, septicemia
Paratyphoid	*S. paratyphi* and *S. schottmülleri* (formerly *S. paratyphi B*). Incubation period, 3 weeks or more.	Fever and transient diarrhea; generally resembles typhoid but less severe
Bacteremia	Any *Salmonella* species, but most commonly *S. choleraesuis*. Incubation period varies.	Fever, chills, anorexia, weight loss (without gastrointestinal symptoms), joint pains
Localized infections	Usually follows bacteremia caused by *Salmonella* species.	Site of localization determines symptoms; localized abscesses may cause osteomyelitis, endocarditis, bronchopneumonia, pyelonephritis, and arthritis.
Typhoid fever	*S. typhi* enters GI tract and invades the bloodstream via the lymphatics, setting up intracellular sites. During this phase, infection of biliary tract leads to intestinal seeding with millions of bacilli. Involved lymphoid tissues (especially Peyer's patches in ilium) enlarge, ulcerate, and necrose, resulting in hemorrhage. Incubation period, usually 1 to 2 weeks.	Symptoms of enterocolitis may develop within hours of ingestion of *S. typhi;* they usually subside before onset of typhoid fever symptoms. **First week:** gradually increasing fever, anorexia, myalgia, malaise, headache **Second week:** remittent fever up to 104° F. (40° C.) usually in the evening, chills, diaphoresis, weakness, delirium, increasing abdominal pain and distention, diarrhea or constipation, cough, moist rales, tender abdomen with enlarged spleen, maculopapular rash (especially on abdomen) **Third week:** persistent fever, increasing fatigue and weakness; usually subsides end of third week, although relapses may occur **Complications:** intestinal perforation or hemorrhage, abscesses, thrombophlebitis, cerebral thrombosis, pneumonia, osteomyelitis, myocarditis, acute circulatory failure, chronic carrier state

tions of a carrier. Most typhoid patients are under age 30; most carriers are women over age 50. Incidence of typhoid in the United States is increasing as a result of travelers returning from endemic areas.

Signs and symptoms

Clinical manifestations of salmonellosis vary but usually include fever, abdominal pain, and severe diarrhea with enterocolitis. Headache, increasing fever, and constipation are more common with typhoidal infection.

Diagnosis

Generally, diagnosis depends on isolation of the organism in a culture, particularly blood (in typhoid, paratyphoid, and bacteremia) or feces (in enterocolitis, paratyphoid, and typhoid). Other appropriate culture specimens include urine, bone marrow, pus, and vomitus. In endemic areas, clinical symptoms of

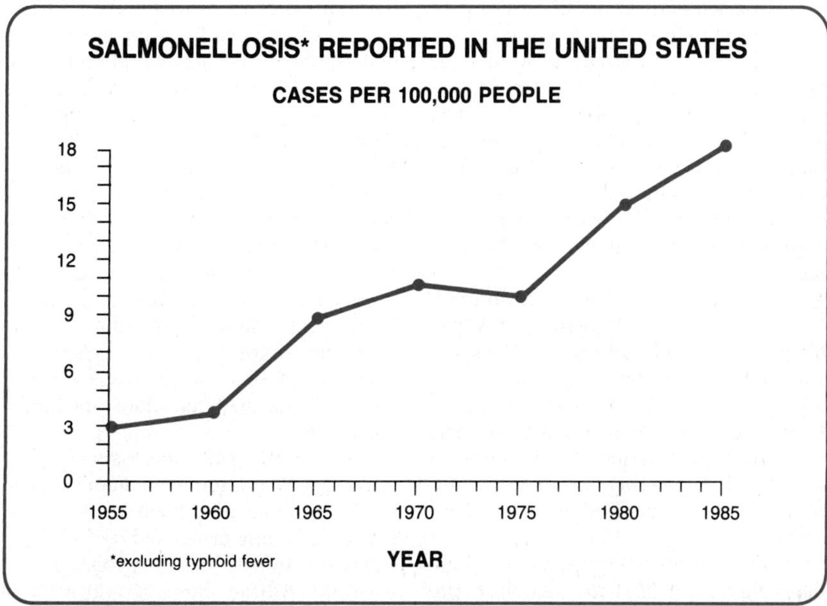

enterocolitis allow a working diagnosis before the cultures are positive. Presence of *S. typhi* in stool 1 or more years after treatment indicates that the patient is a carrier, which is true of 3% of patients.

Widal's test, an agglutination reaction against somatic and flagellar antigens, may suggest typhoid with a fourfold rise in titer. However, drug use or hepatic disease can also increase these titers and invalidate test results. Other supportive laboratory values may include transient leukocytosis during the first week of typhoidal salmonellosis, leukopenia during the third week, and leukocytosis in local infection.

Treatment

Antimicrobial therapy for typhoid, paratyphoid, and bacteremia depends on organism sensitivity. It may include ampicillin, amoxicillin, chloramphenicol, and, in the severely toxemic patient, trimethoprim-sulfamethoxazole. Localized abscesses may also need surgical drainage. Enterocolitis requires a short course of antibiotics only if it causes septicemia or prolonged fever. Symptomatic treatment includes bed rest and, most important, replacement of fluids and electrolytes. Camphorated opium tincture, kaolin with pectin, diphenoxylate hydrochloride, codeine, or small doses of morphine may be necessary to relieve diarrhea and control cramps for patients who must remain active.

Special considerations

- Follow enteric precautions. Always wash your hands thoroughly before and after any contact with the patient, and advise other hospital personnel to do the same. Teach the patient to use proper handwashing technique, especially after defecating and before eating or handling food. Wear gloves and a gown when disposing of feces or fecally contaminated objects. Continue enteric precautions until three consecutive stool cultures are negative—the first one 48 hours after antibiotic treatment ends, followed by two more at 24-hour intervals.
- Observe the patient closely for signs of bowel perforation: sudden pain in the lower right abdomen, possibly after one or more rectal bleeding episodes; sudden fall in temperature or blood pressure; and rising pulse rate.

• During acute infection, plan your care and other activities to allow the patient as much rest as possible. Raise the side rails and use other safety measures because the patient may become delirious. Assign him a room close to the nurses' station so you can check on him often. Use a room deodorizer (preferably electric) to minimize odor from diarrhea and to provide a comfortable atmosphere for rest.

• Accurately record intake and output. Maintain adequate I.V. hydration. When the patient can tolerate oral feedings, encourage high-calorie fluids, such as milkshakes. Watch for constipation.

• Provide good skin and mouth care. Turn the patient frequently, and perform mild passive exercises, as indicated. Apply mild heat to the abdomen to relieve cramps.

• *Don't* administer antipyretics. These mask fever and lead to possible hypothermia. Instead, to promote heat loss through the skin without causing shivering (which keeps fever high by vasoconstriction), apply tepid, wet towels (don't use alcohol or ice) to the patient's groin and axillae. To promote heat loss by vasodilation of peripheral blood vessels, use additional wet towels on the arms and legs, wiping with long, vigorous strokes.

• After draining the abscesses of a joint, provide heat, elevation, and passive range-of-motion exercises to decrease swelling and maintain mobility.

• If the patient has positive stool cultures on discharge, tell him to use a different bathroom than other family members, if possible (while he's on antibiotics), and to avoid preparing uncooked foods, such as salads, for family members.

• To prevent salmonellosis, advise prompt refrigeration of meat and cooked foods (avoid keeping them at room temperature for any prolonged period), and teach the importance of proper handwashing. Advise those at high risk of contracting typhoid (lab workers, travelers) to seek vaccination.

Shigellosis

(Bacillary dysentery)

Shigellosis is an acute intestinal infection caused by the bacteria Shigella, *a short, nonmotile, gram-negative rod.* Shigella *can be classified into four groups, all of which may cause shigellosis: group A* (Shigella dysenteriae), *which is most common in Central America and causes particularly severe infection and septicemia; group B* (Shigella flexneri); *group C* (Shigella boydii); *and group D* (Shigella sonnei). *Typically, shigellosis causes a high fever (especially in children), acute self-limiting diarrhea with tenesmus (ineffectual straining at stool), and possibly electrolyte imbalance and dehydration. It's most common in children ages 1 to 4; however, adults often acquire the illness from children.*

Prognosis is good. Usually, mild infections subside within 10 days; severe infections may persist for 2 to 6 weeks. With prompt treatment, shigellosis is fatal in only 1% of cases, although in severe Shigella dysenteriae *epidemics, mortality may reach 8%.*

Causes and incidence

Shigellosis is endemic in North America, Europe, and the tropics. In the United States, about 23,000 cases appear annually, usually in children or in elderly, debilitated, or malnourished persons. Shigellosis commonly occurs among confined populations, such as those in mental institutions; it's also common in hospitals. In Great Britain, incidence of shigellosis is rising, despite improved sanitation and infection control.

Transmission is through the fecal-oral route, by direct contact with contaminated objects, or through ingestion of contaminated food or water. Occasionally, the housefly is a vector.

Signs and symptoms

After an incubation period of from 1 to 4 days, *Shigella* organisms invade the intestinal mucosa and cause inflammation. In children, shigellosis usually produces high fever, diarrhea with tenesmus, nausea, vomiting, irritability, drowsiness, and abdominal pain and distention. Within a few days, the child's stool may contain pus, mucus, and—from the superficial intestinal ulceration typical of this infection—blood. Without treatment, dehydration and weight loss are rapid and overwhelming.

In adults, shigellosis produces sporadic, intense abdominal pain, which may be relieved at first by passing formed stools. Eventually, however, it causes rectal irritability, tenesmus, and in severe infection, headache and prostration. Stools may contain pus, mucus, and blood. In adults, shigellosis doesn't usually cause fever.

Complications of shigellosis are not common but may be fatal in children and debilitated patients and include electrolyte imbalance (especially hypokalemia), metabolic acidosis, and shock. Less common complications include conjunctivitis, iritis, arthritis, rectal prolapse, secondary bacterial infection, acute blood loss from mucosal ulcers, and toxic neuritis.

Diagnosis

Fever (in children) and diarrhea with stools containing blood, pus, and mucus point to this diagnosis; microscopic bacteriologic studies and culture help confirm it. Microscopic examination of a fresh stool may reveal mucus, RBCs, and polymorphonuclear leukocytes; direct immunofluorescence with specific antisera, *Shigella*. Severe infection increases hemagglutinating antibodies. Sigmoidoscopy/proctoscopy may reveal typical superficial ulcerations.

Diagnosis must rule out other causes of diarrhea, such as enteropathogenic *Escherichia coli* infection, malabsorption diseases, and amebic or viral diseases.

Treatment

Treatment of shigellosis includes enteric precautions, low-residue diet, and most importantly, replacement of fluids and electrolytes with I.V. infusions of normal saline solution (with electrolytes) in sufficient quantities to maintain a urine output of 40 to 50 ml/hour. Antibiotics are of questionable value, but may be used in an attempt to eliminate the pathogen and thereby prevent further spread. Ampicillin, tetracycline, or sulfamethoxazole with trimethoprim may be useful in severe cases, especially in children with overwhelming fluid and electrolyte loss. Antidiarrheals that slow intestinal motility are contraindicated in shigellosis, since they delay fecal excretion of *Shigella* and prolong fever and diarrhea. An investigational vaccine containing attenuated strains of *Shigella* appears promising in preventing shigellosis.

Special considerations

Supportive care can minimize complications and increase patient comfort.

- To prevent dehydration, administer I.V. fluids, as ordered. Measure intake and output (including stools) carefully.
- Correct identification of *Shigella* requires examination and culture of fresh stool specimens. Therefore hand-carry specimens directly to the laboratory. Since shigellosis is suspected, include this information on the lab slip.
- Use a disposable hot-water bottle to relieve abdominal discomfort, and schedule care to conserve patient strength.
- To help prevent spread of this disease, maintain enteric precautions until the stool specimen is negative. Before entering the patient's room, wash your hands and put on a gown and gloves. Also, wash your hands after removing the gown and gloves. Keep the patient's (and

your own) nails short to avoid harboring organisms. Change soiled linen promptly and store in an isolation container.

• During shigellosis outbreaks, obtain stool specimens from all potentially infected staff, and instruct those infected to remain away from work until two stool specimens are negative.

Escherichia coli and Other Enterobacteriaceae Infections

Enterobacteriaceae—a group of mostly aerobic, gram-negative bacilli—cause local and systemic infections, including an invasive diarrhea resembling shigella and, more often, a noninvasive toxin-mediated diarrhea resembling cholera. With other Enterobacteriaceae, Escherichia coli *causes most nosocomial infections. Noninvasive, enterotoxin-producing* E. coli *infections may be a major cause of diarrheal illness in children in the United States.*

Prognosis in cases of mild to moderate infection is good. But severe infection requires immediate fluid and electrolyte replacement to avoid fatal dehydration, especially among children, in whom mortality may be quite high.

Causes and incidence

Although some strains of *E. coli* exist as part of the normal gastrointestinal flora, infection results from certain nonindigenous strains. For example, noninvasive diarrhea results from two toxins produced by strains called enterotoxic or enteropathogenic *E. coli*. These toxins interact with intestinal juices and promote excessive loss of chloride and water. In the invasive form, *E. coli* directly invades the intestinal mucosa without producing enterotoxins, thereby causing local irritation, inflammation, and diarrhea.

Transmission can occur directly from an infected person or indirectly by ingestion of contaminated food or water or contact with contaminated utensils. Incubation takes 12 to 72 hours.

Incidence of *E. coli* infection is highest among travelers returning from other countries, particularly Mexico (noninvasive), Southeast Asia, and South America (invasive). *E. coli* infection also induces other diseases, especially in persons whose resistance is low.

Signs and symptoms

Clinical effects of noninvasive diarrhea depend on the toxin causing the infection but generally include the abrupt onset of watery diarrhea with cramping abdominal pain and, in severe illness, symptoms of acidosis (hypotension and mental lethargy).

Invasive infection produces chills, abdominal cramps, and diarrheal stools that may contain blood and pus.

Infantile diarrhea from an *E. coli* infection is usually noninvasive; it begins with loose, watery stools that change from yellow to green and contain little mucus or blood. Vomiting, listlessness, irritability, and anorexia often precede diarrhea. This condition can progress to fever, severe dehydration, acidosis, and shock.

Diagnosis

Because certain strains of *E. coli* normally reside in the gastrointestinal tract, culturing is of little value; a working diagnosis depends on clinical observation alone.

Firm diagnosis requires sophisticated identification procedures, such as bioassays, that are expensive, time-consuming, and, consequently, not widely available. Diagnosis must rule out salmonellosis and shigellosis, other common infections that produce similar signs and symptoms.

Treatment

Treatment consists of isolation, correction of fluid and electrolyte imbalance, and, in an infant, I.V. antibiotics based on the organism's drug sensitivity. For cramping and diarrhea, bismuth subsalicylate may be ordered.

Special considerations

- Keep accurate intake and output records. Measure stool volume and note presence of blood and pus. Replace fluids and electrolytes, as needed, monitoring for decreased serum sodium and chloride levels and signs of gram-negative shock. Watch for signs of dehydration, such as poor skin turgor and dry mouth.
- For infants, provide isolation, give nothing by mouth, administer antibiotics, as ordered, and maintain body warmth.

To prevent spread of this infection:

- Screen all hospital personnel and visitors for diarrhea, and prevent them from making direct patient contact during epidemics. Report cases to local public health authorities.
- Use proper handwashing technique. Teach personnel, patients, and their families to do the same.
- Use enteric precautions: private room, gown and gloves while handling feces, and handwashing before entering and after leaving the patient's room.
- Advise travelers to foreign countries to avoid unbottled water and uncooked vegetables.
- To prevent accumulation of these water-loving organisms, discard suction bottles, irrigating fluid, and open bottles of saline solution every 24 hours. Be sure to change I.V. tubing according to hospital policy and empty ventilator water reservoirs before refilling with sterile water. Remember to use suction catheters only once.

ENTEROBACTERIAL INFECTIONS

The Enterobacteriaceae include *Escherichia coli, Arizona, Citrobacter, Enterobacter, Erwinia, Hafnia, Klebsiella, Morganella, Proteus, Providencia, Salmonella, Serratia, Shigella,* and *Yersinia.*

Enterobacterial infections are exogenous (from other people or the environment), endogenous (from one part of the body to another), or a combination of both. Enterobacteriaceae infections may cause any of a long list of bacterial diseases: bacterial (gram-negative) pneumonia, empyema, endocarditis, osteomyelitis, septic arthritis, urethritis, cystitis, bacterial prostatitis, urinary tract infection, pyelonephritis, perinephric abscess, abdominal abscesses, cellulitis, skin ulcers, appendicitis, gastroenterocolitis, diverticulitis, eyelid and periorbital cellulitis, corneal conjunctivitis, meningitis, bacteremia, and intracranial abscesses.

Appropriate antibiotic therapy depends on the results of culture and sensitivity tests. Generally, the aminoglycosides, cephalosporins, and penicillins—such as ampicillin, mezlocillin, and piperacillin—are most effective.

Pseudomonas Infections

Pseudomonas is a small gram-negative bacillus that produces nosocomial infections, superinfections of various parts of the body, and a rare disease called melioidosis. This bacillus is also associated with bacteremia, endocarditis, and osteomyelitis in drug addicts. In local pseudomonas infections, treatment is usually successful and complications rare. However, in patients with poor immunologic resistance—premature infants, the elderly, or those with debilitating disease, burns, or wounds—septicemic pseudomonas infections are serious and sometimes fatal.

Causes

The most common species of pseudomonas is *Pseudomonas aeruginosa*. Other species that typically cause disease in humans include *Pseudomonas maltophilia*, *Pseudomonas cepacia*, *Pseudomonas fluorescens*, *Pseudomonas testosteroni*, *Pseudomonas acidovorans*, *Pseudomonas alcaligenes*, *Pseudomonas stutzeri*, *Pseudomonas putrefaciens*, and *Pseudomonas putida*. These organisms are frequently found in hospital liquids that have been allowed to stand for a long time, such as benzalkonium chloride, hexachlorophene soap, saline solution, penicillin, water in flower vases, and fluids in incubators, humidifiers, and inhalation therapy equipment. In elderly patients, pseudomonas infection usually enters through the genitourinary tract; in infants, through the umbilical cord, skin, and gastrointestinal tract.

MELIOIDOSIS

Melioidosis results from wound penetration, inhalation, or ingestion of the gram-negative bacteria *Pseudomonas pseudomallei*. Once confined to Southeast Asia, Central America, South America, Madagascar, and Guam, incidence in the United States is rising due to the recent influx of Southeast Asians.

Melioidosis occurs in two forms: chronic melioidosis, causing osteomyelitis and lung abscesses; and acute melioidosis, which is rare, causing pneumonia, bacteremia, and prostration. Acute melioidosis is often fatal. However, most infections are chronic and asymptomatic, producing clinical symptoms only with accompanying malnutrition, major surgery, or severe burns.

Diagnostic measures consist of isolation of *P. pseudomallei* in a culture of exudate, blood, or sputum; serology tests (complement fixation, passive hemagglutination); and chest X-ray (findings resemble tuberculosis). Treatment includes oral tetracycline—and a sulfonamide, abscess drainage, and in severe cases, chloramphenicol—until X-ray shows resolution of primary abscesses.

Prognosis is good, since most patients have mild infections and acquire permanent immunity; aggressive use of antibiotics and sulfonamides has improved the prognosis in acute melioidosis.

Signs and symptoms

The most common infections associated with pseudomonas include skin infections (such as burns and decubitus ulcers), urinary tract infections, infant epidemic diarrhea and other diarrheal illnesses, bronchitis, pneumonia, bronchiectasis, meningitis, corneal ulcers, mastoiditis, otitis externa, otitis media, endocarditis, and bacteremia.

Drainage in pseudomonas infections has a distinct, sickly sweet odor and a greenish blue pus that forms a crust on wounds. Other symptoms depend on the site of infection. For example, when it invades the lungs, pseudomonas causes pneumonia with fever, chills, and a productive cough.

Diagnosis

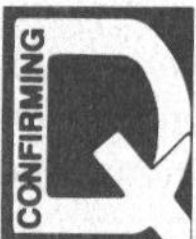

Diagnosis requires isolation of the *Pseudomonas* organism in blood, spinal fluid, urine, exudate, or sputum culture.

Treatment

In the debilitated or otherwise vulnerable patient with clinical evidence of pseudomonas infection, treatment should begin immediately, without waiting for results of laboratory tests. Antibiotic treatment includes aminoglycosides, such as gentamicin or tobramycin, combined with a *Pseudomonas*-sensitive penicillin, such as carbenicillin disodium or ticarcillin. An alternative combination is amikacin and a similar penicillin. Such combination therapy is necessary because *Pseudomonas* quickly becomes resistant to carbenicillin alone. However, in urinary tract infections, carbenicillin indanyl sodium can be used alone if the organism is susceptible and the infection doesn't have systemic effects; it is excreted in the urine and builds up high urine levels that prevent resistance.

Local pseudomonas infections or septicemia secondary to wound infection requires 1% acetic acid irrigations, topical applications of colistimethate sodium and polymyxin B, and debridement or drainage of the infected wound.

Special considerations

- Observe and record the character of wound exudate and sputum.
- Before administering antibiotics, ask the patient about a history of allergies, especially to penicillin. If combinations of carbenicillin or ticarcillin and an aminoglycoside are ordered, schedule the doses 1 hour apart (carbenicillin and ticarcillin may decrease the antibiotic effect of the aminoglycoside). *Don't* give both antibiotics through the same administration set.
- Monitor the patient's renal function (output, BUN, specific gravity, urinalysis, creatinine) during treatment with aminoglycosides.
- Protect immunocompromised patients from exposure to this infection. Attention to handwashing and aseptic techniques prevent further spread.
- To prevent pseudomonas infection, maintain proper endotracheal/tracheostomy suctioning technique: use strict sterile technique when caring for I.V.s, catheters, and other tubes; dispose of suction bottle contents properly; and label and date solution bottles, and change them frequently, according to policy.

Cholera

(Asiatic cholera, epidemic cholera)

Cholera is an acute enterotoxin-mediated gastrointestinal infection caused by the gram-negative rod Vibrio cholerae. *It produces profuse diarrhea, vomiting, massive fluid and electrolyte loss, and possibly hypovolemic shock, metabolic acidosis, and death. A similar bacterium,* Vibrio parahaemolyticus, *causes food poisoning.*

Even with prompt diagnosis and treatment, cholera is fatal in up to 2% of children because of difficulty with fluid replacement; in adults, it is fatal in fewer than 1%. However, untreated cholera may be fatal in as many as 50% of victims. Cholera infection confers only transient immunity.

Causes

Humans are the only documented hosts and victims of *V. cholerae*, a motile, aerobic rod. It's transmitted directly through food and water contaminated with fecal material from carriers or persons with active infections. Cholera is most common in Africa, southern and Southeast Asia, and the Middle East, although isolated outbreaks have occurred in Japan, Australia, and Europe. It usually occurs during the warmer months, and is most prevalent among lower socioeconomic groups. In India, cholera is especially common among children aged 1 to 5, but in other endemic areas, it's equally distributed among all age-groups. Deficiency or absence of hydrochloric acid in gastric juices may increase susceptibility to cholera.

Signs and symptoms

After an incubation period ranging from several hours to 5 days, cholera produces acute, painless, profuse, watery diarrhea and effortless vomiting (without preceding nausea). As the number of stools increases, the stools contain white flecks of mucus ("rice water stools"). Because of massive fluid and electrolyte loss from diarrhea and vomiting (fluid loss in adults may reach 1 liter per hour),

VIBRIO PARAHAEMOLYTICUS FOOD POISONING

V. parahaemolyticus is a common cause of gastroenteritis in Japan; outbreaks also occur on American cruise ships and in the eastern and southeastern coastal areas of the United States, especially during the summer.

V. parahaemolyticus, which thrives in a salty environment, is transmitted by ingesting uncooked or undercooked contaminated shellfish, particularly crabs and shrimp. After an incubation period of 2 to 48 hours, *V. parahaemolyticus* causes watery diarrhea, moderately severe cramps, nausea, vomiting, headache, weakness, chills, and fever. Food poisoning is usually self-limiting and subsides spontaneously within 2 days. Occasionally, however, it's more severe, and may even be fatal in debilitated or elderly persons.

Diagnosis requires bacteriologic examination of vomitus, blood, stool smears, or fecal specimens collected by rectal swab. Diagnosis must rule out not only other causes of food poisoning but also other acute gastrointestinal disorders.

Treatment is supportive, consisting primarily of bed rest and oral fluid replacement. I.V. replacement therapy is seldom necessary, but oral tetracycline may be prescribed. Thorough cooking of seafood prevents infection.

cholera causes intense thirst, weakness, loss of skin turgor, wrinkled skin, sunken eyes, pinched facial expression, muscle cramps (especially in the extremities), cyanosis, oliguria, tachycardia, tachypnea, thready or absent peripheral pulses, falling blood pressure, fever, and inaudible, hypoactive bowel sounds.

Patients usually remain oriented but apathetic, although small children may become stuporous or develop convulsions. If complications don't occur, the symptoms subside and the patient recovers within a week. But if treatment is delayed or inadequate, cholera may lead to metabolic acidosis, uremia, and possibly coma and death. About 3% of patients who recover continue to carry *V. cholerae* in the gallbladder; however, most patients are free of the infection after about 2 weeks.

Diagnosis

In endemic areas or during epidemics, typical clinical features strongly suggest cholera. A culture of *V. cholerae* from feces or vomitus indicates cholera, but definitive diagnosis requires agglutination and other clear reactions to group- and type-specific antisera. A dark-field microscopic examination of fresh feces showing rapidly moving bacilli (like shooting stars) allows for quick, tentative diagnosis. Immunofluorescence also allows rapid diagnosis. Diagnosis must rule out *Escherichia coli* infection, salmonellosis, and shigellosis.

Treatment

Improved sanitation and the administration of cholera vaccine to travelers in endemic areas can control this disease. Unfortunately, the vaccine now available confers only 60% to 80% immunity and is effective for only 3 to 6 months. Consequently, vaccination is impractical for residents of endemic areas.

Treatment requires rehydration by rapid I.V. infusion of large amounts (50 to 100 ml/minute) of isotonic saline solution, alternating with isotonic sodium bicarbonate or sodium lactate. Potassium replacement may be added to the I.V. solution.

When I.V. infusions have corrected hypovolemia, fluid infusion decreases to quantities sufficient to maintain normal pulse and skin turgor or to replace fluid loss through diarrhea. An oral glucose-electrolyte solution can substitute for I.V. infusions. In mild cholera, oral fluid replacement is adequate. If symptoms persist despite fluid and electrolyte replacement, treatment includes tetracycline.

Special considerations

A cholera patient requires enteric precautions, supportive care, and close observation during the acute phase.

- Wear a gown and gloves when giving

physical care, and wash your hands before entering and after leaving the patient's room.

• Monitor output (including stool volume) and I.V. infusion accurately. To detect overhydration, carefully observe neck veins and auscultate the lungs (fluid loss in cholera is massive, and improper replacement may cause potentially fatal renal insufficiency).

• Protect the patient's family by administering oral tetracycline, if ordered.

• Advise anyone traveling to an endemic area to boil all drinking water and avoid uncooked vegetables. If the doctor orders a cholera vaccine, tell the patient that he'll need a booster 3 to 6 months later for continuing protection.

Septic Shock

Second only to cardiogenic shock as the leading cause of shock-death, septic shock (usually a result of bacterial infection) causes inadequate blood perfusion and circulatory collapse. It occurs most often among hospitalized patients, especially men over age 40 and women ages 25 to 45. About 25% of patients who develop gram-negative bacteremia go into shock. Unless vigorous treatment begins promptly, preferably before symptoms fully develop, septic shock rapidly progresses to death (often within a few hours) in up to 80% of these patients.

Causes

In two thirds of patients, septic shock results from infection with gram-negative bacteria: *Escherichia coli, Klebsiella, Enterobacter, Proteus, Pseudomonas,* and *Bacteroides;* in others, from gram-positive bacteria: *Streptococcus pneumoniae, Streptococcus pyogenes,* and *Actinomyces.* Infections with viruses, rickettsiae, chlamydiae, and protozoa may be complicated by shock.

These organisms produce septicemia in persons whose resistance is already compromised by an existing condition; infection also results from transplantation of bacteria from other areas of the body through surgery, I.V. therapy, and catheters. Septic shock often occurs in patients hospitalized for primary infection of the genitourinary, biliary, gastrointestinal, and gynecologic tracts. Other predisposing factors include immunodeficiency, advanced age, trauma, burns, diabetes mellitus, cirrhosis, and disseminated cancer.

Signs and symptoms

The symptoms of septic shock vary according to the stage of the shock, the organism causing it, and the age of the patient.

• *Early stage:* oliguria, sudden fever (over 101° F. [38.3° C.]), and chills; nausea, vomiting, diarrhea, and prostration.

• *Late stage:* restlessness, apprehension, irritability, thirst from decreased cerebral tissue perfusion, tachycardia, tachypnea. Hypotension, altered consciousness, and hyperventilation may be the *only* signs among infants and the elderly.

Hypothermia and anuria are common late signs. Complications of septic shock include disseminated intravascular coagulation (DIC), renal failure, heart failure, gastrointestinal ulcers, and abnormal hepatic function.

Diagnosis

Observation of one or more typical symptoms (fever, confusion, nausea, vomiting, hyperventilation) in a patient suspected of having an infection suggests septic shock and necessitates immediate treatment.

In early stages, arterial blood gases indicate respiratory alkalosis (low PCO_2, low or normal bicarbonate, high pH); as shock progresses, metabolic acidosis develops with hypoxemia indicated by decreasing PCO_2 (may increase as respiratory failure ensues), PO_2, HCO_3-, and pH. The following laboratory tests support the diagnosis and determine the treatment:

- blood cultures to isolate the organism
- decreased platelet count and leukocytosis (15,000 to 30,000/mm³)
- increased BUN and creatinine, decreased creatinine clearance
- abnormal prothrombin consumption and partial thromboplastin time
- simultaneous measurement of urine and plasma osmolalities for renal failure (urine osmolality below 400 milliosmoles, with a ratio of urine to plasma below 1.5)
- decreased central venous pressure (CVP), pulmonary artery and wedge pressures, decreased cardiac output (in early septic shock, cardiac output increases)
- EKG—S-T segment depression, inverted T waves, and dysrhythmias resembling myocardial infarction.

Treatment

The first goal of treatment is to monitor and reverse shock through volume expansion with I.V. fluids and insertion of a pulmonary artery catheter to check pulmonary circulation and pulmonary wedge pressure (PWP). Administration of whole blood or plasma can then raise the PWP to a satisfactory level of 14 to 18 mm Hg. A respirator may be necessary for proper ventilation to overcome hypoxia. Urinary catheterization allows accurate measurement of hourly urine output.

Treatment also requires immediate administration of I.V. antibiotics to control the infection. Depending on the organism, the antibiotic combination usually includes an aminoglycoside, such as gentamicin or tobramycin for gram-negative bacteria, combined with a penicillin, such as carbenicillin or ticarcillin. Sometimes treatment includes a cephalosporin, such as cefazolin, and nafcillin for suspected staphylococcal infection instead of carbenicillin or ticarcillin. Therapy may include chloramphenicol for nonsporulating anaerobes (*Bacteroides*), although it may cause bone marrow depression, and clindamycin, which may produce pseudomembranous enterocolitis. Appropriate anti-infectives for other causes of septic shock depend on the suspected organism. Other measures to combat infections include surgery to drain and excise abscesses, and debridement.

If shock persists after fluid infusion, treatment with vasopressors, such as dopamine, maintains adequate blood perfusion in the brain, liver, digestive tract, kidneys, and skin. Other treatment includes I.V. bicarbonate to correct acidosis, and I.V. corticosteroids, which may improve blood perfusion and increase cardiac output.

Special considerations

Determine which of your patients are at high risk of developing septic shock. Know the signs of impending septic shock, but don't rely solely on technical aids to judge the patient's status. Consider any change in mental status and urinary output as significant as a change in CVP. Report such changes promptly.

- Carefully maintain the pulmonary artery catheter. Check blood gases for adequate oxygenation or gas exchange, and report any changes immediately.
- Keep accurate intake and output records. Maintain urine output (0.5 to 1 ml/kg/hour) and adequate systolic pressure. Be careful to avoid fluid overload.
- Monitor serum gentamicin, and administer drugs, as ordered.

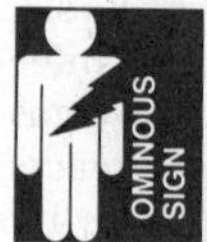

- Watch closely for complications of septic shock: DIC (abnormal bleeding), renal failure (oliguria, increased specific gravity), heart failure (dyspnea, edema, tachycardia, distended neck veins), gastrointestinal ulcers (hematemesis, melena), and hepatic abnormality (jaundice, hypoprothrombinemia, and hypoalbuminemia).

Hemophilus influenzae Infection

Hemophilus influenzae *is a small, gram-negative, pleomorphic aerobic bacillus that appears predominantly coccobacillarly in exudates. It causes diseases in many organ systems but most frequently attacks the respiratory system. It's a common cause of epiglottitis, laryngotracheobronchitis, pneumonia, bronchiolitis, otitis media, and meningitis. Less often, it causes bacterial endocarditis, conjunctivitis, facial cellulitis, septic arthritis, and osteomyelitis.* H. influenzae *pneumonia is an increasingly common nosocomial infection. It infects about half of all children before age 1, and virtually all children by age 3, although a promising new vaccine may reduce this number.*

Signs and symptoms

H. influenzae provokes a characteristic tissue response—acute suppurative inflammation.

When *H. influenzae* infects the larynx, the trachea, and the bronchial tree, it leads to mucosal edema and thick exudate; when it invades the lungs, it leads to bronchopneumonia. In the pharynx, *H. influenzae* usually produces no remarkable changes, except when it causes epiglottitis, which generally affects both the laryngeal and the pharyngeal surfaces. The pharyngeal mucosa may be reddened, rarely with soft yellow exudate. More likely, however, it appears normal or shows only slight diffuse redness, even while severe pain makes swallowing difficult or impossible. These infections typically cause high fever and generalized malaise.

Diagnosis

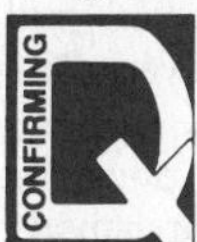

Isolation of the organism confirms *H. influenzae* infection, usually with a blood culture. Other laboratory findings include:

- polymorphonuclear leukocytosis (15,000 to 30,000/mm³)
- leukopenia (2,000 to 3,000/mm³), in young children with severe infection
- *H. influenzae* bacteremia, found frequently in patients with meningitis.

Treatment

H. influenzae infections usually respond to a 2-week course of ampicillin (resistant strains are becoming more common) or chloramphenicol.

Special considerations

- Maintain adequate respiratory function through proper positioning, humidification (croup tent) in children, and suctioning, as needed. Monitor rate and type of respirations. Watch for signs of cyanosis and dyspnea, as they necessitate intubation or a tracheotomy. For home treatment, suggest using a room humidifier or breathing moist air from a shower or bath, as necessary.
- Check the patient's history for drug allergies before administering antibiotics. Monitor CBC for signs of bone marrow depression when therapy includes chloramphenicol.
- Monitor intake (including I.V. infusions) and output. Watch for signs of dehydration, such as decreased skin turgor, parched lips, concentrated urine, decreased urine output, and increased pulse.
- Organize your physical care measures beforehand, and do them quickly so as not to disrupt the patient's rest.
- Take preventive measures, such as giving the *H. influenzae* vaccine to children aged 2 (or younger) to 6, maintaining respiratory isolation, using proper handwashing technique, properly disposing of respiratory secretions, placing soiled tissues in a plastic bag, and decontaminating all equipment.

Whooping Cough

(Pertussis)

Whooping cough is a highly contagious respiratory infection usually caused by the nonmotile, gram-negative coccobacillus Bordetella pertussis, *and, occasionally, by the related similar bacteria* Bordetella parapertussis *and* Bordetella bronchiseptica. *Characteristically, whooping cough produces an irritating cough that becomes paroxysmal and often ends in a high-pitched inspiratory whoop.*

Since the 1940s, immunization and aggressive diagnosis and treatment have significantly reduced mortality from whooping cough in the United States. Whooping cough mortality in children under age 1 is usually a result of pneumonia and other complications. It's also dangerous in the elderly but tends to be less severe in older children and adults.

Causes

Whooping cough is usually transmitted by the direct inhalation of contaminated droplets from a patient in the acute stage; it may also be spread indirectly through soiled linen and other articles contaminated by the patient.

Microscopic enlargement shows *Bordetella pertussis,* the nonmotile, gram-negative coccobacillus that commonly causes whooping cough. After entering the tracheobronchial tree, *B. pertussis* causes mucus to become increasingly tenacious. Classic 6-week course of whooping cough then follows.

Whooping cough is endemic throughout the world, and usually occurs in early spring and late winter. About half the time it strikes unimmunized children under the age of 2, probably because women of childbearing age don't usually have high serum levels of *B. pertussis* antibodies to transmit to their offspring.

Signs and symptoms

After an incubation period of about 7 to 10 days, *B. pertussis* enters the tracheobronchial mucosa, where it produces progressively tenacious mucus. Whooping cough follows a classic 6-week course that includes three stages, each of which lasts about 2 weeks.

First, the *catarrhal stage* characteristically produces an irritating hacking, nocturnal cough, anorexia, sneezing, listlessness, infected conjunctiva, and, occasionally, a low-grade fever. This stage is highly communicable.

After a period of 7 to 14 days, the *paroxysmal stage* produces spasmodic and recurrent coughing that may expel tenacious mucus. Each cough characteristically ends in a loud, crowing inspiratory whoop, and choking on mucus causes vomiting. (Very young infants, however, might not develop the typical whoop.) Paroxysmal coughing may induce complications, such as increased venous pressure, nosebleed, periorbital edema, conjunctival hemorrhage, hemorrhage of the anterior chamber of the eye, detached retina (and blindness), rectal prolapse, inguinal or umbilical hernia, convulsions, atelectasis, and pneumonitis. In infants, choking spells may cause apnea, anoxia, and disturbed acid-base balance. During this stage, patients are highly vulnerable to fatal secondary bacterial or viral infections. Suspect such secondary infection (usually otitis media or pneumonia) in any whooping cough patient with a fever during this stage, since whooping cough itself seldom causes fever.

During the *convalescent stage,* paroxysmal coughing and vomiting gradually subside. However, for months afterward, even a mild upper respiratory infection may trigger paroxysmal coughing.

Diagnosis

Classic clinical findings, especially during the paroxysmal stage, suggest this diagnosis; laboratory studies confirm it. Nasopharyngeal swabs and sputum cultures show *B. pertussis* only in the early stages of this disease; fluorescent antibody screening of nasopharyngeal smears provides quicker results than cultures but is less reliable. In addition, WBC is usually increased, especially in children older than 6 months and early in the paroxysmal stage. Sometimes, the WBC may reach 175,000 to 200,000/mm^3, with 60% to 90% lymphocytes.

Treatment

Vigorous supportive therapy requires hospitalization of infants (often in the ICU), and fluid and electrolyte replacement. Other treatment includes adequate nutrition, codeine and mild sedation to decrease coughing, oxygen therapy in apnea, and antibiotics, such as erythromycin and, possibly, ampicillin, to shorten the period of communicability and prevent secondary infections.

Because very young infants are particularly susceptible to pertussis, immunization—usually with diphtheria and tetanus toxoids (DPT)—begins at 2, 4, and 6 months. Boosters follow at 18 months and at 4 to 6 years. The risk of pertussis is greater than the risk of vaccine complications, such as neurologic damage. However, if such vaccination causes convulsions or unusual and persistent crying, this may be a sign of severe neurologic reaction and the doctor may not order the other doses. The vaccine is contraindicated in children over age 6, because it can cause a severe fever.

Special considerations

Whooping cough calls for aggressive, supportive care and respiratory isolation throughout the illness.

- Monitor acid-base, fluid, and electrolyte balances.
- Carefully suction secretions, and monitor oxygen therapy. Remember: Suctioning removes oxygen as well as secretions.
- Create a quiet environment to decrease coughing stimulation. Provide small, frequent meals, and treat constipation or nausea caused by codeine.
- Offer emotional support to parents of children with whooping cough.
- To decrease exposure to organisms, change soiled linen, empty the suction bottle, and change the trash bag at least once each shift.

Plague

(Black death)

Plague is an acute infection caused by the gram-negative, nonmotile, nonsporulating bacillus Yersinia pestis *(formerly called* Pasteurella pestis*).*

Plague occurs in several forms. Bubonic plague, *the most common, causes the characteristic swollen, and sometimes suppurating, lymph glands (buboes) that give this infection its name. Other forms include* septicemic plague, *a severe, rapid systemic form, and* pneumonic plague, *which can be primary or secondary to the other two forms.* Primary pneumonic plague *is an acutely fulminant, highly contagious form that causes acute prostration, respiratory distress, and death—often within 2 to 3 days after onset.*

Without treatment, mortality is about 60% in bubonic plague, and approaches 100% in both septicemic and pneumonic plagues. With treatment, reported mortality is approximately 18%, and is related to the delay between onset and treatment and to the patient's age and physical condition.

Causes and incidence

Plague is usually transmitted to a human through the bite of a flea from an infected rodent host, such as a rat, squirrel, prairie dog, or hare. Occasionally, transmission occurs when infected animals or their tissues are handled. Bubonic plague is notorious for the historic pandemics in Europe and Asia during the Middle Ages, which in some areas killed up to two thirds of the population. This form is rarely transmitted from person to person. However, the untreated bubonic form may progress to a secondary pneumonic form, which is transmitted by contaminated respiratory droplets (coughing) and is highly contagious. In the United States, the primary pneumonic form usually occurs after inhalation of *Y. pestis* in a laboratory.

Sylvatic (wild rodent) plague remains endemic to South America, the Near East, central and Southeast Asia, north central and southern Africa, Mexico, and the western United States and Canada. In the United States, its incidence has been rising, a possible reflection of different bacterial strains or environmental changes that favor rodent growth in certain areas. Plague tends to occur between May and September; between October and February it usually occurs in hunters who skin wild animals. One attack confers permanent immunity.

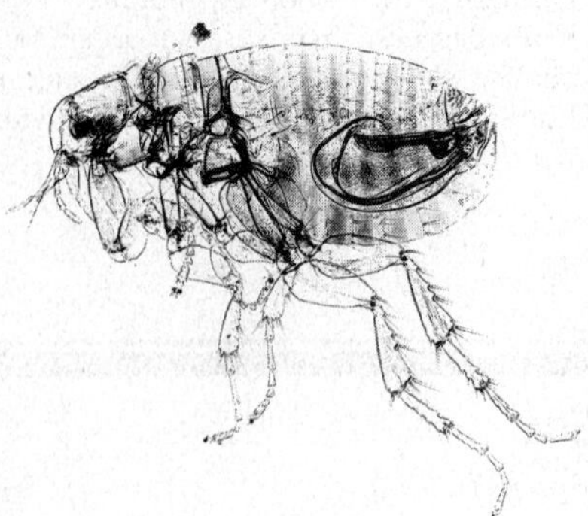

Bubonic plague is transmitted to a human through the bite of a flea—*Xenopsylla cheopis* (bubonic plague flea).

Signs and symptoms

The incubation period, early symptoms, severity at onset, and clinical course vary in the three forms of plague. In *bubonic plague,* the incubation period is 2 to 6 days. The milder form begins with malaise, fever, and pain or tenderness in regional lymph nodes, possibly associated with swelling. Lymph node damage (usually axillary or inguinal) eventually produces painful, inflamed, and possibly suppurative buboes. The classic sign of plague is an excruciatingly painful bubo. Hemorrhagic areas may become necrotic; in the skin, such areas appear dark—hence the name "black death." This infection can progress extremely rapidly: a seemingly mildly ill person with symptoms limited to fever and adenitis may become moribund within hours. Plague may also begin dramatically, with a sudden high temperature of 103° to 106° F. (39.5° to 41.1° C.), chills, myalgia, headache, prostration, restlessness, disorientation, delirium, toxemia, and staggering gait. Occasionally, it causes abdominal pain, nausea, vomiting, and constipation, followed by diarrhea (frequently bloody), skin mottling, petechiae, and circulatory collapse.

In *primary pneumonic plague,* the incubation period is 2 to 3 days, followed by a typically acute onset, with high fever, chills, severe headache, tachycardia, tachypnea, dyspnea, and a productive cough (first mucoid sputum, later frothy pink or red).

Secondary pneumonic plague, the pulmonary extension of the bubonic form, complicates about 5% of untreated plague. A cough producing bloody sputum signals this complication. Primary and secondary pneumonic plagues rapidly cause severe prostration, respiratory distress, and possibly death.

Septicemic plague usually develops without overt lymph node enlargement. In this form, the patient shows toxicity, hyperpyrexia, convulsions, prostration, shock, and disseminated intravascular coagulation (DIC). Septicemic plague causes widespread nonspecific tissue damage—such as peritoneal or pleural effusions, pericarditis, and meningitis—and is rapidly fatal unless promptly and correctly treated.

Diagnosis

Since plague is rare in the United States, it's often overlooked until after the patient dies or multiple cases develop. Characteristic buboes and a history of exposure to rodents strongly suggest bubonic plague.

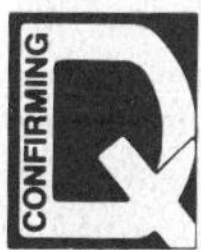

Stained smears and cultures of *Y. pestis* obtained from a needle aspirate of a small amount of fluid from skin lesions confirm this diagnosis.

Postmortem examination of a guinea pig inoculated with a sample of blood or purulent drainage allows isolation of the organism. Other laboratory studies include WBC increased to over 20,000 per mm^3 with increased polymorphonuclear leukocytes, and hemoagglutination reaction (antibody titer) studies. Diagnosis should rule out tularemia, typhus, and typhoid.

In pneumonic plague, diagnosis requires a chest X-ray to show fulminating pneumonia, and stained smear and culture of sputum to identify *Y. pestis.* Other bacterial pneumonias and psittacosis must be ruled out. Stained smear and blood culture containing *Y. pestis* are diagnostic in septicemic plague. However, cultures of *Y. pestis* grow slowly; so, in suspected plague (especially pneumonic and septicemic plagues), treatment should begin without waiting for laboratory confirmation. For a presumptive diagnosis of plague, a fluorescent antibody test may be ordered.

Treatment

Antimicrobial treatment of suspected plague must begin immediately after blood specimens have been taken for culture and shouldn't be delayed for laboratory confirmation. Generally, treatment consists of large doses of streptomycin, the drug proven most effective against *Y. pestis.* Other effective drugs include tetracycline, chloramphenicol, kanamycin, and possibly trimethoprim-sulfamethoxazole. Penicillins are ineffective against plague.

In both septicemic and pneumonic plagues, life-saving antimicrobial treatment must begin within 18 hours of onset. Supportive management aims to control fever, shock, and convulsions and to maintain fluid balance.

After antimicrobial therapy has begun, glucocorticoids can combat life-threatening toxemia and shock; diazepam relieves restlessness; and if the patient develops DIC, treatment may include heparin.

Special considerations

Patients with plague infections require strict isolation, which may be discontinued 48 hours after antimicrobial therapy begins unless respiratory symptoms develop.

- Carefully dispose of soiled dressings, feces, and sputum, and launder soiled linens. When caring for a patient with pneumonic plague, always wear a gown, mask, and gloves. Handle all exudates, purulent discharge, and laboratory specimens with rubber gloves. For further information on precautions, consult your infection control officer.

• Give drugs and treat complications, as ordered.
• Treat buboes with hot, moist compresses. Never excise or drain them, since this may spread the infection.
• When septicemic plague causes peripheral tissue necrosis, prevent further injury to necrotic tissue. Avoid using restraints or armboards, and pad the side rails.
• Obtain a history of patient contacts for a quarantine of 6 days of observation. Administer prophylactic tetracycline, as ordered.
• Report suspected cases to local public health department officials so they can identify the source of infection.
• To help prevent plague, discourage contact with wild animals (especially those that are sick or dead), and support programs aimed at reducing insect and rodent populations. Recommend immunization with plague vaccine to travelers to or residents of endemic areas, even though the effect of immunization is transient.

Brucellosis

(Undulant fever, Malta fever, Bang's disease)

Brucellosis is an acute febrile illness transmitted to humans from animals, and is caused by the nonmotile, nonsporeforming, gram-negative coccobacilli Brucella *bacteria, notably* Brucella suis *(found in swine),* Brucella melitensis *(in goats),* Brucella abortus *(in cattle), and* Brucella canis *(in dogs). Brucellosis causes fever, profuse sweating, anxiety, general aching, and bone, spleen, liver, kidney, or brain abscesses. Prognosis is good. With treatment, brucellosis is rarely fatal, although complications may cause permanent disability.*

Causes

Brucellosis is transmitted through the consumption of unpasteurized dairy products, or uncooked or undercooked contaminated meat, and through contact with infected animals or their secretions or excretions. It's most common among farmers, stock handlers, butchers, and veterinarians. Because of such occupational risks, brucellosis infects men six times more often than it does women, especially those between ages 20 and 50; it's less common in children. Since hydrochloric acid in gastric juices kills *Brucella* bacteria, persons with achlorhydria are particularly susceptible to this disease. While brucellosis occurs throughout the world, it's most prevalent in the Middle East, Africa, the Soviet Union, India, South America, and Europe; it is rarely found in the United States. The incubation period is usually from 5 to 35 days, but in some cases it can last for months.

Signs and symptoms

Onset of brucellosis is usually insidious, but the disease course falls into two distinct phases. Characteristically, the acute phase causes fever, chills, profuse sweating, fatigue, headache, backache, enlarged lymph nodes, hepatosplenomegaly, weight loss, and abscess and granuloma formulation in subcutaneous tissues, lymph nodes, the liver, and the spleen. Despite this disease's common name, few patients have a truly intermittent (undulant) fever; in fact, fever is often insignificant.

The chronic phase produces recurrent depression, sleep disturbances, fatigue, headache, sweating, and sexual impotence; hepatosplenomegaly and enlarged lymph nodes persist. In addition, abscesses may form in the testes, ovaries, kidneys, and brain (meningitis and encephalitis). About 10% to 15% of patients with such brain abscesses develop hearing and visual disorders, hemiplegia, and ataxia. Other complications include osteomyelitis, orchitis, and rarely, subacute bacterial endocarditis, which is difficult to treat.

Diagnosis

In persons with characteristic clinical features, a history of exposure to animals suggests brucellosis. Multiple agglutination tests help to confirm the diagnosis.

• Approximately 90% of patients with brucellosis have agglutinin titers of 1:160 or more within 3 weeks of developing this disease. However, elevated agglutinin titers also follow vaccination against tularemia, *Yersinia* infection, or cholera; skin tests; or relapse. Agglutinin titers testing can also monitor effectiveness of treatment.

• Multiple (three to six) cultures of blood and bone marrow and biopsies of infected tissue (for example, the spleen) provide definite diagnosis. Culturing is best done during the acute phase.

• Blood studies indicate increased erythrocyte sedimentation rate (ESR) and normal or reduced WBC count.

Diagnosis must rule out infectious diseases that produce similar symptoms, such as typhoid and malaria.

Treatment

Treatment consists of bed rest during the febrile phase; a 3-week course of oral tetracycline, with a 2-week course of streptomycin I.M.; and, in severe cases, corticosteroids I.V. for 3 days, followed by oral corticosteroids. Secretion precautions are required until lesions stop draining.

Special considerations

In suspected brucellosis, take a full history. Ask the patient about his occupation and if he has recently traveled or eaten unprocessed food, such as goat's milk.

• During the acute phase, monitor and record the patient's temperature every 4 hours. Be sure to use the same route (oral or rectal) every time. Ask the dietary department to provide between-meal milk shakes and other supplemental foods to counter weight loss. Watch for heart murmurs, muscle weakness, vision loss, and joint inflammation—all may point to complications.

• During the chronic phase, watch for depression and disturbed sleep patterns. Administer sedatives, as ordered, and plan your care to allow adequate rest.

• Keep suppurative granulomas and abscesses dry. Double-bag and properly dispose of all secretions and soiled dressings. Give reassurance that this infection *is* curable.

• Before discharge, stress the importance of continuing medication for the prescribed duration. To prevent recurrence, advise patients to cook meat thoroughly and avoid using unpasteurized milk. Warn meat packers and other persons at risk of occupational exposure to wear rubber gloves and goggles.

SPIROCHETES AND MYCOBACTERIA

Lyme Disease

A multisystemic disorder, Lyme disease is caused by the spirochete, Borrelia burgdorferi, *which is carried by the minute tick* Ixodes dammini *or another tick in the Ixodidae family. It often begins in the summer with the classic skin lesion called erythema chronicum migrans (ECM). Weeks or months later, cardiac or neurologic abnormalities sometimes develop, possibly followed by arthritis.*

Initially, Lyme disease was identified in a group of children in Lyme, Connecticut. Now Lyme disease is known to occur primarily in three parts of the United States: in the northeast, from Massachusetts to Maryland; in the midwest, in Wisconsin and Minnesota; and in the west, in California and Oregon. Although it's endemic to these areas, cases have been reported in 24 states and 18 other countries, including Germany, Switzerland, France, and Australia.

Causes

Lyme disease occurs when a tick injects spirochete-laden saliva into the bloodstream or deposits fecal matter on the skin. After incubating for 3 to 32 days, the spirochetes migrate out to the skin, causing ECM. Then they disseminate to other skin sites or organs by the bloodstream or lymph system. The spirochetes' life cycle isn't completely clear: they may survive for years in the joints or they may trigger an inflammatory response in the host and then die.

Signs and symptoms

Typically, Lyme disease has three stages. ECM heralds stage one with a red macule or papule, often at the site of a tick bite. This lesion often feels hot and itchy and may grow to over 50 cm in diameter. Within a few days, more lesions may erupt along with a malar rash, conjunctivitis, or diffuse urticaria. In 3 to 4 weeks, lesions are replaced by small red blotches, which persist for several more weeks. Malaise and fatigue are constant, but other findings are intermittent: headache, fever, chills, achiness, and regional lymphadenopathy. Less common effects are meningeal irritation, mild encephalopathy, migrating musculoskeletal pain, and hepatitis. A persistent sore throat and dry cough may appear several days before ECM.

Weeks to months later, the second stage begins with neurologic abnormalities—fluctuating meningoencephalitis with peripheral and cranial neuropathy—that usually resolve after days or months. Facial palsy is especially noticeable. Cardiac abnormalities, such as a brief, fluctuating atrioventricular heart block, may also develop.

Stage three begins weeks or years later and is characterized by arthritis. Migrating musculoskeletal pain leads to frank arthritis with marked swelling, especially in the large joints. Recurrent attacks may precede chronic arthritis with severe cartilage and bone erosion.

Diagnosis

Because isolation of *B. burgdorferi* is unusual in humans and because indirect immunofluorescent antibody tests are marginally sensitive, diagnosis often rests on the characteristic ECM lesion and related clinical findings, especially in endemic areas. Mild anemia and an elevated erythrocyte sedimentation rate, leukocyte count, serum IgM, and SGOT support the diagnosis.

Treatment

A 10- to 20-day course of oral tetracycline is the treatment of choice for adults. Penicillin and erythromycin are alternates. Oral penicillin is usually prescribed for children. When given in the early stages, these drugs can minimize later complications. When given during the late stages, high-dose penicillin I.V. may be a successful treatment.

Special considerations

- Take a detailed patient history, asking about travel to endemic areas and exposure to ticks.
- Check for drug allergies, and administer antibiotics carefully.
- For a patient with arthritis, help with range-of-motion and strengthening exercises, but avoid overexertion.
- Assess the patient's neurologic function and level of consciousness frequently. Watch for signs of increased intracranial pressure and cranial nerve involvement, such as ptosis, strabismus, and diplopia. Also check for cardiac abnormalities, such as dysrhythmias and heart block.

Relapsing Fever

(Tick, fowl-nest, cabin, or vagabond fever; or bilious typhoid)

An acute infectious disease caused by spirochetes of the genus Borrelia, *relapsing fever is transmitted to humans by lice or ticks, and is characterized by relapses and remissions. Rodents and other wild animals serve as the primary reservoirs for the* Borrelia *spirochetes. Humans can become secondary reservoirs but cannot transmit this infection by ordinary contagion; however, congenital infection and transmission by contaminated blood are possible. Untreated louse-borne relapsing fever normally carries a mortality rate of more than 10%. However, during an epidemic, the mortality rate may rise to as high as 50%. The victims are usually indigent people who are already suffering from other infections and malnutrition. With treatment, however, prognosis for both louse- and tick-borne relapsing fevers is excellent.*

Causes and incidence

The body louse *(Pediculus humanis* var. *corporis)* carries louse-borne relapsing fever, which often erupts epidemically during wars, famines, and mass migrations. Cold weather and crowded living conditions also favor the spread of body lice.

Inoculation takes place when the victim crushes the louse, causing its infected blood or body fluid to soak into the victim's bitten or abraded skin, or mucous membranes.

Louse-borne relapsing fever occurs most often in North and Central Africa, Europe, Asia, and South America. No cases of louse-borne relapsing fever have been reported in the United States since 1900.

Tick-borne relapsing fever, however, is found in the United States, and is caused by three species of *Borrelia* most closely identified with tick carriers: hermsii with *Ornithodoros hermsi*, turicatae with *Ornithodoros turicata*, and parkeri with *Ornithodoros parkeri*.

This disease is most prevalent in Texas and in other western states, usually during the summer, when ticks and their hosts (chipmunks, goats, prairie dogs) are most active. However, cold-weather outbreaks sometimes afflict persons, such as campers, who sleep in tick-infested cabins.

Because tick bites are virtually painless, and *Ornithodoros* ticks frequently feed at night but do not imbed themselves in the victim's skin, many people are bitten unknowingly.

Signs and symptoms

The incubation period for relapsing fever is 5 to 15 days (the average is 7 days). Clinically, tick- and louse-borne diseases are similar. Both begin suddenly, with a temperature approaching 105° F. (40.5° C.), prostration, headache, severe myalgia, arthralgia, diarrhea, vomiting, coughing, and eye or chest pains. Splenomegaly is common; hepatomegaly and lymphadenopathy are possible. During febrile periods, the victim's pulse rate and respiration rate rises, and a transient, macular rash may develop over his torso.

The first attack usually lasts from 3 to 6 days; then the patient's temperature drops quickly, and is accompanied by profuse sweating. About 5 to 10 days later, a second febrile, symptomatic period begins. In louse-borne infection, additional relapses are unusual; but in tick-borne cases, a second or third relapse is common. As the afebrile intervals become longer, relapses become shorter and milder because of antibody accumulation. Relapses are possibly due to antigenic changes in the *Borrelia* organism.

Complications from relapsing fever

include nephritis, bronchitis, pneumonia, endocarditis, seizures, cranial nerve lesions, paralysis, and coma.

Death may occur from hyperpyrexia, massive bleeding, circulatory failure, splenic rupture, or a secondary infection.

Diagnosis

Diagnosis requires demonstration of the spirochetes in blood smears during febrile periods, using Wright's or Giemsa stain. *Borrelia* spirochetes may be harder to detect in later relapses, because their number in the blood declines. In such cases, injecting the patient's blood or tissue into a young rat and incubating the organism in the rat's blood for 1 to 10 days often facilitates spirochete identification.

In severe infection, spirochetes are found in the urine and cerebrospinal fluid. Other abnormal laboratory results include WBC as high as 25,000/mm^3, with increases in lymphocytes and erythrocyte sedimentation rate; however, WBC may be within normal limits. Because the *Borrelia* organism is a spirochete, relapsing fever may cause a false-positive test for syphilis.

Treatment

Oral tetracycline is the treatment of choice; it may be given I.V., if necessary, and should continue for 4 to 5 days. In cases of tetracycline allergy or resistance, penicillin G may be administered as an alternative. However, neither drug should be given at the height of a severe febrile attack. If they are given, Jarisch-Herxheimer reaction may occur, causing malaise, rigors, leukopenia, flushing, fever, tachycardia, rising respiration rate, and hypotension. This reaction, which is caused by toxic by-products from massive spirochete destruction, can mimic septic shock and may prove fatal. Antimicrobial therapy should be postponed until the fever subsides. Until then, supportive therapy (consisting of parenteral fluids and electrolytes) should be given instead.

When neither tetracycline nor penicillin G controls relapsing fever, chloramphenicol may be given with caution. A complete blood count should be done regularly during treatment with chloramphenicol, because a fatal granulocytopenia, thrombocytopenia, or even aplastic anemia may develop.

Special considerations

- During the initial evaluation period, obtain a complete history of the patient's travels.
- Throughout febrile periods, monitor vital signs, level of consciousness, and temperature every 4 hours. Watch for and immediately report any signs of neurologic complications, such as decreasing level of consciousness or seizures. To reduce fever, give tepid sponge baths and antipyretics, as ordered.
- Maintain adequate fluid intake to prevent dehydration. Provide I.V. fluids as ordered. Measure intake and output accurately, especially if the patient is vomiting and has diarrhea.
- Administer antibiotics carefully. Document and report any hypersensitive reactions (rash, fever, anaphylaxis), especially a Jarisch-Herxheimer reaction.
- Treat flushing, hypotension, or tachycardia with vasopressors or fluids, as ordered.
- Look for symptoms of relapsing fever in family members and in others who may have been exposed to ticks or lice along with the victim.
- Use proper handwashing technique, and teach it to the patient. Isolation is unnecessary because the disease isn't transmitted from person to person.
- Report all cases of louse- or tickborne relapsing fever to the local public health department, as required by law.
- To prevent relapsing fever, suggest to anyone traveling to tick-infested areas (Asia, North and Central Africa, South America) that they wear clothing that covers as much skin as possible. Sleeves and collars should be worn snugly and pant legs should be tucked into boots or socks.

Leprosy

(Hansen's disease)

Leprosy is a chronic, systemic infection characterized by progressive cutaneous lesions. It's caused by Mycobacterium leprae, *an acid-fast bacillus that attacks cutaneous tissue and peripheral nerves, producing skin lesions, anesthesia, infection, and deformities.*

With timely and correct treatment, leprosy has a good prognosis and is rarely fatal. Untreated, however, it can cause severe disability. The lepromatous type may lead to blindness and deformities.

Leprosy occurs in three distinct forms:

- *Lepromatous leprosy,* the most serious type, causes damage to the upper respiratory tract, eyes, and testes, as well as the nerves and skin.
- *Tuberculoid leprosy* affects peripheral nerves and sometimes the surrounding skin, especially on the face, arms, legs, and buttocks.
- *Borderline (dimorphous) leprosy* has characteristics of both lepromatous and tuberculoid leprosies. Skin lesions in this type of leprosy are diffuse and poorly defined.

Causes and incidence

Contrary to popular belief, leprosy is not highly contagious. Rather, continuous, close contact is needed to transmit it. In fact, 9 out of 10 persons have a natural immunity to it. Susceptibility appears highest during childhood and seems to decrease with age. Presumably, transmission occurs through airborne respiratory droplets containing *M. leprae* or by inoculation through skin breaks (with a contaminated hypodermic or tattoo needle, for example). The incubation period is unusually long—6 months to 8 years.

Leprosy is most prevalent in the underdeveloped areas of Asia (especially India and China), Africa, South America, and the islands of the Caribbean and Pacific. About 15 million people worldwide suffer from this disease; approximately 4,000 are in the United States, mostly in California, Texas, Louisiana, Florida, New York, and Hawaii.

Signs and symptoms

M. leprae attacks the peripheral nervous system, especially the ulnar, radial, posterior-popliteal, anterior-tibial, and facial nerves. The central nervous system appears highly resistant. When the bacilli damage the skin's fine nerves, they cause anesthesia, anhidrosis, and dryness; if they attack a large nerve trunk, motor nerve damage, weakness, and pain occur, followed by peripheral anesthesia, muscle paralysis, or atrophy. In later stages, clawhand, footdrop, and ocular complications—such as corneal insensitivity and ulceration, conjunctivitis, photophobia, and blindness—can occur. Injury, ulceration, infection, and disuse of the deformed parts cause scarring and contracture. Neurologic complications occur in both lepromatous and tuberculoid leprosies but are less extensive and develop more slowly in the lepromatous form. Lepromatous leprosy can invade tissue in virtually every organ of the body, but the organs generally remain functional.

Lepromatous and tuberculoid leprosies affect the skin in markedly different ways. In lepromatous disease, early lesions are multiple, symmetrical, and erythematous, sometimes appearing as macules or papules with smooth surfaces. Later, they enlarge and form plaques or nodules called lepromas on the earlobes, nose, eyebrows, and forehead, giving the patient a characteristic leonine appearance. In advanced stages, *M. leprae* may infiltrate the entire skin surface. Lepromatous leprosy also causes loss of eyebrows, eyelashes, and sebaceous and sweat gland function; and, in advanced stages, conjunctival and scleral nodules. Upper respiratory lesions cause epistaxis, ulceration of the uvula and tonsils, septal perforation, and nasal collapse. Lepromatous leprosy can lead to hepatosplenomegaly and orchitis. Fingertips and toes deteriorate as bone resorption follows trauma and infection in these insensitive areas.

When tuberculoid leprosy affects the skin—sometimes its effect is strictly neural—it produces raised, large, erythematous plaques or macules with clearly defined borders. As they grow, they become rough, hairless, and hypopigmented, and leave anesthetic scars.

In borderline leprosy, skin lesions are numerous, but smaller, less anesthetic, and less sharply defined than tuberculoid lesions. Untreated, borderline leprosy may deteriorate into lepromatous disease.

Complications

Occasionally, acute episodes intensify leprosy's slowly progressing course. It remains a matter of dispute whether such exacerbations are part of the disease process or a reaction to therapy. *Erythema nodosum leprosum* (ENL), seen in lepromatous leprosy, produces fever, malaise, lymphadenopathy, and painful red skin nodules, usually during antimicrobial treatment, although it may occur in untreated persons. In Mexico and other Central American countries, some patients with lepromatous disease develop *Lucio's phenomenon,* which produces generalized punched-out ulcers that may extend into muscle and fascia. Leprosy may also lead to complications, such as tuberculosis, malaria, secondary bacterial infection of skin ulcers, and amyloidosis.

Diagnosis

Early clinical indications of skin lesions, and muscular and neurologic deficits are usually sufficiently diagnostic in patients from endemic areas. Biopsies of skin lesions are also diagnostic. Biopsies of peripheral nerves, or smears of the skin or of ulcerated mucous membranes, help confirm the diagnosis. Blood tests show increased erythrocyte sedimentation rate; decreased albumin, calcium, and cholesterol levels; and possibly anemia.

Treatment

Treatment consists of antimicrobial therapy using sulfones, primarily oral dapsone, which may cause hypersensitivity reactions. Hepatitis and exfoliative dermatitis, although uncommon, are especially dangerous reactions. If these reactions do occur, sulfone therapy should be stopped immediately.

Failure to respond to sulfone, or the occurrence of respiratory involvement or other complications, requires use of alternative therapy, such as rifampin in combination with the investigational agent clofazimine or ethionamide. Clawhand, wristdrop, or footdrop may require surgical correction.

When a patient's disease becomes inactive, as determined by the morphologic and bacterial index, treatment is discontinued according to the following schedule: tuberculoid—3 years; borderline—depends on the severity of the disease, but may be as long as 10 years; lepromatous—lifetime therapy.

Since ENL is often considered a sign that the patient is responding to treatment, antimicrobial therapy should be continued. Thalidomide and clofazimine have been used successfully to treat ENL at the National Hansen's Disease Center (NHDC). However, this treatment requires a signed consent form and strict adherence to established NHDC protocols. Corticosteroids may also be given as part of ENL therapy.

Any patient suspected of having Hansen's disease may be referred to the NHDC at Carville, La. At this international research and educational center, patients undergo diagnostic studies and treatment and are educated about their disease. Patients are encouraged to return home as soon as their medical condition permits. The federal government pays the full cost of their medical and nursing care.

Special considerations

Patient care is supportive and consists of measures to control acute infection, prevent complications, speed rehabilitation and recovery, and provide psychological support.

- Give antipyretics, analgesics, and sedatives, as needed. Watch for and report ENL or Lucio's phenomenon.
- Although leprosy isn't highly contagious, take precautions against the possible spread of infection. Tell patients to cover coughs or sneezes with a paper tissue and to dispose of it properly. Take infection precautions when handling clothing or articles that have been in contact with open skin lesions.
- Patients with borderline or lepromatous leprosy may suffer associated eye complications, such as iridocyclitis and glaucoma. Decreased corneal sensation and lacrimation may also occur, requiring patients to use a tear substitute daily and protect their eyes to prevent corneal irritation and ulceration.
- Stress the importance of adequate nutrition and rest. Watch for fatigue, jaundice, and other signs of anemia and hepatitis.
- Tell the patient to be careful not to injure an anesthetized leg by putting too much weight on it. Advise testing bath water carefully to prevent scalding. To prevent ulcerations, suggest the use of sturdy footwear and soaking feet in warm water after any kind of exercise, even a short walk. Advise rubbing the feet with petrolatum, oil, or lanolin.
- For patients with deformities, an interdisciplinary rehabilitation program employing a physiotherapist and plastic surgeon may be necessary. Teach the patient and help him with prescribed therapies.
- Provide emotional support throughout treatment. Communicating accurate information about Hansen's disease to the general public, and especially to health-care professionals, is a function of primary importance for the entire staff at the NHDC.

MYCOSES

Candidiasis

(Candidosis, moniliasis)

Candidiasis is usually a mild, superficial fungal infection caused by the Candida *genus. Most often, it infects the nails (paronychial), skin (diaper rash), or mucous membranes, especially the oropharynx (thrush), vagina (moniliasis), esophagus, and gastrointestinal tract. Rarely, these fungi enter the bloodstream and invade the kidneys, lungs, endocardium, brain, or other structures, causing serious infections. Such systemic infection is most prevalent among drug addicts and patients already hospitalized, particularly diabetics and immunosuppressed patients. Prognosis varies and depends on the patient's resistance.*

Causes

Most cases of *Candida* infection result from *Candida albicans* and *Candida tropicalis*. Other infective strains include *Candida parapsilosis* (cutaneous infection, endocarditis) and *Candida guillermondii* (endocarditis). These fungi are part of the normal flora of the gastrointestinal tract, mouth, vagina, and skin. They cause infection when some change in the body permits their sudden proliferation: rising glucose levels from diabetes mellitus; lowered resistance from a disease such as a carcinoma, an immunosuppressive drug, radiation, aging, or irritation from dentures; or systemic introduction from I.V. or urinary catheters, drug abuse, hyperalimentation, or surgery. However, the most common predisposing factor remains the use of broad-spectrum antibiotics, such as tetracycline, or a combination of drugs that decreases the normal flora and permits an increase of *Candida*. If the mother has vaginal moniliasis, an infant can contract oral thrush while passing through the birth canal. Incidence of candidiasis is rising, particularly because of increasing use of I.V. therapy.

Signs and symptoms

Symptoms of superficial candidiasis correspond to the site of infection:

- Skin: scaly, erythematous, papular rash, sometimes covered with exudate, appearing below the breast, between fingers, and at the axillae, groin, and umbilicus. In diaper rash, papules appear at the edges of the rash.
- Nails: red, swollen, darkened nailbed; occasionally, purulent discharge and the separation of a pruritic nail from the nailbed
- Oropharyngeal mucosa (thrush): cream-colored or bluish white patches of exudate on the tongue, mouth, or pharynx that reveal bloody engorgement when scraped. They may swell, causing respiratory distress in infants. They are only occasionally painful but cause a burning sensation in the throats and mouths of adults.
- Esophageal mucosa: dysphagia, retrosternal pain, regurgitation, and, occasionally, scales in the mouth and throat
- Vaginal mucosa: white or yellow discharge, with pruritus and local excoriation; white or gray raised patches on vaginal walls, with local inflammation; dyspareunia.

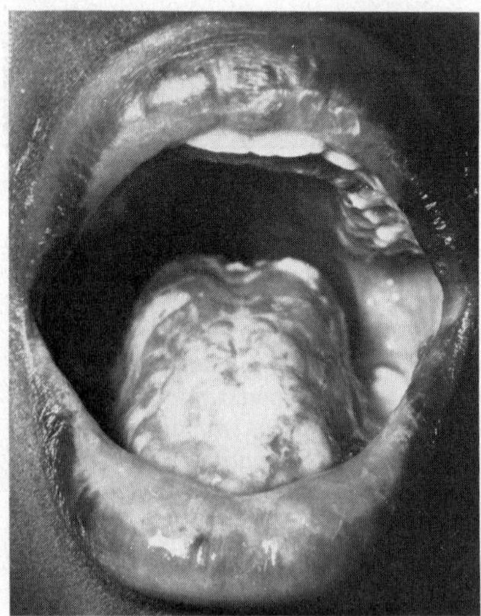

Candidiasis of the oropharyngeal mucosa (thrush) causes cream-colored or bluish-white pseudomembranous patches on the tongue, mouth, or pharynx. Fungal invasion may extend to circumoral tissues.

Systemic infection produces chills; high, spiking fever; hypotension; prostration; and occasional rash. Specific symptoms depend on the site of infection:

- Pulmonary: hemoptysis, cough, fever
- Renal: fever, flank pain, dysuria, hematuria, pyuria
- Brain: headache, nuchal rigidity, seizures, focal neurologic deficits
- Endocardium: systolic or diastolic murmur, fever, chest pain, embolic phenomena
- Eye: endophthalmitis, blurred vision, orbital or periorbital pain, scotoma, and exudate.

Diagnosis

Diagnosis of superficial candidiasis depends on evidence of *Candida* on a Gram stain of skin, vaginal scrapings, pus, or sputum, or on skin scrapings prepared in potassium hydroxide solution. Systemic infections require obtaining a specimen for blood or tissue culture.

Treatment

Treatment first aims to improve the underlying condition that predisposes the patient to candidiasis, such as controlling diabetes or discontinuing antibiotic therapy and catheterization, if possible. Nystatin is an effective antifungal for superficial candidiasis. Topical amphotericin B is effective for candidiasis of the skin and nails; so is gentian violet, which is also effective for thrush and vaginal infections, but is rarely used because it stains the skin. Clotrimazole and miconazole are effective in mucous membrane and vaginal *Candida* infections. Ketoconazole is the treatment of choice for chronic candidiasis of the mucous membranes. Treatment for systemic infection consists of I.V. amphotericin B, flucytosine, or miconazole.

Special considerations

- Instruct a patient using nystatin solution to swish it around his mouth for several minutes before swallowing. Swab nystatin on oral mucosa of an infant with thrush. Provide a nonirritating mouthwash to loosen tenacious secretions and a soft toothbrush to avoid irritation. Relieve mouth discomfort with a topical anesthetic, such as lidocaine, at least 1 hour before meals. (It may suppress the gag reflex and cause aspiration.)
- Provide a soft diet for the patient with severe dysphagia. Tell the patient with mild dysphagia to chew food thoroughly, and make sure he doesn't choke.
- Use cornstarch or dry padding in intertriginous areas of obese patients to prevent irritation.
- Note dates of insertion of I.V. catheters, and replace them according to your hospital's policy, to prevent phlebitis.
- Assess the patient with candidiasis for underlying systemic causes, such as diabetes mellitus. If the patient is receiving amphotericin B for systemic candidiasis, he may have severe chills, fever, anorexia, nausea, and vomiting. Premedicate with aspirin, antihistamines, or antiemetics to help reduce side effects.
- Frequently check vital signs of patients with systemic infections. Provide appropriate supportive care. In patients with renal involvement, carefully monitor intake and output, and urine blood and protein.
- Daily check high-risk patients, especially those receiving antibiotics, for patchy areas, irritation, sore throat, bleeding of mouth or gums, or other signs of superinfection. Check for vaginal discharge; record color and amount.
- Encourage women in their third trimester of pregnancy to be examined for vaginal candidiasis to protect their infants from infection at birth.

Cryptococcosis

(Torulosis, European blastomycosis)

Cryptococcosis is caused by the fungus Cryptococcus neoformans. *It usually begins as an asymptomatic pulmonary infection but disseminates to extrapulmonary sites, usually to the CNS, but also to the skin, bones, prostate gland, liver, or kidneys.*

With treatment, prognosis in pulmonary cryptococcosis is good. However, untreated pulmonary disease may lead to CNS infection, which is invariably fatal within 3 years of diagnosis. Treatment dramatically reduces mortality but does not always reverse neurologic deficit, such as paralysis and hydrocephalus.

Causes and incidence

Transmission is through inhalation of *C. neoformans* in particles of dust contaminated by pigeon feces that harbor this organism. Therefore, cryptococcosis is primarily an urban infection. It is most prevalent in men, usually those between ages 30 and 60 and is rare in children. It's especially likely to develop in immunologically compromised persons, particularly those with Hodgkin's disease, sarcoidosis, leukemia, lymphomas, and those receiving immunosuppressives. In the United States, cryptococcosis is most common in the central and western states.

Signs and symptoms

Typically, pulmonary cryptococcosis is asymptomatic. Onset of CNS involvement is gradual (cryptococcal meningitis), and causes progressively severe frontal and temporal headache, diplopia, blurred vision, dizziness, ataxia, aphasia, vomiting, tinnitus, memory changes, inappropriate behavior, irritability, psychotic symptoms, convulsions, and fever. If untreated, symptoms progress to coma and death, usually a result of cerebral edema or hydrocephalus. Complications include optic atrophy, ataxia, hydrocephalus, deafness, paralysis, chronic brain syndrome, and personality changes.

Skin involvement produces red facial papules and other skin abscesses, with or without ulcerations; bone involvement produces painful osseous lesions of the long bones, skull, spine, and joints.

Diagnosis

Although a routine chest X-ray showing a pulmonary lesion may point to pulmonary cryptococcosis, this infection usually escapes diagnosis until it disseminates. Firm diagnosis requires identification of *C. neoformans* by culture of sputum, urine, prostatic secretions, bone marrow aspirate or biopsy, or pleural biopsy; and in CNS infection, by an India ink preparation of CSF and culture. Blood cultures are positive only in severe infection.

Supportive values include increased antigen titer in serum and CSF in disseminated infection; increased CSF pressure, protein, and white blood cell count in CNS infection; and moderately decreased CSF glucose in about half these patients. Diagnosis must rule out cancer and tuberculosis.

Treatment

Pulmonary cryptococcosis requires close medical observation for a year after diagnosis. Treatment is unnecessary unless extrapulmonary lesions develop or pulmonary lesions progress.

Treatment of disseminated infection calls for I.V. amphotericin B (or, in CNS infection, intrathecal) for 3 to 6 months, or a 6-week course of oral flucytosine with amphotericin B. Supportive measures and acetazolamide can decrease CSF pressure.

Special considerations

Cryptococcosis doesn't necessitate isolation. However, amphotericin B administered intrathecally requires strict aseptic technique.

- Check vital functions, and note changes in mental status, orientation, pupillary response, and motor function. Watch for headache, vomiting, and nuchal rigidity.
- Before giving I.V. amphotericin B, check for phlebitis. Infuse slowly and dilute as ordered—rapid infusion may cause circulatory collapse. Before therapy, draw serum electrolytes to determine baseline renal status. During drug therapy, watch for decreased urinary output, elevated BUN and creatinine levels, and hypokalemia. Monitor CBC, urinalysis, magnesium, potassium, and hepatic function. Ask the patient to report hearing loss, tinnitus, or dizziness.
- Give analgesics and antiemetics, as ordered.
- Provide psychological support to help cope with long-term hospitalization.
- Advise patients to avoid pigeons. Support programs for pigeon control.

Aspergillosis

Aspergillosis is a rare, opportunistic infection caused by fungi of the genus Aspergillus, *usually* Aspergillus fumigatus, Aspergillus flavus, *and* Aspergillus niger. *It occurs in four major forms:* aspergilloma, *which produces a fungus ball in the lungs, called mycetoma, caused by* A. fumigatus; allergic aspergillosis, *a hypersensitive asthmatic reaction to aspergilli antigens;* aspergillosis endophthalmitis, *an infection of the anterior and posterior chambers of the eye that can lead to blindness; and* disseminated aspergillosis, *a rare, acute, and usually fatal infection that produces septicemia, thrombosis, and infarction of virtually any organ, but especially the heart, lungs, brain, and kidneys.*

Aspergillus *may cause infection of the ear (otomycosis), cornea (mycotic keratitis), and prosthetic heart valves (endocarditis), pneumonia (especially in persons receiving immunosuppressive drugs, such as cyclophosphamide), sinusitis, and brain abscesses. Prognosis varies with each form. Occasionally, aspergilloma causes fatal hemoptysis. Disseminated aspergillosis is almost always fatal.*

Causes

Aspergillus is found worldwide, often in fermenting compost piles and damp hay. It's transmitted through inhalation of fungal spores or, in aspergillosis endophthalmitis, the invasion of spores through a wound or other tissue injury. It's a common laboratory contaminant.

Aspergillus is normally present in the mouth and sputum and only produces clinical infection in persons who become especially vulnerable to it. Such debilitation can result from excessive or prolonged use of antibiotics, and from glucocorticoids or other immunosuppressive therapy; also, from Hodgkin's disease, irradiation, leukemia, azotemia, alcoholism, sarcoidosis, organ transplant, bronchitis, or bronchiectasis; or in aspergilloma, from tuberculosis or some other cavitary lung disease.

Signs and symptoms

The incubation period in aspergillosis ranges from a few days to weeks. In aspergilloma, colonization of the bronchial tree with *Aspergillus* produces plugs and atelectasis, and forms a tangled ball of hyphae (fungal filaments), fibrin, and exudate in a cavity left by a previous illness, such as tuberculosis. Characteristically, aspergilloma either causes no symptoms or mimics tuberculosis, with a productive cough and purulent or blood-tinged sputum, dyspnea, empyema, and lung abscesses.

Allergic aspergillosis causes wheezing, dyspnea, cough with some sputum production, pleural pain, and fever.

Aspergillosis endophthalmitis appears 2 to 3 weeks after an eye injury or surgery, and accounts for half of all cases of endophthalmitis. It causes clouded vision, pain, and reddened conjunctiva. Eventually, *Aspergillus* infects the anterior and posterior chambers, where it produces purulent exudate.

In disseminated aspergillosis, *Aspergillus* invades blood vessels, and causes thrombosis, infarctions, and the typical signs of septicemia (chills, fever, hypotension, delirium), with azotemia, hematuria, urinary tract obstruction, headaches, seizures, bone pain and tenderness, and soft-tissue swelling. It's rapidly fatal.

Diagnosis

Aspergillosis is difficult to diagnose. In patients with aspergilloma, a chest X-ray reveals a crescent-shaped radiolucency surrounding a circular mass, but this is not definitive for aspergillosis. In aspergillosis endophthalmitis, a history of ocular trauma or surgery and a culture or exudate showing *Aspergillus* is diagnostic. In allergic aspergillosis, sputum examination shows eosinophils. Culture of mouth scrapings or sputum showing *Aspergillus* is inconclusive, since even healthy persons harbor this fungus. In disseminated aspergillosis, culture and microscopic examination of affected tissue can confirm diagnosis, but this form is usually diagnosed at autopsy.

Treatment and special considerations

Aspergillosis doesn't require isolation. Treatment of aspergilloma necessitates local excision of the lesion and supportive therapy, such as chest physiotherapy and coughing, to improve pulmonary function. Allergic aspergillosis requires desensitization and, possibly, steroids. Disseminated aspergillosis and aspergillosis endophthalmitis require a 2- to 3-week course of I.V. amphotericin B (as well as prompt cessation of immunosuppressive therapy) and possibly flucytosine. However, the disseminated form of aspergillosis often resists amphotericin B therapy and rapidly progresses to death.

Histoplasmosis

(Ohio Valley disease, Central Mississippi Valley disease, Appalachian Mountain disease, Darling's disease)

Histoplasmosis is a fungal infection caused by Histoplasma capsulatum. *In the United States, it occurs in three forms: primary acute histoplasmosis, progressive disseminated histoplasmosis (acute disseminated or chronic disseminated disease), and chronic pulmonary (cavitary) histoplasmosis, which produces cavitations in the lung similar to those in pulmonary tuberculosis.*

A fourth form, African histoplasmosis, occurs only in Africa and is caused by the fungus Histoplasma capsulatum *var.* duboisii.

Prognosis varies with each form. The primary acute disease is benign; the progressive disseminated disease is fatal in approximately 90% of patients; and without proper chemotherapy, chronic pulmonary histoplasmosis is fatal in 50% of patients within 5 years.

Causes

H. capsulatum is found in the feces of birds and bats or in soil contaminated by their feces, such as that near roosts, chicken coops, barns, or caves or underneath bridges. Histoplasmosis occurs worldwide, especially in the temperate areas of Asia, Africa, Europe, and North and South America. In the United States, it's most prevalent in the central and eastern states, especially in the Mississippi and Ohio River valleys.

Transmission is through inhalation of *H. capsulatum* or *H. duboisii* spores or through the invasion of spores after minor skin trauma. Probably because of occupational exposure, histoplasmosis is more common in adult males. Fatal disseminated disease, however, is more common in infants and elderly men.

The incubation period is from 5 to 18 days, although chronic pulmonary histoplasmosis may progress slowly for many years.

Signs and symptoms

Symptoms vary with each form of this disease. Primary acute histoplasmosis may be asymptomatic or may cause symptoms of a mild respiratory illness similar to a severe cold or influenza. Typical clinical effects may include fever, malaise, headache, myalgia, anorexia, cough, and chest pain.

Progressive disseminated histoplasmosis causes hepatosplenomegaly, general lymphadenopathy, anorexia, weight loss, fever, and possibly ulceration of the tongue, palate, epiglottis, and larynx, with resulting pain, hoarseness, and dysphagia. It may also cause endocarditis, meningitis, pericarditis, and adrenal insufficiency.

Chronic pulmonary histoplasmosis mimics pulmonary tuberculosis and causes a productive cough, dyspnea, and occasional hemoptysis. Eventually, it produces weight loss, extreme weakness, breathlessness, and cyanosis.

African histoplasmosis produces cutaneous nodules, papules, and ulcers; lymphadenopathy; lesions of the skull and long bones; and visceral involvement without pulmonary lesions.

Diagnosis

A history of exposure to contaminated soil in an endemic area, miliary calcification in the lung or spleen, and a positive histoplasmin skin test indicate exposure to histoplasmosis. Rising complement fixation and agglutination titers (more than 1:32) strongly suggest histoplasmosis.

The diagnosis of histoplasmosis requires a morphologic examination of tissue biopsy and culture of *H. capsulatum* from sputum in acute primary and chronic pulmonary histoplasmosis; and from bone marrow, lymph node, blood, and infection sites in disseminated histoplasmosis. However, cultures take several weeks to grow these organisms. Faster diagnosis is possible with stained biopsies using Gomori's stains (methenamine silver) or periodic acid-Schiff reaction. Findings must rule out tuberculosis and other diseases that produce similar symptoms.

The diagnosis of histoplasmosis caused by *H. duboisii* necessitates examination of tissue biopsy and culture of the affected site.

Treatment

Treatment consists of antifungal therapy, surgery, and supportive care.

- Antifungal therapy is most important. Except for asymptomatic primary acute histoplasmosis (which resolves spontaneously) and the African form, histoplasmosis requires high-dose or long-term (10-week) therapy with amphotericin B or ketoconazole.
- Surgery includes lung resection to remove pulmonary nodules, a shunt for increased intracranial pressure, and cardiac repair for constrictive pericarditis.
- Supportive care includes oxygen for respiratory distress, glucocorticoids for adrenal insufficiency, and parenteral fluids for dysphagia due to oral or laryngeal ulcerations. Histoplasmosis doesn't require isolation.

Special considerations

Patient care is primarily supportive.

- Give drugs, as ordered, and teach patients about possible side effects. Since amphotericin B may cause chills, fever, nausea, and vomiting, give appropriate antipyretics and antiemetics, as ordered.
- Patients with chronic pulmonary or disseminated histoplasmosis also need psychological support because of long-term hospitalization. As needed, refer to a social worker or occupational therapist. Help parents of children with this disease arrange for a visiting teacher.
- To help prevent histoplasmosis, teach persons in endemic areas to watch for early signs of this infection and to seek treatment promptly. Instruct persons who risk occupational exposure to contaminated soil to wear face masks.

Blastomycosis

(North American blastomycosis, Gilchrist's disease)

Blastomycosis is caused by the yeastlike fungus Blastomyces dermatitidis, *which usually infects the lungs and produces bronchopneumonia. Less frequently, this fungus may disseminate through the blood and cause osteomyelitis and CNS, skin, and genital disorders. Untreated blastomycosis is slowly progressive and usually fatal; however, spontaneous remissions occasionally occur. With antifungal drug therapy and supportive treatment, the prognosis for patients with blastomycosis is good.*

Causes and incidence

Blastomycosis is generally found in North America (where *B. dermatitidis* normally inhabits the soil) and is endemic to the southeastern United States. Sporadic cases have also been reported in Africa. Blastomycosis usually infects men aged 30 to 50, but no occupational link has been found. *B. dermatitidis* is probably inhaled by people who are in close contact with the soil. The incubation period may range from weeks to months.

Signs and symptoms

Initial signs and symptoms of pulmonary blastomycosis mimic those of a viral upper respiratory infection. These findings typically include a dry, hacking, or productive cough (occasionally hemoptysis), pleuritic chest pain, fever, shaking, chills, night sweats, malaise, anorexia, and weight loss.

Cutaneous blastomycosis causes small, painless, nonpruritic, and nondistinctive macules or papules on exposed body parts. These lesions become raised and reddened, and occasionally progress to draining skin abscesses or fistulas.

Dissemination to the bone causes soft-tissue swelling, tenderness, and warmth over bony lesions, which generally occur in the thoracic, lumbar, and sacral regions; long bones of the legs; and, in children, the skull.

Genital dissemination produces painful swelling of the testes, the epididymis, or the prostate; deep perineal pain; pyuria; and hematuria. CNS dissemination causes meningitis or cerebral abscesses, and resulting decreased level of consciousness, lethargy, and change in mood or affect. Other dissemination may result in Addison's disease (adrenal insufficiency), pericarditis, and arthritis.

Diagnosis

Diagnosis of blastomycosis requires:

- culture of *B. dermatitidis* from skin lesions, pus, sputum, or pulmonary secretions
- microscopic examination of tissue biopsy from the skin or the lungs, or of bronchial washings, sputum, or pus, as the doctor finds appropriate
- complement fixation testing. While such testing isn't conclusive, a high titer in extrapulmonary disease is a poor prognostic sign
- immunodiffusion testing. This specific study detects antibodies for the A and B antigen of blastomycosis.

In addition, suspected pulmonary blastomycosis requires a chest X-ray, which may show pulmonary infiltrates. Other abnormal laboratory findings include increased WBC and erythrocyte sedimentation rate, slightly increased serum globulin, mild normochromic anemia, and, with bone lesions, increased alkaline phosphatase.

Treatment and special considerations

All forms of blastomycosis respond to amphotericin B; primary skin lesions usually respond to hydroxystilbamidine isethionate. Care is mainly supportive.

- In severe pulmonary blastomycosis, check for hemoptysis. If the patient is febrile, provide a cool room and give tepid sponge baths.
- If blastomycosis causes joint pain or swelling, elevate the joint and apply heat. In CNS infection, watch the patient carefully for decreasing level of consciousness and unequal pupillary response. In men with disseminated disease, watch for hematuria.
- Infuse I.V. amphotericin B slowly (too rapid infusion may cause circulatory collapse). During infusion, monitor vital signs (temperature may rise but should subside within 1 to 2 hours). Watch for decreased urinary output and monitor laboratory results for increased BUN, increased creatinine, and hypokalemia, which may indicate kidney toxicity. Report any hearing loss, tinnitus, or dizziness immediately. To relieve side effects of amphotericin B, give antiemetics and antipyretics, as ordered.
- Protect hydroxystilbamidine isethionate from light during infusion.

Coccidioidomycosis

(Valley fever, San Joaquin Valley fever)

Coccidioidomycosis is caused by the fungus Coccidioides immitis *and occurs primarily as a respiratory infection, although generalized dissemination may occur. The* primary *pulmonary form is usually self-limiting and rarely fatal. The rare* secondary *(progressive, disseminated) form produces abscesses throughout the body and carries a mortality of up to 60%, even with treatment. Such dissemination is more common in dark-skinned men, pregnant women, and patients who are receiving immunosuppressives.*

Causes

Coccidioidomycosis is endemic to the southwestern United States, especially between the San Joaquin Valley in California and southwestern Texas; it also is found in Mexico, Guatemala, Honduras, Venezuela, Colombia, Argentina, and Paraguay. It may result from inhalation of *C. immitis* spores found in the soil in these areas, or from inhalation of spores from dressings or plaster casts of infected persons. It's most prevalent during warm, dry months.

Because of population distribution and an occupational link (it's common in migrant farm laborers), coccidioidomycosis generally strikes Philippine Americans, Mexican Americans, American Indians, and blacks. In primary infection, the incubation period is from 1 to 4 weeks.

Signs and symptoms

Primary coccidioidomycosis usually produces acute or subacute respiratory symptoms (dry cough, pleuritic chest pain, pleural effusion), fever, sore throat, chills, malaise, headache, and an itchy macular rash. Occasionally, the sole symptom is a fever that persists for weeks. From 3 days to several weeks after onset, some patients, particularly Caucasian women, may develop tender red nodules (erythema nodosum) on their legs, especially the shins, with joint pain in the knees and ankles. Generally, primary disease heals spontaneously within a few weeks.

In rare cases, coccidioidomycosis disseminates to other organs several weeks or months after the primary infection. Disseminated coccidioidomycosis causes fever and abscesses throughout the body, especially in skeletal, CNS, splenic, hepatic, renal, and subcutaneous tissues. Depending on the location of these abscesses, disseminated coccidioidomycosis may cause bone pain and meningitis. Chronic pulmonary cavitation, which can occur in both the primary and the disseminated forms, causes hemoptysis with or without chest pain.

Diagnosis

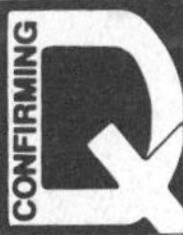

Typical clinical features and skin and serologic studies confirm this diagnosis. The primary form—and sometimes the disseminated form—produces a positive coccidioidin skin test. In the first week of illness, complement fixation for IgG antibodies, or in the first month, positive serum precipitins (immunoglobulins) also establish this diagnosis. Examination or, more recently, immunodiffusion testing of sputum, pus from lesions, and a tissue biopsy may show *C. immitis* spores. The presence of antibodies in pleural and joint fluid, and a rising serum or body fluid antibody titer indicate dissemination.

Other abnormal laboratory results include increased WBC count, eosinophilia, increased erythrocyte sedimentation rate, and a chest X-ray showing bilateral diffuse infiltrates.

In coccidioidal meningitis, examination of CSF shows WBC increased to more than 500/mm³ (due primarily to mononuclear leukocytes), increased protein, and decreased glucose. Ventricular fluid obtained from the brain may contain complement fixation antibodies.

After diagnosis, the results of serial skin tests, blood cultures, and serologic testing may document the effectiveness of therapy.

Treatment

Usually, mild primary coccidioidomycosis requires only bed rest and relief of symptoms. Severe primary disease and dissemination, however, also require long-term I.V. infusion or, in CNS dissemination, intrathecal administration of amphotericin B, and, possibly, excision or drainage of lesions. Severe pulmonary lesions may require lobectomy. Miconazole and ketoconazole show promise.

Special considerations

- Don't wash off the circle marked on the skin for serial skin tests, since this aids in reading test results.
- In mild primary disease, encourage bed rest and adequate fluid intake. Record the amount and color of sputum. Watch for shortness of breath that may point to pleural effusion. In patients with arthralgia, provide analgesics, as ordered.
- Coccidioidomycosis requires strict secretion precautions if the patient has draining lesions. "No touch" dressing technique and careful handwashing are essential.
- In CNS dissemination, monitor carefully for decreased level of consciousness or change in mood or affect.
- Before intrathecal administration of amphotericin B, explain the procedure to the patient, and reassure him that he'll receive analgesics before a lumbar puncture. If the patient is to receive amphotericin B intravenously, infuse it slowly, as ordered, since rapid infusion may cause circulatory collapse. During infusion, monitor vital signs (temperature may rise but should return to normal within 1 to 2 hours). Watch for decreased urinary output, and monitor laboratory results for elevated BUN, elevated creatinine, and hypokalemia. Tell the patient to immediately report hearing loss, tinnitus, dizziness, and all signs of toxicity. To ease side effects of amphotericin B, give antiemetics and antipyretics, as ordered.

Sporotrichosis

Sporotrichosis is a chronic disease caused by the fungus Sporothrix schenckii. *It occurs in three forms:* cutaneous lymphatic, *which produces nodular erythematous primary lesions and secondary lesions along lymphatic channels;* pulmonary, *a rare form that produces a productive cough and pulmonary lesions; and* disseminated, *another rare form, which may cause arthritis or osteomyelitis. The course of sporotrichosis is slow, prognosis is good, and fatalities are rare. However, untreated skin lesions may cause secondary bacterial infection.*

Causes

S. schenckii is found in soil, wood, sphagnum moss, and decaying vegetation throughout the world. Since this fungus usually enters through broken skin (the pulmonary form through inhalation), sporotrichosis is more common in horticulturists, agricultural workers, and home gardeners. Perhaps because of occupational exposure, it's more prevalent in adult men than in women and children. The typical incubation period lasts from 1 week to 3 months.

Signs and symptoms

Cutaneous lymphatic sporotrichosis produces characteristic skin lesions, usually on the hands or fingers. Each lesion begins as a small, painless, movable subcutaneous nodule, but grows progressively larger, discolors, and eventually ulcerates. Later, additional lesions form along the adjacent lymph node chain.

Pulmonary sporotrichosis causes a productive cough, lung cavities and nodules, hilar adenopathy, pleural effusion, fibrosis, and the formation of a fungus ball. It's often associated with sarcoidosis and tuberculosis.

Disseminated sporotrichosis produces multifocal lesions that spread from the primary lesion in the skin or lungs. Onset is insidious. Typically, it causes weight loss, anorexia, synovial or bony lesions, and possibly arthritis or osteomyelitis.

Diagnosis

Typical clinical findings and culture of *S. schenckii* in sputum, pus, or bone drainage confirm this diagnosis. Histologic identification is difficult. Diagnosis must rule out tuberculosis, sarcoidosis, and, in patients with the disseminated form, bacterial osteomyelitis and neoplasm.

Treatment

Sporotrichosis doesn't require isolation. The cutaneous lymphatic form usually responds to application of a saturated solution of potassium iodide, generally continued for 1 to 2 months after lesions heal. Occasionally, cutaneous lesions must be excised or drained. The disseminated form responds to intravenous amphotericin B but may require several weeks of treatment. Local heat application relieves pain. Cavitary pulmonary lesions may require surgery.

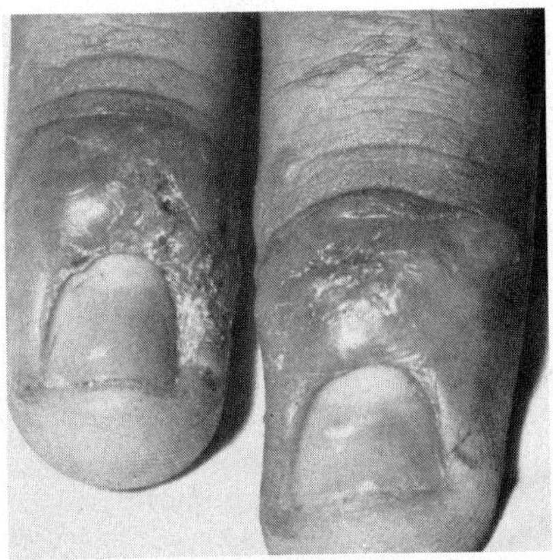

Ulceration, swelling, and crusting of nodules on fingers is characteristic of cutaneous-lymphatic sporotrichosis.

Special considerations

- Keep lesions clean, make the patient as comfortable as possible, and carefully dispose of contaminated dressings.
- Warn patients about possible adverse effects of drugs. Because amphotericin B may cause fever, chills, nausea, and vomiting, give antipyretics and antiemetics, as ordered.
- To help prevent sporotrichosis, advise horticulturists and home gardeners to wear gloves while working.

RESPIRATORY VIRUSES

Common Cold

The common cold is an acute, usually afebrile viral infection that causes inflammation of the upper respiratory tract. It accounts for more time lost from school or work than any other cause, and is the most common infectious disease. Although it's benign and self-limiting, it can lead to secondary bacterial infections.

Causes and incidence

The common cold is more prevalent in children than in adults; in adolescent boys than in girls; and in women than in men. In temperate zones, it occurs more often in the colder months; in the tropics, during the rainy season.

About 90% of colds stem from a viral infection of the upper respiratory passages and consequent mucous membrane inflammation; occasionally, colds result from mycoplasma. Over a hundred viruses can cause the common cold. Major offenders include rhinoviruses, coronaviruses, myxoviruses, adenoviruses, coxsackieviruses, and echoviruses.

Transmission occurs through airborne respiratory droplets, contact with contaminated objects, and hand-to-hand transmission. Children acquire new strains from their schoolmates and pass them on to family members. Fatigue or drafts doesn't increase susceptibility.

Signs and symptoms

After a 1- to 4-day incubation period, the common cold produces pharyngitis, nasal congestion, coryza, headache, and burning, watery eyes; there may be fever (in children), chills, myalgia, arthralgia, malaise, lethargy, and a hacking, nonproductive, or nocturnal cough.

As the cold progresses, clinical features develop more fully. After a day, symptoms include a feeling of fullness with a copious nasal discharge that often irritates the nose, adding to discomfort. About 3 days after onset, major signs diminish, but the "stuffed up" feeling often persists for a week. Reinfection (with productive cough) is common, but complications (sinusitis, otitis media, pharyngitis, lower respiratory tract infection) are rare. A cold is communicable for 2 to 3 days after the onset of symptoms.

Diagnosis

No explicit diagnostic test exists to isolate the specific organism responsible for the common cold. Consequently, diagnosis rests on the typically mild, localized and afebrile upper respiratory symptoms. Despite infection, WBC and differential are within normal limits. Diagnosis must rule out allergic rhinitis, measles, rubella, and other disorders that produce similar early symptoms. A temperature higher than 100° F. (37.8° C.), severe malaise, anorexia, tachycardia, exudate on the tonsils or throat, petechiae, and tender lymph glands may point to more serious disorders and require additional diagnostic tests.

Treatment

The primary treatment—aspirin or acetaminophen, fluids, and rest—is purely symptomatic, as the common cold has no cure. Aspirin eases myalgia and headache; fluids help loosen accumulated respiratory secretions and maintain hydration; and rest combats fatigue and weakness. In a child with a fever, acetaminophen is the drug of choice.

Decongestants can relieve congestion. Throat lozenges relieve soreness. Steam encourages expectoration. Nasal douching, sinus drainage, and antibiotics aren't necessary except in complications or chronic illness. Pure antitussives relieve severe coughs but are contraindicated with productive coughs, when cough suppression is harmful. The role of vitamin C remains controversial. In infants, saline nose drops and mucus aspiration with a bulb syringe may be beneficial.

Currently, no known measure can prevent the common cold. Vitamin therapy, interferon administration, and ultraviolet irradiation are under investigation.

Special considerations

- Emphasize that antibiotics do not cure the common cold.
- Tell the patient to maintain bed rest during the first few days; to use a lubricant on his nostrils to decrease irritation; to relieve throat irritation with hard candy or cough drops; to increase fluid intake; and to eat light meals.
- Warm baths or heating pads can reduce aches and pains but won't hasten a cure. Suggest hot or cold steam vaporizers. Commercial expectorants are

available, but their effectiveness is questionable.

- Advise against overuse of nose drops or sprays, since these may cause rebound congestion.
- To help prevent colds, warn the patient to minimize contact with people who have colds. To avoid spreading colds, teach patient to wash hands often, to cover coughs and sneezes, and to avoid sharing towels and drinking glasses.

Respiratory Syncytial Virus Infection

Respiratory syncytial virus (RSV) infection results from a subgroup of the myxoviruses resembling paramyxovirus. RSV is the leading cause of lower respiratory tract infections in infants and young children; it's the major cause of pneumonia, tracheobronchitis, and bronchiolitis in this age-group, and a suspected cause of the fatal respiratory diseases of infancy.

Causes and incidence

Antibody titers seem to indicate that few children under age 4 escape contracting some form of RSV, even if it's mild. In fact, RSV is the only viral disease that has its maximum impact during the first few months of life (incidence of RSV bronchiolitis peaks at age 2 months).

This virus creates annual epidemics that occur during the late winter and early spring in temperate climates, and during the rainy season in the Tropics. The organism is transmitted from person to person by respiratory secretions, and has an incubation period of 4 to 5 days.

Reinfection is common, producing milder symptoms than the primary infection. School-age children, adolescents, and young adults with mild reinfections are probably the source of infection for infants and young children.

Signs and symptoms

Clinical features of RSV infection vary in severity, ranging from mild coldlike symptoms to bronchiolitis or bronchopneumonia, and in a few patients, severe, life-threatening lower respiratory tract infections. Generally, symptoms include coughing, wheezing, malaise, pharyngitis, dyspnea, and inflamed mucous membranes in the nose and throat.

Otitis media is a common complication of RSV in infants. RSV has also been identified in patients with a variety of CNS disorders, such as meningitis and myelitis.

Diagnosis

Diagnosis is usually made on the basis of clinical findings and epidemiologic information.

- Cultures of nasal and pharyngeal secretions may show RSV; however, the virus is very labile, so cultures aren't always reliable.
- Serum antibody titers may be elevated, but before 6 months of age, maternal antibodies may impair test results.
- Two recently developed serologic techniques are the indirect immunofluorescent and the enzyme-linked immunosorbent assay (ELISA) methods.
- Chest X-rays help detect pneumonia.

Treatment

Treatment aims to support respiratory function, maintain fluid balance, and relieve symptoms.

Special considerations

Your care plan should provide support and relief of symptoms.

- Monitor respiratory status. Observe the rate and pattern; watch for nasal flaring or retraction, cyanosis, pallor, and dyspnea; listen for or auscultate for wheezing, rhonchi, or other signs of respiratory distress. Monitor arterial blood gases.

• Maintain a patent airway, and be especially watchful when the patient has periods of acute dyspnea. Perform percussion, and provide drainage and suction, when necessary. Use a croup tent to provide a high-humidity atmosphere. Semi-Fowler's position may help prevent aspiration of secretions.
• Monitor intake and output carefully. Observe for signs of dehydration, such as decreased skin turgor. Encourage the patient to drink plenty of high-calorie fluids. Administer I.V. fluids, as needed.
• Promote bed rest. Plan your nursing care to allow uninterrupted rest.
• Hold and cuddle infants; talk to and play with toddlers. Offer suitable diversional activities to the child's condition and age. Foster parental visits and cuddling. Restrain child only as necessary.
• Impose oral secretion precautions. Enforce strict handwashing, since RSV may be transmitted from fomites.
• Staff members with respiratory illnesses should not care for infants.

Parainfluenza

Parainfluenza refers to any of a group of respiratory illnesses caused by paramyxoviruses, a subgroup of the myxoviruses. Affecting both the upper and lower respiratory tracts, these self-limiting diseases resemble influenza but are milder and seldom fatal. Parainfluenza is rare among adults, but it's widespread among children. Incidence of parainfluenza in children rises in the winter and spring.

Causes

Parainfluenza is transmitted by direct contact or by inhalation of contaminated airborne droplets. Paramyxoviruses occur in four forms—Para 1 to 4—that are linked to several diseases: croup (Para 1, 2, 3), acute febrile respiratory illnesses (1, 2, 3), the common cold (1, 3, 4), pharyngitis (1, 3, 4), bronchitis (1, 3), and bronchopneumonia (1, 3). Para 3 ranks second to respiratory syncytial viruses (RSV) as the infecting organism in lower respiratory tract infections in children. Para 4 rarely causes symptomatic infections in humans.

By age 8, most children demonstrate antibodies to Para 1 and Para 3. Most adults have antibodies to all four types as a result of childhood infections and subsequent multiple exposures. Reinfection is usually less severe and affects only the upper respiratory tract.

Signs and symptoms

After a short incubation period (usually 3 to 6 days), symptoms emerge that are similar to those of other respiratory diseases: sudden fever, nasal discharge, reddened throat (with little or no exudate), chills and muscle pain. Bacterial complications are uncommon, but in infants and very young children, parainfluenza may lead to croup or laryngotracheobronchitis.

Diagnosis

Parainfluenza infections are usually clinically indistinguishable from similar viral infections. Isolation of the virus and serum antibody titers differentiate parainfluenza from other respiratory illness but are rarely done.

Treatment and special considerations

Parainfluenza may require no treatment, or may require bed rest, antipyretics, analgesics, and antitussives, depending on the severity of the symptoms. Complications, such as croup and pneumonia, require appropriate treatment. No vaccine is effective against parainfluenza. Throughout this illness, monitor respiratory status and temperature, and ensure adequate fluid intake and rest.

Adenovirus Infection

Adenoviruses cause acute self-limiting febrile infections, with inflammation of the respiratory or the ocular mucous membranes, or both.

Causes and incidence

Adenovirus has 35 known serotypes; it causes five major infections, all of which occur in epidemics. These organisms are common and can remain latent for years; they infect almost everyone early in life (though maternal antibodies offer some protection during the first 6 months of life).

Transmission of adenovirus can occur by direct inoculation into the eye, by the fecal-oral route (adenovirus may persist in the GI tract for years after infection), or by inhalation of an infected droplet. The incubation period is usually less than 1 week; acute illness lasts less than 5 days and can be followed by prolonged asymptomatic reinfection.

Signs and symptoms

Clinical features vary. (See chart below.)

Diagnosis

Definitive diagnosis requires isolation of the virus from respiratory or ocular secretions, or fecal smears; during epidemics, however, typical symptoms alone can confirm diagnosis. Since adenoviral illnesses resolve rapidly, serum antibody titers aren't useful for diagnosis. Adenoviral diseases cause lymphocytosis in children. When they cause respiratory disease, chest X-ray may show pneumonitis.

Treatment

Supportive treatment includes bed rest,

MAJOR ADENOVIRAL INFECTIONS

DISEASE	AGE-GROUP	CLINICAL FEATURES
Acute febrile respiratory illness (AFRI)	Children	Nonspecific coldlike symptoms, similar to other viral respiratory illness: fever, pharyngitis, tracheitis, bronchitis, pneumonitis
Acute respiratory disease (ARD)	Adults (usually military recruits)	Malaise, fever, chills, headache, pharyngitis, hoarseness, and dry cough
Viral pneumonia	Children and adults	Sudden onset of high fever, rapid infection of upper and lower respiratory tracts, skin rash, diarrhea, intestinal intussusception
Acute pharyngoconjunctival fever (APC)	Children (particularly after swimming in pools or lakes)	Spiking fever lasting several days, headache, pharyngitis, conjunctivitis, rhinitis, cervical adenitis
Acute follicular conjunctivitis	Adults	Unilateral tearing and mucoid discharge; later, milder symptoms in other eye
Epidemic keratoconjunctivitis (EKC)	Adults	Unilateral or bilateral ocular redness and edema, preorbital swelling, local discomfort, superficial opacity of the cornea without ulceration
Hemorrhagic cystitis	Children (boys)	Adenoviruria, hematuria, dysuria, urinary frequency

antipyretics, and analgesics. Ocular infections may require corticosteroids and direct supervision by an ophthalmologist. Hospitalization is required in cases of pneumonia (in infants) to prevent death and in epidemic keratoconjunctivitis (EKC) to prevent blindness.

Special considerations

During the acute illness, monitor respiratory status, and intake and output. Give analgesics and antipyretics, as needed. Stress the need for bed rest.

To help minimize the incidence of adenoviral disease, instruct all patients in proper handwashing to reduce fecal-oral transmission. EKC can be prevented by sterilization of ophthalmic instruments, adequate chlorination in swimming pools, and avoidance of swimming pools during EKC epidemics. Killed virus vaccine (not widely available) and a live oral virus vaccine can prevent adenoviral infection and are recommended for high-risk groups.

Influenza

(Grippe, flu)

Influenza, an acute, highly contagious infection of the respiratory tract, results from three different types of Myxovirus influenzae. *It occurs sporadically or in epidemics (usually during the colder months). Epidemics tend to peak within 2 to 3 weeks after initial cases and subside within a month.*

Although influenza affects all age-groups, its incidence is highest in schoolchildren. However, its severity is greatest in the very young, the elderly, and those with chronic diseases. In these groups, influenza may even lead to death. The catastrophic pandemic of 1918 was responsible for an estimated 20 million deaths. The most recent pandemics—in 1957, 1968, and 1977—began in mainland China.

Causes

Transmission of influenza occurs through inhalation of a respiratory droplet from an infected person or by indirect contact, such as the use of a contaminated drinking glass. The influenza virus then invades the epithelium of the respiratory tract, causing inflammation and desquamation.

One of the remarkable features of the influenza virus is its capacity for antigenic variation. Such variation leads to infection by strains of the virus to which little or no immunologic resistance is present in the population at risk. Antigenic variation is characterized as *antigenic drift* (minor changes that occur yearly or every few years) and *antigenic shift* (major changes that lead to pandemics). Influenza viruses are classified into three groups:

- Type A, the most prevalent, strikes every year, with new serotypes causing epidemics every 3 years.
- Type B also strikes annually, but only causes epidemics every 4 to 6 years.
- Type C is endemic and causes only sporadic cases.

Signs and symptoms

Following an incubation period of from 24 to 48 hours, flu symptoms begin to appear: sudden onset of chills, temperature of 101° to 104° F. (38.3° to 40° C.), headache, malaise, myalgia (particularly in the back and limbs), a nonproductive cough, and, occasionally, laryngitis, hoarseness, conjunctivitis, rhinitis, and rhinorrhea. These symptoms usually subside in 3 to 5 days, but cough and weakness may persist. Fever is usually higher in children than in adults. Also, cervical adenopathy and croup are likely to be associated with influenza in children. In some patients (especially the elderly), lack of energy and easy fatigability may persist for several weeks.

Fever that persists longer than 3 to 5 days signals the onset of complications. The most common complication is pneumonia, which can be primary influenza viral pneumonia or secondary to bacterial infection. Influenza may also cause myositis, exacerbation of chronic obstructive pulmonary disease (COPD), Reye's syndrome, and, rarely, myocarditis, pericarditis, transverse myelitis, and encephalitis.

Diagnosis

At the beginning of an influenza epidemic, early cases are usually mistaken for other respiratory disorders. Since signs and symptoms are not pathognomonic,

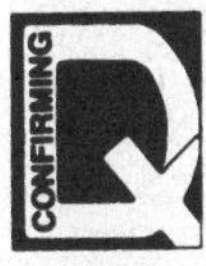

isolation of *M. influenzae* through inoculation of chicken embryos (with nasal secretions from infected patients) is essential at the first sign of an epidemic. In addition, nose and throat cultures and increased serum antibody titers help confirm this diagnosis.

After these measures confirm an influenza epidemic, diagnosis requires only observation of clinical signs and symptoms. Uncomplicated cases show decreased WBCs with an increase in lymphocytes.

Treatment

Treatment of uncomplicated influenza includes bed rest, adequate fluid intake, aspirin or acetaminophen (in children) to relieve fever and muscle pain, and guaifenesin or another expectorant to relieve nonproductive coughing. Prophylactic antibiotics aren't recommended, because they have no effect on the influenza virus.

Amantadine (an antiviral agent) has proven to be effective in reducing the duration of signs and symptoms in influenza A infection. In influenza complicated by pneumonia, supportive care (fluid and electrolyte supplements, oxygen, assisted ventilation) and treatment of bacterial superinfection with appropriate antibiotics are necessary. No specific therapy exists for cardiac, CNS, or other complications.

Special considerations

Unless complications occur, influenza doesn't require hospitalization. Like treatment, patient care focuses on relief of symptoms:

- Advise the patient to use mouthwashes and increase his fluid intake. Warm baths or heating pads may relieve myalgia. Give him nonnarcotic analgesics-antipyretics, as ordered.
- Screen visitors to protect the patient from bacterial infection and the visitor from influenza. Use respiratory precautions.
- Teach the patient proper disposal of tissues and proper handwashing technique to prevent the virus from spreading.
- Watch for signs and symptoms of developing pneumonia, such as rales, another temperature rise, or coughing accompanied by purulent or bloody sputum. Assist the patient in a gradual return to his normal activities.

Educate patients about influenza immunizations. For high-risk patients and health-care personnel, suggest annual inoculations at the start of the flu season (late autumn). Remember, however, that such vaccines are made from chicken embryos and must not be given to persons who are hypersensitive to eggs, feathers, or chickens. The vaccine administered is based on the previous year's virus and is usually about 75% effective.

All persons receiving the vaccine should be made aware of possible side effects (discomfort at the vaccination site, fever, malaise, and rarely Guillain-Barré syndrome). Although the vaccine has not been proven harmful to the fetus, it is not recommended for pregnant women, except those who are highly susceptible to influenza, such as those with chronic diseases. For people who are hypersensitive to eggs, amantadine is an effective alternative to the vaccine.

—LINDA LASS-SCHUHMACHER, RN, MED

RASH-PRODUCING VIRUSES

Varicella

(Chicken pox)

Varicella is a common, acute, and highly contagious infection caused by the herpesvirus varicella-zoster (V-Z), the same virus that, in its latent stage, causes herpes zoster (shingles).

Causes and incidence

Chicken pox can occur at any age, but it's most common in 2- to 8-year-olds. Congenital varicella may affect infants whose mothers had acute infections in their first or early second trimester. Neonatal infection is rare, probably due to transient maternal immunity. Second attacks are also rare. This infection is transmitted by direct contact (primarily with respiratory secretions; less often, with skin lesions) and indirect contact (air waves). The incubation period lasts from 13 to 17 days. Chicken pox is probably communicable from 1 day before lesions erupt to 6 days after vesicles form (it's most contagious in the early stages of eruption of skin lesions).

Chicken pox occurs worldwide and is endemic in large cities. Outbreaks occur sporadically, usually in areas with large groups of susceptible children. It affects all races and both sexes equally. Seasonal distribution varies; in temperate areas, incidence is higher during late autumn, winter, and spring.

Most children recover completely. Potentially fatal complications may affect children receiving corticosteroids, antimetabolites, or other immunosuppressives, and those with leukemia, other neoplasms, or immunodeficiency disorders. Congenital and adult varicella may also have severe effects.

Signs and symptoms

Chicken pox produces distinctive signs and symptoms, notably a pruritic rash. During the prodromal phase, the patient has slight fever, malaise, and anorexia. Within 24 hours, the rash typically begins as crops of small, erythematous macules on the trunk or scalp that progress to papules and then clear vesicles on an erythematous base (the so-called "dewdrop on a rose petal"). The vesicles become cloudy and break easily; then scabs form. The rash spreads to the face and, rarely, to the extremities. New vesicles continue to appear for 3 or 4 days, so the rash contains a combination of red papules, vesicles, and scabs in various stages. Occasionally, chicken pox also produces shallow ulcers on mucous membranes of the mouth, conjunctivae, and genitalia.

Congenital varicella causes hypoplastic deformity and scarring of a limb, retarded growth, and CNS and eye manifestations. In progressive varicella, an immunocompromised patient will have lesions and a high fever for over 7 days.

Severe pruritus with this rash may provoke persistent scratching, which can lead to infection, scarring, impetigo, furuncles, and cellulitis. Rare complications include pneumonia, myocarditis, fulminating encephalitis (Reye's syndrome), bleeding disorders, arthritis, nephritis, hepatitis, and acute myositis.

Diagnosis

Diagnosis rests on the characteristic clinical signs and usually doesn't require laboratory tests. However, the virus can be isolated from vesicular fluid within the first 3 or 4 days of the rash; Giemsa stain distinguishes V-Z from vaccinia-variola viruses. Serum contains antibodies 7 days after onset.

Treatment

Chicken pox calls for strict isolation until all the vesicles and most of the scabs disappear (usually for 1 week after the onset of the rash). Children can go back to school, however, if just a few scabs remain since, at this stage, chicken pox is no longer contagious. Congenital chicken pox requires no isolation.

Generally, treatment consists of local or systemic antipruritics: cool bicarbonate of soda baths, calamine lotion, or diphenhydramine or another antihistamine. Antibiotics are unnecessary unless bacterial infection develops. Salicylates are contraindicated because of their link with Reye's syndrome.

Susceptible patients may need special treatment. When given up to 72 hours after exposure to varicella, zoster immune globulin may provide passive immunity. Vidarabine may slow vesicle formation, speed skin healing, and control the systemic spread of infection.

Special considerations

Care is supportive and emphasizes patient and family teaching and preventive measures.

- Teach the child and his family how to apply topical antipruritic medications correctly. Stress the importance of good hygiene.
- Tell the patient not to scratch the lesions. However, because the need to scratch may be overwhelming, parents should trim the child's fingernails or tie mittens on his hands.
- Warn parents to watch for and immediately report signs of complications. Severe skin pain and burning may indicate a serious secondary infection and require prompt medical attention.

To help prevent chicken pox, don't admit a child exposed to chicken pox to a unit that contains children who receive immunosuppressives or who have leukemia or immunodeficiency disorders. A vulnerable child who's been exposed to chicken pox should receive varicella-zoster immunoglobulin, to lessen its severity.

Rubella

(German measles)

Rubella is an acute, mildly contagious viral disease that produces a distinctive, 3-day rash and lymphadenopathy. It occurs most often among children aged 5 to 9, adolescents, and young adults. Worldwide in distribution, rubella flourishes during the spring (particularly in big cities) and epidemics occur sporadically. This disease is self-limiting, and the prognosis is excellent.

Causes

The rubella virus is transmitted through contact with the blood, urine, stools, or nasopharyngeal secretions of infected persons, and possibly by contact with contaminated articles of clothing. Transplacental transmission, especially in the first trimester of pregnancy, can cause serious birth defects. Humans are the only known hosts for the rubella virus. The period of communicability lasts from about 10 days before until 5 days after the rash appears.

Signs and symptoms

In children, after an incubation period of from 16 to 18 days, an exanthematous, maculopapular rash erupts abruptly. In adolescents and adults, prodromal symptoms—headache, malaise, anorexia, low-grade fever, coryza, lymphadenopathy, and sometimes conjunctivitis—appear first. Suboccipital, postauricular, and postcervical lymph node enlargement is a hallmark of rubella.

Typically, the rubella rash begins on the face. This maculopapular eruption spreads rapidly, often covering the trunk and extremities within hours. Small, red, petechial macules on the soft palate (Forschheimer spots) may precede or accompany the rash. By the end of the second day, the facial rash begins to fade, but the rash on the trunk may be confluent and may be mistaken for scarlet fever. The rash continues to fade in the downward order in which it appeared. The rash generally disappears on the third day, but it may persist for 4 or 5 days—sometimes accompanied by mild coryza and conjunctivitis. The rapid appearance and disappearance of the rubella rash distinguishes it from rubeola. Rubella can occur without a rash, but this is rare. Low-grade fever may accompany the rash (99° to 101° F. [37.2° to 38.3° C.]), but it usually doesn't persist after the first day of the rash; rarely, temperature may reach 104° F. (40° C.).

Complications seldom occur in children with rubella, but when they do, they often appear as hemorrhagic problems, such as thrombocytopenia. Young women, however, often experience transient joint pain or arthritis, usually just as the rash is fading. Fever may then recur. These complications usually subside spontaneously within 5 to 30 days.

Diagnosis

The rubella rash, lymphadenopathy, other characteristic signs, and a history of exposure to infected persons usually permit clinical diagnosis without lab tests. However, cell cultures of the throat, blood, urine, and cerebrospinal fluid can confirm the virus' presence. Convalescent serum that shows a fourfold rise in antibody titers confirms the diagnosis.

Treatment

Since the rubella rash is self-limiting and only mildly pruritic, it doesn't require topical or systemic medication. Treatment consists of aspirin for fever and joint pain. Bed rest isn't necessary, but the patient should be isolated until the rash disappears.

Immunization with live virus vaccine RA27/3, the only rubella vaccine available in the United States, is necessary for prevention and appears to be more immunogenic than previous vaccines. The rubella vaccine should be given with measles and mumps vaccines at age 15 months to decrease the cost and the num-

EXPANDED RUBELLA SYNDROME

Congenital rubella is by far the most serious form of the disease. Intrauterine rubella infection, especially during the first trimester, can lead to spontaneous abortion or stillbirth, as well as single or multiple birth defects. (As a rule, the earlier the infection occurs during pregnancy, the greater the damage to the fetus.) The combination of cataracts, deafness, and cardiac disease comprises the classic rubella syndrome. Low birth weight, microcephaly, and mental retardation are other common manifestations. However, researchers now believe that congenital rubella can cause several more disorders, many of which don't appear until later in life. These include dental abnormalities, thrombocytopenic purpura, hemolytic and hypoplastic anemia, encephalitis, giant-cell hepatitis, seborrheic dermatitis, and diabetes mellitus. Indeed, it now appears that congenital rubella may be a lifelong disease. This theory is supported by the fact that the rubella virus has been isolated from urine 15 years after its acquisition in the uterus.

Infants born with congenital rubella should be isolated immediately, because they excrete the virus for a period of from several months to a year after birth. Cataracts and cardiac defects may require surgery. Prognosis depends on the particular malformations that occur. The overall mortality for rubella infants is 6%, but it's higher for babies born with thrombocytopenic purpura, congenital cardiac disease, or encephalitis. Parents of affected children need emotional support and guidance in finding help from community resources and organizations.

ber of injections needed.

Special considerations

- Make the patient with active rubella as comfortable as possible. Give children books to read or games to play to keep them occupied.
- Explain why respiratory isolation is necessary. Make sure the patient understands how important it is to avoid exposing pregnant women to this disease.
- Report confirmed cases of rubella to local public health officials.

Know how to manage rubella immunization before giving the vaccine:

- Obtain a history of allergies, especially to neomycin. If the patient has this allergy or if he's had a reaction to immunization in the past, check with the doctor before giving the vaccine.
- Ask women of childbearing age if they're pregnant. If they are or think they may be, *don't* give the vaccine. Warn women who receive rubella vaccine to use an effective means of birth control for at least 3 months after immunization.
- Give the vaccine at least 3 months after any administration of immune globulin or blood, which could have antibodies that neutralize the vaccine.
- Don't vaccinate any immunocompromised patients, patients with immunodeficiency diseases, or those receiving immunosuppressive, radiation, or corticosteroid therapy. Instead, administer immune serum globulin, as ordered, to prevent or reduce infection in susceptible patients.
- After giving the vaccine, observe for signs of anaphylaxis for at least 30 minutes. Keep epinephrine 1:1,000 handy.
- Warn about possible mild fever, slight rash, transient arthralgia (in adolescents), and arthritis (in the elderly). Suggest aspirin or acetaminophen for fever.
- Advise the patient to apply warmth to the injection site for 24 hours after immunization (to help the body absorb the vaccine). If swelling persists after the initial 24 hours, suggest a cold compress to promote vasoconstriction and prevent antigenic cyst formation.

Rubeola

(Measles, morbilli)

Rubeola is an acute, highly contagious paramyxovirus infection that may be one of the most common and the most serious of all communicable childhood diseases. Use of the vaccine has reduced the occurrence of measles during childhood; as a result, measles is becoming more prevalent in adolescents and adults. In the United States, prognosis is usually excellent. However, measles is a major cause of death in children in underdeveloped countries.

Causes and incidence

Measles is spread by direct contact or by contaminated airborne respiratory droplets. The portal of entry is the upper respiratory tract. In temperate zones, incidence is highest in late winter and early spring. Before the availability of measles vaccine, epidemics occurred every 2 to 5 years in large urban areas.

Signs and symptoms

Incubation is from 10 to 14 days. Initial symptoms begin and greatest communicability occurs during a prodromal phase, about 11 days after exposure to the virus. This phase lasts from 4 to 5 days; symptoms include fever, photophobia, malaise, anorexia, conjunctivitis, coryza, hoarseness, and hacking cough.

At the end of the prodrome, Koplik's spots, the hallmark of the disease, appear. These spots look like tiny, bluish gray specks surrounded by a red halo.

They appear on the oral mucosa opposite the molars and occasionally bleed. About 5 days after Koplik's spots appear, temperature rises sharply, spots slough off, and a slightly pruritic rash appears. This characteristic rash starts as faint macules behind the ears and on the neck and cheeks. These macules become papular and erythematous, rapidly spreading over the entire face, neck, eyelids, arms, chest, back, abdomen, and thighs. When the rash reaches the feet (2 to 3 days later), it begins to fade in the same sequence it appeared, leaving a brownish discoloration that disappears in 7 to 10 days.

The disease climax occurs 2 to 3 days after the rash appears, and is marked by a temperature of 103° to 105° F. (39.4° to 40.6° C.), severe cough, puffy red eyes, and rhinorrhea. About 5 days after the rash appears, other symptoms disappear and communicability ends. Symptoms are usually mild in patients with partial immunity (conferred by administration of gamma globulin) or infants with transplacental antibodies. More severe symptoms and complications are more likely to develop in young infants, adolescents, adults, and immunocompromised patients than in young children.

Atypical measles may appear in patients who received the killed measles vaccine. These patients are acutely ill

ADMINISTERING MEASLES VACCINE

Warn the patient or his parents that possible side effects are anorexia, malaise, rash, mild thrombocytopenia or leukopenia, and fever. Advise that the vaccine may produce slight reactions, usually within 7 to 10 days.

- Ask the patient about known allergies, especially to neomycin (each dose contains a small amount). However, a patient who's allergic to eggs may receive the vaccine, because it contains only minimal amounts of albumin and yolk components.
- Avoid giving the vaccine to a pregnant woman (ask for date of last menstrual period). Warn female patients to avoid pregnancy for at least 3 months following vaccination.
- Don't vaccinate children with untreated tuberculosis, immunodeficiencies, leukemia, or lymphoma, or those receiving immunosuppressives. If such children are exposed to the virus, recommend they receive gamma globulin (gamma globulin won't prevent measles but will lessen its severity). Older unimmunized children who have been exposed to measles for more than 5 days may also require gamma globulin. Be sure to immunize them 3 months later.
- Delay vaccination for 8 to 12 weeks after administration of whole blood, plasma, or gamma globulin, since measles antibodies in these components may neutralize the vaccine.
- Watch for signs of anaphylaxis for 30 minutes after vaccination. Keep epinephrine 1:1,000 handy.
- Advise application of a warm compress to the vaccination site to facilitate absorption of the vaccine. If swelling occurs within 24 hours after vaccination, tell patient to apply cold compresses to promote vasoconstriction and to prevent antigenic cyst formation.

Generally, one bout of measles renders immunity (a second infection is extremely rare and may represent misdiagnosis); infants under age 4 months may be immune because of circulating maternal antibodies. Under normal conditions, measles vaccine isn't administered to children younger than age 15 months. However, during an epidemic, infants as young as 6 months may receive the vaccine; they must be reimmunized at age 15 months. An alternate approach calls for administration of gamma globulin to infants between ages 6 and 15 months who are likely to be exposed to measles.

with a fever and maculopapular rash that's most obvious in the arms and legs, or with pulmonary involvement and no skin lesions.

Severe infection may lead to secondary bacterial infection and to autoimmune reaction or organ invasion by the virus, resulting in otitis media, pneumonia, and encephalitis. Subacute sclerosing panencephalitis (SSPE), a rare and invariably fatal complication, may develop several years after measles. SSPE is less common in patients who have received the measles vaccine.

Diagnosis

Diagnosis rests on distinctive clinical features, especially the pathognomonic Koplik's spots. Mild measles may resemble rubella, roseola infantum, enterovirus infection, toxoplasmosis, and drug eruptions; laboratory tests are required for a differential diagnosis. If necessary, measles virus may be isolated from the blood, nasopharyngeal secretions, and urine during the febrile period. Serum antibodies appear within 3 days after onset of the rash, and reach peak titers 2 to 4 weeks later.

Treatment and special considerations

Treatment for measles requires bed rest, relief of symptoms, and respiratory isolation throughout the communicable period. Vaporizers and a warm environment help reduce respiratory irritation, but cough preparations and antibiotics are generally ineffective; antipyretics can reduce fever. Therapy must also combat complications.

- Teach parents supportive measures, and stress the need for isolation, plenty of rest, and increased fluid intake. Advise them to cope with photophobia by darkening the room or providing sunglasses, and to reduce fever with antipyretics and tepid sponge baths.
- Warn parents to watch for and report the early signs and symptoms of complications, such as encephalitis, otitis media, and pneumonia.

Herpes Simplex

Herpes simplex, a recurrent viral infection, is caused by Herpesvirus hominis (HVH), *a most widespread infectious agent. Herpes Type I, which is transmitted by oral and respiratory secretions, affects the skin and mucous membranes and commonly produces cold sores and fever blisters. Herpes Type II primarily affects the genital area and is transmitted by sexual contact. However, cross-infection may result from orogenital sex.*

Causes and incidence

About 85% of all HVH infections are subclinical. The others produce localized lesions and systemic reactions. After the first infection, a patient is a carrier susceptible to recurrent infections, which may be provoked by fever, menses, stress, heat, and cold. However, in recurrent infections, the patient usually has no constitutional signs and symptoms.

Primary HVH is the leading cause of childhood gingivostomatitis in children aged 1 to 3. It causes the most common nonepidemic encephalitis and is the second most common viral infection in pregnant women. It can pass to the fetus transplacentally and, in early pregnancy, may cause spontaneous abortion or premature birth. Herpes is equally common in males and females. Worldwide in distribution, it is most prevalent among children in lower socioeconomic groups who live in crowded environments. Saliva, stool, skin lesions, purulent eye exudate, and urine are potential sources of infection.

Signs and symptoms

In neonates, HVH symptoms usually appear a week or two after birth. They range from localized skin lesions to a disseminated infection of such organs as the liver, lungs, or brain. Common complications include seizures, mental retardation, blindness, chorioretinitis, deafness, microcephaly, diabetes insipidus, and spasticity. Up to 90% of infants with disseminated disease will die.

Primary infection in childhood may be generalized or localized. After an incubation period of from 2 to 12 days, onset of generalized infection begins with fever, pharyngitis, erythema, and edema. After brief prodromal tingling and itching, typical primary lesions erupt as vesicles on an erythematous base, eventually rupturing and leaving a painful ulcer, followed by a yellowish crust. Healing begins 7 to 10 days after onset and is complete in 3 weeks. Vesicles may form on any part of the oral mucosa, especially the tongue, gingiva, and cheeks. In generalized infection, vesicles occur with submaxillary lymphadenopathy, increased salivation, halitosis, anorexia, and fever of up to 105° F. (40.6° C.). Herpetic stomatitis may lead to severe dehydration in children. A generalized infection usually runs its course in 4 to 10 days. In this form, virus reactivation causes cold sores—single or grouped vesicles in and around the mouth.

Genital herpes usually affects adolescents and young adults. Typically painful, the initial attack produces fluid-filled vesicles that ulcerate and heal in 1 to 3 weeks. Fever, regional lymphadenopathy, and dysuria may also occur.

Usually, herpetic keratoconjunctivitis is unilateral and causes only local symptoms: conjunctivitis, regional adenopathy, blepharitis, and vesicles on the lid. Other ocular symptoms may be excessive lacrimation, edema, chemosis, photophobia, and purulent exudate.

Both types of HVH can cause acute sporadic encephalitis with an altered level of consciousness, personality changes, and convulsions. Other effects may include smell and taste hallucinations and neurologic and mental abnormalities, such as seizures and aphasia.

Herpetic whitlow, an HVH finger infection, commonly affects nurses. First the finger tingles and then it becomes red, swollen, and painful. Vesicles with a red halo erupt and may ulcerate or coalesce. Other effects may include satellite vesicles, fever, chills, malaise, and a red streak up the arm.

Diagnosis

Typical lesions may suggest HVH infection. However, confirmation requires isolation of the virus from local lesions and histologic biopsy. A rise in antibodies and moderate leukocytosis may support the diagnosis.

Treatment

Symptomatic and supportive therapy is essential. Generalized primary infection usually requires an analgesic-antipyretic to reduce fever and relieve pain. Anesthetic mouthwashes, such as viscous lidocaine, may reduce the pain of gingivostomatitis, enabling the patient to eat and preventing dehydration. Drying agents, such as calamine lotion, make labial lesions less painful.

Refer patients with eye infections to an ophthalmologist. Topical corticosteroids are contraindicated in active infection, but idoxuridine, trifluridine, and vidarabine are effective.

A 5% acyclovir ointment may bring relief to patients with genital herpes or to immunosuppressed patients with HVH skin infections. Acyclovir I.V. helps treat more severe infections.

Special considerations

- Teach the patient with genital herpes to use warm compresses or take sitz baths several times a day. Tell him to use a drying agent, such as povidone-iodine solution; to increase his fluid intake; and to avoid all sexual contact during the active stage.
- For pregnant women with HVH infection, recommend weekly viral cultures of the cervix and external genitalia start-

ing at 32 weeks' gestation.

- Instruct patients with herpetic whitlow not to share towels or utensils with uninfected people. Educate staff members and other susceptible people about the risk of contracting the disease.
- Tell patients with cold sores not to kiss infants or people with eczema. (Those with genital herpes pose no risk to infants if their hygiene is meticulous.)
- Abstain from direct patient care if you have herpetic whitlow.
- Patients with central nervous system infection alone need no isolation.

Herpes Zoster

(Shingles)

Herpes zoster is an acute unilateral and segmental inflammation of the dorsal root ganglia caused by infection with the herpesvirus varicella-zoster (V-Z), which also causes chicken pox. This infection usually occurs in adults; it produces localized vesicular skin lesions confined to a dermatome, and severe neuralgic pain in peripheral areas innervated by the nerves arising in the inflamed root ganglia.

Prognosis is good unless the infection spreads to the brain. Eventually, most patients recover completely, except for possible scarring and, in corneal damage, visual impairment. Occasionally, neuralgia may persist for months or years.

Causes

Herpes zoster results from reactivation of varicella virus that has lain dormant in the cerebral ganglia (extramedullary ganglia of the cranial nerves) or the ganglia of posterior nerve roots since a previous episode of chicken pox. Exactly how or why this reactivation occurs isn't clear. Some believe that the virus multiplies as it's reactivated and that it's neutralized by antibodies remaining from the initial infection. But if effective antibodies aren't present, the virus continues to multiply in the ganglia, destroy the host neuron, and spread down the sensory nerves to the skin.

Herpes zoster is found primarily in adults, especially those past age 50. It seldom recurs.

Signs and symptoms

Onset of herpes zoster is characterized by fever and malaise. Within 2 to 4 days, severe deep pain, pruritus, and paresthesia or hyperesthesia develops, usually on the trunk and occasionally on the arms and legs. Such pain may be continuous or intermittent and usually lasts from 1 to 4 weeks. Up to 2 weeks after the first symptoms, small red nodular skin lesions erupt on the painful areas (such lesions commonly spread unilaterally around the thorax or vertically over the arms or legs). Sometimes nodules don't appear at all, but when they do, they quickly become vesicles filled with clear fluid or pus. About 10 days after

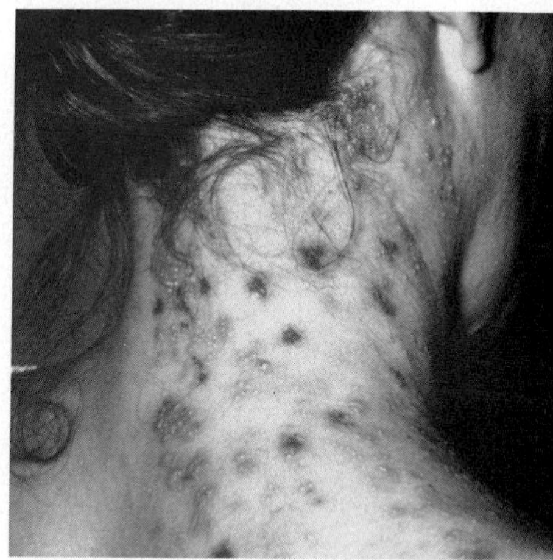

Characteristic skin lesions in herpes zoster are fluid-filled vesicles that dry and form scabs after about 10 days.

they appear, the vesicles dry and form scabs. When ruptured, such lesions often become infected and, in severe cases, may lead to the enlargement of regional lymph nodes; lesions may even become gangrenous. Intense pain may occur before the rash appears and after the scabs form.

Occasionally, herpes zoster involves the cranial nerves, especially the trigeminal and geniculate ganglia or the oculomotor nerve. Geniculate zoster may cause vesicle formation in the external auditory canal, ipsilateral facial palsy, hearing loss, dizziness, and loss of taste. Trigeminal ganglion involvement causes eye pain and, possibly, corneal and scleral damage and impaired vision. Rarely, oculomotor involvement causes conjunctivitis, extraocular weakness, ptosis, and paralytic mydriasis.

In rare cases, herpes zoster leads to generalized CNS infection, muscle atrophy, motor paralysis (usually transient), acute transverse myelitis, and ascending myelitis. More often, generalized infection causes acute retention of urine and unilateral paralysis of the diaphragm. In postherpetic neuralgia, a complication most common in the elderly, intractable neurologic pain may persist for years. Scars may be permanent.

Diagnosis

Diagnosis of herpes zoster usually isn't possible until the characteristic skin lesions develop. Before then, the pain may mimic appendicitis, pleurisy, or other conditions. Examination of vesicular fluid and infected tissue shows eosinophilic intranuclear inclusions and varicella virus. Also, a lumbar puncture shows increased pressure; examination of cerebrospinal fluid shows increased protein levels and, possibly, pleocytosis. Differentiation of herpes zoster from localized herpes simplex requires staining antibodies from vesicular fluid and identification under fluorescent light.

Treatment

The primary goal of treatment is to relieve itching and neuralgic pain with calamine lotion or another antipruritic; aspirin, possibly with codeine or another analgesic; and occasionally, application of collodion or tincture of benzoin to unbroken lesions. If bacteria have infected ruptured vesicles, treatment includes an appropriate systemic antibiotic.

Trigeminal zoster with corneal involvement calls for instillation of idoxuridine ointment or another antiviral agent. To help a patient cope with the intractable pain of postherpetic neuralgia, the doctor may order a systemic corticosteroid—such as cortisone or, possibly, corticotropin—to reduce inflammation, tranquilizers, sedatives, or tricyclic antidepressants with phenothiazines.

Researchers are studying two other drugs that can help treat herpes zoster. Acyclovir seems to stop progression of the skin rash and prevent visceral complications. Vidarabine reportedly speeds healing of lesions, decreases pain, and prevents the disease from spreading and developing complications.

As a last resort, transcutaneous peripheral nerve stimulation, cordotomy (used with limited success in "suicidal pain"), or a small dose of radiotherapy may also be considered.

Special considerations

Your care plan should emphasize keeping the patient comfortable, maintaining meticulous hygiene, and preventing infection. During the acute phase, adequate rest and supportive care can promote proper healing of lesions.

- If calamine lotion has been ordered, apply it liberally to the lesions. If lesions are severe and widespread, apply a wet dressing.
- Instruct the patient to avoid scratching the lesions.
- If vesicles rupture, apply a cold compress, as ordered.
- To decrease the pain of oral lesions, tell the patient to use a soft toothbrush, eat a soft diet, and use saline mouthwash.
- To minimize neuralgic pain, never

withhold or delay administration of analgesics. Give them exactly on schedule, because the pain of herpes zoster can be severe. In postherpetic neuralgia, avoid narcotic analgesics because of the danger of addiction.

- Repeatedly reassure the patient that herpetic pain will eventually subside. Provide diversionary activity to take his mind off the pain and pruritus.

Variola

(Smallpox)

Variola was an acute, highly contagious infectious disease caused by the poxvirus variola. After a global eradication program, begun in 1967, the World Health Organization pronounced smallpox eradicated on October 26, 1979, 2 years after the last naturally occurring case was reported in Somalia. The last known case of smallpox in the United States was reported in 1949. Although naturally occurring smallpox has been eradicated, variola virus preserved in laboratories remains a possible though unlikely source of infection.

Smallpox developed in three major forms: variola major *(classic smallpox), which carried a high mortality;* variola minor, *a mild form that occurred in nonvaccinated persons and resulted from a less virulent strain; and* varioloid, *a mild variant of smallpox that occurred in previously vaccinated persons who had only partial immunity.*

Causes

Smallpox affected people of all ages. In temperate zones, incidence was highest during the winter; in the tropics, during the hot, dry months. Smallpox was transmitted directly by respiratory droplets or dried scales of virus-containing lesions, or indirectly through contact with contaminated linens or other objects. Variola major was contagious from onset until after the last scab was shed.

Signs and symptoms

Characteristically, after an incubation period of from 10 to 14 days, smallpox caused an abrupt onset of chills (and possible convulsive seizures in children), high fever (temperature rose above 104° F. [40° C.]), headache, backache, severe malaise, vomiting (especially in children), marked prostration, and occasionally violent delirium, stupor, or coma. Two days after onset, symptoms became more severe, but by the third day the patient began to feel better.

However, he soon developed a sore throat and cough, and lesions appeared on the mucous membranes of the mouth, throat, and respiratory tract. Within days, skin lesions also appeared, and progressed from macular to papular, vesicular, and pustular (pustules were as large as ⅓″ [8 mm] in diameter). During the pustular stage, the patient's temperature again rose, and early symptoms returned. By day 10, the pustules began to rupture, and eventually dried and formed scabs. Symptoms finally subsided about 14 days after onset. Desquamation of the scabs took another 1 to 2 weeks, caused intense pruritus, and often left permanently disfiguring scars. In fatal cases, a diffuse dusky appearance came over the patient's face and upper chest. Death was the result of encephalitic manifestations, extensive bleeding from any or all orifices, or secondary bacterial infections.

Diagnosis

Smallpox was readily recognizable, especially during an epidemic or after known contact.

The most conclusive laboratory test was a culture of variola virus isolated from an aspirate of vesicles and pustules. Other laboratory tests included microscopic examination of smears from lesion scrapings, and complement fixation to detect virus or antibodies to the virus in the patient's blood.

Treatment and special considerations

Treatment required hospitalization, with strict isolation, antimicrobial therapy to treat bacterial complications, vigorous supportive measures, and symptomatic treatment of lesions with antipruritics, starting during the pustular stage. Aspirin, codeine, or (as needed) morphine relieved pain; I.V. infusions and gastric tube feedings provided fluids, electrolytes, and calories, since pharyngeal lesions made swallowing difficult.

Roseola Infantum

(Exanthema subitum)

Roseola infantum, an acute, benign, presumably viral infection, usually affects infants and young children (ages 6 months to 3 years). Characteristically, it first causes a high fever and then a rash that accompanies an abrupt drop to normal temperature.

Causes and incidence

Roseola affects boys and girls alike. It occurs year-round but is most prevalent in the spring and fall. Overt roseola, the most common exanthem in infants under age 2, affects 30% of all children; inapparent roseola (febrile illness without a rash) may affect the rest. The mode of transmission isn't known. Only rarely does an infected child transmit roseola to a sibling.

Signs and symptoms

After a 10- to 15-day incubation period, the infant with roseola develops an abruptly rising, unexplainable fever and, sometimes, seizures. Temperature peaks at 103° to 105° F. (39.4° to 40.6° C.) for 3 to 5 days, then drops suddenly. In the early febrile period, the infant may be anorexic, irritable, and listless but doesn't seem particularly ill. Simultaneously with an abrupt drop in temperature, a maculopapular, nonpruritic rash develops, which blanches on pressure. The rash is profuse on the infant's trunk, arms, and neck, and is mild on the face and legs. It fades within 24 hours. Although possible, complications are extremely rare.

INCUBATION AND DURATION OF COMMON RASH-PRODUCING INFECTIONS

INFECTION	INCUBATION (DAYS)	DURATION (DAYS)
Roseola	10-15	3-6
Varicella	10-14	7-14
Rubeola	13-17	5
Rubella	16-18	3
Herpes simplex	2-12	7-21

Diagnosis

Diagnosis requires observation of the typical rash that appears about 48 hours after fever subsides.

Treatment and special considerations

Because roseola is self-limiting, treatment is supportive and symptomatic: antipyretics to lower fever and, if necessary, anticonvulsants to relieve seizures.

Teach parents how to lower their infant's fever by giving tepid baths, keeping him in lightweight clothes, and maintaining normal room temperature. Stress the need for adequate fluid intake. Strict bed rest and isolation are unnecessary. Tell parents that a short febrile convulsion will not cause brain damage. Explain that convulsions will cease after fever subsides and that phenobarbital is likely to cause drowsiness; if it causes stupor, parents should call their doctor immediately.

ENTEROVIRUSES

Herpangina

Herpangina is an acute infection caused by group A coxsackieviruses (usually types 1 through 10, 16, and 23) and, less commonly, by group B coxsackieviruses and echoviruses. The disease characteristically produces vesicular lesions on the mucous membranes of the soft palate, tonsillar pillars, and throat.

Causes

Because fecal-oral transfer is the main mode of transmission, herpangina usually affects children under age 10 (except newborns, because of maternal antibodies). It occurs slightly more often in late summer and fall, and can be sporadic, endemic, or epidemic. Herpangina generally subsides in 4 to 7 days.

Signs and symptoms

After a 2- to 9-day incubation period, herpangina begins abruptly with a sore throat, pain on swallowing, a temperature of 100° to 104° F. (37.8° to 40° C.) that persists for 1 to 4 days and may cause convulsions, headache, anorexia, vomiting, malaise, diarrhea, and pain in the stomach, back of the neck, legs, and arms. After this, up to 12 grayish white papulovesicles appear on the soft palate and, less frequently, on the tonsils, uvula, tongue, and larynx. These lesions grow from 1 to 2 mm in diameter to large, punched out ulcers surrounded by small, inflamed margins.

Diagnosis

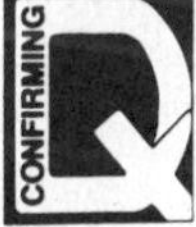

Characteristic oral lesions suggest this diagnosis; isolation of the virus from mouth washings or feces, and elevated specific antibody titer confirm it. Other routine test results are

ENTEROVIRUS FACTS

Enteroviruses (polioviruses, coxsackieviruses, echoviruses) inhabit the gastrointestinal tract. These viruses, among the smallest viruses that affect humans, include 3 known polioviruses, 23 group A coxsackieviruses, 6 group B coxsackieviruses, and 34 echoviruses. They usually infect humans as a result of ingestion of fecally contaminated material, causing a wide range of diseases (hand, foot, and mouth disease; aseptic meningitis; myocarditis; pericarditis; gastroenteritis; poliomyelitis). They can show up in the pharynx, feces, blood, CSF, and CNS tissue. Enterovirus infections are more prevalent in the summer and fall.

normal except for slight leukocytosis.

Diagnosis requires distinguishing the mouth lesions in herpangina from those in streptococcal tonsillitis (no ulcers; lesions confined to tonsils).

Treatment and special considerations

Treatment for herpangina is entirely symptomatic, emphasizing measures to reduce fever and prevent convulsions and possible dehydration. Herpangina doesn't require isolation or hospitalization but does require careful handwashing and sanitary disposal of excretions.

Teach parents to give adequate fluids, enforce bed rest, and administer tepid sponge baths and antipyretics.

Poliomyelitis

(Polio, infantile paralysis)

Poliomyelitis is an acute communicable disease caused by the poliovirus and ranges in severity from inapparent infection to fatal paralytic illness. First recognized in 1840, poliomyelitis became epidemic in Norway and Sweden in 1905. Outbreaks reached pandemic proportions in Europe, North America, Australia, and New Zealand during the first half of this century. Incidence peaked during the 1940s and early 1950s, and led to the development of the Salk vaccine.

Minor polio outbreaks still occur, usually among nonimmunized groups, as among the Amish of Pennsylvania in 1979. The disease strikes most often during the summer and fall. Once confined mainly to infants and children, poliomyelitis occurs more often today in people over age 15. Among children, it paralyzes boys most often; adults and girls are at greater risk of infection but not of paralysis.

Prognosis depends largely on the site affected. If the central nervous system is spared, prognosis is excellent. However, CNS infection can cause paralysis and death. The mortality for all types of poliomyelitis is 5% to 10%.

Causes

The poliovirus has three antigenically distinct serotypes—types I, II, and III—all of which cause poliomyelitis. These polioviruses are found worldwide and are transmitted from person to person by direct contact with infected oropharyngeal secretions or feces. The incubation period ranges from 5 to 35 days—7 to 14 days on the average. The virus usually enters the body through the alimentary tract, multiplies in the oropharynx and lower intestinal tract, then spreads to regional lymph nodes and the blood. Factors that increase the probability of paralysis include pregnancy; old age; localized trauma, such as a recent tonsillectomy, tooth extraction, or inoculation; and unusual physical exertion at or just before clinical onset of poliomyelitis.

Signs and symptoms

Manifestations of poliomyelitis follow three basic patterns. Inapparent (subclinical) infections constitute 95% of all poliovirus infections. Abortive poliomyelitis (minor illness), which makes up between 4% and 8% of all cases, causes slight fever, malaise, headache, sore throat, inflamed pharynx, and vomiting. The patient usually recovers within 72 hours. Most inapparent and abortive cases of poliomyelitis go unnoticed.

Major poliomyelitis, however, involves the CNS and takes two forms: nonparalytic and paralytic. Children often show a biphasic course, in which the onset of major illness occurs after recovery from the minor illness stage. Nonparalytic poliomyelitis produces moderate fever, headache, vomiting, lethargy, irritability, and pains in the neck, back, arms, legs, and abdomen. It also causes muscle tenderness and spasms in the extensors of the neck and back, and sometimes in the hamstring and other muscles. (These spasms may be observed during maximum range-of-motion exercises.) Nonparalytic polio usually lasts about a week, with meningeal irritation persisting for about 2 weeks.

Paralytic poliomyelitis usually develops within 5 to 7 days of the onset of fever. The patient displays symptoms similar to those of nonparalytic poliomyelitis, with asymmetrical weakness of various muscles, loss of superficial and deep reflexes, paresthesia, hypersensitivity to touch, urine retention, constipation, and abdominal distention. The extent of paralysis depends on the level of the spinal cord lesions, which may be cervical, thoracic, or lumbar.

Resistance to neck flexion is characteristic in nonparalytic and paralytic poliomyelitis. The patient will "tripod"—extend his arms behind him for support—when he sits up. He'll display Hoyne's sign—his head will fall back when he is supine and his shoulders are elevated. From a supine position, he won't be able to raise his legs a full 90°. Paralytic poliomyelitis also causes positive Kernig's and Brudzinski's signs.

When the disease affects the medulla of the brain, it's called bulbar paralytic poliomyelitis, which is the most perilous type. Bulbar paralytic poliomyelitis weakens the muscles supplied by the cranial nerves (particularly the ninth and tenth) and produces symptoms of encephalitis. Other symptoms include facial weakness, dysphasia, difficulty in chewing, inability to swallow or expel saliva, regurgitation of food through the nasal passages, dyspnea, as well as abnormal respiratory rate, depth, and rhythm, which may lead to respiratory arrest. Fatal pulmonary edema and shock are possible.

Complications—many of which result from prolonged immobility and respiratory muscle failure—include hypertension, urinary tract infection, urolithiasis, atelectasis, pneumonia, myocarditis, cor pulmonale, skeletal and soft-tissue deformities, and paralytic ileus.

POLIO PROTECTION

Dr. Jonas Salk's poliomyelitis vaccine, which became available in 1955, has been rightly called one of the miracle drugs of modern medicine. The vaccine contains dead (formalin-inactivated) polioviruses that stimulate production of circulating antibodies in the human body. This vaccine so effectively eliminated poliomyelitis that today it's hard to appreciate how feared the disease once was.

However, even miracle drugs can be improved. Today, the Sabin vaccine, which can be taken orally and is more than 90% effective, is the vaccine of choice in preventing poliomyelitis. The Sabin vaccine is available in trivalent and monovalent forms. The trivalent form (TOPV) contains live but weakened organisms of all three poliovirus serotypes in one solution. TOPV is generally preferred to the monovalent form (MOPV), which contains only one viral type and is useful only when the particular serotype is known.

All infants should be immunized with the Sabin vaccine; pregnant women may be vaccinated without risk. However, because of the risk of contracting poliomyelitis from the vaccine, it's contraindicated in patients with immunodeficiency diseases, leukemia, or lymphoma, and in those receiving corticosteroids, antimetabolites, other immunosuppressives, or radiation therapy. These patients are usually immunized with the Salk vaccine. When possible, immunodeficient patients should avoid contact with family members who are receiving the Sabin vaccine for at least 2 weeks after vaccination. Sabin vaccine is no longer routinely advised for adults unless they're apt to be exposed to this disease or plan travel to endemic areas.

Diagnosis

Diagnosis requires isolation of the poliovirus from throat washings early in the disease, from stools throughout the disease, and from CSF cultures in CNS infection. Coxsackievirus and echovirus infections must be ruled out. Convalescent serum antibody titers four times greater than acute titers support a diagnosis of poliomyelitis. Routine laboratory tests are usually within normal limits, though CSF pressure and protein levels may be slightly increased and WBC elevated initially, mostly due to polymorphonuclear leukocytes, which constitute 50% to 90% of the total count. Thereafter, mononuclear cells constitute most of the diminished number of cells.

Treatment

Treatment is supportive and includes analgesics to ease headache, back pain, and leg spasms; morphine is contraindicated because of the danger of additional respiratory suppression. Moist heat applications may also reduce muscle spasm and pain.

Bed rest is necessary only until extreme discomfort subsides; in paralytic poliomyelitis, this may take a long time. Paralytic polio also requires long-term rehabilitation using physical therapy, braces, corrective shoes and, in some cases, orthopedic surgery.

Special considerations

Your patient care plan must be comprehensive to help prevent complications and to assist polio patients—physically and emotionally—during their prolonged convalescence.

- Observe the patient carefully for signs of paralysis and other neurologic damage, which can occur rapidly. Maintain a patent airway, and watch for respiratory weakness and difficulty in swallowing. A tracheotomy is often done at the first sign of respiratory distress. Following this, the patient is then placed on a mechanical ventilator. Remember to reassure the patient that his breathing is being supported. Practice strict aseptic technique during suctioning. Be sure to use only sterile solutions to nebulize medications.
- Perform a brief neurologic assessment at least once a day, but don't demand any vigorous muscle activity. Encourage a return to mild activity as soon as the patient is able.
- Check blood pressure frequently, especially with bulbar poliomyelitis, which can cause hypertension or shock because of its effect on the brain stem.
- Watch for signs of fecal impaction (due to dehydration and intestinal inactivity). To prevent this, give sufficient fluids to ensure an adequate daily output of low specific gravity urine (1.5 to 2 liters/day for adults).
- Monitor the bedridden patient's food intake for an adequate, well-balanced diet. If tube feedings are required, give liquid baby foods, juices, lactose, and vitamins.
- To prevent pressure sores, give good skin care, reposition the patient often, and keep the bed dry. Remember, muscle paralysis may cause bladder weakness or transient bladder paralysis.
- Apply high-top sneakers or use a footboard to prevent footdrop. To alleviate discomfort, use foam rubber pads and sandbags, as needed, and light splints, as ordered.
- To control the spread of poliomyelitis, wash your hands thoroughly after contact with the patient, especially after contact with excretions. Instruct the ambulatory patient to do the same. (Only hospital personnel who have been vaccinated against poliomyelitis may have direct contact with the patient.)
- Provide emotional support to the patient and his family. Reassure the nonparalytic patient that his chances for recovery are good. Long-term support and encouragement are essential for maximum rehabilitation.
- When caring for a paralytic patient, help set up an interdisciplinary rehabilitation program. Such a program should include physical and occupational therapists, doctors, and, if necessary, a psychiatrist to help manage the emotional problems that develop in a patient suddenly facing severe physical disabilities.

ARBOVIRUS

Colorado Tick Fever

Colorado tick fever is a benign infection that results from the Colorado tick fever virus, an arbovirus, and is transmitted to humans by a hard-shelled wood tick called Dermacentor andersoni. *The adult tick acquires the virus when it bites infected rodents, and remains permanently infective. Colorado tick fever occurs in the Rocky Mountain region of the United States, mostly in April and May at lower altitudes and in June and July at higher altitudes. Because of occupational or recreational exposure, it's more common in men than in women. Colorado tick fever apparently confers long-lasting immunity against reinfection.*

Signs and symptoms

After a 3- to 6-day incubation period, Colorado tick fever begins abruptly with chills; temperature of 104° F. (40° C.); severe aching of back, arms, and legs; lethargy; and headache with eye movement. Photophobia, abdominal pain, nausea, and vomiting may occur. Rare effects include petechial or maculopapular rashes and CNS involvement. After several days, symptoms subside but return within 2 to 3 days and continue for 3 more days before slowly disappearing. Complete recovery usually follows.

Diagnosis

A history of recent exposure to ticks, and moderate to severe leukopenia, complement fixation tests, or virus isolation confirm the diagnosis.

Treatment and special considerations

After correct removal of the tick, supportive treatment relieves symptoms, combats secondary infection, and maintains fluid balance.

- Carefully remove the tick by grasping it with forceps or gloved fingers and pulling gently. Be careful not to crush the tick's body. Keep it for identification. Thoroughly wash the wound with soap and water. If the tick's head remains embedded, surgical removal is necessary. Give a tetanus-diphtheria booster, as ordered.
- Be alert for secondary infection.
- Monitor fluid and electrolyte balance, and provide replacement accordingly.
- Reduce fever with antipyretics and tepid sponge baths.
- To prevent tickborne infection, tell the patient to avoid tick bites by wearing protective clothing (long pants tucked into boots) and carefully checking his body and scalp for ticks several times a day whenever in infested areas.

MISCELLANEOUS VIRUSES

Mumps

(Infectious or epidemic parotitis)

Mumps is an acute viral disease caused by a paramyxovirus. It is most prevalent in children older than age 5 but younger than age 9. Infants less than 1 year old seldom get this disease because of passive immunity from maternal antibodies. Peak incidence occurs during late winter and early spring. Prognosis for complete recovery is good, although mumps sometimes causes complications.

Causes

The mumps paramyxovirus is found in the saliva of an infected person and is transmitted by droplets or by direct contact. The virus is present in the saliva 6 days before to 9 days after onset of parotid gland swelling; the 48-hour period immediately preceding onset of swelling is probably the time of highest communicability. The incubation period ranges from 14 to 25 days (the average is 18). One attack of mumps (even if unilateral) almost always confers lifelong immunity.

Signs and symptoms

The clinical features of mumps vary widely. An estimated 30% of susceptible people have subclinical illness.

Mumps usually begins with prodromal symptoms that last for 24 hours and include myalgia, anorexia, malaise, headache, and low-grade fever, followed by an earache that's aggravated by chewing, parotid gland tenderness and swelling, a temperature of 101° to 104° F. (38.3° to 40° C.), and pain when chewing or when drinking sour or acidic liquids. Simultaneously with the swelling of the parotid gland or several days later, one or more of the other salivary glands may become swollen.

Complications include epididymoorchitis and mumps meningitis.

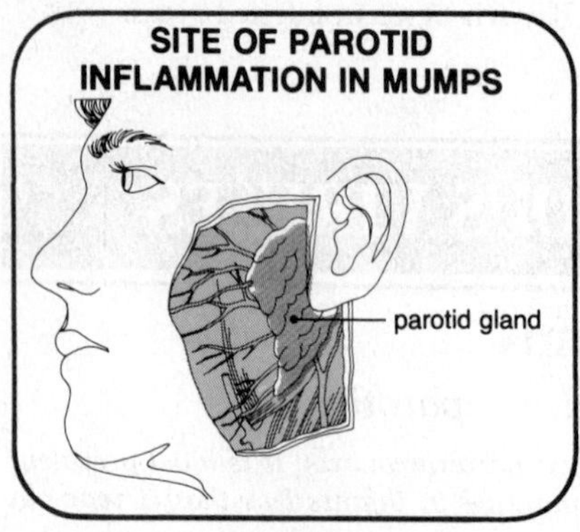

SITE OF PAROTID INFLAMMATION IN MUMPS

Epididymoorchitis occurs in approximately 25% of postpubertal males who contract mumps, and produces abrupt onset of testicular swelling and tenderness, scrotal erythema, lower abdominal pain, nausea, vomiting, fever, and chills. Swelling and tenderness may last for several weeks; epididymitis may precede or accompany orchitis. In 50% of men with mumps-induced orchitis, the testicles show some atrophy, but *sterility is extremely rare.*

Mumps meningitis complicates mumps in 10% of patients and affects males three to five times more often than females. Symptoms include fever, meningeal irritation (nuchal rigidity, headache, and irritability), vomiting, drowsiness, and a CSF lymphocyte count ranging from 500 to 2,000/mm³. Recovery is usually complete. Less common effects are pancreatitis, deafness, arthritis, myocarditis, encephalitis, pericarditis, oophoritis, and nephritis.

Diagnosis

Diagnosis is usually made after the characteristic signs and symptoms develop, especially parotid gland enlargement with a history of exposure to mumps. Serologic antibody testing can verify the diagnosis when parotid or other salivary gland enlargement is absent. If comparison between a blood specimen obtained during the acute phase of illness and another specimen obtained 3 weeks later shows a fourfold rise in antibody titer, the patient most likely had mumps.

Treatment

Treatment includes analgesics for pain, antipyretics for fever, and adequate fluid intake to prevent dehydration from fever and anorexia. If the patient can't swallow, consider I.V. fluid replacement.

Special considerations

Stress the need for bed rest during the febrile period. Give analgesics, and apply warm or cool compresses to the neck to relieve pain. Give antipyretics and tepid sponge baths for fever. To prevent dehydration, encourage the patient to drink fluids; to minimize pain and anorexia, advise him to avoid spicy, irritating foods and those that require a lot of chewing. During the acute phase, observe the patient closely for signs of CNS involvement, such as altered level of consciousness and nuchal rigidity.

Because the mumps virus is present in the saliva throughout the course of the disease, respiratory isolation is recommended until symptoms subside.

Emphasize the importance of routine immunization with live attenuated mumps virus (paramyxovirus) at age 15 months and for susceptible patients (especially males) who are approaching or are past puberty. Remember, immunization within 24 hours of exposure may prevent or attenuate the actual disease. Immunity against mumps lasts at least 12 years.

Report all cases of mumps to local public health authorities.

Infectious Mononucleosis

Infectious mononucleosis is an acute infectious disease caused by the Epstein-Barr virus (EBV), a member of the herpes group. It primarily affects young adults and children, although in children it's usually so mild that it's often overlooked. Characteristically, infectious mononucleosis produces fever, sore throat, and cervical lymphadenopathy (the hallmarks of the disease), as well as hepatic dysfunction, increased lymphocytes and monocytes, and development and persistence of heterophil antibodies. Prognosis is excellent, and major complications are uncommon.

Causes and incidence

Apparently, the reservoir of EBV is limited to humans. Infectious mononucleosis probably spreads by the oral-pharyngeal route, since about 80% of patients carry EBV in the throat during the acute infection and for an indefinite period afterward. It can also be transmitted by blood transfusion, and has been reported after cardiac surgery as the "post-pump perfusion" syndrome. Infectious mononucleosis is probably contagious from before symptoms develop until the fever subsides and oral-pharyngeal lesions disappear.

Infectious mononucleosis is fairly common in the United States, Canada, and Europe, and both sexes are affected equally. Incidence varies seasonally among college students (most common in the early spring and early fall) but not among the general population.

Signs and symptoms

The symptoms of mononucleosis mimic those of many other infectious diseases, including hepatitis, rubella, and toxoplasmosis. Typically, after an incubation period of about 10 days in children and from 30 to 50 days in adults, infectious mononucleosis produces prodromal symptoms, such as headache, malaise, and fatigue. After 3 to 5 days, patients typically develop a triad of symptoms: sore throat, cervical lymphadenopathy, and temperature fluctuations, with an evening peak of 101° to 102° F. (38.3° to 38.9° C.). Splenomegaly, hepatomegaly, stomatitis, exudative tonsillitis, or pharyngitis may also develop.

Sometimes, early in the illness, a maculopapular rash that resembles rubella develops; also, jaundice occurs in about 5% of patients. Major complications are rare but may include splenic rupture, aseptic meningitis, encephalitis, hemolytic anemia, and Guillain-Barré syndrome. Symptoms usually subside about 6 to 10 days after onset of the disease but may persist for weeks.

Diagnosis
Physical examination demonstrating the clinical triad suggests infectious mononucleosis. The following abnormal laboratory results confirm it:
- Leukocyte count increases 10,000 to 20,000/mm³ during the second and third weeks of illness. Lymphocytes and monocytes account for 50% to 70% of the total white blood cell (WBC) count; 10% of the lymphocytes are atypical.
- Heterophil antibodies (agglutinins for sheep RBCs) in serum drawn during the acute illness and at 3- to 4-week intervals rise to four times normal.
- Indirect immunofluorescence shows antibodies to EBV and cellular antigens. Such testing is usually more definitive than heterophil antibodies.
- Liver function studies are abnormal.

Treatment
Infectious mononucleosis resists prevention and antimicrobial treatment. Thus, therapy is essentially supportive: relief of symptoms, bed rest during the acute febrile period, and aspirin or another salicylate for headache and sore throat. If severe throat inflammation causes airway obstruction, steroids can be used to relieve swelling and avoid tracheotomy. Splenic rupture, marked by sudden abdominal pain, requires splenectomy. About 20% of patients with infectious mononucleosis will also have streptococcal pharyngotonsillitis; these patients should receive antibiotic therapy for at least 10 days.

Special considerations
Since uncomplicated infectious mononucleosis doesn't require hospitalization, patient teaching is essential. Convalescence may take several weeks, usually until the patient's WBC count returns to normal.
- During the acute illness, stress the need for bed rest. If the patient is a student, tell him he may continue less demanding school assignments and see his friends but should avoid long, difficult projects until after recovery.
- To minimize throat discomfort, encourage the patient to drink milk shakes, fruit juices, and broths, and also to eat cool, bland foods. Advise the use of saline gargles and aspirin, as needed.

Rabies
(Hydrophobia)

Rabies, usually transmitted by an animal bite, is an acute CNS infection caused by an RNA virus. If symptoms occur, rabies is almost always fatal. Treatment soon after a bite, however, may prevent fatal CNS invasion.

Causes and incidence
Generally, the rabies virus is transmitted to a human through the bite of an infected animal that introduces the virus through the skin or mucous membrane. The virus begins to replicate in the striated muscle cells at the bite site. Then it spreads up the nerve to the central nervous system and replicates in the brain. Finally, it moves through the nerves into other tissues, including the salivary glands. Occasionally, airborne droplets and infected tissue transplants can transmit the virus.

If the bite is on the face, the risk of developing rabies is about 60%; on the upper extremities, 15% to 40%; and on the lower extremities, about 10%. In the United States, dog vaccinations have reduced rabies' transmission to humans. Wild animals, such as skunks, foxes, and bats, account for 70% of rabies cases.

Signs and symptoms
Typically, after an incubation period of from 1 to 3 months, rabies produces local

or radiating pain or burning, a sensation of cold, pruritus, and tingling at the bite site. It also produces prodromal symptoms, such as a slight fever (100° to 102° F. [37.8° to 38.9° C.]), malaise, headache, anorexia, nausea, sore throat, and persistent loose cough. After this, the patient begins to show nervousness, anxiety, irritability, hyperesthesia, photophobia, sensitivity to loud noises, pupillary dilation, tachycardia, shallow respirations, and excessive salivation, lacrimation, and perspiration.

About 2 to 10 days after onset of prodromal symptoms, a phase of excitation begins. It's characterized by agitation, marked restlessness, anxiety and apprehension, and cranial nerve dysfunction that causes ocular palsies, strabismus, asymmetrical pupillary dilation or constriction, absence of corneal reflexes, weakness of facial muscles, and hoarseness. Severe systemic symptoms include tachycardia or bradycardia, cyclic respirations, urinary retention, and a temperature of about 103° F. (39.4° C.).

About 50% of affected patients exhibit hydrophobia (literally, "fear of water"), during which forceful, painful pharyngeal muscle spasms expel liquids from the mouth and cause dehydration and, possibly, apnea, cyanosis, and death. Difficulty swallowing causes frothy saliva to drool from the patient's mouth. Eventually, even the sight, mention, or thought of water causes uncontrollable pharyngeal muscle spasms and excessive salivation. Between episodes of excitation and hydrophobia, the patient commonly is cooperative and lucid. After about 3 days, excitation and hydrophobia subside and the progressively paralytic, terminal phase of this illness begins.

The patient experiences progressive, generalized, flaccid paralysis that ultimately leads to peripheral vascular collapse, coma, and death.

Diagnosis

Because rabies is fatal unless treated promptly, always suspect rabies in any

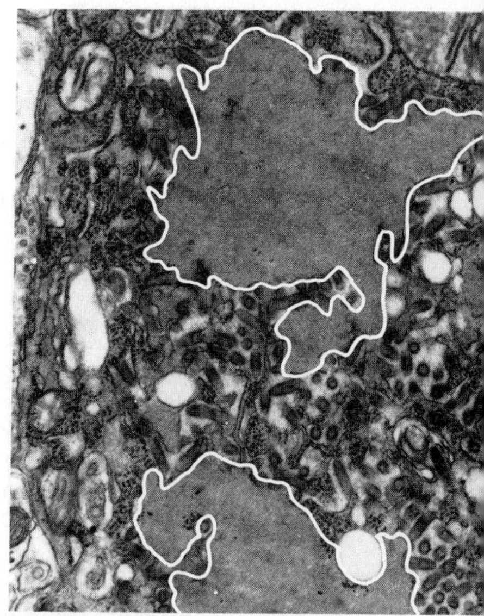

Negri bodies (outlined above) in the brain tissue of an animal suspected to be rabid conclusively confirm rabies. This electron micrograph also shows the rabies virus. Negri bodies are the areas of viral inclusion.

person who suffers an unprovoked animal bite until you can prove otherwise.

Virus isolation from the patient's saliva or throat and examination of his blood for fluorescent rabies antibody (FRA) are considered the most diagnostic tests. Other results typically include elevated WBC count, with increased polymorphonuclear and large mononuclear cells, and elevated urinary glucose, acetone, and protein.

Confinement of the suspected animal for 10 days of observation by a veterinarian also helps support this diagnosis. If the animal appears rabid, it should be killed and its brain tissue tested for FRA and Negri bodies (oval or round masses that conclusively confirm rabies).

Treatment

Treatment consists of wound treatment and immunization as soon as possible after exposure. Thoroughly wash all bite wounds and scratches with soap and wa-

FIRST AID IN ANIMAL BITES

Immediately wash the bite vigorously with soap and water for at least 10 minutes to remove the animal's saliva. As soon as possible, flush the wound with a viricidal agent, followed by a clear-water rinse. After cleansing the wound, apply a sterile dressing. If possible, don't suture the wound, and don't immediately stop the bleeding (unless it's massive), since blood flow helps to cleanse the wound.

Question the patient about the animal bite. Ask if he provoked the animal (if so, chances are it's not rabid) and if he can identify it or its owner (since the animal may need to be confined for observation).

ter. Check the patient's immunization status, and administer tetanus-diphtheria prophylaxis, if needed. Take measures to control bacterial infection, as ordered. If the wound requires suturing, special treatment and suturing techniques must be used to allow proper wound drainage.

After rabies exposure, a patient who has not been immunized before must receive passive immunization with rabies immune globulin (RIG) and active immunization with human diploid cell vaccine (HDCV). If the patient has received HDCV before and has an adequate rabies antibody titer, he doesn't need RIG immunization, just an HDCV booster.

Special considerations

- When injecting rabies vaccine, rotate injection sites on the upper arm or thigh. Watch for and symptomatically treat redness, itching, pain, and tenderness at the injection site.
- Cooperate with public health authorities to determine the vaccination status of the animal. If the animal is proven rabid, help identify others at risk.

If rabies develops, aggressive supportive care (even after onset of coma) can make probable death less agonizing.

- Monitor cardiac and pulmonary function continuously.
- Isolate the patient. Wear a gown, gloves, and protection for the eyes and mouth when handling saliva and articles contaminated with saliva. Take precautions to avoid being bitten by the patient during the excitation phase.
- Keep the room dark and quiet.
- Establish communication with the patient and his family. Provide psychological support to help them cope with the patient's symptoms and probable death.

To help prevent this dreaded disease, stress the need for vaccination of household pets that may be exposed to rabid wild animals. Warn persons not to try to touch wild animals, especially if they appear ill or overly docile (a possible sign of rabies). Assist in the prophylactic administration of rabies vaccine to high-risk persons, such as farm workers, forest rangers, spelunkers (cave explorers), and veterinarians.

Cytomegalovirus Infection

(Generalized salivary gland disease, cytomegalic inclusion disease [CID])

Cytomegalovirus (CMV) infection is caused by the cytomegalovirus, which is a DNA, ether-sensitive virus belonging to the herpes family. The disease occurs worldwide and is transmitted by human contact. About four out of five people over age 35 have been infected with cytomegalovirus, usually during childhood or early adulthood. In most of these people, the disease is so mild that it's overlooked. However, CMV infection during pregnancy can be hazardous to the fetus, possibly leading to stillbirth, brain damage, and other birth defects, or to severe neonatal illness.

Causes

Cytomegalovirus has been found in the saliva, urine, semen, breast milk, feces, blood, and vaginal and cervical secretions of infected persons.

Transmission usually takes place through contact with these infected secretions, which harbor the virus for months or even years. It may be transmitted by sexual contact and can travel across the placenta of a pregnant woman, causing a congenital infection. Immunodeficient patients, especially those who have received transplanted organs, run a 90% chance of contracting CMV infection. Recipients of blood transfusions from donors with positive CMV antibodies are at some risk.

Signs and symptoms

Cytomegalovirus probably spreads through the body in lymphocytes or mononuclear cells to the lungs, liver, and central nervous system where it often produces inflammatory reactions.

Most patients with CMV infection, however, exhibit mild, nonspecific clinical signs and symptoms, or none at all, even though antibody titers show they have been infected. In these patients, the disease usually runs a benign, self-limiting course. However, immunodeficient patients and those receiving immunosuppressives may develop pneumonia or other secondary infections. Infected infants aged 3 to 6 months usually appear asymptomatic but may develop hepatic dysfunction, hepatosplenomegaly, and spider angiomas, as well as pneumonitis, and lymphadenopathy.

Congenital CMV infection is often not apparent at birth, although the infant's urine contains the cytomegalovirus. About 1% of all newborns have CMV infection. The virus can cause serious brain damage that may not show up for weeks or months after birth. It can also produce a rapidly fatal neonatal illness characterized by jaundice, petechial rash, hepatosplenomegaly, thrombocytopenia, hemolytic anemia, microcephaly, psychomotor retardation, mental deficiency, and hearing loss.

In some adults, CMV may cause cytomegalovirus mononucleosis, with 3 weeks or more of irregular, high fever. Other findings may include normal or elevated WBC count, lymphocytosis, and increased atypical lymphocytes.

Diagnosis

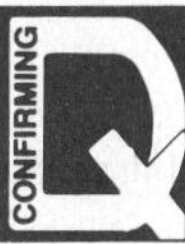

Although virus isolation in urine is the most sensitive laboratory method, diagnosis can also rest on virus isolation from saliva, throat, cervix, WBC, and biopsy specimens.

Other laboratory tests support the diagnosis, including complement fixation studies, hemagglutination inhibition antibody tests, and, for congenital infections, indirect immunofluorescent tests for CMV immunoglobulin M antibody.

Treatment

Treatment aims to relieve symptoms and prevent complications. Most important, parents of children with severe congenital CMV infection need emotional support and counseling to help them accept and cope with the possibility of brain damage or death.

Special considerations

To help prevent CMV infection:

- Warn immunodeficient patients and pregnant women to avoid any individuals with confirmed or suspected CMV infection. (A maternal CMV infection can cause fetal abnormalities, such as hydrocephaly, microphthalmia, seizures, encephalitis, hepatosplenomegaly, hematologic changes, microcephaly, and blindness.)
- Urge patients with CMV infection to wash their hands thoroughly to prevent spreading it. It is especially important to stress this with young children, who are usually unconcerned with personal hygiene.
- Be careful when handling urine and saliva or articles contaminated with these or other body secretions. Dispose of such articles properly. Mark contaminated linens for special handling.

Lassa Fever

Lassa fever is an epidemic hemorrhagic fever caused by the Lassa virus, an extremely virulent arenavirus. As many as 100 cases occur annually in western Africa; the disease is rare in the United States. This highly fatal disorder kills 10% to 50% of its victims, but those who survive its early stages usually recover and acquire immunity to secondary attacks.

Causes

A chronic infection in rodents, Lassa virus is transmitted to humans by contact with infected rodent urine, feces, and saliva. (This is the reason why Lassa fever sometimes strikes laboratory workers.) Then the virus enters the bloodstream, lymph vessels, and respiratory and digestive tracts. Following this, it multiplies in cells of the reticuloendothelial system. In the early stages of this illness, when the virus is in the throat, human transmission may occur through inhalation of infected droplets.

Signs and symptoms

After a 7- to 15-day incubation period, this disease produces a fever that persists for 2 to 3 weeks, exudative pharyngitis, oral ulcers, lymphadenopathy with swelling of the face and neck, purpura, conjunctivitis, and bradycardia. Severe infection may also cause hepatitis, myocarditis, pleural infection, encephalitis, and permanent unilateral or bilateral deafness. Virus multiplication in reticuloendothelial cells causes capillary lesions that lead to erythrocyte and platelet loss, mild to moderate thrombocytopenia (with a tendency to bleeding), and secondary bacterial infection. Capillary lesions also cause focal hemorrhage in the stomach, small intestine, kidneys, lungs, and brain and, possibly, hemorrhagic shock and peripheral vascular collapse.

Diagnosis

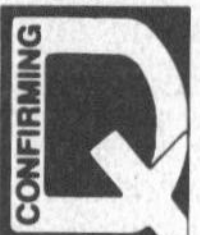

Isolation of the Lassa virus from throat washings, pleural fluid, or blood confirms the diagnosis. Recent travel to an endemic area and specific antibody titer support this diagnosis.

Treatment

Treatment of Lassa fever is primarily supportive. It includes administration of antibiotics (depending on the organism cultured) for secondary bacterial infection, I.V. colloids for shock, analgesics for pain, and antipyretics for fever. Infusion of immune plasma from patients who've recovered from Lassa fever may be useful in treatment, but test results on the benefits of this type of therapy are inconclusive.

Special considerations

- Carefully monitor fluid and electrolytes, vital signs, and intake and output. Watch for and immediately report signs of infection or shock.
- Strict isolation is necessary for at least 3 weeks, until the patient's throat washings and urine are free of the virus. To prevent the spread of this contagious disease, carefully dispose of or disinfect all materials contaminated with the infected patient's urine, feces, respiratory secretions, or exudates. Watch known contacts closely for at least 3 weeks for signs of the disease.
- Provide good mouth care. Remember to clean the patient's mouth with a soft-bristled brush to avoid irritating his mouth ulcers. Ask your hospital's dietary department to supply a soft, bland, nonirritating diet.
- Immediately report all cases of Lassa fever to the public health authorities in your area.
- Immediately contact the Viral Diseases Division of the Centers for Disease Control in Atlanta to get specific guidelines for managing suspected or confirmed cases of Lassa fever.

RICKETTSIA

Rocky Mountain Spotted Fever

Rocky Mountain spotted fever (RMSF) is a febrile, rash-producing illness caused by Rickettsia rickettsii *and is transmitted through a tick bite. Endemic throughout the continental United States, RMSF is particularly prevalent in the southeast and southwest. RMSF is becoming more common because of the increasing popularity of outdoor activities, such as camping and backpacking. Because it's associated with such activities, the incidence of this illness is usually higher in the spring and summer.*

RMSF is fatal in about 5% of patients. Mortality rises when treatment is delayed; it also increases in older patients.

Causes

R. rickettsii is transmitted by the wood tick (*Dermacentor andersoni*) in the west and by the dog tick (*Dermacentor variabilis*) in the east. RMSF is transmitted to a human or small animal by a prolonged bite (4 to 6 hours) of an adult tick. Occasionally, this disease is acquired through inhalation or through contact of abraded skin with tick excreta or tissue juices. (This explains why people shouldn't crush ticks between their fingers when removing them from others.) In most tick-infested areas, 1% to 5% of the ticks harbor *R. rickettsii.*

Signs and symptoms

The incubation period is usually about 7 days, but it can range anywhere from 2 to 14 days. Generally, the shorter the incubation time, the more severe the infection. Onset of symptoms is usually abrupt, producing a persistent temperature of 102° to 104° F. (38.9° to 40° C.); a generalized, excruciating headache; and aching in the bones, muscles, joints, and back. In addition, the tongue is covered with a thick white coating that gradually turns brown as the fever persists and rises.

Initially, the skin may simply appear flushed. But between days 2 and 5, eruptions begin about the wrists, ankles, or forehead and, within 2 days, cover the entire body, including the scalp, palms, and soles. The rash consists of erythematous macules 1 to 5 mm in diameter that blanch on pressure; if untreated, the rash may become petechial and maculopapular. By the third week, the skin peels off and may become gangrenous over the elbows, fingers, and toes.

At onset, the pulse is strong, but it gradually becomes rapid (possibly reaching 150 beats/minute) and thready.

OMINOUS SIGN

Rapid pulse and hypotension (less than 90 mm Hg systolic) herald imminent death from vascular collapse.

Other clinical signs and symptoms include a bronchial cough, rapid respirations (as many as 60 breaths/minute), anorexia, nausea, vomiting, constipation, abdominal pain, hepatomegaly, splenomegaly, insomnia, restlessness, and, in extreme cases, de-

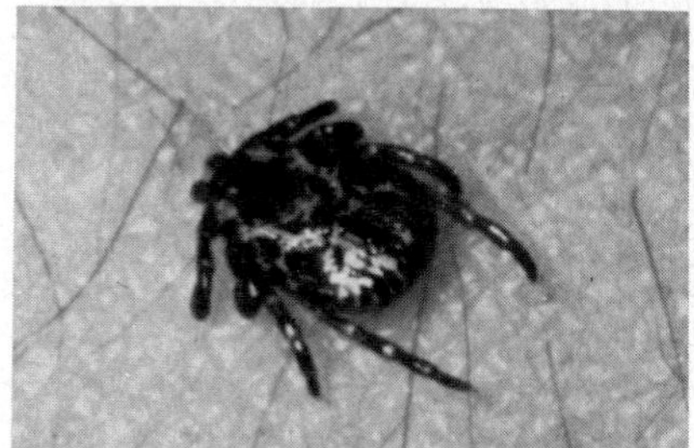

Rocky Mountain spotted fever is transmitted by the prolonged bite of an adult tick.

PATIENT TEACHING AID

Prevent Rocky Mountain Spotted Fever

Dear Patient:
You can prevent Rocky Mountain spotted fever by taking the following precautions:

- Avoid tick-infested areas, if possible. If you must go to a tick-infested area, check your entire body, including scalp, every 3 to 4 hours for attached ticks. Wear protective clothing, such as a long-sleeved shirt, and slacks tucked into firmly laced boots.
- Apply insect repellent to clothes and exposed skin.
- If you find a tick attached to your body, don't crush it, as this may contaminate the bite wound. To detach the tick, place a drop of oil, alcohol, gasoline, or kerosene on it or hold a lighted cigarette near it.
- If you're at high risk (for instance, if you work in a laboratory with rickettsiae, or if you're planning an extended camping trip and will be far from adequate medical facilities), you should receive vaccination against this disease.

This patient teaching aid may be reproduced by office copier for distribution to patients.

lirium. Urinary output falls to half or less of the normal level, and the urine is dark and contains albumin. Complications, although uncommon, include lobar pneumonia, otitis media, parotitis, disseminated intravascular coagulation (DIC), and possibly renal failure. In rare cases, Rocky Mountain spotted fever leads to death.

Diagnosis

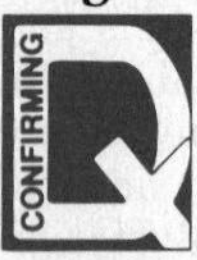

Diagnosis generally rests on a history of a tick bite or travel to a tick-infested area and a positive complement fixation test (which shows a fourfold increase in convalescent antibody titer compared with acute titers). Blood cultures should be performed to isolate the organism and confirm the diagnosis. Another common but less reliable antibody test is the Weil-Felix reaction, which also shows a fourfold increase between the acute and convalescent sera titer levels. Increased titers usually develop after 10 to 14 days and persist for several months.

Additional recommended laboratory tests consist of a platelet count for thrombocytopenia (12,000 to 150,000/mm^3) and a white blood cell count (elevation to 11,000 to 33,000/mm^3) during the second week of illness.

Treatment

Treatment requires careful removal of the tick and administration of antibiotics, such as chloramphenicol or tetracycline, until 3 days after the fever subsides. Treatment also includes symptomatic measures and, in DIC, heparin and platelet transfusion.

Special considerations

- Carefully monitor intake and output. Watch closely for decreased urinary output—a possible indicator of renal failure. Also watch for signs of dehydration, such as poor skin turgor and dry mouth. Give antipyretics, as ordered, and tepid sponge baths to reduce fever.
- Monitor vital signs, and watch for profound hypotension and shock. Also, be prepared to give oxygen therapy and assisted ventilation for pulmonary complications.
- Turn the patient frequently to prevent decubitus ulcers and pneumonia.
- Pay attention to the patient's nutritional needs, as vomiting may necessitate intravenous nutrition or frequent small meals.
- Give meticulous mouth care.

PROTOZOA

Malaria

Malaria, an acute infectious disease, is caused by protozoa of the genus Plasmodium: Plasmodium falciparum, Plasmodium vivax, Plasmodium malariae, *and* Plasmodium ovale, *all of which are transmitted to humans by mosquito vectors. Falciparum malaria is the most severe form of the disease. When treated, malaria is rarely fatal; untreated, it's fatal in 10% of victims, usually as a result of complications, such as disseminated intravascular coagulation (DIC). Untreated primary attacks last from a week to a month, or longer. Relapses are common and can recur sporadically for several years. Susceptibility to the disease is universal.*

Causes and incidence

Malaria literally means "bad air" and for centuries was thought to result from the inhalation of swamp vapors. It is now known that malaria is transmitted by the bite of female *Anopheles* mosquitoes, which abound in humid, swampy areas. When an infected mosquito bites, it injects *Plasmodium* sporozoites into the wound. The infective sporozoites migrate by blood circulation to parenchymal cells of the liver; there they form cystlike structures containing thousands of merozoites.

Upon release, each merozoite invades an erythrocyte and feeds on hemoglobin. Eventually, the erythrocyte ruptures, releasing heme (malaria pigment), cell debris, and more merozoites that, unless destroyed by phagocytes, enter other erythrocytes. At this point, the infected person becomes a reservoir of malaria who infects any mosquito that feeds on him, thus beginning a new cycle of transmission. Hepatic parasites (*P. vivax, P. ovale,* and *P. malariae*) may persist for years in the liver and are responsible for the chronic carrier state. Since blood transfusions and street-drug paraphernalia can also spread malaria, drug addicts have a higher incidence of the disease.

Malaria is a tropical as well as a subtropical disease and is most prevalent in Asia, Africa, and Latin America. Incidence in the United States during the last 15 years has ranged from a high of 4,230 cases in 1970 (mainly among military personnel returning from Vietnam) to a low of 222 cases in 1973. Rarely have cases of malaria actually been contracted in the United States within the last 15 years; those resulted from blood transfusions or the use of contaminated needles by drug addicts.

Signs and symptoms

After an incubation period of 12 to 30 days, malaria produces chills, fever, headache, and myalgia interspersed

HOW TO PREVENT MALARIA

- Drain, fill, and eliminate breeding areas of the *Anopheles* mosquito.
- Install screens in living and sleeping quarters in endemic areas.
- Use a residual insecticide on clothing and skin to prevent mosquito bites.
- Seek treatment for known cases.
- Question blood donors about a history of malaria or possible exposure to malaria. They *may* give blood if: they haven't taken any antimalarial drugs and are asymptomatic after 6 months outside an endemic area; they were asymptomatic after treatment for malaria over 3 years ago; or they were asymptomatic after receiving malaria prophylaxis over 3 years ago.
- Seek prophylactic drug therapy before traveling to an endemic area.

with periods of well-being (the hallmark of the benign form of malaria). Acute attacks (paroxysms) occur when erythrocytes rupture and have three stages:

- *cold stage,* lasting 1 to 2 hours, ranging from chills to extreme shaking
- *hot stage,* lasting 3 to 4 hours, characterized by a high fever (temperature up to 107° F. [41.7° C.])
- *wet stage,* lasting 2 to 4 hours, characterized by profuse sweating.

Paroxysms occur every 48 to 72 hours when caused by *P. malariae*, and every 42 to 50 hours with *P. vivax* and *P. ovale*. All three types have low levels of parasitosis and are self-limiting as a result of early acquired immunity. Vivax and ovale malaria also produce hepatosplenomegaly. Hemolytic anemia is present in all but the mildest infections.

The most severe form of malaria is caused by *P. falciparum*, the only life-threatening strain. This species produces persistent high fever, orthostatic hypotension, and massive erythrocytosis that leads to capillary obstruction at various sites:

- *cerebral:* hemiplegia, convulsions, delirium, coma
- *pulmonary:* coughing, hemoptysis
- *splanchnic:* vomiting, abdominal pain, diarrhea, melena
- *renal:* oliguria, anuria, uremia.

Because it produces these severe systemic complications, falciparum malaria prevents the respites of well-being common to other malarial infections. During blackwater fever (a complication of *P. falciparum* infection), massive intravascular hemolysis causes jaundice, hemoglobinuria, a tender and enlarged spleen, acute renal failure, and uremia. This dreaded complication is fatal in about 20% of patients.

Diagnosis

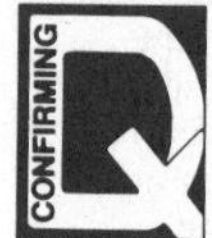

A history showing travel to endemic areas, recent blood transfusion, or drug abuse in a person with high fever of unknown origin strongly suggests malaria. But because symptoms of malaria mimic other diseases, unequivocal diagnosis depends on laboratory identification of the parasites in RBCs of peripheral blood smears. The CDC can identify donors responsible for transfusion malaria through indirect fluorescent serum antibody tests. These tests are unreliable in the acute phase, because antibodies can be undetectable for 2 weeks after onset.

Supplementary laboratory values that support this diagnosis include decreased hemoglobin, normal to decreased leukocyte count (as low as 3,000/mm^3), and protein and leukocytes in urine sediment. In falciparum malaria, serum values reflect DIC: reduced number of platelets (20,000 to 50,000/mm^3), prolonged prothrombin time (18 to 20 seconds), prolonged partial thromboplastin time (60 to 100 seconds), and decreased plasma fibrinogen.

Treatment

Malaria is best treated with chloroquine P.O. in all but chloroquine-resistant *P. falciparum*. Within 24 hours after such therapy begins, symptoms and parasitosis decrease, and the patient usually recovers within 3 to 4 days. If the patient is comatose or vomiting frequently, chloroquine is given I.M. instead. Although rare, toxic reactions include gastrointestinal upset, pruritus, headache, and visual disturbances.

Malaria due to *P. falciparum*, which is resistant to chloroquine, requires treatment with quinine P.O. for 10 days, given concurrently with pyrimethamine and a sulfonamide, such as sulfadiazine. Relapses require the same treatment, or quinine alone, followed by tetracycline.

The only drug effective against the hepatic stage of the disease that is available in the United States is primaquine phosphate, given daily for 14 days. This drug can induce DIC from increased hemolysis of RBCs; consequently, it's contraindicated during an acute attack.

For travelers spending less than 3 weeks in areas where malaria exists, weekly prophylaxis includes chloroquine P.O. beginning 2 weeks before and ending 6 weeks after the trip. Chloroquine and sulfadoxine/pyrimethamine (Fansidar) may be ordered for those staying longer than 3 weeks, although combination treatment can have severe side effects. If the traveler isn't sensitive to either component of Fansidar, he may be given a single dose to take if he has a febrile episode. Any traveler who develops an acute febrile illness should seek prompt medical attention, regardless of prophylaxis taken.

Special considerations

- Obtain a detailed patient history, noting any recent travel, foreign residence, blood transfusion, or drug addiction. Record symptom pattern, fever, type of malaria, and any systemic signs.
- Assess the patient on admission and daily thereafter for fatigue, fever, orthostatic hypotension, disorientation, myalgia, and arthralgia. Enforce bed rest during periods of acute illness.
- Protect the patient from secondary bacterial infection by following proper handwashing and aseptic techniques. Protect yourself by wearing gloves when handling blood or body fluids containing blood. If DIC occurs, wear a gown and gloves while in contact with the patient. Discard needles and syringes in an impervious container designated for incineration. Double-bag all contaminated linen, and send it to the laundry as an isolation item.
- To reduce fever, administer antipyretics, as ordered. Document onset of fever and its duration, and symptoms before and after episodes.
- Fluid balance is fragile, so keep a strict record of intake and output. Monitor I.V. fluids closely. Avoid fluid overload (especially with *P. falciparum*), since it can lead to pulmonary edema and the aggravation of cerebral symptoms. Observe blood chemistry levels for hyponatremia and increased BUN, creatinine, and bilirubin levels. Monitor urine output hourly, and maintain it at 40 to 60 ml/hour for an adult and at 15 to 30 ml/hour for a child. Immediately report any decrease in urine output or the onset of hematuria as a possible sign of renal failure; be prepared to do peritoneal dialysis for uremia caused by renal failure. For oliguria, administer furosemide or mannitol I.V., as ordered.
- Slowly administer packed RBCs or whole blood while checking for rales,

NURSING CONSIDERATIONS FOR ANTIMALARIAL DRUGS

Chloroquine and amodiaquine

- Perform baseline and periodic ophthalmologic examinations, and report blurred vision, increased sensitivity to light, and muscle weakness to the doctor.
- Consult with the doctor about altering therapy if muscle weakness appears in a patient on long-term therapy.
- Suggest an audiometric examination before, during, and after therapy, particularly in long-term therapy.
- Caution the patient to avoid excessive exposure to the sun to prevent exacerbating drug-induced dermatoses.

Primaquine

- Give with meals or antacids.
- Discontinue administration if you observe a sudden fall in hemoglobin concentration or in erythrocyte or leukocyte count, or marked darkening of the urine, suggesting impending hemolytic reaction.

Pyrimethamine

- Administer with meals to minimize gastrointestinal distress.
- Check blood counts (including platelets) twice a week. If signs of folic or folinic acid deficiency develop, reduce or discontinue dosage while patient receives parenteral folinic acid until blood counts become normal.

Quinine

- Use with caution in patient with a cardiovascular condition. Discontinue dosage if you see any signs of idiosyncrasy or toxicity, such as headache, epigastric distress, diarrhea, rashes, and pruritus, in a mild reaction; or delirium, convulsions, blindness, cardiovascular collapse, asthma, hemolytic anemia, and granulocytosis, in a severe reaction.
- Monitor blood pressure frequently while administering quinine I.V. Rapid administration causes marked hypotension.

tachycardia, and shortness of breath.
• If humidified oxygen is ordered because of anemia, note the patient's response, particularly any changes in rate or character of respirations, or improvement in mucous membrane color.
• Watch for and immediately report signs of internal bleeding, such as tachycardia, hypotension, and pallor.
• Encourage frequent coughing and deep breathing, especially if the patient is on bed rest or has pulmonary complications. Record the amount and color of sputum.
• Watch for side effects of drug therapy, and take measures to relieve them.
• If the patient is comatose, make frequent, gentle changes in his position, and give passive range-of-motion exercises every 3 to 4 hours. If the patient is unconscious or disoriented, use restraints, as needed, and keep an airway or padded tongue blade available.
• Provide emotional support and reassurance, especially in critical illness. Explain the procedures and treatment to the patient and his family. Listen sympathetically, and answer questions clearly. Suggest that other family members be tested for malaria. Emphasize the need for follow-up care to check the effectiveness of treatment and to manage residual problems.
• Report all cases of malaria to the local public health authorities.

Amebiasis

(Amebic dysentery)

Amebiasis is an acute or chronic protozoal infection caused by Entamoeba histolytica. *This infection produces varying degrees of illness, from no symptoms at all or mild diarrhea to fulminating dysentery. Extraintestinal amebiasis can induce hepatic abscess and infections of the lungs, pleural cavity, pericardium, peritoneum, and, rarely, the brain.*

Amebiasis occurs worldwide but is most common in the tropics, subtropics, and other areas with poor sanitation and health practices. Incidence in the United States averages between 1% and 3% but may be higher among homosexuals and institutionalized groups, in whom fecal-oral contamination is common.

Prognosis is generally good, although complications—such as ameboma, intestinal stricture, hemorrhage or perforation, intussusception, or abscess—increase mortality. Brain abscess, a rare complication, is usually fatal.

Causes

E. histolytica exists in two forms: a cyst (which can survive outside the body), and a trophozoite (which can't survive outside the body). Transmission occurs through ingesting feces-contaminated food or water. The ingested cysts pass through the intestine, where digestive secretions break down the cysts and liberate the motile trophozoites within. The trophozoites multiply, and either invade and ulcerate the mucosa of the large intestine, or simply feed on intestinal bacteria. As the trophozoites are carried slowly toward the rectum, they are encysted and then excreted in feces. Man is the principal reservoir of infection.

Signs and symptoms

The clinical effects of amebiasis vary with the severity of the infestation. *Acute amebic dysentery* causes a sudden high fever of 104° to 105° F. (40° to 40.6° C.) accompanied by chills and abdominal cramping; profuse, bloody diarrhea with tenesmus; and diffuse abdominal tenderness due to extensive rectosigmoid ulcers. *Chronic amebic dysentery* produces intermittent diarrhea that lasts for 1 to 4 weeks, and recurs several times a year.

Such diarrhea produces 4 to 8 (or, in severe diarrhea, up to 18) foul-smelling mucus- and blood-tinged stools daily in a patient with a mild fever, vague abdominal cramps, possible weight loss, tenderness over the cecum and ascending colon, and occasionally hepatomegaly. Amebic granuloma (ameboma), often mistaken for cancer, can be a complication of the chronic infection. Amebic granuloma produces blood and mucus in the stool and, when granulomatous tissue covers the entire circumference of the bowel, causes partial or complete obstruction.

Parasitic and bacterial invasion of the appendix may produce typical signs of subacute appendicitis (abdominal pain and tenderness). Occasionally, *E. histolytica* perforates the intestinal wall and spreads to the liver. When it perforates the liver and diaphragm, it spreads to the lungs, pleural cavity, peritoneum, and, rarely, the brain.

Diagnosis

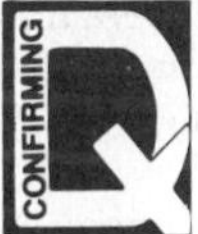

Isolating *E. histolytica* (cysts and trophozoites) in fresh feces or aspirates from abscesses, ulcers, or tissue confirms acute amebic dysentery.

Diagnosis must distinguish between cancer and ameboma with X-rays, sigmoidoscopy, stool examination for amebae, and cecum palpation. In those with amebiasis, exploratory surgery is hazardous; it can lead to peritonitis, perforation, and pericecal abscess.

Other lab tests that support the diagnosis of amebiasis include:

- indirect hemagglutination test—positive with current or previous infection
- complement fixation—usually positive only during active disease
- barium studies—rule out nonamebic causes of diarrhea, such as polyps and cancer
- sigmoidoscopy—detects rectosigmoid ulceration; a biopsy may be helpful.

Patients with amebiasis shouldn't have preparatory enemas, since these may remove exudates and destroy the trophozoites, thus interfering with test results.

Treatment and special considerations

Drugs used to treat amebic dysentery include metronidazole, an amebicide at intestinal and extraintestinal sites; emetine hydrochloride, also an amebicide at intestinal and extraintestinal sites, including the liver and lungs; iodoquinol (diiodohydroxyquin), an effective amebicide for asymptomatic carriers; chloroquine, for liver abscesses, not intestinal infections; and tetracycline (in combination with emetine hydrochloride, metronidazole, or paromomycin), which supports the antiamebic effect by destroying intestinal bacteria on which the amebae normally feed.

Tell patients with amebiasis to avoid drinking alcohol when taking metronidazole. The combination may cause nausea, vomiting, and headache.

Giardiasis

(Giardia *enteritis, lambliasis)*

Giardiasis is an infection of the small bowel caused by the symmetrical flagellate protozoan Giardia lamblia. *A mild infection may not produce intestinal symptoms. In untreated giardiasis, symptoms wax and wane; with treatment, recovery is complete.*

Causes

G. lamblia has two stages: the cystic stage and the trophozoite stage. Ingestion of *G. lamblia* cysts in fecally contaminated water or the fecal-oral transfer of cysts by an infected person results in giardiasis. When cysts enter the small bowel, they become trophozoites and attach themselves with their sucking disks to the bowel's epithelial surface. Following this, the trophozoites encyst again, travel down the colon, and are excreted. Unformed feces that pass quickly through the intestine may contain trophozoites as well as cysts.

Giardiasis occurs worldwide but is most common in developing countries and other areas where sanitation and hygiene are poor. In the United States, giardiasis is most common in travelers who've recently returned from endemic areas and in campers who drink unpurified water from contaminated streams. Probably because of frequent hand-to-mouth activity, children are more likely to become infected with *G. lamblia* than adults. In addition, hypogammaglobulinemia also appears to predispose persons to this disorder. Giardiasis doesn't confer immunity, so reinfections may occur.

Signs and symptoms

Attachment of *G. lamblia* to the intestinal lumen causes superficial mucosal invasion and destruction, inflammation, and irritation. All of these destructive effects decrease food transit time through the small intestine and result in malabsorption. Such malabsorption produces chronic gastrointestinal complaints—such as abdominal cramps—and pale, loose, greasy, malodorous, and frequent stools (from 2 to 10 daily), with concurrent nausea. Stools may contain mucus but not pus or blood. Chronic giardiasis may produce fatigue and weight loss in addition to these typical signs and symptoms.

Diagnosis

Suspect giardiasis when travelers to endemic areas or campers who may have drunk unpurified water develop symptoms.

Actual diagnosis requires laboratory examination of a fresh stool specimen for cysts or examination of duodenal aspirate for trophozoites. A barium X-ray of the small bowel may show mucosal edema and barium segmentation. Diagnosis must also rule out other causes of diarrhea and malabsorption.

Treatment

Giardiasis responds readily to a 10-day course of metronidazole or a 7-day course of quinacrine and furazolidone P.O. Severe diarrhea may require parenteral fluid replacement to prevent dehydration if oral fluid intake is inadequate.

Special considerations

- Inform the patient receiving metronidazole of the expected side effects of this drug: commonly headache, anorexia, and nausea; and less commonly vomiting, diarrhea, and abdominal cramps. Warn against drinking alcoholic beverages, since these may provoke a disulfiram-like reaction. If the patient is a woman, ask if she's pregnant, since metronidazole is contraindicated during pregnancy.
- When talking to family members and other suspected contacts, emphasize the importance of stool examinations for *G. lamblia* cysts.
- Hospitalization may be required. If so, apply enteric precautions. The patient will require a private room if he's a child or an incontinent adult. When caring for such a patient, pay strict attention to hand washing, particularly after handling feces. Quickly dispose of fecal material. (Normal sewage systems can remove and process infected feces adequately.)
- Teach good personal hygiene, particularly proper hand washing technique.
- To help prevent giardiasis, warn travelers to endemic areas not to drink water or eat uncooked and unpeeled fruits or vegetables (they may have been rinsed in contaminated water). Prophylactic drug therapy isn't recommended. Advise campers to purify all stream water before drinking it.
- Report epidemic situations to the public health authorities.

Toxoplasmosis

Toxoplasmosis, one of the most common infectious diseases, results from the protozoa Toxoplasma gondii. *Distributed worldwide, it's less common in cold or hot, arid climates and at high elevations. It usually causes localized infection but may produce significant generalized infection, especially in immunodeficient patients or newborns. Congenital toxoplasmosis, characterized by lesions in the central nervous system, may result in stillbirth or serious birth defects.*

Causes

T. gondii exists in trophozoite forms in the acute stages of infection and in cystic forms (tissue cysts and oocysts) in the latent stages. Ingestion of tissue cysts in raw or uncooked meat (heating, drying, or freezing destroys these cysts) or fecal-oral contamination from infected cats transmits toxoplasmosis. However, toxoplasmosis also occurs in vegetarians who aren't exposed to cats, so other means of transmission may exist. Congenital toxoplasmosis follows transplacental transmission from a chronically infected mother or one who acquired toxoplasmosis shortly before or during pregnancy.

Signs and symptoms

Toxoplasmosis acquired in the first trimester of pregnancy often results in stillbirth. About one third of infants who survive have congenital toxoplasmosis. The later in pregnancy maternal infection occurs, the greater the risk of congenital infection in the infant. Obvious signs of congenital toxoplasmosis include retinochoroiditis, hydrocephalus or microcephalus, cerebral calcification, convulsions, lymphadenopathy, fever, hepatosplenomegaly, jaundice, and rash. Other defects, which may become apparent months or years later, include strabismus, blindness, epilepsy, and mental retardation.

Acquired toxoplasmosis may cause localized (mild lymphatic) or generalized (fulminating, disseminated) infection. Localized infection produces fever and a mononucleosis-like syndrome (malaise, myalgia, headache, fatigue, sore throat) and lymphadenopathy. Generalized infection produces encephalitis, fever, headache, vomiting, delirium, convulsions, and a diffuse maculopapular rash (except on the palms, soles, and scalp). Generalized infection may lead to myocarditis, pneumonitis, hepatitis, and polymyositis.

Diagnosis

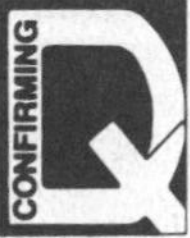

Isolation of *T. gondii* in mice after their inoculation with specimens of body fluids, blood, and tissue, or *T. gondii* antibodies in such specimens confirms toxoplasmosis.

Treatment

Treatment is most effective during the acute stage and consists of drug therapy with sulfonamides and pyrimethamine for approximately 4 weeks and, possibly, folinic acid to control pyrimethamine side effects.

OCULAR TOXOPLASMOSIS

Ocular toxoplasmosis (active retinochoroiditis), characterized by focal necrotizing retinitis, accounts for about 25% of all granulomatous uveitis. It is usually the result of congenital infection, but may not appear until adolescence or young adulthood, when infection is reactivated. Symptoms include blurred vision, scotoma, pain, photophobia, and impairment or loss of central vision. Vision improves as inflammation subsides but usually without recovery of lost visual acuity. Ocular toxoplasmosis may subside after treatment with prednisone.

No safe, effective treatment exists for chronic toxoplasmosis or toxoplasmosis occurring during the first trimester of a patient's pregnancy.

Special considerations

When caring for patients with toxoplasmosis, monitor drug therapy carefully and emphasize thorough patient teaching to prevent complications and control spread of the disease.

- Since sulfonamides cause blood dyscrasias and pyrimethamine depresses bone marrow, closely monitor the patient's hematologic values. Also emphasize the importance of regularly scheduled follow-up care.
- Teach all persons to wash their hands after working with soil (since it may be contaminated with cat oocysts); to cook meat thoroughly and freeze it promptly if it's not for immediate use; to change cat litter daily (cat oocysts don't become infective until 1 to 4 days after excretion); to cover children's sand boxes; and to keep flies away from food (flies transport oocysts).
- Report all cases of toxoplasmosis to your local public health department.

HELMINTHS

Trichinosis

(Trichiniasis, trichinellosis)

Trichinosis is an infection caused by larvae of the intestinal roundworm Trichinella spiralis. *It occurs worldwide, especially in populations that eat pork or bear meat. Trichinosis may produce multiple symptoms; respiratory, CNS, and cardiovascular complications; and, rarely, death.*

Causes

Transmission is through ingestion of uncooked or undercooked meat that contains *T. spiralis* cysts. Such cysts are found primarily in swine, less often in dogs, cats, bears, foxes, wolves, and marine animals. These cysts result from the animals' ingestion of similarly contaminated flesh. In swine, such infection results from eating table scraps or raw garbage.

After gastric juices free the worm from the cyst capsule, it reaches sexual maturity in a few days. The female roundworm burrows into the intestinal mucosa and reproduces. Larvae are then transported through the lymphatic system and the bloodstream. They become embedded as cysts in striated muscle, especially in the diaphragm, chest, arms, and legs. Human-to-human transmission does not take place.

Signs and symptoms

In the United States, trichinosis is usually mild and seldom produces symptoms. When symptoms do occur, they vary with the stage and degree of infection:

- *Stage 1*—Invasion: occurs 1 week after ingestion. Release of larvae and reproduction of adult *T. spiralis* cause anorexia, nausea, vomiting, diarrhea, abdominal pain, and cramps.
- *Stage 2*—Dissemination: occurs 7 to 10 days after ingestion. *T. spiralis* penetrates the intestinal mucosa and begins to migrate to striated muscle. Symptoms include edema, especially of the eyelids or face; muscle pain, particularly in extremities; and, occasionally, itching and burning skin, sweating, skin lesions, a temperature of 102° to 104° F. (38.9° to 40° C.), and delirium; and, in severe respiratory, cardiovascular, or CNS infections, palpitations and lethargy.

• *Stage 3*—Encystment: occurs during convalescence, generally 1 week later. *T. spiralis* larvae invade muscle fiber and become encysted.

Diagnosis

A history of ingestion of raw or improperly cooked pork or pork products, with typical clinical features, suggests trichinosis; but infection may be difficult to prove. Stools may contain mature worms and larvae during the invasion stage. Skeletal muscle biopsies can show encysted larvae 10 days after ingestion; and, if available, analyses of contaminated meat also show larvae.

Skin testing may show a positive histamine-like reactivity 15 minutes after intradermal injection of the antigen (within 17 to 20 days after ingestion). However, such a result may remain positive for up to 5 years after exposure. Elevated acute and convalescent antibody titers (determined by flocculation tests 3 to 4 weeks after infection) confirm this diagnosis.

Other abnormal results include elevated SGOT, SGPT, CPK, and LDH levels during the acute stages and an elevated eosinophil count (up to 15,000/mm^3). A normal or increased CSF lymphocyte level (to 300/mm^3) and increased protein levels indicate CNS involvement.

Treatment and special considerations

Thiabendazole effectively combats this parasite during the intestinal stage; severe infection (especially CNS invasion) may warrant glucocorticoids to fight against possible inflammation.

• Question the patient about recent ingestion of pork products and the methods used to store and cook them.

• Reduce fever with alcohol rubs, tepid baths, cooling blankets, or antipyretics; relieve muscular pain with analgesics, enforced bed rest, and proper body alignment.

• Avoid touching painful muscle areas when giving patient care.

• To prevent decubitus ulcers, frequently reposition the patient, and gently massage bony prominences.

• Tell the patient that possible side effects of thiabendazole are nausea, vomiting, dizziness, dermatitis, and fever.

• Explain the importance of bed rest. Sudden death from cardiac involvement may occur in a patient with moderate to severe infection who has resumed activity too soon. Warn the patient to continue bed rest into the convalescent stage to avoid a serious relapse and possible death.

To help prevent trichinosis:

• Educate the public about proper cooking and storing methods not only for pork and pork products, but also for meat from carnivores. To kill trichinae, internal meat temperatures should reach 131° F. (55° C.) unless the meat has been cured or frozen.

• Warn travelers to foreign countries or to very poor areas in the United States to avoid eating pork; swine in these areas are often fed raw garbage.

• Report all cases of trichinosis to local public health authorities.

Hookworm Disease

(Uncinariasis)

Hookworm disease is an infection of the upper intestine caused by Ancylostoma duodenale *(found in the eastern hemisphere) or* Necator americanus *(in the western hemisphere). Sandy soil, high humidity, a warm climate, and failure to wear shoes all favor its transmission. In the United States, hookworm disease is most common in the southeast. Although this disease can cause cardiopulmonary complications, it's rarely fatal, except in debilitated persons or infants under age 1.*

Causes

Both forms of hookworm disease are transmitted to humans through direct skin penetration (usually in the foot) by hookworm larvae in soil contaminated with feces containing hookworm ova. These ova develop into infectious larvae in 1 to 3 days. Larvae travel through the lymphatics to the pulmonary capillaries, where they penetrate alveoli and move up the bronchial tree to the trachea and epiglottis. There they are swallowed and enter the gastrointestinal tract. When they reach the small intestine, they mature, attach to the jejunal mucosa, and suck blood, oxygen, and glucose from the intestinal wall. These mature worms then deposit ova, which are excreted in the stool, starting the cycle anew. Hookworm larvae mature in approximately 5 to 6 weeks.

Signs and symptoms

Most cases of hookworm disease produce few symptoms and may be overlooked until worms are passed in the stool. The earliest signs and symptoms include irritation, pruritus, and edema at the site of entry, which are sometimes accompanied by secondary bacterial infection with pustule formation.

When the larvae reach the lungs, they may cause pneumonitis and hemorrhage with fever, sore throat, rales, and cough. Finally, intestinal infection may cause fatigue, nausea, weight loss, dizziness, melena, and uncontrolled diarrhea.

In severe and chronic infection, anemia from blood loss may lead to cardiomegaly (a result of increased oxygen demands), heart failure, and generalized massive edema.

Diagnosis

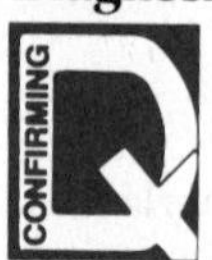

Identification of hookworm ova in the stool confirms the diagnosis. Anemia suggests severe chronic infection. In infected patients, blood studies show:

- hemoglobin 5 to 9 g (in severe case)
- leukocyte count as high as 47,000/mm³
- eosinophil count of 500 to 700/mm³.

Treatment

Treatment for hookworm infection includes administering mebendazole or pyrantel and providing an iron-rich diet or iron supplements to prevent or correct anemia.

Special considerations

- Obtain a complete history, with special attention to travel or residency in endemic areas. Note the sequence and onset of symptoms. Interview the family and other close contacts to see if they too have any symptoms.
- Carefully assess the patient, noting signs of entry, lymphedema, and respiratory status.

If the patient has confirmed hookworm infestation:

- Segregate the incontinent patient.
- Wash your hands thoroughly after every patient contact.
- For severe anemia, administer oxygen, if ordered, at low to moderate flow. Be sure the oxygen is humidified, because the patient may already have upper airway irritation from the parasites. Encourage coughing and deep breathing to stimulate removal of blood or secretions from involved lung areas and to prevent secondary infection. Plan your care to allow frequent rest periods, since the patient may tire easily. If anemia causes immobility, reposition the patient often to prevent skin breakdown.
- Closely monitor intake and output. Note quantity and frequency of diarrheal stools. Dispose of feces promptly, and wear gloves when doing so.
- To help assess nutritional status, weigh the patient daily. To combat malnutrition, emphasize the importance of good nutrition, with particular attention to foods high in iron and protein. If the patient receives iron supplements, explain that they will darken stools. Administer anthelmintics on an empty stomach, but without a purgative.
- To help prevent reinfection, educate the patient in proper handwashing technique and sanitary disposal of feces. Tell him to wear shoes in endemic areas.

Ascariasis

(Roundworm infection)

Ascariasis, an infection caused by Ascaris lumbricoides, *occurs worldwide but is most common in tropical areas with poor sanitation and in the Orient, where farmers use human feces as fertilizer. In the United States, it's more prevalent in the south, particularly among 4- to 12-year-olds.*

Causes and incidence

A. lumbricoides is a large roundworm resembling an earthworm. It's transmitted to humans by ingestion of soil contaminated with human feces that harbor *A. lumbricoides* ova. Such ingestion may occur directly (by eating contaminated soil) or indirectly (by eating poorly-washed raw vegetables grown in contaminated soil). Ascariasis never passes directly from person to person. After ingestion, *A. lumbricoides* ova hatch and release larvae, which penetrate the intestinal wall and reach the lungs through the bloodstream. After about 10 days in pulmonary capillaries and alveoli, the larvae migrate to the bronchioles, bronchi, trachea, and epiglottis. There they are swallowed and return to the intestine to mature into worms.

Signs and symptoms

Ascariasis produces two phases: early pulmonary and prolonged intestinal. Mild intestinal infection may cause only vague stomach discomfort. The first clue may be vomiting a worm or passing a worm in the stool. Severe infection, however, effects stomach pain, vomiting, restlessness, disturbed sleep, and, in extreme cases, intestinal obstruction. Larvae migrating by the lymphatic and the circulatory systems cause symptoms that vary; for instance, when they invade the lungs, pneumonitis may result.

Diagnosis

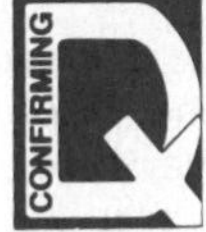

The key to diagnosis is identifying ova in the stool or adult worms, which may be passed rectally or by mouth. When migrating larvae invade alveoli, other conclusive tests include X-rays that show characteristic bronchovascular markings: infiltrates, patchy areas of pneumonitis, and widening of hilar shadows. In a patient with ascariasis, these findings usually accompany a complete blood count that shows eosinophilia.

Treatment

Anti-ascaris drug therapy, the primary treatment, uses pyrantel or piperazine to temporarily paralyze the worms, permitting peristalsis to expel them. Mebendazole is also used to block helminth nutrition. These drugs are up to 95% effective, even after a single dose. In multiple helminth infection, one of these drugs must be the first treatment; using some other anthelmintic first may stimulate *A. lumbricoides* perforation into other organs. No specific treatment exists for migratory infection, since anthelmintics affect only mature worms.

In intestinal obstruction, nasogastric suctioning controls vomiting. When suctioning can be discontinued, instill piperazine and clamp the tube. If vomiting does not occur, give a second dose of piperazine orally 24 hours later, as ordered. If this is ineffective, treatment probably requires surgery.

Special considerations

- Although isolation is unnecessary, properly dispose of feces and soiled linen, and carefully wash your hands after patient contact.
- If the patient is receiving nasogastric suction, be sure to give him good mouth care.
- Teach the patient to prevent reinfection by washing hands thoroughly, especially before eating and after

defecation, and by bathing and changing underwear and bed linens daily.

- Inform the patient of drug side effects. Tell him piperazine may cause stomach upset, dizziness, and urticaria. Remember, piperazine is contraindicated in convulsive disorders. Pyrantel produces red stools and vomit and may cause stomach upset, headache, dizziness, and skin rash; and mebendazole, abdominal pain and diarrhea.

Taeniasis

(Tapeworm disease, cestodiasis)

Taeniasis is a parasitic infestation by Taenia saginata *(beef tapeworm),* Taenia solium *(pork tapeworm),* Diphyllobothrium latum *(fish tapeworm), or* Hymenolepis nana *(dwarf tapeworm). Taeniasis is usually a chronic, benign intestinal disease; however, infestation with* T. solium *may cause dangerous systemic and CNS symptoms if larvae invade the brain and striated muscle of vital organs.*

Causes

T. saginata, T. solium, and *D. latum* are transmitted to humans by ingestion of beef, pork, or fish that contains tapeworm cysts. Gastric acids break down these cysts in the stomach, liberating them to mature. Mature tapeworms fasten to the intestinal wall and produce ova that are passed in the feces. Transmission of *H. nana* is direct from person to person and requires no intermediate host; it completes its life cycle in the intestine.

Diagnosis

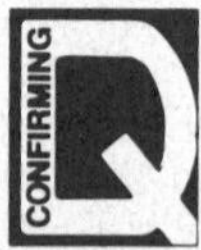

Diagnosis of tapeworm infestations requires laboratory observation of tapeworm ova or body segments in feces. Since ova aren't excreted continuously, confirmation may require multiple specimens. A supporting dietary or travel history aids confirmation.

Treatment

Treatment with niclosamide offers a cure in up to 95% of patients. In beef, pork, and fish tapeworm infestation, the drug is given once; in severe dwarf tapeworm infestation, twice (5 to 7 days each spaced 2 weeks apart).

In beef tapeworm disease, absence of strobilae (multiple tapeworm segments) in feces within 2 to 3 hours after such treatment necessitates administration of a laxative. During treatment for pork tapeworm, a laxative or induced vomiting is contraindicated because of the danger of autoinfection and systemic disease. After drug treatment, all types of tapeworm infestation require follow-up stool specimens during the next 3 to 5 weeks to check for remaining ova or worm segments. Persistent infestation often requires a second course of medication.

Special considerations

- Obtain a complete history, including recent travel to endemic areas, dietary habits, and physical symptoms.
- Dispose of the patient's excretions carefully. Wear gloves when giving personal care and handling fecal excretions, bedpans, and bed linens; wash your hands thoroughly and instruct the patient to do the same.
- Tell the patient not to consume anything after midnight on the day niclosamide therapy is to start, as the drug must be given on an empty stomach. After administering the drug, document passage of strobilae.
- In pork tapeworm infestation, use enteric and secretion precautions. Avoid procedures and drugs that may cause vomiting or gagging. If the patient is a child or is incontinent, he requires a pri-

COMMON TAPEWORM INFESTATION

TYPE	SOURCE OF INFECTION	INCIDENCE	CLINICAL FEATURES
Taenia saginata (beef tapeworm)	Uncooked or undercooked infected beef	Worldwide but prevalent in Europe and East Africa	Crawling sensation in the perianal area caused by worm segments that have been passed rectally; intestinal obstruction and appendicitis due to long worm segments that have twisted in the intestinal lumen
Taenia solium (pork tapeworm)	Uncooked or undercooked infected pork	Highest in Mexico, Latin America; lowest among Muslims and Jews	Seizures, headaches, personality changes; often overlooked in adults
Diphyllobothrium latum (fish tapeworm)	Uncooked or undercooked infected freshwater fish, such as pike, trout, salmon, and turbot	Finland, northern U.S.S.R., Japan, Alaska, Australia, the Great Lakes region (U.S.), Switzerland, Chile, and Argentina	Anemia (hemoglobin as low as 6 to 8 g)
Hymenolepis nana (dwarf tapeworm)	No intermediate host; parasite passes directly from person to person via ova passed in stool; inadequate handwashing facilitates its spread	Most common tapeworm in humans; particularly prevalent among institutionalized mentally retarded children and in underdeveloped countries	Dependent on patient's nutritional status and number of parasites; often no symptoms with mild infestation; with severe infestation, anorexia, diarrhea, restlessness, dizziness, and apathy

vate room. Obtain a list of contacts.

• Document level of consciousness, and report any changes immediately. If CNS symptoms appear, keep an artificial airway or padded tongue blade close at hand, raise side rails, keep the bed low, and help with walking, as needed.

• To prevent reinfection, teach proper handwashing technique and the need to cook meat and fish thoroughly. Stress the need for follow-up evaluations to monitor the success of therapy and to detect possible reinfection.

Enterobiasis

(Pinworm, seatworm, or threadworm infection, oxyuriasis)

Enterobiasis is a benign intestinal disease caused by the nematode Enterobius vermicularis. *Found worldwide, it's common even in temperate regions with good sanitation. It's the most prevalent helminthic infection in the United States.*

Causes

Adult pinworms live in the intestine; female worms migrate to the perianal region to deposit their ova. *Direct transmission* occurs when the patient's hands transfer infective eggs from the anus to the mouth. *Indirect transmission* occurs when he comes in contact with contaminated articles, such as linens and clothing. Enterobiasis infection and reinfection occurs most often in children between ages 5 and 14 and in certain institutionalized groups because of poor hygiene and frequent hand-to-mouth activity. Crowded living conditions often enhance its spread to several members of a family.

Signs and symptoms

Asymptomatic enterobiasis is often overlooked. However, intense perianal pruritus may occur, especially at night, when the female worm crawls out of the anus to deposit ova. Pruritus disturbs sleep and causes irritability, scratching, skin irritation, and sometimes, vaginitis. Rarely, complications include appendicitis, salpingitis, and pelvic granuloma.

Diagnosis

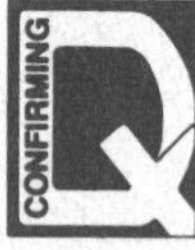

A history of pruritus ani suggests enterobiasis; identification of *Enterobius* ova recovered from the perianal area with a cellophane tape swab confirms it. In this test, cellophane tape is placed sticky side out on the base end of a test tube, and the tube is rolled around the perianal region. The tape is then examined under a microscope. This test should be done before the patient bathes and defecates in the morning. A stool sample is generally ova- and worm-free, because these worms deposit the ova outside the intestine and die after migration to the anus.

Treatment

Drug therapy with pyrantel, piperazine, or mebendazole destroys these parasites. Effective eradication requires simultaneous treatment of family members and, in institutions, other patients.

Special considerations

- If the patient receives pyrantel, tell him and his family that this drug colors the stool bright red and may cause vomiting (vomitus will also be red). The tablet form of this drug is coated with aspirin and shouldn't be given to aspirin-sensitive patients.
- Before giving piperazine, obtain a history of convulsive disorders. Piperazine may aggravate these disorders and is contraindicated in a patient with such a history.
- To help prevent this disease, tell parents to bathe children daily (showers are preferable to tub baths) and to change underwear and bed linens daily. Educate children in proper personal hygiene, and stress the need for handwashing after defecation and before handling food. Discourage nail biting. If the child can't stop, suggest that he wear gloves until the infection clears.
- Report *all* outbreaks of enterobiasis to school authorities.

Schistosomiasis

(Bilharziasis)

Schistosomiasis is a slowly progressive disease caused by blood flukes of the class Trematoda. These parasites are of three major types: Schistosoma mansoni *and* S. japonicum *infect the intestinal tract;* S. haematobium *infects the urinary tract. The degree of infection determines the intensity of illness. Complications—such as portal hypertension, pulmonary hypertension, heart failure, ascites, hematemesis from ruptured esophageal varices, and renal failure—can be fatal.*

Causes

The mode of transmission is bathing, swimming, wading, or working in water contaminated with *Schistosoma* larvae, known (while infective) as cercariae. These cercariae penetrate the skin or mucous membranes and eventually work their way to the liver's venous portal circulation. There, they mature in 1 to 3 months. The adults then migrate to other parts of the body.

The female cercariae lay spiny eggs in blood vessels surrounding the large intestine or bladder. After penetrating the mucosa of these organs, the eggs are excreted in feces or urine. If the eggs hatch in fresh water, the first-stage larvae (miracidia) penetrate freshwater snails, which act as passive intermediate hosts. Cercariae produced in snails escape into water and begin a new life cycle.

Signs and symptoms

Signs and symptoms of schistosomiasis depend on the site of infection and the stage of the disease. Initially, a transient, pruritic rash develops at the site of cercariae penetration, along with fever, myalgia, and cough. Worm migration and egg deposition may cause such complications as flaccid paralysis, seizures, and skin abscesses.

Diagnosis

Typical symptoms and a history of travel to endemic areas suggest the diagnosis; ova in the urine or stool or a mucosal lesion biopsy confirms it. WBC count shows eosinophilia.

TYPES OF SCHISTOSOMES

SPECIES AND INCIDENCE	SIGNS AND SYMPTOMS	TREATMENT	SIDE EFFECTS
S. mansoni Western hemisphere, particularly Puerto Rico, Lesser Antilles, Brazil, and Venezuela; also Nile delta, Sudan, and central Africa	Irregular fever, malaise, weakness, abdominal distress, weight loss, diarrhea, ascites, hepatosplenomegaly, portal hypertension, fistulas, intestinal stricture	Niridazole P.O. (available from Center for Disease Control); antimony sodium dimercapto succinate I.M. once a week for 5 weeks	Vomiting, abdominal pain, anorexia, weakness, diarrhea, headache, lassitude, myalgia
S. japonicum Affects men more than women; particularly prevalent among farmers in Japan, China, and the Philippines	Irregular fever, malaise, weakness, abdominal distress, weight loss, diarrhea, ascites, hepatosplenomegaly, portal hypertension, fistulas, intestinal stricture	Antimony potassium tartrate by slow I.V.; usually for 15 doses	Thrombocytopenia, hypotension, syncope, bradycardia, EKG changes, nausea, vomiting, diarrhea, colic, hepatic necrosis, dyspnea, severe arthralgia, albuminuria, fever, dermatitis
S. haematobium Africa, Cyprus, Greece, India	Terminal hematuria, dysuria, ureteral colic; with secondary infection—colicky pain, intermittent flank pain, vague GI complaints, total renal failure	Metrifonate P.O.; niridazole P.O. (available from Center for Disease Control)	Nausea, vomiting, diarrhea, anorexia, dizziness, headache, abdominal pain, insomnia, cardiac arrhythmia, anxiety, confusion, hallucinations, convulsions

SCHISTOSOMAL DERMATITIS

This form of dermatitis, also known as swimmer's itch or clam digger's itch, affects those who bathe in and camp along freshwater lakes in the eastern and western United States. It's caused by a schistosomal cercariae that is harbored by migratory birds and can penetrate the skin, causing a pruritic papular rash. Initially mild, the reaction grows more severe with repeated exposure. Treatment consists of 5% copper sulfate solution as an antipruritic and 2% methylene blue as an antibacterial agent.

Treatment

The treatment of choice is the anthelmintic drug praziquantel. Three to six months after treatment, the patient will need to be examined again. If this checkup detects any living eggs, treatment may be resumed.

Special considerations

To help prevent schistosomiasis, teach those in endemic areas to work for a pure water supply and to avoid contaminated water. If they must enter this water, tell them to wear protective clothing and to dry themselves afterward.

Strongyloidiasis

(Threadworm infection)

Strongyloidiasis is a parasitic intestinal infection caused by the helminth Strongyloides stercoralis. *Occurring worldwide, this infection is endemic in the tropics and subtropics. Susceptibility to strongyloidiasis is universal; infection doesn't confer immunity. Since the reproduction cycle of the threadworm may continue in the untreated host for as long as 45 years after the initial infection, autoinfection is highly probable. Most patients with strongyloidiasis recover completely, but debilitation from protein loss is occasionally fatal.*

Causes

Transmission to humans usually occurs through contact with soil that contains infective *S. stercoralis* filariform larvae; such larvae develop from noninfective rhabdoid (rod-shaped) larvae in human feces. The filariform larvae penetrate the human skin, usually at the feet, then migrate by way of the lymphatic system to the bloodstream and the lungs.

Once they enter into pulmonary circulation, the filariform larvae break through the alveoli and migrate upward to the pharynx, where they are swallowed. Then, they lodge in the small intestine, where they deposit eggs that mature into noninfectious rhabdoid larvae. Next, these larvae migrate into the large intestine and are excreted in feces, starting the cycle again. The threadworm life cycle—which begins with penetration of the skin and ends with excretion of rhabdoid larvae—takes 17 days.

In autoinfection, rhabdoid larvae mature within the intestine to become infective filariform larvae.

Signs and symptoms

The patient's resistance and the extent of infection determine the severity of symptoms. Some patients have no symptoms, but many develop an erythematous maculopapular rash at the site of penetration that produces swelling and pruritus and that may be confused with an insect bite. As the larvae migrate to the lungs, pulmonary signs develop, including minor hemorrhage, pneumonitis, and pneumonia; later, intestinal infection produces frequent, watery, and bloody diarrhea, accompanied by intermittent abdominal pain. Severe infection can cause malnutrition from substantial fat and protein loss, anemia, and lesions resembling ulcerative colitis, all of which invite secondary bacterial infection. Ulcerated intestinal mucosa may lead to perforation and, possibly, potentially fatal dissemination, especially in patients with malignancy or immunodeficiency diseases or in those who receive immunosuppressives.

Diagnosis

Diagnosis requires observation of *S. stercoralis* larvae in a fresh stool specimen (2 hours after excretion, rhabdoid larvae look like hookworm larvae). During the pulmonary phase, sputum may show many eosinophils and larvae; marked eosinophilia also occurs in disseminated strongyloidiasis.

Other helpful tests include:
- *chest X-ray* (positive during pulmonary phase of infection)
- *hemoglobin* (as low as 6 to 10 g)
- *WBC with differential* (eosinophils 450 to 700/mm^3).

Treatment

Because of potential autoinfection, treatment with thiabendazole is required for 2 to 3 days (total dose not to exceed 3 g). Patients also need protein replacement, blood transfusions, and I.V. fluids. Retreatment is necessary if *S. stercoralis* remains in stools after therapy. Glucocorticoids are contraindicated because they increase the risk of autoinfection and dissemination.

Special considerations

- Keep accurate intake and output records, especially if treatment includes blood transfusions and I.V. fluids. Ask the dietary department to provide a high-protein diet. The patient may need tube feedings to increase caloric intake.
- Wear gloves when handling bedpans or giving perineal care, and dispose of feces promptly.
- Since direct person-to-person transmission doesn't occur, isolation is not required. Label stool specimens for laboratory as contaminated.
- Warn the patient that thiabendazole may cause mild nausea, vomiting, drowsiness, and giddiness.
- In pulmonary infection, reposition the patient frequently, encourage coughing and deep breathing, and administer oxygen, as ordered.
- To prevent reinfection, teach the patient proper handwashing technique. Stress the importance of washing hands before eating and after defecating, and of wearing shoes when in endemic areas. Check the patient's family and close contacts for signs of infection. Emphasize the need for follow-up stool examination, continuing several weeks after treatment.

MISCELLANEOUS INFECTIONS

Ornithosis

(Psittacosis, parrot fever)

Ornithosis is caused by the gram-negative intracellular parasite Chlamydia psittaci *and is transmitted by infected birds. This disease occurs worldwide and is mainly associated with occupational exposure to birds (such as poultry farming). Incidence is higher in women and in persons aged 20 to 50 years. With adequate antimicrobial therapy, ornithosis is fatal in less than 4% of patients.*

Causes

Psittacine birds (parrots, parakeets, cockatoos), pigeons, and turkeys may harbor *C. psittaci* in their blood, feathers, tissues, nasal secretions, liver, spleen, and feces. Transmission to humans occurs primarily through inhalation of dust containing *C. psittaci* from bird droppings; less often, through direct contact with infected secretions or body tissues, as in laboratory personnel who work with birds. Rarely, person-to-person transmission occurs, usually causing severe ornithosis.

Signs and symptoms

After an incubation period of 4 to 15 days, onset of symptoms may be insidious or sudden. Clinical effects include chills and a low-grade fever that increases to 103° to 105° F. (39.4° to 40.6° C.) for 7 to 10 days, then, with treatment, declines during the second or third week. Other signs include headache, myalgia, sore throat, cough (may be dry, hacking, and nonproductive, or may produce blood-tinged sputum), abdominal distention and tenderness, nausea, vomiting, photophobia, decreased pulse rate, slightly increased respirations, secondary purulent lung infection, and a faint macular rash. Severe infection also produces delirium, stupor, and, in extensive pulmonary infiltration, cyanosis. Ornithosis may recur, but is usually milder.

Diagnosis

These symptoms and a recent history of exposure to birds suggest ornithosis.

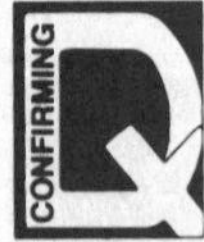

Firm diagnosis requires recovery of *C. psittaci* from mice, eggs, or tissue culture inoculated with the patient's blood or sputum. Comparison of acute and convalescent serum shows a fourfold rise in *Chlamydia* antibody titers. In addition, a patchy lobar infiltrate appears on chest X-rays during the first week of illness.

Treatment

Ornithosis calls for treatment with tetracycline. If the infection is severe, tetracycline may be given I.V. until the fever subsides. Fever and other symptoms should begin to subside 48 to 72 hours after antibiotic treatment begins; but treatment must continue for 2 weeks after temperature returns to normal. If the patient can't tolerate tetracycline, penicillin G procaine or chloramphenicol is an alternative.

Special considerations

- Monitor fluid and electrolyte balance. Give I.V. fluids, as needed.
- Carefully monitor vital signs. Watch for signs of overwhelming infection.
- Reduce fever with tepid alcohol or sponge baths and a cooling blanket.
- Reposition the patient often.
- Observe secretion precautions. During the acute, febrile stage, if the patient has a cough, wear a face mask and wash your hands carefully. Instruct him to use tissues when he coughs and to dispose of them in a closed plastic bag.
- To prevent ornithosis, those who raise birds for sale should feed them tetracycline-treated birdseed and follow regulations on bird importation. They should segregate infected or possibly infected birds from healthy birds, and disinfect structures that housed infected ones.
- Report all cases of ornithosis.

Toxic Shock Syndrome

Toxic shock syndrome (TSS) is an acute bacterial infection caused by penicillin-resistant Staphylococcus aureus, *generally in association with continuous use of tampons during the menstrual period. It usually affects menstruating women under age 30. (Of the reported cases, 96% involve women, and 92% of these cases begin during menstruation.) A strong correlation exists between TSS and use of super-absorbent tampons. Incidence is rising, and the recurrence rate is about 30%.*

Causes

Although tampons are clearly implicated in TSS, their exact role is uncertain. Theoretically, tampons may contribute to development of TSS by:
- introducing *S. aureus* into the vagina during insertion.
- absorbing toxin from the vagina.
- traumatizing the vaginal mucosa during insertion, thus leading to infection.
- providing a favorable environment for the growth of *S. aureus*.

When TSS isn't related to menstruation, it seems to be linked to *S. aureus* infections, such as abscesses, osteomyelitis, and postsurgical infections.

Signs and symptoms

Typically, TSS produces intense myalgias, fever over 104° F. (40° C.), vomiting, diarrhea, headache, decreased level of consciousness, rigors, conjunctival hyperemia, and vaginal hyperemia and discharge. Severe hypotension occurs with hypovolemic shock. Within a few hours of onset, a deep red rash develops—especially on the palms and soles—and later desquamates.

Major complications include persistent neuropsychological abnormalities, mild renal failure, rash, and cyanotic arms and legs.

Diagnosis

Diagnosis will be based on clinical findings and the presence of at least three of the following:
- gastrointestinal effects, including vomiting and profuse diarrhea
- muscular effects, with severe myalgias or a fivefold or greater increase in creatine phosphokinase
- mucous membrane effects, such as frank hyperemia
- renal involvement with elevated BUN or creatinine levels (at least twice the normal levels)
- liver involvement with elevated bilirubin, SGOT, or SGPT levels (at least twice the normal levels)
- blood involvement with signs of thrombocytopenia and a platelet count of less than 100,000/mm^3
- central nervous system effects, such as disorientation without focal signs.

In addition, isolation of *S. aureus* from vaginal discharge or lesions helps support the diagnosis. Negative results on blood tests for Rocky Mountain spotted fever, leptospirosis, and measles help rule out these disorders.

Treatment

Treatment consists of I.V. antistaphylococcal antibiotics that are beta-lactamase–resistant, such as oxacillin, nafcillin, and methicillin. To reverse shock, expect to replace fluids with saline solution and colloids, as ordered.

Special considerations

- Monitor the patient's vital signs frequently.
- Administer antibiotics slowly and strictly on time. Be sure to watch for signs of penicillin allergy.
- Check the patient's fluid and electrolyte balance.
- Obtain specimens of vaginal and cervical secretions for culture of *S. aureus*.
- Tell the patient to avoid tampons.
- Take secretion precautions for all vaginal and lesion drainage.

Selected References

Christensen, Mary L. *Microbiology for Nursing and Allied Health Students*. Springfield, Ill.: Charles C. Thomas, 1982.

Larson, Elaine. *Clinical Microbiology and Infection Control*. Boston: Blackwell Scientific Publications, 1984.

Mandell, G., et al, eds. *Principles and Practice of Infectious Diseases*. New York: John Wiley & Sons, 1979.

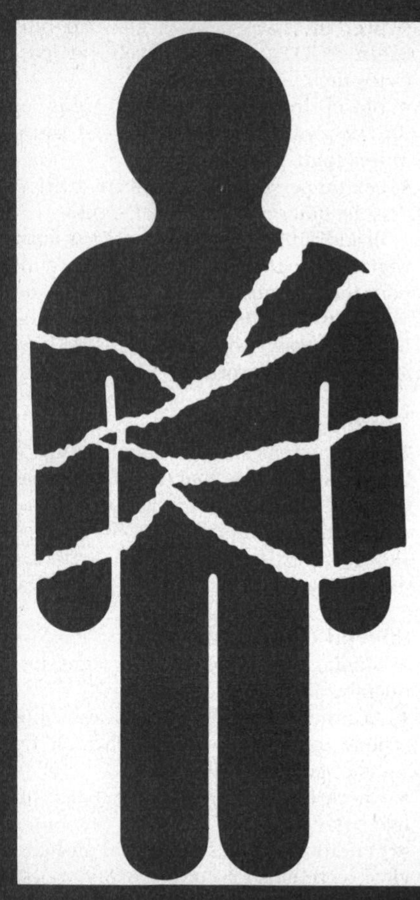

4 Trauma

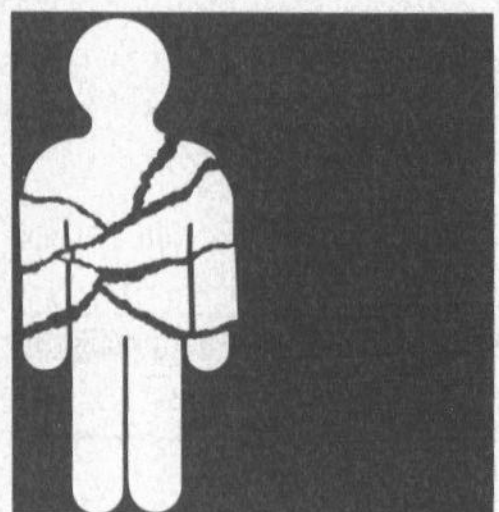

Trauma

Introduction

Trauma is the third leading cause of death in the United States, outranked only by cardiovascular disease and cancer. In people under age 35, it's *the* leading cause of death. Trauma care basics include triage; assessing and maintaining airway, breathing, and circulation (the ABCs); protecting the cervical spine; assessing the level of consciousness; and, as necessary, preparing the patient for transport and possibly surgery.

Three types of trauma exist: blunt trauma, which leaves the body surface intact; penetrating trauma, which disrupts the body surface; and perforating trauma, which leaves entrance and exit wounds as an object passes through the body.

Triage: First things first

Basically, triage is the setting of medical priorities for emergency care by making sound, rapid assessments. The need for triage often arises at the scene of injury and continues in the emergency department. Following hospital protocol, you'll decide which patient to treat first, which injury to treat first, how to best utilize other members of the medical team, and how to control patient and staff traffic.

Generally, victims are assigned to the following categories:

1. Emergent—Life-threatening injury requiring treatment within a few minutes to prevent death or further injury. This includes patients with respiratory distress or cardiopulmonary arrest, and severe hemorrhage or shock.

2. Urgent—Serious but not immediately life-threatening injury that should receive treatment within 1 hour; for example, stable head, chest, or abdominal injuries and long bone fractures.

3. Delayed—Minor injuries, such as lacerations or abrasions, that can wait 4 to 6 hours for treatment.

4. Indefinite—Treatment can wait indefinitely; patient can be referred to a clinic. In disaster or military situations, this applies to patients with massive injuries who have marginal chance for recovery even with immediate, vigorous care.

5. Deceased.

Trauma care generates a great deal of stress, and much of it falls on your shoulders. Often, you must deal with patients and families who are emotionally upset, angry, belligerent, intoxicated, or frightened; some may speak only a foreign language. Therefore, you must work calmly and rationally and must avoid becoming easily upset or angered. You can help the patient a great deal by talking to him while giving him care. Be sure to tell him what you're going to do before you touch him. You must also handle difficult situations diplomatically and intelligently, recognize your limitations, and ask for help when you need it.

Begin with the ABCs

Always begin your care of an injured patient with a brief assessment of the ABCs: airway, breathing, and circulation. Obtain a brief history from the patient, family, or friends.

To assess airway patency, routinely check for respiratory distress or signs of obstruction, such as stridor, choking, or cyanosis. Be especially alert for respiratory distress in a patient who inhaled chemicals, was in a fire, or has upper body burns. If the airway's obstructed, remove vomitus, dentures, blood clots, or foreign bodies from the patient's mouth.

To open the airway, use a jaw thrust maneuver. (*Don't* use the head-tilt maneuver for a trauma patient. Suspect cervical spine injury until X-rays rule it out.) Then, insert an oropharyngeal or nasopharyngeal airway. As necessary, assist with the insertion of an endotracheal tube. If rescue personnel have inserted an esophageal obturator airway, leave it in place until the patient has been tracheally intubated. This will prevent him from vomiting and possibly aspirating.

Next, make sure the patient's breathing is adequate. Look, listen, and feel for respirations. If the patient isn't breathing, call for help immediately and begin mouth-to-mouth or bag/valve/mask respiration. Give supplemental oxygen.

To assess circulation, check for carotid and peripheral pulses. If a carotid pulse is absent, apply external cardiac massage. If external hemorrhage is evident, apply direct pressure to the bleeding site, and if the wound is on an extremity, elevate it above heart level, if possible. Apply a tourniquet only if hemorrhage is life-threatening.

Immobilize the patient's head and neck with an immobilization device, sandbags, backboard, and tape, if this hasn't been done. Obtain cervical spine X-rays and rule out cervical spine injury before moving the patient again.

Assess vital signs

Monitor vital signs even if the patient appears stable. Because vital signs may change rapidly, taking them serially can point out subtle and overt changes. Document baseline readings, and obtain new readings every 5 to 15 minutes, until the patient is stable. Place him on a cardiac monitor.

Your assessment should also include level of consciousness, and pupillary and motor response to assess neurologic status. Determine and report level of consciousness by using a stimulus-response method of reporting, rather than categorizing; don't use words like "semiconscious" or "stuporous." Report decorticate or decerebrate responses immediately. The patient need not have a head injury to show abnormal neuro-

MANAGING TETANUS PROPHYLAXIS

HISTORY OF TETANUS IMMUNIZATION (number of doses)	TETANUS-PRONE WOUNDS		NON-TETANUS-PRONE WOUNDS	
	Td*	TIG**	Td	TIG
Uncertain	Yes	Yes	Yes	No
0 to 1	Yes	Yes	Yes	No
2	Yes	No (*yes* if 24 hours since wound was inflicted)	Yes	No
3 or more	No (*yes* if more than 5 years since last dose)	No	No (*yes* if more than 10 years since last dose)	No

*Td = Tetanus and diphtheria toxoids adsorbed (for adult use), 0.5 ml
**TIG = Tetanus immune globulin (human), 250 units

When Td and TIG are given concurrently, separate syringes and separate sites should be used.

NOTE: For children under age 7, tetanus and diphtheria toxoids and pertussis vaccine adsorbed (DPT) are preferred to tetanus toxoid alone. If pertussis vaccine is contraindicated, administer tetanus and diphtheria toxoids adsorbed (DT).

Adapted from American College of Surgeons, Committee on Trauma, *Prophylaxis against Tetanus in Wound Management*, April 1984.

logic response. Any injury that impairs ventilation or perfusion can cause cerebral edema and can raise intracranial pressure. If the patient has neurologic symptoms and is *hypotensive*, look for an extracranial cause, since intracranial bleeding is usually not the cause of hypotension.

Give the patient oxygen. Then draw samples for arterial blood gas measurement and calculate the effects of the supplemental oxygen, to establish a baseline for oxygen and acid-base therapy. Multiple injuries always create a need for supplementary oxygen because of blood loss and overwhelming physiologic stress. Actually, the conscious multiple-injury patient should show compensatory hyperventilation. If he doesn't, expect neurologic involvement or chest injury.

Draw blood for type and cross match, complete blood count, prothrombin time, partial thromboplastin time, platelets, and routine blood studies, including amylase. Begin at least two I.V. lines with 14G or 16G catheters for fluid resuscitation with normal saline or Ringer's lactate solution. As ordered, administer tetanus prophylaxis. (See *Managing Tetanus Prophylaxis.*)

Quickly and carefully look for multiple injuries by systematically examining the patient. If no spine injury exists, carefully roll the patient over to examine his back for other wounds.

In chest trauma, assess for open wounds, tension pneumothorax, hemothorax, cardiac tamponade, bruises and hematomas, flail chest, and fractured larynx. Cover open wounds and, as necessary, apply direct pressure to the wound. Be ready to assist with insertion of chest tubes, needle thoracotomy, pericardiocentesis, cricothyrotomy, or tracheotomy.

As indicated, insert a Foley catheter and a nasogastric tube, give prophylactic antibiotics, obtain an order for appropriate diagnostic studies—such as peritoneal lavage or intravenous pyelography—and notify medical or surgical specialists.

Combat shock

Since severe injuries often lead to shock, check skin temperature, color, and moisture. To control shock, administer I.V. fluids (Ringer's lactate or normal saline solution) followed by blood or blood products, and use medical antishock trousers (MAST) suit, as ordered.

In all massive external bleeding or suspected internal bleeding, watch for hypovolemia and estimate blood loss. Remember, however, that a blood loss of 500 to 1,000 ml might not change systolic blood pressure, but it may elevate the pulse rate. Stay alert for signs of occult bleeding, common in the chest, abdomen, and thigh. Assess for such bleeding by taking serial girth measurements at these sites. Use a tape measure, and mark its placement on the body with a marking pen, so you measure in exactly the same place each time. This way you can accurately detect any enlargement. Increased diameter of the legs or abdomen often means leakage of blood into these tissues (as much as 4,000 ml into the abdomen, 3,000 ml into the chest, and 500 ml into a thigh). Such blood loss will induce textbook signs of hypovolemic shock (tachycardia, tachypnea, hypotension, restlessness, falling urinary output, delayed capillary refill, and cold, clammy skin).

If the patient has renal injuries or a fractured pelvis, look for the classic sign of retroperitoneal hematoma—numbness or pain in the leg on the affected side, which is the result of pressure on the lateral femoral cutaneous nerve in L1 to L3. Retroperitoneal bleeding may not cause abdominal tenderness. If the patient shows clinical signs of hypovolemia, immediately begin I.V. therapy with two or more large-bore catheters and regulate fluids according to the severity of hypovolemia. Assist with insertion of a central venous pressure or pulmonary artery catheter to monitor circulating blood volume.

Splinting for transport

Look for limb fractures and dislocations, and check circulation and neurovascular status distal to injury by palpating pulses distal to the injury and looking for the classic signs of arterial insufficiency: decreased or absent pulse, pallor, paresthesia, pain, and paralysis. Splint and apply traction, as needed.

Prepare the victim for transport. Use special care in suspected cervical spinal injury. If necessary, after splinting the injury site, also splint the areas above and below it, to prevent further soft-tissue and neurovascular damage and to minimize pain. Example: if the forearm is injured, splint wrist and elbow too.

Types of splints include:

- *soft splint*—a nonrigid splint (examples: pillow or blanket)
- *hard splint*—rigid splint with a firm surface (examples: long or short board, aluminum ladder splint, cardboard splint)
- *air splint*—inflatable splint
- *traction splint*—uses traction to decrease angulation and reduce pain (examples: Hare and Thomas splints).

Tips on applying a splint

- Splint most injuries "as they lie," except when the neurovascular status is compromised.
- Whenever possible, have one person support the injured part while another applies padding and the splint.
- Secure the splint with straps or gauze, *not* an elastic bandage.
- To apply an air splint, slide the splint backward over your arm, and grasp the distal portion of the injured limb. Then, slip the splint from your arm onto the injured extremity, and inflate the splint.

HEAD INJURIES

Concussion

By far the most common head injury, concussion results from a blow to the head—a blow hard enough to jostle the brain and make it hit against the skull, causing temporary neural dysfunction, but not hard enough to cause a cerebral contusion. Most concussion victims recover completely within 24 to 48 hours. Repeated concussions, however, exact a cumulative toll on the brain.

Causes

The blow that causes a concussion is usually sudden and forceful—a fall to the ground, a punch to the head, an automobile accident. Also, such a blow sometimes results from child abuse. Whatever the cause, the resulting injury is mild compared to the damage done by cerebral contusions or lacerations.

Signs and symptoms

Concussion may produce a short-term loss of consciousness, vomiting, and both anterograde and retrograde amnesia; the patient not only can't recall what happened immediately after the injury, but also has difficulty recalling events that led up to the traumatic incident. The presence of anterograde amnesia and the duration of retrograde amnesia reliably correlate with the severity of the injury. The injury often causes adults to behave irritably, lethargically, or simply out of character, and usually brings complaints of dizziness, nausea, or severe headache. Some children have no apparent ill effects, but many grow lethargic and somnolent in a few hours. All these signs occur normally with a concussion, and don't necessarily indicate a serious injury. Postconcussion syndrome—headache, dizziness, vertigo, anxiety, fatigue—may persist for several weeks after the injury.

Diagnosis

Differentiating between concussion and more serious head injuries requires a

PATIENT TEACHING AID

What to Do After Concussion

Dear Patient:

You have suffered a concussion, which does not appear to have caused any serious brain injury. For safety's sake, however, follow these instructions:

- Return to the hospital immediately if you experience a persistent or worsening headache, forceful or constant vomiting, blurred vision, any change in personality, abnormal eye movements, staggering gait, or twitching.
- Don't take anything stronger than aspirin or acetaminophen for a headache.
- If vomiting occurs, eat lightly until it stops. (*Occasional* vomiting is normal after concussion.)
- Relax for 24 hours. Then, if you feel well, resume normal activities.
- Give this note to your parents, guardian, spouse, or roommate: *Wake the patient every 2 hours during the night, and ask him his name, where he is, and whether he can identify you. If you can't awaken him, or he can't answer these questions, or if he has convulsions, bring him back to the hospital immediately.*

thorough history of the trauma and a neurologic examination. Such an examination must evaluate the level of consciousness, mental status, cranial nerve and motor functions, deep tendon and abdominal reflexes, and orientation as to time, place, and person. If no abnormalities are found, the patient has probably suffered nothing worse than a concussion but should be observed for signs of more severe cerebral trauma. Observation provides a baseline for gauging any deterioration in the patient's condition. Skull X-rays and computerized tomography scans may rule out fractures and more serious injuries.

Treatment and special considerations

- Obtain a thorough history of the trauma from the patient (if he's not suffering from amnesia), his family, eyewitnesses, or ambulance personnel. Ask whether the patient lost consciousness and, if so, for how long.
- Monitor vital signs, and check for additional injuries. Palpate the skull for tenderness or hematomas.
- If the patient has an altered state of consciousness or if a neurologic examination reveals abnormalities, the injury may be more severe than a concussion; the patient should be admitted for neurologic consultation. If a neurologic examination reveals no abnormalities, observe the patient in the emergency room. Check vital signs, level of consciousness, and pupil size every 15 minutes. If his condition worsens or fluctuates, he should be admitted for neurosurgical consultation. The patient who is stable after 4 or more hours of observation can be discharged (with a head injury instruction sheet) in the care of a responsible adult.

Cerebral Contusion

Cerebral contusion is a bruising of brain tissue as a result of a severe blow to the head. More serious than a concussion, contusion disrupts normal nerve functions in the bruised area, and may cause loss of consciousness, hemorrhage, edema, and even death.

Causes

Cerebral contusion results from acceleration-deceleration or coup-contrecoup injuries. Such injuries can occur directly beneath the site of impact when the brain rebounds against the skull from the force of a blow (a beating with a blunt instrument, for example), when the force of the blow drives the brain against the opposite side of the skull, or when the head is hurled forward and stopped abruptly (as in an automobile accident when a driver's head strikes the windshield). The brain continues moving and slaps against the skull (acceleration), then rebounds (deceleration). These injuries can also cause the brain to strike against bony prominences inside the skull (especially the sphenoidal ridges), causing intracranial hemorrhage or hematoma that may result in tentorial herniation.

Signs and symptoms

With cerebral contusion, the patient may have severe scalp wounds and labored respirations. He may lose consciousness for a few minutes or for an hour. If conscious, he may be drowsy, confused, and/or disoriented, agitated, or even violent. He may display hemiparesis and decorticate or decerebrate posturing, and unequal pupillary response. Eventually, he should return to a relatively alert state, perhaps with temporary aphasia, slight hemiparesis, or unilateral numbness. A lucid period followed by rapid deterioration suggests epidural hematoma.

Diagnosis

A history of the trauma and a neurologic examination are the principal diagnostic tools. Skull X-rays rule out fractures and may help to show a shift in brain tissue. Cerebral angiography outlines vasculature, and a CT scan shows ischemic or necrotic tissue and subdural, epidural, and intracerebral hematomas. Intracranial hemorrhage contraindicates lumbar puncture.

Treatment and special considerations

- Establish a patent airway. As ordered, assist with a tracheotomy or an endotracheal intubation (for an unconscious patient with no cervical spine fracture). Perform a neurologic examination, focusing on the level of consciousness, motor responses, and intracranial pressure.
- Start I.V. fluids with 5% dextrose in .45 normal saline solution. Hypotonic fluids are not indicated; they may aggravate cerebral edema. Mannitol I.V. may be given to reduce cerebral edema. Dexamethasone I.V. or I.M. will be given for several days to control cerebral edema.
- Type and cross match blood for a patient suspected of having intracerebral hemorrhage. A blood transfusion may be needed and possibly a craniotomy, to control bleeding and to aspirate blood.
- Insert a Foley catheter, as ordered. Monitor intake and output. With unconscious patients, insert a nasogastric tube to prevent aspiration.
- Enforce absolute bed rest. Observe for cerebrospinal fluid (CSF) leaks. Check bed sheets for a blood-tinged spot surrounded by a lighter ring (halo sign). If CSF leaks develop, raise the head of the bed 30°. If you detect CSF leaks from the

HEMORRHAGE, HEMATOMA, AND TENTORIAL HERNIATION

Among the most serious consequences of a head injury are hemorrhage, hematoma, and tentorial herniation. An epidural hemorrhage or hematoma results from a rapid accumulation of blood between the skull and the dura mater; a subdural hemorrhage or hematoma, from a slow accumulation of blood between the dura mater and the subarachnoid membrane. Intracerebral hemorrhage or hematoma occurs within the cerebrum itself. Tentorial herniation occurs when injured brain tissue swells and squeezes itself through the tentorial notch, constricting the brain stem.

Epidural hemorrhage or hematoma can cause immediate loss of consciousness, followed by a lucid interval lasting minutes to hours, which eventually gives way to a rapidly progressive decrease in the level of consciousness. Other effects are contralateral hemiparesis, progressively severe headache, ipsilateral pupillary dilation, and signs of increased intracranial pressure (ICP): decreasing pulse and respirations and increasing systolic blood pressure. With a subacute or chronic subdural hemorrhage or hematoma, blood accumulates slowly so symptoms may not occur until days after the injury. In an acute subdural hematoma, symptoms appear earlier because blood accumulates within 24 hours of the injury. Loss of consciousness occurs, often with weakness or paralysis. Intracerebral hemorrhage or hematoma usually causes nuchal rigidity, photophobia, nausea, vomiting, dizziness, convulsions, decreased respiratory rate, and progressive obtundation.

Tentorial herniation causes drowsiness, confusion, dilation of one or both pupils, hyperventilation, nuchal rigidity, bradycardia, and decorticate or decerebrate posturing. Irreversible brain damage or death can occur rapidly.

Intracranial hemorrhage may require a craniotomy, to locate and control bleeding and to aspirate blood. Epidural and subdural hematomas are usually drained by aspiration through burr holes in the skull. Increased ICP may be controlled with mannitol I.V., steroids, or diuretics, but emergency surgery is usually required.

nose, place a gauze pad under the nostrils. Be sure to tell the patient not to blow his nose, but to wipe it instead. If CSF leaks from the ear, position the patient so that the ear drains naturally, and don't pack the ear or nose.

- Monitor vital signs and respirations regularly (usually every 15 minutes). Abnormal respirations could indicate a breakdown in the respiratory center in the brain stem and a possible impending tentorial herniation—a critical neurologic emergency.
- Perform frequent neurologic checks. Assess for restlessness, level of consciousness, and orientation.
- After the patient is stabilized, clean and dress any superficial scalp wounds. (If the skin has been broken, tetanus prophylaxis may be in order.) Assist with suturing, if necessary.

Skull Fractures

A skull fracture is considered a neurosurgical condition, since possible damage to the brain is the first concern, rather than the fracture itself. Skull fractures may be simple (closed) or compound (open) and may or may not displace bone fragments. Skull fractures are further described as linear, comminuted, or depressed. A linear fracture is a common hairline break, without displacement of structures; a comminuted fracture splinters or crushes the bone into several fragments; a depressed fracture pushes the bone toward the brain. Depressed fractures are of significance only if they compress underlying structures. In children, thinness and elasticity of the skull allow a depression without fracture (linear fracture across a suture line in an infant increases the possibility of epidural hematoma). Skull fractures are also classified according to location, such as a cranial vault fracture; a basilar fracture is at the base of the skull and involves the cribriform plate and the frontal sinuses. Because of the danger of grave cranial complications and meningitis, basilar fractures are usually far more serious than vault fractures.

Causes

Like concussions and cerebral contusions or lacerations, skull fractures invariably result from a traumatic blow to the head. Motor vehicle accidents, bad falls, and severe beatings (especially in children) top the list of causes.

Signs and symptoms

Skull fractures are often accompanied by scalp wounds—abrasions, contusions, lacerations, or avulsions. If the scalp has been lacerated or torn away, bleeding may be profuse, because the scalp contains many blood vessels. Bleeding is rarely heavy enough to induce hypovolemic shock, although the patient may be in shock from other injuries or from medullary failure in severe head injuries. Linear fractures associated only with concussion don't produce loss of consciousness (although the patient may appear dazed) and don't require treatment. A fracture that results in cerebral contusion or laceration, however, may cause the classic signs of brain injury: agitation and irritability, loss of consciousness, changes in respiratory pattern (labored respirations), abnormal deep tendon reflexes, and altered pupillary and motor response.

If the patient with a skull fracture remains conscious, he is apt to complain of persistent, localized headache. Skull fracture also may result in cerebral edema, which may "jam" the reticular activating system, cutting off the normal flow of impulses to the brain and resulting in possible respiratory distress. The patient may have alterations in level of consciousness or may lose consciousness for hours, days, weeks, or indefinitely. When jagged bone fragments pierce the dura mater or the cerebral cortex, skull fractures may cause subdural, epidural, or intracerebral hemorrhage or hematoma. With the resulting space-occupying lesions, clinical findings may include hemiparesis, dizziness, convulsions, projectile vomiting, decreased pulse and respirations, and progressive unresponsiveness. Sphenoidal fractures may also damage the optic nerve, causing blindness, whereas temporal fractures can cause unilateral deafness or facial paralysis. Symptoms reflect the severity and the extent of the head injury. However, some elderly patients may have brain atrophy; therefore, they have more space for brain swelling under the cranium and, as a result, may not show signs of increased intracranial pressure (ICP).

A vault fracture often produces soft-tissue swelling near the fracture, making it hard to detect without X-rays.

A basilar fracture often produces hemorrhage from the nose, pharynx, or ears; blood under the periorbital skin ("raccoon's eyes") and under the conjunctiva; and Battle's sign (supramastoid ecchymosis), sometimes with bleeding behind the eardrum. This type of fracture may also cause cerebrospinal fluid (CSF) or even brain tissue to leak from the nose or ears.

Depending on the extent of brain damage, the patient could suffer residual effects, such as convulsive disorders (epilepsy), hydrocephalus, and organic brain syndrome. Children may develop headaches, giddiness, easy fatigability, neuroses, and behavior disorders.

Diagnosis

Suspect brain injury in all skull fractures until clinical evaluation proves otherwise. Therefore, every suspected skull injury calls for a thorough history of the trauma and skull X-rays to attempt to locate the fracture (vault fractures often aren't visible or palpable).

A fracture also requires a neurologic examination, to check cerebral function (mental status and orientation to time, place, and person), level of consciousness, pupillary response, motor function, and deep tendon and abdominal reflexes. Using reagent strips, dipstick test the draining nasal or ear fluid for CSF. The tape turns blue if CSF is present; there is no change in the presence of blood alone. However, the tape will also turn blue if the patient is hyperglycemic. Also check the patient's bedsheets for the "halo sign"—a blood-tinged spot surrounded by a lighter ring—from leakage of CSF.

Brain damage can be assessed through:

- cerebral angiography, which reveals vascular disruptions from internal pressure or injury.
- computed tomography scan, echoencephalography, air encephalography, magnetic resonance imaging, and radioactive scan, which disclose intracranial hemorrhage from ruptured blood vessels (carotid arteries, venous sinuses) or cranial nerve injury, or will serve to indicate or localize subdural or intracerebral hematomas. Expanding lesions contraindicate lumbar puncture.

Treatment

Although occasionally even a simple linear skull fracture can tear an underlying blood vessel or cause a CSF leak, linear fractures generally require only supportive treatment, including mild analgesics (aspirin or acetaminophen), and cleansing and debridement of any wounds after a local injection of procaine and shaving of the scalp around the wound. If the patient hasn't lost consciousness, he should be observed in the emergency room for at least 4 to 6 hours. Following this observation period, if vital signs are stable, the patient can be discharged and should be given an instruction sheet for 24 to 48 hours of observation at home.

More severe vault fractures, especially depressed fractures, usually require a craniotomy to elevate or remove fragments that have been driven into the brain and to extract foreign bodies and necrotic tissue, thereby reducing the risk of infection and further brain damage. Cranioplasty follows the use of tantalum mesh or acrylic plates to replace the removed skull section. Antibiotic therapy and, in profound hemorrhage, blood transfusions are often required.

Basilar fractures call for immediate prophylactic antibiotics to prevent the onset of meningitis from CSF leaks, and close observation for secondary hematomas and hemorrhages. Surgery may be necessary. In addition, both basilar and vault fractures require dexamethasone I.V. or I.M. to reduce cerebral edema and minimize brain tissue damage.

Special considerations

- Establish and maintain a patent airway; intubation may be necessary. Suction through the mouth, not the nose, to prevent introduction of bacteria in case a CSF leak is present.
- Obtain a complete history of the trauma from the patient, his family, eyewitnesses, and ambulance personnel. Ask whether the patient lost consciousness and, if so, for how long. Assist with diagnostic tests, including a complete neurologic examination, skull X-rays, and other studies. Check for abnormal reflexes, such as Babinski's reflex.
- Look for CSF draining from the ears, nose, or mouth. Check pillowcases and linens for CSF leaks and look for a halo sign. If the patient's nose is draining CSF, wipe it—*don't* let him blow it. If an ear is draining, cover it lightly with sterile gauze—*don't* pack it.
- Position a patient with a head injury so secretions can drain properly. With CSF leaks, elevate the head of the bed 30°; without CSF leaks, leave the head of the bed flat, but position the patient on his side or abdomen. Remember, however, that such a patient risks jugular compression leading to increased ICP, if he's not positioned on his back, so be sure to keep his head properly aligned. Cover scalp wounds carefully with a sterile dressing; control any bleeding, as necessary.
- Take seizure precautions, but don't restrain the patient. Agitated behavior may be due to hypoxia or increased ICP, so check for these. Speak in a calm, reassuring voice, and touch the patient gently. Don't make any sudden, unexpected moves.
- Don't give narcotics or sedatives, because they may depress respirations, increase CO_2, and lead to increased ICP, as well as mask changes in neurologic status. Give aspirin or another mild analgesic for pain, as ordered.

When a skull fracture requires surgery:

- Obtain consent, as needed, to shave the patient's head. Explain that you're doing this to provide a clean area for surgery. Type and cross match blood. Obtain orders for baseline laboratory studies, such as complete blood count, electrolytes, and urinalysis.
- After surgery, monitor vital signs and neurologic status often (usually every 5 minutes until stable, and then every 15 minutes for 1 hour), and report any changes in level of consciousness. Since skull fractures and brain injuries heal slowly, don't expect dramatic postop improvement.
- Monitor intake and output frequently, and maintain Foley catheter patency. Take special care with fluid intake. Hypotonic fluids (even 5% dextrose in water) can increase cerebral edema. Their use should be restricted; give only as ordered.
- If the patient is unconscious, provide parenteral nutrition. (Remember, the patient may regurgitate and aspirate food if you use a nasogastric tube.)

If the fracture doesn't require surgery:

- Wear sterile gloves to examine the scalp laceration. With your finger, probe the wound for foreign bodies and palpable fracture. Gently cleanse lacerations and surrounding area. Cover with sterile gauze. Assist with suturing, if necessary.
- Provide emotional support for the patient and his family. Explain the need for procedures to reduce the risk of brain injury.
- Before discharge, instruct the patient's family to watch closely for changes

in mental status, level of consciousness, or respirations, and to relieve the patient's headache with aspirin or acetaminophen. Tell the patient's family to return him to the hospital immediately if level of consciousness decreases, if headache persists after several doses of mild analgesics, if he vomits more than once, or if weakness develops in arms or legs. Teach the patient and his family how to care for his scalp wound. Emphasize the need to return for suture removal and follow-up evaluation.

Fractured Nose

The most common facial fracture, a fractured nose usually results from blunt injury and is often associated with other facial fractures. The severity of the fracture depends on the direction, force, and type of the blow. Severe, comminuted fracture may cause extreme swelling or bleeding that may jeopardize the airway and require tracheotomy during early treatment. Inadequate or delayed treatment may cause permanent nasal displacement, septal deviation, and obstruction.

Signs and symptoms

Immediately after injury, nosebleed may occur (ranging from minimal trickling to full nasal hemorrhage), and soft-tissue swelling may quickly obscure the break. After several hours, pain, periorbital ecchymoses, and nasal displacement and deformity are prominent. Possible complications are septal hematoma, which may lead to abscess formation, resulting in avascular and septic necrosis.

Diagnosis

Palpation, X-rays, and clinical findings, such as a deviated septum, confirm a nasal fracture. Diagnosis also requires a full patient history, including the cause of the injury and the amount of nasal bleeding. Watch for clear fluid drainage, which may suggest a cerebrospinal fluid (CSF) leak.

Treatment

Treatment restores normal facial appearance and reestablishes bilateral nasal passage after swelling subsides. Reduction of the fracture corrects alignment; immobilization (intranasal packing and an external splint shaped to the nose and taped) maintains it. Such reduction is best accomplished in the operating room, with local anesthetic for adults and general anesthetic for children. Severe swelling may delay treatment for several days to a week. In addition, CSF leakage calls for close observation and antibiotic therapy; septal hematoma requires incision and drainage to prevent necrosis.

Special considerations

- Start treatment immediately. While waiting for X-rays, apply ice packs to the nose to minimize swelling. Wrap the ice packs in a light towel to prevent ice from directly contacting the skin. To control anterior bleeding, gently apply local pressure. Posterior bleeding is rare and requires an internal tamponade applied in the emergency department.
- Since the patient will find breathing more difficult as the swelling increases, instruct him to breathe slowly through his mouth. To warm the inhaled air during cold weather, tell him to cover his mouth with a handkerchief or scarf. To prevent subcutaneous emphysema or intracranial air penetration (and potential meningitis), warn him not to blow his nose.
- After packing and splinting, apply ice in a plastic bag.
- Before discharge, tell the patient that ecchymoses should fade after about 2 weeks.

Dislocated or Fractured Jaw

Dislocation of the jaw is a displacement of the temporomandibular joint. A fracture of the jaw is a break in one or both of the two maxillae (upper jawbones) or the mandible (lower jawbone). Treatment can usually restore jaw alignment and function.

Causes

Simple fractures or dislocations are usually caused by a manual blow along the jawline; more serious compound fractures often result from car accidents.

Signs and symptoms

Malocclusion is the most obvious sign of dislocation or fracture. Other signs include mandibular pain, swelling, ecchymosis, loss of function, and asymmetry. In addition, mandibular fractures that damage the alveolar nerve produce paresthesia or anesthesia of the chin and lower lip. Maxillary fractures produce infraorbital paresthesia and often accompany fractures of the nasal and orbital complex.

Diagnosis

Abnormal maxillary or mandibular mobility during physical examination and a history of trauma suggest fracture or dislocation; X-rays confirm it.

Treatment

As in all trauma, check first for a patent airway, adequate ventilation, and pulses; then, control hemorrhage, and check for other injuries. As necessary, maintain an airway with an oropharyngeal airway, nasotracheal intubation, or a tracheotomy. Relieve pain with analgesics, as needed. After the patient stabilizes, surgical reduction and fixation by wiring restores mandibular and maxillary alignment. Maxillary fractures may also require reconstruction and repair of soft-tissue injuries. Teeth or bone are never removed during surgery unless unavoidable. If the patient has lost teeth due to trauma, the surgeon will decide whether they can be reimplanted. If they can, he will reimplant them within 6 hours, while they're still viable. Dislocations are usually manually reduced under anesthesia.

Special considerations

After reconstructive surgery:

- Position the patient on his side, with his head slightly elevated. A nasogastric tube is usually in place, with low suction to remove gastric contents and prevent nausea, vomiting, and aspiration of vomitus. As necessary, suction the nasopharynx through the nose, or by pulling the cheek away from the teeth and inserting a small suction catheter through any natural gap between teeth.
- If the patient isn't intubated, provide nourishment through a straw. If a natural gap occurs between teeth, insert the straw there; if not, one or two teeth may have to be extracted. However, such extraction is avoided when possible. Start with clear liquids; after the patient can tolerate fluids, offer milk shakes, eggnog, broth, juices, blenderized foods, and commercial nutritional supplements.
- If the patient is unable to tolerate oral fluids, I.V. therapy can maintain hydration postoperatively.
- Administer antiemetics, as ordered, to minimize nausea and prevent aspiration of vomitus (a very real danger in a patient whose jaw is wired). Keep a pair of wire cutters at the bedside to snip the wires should the patient vomit.
- A dental water-pulsator may be used for mouth care while the wires are intact.
- Since the patient will have difficulty talking while his jaw is wired, provide a Magic Slate or pencil and paper, and suggest appropriate diversions.

Perforated Eardrum

Perforation of the eardrum is a rupture of the tympanic membrane. Such injury may cause otitis media and hearing loss.

Causes

The usual cause of perforated eardrum is trauma: the deliberate or accidental insertion of sharp objects (cotton swabs, bobby pins) or sudden excessive changes in pressure (explosion, a blow to the head, flying, or diving). The injury may also result from untreated otitis media and, in children, from acute otitis media.

Signs and symptoms

Sudden onset of severe earache and bleeding from the ear are the first signs of a perforated eardrum. Other symptoms include hearing loss, tinnitus, and vertigo. Purulent otorrhea within 24 to 48 hours of injury signals infection.

Diagnosis

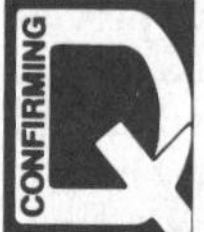

Severe earache and bleeding from the ear with a history of trauma strongly suggest perforated eardrum; direct visualization of the perforated tympanic membrane with an otoscope confirms it. Additional diagnostic measures include audiometric testing and a check of voluntary facial movements to rule out facial nerve damage.

Treatment and special considerations

If there is bleeding from the ear, use a sterile, cotton-tipped applicator to absorb the blood, and check for purulent drainage or evidence of cerebrospinal fluid leakage. A culture of the specimen may be ordered. *Irrigation of the ear is absolutely contraindicated.*

Apply a sterile dressing over the outer ear, and refer the patient to an ear specialist. A large perforation with uncontrolled bleeding may require immediate surgery to approximate the ruptured edges. Treatment may include a mild analgesic, a sedative to decrease anxiety, and an oral antibiotic.

Find out the cause of the injury, and report suspected child abuse. Before discharge, tell the patient not to blow his nose or get water in his ear canal until the perforation heals.

NECK & SPINAL INJURIES

Acceleration-Deceleration Cervical Injuries

(Whiplash)

Acceleration-deceleration cervical injuries result from sharp hyperextension and flexion of the neck that damage muscles, ligaments, disks, and nerve tissue. Prognosis is excellent; symptoms usually subside with symptomatic treatment.

Causes

Commonly, whiplash results from rear-end automobile accidents. Fortunately, the padded headrests and seat belts with shoulder harnesses required in new cars have reduced the risk of this type of trauma.

Signs and symptoms

Although symptoms may develop immediately, if the injury is mild they're often delayed 12 to 24 hours. Whiplash produces moderate to severe anterior and posterior neck pain. Within several days, the anterior pain diminishes, but posterior pain persists or even intensifies, causing patients to seek medical attention if they didn't do so before. Whiplash may also cause dizziness, gait disturbances, vomiting, headache, nuchal rigidity, neck muscle asymmetry, and rigidity or numbness in the arms.

Diagnosis

Full cervical spine X-rays are required to rule out cervical fractures. If the X-rays are negative, examination emphasizes motor ability and sensation below the cervical spine to detect signs of nerve root compression.

Treatment and special considerations

In all suspected spinal injuries, assume the spine is injured until proven otherwise. Any patient with suspected whiplash or other injuries requires careful transportation from the accident scene. To do this, place him in a supine position on a spine board and immobilize his neck with tape and a hard cervical collar or sandbags. Until an X-ray rules out cervical fracture, move the patient as little as possible. Before the X-ray is taken, remove neck jewelry carefully. Don't undress the patient. Warn him against movements that could injure his spine.

Symptomatic treatment includes:

- mild analgesic—such as aspirin with codeine or ibuprofen—and possibly a muscle relaxant—such as diazepam, cyclobenzaprine (Flexeril), or chlorzoxazone with acetaminophen
- hot showers or warm compresses to the neck to relieve pain
- immobilization with a soft, padded cervical collar for several days or weeks
- in severe muscle spasms, short-term cervical traction.

Most whiplash patients are discharged immediately. Before discharge, teach patients to watch for possible drug side effects, to avoid alcohol if they're receiving diazepam or narcotics, and to rest for a few days and avoid lifting heavy objects. Warn them to return immediately if they experience persistent pain or if they develop numbness, tingling, or weakness on one side.

Spinal Injuries

(Without cord damage)

Spinal injuries include fractures, contusions, and compressions of the vertebral column, usually the result of trauma to the head or neck. The real danger lies in possible spinal cord damage. Spinal fractures most commonly occur in the fifth, sixth, and seventh cervical, twelfth thoracic, and first lumbar vertebrae.

Causes

Most serious spinal injuries result from motor vehicle accidents, falls, diving into shallow water, and gunshot wounds; less serious injuries, from lifting heavy objects and minor falls. Spinal dysfunction may also result from hyperparathyroidism and neoplastic lesions.

Signs and symptoms

The most obvious symptom of spinal injury is muscle spasm and back pain that worsens with movement. In cervical fractures, pain may produce point tenderness; in dorsal and lumbar fractures, it may radiate to other body areas, such as the legs. If the injury damages the spinal cord, clinical effects range from mild paresthesia to quadriplegia and shock. After milder injuries, such symptoms may be delayed for several days or weeks.

Diagnosis

Typically, diagnosis is based on patient history, physical examination, X-rays, and, possibly, lumbar puncture, myelography, and computed tomography scan.

- *Patient history* may reveal trauma, metastatic lesion, infection that could produce a spinal abscess, or endocrine disorder.
- *Physical examination* (including a neurologic evaluation) locates the level of injury and detects cord damage.
- *Spinal X-rays*, the most important diagnostic measure, locate the fracture.
- In spinal compression, a *lumbar puncture* may show increased cerebrospinal fluid pressure from a lesion or trauma; *myelography* locates the spinal mass.

Treatment

The primary treatment after spinal injury is immediate immobilization to stabilize the spine and prevent cord damage; other treatment is supportive. Cervical injuries require immobilization, using sandbags on both sides of the patient's head, a plaster cast, hard cervical collar, or skeletal traction with skull tongs (Crutchfield, Barton, Vinke) or a halo device.

Treatment of stable lumbar and dorsal fractures consists of bed rest on firm support (such as a bed board), analgesics, and muscle relaxants until the fracture stabilizes (usually 10 to 12 weeks). Later treatment includes exercises to strengthen the back muscles and a back brace or corset to provide support while walking.

An unstable dorsal or lumbar fracture requires a plaster cast, a turning frame, and, in severe fracture, a laminectomy and spinal fusion.

When the damage results in compression of the spinal column, neurosurgery may relieve the pressure. If the cause of compression is a metastatic lesion, chemotherapy and radiation may relieve it. Surface wounds accompanying the spinal injury require tetanus prophylaxis unless the patient has had recent immunization.

Special considerations

In all spinal injuries, suspect cord damage until proven otherwise.

- During initial assessment and during X-rays, immobilize the patient on a firm surface, with sandbags on both sides of his head. Tell him not to move; avoid moving him, since hyperflexion can damage the cord. If you must move the patient, get at least one other member of the staff to help you logroll him, to avoid disturbing body alignment.
- Throughout assessment, offer comfort and reassurance. Remember, the fear of possible paralysis will be overwhelming. Allow a family member who isn't too distraught to accompany him and talk to him quietly and calmly.
- If the injury necessitates surgery, administer prophylactic antibiotics, as ordered. Catheterize the patient, as ordered, to avoid urinary retention, and monitor defecation patterns to avoid impaction.
- Explain traction methods to the patient and his family, and reassure them that traction devices don't penetrate the brain. If the patient has a halo or skull-tong traction device, cleanse pin sites daily, trim hair short, and provide analgesics for persistent headaches. During traction, turn the patient often to prevent pneumonia, embolism, and skin breakdown; perform passive range-of-motion exercises to maintain muscle tone. If available, use a CircOlectric bed or Stryker frame to facilitate turning and to avoid spinal cord injury.
- Turn the patient on his side during feedings, to prevent aspiration. Create a relaxed atmosphere at mealtimes.
- Suggest appropriate diversionary activities to fill the hours of immobility. Offer prism glasses for reading.
- Watch closely for neurologic changes. Immediately report changes in skin sensation and loss of muscle strength—either could point to pressure on the spinal cord, possibly as a result of edema or shifting bone fragments.
- Help the patient walk as soon as the doctor allows; it'll probably be necessary for him to wear a back brace.

- Before discharge, instruct the patient about continuing analgesics or other medication, and stress the importance of regular follow-up examinations.
- To help prevent spinal injury from becoming spinal *cord* injury, educate firemen, policemen, paramedics, and the general public about the proper way to handle such injuries.

THORACIC INJURIES

Blunt Chest Injuries

Chest injuries account for one fourth of all trauma deaths in the United States. Many are blunt chest injuries, which include myocardial contusion, and rib and sternal fractures that may be simple, multiple, displaced, or jagged. Such fractures may cause potentially fatal complications, such as hemothorax, pneumothorax, hemorrhagic shock, and diaphragmatic rupture.

Causes

Most blunt chest injuries result from automobile accidents. Other common causes include sports and blast injuries.

Signs and symptoms

Rib fractures produce tenderness, slight edema over the fracture site, and pain that worsens with deep breathing and movement; this painful breathing causes the patient to display shallow, splinted respirations that may lead to hypoventilation. Sternal fractures, which are usually transverse and located in the middle or upper sternum, produce persistent chest pains, even at rest. If a fractured rib tears the pleura and punctures a lung, it causes pneumothorax, which usually produces severe dyspnea, cyanosis, agitation, extreme pain, and, when air escapes into chest tissue, subcutaneous emphysema.

Multiple rib fractures may cause flail chest: a portion of the chest wall "caves" in, which causes a loss of chest wall integrity and prevents adequate lung inflation. Bruised skin, extreme pain caused by rib fracture and disfigurement, paradoxical chest movements, and rapid, shallow respirations are all signs of flail chest, as are tachycardia, hypotension, respiratory acidosis, and cyanosis. Flail chest can also cause tension pneumothorax, a condition in which air enters the chest but can't be ejected during exhalation; life-threatening thoracic pressure buildup causes lung collapse and subsequent mediastinal shift. The cardinal symptoms of tension pneumothorax include tracheal deviation (away from the affected side), cyanosis, severe dyspnea, absent breath sounds (on the affected side), agitation, distended jugular veins, and shock.

Hemothorax occurs when a rib lacerates lung tissue or an intercostal artery, causing blood to collect in the pleural cavity, thereby compressing the lung and limiting respiratory capacity. It can also result from rupture of large or small pulmonary vessels. Massive hemothorax is the most common cause of shock following chest trauma. Although slight bleeding occurs even with mild pneumothorax, such bleeding resolves very quickly, usually without changing the patient's condition. Rib fractures may also cause pulmonary contusion (resulting in hemoptysis, hypoxia, dyspnea, and possible obstruction), large myocardial tears (rapidly fatal), and small myocardial tears (causing pericardial effusion). Myocardial contusions produce tachycardia, arrhythmia, conduction abnormalities, and ST-T segment changes. Laceration or rupture of

FLAIL CHEST: PARADOXICAL BREATHING

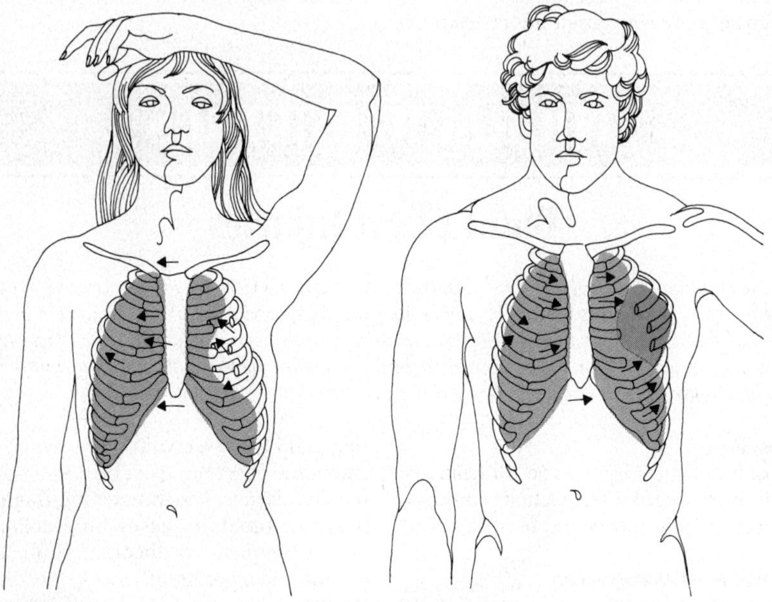

Inhalation
- Injured chest wall collapses in
- Uninjured chest wall moves out

Exhalation
- Injured chest wall moves out
- Uninjured chest wall moves in

the aorta is nearly always immediately fatal. Rarely, aortic laceration may develop 24 hours after blunt injury, so patient observation is critical. Diaphragmatic rupture (usually on the left side) causes severe respiratory distress. Unless treated early, abdominal viscera may herniate through the rupture into the thorax, compromising both circulation and the lungs' vital capacity.

Other complications of blunt chest trauma may be cardiac tamponade, pulmonary artery tears, ventricular rupture, and bronchial, tracheal, or esophageal tears or rupture.

Diagnosis

History of trauma with dyspnea, chest pain, and other typical clinical features suggest a blunt chest injury. To determine its extent, a physical examination and diagnostic tests are needed.

- Chest X-rays may confirm rib and sternal fractures, pneumothorax, flail chest, pulmonary contusions, lacerated or ruptured aorta, tension pneumothorax (mediastinal shift), diaphragmatic rupture, lung compression, or atelectasis with hemothorax.
- In hemothorax, percussion reveals a dullness that shifts when the patient changes position. In tension pneumothorax, percussion reveals tympany; auscultation may reveal a change in position of the loudest heart sound, indicating possible mediastinal shift.
- With cardiac damage, EKG changes may show a right bundle branch block.
- Serial SGOT, SGPT, LDH, creatine phosphokinase, and MB fraction are elevated.
- Retrograde aortography reveals aortic laceration or rupture.
- Contrast studies and liver and spleen

scans detect diaphragmatic rupture.

- Other studies, such as echocardiography, computed tomography, and cardiac and lung scans, show the injury's extent.

Treatment and special considerations

Blunt chest injuries call for immediate physical assessment, control of bleeding, maintenance of a patent airway, adequate ventilation, and fluid and electrolyte balance. In addition:

- Check pulses (including peripheral pulses) and level of consciousness. Also evaluate color and temperature of skin, depth of respiration, use of accessory muscles, and length of inhalation compared to exhalation.
- Observe tracheal position. Look for distended jugular veins and paradoxical chest motion. Listen to heart and lung sounds carefully; palpate for subcutaneous emphysema (crepitation) or structural disintegrity of the ribs.
- Obtain a thorough history of the injury. Unless severe dyspnea is present, ask the patient to locate the pain, and ask if he's having trouble breathing. Obtain an order for appropriate lab studies (arterial blood gas analysis, cardiac enzyme studies, complete blood count, type and cross match).
- For simple rib fractures, give mild analgesics, encourage bed rest, and apply heat. Do not strap or tape the chest.
- For more severe fractures, assist with administration of intercostal nerve blocks. (Obtain X-rays both before and after to rule out pneumothorax.) Intubate the patient in the event of excessive bleeding or hemopneumothorax. Chest tubes may be inserted, especially if bleeding is prolonged. To prevent atelectasis, turn the patient frequently, and encourage coughing and deep breathing.
- For pneumothorax, assist during placement of a large-bore needle into the second intercostal space—in the midclavicular line on the affected side or in the midaxillary line at the fourth intercostal space—to aspirate as much air as possible from the pleural cavity and to reexpand the lungs. When time permits, insert chest tubes attached to water-seal drainage and suction.
- For flail chest, place the patient in semi-Fowler's position. Wrap the affected area with an elastic bandage, or pad it with a thick dressing. Then, tape it with wide adhesive, to stabilize the chest wall. As temporary first aid, place sandbags on the affected side, or exert manual pressure over the flail segment on exhalation. Using an endotracheal tube, give oxygen at a high flow rate under positive pressure. Reposition the patient, suction frequently, give postural drainage, maintain acid-base balance, and provide controlled mechanical ventilation until paradoxical motion of the chest wall ceases. Observe for signs of tension pneumothorax. Start I.V. therapy, using Ringer's lactate or normal saline solution.
- For hemothorax, treat shock with I.V. infusions of Ringer's lactate or normal saline solution. Administer oxygen, and assist with insertion of chest tubes into the fifth or sixth intercostal space at the midaxillary line to remove blood. Monitor vital signs and blood loss. Watch for and immediately report falling blood pressure, rising pulse rate, and uncontrolled hemorrhage—all mandate thoracotomy to stop bleeding.
- For pulmonary contusions, give limited amounts of colloids (salt-poor albumin, whole blood, or plasma), as ordered, to replace volume and maintain oncotic pressure. Give analgesics, diuretics, and, if necessary, corticosteroids, as ordered (the use of steroids is controversial). Monitor blood gases to ensure adequate ventilation. Provide oxygen therapy, mechanical ventilation, and chest tube care, as needed.
- For suspected cardiac damage, close intensive care or telemetry may detect arrhythmias and prevent cardiogenic shock. Impose bed rest in semi-Fowler's position (unless the patient requires shock position); as needed, administer oxygen, analgesics, and supportive drugs, such as digitalis, to control heart failure or supraventricular arrhythmia.

Watch for cardiac tamponade, which calls for pericardiocentesis. Essentially, provide the same care as for a patient who has suffered a myocardial infarction.

- For myocardial rupture, septal perforations, and other cardiac lacerations, immediate surgical repair is mandatory; less severe ventricular wounds require a digital or balloon catheter; atrial wounds, a clamp or balloon catheter.
- For the few patients with aortic rupture or laceration who reach the hospital alive, immediate surgery is mandatory, using synthetic grafts or anastomosis to repair the damage. Give large volumes of I.V. fluids (Ringer's lactate or normal saline solution) and whole blood, along with oxygen at very high flow rates; apply medical antishock trousers (MAST) suit and transport promptly to the operating room.
- For tension pneumothorax, expect to assist with insertion of a spinal or 14G to 16G needle into the second intercostal space at the midclavicular line, to release pressure in the chest. Following this, insert a chest tube to normalize pressure and reexpand the lung. Administer oxygen under positive pressure, along with I.V. fluids.
- For a diaphragmatic rupture, insert a nasogastric tube to temporarily decompress the stomach, and prepare the patient for surgical repair.

Penetrating Chest Wounds

Penetrating chest wounds, depending on their size, may cause varying degrees of damage to bones, soft tissue, blood vessels, and nerves. Mortality and morbidity from a chest wound depend on the size and severity of the wound. Gunshot wounds are usually more serious than stab wounds, both because they cause more severe lacerations and cause rapid blood loss and because ricochet often damages large areas and multiple organs. With prompt, aggressive treatment, up to 90% of patients with penetrating chest wounds recover.

Causes

Stab wounds from a knife or ice pick are the most common penetrating chest wounds; gunshot wounds are a close second. Wartime explosions or firearms fired at close range are the usual source of large, gaping wounds.

Signs and symptoms

In addition to the obvious chest injuries, penetrating chest wounds can also cause:

- a sucking sound, as the diaphragm contracts and air enters the chest cavity through the opening in the chest wall.
- varying levels of consciousness, depending on the extent of the injury. If the patient is awake and alert, he may be in severe pain, which will make him splint his respirations, thereby reducing his vital capacity.
- tachycardia, which is caused by anxiety and blood loss.
- weak, thready pulse, which results from massive blood loss and hypovolemic shock.

Penetrating chest wounds may also cause lung lacerations (bleeding and substantial air leakage through the chest tube); arterial lacerations (loss of more than 100 ml blood/hour through the chest tube); exsanguination; pneumothorax (air in pleural space causes loss of negative intrathoracic pressure and lung collapse); tension pneumothorax (intrapleural air accumulation causes potentially fatal mediastinal shift); and hemothorax. Other effects may include arrhythmias, cardiac tamponade, mediastinitis, subcutaneous emphysema, esophageal perforation, bronchopleural fistula, and tracheobronchial, abdominal, or diaphragmatic injuries.

Diagnosis

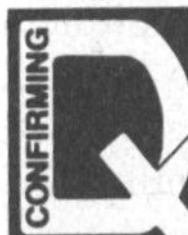

An obvious chest wound and a sucking sound during breathing confirm the diagnosis. Consider any lower thoracic chest injury a thoracicoabdominal injury until proven otherwise. Baseline data include:

- arterial blood gases to assess respiratory status
- chest X-rays before and after chest tube placement to evaluate injury and tube placement
- CBC, including hemoglobin, hematocrit, and differential; low hemoglobin and hematocrit reflect severe blood loss
- palpation and auscultation of chest and abdomen to evaluate damage to adjacent organs and structures.

Treatment and special considerations

Penetrating chest wounds require immediate support of respiration and circulation, prompt surgical repair of tissue injury, and appropriate measures to prevent complications.

- Immediately assess airway, breathing, and circulation (ABCs). Establish a patent airway, and support ventilation, as needed. Monitor pulses frequently for rate and quality.
- Place an occlusive dressing (for example, petrolatum-impregnated gauze) over the sucking wound. Monitor for signs of tension pneumothorax (tracheal shift, respiratory distress, tachycardia, tachypnea, and diminished or absent breath sounds on the affected side); if tension pneumothorax develops, temporarily remove the occlusive dressing to create a simple pneumothorax.
- Control blood loss (also remember to look *under* the patient to estimate loss), type and cross match blood, and replace blood and fluids, as necessary.
- Assist with chest X-ray and placement of chest tubes (using water-seal drainage) to reestablish intrathoracic pressure and to drain blood in hemothorax. A second X-ray will evaluate the position of tubes and their function.
- After the patient's condition has stabilized, surgery can repair the damage caused by the wound.
- Throughout treatment, monitor central venous pressure and blood pressure to detect hypovolemia, and assess vital signs. Provide analgesics as appropriate. Tetanus and antibiotic prophylaxis may be necessary.
- Reassure the patient, especially if he's been the victim of a violent crime. Report the incident to the police in accordance with local laws. Help contact the patient's family, and offer them reassurance, as well.

ABDOMINAL INJURIES

Blunt and Penetrating Abdominal Injuries

Blunt and penetrating abdominal injuries may damage major blood vessels and internal organs. Their most immediate life-threatening consequences are hemorrhage and hypovolemic shock; later threats include infection. Prognosis depends on the extent of injury and the organs damaged but is generally improved by prompt diagnosis and surgical repair.

Causes

Blunt (nonpenetrating) abdominal injuries usually result from automobile accidents, falls from heights, or athletic injuries; penetrating abdominal injuries, from stab and gunshot wounds.

Signs and symptoms

Symptoms vary with the degree of injury and the organs damaged. Penetrating abdominal injuries cause obvious wounds (gunshots often produce both entrance and exit wounds), with variable blood loss, pain, and tenderness. These injuries often cause pallor, cyanosis, tachycardia, shortness of breath, and hypotension.

Blunt abdominal injuries cause severe pain (such pain may radiate beyond the abdomen, for instance, to the shoulders), bruises, abrasions, contusions, or distention. They may also result in tenderness, abdominal splinting or rigidity, nausea, vomiting, pallor, cyanosis, tachycardia, and shortness of breath. Rib fractures often accompany blunt injuries.

In both blunt and penetrating injuries, massive blood loss may cause hypovolemic shock. In general, damage to solid abdominal organs (liver, spleen, pancreas, and kidneys) causes hemorrhage; damage to hollow organs (stomach, intestine, gallbladder, and bladder) causes rupture and release of the organs' contents (including bacteria) into the abdomen, which, in turn, produces inflammation.

PROJECTILE PATHWAY

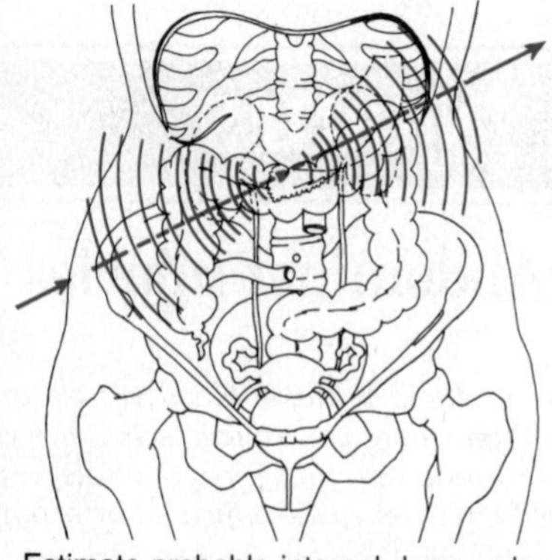

Estimate probable internal damage by determining the organs lying on the pathway between the entry and exit sites.

Diagnosis

A history of abdominal trauma, clinical features, and laboratory results confirm the diagnosis and determine organ damage. Consider any upper abdominal injury a thoracicoabdominal injury until proven otherwise. Laboratory studies vary with the patient's condition but usually include:

- chest X-rays (preferably done with the patient upright, to show free air)
- abdominal films
- examination of the stool and stomach aspirate for blood
- blood studies (decreased hematocrit and hemoglobin levels point to blood loss; coagulation studies evaluate hemostasis; white blood cell count is usually elevated but doesn't necessarily point to infection; type and cross match to prepare for blood transfusion)
- arterial blood gas analysis to evaluate respiratory status
- serum amylase levels, which often may be elevated in pancreatic injury
- SGOT and SGPT levels, which increase with tissue injury and cell death
- ultrasound examination
- intravenous pyelography and cystourethrography to detect renal and urinary tract damage
- radioisotope scanning and ultrasound to detect liver, kidney, or spleen injury
- angiography to detect specific injuries, especially to the kidneys
- peritoneal lavage, with insertion of a lavage catheter to check for blood, urine, pus, ascitic fluid, bile, and chyle (a milky fluid absorbed by the intestinal lymph vessels during digestion). In blunt trauma with equivocal abdominal findings, this procedure helps establish the need for exploratory surgery.
- computed tomography scan to detect abdominal, head, or other injuries
- exploratory laparotomy to detect specific injuries when other clinical evidence is incomplete
- other lab studies to rule out associated injuries.

Treatment

Emergency treatment of abdominal injuries controls hemorrhage and prevents hypovolemic shock by the infusion of I.V. fluids and blood components. After stabilization, most abdominal injuries require surgical repair. Analgesics and antibiotics increase patient comfort and prevent infection. Most patients require hospitalization; if they're asymptomatic, they may require observation for only 6 to 24 hours.

Special considerations

Emergency care in patients with abdominal injuries supports vital functions by maintaining airway, breathing, and circulation. At admission, immediately evaluate respiratory and circulatory status and, if possible, obtain a history of the trauma.

- To maintain airway and breathing, intubate the patient and provide mechanical ventilation, as necessary; otherwise, provide supplemental oxygen.
- Using a large-bore needle, start one or more I.V. lines for monitoring and rapid fluid infusion, using a normal saline solution. Then, draw a blood sample for laboratory studies. Also, insert a nasogastric tube and, if necessary, a Foley catheter; monitor stomach aspirate and urine for blood.
- Obtain vital signs for baseline data; continue to monitor every 15 minutes.
- Apply a sterile dressing to open wounds. Splint a suspected pelvic injury on arrival by tying the patient's legs together with a pillow between them. Move such a patient as little as possible.
- Give analgesics, as ordered. Usually, narcotics aren't recommended; but if the pain is severe, give narcotics in small titrated I.V. doses.
- Give tetanus prophylaxis and prophylactic I.V. antibiotics, as ordered.
- Prepare the patient for surgery. Get a consent form signed by the patient or a responsible relative. Remove dentures. Type and cross match blood.
- If the injury was caused by a motor vehicle accident, find out if the police were notified, and if not, notify them. If the patient suffered a gunshot or stab wound, notify the police, place all his clothes in a bag, and retain them for the police. Document the number and sites of the wounds. Contact the patient's family and offer them reassurance.

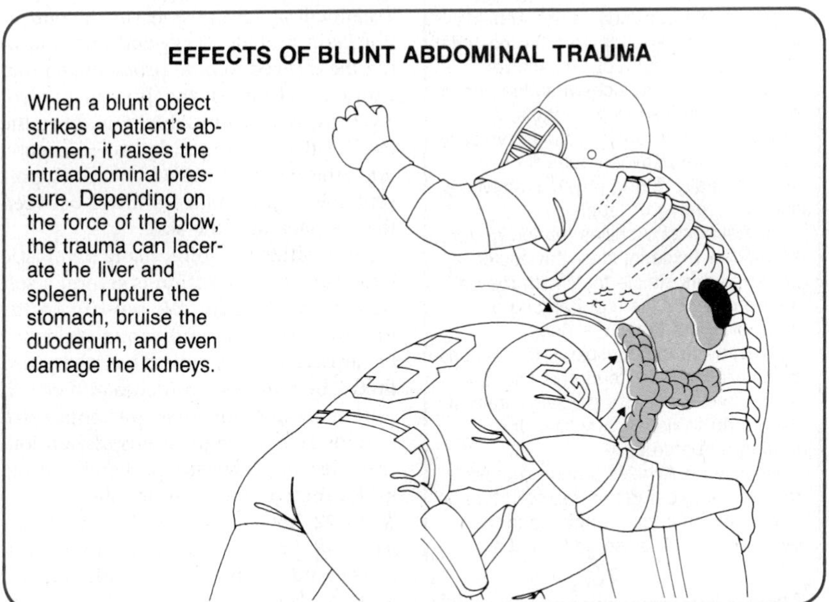

EFFECTS OF BLUNT ABDOMINAL TRAUMA

When a blunt object strikes a patient's abdomen, it raises the intraabdominal pressure. Depending on the force of the blow, the trauma can lacerate the liver and spleen, rupture the stomach, bruise the duodenum, and even damage the kidneys.

INJURIES OF THE EXTREMITIES

Sprains and Strains

A sprain *is a complete or incomplete tear in the supporting ligaments surrounding a joint that usually follows a sharp twist. A* strain *is an injury to a muscle or tendinous attachment. Both injuries usually heal without surgical repair.*

Signs and symptoms

A sprain causes local pain (especially during joint movement), swelling, loss of mobility (which may not occur until several hours after the injury), and a black-and-blue discoloration, from blood extravasating into surrounding tissues. A sprained ankle is the most common joint injury.

A strain may be acute (an immediate result of vigorous muscle overuse or overstress) or chronic (a result of repeated overuse). An acute strain causes a sharp, transient pain (the patient may say he heard a snapping noise) and rapid swelling. When severe pain subsides, the muscle is tender; after several days, ecchymoses appear. A chronic strain causes stiffness, soreness, and generalized tenderness; these conditions appear several hours after the injury.

Diagnosis

History of recent injury or chronic overuse, clinical findings, and an X-ray to rule out fractures establish the diagnosis.

Treatment and special considerations

Treatment of sprains consists of controlling pain and swelling, and immobilizing the injured joint to promote healing. Immediately after the injury, control swelling by elevating the joint above the level of the heart, and by intermittently applying ice for 12 to 48 hours. To prevent cold injury, place a towel between the ice pack and the skin.

Immobilize the joint, using an elastic bandage, or if the sprain is severe, a soft cast. Depending on the severity of the injury, codeine or another analgesic may be necessary. If the patient has a sprained ankle, he may need crutches and crutch gait training. Because patients with sprains seldom require hospitalization, provide comprehensive patient teaching.

- Tell the patient to elevate the joint for 48 to 72 hours after the injury (while sleeping, joint can be elevated with pillows), and to apply ice intermittently for 12 to 48 hours.

MUSCLE-TENDON RUPTURES

Perhaps the most serious muscle-tendon injury is a rupture of the muscle-tendon junction. These ruptures may occur at any such junction, but they're most common at the Achilles tendon, which extends from the posterior calf muscle to the foot. An Achilles tendon rupture produces a sudden sharp pain, and until swelling begins, a palpable defect. Such ruptures typically occur in men between ages 35 and 40, especially during physical activities such as jogging or tennis.

To distinguish Achilles tendon rupture from other ankle injuries, the doctor performs this simple test: With the patient prone and his feet hanging off the foot of the table, the doctor squeezes the calf muscle. If this causes plantar flexion, the tendon is intact; if ankle dorsiflexion, it's partially intact; if there's no flexion of any kind, the tendon is ruptured.

Usually an Achilles tendon rupture requires surgical repair, followed first by a long leg cast for 4 weeks, and then by a short cast for an additional 4 weeks.

• If an elastic bandage has been applied, teach the patient to reapply it by wrapping from below to above the injury, forming a figure eight. For a sprained ankle, apply the bandage from the toes to midcalf. Tell the patient to remove the bandage before going to sleep, and to loosen it if it causes the leg to become pale, numb, or painful.
• Instruct the patient to call the doctor if pain worsens or persists (if so, an additional X-ray may detect a fracture originally missed).

An immobilized sprain usually heals in 2 to 3 weeks, and the patient can then gradually resume normal activities. Occasionally, however, torn ligaments don't heal properly and cause recurrent dislocation, necessitating surgical repair. Some athletes may request immediate surgical repair to hasten healing; to prevent sprains, they may tape their wrists and ankles before sports activities.

Acute strains require analgesics and immediate application of ice for up to 48 hours, followed by heat application. Complete muscle rupture may require surgical repair. Chronic strains usually don't require treatment, but local heat application, aspirin, or an analgesic-muscle relaxant relieves discomfort.

Arm and Leg Fractures

Arm and leg fractures usually result from trauma and often cause substantial muscle, nerve, and other soft-tissue damage. Prognosis varies with extent of disablement or deformity, amount of tissue and vascular damage, adequacy of reduction and immobilization, and the patient's age, health, and nutrition. Children's bones usually heal rapidly and without deformity. Bones of adults in poor health and with impaired circulation may never heal properly. Severe open fractures, especially of the femoral shaft, may cause substantial blood loss and life-threatening hypovolemic shock.

Causes

Most arm and leg fractures result from major trauma; for example, a fall on an outstretched arm, a skiing accident, or child abuse (shown by multiple or repeated episodes of fractures). However, in a person with a pathologic bone-weakening condition, such as osteoporosis, bone tumors, or metabolic disease, a mere cough or sneeze can also produce a fracture. Prolonged standing, walking, or running can cause stress fractures of the foot and ankle—usually in nurses, postal workers, soldiers, and joggers.

Signs and symptoms

Arm and leg fractures may produce any or all of the "5 Ps": pain and point tenderness, pallor, pulse loss, paresthesia, and paralysis. (The last three are distal to the fracture site.) Other signs include deformity, swelling, discoloration, crepitus, and loss of limb function. Numbness and tingling, mottled cyanosis, cool skin at the end of the extremity, and loss of pulses distal to the injury indicate possible arterial compromise or nerve damage. Open fractures also produce an obvious skin wound.

Complications of arm and leg fractures include:
• permanent deformity and dysfunction if bones fail to heal (nonunion) or heal improperly (malunion)
• aseptic necrosis of bone segments from impaired circulation
• hypovolemic shock as a result of blood vessel damage (this is especially likely to develop in patients with fractured femur)
• muscle contractures
• renal calculi from decalcification (produced by prolonged immobility)
• fat embolism.

Diagnosis

History of trauma and physical examination, including gentle palpation and a cautious attempt by the patient to move parts distal to the injury, suggest an arm or leg fracture. (Physical examination should also check for other injuries.)

Anteroposterior and lateral X-rays of the suspected fracture, as well as X-rays of the joints above and below it, confirm the diagnosis.

Treatment

Emergency treatment consists of splinting the limb above and below the suspected fracture, applying a cold pack, and elevating the limb, to reduce edema and pain. In severe fractures that cause blood loss, direct pressure should be applied to control bleeding, and fluid replacement (including blood products) should be administered to prevent or treat hypovolemic shock.

After confirming diagnosis of a fracture, treatment begins with reduction (restoring displaced bone segments to their normal position), followed by immobilization by splint, cast, or traction. In closed reduction (manual manipulation), a local anesthetic—such as lidocaine—and an analgesic—such as

TYPES OF FRACTURES

Incomplete: Break extends only partially through the bone; for example, in a greenstick fracture (more common in children), bone splinters fibers on one side of the bone, leaving the other side intact
Complete: Bone breaks into two or more pieces
Simple (closed): Overlying skin remains unbroken
Compound (open): Overlying skin is broken, creating the risk of infection
Nondisplaced: Fractured bones remain in alignment
Displaced: Break knocks bone ends out of alignment, creating the risk of muscle contractures and deformities
Transverse: Break runs transversely across the bone shaft
Oblique: Break runs across the bone on an angle
Spiral: Break winds around bone like a coil
Linear: Break runs the length of the bone
Comminuted: Bone shatters or is compressed into fragments
Impacted: Bone ends are driven into each other
Compression: Bone collapses (vertebrae) under excessive pressure
Avulsion: Overexertion tears a muscle or ligament away from a bone, pulling a small bone fragment with it
Depression: Trauma drives bone fragments inward

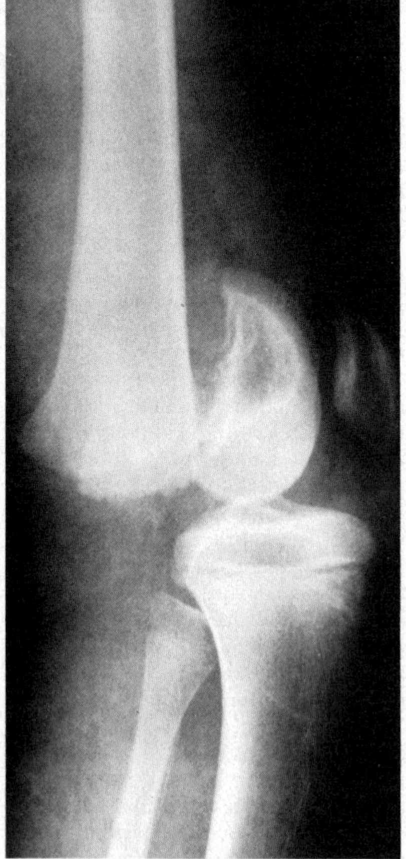

This X-ray shows a complete, displaced fracture at the epiphyseal line at the distal end of the femur.

meperidine I.M.—minimize pain, whereas a muscle relaxant—such as diazepam I.V.—facilitates muscle stretching necessary to realign the bone. (An X-ray confirms reduction and proper bone alignment.) When closed reduction is impossible, open reduction during surgery reduces and immobilizes the fracture by means of rods, plates, or screws. Afterward, a plaster cast is usually applied.

When a splint or cast fails to maintain the reduction, immobilization requires skin or skeletal traction, using a series of weights and pulleys. In skin traction, elastic bandages and moleskin coverings are used to attach traction devices to the patient's skin. In skeletal traction, a pin or wire inserted through the bone distal to the fracture and attached to a weight allows more prolonged traction.

Treatment for open fractures also requires careful wound cleansing, tetanus prophylaxis, prophylactic antibiotics, and, possibly, surgery to repair soft-tissue damage.

Special considerations

- Watch for signs of shock in the patient with a severe open fracture of a large bone, such as the femur. Monitor vital signs (rapid pulse, decreased blood pressure, cool clammy skin, and pallor may indicate shock). Administer I.V. fluids, as ordered.
- Offer reassurance. With any fracture the patient is apt to be frightened and in pain. Ease pain with analgesics, as needed. Help the patient set realistic goals for recovery.
- If the fracture requires long-term immobilization with traction, reposition the patient often to increase comfort and prevent decubitus ulcers. Assist with active range-of-motion exercises to prevent muscle atrophy. Encourage deep breathing and coughing to avoid hypostatic pneumonia.
- Urge adequate fluid intake to prevent urinary stasis and constipation. Watch for signs of renal calculi (flank pain, nausea, and vomiting).
- Give good cast care. While the cast is wet, support it with pillows. Observe for skin irritation near cast edges; check for foul odors or discharge. Tell the patient to report signs of impaired circulation (skin coldness, numbness, tingling, or discoloration) immediately. Warn against getting the cast wet, and instruct the patient not to insert foreign objects under the cast.
- Encourage the patient to start moving around as soon as he is able. Help with walking. (Remember, the patient who's been bedridden for some time may be dizzy at first.) Demonstrate how to use crutches properly.
- After cast removal, refer for physical therapy to restore limb mobility.

FAT EMBOLISM

A complication of long bone fracture, fat embolism may also follow severe soft-tissue bruising and fatty liver injury. Posttraumatic embolization may occur as bone marrow releases fat into the veins. The fat can lodge in the lungs, obstructing the pulmonary vascular bed, or pass into the arteries, eventually disturbing the central nervous system.

Fat embolism occurs 12 to 48 hours after injury, typically producing fever, tachycardia, tachypnea, blood-tinged sputum, cyanosis, anxiety, restlessness, altered level of consciousness, convulsions, coma, and a rash. Studies reveal decreased hemoglobin, increased serum lipase, leucocytosis, thrombocytopenia, hypoxemia, and fat globules in urine and sputum. A chest X-ray may show mottled lung fields and right ventricular dilation: an EKG; large S waves in lead I, large Q waves in lead III, and right axis deviation.

Although treatment is controversial, it may include steroids to reduce inflammation, heparin to clear lipemia, diazepam for sedation, and oxygen to correct hypoxemia. Expect to immobilize fractures early. As ordered, assist with endotracheal intubation and ventilation.

Dislocations and Subluxations

Dislocations displace joint bones so their articulating surfaces totally lose contact; subluxations partially displace the articulating surfaces. Dislocations and subluxations occur at the joints of the shoulders, elbows, wrists, digits, hips, knees, ankles, and feet; the injury may accompany fractures of these joints or result in deposition of fracture fragments between joint surfaces. Prompt reduction can limit the resulting damage to soft tissue, nerves, and blood vessels.

Causes

A dislocation or subluxation may be congenital (as in congenital dislocation of the hip), or it may follow trauma or disease of surrounding joint tissues (for example, Paget's disease).

Signs and symptoms

Dislocations and subluxations produce deformity around the joint, change the length of the involved extremity, impair joint mobility, and cause point tenderness. When the injury results from trauma, it is extremely painful and often accompanies joint surface fractures. Even in the absence of concomitant fracture, the displaced bone may damage surrounding muscles, ligaments, nerves, and blood vessels, and may cause bone necrosis, especially if reduction is delayed.

Diagnosis

Patient history, X-rays, and clinical examination rule out or confirm fracture.

Treatment

Immediate reduction (before tissue edema and muscle spasm make reduction difficult) can prevent additional tissue damage and vascular impairment. Closed reduction consists of manual traction, under general anesthetic, or local anesthetic and sedatives. During such reduction, meperidine I.V. controls pain; diazepam I.V. controls muscle spasm and facilitates muscle-stretching during traction. Occasionally, such injuries require open reduction under regional block or general anesthetic. Such surgery may include wire fixation of the joint, skeletal traction, and ligament repair.

After reduction, a splint, cast, or traction immobilizes the joint. Generally, immobilizing the digits for 2 weeks, hips for 6 to 8 weeks, and other dislocated joints for 3 to 6 weeks allows surrounding ligaments to heal.

Special considerations

- Until reduction immobilizes the dislocated joint, do not attempt manipulation. Apply ice to ease pain and edema. Splint the extremity "as it lies," even if the angle is awkward. If severe vascular compromise is present or is indicated by pallor, pain, loss of pulses, paralysis, and paresthesia—then an immediate orthopedic examination is necessary.
- When a patient receives meperidine I.V. or diazepam I.V., he may develop respiratory depression or even respiratory arrest. So during reduction, keep an airway and hand-held resuscitator (AMBU bag) in the room, and monitor respirations closely.
- To avoid injury from a dressing that is too tight, instruct the patient to report numbness, pain, cyanosis, or coldness of the extremity below the cast or splint.
- To avoid skin damage, watch for signs

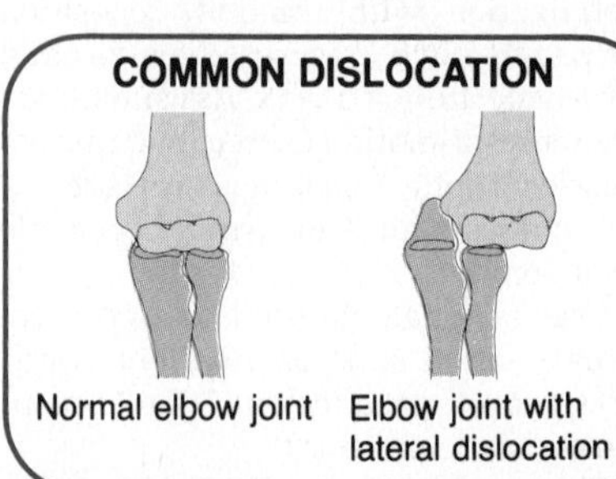

of pressure injury (pressure, pain, or soreness) both inside and outside the dressing.

• After removal of the cast or splint, inform the patient that he may gradually return to normal joint activity.

• A dislocated hip needs immediate reduction. At discharge, stress the need for follow-up visits to detect aseptic femoral head necrosis from vascular damage.

Traumatic Amputation

Traumatic amputation is the accidental loss of a body part, usually a finger, toe, arm, or leg. In complete amputation, the member is totally severed; in partial amputation, some soft-tissue connection remains. Prognosis has improved as a result of early improved emergency and critical care management, new surgical techniques, early rehabilitation, prosthesis fitting, and new prosthesis design. New limb reimplantation techniques have been moderately successful, but incomplete nerve regeneration remains a major limiting factor.

Causes

Traumatic amputations usually result directly from factory, farm, or power tools or from motor vehicle accidents.

Assessment

Every traumatic amputee requires careful monitoring of vital signs. If amputation involves more than just a finger or toe, assessment of airway, breathing, and circulation is also required. Since profuse bleeding is likely, watch for signs of hypovolemic shock, and draw blood for hemoglobin, hematocrit, and type and cross match. In partial amputation, check for pulses distal to the amputation. After any traumatic amputation, assess for other traumatic injuries, as well.

Treatment

Because the greatest immediate threat after traumatic amputation is blood loss and hypovolemic shock, emergency treatment consists of local measures to control bleeding, fluid replacement with normal saline solution and colloids, and blood replacement, as needed. Reimplantation remains controversial, but it's becoming more common and successful because of advances in microsurgery. If reconstruction or reimplantation is possible, surgical intervention attempts to preserve usable joints. When arm or leg amputations are done, the surgeon creates a stump to be fitted with a prosthesis. A rigid dressing permits early prosthesis fitting and rehabilitation.

Special considerations

During emergency treatment, monitor vital signs (especially in hypovolemic shock); cleanse the wound; and give tetanus prophylaxis, analgesics, and antibiotics, as ordered. After complete amputation, flush the amputated part with sterile saline solution, wrap it in a moist sterile towel or gauze, and put it in a plastic bag. Then place the bag in a container on ice. Flush the wound with sterile saline solution, apply a sterile pressure dressing, and elevate the limb. Notify the reimplantation team. After partial amputation, position the limb in normal alignment, and drape it with towels or dressings soaked in sterile normal saline solution.

Preoperative care includes thorough wound irrigation and debridement (using a local block). Postoperative dressing changes using sterile technique help prevent skin infection and ensure skin graft viability. Help the amputee cope with his altered body image. Reinforce exercises and prevent stump trauma.

WHOLE BODY INJURIES

Burns

A major burn is a horrifying injury, necessitating painful treatment and a long period of rehabilitation. It is often fatal or permanently disfiguring and incapacitating (both emotionally and physically). In the United States, about 2 million persons annually suffer burns. Of these, 300,000 are burned seriously and over 6,000 are fatalities, making burns this nation's third largest cause of accidental death.

Causes

Thermal burns, the most common type, are frequently the result of residential fires, automobile accidents, playing with matches, improperly stored gasoline, space heater or electrical malfunctions, or arson. Other causes include improper handling of firecrackers, scalding accidents, and kitchen accidents (such as a child climbing on top of a stove or grabbing a hot iron). Burns in children are sometimes traced to parental abuse.

Chemical burns result from the contact, ingestion, inhalation, or injection of acids, alkalis, or vesicants. Electrical burns usually occur after contact with faulty electrical wiring or with high-voltage power lines, or when electric cords are chewed (by young children). Friction, or abrasion, burns happen when the skin is rubbed harshly against a coarse surface. Sunburn, of course, follows excessive exposure to sunlight.

Assessment

One goal of assessment is to determine the *depth* of skin and tissue damage. A partial-thickness burn damages the epidermis and part of the dermis, while a full-thickness burn affects the epidermis, dermis, and subcutaneous tissue. However, a more traditional method gauges burn depth by degrees, although most burns are a combination of different degrees and thicknesses.

- *First degree*—Damage is limited to the epidermis, causing erythema and pain.
- *Second degree*—The epidermis and part of the dermis are damaged, producing blisters and mild-to-moderate edema and pain.
- *Third degree*—Epidermis and the dermis are damaged. No blisters appear, but white, brown, or black leathery tissue and thrombosed vessels are visible.
- *Fourth degree*—Damage extends through deeply charred subcutaneous tissue to muscle and bone.

Another assessment goal is to estimate the *size* of a burn. This is usually expressed as the percentage of body surface area (BSA) covered by the burn. The Rule of Nines chart most commonly provides this estimate, although the Lund and Browder chart is more accurate, because it allows for BSA changes with age. A correlation of the burn's depth and size permits an estimate of its severity.

- *Major*—third-degree burns on more than 10% of BSA; second-degree burns on more than 25% of adult BSA (more than 20% in children); burns of hands, face, feet, or genitalia; burns complicated by fractures or respiratory damage; electrical burns; all burns in poor-risk patients
- *Moderate*—third-degree burns on 2% to 10% of BSA; second-degree burns on 15% to 25% of adult BSA (10% to 20% in children)
- *Minor*—third-degree burns on less than 2% of BSA; second-degree burns on less than 15% of adult BSA (10% in children).

Here are other important factors in assessing burns:

- Location—Burns on the face, hands, feet, and genitalia are most serious, because of possible loss of function.
- Configuration—Circumferential burns can cause total occlusion of circulation in an extremity as a result of edema. Burns on the neck can produce airway obstruction whereas burns on the chest can lead to restricted respiratory expansion.
- History of complicating medical problems—Note disorders that impair peripheral circulation, especially diabetes, peripheral vascular disease, and chronic alcohol abuse.
- Other injuries sustained at the time of the burn.
- Patient age—Victims under age 4 or over age 60 have a higher incidence of complications and, consequently, a higher mortality.
- Pulmonary injury can result from smoke inhalation.

FLUID REPLACEMENT: THE FIRST 24 HOURS POSTBURN

Use one of these two formulas as a general guideline for the amount of fluid replacement, but vary the specific infusions according to the patient's response, especially urinary output.

- *Baxter formula*:
4 ml Ringer's lactate solution/kg/% BSA/24 hours. Give one half of total over first 8 hours postburn and remainder over next 16 hours.
- *Brooke formula*:
Colloids (plasma, plasmanate, dextran) 0.5 ml/kg/% BSA + Ringer's lactate solution 1.5 ml/kg/% BSA + 2,000 ml dextrose in water for adults (less for children). Give one half of total over first 8 hours postburn and remainder over next 16 hours.

Treatment and special considerations

Immediate, aggressive burn treatment increases the patient's chance for survival. Later, supportive measures and strict aseptic technique can minimize infection. Because burns necessitate such comprehensive care, good nursing can make the difference between life and death.

If the burns are minor, immerse the burned area in cool saline solution (55° F. [12.8° C.]) or apply cool compresses. Next, soak the wound in a mild antiseptic solution to cleanse it, and give pain medication, as ordered. Debride the devitalized tissue, taking care not to break any blisters. Cover the wound with an antimicrobial agent and a nonstick bulky dressing; administer tetanus prophylaxis, as ordered. Provide aftercare instructions for the patient. Stress the importance of keeping the dressing dry and clean, elevating the burned extremity for the first 24 hours, taking analgesics as ordered, and returning for a wound check in 2 days.

In moderate and major burns, immediately assess the patient's airway, breathing, and circulation. Be especially alert for signs of smoke inhalation and pulmonary damage: singed nasal hairs, mucosal burns, voice changes, coughing, wheezing, soot in the mouth or nose, and darkened sputum. As ordered, assist with endotracheal intubation and administer 100% oxygen. When you have assured the patient's ABCs, take a brief history about the burn. Draw blood samples for complete blood count, electrolytes, glucose, blood urea nitrogen, creatinine, arterial blood gases, and type and cross match.

Control bleeding, and remove smoldering clothing (soak it first in saline solution if it's stuck to the patient's skin), rings, and other constricting items. Be sure to cover burns with a clean, dry, sterile bed sheet. (*Never* cover large burns with saline-soaked dressings, since they can drastically lower body temperature.)

Begin I.V. therapy immediately to prevent hypovolemic shock and maintain cardiac output. Use Ringer's lactate solution or a fluid replacement formula, as ordered. (See *Fluid Replacement: The First 24 Hours Postburn.*) Closely monitor intake and output, and frequently

MANAGING BURNS WITH SKIN GRAFTS

When a patient has a limited, well-defined burn, he may need a *temporary graft* to minimize fluid and protein loss from the burn surface, prevent infection, and reduce pain. Types of temporary grafts include:
• allografts (homografts), which are usually cadaver skin
• xenografts (heterografts), which are typically pigskin
• biosynthetic grafts, which are a combination of collagen and synthetics.

To treat a full-thickness burn, a patient may need an *autograft*. This method uses the patient's own skin—usually a split-thickness graft—to replace the burned skin. For areas where appearance or joint movement is important, the autograft will be transplanted intact. In flat areas where appearance is less critical, the graft may be meshed (fenestrated) to cover up to three times its original size.

When burns cover the entire body surface, a new method—the *test-tube skin graft*—may provide lifesaving treatment. In this method, a small full-thickness biopsy yields epidermal cells that are cultured into sheets and then grafted onto the burns. According to its developers, this smooth, supple test-tube skin represents a major advance in the treatment of extensive burns.

check vital signs. Although it may make you nervous, don't be afraid to take the patient's blood pressure because of burned limbs.

In the hospital, a central venous pressure line and additional I.V. lines (using venous cutdown, if necessary), and a Foley catheter may be inserted. To combat fluid evaporation through the burn and the release of fluid into interstitial spaces (possibly resulting in hypovolemic shock), continue fluid therapy, as ordered.

Check vital signs every 15 minutes (the doctor may insert an arterial line if blood pressure is unobtainable with a cuff). Send a urine specimen to the laboratory to check for myoglobinuria and hemoglobinuria.

Insert a nasogastric tube to decompress the stomach and avoid aspiration of stomach contents.

Electrical and chemical burns demand special attention. Tissue damage from electrical burns is difficult to assess, because internal destruction along the conduction pathway is usually greater than the surface burn would indicate. Electrical burns that ignite the patient's clothes may cause thermal burns as well. If the electric shock caused ventricular fibrillation and cardiac and respiratory arrest, begin cardiopulmonary resuscitation at once. Get an estimate of the voltage. (For more details, see ELECTRIC SHOCK.)

In a chemical burn, irrigate the wound with copious amounts of water or normal saline solution. Using a weak base ($NaHCO_3$) to neutralize hydrofluoric acid, hydrochloric acid, or sulfuric acid on skin or mucous membrane is controversial, particularly in the emergency phase, since the neutralizing agent can produce more heat and tissue damage.

If the chemical entered the patient's eyes, flush them with large amounts of water or saline solution for at least 30 minutes; in an alkali burn, irrigate until the pH of the cul-de-sacs returns to 7. Have the patient close his eyes, and cover them with a dry, sterile dressing. Note the type of chemical causing the burn and the presence of any noxious fumes. The patient will need an ophthalmologic examination.

Don't treat the burn wound itself in the emergency department if the patient is to be transferred to a specialized burn care unit within 4 hours after the burn. Instead, prepare the patient for transport by wrapping him in a sterile sheet and a blanket for warmth and elevating the burned extremity to decrease edema. Then, transport immediately.

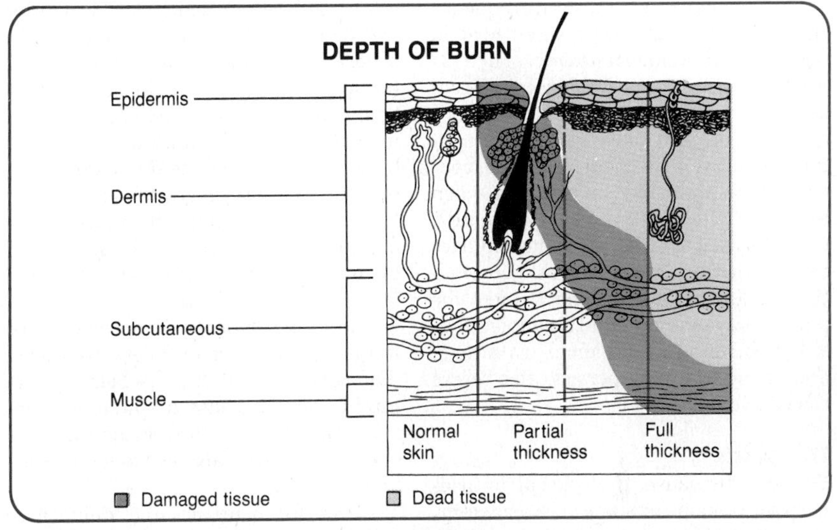

Electric Shock

When an electric current passes through the body, the damage it does depends on the intensity of the current (amperes, milliamperes, or microamperes); the resistance of the tissues it passes through; the kind of current (AC, DC, or mixed); and the frequency and duration of current flow. Electric shock may cause ventricular fibrillation, respiratory paralysis, burns, and death. Prognosis depends on the site and extent of damage, the patient's state of health, and the speed and adequacy of treatment. In the United States, each year about 1,000 people die of electric shock.

Causes

Electric shock usually follows accidental contact with exposed parts of electrical appliances or wiring, but it may also result from lightning or the flash of electric arcs from high-voltage power lines or machines. The increased use of electrical medical devices in the hospital, many of which are connected directly to the patient, has raised serious concern for electrical safety and has led to the development of electrical safety standards. But even well-designed equipment with reliable safety features can cause electric shock if mishandled.

Electric current can cause injury in three ways: true electrical injury as the current passes through the body; arc or flash burns from current that doesn't pass through the body; and thermal surface burns caused by associated heat and flames.

Signs and symptoms

Severe electric shock usually causes muscle contraction, followed by unconsciousness and loss of reflex control, sometimes with respiratory paralysis (by way of prolonged contraction of respiratory muscles, or a direct effect on the respiratory nerve center). After momentary shock, hyperventilation may follow initial muscle contraction. Passage of even the smallest electric current—if it passes through the heart—may induce ventricular fibrillation or other arrhythmia that progresses to fibrillation or myocardial infarction.

Electric shock from a high-frequency current (which generates more heat in tissues than a low-frequency current) usually causes burns and local tissue coagulation and necrosis. Low-frequency currents can also cause serious burns if the contact with the current is concentrated in a small area (for example, when a toddler bites into an electrical cord). Contusions, fractures, and other injuries can result from violent muscle contractions or falls during the shock; later, the patient may develop renal shutdown. Residual hearing impairment, cataracts, and vision loss may persist after severe electric shock.

Diagnosis

Usually, the cause of electrical injuries is either obvious or suspected. However, an accurate history can define the voltage and the length of contact.

Treatment and special considerations

Immediate emergency treatment includes separating the victim from the current source, quick assessment of vital functions, and emergency measures, such as cardiopulmonary resuscitation (CPR) and defibrillation.

To separate the victim from the current source, immediately turn it off or unplug it. If this isn't possible, pull the victim free with a nonconductive device, such as a loop of dry cloth or rubber, a dry rope, or a leather belt.

Then begin emergency treatment:

- Quickly assess vital functions. If you don't detect a pulse or breathing, start CPR at once. Continue until vital signs return or emergency help arrives with a defibrillator and other life-support equipment. Then monitor the patient's cardiac rhythm continuously and obtain a 12-lead EKG.
- Since internal tissue destruction may be much greater than skin damage leads one to believe, give I.V. Ringer's lactate solution, as ordered, to maintain a urine output of 50 to 100 ml/hour. Insert an indwelling urinary catheter and send the first specimen to the laboratory. Measure intake and output hourly and watch for tea- or port wine–colored urine, which occurs when coagulation necrosis and tissue ischemia liberate myoglobin and hemoglobin. These proteins can precipitate in the renal tubules, causing tubular necrosis and renal shutdown. To prevent this, give mannitol, as ordered.
- Administer sodium bicarbonate, as directed, to counteract acidosis caused by widespread tissue destruction and anaerobic metabolism.
- Assess the patient's neurologic status frequently, since central nervous system damage may result from ischemia or demyelination. Because a spinal cord injury may follow cord ischemia or a compression fracture, watch for sensorimotor deficits.
- Check for neurovascular damage in the extremities by assessing peripheral pulses and capillary refill and by asking about numbness, tingling, or pain. Elevate any injured extremities.
- Apply a temporary sterile dressing and admit the patient for surgical debridement and observation, as needed. Frequent debridement and use of topical and systemic antibiotics can help reduce the risk of infection. As ordered, prepare the patient for grafting or, if his injuries are extreme, for amputation.

Prevent electric shock by being alert for electrical hazards:

- Check for cuts, cracks, or frayed insulation on electric cords, call buttons (also check for warm call buttons), and electric devices attached to the patient's bed; keep these away from hot or wet surfaces and sharp corners. Don't set glasses of water, damp towels, or other wet items on electrical equipment. Wipe up accidental spills before they leak into electrical equipment. Avoid using extension cords, since they may circumvent the ground; if they're absolutely necessary, don't place them under carpeting or in areas where they'll be walked on.
- Make sure ground connections on electrical equipment are intact. Line cord plugs should have three prongs; the prongs should be straight and firmly fixed. Check that prongs fit wall outlets

properly, and that outlets aren't loose or broken. Don't use adapters on plugs.

- Report faulty equipment promptly to maintenance personnel. If a machine sparks, smokes, seems unusually hot, or gives you or your patient a slight shock, unplug it immediately, if doing so won't endanger the patient's life. Check inspection labels, and report equipment overdue for inspection.
- Be especially careful when using electrical equipment near patients with pacemakers or direct cardiac lines, since a cardiac catheter or pacemaker can create a direct, low-resistance path to the heart; even a small shock may cause ventricular fibrillation.
- Remember: Dry, calloused, unbroken skin offers more resistance to electric current than mucous membrane, an open wound, or thin, moist skin.
- Make sure defibrillator paddles are free of dry, caked gel before applying fresh gel, since poor electrical contact can cause burns. Also, don't apply too much gel. If the gel runs over the edge of the paddle and touches your hand, you'll receive some of the defibrillator shock, while the patient loses some of the energy in the discharge.
- Tell patients how to avoid electrical hazards at home and at work. Advise parents of small children to put safety guards on all electrical outlets and keep children away from electrical devices. Warn all patients not to use electrical appliances while showering or wet. Also warn them *never* to touch electrical appliances while touching faucets or cold water pipes in the kitchen, since these pipes often provide the ground for all circuits in the house.

Cold Injuries

Cold injuries result from overexposure to cold air or water and occur in two major forms: localized injuries (such as frostbite) and systemic injuries (such as hypothermia). Untreated or improperly treated frostbite can lead to gangrene and may necessitate amputation; severe hypothermia can be fatal.

Causes

Localized cold injuries occur when ice crystals form in the tissues and expand extracellular spaces. With compression of the tissue cell, the cell membrane ruptures, interrupting enzymatic and metabolic activities. Increased capillary permeability accompanies the release of histamine, resulting in aggregation of red blood cells and microvascular occlusion. Hypothermia effects chemical changes that slow the functions of most major organ systems, such as decreased renal blood flow and decreased glomerular filtration. Frostbite results from prolonged exposure to dry temperatures far below freezing; hypothermia, from cold-water near-drowning and prolonged exposure to cold temperatures.

The risk of serious cold injuries, especially hypothermia, is increased by youth, lack of insulating body fat, wet or inadequate clothing, old age, drug abuse, cardiac disease, smoking, fatigue, hunger and depletion of caloric reserves, and excessive alcohol intake (which draws blood into capillaries and away from body organs).

Signs and symptoms

Frostbite may be deep or superficial. Superficial frostbite affects skin and subcutaneous tissue, especially of the face, ears, extremities, and other exposed body areas. Although it may go unnoticed at first, upon returning to a warm place, frostbite produces burning, tingling, numbness, swelling, and a mot-

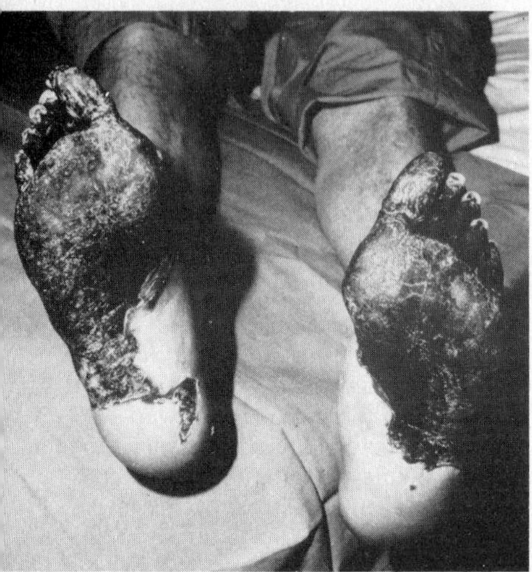

Frostbite of the feet. Blackened areas in photo show tissue necrosis and gangrene—the result of deep frostbite that extends beyond subcutaneous tissue.

tled, blue-gray skin color.

Deep frostbite extends beyond subcutaneous tissue and usually affects the hands or feet. The skin becomes white until it's thawed; then it turns purplish blue. Deep frostbite also produces pain, skin blisters, tissue necrosis, and gangrene.

Indications of hypothermia—a core body temperature below 95° F. (35° C.)—vary with severity:

• *Mild hypothermia*: Drop to 89.6° to 95° F. (32° to 35° C.), severe shivering, slurred speech, and amnesia
• *Moderate hypothermia*: Drop to 82.4° to 89.6° F. (28° to 32° C.), unresponsiveness, muscle rigidity, peripheral cyanosis, and, with improper rewarming, signs of shock
• *Severe hypothermia*: Drop to 77° to 82.4° F. (25° to 28° C.), loss of deep tendon reflexes and ventricular fibrillation. The patient may appear dead, with no palpable pulse or audible heart sounds. His pupils may dilate, and he appears to be in a state of rigor mortis. Body temperature drop below 77° F. (25° C.) causes cardiopulmonary arrest and death.

Diagnosis

A history of severe and prolonged exposure to cold may make this diagnosis obvious. But hypothermia can be overlooked if outdoor temperatures are above freezing or if the patient is comatose.

Treatment and special considerations

In a localized cold injury, treatment consists of rewarming the injured part, supportive measures, and sometimes a fasciotomy to increase circulation by lowering edematous tissue pressure. However, if gangrene occurs, amputation may be necessary. In hypothermia, therapy consists of immediate resuscitative measures, careful monitoring, and gradual rewarming of the body. Cold injuries in children suggest neglect or abuse and need a thorough history.

To treat localized cold injuries:

• Remove constrictive clothing and jewelry. Slowly rewarm the affected part in tepid water (about 100° to 108° F. [37.8° to 42.2° C.]). Give the patient warm fluids to drink. *Never* rub the injured area—this aggravates tissue damage.
• When the affected part begins to rewarm, the patient will feel pain, so give analgesics, as ordered. Check for a pulse. Be careful not to rupture any blebs. If the injury is on the foot, place cotton or gauze sponges between the toes to prevent maceration. Instruct the patient not to walk.
• If the injury has caused an open skin wound, give antibiotics and tetanus prophylaxis, as ordered.
• If pulse fails to return, the patient may develop compartment syndrome and need fasciotomy to restore circulation. If pain and edema persist, expect to give tolazoline intraarterially to create a temporary sympathectomy. If gangrene occurs, prepare for amputation.
• Before discharge, tell the patient about possible long-term effects: increased sensitivity to cold, burning and tingling, and increased sweating. Warn against smoking, since this causes vasoconstriction and slows healing.

To treat systemic hypothermia:

• If there's no pulse or respiration, begin cardiopulmonary resuscitation (CPR) immediately and, if necessary, continue it for 2 to 3 hours. (Remember: Hypothermia helps protect the brain from anoxia, which normally accompanies prolonged cardiopulmonary arrest. Therefore, even after the patient has been unresponsive for a long time, resuscitation may be possible, especially after cold-water near-drownings.) Perform CPR until the patient is adequately rewarmed.
• Move the patient to a warm area, remove wet clothing, and keep him dry. If he's conscious, give warm fluids with high sugar content, such as tea with sugar. If the patient's core temperature is above 89.6° F. (32° C.), use external warming techniques. Bathe him in water that is 104° F. (40° C.), cover him with a heating blanket set at 97.9° to 99.9° F. (36.6° to 37.7° C.), and cautiously apply hot water bottles at 104° F. to groin and axillae, guarding against burns.
• If the patient's core temperature is below 89.6° F. (32° C.), use internal and external warming methods. Rewarm his body core and surface 1 F. to 2 F. degrees per hour concurrently. (If you rewarm the surface first, rewarming shock can cause potentially fatal ventricular fibrillation.) To warm inhalations, provide oxygen heated to 107.6° to 114.8° F. (42° to 46° C.). Infuse I.V. solutions that have passed through a warming coil at 98.6° F. (37° C.), and give nasogastric lavage with normal saline solution that has been warmed to the same temperature. Assist with peritoneal lavage, using a normal saline solution (full or half strength) warmed to 98.6° F.; in severe hypothermia, assist with heart/lung bypass at controlled temperatures and thoracotomy with direct cardiac warm-saline bath.
• Throughout treatment, monitor arterial blood gases, intake and output, central venous pressure, temperature, and cardiac and neurologic status every half hour. Monitor lab results such as CBC, BUN, electrolytes, prothrombin time, and partial thromboplastin time.

Teach your patient how to prevent cold injuries:
• In cold weather, wear mittens (not gloves); windproof, water-resistant, many-layered clothing; two pairs of socks (cotton next to skin, then wool); and a scarf and a hat that cover the ears (to avoid substantial heat loss through the head).
• Before anticipated prolonged exposure to cold, don't drink alcohol or smoke, and get adequate food and rest.
• If caught in a severe snowstorm, find shelter early or increase physical activity to maintain body warmth.

Patients who have developed cold injuries because of inadequate clothes or housing may need referral to a community social service agency.

Heat Syndrome

Heat syndrome may result from environmental or internal conditions that increase heat production or impair heat dissipation. Heat syndromes fall into three categories: heat cramps, heat exhaustion, and heatstroke.

Causes

Normally, humans adjust to excessive temperatures by complex cardiovascular and neurologic changes, which are coordinated by the hypothalamus. Heat loss offsets heat production to regulate the body temperature. It does this by evaporation (sweating) or vasodilation, which cools the body's surface by radiation, conduction, and convection.

HOW TO MANAGE HEAT SYNDROME

TYPE AND PREDISPOSING FACTORS	SIGNS AND SYMPTOMS	MANAGEMENT
Heat cramps		
• Commonly affect young adults • Strenuous activity without training or acclimatization • Normal to high temperature or high humidity	• Muscle twitching and spasms, weakness, severe muscle cramps • Nausea • Normal temperature or slight fever • Normal CNS findings • Diaphoresis	• Hospitalization usually unnecessary. • To replace fluid and electrolytes, give salt tablets and balanced electrolyte drink. • Loosen patient's clothing, and have him lie down in a cool place. Massage his muscles. If muscle cramps are severe, start an I.V. infusion with normal saline solution.
Heat exhaustion		
• Commonly affects young people • Physical activity without acclimatization • Decreased heat dissipation • High temperature and humidity	• Muscle cramps (infrequent) • Nausea and vomiting • Decreased blood pressure • Thready, rapid pulse • Cool, pallid skin • Headache, mental confusion, syncope, giddiness • Oliguria, thirst • No fever	• Hospitalization usually unnecessary. • *Immediately* give salt tablets and balanced electrolyte drink. • Loosen patient's clothing, and put him in a shock position in a cool place. Massage his muscles. If cramps are severe, start an I.V. infusion, as ordered. • If needed, give oxygen.
Heatstroke		
• Exertional heatstroke commonly affects young, healthy people who are involved in strenuous activity. • Classical heatstroke commonly affects elderly, inactive people who have cardiovascular disease or who take drugs that influence temperature regulation. • High temperature and humidity without any wind	• Hypertension, followed by hypotension • Atrial or ventricular tachycardia • Hot, dry, red skin, which later turns gray; no diaphoresis • Confusion, progressing to seizures and loss of consciousness • Temperature higher than 104° F. (40° C.) • Dilated pupils • Slow, deep respiration; then Cheyne-Stokes	• Initiate ABCs of life support. • To lower body temperature, cool rapidly with ice packs on arterial pressure points and hypothermia blankets. • To replace fluids and electrolytes, start an I.V. infusion, as ordered. • Hospitalization needed. • Insert nasogastric tube to prevent aspiration. • Give diazepam to control seizures; chlorpromazine I.V. to reduce shivering; or mannitol to maintain urine output, as ordered. • Monitor temperature, intake, output, and cardiac status. Give dobutamine, as ordered, to correct cardiogenic shock. (Vasoconstrictors are contraindicated.)

However, heat production increases with exercise, infection, and drugs, such as amphetamines. Heat loss decreases with high temperatures or humidity, lack of acclimatization, excess clothing, obesity, dehydration, cardiovascular disease, sweat gland dysfunction, and drugs, such as phenothiazines and anticholinergics. So when heat loss mechanisms fail to offset heat production, the body retains heat and may develop heat syndrome.

Special considerations

Heat illnesses are easily preventable, so it's important to educate the public about the various factors that cause them. This information is especially vital for athletes, laborers, and soldiers in field training.

- Advise your patients to avoid heat syndrome by taking the following precautions in hot weather: wear loose-fitting, lightweight clothing; rest frequently; avoid hot places; and drink adequate fluids.
- Advise patients who are obese, elderly, or taking drugs that impair heat regulation to avoid overheating.
- Tell patients who've had heat cramps or heat exhaustion to exercise gradually and to increase their salt and water intake.
- Tell patients with heatstroke that residual hypersensitivity to high temperatures may persist for several months.

Asphyxia

A condition of insufficient oxygen and accumulating carbon dioxide in the blood and tissues due to interference with respiration, asphyxia results in cardiopulmonary arrest. Without prompt treatment it is fatal.

Causes

Asphyxia results from any internal or external condition or substance that inhibits respiration. Some examples:

- hypoventilation as result of narcotic abuse, medullary disease or hemorrhage, respiratory muscle paralysis, or cardiopulmonary arrest
- intrapulmonary obstruction, as in airway obstruction, pulmonary edema, pneumonia, and near-drowning
- extrapulmonary obstruction, as in tracheal compression from a tumor, strangulation, trauma, or suffocation
- inhalation of toxic agents, as in carbon monoxide poisoning, smoke inhalation, and excessive oxygen inhalation.

Signs and symptoms

Depending on the duration and degree of asphyxia, common symptoms include anxiety, dyspnea, agitation and confusion leading to coma, altered respiratory rate (apnea, bradypnea, occasional tachypnea), decreased breath sounds, central and peripheral cyanosis (cherry-red mucous membranes in late-stage carbon monoxide poisoning), convulsions, and fast, slow, or absent pulse.

Diagnosis

Diagnosis rests on patient history and laboratory results. Arterial blood gas measurement, the most important test, indicates decreased PO_2 (less than 60 mm Hg) and increased PCO_2 (more than 50 mm Hg) levels. Chest X-rays may show a foreign body, pulmonary edema, or atelectasis. Toxicology tests may show drugs, chemicals, or abnormal hemoglobin. Pulmonary function tests may indicate respiratory muscle weakness.

Treatment and special considerations

Asphyxia requires immediate respiratory support—with cardiopulmonary resuscitation, endotracheal intubation, and supplemental oxygen, as needed—and removal of the underlying cause: bronchoscopy for extraction of a foreign body, a narcotic antagonist like naloxone for narcotic overdose, gastric lavage for poisoning, and withholding of supplemental oxygen for CO_2 narcosis caused by excessive oxygen therapy.

Respiratory distress is frightening, so reassure the patient during treatment. Give drugs, as ordered. Suction carefully, as needed, and encourage deep breathing. Closely monitor vital signs and lab results. To prevent drug-induced asphyxia, warn patients about the danger of taking alcohol with other central nervous system depressants.

Near-drowning

Near-drowning refers to surviving—temporarily, at least—the physiologic effects of hypoxemia and acidosis that result from submersion in fluid. Hypoxemia and acidosis are the primary problems in victims of near-drowning.

Near-drowning occurs in three forms: (1) "dry"—the victim doesn't aspirate fluid but suffers respiratory obstruction or asphyxia (10% to 15% of patients); (2) "wet"—the victim aspirates fluid and suffers from asphyxia or secondary changes due to fluid aspiration (about 85% of patients); (3) secondary—the victim suffers recurrence of respiratory distress (usually aspiration pneumonia or pulmonary edema) within minutes or 1 to 2 days after a near-drowning incident.

Causes and incidence

In the United States, drowning claims nearly 8,000 lives annually. No statistics are available for near-drowning incidents. Near-drowning results from an inability to swim or, in swimmers, from panic, a boating accident, a heart attack or a blow to the head while in the water, drinking heavily before swimming, or a suicide attempt.

Regardless of the tonicity of the fluid aspirated, hypoxemia is the most serious consequence of near-drowning, followed by metabolic acidosis. Other consequences depend on the kind of water aspirated. After fresh water aspiration, changes in the character of lung surfactant result in exudation of protein-rich plasma into the alveoli. This, plus increased capillary permeability, leads to pulmonary edema and hypoxemia. After saltwater aspiration, the hypertonicity of sea water exerts an osmotic force, which pulls fluid from pulmonary capillaries into the alveoli. The resulting intrapulmonary shunt causes hypoxemia. Also, the pulmonary capillary membrane may be injured and induce pulmonary edema. In both kinds of near-drowning, pulmonary edema and hypoxemia are secondary to aspiration.

Signs and symptoms

Near-drowning victims can display a host of clinical problems: apnea, shallow or gasping respirations, substernal chest pain, asystole, tachycardia, bradycardia, restlessness, irritability, lethargy, fever, confusion, unconsciousness, vomiting, abdominal distention, and a cough that produces a pink, frothy fluid.

Diagnosis

Diagnosis requires a history of near-drowning, along with characteristic features and auscultation of rales and rhonchi. Supportive tests include:

- blood tests: arterial blood gases show decreased oxygen content, low HCO_3-, and low pH. Leukocytosis may occur.
- EKG: supraventricular tachycardia, occasional premature contractions, nonspecific ST segment, and T wave abnormalities may occur.

Treatment and special considerations

Emergency treatment begins with immediate cardiopulmonary resuscitation (CPR) and administration of oxygen (100%).

• When the patient arrives at the hospital, assess for a patent airway. Establish one, if necessary. Continue CPR, intubate the patient, and provide respiratory assistance, such as mechanical ventilation with positive end expiratory pressure, if needed.
• Assess arterial blood gases.
• If the patient's abdomen is distended, insert a nasogastric tube. (Intubate the patient first if he's unconscious.)
• Start I.V. lines; insert a Foley catheter.
• Give medications, as ordered. Much controversy exists about the benefits of drug treatment of near-drowning victims. However, such treatment may include sodium bicarbonate for acidosis, corticosteroids for cerebral edema, antibiotics to prevent infections, and bronchodilators to ease bronchospasms.
• Remember, all near-drowning victims should be admitted for an observation period of 24 to 48 hours because of the possibility of delayed drowning.
• Observe for pulmonary complications and signs of delayed drowning (confusion, substernal pain, adventitious breath sounds). Suction often. Pulmonary artery catheters may be useful in assessing cardiopulmonary status. Monitor vital signs, intake and output, and peripheral pulses. Check for skin perfusion. Watch for signs of infection.
• To facilitate breathing, raise the head of the bed slightly.
• To prevent near-drowning, advise swimmers to avoid drinking alcohol before swimming, to observe water safety measures, and to take a water safety course sponsored by the Red Cross, YMCA, or YWCA.

Decompression Sickness

("The bends," caisson disease)

Decompression sickness is a painful condition that results from too rapid change from high- to low-pressure environments (decompression). Usually, victims are scuba divers who ascend too quickly from water deeper than 33' and pilots and passengers of unpressurized aircraft who ascend too quickly to high altitudes.

Causes

Decompression sickness results from an abrupt change in air or water pressure that causes nitrogen to spill out of tissues faster than it can be diffused through respiration. It causes gas bubbles to form in blood and body tissues, which produce excruciating joint and muscle pain, neurologic and respiratory distress, and skin changes.

Signs and symptoms

Usually, symptoms appear during or within 30 minutes of rapid decompression, although they may be delayed up to 24 hours. Typically, decompression sickness results in:

• "the bends," which is deep and usually constant joint and muscle pain so severe that it may be incapacitating
• transitory neurologic disturbances, such as difficult urination (from bladder paralysis), hemiplegia, deafness, visual disturbances, dizziness, aphasia, paresthesia and hyperesthesia of the legs, unsteady gait, and, possibly, coma
• respiratory distress, known as the "chokes," which includes chest pain, retrosternal burning, and a cough that may become paroxysmal and uncontrollable.

Such symptoms may persist for days and result in dyspnea, cyanosis, fainting, and, occasionally, shock. Other symptoms include decreased temperature, pallor, itching, burning, mottled skin, and fatigue. In some patients, tachypnea may occur.

Diagnosis

History of rapid decompression and a physical examination showing characteristic clinical features confirm the diagnosis.

Treatment and special considerations

Treatment consists of supportive measures, with recompression and oxygen administration, followed by gradual decompression. Recompression takes place in a hyperbaric chamber (not available in all hospitals), in which air pressure is increased to 2.8 absolute atmospheric pressure over 1 to 2 minutes. This rapid rise in pressure reduces the size of the circulating nitrogen bubbles, and relieves pain and other clinical effects. During recompression, intermittent oxygen administration, with periodic maximal exhalations, promotes gas bubble diffusion. Once symptoms subside and diffusion is complete, a slow air pressure decrease in the chamber allows for gradual, safe decompression.

Supportive measures include fluid replacement in hypovolemic shock and sometimes corticosteroids to reduce the risk of spinal edema. Narcotics are contraindicated, since they further depress impaired respiration.

- To avoid oxygen toxicity during recompression, tell the patient to alternate breathing oxygen for 5 minutes with breathing air for 5 minutes.
- During oxygen administration, make sure all electrical equipment is grounded. Prohibit smoking and the use of electric razors and other electrical appliances in the patient's room, and don't use wool or other static electricity–producing blankets.
- If the patient with bladder paralysis needs catheterization, monitor intake and output accurately.
- To prevent decompression sickness, advise divers and fliers to follow the U.S. Navy's ascent guidelines.

Radiation Exposure

Expanded use of ionized radiation has vastly increased the incidence of radiation exposure. Cancer patients receiving radiation therapy and nuclear power plant workers are the most likely victims of this modern anomaly. The amount of radiation absorbed by a human body is measured in radiation absorbed doses (rads), not to be confused with roentgens, which are used to measure radiation emissions. A person can absorb up to 200 rads without fatal consequences. A dose of 450 rads is fatal in about half the cases; more than 600 rads is nearly always fatal. However, when radiation is focused on a small area, the body can absorb and survive many thousands of rads, if they are administered in carefully controlled doses over a long period of time. This basic principle is the key to safe and successful radiation therapy.

Causes

Exposure to radiation can occur by inhalation, ingestion, or direct contact. The existence and severity of tissue damage depend on the amount of body area exposed (the smaller, the better), length of exposure, dosage absorbed, distance from the source, and presence of protective shielding. Ionized radiation (X-rays, protons, neutrons, and alpha, beta, and gamma rays) may cause immediate cell necrosis or disturbed DNA synthesis, which impairs cell function and division. Rapidly dividing cells—bone marrow, hair follicles, gonads, lymph tissue—are most susceptible to radiation damage; highly differentiated cells—nerve, bone, muscle—resist radiation more successfully.

Signs and symptoms

The effects of ionized radiation can be immediate and acute, or delayed and chronic. Acute effects may be hematopoietic (after 200 to 500 rads), gastrointestinal (after 400 rads or more), cerebral (after 1,000 rads or more), or cardiovascular (gross after 5,000 rads). They depend strictly on the *amount* of radiation absorbed.

Acute hematopoietic radiation exposure induces nausea, vomiting, diarrhea, and anorexia, which subside after 24 to 48 hours. During the latent period that follows, pancytopenia develops. Within 2 to 3 weeks, thrombocytopenia, leukopenia, lymphopenia, and anemia produce nosebleeds, hemorrhage, petechiae, pallor, weakness, oropharyngeal abscesses, and increased susceptibility to infection because of impaired immunologic response.

Gastrointestinal radiation exposure causes ulceration, infection, intractable nausea, vomiting, and diarrhea, resulting in severe fluid and electrolyte imbalance. Breakdown of intestinal villi later causes plasma loss, which can lead to circulatory collapse and death.

Cerebral radiation poisoning after brief exposure to large amounts of radiation causes nausea, vomiting, and diarrhea within hours. Then lethargy, tremors, convulsions, confusion, coma, and even death may follow within hours or days.

Delayed or chronic effects from repeated, prolonged exposure to small doses of radiation over a long time can seriously damage skin, causing dryness, erythema, atrophy, and malignant lesions. (Such damage can also follow acute exposure.) Other delayed effects include alopecia, brittle nails, hypothyroidism, amenorrhea, cataracts, decreased fertility, anemia, leukopenia, thrombocytopenia, malignant neoplasms, bone necrosis and fractures, and a shortened life span. Long-term exposure to radiation may retard fetal growth or may cause genetic defects.

Diagnosis

An accurate history offers the best clues to radiation exposure. Supportive lab findings show decreased hematocrit, hemoglobin, white blood cell, platelet, and lymphocyte counts and decreased serum electrolytes (K and Cl) from vomiting and diarrhea. Bone marrow studies show blood dyscrasia; X-rays may reveal bone necrosis. A Geiger counter may help determine the amount of radiation in open wounds.

Treatment

Treatment is essentially symptomatic and includes antiemetics to counter nausea and vomiting, fluid and electrolyte replacement, antibiotics, and possibly sedatives, if convulsions occur. Transfusions of plasma, platelets, and red blood cells may be necessary. Bone marrow transplant is a controversial treatment but may be the only recourse in extreme cases. When radiation exposure results from inhalation or ingestion of large amounts

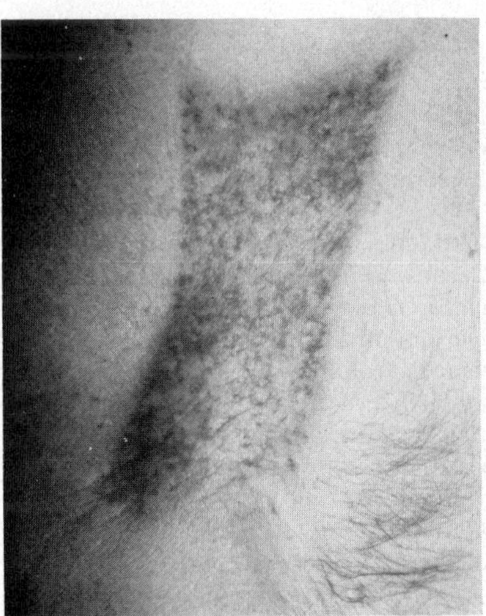

Radiation dermatitis of the axilla. Repeated prolonged exposure to radiation—even small doses—often induces erythematous dermatitis and atrophy of skin at site of radiation treatment.

of radioiodine, potassium iodide or a strong iodine solution may be given to block thyroid uptake.

Special considerations

- To minimize radiation exposure, dispose of contaminated clothing properly. If the patient's skin is contaminated, wash his body thoroughly with a chelating solution (calcium trisodium pentetate or calcium disodium edetate) and water. Debride and irrigate open wounds. If he recently ingested radioactive material, induce vomiting and start lavage.
- Monitor intake and output, and maintain fluid and electrolyte balance. Give I.V. fluids and electrolytes, as ordered. If the patient can take oral feedings, encourage a high-protein, high-calorie diet. Tell him to use a soft toothbrush to minimize gum bleeding. Offer lidocaine to soothe painful mouth ulcers.
- To prevent skin breakdown, make sure the patient avoids extreme temperatures, tight clothing, and drying soaps. Use rigid aseptic technique.
- Prevent complications. Monitor vital signs and watch for signs of hemorrhage.
- Provide emotional support for the patient and his family, especially after severe exposure. Suggest genetic counseling and screening, as needed.

Hospital personnel can avoid exposure to radiation by wearing proper shielding devices when supervising X-ray and radiation treatments. If you work in these vulnerable areas, wear radiation detection badges and turn them in periodically for readings.

MISCELLANEOUS INJURIES

Poisoning

Inhalation, ingestion, or injection of, or skin contamination with, any harmful substance is a common problem. In fact, in the United States, approximately 10 million persons are poisoned annually, 4,000 of them fatally. Prognosis depends on the amount of poison absorbed, its toxicity, and the time interval between poisoning and treatment.

Causes

Because of their curiosity and ignorance, children are the most common poison victims. In fact, accidental poisoning—usually from the ingestion of salicylates (aspirin), cleaning agents, insecticides, paints, and cosmetics—is the fourth leading cause of death in children.

In adults, poisoning is most common among chemical company employees, particularly those in companies that use chlorine, carbon dioxide, hydrogen sulfide, nitrogen dioxide, and ammonia, and in companies that ignore safety standards. Other causes of poisoning in adults include improper cooking, canning, and storage of food; ingestion of, or skin contamination from, plants; and accidental or intentional drug overdose (usually barbiturates).

Signs and symptoms

Symptoms vary according to the poison.

Diagnosis

A history of ingestion, inhalation, or injection of, or skin contact with, a poisonous substance and typical clinical features suggest the diagnosis. Suspect poisoning in any unconscious patient with no history of diabetes, seizure disorders, or trauma.

Toxicologic studies (including drug screens) of poison levels in the mouth,

COMMON POISONOUS PLANTS

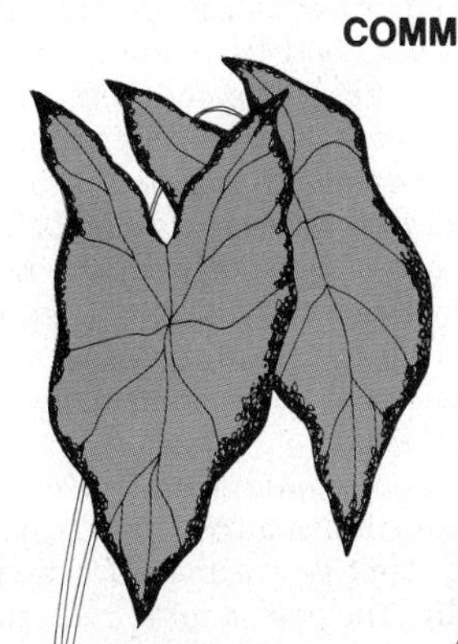

ELEPHANT EAR PHILODENDRON
Sx: burning throat and GI distress
Rx: gastric lavage or emesis; antihistamines and lime juice; symptomatic treatment

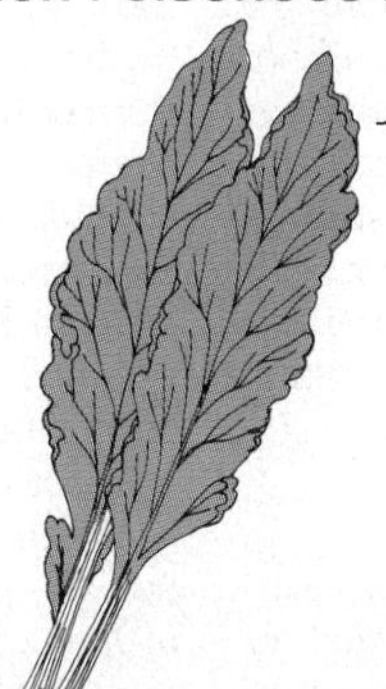

RHUBARB LEAVES
Sx: GI and respiratory distress, internal bleeding, coma
Rx: gastric lavage or emesis with lime water; calcium gluconate and force fluids

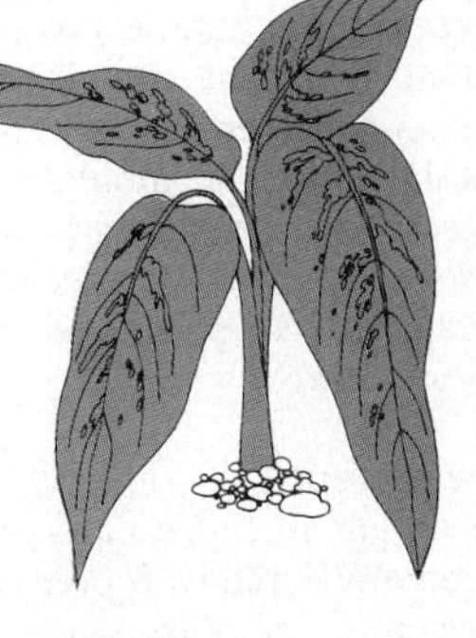

DIEFFENBACHIA
Sx: burning throat, edema, GI distress
Rx: gastric lavage or emesis; antihistamines and lime juice; symptomatic treatment

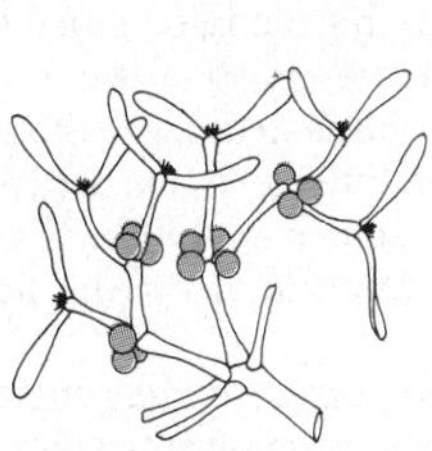

MISTLETOE
Sx: GI distress and slow pulse
Rx: gastric lavage or emesis; cardiac drugs, potassium, and sodium

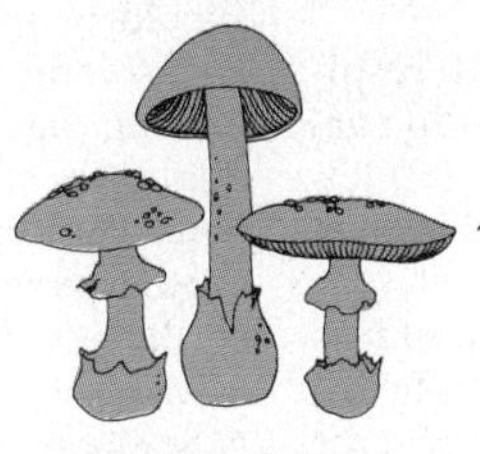

MUSHROOMS
Sx: GI, respiratory, CNS, parasympathomimetic effects
Rx: lavage with potassium permanganate; saline catharsis; atropine

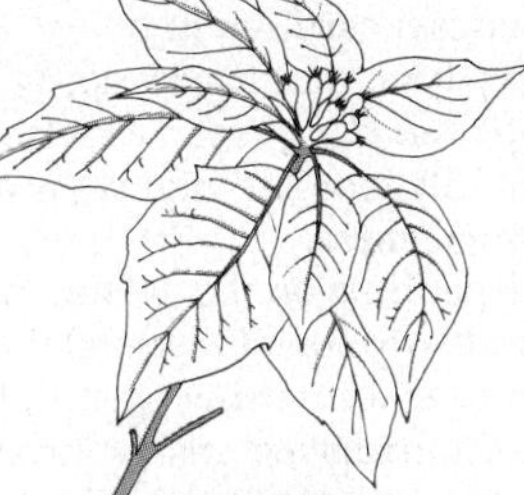

POINSETTIA
(milky juice)
Sx: inflammation and blisters
Rx: none; condition will disappear after several days

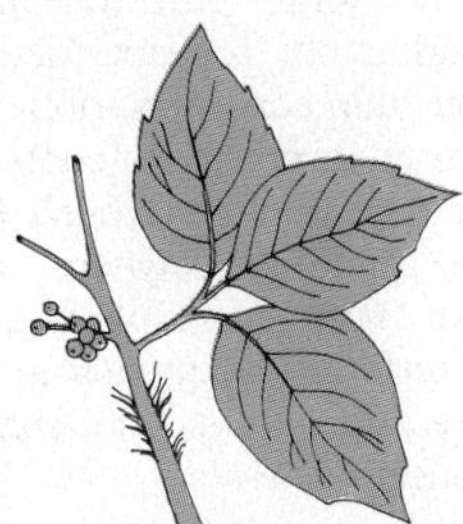

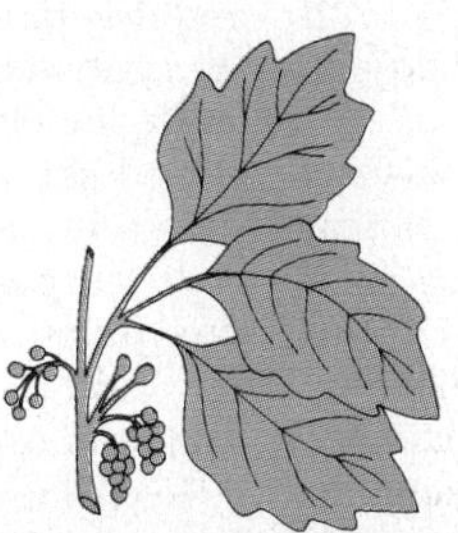

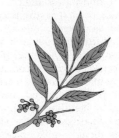

POISON IVY, POISON SUMAC, POISON OAK (sap)
Sx: allergic skin reactions; if ingested, GI distress, liver and kidney damage
Rx: if ingested: demulcents, morphine, fluids; high-protein low-fat diet. For skin reactions: antihistamine, topical antipyretics.

Poisonous parts of the plant appear in color. If the poisonous part can't be shown, it appears in parentheses after the plant's name.

vomitus, urine, feces, or blood or on the victim's hands or clothing confirm the diagnosis. If possible, have the family or patient bring the container holding the poison to the emergency room for comparable study. In inhalation poisoning, chest X-rays may show pulmonary infiltrates or edema; in petroleum distillate inhalation, X-rays may show aspiration pneumonia.

Treatment

Treatment includes emergency resuscitation and support, prevention of further absorption of poison, continuing supportive or symptomatic care, and, when possible, a specific antidote. If barbiturate, glutethimide, or tranquilizer poisoning causes hypothermia, use a hyperthermia blanket to control the patient's temperature.

Special considerations

- Assess cardiopulmonary and respiratory function. If necessary, begin cardiopulmonary resuscitation (CPR). Carefully monitor vital signs and level of consciousness.
- Depending on the poison, prevent further absorption of ingested poison by inducing emesis using syrup of ipecac or by administering gastric lavage and cathartics (magnesium sulfate). The treatment's effectiveness depends on the speed of absorption and the time elapsed between ingestion and removal. With syrup of ipecac, give warm water (usually less than 1 quart [less than 1 liter]) until vomiting occurs, or give another dose of ipecac, as ordered.
- Never induce emesis if you suspect corrosive acid poisoning, if the patient is unconscious or has convulsions, or if the gag reflex is impaired even in a conscious patient. Instead, neutralize the poison by instilling the appropriate antidote by nasogastric tube. Common antidotes include milk, magnesium salts (milk of magnesia), activated charcoal, or other chelating agents (deferoxamine, edetate disodium [EDTA]). When possible, add the antidote to water or juice. (Note: The removal of hydrocarbon poisoning is controversial. In the conscious patient, since there is a lower risk of aspiration with ipecac-induced emesis than with lavage, emesis is becoming the preferred treatment, but some doctors still use lavage. Moreover, some believe that because of poor absorption, kerosene [a hydrocarbon] does not require removal from the gastrointestinal tract; others believe removal depends on the amount ingested.)
- When you do want to induce emesis and the patient has already taken syrup of ipecac, don't give activated charcoal to neutralize the poison until *after* emesis. Activated charcoal absorbs ipecac.
- To perform gastric lavage, instill 30 ml fluid by nasogastric tube; then aspirate the liquid. Repeat until aspirate is clear. Save vomitus and aspirate for analysis. (To prevent aspiration in the unconscious patient, an endotracheal tube should be in place before lavage.)
- If several hours have passed since the patient ingested the poison, use large quantities of I.V. fluids to diurese the patient. The kind of fluid you'll use depends on the patient's acid-base balance and cardiovascular status, and on the flow rate.
- Severe ingested poisoning may call for peritoneal dialysis or hemodialysis.
- To prevent further absorption of inhaled poison, remove the patient to fresh or uncontaminated air. Alert the anesthesia department and provide supplemental oxygen. Some patients may require intubation. To prevent further absorption from skin contamination, remove the clothing covering the contaminated skin, and immediately flush the area with large amounts of water.
- If the patient is in severe pain, give analgesics, as ordered; frequently monitor fluid intake and output, vital signs, and level of consciousness.
- Keep the patient warm, and provide support in a quiet environment.
- If the poison was ingested intentionally, refer the patient for counseling to prevent future suicide attempts.
- For more specific treatment, contact the local poison center.

• To prevent accidental poisoning, instruct patients to read the label before they take medicine. Tell them to store all medications and household chemicals properly, keep them out of reach of children, and discard old medications. Warn them not to take medicines prescribed for someone else, not to transfer medicines from their original bottles to other containers without labeling them properly, and never to transfer poisons to food containers. Parents should not take medicine in front of their young children or call medicine "candy" to get children to take it. Stress the importance of using toxic sprays only in well-ventilated areas and of following instructions carefully. Tell patients to use pesticides carefully and to keep the number of their poison control center handy.

Poisonous Snakebites

Each year, poisonous snakes bite about 7,000 persons in the United States. Such bites are most common during summer afternoons, in grassy or rocky habitats. Poisonous snakebites are medical emergencies. With prompt, correct treatment, they need not be fatal.

Causes

The only poisonous snakes in the United States are pit vipers (Crotalidae) and coral snakes (Elapidae). Pit vipers include rattlesnakes, water moccasins (cottonmouths), and copperheads. They have a pitted depression between their eyes and nostrils, and two fangs ¾" to 1¼" (2 to 3 cm) long. Since fangs may break off or grow behind old ones, some snakes may have one, three, or four fangs.

Since coral snakes are nocturnal and placid, their bites are less common than pit viper bites; pit vipers are also nocturnal but are more active. The fangs of coral snakes are short but have teeth behind them. Coral snakes have distinctive red, black, and yellow bands (yellow bands always border red ones), tend to bite with a chewing motion, and may leave multiple fang marks, small lacerations, and much tissue destruction.

Signs and symptoms

Most snakebites happen on the arms and legs, below the elbow or knee. Bites to the head or trunk are most dangerous, but any bite into a blood vessel is dangerous, regardless of location.

Most pit viper bites that result in envenomation cause immediate and progressively severe pain and edema (the entire extremity may swell within a few hours), local elevation in skin temperature, fever, skin discoloration, petechiae, ecchymoses, blebs, blisters, bloody wound discharge, and local necrosis.

Because pit viper venom is neurotoxic, pit viper bites may cause local and facial numbness and tingling, fasciculation and twitching of skeletal muscles, convulsions (especially in children), extreme anxiety, difficulty in speaking, fainting, weakness, dizziness, excessive sweating, occasional paralysis, mild to severe respiratory distress, headache, blurred vision, marked thirst, and, in severe envenomation, coma and death. Pit viper venom may also impair coagulation and cause hematemesis, hematuria, melena, bleeding gums, and internal bleeding. Other symptoms of pit viper bites include nausea, vomiting, diarrhea, tachycardia, lymphadenopathy, hypotension, and shock.

The reaction to coral snakebite is usually delayed—perhaps up to several hours. These snakebites cause little or no local tissue reaction (local pain, swelling, or necrosis). However, because their venom is neurotoxic, a reaction can progress swiftly, producing such effects as local paresthesia, weakness, euphoria, drowsiness, nausea, vomiting, difficulty swallowing, marked salivation, dysphonia, ptosis, blurred vision, miosis, respiratory distress and possible respiratory failure, loss of muscle coordination, abnormal reflexes, peripheral paralysis, and, possibly, shock with cardiovascular collapse and death. Coral snakebites can also cause coagulotoxicity.

Diagnosis

Patient history, observation of fang marks, snake identification (when possible), and progressive symptoms of envenomation all point to poisonous snakebite. Lab values help identify the extent of envenomation and provide guidelines for supportive treatment. Abnormal lab results may include prolonged bleeding time and partial thromboplastin time, decreased hemoglobin and hematocrit, sharply decreased platelet count (less than 200,000/mm^3), urinalysis showing hematuria, and, in infection (snake mouths contain gram-negative bacteria), increased white blood cell count. Chest X-ray may show pulmonary edema or emboli, an EKG may show tachycardia and ectopic beats, and severe envenomation may produce an abnormal EEG. (Usually, an EKG is necessary only in severe envenomation for a patient over age 40.)

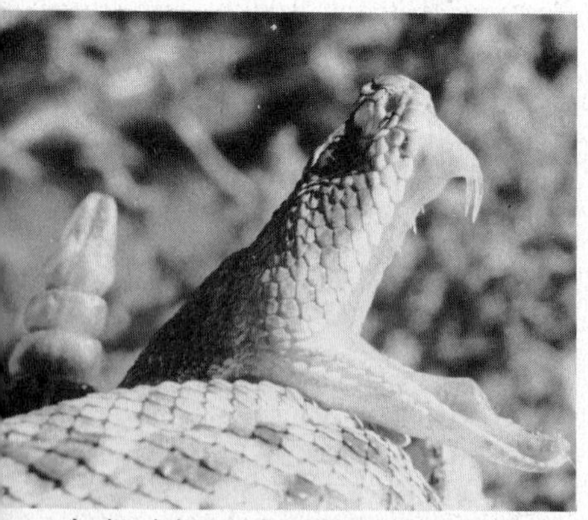

A pitted depression between eyes and nostrils, and two long fangs are characteristic of pit vipers, the most common poisonous snakes.

Treatment

Prompt, appropriate first aid can reduce venom absorption and prevent severe symptoms.

- If possible, identify the snake, but don't waste time trying to find it.
- Immediately immobilize the limb below heart level, and instruct the victim to remain as quiet as possible.
- Apply a slightly *constrictive tourniquet* (one that obstructs only lymphatic and superficial venous blood flow) about 4″ (10 cm) above the fang marks, or just above the first joint proximal to the bite. Caution: Do not apply this constrictive tourniquet if more than 30 minutes has elapsed since the bite. Also, total constrictive tourniquet time should not exceed 2 hours; nor should it delay antivenin administration. Release the tourniquet for 60 to 90 seconds every 30 minutes, but consider that most feel release is only necessary if swelling progresses rapidly. Apply a *tight tourniquet* only for extremely severe envenomation by a coral snake. In this case, apply a tight tourniquet, and release it every 10 minutes for 90 seconds until you can administer antivenin. Remember: Loss of limb is possible if a tourniquet is too tight or if tourniquet time is too long.
- Wash the skin over the fang marks. Within 30 minutes of pit viper bites, make an incision through the marks approximately ½″ (1.27 cm) long and ⅛″ (3 mm) deep. Be especially careful if the bite is on the hand, where blood vessels and tendons are close to the skin surface. Using a bulb syringe—or, if no other means is available, mouth suction—apply suction for 20 to 30 minutes and for up to 2 hours in the absence of antivenin administration. Remember: An incision and suction are effective only in pit viper bites and only within 30 minutes of the bite; also, mouth suction is contraindicated if the rescuer has oral ulcers.
- Never give the victim alcoholic drinks or stimulants, since these speed venom absorption. Never apply ice to a snake-

bite: it increases tissue damage.

• Transport the victim as quickly as possible, keeping him warm and at rest. Record the signs and symptoms of progressive envenomation and when they develop. Most snakebite victims are hospitalized for only 24 to 48 hours, but some remain longer after severe envenomation. Usually, treatment consists of antivenin administration, though minor snakebites may not require antivenin. Other treatment includes tetanus toxoid or tetanus immune globulin, human; broad-spectrum antibiotics; and, depending on respiratory status, severity of pain, and type of snakebite (narcotics are contraindicated in coral snakebites), aspirin, codeine, morphine, or meperidine. Usually, necrotic snakebites need surgical debridement after 3 or 4 days. Intense, rapidly progressive edema requires fasciotomy within 2 or 3 hours of the bite; extreme envenomation may require limb amputation and subsequent reconstructive surgery, rehabilitation, and physical therapy.

Special considerations

When the patient arrives at the hospital, immobilize the extremity if this hasn't already been done. If a tight tourniquet has been applied within the past hour, apply a loose tourniquet proximally and remove the first tourniquet. Release the second tourniquet gradually during antivenin administration, as ordered. A sudden release of venom into the bloodstream can cause cardiorespiratory collapse, so keep emergency equipment handy.

• On a flow sheet, document vital signs, level of consciousness, skin color, swelling, respiratory status, description of the bite, surrounding area, and symptoms. Monitor vital signs every 15 minutes and check for a pulse in the affected limb.

• Start an I.V. with a large-bore needle for antivenin administration. Severe bites that result in coagulotoxic signs and symptoms may require two I.V. lines: one for antivenin, the second for blood products.

• Before antivenin administration, obtain a patient history of allergies (especially to horse serum) and other medical problems. Do hypersensitivity tests, as ordered, and assist with desensitization, as needed. During antivenin administration, keep epinephrine, oxygen, and vasopressors available to combat anaphylaxis from horse serum.

• Give packed cells, whole blood, I.V. fluids, and, possibly, fresh frozen plasma or platelets, as ordered, to counteract coagulotoxicity and maintain blood pressure. If the patient develops respiratory distress and requires endotracheal intubation or tracheotomy, give good tracheostomy care.

• Give analgesics, as needed. *Don't* give narcotics to victims of coral snakebites. Clean the snakebite using sterile technique. Open, debride, and drain any blebs and blisters, since they may contain venom. Be sure to change dressings daily.

• If the patient requires hospitalization for longer than 24 to 48 hours, position him carefully to avoid contractures. Give passive exercises until the fourth day after the bite, then active exercises and whirlpool treatments, as ordered.

• Encourage hikers and campers to carry a snakebite kit if they'll be more than a half hour from the nearest hospital.

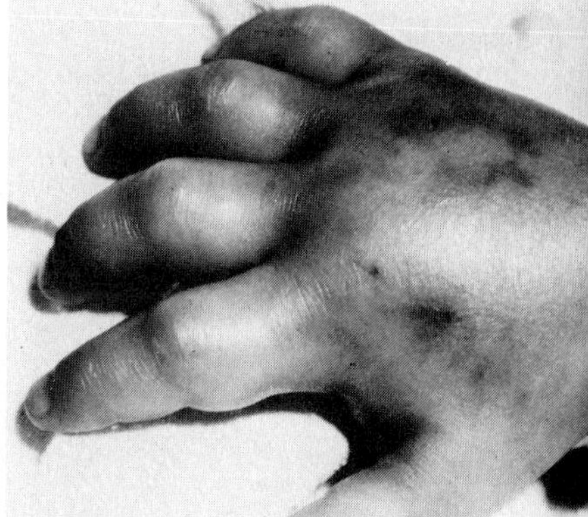

After snakebite, severe edema of the affected extremity occurs within hours.

Insect Bites and Stings

Among the most common traumatic complaints are insect bites and stings, the more serious of which include those of a tick, brown recluse spider, black widow spider, scorpion, bee, wasp, or yellow jacket.

GENERAL INFORMATION	CLINICAL FEATURES
Tick • Common in woods and fields throughout the United States • Attaches to host in any of its life stages (larva, nymph, adult). Fastens to host with its teeth, then secretes a cementlike material to reinforce attachment. • Flat, brown, speckled body about 0.25″ (6.25 mm) long; has eight legs • Also transmits diseases such as Rocky Mountain spotted fever.	• Itching may be sole symptom; or after several days, host may develop tick paralysis (acute flaccid paralysis, starting as paresthesia and pain in legs and resulting in respiratory failure from bulbar paralysis).
Brown recluse (violin) spider • Common to south-central United States; usually found in dark areas (outdoor privy, barn, woodshed) • Dark brown violin on its back, three pairs of eyes; female more dangerous than male • Most bites occur between April and October. 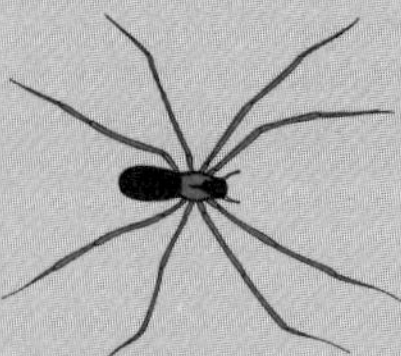	Venom is coagulotoxic. Reaction begins within 2 to 8 hours after bite. • Localized vasoconstriction causes ischemic necrosis at bite site. Small, reddened puncture wound forms a bleb and becomes ischemic. In 3 to 4 days, center becomes dark and hard. Within 2 to 3 weeks, an ulcer forms. • Minimal initial pain increases over time. • Other symptoms: fever, chills, malaise, weakness, nausea, vomiting, edema, convulsions, joint pains, petechiae, cyanosis, phlebitis • Rarely, thrombocytopenia and hemolytic anemia develop and lead to death within first 24 to 48 hours (usually in a child or patient with previous history of cardiac disease). Prompt and appropriate treatment results in recovery.
Black widow spider • Common throughout the United States, particularly in warmer climates; usually found in dark areas (outdoor privy, barn, woodshed) • Female is coal black with a red or orange hourglass on her ventral side; she is larger than male (male does not bite). • Mortality less than 1% (increased risk among the elderly, infants, and those with allergies). 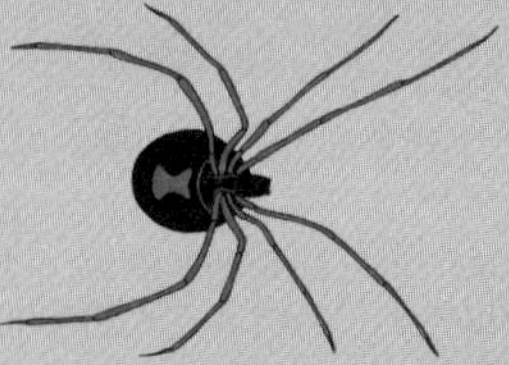	Venom is neurotoxic. Age, size, and sensitivity of patient determines severity and progression of symptoms • Pinprick sensation, followed by dull, numbing pain (may go unnoticed) • Edema and tiny, red bite marks • Rigidity of stomach muscles and severe abdominal pain (10 to 40 minutes after bite) • Muscle spasms in extremities • Ascending paralysis, causing difficulty in swallowing and labored, grunting respirations • Other symptoms: extreme restlessness, vertigo, sweating, chills, pallor, convulsions (especially in children), hyperactive reflexes, hypertension, tachycardia, thready pulse, circulatory collapse, nausea, vomiting, headache, ptosis, eyelid edema, urticaria, pruritus, and fever

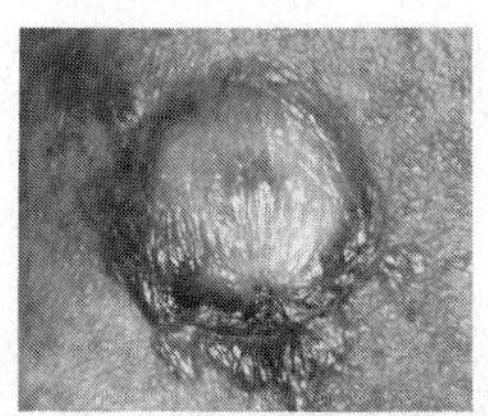

After brown recluse (violin) spider bite, localized vasoconstriction causes ischemic necrosis at bite site. Small, reddened puncture wound forms a bleb and becomes ischemic.

TREATMENT	SPECIAL CONSIDERATIONS
• Removal of tick • Local antipruritics for itching papule • Mechanical ventilation for respiratory failure	• To remove tick, cover it with mineral, salad, or machine oil, or alcohol on a tissue or gauze pad. This blocks the tick's breathing pores and causes it to withdraw from the skin. If the tick doesn't disengage after the pad has been in place for ½ hour, carefully remove it with tweezers, taking care to remove all parts. • To reduce risk of being bitten, teach the patient to keep away from wooded areas, to wear protective clothes, and to carefully examine body for ticks after being outdoors. • Teach patients how to safely remove ticks.
• No known specific treatment • Combination therapy with corticosteroids, antibiotics, antihistamines, tranquilizers, I.V. fluids, and tetanus prophylaxis • Lesion excision in first 10 to 12 hours relieves pain. A split-thickness skin graft closes the wound. Without grafting, healing may take 6 to 8 weeks. • A large chronic ulcer may require skin grafting.	• Cleanse the lesion with a 1:20 Burow's aluminum acetate solution, and as ordered, apply antibiotic ointment. • Take complete patient history, including allergies and other preexisting medical problems. • Monitor vital signs, patient's general appearance, and any changes at bite site. • Reassure patient with disfiguring ulcer that skin grafting can improve appearance. • To prevent brown recluse bites, tell patients to spray areas of infestation with creosote at least every 2 months, to wear gloves and heavy clothes when working around woodpiles or sheds, to inspect outdoor working clothes for spiders before use, and to discourage children from playing near infested areas.
• Neutralization of venom using antivenin I.V., preceded by desensitization when skin or eye tests show sensitivity to horse serum • Calcium gluconate I.V. to control muscle spasms. • Muscle relaxants like diazepam for severe muscle spasms • Adrenalin or antihistamines • Oxygen by nasal cannula or mask • Tetanus immunization • Antibiotics to prevent infection	• Take complete patient history, including allergies and other preexisting medical problems. • Have epinephrine and emergency resuscitation equipment on hand in case of anaphylactic reaction to antivenin. • Keep patient quiet and warm, and the affected part immobile. • Cleanse bite site with antiseptic, and apply ice to relieve pain and swelling, and to slow circulation. • Check vital signs frequently during first 12 hours after bite. Report any changes to doctor. Symptoms usually subside in 3 to 4 hours. • When giving analgesics, monitor respiratory status. • To prevent black widow spider bites, tell patient to spray areas of infestation with creosote at least every 2 months, to wear gloves and heavy clothing when working around woodpiles or sheds, to inspect outdoor working clothes for spiders before putting them on, and to discourage children from playing near infested areas.

GENERAL INFORMATION	CLINICAL FEATURES
Scorpion • Common throughout the United States (30 different species); two deadly species in southwestern states • Curled tail with stinger on end; eight legs; 3″ (7.5 cm) long • Most stings occur during warmer months. • Mortality less than 1% (increased risk among the elderly and children).	*Nonlethal reaction:* anaphylaxis (rare) • Local swelling and tenderness, sharp burning sensation, skin discoloration, paresthesia, lymphangitis with regional gland swelling *Lethal reaction* (neurotoxic): immediate sharp pain; hyperesthesia; drowsiness; itching of nose, throat, and mouth; impaired speech (due to sluggish tongue); generalized muscle spasms (including jaw muscle spasms, laryngospasms, incontinence, convulsions, nausea, vomiting, drooling) • Symptoms last from 24 to 78 hours. Bite site recovers last. • Death may follow cardiovascular or respiratory failure. • Prognosis is poor if symptoms progress rapidly in first few hours.
Bee, wasp, and yellow jacket • When a honeybee (rounded abdomen) or a bumblebee (over 1″ [2.5 cm] long; furry, rounded abdomen) stings, its stinger remains in the victim; the bee flies away and dies. • A wasp or yellow jacket (slender body with elongated abdomen) retains its stinger and can sting repeatedly.	*Localized reaction:* painful wound (protruding stinger from bees), edema, urticaria, pruritus *Systemic reaction* (anaphylaxis): symptoms of hypersensitivity usually appear within 20 minutes and may include weakness, chest tightness, dizziness, nausea, vomiting, abdominal cramps, and throat constriction. The shorter the interval between the sting and systemic symptoms, the worse the prognosis. Without prompt treatment, symptoms may progress to cyanosis, coma, and death.

Open Trauma Wounds

(Abrasions, avulsions, crush wounds, lacerations, missile injuries, punctures)

Open trauma wounds are injuries that often result from home, work, or motor vehicle accidents and from acts of violence. For information on specific types of wounds, see the chart on page 308.

Assessment

In all open wounds, assess the extent of injury, vital signs, level of consciousness, obvious skeletal damage, local neurologic deficits, and general patient condition. Obtain an accurate history of the injury from the patient or witnesses, including such details as the mechanism and time of injury and any treatment already provided. If the injury involved a weapon, notify the police.

Also assess for peripheral nerve damage—a common complication in lacerations and other open trauma wounds, as well as fractures and dislocations. Signs of peripheral nerve damage vary with location.

• *Radial nerve:* weak forearm dorsiflexion, inability to extend thumb in a hitchhiker's sign
• *Median nerve:* numbness in tip of index finger; inability to place forearm in

TREATMENT	SPECIAL CONSIDERATIONS
• Antivenin (made from cat serum), if available. (Contact Antivenin Lab, Arizona State University, Tempe, Arizona.) • Calcium gluconate I.V. for muscle spasm • Phenobarbital I.M. for convulsions • Emetine subcutaneously to relieve pain (opiates such as morphine and codeine are contraindicated because they enhance the venom's effects).	• Take complete patient history, including allergies and other preexisting medical conditons. • Immobilize patient, and apply tourniquet proximal to sting. • Pack area extending beyond tourniquet in ice. After 5 minutes of ice pack, remove tourniquet. • Monitor vital signs. Watch closely for signs of respiratory distress. (Keep emergency resuscitation equipment available.)
• Antihistamines and corticosteroids (in urticaria) • Tetanus prophylaxis *In anaphylaxis:* • Oxygen by nasal cannula or mask • Epinephrine 1:1,000 subcutaneously or I.M. • In bronchospasm, aminophylline and hydrocortisone • In hypotension, epinephrine and isoproterenol	If stinger is in place, scrape it off. Don't pull it; this action releases more toxin. • Cleanse the site and apply ice. • Watch the patient carefully for signs of anaphylaxis. Keep emergency resuscitation equipment available. • Tell patient who is allergic to bee stings to wear a medical identification bracelet or carry a card, and to carry an anaphylaxis kit. Teach him how to use the kit, and refer him to an allergist for hyposensitization. • To prevent bee stings, tell patient not to wear fragrant cosmetics during insect season, to avoid wearing bright colors and going barefoot, to avoid flowers and fruit that attract bees, and to use insect repellent.

prone position; weak forearm, thumb, and index finger flexion
• *Ulnar nerve:* numbness in tip of little finger, clawing of hand
• *Peroneal nerve:* inability to extend the foot or big toe, footdrop
• *Sciatic and tibial nerves:* paralysis of ankles and toes, footdrop, weakness in leg, numbness in sole.

Most open wounds require emergency treatment. In those with suspected nerve involvement, however, electromyography, nerve conduction, and electrical stimulation tests can provide more detailed information about possible peripheral nerve damage.

Treatment and special considerations

• If hemorrhage occurs, stop bleeding by applying direct pressure on the wound and, if necessary, on arterial pressure points. If the wound is on an extremity, elevate it, if possible. Don't apply a tourniquet except in life-threatening hemorrhage. If you must do so, be aware that resulting lack of perfusion to tissue could necessitate limb amputation.
• Frequently assess vital signs in patients with major wounds. Be alert for a 20 mm Hg drop in blood pressure and a 20 beat increase in pulse (compare the patient's blood pressure and pulse when he's sitting with his blood pressure and pulse when he's lying down), increased respirations, decreasing level of consciousness, thirst, and cool, clammy skin—all indicate blood loss and hypovolemic shock.
• Administer oxygen.
• Send blood specimens to the laboratory for type and cross match, complete blood count (including hematocrit and hemoglobin levels), and prothrombin

HOW TO MANAGE OPEN TRAUMA

TYPE	CLINICAL ACTION
Abrasion Open surface wounds (scrapes) of epidermis and possibly the dermis, resulting from friction. Nerve endings exposed. Diagnosis based on scratches, reddish welts, bruises, pain, and history of friction injury.	• Obtain a history to distinguish injury from second-degree burn. • Cleanse gently with topical germicide, and irrigate. Too vigorous scrubbing of abrasions will increase tissue damage. • Remove all imbedded foreign objects. Apply local anesthetic if cleansing is very painful. • Apply light, water-soluble antibiotic cream to prevent infection. • If wound is severe, apply loose protective dressing that allows air to circulate. • Administer tetanus prophylaxis, if necessary.
Avulsion Complete tissue loss that prevents approximation of wound edges, resulting from cutting, gouging, or complete tearing of skin. Frequently affects nose tip, earlobe, fingertip, and penis. Diagnosis based on full-thickness skin loss, hemorrhage, pain, history of trauma. X-ray required to rule out bone damage; CBC and differential before surgery.	• Check history for bleeding tendencies and use of anticoagulants. • Record time of injury to help determine if tissue is salvageable. Preserve tissue (if available) in cool saline solution for possible split-thickness graft or flap. • Control hemorrhage with pressure, absorbable gelatin sponge, or topical thrombin. • Cleanse gently, irrigate with saline solution, and debride, if necessary. Cover with a bulky dressing. • Tell patient to leave dressing in place until return visit, to keep area dry, and to watch for signs of infection (pain, fever, redness, swelling). • Administer analgesic and tetanus prophylaxis, if necessary.
Crush wound Heavy falling object splits skin and causes necrosis along split margins and damages tissue underneath. May look like laceration. Diagnosis based on history of trauma, edema, hemorrhage, massive hematomas, damage to surrounding tissues (fractures, nerve injuries, loss of tendon function), shock, pain, history of trauma. X-rays required to determine extent of injury to surrounding structures. CBC and differential, and electrolyte count also required.	• Check history for bleeding tendencies and use of anticoagulants. • Cleanse open areas gently with soap and water. • Control hemorrhage with pressure and cold pack. • Apply dry, sterile bulky dressing; wrap entire extremity in compression dressing. • Immobilize injured extremity, and encourage patient to rest. Monitor vital signs, and check peripheral pulses and circulation often. • Administer tetanus prophylaxis, if necessary. • Severe injury may require I.V. infusion of lactated Ringer's or saline solution with large-bore catheter, and surgical exploration, debridement, and repair.
Puncture wound Small-entry wounds that probably damage underlying structures, resulting from sharp, pointed objects. Diagnosis based on hemorrhage (rare), deep hematomas (in chest or abdominal wounds), ragged wound edges (in bites), small-entry wound (in very sharp object), pain, and history of trauma. X-rays can detect retention of injuring object.	• Check history for bleeding tendencies and use of anticoagulants. • Obtain description of injury, including force of entry. • Assess extent of injury. • Don't remove impaling objects until injury is completely evaluated. (If the eye is injured, call ophthalmologist immediately.) • Thoroughly cleanse injured area with soap and water. Irrigate all minor wounds with saline solution after removing foreign object. • Leave human bite wounds open. Apply dry, sterile dressing to other minor puncture wounds. • Tell patient to apply warm soaks daily. • Administer tetanus prophylaxis and, if necessary, rabies vaccine. • Deep wounds that damage underlying tissues may require exploratory surgery; retention of injuring object requires surgical removal.

TYPE	CLINICAL ACTION
Laceration Open wound, possibly extending into deep epithelium, resulting from penetration with knife or other sharp object or from a severe blow with a blunt object. Diagnosis based on hemorrhage, torn or destroyed tissues, pain, and history of trauma.	*In laceration less than 8 hours old, and in all lacerations of face and areas of possible functional disability* (such as the elbow): • Apply pressure and elevate injured extremity to control hemorrhage. • Cleanse wound gently with soap and water; irrigate with normal saline solution. • As necessary, debride necrotic margins, and close wound, using strips of tape or sutures. • Severe laceration with underlying structural damage may require surgery. *In grossly contaminated laceration or laceration more than 8 hours old* (except laceration of face and areas of possible functional disability): • Administer broad-spectrum antibiotic, such as tetracycline, for at least a 5-day course, as ordered. • *Don't* close wound immediately. • Instruct patient to elevate injured extremity for 24 hours after injury to reduce swelling. • Tell patient to keep dressing clean and dry and to watch for signs of infection. • After 5 to 7 days, close wound with sutures or butterfly dressing if it appears uninfected and contains healthy granulated tissue. • Apply sterile dressing and splint, as necessary. *In all lacerations:* • Check history for bleeding tendencies and anticoagulant use. • Determine approximate time of injury, and estimate blood loss. • Assess for neuromuscular, tendon, and circulatory damage. • Administer tetanus prophylaxis, as necessary. • Stress the need for follow-up and suture removal. • If sutures become infected, culture the wound and scrub with surgical soap preparation. Remove some or all sutures, and give broad-spectrum antibiotic, as ordered. Instruct patient to soak wound in warm, soapy water for 15 minutes, three times daily, and to return for follow-up every 2 to 3 days, until the wound until the wound heals. • If injury is the result of foul play, report it to police department.
Missile injury High velocity tissue penetration, such as a gunshot wound. Diagnosis based on entry and possibly exit wounds, signs of hemorrhage, shock, pain, and history of trauma. X-ray, CBC, and differential and electrolyte levels required to assess extent of injury and estimate blood loss.	• Check history for bleeding tendencies and use of anticoagulant. • Control hemorrhage with pressure, if possible. If injury is near vital organs, use large-bore catheters to start two I.V.s using lactated Ringer's or normal saline solution for volume replacement and prepare for possible exploratory surgery. • Maintain airway, and monitor for signs of hypovolemia, shock, and cardiac arrhythmias. Check vital signs and neurovascular response often. • Cover sucking chest wound during exhalation with petrolatum gauze and an occlusive dressing. • Cleanse wound gently with soap and water; debride as necessary. • If damage is minor, apply dry sterile dressing. • Administer tetanus prophylaxis, if necessary. • Obtain X-rays to detect retained fragments. • If possible, determine caliber of weapon. • Report to police department.

and partial thromboplastin times.

• Prepare the patient for surgery. Start I.V. lines, using two large-bore catheters, and infuse Ringer's lactate or normal saline solution or whole blood, as ordered. Insert a central venous pressure line, and place the patient in a modified V position (head flat, legs elevated). If modified V position doesn't help and medical antishock trousers (MAST) suit isn't available, the Trendelenburg position is a possible alternative.

• In suspected internal bleeding, insert a nasogastric tube; if systolic blood pressure is less than 90 mm Hg, apply a MAST suit, when available, to *temporarily* restore blood volume to vital organs.

Rape Trauma Syndrome

The term rape refers to illicit sexual intercourse without consent. It's a violent assault, in which sex is used as a weapon. Rape inflicts varying degrees of physical and psychological trauma. Rape trauma syndrome occurs during the period following the rape or attempted rape; it refers to the victim's short-term and long-term reactions and to the methods she uses to cope with this trauma.

In the United States, a rape is reported every 7 minutes (200 per day, 62,500 per year). Incidence of reported rape is highest in large cities and is rising. However, possibly over 90% of assaults are never reported.

Known victims of rape range in age from 2 months to 97 years. The age-group most affected are the 10- to 19-year-olds; the average victim's age is 13½. About one out of seven reported rapes involves a prepubertal child. Over 50% of rapes occur in the home; about one third of these involve a male intruder, who forces his way into a home. Approximately half the time, the victim has some casual acquaintance with the attacker. Most rapists are 15 to 24 years old. Usually, the attack is planned.

In most cases, the rapist is a man and the victim is a woman. However, rapes do occur between persons of the same sex, especially in prisons, schools, hospitals, and other institutions. Also, children are often the victims of rape; most of the time these cases involve manual, oral, or genital contact with the child's genitals. Usually, the rapist is a member of the child's family. In rare instances, a man or child is sexually abused by a woman.

Prognosis is good if the rape victim receives physical and emotional support and counseling to help her deal with her feelings. Victims who articulate their feelings are able to cope with fears, interact with others, and return to normal routines faster than those who do not.

Causes

Some of the cultural, sociologic, and psychological factors that contribute to rape are increasing exposure to sex, permissiveness, cynicism about relationships, feelings of anger, and powerlessness amid social pressures. The rapist often has feelings of violence or hatred toward women, or sexual problems, such as impotence or premature ejaculation. Often he feels socially isolated and unable to form warm, loving relationships. Some rapists may be psychopaths who need violence for physical pleasure, no matter how it affects their victims; others rape to satisfy a need for power. Some were abused as children.

Assessment

When a rape victim arrives in the emergency department, assess her physical injuries. If she's not *seriously* injured, allow her to remain clothed and take her to a private room, where she can talk with you or a counselor before the necessary physical examination. Remember, immediate reactions to rape differ and include crying, laughing, hostility, confusion, withdrawal, or outward calm; often anger and rage don't surface until later. During the assault, the victim may have felt demeaned, helpless, and afraid for her life; afterward, she may feel ashamed, guilty, shocked, and vulnerable, and have a sense of disbelief and lowered self-esteem. Offer support and reassurance. Help her explore her feelings; listen, convey trust and respect, and remain nonjudgmental. Don't leave her alone unless she asks you to.

Being careful to upset the victim as little as possible, obtain an accurate history of the rape, pertinent to physical assessment. (Remember: Your notes may be used as evidence if the rapist is tried.) Record the victim's statements in the first person, using quotation marks. Also document objective information provided by others. Never speculate as to what may have happened or record subjective impressions or thoughts. Include in your notes the time the victim arrived at the hospital, the date and time of the alleged rape, and the time the victim was examined. Ask the victim about allergies to penicillin and other drugs, if she's had recent illnesses (especially venereal disease), if she was pregnant before the attack, the date of her last menstrual period, and details of her obstetric/gynecologic history.

Thoroughly explain the examination she'll have, and tell her why it's necessary (to rule out internal injuries and obtain a specimen for venereal disease testing). Obtain her informed consent for treatment and for the police report. Allow her some control, if possible; for instance, ask her if she's ready to be examined or if she'd rather wait a bit.

Before the examination, ask the victim whether she douched, bathed, or washed before coming to the hospital. Note this on her chart. Have her change into a hospital gown, and place her clothing in *paper bags*. (*Never* use plastic bags, because secretions and seminal stains will mold, destroying valuable evidence.) La-

IF THE RAPE VICTIM IS A CHILD

Carefully interview the child to assess how well he or she will be able to deal with the situation after going home. Interview the child alone, away from the parents. Tell parents this is being done for the child's comfort, not to keep secrets from them. Ask them what words the child is comfortable with when referring to parts of the anatomy. A young child will place only as much importance on an experience as others do unless there is physical pain. A good question to ask is, "Did someone touch you when you didn't want to be touched?" As with other rape victims, record information in the child's own words. A complete pelvic examination is necessary only if penetration has occurred; such an examination requires parental consent and an analgesic or local anesthetic.

The child and the parents need counseling to minimize possible emotional disturbances. Encourage the child to talk about the experience, and try to alleviate any confusion. A young victim may regress; an older child may become fearful about being left alone. The child's behavior may change at school or at home.

Help parents understand that it's normal for them to feel angry and guilty, but warn them against displacing or projecting these feelings onto the child. Instruct them to assure the child that they're not angry with her or him; that the child is good and did not cause the incident; that they're sorry it happened but glad the child's all right; and that the family will work the problems out together.

LEGAL CONSIDERATIONS

If your hospital observes a protocol for emergency care of the rape victim, it may include a rape evidence kit. If it does, follow the kit's instructions carefully. Include only medically relevant information in your notes.

If you're called as a witness during the trial, try to provide the judge and jury with pertinent facts, while maintaining your own credibility.

Tips for the courtroom

- Go to court tastefully dressed and well groomed.
- Maintain a confident manner.
- Keep your posture erect, and project a quiet confidence.
- Look the prosecuting and the defense attorneys in the eye when answering their questions, but avoid long eye contact with the victim—this may cause you to appear biased.
- Don't offer speculations about the rape or volunteer information. Just answer questions that you're asked. If you don't know an answer, don't be afraid to say so.

bel each bag and its contents.

Tell the victim she may urinate, but warn her not to wipe or otherwise cleanse the perineal area. Stay with her, or ask a counselor to stay with her, throughout the examination.

Even if the victim wasn't beaten, physical examination (including a pelvic examination by a gynecologist) will probably show signs of physical trauma, especially if the assault was prolonged. Depending on specific body areas attacked, a patient may have a sore throat, mouth irritation, difficulty swallowing, ecchymoses, or rectal pain and bleeding.

If additional physical violence accompanied the rape, the victim may have hematomas, lacerations, bleeding, severe internal injuries, and hemorrhage; and if the rape occurred outdoors, she may suffer from exposure. X-rays may reveal fractures. If severe injuries require hospitalization, introduce the victim to her primary nurse, if possible.

Assist throughout the examination, providing support and reassurance, and carefully labeling all possible evidence. Before the victim's pelvic area is examined, take vital signs, and if the patient is wearing a tampon, remove it, wrap it, and label it as evidence. This exam is often very distressing to the rape victim. Reassure her, and allow her as much control as possible. During the exam, assist in specimen collection, including those for semen and gonorrhea. Carefully label all specimens with the patient's name, the doctor's name, and the location from which the specimen was obtained. List all specimens in your notes. If the case comes to trial, specimens will be used for evidence, so accuracy is vital.

Carefully collect and label fingernail scrapings and foreign material obtained by combing the victim's pubic hair; these also provide valuable evidence. Note to whom these specimens are given.

For a male victim, be especially alert for injury to the mouth, perineum, and anus. As ordered, obtain a pharyngeal sample for a gonorrhea culture and rectal aspirate for acid phosphatase or sperm analysis.

Assist in photographing the patient's injuries (this may be delayed for a day or repeated when bruises and ecchymoses are more apparent).

Most states require the hospital to report all incidents of rape. The patient may elect not to press charges and not to assist the police investigation. If the patient does *not* go to the hospital, she may not report the rape.

If the police interview the patient in the hospital, be supportive and encourage her to recall details of the rape. Your kindness and empathy are invaluable.

The patient may also want you to call her family. Help her to verbalize anticipation of her family's response.

Treatment and special considerations

Treatment consists of supportive measures and protection against venereal disease and, if the patient wishes, against pregnancy. Give probenecid P.O., with penicillin G procaine I.M., as ordered, to prevent venereal disease.

Since cultures can't detect gonorrhea for 5 to 6 days after the rape, or syphilis for 6 weeks, stress the importance of returning for follow-up venereal disease testing. If the victim wishes to prevent possible pregnancy as a result of the rape, she may be given large doses of oral diethylstilbestrol (DES) for 5 consecutive days. Immediately inserting an intrauterine device (IUD) may prevent pregnancy but cause an infection. Adverse effects of DES usage and IUD insertion should be explained. The victim may wait 3 to 4 weeks and have a dilatation and curettage or a vacuum aspiration to abort a pregnancy.

If the patient has vulvar lacerations and hair cuts, the doctor will clean the area and repair the lacerations after all the evidence is obtained. Topical use of ice packs may reduce vulvar swelling.

Recovery from rape, which may be prolonged, consists of the acute phase (immediate reaction) and the reorganization phase. During the acute phase, physical aspects include pain, loss of appetite, and wound healing; emotional reactions typically include shaking, crying, and mood swings. Feelings of grief, anger, fear, or revenge may color the victim's social interactions. Counseling helps the victim identify her coping mechanisms. She may relate more easily to a counselor of the same sex.

During the reorganization phase, which usually begins a week after the rape and may last months or years, the victim is concerned with restructuring her life. Initially, she often has nightmares in which she's powerless; later dreams show her gradually gaining more control. When she's alone, she may also suffer from "daymares"—frightening thoughts about the rape. She may have reduced sexual desire or may develop fear of intercourse or mistrust of men.

Legal proceedings during this time force the victim to relive the trauma, leaving her feeling lonely and isolated, perhaps even temporarily halting her emotional recovery. To help her cope, encourage her to write her thoughts, feelings, and reactions in a daily diary, and refer her to organizations such as Women Organized Against Rape or a local rape crisis center for empathy and advice.

Selected References

Alexy, Betty J. "Problems Due to Cold," *Journal of Emergency Nursing* 6(1):22-24, January/February 1980.

Connolly, John F., ed. *DePalma's the Management of Fractures and Dislocations: An Atlas*, 3rd ed., 2 vols. Philadelphia: W.B. Saunders Co., 1981.

Critical Care Quarterly Issue on Poisonings and Overdose. 4(4): April 1982.

Kaye, Donald, and Rose, Louis F. *Fundamentals of Internal Medicine*. St. Louis: C.V. Mosby Co., 1983.

Kinney, Marguerite, et al. *AACN's Clinical Reference for Critical Care Nursing*. New York: McGraw-Hill Book Co., 1981.

Miller, Robert H. *Textbook of Basic Emergency Medicine*, 2nd ed. St. Louis: C.V. Mosby Co., 1980.

Rosen, Peter, et al. *Emergency Medicine: Concepts and Clinical Practice*, vol. 1. St. Louis: C.V. Mosby Co., 1983.

Salisbury, Roger E., and Newman, Nancy. *Manual of Burn Therapeutics*. Boston: Little, Brown & Co., 1983.

Wachtel, Tom, et al. *Current Topics in Burn Care*. Rockville, Md.: Aspen Systems Corp., 1983.

Warner, Carmen G. *Emergency Care: Assessment and Intervention*, 3rd ed. St. Louis: C.V. Mosby Co., 1982.

Warner, Carmen G. *Rape and Sexual Assault: Management and Intervention*. Rockville, Md.: Aspen Systems Corp., 1980.

Wilkins, Earle W., Jr. *MGH Textbook of Emergency Medicine*, 2nd ed. Baltimore: Williams & Wilkins Co., 1983.

Wingate, Elizabeth. "A Nursing Perspective on Frostbite," *Critical Care Update* 10(1):8-15, January 1983.

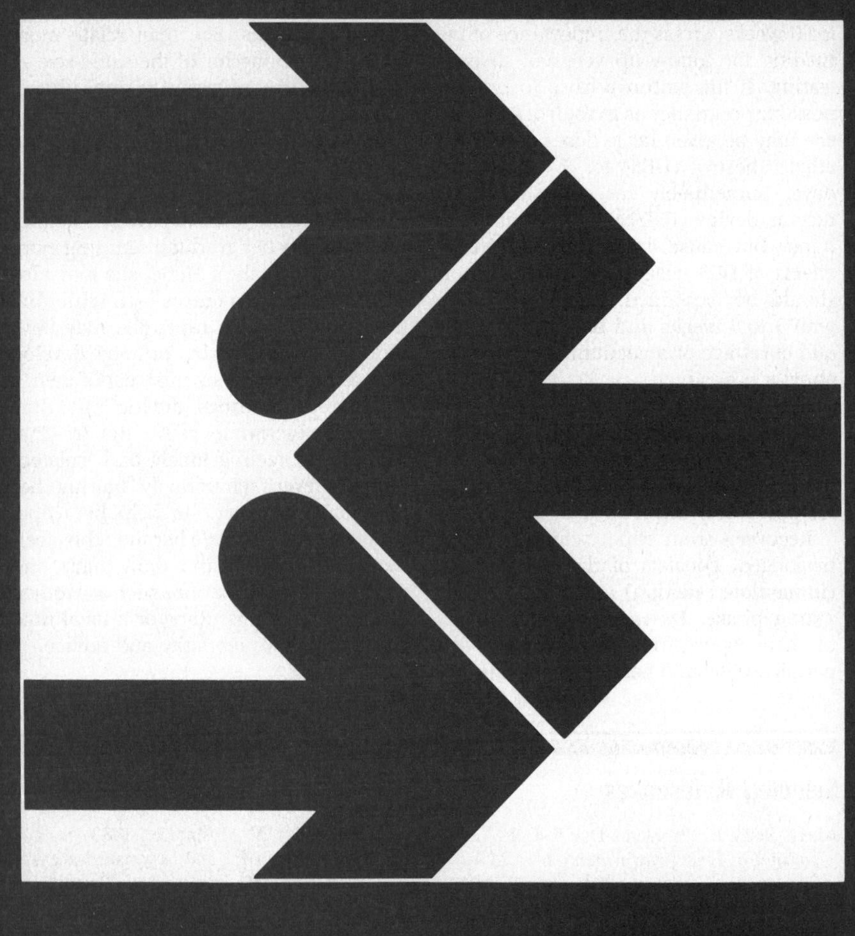

5 Immune Disorders

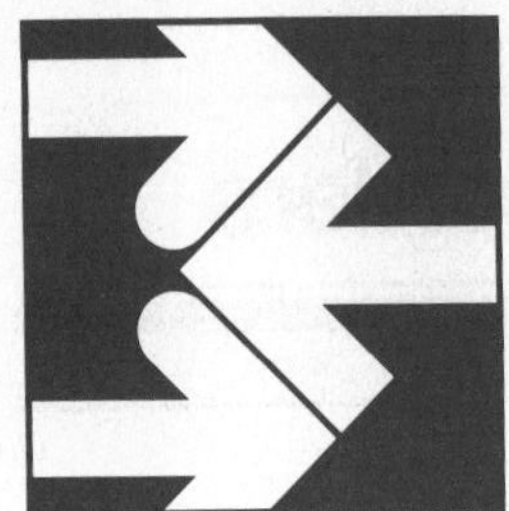

Immune Disorders

Introduction

The environment contains thousands of pathogenic organisms—viruses, bacteria, fungi, and parasites. Ordinarily, though, these organisms pose little threat to us. We normally protect ourselves from infectious organisms and other harmful invaders through an elaborate network of safeguards—the host defense system. Understanding how this system functions provides the framework for studying various immune disorders.

The host defense system

The host defense system includes physical and chemical barriers to infection, the inflammatory response, and the immune response. Physical barriers, such as the skin and mucous membranes, prevent invasion by most organisms. Those organisms that do penetrate this first line of defense simultaneously trigger the inflammatory and immune responses. Both responses involve cells derived from a hematopoietic stem cell in the bone marrow. The immune response primarily involves the interaction of lymphocytes (T and B), macrophages, and macrophage-like cells and their products. These cells are localized in the tissues and organs of the immune system, including the thymus, lymph nodes, spleen, tonsils, Peyer's patches, and appendix. The thymus participates in the maturation of T lymphocytes; here, these cells are "educated" to differentiate self and nonself. In contrast, B lymphocytes probably mature in the bone marrow. The lymph nodes, spleen, and intestinal lymphoid tissue help remove and destroy circulating antigen in the blood and lymph. The inflammatory response involves polymorphonuclear leukocytes, basophils, mast cells, and platelets. The key humoral effector mechanism, however, is the complement cascade.

Antigens

Fundamental to an understanding of the immune response is an understanding of antigens and of the concepts of specificity and memory. An antigen is any substance that can induce an immune response. T and B lymphocytes recognize and respond to antigens through specific cell surface receptors. These antigen receptors are characterized by variable and constant regions. In B cells, the antigen receptor is a form of immunoglobulin M called surface immunoglobulin (SIg). The more complex T cell antigen receptor recognizes antigen only in association with specific cell surface antigen determinants, known as the major histocompatibility complex (MHC). Slightly different antigen receptors can recognize a phenomenal number of distinct antigens coded for by distinct, variable region genes.

Groups, or clones, of lymphocytes exist with identical receptors for a specific an-

THE MAJOR HISTOCOMPATIBILITY COMPLEX

The major histocompatibility complex (MHC) is a cluster of genes on human chromosome 6 that plays a pivotal role in the immune response. Also known as human leukocyte antigen (HLA) genes, these genes are inherited in an autosomal codominant manner. That is, each individual receives one set of MHC genes (haplotype) from each parent and both sets of genes are expressed on the individual's cells. These genes play an essential role in the recognition of self versus nonself and the interaction of immunologically active cells by coding for cell-surface proteins.

HLA antigens are divided into three classes. Class I antigens appear on nearly all of the body's cells and include HLA-A, -B, and -C antigens. During tissue graft rejection, they are the chief antigens recognized by the host. When killer T cells lyse a virally infected antigen, they recognize it in the context of a Class I antigen. Class II antigens only appear on B cells, macrophages, and activated T cells. They include the HLA-D and -DR antigens. Class II antigens promote efficient collaboration between immunocompetent cells. T cells require that antigen be presented in the context of a Class II antigen. Because these antigens also determine whether an individual responds to a particular antigen, they're also known as immune response genes. Class III antigens include certain complement proteins (C2, C4, and Factor B).

tigen. The clone of lymphocytes rapidly proliferates when exposed to the specific antigen. Some of these lymphocytes further differentiate, and others become memory cells, which enable a more rapid response—the memory or anamnestic response—to subsequent challenge by the antigen.

Many factors influence antigenicity. Among them are the physical/chemical characteristics of the antigen, its relative foreignness, and the individual's genetic makeup. Most antigens are large molecules—greater than 10,000 daltons—such as proteins or polysaccharides. (Smaller molecules, such as drugs, that aren't antigenic by themselves are known as haptens. These haptens can bind with larger molecules, or carriers, and become antigenic or immunogenic.) The relative foreignness of the antigen influences the intensity of the immune response. For example, little or no immune response may follow transfusion of

STRUCTURE OF THE IMMUNOGLOBULIN MOLECULE

The Ig molecule consists of four polypeptide chains—two heavy (H) and two light (L) chains—held together by disulfide bonds. The H chain has one variable (V) and at least three constant (C) regions. The L chain has one V and one C region. Together, the V regions of the H and L chains form a pocket known as the antigen-binding site. This site is located within the antigen-binding fragment (Fab) region of the molecule. Part of the C region of the H chains forms the crystallizable fragment (Fc) region of the molecule. This region mediates effector mechanisms, such as complement activation, and is the portion of the Ig molecule bound by Fc receptors on phagocytic cells, mast cells, and basophils. Each Ig molecule also has two antibody-combining sites (except for the IgM molecule, which has ten).

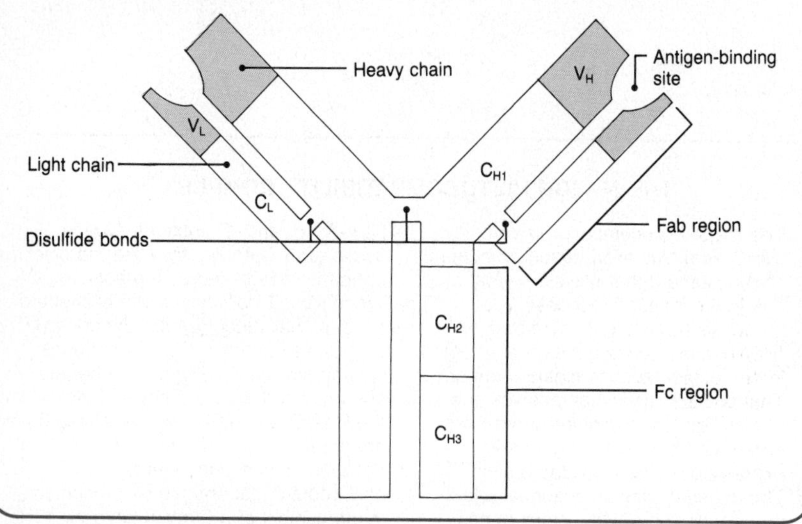

serum proteins between humans; however, a vigorous immune response (serum sickness) often follows transfusion of horse serum proteins to a human. Genetic makeup may also determine why some individuals respond to certain antigens while others do not. The genes responsible for this phenomenon—the immune response genes—are located within the MHC.

B lymphocytes

B lymphocytes and their product immunoglobulin (Ig) comprise humoral immunity. The binding of soluble antigen with B cell antigen receptors initiates the humoral immune response. The activated B cells differentiate into plasma cells that secrete immunoglobulins, or antibodies. This response is regulated by T lymphocytes and their products, such as B cell growth factor and B cell differentiating factor.

The Ig secreted by plasma cells are four-chain molecules with two heavy and two light chains. Each chain has a variable (V) region and one or more constant (C) regions coded for by separate genes. The V regions of both light and heavy chains participate in the binding of an antigen. The C regions of the heavy chain provide a binding site for Fc receptors on cells and govern other mechanisms, such as complement activation.

Any clone of B cells has one antigen specificity determined by the V regions of its light and heavy chains. However, the clone can change the class of immunoglobulin that it makes by changing the association between its V region genes and heavy chain C region genes (a process known as isotype switching). For example, a clone of B cells genetically preprogrammed to recognize tetanus toxoid will first make an IgM antibody against tetanus toxoid and later an IgG or other antibody against it.

T lymphocytes

T lymphocytes and macrophages are the chief participants in cell-mediated immunity. Like B lymphocytes, T lymphocytes derive from the bone marrow but then migrate to the thymus. Within the thymus, T cells are "educated" to distinguish self and nonself. This maturation appears linked to products of the MHC, human leukocyte antigen (HLA) genes. Also within the thymus, T cells acquire certain surface molecules, or markers. The T_3 protein molecule marks all mature T cells and, together with the T cell antigen receptor, promotes activation of T cells. Suppressor T cells and cytotoxic (killer) T cells also have the marker known as T_8, and helper T cells have the marker known as T_4. Helper T cells promote B cell production of immunoglobulin, whereas suppressor T cells dampen this response. Cytotoxic T cells lyse foreign cells and virally infected autologous cells. T cell activation requires presentation of antigen in the context of a specific HLA antigen. Helper T cells require Class II HLA antigen; cytotoxic T cells require Class I HLA antigen. Interleukin-1, produced by macrophages, and interleukin-2, produced by T cells, are also involved in T cell activation.

Macrophages: Key antigen-presenting cells

Important cells of the reticuloendothelial system, macrophages influence both immune and inflammatory responses. These cells may circulate in the blood or collect in various tissues and organs, such as the liver, spleen, lung, and connective tissue. Unlike B and T lymphocytes, macrophages lack surface receptors for specific antigens; instead, they have receptors for the C region of the heavy chain (Fc region) of immunoglobulin, for fragments of the third component of complement (C3), and for nonimmunologic factors, such as carbohydrate molecules.

One of the most important functions of macrophages is the presentation of antigen to T lymphocytes. Macrophages ingest and process antigen, then deposit it on their own surfaces in association with HLA antigen. T lymphocytes become activated upon recognizing this complex. Macrophages also function in the inflammatory response by producing interleukin-1, which generates fever, and by synthesizing complement proteins and other mediators with phagocytic, microbicidal, and tumoricidal effects.

The complement system

The chief humoral effector of the inflammatory response, the complement system consists of more than 20 serum proteins. When activated, these proteins interact in a cascadelike process that has profound biologic effects. Complement activation takes place through one of two pathways. In the classical pathway, binding of immunoglobulin (IgM or IgG) and antigen forms antigen-antibody complexes that activate the first complement component, C1. This, in turn, activates C4, C2, and C3. In the alternate pathway, activating surfaces, such as bacterial membranes, directly amplify spontaneous cleavage of C3. Once C3 is activated in either pathway, activation of the terminal components—C5 to C9—follows.

The major biological effects of complement activation include phagocyte attraction (chemotaxis) and activation, histamine release, viral neutralization, promotion of phagocytosis by opsonization, and lysis of cells and bacteria. Other mediators of inflammation derived from the kinin and coagulation pathways interact with the complement system.

Polymorphonuclear leukocytes

Besides macrophages and complement, other key participants in the inflam-

GELL AND COOMBS CLASSIFICATION OF HYPERSENSITIVITY REACTIONS

TYPE I

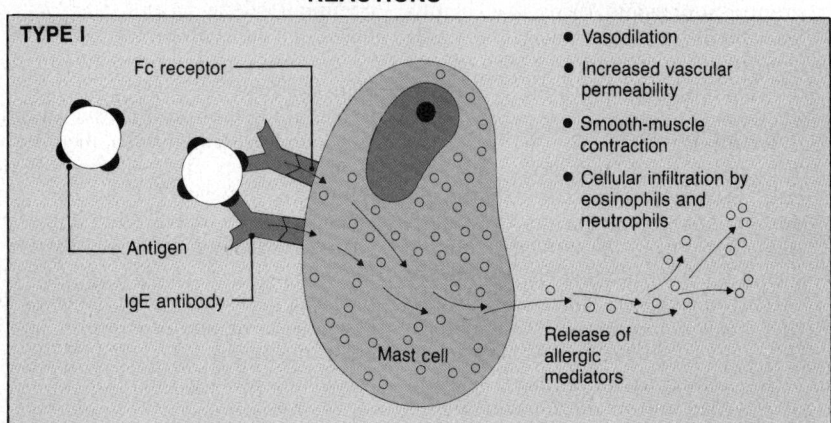

REACTIONS	PATHOPHYSIOLOGY	SIGNS AND SYMPTOMS	CLINICAL EXAMPLES
Anaphylactic (immediate, atopic, IgE-mediated, reaginic)	Binding of antigens to IgE antibodies on mast cell surfaces releases allergic mediators, causing vasodilation, increased capillary permeability, smooth-muscle contraction, and eosinophilia.	Systemic: angioedema; hypotension; bronchospasm, GI or uterine spasm; stridor Local: urticaria, pruritus	Extrinsic asthma, seasonal allergic rhinitis, systemic anaphylaxis, reactions to stinging insects, some food and drug reactions, some cases of urticaria, infantile eczema

TYPE II

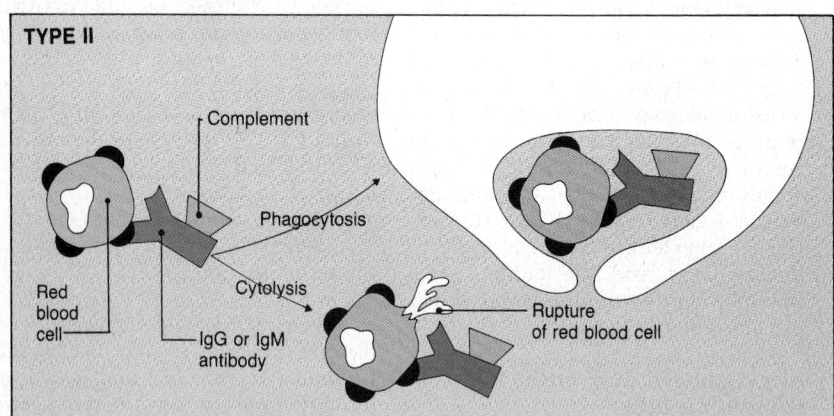

REACTIONS	PATHOPHYSIOLOGY	SIGNS AND SYMPTOMS	CLINICAL EXAMPLES
Cytotoxic (cytolytic, complement-dependent cytotoxicity)	Binding of IgG or IgM antibodies to cellular or exogenous antigens activates the complement cascade, resulting in phagocytosis or cytolysis.	Varies with disease; can include dyspnea, hemoptysis, fever	Goodpasture's syndrome, autoimmune hemolytic anemia, thrombocytopenia, pernicious anemia, hyperacute renal allograft rejection, transfusion reaction, hemolytic disease of the newborn, some drug reactions

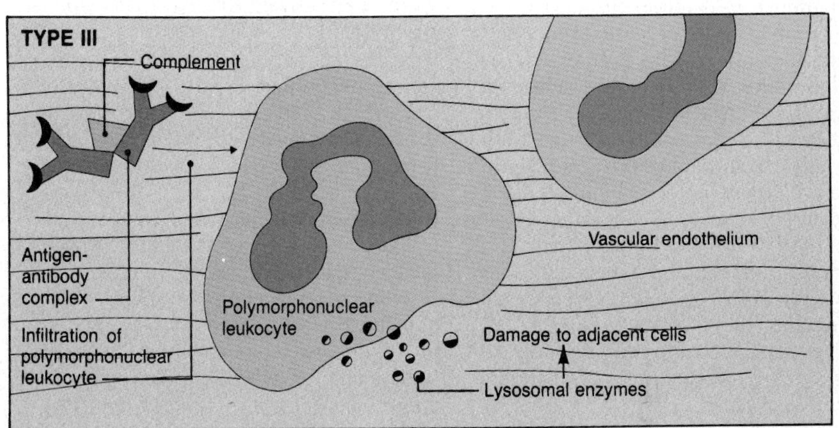

REACTIONS	PATHOPHYSIOLOGY	SIGNS AND SYMPTOMS	CLINICAL EXAMPLES
Immune complex disease	Activation of complement by immune complexes causes infiltration of polymorphonuclear leukocytes and release of lysosomal enzymes and permeability factors, producing an inflammatory reaction.	Urticaria, palpable purpura, adenopathy, joint pain, fever, serum sickness–like syndrome	Serum sickness due to serum, drugs, or viral hepatitis antigen; membranous glomerulonephritis; systemic lupus erythematosus; rheumatoid arthritis; polyarteritis; cryoglobulinemia

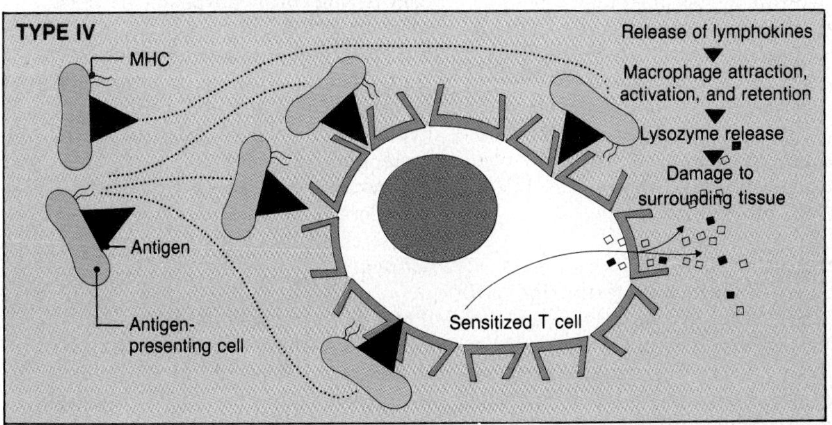

REACTIONS	PATHOPHYSIOLOGY	SIGNS AND SYMPTOMS	CLINICAL EXAMPLES
Delayed (cell-mediated)	An antigen-presenting cell presents antigen to T cells in association with MHC. The sensitized T cells release lymphokines, which stimulate macrophages; lysozymes are released, and surrounding tissue is damaged.	Varies with disease; can include fever, erythema, and pruritus.	Contact dermatitis, graft-versus-host disease, allograft rejection, granuloma due to intracellular organisms, some drug sensitivities, Hashimoto's thyroiditis, tuberculosis, sarcoidosis

matory response are the polymorphonuclear leukocytes—neutrophils, eosinophils, and basophils. Neutrophils, the most numerous of these cells, derive from bone marrow and increase dramatically in number in response to infection and inflammation. Highly mobile cells, neutrophils are attracted to areas of inflammation (chemotaxis); in fact, they're the primary constituent of pus. Neutrophils have surface receptors for immunoglobulin and complement fragments, and avidly ingest opsonized particles such as bacteria. Ingested organisms are then promptly killed by toxic oxygen metabolites and enzymes such as lysozyme. Unfortunately, neutrophils not only kill invading organisms, but may also damage host tissues.

Also derived from bone marrow, eosinophils multiply in allergic disorders and parasitic infestations. Although their phagocytic function isn't entirely clear, evidence suggests that they participate in host defense against parasites. Their products may also dampen the inflammatory response in allergic disorders.

Two other cells that function in allergic disorders are basophils and mast cells. Basophils circulate in peripheral blood, whereas mast cells accumulate in connective tissue, particularly in the lungs, gut, and skin. Both cells have surface receptors for IgE. When cross-linked by an IgE-antigen complex, they release allergic mediators.

Immune disorders

Because of their complexity, the processes involved in host defense and immune response may malfunction. When the body's defenses are exaggerated, misdirected, absent, or depressed, the result may be a hypersensitivity disorder, autoimmunity, or immunodeficiency, respectively.

Hypersensitivity disorders

An exaggerated or inappropriate immune response may lead to various hypersensitivity disorders. Such disorders are classified as Type I through Type IV, although some overlap exists. (See *Gell and Coombs Classification of Hypersensitivity Reactions, pages 320 and 321.*)

Type I hypersensitivity (allergic disorders)

In some individuals, certain antigens (allergens) induce B cell production of IgE, which binds to the Fc receptors on the surface of mast cells. When these cells are re-exposed to the same antigen, the antigen binds with the surface IgE, cross-links the Fc receptors, and causes mast cell degranulation with release of various mediators. (Degranulation may also be triggered by complement-derived anaphylatoxins—C3a and C5a—or by certain drugs, such as morphine.) Some of these mediators are preformed, whereas others are newly synthesized upon activation of mast cells. Preformed mediators include heparin, histamine, proteolytic and other enzymes, and chemotactic factors for eosinophils and neutrophils. Newly synthesized mediators include prostaglandins and leukotrienes. The effects of these mediators include vasodilation, smooth-muscle contraction, bronchospasm, increased vascular permeability, edema, mucous secretion, and cellular infiltration by eosinophils and neutrophils. Among classic associated signs and symptoms are hypotension, wheezing, swelling, urticaria, and rhinorrhea.

Examples of Type I hypersensitivity disorders are anaphylaxis, hay fever (allergic rhinitis), and, in some cases, asthma.

Type II hypersensitivity (antibody-dependent cytotoxicity)

In this form of hypersensitivity, antibody is directed against cell surface antigens. (Alternately, though, antibody may be directed against small molecules adsorbed to cells or against cell surface receptors, rather than against cell constituents themselves.) Type II hypersensitivity then causes tissue damage through several mechanisms. Binding of antigen and antibody activates complement, which ultimately disrupts cellular membranes. Another mechanism is mediated by various phagocytic cells with receptors for immunoglobulin (Fc region) and complement fragments. These cells envelop and destroy (phagocytose) opsonized targets, such as red blood cells, leukocytes, and platelets. Antibody against these cells may be visualized by immunofluorescence. Cytotoxic T cells and natural killer cells also contribute to tissue damage in Type II hypersensitivity.

Examples of Type II hypersensitivity include transfusion reactions, hemolytic disease of the newborn, autoimmune hemolytic anemia, Goodpasture's syndrome, and myasthenia gravis.

Type III hypersensitivity (immune complex disease)

In Type III hypersensitivity, excessive circulating antigen results in the deposition of immune complexes in tissue—most commonly in the kidneys, joints, skin, and blood vessels. (Normally, immune complexes are effectively cleared by the reticuloendothelial system). These deposited immune complexes activate the complement cascade, resulting in local inflammation. They also trigger platelet release of vasoactive amines that increase vascular permeability, augmenting deposition of immune complexes in vessel walls.

Type III hypersensitivity may be associated with infections, such as hepatitis B and bacterial endocarditis; malignancies, in which a serum sickness–like syndrome may occur; and autoimmune disorders, such as lupus erythematosus. This hypersensitivity reaction may also follow drug or serum therapy.

Type IV hypersensitivity (delayed hypersensitivity)

In this form of hypersensitivity, antigen is processed by macrophages and presented to T cells. The sensitized T cells then release lymphokines, which recruit and activate other lymphocytes, monocytes, macrophages, and polymorphonuclear leukocytes. The coagulation, kinin, and complement pathways also contribute to tissue damage in this type of reaction.

Examples of Type IV hypersensitivity include tuberculin reactions, contact hypersensitivity, and sarcoidosis.

Autoimmune disorders

Autoimmunity is characterized by a misdirected immune response, in which the body's defenses become self-destructive. What causes this abnormal response remains puzzling. Recognition of self through the MHC is known to be of primary importance in an immune response. However, just how an immune response against self is prevented, and which cells are primarily responsible, isn't well understood.

Autoimmunity likely results from a combination of factors. Characteristic of many autoimmune disorders is B cell hyperactivity, marked by proliferation of B cells and autoantibodies and by hypergammaglobulinemia. T cell abnormalities—especially suppressor T cell deficiency—are also common. Viruses may contribute to autoimmunity by causing proliferation (Epstein-Barr virus) or destruction (HTLV-III) of lymphocytes; so may macrophage abnormalities, which interfere with processing and presentation of antigen. Hormonal and genetic factors strongly influence the incidence of autoimmune disorders; for example, lupus erythematosus predominantly affects women of childbearing age, and certain HLA haplotypes are associated with increased risk of specific autoimmune disorders.

Immunodeficiency

In immunodeficiency, the immune response is absent or depressed, resulting in increased susceptibility to infection. This disorder may be classified as primary or secondary. Primary immunodeficiency reflects a defect involving T cells, B cells, or lymphoid tissues, such as the thymus. Secondary immunodeficiency results from an underlying disease or factor that depresses or blocks the immune response.

ALLERGY

Asthma

Asthma is a chronic reactive airway disorder that produces episodic, reversible airway obstruction via bronchospasms, increased mucous secretion, and mucosal edema. Its symptoms range from mild wheezing and dyspnea to life-threatening respiratory failure. Symptoms of bronchial airway obstruction may or may not persist between acute episodes.

Causes and incidence

Although this common condition can strike at any age, half of all cases occur in children under age 10; in this age-group, asthma affects twice as many boys as girls. In another third, asthma begins between ages 10 and 30; in this age-group, incidence is equal between the sexes. Underlining the significance of hereditary predisposition, about one third of all asthmatics share the disease with at least one member of their immediate family, and three fourths of the children with two asthmatic parents also have asthma.

Asthma may result from sensitivity to specific external allergens (extrinsic) or from internal, nonallergenic factors (intrinsic). Allergens, which cause extrinsic asthma, include pollen, animal dander, house dust or mold, kapok or feather pillows, food additives containing sulfites, or any other sensitizing substance. Most *extrinsic asthma* (atopic asthma) begins in children and is usually accompanied by other manifestations of atopy (Type I—IgE-mediated allergy), such as eczema and allergic rhinitis. In *intrinsic asthma* (nonatopic asthma), no extrinsic substance can be identified. Most cases are preceded by a severe respiratory infection (especially in adults). Irritants, emotional stress, fatigue, endocrine changes, temperature and humidity changes, and exposure to noxious fumes may aggravate intrinsic asthma attacks. In many asthmatics, especially children, intrinsic and extrinsic asthma coexist.

Several drugs and chemicals may provoke an asthmatic attack without using the IgE pathway. Apparently, they trigger release of mast cell mediators via prostaglandin inhibition. Examples of these substances include aspirin, various nonsteroidal anti-inflammatory drugs (such as indomethacin and mefenamic acid), and tartrazine, a yellow food dye. Exercise may also provoke an asthmatic attack. In exercise-induced asthma, bronchospasm may follow heat and moisture loss in the upper airways. Certain exercises, such as jogging in cold weather, are more likely to precipitate attacks than others. Occupational exposure to various allergenic and nonallergenic factors may also be linked with asthma. For example, many persons who work with platinum develop asthma.

What causes the fundamental reaction in asthma is still unclear. Presumably, it occurs as follows: When the patient inhales an allergenic substance, sensitized IgE antibodies trigger mast cell degranulation in the lung interstitium, releasing histamine and leukotrienes, or slow-reacting substance of anaphylaxis (SRS-A). Histamine then attaches to receptor sites in the larger bronchi, causing irritation, inflammation, and edema. Leukotrienes attach to receptor sites in the smaller bronchi, causing edema and attracting prostaglandins, which enhance the effects of histamine in the lungs.

Signs and symptoms

An asthma attack may begin dramatically, with simultaneous onset of severe, multiple symptoms, or insidiously, with gradually increasing respiratory distress. Typically, an acute asthmatic attack causes sudden dyspnea, wheezing, tightness in the chest, and cough with thick, clear or yellow sputum. The patient may feel as if he is suffocating. During a severe attack, he may be unable to speak more than a few words without pausing for breath.

When examining such a patient, you'll find tachypnea, though respiratory rate is frequently normal; audible wheezing; obvious use of accessory respiration muscles; rapid pulse; profuse perspiration; hyperresonant lung fields; and diminished breath sounds with wheezes and rhonchi. Cyanosis, confusion, and lethargy indicate the onset of life-threatening status asthmaticus and respiratory failure.

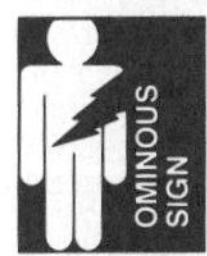

Diagnosis

Laboratory studies in patients with asthma often show these abnormalities:

• *Pulmonary function studies:* signs of airway obstructive disease (decreased flow rates and forced expiratory volume in 1 second [FEV_1]), low normal or decreased vital capacity, and increased total lung and residual capacity. However, pulmonary function studies may be normal between attacks. Typically, the patient has decreased PaO_2 and $PaCO_2$ levels. However, in severe asthma, the $PaCO_2$ may be normal or increased, indicating severe bronchial obstruction. In fact, the FEV will probably be less than 25% of the predicted value. Initiating treatment tends to decrease the PaO_2 level, making frequent arterial blood gas analysis mandatory. Even when the asthmatic attack appears under control, the spirometric values (FEV, and forced expiratory flow between 25% and 75% of vital capacity) remain abnormal. Residual volume remains abnormal for the longest period—up to 3 weeks after the attack.

• *Complete blood count with differential:* increased eosinophil count.

BREATHING EXERCISES FOR ASTHMA

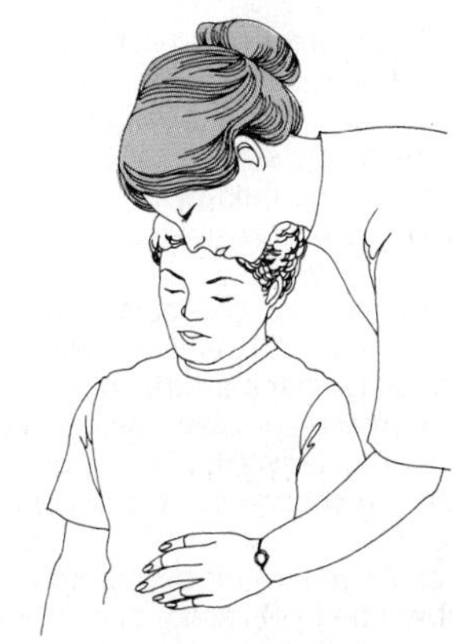

To promote diaphragmatic breathing, firmly put your hand on the patient's abdomen, just below his ribs. His stomach should swell as he inhales and return to a relaxed position when he exhales.

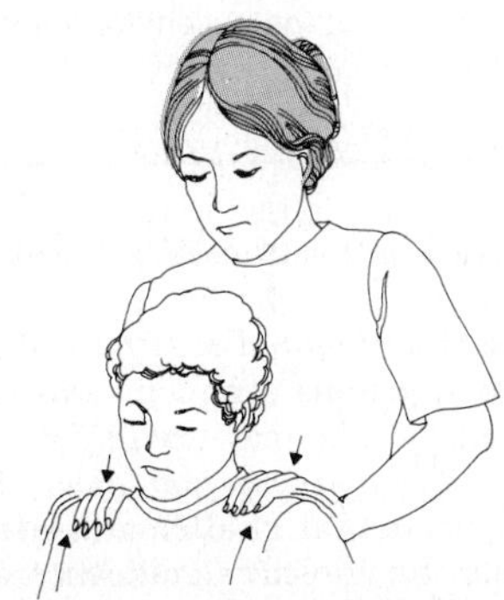

To promote relaxation, put your hands on the patient's shoulders, and ask him to push up against the pressure of your hands. Have him relax at regular intervals.

To best use these techniques with a child, have him:

- blow up balloons
- blow out candles
- blow Ping-Pong balls across a table
- blow butterflies made from facial tissues across a table.

HOW TO TREAT STATUS ASTHMATICUS

Unless it is promptly and correctly treated, status asthmaticus may lead to fatal respiratory failure. The patient with increasingly severe asthma unresponsive to drug therapy is usually admitted to the intensive care unit for the following care:

- As ordered, give corticosteroids, epinephrine, and I.V. aminophylline.
- Frequently check arterial blood gas measurements to assess respiratory status, particularly after ventilator therapy or a change in oxygen concentration.
- Carefully administer oxygen (the patient will be hypoxemic) and, if necessary, assist in endotracheal intubation and mechanical ventilation (when he has an elevated Pco_2).
- Administer I.V. fluids according to the patient's clinical status and age. (Dehydration is likely because of inadequate fluid intake and increased insensible loss.)
- Help position the patient for frequent chest X-rays.

- *Chest X-ray:* possible hyperinflation, with areas of focal atelectasis (mucous plugging).
- *History of familial allergy:* If the patient with asthma symptoms has no allergic history, he may need s' [illegible] testing for specific allergens and, later, inhalation bronchial challenge testing to evaluate the clinical significance of allergens identified by skin testing.

Before testing for asthma, rule out other causes of airway obstruction and wheezing. In children, such causes include cystic fibrosis; aspiration; congenital anomaly; benign or malignant tumors of the bronchi, thyroid, thymus, or mediastinum; and acute viral bronchitis; in adults, obstructive pulmonary disease and congestive heart failure.

Treatment

The best treatment for asthma is prevention, by identifying and avoiding precipitating factors such as allergens or irritants. Usually, such stimuli can't be removed entirely, so desensitization to specific antigens may be helpful but is rarely totally effective or persistent.

Drug treatment for asthma usually includes some form of bronchodilator and is more effective when begun soon after onset of symptoms. Drugs used include rapid-acting epinephrine; epinephrine in oil, which is not recommended for infants; terbutaline; aminophylline; theophylline and theophylline-containing oral preparations; oral sympathomimetics; corticosteroids; or aerosolized sympathomimetics such as isoproterenol or albuterol. Arterial blood gases help determine the severity of an asthmatic attack and the patient's response to treatment.

Special considerations

During an acute attack:

- First, maintain respiratory function and relieve bronchoconstriction, while allowing mucous plug expulsion.
- If the attack is induced by exercise, you may be able to control it by having the patient sit down, rest, and sip warm water. This helps slow breathing, promotes bronchodilation, and loosens secretions. (Before exercising, asthmatic children should use an oral bronchodilator for 30 to 60 minutes or an inhaled bronchodilator for 15 to 20 minutes. Cromolyn sodium can also be used to prevent exercise-induced bronchospasm; have the patient inhale one capsule no more than 1 hour before exercising.)
- Find out if the patient has a nebulizer and if he has used it. The asthmatic should have access to an isoproterenol or isoetharine nebulizer at all times. But, he should take no more than two or three whiffs every 4 hours. If he needs the nebulizer again in less than 4 hours, give it and call the doctor for further instruction. (Overuse of a nebulizer can progressively weaken the patient's response until it has no effect at all. Extended overuse can even lead to cardiac arrest and death, although this is rare.)

• Loss of breath is terrifying, so reassure the patient that you'll help him. Then, place him in a semi-Fowler's position, encourage diaphragmatic breathing, and urge him to relax as much as possible.
• Consider status asthmaticus unrelieved by epinephrine a medical emergency.
• Administer humidified oxygen by nasal cannula at 2 liters/minute to ease difficulty in breathing and to increase arterial oxygen saturation. Later, adjust oxygen according to the patient's vital functions and arterial blood gas measurements.
• Administer drugs and I.V. fluids as ordered. Continue epinephrine, and administer aminophylline I.V. as a loading dose, followed by I.V. drip. (Caution: Elderly patients with hepatic or cardiac insufficiency or those taking erythromycin are predisposed to aminophylline toxicity.) Young patients and those who smoke or who are receiving barbiturates have increased aminophylline metabolism and require a larger dose. Monitor the drip rate, and, when possible, use an I.V. infusion pump. Simultaneously, a loading dose of corticosteroids can be given I.V. or I.M. Combat dehydration with I.V. fluids until the patient can tolerate oral fluids, which will help loosen secretions.

During long-term care:
• Supervise the patient's drug regimen. Make sure he knows how to use aerosolized bronchodilator drugs properly. When the patient is using an aminophylline bronchodilator, monitor his blood levels, as oral absorption of aminophylline can be erratic. With long-term steroid therapy, watch for cushingoid side effects. Minimize them by alternate-day dosage or use of the orally inhalable steroid beclomethasone. Because of their respiratory depressant effect, sedatives and narcotics are not recommended.

To prevent recurring attacks:
• Instruct the patient to breathe deeply, cough up secretions accumulated overnight, and allow time for medication to work. He can best loosen secretions by coughing correctly—inhaling fully and gently, then bending over with arms crossed over the abdomen before coughing—and by drinking 3 quarts of liquid daily. Also tell the patient and his family that the patient should avoid known allergens, irritating fumes of any kind, aerosol spray, smoke, and automobile exhaust. Refer the patient to community resources such as the American Lung Association and the Asthma and Allergy Foundation.

Allergic Rhinitis

Allergic rhinitis is a reaction to airborne (inhaled) allergens. Depending on the allergen, the resulting rhinitis and conjunctivitis may be seasonal (hay fever) or occur year round (perennial allergic rhinitis). Allergic rhinitis is the most common atopic allergic reaction, affecting over 20 million Americans. It's most prevalent in young children and adolescents, but can occur in all age-groups.

Causes

Hay fever reflects an IgE-mediated Type I hypersensitivity response to an environmental antigen (allergen) in a genetically susceptible individual. It's usually induced by wind-borne pollens: in spring by tree pollens (oak, elm, maple, alder, birch, cottonwood); in summer by grass pollens (sheep sorrel, English plantain); and in the fall by weed pollens (ragweed). Occasionally, in summer and fall, hay fever is induced by allergy to mold (fungal spores).

In perennial allergic rhinitis, inhalant allergens provoke antigen responses that produce recurring symptoms year round.

The major perennial allergens and irritants are house dust, feather pillows, mold, cigarette smoke, upholstery, and animal danders. Seasonal pollen allergy may exacerbate symptoms of perennial rhinitis.

Signs and symptoms

In hay fever, the key signs and symptoms are paroxysmal sneezing, profuse watery rhinorrhea, nasal obstruction or congestion, and pruritus of the nose and eyes, sometimes accompanied by malaise and fever but usually by pale, cyanotic, edematous nasal mucosa; red and edematous eyelids and conjunctivae; excessive lacrimation; and headache or sinus pain. Some patients also complain of itching in the throat.

In perennial allergic rhinitis, conjunctivitis and other extranasal effects are rare, but chronic nasal obstruction is common and often extends to eustachian tube obstruction, particularly in children. In both conditions, dark circles may appear under the patient's eyes ("allergic shiners") because of venous congestion in the maxillary sinuses. The severity of signs and symptoms may vary from year to year.

Diagnosis

Microscopic examination of sputum and nasal secretions reveals large numbers of eosinophils. Blood chemistry shows normal or elevated IgE. Firm diagnosis rests on the patient's personal and family history of allergies and on physical findings during a symptomatic phase. Skin testing, paired with tested responses to environmental stimuli, can pinpoint the responsible allergens when interpreted in light of the patient's history.

To distinguish between allergic rhinitis and other disorders of the nasal mucosa, remember these differences. In chronic vasomotor rhinitis, eye symptoms are absent, rhinorrhea is mucoid, and seasonal variation is absent. In infectious rhinitis (common cold), the nasal mucosa is beet red; nasal secretions contain polymorphonuclear, not eosinophilic, exudate; and signs and symptoms include fever and sore throat. In rhinitis medicamentosa, which results from excessive use of nasal sprays or drops, nasal drainage and mucosal redness and swelling disappear when such medication is withheld. In children, differential diagnosis should rule out a nasal foreign body.

Treatment and special considerations

Treatment aims to control symptoms by eliminating the environmental antigen, if possible, and by drug therapy and immunotherapy. Antihistamines effectively block histamine effects but commonly produce anticholinergic side effects (sedation, dry mouth, nausea, dizziness, blurred vision, and nervousness). However, new antihistamines, such as terfenadine (Seldane), produce fewer side effects, and are much less likely to cause sedation. Topical intranasal steroids produce local anti-inflammatory effects with minimal systemic side effects. The most commonly used drugs are flunisolide (Nasalide) and beclomethasone (Beconase, Vancenase). Generally, these drugs aren't effective for acute exacerbations; nasal decongestants and oral antihistamines may be needed instead. Advise the patient to use intranasal steroids regularly, as prescribed, for optimal effectiveness. Cromolyn sodium (Nasalcrom) may be helpful in preventing allergic rhinitis. However, this drug may take up to 4 weeks to produce a satisfactory effect and must be taken regularly during allergy season.

When caring for the patient with allergic rhinitis, monitor his compliance with prescribed drug treatment regimens and note any changes in symptom control or signs of drug misuse.

Long-term management includes immunotherapy, or desensitization with injections of extracted allergens, administered preseasonally, coseasonally, or perennially. Seasonal allergies require particularly close dosage regulation. Before such injections, assess the patient's symptom status. Afterward, watch for adverse reactions, including anaphylaxis and severe localized erythema. Keep epinephrine and emergency resuscitative equipment available. Observe the patient for 30 minutes after the injection. Tell him to call the doctor if a delayed reaction occurs.

Patients can reduce environmental exposure to airborne allergens in several ways: by sleeping with the windows closed, by avoiding the countryside during pollination seasons, by using air conditioning to filter allergens and keep down moisture and dust, and by eliminating dust-collecting items, such as wool blankets, deep-pile carpets, and heavy drapes, from the home. Occasionally, in severe and resistant cases, patients may have to consider drastic changes in life-style, such as relocation to a pollen-free area either seasonally or year round.

Atopic Dermatitis

This chronic skin disorder is characterized by superficial skin inflammation and intense itching. Although atopic dermatitis may appear at any age, it typically begins during infancy or early childhood. It may then subside spontaneously, followed by exacerbations in late childhood, adolescence, or early adulthood. Atopic dermatitis affects approximately 0.7% of the population.

Causes

The cause of atopic dermatitis is still unknown. However, several theories attempt to explain its pathogenesis. One theory suggests an underlying metabolic- or biochemical-induced skin disorder genetically linked to elevated serum IgE levels; another suggests defective T cell function.

Exacerbating factors of atopic dermatitis include irritants, infections (commonly caused by *Staphylococcus aureus*), and some allergens. Although no reliable link exists between atopic dermatitis and exposure to inhalant allergens (such as house dust and animal dander), exposure to food allergens (such as soybeans, fish, or nuts) may coincide with flare-ups of atopic dermatitis.

Signs and symptoms

Scratching the skin causes vasoconstriction and intensifies pruritus, resulting in erythematous, weeping lesions. Eventually, the lesions become scaly and lichenified. Usually, they're located in areas of flexion and extension such as the neck, antecubital fossa, popliteal folds, and behind the ears. Patients with atopic dermatitis are prone to unusually severe viral infections, bacterial and fungal skin infections, ocular complications, and allergic contact dermatitis.

Diagnosis

Typically, the patient has a history of atopy such as asthma, hay fever, or urticaria; his family may have a similar history. Laboratory tests reveal eosinophilia and elevated serum IgE levels.

Treatment

Measures to ease this chronic disorder include meticulous skin care, environmental control of offending allergens, and drug therapy. Because dry skin aggravates itching, frequent application of nonirritating topical lubricants is important, especially after bathing or showering. Minimizing exposure to allergens and irritants, such as wools and harsh detergents, also helps control symptoms.

Drug therapy involves corticosteroids and antipruritics. Active dermatitis responds well to topical corticosteroids such as fluocinolone acetonide (Synalar) and flurandrenolide (Cordran). These drugs should be applied immediately after bathing for optimal penetration. Oral antihistamines, especially the phenothiazine derivatives such as methdilazine (Tacaryl) and trimeprazine (Temaril), help control itching. A bedtime dose of antihistamines may reduce involuntary scratching during sleep. If secondary infection develops, antibiotics are necessary.

Because this disorder may frustrate the patient and strain family ties, counseling may play a role in treatment.

Special considerations

- Monitor the patient's compliance with drug therapy.
- Teach the patient when and how to apply topical corticosteroids.
- Emphasize the importance of good personal hygiene.
- Be alert for signs and symptoms of secondary infection; teach the patient how to recognize them as well.
- If the patient's diet is modified to exclude food allergens, monitor his nutritional status.
- Offer support to help the patient and his family cope with this chronic disorder.

Anaphylaxis

Anaphylaxis is a dramatic, acute atopic reaction marked by the sudden onset of rapidly progressive urticaria and respiratory distress. A severe reaction may precipitate vascular collapse, leading to systemic shock and, sometimes, death.

Causes and incidence

The source of anaphylactic reactions is ingestion of or other systemic exposure to sensitizing drugs or other substances. Such substances may include serums (usually horse serum), vaccines, allergen extracts, enzymes (L-asparaginase), hormones, penicillin and other antibiotics, sulfonamides, local anesthetics, salicylates, polysaccharides, diagnostic chemicals (sulfobromophthalein, sodium dehydrocholate, and radiographic contrast media), foods (legumes, nuts, berries, seafoods, and egg albumin) and sulfite-containing food additives, insect venom (honeybees, wasps, hornets, yellow jackets, fire ants, mosquitoes, and certain spiders), and, rarely, ruptured hydatid cyst.

The single most common cause of anaphylaxis is penicillin, which induces anaphylaxis in 1 to 4 of every 10,000 patients treated with it. Penicillin is most likely to induce anaphylaxis after parenteral administration or prolonged therapy and in atopic patients with an allergy to other drugs or foods.

An anaphylactic reaction requires previous sensitization or exposure to the specific antigen, resulting in the production of specific IgE antibodies by plasma cells. This antibody production takes place in the lymph nodes and is enhanced by helper T cells. IgE antibodies then bind to membrane receptors on mast cells (found throughout connective tissue) and basophils.

On reexposure, the antigen binds to adjacent IgE antibodies or cross-linked IgE receptors, activating a series of cellular reactions that trigger degranulation—the release of powerful chemical mediators (such as histamine, ECF-A and PAF) from mast cell stores. IgG or IgM enters into the reaction and activates the release of complement fractions.

At the same time, two other chemical mediators, bradykinin and leukotrienes, induce vascular collapse by stimulating contraction of certain groups of smooth muscles and by increasing vascular permeability. In turn, increased vascular permeability leads to decreased peripheral resistance and plasma leakage from the circulation to extravascular tissues (which lowers blood volume, causing

PATIENT TEACHING AID

How to use an anaphylaxis kit

Dear Patient:

1. Contact doctor, if possible; then proceed with emergency kit.
2. Remove insect stinger if it's still there. Be careful not to push, pinch, squeeze, or imbed stinger farther into skin.
3. If you were stung on an arm or leg, apply tourniquet between sting and body. To tighten, pull end of one string. Release tourniquet every 10 minutes by pulling metal ring. If you were stung on the body, neck, or face, apply ice to the affected area.

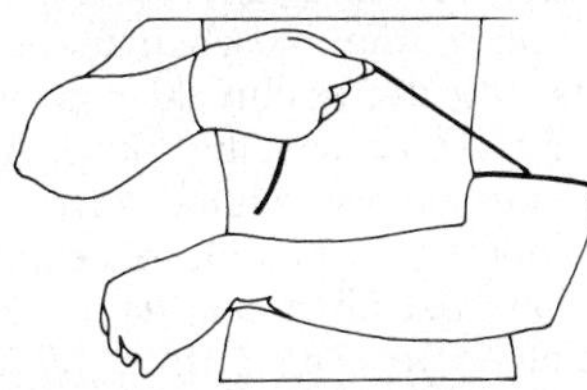

4. Using an alcohol swab, cleanse a 4" (10 cm) area on your arm or thigh (above tourniquet).
5. Prepare prefilled syringe. First, remove needle cover. Then, expel air from syringe by holding syringe with needle pointing up and carefully pushing plunger.
6. Inject epinephrine. Insert whole needle straight down into cleansed skin area. When this is done, pull back on plunger. If blood enters syringe, the needle is in a blood vessel. Withdraw needle, and reinsert in another site. For adults, and children over 12 years, push plunger until it stops (0.3 ml). Do not force farther. Remove the needle, and replace the needle cover. A second injection of 0.3 ml remains in the syringe. Children 12 years and younger: H-S Epinephrine 1:1,000 syringe has graduations of 0.1 ml so that doses less than 0.3 ml can be measured for children: 6 to 12 years, 0.2 ml; 2 to 6 years, 0.15 ml; infants to 2 years, 0.05 to 0.1 ml.

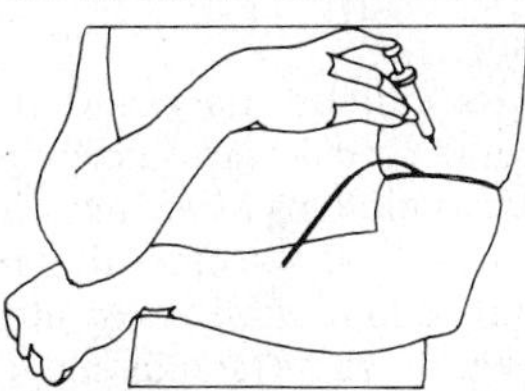

7. Chew and swallow Chlo-Amine (antihistamine) tablets. Adults and children over 12 years should take four tablets; children 12 years or younger, two tablets.
8. Apply ice packs, if available.
9. Keep warm. Avoid exertion.
10. Prepare prefilled syringe for second injection. Turn rectangular plunger one quarter turn to right, to line up with rectangular slot in syringe. Do not depress plunger until ready for second injection.
11. Second injection: If no noticeable improvement in 10 minutes, repeat steps 4, 5, and 6.

hypotension, hypovolemic shock, and cardiac dysfunction).

Signs and symptoms

Anaphylactic reaction produces sudden physical distress within seconds or minutes (although a delayed or persistent reaction may occur for up to 24 hours) after exposure to an allergen. Severity of the reaction is inversely related to the interval between exposure to the allergen and the onset of symptoms. Usually, the first symptoms include a feeling of impending doom or fright, weakness, sweating, sneezing, shortness of breath, nasal pruritus, urticaria, and angioedema, followed rapidly by symptoms in one or more target organs. Cardiovascular symptoms include hypotension, shock, and sometimes cardiac dysrhythmias, which, if untreated, may precipitate circulatory collapse. Respiratory symptoms can occur at any level in the respiratory tract and commonly include nasal mucosal edema, profuse watery rhinorrhea, itching, nasal congestion, and sudden sneezing attacks. Edema of the upper respiratory tract, resulting in hypopharyngeal and laryngeal obstruction (hoarseness, stridor, and dyspnea), is an early sign of acute respiratory failure, which can be fatal. Gastrointestinal and genitourinary symptoms include severe stomach cramps, nausea, diarrhea, and urinary urgency and incontinence.

Diagnosis

Anaphylaxis can be diagnosed by the rapid onset of severe respiratory or cardiovascular symptoms after ingestion or injection of a drug, vaccine, diagnostic agent, food, or food additive or after an insect sting. If these symptoms occur without a known allergic stimulus, rule out other possible causes of shock (acute myocardial infarction, status asthmaticus, congestive heart failure).

Treatment and special considerations

Anaphylaxis is always an emergency. It requires an *immediate* injection of epinephrine 1:1,000 aqueous solution, 0.1 to 0.5 ml, repeated every 5 to 20 minutes, as necessary.

In the early stages of anaphylaxis, when the patient has not lost consciousness and is normotensive, give epinephrine intramuscularly or subcutaneously, and help it move into circulation faster by massaging the site of injection. In severe reactions, when the patient has lost consciousness and is hypotensive, give epinephrine I.V.

Maintain airway patency. Observe for early signs of laryngeal edema (stridor, hoarseness, and dyspnea), which will probably necessitate endotracheal tube insertion or a tracheotomy and oxygen therapy.

In case of cardiac arrest, begin cardiopulmonary resuscitation, including closed-chest heart massage, assisted ventilation, and sodium bicarbonate; other therapy is indicated by clinical response.

Watch for hypotension and shock, and maintain circulatory volume with volume expanders (plasma, plasma expanders, saline, and albumin), as needed. Stabilize blood pressure with the I.V. vasopressors norepinephrine and dopamine. Monitor blood pressure, central venous pressure, and urinary output as a response index.

After the initial emergency, administer other medications as ordered: subcutaneous epinephrine, longer-acting epinephrine, corticosteroids, and diphenhydramine I.V. for long-term management; and aminophylline I.V. over 10 to 20 minutes for bronchospasm. (Caution: Rapid infusion of aminophylline may cause or aggravate severe hypotension.)

To prevent anaphylaxis, teach the patient to avoid exposure to known aller-

PENICILLIN WITH CAUTION

When administering penicillin or its derivatives, such as ampicillin or carbenicillin, follow these recommendations of the World Health Organization to prevent allergic response:

- Have an emergency kit available to treat allergic reactions.
- Take a detailed patient history, including penicillin allergy and other allergies. In an infant younger than 3 months old, check for penicillin allergy in the mother.
- Never give penicillin to a patient who has had an allergic reaction to it.
- Before giving penicillin to a patient with suspected penicillin allergy, refer the patient for skin and immunologic tests to confirm it.
- Always tell a patient he is going to receive penicillin before he takes the first dose.
- Observe carefully for adverse effects for at least one half hour after penicillin administration.
- Be aware that penicillin derivatives also elicit an allergic reaction.

gens. In food or drug allergy, the sensitized person must learn to avoid the offending food or drug in all its forms. With allergy to insect stings, he should avoid open fields and wooded areas during the insect season and should carry an anaphylaxis kit (epinephrine, antihistamine, tourniquet) whenever he must go outdoors. In addition, every patient prone to anaphylaxis should wear a Medic Alert bracelet identifying his allergy or allergies.

If a patient must receive a drug to which he is allergic, prevent a severe reaction by making sure he receives careful desensitization with gradually increasing doses of the antigen or advance administration of steroids. Of course, a person with a known allergic history should receive a drug with a high anaphylactic potential only after cautious pre-testing for sensitivity. Closely monitor the patient during testing, and make sure you have resuscitative equipment and epinephrine ready. When any patient needs a drug with a high anaphylactic potential (particularly parenteral drugs), make sure he receives each dose under close medical observation.

Closely monitor a patient undergoing diagnostic tests, such as intravenous pyelography (IVP), cardiac catheterization, and angiography, that use radiographic contrast media.

Urticaria and Angioedema

(Hives)

Urticaria is an episodic, usually self-limited skin reaction characterized by local dermal wheals surrounded by an erythematous flare. Angioedema is a subcutaneous and dermal eruption that produces deeper, larger wheals (usually on the hands, feet, lips, genitals, and eyelids) and a more diffuse swelling of loose subcutaneous tissue. Urticaria and angioedema can occur simultaneously, but angioedema may last longer.

Causes and incidence

Urticaria and angioedema are common allergic reactions that may occur in 20% of the general population at some time or other. The causes of these reactions include allergy to drugs, foods, insect stings, and, occasionally, inhalant allergens (animal danders, cosmetics) that provoke an IgE-mediated response to protein allergens. However, certain drugs may cause urticaria without an IgE response. When urticaria and angioedema are part of an anaphylactic reaction, they almost always persist long after the systemic response has subsided. This occurs because circulation to the skin is the last to be restored after an allergic reaction, which results in slow histamine reabsorption at the reaction site.

Nonallergic urticaria and angioedema are probably also related to histamine release by some still-unknown mechanism. External physical stimuli, such as cold (usually in young adults), heat, water, or sunlight, may also provoke urticaria and angioedema. *Dermographism urticaria*, which develops after stroking or scratching the skin, occurs in as many as 20% of the population. Such urticaria develops with varying pressure, most often under tight clothing, and is aggravated by scratching.

Several different mechanisms and underlying disorders may provoke urticaria and angioedema: these include IgE-induced release of mediators from cutaneous mast cells; binding of IgG or IgM to antigen, resulting in complement activation; and disorders such as localized or secondary infection (respiratory infection), neoplastic disease (Hodgkin's

HEREDITARY ANGIOEDEMA

A nonallergenic type of angioedema, hereditary angioedema results from an autosomal dominant trait—a hereditary deficiency of an alpha globulin, the normal inhibitor of C1 esterase (a component of the complement system). This deficiency allows uninhibited C1 esterase release, resulting in the vascular changes common to angioedema.

The clinical effects of hereditary angioedema usually appear in childhood with recurrent episodes of subcutaneous or submucosal edema at irregular intervals of weeks, months, or years, often following trauma or stress. Hereditary angioedema is unifocal, without urticarial pruritus but associated with recurrent edema of the skin and mucosa (especially of the GI and respiratory tracts). GI tract involvement may cause nausea, vomiting, and severe abdominal pain. Laryngeal angioedema may cause fatal airway obstruction.

Treatment for acute hereditary angioedema may require androgens, such as danazol. Tracheotomy may be necessary to relieve airway obstruction resulting from laryngeal angioedema.

lymphoma), connective tissue diseases (systemic lupus erythematosus), collagen vascular disease, and psychogenic disease.

Signs and symptoms

The characteristic features of urticaria are distinct, raised, evanescent dermal wheals surrounded by an erythematous flare. These lesions may vary in size. In cholinergic urticaria, the wheals may be tiny and blanched, surrounded by erythematous flares.

Angioedema characteristically produces nonpitted swelling of deep subcutaneous tissue, usually on the eyelids, lips, genitalia, and mucous membranes. These swellings don't usually itch but may burn and tingle.

Diagnosis

An accurate patient history can help determine the cause of hives. Such a history should include:

- drug history, including over-the-counter preparations (vitamins, aspirin, antacids)
- frequently ingested foods (strawberries, milk products, fish)
- environmental influences (pets, carpet, clothing, soap, inhalants, cosmetics, hair dye, insect bites and stings).

Diagnosis also requires physical assessment to rule out similar conditions, and complete blood count, urinalysis, erythrocyte sedimentation rate, and chest X-ray to rule out inflammatory infections. Skin testing, an elimination diet, and a food diary (recording time and amount of food eaten, and circumstances) can pinpoint provoking allergens. The food diary may also suggest other allergies. For instance, a patient allergic to fish may also be allergic to iodine contrast materials.

Recurrent angioedema without urticaria, along with a familial history, points to hereditary angioedema. Decreased serum levels of C4 and C1 esterase inhibitor confirm this diagnosis.

Treatment and special considerations

Treatment aims to prevent or limit contact with triggering factors or, if this is impossible, to desensitize the patient to them and to relieve symptoms. Once the triggering stimulus has been removed, urticaria usually subsides in a few days—except for drug reactions, which may persist as long as the drug is in the bloodstream.

During desensitization, progressively larger doses of specific antigens (determined by skin testing) are injected intradermally.

Diphenhydramine or another antihistamine can ease itching and swelling with every kind of urticaria. Inform patients receiving antihistamines of the possibility of drowsiness.

Blood Transfusion Reaction

Mediated by immune or nonimmune factors, a transfusion reaction accompanies or follows I.V. administration of blood components. Its severity varies from mild (fever and chills) to severe (acute renal failure or complete vascular collapse and death), depending on the amount of blood transfused, the type of reaction, and the patient's general health.

Causes and types

Hemolytic reactions follow transfusion of mismatched blood. Transfusion with serologically incompatible blood triggers the most serious reaction, marked by intravascular agglutination of red blood cells (RBCs). The recipient's antibodies (IgG or IgM) attach to the donated RBCs, leading to widespread clumping and destruction of the recipient's RBCs and possibly the development of disseminated intravascular coagulation and other serious effects.

Transfusion with Rh-incompatible blood triggers a less serious reaction within several days to 2 weeks. Rh reactions are most likely in women sensitized to RBC antigens by prior pregnancy or by unknown factors such as bacterial or viral infection, and in persons who have received more than five transfusions.

Allergic reactions are fairly common but only occasionally serious. In this type of reaction, transfused soluble antigens react with surface IgE molecules on mast cells and basophils, causing degranulation and release of allergic mediators. Antibodies against IgA in an IgA-deficient recipient can also trigger a severe allergic reaction (anaphylaxis).

Febrile nonhemolytic reactions, the most common type of reaction, apparently develop when cytotoxic or agglutinating antibodies in the recipient's plasma attack antigens on transfused lymphocytes, granulocytes, or plasma cells.

Although fairly uncommon, *bacterial contamination* of donor blood can occur during donor phlebotomy. Offending organisms are usually gram-negative, especially *Pseudomonas* species, *Citrobacter freundii*, and *Escherichia coli*.

Also possible is contamination of donor blood with viruses such as hepatitis, cytomegalovirus, and malaria.

Signs and symptoms

Immediate effects of hemolytic transfusion reaction develop within a few minutes or hours after the start of transfusion and may include chills, fever, urticaria, tachycardia, dyspnea, nausea, vomiting, tightness in the chest, chest and back pain, hypotension, bronchospasm, angioedema, and signs and symptoms of anaphylaxis, shock, pulmonary edema, and congestive heart failure. In a surgical patient under anesthesia, these symptoms are masked, but blood oozes from mucous membranes or the incision site.

Delayed hemolytic reactions can occur up to several weeks after transfusion, causing fever, an unexpected fall in serum hemoglobin level, and jaundice.

Allergic reactions are typically afebrile and characterized by urticaria and angioedema, possibly progressing to cough, respiratory distress, nausea and vomiting, diarrhea, abdominal cramps, vascular instability, shock, and coma.

The hallmark of febrile nonhemolytic reactions is mild to severe fever that may begin at the start of transfusion or within 2 hours after its completion.

Bacterial contamination causes high fever, nausea and vomiting, diarrhea, abdominal cramps, and possibly shock.

Symptoms of viral contamination may not appear for several weeks after transfusion.

Diagnosis

Confirming a hemolytic transfusion re-

Rh SYSTEM

The Rh system contains more than 30 antibodies and antigens. Eighty-five percent of the world's population are Rh-positive, which means their red blood cells carry the D or Rh antigen. The remaining 15% of the population who are Rh-negative do not carry this antigen.

When Rh-negative persons receive Rh-positive blood for the first time, they become sensitized to the D antigen but show no immediate reaction to it. If they receive Rh-positive blood a second time, they then develop a massive hemolytic reaction. For example, an Rh-negative mother who delivers an Rh-positive baby is sensitized by the baby's Rh-positive blood. During her next Rh-positive pregnancy, her sensitized blood would cause a hemolytic reaction in fetal circulation. Thus, the Rh-negative mother should receive Rh_o (D) immune globulin (human) I.M. within 72 hours after delivering an Rh-positive baby to prevent formation of antibodies against Rh-positive blood.

action requires proof of blood incompatibility and evidence of hemolysis, such as hemoglobinuria, anti-A or anti-B antibodies in the serum, low serum hemoglobin, and elevated bilirubin levels. When you suspect such a reaction, have the patient's blood retyped and cross matched with the donor's blood. After a hemolytic transfusion reaction, laboratory tests will show increased indirect bilirubin, decreased haptoglobin, increased serum hemoglobin, and hemoglobin in urine. As the reaction progresses, tests may show signs of disseminated intravascular coagulation (thrombocytopenia, increased prothrombin time, decreased fibrinogen level) and acute tubular necrosis (increased serum BUN and creatinine).

Blood culture to isolate the causative organism should be done when bacterial contamination is suspected.

Treatment and special considerations

At the first sign of a hemolytic reaction, *stop the transfusion immediately*. Depending on the nature of the patient's reaction, prepare to:

- Monitor vital signs every 15 to 30 minutes, watching for signs of shock.
- Maintain a patent I.V. line with normal saline, and insert an indwelling catheter and monitor intake and output.
- Cover the patient with blankets to ease chills, and explain what is happening.
- Deliver supplemental oxygen at low flow rates through a nasal cannula or bag-valve-mask (Ambu bag).
- Give drugs as ordered: an I.V. antihypotensive drug and normal saline solution to combat shock, epinephrine to treat dyspnea and wheezing, diphenhydramine to combat cellular histamine released from mast cells, corticosteroids to reduce inflammation, and mannitol or furosemide to maintain urinary function. Administer parenteral antihistamines and corticosteroids for allergic reactions. (Severe reactions—anaphylaxis—may require epinephrine.) Administer antipyretics for nonhemolytic febrile reactions and appropriate I.V. antibiotics for bacterial contamination.
- Remember to fully document the transfusion reaction on the patient's chart, noting the duration of the transfusion, the amount of blood absorbed, and a complete description of the reaction and of any interventions.

To prevent a hemolytic transfusion reaction: Before giving a blood transfusion, be sure you know your hospital's policy about giving blood. Then make sure you have the right blood and the right patient. Check and double-check the patient's name, hospital number, ABO group, and Rh status. If you find even a small discrepancy, don't give the blood. Notify the blood bank immediately and return the unopened unit.

AUTOIMMUNITY

Rheumatoid Arthritis

A chronic, systemic, inflammatory disease, rheumatoid arthritis (RA) primarily attacks peripheral joints and surrounding muscles, tendons, ligaments, and blood vessels. Spontaneous remissions and unpredictable exacerbations mark the course of this potentially crippling disease. Rheumatoid arthritis usually requires lifelong treatment and, sometimes, surgery. In most patients, the disease follows an intermittent course and allows normal activity, although 10% suffer total disability from severe articular deformity or associated extraarticular symptoms, or both. Prognosis worsens with the development of nodules, vasculitis, and high titers of rheumatoid factor (RF).

Causes and incidence

RA occurs worldwide, striking females three times more often than males. Although RA can occur at any age, the peak onset period for women is between ages 30 and 60. It affects more than 6.5 million people in the United States alone.

What causes the chronic inflammation characteristic of RA isn't known, but various theories point to infectious, genetic, and endocrine factors. Currently, it's believed that a genetically susceptible individual develops abnormal or altered IgG antibodies when exposed to an antigen. This altered IgG antibody is not recognized as "self", and the individual forms an antibody against it—an antibody known as RF. By aggregating into complexes, RF generates inflammation. Eventually, cartilage damage by inflammation triggers additional immune responses, including activation of complement. This in turn attracts polymorphonuclear leukocytes and stimulates release of inflammatory mediators, which enhance joint destruction.

Much more is known about the pathogenesis of RA than about its causes. If unarrested, the inflammatory process within the joints occurs in four stages. First, synovitis develops from congestion and edema of the synovial membrane and joint capsule. Formation of pannus—thickened layers of granulation tissue—marks the onset of the second stage. Pannus covers and invades cartilage, and eventually destroys the joint capsule and bone. Progression to the third stage is characterized by fibrous ankylosis—fibrous invasion of the pannus and scar formation that occludes the joint space. Bone atrophy and malalignment cause visible deformities and disrupt the articulation of opposing bones, causing muscle atrophy and imbalance and, possibly, partial dislocations or subluxations. In the fourth stage, fibrous tissue calcifies, resulting in bony ankylosis and total immobility.

Signs and symptoms

RA usually develops insidiously, and initially produces nonspecific symptoms such as fatigue, malaise, anorexia, persistent low-grade fever, weight loss, lymphadenopathy, and vague articular symptoms. Later, more specific localized articular symptoms develop, frequently in the fingers at the proximal interphalangeal (PIP), metacarpophalangeal (MCP), and metatarsophalangeal (MTP) joints. These symptoms usually occur bilaterally and symmetrically, and may extend to the wrists, knees, elbows, and ankles. The affected joints stiffen after inactivity, especially upon rising in the morning. The fingers may assume a spindle shape from marked edema and congestion in the joints. The joints become tender and painful, at first only when

WHEN ARTHRITIS REQUIRES SURGERY

Arthritis severe enough to necessitate total knee or total hip arthroplasty calls for comprehensive preoperative teaching and postoperative care.

Before surgery:

- Explain surgical procedures and show the patient the prosthesis to be used, if available. Also, explain preoperative procedures (skin scrubs, prophylactic antibiotics).
- Teach the patient postoperative exercises (such as isometrics), and supervise his practice. Also, teach deep-breathing and coughing exercises.
- Explain that total hip or knee arthroplasty requires frequent range-of-motion exercises of the leg after surgery; total knee arthroplasty requires frequent leg-lift exercises.
- Show the patient how to use a trapeze to move himself about in bed after surgery, and make sure he has a fracture bedpan handy.
- Tell the patient what kind of dressings to expect after surgery. After total knee arthroplasty, he may have a cast, compression dressing, or dressing with a posterior splint. After total hip arthroplasty, he'll have an abduction pillow between the legs to help keep the hip prosthesis in place.

After surgery:

- Closely monitor and record vital signs. Watch for complications, such as steroid crisis and shock in patients receiving steroids. Measure distal leg pulses often, marking them with a waterproof marker to make them easier to find.
- As soon as the patient awakens, have him do active dorsiflexion; if he can't, report this immediately. Supervise isometrics every 2 hours. After total hip arthroplasty, check traction for pressure areas and keep the head of the bed raised between 30° and 45°.
- Change or reinforce dressings, as needed, using aseptic technique. Check wounds for hematoma, excessive drainage, color changes, or foul odor—all possible signs of infection. (Wounds on RA patients may heal slowly.) Avoid contaminating dressings while helping the patient use the urinal or bedpan.
- Administer blood replacement products, antibiotics, and pain medication, as ordered. Monitor serum electrolytes, hemoglobin, and hematocrit.
- Have the patient turn, cough, and deep breathe every 2 hours; then percuss his chest.
- After total knee arthroplasty, keep the patient's leg extended and slightly elevated.
- After total hip arthroplasty, keep the patient's hip in abduction to prevent dislocation. Watch for and immediately report any inability to rotate the hip or bear weight on it, increased pain, or a leg that appears shorter—all may indicate dislocation.
- As soon as allowed, help the patient get out of bed and sit in a chair, keeping his weight on the unaffected side. When he's ready to walk, consult with the physical therapist for walking instruction and aids.

the patient moves them, but eventually even at rest. They often feel hot to the patient. Ultimately, joint function is diminished.

Deformities are common if active disease continues. PIP joints may develop flexion deformities or become hyperextended. MCP joints may swell dorsally, and volar subluxation and stretching of tendons may pull the fingers to the ulnar side ("ulnar drift"). The fingers may become fixed in a characteristic "swan's neck" appearance, or "boutonnière" deformity. The hands appear foreshortened, the wrists boggy; carpal tunnel syndrome from synovial pressure on the median nerve causes tingling paresthesias in the fingers.

The most common extraarticular finding is the gradual appearance of rheumatoid nodules—subcutaneous, round or oval, nontender masses—usually on pressure areas such as the elbows. Vasculitis can lead to skin lesions, leg ulcers, and multiple systemic complications. Peripheral neuropathy may produce numbness or tingling in the feet or weakness and loss of sensation in the fingers. Stiff, weak, or painful muscles are common. Other common extraarticular effects include pericarditis, pulmonary nodules or fibrosis, pleuritis, scleritis, and episcleritis.

Another complication is destruction of the odontoid process, part of the second cervical vertebra. Rarely, cord compression may occur, particularly in patients with long-standing deforming RA. Upper motor neuron signs, such as a positive Babinski's sign and muscle weakness, may also develop.

RA can also cause temporomandibular joint disease, which impairs chewing and causes earaches. Other extraarticular findings may include infection, osteoporosis, myositis, cardiopulmonary lesions, lymphadenopathy, and peripheral neuritis.

Diagnosis

Typical clinical features suggest RA, but firm diagnosis relies on laboratory and other test results:

- *X-rays*: in early stages, show bone demineralization and soft-tissue swelling; later, loss of cartilage and narrowing of joint spaces; finally, cartilage and bone destruction, and erosion, subluxations, and deformities
- *rheumatoid factor (RF) test*: positive in 75% to 80% of patients, as indicated by a titer of 1:160 or higher
- *synovial fluid analysis*: increased volume and turbidity, but decreased viscosity and complement (C3 and C4) levels; WBC often more than 10,000/mm^3
- *serum protein electrophoresis*: may show elevated serum globulins
- *erythrocyte sedimentation rate:* elevated in 85% to 90% of patients (may be useful to monitor response to therapy, since elevation frequently parallels disease activity)
- *complete blood count*: usually moderate anemia and slight leukocytosis.

A C-reactive protein test can help monitor response to therapy.

Treatment

Salicylates, particularly aspirin, are the mainstay of RA therapy, since they decrease inflammation and relieve joint pain. Other useful medications include nonsteroidal anti-inflammatory agents (such as indomethacin, fenoprofen, and ibuprofen), antimalarials (chloroquine and hydroxychloroquine), gold salts, penicillamine, and corticosteroids (prednisone). Immunosuppressives, such as cyclophosphamide and azathioprine, are also therapeutic.

Supportive measures include 8 to 10 hours of sleep every night, frequent rest periods between daily activities, and splinting to rest inflamed joints. A physical therapy program including range-of-motion exercises and carefully individualized therapeutic exercises forestalls loss of joint function; application of heat relaxes muscles and relieves pain. Moist heat (hot soaks, paraffin baths, whirlpool) usually works best for patients with chronic disease. Ice packs are effective during acute episodes.

Advanced disease may require synovectomy, joint reconstruction, or total joint arthroplasty.

Useful surgical procedures in RA in-

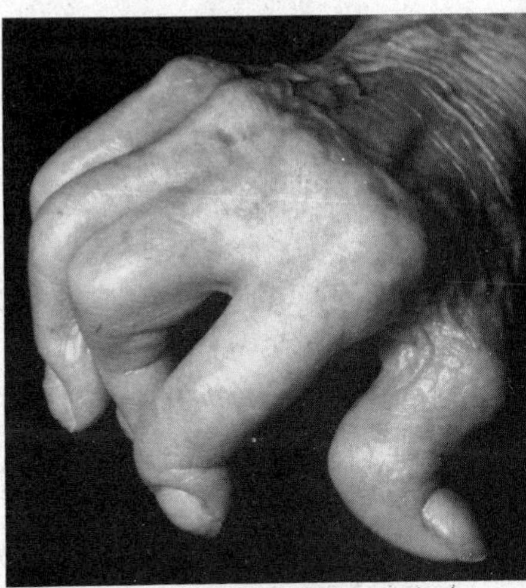

In advanced rheumatoid arthritis, marked edema and congestion cause spindle-shaped interphalangeal joints and severe flexion deformities.

DRUG THERAPY FOR ARTHRITIS

DRUG AND SIDE EFFECTS	CLINICAL CONSIDERATIONS
Aspirin • Prolonged bleeding time; GI disturbances including nausea, dyspepsia, anorexia, ulcers, and hemorrhage; hypersensitivity reactions ranging from urticaria to anaphylaxis; salicylism (mild toxicity: tinnitus, dizziness; moderate toxicity: restlessness, hyperpnea, delirium, marked lethargy; and severe toxicity: coma, convulsions, severe hyperpnea)	• Don't use in patients with GI ulcers, bleeding, or hypersensitivity or in newborns. • Give with food, milk, antacid, or large glass of water to reduce GI side effects. • Remember that toxicity can develop rapidly in febrile, dehydrated children. • Monitor salicylate level. • Teach patient to reduce dose, one tablet at a time, if tinnitus occurs. • Teach patient to watch for signs of bleeding, such as bruising, melena, and petechiae.
Fenoprofen, ibuprofen, naproxen, piroxicam, sulindac, and tolmetin • Prolonged bleeding time, CNS abnormalities (headache, drowsiness, restlessness, dizziness, tremor), GI disturbances including hemorrhage and peptic ulcer, increased blood urea nitrogen and liver enzymes	• Don't use in patients with renal disease, in asthmatics with nasal polyps, or in children. • Use cautiously in GI disorders and cardiac disease or when patient is allergic to other nonsteroidal anti-inflammatory drugs. • Give with milk or meals to reduce GI side effects. • Tell patient that therapeutic effect may be delayed for 2 to 3 weeks. • Monitor kidney, liver, and auditory functions in long-term therapy. Stop drug if abnormalities develop.
Indomethacin • Blood dyscrasias; hemolytic, aplastic, and iron deficiency anemia; blurred vision; corneal and retinal damage; hearing loss; tinnitus; GI disturbances including GI ulcer, hematuria	• Don't use in children under age 14 or in patients with aspirin intolerance or GI disorders. • Severe headache may occur within 1 hour. Stop drug if headache persists. • Tell patient to report any visual changes. Stress the need for regular eye examinations during long-term therapy. • Always give with food or milk. • A single dose at bedtime may alleviate morning stiffness.
Gold (oral and parenteral) • Dermatitis, pruritus, rash, stomatitis, nephrotoxicity, blood dyscrasias, and, with oral form, GI distress and diarrhea	• Watch for and report side effects. Observe for nitritoid reaction (flushing, fainting, sweating). • Check urine for blood and albumin before each dose. If positive, hold drug and notify doctor. Stress the need for regular follow-up examinations, including blood and urine testing. • To avoid local nerve irritation, mix drug well and give deep I.M. injection in buttock. • Advise patient not to expect improvement for 3 to 6 months. • Instruct patient to report rash, bruising, bleeding, hematuria, or oral ulcers
Penicillamine • Blood dyscrasias, glomerulonephropathy	• Give on empty stomach, before meals, and separately from other drugs or milk. • Tell patient to report fever, sore throat, chills, bruising, or bleeding. • Monitor urine (for protein and blood), liver function, and complete blood count.

Other drugs that may be used in resistant cases include prednisone, chloroquine, azathioprine, cyclophosphamide, and methotrexate.

clude metatarsal head and distal ulnar resectional arthroplasty, insertion of a Silastic prosthesis between MCP and PIP joints, and arthrodesis (joint fusion). Arthrodesis sacrifices joint mobility for stability and relief of pain. Synovectomy (removal of destructive, proliferating synovium, usually in the wrists, knees, and fingers) may halt or delay the course of this disease. Osteotomy (the cutting of bone or excision of a wedge of bone) can realign joint surfaces and redistribute stresses. Tendons may rupture spontaneously, requiring surgical repair. Tendon transfers may prevent deformities or relieve contractures.

Special considerations

- Assess all joints carefully. Look for deformities, contractures, immobility, and inability to perform everyday activities.
- Monitor vital signs, and note weight changes, sensory disturbances, and level of pain. Administer analgesics, as ordered, and watch for side effects.
- Give meticulous skin care. Check for rheumatoid nodules, as well as pressure sores and breakdowns due to immobility, vascular impairment, corticosteroid treatment, or improper splinting. Use lotion or cleansing oil, not soap, for dry skin.
- Explain all diagnostic tests and procedures. Tell the patient to expect multiple blood samples to allow firm diagnosis and accurate monitoring of therapy.
- Monitor the duration, not the intensity, of morning stiffness, because duration more accurately reflects the severity of the disease. Encourage the patient to take hot showers or baths at bedtime or in the morning to reduce the need for pain medication.
- Apply splints carefully and correctly. Observe for pressure sores if the patient is in traction or wearing splints.
- Explain the nature of RA. Make sure the patient and his family understand that RA is a chronic disease that requires major changes in life-style. Emphasize that there are no miracle cures, despite claims to the contrary.
- Encourage a balanced diet, but make sure the patient understands that special diets won't cure RA. Stress the need for weight control, since obesity adds further stress to joints.
- Urge the patient to perform activities of daily living, such as dressing and feeding himself (supply easy-to-open cartons, lightweight cups, and unpackaged silverware). Allow the patient enough time to calmly perform these tasks.
- Provide emotional support. Remember that the patient with chronic illness easily becomes depressed, discouraged, and irritable. Encourage the RA patient to discuss his fears concerning dependency, sexuality, body image, and self-esteem. Refer him to an appropriate social service agency, as needed.
- Discuss sexual aids: alternative positions, pain medication, and moist heat to increase mobility.
- Before discharge, make sure the patient knows how and when to take prescribed medication and how to recognize possible side effects.
- Teach the patient how to stand, walk, and sit correctly: upright and erect. Tell him to sit in chairs with high seats and armrests; he'll find it easier to get up from a chair if his knees are lower than his hips. If he doesn't own a chair with a high seat, recommend putting blocks of wood under the legs of a favorite chair. Suggest an elevated toilet seat.
- Instruct the patient to pace daily activities, resting for 5 to 10 minutes out of each hour and alternating sitting and standing tasks. Adequate sleep is important, and so is correct sleeping posture. He should sleep on his back on a firm mattress and should avoid placing a pillow under his knees, which encourages flexion deformity.
- Teach him to avoid putting undue stress on joints and to use the largest joint available for a given task; to support weak or painful joints as much as possible; to avoid positions of flexion and promote positions of extension; to hold objects parallel to the knuckles as briefly as possible; to always use his hands toward the center of his body; and to

slide—not lift—objects, whenever possible. Enlist the aid of the occupational therapist to teach how to simplify activities and protect arthritic joints. Stress the importance of shoes with proper support.

- Suggest dressing aids—long-handled shoehorn, reacher, elastic shoelaces, zipper-pull, and buttonhook—and helpful household items, such as easy-to-open drawers, hand-held shower nozzle, handrails, and grab bars. The patient who has trouble maneuvering fingers into gloves should wear mittens. Tell him to dress while in a sitting position as often as possible.
- For more information on coping with RA, refer the patient to the Arthritis Foundation.

Juvenile Rheumatoid Arthritis

Affecting children under age 16, juvenile rheumatoid arthritis (JRA) is an inflammatory disorder of the connective tissues characterized by joint swelling and pain or tenderness. It may also involve organs such as the skin, heart, lungs, liver, spleen, and eyes, producing extraarticular signs and symptoms. JRA has three major types: systemic (Still's disease or acute febrile type), polyarticular, and pauciarticular. Depending on the type, this disease can occur as early as age 6 weeks—although rarely before 6 months—with peaks of onset between ages 1 and 3, and 8 and 12. Considered the major chronic rheumatic disorder of childhood, JRA affects an estimated 150,000 to 250,000 children in the United States; overall incidence is twice as high in girls, with variation among the types.

Causes

The cause of JRA remains puzzling. Research continues to test several theories, such as those linking JRA to genetic factors or to an abnormal immune response. Viral or bacterial (particularly streptococcal) infection, trauma, and emotional stress may be precipitating factors, but their relationship to JRA remains unclear.

Signs and symptoms

Signs and symptoms vary with the type of JRA. Affecting boys and girls almost equally, systemic JRA accounts for approximately 20% to 30% of cases. The affected children may have mild, transient arthritis or frank polyarthritis associated with fever and rash. Joint involvement may not be evident at first, but the child's behavior may clearly suggest joint pain. Such a child may want to constantly sit in a flexed position, may not walk much, or may refuse to walk at all. Young children with JRA are noticeably irritable and listless.

Fever in systemic JRA occurs suddenly and spikes to 103° F. (39.4° C.) or higher once or twice daily, usually in the late afternoon, then rapidly returns to normal or subnormal. (This "sawtooth" or intermittent spiking fever pattern helps differentiate JRA from other inflammatory disorders.) When fever spikes, an evanescent rheumatoid rash often appears, consisting of small, pale, or salmon pink macules, most commonly on the trunk and proximal extremities and occasionally on the face, palms, and soles. Massaging or applying heat intensifies this rash, which is usually most conspicuous where the skin has been rubbed or subjected to pressure, such as that from underclothing.

Other signs and symptoms of systemic JRA may include hepatosplenomegaly, lymphadenopathy, pleuritis, pericarditis, myocarditis, and nonspecific abdominal pain.

Polyarticular JRA affects girls three times more often than boys and may be seronegative or seropositive for rheumatoid factor (RF). It involves five or more joints, and usually develops insidiously. Most commonly involved joints are the wrists, elbows, knees, ankles, and small joints of the hands and feet. Polyarticular JRA can also affect larger joints, including the temporomandibular joints and those of the cervical spine, hips, and shoulders. These joints become swollen, tender, and stiff. Usually, the arthritis is symmetric; it may be remittent or indolent. The patient may run a low-grade fever with daily peaks. Listlessness and weight loss can occur, possibly with lymphadenopathy and hepatosplenomegaly. Other signs of polyarticular JRA include subcutaneous nodules on the elbows or heels and noticeable developmental retardation.

Seropositive polyarticular JRA, the more severe type, usually occurs late in childhood and can cause destructive arthritis that mimics adult RA.

Pauciarticular JRA involves few joints (usually no more than four) and most often affects the knees and other large joints. It accounts for 45% of cases. Three major subtypes exist. The first, pauciarticular JRA with chronic iridocyclitis, most commonly strikes girls under age 6 and involves the knees, elbows, ankles, or iris. Inflammation of the iris and ciliary body is often asymptomatic but may produce pain, redness, blurred vision, and photophobia. The second subtype, pauciarticular JRA with sacroiliitis, usually strikes boys (9:1) over age 8, who tend to be HLA-B27 positive. This subtype is characterized by lower extremity arthritis that produces hip, sacroiliac, heel, and foot pain and Achilles tendinitis. These patients may later develop the sacroiliac and lumbar arthritis characteristic of ankylosing spondylitis. Some also experience acute iritis, but not as frequently as those with the first subtype. The third subtype includes patients with joint involvement who are antinuclear antibody (ANA) and HLA-B27 negative and do not develop iritis. These patients have a better prognosis than those with the first or second subtype.

Common to all types of JRA is joint stiffness in the morning or after periods of inactivity. Growth disturbances may also occur, resulting in overgrowth or undergrowth adjacent to inflamed joints.

Diagnosis

Persistent joint pain and the rash and fever clearly point to JRA. Laboratory tests are useful for ruling out other inflammatory or even malignant diseases that can mimic JRA and for monitoring disease activity and response to therapy.

- Complete blood count shows decreased hemoglobin, neutrophilia, and thrombocytosis.
- Erythrocyte sedimentation rate, C-reactive protein, haptoglobin, immunoglobulins, and C3 complement may be elevated.
- ANA test may be positive in patients who have pauciarticular JRA with chronic iridocyclitis.
- RF is present in 15% of JRA cases, as compared with 85% of RA cases.
- Positive HLA-B27 may forecast later development of ankylosing spondylitis.
- Early X-ray changes include soft-tissue swelling, effusion, and periostitis in affected joints. Later, osteoporosis and accelerated bone growth may appear, followed by subchondral erosions, joint space narrowing, bone destruction, and fusion.

Treatment and special considerations

Successful management of JRA usually involves administration of anti-inflammatory drugs, physical therapy, carefully planned nutrition and exercise, and regular eye examinations. Both child and parents must be involved in therapy.

Aspirin is the initial drug of choice, with dosage based on the child's weight. However, other nonsteroidal anti-inflammatory drugs (NSAIDs) may also be used. If these prove ineffective, gold salts, hydroxychloroquine, and penicillamine may be tried. Because of adverse effects, steroids are generally reserved for treatment of systemic complications, such as pericarditis or iritis, that are resistant to

NSAIDs. Corticosteroids and mydriatic drugs are commonly used for iridocyclitis. Low-dose cytotoxic drug therapy is currently being investigated.

Physical therapy promotes regular exercise to maintain joint mobility and muscle strength, thereby preventing contractures, deformity, and disability. Good posture, gait training, and joint protection are also beneficial. Splints help reduce pain, prevent contractures, and maintain correct joint alignment.

Parents and health care professionals should encourage the child to be as independent as possible and to develop a positive attitude toward school, social development, and vocational planning.

Regular slit-lamp examinations help ensure early diagnosis and treatment of iridocyclitis. Children with pauciarticular JRA with chronic iridocyclitis should be checked every 3 months during periods of active disease and every 6 months during remissions.

Generally, the prognosis for JRA is good, although disabilities can occur. Surgery is usually limited to soft-tissue releases to improve joint mobility. Joint replacement is delayed until the child has matured physically and can handle vigorous rehabilitation.

Psoriatic Arthritis

Psoriatic arthritis is a syndrome of rheumatoidlike joint disease associated with psoriasis of nearby skin and nails. Although the arthritis component of this syndrome may be clinically indistinguishable from rheumatoid arthritis, the rheumatoid nodules are absent, and serologic tests for rheumatoid factor are negative. Psoriatic arthritis usually is mild, with intermittent flare-ups, but rarely may progress to crippling arthritis mutilans. This disease affects both men and women equally; usually, onset occurs between ages 30 and 35.

Causes

Evidence suggests that predisposition to psoriatic arthritis is hereditary; 20% to 50% of patients are HLA-B27 positive. However, onset is usually precipitated by streptococcal infection or trauma.

Signs and symptoms

Psoriatic lesions usually precede the arthritic component. However, once the full syndrome is established, joint and skin lesions recur simultaneously. Arthritis (swelling, tenderness, warmth, and restricted movement) may involve a single joint or several joints symmetrically. It can develop in any peripheral joint but is most common in the distal interphalangeal joints of the hands. Characteristic nail changes include pitting, transverse ridging, onycholysis, keratosis, yellowing, and destruction of the entire nail. Psoriatic arthritis may also produce general malaise and fever.

Diagnosis

Inflammatory arthritis in a patient with psoriatic skin lesions suggests psoriatic arthritis.

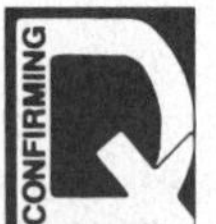

X-rays confirm joint involvement and show:

- erosion of terminal phalangeal tufts
- "whittling" of the distal end of the terminal phalanges
- "pencil-in-cup" deformity of the distal interphalangeal joints
- relative absence of osteoporosis
- sacroiliitis
- atypical spondylitis with syndesmophyte formation, resulting in hyperostosis and paravertebral ossification, which may lead to vertebral fusion.

Typical serum values include negative rheumatoid factor and elevated ESR.

Treatment

In mild psoriatic arthritis, treatment is

supportive and consists of immobilization through bed rest or splints, isometric exercises, paraffin baths, heat therapy, and aspirin and other nonsteroidal anti-inflammatory drugs. Some patients respond well to low-dose systemic corticosteroids; topical steroids may help control skin lesions. Gold salt and—most commonly—methotrexate therapy are effective in treating both the articular and cutaneous effects of psoriatic arthritis. Antimalarials are contraindicated, because these drugs can provoke exfoliative dermatitis.

Special considerations

- Explain the disease and its treatment to the patient and his family.
- Reassure the patient that psoriatic plaques aren't contagious. Avoid showing any revulsion to unsightly psoriatic patches—doing so will only reinforce the patient's fear of rejection.
- Encourage exercise, particularly swimming, to maintain strength and range of motion.
- Teach the patient how to apply skin care products and medications correctly; explain possible side effects.
- Stress the importance of adequate rest and protection of affected joints.
- Encourage regular, moderate exposure to the sun.
- Consider referral to the Arthritis Foundation for self-help and support groups.

Ankylosing Spondylitis

(Rheumatoid spondylitis, Marie-Strümpell disease)

A chronic, usually progressive inflammatory disease, ankylosing spondylitis primarily affects the sacroiliac, apophyseal, and costovertebral joints and adjacent soft tissue. Generally, the disease begins in the sacroiliac joints and gradually progresses to the lumbar, thoracic, and cervical regions of the spine. Deterioration of bone and cartilage can lead to fibrous tissue formation and eventual fusion of the spine or peripheral joints. Ankylosing spondylitis may be equally prevalent in both sexes. Progressive disease is well-recognized in men, but diagnosis is often overlooked or missed in women, who tend to have more peripheral joint involvement.

Causes

Recent evidence strongly suggests a familial tendency in ankylosing spondylitis. The presence of histocompatibility antigen HLA-B27 (positive in over 90% of patients with this disease) and circulating immune complexes suggests immunologic activity.

Signs and symptoms

The first indication is intermittent low back pain that's usually most severe in the morning or after a period of inactivity. Other symptoms depend on the disease stage and may include:

- stiffness and limited motion of the lumbar spine
- pain and limited expansion of the chest due to involvement of the costovertebral joints
- peripheral arthritis involving shoulders, hips, and knees
- kyphosis in advanced stages, caused by chronic stooping to relieve symptoms
- hip deformity and associated limited range of motion
- tenderness over the site of inflammation
- mild fatigue, fever, anorexia, or loss of weight; occasional iritis; aortic regurgitation and cardiomegaly; upper lobe pulmonary fibrosis (mimics tuberculosis).

These symptoms progress unpredictably, and the disease can go into remission, exacerbation, or arrest at any stage.

Diagnosis

Typical symptoms, familial history, and demonstration of positive HLA-B27 histocompatibility antigen strongly suggest ankylosing spondylitis. However, confirmation requires characteristic X-ray findings:

- blurring of the bony margins of joints in the early stage
- bilateral sacroiliac involvement
- patchy sclerosis with superficial bony erosions
- eventual squaring of vertebral bodies
- "bamboo spine" with complete ankylosis.

Erythrocyte sedimentation rate and alkaline phosphatase and creatinine phosphokinase levels may be slightly elevated. A negative rheumatoid factor helps rule out rheumatoid arthritis, which produces similar symptoms.

Treatment

No treatment reliably stops progression of this disease, so management aims to delay further deformity by good posture, stretching and deep-breathing exercises, and, in some patients, braces and lightweight supports. Anti-inflammatory analgesics, such as aspirin, indomethacin, and sulindac, control pain and inflammation.

Severe hip involvement usually necessitates surgical hip replacement. Severe spinal involvement may require a spinal wedge osteotomy to separate and reposition the vertebrae. This surgery is performed only on selected patients because of the risk of spinal cord damage and the long convalescence involved.

Special considerations

Ankylosing spondylitis can be an extremely painful and crippling disease, so your main responsibility is to promote the patient's comfort. When dealing with such a patient, keep in mind that limited range of motion makes simple tasks difficult. Offer support and reassurance.

Administer medications, as ordered. Apply local heat and provide massage to relieve pain. Assess mobility and degree of discomfort frequently. Teach and assist with daily exercises, as needed, to maintain strength and function. Stress the importance of maintaining good posture.

If treatment includes surgery, provide good postoperative nursing care. Since ankylosing spondylitis is a chronic, progressively crippling condition, a comprehensive treatment plan should also reflect counsel from a social worker, visiting nurse, and dietitian. To minimize deformities, advise the patient to:

- avoid any physical activity that places undue stress on the back, such as lifting heavy objects
- stand upright; to sit upright in a high, straight chair; and to avoid leaning over a desk
- sleep in a prone position on a hard mattress and to avoid using pillows under neck or knees
- avoid prolonged walking, standing, sitting, or driving
- perform regular stretching and deep-breathing exercises and to swim regularly, if possible
- have height measured every 3 to 4 months to detect any tendency toward kyphosis
- seek vocational counseling if work requires standing or prolonged sitting at a desk
- contact the local Arthritis Foundation chapter for a support group.

Sjögren's Syndrome

The second most common autoimmune rheumatic disorder after rheumatoid arthritis, Sjögren's syndrome (SS) is characterized by diminished lacrimal and salivary gland secretion (sicca complex). This syndrome occurs mainly in women (90% of patients); mean age of occurrence is 50. SS may be a primary disorder or associated with connective tissue disorders such as rheumatoid arthritis, scleroderma, systemic lupus erythematosus, and polymyositis. In some patients, the disorder is limited to the exocrine glands (glandular SS); in others, it also involves other organs, such as the lung and kidney (extraglandular SS).

Causes

The cause of SS is unknown. Most likely, both genetic and environmental factors contribute to its development. Viral or bacterial infection or perhaps exposure to pollen may trigger SS in a genetically susceptible individual. Tissue damage results from infiltration by lymphocytes or from the deposition of immune complexes. Lymphocytic infiltration may be classified as benign, malignant, or pseudolymphoma (nonmalignant, but tumorlike aggregates of lymphoid cells).

Signs and symptoms

About 50% of patients with SS have confirmed rheumatoid arthritis and a history of slowly developing sicca complex. However, some seek medical help for rapidly progressive and severe oral and ocular dryness, often accompanied by periodic parotid gland enlargement. Ocular dryness (xerophthalmia) leads to foreign body sensation (gritty, sandy eye), redness, burning, photosensitivity, eye fatigue, itching, and mucoid discharge. The patient may also complain of a film across his field of vision.

Oral dryness (xerostomia) leads to difficulty swallowing and talking; abnormal taste or smell sensation, or both; thirst; ulcers of the tongue, buccal mucosa, and lips (especially at the corners of the mouth); and severe dental caries. Dryness of the respiratory tract leads to epistaxis, hoarseness, chronic nonproductive cough, recurrent otitis media, and increased incidence of respiratory infections.

Other effects of SS may include dyspareunia and pruritus (associated with vaginal dryness), generalized itching, fatigue, recurrent low-grade fever, and arthralgia or myalgia. Lymph node enlargement may be the first sign of malignant lymphoma or pseudolymphoma.

Specific extraglandular findings in SS include interstitial pneumonitis; interstitial nephritis, resulting in renal tubular acidosis in 25% of patients; chronic thyroiditis, resulting in hypothyroidism (50%); Raynaud's phenomenon (20%); and vasculitis, usually limited to the skin and characterized by palpable purpura on the legs (20%). An occasional patient develops systemic necrotizing vasculitis, involving the skin, peripheral nerves, and gastrointestinal tract.

Diagnosis

Diagnosis of SS rests on the detection of two of the following three conditions: xerophthalmia, xerostomia (with salivary gland biopsy showing lymphocytic infiltration), and an associated autoimmune or lymphoproliferative disorder. Diagnosis must rule out other causes of oral and ocular dryness including sarcoidosis, endocrine disorders, anxiety or depression, and effects of therapy, such as radiation to the head and neck. Over 200 commonly used drugs also produce dry mouth as a side effect. In patients with salivary gland enlargement and severe lymphoid infiltration, diagnosis must rule out malignancy.

Laboratory values in SS show elevated erythrocyte sedimentation rate in more than 90% of patients, mild anemia and leukopenia in 30%, and hypergammaglobulinemia in 50%. Various autoantibodies are also common, including antisalivary duct antibodies. Typically, 75% to 90% of patients have positive rheumatoid factor; 50% to 80%, positive antinuclear antibodies.

Other tests help support this diagnosis. Schirmer's tearing test and slit-lamp examination with rose bengal dye are used to measure eye involvement. Salivary gland involvement is evaluated by measuring the volume of parotid saliva and by secretory sialography and salivary scintigraphy. Lower lip biopsy shows salivary gland infiltration by lymphocytes.

Treatment and special considerations

Treatment is usually symptomatic and includes conservative measures to relieve ocular or oral dryness. Mouth dryness can be relieved by using a methylcellulose swab or spray and by drinking plenty of fluids, especially at mealtime. Meticulous oral hygiene is essential, including regular flossing, brushing, and fluoride treatment at home and frequent dental checkups. Advise the patient to avoid drugs that decrease saliva production, such as atropine derivatives, antihistamines, anticholinergics, and antidepressants. If mouth lesions make eating painful, suggest high-protein, high-calorie liquid supplements to prevent malnutrition. Advise the patient to avoid sugar, which contributes to dental caries, and tobacco, alcohol, and spicy, salty, or highly acidic foods, which cause mouth irritation.

Instill artificial tears as often as every half hour to prevent eye damage (corneal ulcerations, corneal opacifications) from insufficient tear secretions. Some patients may also benefit from instillation of an eye ointment at bedtime, or from twice-a-day use of sustained-release cellulose capsules (Lacrisert). Suggest the use of sunglasses to protect the patient's eyes from dust, wind, and strong light. Moisture chamber spectacles may also be helpful. Because dry eyes are more suseptible to infection, advise the patient to keep his face clean and to avoid rubbing his eyes. If infection develops, antibiotics should be given immediately; topical steroids should be avoided.

To help relieve respiratory dryness, stress the need to humidify home and work environments. Suggest normal saline solution drops or aerosolized spray for nasal dryness. Advise the patient to avoid prolonged hot showers and baths and to use moisturizing lotions to help ease dry skin. Suggest K-Y Lubricating Jelly as a vaginal lubricant.

Other treatment measures vary with associated extraglandular findings. Parotid gland enlargement requires local heat and analgesics; pulmonary and renal interstitial disease, corticosteroids; accompanying lymphoma, a combination of chemotherapy, surgery, or radiation.

Refer the patient to the Sjögren's Syndrome Foundation for additional information and support.

Lupus Erythematosus

A chronic inflammatory disorder of the connective tissues, lupus erythematosus appears in two forms: discoid lupus erythematosus *(DLE), which affects only the skin, and* systemic lupus erythematosus *(SLE), which affects multiple organ systems (as well as the skin) and can be fatal. Like rheumatoid arthritis, SLE is characterized by recurring remissions and exacerbations, especially common during the spring and summer. The annual incidence of SLE averages 75 cases per 1 million people. It strikes women 8 times as often as men, increasing to 15 times as often during childbearing years. SLE occurs worldwide but is most prevalent among Asians and blacks. Prognosis improves with early detection and treatment but remains poor for patients who develop cardiovascular, renal, or neurologic complications or severe bacterial infections.*

Causes

The exact cause of SLE remains a mystery, but evidence points to interrelated immunologic, environmental, hormonal, and genetic factors. Immune dysregulation, in the form of autoimmunity, is thought to be the prime causative mechanism. In autoimmunity, the body produces antibodies, such as antinuclear antibody (ANA), which form antigen-antibody complexes that suppress the body's normal immunity.

Certain predisposing factors may make a person susceptible to SLE. Physical or mental stress, streptococcal or viral infections, exposure to sunlight or ultraviolet light, immunization, pregnancy, and abnormal estrogen metabolism may all affect the development of this disease. Because SLE has been found in certain families for several generations, genetic predisposition is also suspected.

SLE also may be triggered or aggravated by certain drugs—procainamide, hydralazine, anticonvulsants, and, less frequently, penicillins, sulfa drugs, and oral contraceptives.

Signs and symptoms

Primary clinical features include nondeforming arthritis, a characteristic "butterfly rash," and photosensitivity. The first and most common symptom is joint pain and stiffness, which is rarely deforming and usually involves the hands, feet, and large joints. Joints may show redness, warmth, tenderness, and synovial effusions, with associated muscle weakness and tenderness.

Perhaps the most distinctive feature of SLE is the "butterfly rash" that appears in a malar distribution across the nose and cheeks (in about 40% of patients). This rash may range from malar erythema to discoid lesions (plaques), most commonly on the face, neck, and scalp. Similar rashes may appear on other body surfaces, especially exposed areas. Ultraviolet rays often provoke or aggravate skin eruptions. Vasculitis can occur (especially in the digits), possibly leading to infarctive lesions, necrotic leg ulcers, or digital gangrene. Raynaud's phenomenon appears in about 20% of patients. Patchy alopecia and painless ulcers of the mucous membranes are common.

Constitutional symptoms of SLE include aching, malaise, fatigue, low-grade or spiking fever, chills, anorexia, and weight loss. Lymph node enlarge-

DISCOID LUPUS ERYTHEMATOSUS

Discoid lupus erythematosus (DLE) is a form of lupus erythematosus marked by chronic skin eruptions that, if untreated, can lead to scarring and permanent disfigurement. About 1 out of 20 patients with DLE later develops SLE. The exact cause of DLE is unknown, but some evidence suggests an autoimmune defect. An estimated 60% of patients with DLE are women in their late twenties or older. This disease is rare in children.

DLE lesions are raised, red, scaling plaques, with follicular plugging and central atrophy. The raised edges and sunken centers give them a coin-like appearance. Although these lesions can appear anywhere on the body, they usually erupt on the face, scalp, ears, neck, and arms or on any part of the body that's exposed to sunlight. Such lesions can resolve completely or may cause hypopigmentation or hyperpigmentation, atrophy, and scarring. Facial plaques sometimes assume the butterfly pattern characteristic of SLE. Hair tends to become brittle or may fall out in patches.

As a rule, patient history and the appearance of the rash itself are diagnostic. LE cell test is positive in less than 10% of patients. Skin biopsy of lesions reveals immunoglobulins or complement components. SLE must be ruled out.

Patients with DLE should avoid prolonged exposure to the sun, fluorescent lighting, or reflected sunlight. They should wear protective clothing, use sunscreening agents, avoid engaging in outdoor activities during periods of most intense sunlight (between 10 a.m. and 2 p.m.), and report any changes in the lesions. Drug treatment consists of topical, intralesional, or systemic medication, as in SLE.

SIGNS OF SYSTEMIC LUPUS ERYTHEMATOSUS

Diagnosing systemic lupus erythematosus is far from easy, because SLE often mimics other diseases; symptoms may be vague and vary greatly from patient to patient. For these reasons, the American Rheumatism Association has issued a list of criteria for classification of SLE, to be used primarily for consistency in epidemiologic surveys. Usually, four or more of these symptoms are present some time during the course of the disease:

- facial erythema (butterfly rash)
- discoid rash
- photosensitivity
- oral or nasopharyngeal ulcerations
- nonerosive arthritis
- pleuritis or pericarditis
- profuse proteinuria (greater than 0.5 g/day)
- excessive cellular casts in the urine
- seizures or psychoses
- hemolytic anemia, leukopenia, lymphopenia, or thrombocytopenia
- positive LE cell, anti-DNA, or anti-Sm test
- chronic false-positive serologic test for syphilis
- abnormal titer of ANA.

Tan, E.M., et al. The 1982 revised criteria for the classification of systemic lupus erythematosus.

ment (diffuse or local, and nontender), abdominal pain, nausea, vomiting, diarrhea, and constipation may occur. Women may experience irregular menstrual periods or amenorrhea, particularly during the active phase of this disease.

About 50% of SLE patients develop signs of cardiopulmonary abnormalities, such as pleuritis, pericarditis, and dyspnea. Myocarditis, endocarditis, tachycardia, parenchymal infiltrates, and pneumonitis may occur. Renal effects include hematuria, proteinuria, urine sediment, and cellular casts; renal involvement may progress to total kidney failure. Urinary tract infections may result from heightened susceptibility to infection. Convulsive disorders and mental dysfunction may indicate neurologic damage. CNS involvement may produce emotional instability, psychosis, and organic brain syndrome. Headaches, irritability, and depression are especially common.

Diagnosis

Diagnostic tests for patients with SLE include a CBC with differential, which may show anemia and decreased WBC; platelet count, which may be decreased; ESR, which is often elevated; and serum electrophoresis, which may show hypergammaglobulinemia.

Specific tests for SLE include:

- *antinuclear antibody (ANA), anti-DNA,* and *lupus erythematosus (LE) cell tests:* positive in most patients with active SLE; since the anti-DNA test is rarely positive in other conditions, it's the most specific test for SLE. However, if the patient is in remission, anti-DNA may be reduced or absent. (This test correlates well with disease activity, especially with renal involvement, and helps monitor response to therapy.)
- *urine studies:* may show RBCs and WBCs, urine casts and sediment, and significant protein loss (more than 3.5 g/ 24 hours).
- *blood studies:* decreased serum complement (C3 and C4) levels indicate active disease.
- *chest X-ray:* may show pleurisy or lupus pneumonitis.
- *EKG:* may show conduction defect with cardiac involvement or pericarditis.
- *kidney biopsy:* determines disease stage and extent of renal involvement.

Treatment

Patients with mild disease require little or no medication. Nonsteroidal anti-inflammatory compounds, including aspirin, often control arthritis symptoms. Skin lesions need topical treatment. Corticosteroid creams, such as flurandrenolide, are recommended for acute lesions.

Refractory skin lesions are treated with intralesional corticosteroids or antimalarials, such as hydroxychloroquine and chloroquine. Because hydroxychloroquine and chloroquine can cause retinal damage, such treatment requires ophthalmologic examination every 6 months.

Corticosteroids remain the treatment of choice for systemic symptoms of SLE, for acute generalized exacerbations, or for serious disease related to vital organ systems, such as pleuritis, pericarditis, lupus nephritis, vasculitis, and CNS involvement. Initial doses equivalent to 60 mg or more of prednisone often bring noticeable improvement within 48 hours. As soon as symptoms are under control, steroid dosage is tapered down slowly. (Rising serum complement levels and decreasing anti-DNA titers indicate patient response.) Diffuse proliferative glomerulonephritis, a major complication of SLE, requires treatment with large doses of steroids. If renal failure occurs, dialysis or kidney transplant may be necessary. In some patients, cytotoxic drugs—such as azathioprine and cyclophosphamide—may delay or prevent deteriorating renal status. Antihypertensive drugs and dietary changes may also be warranted in renal disease.

The photosensitive patient should wear protective clothing (hat, sunglasses, long sleeves, slacks) and use a screening agent containing para-aminobenzoic acid when out in the sun. Since SLE usually strikes women of childbearing age, questions associated with pregnancy often arise. The best evidence available indicates that a woman with SLE can have a safe, successful pregnancy if she has no serious renal or neurologic impairment.

BUTTERFLY RASH

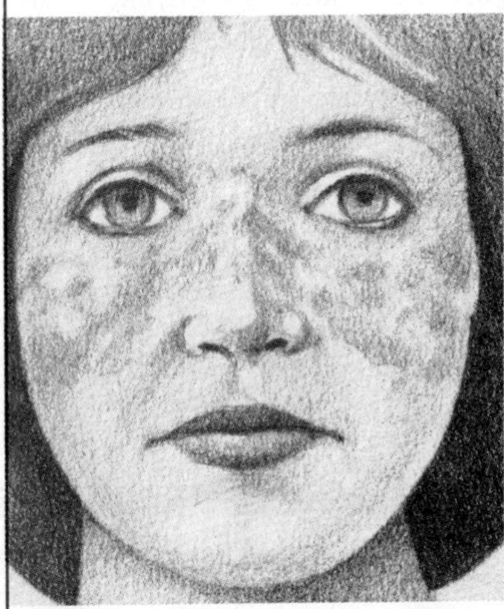

In classic butterfly rash, lesions appear on the cheeks and the bridge of the nose, creating a characteristic butterfly pattern. The rash may vary in severity from malar erythema to discoid lesions (plaque).

Special considerations

Careful assessment, supportive measures, emotional support, and patient teaching are all important parts of the care plan for patients with SLE.

- Watch for constitutional symptoms: joint pain or stiffness, weakness, fever, fatigue, and chills. Observe for dyspnea, chest pain, and any edema of the extremities. Note the size, type, and location of skin lesions. Check urine for hematuria, scalp for hair loss, and skin and mucous membranes for petechiae, bleeding, ulceration, pallor, and bruising.
- Provide a balanced diet. Renal involvement may mandate a low-sodium, low-protein diet.
- Urge the patient to get plenty of rest. Schedule diagnostic tests and procedures to allow adequate rest. Explain all tests and procedures. Tell the patient that several blood samples are needed initially, then periodically, to monitor progress.
- Apply heat packs to relieve joint pain and stiffness. Encourage regular exercise to maintain full range of motion and prevent contractures. Teach range-of-motion exercises, as well as body alignment and postural techniques. Arrange for physical therapy and occupational counseling, as appropriate.
- Explain the expected benefit of prescribed medications, and watch for side effects, especially when the patient is taking high doses of corticosteroids.

- Monitor vital signs, intake and output, weight, and laboratory reports closely. Check pulse rates regularly, and observe for orthopnea. Check stools and GI secretions for blood.
- Observe for hypertension, weight gain, and other signs of renal involvement.
- Assess for signs of neurologic damage: personality change, paranoid or psychotic behavior, ptosis, or diplopia. Take seizure precautions. If Raynaud's phenomenon is present, warm and protect the patient's hands and feet.
- Support the female patient's self-image by offering helpful cosmetic tips, such as suggesting the use of hypoallergenic makeup, and by referring her to a hairdresser who specializes in scalp disorders. Encourage her to take an interest in her appearance.
- Advise the patient to purchase medications in quantity, if possible. Warn against "miracle" drugs for relief of arthritis symptoms.
- Refer the patient to the Lupus Foundation of America and the Arthritis Foundation, as necessary.

Goodpasture's Syndrome

In Goodpasture's syndrome, hemoptysis and rapidly progressive glomerulonephritis follow the deposition of antibody against the alveolar and glomerular basement membranes. This syndrome may occur at any age but is most common in men between ages 20 and 30. Prognosis improves with aggressive immunosuppressive and antibiotic therapy and with dialysis or renal transplantation.

Causes

The cause of Goodpasture's syndrome is unknown. Although some cases have been associated with exposure to hydrocarbons or type 2 influenza, many have no precipitating events. The high incidence of HLA-DRw2 in these patients suggests a genetic predisposition. Abnormal production and deposition of antibody against glomerular basement membrane (GBM) and alveolar basement membrane activates the complement and inflammatory responses, resulting in glomerular and alveolar tissue damage.

Signs and symptoms

Goodpasture's syndrome may initially cause malaise, fatigue, and pallor associated with severe iron deficiency anemia. Pulmonary findings range from slight dyspnea and cough with blood-tinged sputum to hemoptysis and frank pulmonary hemorrhage. Subclinical pulmonary bleeding may precede overt hemorrhage and renal disease by months or years. Usually, renal findings are more subtle, although some patients note hematuria and peripheral edema.

Diagnosis

Confirmation of Goodpasture's syndrome requires measurement of circulating anti-GBM antibody by radioimmunoassay and linear staining of GBM and alveolar basement membrane by immunofluorescence.

Immunofluorescence of alveolar basement membrane shows linear deposition of immunoglobulin, as well as C3 and fibrinogen. Immunofluorescence of GBM also shows linear deposition of immunoglobulin combined with detection of circulating anti-GBM antibody, this finding distinguishes Goodpasture's from other pulmonary-renal syndromes such as Wegener's granulomatosis, polyarteritis, and systemic lupus erythematosus.

Lung biopsy shows interstitial and intraalveolar hemorrhage with hemosiderin-laden macrophages. Chest X-ray reveals pulmonary infiltrates in a diffuse, nodular pattern, and renal biopsy frequently shows focal necrotic lesions and cellular crescents.

Creatinine and BUN levels typically increase two to three times normal. Urinalysis may reveal red blood cells and cellular casts, which typify glomerular inflammation. Granular casts and proteinuria may also be observed.

Treatment

Treatment aims to remove antibody by plasmapheresis and to suppress antibody production with immunosuppressive drugs. Patients with renal failure may benefit from dialysis or transplantation. Aggressive ultrafiltration helps relieve pulmonary edema that may aggravate pulmonary hemorrhage. High-dose I.V. steroids also help control pulmonary hemorrhage.

Special considerations

- Promote adequate oxygenation by elevating the head of the bed and administering humidified oxygen. Encourage the patient to conserve his energy. Assess respirations and breath sounds regularly; note sputum quantity and quality.
- Monitor vital signs, arterial blood gases, hematocrit, and coagulation studies.
- Transfuse blood and administer steroids, as ordered. Observe closely for drug side effects.
- Assess renal function by monitoring symptomatology, intake and output, daily weights, creatinine clearance, and BUN and creatinine levels.
- Teach the patient and his family what signs and symptoms to expect and how to relieve them. Carefully describe other treatment measures, such as dialysis.

Reiter's Syndrome

A self-limiting syndrome associated with polyarthritis (dominant feature), urethritis, balanitis, conjunctivitis, and mucocutaneous lesions, Reiter's syndrome appears to be related to infection, either venereal or enteric. This disease usually affects young men (aged 20 to 40); it's rare in women and children.

Causes

While the exact cause of Reiter's syndrome is unknown, most cases follow venereal or enteric infection. Since 75% to 85% of patients with Reiter's syndrome are positive for the HLA-B27 antigen, genetic susceptibility is likely. Reiter's syndrome has followed infections caused by *Mycoplasma*, *Shigella*, *Salmonella*, *Yersinia*, and *Chlamydia* organisms.

Signs and symptoms

The patient with Reiter's syndrome may complain of dysuria, hematuria, urgent and frequent urination, and mucopurulent penile discharge, with swelling and reddening of the urethral meatus. Small painless ulcers may erupt on the glans penis (balanitis) and coalesce to form irregular patches that cover the penis and scrotum. He may also experience suprapubic pain, fever, and anorexia with weight loss. This disorder may also cause other genitourinary complications, such as prostatitis and hemorrhagic cystitis.

Arthritic symptoms usually follow genitourinary or enteric symptoms and often last from 2 to 4 months. Asymmetric and extremely variable polyarticular arthritis occurs most often and tends to develop in weight-bearing joints of the legs and sometimes in the low back or sacroiliac joints. The arthritis is usually acute, with warm, erythematous, and painful joints; but it may be mild, with minimal synovitis. Muscle wasting is common near affected joints. Fingers and toes may swell and appear sausagelike.

Ocular symptoms include mild bilateral conjunctivitis, possibly complicated by keratitis, iritis, retinitis, or optic neuritis. In severe cases, burning, itching, and profuse mucopurulent discharge are possible.

In 30% of patients, skin lesions (keratoderma blennorrhagicum) develop 4 to 6 weeks after onset of other symptoms and may last for several weeks. These macular to hyperkeratotic lesions often resemble those of psoriasis. They occur most commonly on the palms and soles but can develop anywhere on the trunk, extremities, or scalp. Nails become thick, opaque, and brittle; keratic debris accumulates under the nails. In many patients, painless, transient ulcerations erupt on the buccal mucosa, palate, and tongue.

Diagnosis

Nearly all patients with Reiter's syndrome are positive for the HLA-B27 antigen and have an elevated white blood cell (WBC) count and erythrocyte sedimentation rate. Mild anemia may develop. Urethral discharge and synovial fluid contain many WBCs, mostly polymorphonuclear leukocytes; synovial fluid is high in complement and protein and is grossly purulent. Cultures of discharge and synovial fluid rule out other causes such as gonococci.

During the first few weeks, X-rays are normal and may remain so, but some patients may show osteoporosis in inflamed areas. If inflammation persists, X-rays may show erosions of the small joints, periosteal proliferation (new bone formation) of involved joints, and calcaneal spurs.

Treatment

No specific treatment exists for Reiter's syndrome. Most patients recover in 2 to 16 weeks. About 50% of patients have recurring acute attacks, while the rest follow a chronic course, experiencing continued synovitis and sacroiliitis. In acute stages, limited weight-bearing or complete bed rest may be necessary.

Anti-inflammatory agents can be given for relief of discomfort and fever. Steroids may be used for persistent skin lesions; gold therapy, for bony erosion. Physical therapy includes range-of-motion and strengthening exercises and the use of padded or supportive shoes to prevent contractures and deformities of the feet.

Special considerations

- Communicate an accepting, nonjudgmental attitude, since the patient may be embarrassed if attacks are associated with sexual activity.
- Explain Reiter's syndrome to the patient. Discuss the recommended medications and their possible side effects. Warn the patient to take medications with meals or milk to prevent gastrointestinal bleeding.
- Encourage normal daily activity and moderate exercise. Suggest a firm mattress and encourage good posture and body mechanics.
- Arrange for occupational counseling if the patient has severe or chronic joint impairment.

Progressive Systemic Sclerosis

(CREST Syndrome, Scleroderma)

Progressive systemic sclerosis (PSS) is a diffuse connective tissue disease characterized by fibrotic, degenerative, and occasionally inflammatory changes in skin, blood vessels, synovial membranes, skeletal muscles, and internal organs (especially the esophagus, intestinal tract, thyroid, heart, lungs, and kidneys). It affects women more frequently than men, especially between ages 30 and 50. Approximately 30% of patients with PSS die within 5 years of onset.

Causes

The cause of PSS is unknown. This disease occurs in four distinctive forms:

- *CREST syndrome:* the more benign form, characterized by calcinosis, Raynaud's phenomenon, esophageal dysfunction, sclerodactyly, and telangiectasia
- *diffuse systemic sclerosis:* characterized by generalized skin thickening and invasion of internal organ systems
- *localized scleroderma:* characterized by patchy skin changes with a droplike appearance known as morphea
- *linear scleroderma:* characterized by a band of thickened skin on the face or extremities which severely damages underlying tissues, causing atrophy and deformity (most common in childhood).

Signs and symptoms

PSS typically begins with Raynaud's phenomenon—blanching, cyanosis, and erythema of the fingers and toes in response to stress or exposure to cold. Progressive phalangeal resorption may shorten the fingers. Compromised circulation may cause slowly healing ulcerations on the tips of the fingers or toes that may lead to gangrene. This compromised circulation results from thickening of the arterial intima from the normal one- to two-cell thickness to many cells thick. Raynaud's phenomenon may precede diagnosis of PSS by months or even years.

Later symptoms include pain, stiffness, and swelling of fingers and joints. Skin thickening produces taut, shiny skin over the entire hand and forearm. Facial skin also becomes tight and inelastic, causing a masklike appearance (no wrinkles) and "pinching" of the mouth. As tightening progresses, contractures may develop.

Gastrointestinal dysfunction causes frequent reflux, heartburn, dysphagia, and bloating after meals, all of which may cause the patient to decrease food intake and lose weight. Other common gastrointestinal complaints include abdominal distention, diarrhea, constipation, and malodorous floating stools.

In advanced disease, cardiac and pulmonary fibrosis produce dysrhythmias and dyspnea. Renal involvement is usually accompanied by malignant hypertension, which is the major cause of death.

Diagnosis

Typical cutaneous changes provide the first clue to diagnosis. Results of diagnostic tests include:

- *blood studies:* slightly elevated erythrocyte sedimentation rate, positive rheumatoid factor in 25% to 35% of patients, and positive antinuclear antibody (low titer, speckled pattern)
- *urinalysis:* proteinuria, microscopic hematuria, and casts (with renal involvement)
- *hand X-rays:* terminal phalangeal tuft resorption, subcutaneous calcification, joint space narrowing and erosion
- *chest X-rays:* bilateral basilar pulmonary fibrosis
- *gastrointestinal X-rays:* distal esophageal hypomotility and stricture, duodenal loop dilation, small bowel malabsorption pattern, and large diverticula
- *pulmonary function studies:* decreased diffusion and vital capacity
- *EKG:* possible nonspecific abnormalities related to myocardial fibrosis
- *skin biopsy:* may show changes consistent with the progress of the disease, such as marked thickening of the dermis and occlusive vessel changes.

Treatment

Currently, no cure exists for PSS. Treatment aims to preserve normal body functions and minimize complications. Use of immunosuppressives, such as chlorambucil, is a common palliative measure. Corticosteroids and colchicine have been used experimentally and seem to stabilize symptoms; D-penicillamine may be helpful. Blood platelet levels need to be monitored throughout drug and immunosuppressive therapy. Other treatment varies according to symptoms:

- *Raynaud's phenomenon:* various vasodilators and antihypertensive agents

(such as methyldopa and reserpine), intermittent cervical sympathetic blockade, or, rarely, thoracic sympathectomy.
• *chronic digital ulcerations:* a digital plaster cast to immobilize the affected area, minimize trauma, and maintain cleanliness; possibly surgical debridement.
• *esophagitis with stricture:* antacids, cimetidine, a soft, bland diet, and periodic ésophageal dilation.
• *small-bowel involvement* (diarrhea, pain, malabsorption, weight loss): broad-spectrum antibiotics, such as erythromycin or tetracycline, to counteract bacterial overgrowth in the duodenum and jejunum related to hypomotility.
• *scleroderma kidney* (with malignant hypertension and impending renal failure): dialysis, antihypertensives, and calcium blockers.
• *hand debilitation:* physical therapy to maintain function and promote muscle strength, heat therapy to relieve joint stiffness, and patient teaching to make performance of daily activities easier.

Special considerations

• Assess motion restrictions, pain, vital signs, intake and output, respiratory function, and daily weight.
• Because of compromised circulation, warn against finger-stick blood tests.
• Remember that air conditioning may aggravate Raynaud's phenomenon.
• Help the patient and family adjust to the patient's new body image and to the limitations and dependency these changes cause. Teach the patient to avoid fatigue by pacing activities and organizing schedules to include necessary rest. The patient and family need to accept the fact that this condition is incurable. Encourage them to express their feelings, and help them cope with their fears and frustrations by offering information about the disease, its treatment, and relevant diagnostic tests. Whenever possible, let the patient participate in treatment by measuring his own intake and output, planning his own diet, assisting in dialysis, giving himself heat therapy, and doing prescribed exercises.

Polymyositis and Dermatomyositis

Diffuse, inflammatory myopathies of unknown cause, polymyositis and dermatomyositis produce symmetrical weakness of striated muscle—primarily proximal muscles of the shoulder and pelvic girdles, neck, and pharynx. In dermatomyositis, such muscle weakness is accompanied by cutaneous involvement. These diseases usually progress slowly, with frequent exacerbations and remissions. They occur twice as often in women as in men (with the exception of dermatomyositis with malignancy, which is most common in men over age 40).

Generally, prognosis worsens with age. The 7-year survival rate for adults is approximately 60%, with death often occurring from associated malignancy, respiratory disease, heart failure, or side effects of therapy (corticosteroids and immunosuppressives). On the other hand, 80% to 90% of affected children regain normal function if properly treated; but, if untreated, childhood dermatomyositis may progress rapidly to disabling contractures and muscular atrophy.

Causes

Although the cause of polymyositis remains puzzling, it may result from autoimmunity, perhaps combined with defective T cell function. Presumably, the patient's T cells inappropriately recognize muscle fiber antigens as foreign and release lymphotoxins that cause diffuse or focal muscle fiber degeneration. (Regeneration of new muscle cells then follows, producing remission.) Polymyositis and dermatomyositis may be associated with other disorders such as allergic reactions; systemic lupus erythematosus (SLE); scleroderma; rheumatoid arthritis; Sjögren's syndrome; carcinomas of the lung, breast, or other organs; penicillamine administration; or systemic viral infection.

Signs and symptoms

Polymyositis begins acutely or insidiously with muscle weakness, tenderness, and discomfort. It affects proximal muscles (shoulder, pelvic girdle) more often than distal muscles. Muscle weakness impairs performance of ordinary activities. The patient may have trouble getting up from a chair, combing his hair, reaching into a high cupboard, climbing stairs, or even raising his head from a pillow. Other muscular symptoms include inability to move against resistance, proximal dysphagia (regurgitation of fluid through nose), and dysphonia (nasal voice).

In dermatomyositis, an erythematous rash usually erupts on the face, neck, upper back, chest, and arms and around the nail beds. A characteristic heliotropic rash appears on the eyelids, accompanied by periorbital edema. Grotton's papules (violet, flat-topped lesions) may appear on the interphalangeal joints.

Diagnosis

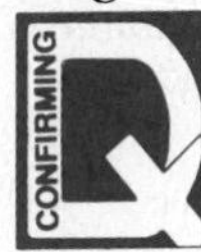

Diagnosis requires muscle biopsy that shows necrosis, degeneration, regeneration, and interstitial chronic lymphocytic infiltration. Appropriate laboratory tests differentiate polymyositis from diseases that cause similar muscular or cutaneous symptoms, such as muscular dystrophy, advanced trichinosis, psoriasis, seborrheic dermatitis, and SLE.

Typical laboratory results in polymyositis include: elevated erythrocyte sedimentation rate; elevated white blood cell count; elevated muscle enzymes (creatine phosphokinase, aldolase, serum glutamic-oxaloacetic transaminase) not attributable to hemolysis of red blood cells or hepatic or other diseases; increased urine creatine (more than 150 mg/24 hours); decreased creatinine; electromyography showing polyphasic short-duration potentials, fibrillation (positive spike waves), and bizarre high-frequency repetitive changes; and positive antinuclear antibodies.

Treatment

High-dose corticosteroid therapy relieves inflammation and lowers muscle enzyme levels. Within 2 to 6 weeks following treatment, serum muscle enzyme levels usually return to normal and muscle strength improves, permitting a gradual tapering down of corticosteroid dosage. If the patient responds poorly to corticosteroids, treatment may include cytotoxic or immunosuppressive drugs, such as cyclophosphamide intermittent I.V. or daily P.O. Supportive therapy includes bed rest during the acute phase, range-of-motion exercises to prevent contractures, analgesics and application of heat to relieve painful muscle spasms, and diphenhydramine to relieve itching. Patients over age 40 need thorough assessment for coexisting malignancies.

Special considerations

- Assess level of pain, muscular weakness, and range of motion daily. Administer analgesics, as needed.
- If the patient is confined to bed, prevent decubitus ulcers by giving good skin care. To prevent footdrop and contractures, apply high-topped sneakers, and assist with passive range-of-motion exercises at least four times daily. Teach the patient's family how to perform these exercises on the patient.
- If 24-hour urine collection for creatine/creatinine is necessary, make sure your co-workers understand the procedure. When you assist with muscle biopsy, make sure the biopsy is not taken from an area of recent needle insertion, such as an injection or electromyography site.
- If the patient has a skin rash, warn him against scratching, which may cause infection. If antipruritic medication

doesn't relieve severe itching, apply tepid sponges or compresses.

- Encourage the patient to feed and dress himself to the best of his ability but to ask for help when needed. Advise him to pace his activities to counteract muscle weakness. Encourage him to express his anxiety. Ease his fear of dependence by giving reassurance that muscle weakness is probably temporary.
- Explain the disease to the patient and his family. Prepare them for diagnostic procedures and possible side effects of corticosteroid therapy (weight gain, hirsutism, hypertension, edema, amenorrhea, purplish striae, glycosuria, acne, easy bruising). Advise a low-sodium diet to prevent fluid retention. Emphatically warn against abruptly discontinuing corticosteroids. Reassure the patient that steroid-induced weight gain will diminish when the drug is discontinued.

Vasculitis

Vasculitis includes a broad spectrum of disorders characterized by inflammation and necrosis of blood vessels. Its clinical effects depend on the vessels involved and reflect tissue ischemia caused by blood flow obstruction. Prognosis is also variable. For example, hypersensitivity vasculitis is usually a benign disorder limited to the skin, but more extensive polyarteritis nodosa can be rapidly fatal. Vasculitis can occur at any age, except for mucocutaneous lymph node syndrome, which occurs only during childhood. Vasculitis may be a primary disorder or secondary to other disorders such as rheumatoid arthritis (RA) or systemic lupus erythematosus (SLE).

Causes

Exactly how vascular damage develops in vasculitis isn't well understood. Current theory holds that it's initiated by excessive antigen in the circulation, which triggers the formation of soluble antigen-antibody complexes. These complexes cannot be effectively cleared by the reticuloendothelial system and so are deposited in blood vessel walls (Type III hypersensitivity). Increased vascular permeability associated with release of vasoactive amines by platelets and basophils enhances such deposition. The deposited complexes activate the complement cascade, resulting in chemotaxis of neutrophils, which release lysosomal enzymes. In turn, these enzymes cause vessel damage and necrosis, which may precipitate thrombosis, occlusion, hemorrhage, and tissue ischemia.

Another mechanism that may contribute to vascular damage is the cell-mediated (T cell) immune response. In this response, circulating antigen triggers the release of soluble mediators by sensitized lymphocytes, which attracts macrophages. The macrophages release intracellular enzymes, which cause vascular damage. They can also transform into the epithelioid and multinucleated giant cells that typify the granulomatous vasculitides. Phagocytosis of immune complexes by macrophages enhances granuloma formation.

Signs and symptoms and diagnosis

Clinical effects of vasculitis and laboratory procedures used to confirm diagnosis depend on the blood vessels involved. See the chart on pages 360 and 361 for signs and symptoms and diagnostic criteria specific to each type of vasculitis.

Treatment

Treatment of vasculitis aims to minimize irreversible tissue damage associated with ischemia. In primary vasculitis, treatment may involve removal of an offending antigen or use of anti-inflammatory or immunosuppressive drugs. For example, antigenic drugs, food, and other environmental substances should be identified and eliminated, if possible. Drug therapy in primary vasculitis frequently involves low-dose cyclophosphamide (2 mg/kg P.O. daily) with daily corticosteroids. In rapidly fulminant vasculitis, cyclophosphamide dosage may be increased to 4 mg/kg daily for the first 2 to 3 days, followed by the regular dose. Prednisone should be given in a dose of 1 mg/kg daily in divided doses for 7 to 10 days, with consolidation to a single morning dose by 2 to 3 weeks. When the vasculitis appears to be in remission or when prescribed cytotoxic drugs take full effect, corticosteroids are tapered down to a single daily dose and then to an alternate-day schedule that may continue for 3 to 6 months before steroids are slowly discontinued.

In secondary vasculitis, treatment focuses on the underlying disorder.

Special considerations

- Assess for dry nasal mucosa in patients with Wegener's granulomatosis. Instill nose drops to lubricate the mucosa and help diminish crusting. Or irrigate the nasal passages with warm normal saline solution.
- Monitor vital signs. Use a Doppler ultrasonic flowmeter, if available, to auscultate blood pressure in patients with Takayasu's arteritis, whose peripheral pulses are frequently difficult to palpate.
- Monitor intake and output. Check daily for edema. Keep the patient well-hydrated (3 liters daily) to reduce the risk of hemorrhagic cystitis associated with cyclophosphamide therapy.
- Provide emotional support to help the patient and his family cope with an altered body image—the result of the disorder or its therapy. (For example, Wegener's granulomatosis may be associated with saddle nose, steroids may cause weight gain, and cyclophosphamide may cause alopecia.)
- Teach the patient how to recognize drug side effects. Monitor the patient's white blood cell count during cyclophosphamide therapy to prevent severe leukopenia.

IMMUNODEFICIENCY

X-linked Infantile Hypogammaglobulinemia

(Bruton's agammaglobulinemia)

X-linked infantile hypogammaglobulinemia is a congenital disorder in which all five immunoglobulins—IgM, IgG, IgA, IgD, and IgE—and circulating B cells are absent or deficient. Affecting males almost exclusively, this disorder occurs in 1 in 50,000 to 100,000 births and causes severe, recurrent infections during infancy. Prognosis is good with early treatment, except in infants who develop polio or persistent viral infection. Infection usually causes some permanent damage, especially in the neurologic or respiratory system.

Causes

In X-linked infantile hypogammaglobulinemia, B cells and B cell precursors may be present in the bone marrow and peripheral blood, but for unknown reasons they fail to mature and to secrete immunoglobulin.

Signs and symptoms

Typically, the infant with X-linked hypogammaglobulinemia is asymptomatic until age 6 months, when transplacental maternal immunoglobulins that provided immune response have been depleted. Then he develops recurrent

TYPES OF VASCULITIS

TYPE	VESSELS INVOLVED
Polyarteritis nodosa	Small- to medium-sized arteries throughout body. Lesions tend to be segmental, occur at bifurcations and branchings of arteries, and spread distally to arterioles. In severe cases, lesions circumferentially involve adjacent veins.
Allergic angiitis and granulomatosis (Churg-Strauss syndrome)	Small- to medium-sized arteries and small vessels (arterioles, capillaries, and venules), mainly of the lung but also other organs
Polyangiitis overlap syndrome	Small- to medium-sized arteries and small vessels (arterioles, capillaries, venules) of lung and other organs
Wegener's granulomatosis	Small- to medium-sized vessels of the respiratory tract and kidney
Temporal arteritis	Medium- to large-sized arteries, most commonly branches of the carotid artery
Takayasu's arteritis (aortic arch syndrome)	Medium- to large-sized arteries, particularly the aortic arch and its branches and, possibly, the pulmonary artery
Hypersensitivity vasculitis	Small vessels, especially of the skin
Mucocutaneous lymph node syndrome (Kawasaki disease)	Small- to medium-sized vessels, primarily of the lymph nodes; may progress to involve coronary arteries
Behçet's disease	Small vessels, primarily of the mouth and genitalia but also of the eyes, skin, joints, GI tract, and central nervous system

SIGNS & SYMPTOMS	DIAGNOSIS
Hypertension, abdominal pain, myalgias, headache, joint pain, weakness	History of symptoms. Elevated ESR; leukocytosis; anemia; thrombocytosis; depressed C3 complement; rheumatoid factor >1:60; circulating immune complexes. Tissue biopsy shows necrotizing vasculitis.
Resembles polyarteritis nodosa with hallmark of severe pulmonary involvement	History of asthma. Eosinophilia; tissue biopsy shows granulomatous inflammation with eosinophilic infiltration.
Combines symptoms of polyarteritis nodosa and allergic angiitis and granulomatosis	Possible history of allergy. Eosinophilia; tissue biopsy shows granulomatous inflammation with eosinophilic infiltration.
Fever, pulmonary congestion, cough, malaise, anorexia, weight loss, mild to severe hematuria	Tissue biopsy shows necrotizing vasculitis with granulomatous inflammation. Leukocytosis; elevated ESR, IgA, and IgG; low titer rheumatoid factor; circulating immune complexes.
Fever, myalgia, jaw claudication, visual changes, headache (associated with polymyalgia rheumatica syndrome)	Decreased hemoglobin; elevated ESR; tissue biopsy shows panarteritis with infiltration of mononuclear cells, giant cells within vessel wall, fragmentation of internal elastic lamina, and proliferation of intima.
Malaise, pallor, nausea, night sweats, arthralgias, anorexia, weight loss, pain or paraesthesia distal to affected area, bruits, loss of distal pulses, syncope, and, if carotid artery is involved, diplopia and transient blindness. May progress to congestive heart failure or cerebrovascular accident.	Decreased hemoglobin; leukocytosis; positive LE cell preparation and elevated ESR. Arteriography shows calcification and obstruction of affected vessels. Tissue biopsy shows inflammation of adventitia and intima of vessels, and thickening of vessel walls.
Palpable purpura, papules, nodules, vesicles, bullae, ulcers, or chronic or recurrent urticaria	History of exposure to antigen, such as a microorganism or drug. Tissue biopsy shows leukocytoblastic angiitis, usually in postcapillary venules, with infiltration of polymorphonuclear leukocytes, fibrinoid necrosis, and extravasation of erthyrocytes.
Fever; nonsuppurative cervical adenitis; edema; congested conjunctivae; erythema of oral cavity, lips and palms; and desquamation of fingertips. May progress to myocarditis, pericarditis, myocardial infarction, and cardiomegaly.	History of symptoms. Tissue biopsy shows intimal proliferation and infiltration of vessel walls with mononuclear cells.
Recurrent oral ulcers, eye lesions, genital lesions, and cutaneous lesions	History of symptoms.

bacterial otitis media, pneumonia, dermatitis, bronchitis, and meningitis—usually caused by pneumococci, streptococci, or *Hemophilus influenzae* or other gram-negative organisms. Purulent conjunctivitis, abnormal dental caries, and polyarthritis resembling rheumatoid arthritis may also occur. Severe malabsorption associated with infestation by *Giardia lamblia* may result in retarded development. Despite recurrent infections, lymphadenopathy and splenomegaly are usually absent.

Diagnosis

Diagnosis of X-linked hypogammaglobulinemia may be especially difficult, since recurrent infections are common even in normal infants (many of whom don't start producing their own antibodies until age 18 to 20 months). It rests on the detection of absent or decreased IgM, IgA, and IgG in the serum by immunoelectrophoresis. However, diagnosis by this method usually isn't possible until the infant is 9 months old. Antigenic stimulation confirms an inability to produce specific antibodies, although cellular immunity remains intact.

Treatment and special considerations

Treatment aims to prevent or control infections and to boost the patient's immune response. Injection of immune globulin helps maintain immune response. Since these injections are very painful, give them deep into a large muscle mass, such as the gluteal or thigh muscles, and massage well. If the dosage is more than 1.5 ml, divide it and inject it into more than one site; for frequent injections, rotate the injection sites. Because immune globulin is composed primarily of IgG, the patient may also need fresh frozen plasma infusions to provide IgA and IgM. Unfortunately, mucosal secretory IgA cannot be replaced by therapy, resulting in frequent crippling pulmonary disease.

Judicious use of antibiotics also helps combat infection; in some cases, chronic broad-spectrum antibiotics may be indicated. To help prevent severe infection, teach the patient and his family how to recognize its early signs and to report them promptly. Advise them to have cuts and scrapes cleaned immediately. Warn them to avoid crowds and persons who have active infections.

During acute infection, monitor the patient closely. Maintain adequate nutrition and hydration, and perform chest physiotherapy if required. As always, carefully explain all treatment measures and make sure the patient and his family understand the disorder. Suggest genetic counseling if parents have questions about vulnerability of future offspring.

Common Variable Immunodeficiency

(Acquired hypogammaglobulinemia, Agammaglobulinemia with Ig-bearing B cells)

Common variable immunodeficiency is characterized by progressive deterioration of B cell (humoral) immunity, resulting in increased susceptibility to infection. Unlike X-linked hypogammaglobulinemia, this disorder usually causes symptoms after infancy and childhood, between ages 25 and 40. It affects males and females equally and usually doesn't interfere with normal life span or with normal pregnancy and offspring.

Causes

The cause of common variable immunodeficiency is unknown. Most patients have a normal circulating B cell count but defective synthesis or release of immunoglobulins. Many also exhibit progressive deterioration of T cell (cell-mediated) immunity revealed by delayed hypersensitivity skin testing.

Signs and symptoms

In common variable immunodeficiency, pyogenic bacterial infections are characteristic, but tend to be chronic rather than acute (as in X-linked hypogammaglobulinemia). Recurrent sinopulmonary infections, chronic bacterial conjunctivitis, and malabsorption (often associated with infestation by *Giardia lamblia*) are usually the first clues to immunodeficiency.

Common variable immunodeficiency may be associated with autoimmune diseases, such as systemic lupus erythematosus, rheumatoid arthritis, hemolytic anemia, and pernicious anemia, and with malignancy, such as leukemia and lymphoma.

Diagnosis

Characteristic diagnostic markers in this disorder are decreased serum IgM, IgA, and IgG detected by immunoelectrophoresis, along with a normal circulating B cell count. Antigenic stimulation confirms an inability to produce specific antibodies; cell-mediated immunity may be intact or delayed. X-rays usually show signs of chronic lung disease or sinusitis.

Treatment and special considerations

Treatment and care for patients with common variable immunodeficiency are essentially the same as for X-linked hypogammaglobulinemia.

Injection of immune globulin (usually weekly to monthly) helps maintain immune response. Since these injections are very painful, give them deep into a large muscle mass, such as the gluteal or thigh muscles, and massage well. If the dosage is more than 1.5 ml, divide the dose and inject it into more than one site; for frequent injections, rotate the injection sites. Because immune globulin is composed primarily of IgG, the patient may also need fresh frozen plasma infusions to provide IgA and IgM.

Antibiotics are the mainstay for combating infection. Regular X-rays and pulmonary function studies help monitor infection in the lungs; chest physiotherapy may be ordered to forestall or help clear such infection.

To help prevent severe infection, teach the patient and his family how to recognize its early signs. Warn them to avoid crowds and persons who have active infections. Also stress the importance of good nutrition and regular follow-up care.

IgA Deficiency

(Janeway Type 3 dysgammaglobulinemia)

Selective deficiency of IgA is the most common immunoglobulin deficiency, appearing in as many as 1 in 800 persons. IgA—the major immunoglobulin in human saliva, nasal and bronchial fluids, and intestinal secretions—guards against bacterial and viral reinfections. Consequently, IgA deficiency leads to chronic sinopulmonary infections, gastrointestinal diseases, and other disorders. Prognosis is good for patients who receive correct treatment, especially if they are free of associated disorders. Such patients have been known to survive to age 70.

Causes

IgA deficiency seems to be linked to autosomal dominant or recessive inheritance. The presence of normal numbers of peripheral blood lymphocytes carrying IgA receptors and of normal amounts of other immunoglobulins suggests that B cells may not be secreting IgA. In an occasional patient, suppressor T cells appear to inhibit IgA. IgA deficiency also seems related to autoimmune disorders, since many patients with rheumatoid arthritis or systemic lupus erythematosus are also IgA deficient. Some drugs, such as anticonvulsants, may cause transient IgA deficiency.

Signs and symptoms

Some IgA-deficient patients have no symptoms, possibly because they have extra amounts of low-molecular-weight IgM (7s), which takes over IgA function and helps maintain immunologic defenses. Among patients who do develop symptoms, chronic sinopulmonary infection is most common. Other effects are respiratory allergy, often triggered by infection; gastrointestinal tract diseases, such as celiac disease, ulcerative colitis, and regional enteritis; autoimmune diseases, such as rheumatoid arthritis, systemic lupus erythematosus, immunohemolytic anemia, and chronic hepatitis; and malignant tumors, such as squamous cell carcinoma of the lungs, reticulum cell sarcoma, and thymoma. Age of onset varies. Some IgA-deficient children with recurrent respiratory disease and middle-ear inflammation may begin to synthesize IgA spontaneously as recurrent infections subside and their condition improves.

Diagnosis

Immunologic analyses of IgA-deficient patients show serum IgA levels below 5 mg/dl. While IgA is usually absent from secretions in IgA-deficient patients, levels may be normal in rare cases. IgE is normal, while IgM may be normal or elevated in serum and secretions. Normally absent low-molecular-weight IgM (7S) may be present.

Tests may also indicate autoantibodies and antibodies against IgG (rheumatoid factor), IgM, and bovine milk. Cell-mediated immunity and secretory piece (the glycopeptide that transports IgA) are usually normal, and most circulating B cells appear normal.

Treatment and special considerations

Selective IgA deficiency has no known cure. Treatment aims to control symptoms of associated diseases, such as respiratory and gastrointestinal infections, and is generally the same as for a patient with normal IgA, with one exception: *Don't* give an IgA-deficient patient immune globulin, because sensitization may lead to anaphylaxis during future administration of blood products.

If transfusion with blood products is necessary, minimize the risk of adverse reaction by using washed red blood cells or avoid the reaction completely by cross matching the patient's blood with that of an IgA-deficient donor.

Since this is a lifelong disorder, teach the patient to prevent infection, to recognize its early signs, and to seek treatment promptly.

DiGeorge's Syndrome

(Congenital thymic hypoplasia or aplasia)

DiGeorge's syndrome is a disorder known typically by the partial or total absence of cell-mediated immunity that results from a deficiency of T lymphocytes. It characteristically produces life-threatening hypocalcemia that may be associated with cardiovascular and facial anomalies. Patients rarely live beyond age 2 without fetal thymic transplant; however, prognosis improves when fetal thymic transplant, correction of hypocalcemia, and repair of cardiac anomalies are possible.

Causes

DiGeorge's syndrome is probably caused by abnormal fetal development of the third and fourth pharyngeal pouches

(12th week of gestation) that interferes with the formation of the thymus. As a result, the thymus is completely or partially absent and abnormally located, causing deficient cell-mediated immunity. This syndrome has been associated with maternal alcoholism and resultant fetal alcohol syndrome.

Signs and symptoms

Symptoms are usually obvious at birth or shortly thereafter. An infant with DiGeorge's syndrome may have low-set ears, notched ear pinnae, a fish-shaped mouth, an undersized jaw, and abnormally wide-set eyes (hypertelorism) with antimongoloid eyelid formation (downward slant). Cardiovascular abnormalities include great blood vessel anomalies (these may also develop soon after birth) and tetralogy of Fallot. The thymus may be absent or underdeveloped, and abnormally located. An infant with thymic hypoplasia (rather than aplasia) may experience a spontaneous return of cell-mediated immunity but can develop severe T cell deficiencies later in life, allowing exaggerated susceptibility to viral, fungal, or bacterial infections, which may be overwhelming. Typically, hypoparathyroidism, usually associated with DiGeorge's syndrome, causes tetany, hyperphosphoremia, and hypocalcemia. Hypocalcemia develops early and is both life-threatening and unusually resistant to treatment. It can lead to seizures, central nervous system damage, and early congestive heart failure.

Diagnosis

Immediate diagnosis is difficult unless the infant shows typical facial anomalies—normally the first clues to the disorder. Definitive diagnosis depends on successful treatment of hypocalcemia and other life-threatening birth defects during the first few weeks of life. Such diagnosis rests on proof of decreased or absent T lymphocytes (sheep cell test, lymphopenia) and of an absent thymus (chest X-ray). Immunoglobulin assays are useless, because antibodies present are usually from maternal circulation.

ROLE OF THE THYMUS IN IMMUNE RESPONSE

Although the exact relationship between the thymus and the immune system remains unclear, possible thymic functions include:

- destruction of T cells that would have "mistaken" components of the human organism as foreign during the fetal stage. This establishes immunologic differentiation between self and nonself.
- maturation of T cells in the thymic epithelium or mesenchymal cells. These mature cells help regulate the humoral immune response.

Additional tests showing low serum calcium, elevated serum phosphorus, and missing parathyroid hormone confirm hypoparathyroidism.

Treatment and special considerations

Life-threatening hypocalcemia must be treated immediately, but it's unusually resistant and requires aggressive treatment; for example, with a rapid I.V. infusion of 10% solution of calcium gluconate. During such an infusion, monitor heart rate and watch carefully to avoid infiltration. Remember that calcium supplements *must* be given with vitamin D, or sometimes also with parathyroid hormone, to ensure effective calcium utilization. After hypocalcemia is under control, fetal thymic transplant may restore normal cell-mediated immunity. Cardiac anomalies require surgical repair when possible.

A patient with DiGeorge's syndrome also needs a low-phosphorus diet and careful preventive measures for infection. Teach the mother of such an infant to watch for signs of infection and have it treated immediately; to keep the infant away from crowds or any other potential sources of infection; and to provide good hygiene and adequate nutrition and hydration.

Acquired Immunodeficiency Syndrome (AIDS)

Currently one of the most widely publicized diseases, AIDS is characterized by progressively weakened cell-mediated (T cell) immunity, which makes the patient susceptible to opportunistic infections and unusual cancers (see Common Infectious Organisms in AIDS*). The syndrome was first defined by the Centers for Disease Control (CDC) in 1981. Recent studies point overwhelmingly to a retrovirus—the human T cell leukemia/lymphoma virus (HTLV-III)—as the cause of AIDS. The population most at risk for contracting AIDS consists of homosexual and bisexual men who are sexually active with many partners. Other risk groups include intravenous drug abusers and hemophiliacs. Most recently, heterosexual partners and children of patients with AIDS or of those in high-risk groups and persons receiving multiple blood transfusions have been added to the high-risk category. More than 75% of AIDS victims die within 2 years of diagnosis. To date, no effective therapy has been found to stop growth of the virus or to correct the immune defect.*

The CDC has also defined an AIDS-related complex (ARC), in which the patient develops some of the nonspecific symptoms of AIDS but not the typical opportunistic infections. Occasionally, this complex is mistakenly labeled pre-AIDS; some, but not all, cases progress to AIDS.

COMMON INFECTIOUS ORGANISMS IN AIDS

Protozoa

Pneumocystis carinii
Cryptosporidium
Toxoplasma gondii
Entamoeba histolytica
Giardia lamblia

Fungi

Candida species
Cryptococcus neoformans

Mycobacteria

Mycobacterium avium-intracellularis

Viruses

Cytomegalovirus
Epstein-Barr virus
Herpes simplex virus
Herpes zoster
Poxvirus
Polyomavirus

Causes

AIDS results from infection with the HTLV-III virus, which selectively strikes T_4 (helper) lymphocytes, gradually depleting their number and impairing their function. The resultant decrease in the T_4:T_8 (helper:suppressor) lymphocyte ratio profoundly impairs cell-mediated immunity. Natural killer cells and cytotoxic T cells also display limited activity. Although B cell production of immunoglobulin increases, these cells respond poorly to new antigens. (T_4 lymphocytes normally enhance B cell recognition of antigen.) The HTLV-III virus appears to be transmitted by direct inoculation alone via intimate sexual contact, especially associated with rectal mucosal trauma; transfusion of blood or blood products; contaminated needles; or transplacental contact between mother and fetus. The time between probable exposure to the virus and diagnosis averages 1 to 3 years.

Signs and symptoms

Some patients with AIDS are asymptomatic until they abruptly develop an opportunistic infection or the purple skin nodules that typify Kaposi's sarcoma. But more often, patients have a recent history of nonspecific signs and symptoms, such as fatigue, afternoon fevers, night sweats, weight loss, diarrhea, or cough. Soon after these appear, the patient typically develops several concurrent infections.

This clinical course varies slightly in children with AIDS. First, incubation time appears to be shorter, with a mean of 8 months. In children, signs and symptoms resemble those of adult AIDS, except for those findings related to venereal disease. Finally, in children, the most common manifestation—and cause of death—is diffuse interstitial pneumonitis, not *Pneumocystis carinii* pneumonia as in adults.

Patients with ARC display some of the nonspecific symptoms of AIDS but not the typical opportunistic infections. Most of these patients have a history of unexplained fever, lymphadenopathy, weight loss, diarrhea, sore throat, fatigue, and night sweats.

Diagnosis

The CDC defines AIDS as the presence of an opportunistic infection or unusual cancer (such as Kaposi's sarcoma) in a patient with no known cause of immunodeficiency. Diagnosis rests on careful correlation of the patient's history and clinical features with this definition. To date, presence of the HTLV-III virus or antibody is not considered diagnostic of AIDS.

Several blood tests help evaluate immunity and support the diagnosis, including complete blood count with differential, fluorescent activated cell sorter (FACS) analysis of total T cell and B cell number, and the T_4:T_8 ratio. A decreased T_4:T_8 ratio associated with a severely depleted T_4 lymphocyte population is characteristic. Skin testing with common antigens confirms impaired cell-mediated immunity.

Treatment

Currently, no cure exists for the immunodeficiency of AIDS. However, researchers continue to explore methods to arrest growth of the HTLV-III virus or to restore lost immune function. Although bone marrow transplant has failed to improve immune function, I.V. infusion of interleukin-2 and interferon has shown limited effectiveness. New antiviral drugs also offer some hope.

Supportive measures in AIDS aim to reduce the risk of infection, to treat existing infections and malignancies, to maintain adequate nutrition, and to provide emotional support.

Drug treatment for AIDS varies. Although many of the causative infectious organisms are responsive to drugs, infection tends to recur when treatment is discontinued. The drug of choice for *P. carinii* pneumonia is an oral or I.V. preparation of co-trimoxazole (Bactrim, Septra). If treatment fails or if toxicity occurs, pentamidine (Pentam 300) may be substituted; however, this drug may cause side effects such as azotemia, liver dysfunction, tachycardia, hypotension, hypoglycemia, and skin rashes.

Antineoplastic drugs, such as vincristine and VP-16, may be used to treat Kaposi's sarcoma; however, aggressive treatment increases the likelihood of infection. Alpha-interferon is also being used to treat Kaposi's sarcoma. Radiation and laser therapy are palliative mea-

KAPOSI'S SARCOMA

Kaposi's sarcoma (KS) is a vascular tumor that was rare in the U.S. and Europe until the recent outbreak of AIDS. This rare tumor formerly affected elderly Jewish and Italian men, young black Africans, and patients with depressed immune function. It commonly produced purple and brown plaques or nodules on the lower legs. The KS associated with AIDS, although histiologically identical to the rarer form, is more rapidly progressive and often involves many body sites (instead of just the lower extremities), including the oral cavity, hard palate, gastrointestinal tract, lymph nodes, and lungs.

sures for local lesions.

To reduce the risk of contracting AIDS, the U.S. Public Health Service recommends avoiding sexual contact with persons known to have or suspected of having AIDS. It also advises that members of high-risk groups refrain from donating blood.

Special considerations

Although AIDS is not thought to be transmitted by casual contact, you should observe special precautions when caring for an AIDS patient. Wear gloves and a gown when handling blood, other body fluids, or excretions—or potentially contaminated objects or surfaces. If such contact occurs, wash your hands immediately with soap and water. Of course, thorough hand washing is necessary before and after any contact with suspected AIDS patients, as well as those diagnosed as having AIDS. Generally, follow precautions appropriate for hepatitis B: properly labeling all specimens collected from the patient; placing soiled linen in a labeled, impervious bag; and disposing of needles (unsheathed) in a puncture-resistant container.

- Monitor the patient for fever, noting its pattern. Also assess for tender, swollen lymph nodes and check laboratory values regularly. Be alert for signs of infection, such as skin breakdown, cough, sore throat, and diarrhea.
- Encourage daily oral rinsing with normal saline or bicarbonate solution. To relieve oral *Candida* or stomatitis, offer the patient hydrogen peroxide or Benadryl-Kaopectate solution (swish and spit). Avoid glycerin swabs, which dry mucous membranes.
- Record the patient's caloric intake. Total parenteral nutrition may be necessary to maintain adequate caloric intake, although it provides a potential route for infection.
- If the patient develops Kaposi's sarcoma, monitor the progression of lesions. Provide meticulous skin care, especially in the debilitated patient.
- Recognize that diagnosis of AIDS is typically emotionally charged because of the disease's social impact and discouraging prognosis. The patient may face the loss of his job and financial security, as well as the support of his family and friends. Coping with an altered body image and the emotional burden of untimely death may also overwhelm the patient. Be as supportive as possible.

Chronic Mucocutaneous Candidiasis

Chronic mucocutaneous candidiasis is a form of candidiasis (moniliasis) that usually develops during the first year of life but occasionally may occur as late as the twenties. Affecting males and females, it's characterized by repeated infection with Candida albicans *that may result from an inherited defect in the cell-mediated (T cell) immune system. (The humoral immune system, mediated by B cells, is intact and gives a normal antibody response to* C. albicans.*) In some patients, an autoimmune response affecting the endocrine system may induce various endocrinopathies.*

Despite chronic candidiasis, these patients rarely die of systemic infection. Instead, they usually die of hepatic or endocrine failure. Prognosis for chronic mucocutaneous candidiasis depends on the severity of the associated endocrinopathy. Indeed, patients with associated endocrinopathy rarely live beyond their thirties.

Causes

Although no characteristic immunologic defects have been identified in this infection, many patients are anergic to various antigens or to *Candida* alone. In some patients, anergy may result from deficient migration inhibition factor, a mediator normally produced by lymphocytes.

Signs and symptoms

Chronic candidal infections can affect the skin, mucous membranes, nails, and vagina, usually causing large, circular lesions. These infections rarely produce systemic symptoms, but in late stages may be associated with recurrent respiratory tract infections. Other associated conditions include severe viral infections that may precede the onset of endocrinopathy and, sometimes, hepatitis. Involvement of the mouth, nose, and palate may cause speech and eating difficulties.

Symptoms of endocrinopathy are peculiar to the organ involved. Tetany and hypocalcemia are most common and are associated with hypoparathyroidism. Addison's disease, hypothyroidism, diabetes, and pernicious anemia are also connected with chronic mucocutaneous candidiasis. Psychiatric disorders are likely because of disfigurement and multiple endocrine aberrations.

Diagnosis

Laboratory findings usually show a normal circulating T cell count, although it may be decreased. Most patients don't have delayed hypersensitivity skin tests to *Candida*, even during the infectious stage. Migration inhibiting factor that indicates the presence of activated T cells may not respond to *Candida*.

Nonimmunologic abnormalities result from endocrinopathy and may include hypocalcemia, abnormal hepatic function studies, hyperglycemia, iron deficiency, and abnormal vitamin B_{12} absorption (pernicious anemia). Diagnosis must rule out other immunodeficiency disorders associated with chronic *Candida* infection, especially DiGeorge's syndrome, ataxia-telangiectasia, and severe combined immunodeficiency disease (SCID), all of which produce severe immunologic defects. After diagnosis, the patient needs evaluation of adrenal, pituitary, thyroid, gonadal, pancreatic, and parathyroid functions, with careful follow-up. The disease is progressive, and most patients eventually develop endocrinopathy.

Treatment and special considerations

Treatment aims to control infection but isn't always successful. Topical antifungal agents are often ineffective against chronic mucocutaneous candidiasis. Miconazole and nystatin are sometimes useful, but ultimately fail to control this infection.

Systemic infections may not be fatal, but they're serious enough to warrant vigorous treatment. Oral ketaconazole and injected thymosin and levamisole have had some positive effect. Oral or intramuscular iron replacement may also be necessary.

Teach the patient about the progressive manifestations of the disease and emphasize the importance of seeing an endocrinologist for regular checkups. Treatment may also include plastic surgery, when possible, and counseling to help patients cope with their disfigurement.

Immunodeficiency with Eczema and Thrombocytopenia

(Wiskott-Aldrich syndrome)

Wiskott-Aldrich syndrome is an X-linked recessive immunodeficiency disorder in which both B cell and T cell functions are defective. Its clinical features include thrombocytopenia with severe bleeding, eczema, recurrent infection, and an in-

creased risk of lymphoid malignancy. Prognosis is poor. This syndrome causes early death (average life span is 4 years; rarely, affected children survive to their teens), usually from massive bleeding during infancy or from malignancy or severe infection in early childhood.

Causes

Because Wiskott-Aldrich syndrome results from an X-linked recessive trait, it affects only males. Children with this genetic defect are born with a normal thymus gland and normal plasma cells and lymphoid tissues. But an inherited defect in both B cell and T cell functions compromises the child's immune system response and increases his vulnerability to infection. These children also have a metabolic defect in platelet synthesis that causes them to produce only small, short-lived platelets, resulting in thrombocytopenia.

Signs and symptoms

Characteristically, newborns with Wiskott-Aldrich syndrome develop bloody stools, bleeding from a circumsion site, petechiae, and purpura as a result of thrombocytopenia. As these infants get older, thrombocytopenia subsides. But beginning at about 6 months, they typically develop recurrent systemic infections, such as chronic pneumonia, sinusitis, otitis media, and herpes simplex of the skin and eyes (which may cause keratitis and vision loss), with hepatosplenomegaly. Usually, *Streptococcus pneumoniae,* meningococci, and *Hemophilus influenzae* are the infecting organisms. At about 1 year, eczema develops and becomes progressively more severe. Skin is easily infected because of persistent scratching. These children are also highly vulnerable to malignancy, especially leukemia and lymphoma.

Diagnosis

The most important clues to diagnosis of Wiskott-Aldrich syndrome are thrombocytopenia (demonstrated by coagulation tests showing a platelet count below 100,000/mm^3 and prolonged bleeding time) and bleeding disorders at birth. Laboratory tests may show normal or elevated IgE and IgA levels, decreased IgM levels, normal IgG levels, and low levels or absence of isohemagglutinins. In newborns, T cell immunity may be normal, but it gradually declines with age.

Treatment

Treatment aims to limit bleeding through the use of fresh, cross-matched platelet transfusions; to prevent or control infection with prophylactic or early and aggressive antibiotic therapy, as appropriate; to supply passive immunity with immune globulin infusion; and to control eczema with topical corticosteroids. (Systemic corticosteroids are contraindicated, since they further compromise immunity.) An antipruritic may relieve itching.

Treatment with transfer factor has had limited success. However, bone marrow transplantation has been remarkably successful in some patients.

Special considerations

• Physical and psychological support and patient teaching can help these children and their families cope with this disorder. As soon as the child is old enough, begin teaching him about his disease and his limitations.

• Teach parents of an affected child to watch him for signs of bleeding, such as easy bruising, bloody stools, swollen joints, and tenderness in the trunk area. Help them plan their child's activity levels to ensure normal development. Although the child must avoid contact sports, he is allowed to ride a bike (while wearing protective football gear) and swim.

• Before giving platelet transfusions, establish the child's baseline platelet count. Be sure to check the platelet count often during therapy; each platelet unit transfused should raise the count by 10,000/mm^3.

• Instruct parents to observe the child for signs of infection, such as fever, cold-

HOSPITAL MANAGEMENT OF BONE MARROW TRANSPLANT

The patient who undergoes bone marrow transplant needs special care before, during, and after this difficult procedure.

Before the transplant

- Assist, as needed, as the patient receives various blood tests for baseline hematologic studies and histocompatibility (human leukocyte antigen [HLA] typing and mixed leukocyte culture [MLC]).
- Carefully monitor the patient during pharmacologic or radiologic treatment to suppress the immune system.
- Impose use of sterile clothing, sheets, food, and equipment; implement reverse isolation or use of laminar flow. Help the patient adjust to the sterile environment, which will protect him from his own flora during extreme immunosuppression.
- During decontamination, provide regular baths with Hibiclens Liquid or Betadine, as ordered; administer oral nonabsorbable antibiotics to sterilize the patient's GI tract.
- Monitor vital signs, EKGs, intake and output, and blood chemistries.
- Teach patient and his family what they need to know about the transplant procedure and the preparations for it. Offer them reassurance and support.

During bone marrow infusion

- Monitor for possible allergic reactions and pulmonary overload.
- Provide meticulous care of the I.V. line and the infusion site.

After the transplant

- Provide meticulous supportive care to avoid complications and promote successful engraftment.
- During the early weeks of post-transplant pancytopenia, carefully administer ordered transfusions of red blood cells, platelets, or granulocytes.
- Maintain a sterile environment. Assess carefully for signs of infection and monitor vital signs. Take weekly samples for cultures of stool, urine, throat, and catheter sites.
- Take special care to protect venous access devices such as a Hickman or Broviac catheter.
- Watch for signs of graft-versus-host disease; administer immunosuppressive drugs as ordered.
- Provide good skin care to prevent breakdown, which provides an avenue for infection.
- Ensure adequate nutrition and fluid balance; provide I.V. fluid replacement and total parenteral nutrition, as needed.
- Watch for opportunistic infections. Monitor closely for signs of respiratory infection. Check respiration and temperature regularly. At the first sign of a fever, obtain chest X-rays and cultures. (Commonly, treatment for suspected bacterial infection begins with administration of broad-spectrum antibiotics without waiting for the results of culture tests.) Treatment for fungal infection usually includes I.V. amphotericin B; for *Pneumocystis carinii* pneumonia, co-trimoxazole (Bactrim, Septra). No effective therapy is currently available for cytomegalovirus infections.
- Provide continuing emotional support and reassurance.

like symptoms, or drainage and redness around any superficial wound, and to report such signs promptly. Emphasize the importance of meticulous mouth and skin care (including careful cleansing of all skin wounds, no matter how superficial), good nutrition, and adequate hydration. Stress the need to avoid exposing the child to crowds or to persons who have active infections.

- As appropriate, arrange for the parents of children with Wiskott-Aldrich syndome to receive genetic counseling to answer any questions they may have about the potential vulnerability of future offspring.

Nezelof's Syndrome

Nezelof's syndrome is a primary immunodeficiency disease characterized by absent T cell function and variable B cell function, with fairly normal immunoglobulin levels and little or no specific antibody production. The degree of B cell deficiency varies. Nezelof's syndrome causes early onset of recurrent, progressively severe, and eventually fatal infections.

Causes

The cause of Nezelof's syndrome is unknown. It may be a genetic disorder transmitted as an autosomal recessive trait, because it affects both male and female siblings. However, not all patients with Nezelof's syndrome have a positive family history, so alternative explanations are possible. For example, the syndrome could result from a stem cell deficiency that causes T cell and B cell deficiencies; it could result from an underdeveloped thymus gland that inhibits T lymphocyte development or from failure to produce or secrete thymic humoral factors, particularly thymosin.

Signs and symptoms

Clinical signs of Nezelof's syndrome may appear in infants or in toddlers up to 4 years and usually include recurrent pneumonia, otitis media, chronic fungal infections, upper respiratory tract infections, hepatosplenomegaly, diarrhea, and failure to thrive. Lymph nodes and tonsils may be absent or enlarged; a tendency toward malignancy is common. Eventually, infection may cause sepsis, which is the usual cause of death in patients with this disorder.

Diagnosis

Failure to thrive, poor eating habits, weight loss, and recurrent infections in children may all suggest Nezelof's syndrome. But definitive diagnosis requires evidence of defective T cell immunity and moderate-to-marked decrease in T cell count. Other laboratory findings are less conclusive: B cell count and function vary; 50% of patients have normal B cells. Immunoglobulin levels also vary. Isohemagglutinins are absent or normal, and eosinophilia may be present.

Treatment

Initial treatment is primarily supportive and includes use of antibiotics to fight infection and monthly immune globulin or fresh frozen plasma infusions (or, rarely, immune globulin injections), especially if the patient can't produce specific antibodies.

Fetal thymus transplant can fully restore T cell immunity within weeks, but its effect is transient, necessitating repeated transplants. Both transfer factor therapy and repeated injections of thymosin are only partially effective in restoring T cell immunity. Although difficult and somewhat risky, histocompatible bone marrow transplants have proven effective in restoring immunity.

Special considerations

- When administering immune globulin I.V., infuse the first 50 cc very slowly, observing the patient for signs of hypersensitivity reaction.
- If you do give immune globulin injections, prevent tissue damage by rotating injection sites and by injecting immune globulin deeply into a large muscle mass. If the child is to receive more than 1.5 ml of immune globulin, divide the dose and use more than one injection site.
- When caring for a patient with Nezelof's syndrome, continuously monitor for signs of infection.
- Teach the parents of a child with Nezelof's syndrome to recognize signs of infection, and warn them that their child must avoid crowds and persons who have active infections.

Ataxia-telangiectasia

Inherited as an autosomal recessive disorder, ataxia-telangiectasia is characterized by progressively severe ataxia; telangiectasia, particularly of the face, earlobes, and conjunctivae; and chronic, recurrent sinopulmonary infections that may reflect both humoral (B cell) and cell-mediated (T cell) immunodeficiencies. At one time, ataxia-telangiectasia was considered a neurologic disease, because its dominant sign is cerebellar ataxia. It's now known to have associated endocrine and vascular aspects. Ataxia usually appears within 2 years after birth, but may develop as late as age 9. The degree of immunodeficiency determines the rate of deterioration. Some patients die within several years; others survive until their thirties. Severe abnormalities cause rapid clinical deterioration and premature death due to overwhelming sinopulmonary infection or malignancy.

Causes

In this autosomal recessive disorder, immunodeficiency may result from defective embryonic development of the mesoderm, hormone deficiency, or defective DNA repair.

Signs and symptoms

The earliest and most dominant signs of cerebellar ataxia usually develop by the time the infant begins to use his motor skills. They typically include continual and involuntary jerky (choreoathetoid) movements, nystagmus, extrapyramidal symptoms (pseudoparkinsonism, motor restlessness, dystonias), and posterior column signs (unsteady gait, with forward leaning to maintain balance; decreased arm movements; and purposeless tremors). The associated telangiectasia usually appears later and may not develop until age 9, appearing first as a vascular lesion on the sclera and later on the bridge or side of the nose, the ear, or the antecubital or popliteal areas. Approximately 80% of affected children develop recurrent or chronic respiratory infections because of IgA deficiency early in life, but some may be symptom-free for 10 years or more. These children are unusually vulnerable to lymphomas, particularly lymphosarcomas and lymphoreticular malignancies, and may also develop leukemia, adenocarcinoma, dysgerminoma, or medulloblastoma. They may fail to develop secondary sex characteristics during puberty and eventually may become mentally retarded. Rarely, a patient shows signs of progeria: premature graying, senile keratoses, and vitiligo.

Diagnosis

If a patient has the complete syndrome (ataxia, telangiectasia, and recurrent sinopulmonary infection), the diagnosis can be made on these clinical facts alone. However, the complete syndrome may not be apparent, and ataxia may be the only symptom for 6 years or longer. So, early diagnosis usually depends on immunologic tests. A patient with ataxia-telangiectasia usually shows:

- selective absence of IgA (in 60% to 80%) or deficient IgA and IgE
- normal B cell count but diminished antibody responses
- absence of Hassall's corpuscles on examination of thymic tissue
- high serum levels of oncofetal proteins
- decreased T cells.

Physical examination reveals degenerative neurologic changes; these can also be demonstrated by computed tomography scan, magnetic resonance imaging, and pneumoencephalography.

Treatment and special considerations

No treatment is yet available to stop progression of ataxia-telangiectasia. However, prophylactic or early and aggressive therapy with broad-spectrum antibiotics is essential to prevent or control recurrent infections.

To help parents protect their child from infections, advise them to avoid crowds and persons who have infections, and teach them to recognize early signs of infection. Also teach physical therapy and postural drainage techniques if their child has chronic bronchial infections. As always, stress proper nutrition and adequate hydration.

Immune globulin infusion or injection can passively replace missing antibodies in an IgG-deficient patient and may also help prevent infection. (This treatment may not help an IgA-deficient patient, however.) The effectiveness of other forms of immunotherapy—such as fetal thymus transplant or histocompatible bone marrow transplant—is unproven.

Parents of a child with ataxia-telangiectasia may have questions about the vulnerability of future offspring and may need genetic counseling. They may also need psychological therapy to help them cope with their child's long-term illness and inevitable early death.

Chronic Granulomatous Disease (CGD)

In CGD, abnormal neutrophil metabolism impairs phagocytosis—one of the body's chief defense mechanisms—resulting in increased susceptibility to low-virulent or nonpathogenic organisms, such as Staphylococcus epidermidis, Escherichia coli, Aspergillus, *and* Nocardia. *Phagocytes attracted to sites of infection can engulf these invading organisms but are unable to destroy them. Patients with CGD may develop granulomatous inflammation, which leads to ischemic tissue damage.*

Causes

CGD is usually inherited as an X-linked trait, although a variant form—probably autosomal recessive—also exists. The genetic defect may be linked to deficiency of the enzyme NADH, NADPH oxidase, or NADH reductase.

Signs and symptoms

Usually, the patient with CGD displays signs and symptoms by age 2, associated with infections of the skin, lymph nodes, lung, liver, and bone. Skin infection is characterized by small, well-localized areas of tenderness. Seborrheic dermatitis of the scalp and axilla is also common. Lymph node infection typically causes marked lymphadenopathy with draining lymph nodes and hepatosplenomegaly. Many patients develop liver abscess, which may be recurrent and multiple; abdominal tenderness, fever, anorexia, and nausea point to abscess formation. Other common infections include osteomyelitis, which causes localized pain and fever; pneumonia; and gingivitis with severe periodontal disease.

Diagnosis

Clinical features of osteomyelitis, pneumonia, liver abscess, or chronic lymphadenopathy in a young child provide the first clues to diagnosis of CGD. An important tool for confirming this diagnosis is the nitroblue tetrazolium (NBT) test. A clear yellow dye, NBT is normally reduced by neutrophil metabolism, resulting in a color change from yellow to blue. Quantifying this color change estimates the degree of neutrophil metabolism. Patients with CGD show impaired NBT reduction, indicating abnormal neutrophil metabolism. Another test measures the rate of intracellular killing by neutrophils; in CGD, killing is delayed or absent.

Other laboratory values may support the diagnosis or help monitor disease activity. Osteomyelitis typically causes elevated white blood cell count and erythrocyte sedimentation rate; bone scans help locate and size such infections. Recurrent liver or lung infection may eventually cause abnormal function studies. Cell-mediated and humoral immunity are usually normal in CGD, although some patients have hypergammaglobulinemia.

Treatment and special considerations

Early, aggresssive treatment of infection is the chief goal in caring for a patient with CGD. Areas of suspected infection should be biopsied or cultured, with broad-spectrum antibiotics usually started immediately—without waiting for results of cultures. Confirmed abscesses may be drained or surgically removed. Provide meticulous wound care after such treatment, including irrigation or packing.

Many patients with CGD receive a combination of I.V. antibiotics, often extended beyond the usual 10- to 14-day course. However, for fungal infections with *Aspergillus* or *Nocardia,* treatment involves amphotericin B in gradually increasing doses to achieve a maximum cumulative dose. During I.V. drug therapy, monitor the patient's vital signs frequently. Rotate the I.V. site every 48 to 72 hours.

To help treat life-threatening or antibiotic-resistant infection or to help localize infection, the patient may receive granulocyte transfusions—usually once daily until the crisis has passed. During such transfusions, watch for fever and chills (these effects can sometimes be prevented by premedication with acetaminophen). Transfusions should not be given within 6 hours before or after amphotericin B to avoid severe pulmonary edema and possibly respiratory arrest.

If prophylactic antibiotics are ordered, teach the patient and his family how to administer them properly and how to recognize side effects. Advise them to promptly report any signs or symptoms of infection. Stress the importance of good nutrition and hygiene, especially meticulous skin and mouth care.

During hospitalizations, encourage the patient to continue his activities of daily living as much as possible. Try to arrange for a tutor to help the child keep up with his school work.

Chédiak-Higashi Syndrome (CHS)

CHS is characterized by morphologic changes in granulocytes that impair their ability to respond to chemotaxis and to digest or "kill" invading organisms. This rare syndrome has been documented in about 100 cases worldwide. It also affects certain animals, including cows, mice, whales, tigers, and minks. Partial albinism is typically associated with CHS.

Causes

CHS is transmitted as an autosomal recessive trait. In many cases, it seems linked to consanguinity. The genetic defect is expressed by morphologic changes in the granulocytes, which contain giant granules with abnormal lysosomal enzymes. These abnormal granulocytes display delayed chemotaxis and impaired intracellular digestion of organisms, both of which diminish the inflammatory response.

Signs and symptoms

The child with CHS has recurrent bacterial infections, most commonly caused by *Staphylococcus aureus* but also by streptococci and pneumococci. These infections occur primarily in the skin, subcutaneous tissue, and lungs and may be accompanied by fever, thrombocytopenia, neutropenia, and hepatosplenomegaly.

Partial albinism in CHS involves the ocular fundi, skin, and hair, which has a characteristic silvery sheen. Most patients also have significant photophobia. Progressive motor and sensory neuropathy may eventually cause debilitation and inability to walk or perform activities of daily living. Patients who survive recurrent bouts of infection commonly develop marked proliferation of granulocytes or lymphocytes, resembling lymphoreticular malignancy. These cells infiltrate the liver, spleen, and bone marrow, causing progressively severe hepatosplenomegaly, thrombocytopenia, neutropenia, and anemia. Eventually, this cellular proliferation is fatal.

Diagnosis

Diagnosis of CHS rests on detection of characteristic morphologic changes in granulocytes on a peripheral smear. Functional studies confirm delayed chemotaxis of granulocytes and impaired intracellular digestion of organisms.

Treatment

When prevention of infection fails, the next best step is early detection and vigorous treatment of infection with antimicrobials and surgical drainage, if indicated.

In a few patients, large doses of vitamin C (ascorbic acid) have helped enhance chemotaxis of abnormal granulocytes, although without associated clinical improvement.

Special considerations

- Provide meticulous skin care to maintain skin integrity and prevent infection.
- Teach the patient and his family how to prevent and recognize infection, especially in areas of decreased sensation.
- After surgical drainage of infection, provide diligent wound care. Irrigate draining or open wounds and change sterile dressings frequently.
- Administer antimicrobials, as ordered, and monitor the patient for drug side effects. Also check the I.V. site frequently.
- Suggest sunglasses or a visor, or both, to minimize discomfort from photophobia. Also teach the patient how to avoid injury associated with decreased sensation or motor coordination.
- Offer emotional support to help the patient and his family cope with this difficult disorder and maintain as normal a life-style as possible.

Severe Combined Immunodeficiency Disease (SCID)

In SCID, both cell-mediated (T cell) and humoral (B cell) immunity are deficient or absent, resulting in susceptibility to infection from all classes of microorganisms during infancy. At least three types of SCID exist: reticular dysgenesis, the most severe type, in which the hematopoietic stem cell fails to differentiate into lymphocytes and granulocytes; Swiss-type agammaglobulinemia, in which the hematopoietic stem cell fails to differentiate into lymphocytes alone; and enzyme deficiency, such as adenosine deaminase (ADA) deficiency, in which the buildup of toxic products in the lymphoid tissue causes damage and subsequent dysfunction. SCID affects more males than females; its estimated incidence is 1 in every 100,000 to 500,000 births. Most untreated patients die from infection within 1 year of birth.

Causes

SCID is usually transmitted as an autosomal recessive trait, although it may be X-linked. In most cases, the genetic defect seems associated with failure of the stem cell to differentiate into T and B lymphocytes. Less commonly, it results from enzyme deficiency.

Signs and symptoms

An extreme susceptibility to infection becomes obvious in the infant with SCID in the first few months of life. Commonly, such an infant fails to thrive and develops chronic otitis; sepsis; watery diarrhea (associated with *Salmonella* or *Escherichia coli*); recurrent pulmonary infections (usually caused by *Pseudomonas*, cytomegalovirus, or *Pneumocystis carinii*); persistent oral candidiasis, sometimes with esophageal erosions; and common viral infections (such as chicken pox) that are often fatal.

Pneumocystis carinii pneumonia usually strikes a severely immunodeficient infant in the first 3 to 5 weeks of life. Onset is typically insidious, with gradually worsening cough, low-grade fever, tachypnea, and respiratory distress. Chest X-ray characteristically shows bilateral pulmonary infiltrates.

Because of protection by maternal IgG, gram-negative infections don't usually appear until the infant is about 6 months old.

Diagnosis

Diagnosis is generally made clinically, since most SCID infants suffer recurrent overwhelming infections within 1 year of birth. Some infants are diagnosed after a severe reaction to vaccination.

Defective humoral immunity is difficult to detect before an infant is 5 months old. Before age 5 months, even normal infants have very small amounts of serum immunoglobulins IgM and IgA, and normal IgG levels merely reflect maternal IgG. However, severely diminished or absent T cell number and function and lymph node biopsy showing absence of lymphocytes can confirm diagnosis of SCID.

Treatment

Treatment aims to restore immune response and prevent infection. Histocompatible bone marrow transplant is the only satisfactory treatment available to correct immunodeficiency. Since bone marrow cells must be HLA- (human leukocyte antigen) and MLC- (mixed leukocyte culture) matched, the most common donors are histocompatible siblings. But because bone marrow transplant can produce a potentially fatal graft-versus-host (GVH) reaction, newer methods of bone marrow transplant that eliminate GVH reaction (such as lectin separation and the use of monoclonal antibodies) are being evaluated.

Fetal thymus and liver transplants have achieved limited success. Administration of immune globulin may also play a role in treatment. Some SCID infants have received long-term protection by being isolated in a completely sterile environment. However, this approach isn't effective if the infant already has had recurring infections.

Special considerations

Patient care is primarily preventive and supportive. Constantly monitor the infant for early signs of infection; if infection develops, provide prompt and aggressive drug therapy, as ordered. Also, watch for side effects of any medications given. Avoid vaccinations, and give only irradiated blood products if transfusion is ordered.

Although SCID infants must remain in strict protective isolation, try to provide a stimulating atmosphere to promote growth and development. Encourage parents to visit their child often, to hold him, and to bring him toys that can be easily sterilized. Explain all procedures, medications, and precautions to them. Maintain a normal day/night routine, and talk to the child as much as possible. If parents cannot visit, call them often to report on the infant's condition.

Since parents will have questions about the vulnerability of future offspring, refer them for genetic counseling. Parents and siblings need psychological and spiritual support to help them cope with the child's inevitable long-term illness and early death. They may also need a social service referral for assistance in coping with the financial burden of the child's long-term hospitalization.

IATROGENIC IMMUNODEFICIENCY

Iatrogenic immunodeficiency may be a complicating side effect of chemotherapy or other treatment. At times, though, it's the very goal of therapy—for example, to suppress immune-mediated tissue damage in autoimmune disorders or to prevent rejection of an organ transplant.

As explained below, iatrogenic immunodeficiency may be induced by immunosuppressive drugs, radiation therapy, or splenectomy.

Immunosuppressive drug therapy

Immunosuppressive drugs fall into several categories:

• **Cytotoxic drugs.** These drugs kill immunocompetent cells while they're replicating. However, most cytotoxic drugs aren't selective and thus interfere with all rapidly proliferating cells. As a result, they reduce the number of lymphocytes as well as of phagocytes. Besides depleting their number, cytotoxic drugs interfere with lymphocyte synthesis and release of immunoglobulins and lymphokines.

Cyclophosphamide, a potent and frequently used immunosuppressant, initially depletes the number of B cells, suppressing humoral immunity. However, chronic therapy also depletes T cells, suppressing cell-mediated immunity as well. Cyclophosphamide may be used in systemic lupus erythematosus, Wegener's granulomatosis, and other systemic vasculitides, and in certain autoimmune disorders. Because it non-selectively destroys rapidly dividing cells, this drug can cause severe bone marrow suppression with neutropenia, anemia, and thrombocytopenia; gonadal suppression with sterility; alopecia; hemorrhagic cystitis; and nausea, vomiting, and stomatitis. It may also increase the risk of lymphoproliferative malignancy.

Among other cytotoxic drugs used for immunosuppression are azathioprine, which is frequently used in kidney transplantation, and methotrexate, which is occasionally used in rheumatoid arthritis and other autoimmune disorders.

When caring for a patient who's receiving cytotoxic drugs, carefully monitor his white blood cell count; if it falls too low, the drug dosage may need to be adjusted. Also, monitor urine output and watch for signs of cystitis, especially if the patient is taking cyclophosphamide. Ensure adequate fluid intake (approximately 2 liters per day). Provide antiemetics to relieve nausea and vomiting, as ordered. Give meticulous oral hygiene and promptly report signs of stomatitis. Warn the patient about his increased risk of infection; be sure he recognizes its early signs and symptoms. Suggest a scarf, hat, or wig to hide temporary alopecia; assure the patient that his hair will grow back. Make sure the male patient understands the risk of sterility; advise sperm banking, if appropriate. Generally, young women are advised to take oral contraceptives to minimize ovarian dysfunction and to prevent pregnancy during administration of these potentially teratogenic drugs.

• **Corticosteroids.** These adrenocortical hormones are widely used to treat immune-mediated disorders because of their potent anti-inflammatory and immunosuppressive effects. Corticosteroids stabilize the vascular membrane, blocking tissue infiltration by neutrophils and monocytes and thus inhibiting inflammation. They also "kidnap" T cells in the bone marrow, causing lymphopenia. However, because these drugs aren't cytotoxic, lymphocyte concentration can quickly return to normal within 24 hours after they are withdrawn. Corticosteroids also appear to inhibit immunoglobulin synthesis and to interfere with the binding of immunoglobulin to antigen or to cells with Fc receptors.

The most commonly used oral corticosteroid is prednisone. For long-term therapy, prednisone is best given early in the morning to minimize exogenous suppression of cortisol production and with food or milk to minimize gastric irritation. After the acute phase, it's usually reduced to an alternate-day schedule and then gradually withdrawn to minimize potentially harmful side effects. Other corticosteroids used for immunosuppression include hydrocortisone, methylprednisolone, and dexamethasone.

Chronic corticosteroid therapy can cause numerous side effects, which are sometimes more harmful than the disease itself. Neurologic side effects include euphoria, insomnia, or psychosis; cardiovascular effects inlude hypertension and edema; and GI effects include gastric irritation, ulcers, and increased appetite with weight gain. Other possible effects are cataracts, hyperglycemia, glucose intolerance, muscle weakness, osteoporosis, delayed wound healing, and increased susceptibility to infection.

During corticosteroid therapy, monitor the patient's blood pressure, weight, and intake and output. Instruct the patient to eat a well-balanced, low-salt diet or to follow the specially prescribed diet to prevent excessive weight gain. Remember that even though the patient is more susceptible to infection, he'll show fewer or less dramatic signs of inflammation.

- **Cyclosporine.** A relatively new immunosuppressive drug, cyclosporine selectively suppresses the proliferation and development of helper T cells, resulting in depressed cell-mediated immunity. This drug is used primarily to prevent rejection of kidney, liver, and heart transplants but is also being investigated for use in several other disorders. Significant toxic effects of cyclosporine primarily involve the liver and kidney, so treatment with this drug requires regular evaluation of renal and hepatic function. Some studies also link cyclosporine with increased risk of lymphoma. Adjusting the dose or the duration of therapy helps minimize certain side effects.
- **Antilymphocyte serum or antithymocyte globulin (ATG).** This anti–T cell antibody reduces T cell number and function, thus suppressing cell-mediated immunity. It has been used effectively to prevent cell-mediated rejection of tissue grafts or transplants. Usually, ATG is administered immediately before the transplant and continued for some time afterward. Potential side effects include anaphylaxis and serum sickness. Occurring 1 to 2 weeks after injection of ATG, serum sickness is characterized by fever, malaise, rash, arthralgias, and occasionally glomerulonephritis or vasculitis. It presumably results from the deposition of immune complexes throughout the body.

Radiation therapy

Because irradiation is cytotoxic to proliferating and intermitotic cells, including most lymphocytes, radiation therapy may induce profound lymphopenia, resulting in immunosuppression. Irradiation of all major lymph node areas—a procedure known as total nodal irradiation (TNI)—is used to treat certain disorders, such as Hodgkin's lymphoma. Its effectiveness in severe rheumatoid arthritis, lupus nephritis, and prevention of kidney transplant rejection is still under investigation.

Splenectomy

After splenectomy, the patient has increased susceptibility to infection, especially with pyogenic bacteria such as *Streptococcus pneumoniae.* This risk of infection is even greater when the patient is very young or has an underlying reticuloendothelial disorder. The incidence of fulminant, rapidly fatal bacteremia is especially high in splenectomized patients and often follows trauma. These patients should receive Pneumovax immunization for prophylaxis and be warned to avoid exposure to infection and trauma.

Complement Deficiencies

Complement is a series of circulating enzymatic serum proteins with nine functional components, labeled C1 through C9. (Historically, the first four complement components are numbered out of sequence—C1, C4, C2, and C3—but the remaining five are numbered sequentially.) When the immunoglobulins IgG or IgM react with antigens as part of an immune response, they activate C1, which then combines with C4, initiating the classic complement pathway, or cascade. (An alternative complement pathway involves the direct activation of C3 by the serum protein properdin, bypassing the initial components [C1, C4, C2] of the classic pathway.) Complement then combines with the antigen-antibody complex and undergoes a sequence of complicated reactions that amplify the immune response against the antigen. This complex process is called complement fixation.

Complement deficiency or dysfunction may increase susceptibility to infection and also seems related to certain autoimmune disorders. Theoretically, any complement component may be deficient or dysfunctional, and many such disorders are under investigation. Primary complement deficiencies are rare. The most common ones are C2, C6, and C8 deficiencies and C5 familial dysfunction. More common secondary complement abnormalities have been confirmed in patients with lupus erythematosus, in some with dermatomyositis, in one with scleroderma (and in his family), and in a few with gonococcal and meningococcal infections. Prognosis varies with the abnormality and the severity of associated diseases.

Causes

Primary complement deficiencies are inherited as autosomal recessive traits, except for deficiency of C1 esterase inhibitor, which is autosomal dominant. Secondary deficiencies may follow complement-fixing (complement-consuming) immunologic reactions, such as drug-induced serum sickness, acute streptococcal glomerulonephritis, and acute active systemic lupus erythematosus.

Signs and symptoms

Clinical effects vary with the specific deficiency. C2 and C3 deficiencies and C5 familial dysfunction increase susceptibility to bacterial infection (which may involve several body systems simultaneously). C2 deficiency is also related to collagen vascular disease, such as lupus erythematosus, and chronic renal failure. C5 dysfunction, a familial defect in infants, causes failure to thrive, diarrhea, and seborrheic dermatitis. C1 esterase inhibitor deficiency (hereditary angioedema) may cause periodic swelling in the face, hands, abdomen, or throat, with potentially fatal laryngeal edema.

Diagnosis

Diagnosis of a complement deficiency is difficult and requires careful interpretation of both clinical features and laboratory results. Total serum complement level (CH50) is low in various complement deficiencies. In addition, specific assays may be done to confirm deficiency of specific complement components. For example, detection of complement components and IgG by immunofluorescent examination of glomerular tissues in glomerulonephritis strongly suggests complement deficiency.

Treatment

Primary complement deficiencies have no known cure. Associated infection, collagen vascular disease, or renal disease requires prompt, appropriate treatment. Transfusion of fresh frozen plasma to provide replacement of complement components is controversial, because replacement therapy doesn't cure complement deficiencies and any beneficial effects are transient. Bone marrow transplant may be helpful but can cause a potentially fatal graft-versus-host (GVH) reaction. Anabolic steroids and antifibrinolytic agents are often used to reduce acute swelling in patients with C1 esterase inhibitor deficiency.

Special considerations

- Teach the patient (or his family, if he's a child) the importance of avoiding infection, how to recognize its early signs and symptoms, and the need for prompt treatment if it occurs.
- After bone marrow transplant, monitor the patient closely for signs of transfusion reaction and GVH reaction.
- Meticulous patient care can speed recovery and prevent complications. For example, a patient with renal infection needs careful monitoring of intake and output, tests for serum electrolytes and acid-base balance, and observation for signs of renal failure.
- When caring for a patient with hereditary angioedema, be prepared for emergency management of laryngeal edema; keep airway equipment on hand.

Selected References

Alexander, E.L., and Provost, T.T. "Cutaneous Manifestations of Sjögren's Syndrome: A Reflection of Vasculitis and Association with Anti-RO (SSA) Antibodies," *The Journal of Investigative Dermatology* 80:386-91, 1983.

Duane, Thomas D., ed. *Clinical Ophthalmology*, vol. 5. New York: Harper & Row Publishers, 1976.

Eisen, Herman. *Immunology*, 2nd ed. New York: Harper & Row Publishers, 1980.

Fox, P., et al. "Xerostomia: Evaluation of a Symptom with Increasing Significance," *The Journal of the American Dental Association* 110:519-25, April 1985.

Golub, Edward S. *The Cellular Basis of the Immune Response*, 2nd ed. Sunderland, Mass.: Sinauer Assoc., 1981.

JAMA. *Primer on Allergic and Immunologic Diseases*. November 26, 1982.

Lichtenstein, Lawrence M., and Fauci, Anthony S. *Current Therapy in Allergy and Immunology 1983-1984*. St. Louis: C.V. Mosby Co., 1983.

McCarty, Daniel J. *Arthritis and Allied Conditions: A Textbook of Rheumatology*, 10th ed. Philadelphia: Lea & Febiger, 1985.

Milgrom, F., et al. *Principles of Immunological Diagnosis in Medicine*. Philadelphia: Lea & Febiger, 1981.

Moutsopoulos, H.M., et al. "Sjögren's Syndrome (Sicca Syndrome): Current Issues," *Annals of Internal Medicine* 92(2, Part 1):212-26, February 1980.

Oppenheim, J.J., and Rosenstreich, D.L., eds. *Cellular Functions in Immunity and Inflammation*. New York: Elsevier Science Publishing Co., 1981.

Parker, C. *Clinical Immunology*. Philadelphia: W.B. Saunders Co., 1980.

Patterson, Roy. *Allergic Diseases: Diagnosis and Management*, 2nd ed. Philadelphia: J.B. Lippincott Co., 1980.

Roitt, Ivan M., ed. *Essential Immunology*, 3rd ed. St. Louis: C.V. Mosby Co., 1981.

Stites, Daniel P., et al., eds. *Basic and Clinical Immunology*, 5th ed. Los Altos, Calif.: Lange Medical Pubns., 1984.

Strand, V., and Talal, N. "Advances in the Diagnosis and Concept of Sjögren's Syndrome (Autoimmune Exocrinopathy)," *Bulletin on the Rheumatic Diseases* 30(9):1046-52, 1980.

Talal, N. "How to Recognize and Treat Sjögren's Syndrome," *Drug Therapy* 14:48-54, February 1984.

Twomey, Jeremiah J. *The Pathophysiology of Human Immunologic Disorders*. Baltimore: Urban & Schwarzenberg, 1982.

U.S. Dept. of Health and Human Services Task Force. *Immunology—Its Role in Disease and Health*. Bethesda, Md.: National Institutes of Health, 1980.

Weir, D.M. *Immunology: An Outline for Students of Medicine and Biology*, 5th ed. New York: Churchill Livingstone, 1983.

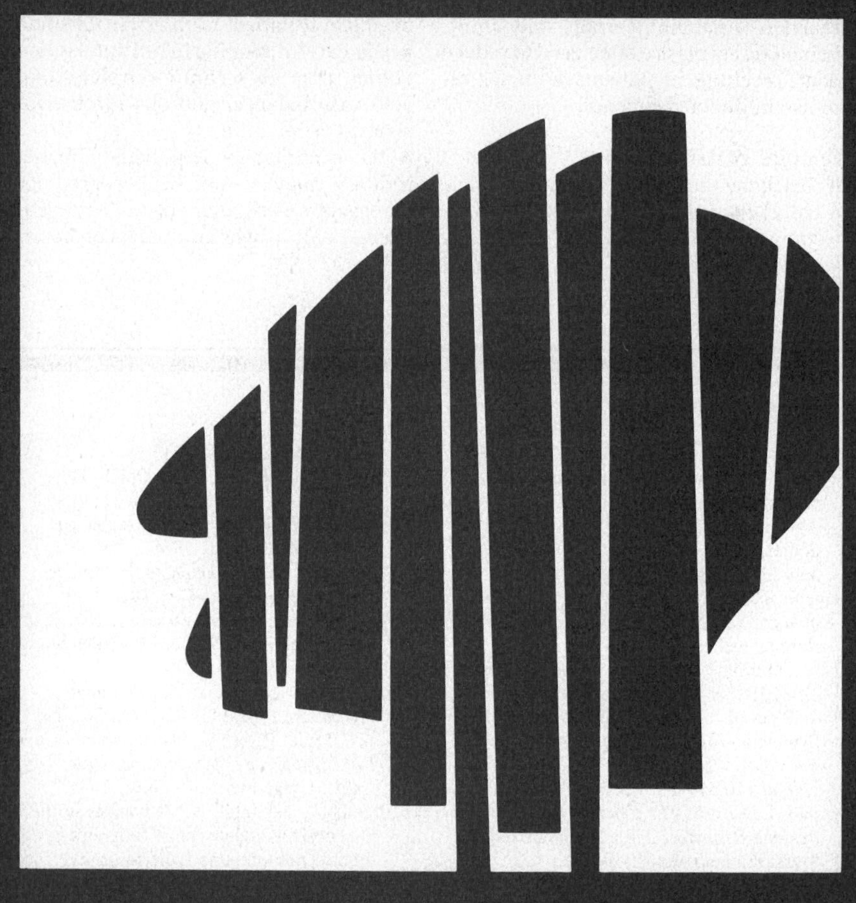

6 Mental and Emotional Disorders

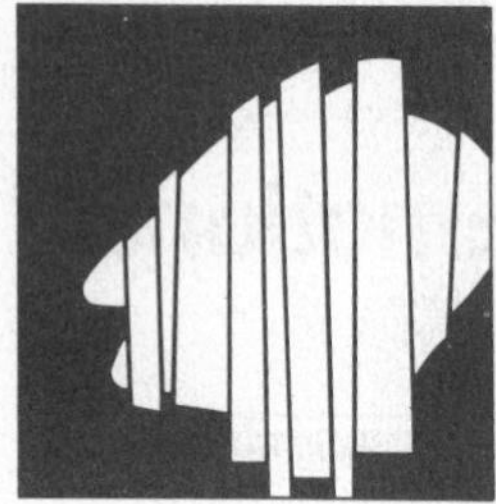

Mental and Emotional Disorders

Introduction

In recent years, social, economic, and professional forces have come together to impose massive changes in the mental health field. Building on the progress in treatment of mental disorders that started in the 1950s with the discovery of neuroleptic drugs, both public and professional interest has now focused on *prevention*—on maintenance of mental and emotional wellness, not just on treatment of established disease.

To work toward this goal, community and professional organizations have established family advocacy programs, parenting classes, stress management workshops, bereavement groups, victim assistance programs, and violence shelters. And the public education system has established widespread information programs about mental health issues. This new emphasis reflects growing public acceptance of primary responsibility for personal wellness. Witness the proliferation of self-help and coping books, as well as the general interest in physical fitness.

Economic forces

Recent cuts in federal funding of mental health programs will place future control of mental health services at the state and local community levels; it may also drastically reduce the funds available for training new professionals for this field. This squeeze in funding, as well as other considerations, has forced increased collaboration between community psychiatric facilities (short-term inpatient, outpatient, and auxiliary services) and long-term inpatient state facilities.

Professional changes

Mental health professionals have experienced enormous changes in perspective, focus, and direction. These changes are documented in the American Psychiatric Association's *Diagnostic and Statistical Manual of Mental Disorders*, 3rd ed. *(DSM-III)*—a document that imposed a whole new system of classifying mental disorders. This system requires the clinician to consider many aspects of the patient's behavior, mental performance, and history; it emphasizes observable data and deemphasizes subjective and theoretical impressions. *DSM-III* defines mental disorders as a "clinically significant behavioral or psychologic syndrome or pattern that occurs in an individual and that is typically associated with either a painful symptom (distress) or impairment in one or more important areas of functioning (disability)."

The *DSM-III* system adds diagnostic detail through a multiaxial approach. (See *DSM-III Multiaxial Evaluation.*) This system recognizes five diagnostic axes: (I) clinical syndromes and conditions, (II) personality and developmental disorders, (III) physical disorders and conditions, (IV) severity of psychosocial stressors, and (V) level of adaptive function.

The first three axes, which constitute the official diagnostic assessment, take in the entire spectrum of mental and physical disorders, ensuring consideration of disorders that are frequently overlooked. This system requires multiple diagnoses whenever necessary. For example, on Axis I, a patient may have both substance use disorder and an affective disorder. He may even have multiple diagnoses within the same class, as in major depression superimposed on cyclothymic disorders. A patient may also have a disorder on Axes I, II, and III simultaneously.

This multiaxial approach ensures consideration of many influencing facts, such as precipitating life stresses or physical illness, and inclusion of these facts in the diagnosis. This flexible ap-

DSM-III MULTIAXIAL EVALUATION

According to the diagnostic criteria listed in the American Psychiatric Association's *Diagnostic and Statistical Manual of Mental Disorders,* 3rd ed. *(DSM-III),* multiaxial evaluation requires that every case be assessed on each of the following axes:

Axis I Clinical syndromes; conditions not attributable to a mental disorder that are a focus of attention or treatment; additional codes

Axis II Personality disorders; specific developmental disorders

Axis III Physical disorders and conditions

Axis IV Severity of psychosocial stressors

Axis V Highest level of adaptive functioning during the past year.

For example, a patient's diagnosis might read as follows:

Axis I: adjustment disorder with anxious mood

Axis II: obsessive-compulsive personality

Axis III: Crohn's disease, acute bleeding episode

Axis IV: 5 to 6 (moderately severe); recent remarriage, death of father

Axis V: very good; patient has been a successful single parent, new wife, school teacher, part-time journalist.

MENTAL STATUS EXAMINATION

This examination formally organizes observations about a patient's behavior, thoughts, and feelings. The examiner's assessment should also include data from the patient's medical, social, and psychological history as well as the patient's description of his problem. This examination should evaluate the following areas:

- *appearance and behavior*—posture and motor behavior; dress, grooming, and personal hygiene; facial expressions and body language; speech (quality, quantity, and organization) and general manner.
- *mood and affect*—appropriateness to situation; range of expressions and ability to function; energy level; signs of depression or anxiety. The examiner should elicit specific and detailed emotional content by asking questions like "How do you feel about...?"
- *thought processes and perceptions*—coherence and relevance of thought; thought content ("What do you think about times like these?"); presence of suicidal or homicidal thoughts. Incongruencies are important signs of schizophrenic or paranoid disorders.
- *cognitive functions*—orientation to time, place, person, and situation; attention and concentration (saying serial 7s or the alphabet backwards); memory (remote and recent); intelligence (information and vocabulary); abstract reasoning (interpretation of proverbs); judgment ("What would you do if...?"); and sensory perception and coordination (handwriting and figure drawing). Abnormal cognitive responses are important signs of organic brain syndromes.

proach to diagnosis offers a more complete and realistic picture of the patient, which should promote better, more individualized treatment.

Improved treatment of psychiatric illness

Management of the acutely ill psychiatric patient continues to require early and accurate diagnosis and treatment—of course, with attention to these patients' legal rights. The immediate use of psychopharmacologic agents is considered effective, positive treatment. For example, to quickly reduce psychotic symptoms, high potency antipsychotic drugs may be administered every 30 to 60 minutes until symptoms subside. Because of such aggressive treatment, patients with acute psychiatric illness are experiencing much shorter hospitalizations.

Psychiatric management of chronic illness has changed as well. Notably, the movement toward deinstitutionalization—begun in the 1960s and overdone in the 1970s—is now being reversed. This well-intentioned movement unfortunately thrust into the mainstream many patients who could not live independently and truly needed the protection of institutional care. Many became our pathetic "street people," suffering a homeless, hungry, and sometimes fatally psychotic existence. The current consensus recognizes that community psychiatry is inadequate for some mental patients, so the trend is to allow intermediate to long-term institutional care for the patients who need it.

Related professional forces

This new emphasis on a holistic approach has promoted a closer affiliation between psychiatry and medicine. Witness the greater effort toward clinical use of psychosomatic concepts, increased use of psychiatric consultation for hospital patients, and growing understanding of the physiologic basis of mental function. For example, biophysical research has provided biologic markers and physiologic indices that help identify several severe mental disorders. And, with the continuing improvement of psychopharmacologic agents, clinicians can provide earlier and more complete control of distressing psychiatric symptoms for many patients. This collaboration of psychia-

CARE STRATEGIES FOR PATIENTS WITH MENTAL AND EMOTIONAL DISORDERS

Social isolation
- Set specific times to visit with the patient.
- Encourage a gradual increase in social interaction.
- Reinforce positive behavior.
- Help the patient practice social skills (group therapy, role playing) and define problem areas in social relationships.

Anxiety
- Control environmental stimuli (visitors, noise, and so forth).
- Encourage noncompetitive activities that can be completed quickly.
- Control caffeine intake.
- Teach relaxation techniques.
- Administer sedatives ordered.
- Help the patient to express feelings, thoughts, and concerns and to identify coping mechanisms.
- Teach the patient to concentrate on positive affirmations, such as "I am good, able, and strong."
- Stay with the patient who's in a panic state until his distress subsides.
- Teach the hyperventilating patient to control symptoms by breathing into a paper bag.

Dependency
- Don't accept dependent behavior.
- Assist with problem solving and reinforce decision making.
- Provide opportunities for the patient to make increasingly difficult decisions.

Suspicion
- Give clear, concise explanations of routines and procedures.
- Don't whisper or act secretive in the patient's presence.
- Don't discuss the patient's condition with his family or others unless he's present or gives permission to do so.
- Don't argue or disagree; avoid a power struggle.
- Expect hostile remarks and react to them neutrally, not defensively.
- Encourage expression of feelings.
- Provide a harmless outlet for anger and hostility in appropriate activities.

Low self-esteem
- Emphasize strengths and attributes.
- Encourage activities in which the patient can succeed.
- Praise achievements; don't criticize.
- Encourage increasing interaction with one person, then with more people.

Manipulative behavior
- Set consistent, firm limits.
- Allow choices whenever possible.
- Consult with other staff members to provide consistent management.
- Be alert to manipulative patterns; confront such behavior without anger.
- Reinforce positive behavior.

Somatic behavior
- Accept the behavior; symptoms are real to the patient.
- Help the patient accept his feelings and deal with them more effectively.
- Minimize the patient's sick role.

Depression
- Help the patient express painful thoughts and feelings.
- Check on the patient frequently.
- Spend some time visiting with the patient even if he doesn't respond.
- Keep the patient involved in hospital routines (self-care, recreation).
- Help the patient work through the grieving process.
- Encourage and help with increasingly complex decision making.
- Encourage social interaction.

Compulsive behavior
- Help the patient recognize his compulsive behavior as abnormal, but don't judge or criticize.
- If compulsive behavior is linked to exaggerated perfectionism, help the patient form more realistic expectations.
- Show the patient how he can control compulsive behavior by setting achievable limits on his compulsions, reviewing priorities, and analyzing his behavior in terms of energy expended compared to the worth of outcome.
- Support the patient's self-esteem.

ADVERSE EFFECTS OF NEUROLEPTIC DRUGS

EFFECT	ONSET	SYMPTOMS	TREATMENT
Drug-induced parkinsonism	1 to 2 weeks	• Rigidity • Bradykinesia • Decreased facial expression • Absence of blinking • Loss of coordination • Tremors	• Anticholinergic drugs if symptoms are incapacitating
Acute dystonia	Within 1 week	• Slow, sustained, twisting movements of tongue, face, neck, or trunk • Oculogyric crisis; symptoms may be mistaken for seizures.	• Diphenhydramine (Benadryl) or benztropine (Cogentin)
Akathisia	May be immediate	• Inability to sit or stand still: rocking, foot tapping, pacing, shifting from foot to foot • Purposeless limb movement • Coarse tremors • Myoclonic jerks • Complaints of feeling "tightened up," wanting to jump out of skin • Intensifies patient's feelings of being out of control • Often mistaken for increased anxiety	• Reduce dose or discontinue drug.
Akinesia	1 to 4 weeks	• "Zombie" look • Motor and psychic hypoactivity	• Anticholinergic drug if symptoms are incapacitating
Tardive dyskinesia	In most patients, within 3 years of continuous therapy; irreversible	• Various involuntary movements of mouth and jaw: lip smacking, chewing, sucking, tongue thrusting • Flapping or writhing wormlike movements of extremities that are irregular, variable, purposeless, rapid, jerky, fidgety • Dystonic postures of neck and trunk • The National Institute of Mental Health's Abnormal Involuntary Movement Scale (AIMS) may be used to assess these symptoms.	• None proven effective • Anticholinergic drugs worsen symptoms. • Increasing dose temporarily reduces symptoms; reducing dose increases symptoms.
Neuroleptic malignant syndrome	Variable; appears after starting therapy or increasing dose; few prodromal signs	• Muscular rigidity • Altered level of consciousness; stupor/coma • Hyperthermia in absence of infection; fever follows extrapyramidal symptoms. • Autonomic dysfunction, including pallor, diaphoresis, salivation, blood pressure instability, tachycardia, pulmonary congestion, and tachypnea	• Symptomatic • Potentially fatal reaction may mimic catatonia. Evaluate patient carefully.

COMMON DEFENSE MECHANISMS

- Denial—completely blocking out a painful reality
- Displacement—transferring feelings, emotions, or drives to a substitute object or person
- Projection—attributing one's own feelings to another
- Rationalization—using an acceptable, logical reason to explain unacceptable feelings or behavior
- Regression—returning (in the mind) to an earlier, safer mode of adapting (developmental stage) in response to severe anxiety
- Compensation—covering up inadequate aspects of character by overemphasizing other aspects to maintain self-respect and gain recognition
- Conversion—redirecting emotional reactions or anxiety to symbolic somatic complaints
- Identification—imitating a person who has the attributes one considers admirable
- Introjection—internalizing the feelings, values, and attitudes of another person, or using the hostility felt toward others against oneself
- Isolation—effectively separating emotions from a painful memory, thought, or experience
- Reaction formation—substituting an attitude with its opposite
- Sublimation—redirecting unacceptable impulses or energy into socially acceptable, constructive activities
- Fantasy—daydreaming as a temporary escape from a painful situation

try and medicine has focused more attention on organic mental disorders, not only in elderly patients but also in medical/surgical patients. Health-care professionals of all levels and specialties now recognize that psychiatric disorders include physical factors, and physical disorders include psychiatric factors.

Nursing involvement

Nurses function as valued members of the treatment team, aiding management of patients with mental and emotional disorders in both inpatient and outpatient programs. Psychiatric nurses serve as milieu managers and primary therapists for hospitalized patients; provide various services, such as psychotherapy and crisis intervention in community mental health centers; and offer consultations in the general hospital setting. In some states, nurses with master's and doctorate degrees have established private counseling practices and receive third-party payment for therapy. Many psychiatric nurses see the *DSM-III* Axes III, IV, and V as hallmarks for nursing intervention, identifying areas within the patient's life that are clearly in the nurse's purview. In all settings, nursing's unique systems approach and holistic view of mental health bring benefit to the patient.

DISORDERS OF INFANCY, CHILDHOOD, & ADOLESCENCE

Mental Retardation

Mental retardation is defined by the American Association of Mental Deficiency (AAMD) as "significantly subaverage general intellectual function coexisting with deficits in adaptive behavior and manifested during the developmental period (before age 18)." An estimated 1% to 3% of the population is mentally retarded, showing an IQ below 70 associated with deficits in tasks required for personal independence.

Causes

The AAMD has grouped the causes of mental retardation into 10 categories (see *Causative Factors in Mental Retardation*). But a specific cause is identifiable in only 25% of retarded persons and, of these, only 10% have the potential for cure through medical or surgical intervention. In the remaining 75%, predisposing factors such as deficient prenatal or perinatal care, inadequate nutrition, poor social environment, and poor child-rearing practices contribute significantly to mental retardation. Prenatal screening for genetic defects (such as Tay-Sachs disease) and genetic counseling for families at risk for specific defects have reduced the incidence of genetically transmitted mental retardation.

Signs and symptoms

The observable effects of mental retardation are deviations from normal adaptive behaviors. Such deviations may be present during infancy and early childhood or, in mild retardation, not until school age or later. The earlier a child's adaptive deficit is recognized and he's placed in a special learning program, the more likely he is to achieve age-appropriate adaptive behaviors.

Diagnosis

A score below 70 on a standardized IQ test confirms mental retardation. The recognized levels of mental retardation are as follows:

- mild retardation, IQ 51 to 69
- moderate retardation, IQ 36 to 51
- severe retardation, IQ 20 to 36
- profound retardation, IQ < 20.

These ranges of IQ scores may differ slightly, depending on the IQ test used. The IQ test primarily predicts school performance and must be supplemented by other diagnostic evaluations. For example, the Adaptive Behavior Scale, a test that deals with behaviors important to activities of daily living, determines the patient's adaptive profile. This test evaluates self-help skills (toileting and eating), physical and social development, language, socialization, and time and number concepts. It also examines inappropriate behaviors (such as violent or destructive acts, withdrawal, or self-abusive or sexually aberrant behavior).

Age-appropriate adaptive behaviors are assessed by use of developmental screening tests, such as the Denver Developmental Screening Test. Such tests compare the subject's functional level to the normal level for the same chronological age. The greater the discrepancy between chronological and developmental age, the more severe the retardation. In children, the functional level rests on sensory motor skills, self-help skills, and socialization. In adolescents and adults, it rests on academic skills, reasoning and judgment skills, and social skills. Continuing assessment and review of development are essential for effective management.

Treatment

Effective management of a mentally retarded patient requires an interdisciplinary team approach that provides complete, continuous, and coordinated services. A primary goal is to develop the patient's strengths as fully as possible, taking into account his interests, personal experiences, and resources. Another major goal is the development of social adaptive skills to help the patient function as normally as possible.

Mentally retarded children require special education and training, ideally beginning in infancy. Such education has been enormously beneficial and has been extended in recent years even to the profoundly retarded.

Prognosis for persons with mental retardation is related more to timing and aggressiveness of treatment, personal motivation, training opportunities, and associated conditions than to the mental retardation itself. With good support systems, many mentally retarded persons

CAUSATIVE FACTORS IN MENTAL RETARDATION

- Infection and intoxication (congenital rubella, syphilis, lead poisoning, meningitis, encephalitis, insecticides, drugs, maternal viral infection)
- Trauma or physical agents (mechanical injury, asphyxia, hyperpyrexia)
- Disorders of metabolism or nutrition (phenylketonuria, hypothyroidism, Hurler's disease, galactosemia, Tay-Sachs disease)
- Gross brain disease, postnatal (neurofibromatosis, intracranial neoplasm)
- Diseases and conditions resulting from unknown prenatal influence (hydrocephalus, hydranencephaly, microcephaly)
- Gestational disorders (prematurity)
- Chromosomal abnormalities (Down's syndrome, Klinefelter's syndrome)
- Psychiatric disorders (autism)
- Environmental influences (cultural-familial retardation, poor nutrition, no medical care)
- Other conditions

Adapted from P. Chinn, et. al., *Mental Retardation: A Life Cycle Approach,* 2nd ed., St. Louis: C.V. Mosby Co., 1979, p. 16.

have become productive members of society. Successful management leads to independent functioning for some and a sheltered environment for others. Even those persons whose handicaps require total care benefit from appropriate stimulation and training.

Special considerations

- Carefully assess the retarded person's health needs, plan activities to maximize abilities, and make referrals as needed. Remember that the mentally retarded child has all the ordinary needs of a normal child plus those created by his handicap. Be aware of special health problems, such as lowered resistance to infection, and associated abnormalities (such as cleft lip, congenital heart defects, cerebral palsy). The child also needs affection, acceptance, stimulation, and prudent, consistent discipline; he is less able to cope if rejected, overprotected, or forced beyond his abilities.
- When caring for a hospitalized retarded patient, promote continuity of care by acting as liaison for parents and other health care professionals involved in his care. During hospitalization, continue training programs already in place, but remember that illness may bring on some regression in behavior and skills.
- Teach retarded adolescents how to deal with physical changes and sexual maturation. Encourage participation in appropriate sex education classes. Consider that the retarded person may find it difficult to express his sexual concerns because of limited verbal skills.
- Provide coordinated advice, support, and practical help for the family. Suggest that the family contact the AAMD and the National Association for Retarded Citizens for more information and referral to sources of community support.

Bulimia

(Eating disorder)

Bulimia is marked by recurring episodes of binge-purge behavior, in which eating binges are followed by induced vomiting. Other essential features include an awareness that the eating pattern is abnormal, a fear of inability to control eating binges, and depressed mood and self-deprecating thoughts after a binge-purge episode.

This disorder, of growing concern to health care professionals, primarily affects females of young adult or adolescent age (generally slightly older than those with anorexia nervosa). Bulimia is much less common, but tends to be more severe, in males.

Causes

The exact cause of bulimia is unknown, but various psychosocial factors are thought to contribute to its development. Such factors include family disturbance or conflict, maladaptive learned behavior, struggle for control or self-identity, and cultural overemphasis on physical appearance. Recent psychiatric theory leans strongly toward considering bulimia a syndrome of depression.

Signs and symptoms

Bulimia is marked by episodic binge eating that may occur as often as several times a day. Induced vomiting (purging) allows eating to continue until abdominal pain, sleep, or the presence of another person interrupts it. The preferred food is usually sweet, soft, and high in calories and carbohydrate content. Actually, although the bulimic patient's weight fluctuates frequently, it usually stays within normal range—through the use of diuretics, laxatives, vomiting, and exercise. So, unlike the anorexic, a bulimic patient can usually keep her eating disorder hidden. A bulimic patient is commonly perceived by others as a "perfect" student, mother, or career woman; an adolescent may be distinguished for participation in competitive activities, such as gymnastics, sports, or ballet.

Overt clues to this disorder include hyperactivity, peculiar eating habits or rituals, frequent weighing, and a distorted body image. Repetitive vomiting may cause dental caries, erosion of tooth enamel, and gum infections. The weight loss in bulimia is rarely life-threatening.

Diagnosis

Bulimia may accompany various neurologic abnormalities, such as central nervous system tumors, or endocrine or metabolic diseases. However, the typical bulimic eating pattern is rarely confused with any physical disorder. Bulimic patients may develop an electrolyte imbalance or dehydration and thus may require laboratory tests to rule out hypokalemia and alkalosis.

Treatment

The bulimic patient knows that her eating pattern is abnormal, but can't control it. Therefore, treatment focuses on breaking the binge-purge cycle and helping the patient regain control over eating behavior. Treatment usually occurs in an outpatient setting. It includes behavior modification therapy, possibly in highly structured psychoeducational group meetings. Individual psychotherapy and family therapy, which address the eating disorder as a symptom of unresolved conflict, may also be used. Antidepressant drugs, such as imipramine, may be helpful because bulimia is often associated with depression. The patient may also benefit from participation in self-help groups such as Overeaters Anonymous.

Special considerations

- Help the patient regain control over eating behavior by encouraging her to keep a daily record of everything she has eaten, to eat only at mealtimes and only at the table, and to reduce her access to food by limiting choice or quantity.
- Help the patient develop more adaptive coping skills by encouraging her to recognize and verbalize feelings, by reinforcing realistic perceptions about body weight and appearance, and by encouraging participation in the prescribed therapy program.
- Suggest to the patient and her family the American Anorexia/Bulimia Association, Inc., and Anorexia Nervosa and Associated Disorders (ANAD) as sources of additional information and community support.

Anorexia Nervosa

Anorexia nervosa, probably a mental disturbance, is characterized by self-imposed starvation and consequent emaciation, nutritional deficiency disorders, and atrophic changes. Gorging, vomiting, and purging may occur during starvation or after normal weight is restored, as a means of weight control instead of starvation. This disorder primarily affects adolescent females and young adults but is not uncommon among older women; occasionally, it also affects males. Prognosis varies but is improved if the diagnosis is made early or if the patient voluntarily seeks help and wants to overcome the disorder. Nevertheless, mortality ranges from 5% to 15%, the highest mortality associated with a psychiatric disturbance.

Causes and incidence

No one knows exactly what causes anorexia nervosa. Researchers in neuroendocrinology are seeking a physiologic cause but have found nothing definite. Clearly, however, social attitudes that equate slimness with beauty play some role in provoking this disorder; family factors are also clearly implicated.

Anorexia nervosa most often strikes girls from achievement-oriented, upwardly mobile families, but it can occur among those of lower socioeconomic status. It may have a higher incidence in families that stress the importance of certain foods or who have rituals involving them.

Signs and symptoms

Anorexia nervosa usually develops in a patient whose weight is normal or who may be only 5 lb (2.3 kg) overweight. One of its cardinal symptoms is a 25% *or greater* weight loss for no organic reason, coupled with a morbid dread of being fat and a compulsion to be thin. Commonly, such a patient tends to be angry and ritualistic. The anorexic patient shows multiple and severe sequelae of chronic undernourishment: skeletal muscle atrophy, loss of fatty tissue, hypotension, constipation, dental caries, susceptibility to infection, blotchy or sallow skin, intolerance to cold, lanugo on the face and body, dryness or loss of scalp hair, and amenorrhea. Oddly, the patient usually demonstrates restless activity and vigor (despite undernourishment) and may exercise avidly without apparent fatigue. Paradoxically, even though she may be obsessed with food or cooking, she refuses to eat and is convinced she's too fat, despite all evidence to the contrary. Gorging, followed by spontaneous or self-induced vomiting or self-administration of laxatives or diuretics, may lead to dehydration or metabolic alkalosis or acidosis; induction of vomiting with ipecac may lead to cardiotoxicity. Circulatory collapse (signaled by a drop in systolic pressure below 50 mm Hg) may prove fatal. Cardiac dysrhythmias due to electrolyte imbalance may cause cardiac arrest.

While anorexia nervosa is not necessarily an expression of a death wish, feelings of despair, hopelessness, and worthlessness produce a higher rate of attempted suicide in these patients.

Diagnosis

Diagnosis requires careful interpretation of clinical status to rule out endocrine, metabolic, and central nervous system abnormalities; malignancy; malabsorption syndrome; and other disorders that cause physical wasting. The patient's obvious physical vigor (despite her emaciated appearance) simplifies this task, and a history of compulsive dieting and bulimic episodes helps confirm the diagnosis.

Initial laboratory analysis should probably include a complete blood count; measurement of serum levels of creatinine, blood urea nitrogen, uric acid, cholesterol, total protein, albumin, sodium, potassium, chloride, CO_2 content, calcium, SGOT, and SGPT; determination of fasting blood glucose levels; a urinalysis; and an electrocardiogram. The necessity for periodic repetition of these studies depends on the severity of malnutrition, emesis, and laxative or diuretic abuse, as well as the degree of abnormality of the test results. Laboratory data are usually normal, unless weight loss exceeds 30%.

Treatment

Treatment aims to promote weight gain or control the patient's compulsive gorging and purging, and to correct the underlying dysfunction. Hospitalization in a medical or a psychiatric unit may be required to improve the patient's precarious physical state. Hospitalization may be as brief as 2 weeks or may stretch from a few months to 2 years or longer. Treatment is difficult and results are often discouraging. Fortunately, many clinical centers are now developing programs for managing eating disorders in both inpatients and outpatients.

Treatment approaches may include behavior modification (privileges are dependent on weight gain); curtailing activity for physical reasons (such as cardiac dysrhythmias); vitamin and mineral supplements; a reasonable diet, with or without liquid supplements; hyperalimentation (subclavian, peripheral, or enteral [enteral and peripheral routes carry less risk of infection]); and group, family, or individual psychotherapy.

All forms of psychotherapy, from psychoanalysis to hypnotherapy, have been used in treating anorexia nervosa, with varying success. To be successful, such therapy should address the patient's underlying problems of low self-esteem, guilt, and anxiety; feelings of hopelessness and helplessness; and depression. Most therapists consider task-centered approaches and therapeutic flexibility important requirements for success.

Special considerations

- During hospitalization, regularly monitor vital signs and intake and output. Weigh the patient daily—before breakfast, if possible. However, since such a patient often fears being weighed, the routine for this may differ greatly.
- Frequently offer small portions of food or drinks, if the patient wants them. Often, nutritionally complete liquids are more acceptable, since they eliminate choices between foods—something the anorexic patient often finds difficult.
- If tube feedings or other special feeding measures become necessary, explain these measures completely to the patient and be ready to discuss her fears or reluctance; however, limit the discussion about food itself.
- Discuss the patient's need for food with her matter-of-factly; point out how improved nutrition can correct abnormal laboratory findings.
- If edema or bloating occurs after the patient has returned to normal eating behavior, reassure her that this phenomenon is temporary. She will probably find this condition frightening.
- Encourage the patient to recognize and assert her feelings freely. If she understands that she can be assertive, she may gradually learn that expressing her true feelings will not result in her losing control or love.
- Remember: The anorexic patient uses exercise, preoccupation with food, ritualism, manipulation, and lying as mechanisms that preserve the only control she feels she has in her life.
- The patient's family may need therapy to uncover and correct faulty interactions. Advise family members to avoid discussing food with the patient. The patient's weight may be monitored by someone who is acceptable to the patient, her family, and her therapist. You or the doctor may refer the patient and her family to Anorexia Nervosa and Associated Disorders (ANAD), a national information and support organization. This organization may help them understand what anorexia is, convince them they need help, and help them find a psychotherapist or medical doctor who is experienced in treating this disorder.

Stereotyped Movement Disorders

These disorders, commonly known as "tics," are spasmodic, purposeless, and involuntary movments of isolated groups of muscles that have no organic cause. Tics occur most frequently during later childhood (ages 5 to 12); they may be transient or chronic. Prognosis is good when treatment corrects the underlying psychopathology.

Causes

Tics commonly develop when a child experiences overwhelming anxiety, usually associated with normal maturation. When his ego can no longer balance conflicting influences from his desires, his conscience, and the environment, symptoms can develop.

Signs and symptoms

Usually, tics involve the facial muscles, causing frequent eye blinking, twitching of the mouth, and wrinkling of the forehead. These movements are recurrent, involuntary, and repetitive. Tics may also involve coughing, sniffling, or jerking head movements. Tics become more pronounced when the patient is anxious or under stress. Most patients can, with conscious effort, control them for short periods.

Diagnosis

Diagnosis is based on the patient's symptoms and history, focusing on the time of onset and any anxieties and chronic stresses in the patient's life at that time.

Treatment

Effective treatment requires an attempt to correct the underlying psychopathology by identifying and resolving the sources of the patient's anxiety, stress, and intrapsychic conflict. Without such an attempt, it's no use pressuring the patient to control tics; he can do so only briefly, and then only with intense effort.

Special considerations

Help the patient to identify and eliminate any avoidable stress and to learn positive new ways to deal with anxiety.

TOURETTE'S SYNDROME

This syndrome, the most severe of the stereotyped movement disorders, is now thought to have an organic origin (unlike the rest of these disorders). It is marked by violent twitching or convulsive movements of the face, arms, and other body parts. These movements may be associated with bizarre vocalizations—explosive sounds, a loud, barking cough, or compulsive shouting of obscene words.

Treatment

Because Tourette's syndrome may reflect a neurologic abnormality, its treatment now includes psychotropic drugs as well as psychotherapy. Haloperidol (Haldol) has proven effective in controlling the tics and vocalizations.

Special considerations

Patients with this disorder suffer overwhelming embarrassment and guilt, since their bizarre behavior is likely to provoke sharp criticism.

- Offer such patients reassurance and emotional support. Explain to their families that their abnormal behavior is involuntary.
- Encourage these patients to seek medical attention and to continue drug treatment, as prescribed. Encourage them to contact the Tourette's Syndrome Association in Bayside, N.Y., for more information.

STRESS DISORDERS WITH PHYSICAL MANIFESTATIONS

These disorders are usually outgrown by adolescence. Treatment involves determining the underlying cause, which is usually related to extreme stress in the parent-child relationship stemming from unrealistic demands on the child in terms of his developmental level.

DISORDER AND DEFINITION	CAUSES AND INCIDENCE	ASSOCIATED PROBLEMS	TREATMENT
Stuttering: abnormalities of the rhythm of speech, with repetitions and hesitations at the beginning of words; may involve associated movements of the respiratory muscles, shoulders, and face	• Possibly associated with mental dullness, poor social background, and history of birth trauma • Often occurs in children of average or superior intelligence who fear they can't meet expectations of socially striving success-oriented families	• Low self-esteem • Tension, anxiety • Withdrawal from social situations because of fear of stuttering • Humiliation	• Usually outgrown • Evaluation and treatment by speech pathologist teaches the patient to place equal weight on each syllable in sentence, proper breathing technique and timing, and anxiety control.
Functional enuresis: involuntary voiding of urine, usually during the night (nocturnal enuresis)	• Normal in children until age 3 or 4; occurs in about 40% of children at this age • Persists in 22% at age 5; in 10% at age 10; and in 1% to 2% at age 20 • Persists longer in boys • Possibly related to stress in child's life: birth of sibling, move to new home, divorce, separation, hospitalization; faulty toilet training (inconsistent, demanding, punitive); or unrealistic, not age-appropriate responsibilities	• Low self-esteem • Social withdrawal from peers	• Parents should avoid punitive reactions that burden the child with additional stress and guilt. A matter-of-fact attitude helps the child learn to control his bladder function without undue stress. • If enuresis persists into late childhood, treatment may help. Tofranil can control or reduce enuresis. *Caution:* Tofranil can cause schizophrenia-like symptoms in young children. Dry-bed therapy may include use of a urine alarm apparatus (wet bell pad), social motivation, self-correction of accidents, and positive reinforcement.

Infantile Autism

*Infantile autism (*a pervasive developmental disorder, *according to* DSM-III*) is a severe disorder marked by unresponsiveness to human contact, gross deficits in language development, and bizarre responses to various aspects of the environment. It becomes apparent before the child reaches age 30 months. Infantile autism is rare, affecting 2 to 4 children per 10,000 births. It affects three to four times more males than females, most commonly the first-born male. Prognosis is poor.*

DISORDER AND DEFINITION	CAUSES AND INCIDENCE	ASSOCIATED PROBLEMS	TREATMENT
Functional encopresis: repeated evacuation of feces into clothes or inappropriate receptacles	• Associated with low intelligence, cerebral dysfunction, or other developmental symptoms, such as language lag • Common in anxious children from socially disadvantaged families with hostile, dependent mother-son relationship and distant, uninvolved father	• Repressed anger • Withdrawal from peers in social relationships • Loss of self-esteem	• Encourage child to come to parents when he has an "accident." Encourage parents to help the child by giving him clean clothes without criticism or punishment. • Medical examination should rule out physical disorder. • Child, adult, and family therapy can reduce anger over disappointment in child's development and parenting techniques.
Sleepwalking and sleep terror: In sleepwalking, the child calmly rises from bed in state of altered consciousness and walks about with no subsequent recollection of any dream content. In sleep terror, he wakes terrified, in a state of clouded consciousness, often unable to recognize parents and familiar surroundings. Visual hallucinations are common.	• Sleep terrors are a normal developmental event in 2- to 3-year-olds. • Usually occurring between 30 and 200 minutes of onset of sleep • Tachycardia, tachypnea, diaphoresis, dilated pupils, or piloerection associated with terror	• Fear of being alone	• Usually are self-limiting and subside within a few weeks • Make sure the child has access to his parents at night.

Causes and incidence

The causes of infantile autism remain unclear but are thought to include psychological, physiologic, and sociologic factors. The autistic child's parents are commonly intelligent, educated people of high socioeconomic status. Parents' behavior toward their autistic child may appear distant and lack affection. However, because autistic children are clearly "different" from birth, and because they are unresponsive or respond with rigid, screaming resistance to touch and attention, parental remoteness may be merely a frustrated, helpless reaction to this disorder, not its cause. However, some theorists consider autism related to early understimulation that causes the child to seek contact with the world through self-stimulating behaviors; or to over-

SYMBIOTIC PSYCHOSIS

This *pervasive developmental disorder,* almost opposite in ego structure to infantile autism, becomes manifest at ages 2 to 5 years.

Signs and symptoms
This condition is marked by abnormal development of ego. The child with this psychosis doesn't see himself as a separate person. His ego is fused with that of a significant other, usually his mother. He can express himself verbally but doesn't need language to convey his ideas to her. (They seem to know each other's thoughts.) He functions at an immature level unless his mother is present; then, the two function as one (for example, when one is cold, both mother and child put on sweaters).

Special considerations
- Treatment is characteristically difficult and prolonged. It must involve both members of the symbiotic relationship. Plan your interventions to support the child and mother in developing separate interests, ideas, and goals.
- Help each to develop a separate identity. Encourage separate activities. Point out individual successes.
- Practice reality therapy with both. Point out separate body parts. ("This is your hand. This is your mother's hand." Or, "I'm going to bandage your foot. This is your foot. Your mother's foot has no cut.")

whelming overstimulation that leads to regression, muteness, and unresponsiveness to external stimuli. Some autistic children show abnormal but nonspecific EEG findings that suggest brain dysfunction, possibly resulting from trauma, disease, or structural abnormality.

Signs and symptoms

A primary characteristic of infantile autism is unresponsiveness to people. Parents report that these children beome rigid or flaccid when held, cry when touched, and show little or no interest in human contact. The child's smiling response is delayed or absent; he does not lift his arms in anticipation of being picked up and doesn't "mold" himself to the adult's body when held. The result is mutual withdrawal between parents and child.

The autistic child treats everyone with equal indifference, showing no sign of recognition or affection to parents or caretakers. In later infancy, the child doesn't show the anxiety about strangers that's typical in the 8-month-old. Such a child doesn't learn the usual socialization games (peek-a-boo, pat-a-cake, or bye-bye). He's likely to relate to others only to fill a physical need and then without eye contact or speech (for example, by dragging the adult to the sink when he's thirsty). An autistic child is usually said to "look right through" a person as though he were not physically present.

Severe language impairment is also characteristic. The child may be mute or may use immature speech patterns. For example, he may use a single word to express a series of activities; he may say "ground" when referring to any step in using a playground slide. His speech commonly shows echolalia, meaningless repetition of words or phrases, and pronoun reversal ("you go walk" when he means "I want to go for a walk.") When answering a question, he may simply repeat the question to mean yes and remain silent if he means no.

The autistic child also shows characteristically bizarre behavior patterns, such as screaming fits, rituals, rhythmic rocking, arm flapping, or crying without tears, and disturbed sleeping and eating patterns. His behavior may also be self-destructive, with hand biting, eye gouging, hair pulling, or head banging, or self-stimulating, such as playing with his own saliva, feces, and urine. His bizarre responses to his environment include an extreme compulsion for sameness—for example, the slightest change in the arrangement of furniture can cause the child to return it immediately to its original place or, if he's unsuccessful, to fall into a panic state, marked by head banging, screaming, or biting himself.

In response to sensory stimuli, the autistic child may overreact or underreact; he may totally ignore objects—dropping objects he's given or not looking at them at all—or become excessively absorbed in them—continuously watching the spinning objects or the movement of his own fingers. Commonly, he will respond to stimuli by head banging, rocking, whirling, and hand flapping. He appears to rely more on smell, taste, and touch, which don't require him to reach out to the environment, and tends to avoid using sight and hearing to respond to or interact with the environment.

Diagnosis

For diagnosis of infantile autism, symptoms must develop before age 30 months. The Denver Developmental Screening Test shows the autistic child to have delayed development, especially of social and language skills. IQ testing shows retardation in 70%, but low IQ scores may simply reflect inability to cooperate during the test. In autistic children who do cooperate, IQ tests often show average or superior intelligence.

Treatment

Treatment of autism is difficult and prolonged. It must begin early, continue for years (through adolescence), and involve the child, parents, teachers, and therapists in coordinated efforts to encourage social adjustment and speech development and to reduce self-destructive behavior. Positive reinforcement using food and other rewards can promote language and social skills. Providing pleasurable sensory and motor stimulation (jogging, playing with a ball) encourages appropriate behavior and helps eliminate inappropriate behavior. In children with a biochemical disorder (excessive dopamine blood levels), haloperidol often mitigates withdrawn and stereotypical behavior patterns, making the child more amenable to behavior modification therapies.

Treatment may take place in a psychiatric institution, in a specialized school, or in a day-care program, but the current trend is toward home treatment. Helping family members to develop strong one-to-one relationships with the autistic child often initiates responsive, imitative behavior. Because family members often feel inadequacy and guilt, they may need counseling. Until the causes of infantile autism are known, prevention is not possible.

Special considerations

- Encourage development of self-esteem. Show the child that he's acceptable as a person. If he sits on the floor, sit on the floor with him.
- Reduce self-destructive behaviors. Physically stop the child from harming himself, while firmly saying "no." When he responds to your voice give a primary reward (food); later, substitute a secondary reward (verbal: "good;" or physical: a hug or pat on the back).
- Encourage appropriate use of language. Give positive reinforcement when the child indicates his needs correctly. Give verbal reinforcement at first ("good, O.K., great"). Later, give physical reinforcement (hug him; pat his hand or his shoulder).
- Encourage self-care. For example, place a brush in his hand and guide his hand to brush his hair. Similarly, teach him to wash his hands and face.
- Encourage acceptance of minor environmental changes. Prepare the child for the change by telling him about it. Make the change minor: change the color of his bedspread or the placement of food on his plate. When he's accepted minor changes, move on to bigger ones.
- Support and assist parents. Refer the family to the National Society for Autistic Children for further assistance.

SUBSTANCE USE DISORDERS

Alcoholism

Alcoholism is a chronic disorder marked by uncontrolled intake of alcoholic beverages that interferes with physical or mental health, social and familial relationships, and occupational responsibilities. Alcoholism cuts across all social and economic groups, involves both sexes, and occurs at all stages of the life cycle, beginning as early as elementary school age.

The statistics on alcoholism vary, but it's said to affect approximately 7% of all adults (over age 18) in the U.S., and its prevalence is growing among adolescents. According to some statistics, the abuse of alcohol is a factor in 50% of all automobile accidents. Alcoholism has no known cure.

Causes

No definite cause of alcoholism has been clearly identified. However, various biologic, psychological, and sociocultural factors have been considered. For example, family background seems to play a significant part. An offspring of one alcoholic parent is seven to eight times more likely to become an alcoholic than a peer without such a parent. Why this happens is still unclear. Biologic factors may include genetic or biochemical abnormalities, nutritional deficiencies, endocrine imbalances, or allergic responses. But there's no clear evidence to confirm the influence of any of these factors. Psychological factors may include a need for relief of severe anxiety, a desire to avoid responsibility, unresolved conflict in family relationships, and low self-esteem. Sociocultural factors include availability of alcoholic beverages, social attitudes that approve its frequent use, group or peer pressures, and excessively stressful life-styles. Paradoxically, however, many alcoholics come from families in which the use of alcohol is strictly forbidden.

Signs and symptoms

The following conditions strongly suggest alcoholism: need for daily or episodic use of alcohol for adequate function; inability to discontinue or reduce alcohol intake; episodes of anesthesia or amnesia during intoxication; episodes of violence during intoxication; and interference with social and familial relationships and occupational responsibilities. Various clues can help you identify an alcoholic. For example, watch for alcoholism in a patient with traumatic injuries he can't fully explain or in someone with unexplained mood swings, unresponsiveness to sedatives, or poor personal hygiene. Watch for secretive behavior, which may be an attempt to hide his disease or his alcohol stock. Suspect alcoholism when a patient uses up inordinate amounts of aftershave lotion or mouthwash. Deprived of his usual supply, an alcoholic will consume alcohol in any form he can find.

When confronted about his drinking problem, an alcoholic characteristically becomes hostile and may even sign out of the hospital, against medical advice. In addition to these progressive signs of psychological deterioration, chronic alcohol abuse brings with it a vast array of physical and mental complications: gastritis, acute pancreatitis, anemia, malnutrition and other nutritional deficiencies, hepatitis, cirrhosis, cardiomyopathy, congestive heart failure, organic brain damage, and traumatic injuries due to falls. Indeed, cirrhosis of the liver is common in alcoholics and may be visible in the telltale signs of jaundice, spider telangiectasia, ascites, and edema. Liver damage may lead to hypoglycemia and ultimately to hepatic coma (in persons who have abused alcohol for many years).

Major complications of chronic alcoholism include organic brain damage. *Wernicke-Korsakoff syndrome*, an organic brain disorder stemming from thiamine deficiency, may follow chronic abuse of alcohol. The alcoholic with this disorder is mentally confused, apathetic, listless, and unable to concentrate. He has large memory gaps and can't put time into sequence; he then confabulates to fill the gaps. Wernicke-Korsakoff syndrome also may cause ocular nerve paralysis and ataxia. Prognosis is fair with vitamin replacement, but restoration of memory may take a year or longer.

After abstinence or reduction of alcohol intake, manifestations of withdrawal may vary in severity from a mild form (morning hangover) to its most acute form (delirium tremens [DTs])—a condition of severe distress that follows abrupt withdrawal after prolonged or massive use. (See also *Symptoms of Alcohol Withdrawal,* page 402.)

Diagnosis

To diagnose alcoholism requires a history of chronic and excessive ingestion of alcohol. However, a complete evaluation—including physical examination, pertinent laboratory results, and observation for typical signs and symptoms of alcoholism or alcohol withdrawal—can support the diagnosis. Depending on the presenting symptoms, evaluation must rule out intoxication with barbiturates or other sedatives and tranquilizers, neurologic diseases, hypoglycemia, diabetic ketoacidosis, psychosis, dementia, delirium, and hepatic insufficiency. If the patient is unwilling or unable to give a history, question his family. Ask how much he drinks and how often, when he had his last drink, and if he uses other drugs. Ask if he has any emotional problems, if he has ever attempted suicide, or if he's received counseling, treatment, or hospitalization for alcoholism.

A complete physical examination can identify complications of alcohol abuse and other physical problems related to alcoholism. Assess the patient's gastrointestinal, hepatic, cardiac, and pulmonary systems, and check his skin for changes characteristic of hepatic damage (spider telangiectasia).

Laboratory data can document recent alcohol ingestion. A blood alcohol level of 0.10% weight/volume (200 mg/dl) is generally accepted as the level of intoxication. Of course, it can't confirm alcoholism. However, by knowing how recently the patient has been drinking, you can tell when to expect withdrawal symptoms.

A complete serum electrolyte count may be necessary to identify electrolyte abnormalities (in severe hepatic disease, BUN level is increased and serum glucose level is decreased). Further testing may show increased serum ammonia and serum amylase levels. Urine toxicology may help to determine if the alcoholic with DTs or another acute complication abuses other drugs as well. Hepatic function studies revealing increased serum cholesterol, lactate dehydrogenase, SGOT, SGPT, and creatine phosphokinase levels may all point to hepatic damage, while elevated serum amylase and lipase levels point to acute pancreatitis. A hematologic workup can identify anemia, thrombocytopenia, increased prothrombin time and increased partial thromboplastin time.

Treatment and special considerations

Total abstinence is the only effective treatment. Supportive programs that offer detoxification, rehabilitation, and aftercare (including continued involvement in Alcoholics Anonymous [AA]) produce the best long-term results.

Treatment during acute withdrawal may include administration of I.V. glucose for hypoglycemia, and forcing fluids containing thiamine and other B complex vitamins to correct nutritional deficiencies and help metabolize glucose.

When caring for a patient in alcohol

SYMPTOMS OF ALCOHOL WITHDRAWAL

SYMPTOM	MILD	MODERATE	SEVERE
Motor impairment	Inner tremulousness with hand tremors	Visible tremors	Gross uncontrollable bodily shaking
Anxiety	Mild restlessness	Obvious motor restlessness and painful anxiety	Extreme restlessness and agitation with intense fearfulness
Sleep disturbance	Restless sleep or insomnia	Marked insomnia and nightmares	Total wakefulness
Appetite	Impaired appetite	Marked anorexia	Rejection of all food and fluid except alcohol common
GI symptoms	Nausea	Nausea and vomiting	Dry heaves and vomiting
Confusion	None	Variable	Marked confusion and disorientation
Hallucinations	None	Vague, transient visual and auditory hallucinations and illusions; commonly nocturnal; often with insight	Visual and occasional auditory hallucinations, usually of fearful or threatening content; misidentification of persons and frightening delusions related to hallucinatory experiences
Pulse rate	Tachycardia	Pulse, 100 to 120	Pulse, 120 to 140
Blood pressure	Normal or slightly elevated systolic	Usually elevated systolic	Elevated systolic and diastolic
Sweating	Slight	Obvious	Marked hyperhidrosis
Convulsions	None	Possible	Common

withdrawal, carefully monitor mental status, heart rate, lung sounds, blood pressure, and temperature every ½ to 6 hours, depending on the severity of symptoms. Orient the patient to reality, since he may have hallucinations and may try to harm himself or others. If he's combative or disoriented, you may have to restrain him temporarily. Take seizure precautions. Administer drugs, as ordered, which may include antianxiety agents, anticonvulsants, or antidiarrheal or antiemetic agents. Participate in the plan of care for medical symptoms and complications. Observe for signs of depression or suicide. Also, encourage adequate nutrition.

Once the alcoholic is sober, treatment

aims to help him stay sober. Educate the patient and his family about his illness. Encourage participation in a rehabilitation program. Warn him that he'll be tempted to drink again and won't be able to control himself after the first drink. Therefore, he must abstain from alcohol *totally* for the rest of his life. Two forms of treatment may help him abstain: aversion therapy, if ordered, and supportive counseling. Unfortunately, neither is completely effective.

Aversion or deterrent therapy employs a daily oral dose of disulfiram. This drug interferes with alcohol metabolism and allows toxic levels of acetaldehyde to accumulate in the patient's blood, producing immediate and potentially fatal distress if the patient drinks alcohol up to 2 weeks after taking it. The reaction includes nausea, vomiting, facial flushing, headache, shortness of breath, red eyes, blurred vision, sweating, tachycardia, hypotension, and fainting, and may last from 30 minutes to 3 hours or longer. The patient needs close medical supervision during this time. Warn the patient taking disulfiram that even a small amount of alcohol will induce this adverse reaction and that the longer he takes the drug, the greater will be his sensitivity to alcohol. Because of this, he must avoid even medicinal sources of alcohol, such as mouthwash, cough syrups, liquid vitamins, or cold remedies. Paraldehyde, a sedative, is chemically similar to alcohol and may also provoke a disulfiram reaction.

Aversion therapy is contraindicated during pregnancy and in patients with diabetes, heart disease, severe hepatic disease, or any disorder in which such a reaction could be especially dangerous. Instruct patients taking this drug that they may continue this treatment for months or years and that they should remain under medical supervision.

Another form of deterrent therapy attempts to induce aversion by administering alcohol with an emetic. However, for long-term success with deterrent therapy, the sober alcoholic must learn to fill the place alcohol once occupied in his life with something constructive. Indeed, for patients with abnormal dependency needs or for those who also abuse other drugs, deterrent therapy with disulfiram may only substitute one drug dependency for another; so it should be used prudently.

Supportive counseling or individual, group, or family psychotherapy may improve the alcoholic's ability to cope with stress, anxiety, and frustration and help him gain insight into the personal problems and conflicts that may have led him to alcohol abuse. Occasionally, a doctor may order a tranquilizer to relieve overwhelming anxiety during rehabilitation, but such drugs are dangerous because of their potential for transferring addiction and for inducing coma and death when combined with alcohol.

In AA, a self-help group with more than a million members worldwide, the alcoholic finds emotional support from others with similar problems. Approximately 40% of AA's members stay sober as long as 5 years, and 30% stay sober longer than 5 years. Offer to arrange a visit from an AA member.

Spouses of alcoholics can find encouragement in Al-Anon, another self-help group; children, in Alateen. Family involvement in rehabilitation can reduce family tensions. For alcoholics who've lost all contact with family and friends and who have a long history of unemployment, trouble with the law, or other problems associated with alcohol abuse, rehabilitation may involve job training, sheltered workshops, halfway houses, or other supervised facilities.

Until the primary causes of alcoholism are discovered, prevention isn't possible. Banning alcoholic beverages, as during Prohibition, has proved spectacularly unsuccessful in preventing alcohol abuse. Providing comprehensive treatment for alcoholics can help them maintain sobriety and may limit family disruptions that could contribute to the development of alcoholism in offspring.

Drug Abuse and Dependence

The National Institute of Drug Abuse defines this condition as the use of a legal or illegal drug that causes physical, mental, emotional, or social harm. Drug abuse is a major health problem today and commonly involves the use of cocaine; however, many drugs are being abused by many groups. The age-groups range from young students who experiment with hallucinogens and marijuana to adults who overuse tranquilizers and other prescription drugs. The most dangerous form of drug abuse is that in which users mix several drugs—sometimes with alcohol and various other chemicals. Prognosis varies with the drug and the extent of abuse.

Causes

Persons predisposed to drug abuse tend to have few mental or emotional resources against stress and a low tolerance for frustration. They demand immediate relief of tension or distress, which they receive from taking the abused drug. Taking the drug gives them pleasure by relieving tension, abolishing loneliness, achieving a temporarily peaceful or euphoric state, or simply by relieving boredom.

Drug dependence may follow the use of drugs for relief of physical pain. In young people, it often follows experimentation with drugs that commonly results from peer pressure. Medical professionals are at special risk of dependence and abuse of drugs because of their easy access to them.

Signs and symptoms

Clinical effects vary according to the substance used, duration, and dosage. (See *Signs and Symptoms of Drug Abuse,* page 405.)

Chronic abuse of drugs, especially by intravenous use, can lead to life-threatening complications that may include bacterial endocarditis, hepatitis, thrombophlebitis, pulmonary emboli, gangrene, malnutrition and gastrointestinal disturbances, respiratory infections, musculoskeletal dysfunction, trauma, and psychosis.

Diagnosis

Diagnosis depends largely on a history that shows a pattern of pathologic use of a substance; related impairment in social or occupational function; and duration of abnormal use and impairment for at least 1 month. A urine or blood screen can determine the amount of the substance present.

Treatment

Treatment of acute drug intoxication is symptomatic and depends on the drug ingested. (See *Treatment of Drug Intoxication,* pages 406 and 407.) It includes fluid replacement therapy and nutritional and vitamin supplements, if indicated; detoxification with the same drug or a pharmacologically similar drug (exceptions: cocaine, hallucinogens, and marijuana are not used for detoxification); sedatives to induce sleep; anticholinergics and antidiarrheal agents to relieve GI distress; antianxiety drugs for severe agitation, especially in cocaine abusers; and symptomatic treatment of medical complications.

Treatment of drug dependence commonly involves a triad of care: detoxification, long-term rehabilitation (up to 2 years), and aftercare; the latter means a lifetime of abstinence, usually aided by participation in Narcotics Anonymous or a similar self-help group.

Detoxification, the controlled and gradual withdrawal of an abused drug, is achieved through substitution of a drug with similar action. Such gradual replacement of the abused drug controls the effects of withdrawal, reducing the patient's discomfort and associated risks. Depending on the abused drug, detoxification is managed on an inpatient or an outpatient basis. For example, with-

SIGNS AND SYMPTOMS OF DRUG ABUSE

DRUG	CLINICAL FEATURES	COMPLICATIONS
Opioids Codeine, heroin, meperidine, morphine, opium. Butorphanol and pentazocine, though not narcotics, have similar effects and addictive potential.	• *Acute:* coma, hypotension, tachycardia, pinpoint pupils • *Chronic* (after injection): needle marks, scars from skin abscesses, thrombophlebitis • *Withdrawal:* sweating, nausea, vomiting, diarrhea, anxiety, insomnia, dilated pupils, runny nose, tearing eyes, yawning, goose bumps, persistent back and abdominal pain, anorexia, cold flashes, spontaneous orgasm, fever, tachycardia, rising blood pressure and respiratory rate	• Viral hepatitis (resulting in hepatic dysfunction), osteomyelitis, pulmonary edema, bacterial endocarditis, coma (resulting in organic brain damage or seizures), secondary infection • Physical and psychological dependence
Amphetamines Amphetamine, dextroamphetamine, methamphetamine	• *After high doses:* anxiety, hyperactivity, irritability, muscle tension, aggressive or violent behavior, paranoia, psychotic symptoms resembling schizophrenia, fever, hypertension, dilated pupils, tachycardia, convulsions, cardiovascular collapse, and hallucinations • *After injection:* needle marks, thrombophlebitis • *Withdrawal:* depression, overwhelming fatigue. Long-term use yields a rapidly developing delusional syndrome resembling paranoid schizophrenia.	• Little or no physical dependence, but tolerance and psychological dependence possible
Cocaine	• *Acute intoxication* (after I.V. injection): tremors, seizures, convulsions, delirium, potentially fatal cardiovascular or respiratory failure • *Chronic intoxication:* hallucinations, dilated pupils, tachycardia, tachypnea, muscle twitching, violent behavior, nasal septum damage • *Withdrawal:* depression, irritability, disorientation, tremors, muscle weakness	• Psychological dependence
Barbiturates Amobarbital, pentobarbital, secobarbital. Methaqualone is not a barbiturate, but symptoms and treatment are similar.	• *Acute intoxication:* progressive central nervous system and respiratory depression • *Chronic intoxication:* slurred speech, impaired coordination, decreased mental alertness and attention span, impaired judgment, memory disturbances, depressed pulse rate and tendon reflexes, mood swings, nystagmus or strabismus, diplopia, dizziness, hypotension, dehydration, and aggressive or suicidal behavior • *Withdrawal:* anxiety, irritability, grand mal seizures, status epilepticus, orthostatic hypotension, tachycardia, auditory and visual disturbances	• Apnea, shock, coma, death • Physical dependence and psychological dependence
Phencyclidine (PCP)	• *Acute intoxication:* apnea, status epilepticus, paralysis, numbness, hallucinations, anxiety, dissociative reaction, paranoid or violent behavior, coma, death • *Chronic intoxication:* confusion, fatigue, irritability, depression, hallucinations	• Psychological dependence, but no physical dependence
Cannabis Hashish, marijuana, tetrahydrocannabinol (THC)	• *Acute transient reaction* (rare): panic and paranoid reactions (with first-time use); pseudopsychotic reaction (with THC)	• Psychological dependence, but no physical dependence
Hallucinogens LSD, mescaline, psilocybin	• *Acute intoxication ("bad trip"):* anxiety, frightening hallucinations, and depression (possible suicidal tendencies)	• Psychological dependence, but no physical dependence

TREATMENT OF DRUG INTOXICATION

DRUG	TREATMENT	SPECIAL CONSIDERATIONS
Opioids	• Immediate goal is to prevent shock and maintain respirations by endotracheal intubation and mechanical ventilation and administration of oxygen, I.V. fluids, and plasma expanders. • Naloxone (Narcan) is administered until central nervous system (CNS) depressant effects are reversed.	• Observe the patient continously, and closely monitor for hypoxemia since narcotics may impair respiratory drive. Auscultate the lungs frequently for rales, possibly indicating pulmonary edema in the patient receiving I.V. fluids and plasma expanders. • Before giving naloxone, apply secure restraints. Patient may be disoriented and agitated as he emerges from coma. • Monitor cardiac rate and rhythm, being alert for atrial fibrillation. • Be alert for signs of withdrawal.
Amphetamines	• If the drug was taken orally, vomiting is induced or gastric lavage performed; activated charcoal and a sodium or magnesium sulfate cathartic are also given. • Ammonium chloride or ascorbic acid may be given I.V. to acidify the patient's urine and lower his urine pH to 5. • Therapeutic drugs may include mannitol to force diuresis; a short-acting barbiturate, such as pentobarbital, to control stimulant-induced seizure activity; haloperidol or chlorpromazine to treat agitation or assaultive behavior; and an alpha-adrenergic blocking agent, such as phentolamine (Regitine), for hypertension.	• Restrain the patient to keep him from injuring himself and others—especially if he's paranoid or hallucinating. • Watch for cardiac dysrhythmias. Notify the doctor if these develop, and expect to give propranolol (Inderal) or lidocaine to treat tachydysrhythmias or ventricular dysrhythmias, respectively. • Treat hyperthermia with tepid sponge baths or a *hypothermia* blanket, as ordered. • Provide a quiet environment to avoid overstimulation. • Be alert for signs and symptoms of withdrawal. • Take suicide precautions, especially if the patient shows signs of withdrawal. • Closely monitor neurologic status, since haloperidol and chlorpromazine lower the seizure threshold.
Cocaine	• If cocaine was ingested, treatment includes induction of vomiting, gastric lavage, and activated charcoal followed by a saline cathartic. • An antipyretic may be given to reduce fever; an anticonvulsant, such as diazepam (Valium) to prevent seizures; and propranolol to treat tachycardia.	• Monitor respirations and blood pressure closely. • Monitor cardiac rate and rhythm—ventricular fibrillation and cardiac standstill can occur as a direct cardiotoxic result of cocaine. Defibrillate and initiate CPR, if indicated. • Calm the patient by talking to him in a quiet room. • Observe for seizures, take seizure precautions, and administer ordered medication.
Barbiturates	• Immediate goal is to restore CNS and respiratory function and	• Perform frequent neurologic assessments. Check pulse rate,

DRUG	TREATMENT	SPECIAL CONSIDERATIONS
Barbiturates *(continued)*	prevent shock. • Treatment usually includes induction of vomiting or gastric lavage, if the patient ingested the drug within 4 hours; endotracheal intubation; I.V. fluids to correct hypotension and dehydration; vasopressors for phenobarbital overdose; and I.V. sodium bicarbonate to promote diuresis and counteract intoxication. • Gastric lavage or administration of activated charcoal followed by a cathartic is usually recommended to eliminate the toxic drug. • During detoxification, a pentobarbital-challenge test determines the patient's tolerance level. An appropriate pentobarbital dose lessens withdrawal symptoms until dosage can gradually be reduced and finally totally withdrawn. • Extreme intoxication may require dialysis.	temperature, skin color, and reflexes often. • Notify the doctor if you see signs of respiratory distress or pulmonary edema. • Watch for and report signs of withdrawal. • Protect the patient from injuring himself and provide symptomatic relief of withdrawal symptoms, as ordered.
Phencyclidine (PCP)	• If the drug was taken orally, vomiting is induced or gastric lavage performed; activated charcoal is repeatedly instilled and removed. • Acidic diuresis is performed by acidifying the patient's urine with ascorbic acid to increase excretion of the drug. This is continued for 2 weeks, because signs and symptoms may recur when fat cells release their stores of PCP. • Therapeutic drugs may include diazepam and haloperidol to control agitation or psychotic behavior; diazepam to control seizures; propranolol for hypertension and tachycardia; and nitroprusside for severe hypertension. • If the patient develops renal failure, hemodialysis is performed.	• Provide a quiet, safe environment with dimmed lights. • Be aware that overt attempts to reassure an aggressive patient often provoke more aggressive behavior. • Closely monitor the patient's intake and output; maintain adequate hydration to promote PCP excretion; report diminished urinary output or abnormal renal function tests. • Take suicide precautions as needed.
Hallucinogens	• Diazepam may be given to control seizures. • If the drug was taken orally, vomiting is induced or gastric lavage performed; activated charcoal and a cathartic are given.	• Reorient the patient repeatedly to time, place, and person. • Restrain the patient, as ordered, to protect him from injuring himself and others. • Calm the patient by sequestering him in a quiet room and talking to him in a soothing tone.

DRUG ABUSE OR DEPENDENCE?

For most classes of substances, pathologic use is divided into abuse and dependence, as defined below according to *DSM-III.*

ABUSE	DEPENDENCE
A pattern of pathologic use (as manifested by inability to reduce or control intake despite: • a physical disorder that the user knows is made worse by using the substance • need for daily use of the substance for adequate function • episodes of a complication of intoxication (alcoholic blackouts, opioid overdose) • impairment in social or occupational function due to substance use • minimal duration of disturbance at least 1 month.	A severe form of substance use with physiologic dependence shown by tolerance and withdrawal symptoms: • Tolerance means markedly increased amounts of the addicting substance are needed to achieve the desired effect; or regular use of the same dose produces a markedly diminished effect. • Withdrawal is a substance-specific syndrome provoked by stopping or reducing substance intake.

drawal from general depressants can produce hazardous effects, such as grand mal seizures, status epilepticus, and hypotension; the severity of these effects determines whether the patient can be safely treated as an outpatient or requires hospitalization. Withdrawal from depressants usually doesn't require detoxification. Opioid withdrawal causes severe physical discomfort and can even be life-threatening. To minimize these effects, chronic opioid abusers are frequently detoxified with methadone substitution.

To ease withdrawal from opioids, general depressants, and other drugs, useful nonchemical measures may include psychotherapy, exercise, relaxation techniques, and nutritional support. Sedatives and tranquilizers may be administered temporarily to help the patient cope with insomnia, anxiety, and depression.

After withdrawal, rehabilitation is needed to prevent recurrence of drug abuse. Rehabilitation programs are available for both inpatients and outpatients; they usually last a month or longer and may include individual, group, and family psychotherapy. During and after rehabilitation, participation in a drug-oriented self-help group may be helpful. The largest such group is Narcotics Anonymous. Three new groups were formed recently: Potsmokers Anonymous, Pills Anonymous, and Cocaine Anonymous.

Naltrexone (Trexan), a newly released drug, is used to help outpatient opiate abusers maintain abstinence. By blocking the opiate euphoria, it helps prevent readdiction. It is most useful in a comprehensive rehabilitation program.

Special considerations

Patient care for drug abusers must focus not only on restoring physical health but on educating the patient and his family about drug abuse and dependence, providing support, and encouraging participation in drug treatment programs and self-help groups. Specific interventions may vary, depending on the drug abused, but commonly include the following measures:

• Observe the patient for signs and symptoms of withdrawal.

• During the patient's withdrawal from any drug, maintain a quiet, safe environment. Remove harmful objects from the room and use restraints judiciously. Use side rails for the comatose patient. Reassure the anxious patient that medication will control most symptoms of withdrawal.

• Closely monitor visitors who might

bring the patient drugs from the outside.
- Develop self-awareness and an understanding and positive attitude toward the patient; control your reactions to the patient's undesirable behaviors—commonly, dependency, manipulation, anger, frustration, and alienation.
- Set limits for dealing with demanding, manipulative behavior.
- Carefully monitor and promote adequate nutritional intake.
- Administer medications carefully to prevent hoarding by the patient.
- Refer the patient for detoxification and rehabilitation, as appropriate.
- Encourage family members to seek help whether or not the abuser seeks it. You can suggest private therapy or community mental health clinics.

SCHIZOPHRENIC DISORDERS

Schizophrenic Disorders

This group of disorders is marked mainly by withdrawal into self and failure to distinguish reality from fantasy. DSM-III *recognizes five types of schizophrenia: catatonic, paranoid, disorganized, undifferentiated, and residual. Schizophrenic disorders are equally prevalent among males and females. According to current statistics, an estimated 2 million Americans may suffer from this disease.*

Schizophrenic disorders produce varying degrees of impairment. As many as a third of such patients have just one psychotic episode and no more. Some patients have no disability between periods of exacerbation; others need continuous institutional care. Prognosis worsens with each acute episode.

Causes and incidence

Various theories—both biological and psychological—have been proposed to explain the development of schizophrenia. Some evidence supports a genetic predisposition to this disorder. Close relatives of schizophrenic patients are 2 to 50 times more likely to develop schizophrenia; the closer the degree of biologic relatedness, the higher the risk. One biochemical hypothesis holds that schizophrenia is a hyperdopaminergic condition. Another holds that schizophrenics have a deficiency or disturbance of B endorphins.

Numerous psychological and sociocultural causes, such as disturbed family and interpersonal patterns, have also been proposed. Schizophrenic disorders have a higher incidence among lower socioeconomic groups, possibly related to downward social drift or lack of upward socioeconomic mobility, and to high stress levels, possibly brought on by poverty, social failure, illness, and inadequate social resources. Higher incidence is also linked to low birth weight and congenital deafness.

Signs and symptoms

According to the *DSM-III* classification, schizophrenic disorders have these essential features: presence of psychotic features during the acute phase; deterioration from a previous level of functioning; onset before age 45; and presence of symptoms for at least 6 months, with deterioration in occupational functioning, social relations, or self-care.

Characteristically, symptoms of schizophrenic disorders involve several of the following areas: content and form of thought, sensory perception, affect, sense of self, volition, relationship to the external world, and psychomotor behavior. There must be no symptoms that suggest organic disorder, substance abuse, or af-

OTHER SUBTYPES OF SCHIZOPHRENIA

Besides catatonic and paranoid schizophrenia, *DSM-III* lists three other subtypes of schizophrenia: disorganized, undifferentiated, and residual. This table lists characteristics of these other subtypes and special considerations for all three.

TYPE OF SCHIZOPHRENIA	SPECIAL CONSIDERATIONS FOR ALL TYPES
Disorganized • Marked incoherence; regressive, chaotic speech • Flat, incongruous, or silly affect • Delusions not systematized into coherent theme • Hallucinations fragmented • Unpredictable laughter • Grimaces • Mannerisms • Hypochondriacal complaints • Extreme social withdrawal • Oddities of behavior • Regressive behavior **Undifferentiated** • Prominent psychotic symptoms that meet criteria for more than one subtype **Residual** • Previous history of episode of schizophrenia with prominent psychotic symptoms • Present clinical picture is without prominent psychotic symptoms • Continuing evidence of illness, such as inappropriate affect, social withdrawal, eccentric behavior, illogical thinking, or loosening of associations	• Distinguish adult behavior from regressed behavior; reward adult behavior. Work with patient to increase sense of his own responsibility to improve level of functioning. • Engage patient in reality-oriented activities that involve human contact: inpatient social skills training groups; outpatient day-care, sheltered workshops. Provide reality-based explanations for distorted body images or hypochondriacal complaints. • Avoid promoting dependence. Meet patient's needs, but only do for patient what he can't do for himself. • Remember, institutionalization may produce symptoms and handicaps that are not part of illness, so evaluate symptoms carefully. • Clarify private language, autistic inventions, or neologisms. Give patient feedback that what he says is not understood. • Assist patient to engage in meaningful interpersonal relationships; do not avoid patient; maintain sense of hope for possible improvement and convey this to patient. • Expect patient to put nurse through rigorous period of testing before he shows evidence of trust. • Mobilize all resources to provide support system for patient to reduce his vulnerability to stress. • Encourage compliance with neuroleptic medication regimen. Patients relapse when medication is discontinued. • Involve family in treatment; teach them symptoms associated with relapse and suggest ways to manage symptoms. These include tension, nervousness, insomnia, decreased concentration ability, and loss of interest. • Provide continued support in assisting patient to learn social skills.

fective disorder.

No single symptom or characteristic is present in all schizophrenic disorders. The five subtypes differ markedly. Characteristics of catatonic and paranoid schizophrenia are discussed below; see *Other Subtypes of Schizophrenia* for characteristics of disorganized, undifferentiated, and residual schizophrenia.

Catatonic schizophrenia is most recognizable by its characteristic motor disturbances: stupor, negativism, rigidity, excitement, or posturing. The catatonic patient may be unable to move around or take care of his personal needs. Commonly, he doesn't even feed himself or talk and may show bizarre, stereotyped mannerisms, such as facial grimacing and sucking movements of the mouth. Rarely, he may also exhibit waxy flexibility, in which the body (especially the extremities) will rigidly hold any placed position for prolonged periods. Diminished sensitivity to painful stimuli and rapid swings between excitement and stupor may also be observed. The excitement phase may include extreme psychomotor agitation with excessive, senseless, or incoherent talking or shouting and with increased potential for destructive, violent behavior. This behavior is not influenced by environmental stimuli. Because many medical conditions may induce catatonia, careful differential diagnosis is essential.

Paranoid schizophrenia is characterized by persecutory or grandiose delusional thought content and possible delusional jealousy. This condition may be associated with unfocused anxiety, anger, argumentativeness, and violence. It may also involve gender-identity problems, including fears of being thought of as homosexual or being approached by homosexuals. Paranoid schizophrenia may cause only minimal impairment of function if the patient doesn't act upon the delusional thoughts. His affective responsiveness may remain intact, but interactions with others commonly show stilted formality or intensity. This type of schizophrenia tends to develop in later life; its features tend to be stable over time.

Diagnosis

The diagnosis of schizophrenic disorders remains difficult and controversial. Psychiatrists in the United States have tended to diagnose schizophrenia more often than their English counterparts. Psychiatrists consider the following features important for diagnosing schizophrenic disorders with greater accuracy: developmental background, genetic and family history, current environmental stressors, relationship of patient to interviewer, level of patient's premorbid adjustment, course of illness, and response to treatment. Psychological tests may help, although none clearly confirms this diagnosis.

Some psychiatrists may use the dexamethasone suppression test to aid diagnosis, but others question its accuracy. Computed tomography (CT) scans may help establish an accurate diagnosis. CT scans have shown enlarged ventricles in schizophrenics. The ventricular brain ratio (VBR) determination may also support diagnosis. Some studies have reported an elevated VBR determination in schizophrenics.

Treatment

The goals of treatment for patients with schizophrenic disorders include equipping them with the skills they need to live in an unrestrictive environmental setting that offers opportunity for meaningful interpersonal relationships. Another major aim of treatment is control of this illness through continuous administration of carefully selected neuroleptic drugs. Drug treatment should be continuous because schizophrenic patients relapse when it's discontinued.

Clinicians disagree about the effectiveness of psychotherapy in schizophrenics. Some consider it a useful adjunct through reducing loneliness, isolation, and withdrawal and enhancing productivity.

Special considerations

Patient management varies according to the patient's symptoms and the type of schizophrenia he has.

For catatonic schizophrenia:

- Assess for physical illness. Remember that the mute patient won't complain of pain or physical symptoms; if he's in a bizarre posture, he's consequently at risk for pressure sores or decreased circulation to a body area.
- Meet physical needs for adequate food, fluid, exercise, and elimination; follow orders with respect to nutrition, urinary catheterization, and enema.
- Provide range-of-motion exercises or ambulate the patient every 2 hours.
- Prevent physical exhaustion and injury during periods of hyperactivity.
- Tell the patient directly, specifically, and concisely what needs to be done. Don't offer the negativistic patient a choice. For example, you might say: "It's time to go for a walk. Let's go."
- Spend some time with the patient even if he's mute and unresponsive. The patient is acutely aware of his environment even though he seems not to be. Your presence can be reassuring and supportive. Avoid mutual withdrawal.

CHILDHOOD SCHIZOPHRENIA

Schizophrenic reactions that occur before puberty (age 12 years) are included in this group; some children have these reactions as early as ages 2 to 3.

Schizophrenic children may be confused and anxious but may be responsive to those who are taking care of them and to their environment. Usually, they've learned to talk but don't always feel the need to communicate. When they do speak, their language isn't always meaningful. These children aren't able to differentiate between what's real and what isn't. Those who become ill when very young aren't able to distinguish themselves from others around them (autistic tendency) and are usually hospitalized.

The nurse must work to establish a loving, secure, accepting relationship with the schizophrenic child. She can help him distinguish his own body from those of others. Only after he begins to improve or to develop *some* concept of himself is it advisable to involve him in a daily routine. One goal is to provide regular intervals for the child to rest, work, or play. Another important goal is to have such a child learn to eat, dress, and bathe himself. If his family's life-style has been upset, all members may need psychotherapy as a unit.

- Verbalize for the patient the message his nonverbal behavior seems to convey; encourage him to do so as well.
- Offer reality orientation. You might say: "The leaves on the trees are turning colors and the air is cooler. It's Fall!" Emphasize reality in all contacts to reduce distorted perceptions.
- Stay alert for violent outbursts; get help promptly to intervene safely for yourself and the patient.

For paranoid schizophrenia:

- When the patient is newly admitted, minimize contact with staff.
- Don't crowd the patient physically or psychologically; he may strike out to protect himself.
- Be flexible; allow the patient some control. Approach him in a calm and unhurried manner. Let him talk about anything he wishes initially, but keep conversation light and social, and avoid entering into power struggles.
- Respond to the patient's condescending attitudes (arrogance, put-downs, sarcasm, or open hostility) with neutral remarks; don't let the patient put you on the defensive and don't take his remarks personally. If he tells you to leave him alone, do leave, but return soon. Brief contacts with the patient may be most useful at first.
- Don't try to combat the patient's delusions with logic. Instead, respond to feelings, themes, or underlying needs: "It seems you feel you've been treated unfairly" (persecution).
- Build trust; be honest and dependable. Don't threaten, and don't promise what you can't fulfill.
- Don't tease, joke, argue with, or confront the patient. Remember, his distorted perception will misinterpret such action in a way that's derogatory to himself.
- Make sure the patient's nutritional needs are met. Monitor his weight if he isn't eating. If he feels food is poisoned, let him fix his own food when possible; or offer foods in closed containers he can open. If you give liquid medication in a unit dose container, allow the patient to open the container.
- Monitor the patient carefully for side effects of neuroleptic drugs: drug-induced parkinsonism, acute dystonia, akathisia, tardive dyskinesia, and malignant neuroleptic syndrome (see *Adverse Effects of Neuroleptic Drugs*, page 388). Document and report adverse effects promptly.
- If the patient is hallucinating, explore the content of the hallucinations. If he hears voices, find out if he feels he must

do what they command. Tell the patient you don't hear the voices but you know they're real to him.
• If the patient is expressing suicidal thoughts, institute suicide precautions. Document his behavior and your precautions.
• If he's expressing homicidal thoughts (for example: "I have to kill my mother"), institute homicidal precautions. Notify the doctor and the potential victim. Document the patient's comments and who was notified.
• Decode autistic inventions and other private language; let the patient know when you don't understand what he's saying.
• Don't touch the patient without telling him first exactly what you're going to do. For example: "I'm going to put this cuff on your arm so I can take your blood pressure."
• Postpone procedures that require physical contact with hospital personnel until the patient is less suspicious or agitated.
• For information on management of other forms of schizophrenia, see *Other Subtypes of Schizophrenia,* page 410.

Paranoid Disorders

According to DSM-III, *paranoid disorders are marked by persistent persecutory delusions or delusional jealousy, but without prominent hallucinations. These delusions are less bizarre than those in schizophrenic disorders and usually develop in logical progression. The patient maintains appropriate emotional responses and social behavior, with minimal personality deterioration. Generally, paranoid disorders have better prognoses than schizophrenic disorders.*

Causes

Paranoid disorders of later life strongly suggest a hereditary predisposition. At least one study has linked development of paranoia to inferiority feelings in the family. Some researchers suggest that paranoia is the product of specific early childhood experiences with an authoritarian family structure. Others hold that anyone with a sensitive personality is particularly vulnerable to developing paranoia. Certain medical conditions are also known to exaggerate the risks of paranoid disorders: head injury, chronic alcoholism, and aging. Predisposing factors linked to aging include isolation, lack of stimulating interpersonal relationships, physical illness, and diminished hearing and vision.

Signs and symptoms

The *DSM-III* criteria for paranoid disorders include persistent persecutory delusions or delusional jealousy. The patient's emotions and other behavior are congruent with the delusional content. These delusions are not accompanied by hallucinations, and the rest of the personality remains intact. The patient generally feels inadequate and inferior and defends against these feelings by criticizing and belittling others, commonly resorting to denial and projection. These symptoms must persist for at least 1 week to meet *DSM-III* criteria for paranoid illness.

Elderly patients may have sexual delusions, including bizarre ideas of sexual abuse, irrational accusations of a spouse's infidelity or of ill-defined criminal and assaultive activity against them. Late-life delusional systems commonly focus on domestic issues, such as marriage, food, or the home.

Diagnosis

Diagnostic evaluation for paranoid disorders must rule out delusional syndromes, such as amphetamine-induced psychoses and dementia. For example,

PARANOID STATE OR PARANOID SCHIZOPHRENIA?

DIFFERENTIAL DIAGNOSIS	
Paranoid state	**Paranoid schizophrenia**
• Delusional system reflects reality; well systematized • Based on misinterpretations or elaborations of reality • No hallucinations • Affect and behavior normal	• Delusional system scattered, illogical, and poorly systematized • No relationship to reality or real events • Hallucinations possible • Inconsistent and inappropriate affect • Bizarre behavior

psychological testing and thorough neurologic evaluation may rule out Alzheimer's disease. Endocrine function tests can identify thyroid disorders, such as "myxedemic madness." Such tests may also point to hyperadrenalism, another medical source of paranoid ideation. Blood studies may show altered physiologic states, such as pernicious anemia, which may induce paranoia. The diagnosis should also consider the patient's history, premorbid personality traits, and current life stressors.

Treatment

Effective treatment of paranoia must correct the behavior and mood disturbances that result from the patient's mistaken belief system. Drug treatment with carefully selected neuroleptic medication is similar to that used in schizophrenic disorders. Since paranoia tends to develop in later life, dosage levels must take into account the physiologic changes associated with aging. Treatment may have to include mobilizing a support system for the isolated, aged patient.

Special considerations

• Initially limit the patient's contact with staff; designate a few staff members to develop relationships with him.
• Respect the patient's space and privacy. Observe how much physical closeness the patient can tolerate; don't touch him without first telling him you're going to. The elderly patient may not hear well, so remember to face him while speaking; speak slowly and distinctly.
• Be aware of the potential for impulsive behavior related to fear of closeness and distorted perception of reality; prevent self-destructive behavior.
• Notice what events tend to upset the patient.
• Watch for refusal of medications due to suspicion; explore the patient's reasons for refusing them.
• Enhance the patient's confidence and self-esteem through participation in satisfying activities. Assess his hobbies and refer him to occupational therapy if appropriate.
• In dealing with the patient, be honest, direct, straightforward, trustworthy, and dependable.
• Establish a caring relationship with the patient to reduce his feelings of loneliness. Move slowly, with a matter-of-fact manner; be patient and persistent; respond without anger or defensiveness to his hostile remarks.
• Meet the patient's physical needs and monitor his mental status. Remember, neuroleptic drugs tend to cause more side effects in the older patient.
• Focus on reality; provide feedback to correct distorted perceptions.
• Allow compulsive rituals unless they're physically harmful.
• Help the patient learn to feel comfortable in social interaction. Gradually increase social contacts after the patient has become comfortable with staff.

- Provide the patient with a structured, moderately stimulating environment. Modify the environment to accommodate any physical deficits the patient may have, and keep it predictable; tell the patient what to expect and when. Introduce change slowly.
- Limit intrusive diagnostic studies; too many tests in too short a time tend to increase the patient's confusion.
- Assess recent life stressors.
- Mobilize resources to reduce the patient's loneliness and isolation; explore the possibility of his involvement in a volunteer program or self-help group after discharge.
- Be aware of your own responses to the patient; these patients' critical and belittling attitudes can be distressing.

AFFECTIVE DISORDERS

Bipolar Affective Disorder

Bipolar affective disorder is marked by severe pathologic mood swings from euphoria to sadness, by spontaneous recoveries, and by a tendency to recur. The cyclic (bipolar) form consists of separate episodes of mania (elation) and depression; however, either the manic or the depressive episodes can be predominant, producing few, if any, mood swings; or the two moods can be mixed. When depression is the predominant mood, the patient has the unipolar form of the disease. The overall incidence of unipolar affective disorder is 3 to 4 per 1,000.

Bipolar affective disorder is 1.5 to 2 times more common among women than men; it is more common in higher socioeconomic groups and is associated with high levels of creativity. It can begin any time after adolescence, but first attacks usually occur between ages 20 and 35; approximately 35% of these patients experience onset between ages 35 and 60. The manic form is more prevalent in young patients and the depressive form in older ones. Bipolar disorder recurs in 80% of patients; as they grow older, the attacks of illness recur more frequently and last longer. This illness is associated with a significant mortality; 20% of these patients die as a result of suicide, many just as the depression lifts.

Causes

The cause of bipolar affective disorder is not clearly understood, but hereditary, biologic, and psychological factors may play a part. The incidence of this illness in siblings is 20% to 25%; 66% to 96% in identical twins. The higher incidence in females suggests a socially learned or a sex-linked genetic cause. Other familial influences, especially the early loss of a parent, parental depression, incest, or abuse may predispose to depressive illness. Emotional or physical trauma, such as bereavement, disruption of an important relationship, or severe accidental injury, may precede the onset of bipolar illness but it often appears without identifiable predisposing factors. Before the onset of overt symptoms, many patients with this illness have an energetic and outgoing personality type with a history of wide mood swings.

Although certain biochemical changes accompany mood swings, it's not clear whether these changes cause the mood swings or result from them. In both mania and depression, intracellular sodium concentration increases during illness and returns to normal with recovery. Biochemical research also reports changes in brain catecholamines that accompany adrenal steroid and other metabolic changes. In depression, brain catecholamine levels decrease; in

PRECAUTIONS FOR DRUG THERAPY IN BIPOLAR DISORDER AND DEPRESSION

Tricyclic antidepressants (TCAs)
Examples: amitriptyline HCl (Elavil), desipramine HCl (Norpramin), imipramine HCl (Tofranil), protriptyline HCl (Vivactil)

- Warn the patient that the TCA may cause drowsiness and fatigue. Tell him to take the drug only as prescribed and to avoid hazardous tasks. If drowsiness persists, he may take a single daily dose at bedtime.
- Warn him against using alcohol and to use other central nervous system depressants only as prescribed.
- If he's been taking large doses for a long time, advise him not to discontinue the drug without the doctor's guidance, since abrupt withdrawal may cause severe nausea and headache.
- Tell the patient to expect a lag time of 10 to 14 days, or even a month, before the antidepressant effects begin, but that side effects may develop within 24 hours. Side effects include dry mouth (tell the patient to chew gum or use hard candies), urinary retention or constipation (increase his fluid intake or administer a stool softener), blurred vision, tachycardia, dysrhythmias, diaphoresis, dizziness, and hallucinations.
- TCAs are contraindicated in males with prostatic hypertrophy.
- TCAs are very seldom used with monoamine oxidase inhibitors because of possible drug interactions.

Monoamine oxidase (MAO) inhibitors
Examples: isocarboxazid (Marplan), phenelzine sulfate (Nardil), tranylcypromine sulfate (Parnate)

- Emphatically warn the patient on an MAO inhibitor against eating foods containing tryptophan, tyramine, or caffeine (such as cheese; sour cream; beer, chianti, or sherry; pickled herring; liver; canned figs; raisins, bananas, or avocados; chocolate; soy sauce; fava beans; yeast extracts; meat tenderizers; coffee; or colas); severe hypertensive symptoms may occur.
- Carefully monitor blood pressure throughout MAO inhibitor therapy. Keep phentolamine available for possible hypertensive crisis.
- Warn the patient to sit up for at least a minute before attempting to get out of bed, and then to rise slowly to avoid dizziness. Advise him to lie down or squat if he feels dizzy or faint.
- Warn the patient not to discontinue medication without a doctor's guidance, since abrupt withdrawal may cause severe symptoms; also warn him against taking other medications, especially over-the-counter cold, hay fever, or reducing medications, for 2 to 3 weeks after discontinuing MAO inhibitor therapy.
- Tell the patient to expect a lag time of 1 to 3 weeks before antidepressant effects begin.
- MAO inhibitors are rarely given with TCAs because of possible drug interactions.
- All patients on antidepressants should be supervised for suicidal ideations as the depression lifts.

Lithium carbonate

- Use with extreme caution with haloperidol (monitor carefully for early signs of encephalopathy, such as lethargy or fever), diuretics, sodium bicarbonate, and I.V. solutions containing sodium chloride.
- Keep daily salt intake constant. Monitor for excessive perspiration, vomiting, or diarrhea.
- Monitor intake and output and serum electrolyte levels closely, since lithium interferes with antidiuretic hormone and is contraindicated in fluid or electrolyte imbalance.
- Watch for side effects (fine tremor, orthostatic hypotension, polyuria, nausea, and diarrhea) and early signs of toxicity (tremor, slurred speech, nystagmus, drowsiness, and ataxia).
- Warn the patient to avoid hazardous tasks until drug response is determined and to carry a Medic Alert card.
- Warn the patient not to stop the drug abruptly without a doctor's supervision.

mania, they increase. These changes can accompany abnormal adrenal steroid levels and other metabolic anomalies.

Signs and symptoms

The manic and the depressive phases of bipolar disorder produce characteristic mood swings and other behavioral and physical changes. In the depressive phase, the patient experiences loss of self-esteem, overwhelming inertia, hopelessness, despondency, withdrawal, apathy, sadness, and helplessness. He has increased fatigue, difficulty sleeping (falling asleep, staying asleep, or early morning awakening), and awakes feeling tired. He usually feels worse in the morning. He may also have anorexia, causing a significant weight loss without dieting, and may become constipated. The patient may show psychomotor retardation, with slowed speech movement and thoughts, and may complain of difficulty in concentrating. He is usually not disoriented or intellectually impaired but may offer slow, one-word answers in a monotonic voice. The depressed patient may also express excessive and hypochondriacal concern about body changes and multiple somatic complaints, such as constipation, fatigue, headaches, chest pains, or heaviness in the limbs; he may worry excessively about having cancer or some other severe illness. In an elderly patient, such physical symptoms may be the only clues to his depression.

The depressed patient may feel guilt and self-reproach over past events and, as depression deepens, may feel worthless. He may believe he is wicked and deserves to be punished. His deepening sadness, guilt, negativity, and fatigue place extraordinary burdens on his family. Suicide is an ever-present risk, especially when the depression begins to lift. Then, a rising energy level may give the strength to carry out suicidal ideas. The suicidal patient may also have homicidal ideas, thinking, for example, of killing his family either in anger or to spare them pain and disgrace.

The manic phase of bipolar disorder is marked by recurrent, distinct episodes of persistently euphoric, expansive, or irritable mood. It must be associated with four of the following symptoms that persist for at least 1 week:

- increase in social, occupational, or sexual activity with physical restlessness
- unusual talkativeness or pressure to keep talking
- flight of ideas or the subjective experience that thoughts are racing
- inflated self-esteem, grandiosity
- decreased need for sleep
- distractability, attention too easily drawn to trivial stimuli
- excessive involvement in activities that have a high potential for painful but unrecognized consequences (shopping sprees, reckless driving). The manic patient has little control over incessant pressure of ideas, speech, and activity; he ignores the need to eat, sleep, or relax. Such a patient's constant demands for attention, his high energy level, and his need to test limits and rules can tire even the most energetic nursing staff and frequently cause a major nursing care problem.

Hypomania, more common than acute mania, is marked by a classic triad of symptoms: elated but unstable mood, pressure of speech, and increased motor activity. It, too, causes patients to be elated, hyperactive, easily distracted, talkative, irritable, impatient, impulsive, and full of energy, but it doesn't induce flight of ideas, delusions, or absence of discretion and self-control.

Diagnosis

Diagnosis rests primarily on observation and a psychiatric history of pathologic mood swings from elation to sadness. However, rating scales of increased or decreased activity, speech, or sleep and other psychological tests may support the diagnosis of bipolar affective disorder. A manic patient's dramatic improvement in response to treatment with lithium carbonate further validates this diagnosis. A careful history may identify previous mood swings or a family history of manic-depressive illness. Nevertheless, the patient needs careful physical evaluation to rule out possible medical causes (intraabdominal neoplasm, hypothyroidism, cardiac failure, cerebral arteriosclerosis, parkinsonism, brain tumor, and uremia); amphetamine, alcohol, or phencyclidine (PCP) intoxication; and drug-induced depression.

Treatment

Treatment for an acute manic or depressive episode may require brief hospitalization to provide:

- drug therapy with monoamine oxidase (MAO) inhibitors such as phenelzine (Nardil) and with the tricyclic antidepressant imipramine (Tofranil), which relieves depression without causing the amnesia or confusion that commonly follow electroconvulsive therapy (ECT).
- ECT, in which an electric current is passed through the temporal lobe to produce a controlled grand mal seizure. ECT is a well-known and effective treatment for persistent depression; it's less effective in the manic phase. However, it's the treatment of choice for middle-aged, agitated, and suicidal patients.
- lithium therapy, which can dramatically relieve symptoms of mania and hypomania and may prevent recurrence of depression. In some patients, maintenance therapy with lithium has prevented recurrence of symptoms for decades. Lithium has a narrow therapeutic range, so treatment must include close monitoring of blood levels to avoid dehydration, salt imbalance, and other adverse effects. Because therapeutic doses of lithium produce adverse effects in many patients, compliance may be a problem. In those who fail to respond to lithium, or to treat acute symptoms before onset of lithium effect, haloperidol (Haldol) may be effective. (Onset of lithium effect takes 7 to 10 days.)

Special considerations

For the depressed patient:

The depressed patient needs continual positive reinforcement to improve his self-esteem.

- Encourage him to talk or to write down his feelings if he's having trouble expressing them. Listen attentively and respectfully, and allow him time to formulate his thoughts if he seems sluggish.
- Provide a structured routine, including activities to boost confidence and promote interaction with others (for instance, group therapy), and keep reassuring him that depression will lift.
- To prevent possible self-injury or suicide, remove harmful objects from the patient's environment (glass, belts, rope, bobby pins), observe him closely, and strictly supervise his medications.
- Record all observations and conversations with the patient, since these records are valuable for evaluating his condition.
- Don't forget the patient's physical needs. If he's too depressed to take care of himself, help him with personal hygiene. Encourage him to eat, or feed him, if necessary. If he's constipated, add high-fiber foods to his diet, offer small, frequent meals, and encourage physical activity. To help him sleep, give back rubs or warm milk at bedtime.

For the manic patient:

- Remember the manic patient's physical needs. Encourage him to eat; he may jump up and walk around the room after every mouthful but will sit down again if you remind him.
- Encourage short naps during the day, and assist with personal hygiene.
- Provide emotional support, maintain a calm environment, and set realistic goals for behavior.
- Provide diversional activities suited to a short attention span; firmly discourage him if he tries to overextend himself.
- When necessary, reorient the patient to reality, and tactfully divert conversations when they become intimately involved with other patients or staff members.
- Set limits in a calm, clear, and self-confident manner for the manic patient's demanding, hyperactive, manipulative, and acting-out behaviors. Setting limits tells the patient you'll provide security and protection by refusing inappro-

priate and possibly harmful requests. Avoid leaving an opening for the patient to test or argue.

- Listen to requests attentively and with a neutral attitude, but avoid power struggles if a patient tries to put you on the spot for an immediate answer. Explain that you'll consider the request seriously and will respond later.
- Collaborate with other staff members to provide consistent responses to the patient's manipulations or acting out.
- Watch for early signs of frustration (when the patient's anger escalates from verbal threats to hitting an object). Tell the patient firmly that threats and hitting are unacceptable and that these behaviors show he needs help to control his behavior. Then tell him that staff will help him move to a quiet area and will help him control his behavior so he won't hurt himself or others. Staff who have practiced as a team can work effectively to prevent acting-out behavior or to remove and confine a patient.
- Alert the staff team promptly when acting-out behavior escalates. It's safer to have help available before you need it than to try controlling an anxious or frightened patient by yourself.
- Once the incident is over and the patient is calm and in control, discuss his feelings with him and offer suggestions to prevent recurrence.
- Treatment sometimes includes ECT, but this is less effective for mania than for depression; the results are better with frequent treatments.

Depression

Major depression, a recurring syndrome of persistent sad, dysphoric mood with accompanying symptoms, may be a primary disorder, a response to systemic disease, or a drug reaction. Major depression occurs in about 1 of 10 Americans, affecting all races and ethnic and socioeconomic groups. It affects both sexes but is more common in women. About 50% of depressed persons recover completely; the others experience recurrences. Depression is difficult to treat, especially in children, adolescents, elderly persons, or those with a history of chronic disease, but there's been some improvement in effectiveness of treatment.

Causes

The multiple causes of depression are controversial and not completely understood. Current research suggests possible genetic, familial, biochemical, physical, psychological and social causes. Psychological causes, the focus of many nursing interventions, may include feelings of helplessness and vulnerability, anger, hopelessness and pessimism, and low self-esteem; they may be related to abnormal character and behavior patterns and troubled personal relationships. In many patients, the history identifies a specific personal loss or severe stress that probably interacts with an individual's predisposition to provoke major depression.

Signs and symptoms

According to the *DSM-III* classification, the primary feature of major depression is a relatively persistent and prominent dysphoric mood with loss of interest in usual activities and pastimes. The sad, hopeless, or apathetic mood may shift periodically to anger or anxiety. The second diagnostic requirement is the daily presence of at least four of the following symptoms for at least 2 weeks:

- appetite disturbance (weight loss of at least 1 lb/week without dieting, or significant appetite or weight increase)
- sleep disturbance (insomnia or hypersomnia)
- energy loss, fatigue
- psychomotor agitation or retardation

SUICIDE PREVENTION GUIDELINES

- **Assess for clues to suicide:** suicidal thoughts, threats, and messages; hoarding medication; talking about death and feelings of futility; giving away prized possessions; changing behavior, especially as depression begins to lift.
- **Provide a safe environment:** check patient areas and correct dangerous conditions: exposed pipes, windows without safety glass, access to the roof or open balconies.
- **Remove dangerous objects:** belts, razors, suspenders, light cords, glass, knives, nail files, clippers.
- **Consult with staff:** recognize and document both verbal and nonverbal suicidal behaviors; keep doctor informed; share data with all staff; clarify patient's specific restrictions; assess risk and plan for observation; clarify day and night staff responsibilities and frequency of consultation.
- **Observe suicidal patients:** be alert when patients are using sharp objects (shaving); taking medication; or using the bathroom (to prevent hanging or other injury). Assign patient to a room near nurses' station and with another patient. Observe acutely suicidal patients continuously.
- **Maintain personal contact with patient:** suicidal patients feel alone and without resources or hope. Encourage continuity of care and consistency of primary nurses. Building emotional ties to others is the ultimate technique for preventing suicide.

(hyperactive or slowed behavior)

- loss of interest or pleasure in activities, decreased sex drive
- feelings of worthlessnes, self-reproach, excessive guilt
- difficulty with concentration, decision making, or ability to think
- recurrent suicidal thoughts, suicide attempts, or death wishes.

Acute depression involves recent onset of four or five of these behaviors and dysphoric mood. Chronic depression involves the same symptoms in milder form, present for 2 or more months.

Diagnosis

Diagnosis of major depression rests primarily on observations and history of persistent or recurrent dysphoric mood, with a review of social, personal, family, and neuropsychiatric history for sources of grief and stress, drug toxicity, or medical problems.

Beck's Depression Scale and other psychological tests, as well as the dexamethasone suppression test and EEG evidence of sleep disturbance, may be used to support this diagnosis. Careful assessment of mood and behavior also supports this diagnosis. Obtain an accurate account of the onset, severity, duration, and progression of all feelings, symptoms, and changes in daily activities. Pay special attention to recent changes in diet, appetite, or sleep patterns; sexual activity; constipation; and use of alcohol. Ask about recent losses and unusual stress.

Treatment

The primary treatment methods—psychotherapy, drug and somatic therapy (including electroconvulsive therapy [ECT])—along with possible adjuvant therapies, aim to relieve the depressive symptoms. Research confirms the effectiveness of antidepressant drug therapy, which, when combined with psychotherapy, is more effective than either method alone. Drug therapy usually includes tricyclic antidepressants (TCAs) and monoamine oxidase (MAO) inhibitors. TCAs produce fewer side effects and so are usually the preferred treatment. Drug treatment may include sedatives if the patient suffers insomnia; careful monitoring is required to prevent hoarding of doses.

In severely depressed or suicidal patients who don't respond to other treatments, ECT may improve mood dramatically. However, ECT should be prescribed only after a complete evaluation, including history, physical examination, chest X-ray, and EKG. ECT may cause side effects—dysrhythmias, fractures, confusion, drowsiness, temporary memory loss, sluggish respirations and, occasionally, permanent memory loss or learning difficulties. Consequently, before such treatment, safety, long-term risk, and the patient's rights associated with ECT should be discussed thoroughly with the patient and his family.

Special considerations

The depressed patient needs a therapeutic relationship with encouragement to talk and boost self-esteem.

- Encourage the patient to talk about and write down his feelings. Show him he's important by setting aside uninterrupted time each day to listen attentively and respectfully, allowing time for sluggish responses.
- Provide a structured routine, including noncompetitive activities, to build the patient's self-confidence and encourage interaction with others. Help him avoid isolation by urging him to join group activities and socialize.
- Reassure him that he can help ease his depression by expressing his feelings, participating in pleasurable activities, and improving grooming and hygiene.
- Ask the patient if he thinks of death or suicide. Such thoughts signal an immediate need for consultation and as-

OTHER AFFECTIVE DISORDERS

Dysthymic disorder (depressive neurosis)

This common affliction is marked by feelings of depression that have persisted at least 2 years in adults (and at least 1 year in children and adolescents). It causes persistent depressive symptoms that are not sufficiently severe or prolonged to meet the criteria for major depression.

These symptoms may be relatively continuous or separated by intervening periods of normal mood that last a few days to a few weeks but not longer than a few months. At least three of the following symptoms are present:

- insomnia or hypersomnia
- low energy level or chronic tiredness
- feelings of inadequacy, loss of self-esteem, or self-deprecation
- decreased effectiveness or productivity at home, work, or school
- decreased attention, concentration, or ability to think clearly
- social withdrawal
- loss of interest in or enjoyment of pleasurable activities
- irritability or excessive anger (in children, hostility to parents)
- inability to respond with apparent pleasure to praise or rewards
- less active or talkative than usual, or feelings of sluggishness or restlessness
- pessimistic attitude toward the future, brooding about past events
- tearfulness or crying, self-pity
- recurrent thoughts of death or suicide
- no psychotic features.

Cyclothymic disorder

This disorder describes patients who have moderate or transient symptoms of bipolar disorder, major depression, or mania. These patients have normal moods for months at a time. The essential feature of cyclothymic disorder is a chronic mood disturbance of at least 2 years' duration involving numerous periods of depression and hypomania that aren't sufficiently severe or prolonged to meet the criteria for a major depressive or manic episode.

A cyclothymic disorder commonly precedes a bipolar disorder. Psychotic features, such as delusions and hallucinations, are absent.

Atypical affective disorder

This disorder produces manic symptoms that are less severe and less prolonged than those required for a diagnosis of bipolar or cyclothymic disorders.

sessment. Failure to detect suicidal thoughts early may encourage a patient to attempt suicide.

- Record all observations of and conversations with the patient, because they are valuable for evaluating his response to treatment.
- While caring for the patient's psychological needs, don't forget his physical needs. If he's too depressed to take care of himself, help him with personal hygiene. Encourage him to eat, or feed him if necessary. If he's constipated, add high-fiber foods to his diet, offer small, frequent feedings, and encourage physical activity and fluid intake. Offer warm milk or back rubs at bedtime to improve sleep.
- To prevent possible suicide, watch carefully for signs of suicidal ideations or intent (see *Suicide Prevention Guidelines,* page 420).
- If drug treatment fails, the doctor may order ECT. A course of ECT usually includes two or three treatments per week for 3 to 4 weeks. Before each ECT, give the patient a sedative, and insert a nasal or oral airway. Monitor vital signs. Offer support by talking calmly or by gently touching the patient's arm. Afterward, he may be drowsy and have transient amnesia, but he should be alert, with a good memory, within 30 minutes (or at the latest, 6 to 8 hours).

ANXIETY DISORDERS

Phobias

(Phobic disorder, phobic neurosis)

Classified as a form of anxiety disorder, a phobia is a persistent, irrational fear of places or things that compels the patient to avoid them. Although he knows that his fear is out of proportion to any actual danger, the patient can't control it or explain it away. Many people harbor irrational fears, such as the fear of harmless insects, which make no major impact on their lives. In contrast, the phobic patient's irrational fear causes severe distress and impairment of function.

Three types of phobia exist: agoraphobia, social phobia, and simple phobia. (See Identifying Phobic Disorders.*) Of the milder forms of mental illness, phobias are among the most persistent.*

Causes and incidence

A phobia develops when anxiety about an object or situation compels the patient to avoid it. Phobic disorders may result from drug withdrawal, drug abuse, and anxiety-related behaviors, such as the inability to cope with anger and dependence.

Phobic disorders affect less than 1% of the population and account for less than 5% of all neurotic disorders in patients over age 18. These patients usually have no family history of psychiatric illness or of the same phobia. Because phobias tend to be chronic and resistant to treatment, the prognosis is only fair.

Signs and symptoms

Phobias produce severe anxiety—often panic—and discomfort that's out of proportion to the threat of the feared object or situation. Physically, the patient suffers profuse sweating, poor motor control, tachycardia, and elevated blood pressure.

In a *simple phobia,* the patient anticipates his anxiety and so avoids facing the perceived danger. If he suddenly confronts the object or situation, he may suffer a panic attack. (See *Recognizing a*

Panic Attack, page 425.)

With a *social phobia,* the patient feels shameful, inept, or stupid in social interaction and expects others to criticize or laugh at him. His anxiety isn't focused.

In *agoraphobia,* anxiety causes a patient to restrict his movements to an increasingly smaller area, leading to the inability to leave home without suffering a panic attack. To avoid leaving the familiar setting of his home, his behavior may become pleading, demanding, manipulative, or even infantile. A feeling of helplessness predominates and obsessive behavior often occurs.

When a patient avoids the object of his phobia, he may feel loss of self-esteem and feelings of weakness, cowardice, or ineffectiveness. If he doesn't master the phobia, he may develop mild depression.

Diagnosis

Most often, diagnosis of a phobia is based on careful history taking, observation of the patient, and a description of his behavior by the patient, his family, and friends. Patient interviews and a mental status examination help to confirm the diagnosis of a phobic disorder.

Treatment

The effectiveness of treatment depends on the severity of the patient's phobia. Because phobic behavior may never be completely cured, the goal of treatment is to help the patient function effectively. Although antianxiety drugs may help control phobia, they must be prescribed with caution to prevent addiction. Antidepressants may help relieve symptoms in patients with agoraphobia but they can't cure it completely.

Systematic desensitization, a behavioral therapy, may be more effective than drugs, especially if it includes encouragement, instruction, and suggestion. Such therapy should help the patient understand that his phobia is symbolic of a more fundamental anxiety and that he must deal with it directly.

In some cities, phobia clinics and group therapy are available. People who have recovered from phobias can often help other phobic patients.

Special considerations

- Stay with the patient until he feels comfortable alone.

IDENTIFYING PHOBIC DISORDERS

Phobic disorders can take three forms and can even coexist in some patients. To help identify phobias, review the following information.

Agoraphobia affects 60% of all phobic patients who seek help. This severe phobia commonly affects women and tends to be chronic, with occasional remissions and flare-ups. Patients with agoraphobia fear being alone and losing control in public places where escape is difficult or where help isn't available. Typically, they fear *situations,* such as being in crowds, tunnels, or elevators. These fears can dominate their lives, restricting their normal activities and even confining them to their homes.

Social phobias are similar to agoraphobia. The central fear is one of self-embarrassment, which compels the patient to avoid the scrutiny of others. But most of these fears involve specific *functions,* such as using public lavatories or speaking in public. Characteristically, social phobias affect adolescents.

Simple phobias are the most common, easiest to identify, and most thematic. The patient fears certain objects or situations, such as animals, lightning, or high places. Usually, these fears begin in childhood and follow a chronic course with no remissions. They almost always stem from an actual or anticipated confrontation with the feared object or situation.

MECHANISMS OF ANXIETY DISORDERS

In generalized anxiety disorder or panic disorder, anxiety is the primary feature.

In phobic disorder, anxiety results when the patient *confronts* a threatening situation.

In obsessive-compulsive disorder, anxiety results when the patient *resists* threatening thoughts and feelings.

In posttraumatic stress disorder, the patient *reexperiences* anxiety related to an exceptionally traumatic event.

- Work in an unhurried, reassuring manner. To make the atmosphere conducive to expression of feelings, intervene calmly, listen actively, and reinforce and encourage the patient constantly. Provide privacy, if needed.
- Give feedback and reliable information about the feared object or situation. Support a realistic view of the situation to reduce fear.
- Ask the patient how he normally copes with the fear. When he's able to face the fear, encourage him to verbalize and explore his personal strengths and resources with you.
- Prevent unpleasant surprises that could intensify the patient's fear.
- Avoid enforcing inactivity, which can actually increase fear.
- Reduce demands on the patient, so he has more energy available for coping.
- Teach the patient to use a systematic desensitization technique, such as deep breathing or relaxation exercises. Then bring the feared object closer until he can tolerate it with less anxiety.
- Explain how fatigue can increase stress and fear.
- Suggest ways to channel the patient's energy and relieve stress (such as running and creative activities).
- Recommend relaxation methods, such as listening to music and meditating.
- Because many patients try to relieve their fears with alcohol, barbiturates, or antianxiety medications, teach them about the danger of addiction.
- Educate the patient's family and friends about the phobia and help them become a support system.
- Refer the patient to a doctor for medical intervention, if necessary.

Anxiety States

(Anxiety neuroses)

Anxiety is a feeling of apprehension caused by a threat to a person or his values. Some describe it as an exaggerated feeling of impending doom, dread, or uneasiness. Unlike fear—a reaction to danger from a specific external source—anxiety is a reaction to an internal threat, such as an unacceptable impulse or a repressed thought that's straining to reach a conscious level. Occasional anxiety is a normal part of life as a rational response to a real threat. However, overwhelming anxiety can cause an anxiety state—uncontrollable, unreasonable anxiety that narrows perceptions and interferes with normal functioning.

Anxiety states can be acute or chronic. An acute state, or panic disorder, *often begins between ages 15 and 35. Chronic anxiety that lasts for more than a month is called a* generalized anxiety disorder *and has an uncertain prognosis.*

Causes and incidence

Theorists such as Freud, Horney, and Rank describe the cause of anxiety states in different ways, but they all share a common premise: that conflict, whether intrapsychic, sociopersonal, or interpersonal, promotes an anxiety state.

Panic and generalized anxiety disorders are more widespread than previously thought and are even more common than depression. They affect twice as many women as men.

Research has proven that anxiety states run in families, suggesting genetic predisposition. Studies also show that families of patients with panic disorders have a high incidence of alcoholism and that these patients have increased mortality caused by suicide and heart disease, especially mitral valve prolapse. Some investigators link physiologic symptoms of anxiety to high serum lactate levels.

Signs and symptoms

Psychological or physiologic symptoms of anxiety states vary with the degree of anxiety. Mild anxiety causes mainly psychological symptoms, with unusual self-awareness and alertness to the environment. Moderate anxiety causes selective inattention, yet with the ability to concentrate on a single task. Severe anxiety causes an inability to concentrate on more than scattered details of a task. Panic state with acute anxiety causes a complete loss of concentration, often with unintelligible speech.

In a *generalized anxiety disorder,* mild to moderate signs and symptoms last for a month or more, but no panic attacks occur. Psychological effects vary in severity but may include restlessness, sleeplessness, appetite changes, irritability, repeated questioning, and constant attention- or reassurance-seeking behavior. The patient feels fatigue on awakening and worries about possible misfortunes. Because he has difficulty concentrating, he is unaware of his surroundings. Typically, he's oriented to the past, not the present or future. He may say that he feels apprehensive, helpless, fearful, "keyed up," angry, tearful, withdrawn, or afraid of losing self-confidence or control. In addition, he shows lack of initiative, criticizes himself and others, and is self-deprecating.

Physical effects of a generalized anxiety disorder may include diaphoresis, dilated pupils, dry mouth, difficulty swallowing, frequent urination, dysuria, rapid respirations, flushing or pallor, diarrhea or constipation, nausea, vomiting, belching, sexual dysfunction, and cold, clammy hands. The patient's blood pressure and heart rate rise, and he feels palpitations and weakness. He displays motor tension by trembling, headaches, muscle aches and spasms, inability to relax, twitching eyelids, strained facial expressions, hyperventilation, and over-rapid startle responses.

In a *panic disorder,* acute anxiety causes a panic attack with severe signs and symptoms. (See *Recognizing a Panic Attack.*) After a panic attack, the patient may not remember what precipitated it and may feel depersonalized. Usually, chronic anxiety persists between attacks.

RECOGNIZING A PANIC ATTACK

A panic attack is a brief period of intense apprehension or fear; it may last from minutes to hours. A history of three or more panic attacks within 3 weeks that are unrelated to extreme physical exertion, life-threatening situations, or phobias confirm panic disorder.

During a panic attack, the patient will display four or more of these signs and symptoms:

- chest pains
- palpitations
- dyspnea
- choking or smothering feeling
- vertigo, dizziness, or unsteadiness
- feelings of faintness
- depersonalization or feeling of unreality
- tingling in the hands and feet
- shaking or trembling
- hot and cold flashes
- diaphoresis
- fear of going crazy, dying, or being out of control during a panic attack.

Diagnosis

A thorough patient history confirms an anxiety state when it shows a pattern of failure to cope with past or current stress. However, careful evaluation must rule out organic causes of the patient's symptoms, such as hyperthyroidism, pheochromocytoma, coronary artery disease, paroxysmal tachycardia, and Ménière's disease. For instance, if a patient complains of chest pain or other cardiopulmonary symptoms, he should have an electrocardiogram to rule out myocardial ischemia. Because anxiety is also the central feature of other psychiatric disorders, additional tests must rule out phobias, obsessive-compulsive disorders, depression, and acute schizophrenia. Laboratory tests should include complete blood count, differential, and serum lactate and calcium levels to rule out hypocalcemia.

Treatment

A combination of organic and psychotherapeutic treatments may help a patient with an anxiety disorder. The benzodiazepine antianxiety drugs may relieve mild anxiety and improve the patient's ability to cope with stress. Tricyclic antidepressants or higher doses of benzodiazepines may relieve severe anxiety and panic attacks. These drugs can ease distress and facilitate psychotherapy or psychoanalysis.

Special considerations

When caring for an anxious patient, your role is primarily supportive and protective. Your goal will be to help the patient develop effective coping mechanisms to manage his anxiety. If the patient must take antianxiety drugs or tricyclic antidepressants, you should:

- administer psychotropic medications and evaluate the patient's response.
- stress the importance of taking the medications exactly as prescribed for maximum effectiveness.
- warn the patient and his family that these drugs may cause side effects, such as drowsiness, fatigue, ataxia, blurred vision, slurred speech, tremors, and hypotension.
- tell the patient to avoid simultaneous use of alcohol or any central nervous system depressants. He should also avoid driving and other hazardous tasks until he develops a tolerance for the drug's sedative effects.
- advise him to discontinue medications only with the doctor's approval, because abrupt withdrawal could cause severe symptoms.

If the patient has a panic attack, protect him during the attack. Show him how to take slow, deep breaths if he's hyperventilating. Carefully explain the physiologic reasons for these symptoms. Avoid making judgments or critical comments.

When panic subsides, encourage the patient to face his anxiety, because avoidance only increases it. Help him recognize the symptoms of his anxiety and his coping mechanisms, such as depression, withdrawal, demanding or violent behavior, denial, and manipulation. Explore alternate behaviors; encourage him to take up activities that will distract him from his anxiety. Make referrals for psychiatric treatment, as needed, for such problems as chronic anxiety and disturbed coping mechanisms. Provide telephone numbers for hotlines, psychiatric emergency help, and other emergency agencies.

Obsessive-Compulsive Disorder

*Obsessive thoughts and compulsive behaviors represent recurring efforts to control overwhelming anxiety, guilt, or unacceptable impulses that persistently enter the consciousness (*DSM-III *classifies this as an anxiety disorder).*

The word obsessive or obsession refers to a recurrent idea, thought, or image. Compulsive or compulsion, the action component, refers to a ritualistic, repetitive, and involuntary defensive behavior. This disorder is relatively rare in the general population (0.05%), occurring in both sexes with typical onset in adolescents or young adults. Recent studies indicate a higher incidence in upper-class persons with higher intelligence.

Obsessions and compulsions cause significant distress and may severely impair occupational and social functions. Generally, an obsessive-compulsive disorder is chronic, often with remissions and flare-ups. The prognosis is better than average when symptoms are quickly identified, diagnosed, and treated; and when the resulting environmental stress is recognized and adjusted.

Causes

The cause of obsessive-compulsive disorder is unknown. Some studies suggest the possibility of brain lesions, but the most useful research and clinical studies lead to an explanation based on psychological theories. These studies list four major theories of causation; of these, the psychoanalytic theory is accepted by most psychiatrists. (See *Causes of Obsessive-Compulsive Disorder,* page 428.) In addition, major depression, organic brain syndrome, and schizophrenia may contribute to the onset of obsessive-compulsive disorder.

Signs and symptoms

This disorder may be manifested physically or behaviorally as ideas or impulses, and may refer either to actions completed or to future, anticipated events. These actions or events may be simple, mild, and uncomplicated or dramatic, elaborately complex, and ritualized. Their meanings may be obvious or may reflect inner psychological distortions that are unraveled only through intensive psychotherapy.

Obsessive symptoms are those in which thoughts, words, or mental images persistently and involuntarily invade the conscious awareness. Some common obsessions include: thoughts of violence, thoughts of contamination, and repetitive doubts and worry about a tragic event.

The dominant feature in compulsions is an irrational and recurring impulse to repeat a certain behavior as an expression of anxiety. Common compulsions include repetitive touching; doing and undoing (opening and closing doors, rearranging things); washing (especially hands); and checking (to be sure no tragedy has occurred).

Often, the patient's anxiety is so strong that he will avoid the situation or the object that evokes the impulse. For example, John had the recurring urge to push people down long flights of stairs, so he avoided climbing stairs in any building, lived in a one-story house, and thus controlled his behavior so he wouldn't be tempted to act on this compulsion.

When the obsessive-compulsive phenomena are mental, no one knows that anything unusual is happening unless the patient talks about these private experiences. Or compulsive acts can be evident, although—because of shame, nervousness or embarrassment—the patient usually tries to limit these actions to his own private time.

Obsessive-compulsive states seem to develop in certain personality types and under certain conditions. The obsessional personality is usually rigid and conscientious, and has great aspirations. He has a formal, reserved manner, with precise and careful movements and posture; he takes responsibility seriously and finds decision making difficult. He lacks creativity and the ability to find alternate solutions to his problems. Such a person has a tendency to be painfully accurate and complete—carefully qualifying his statements to avoid making a mistake, and anticipating every move and gesture of the person to whom he speaks. His affect is flat and unemotional, except for controlled anxiety. Self-

CAUSES OF OBSESSIVE-COMPULSIVE DISORDER

PSYCHO-ANALYTIC THEORY	LEARNING THEORY	INTERPERSONAL THEORY	EXISTENTIALIST THEORY
Psychodynamic factors (ego defenses) • Isolation • Undoing • Reaction formation **Psychogenic factors** • Preoccupation with aggression • Preoccupation with dirt • Disturbed growth/development pattern related to anal/sadistic phase **Regression** • Fixation at earlier level of development (anal stage) • Ambivalence • Magical thinking	• Obsession—conditioned stimulus to anxiety • Compulsion—reduced anxiety reinforces behavior • Approach avoidance—reduces conflict • Emphasis on cognitive change to alter behavior	• Irrational coping strategies to handle (inflexible) intense anxiety or guilt • Unrealistic (rigid) view of self (self-hate, self-contempt—"bad me") • Avoidance of anxiety-laden relationships (withdrawal) • Defenses (sublimation, selective inattention, substitution, dissociation) • Inferiority feelings (to gain control of others) • Threat to autonomy and loss of individuality • Family patterns and coping styles that reinforce obsessions • Inability to enjoy life	• Inability to live with uncertainty or ambiguity • Wish to flee situation of great anxiety • Threat of nonexistence • Religious rituals • Excessively high morals

awareness is totally intellectual, without accompanying emotion or feeling.

Diagnosis

Diagnosis rests on evidence of compulsively repetitive patterns of thought or behavior. A careful history may identify previous obsessive-compulsive personality traits. Often, the patient's own description of his behavior offers the best clues to this diagnosis. However, the patient also needs evaluation for other physical or psychiatric disorders. One telling difference between obsessive-compulsive states and schizophrenia, which may produce similar behavioral patterns, is that schizophrenics have lower visible levels of anxiety.

Treatment

Treatment of obsessive-compulsive states aims to reduce anxiety, resolve inner conflicts, relieve depression, and teach more effective ways of dealing with stress. Such treatment (especially during an acute episode) may include tranquilizing and antidepressant drugs. Intensive long-term psychotherapy, brief supportive psychotherapy, or group therapy is the preferred treatment.

Behavioral therapies—aversion therapy, thought stopping, thought switching, flooding, implosion therapy, and response prevention—have also been effective. (See *Behavioral Therapies*.)

Special considerations

Patient care should focus on reducing the associated anxiety, fears, and guilt, building the patient's self-esteem, and helping him understand why he needs the compulsive behavior.

• Approach the patient unhurriedly.
• Provide an accepting atmosphere; don't show shock, amusement, or criticism of the ritualistic behavior.
• Allow the patient time to carry out the ritualistic behavior (unless it's dangerous) until he can be distracted into some other activity. Blocking this behavior raises anxiety to an intolerable level.
• Encourage him to express his feelings about the anxiety that causes the compulsive behavior, especially when he seems fearful.
• Explore patterns leading to the behavior or recurring problems.
• Listen attentively, offering feedback.
• Encourage use of appropriate defense mechanisms to relieve loneliness and isolation.
• Engage the patient in activities to create positive accomplishments and raise his self-esteem and confidence.
• Encourage active diversional resources, such as whistling or humming a tune, to divert attention from the unwanted thoughts and to promote a pleasurable experience.
• Assist the patient with new ways to solve problems and to develop more effective coping skills by setting limits on unacceptable behavior (for example, by limiting the number of times per day he may indulge in obsessive behavior). Gradually shorten the time allowed. Help him focus on other feelings or problems for the remainder of the time.
• Help the patient identify progress and set realistic expectations of himself and others.
• Explain how to channel emotional energy to relieve stress (sports, creative endeavors, etc.).
• Identify insight and improved behavior (reduced compulsive behavior and/or fewer obsessive thoughts). Evaluate behavioral changes by your own and the patient's self-reports.
• Identify disturbing topics of conversation that reflect underlying anxiety or terror.
• Observe when interventions do not work; reevaluate and recommend alternative strategies.

BEHAVIORAL THERAPIES

• **Aversion therapy**—application of a painful stimulus to create an aversion to the obsession that leads to undesirable behavior (compulsion).

• **Thought stopping**—a technique to break the habit of fear-inducing anticipatory thoughts. Patient is taught to stop unwanted thoughts by saying the word "Stop," and then to focus his attention on achieving calmness and muscle relaxation.

• **Thought switching**—a technique to replace fear-inducing self-instructions with competent self-instructions. Patient is taught to replace negative thoughts with positive ones until the positive thoughts become strong enough to overcome the anxiety-provoking ones.

• **Flooding**—frequent full-intensity exposure (through use of imagery) to an object that triggers a symptom. Used with caution because it produces extreme discomfort.

• **Implosion therapy**—a form of desensitization through repeated exposure to a highly feared object.

• **Response prevention**—prevention of compulsive behavior by distraction, persuasion, or redirection of activity. May require hospitalization or involvement of family to be effective.

• Find ways to deal with the anger and frustration that the patient often arouses in you.
• Keep the patient's physical health in mind. For example, compulsive hand washing may cause skin breakdown, and rituals or preoccupations may cause inadequate food and fluid intake and exhaustion.
• Make reasonable demands and set reasonable limits; make their purpose clear. Avoid creating situations that increase frustration and provoke anger, which may interfere with treatment.

Posttraumatic Stress Disorder

The psychological consequences of a traumatic event that occurs outside the range of usual human experience is identified as posttraumatic stress disorder (PTSD). This is classified in DSM-III *as an anxiety disorder.*

Such a disorder can be acute, chronic, or delayed and can follow a natural disaster (flood, tornado), a man-made disaster (war, imprisonment, torture, car accidents, large fires), or an assault or rape. Such extraordinary events produce stress in anyone. Psychological trauma always accompanies physical trauma and involves feelings of intense fear, helplessness, loss of control, and threat of annihilation. The acute subtype of PTSD occurs when symptoms appear within 6 months of the event and persist as long as 6 months. The acute subtype is similar to shell shock or combat fatigue. The chronic or delayed subtype occurs when symptoms persist longer than 6 months (chronic) or appear 6 months after the event (delayed). Chronic PTSD is less common but more debilitating; it has special relevance for veterans of the Vietnam conflict. These war veterans, victims of fires or airplane crashes, and survivors of earthquakes or volcanic eruptions are all vulnerable to this disorder, which often has a concomitant physical aspect to the trauma (direct damage to the central nervous system from malnutrition or head trauma). Apparently, the resulting disorder is more severe and persistent when the precipitating trauma is of human design.

Causes and incidence

PTSD can occur at any age (including childhood), but the very young and very old have more difficulty coping with unusual stressors. Preexisting psychopathology can also predispose to this disorder. Sex-related and familial patterns of incidence are unknown.

In most persons with PTSD, the stressor is a necessary but insufficient cause of the persisting symptoms. Even the most severe stressors do not produce PTSD in everyone, so psychological, physical, genetic, and social factors (for example, a preexisting organic mental disorder such as failing memory, difficulty concentrating, and/or depression with anxiety) may also contribute to it.

Theories of causation include the survivor theory, consisting of a latency or detachment phase, a denial-numbing phase, and an intrusive-repetitive phase in which the survivor must work through the traumatic experiences and put the event into perspective.

In 1981, Arthur Egendorf and others released results of a comprehensive study on veterans and their postwar adjustment. This study encompassed all socioeconomic classes, geographic regions, and ethnic groups and analyzed responses from 1,400 persons directly or indirectly involved in the Vietnam conflict. Results show that unemployment, low educational attainment, minority status, family instability, and the amount and intensity of combat interact to influence the severity of PTSD. Veterans who have strong support systems (wives, friends, family) are less likely to develop PTSD. Over 25% of all Vietnam veterans still show symptoms of PTSD.

Signs and symptoms

Most common effects include pangs of painful emotion and unwelcome thoughts; a traumatic reexperiencing of the tragic event; insomnia, difficulty falling asleep, nightmares of the traumatic event, and aggressive outbursts upon awakening; emotional numbing—diminished or constricted response; and chronic anxiety or panic attacks (with physical symptoms). The patient may also display rage and survivor guilt; use of violence to solve problems; depression and suicidal thoughts; phobic avoidance of situations that arouse memories of trauma (for example, hot weather and tall grasses for the Vietnam veteran); memory impairment or difficulty in concentrating; and feelings of detachment or estrangement that destroy interpersonal relationships. Some patients also experience organic symptoms, fantasies of retaliation, and substance abuse.

Diagnosis

Characteristic symptoms that persist after unusual trauma confirm this diagnosis. A careful history identifies the subtype (acute or chronic). The history should include early life experiences, educational and vocational histories, and relationships with family, peers, and authority figures, as well as a careful military history and an extensive psychosocial history in war veterans.

A psychiatric examination should include a mental status assessment and tests for organic impairment and should focus on other psychiatric syndromes that accompany PTSD, such as depression, generalized anxiety, and phobia.

Treatment

Goals of treatment include reducing the target symptoms, preventing chronic disability, and promoting occupational and social rehabilitation. Specific treatment may emphasize behavioral techniques (relaxation therapy to decrease anxiety and induce sleep, or progressive desensitization); antianxiety and antidepressant drugs, prescribed with caution to avoid possible dependence; or brief psychotherapy (supportive, insight, or cathartic) to minimize the risks of dependency and chronicity.

Support groups are highly effective and are provided through many Veterans Administration Centers and Crisis Clinics. These groups provide a forum in which victims of PTSD can work through their feelings with others who have had similar conflicts. Group settings are appropriate for most degrees of symptoms presented. Some group programs include spouses and families in their treatment process. Rehabilitation in physical, social, and occupational areas is also available for victims of chronic PTSD. Many patients need treatment for depression, alcohol and/or drug abuse, or medical conditions before psychological healing can take place.

Special considerations

The goal of intervention is to encourage the victim of PTSD to express his grief and complete the mourning process so he can go on with his life. Keep in mind that such a patient tends to sharply test your commitment and interest. So first examine your feelings about the event (war or other trauma) so you won't react with disdain and shock. This hampers the working relationship and reinforces the patient's poor self-image and sense of guilt.

To develop an effective therapeutic relationship:

- Know and practice crisis intervention techniques as appropriate.
- Establish trust by accepting the patient's current level of function and assuming a positive, consistent, honest, and nonjudgmental attitude.
- Help the patient to regain control over angry impulses by identifying situations where he lost control and by talking about past and precipitating events (conceptual labeling) to help with later problem-solving skills.
- Give approval as the patient shows a commitment to work on his problem.
- Deal constructively with anger. Encourage joint assessment of angry outbursts (identify how anger escalates, explore preventive measures that family members can take to regain control). Provide a safe, staff-monitored room in which the patient can safely deal with urges to commit physical violence or self-abuse by displacement (such as pounding and throwing clay or destroying selected items). Encourage him to move from physical to verbal expressions of anger.
- Relieve shame and guilt precipitated by real actions—such as killing and mutilation—that violated a consciously held moral code through clarification—putting behavior into perspective; atone-

ment—helping the patient see that he has atoned by social isolation and by engaging in self-destructive behavior; and restitution—having clergy help him conquer guilt (once authority and trust in others is accepted).

- Provide for or refer the patient to group therapy with other victims for peer support and forgiveness.
- Refer the patient to appropriate community resources.

SOMATOFORM DISORDERS

Somatization Disorder

Somatization disorder is present when multiple signs and symptoms that suggest physical disorders exist without a verifiable disease or pathophysiologic condition to account for them. Commonly, the patient with somatization disorder undergoes repeated medical evaluations, which—unlike the symptoms themselves—can be potentially damaging and debilitating. Such a patient can always find just one more hospital or doctor to do another diagnostic workup. However, unlike the hypochondriac, he's not preoccupied with the belief that he has a specific disease.

Causes

This disorder has no specific cause. Its symptoms can begin or worsen after many kinds of losses (job security or personal relationship).

Characteristically, patients with this disorder have a lifelong pattern of sickliness—sometimes beginning in adolescence. They don't relate well to other people except by using their symptoms. They're locked into a pattern of getting attention and meeting their needs through physical complaints.

Signs and symptoms

The essential feature of this disorder is the pattern of recurrent, multiple symptoms and complaints. These complaints can involve any body system but most frequently involve the gastrointestinal tract, with nausea, vomiting, and abdominal pain; the neurologic system, with weakness, paresthesias, and headaches; and the cardiopulmonary system, with dizziness, chest pain, and palpitations. These symptoms can involve multiple body systems or shift from one system to another.

An important clue to somatization disorder is a history of multiple medical evaluations at different institutions without significant findings.

Patients with somatization disorder typically relate their present complaints and their previous evaluations in great detail. They may be quite knowledgeable about tests, procedures, and medical jargon. They don't discuss other aspects of their lives without including their many symptoms. In fact, any attempts to explore areas other than their medical history may cause them to show noticeable anxiety. They tend to disparage previous health care professionals and previous treatment, often with the comment, "No one seems to understand. Everyone thinks I'm imagining these things."

These patients' symptoms are not under voluntary control, and they want to feel better. However, they are never symptom-free. The course of symptoms is chronic, with exacerbations during times of stress.

Diagnosis

No specific test or procedure verifies somatization disorder. The patient's complaints require careful evaluation for organic causes. This does not mean extensive invasive procedures, but rather a thorough history and review of previous evaluations. During this review listen for clues of recent losses or severe stress. Onset of somatization symptoms generally occurs before age 30.

Diagnostic evaluation should rule out physical causes that typically cause vague, confusing symptoms, such as multiple sclerosis, hypothyroidism, systemic lupus erythematosus, or porphyria. Psychological evaluation should rule out depression, schizophrenia with somatic delusions, hypochondriasis, psychogenic pain, and malingering.

Treatment

The goal of treatment is not to eradicate the patient's symptoms, but rather to help him learn to live with them. After diagnostic evaluation has ruled out organic causes, the patient should be told that he has no serious illness but will continue to receive care to ease his symptoms.

The most important aspect of treatment is a continuing, supportive relationship with a sympathetic health care provider who acknowledges the patient's symptoms and is willing to help him live with them. The patient should have regularly scheduled appointments for review of symptoms and basic physical evaluation, but the main aspect of follow-up is review of the patient's coping. Follow-up appointments should last approximately 20 to 30 minutes and should focus on new symptoms or any change in old symptoms to avoid missing a developing physical disease. As many as 30% of patients initially diagnosed with somatization disorder eventually develop an organic disease. Patients with somatization disorder rarely acknowledge any psychological aspect of their illness and reject psychiatric treatment.

Special considerations

- Acknowledge the patient's symptoms and support his efforts to function and cope despite distress. Under no circumstances should you tell the patient his symptoms are imaginary. But do tell him the results and meanings of tests.
- Emphasize the patient's strengths. ("It's good that you can still work with this pain.") Gently point out the time relationship between stress and physical symptoms.
- Help the patient to manage stress, not get rid of symptoms. Typically, his relationships are linked to his symptoms; remedying the symptoms can impair his interactions with others.
- Develop a care plan with some input from the patient. The care plan should include participation of the patient's family. Encourage and help them to understand the patient's need for troublesome symptoms.

The danger in working with these patients is that the anger, irritation, and frustration they understandably generate may interfere with nursing care. It's not unusual to develop an attitude that says: "These people don't want to get better, so why should I waste my time?" Deal with these feelings first by acknowledging them. Consulting a psychiatric clinical nurse specialist can help nursing staff develop effective means of dealing with their feelings.

Conversion Disorder

(Hysterical neurosis, conversion type)

A conversion disorder allows a patient to resolve a psychological conflict through the loss of a specific physical function—for example, by paralysis, blindness, or inability to swallow. The patient's loss of physical function is involuntary, but laboratory tests and diagnostic procedures do not show an organic cause.

Conversion disorder can occur in either sex at any age. The symptom itself is generally not life-threatening, but its complications, such as contractures, muscle wasting, decubitus ulcers, and dramatically altered life-styles, can be severely disruptive and debilitating.

Causes

Typically, the patient quite suddenly develops a physical symptom soon after experiencing traumatic conflict he feels unable to handle. The symptom serves one of two purposes. It can prevent expression or perception of an internal conflict. (For example, the spouse who does not wish to acknowledge her murderous rage develops vocal cord paralysis.) Or, it can help the patient gain support or avoid unpleasant activity. (A soldier may develop blindness when ordered to combat.)

Conversion disorders are more likely to develop in persons with a histrionic or dependent personality.

Signs and symptoms

The most striking characteristic of a conversion disorder is the sudden onset of a debilitating symptom that prevents normal function of the affected body part. The patient doesn't consciously control the symptom. For example, he can't move a leg even though he's trying. The patient will relate a recent and severe psychological stress that preceded the symptom. Generally, only one symptom develops; it's quite specific and dramatic. Oddly, the patient doesn't show the affect and concern that such a severe symptom usually elicits.

Diagnosis

Thorough physical evaluation must rule out any physical cause, especially diseases with vague physical onsets (such as multiple sclerosis or systemic lupus erythematosus). To differentiate conversion disorder from other somatoform disorders, the history must confirm a specific psychological conflict that's resolved through the development of the symptom. Psychological evaluation must also consider somatoform disorder, hy-

FACTITIOUS DISORDERS

Factitious disorders are severely psychopathologic conditions marked by the intentional, repetitious simulation of a physical or mental illness for the purpose of obtaining medical treatment. Factitious illness may or may not be associated with overt mental symptoms.

Chronic factitious illness with physical symptoms (Munchausen's syndrome) has these essential clinical features:

- convincing presentation of feigned physical illness
- voluntary production of symptoms.

Associated features include:

- wandering from hospital to hospital (frequently covering great distances)
- extensive knowledge of medical terminology
- pathologic lying
- evidence of prior treatment, including surgery
- shifting complaints and symptoms
- demanding and disruptive behavior
- drug abuse
- eagerness to undergo hazardous and painful procedures
- discharge against medical advice to avoid detection
- poor interpersonal relationships
- usual refusal of psychiatric examination; many patients have history of deprivation and rejection, and poor identity formation
- patient may be seeking warmth and acceptance but can inspire anger.

Factitious illness with mental symptoms is extremely rare. Its essential features are:

- voluntary production of symptoms suggesting a mental disorder, in the absence of malingering
- actively seeking admission to a mental hospital
- symptoms suggesting simultaneous organic, affective, and schizophrenic disorders.

pochondriasis, somatic delusions in either schizophrenia or depression, or malingering.

Treatment

Effective treatment relieves the symptom and returns the patient to normal function. The patient needs to know that his symptom has no organic cause, though its effect is no less real. He should be helped to understand the time relationship between the stress and the symptom. Psychiatric treatment is strongly indicated to help the patient understand his underlying psychological conflict and to resolve the stress in a more suitable way. When such conflict is resolved, the symptom soon disappears.

Special considerations

- Help the patient maintain integrity of the affected system. Regularly exercise paralyzed limbs to prevent muscle wasting and contractures.
- Change the bedridden patient's position frequently to prevent decubiti.
- Ensure adequate nutrition, even if the patient is complaining of gastrointestinal distress.
- Provide a supportive environment and encourage the patient to discuss the stress that provoked the conversion disorder. Don't force the patient to talk, but convey a caring and concerned attitude to help him share his feelings.
- Don't insist that the patient use the affected system. This will only anger him and prevent a therapeutic relationship.
- Add your support to the recommendation for psychiatric care.
- Include the patient's family in all aspects of care. They may be part of the patient's stress, and they are essential to support the patient and help him regain normal function.

Psychogenic Pain Disorder

The striking feature of psychogenic pain disorder is a persistent complaint of pain without appropriate physical findings. Although psychogenic pain has no physical cause, it's as real to the patient as organic pain. Psychogenic pain can occur in either sex at any age, and is generally related to psychological stress. Such pain is usually chronic, with exacerbations at times of stress. Its complications, including loss of work, interference with interpersonal relationships, drug dependence, extensive evaluations, and surgical procedures, can make prognosis grim.

Causes

Psychogenic pain disorder has no specific cause. Severe psychological stress or conflict is evident, but may not be as clearly time-related to the pain as in conversion disorders. The pain may have special significance, such as leg pain in the same leg a parent lost through amputation. The pain provides the patient with a means to settle upsetting psychological issues. For example, a person with dependency needs may develop psychogenic pain as an acceptable way to receive care and attention. The life history of a patient with psychogenic pain disorder commonly shows aggression, violence, and organic or psychogenic pain. The patient may have learned to gain attention through pain.

Signs and symptoms

The cardinal feature is chronic, consistent complaints of pain without confirming physical disease. Such pain does not follow anatomic pathways. A helpful clue to psychogenic pain is a long history of evaluations and procedures at multiple settings without much pain relief. Such a patient speaks of health care professionals with anger and resentment because they've failed to relieve his pain. Because of frequent hospitalizations, the patient is familiar with pain medications and tranquilizers; he may ask for a specific drug and know its correct dosage and route of administration. He may not show typical nonverbal signs of pain, such as grimacing or guarding, but this isn't necessarily a clue to psychogenic pain, since such reactions are sometimes absent in patients with chronic organic pain.

An important feature in psychogenic pain disorder is secondary gain. The pain may allow the patient to avoid a stressful situation or receive attention not otherwise available. This secondary gain is essential to the persistence of the pain. Unfortunately, the patient does not usually acknowledge any psychological basis for his pain.

Diagnosis

Pain must be the overriding complaint; it must involve some psychological stress, either conscious or unconscious. Diagnosis of psychogenic pain disorder requires complete evaluation to rule out organic causes. Medical evaluation must consider organic diseases that cause persistent pain (such as multiple sclerosis, neuropathy, or tension headaches).

Psychiatric evaluation must rule out malingering, using the complaint to receive narcotics, depressive disorder, somatization disorder, hypochondriasis, schizophrenia, or personality disorders. Pain that subsides with suggestion, hypnosis, or placebo therapy is not necessarily psychogenic, since organic pain may also respond to these measures.

Treatment

The goal of treatment isn't necessarily to eradicate the pain, but rather to ease it and help the patient live with it. Treatment should avoid long, invasive evaluations and surgical interventions. Treatment at a comprehensive pain center may be helpful. Supportive measures for pain relief may include hot or cold packs, physical therapy, distraction techniques, or cutaneous stimulation with massage or transcutaneous electrical nerve stimulation (TENS). Measures to reduce the patient's anxiety may also be helpful. A continuing supportive relationship with an understanding health care professional is essential for effective management; regularly scheduled follow-up appointments are helpful.

Analgesics generally become an issue as the patient feels "I have to fight for everything I get." The patient should clearly be told what medication he will receive and should receive other supportive pain relief measures as well. Regularly scheduled analgesic doses can be more effective than p.r.n. scheduling; regular doses reduce pain by reducing anxiety about asking for medication. The use of placebos will destroy trust when the patient discovers the deceit.

Special considerations

- Provide a caring, accepting atmosphere where the patient's complaints are taken seriously and every effort is made to provide relief. This doesn't mean providing increasing amounts of narcotics on demand; rather, it means communicating to the patient that you'll collaborate in a treatment plan, and clearly stating the limitations. For example, you might say, "I can stay with you now for 15 minutes, but you can't receive another dose until 2 p.m."
- Don't tell the patient he's imagining the pain or can wait longer for medication that's due. Assess his complaints and help him understand what's contributing to the pain. You might ask, "I've noticed you complain of more pain after your doctor visits. What are his visits like for you?" to elicit contributing perceptions and fears.
- Teach the patient noninvasive, drug-free methods of pain control, such as guided imagery, relaxation techniques, or distraction through reading or writing.
- Encourage the patient to maintain independence despite his pain.
- Offer attention at times other than during the patient's complaints of pain, to weaken the link to secondary gain.
- Avoid confronting the patient with the psychogenic nature of his pain; this is

rarely helpful because such pain is his means of avoiding psychological conflict. Psychiatric care can be useful, so consider psychiatric referrals; realize, however, that such patients usually resist psychiatric intervention and don't expect it to replace analgesic measures.

Hypochondriasis

(Hypochondriacal neurosis)

The dominant feature of hypochondriasis is an unrealistic misinterpretation of the severity and significance of physical signs or sensations as abnormal. This leads to preoccupation with fear of having a serious disease, which persists despite medical reassurance to the contrary. Hypochondriasis causes severe social and occupational impairment. It is not due to other mental disorders, such as schizophrenia, affective disorder, or somatization disorder.

Hypochondriasis appears to be equally common in men and women. It involves the danger of overlooking a serious organic disease, given the patient's previously unfounded complaints. It also has potential for significant complications or disabilities resulting from multiple evaluations, tests, and invasive procedures.

Causes

Hypochondriasis is not linked to any specific cause. However, it frequently develops in persons or relatives of those who have experienced an organic disease. Hypochondriasis allows the patient to assume a dependent sick role to ensure his needs are met. Such a patient is unaware of these unmet needs and is not consciously causing his symptoms.

Signs and symptoms

The dominant feature of hypochondriasis is the misinterpretation of symptoms—usually multiple complaints that involve a single organ system—as signs of serious illness; however, as medical evaluation proceeds, complaints may shift and change. These symptoms can range from very specific to general, vague complaints and are often associated with a preoccupation with normal body functions. Symptoms can begin anytime in early to mid-adulthood.

The hypochondriacal patient will relate a chronic history of waxing and waning symptoms. Commonly, he will have undergone multiple evaluations for similar symptoms or complaints of serious illness. His past contacts with health care professionals make him quite informed and knowledgeable about illness, diagnosis, and treatment.

Diagnosis

Hypochondriasis can't be diagnosed easily. Projective psychological testing may show a preoccupation with somatic concerns, but this doesn't itself confirm hypochondriasis. A complete history, including emphasis on current psychological stresses, is the most useful diagnostic tool.

If hypochondriasis is suspected, a thorough physical evaluation must rule out underlying organic disease but should minimize dangerous invasive procedures. Psychological evaluation should rule out schizophrenia with somatic delusions, depression, somatization disorder, panic disorder, and generalized anxiety disorder.

Treatment

The goal of treatment is to help the patient continue to lead a productive life despite distressing symptoms and fears. After medical evaluation is complete, the patient should be told clearly that he doesn't have a serious disease, but that continued medical follow-up will help control his symptoms. Providing a diagnosis won't make hypochondriasis disappear, but it may ease some anxiety.

Regular outpatient follow-up can help the patient deal with his symptoms and is necessary to detect organic illness; up to 30% of these patients later develop an organic disease. Unfortunately, because the patient can be quite demanding and irritating, consistent follow-up is often difficult.

Typically, these patients do not acknowledge any psychological influence on their symptoms and resist psychiatric treatment.

Special considerations

Provide a supportive relationship that lets the patient feel cared for and understood. The patient with hypochondriasis feels real pain and distress, so don't deny his symptoms or challenge his behavior.

- Firmly state that medical tests were negative. Instead of reinforcing his symptoms, encourage him to discuss his other problems, and urge his family to do the same.
- Help the patient and family find new ways to deal with stress other than development of physical symptoms.
- If the patient is receiving a tranquilizer, both he and his family should know dosages, expected effects, and possible side effects (for example, drowsiness, fatigue, blurred vision, and hypotension).
- Warn the patient who's taking tranquilizers to avoid alcohol or other central nervous system depressants, since they may potentiate tranquilizer action. Warn him to take the drug only as prescribed, since larger or more frequent doses may lead to dependence; to avoid hazardous tasks until he has developed a tolerance to the tranquilizer's sedative effects; and to continue the tranquilizer as his doctor directs, since abrupt withdrawal may be hazardous.
- Recognize that the patient will never be symptom-free, and don't become angry when he won't give up his disease. Such anger can drive the patient away to yet another unnecessary medical evaluation.

PSYCHOSEXUAL DISORDERS

Psychosexual Dysfunction

Psychosexual dysfunction is evident by impairment of one or more of the four physiologic phases of the sexual response cycle, also termed the stages of orgasm: 1) appetitive—desire for and fantasies about sexual activity; 2) excitement—the physiologic changes associated with sexual arousal; 3) orgasm—the peak of sexual pleasure with psychological and physiologic effects; and 4) resolution—recovery and relaxation after orgasm. Impairment of sexual response may result from physiologic or psychological factors, or a combination of both.

Psychosexual dysfunction may be lifelong or develop after a period of normal function; generalized or limited to certain situations or partners; and total or partial. The most common age at onset is early adult life; the common age of clinical presentation is the late twenties and early thirties. The course is variable.

Causes

Attitudes toward sex and body image learned in childhood and adolescence contribute heavily toward psychosexual dysfunction. Traumatic experiences related to sexual development and internal conflicts are other important factors.

Impotence may result from lack of sexual attraction to a partner, conflicts with a partner (either conscious or uncon-

PARAPHILIAS

The paraphilias classified in *DSM-III* as psychosexual disorders are marked by unusual or bizarre sexual behaviors that are necessary for sexual arousal and orgasm. Diagnosis should also consider the frequency of the behavior and its interference with function. Some paraphilias that violate social mores or norms are considered sex offenses or sex crimes. Everyone has sexual fantasies, and sexual behavior between two consenting adults that's not physically or psychologically harmful should not be considered a paraphilia.

TYPE OF PARAPHILIA	SOURCE OF SEXUAL AROUSAL
Fetishism	Use of clothing, such as leather or shoes
Transvestism	Recurrent and persistent cross-dressing by a heterosexual male
Frotteurism	Body contact with strangers in public places, such as buses or elevators
Voyeurism	Watching others engaged in sexual activity or undressing
Exhibitionism	Exposure of genitals in public
Sexual sadism	Inflicting physical/mental pain on sexual partner
Sexual masochism	Receiving physical/mental pain from sexual partner
Pedophilia	Sexual activity with children; may be homosexual or heterosexual or incestuous
Necrophilia	Sexual activity with a corpse
Zoophilia	Sexual activity with animals
Gerontophilia	Sexual activity that is not age-appropriate with an elderly person

scious), guilt, shame, anxiety, or depression. However, as many as 50% of cases have a pathophysiologic basis, especially in males over 50. *Frigidity* can be associated with fears of intercourse, such as pain, injury, or pregnancy, or with conflicts with or lack of attraction to a partner. Shame, guilt associated with sexual pleasure, and fears of inadequacy can contribute to *functional dyspareunia* (painful intercourse) and *vaginismus* (vaginal spasms).

Signs and symptoms

Inhibited female orgasm is the delay or absence of orgasm despite sexual stimulation of adequate duration and intensity. Absence of orgasm during intercourse without clitoral stimulation may be a symptom of inhibition or a normal variation of sexual response in the female. Functional dyspareunia occurs predominantly in females, rarely in males. Functional vaginismus inhibits or prevents intercourse.

Inhibited male orgasm is the delay or absence of ejaculation during adequate sexual stimulation. Premature ejaculation occurs before or immediately after penetration or before the wishes of the partners.

Diagnosis

The diagnosis of psychosexual disorders rests on the patient's subjective report of problems of frequency, chronicity, stress, and quality. No true norms exist to define minimum activity and type or quality of sexual function. Great variations are characteristic.

To establish a diagnosis, a careful sexual history must include fantasies, attitudes toward the sexual partner, the environment where sexual activities take place, attitudes toward and desires for sexual foreplay and stimulation, and frequency of sexual activities.

Before confirming a psychosexual disorder, medical evaluation must rule out physical causes of sexual impairment: diabetes, syphilis, multiple sclerosis, and other disorders of the sacral segments of the spinal cord or lumbar innervation of the spine. Many drugs can also inhibit sexual function. Other causes of sexual impairment include psychiatric illnesses such as depression, which often influences sexuality, and aging.

Treatment

Psychosexual disorders can be mild or transient and sometimes quite challenging. Treatment of psychosexual disorders has become increasingly sophisticated. Sex education may be used to correct erroneous sexual notions, to change problematic attitudes, and to impart new information. Topics might include anatomic data, and coital and pleasure-enhancing techniques.

Psychotherapy may include behavioral, supportive, and insight-oriented techniques. These are aimed at encouraging expression of feelings, reduction and control of anxiety, weakening of inhibitions, undoing faulty learning, and promoting assertiveness.

Marital counseling supplements sexual information and advice with an examination of the couple's relationship. Their sexual difficulties may be secondary to other conflicts that, when resolved, lead to improved sexual relations.

Physical therapies and mechanical aids may be of assistance in some cases. Females may be helped by exercises (Kegel exercises) that tone and strengthen the vaginal muscles.

Special considerations

Through meticulous interviewing techniques that follow up on leads from the patient; thorough, nonjudgmental assessments; and expert teaching and counseling techniques, you can influence the patient's improvement. To contribute significantly, you must understand the theory of normal sexual development and function so you can dispel myths and misconceptions of sexual function. Counsel to help overcome guilt, shame, and body image disturbances. As needed, refer the patient for special treatment and counseling.

Gender Identity Disorders

Psychosexual disorders involving gender identity refer to an individual's persistent feelings of gender discomfort and inappropriateness of his or her anatomic sex. Gender identity may be defined as the intimate personal feelings one has about being male or female and includes three components: self-concept, perception of an ideal partner, and external presentation of masculinity and femininity through behavior, dress, and mannerisms.

Persons with gender identity disorder typically behave and present themselves as persons of the opposite sex, which they intensely desire to become. These feelings persist continuously for at least 2 years. In both adults and children, this disorder is rare; it is often referred to as transsexualism in adults. Gender identity disorder should not be confused with the fairly common adult feeling of occasional sexual inadequacy or with the rejection of sexual stereotypes by behavior that's typically called "tomboy" or "sissy."

NORMAL DIFFERENTIATION OF GENDER IDENTITY

VARIABLE	SIGNIFICANCE
Chromosomal	Presence of XX or XY chromosome, the legal and medical definition of sex.
Gonadal	Structure of gonads in utero. With XY, testes differentiate; with XX, ovaries.
Hormonal	Male fetus produces androgen and testosterone; female normally produces none in utero. Drugs and stress may alter the amount and timing of hormone levels in the male and may stimulate hormone production in the female. This produces potential for infinite variety in genital and brain differentiation of the human fetus.
Internal organ formation	Hormones in the male fetus are responsible for disintegrating the müllerian ducts and developing the wolffian ducts into the prostate gland and seminal vesicles. Absence of hormones in the female causes müllerian ducts to develop into the uterus, the inner two thirds of the vagina, and the fallopian tubes.
Formation of external organs	Every human fetus has a clitoris, labia, and vagina. Hormones in the male form the scrotum from the labia minora, and the penis from the labia majora and clitoris.
Sex assignment and rearing	Influence of genital appearance on labeling and psychosocial aspects of gender identity. Core gender identity is formed by age 3.
Self-concept, physiology of orgasm, puberty	Sexual fantasies and first activities associated with orgasm are believed to become "imprinted" on the nervous system, bonding imagery with self-concept. This accounts for individual preferences, normal or abnormal.

Causes

Current theories about the causes of gender identity disorders suggest a combination of predisposing factors: chromosomal anomaly, hormonal imbalance (particularly in utero during brain formation), and pathologic defects in early parent-child bonding and child-rearing practices. For example, parents who consistently and deliberately treat their child as one of the opposite biologic sex significantly contribute to gender identity disorder.

Signs and symptoms

Gender identity disorders may be apparent at an early age. A child may express the desire to be—or insist that he or she is—the opposite sex. Such children sometimes express disgust with their genitals and the belief, often expressed as an ardent hope, that when they grow up they will become the opposite sex. These children, particularly boys, often suffer peer group rejection. They commonly have trouble in school because of this social conflict. (Girls may not experience social difficulties until early adolescence.)

Adults with gender identity disorders are characterized by an overwhelming desire to live as a person of the opposite sex, including the wish to be rid of their own genitals, and by the psychological perception that they *are* a person of the opposite sex. They commonly dress as and engage in activities typical of the opposite sex. Their sexual preference in relationships can be heterosexual or homosexual. Asexuality may also be reported. Depression, isolation, and anxiety often coexist with gender identity disorders.

Diagnosis

Diagnosis rests on a careful history that confirms persistent and severe psychosexual dysphoria and a desire to be the opposite sex.

Treatment

Individual and family therapy are indicated for treatment of childhood gender identity disorders. Ideally, a therapist of the same sex may be useful for role modeling purposes. The earlier this problem is diagnosed and treatment begins, the more hopeful the prognosis.

In adults, individual and couples therapy may help the patient to cope with the decision to live as the opposite sex or to cope with the knowledge that he or she will not be able to live as the opposite sex. Sex reassignment through hormonal and surgical treatment may be an option; however, surgical sex reassignment has not been as beneficial as first hoped. Severe psychological problems may persist after sex reassignment and sometimes lead to suicide. Further, these patients often have gender disorders as part of a larger pattern of depression and personality disorders such as borderline personality.

Female transsexuals have shown more stable patterns of adjustment with or without treatment.

Special considerations

Nursing care of a person with gender identity disorder should include:

- a nonjudgmental approach in facial expression, tone of voice, and choice of words to convey your acceptance of the individual's choices
- respect for the patient's privacy and sense of modesty, particularly during procedures or examinations
- observation for related or compounding problems such as suicidal thought or intent, depression, and anxiety
- the realization that treating such a patient with empathy doesn't threaten your own sexuality
- referral of the patient for therapy, as appropriate.

Ego-Dystonic Homosexuality

Ego-dystonic homosexuality is the preference for a sexual partner of the same sex that causes psychological pain, negative emotions, and the desire for compliance with heterosexual social standards. These homosexuals have a persistent desire to change their sexual orientation rather than a brief difficulty with adjustment to homosexual impulses. Weak or absent heterosexual impulses are found in both adolescents and adults with this disorder.

Causes

The causes of this disorder have not been identified. However, a person with this disorder is strongly influenced by societal norms and negative attitudes.

Signs and symptoms

The ego-dystonic homosexual experiences psychological pain and negative feelings regarding sexual practice; he wishes and strives for heterosexual relationships.

Diagnosis

A history of the client's sexual practices and emotional feelings about them is essential for establishing this diagnosis.

Treatment and special considerations

Psychotherapy directed toward achieving acceptance, building a positive self-image, and learning to build a supportive social network is indicated. Some sources suggest that this disorder is time-limited; that, with maturity, these individuals accept their homosexuality. Good listening and therapeutic techniques help the individual to explore, clarify, and make choices. Encouraging participation in community support groups for homosexuals and working on family acceptance are also useful.

PERSONALITY DISORDERS

Personality Disorders

Personality disorders are individual traits that reflect chronic, inflexible, and maladaptive patterns of behavior that cause discomfort and impair social and occupational function. Personality disorders are widespread, though no actual statistics exist. Patients with personality disorders don't usually receive treatment; when they do, they're usually managed on an outpatient basis.

Personality disorders fall on Axis II of the DSM-III *classification. Personality notations are appropriate and useful for all patients and help give a fuller picture of the patient and a more accurate diagnosis. For example, many features characteristic of personality disorders are apparent during an episode of another mental disorder (such as a major depressive episode in a patient with compulsive personality features).*

Prognosis is variable. Personality disorders are self-limiting, in that most appear at adolescence and wane during middle age.

Causes

Only recently have personality disorders been categorized in detail, and research continues to identify their causes.

Various theories attempt to explain the origin of personality disorders. Biologic theories hold that these disorders may stem from chromosomal and neuronal abnormalities. Social theories hold that the disorders reflect learned responses, having much to do with reinforcement, modeling, and aversive stimuli as contributing factors. Psychodynamic theories hold that personality disorders reflect deficiencies in ego and superego development, and are related to poor mother-child relationships that are fraught with unresponsiveness, overprotectiveness, or early separation.

Signs and symptoms

Signs and symptoms of personality disorders are varied and differ according to the diagnosis. (See *Characteristics of Personality Disorders,* pages 444 and 445.) They differ among individuals and within the same individual at different times. Generally, these disorders produce difficulties in interpersonal relationships, ranging from dependency to avoidant and suspicious behavior, and impair occupational function, with effects ranging from compulsive perfectionism to intentional sabotage. Affected persons may show every shade of self-confidence from total absence of self-esteem to arrogance. They tend to avoid responsibility for the consequences of their behavior, often resorting to projections and blame.

Diagnosis

Central and essential to diagnosis is a history that shows maladaptive personality traits as characteristic of lifelong behavior, and not just occurring during the course of an illness. (During illness, temporary regression causes negative personality traits to become exaggerated.) Symptoms of personality disorder impair social or occupational functioning or cause internal distress. Psychological evaluation must rule out similar personality or psychiatric disorders.

Treatment

Treatment depends on the patient's symptoms but requires a trusting relationship in which the therapist can use a directive approach. Drug therapy is generally ineffective but may be used to relieve severe distress, such as acute anx-

CHARACTERISTICS OF PERSONALITY DISORDERS

Paranoid personality disorder

Suspicion; concern with hidden motives

Inability to relax (hypervigilance), anxiety

Fault-finding with resultant anger

Inability to collaborate

Social isolation

Poor self-image

Coldness, detachment, absence of tender feelings

Need to feel in control

Considered odd or eccentric

Hostility

Argumentativeness, overt antagonism

Conflict with authority

Hypersensitivity

Jealousy

Poor sense of humor

Schizoid and schizotypal personality disorder

Suspicion

Inability to relax

Passive antagonism

Hypersensitivity to criticism

Social withdrawal

Poor self-image

Coldness, absence of warm feelings, detachment, indifference to others' feelings

Considered odd or eccentric

Elaborative, detailed speech

Ideas of reference

Depersonalization

Dependency

Flat or depressed affect

Avoidant

Devastated by separation and loss

Somatic symptoms

Anxiety and fearfulness

Low self-esteem

Dependence in relationships

Social withdrawal: mistrust, fear of rejection, but desire for close relationships

Depression (loneliness)

Dependent

Devastated by separation and loss

Somatic symptoms

Seeks human contact

Self-consciousness and feelings of inadequacy

Overly compliant, clinging behavior; avoids independence, leaves major decisions to others

Depression (inadequacy and helplessness)

Compulsive

Perfectionism

Physical symptoms usually due to overwork

Confident attitude with others

Rigid, cold, businesslike attitude; inability to express affection

Need for control

Depression (worthlessness and low self-esteem)

Procrastination, indecision

Passive-aggressive

Intentional inefficiency (social and occupational), nonadherence to etiquette, forgetfulness; falls asleep at unsuitable times

Complaining and blaming behavior; feelings of confusion and mistreatment

Fear of authority

Chronic lateness, procrastination, dawdling

Resentment, sullenness, stubbornness

No overt hostility or anger

Histrionic

Craving for stimulation and attention

Intolerance of being alone

Manipulative, divisive behavior

Depression (emptiness, loneliness)

Inability to put others' needs first

Attracts attention by dependency, helplessness, obnoxious behavior, or seductive or charming behavior; affect may be very intense

Multiple physical complaints

Tantrums and angry outbursts

Superficial attachments

Dramatic, emotional, or erratic behavior

Narcissistic

Craving for stimulation and attention

Intolerance of being alone

Manipulative behavior

Depression (humiliation, anger)

No capacity for empathy

Exaggeration of achievements and talents: self-centeredness; arrogant behavior ensuring his needs take priority

Grandiosity; preoccupation with fantasies of unlimited success, power, or beauty

Antisocial

Superficial charm, wit, and intelligence, often with manipulative and seductive behavior; inability or refusal to accept guilt for self-serving, destructive behavior

Failure at school and work: school grades markedly below expectations, truancy; delinquency, chronic violations of rules, suspension or expulsion from school, running away from home; inability to keep a job

Promiscuity, casual sexual relationships, desertion, two or more divorces or separations

Repeated substance abuse

Thefts, illegal occupations, multiple arrests, vandalism

Inability to function as a responsible parent (child abuse or neglect)

Fights, assaults, abuse of others

Impulsiveness, recklessness, inability to plan ahead

Borderline

Impulsive and unpredictable behavior in self-damaging areas: spending, sex, gambling, substance abuse, shoplifting, and overeating

Unstable and intense interpersonal relationships: attitude shifts within days or hours; idealization, devaluation, or manipulation

Inappropriate, intense anger

Identity disturbance with uncertain self-image, uncertain gender identity, uncertain relationship commitments, and behavior based on imitation

Unstable affect with mood swings within hours or days

Intolerance of being alone, a sense of emptiness or boredom

Self-destructive behavior: suicidal gestures, self-mutilation, recurrent accidents and physical fights

Fear of abandonment displayed in clinging and distancing maneuvers

Projection

Evaluation of things and people at extremes of good or bad with no gray areas between

Acting out feelings instead of expressing feelings verbally or appropriately

Manipulation: pitting others (including staff) against each other

DISORDERS OF IMPULSE CONTROL

Disorders of impulse control fall into three categories, as outlined below. The three types share these essential features: failure to resist an impulse to perform an act that's harmful to self or others; rising intrapsychic tension before committing the act; and feelings of pleasure, gratification, or release of tension upon committing the act, possibly (but not always) followed by regret or guilt. Patient management is also the same for all three types. When caring for a patient with a disorder of impulse control, remember to: set clear, fair, firm limits on behavior; encourage therapeutic interpersonal relationships with staff; and, as appropriate, refer the patient for psychotherapy and/or to self-help organizations, such as Gambler's Anonymous.

TYPES	MECHANISMS
• Pathological gambling • Kleptomania	• Functions at id level (immediate gratification) • Limited superego strength; ineffective conscience • Lives for the here and now without thought of the future • Unable to plan or work toward realistic, long-range goals
• Pyromania	• Inconsistent parenting • Fire experienced as punishment, becomes acceptable mode of retaliation. • Anger and rage build up and then are released. • Watching fire has a hypnotic and anxiety-reducing effect.
• Intermittent explosive disorder • Isolated explosive disorder	• Difficulty in sharing feelings and in intrapersonal relationships • Acting-out behavior (screaming, breaking objects, physical abuse) occurs intermittently or rarely (isolated) when rising intrapsychic tension becomes intolerable by problems with job, family, finances, intrapsychic conflict. When desires and conscience conflict, severe tension is released in an explosive way. • Impulsive behavior releases tension temporarily but (guilt vs. pleasure causes conflict) an intrapsychic conflict again develops, causing recurring need for release of tension.

iety or depression. Family and group therapy are effective. Hospital inpatient milieu therapy in crisis situations and possibly for long-term treatment of borderline personality disorders can sometimes be effective. However, inpatient treatment is controversial, since patients with personality disorders tend to be noncompliant with extended therapeutic regimes; for such patients, outpatient therapy may be more useful.

Special considerations

First, know your own feelings and reactions as the basis for assessing the patient's overt responses. Keep in mind that many of these patients don't respond well to interviewing, whereas others are charming masters of deceit. Offer patient, persistent, consistent, and flexible care. Take a direct, involved approach to ensure the patient's trust.

Nursing goals for the patient with a personality disorder include teaching social skills; reinforcing appropriate behavior; setting limits on inappropriate behavior; encouraging expression of feelings, self-analysis of behavior, and accountability for actions; and, finally, helping the patient seek appropriate employment.

Selected References

Beck, Cornelia M., and Rawlins, Ruth Parmlee. *Mental Health in Psychiatric Nursing: A Holistic Life-Cycle Approach.* St. Louis: C.V. Mosby Co., 1984.

Burgess, Ann W., and Baldwin, Bruce. *Crisis Intervention Theory and Practice: A Clinical Handbook.* Englewood Cliffs, N.J.: Prentice Hall, 1981.

Cadoret, Remi J., and King, L. *Psychiatry in Primary Care,* 2nd ed. St. Louis: C.V. Mosby Co., 1983.

Carino, C.M., et al. "Disorders of Eating in Adolescence: Anorexia Nervosa and Bulimia," *Nursing Clinics of North America* 18(2):343-52, June 1983.

Estes, Nada J., et al. *Nursing Diagnosis of the Alcoholic Person.* St. Louis: C.V. Mosby Co., 1980.

Furey, J., "Post-traumatic Stress Disorder in Vietnam Veterans. For Some, The War Rages On," *American Journal of Nursing* 82(11):1694-96, November 1982.

Goldstein, William N. "DSM-III and the Diagnosis of Schizophrenia," *American Journal of Psychotherapy* 37(2):168-81, April 1983.

Greist, John H., and Jefferson, James W., eds. *Treatment of Mental Disorders.* New York: Oxford University Press, 1982.

Haber, Judith, et al. *Comprehensive Psychiatric Nursing,* 2nd ed. New York: McGraw-Hill Book Co., 1982.

Hagerty, Bonnie K., and Packard, Karen L. *Psychiatric-Mental Health Assessment.* St. Louis: C.V. Mosby Co., 1984.

Hatton, Corrine, et al. *Suicide: Assessment and Intervention,* 2nd ed. East Norwalk, Conn.: Appleton-Century-Crofts, 1983.

Jakab, Irene, ed., *Mental Retardation.* Karger Continuing Education Series, vol. 2. New York: S. Karger AG, 1982.

Kalkman, Marion E., and Davis, Anne B. *New Dimensions in Mental Health Psychiatric Nursing,* 5th ed. New York: McGraw-Hill Book Co., 1980.

Lamb, H. Richard. "Deinstitutionalization and the Homeless Mentally Ill," *Hospital and Community Psychiatry* 35(9):899-907, September 1984.

Lego, Suzanne. *The American Handbook of Psychiatric Nursing.* Philadelphia: J.B. Lippincott Co., 1984.

Levinson, Boris M., and Osterweil, Lucille. *Autism: Myth or Reality.* Springfield, Ill.: Charles C. Thomas Publishers, 1984.

Magrinat, Gaston, et al. "A Reassessment of Catatonia," *Comprehensive Psychiatry* 24(3):218-28, May/June, 1983.

Martin, Maurice J. "A Brief Review of Organic Diseases Masquerading as Functional Illness," *Hospital and Community Psychiatry* 34(4):328-32, April 1983.

Menoascino, Frank J., and McCann, Brian. *Mental Health and Mental Retardation: Bridging the Gap.* Austin, Tex.: Pro-Ed, 1983.

Mullis, M.R. "Vietnam: The Human Fallout," *Journal of Psychosocial Nursing and Mental Health Services* 22(2):27-31, February 1984.

Murray, Ruth B., and Huelskoetter, Marilyn W. *Psychiatric Mental Health Nursing: Giving Emotional Care.* Englewood Cliffs, N.J.: Prentice-Hall, 1983.

Oxman, T.E., et al. "The Language of Paranoia," *American Journal of Psychiatry* 139(3):275-82, March 1982.

Perry, Samuel W., and Heidrich, George. "Placebo Response: Myth and Matter," *American Journal of Nursing* 81:720-25, April 1981.

Platt-Koch, Lois M. "Borderline Personality Disorder: A Therapeutic Approach," *American Journal of Nursing* 83(12):1666-71, December 1983.

Potts, N.L. "Eating Disorders: The Secret Pattern of Binge/Purge," *American Journal of Nursing* 84(1):32-35, January 1984.

Schultz, Judith, and Dark, Sheila L. *Manual of Psychiatric Nursing Care Plans.* Boston: Little, Brown & Co., 1982.

Stuart, Gail W., and Sundeen, Sandra J. *Principles and Practice of Psychiatric Nursing,* 2nd ed. St. Louis: C.V. Mosby Co., 1983.

Sutterly, Doris C., and Donnelly, Gloria F., eds. *Coping with Stress: A Nursing Perspective.* Rockville, Md.: Aspen Systems Corp., 1982.

Varner, R.V., and Gaitz, C.M. "Schizophrenic and Paranoid Disorders in the Aged," *Psychiatric Clinics of North America* 5(1):107-18, April 1982.

Valente, S.M. "Detecting Depression," *Nursing84* 14(8):63-64, August 1984.

Wilson, Holly S., and Kneisl, Carol Ren. *Psychiatric Nursing,* 2nd ed. Menlo Park, Calif.: Addison-Wesley Publishing Co., Medical/Nursing Division, 1983.

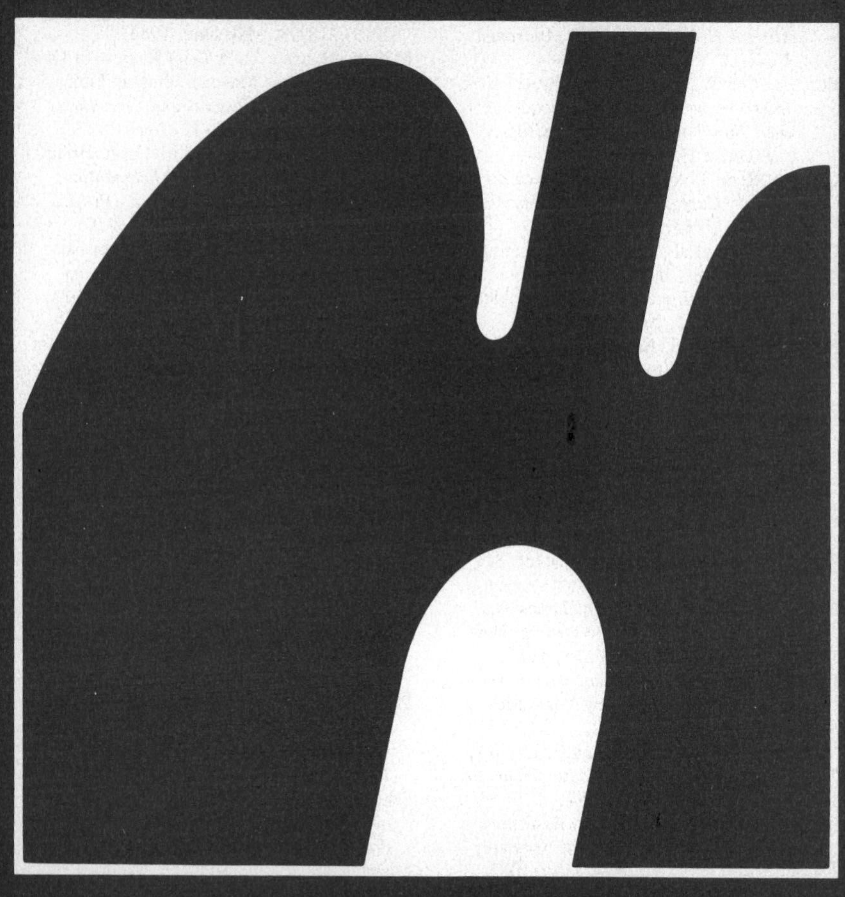

7 Respiratory Disorders

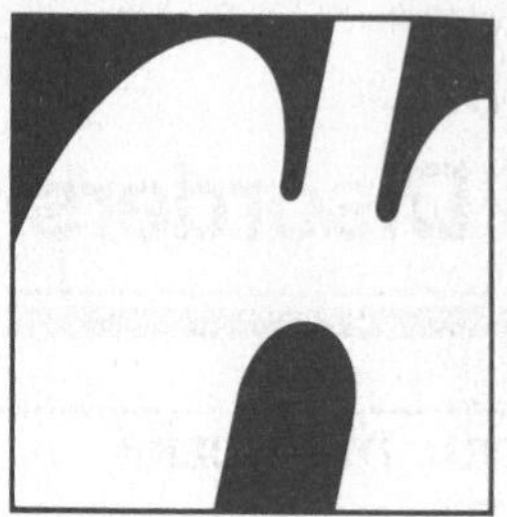

Respiratory Disorders

Introduction

The respiratory system distributes air to the alveoli, where gas exchange—the addition of oxygen (O_2) and the removal of carbon dioxide (CO_2) from pulmonary capillary blood—takes place. Certain specialized structures within this system play a vital role in preparing air for use by the body. The nose, for example, contains vestibular hairs that filter the air and an extensive vascular network that warms it. The nose also contains a layer of goblet cells and a moist mucosal surface; water vapor enters the airstream from this mucosal surface to fully saturate inspired air as it's warmed in the upper airways. Ciliated mucosa in the posterior portion of the nose and nasopharynx, as well as major portions of the tracheobronchial tree, propels particles deposited by impaction or gravity to the oropharynx, where the particles are swallowed. In addition to carbon dioxide, gases such as carbon monoxide may diffuse from pulmonary capillary blood to alveoli, where they are excreted by the lungs.

External respiration

The external component of respiration—ventilation or breathing—delivers inspired gas to the lower respiratory tract and alveoli. Expansion and contraction of the respiratory muscles move air into and out of the lungs. Ventilation begins with the contraction of the inspiratory muscles: the diaphragm—the major muscle of respiration—descends, while external intercostal muscles move the rib cage upward and outward. The accessory muscles of inspiration, which include the scalene and sternocleidomastoid muscles, raise the clavicles, upper ribs, and sternum. The accessory muscles are not used in normal inspiration but are used in certain disease states. As the diaphragm descends and the rib cage expands, pressure in the pleural space becomes more negative, and the lungs adhere to the chest wall. As the thorax expands, the pressure in the lungs falls below atmospheric pressure, and the lungs expand. Air then enters the lungs in response to the pressure gradient between the atmosphere and the lungs.

Normal expiration is passive; the inspiratory muscles cease to contract, and the elastic recoil of the lungs pushes air out. These actions raise the pressure within the lungs above atmospheric pressure, moving air from the lungs to the atmosphere. Active expiration causes the pleural pressure to become less negative.

An adult lung contains an estimated 300 million alveoli; each alveolus is supplied by many capillaries. To reach the capillary lumen, O_2 must cross the alveolar-capillary membrane, which consists of an alveolar epithelial cell, a thin interstitial space, the capillary basement membrane, and the capillary endothelial cell membrane. The oxygen tension of air entering the respiratory tract is approximately 160 mm Hg. In the alveoli, inspired air mixes with CO_2 and water vapor, lowering its pressure to approximately 100 mm Hg. Since alveolar partial pressure of O_2 is higher than that present in mixed venous blood entering the pulmonary capillaries (approximately 40 mm Hg), O_2 diffuses across the alveolar-capillary membrane into the blood.

O_2 and CO_2 transport and internal (cellular) respiration

Circulating blood delivers O_2 to the cells of the body for metabolism and transports metabolic wastes and CO_2 from the tissues back to the lungs. When oxygenated arterial blood reaches tissue capillaries, O_2 diffuses from the blood into the cells again because of an oxygen tension gradient. The amount of O_2 available is determined by the concentration of hemoglobin (the principal carrier of O_2), regional blood flow, arterial oxygen tension, and carboxyhemoglobin tension.

Internal (cellular) respiration occurs as a part of cellular metabolism, which can take place with O_2 (aerobic) or without O_2 (anaerobic). The most efficient method for providing fuel (high-energy compounds such as adenosine triphosphate [ATP]) for cellular reactions is aerobic metabolism, which produces CO_2 and water in addition to ATP. Anaerobic metabolism is less efficient, because a cell produces only a limited amount of ATP and yields lactic acid as well as CO_2 as a metabolic by-product.

Because circulation is continuous, CO_2 does not normally accumulate in tissues. CO_2 produced during cellular respiration diffuses from tissues to regional capillaries and is transported by systemic venous circulation. When CO_2 reaches the alveolar capillaries, it diffuses into the alveoli, where the partial pressure of CO_2 is lower; CO_2 is removed from the alveoli during exhalation.

Mechanisms of control

The central nervous system's control of respiration lies in the respiratory center, located in the lateral medulla oblongata of the brain stem. Impulses travel down the phrenic nerves to the diaphragm, and then down the intercostal nerves to the intercostal muscles, where the impulses change the rate and depth of respiration. The inspiratory and expiratory centers, located in the posterior medulla, establish the involuntary rhythm of the breathing pattern.

Apneustic and pneumotaxic centers in the pons influence the pattern of breathing. Stimulation of the lower pontine apneustic center (by trauma, tumor, or cerebrovascular accident, for example)

EXTERNAL RESPIRATION

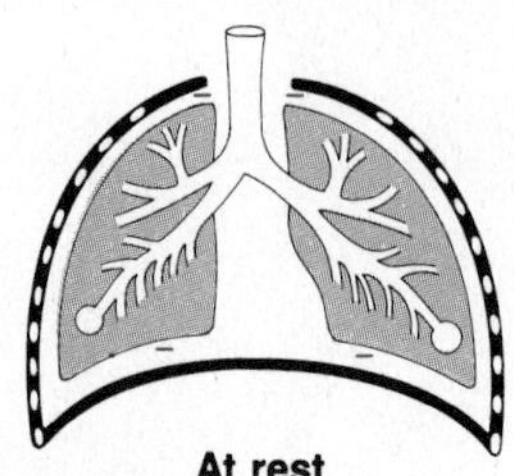

At rest
- resting inspiratory muscles
- atmospheric pressure in tracheobronchial tree
- no airflow

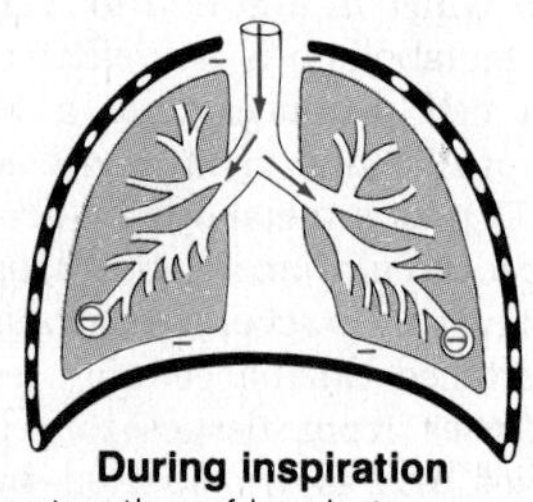

During inspiration
- contraction of inspiratory muscles and chest expansion
- negative alveolar pressure
- airflow into lungs

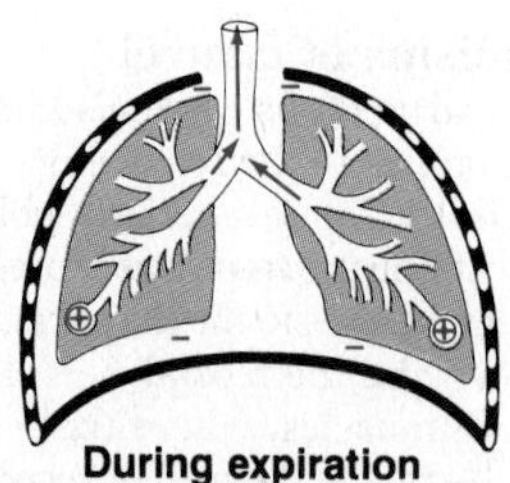

During expiration
- relaxation of inspiratory muscles causes lung recoil
- positive alveolar pressure
- airflow from lungs

KEYS
– negative intrapleural pressure
⊖ negative alveolar pressure
⊕ positive alveolar pressure

produces forceful inspiratory gasps alternating with weak expiration. This pattern does not occur if the vagi are intact. The apneustic center continually excites the medullary inspiratory center and thus facilitates inspiration. Signals from the pneumotaxic center, as well as afferent impulses from the vagus nerve, inhibit the apneustic center and "turn off" inspiration.

Arterial PO_2 and pH, as well as pH of cerebrospinal fluid (CSF), influence output from the respiratory center. When CO_2 enters the CSF, the pH of CSF falls, stimulating central chemoreceptors to increase ventilation.

The respiratory center also receives information from peripheral chemoreceptors in the carotid and aortic bodies, which respond primarily to decreased arterial PO_2 but also to decreased pH. Either change results in increased respiratory drive within minutes.

Several other factors can alter the respiratory pattern. During exercise, stretch receptors in lung tissue and the diaphragm prevent overdistention of the lungs. During eating and drinking, the cortex can interrupt automatic control of ventilation. During sleep, the respiratory drive fluctuates, producing hypoventilation and periods of apnea. External sensations, drugs, chronic hypercapnia, and increased or decreased body heat can also alter the respiratory pattern.

Diagnostic tests

Diagnostic tests evaluate physiologic characteristics and pathologic states within the respiratory tract.

Noninvasive tests:

- *Chest X-ray* shows conditions such as atelectasis, pleural effusion, infiltrates, pneumothorax, lesions, mediastinal shifts, and pulmonary edema.
- *Computed tomography (CT) scan* provides a three-dimensional picture, 100 times more sensitive than chest X-ray.
- *Magnetic resonance imaging (MRI)* identifies obstructed arteries and tissue perfusion.
- *Analysis of sputum specimen* permits study of sputum quantity, color, viscos-

ity, and odor; microbiologic stains and culture of sputum can identify infectious organisms; cytologic preparations can detect respiratory tract malignancy.

• *Pulmonary function tests* measure lung volumes, flow rates, and compliance. Normal values are individualized by body stature and age and are reported in percentage of the normal predicted value. *Static measurements* are volume measurements and include tidal volume (V_T), volume of air contained in a normal breath; functional residual capacity (FRC), volume of air remaining in the lungs after normal expiration; vital capacity (VC), volume of air that can be exhaled after maximal inspiration; residual volume (RV), air remaining in the lungs after maximal expiration; and total lung capacity (TLC), volume of air in the lungs after maximal inspiration. *Dynamic measurements* characterize the movement of air into and out of the lungs and show changes in lung mechanics. They include measurement of forced expiratory volume in 1 second (FEV_1), maximum volume of air that can be expired in 1 second from total lung capacity; maximal voluntary ventilation (MVV), volume of air that can be expired in 1 minute with the patient's maximum voluntary effort; and forced vital capacity (FVC), maximal volume of air that the patient can exhale from TLC.

• *Exercise stress test* evaluates the ability to transport oxygen and remove CO_2 with increasing metabolic demands.

• *Polysomnography* can diagnose sleep disorders.

Invasive tests:

• *Bronchoscopy* permits direct visualization of the trachea, and mainstem, lobar, segmental, and subsegmental bronchi. It may be used to localize the site of lung hemorrhage, visualize masses in these airways, and collect respiratory tract secretions. Brush biopsy may be used to obtain specimens from the lungs for microbiologic stains, culture, and cytology. Lesion biopsies may be performed by using small forceps under direct visualization (when present in the proximal airways) or with the aid of fluoroscopy (when present distal to regions of direct visualization). Bronchoscopy can also be used for therapeutic purposes, such as secretion clearing or foreign body removal.

• *Thoracentesis* permits removal of pleural fluid for analysis.

• *Pleural biopsy* obtains pleural tissue for histologic examination and culture. This test can show neoplasms or granulomatous infections of the pleural space.

• *Lung scan* (scintiphotography) demonstrates ventilation and perfusion patterns and is used primarily to evaluate pulmonary embolus.

• *Transtracheal aspiration* obtains secretions from trachea and proximal bronchi for microbiologic analysis.

• *Arterial blood gas (ABG) measurements* assess gas exchange. Decreased arterial Po_2 may indicate hypoventilation, ventilation-perfusion mismatching, or shunting of blood away from gas exchange sites. Increased Pco_2 reflects hypoventilation or marked ventilation-perfusion mismatching; decreased Pco_2 reflects increased alveolar ventilation. Changes in pH may reflect metabolic or respiratory dysfunction.

Assessment

Complete assessment of the respiratory system helps explore present and potential respiratory problems. Such assessment always begins with a thorough patient *history*. Ask the patient to describe his respiratory problem or difficulty. How long has he had it? How long does each attack last? Does one attack differ from another? Does any activity in particular bring on an attack or make it worse? What relieves the symptoms? Always ask whether the patient was or is a smoker, what and how often he smoked or smokes, and how long he smoked or has been smoking. Record this information in "pack years"—the number of packs of cigarettes per day multiplied by the number of smoking years. Remember to ask about the patient's occupation, hobbies, and travel; some of these activities may involve exposure to toxic or allergenic substances.

If the patient has dyspnea, ask if it occurs during activity or at rest. What position is the patient in when dyspnea occurs? How far can he walk? How many flights of stairs can he climb? Can he relate dyspnea to allergies or environmental conditions? Does it occur only at night, during sleep? If the patient has a cough, ask about its severity, persistence, and duration; ask if it produces sputum and, if so, what kind. Have the patient's cough and sputum habits changed recently?

Next, look for telltale clues to respiratory disease. The patient's general appearance can give you many clues. If he's frail or cachectic, he may have a chronic disease that has impaired his appetite. If he's diaphoretic, restless, or irritable, or protective of a painful body part, he may be in acute distress. Also, look for behavior changes that may indicate hypoxia or hypercapnia. Confusion, lethargy, bizarre behavior, or quiet sleep from which he can't be aroused may point to hypercapnia. Watch for marked cyanosis, indicated by bluish or ashen skin (usually best seen on the lips, tongue, earlobes, and nail beds), which may be due to hypoxemia or poor tissue perfusion.

Check chest configuration at rest and during ventilation. Increased anteroposterior diameter ("barrel chest") characterizes emphysema. Kyphoscoliosis also alters chest configuration, which in turn restricts breathing. To assess the muscles used on inspiration, place the patient in semi-Fowler's or a flat position, and observe which muscles he uses to breathe. If the epigastric area rises during inspiration, he's using his diaphragm. Use of upper chest and neck muscles is normal only during physical stress.

Observe the rate and pattern of breathing. Certain disorders produce characteristic changes in breathing patterns. An acute respiratory disorder, for example, can produce tachypnea (rapid, shallow breathing) or hyperpnea (increased rate and depth of breathing); intracranial lesions—Cheyne-Stokes and Biot's respirations; increased intracranial pressure—central hyperventilation, and apneustic or ataxic breathing; metabolic disorders—Kussmaul's respirations; and airway obstruction—prolonged forceful expiration and pursed lip breathing. Also observe posture and carriage. A patient with chronic obstructive disease, for example, usually supports rib cage movement by placing his arms on the sides of a chair to increase expansion, and leans forward during exhalation to help expel air.

Physical examination

Palpation of the chest wall detects masses, areas of tenderness, changes in fremitus (palpable vocal vibrations), or crepitus (air in subcutaneous tissues). To assess chest excursion and symmetry, place your hands in a horizontal position, bilaterally on the posterior chest, with your thumbs pressed lightly against the spine, creating folds in the skin. As the patient takes a deep breath, your thumbs should move quickly and equally away from the spine. Repeat this with your hands placed anteriorly, at the costal margins (lower lobes) and clavicles (apices). Unequal movement indicates differences in expansion, seen in atelectasis, diaphragm or chest wall muscle disease, or splinting with pain.

Percussion should detect resonance over lung fields that are not covered by bony structures or the heart. A dull sound on percussion may mean consolidation or pleural disease.

Auscultation normally detects soft, vesicular breath sounds throughout most of the lung fields. Absent or adventitious breath sounds may indicate fluid in small airways or interstitial lung disease (rales), secretions in moderate and large airways (rhonchi), and airflow obstruction (wheezes).

Special respiratory care

The hospitalized patient with respiratory disease may require an artificial upper airway, chest tubes, chest physiotherapy, and supervision of mechanical ventilation. In cardiopulmonary arrest, establishing an airway always takes precedence. In a patient with this condition, airway obstruction usually results when the tongue slides back and blocks the posterior pharynx. The head-tilt method or, in suspected or confirmed cervical fracture or arthritis, the jaw-thrust maneuver can immediately push the tongue forward and relieve such obstruction. Endotracheal intubation and, sometimes, a tracheotomy may be necessary.

Chest tubes

An important procedure in patients with respiratory disease is chest tube drainage, which removes air or fluid from the pleural space, allowing the collapsed lung to reexpand to fill the evacuated pleural space. Chest drainage also allows removal of pleural fluid for culture. Chest tubes are commonly used after thoracic surgery, penetrating chest wounds, pleural effusion, and empyema, and for evacuation of pneumothorax, hydrothorax, or hemothorax. Sometimes chest tubes are used to instill sclerosing drugs into the pleural space to prevent recurrent malignant pleural effusions.

Commonly, the chest tube is placed in the sixth or seventh intercostal space, in the axillary region. Occasionally, in pneumothorax, the tube is placed in the second or third intercostal space, in the midclavicular region.

When caring for a patient with chest tubes:

- monitor changes in suction pressure.
- maintain tube patency by milking and draining the tubes every 1 to 2 hours.
- ensure that all connections in the system are tightly connected and secured with tape over insertion sites.
- check for air leaks, and add water to the suction bottle when necessary. Don't clamp the tube if an air leak occurs.
- record the amount, color, and consistency of drainage. Watch for signs of shock, such as tachycardia and hypotension, if drainage is excessive.
- always keep two hemostats at the bedside in case the tube is disconnected.
- tell the patient to cough once an hour, and have him take several deep breaths to enhance drainage and lung function.

Ventilator methods

Mechanical ventilators are used when the normal bellows action usually provided by the diaphragm and rib cage fails. Pressure-cycled ventilators deliver gas until they reach a predetermined airway pressure; they provide no specified tidal volume. Volume-cycled ventilators deliver a preset volume of gas. The tidal volume is set at 10 to 15 ml/kg of body weight. You can use positive end-expiratory pressure (PEEP) to retain a certain amount of pressure in the lungs at the end of expiration, increasing functional residual capacity and improving gas exchange. PEEP is especially beneficial for patients with adult respiratory distress syndrome. High-frequency jet ventilation delivers small tidal volumes at high rates, resulting in low airway and intrathoracic pressures.

You can use several methods to wean a patient from a ventilator. In one method, the patient is disconnected from the ventilator and put on a T piece (endotracheal tube oxygen adapter) that provides supplemental O_2 and humidification. The patient is allowed to breathe spontaneously without the ventilator for gradually increasing periods of time. With intermittent mandatory ventilation (IMV)—another method of weaning—the ventilator provides a specific number of breaths, and the patient is able to breathe spontaneously between ventilator breaths. The frequency of ventilator breaths is gradually decreased until the patient can breathe entirely on his own. Vital signs and arterial blood gases should be monitored periodically during weaning, to assess the patient's status.

Chest physiotherapy

In respiratory conditions marked by excessive accumulation of secretions in the lungs, chest physiotherapy may enhance removal of secretions. Chest physiotherapy includes chest assessment, effective breathing and coughing exercises, postural drainage, percussion, vibration, and evaluation of the therapy's effectiveness. Before initiating treatment, review X-rays to locate areas of consolidation.

• *Deep breathing* maintains use of diaphragm, increases negative intrathoracic pressure, and promotes venous return; it is especially important when pain or dressings restrict chest movement. An incentive spirometer can provide positive visual reinforcement to promote deep breathing.

• *Pursed lip breathing* is used primarily in obstructive disease to slow expiration and prevent large airway collapse. Such breathing funnels air through a narrow opening, creating a positive back pressure on airways to keep them open.

• *Segmental breathing or lateral costal breathing* is used after lung resection and for basilar disorders. Place your hand over the lung area on the affected side. Instruct the patient to try to push that portion of his chest against your hand on deep inspiration. You should be able to feel this with your hand.

• *Coughing* that is controlled and staged gradually increases intrathoracic pressure, reducing pain and bronchospasm of explosive coughing. When wound pain prevents effective coughing, splint the wound with a pillow, towel, or your hand during coughing exercises.

• *Postural drainage* uses gravity to drain secretions into larger airways, where they can be expectorated. This technique is used in patients with copious or tenacious secretions. Before performing postural drainage, auscultate the patient's chest and review chest X-rays to determine the best position for maximum drainage. To prevent vomiting, schedule postural drainage at least 1 hour after meals.

• *Percussion* impacts air against the chest wall, enhancing the effectiveness of postural drainage by loosening lung secretions. Percussion is contraindicated in severe pain, extreme obesity (prevents effective contact with chest wall), cancer that has metastasized to the ribs, crushing chest injuries, bleeding disorders, spontaneous pneumothorax, and spinal compression fractures.

• *Vibration* can be used with percussion or alone when percussion is contraindicated.

Before and after chest physiotherapy, auscultate the patient's lung fields and assess for sputum production to evaluate effectiveness of therapy.

CONGENITAL & PEDIATRIC DISORDERS

Respiratory Distress Syndrome

(Hyaline membrane disease)

Respiratory distress syndrome (RDS) is the most common cause of neonatal mortality. In the United States alone, it causes the death of 40,000 newborns every year. RDS occurs in premature infants and, if untreated, is fatal within 72 hours of birth in up to 14% of infants weighing less than 5.5 lb (2,500 g). Aggressive management using mechanical ventilation can improve prognosis, but a few infants who survive have bronchopulmonary dysplasia. Mild RDS slowly subsides after 3 days.

Causes and incidence

RDS occurs almost exclusively in infants born before the 37th week of gestation (in 60% of those born before the 28th week). It occurs more often in infants of diabetic mothers, those delivered by cesarean section, and those delivered suddenly after antepartum hemorrhage. Although airways and alveoli of an infant's respiratory system are present by the 27th week of gestation, the intercostal muscles are weak and the alveoli and capillary blood supply are immature. In RDS, the premature infant develops widespread alveolar collapse due to lack of surfactant, a lipoprotein present in alveoli and respiratory bronchioles that lowers surface tension and aids in maintaining alveolar patency, preventing collapse, particularly at end expiration. This surfactant deficiency results in widespread atelectasis, which leads to inadequate alveolar ventilation with shunting of blood through collapsed areas of lung, causing hypoxia and acidosis.

Signs and symptoms

While an RDS infant may breathe normally at first, he usually develops rapid, shallow respirations within minutes or hours of birth, with intercostal, subcostal, or sternal retractions, nasal flaring, and audible expiratory grunting. This grunting is a natural compensatory mechanism designed to produce positive end-expiratory pressure (PEEP) and prevent further alveolar collapse. The infant may also display hypotension, peripheral edema, and oliguria; in severe disease, apnea, bradycardia, and cyanosis (from hypoxemia, left-to-right shunting through the foramen ovale, or right-to-left shunting through atelectatic regions of the lung). Other clinical features include pallor, frothy sputum, and low body temperature as a result of an immature nervous system and the absence of subcutaneous fat.

Diagnosis

While signs of respiratory distress in a premature infant during the first few hours of life strongly suggest RDS, chest X-ray and arterial blood gases are necessary to confirm the diagnosis.

- *Chest X-ray* may be normal for the first 6 to 12 hours (in 50% of newborns with RDS), but later shows a fine reticulonodular pattern.
- *Arterial blood gases* show decreased PO_2, with normal, decreased, or increased PCO_2 and decreased pH (a combination of respiratory and metabolic acidosis).
- *Chest auscultation* reveals normal or diminished air entry and rales (rare in early stages).

When a cesarean section is necessary before the 36th week of gestation, amniocentesis enables determination of the lecithin/sphingomyelin (L/S) ratio, which helps to assess prenatal lung development and the risk of RDS.

Treatment

Treatment for an infant with RDS requires vigorous respiratory support. Warm, humidified, oxygen-enriched gases are administered by oxygen hood or, if such treatment fails, by mechanical ventilation. Severe cases may require mechanical ventilation with PEEP or continuous positive airway pressure (CPAP), administered by a tightly fitting face mask or, when absolutely necessary, endotracheal intubation. Treatment also includes:

- a radiant infant warmer or isolette for thermoregulation
- I.V. fluids and sodium bicarbonate to control acidosis and maintain fluid and electrolyte balance
- tube feedings or hyperalimentation to maintain adequate nutrition if the infant is too weak to eat.

Special considerations

Infants with RDS require continual assessment and monitoring in an intensive care nursery.

- Closely monitor blood gases as well as fluid intake and output. If the infant has an umbilical catheter (arterial or venous), check for arterial hypotension or abnormal central venous pressure. Watch for complications such as infection, thrombosis, or decreased circulation to the legs. If the infant has a transcutaneous PO_2 monitor (an accurate method for determining PO_2), change the site of the lead placement every 2 to 4 hours to avoid burning the skin.
- Weigh the infant once or twice daily. To evaluate his progress, assess skin color, rate and depth of respirations, severity of retractions, nostril flaring, frequency of expiratory grunting, frothing

at the lips, and restlessness.

- Regularly assess the effectiveness of oxygen or ventilator therapy. Evaluate every FIO_2 and PEEP or CPAP change by drawing arterial blood gases 20 minutes after each change. Be sure to adjust PEEP or CPAP as indicated by arterial blood gas readings.
- When the infant is on mechanical ventilation, watch carefully for signs of barotrauma (increase in respiratory distress, subcutaneous emphysema) and accidental disconnection from the ventilator. Check ventilator settings frequently. Be alert for signs of complications of PEEP or CPAP therapy, such as decreased cardiac output, pneumothorax, and pneumomediastinum. Mechanical ventilation increases the risk of infection in premature infants, so preventive measures are essential.
- As needed, arrange for follow-up care with a neonatal ophthalmologist to check for retinal damage.
- Teach the parents about their infant's condition and, if possible, let them participate in his care (using aseptic technique), to encourage normal parent-infant bonding. Advise parents that full recovery may take up to 12 months. When the prognosis is poor, prepare the parents for the infant's impending death, and offer emotional support.
- Help reduce mortality in RDS by early detection of respiratory distress. Recognize intercostal retractions and grunting, especially in a premature infant, as signs of RDS, and make sure the infant receives immediate treatment.

Sudden Infant Death Syndrome

(Crib death)

A medical mystery of early infancy, sudden infant death syndrome (SIDS) kills apparently healthy infants, usually between ages 4 weeks and 7 months, for reasons that remain unexplained, even after an autopsy. Typically, parents put the infant to bed and later find him dead, often with no indications of a struggle or distress of any kind. Some infants may have had signs of a cold, but such symptoms are usually absent. SIDS has occurred throughout history, all over the world, and in all climates.

Causes and incidence

SIDS accounts for 7,500 to 8,000 deaths annually in the United States, making it one of the leading causes of infant death. Most of these deaths occur during the winter, in poor families, and among underweight babies and those born to mothers under age 20. Although infants who die from SIDS often appear healthy, research suggests that many may have had undetected abnormalities such as an immature respiratory system and respiratory dysfunction. In fact, the current thinking is that SIDS may result from an abnormality in the control of ventilation, which causes prolonged apneic periods with profound hypoxemia and serious cardiac dysrhythmias. Bottle feeding, instead of breast feeding, and advanced parental age *don't* cause SIDS.

Signs and symptoms

Although parents find some victims wedged in crib corners or with blankets wrapped around their heads, autopsies rule out suffocation as the cause of death. Even when frothy, blood-tinged sputum is found around the infant's mouth or on the crib sheets, autopsy shows a patent airway, so aspiration of vomitus is not the cause of death. Typically, SIDS babies don't cry out and show no signs of having been disturbed in their sleep, although their positions or tangled blankets may suggest movement just before death, perhaps due to terminal spasm.

Depending on how long the infant has been dead, a SIDS baby may have a mottled complexion with extreme cyanosis of the lips and fingertips, or pooling of blood in the legs and feet that may be mistaken for bruises. Pulse and respirations are absent, and the infant's diaper is wet and full of stool.

Diagnosis

Diagnosis of SIDS requires an autopsy to rule out other causes of death. Characteristic histologic findings on autopsy include small or normal adrenal glands and petechiae over the visceral surfaces of the pleura, within the thymus (which is enlarged), and in the epicardium. Autopsy also reveals extremely well-preserved lymphoid structures and certain pathologic characteristics that suggest chronic hypoxemia, such as increased pulmonary artery smooth muscle. Examination also shows edematous, congestive lungs fully expanded in the pleural cavities, liquid (not clotted) blood in the heart, and curd from the stomach inside the trachea.

Treatment and special considerations

If the parents bring the infant to the emergency room, the doctor will decide whether to try to resuscitate him. An "aborted SIDS" is an infant who is found apneic and is successfully resuscitated. Such an infant, or any infant who had a sibling stricken by SIDS, should be tested for infantile apnea. If tests are positive, a home apnea monitor may be recommended.

Since most infants cannot be resuscitated, however, treatment focuses on emotional support for the family.

- Make sure that both parents are present when the child's death is announced. The parents may lash out at emergency room personnel, the babysitter, or anyone else involved in the child's care—even at each other. Stay calm and let them express their feelings. Reassure them that they were not to blame.
- Let the parents see the baby in a private room. Allow them to express their grief in their own way. Stay in the room with them, if appropriate. Offer to call clergy, friends, or relatives.
- After the parents and family have recovered from their initial shock, explain the necessity for an autopsy to confirm the diagnosis of SIDS (in some states, this is mandatory). At this time, provide the family with some basic facts about SIDS and encourage them to give their consent for the autopsy. Make sure they receive the autopsy report promptly.
- Find out whether there's a local counseling and information program for SIDS parents. Participants in such a program will contact the parents, ensure that they receive the autopsy report promptly, put them in touch with a professional counselor, and maintain supportive telephone contact. Also, find out whether there's a local SIDS parents' group; such a group can provide significant emotional support. Contact the National Sudden Infant Death Foundation for information about such local groups.
- If your hospital's policy is to assign a public health nurse to the family, she will provide the continuing reassurance and assistance the parents will need.
- If the parents decide to have another child, they'll need information and counseling to help them deal with the pregnancy and the first year of the new infant's life.

Croup

Croup is a severe inflammation and obstruction of the upper airway, occurring as acute laryngotracheobronchitis (most common), laryngitis, and acute spasmodic laryngitis, and must always be distinguished from epiglottitis. Croup is a childhood disease affecting boys more often than girls (typically between ages 3 months and 3 years), that usually occurs during the winter. Up to 15% of patients have a strong family history of croup. Recovery is usually complete.

Causes

Croup usually results from a viral infection. Parainfluenza viruses cause two thirds of such infections; adenoviruses, respiratory syncytial virus (RSV), influenza and measles viruses, and bacteria (pertussis and diphtheria) account for the rest.

Signs and symptoms

The onset of croup usually follows an upper respiratory tract infection. Clinical features include inspiratory stridor, hoarse or muffled vocal sounds, varying degrees of laryngeal obstruction and respiratory distress, and a characteristic sharp, barklike cough. These symptoms may last only a few hours or persist for a day or two. As it progresses, croup causes inflammatory edema and, possibly, spasm, which can obstruct the upper airway and severely compromise ventilation.

Each form of croup has additional characteristics:

In *laryngotracheobronchitis* (LTB), the symptoms seem to worsen at night. Inflammation causes edema of the bronchi and bronchioles and increasingly difficult expiration which frightens the child. Other characteristic features include fever, diffusely decreased breath sounds, expiratory rhonchi, and scattered rales.

Laryngitis, which results from vocal cord edema, is usually mild and produces no respiratory distress except in infants. Early signs include a sore throat and cough which, rarely, may progress to marked hoarseness, suprasternal and intercostal retractions, inspiratory stridor, dyspnea, diminished breath sounds, restlessness, and in later stages, severe dyspnea and exhaustion.

Acute spasmodic laryngitis affects children between ages 1 and 3, particularly those with allergies and a family history of croup. It typically begins with mild to moderate hoarseness and nasal discharge, followed by the characteristic cough and noisy inspiration (which often awaken the child at night), labored breathing with retractions, rapid pulse, and clammy skin. The child understandably becomes anxious, which may lead to increasing dyspnea and transient cyanosis. These severe symptoms diminish after several hours but reappear in a milder form on the next one or two nights.

Diagnosis

When bacterial infection is the cause, throat cultures may identify organisms and their sensitivity to antibiotics, and also rule out diphtheria. A neck X-ray may show areas of upper airway narrowing and edema in subglottic folds, while laryngoscopy may reveal inflammation and obstruction in epiglottal and laryngeal areas. In evaluating the patient, it is necessary to consider foreign body obstruction (a common cause of croupy cough in young children) as well as masses and cysts.

Treatment

For most children with croup, home care with rest, cool humidification during sleep, and antipyretics, such as aspirin or acetaminophen, relieve symptoms. However, respiratory distress that interferes with oral hydration requires hospitalization and parenteral fluid replacement to prevent dehydration. If bacterial infection is the cause, antibiotic therapy is necessary. Oxygen therapy may also be required.

Special considerations

Monitor and support respiration, and control fever. Because croup is so frightening to the child and his family, you must also provide support and reassurance.

• Carefully monitor cough and breath sounds, hoarseness, severity of retractions, inspiratory stridor, cyanosis, respiratory rate and character (especially prolonged and labored respirations), restlessness, fever, and cardiac rate.

- Keep the child as quiet as possible, but avoid sedation since it may depress respiration. If the patient is an infant, position him in an infant seat or prop him up with a pillow; place an older child in Fowler's position. If an older child requires a cool mist tent to help him breathe, explain why it's needed.
- Isolate patients suspected of having RSV and parainfluenza infections, if possible. Wash your hands carefully before leaving the room, to avoid transmission to other children, particularly infants. Instruct parents and others involved in the care of these children to take similar precautions.
- Control fever with sponge baths and antipyretics. Keep a hypothermia blanket on hand for temperatures above 102° F. (38.9° C.). Watch for seizures in infants and young children with high fevers. Give I.V. antibiotics, as ordered.
- Relieve sore throat with soothing, water-based ices such as fruit sherbet and popsicles. Avoid thicker, milk-based fluids if the child is producing heavy mucus or has great difficulty in swallowing. Apply petrolatum jelly or another ointment around the nose and lips to soothe irritation from nasal discharge and mouth breathing.
- Maintain a calm, quiet environment and offer reassurance. Explain all procedures and answer any questions.

When croup doesn't require hospitalization:

- Provide thorough patient and family teaching for effective home care. Suggest the use of a cool humidifier (vaporizer). To relieve croupy spells, tell parents to carry the child into the bathroom, shut the door, and turn on the hot water. Breathing in warm, moist air quickly eases an acute spell of croup.
- Warn parents that ear infections and pneumonia are complications of croup, which may appear about 5 days after recovery. Stress the importance of reporting earache, productive cough, high fever, or increased shortness of breath immediately.

Epiglottitis

Acute epiglottitis is an acute inflammation of the epiglottis that tends to cause airway obstruction. It typically strikes children between ages 2 and 8. A critical emergency, epiglottitis can prove fatal in 8% to 12% of victims unless it is recognized and treated promptly.

Causes

Epiglottitis usually results from infection with the bacteria *Hemophilus influenzae* type B and, occasionally, pneumococci and group A streptococci.

Signs and symptoms

Sometimes preceded by an upper respiratory infection, epiglottitis may rapidly progress to complete upper airway obstruction within 2 to 5 hours. Laryngeal obstruction occurs due to inflammation and edema of the epiglottis. Accompanying symptoms include high fever, stridor, sore throat, dysphagia, irritability, restlessness, and drooling. To relieve severe respiratory distress, the child with epiglottitis may hyperextend his neck, sit up, and lean forward with his mouth open, tongue protruding, and nostrils flaring as he tries to breathe. He may develop inspiratory retractions and rhonchi.

Diagnosis

In acute epiglottitis, throat examination reveals a large, edematous, bright red epiglottis. Such examination should follow lateral neck X-rays and, generally, should *not* be performed if suspected obstruction is great; special equipment (laryngoscope and endotracheal tubes) should be available, since a tongue depressor can cause sudden complete airway obstruction. Trained personnel (such as an anesthesiologist) should be on hand during throat examination to secure an emergency airway.

Treatment

A child with acute epiglottitis and airway obstruction requires emergency hospitalization; he may need emergency endotracheal intubation or a tracheotomy and should be carefully monitored in an ICU. Respiratory distress that interferes with swallowing necessitates parenteral fluid administration to prevent dehydration. A patient with acute epiglottitis should always receive a 10-day course of parenteral antibiotics—usually ampicillin (if the child is allergic to penicillin or if there is a significant incidence of ampicillin-resistant endemic *H. influenzae*, chloramphenicol or another antibiotic may be substituted). Oxygen therapy and blood gas monitoring may also be desirable.

Special considerations

Keep the following equipment available in case of sudden complete airway obstruction: a tracheotomy tray, endotracheal tubes, Ambu bag, oxygen equipment, and a laryngoscope, with blades of various sizes. Monitor blood gases for hypoxia and hypercapnia.

Watch for increasing restlessness, rising cardiac rate, fever, dyspnea, and retractions, which may indicate a need for emergency tracheotomy.

After tracheotomy, anticipate the patient's needs, since he won't be able to cry or call out, and provide emotional support. Reassure the patient and his family that tracheotomy is a short-term intervention (usually from 4 to 7 days). Monitor the patient for rising temperature and pulse rate and hypotension—signs of secondary infection.

ACUTE DISORDERS

Acute Respiratory Failure in COPD

In patients with essentially normal lung tissue, acute respiratory failure (ARF) usually means PCO_2 *above 50 mm Hg and* PO_2 *below 50 mm Hg. These limits, however, don't apply to patients with chronic obstructive pulmonary disease (COPD), who often have consistently high* PCO_2 *and low* PO_2 *values. In patients with COPD, only acute deterioration in arterial blood gas (ABG) values, with corresponding clinical deterioration, indicates ARF.*

Causes

ARF may develop in COPD patients as a result of any condition that increases the work of breathing and decreases the respiratory drive. Such conditions include respiratory tract infection (such as bronchitis or pneumonia)—the most common precipitating factor—bronchospasm, or accumulating secretions secondary to cough suppression. Other causes of ARF in COPD include:

- *central nervous system (CNS) depression*—head trauma or injudicious use of sedatives, narcotics, tranquilizers, or oxygen
- *cardiovascular disorders*—myocardial infarction, congestive heart failure, or pulmonary emboli
- *airway irritants*—smoke or fumes
- *endocrine and metabolic disorders*—myxedema or metabolic alkalosis
- *thoracic abnormalities*—chest trauma,

pneumothorax, or thoracic or abdominal surgery.

Signs and symptoms

In COPD patients with ARF, increased ventilation-perfusion mismatching and reduced alveolar ventilation decrease arterial PO_2 (hypoxemia) and increase arterial PCO_2 (hypercapnia). This rise in carbon dioxide tension lowers the pH. The resulting hypoxemia and acidemia affect all body organs, especially the central nervous, respiratory, and cardiovascular systems. Specific symptoms vary with the underlying cause of ARF but may include:

- *Respiratory*—Rate may be increased, decreased, or normal depending on the cause; respirations may be shallow, deep, or alternate between the two; air hunger may occur. Cyanosis may or may not be present, depending on the hemoglobin level and arterial oxygenation. Auscultation of the chest may reveal rales, rhonchi, wheezes, or diminished breath sounds.
- *CNS*—The patient shows evidence of restlessness, confusion, loss of concentration, irritability, tremulousness, diminished tendon reflexes, and papilledema; he may slip into coma.
- *Cardiovascular*—Tachycardia, with increased cardiac output and mildly elevated blood pressure secondary to adrenal release of catecholamine, occurs early in response to low PO_2. With myocardial hypoxia, dysrhythmias may develop. Pulmonary hypertension also occurs.

Diagnosis

Progressive deterioration in arterial blood gases (ABGs) and pH, when compared to the patient's "normal" values, strongly suggests ARF in COPD. (In patients with essentially normal lung tissue, pH below 7.35 usually indicates ARF, but COPD patients display an even greater deviation from this normal value, as they do with blood PCO_2 and PO_2.) Other supporting findings include:

- *HCO_3*—Increased levels indicate metabolic alkalosis or reflect metabolic compensation for chronic respiratory acidosis.
- *Hematocrit and hemoglobin*—Abnormally low levels may be due to blood loss, indicating decreased oxygen-carrying capacity.
- *Serum electrolytes*—Hypokalemia may result from compensatory hyperventilation—an attempt to correct alkalosis; hypochloremia often occurs in metabolic alkalosis.
- *White blood cell count*—Count is elevated if ARF is due to bacterial infection; Gram stain and sputum culture can identify pathogens.
- *Chest X-ray*—Findings identify pulmonary pathology, such as emphysema, atelectasis, lesions, pneumothorax, infiltrates, or effusions.
- *EKG*—Dysrhythmias commonly suggest cor pulmonale and myocardial hypoxia.

Treatment

ARF in COPD patients is an emergency that requires cautious oxygen therapy (using nasal prongs or Venturi mask) to raise the patient's PO_2. If significant respiratory acidosis persists, mechanical ventilation through an endotracheal or a tracheostomy tube may be necessary. High-frequency ventilation (HFV) may be used if the patient doesn't respond to conventional mechanical ventilation. Treatment routinely includes antibiotics for infection, bronchodilators, and possibly steroids.

Special considerations

- Since most ARF patients are treated in an ICU, orient them to the environment, procedures, and routines to minimize their anxiety.
- To reverse hypoxemia, administer oxygen at appropriate concentrations to maintain PO_2 at a minimum of 50 to 60 mm Hg. Patients with COPD usually require only small amounts of supplemental oxygen. Watch for a positive response—such as improvement in the patient's breathing and color and in ABG results.
- Maintain a patent airway. If the pa-

UNDERSTANDING HIGH-FREQUENCY VENTILATION

Don't be surprised if you hear the doctor order high-frequency ventilation (HFV) to treat a patient with respiratory failure. HFV is a recently developed mechanical ventilation technique that uses high ventilation rates (60 to 3,000 breaths/minute depending on the type of HFV), low tidal volumes, brief inspiratory time, and low peak airway pressures. HFV has three different delivery forms—high-frequency jet ventilation (HFJV), high-frequency positive-pressure ventilation (HFPPV), and high-frequency oscillation (HFO). You'll probably hear about HFJV most often. Here's a brief summary of how HFJV works:

Mechanics of HFJV

- A humidified, high-pressure gas jet pulses through the narrow lumen gas jet valve on inspiration and accelerates as it flows through the port's narrow lumen and into the patient's endotracheal tube.
- The pressure and velocity of the jet stream cause a drag effect that entrains low pressure gases into the patient's airway.
- These gas flows combine to deliver 100 to 200 breaths per minute to the patient.
- The gas stream moves down the airway in a progressively broader wavefront of decreasing velocity.
- Tidal volume is delivered to airways under constant pressure.
- The gas stream creates turbulence, which causes the gas to vibrate in the airways. Alveolar ventilation increases without raising mean airway pressure or peak inflation pressure.

Uses

- Treatment of bronchopleural fistulae
- Rigid bronchoscopy
- Laryngeal surgery
- Thoracic surgical procedures
- Treatment of infant and adult respiratory distress syndrome (limited clinical experience)

Benefits

- Improved venous return
- Decreased airway pressures and (possibly) improved pulmonary artery pressure
- Improved arterial gas exchange
- Decreased right ventricular afterload
- Reduced chance of pulmonary barotrauma and decreased cardiac output

Special considerations

- Regularly check the mechanical setup, parameter alarms, and tubing connections.
- Assess the patient's respiratory status regularly.
- Suction the patient every hour. During suctioning, disconnect the patient from the ventilator. Turn off the humidification system to prevent fluid from accumulating in the tubing and then being inspired when you restart ventilation. Assess airway secretions: if they're extremely viscous, you may need to increase humidification to prevent formation of mucous plugs.

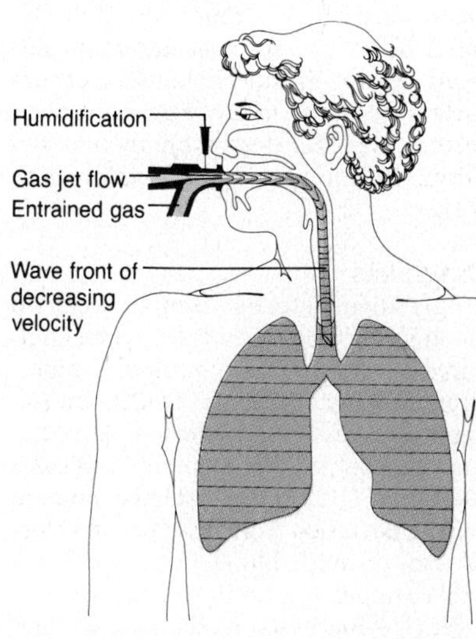

tient is retaining CO_2, encourage him to cough and to breathe deeply with pursed lips. If the patient is alert, have him use an incentive spirometer; if he's intubated and lethargic, turn him every 1 to 2 hours. Use postural drainage and chest physiotherapy to help clear secretions.

• In an intubated patient, suction the trachea p.r.n. after hyperoxygenation. Observe for change in quantity, consistency, and color of sputum. Provide humidification to liquefy secretions.

• Observe the patient closely for respiratory arrest. Auscultate for chest sounds. Monitor ABGs, and report any changes immediately.

• Monitor and record serum electrolytes carefully, and correct imbalances; monitor fluid balance by recording intake and output or daily weights.

• Check cardiac monitor for dysrhythmias.

If the patient requires mechanical ventilation:

• Check ventilator settings and ABG values often since the fraction of inspired oxygen (FIO_2) setting depends on ABGs. Draw specimens for ABGs 20 to 30 minutes after every FIO_2 change.

• Prevent infection by using sterile technique while suctioning and by changing ventilator circuits every 24 hours.

• Since stress ulcers are common in intubated ICU patients, check gastric secretions for evidence of bleeding if the patient has a nasogastric tube or complains of epigastric tenderness, nausea, or vomiting. Monitor hemoglobin and hematocrit levels, and check all stools for occult blood. Administer antacids or cimetidine, as ordered.

• Prevent tracheal erosion that can result from artificial airway cuff overinflation, which compresses tracheal wall vasculature. Use minimal leak technique and a cuffed tube with high residual volume (low pressure cuff), foam cuff, or pressure regulating valve on cuff.

• To prevent nasal necrosis, keep nasotracheal tube midline within the nostrils and provide good hygiene. Loosen tape periodically to prevent skin breakdown. Avoid excessive movement of any tubes and make sure the ventilator tubing is adequately supported.

Adult Respiratory Distress Syndrome

(Shock, stiff, white, wet, or Da Nang lung)

A form of pulmonary edema that causes acute respiratory failure, adult respiratory distress syndrome (ARDS) results from increased permeability of the alveolar capillary membrane. Fluid accumulates in the lung interstitium, alveolar spaces, and small airways, causing the lung to stiffen. Effective ventilation is thus impaired, prohibiting adequate oxygenation of pulmonary capillary blood. Severe ARDS can cause intractable and fatal hypoxemia; however, patients who recover may have little or no permanent lung damage.

Causes

ARDS results from a variety of respiratory and nonrespiratory insults such as:

• aspiration of gastric contents

• sepsis (primarily gram-negative), trauma (lung contusion, head injury, long bone fracture with fat emboli) or oxygen toxicity

• viral, bacterial, or fungal pneumonia or microemboli (fat or air emboli or disseminated intravascular coagulation [DIC])

• drug overdose (barbiturates, glutethimide, narcotics) or blood transfusion

• smoke or chemical inhalation (nitrous oxide, chlorine, ammonia)

• hydrocarbon and paraquat ingestion

• pancreatitis, uremia, or miliary tuberculosis (rare)

• near-drowning.

Altered permeability of the alveolar capillary membranes causes fluid to accumulate in the interstitial space. If the pulmonary lymphatics can't remove this fluid, interstitial edema develops. The fluid collects in the peribronchial and peribronchiolar spaces, producing bronchiolar narrowing. Hypoxemia occurs as a result of fluid accumulation in alveoli and subsequent alveolar collapse, causing the shunting of blood through nonventilated lung regions. In addition, regional differences in compliance and airway narrowing cause regions of low ventilation and inadequate perfusion, which also contribute to hypoxemia.

Signs and symptoms

ARDS initially produces rapid, shallow breathing and dyspnea within hours to days of the initial injury (sometimes after the patient's condition appears to have stabilized). Hypoxemia develops, causing an increased drive for ventilation. Because of the effort required to expand the stiff lung, intercostal and suprasternal retractions result. Fluid accumulation produces rales and rhonchi, and worsening hypoxemia causes restlessness, apprehension, mental sluggishness, motor dysfunction, and tachycardia (possibly with transient increased arterial blood pressure). Severe ARDS causes overwhelming hypoxemia which, if uncorrected, results in hypotension, decreasing urinary output, respiratory and metabolic acidosis, and eventually, ventricular fibrillation or standstill.

Diagnosis

On room air, arterial blood gases (ABGs) initially show decreased PO_2 (less than 60 mm Hg) and PCO_2 (less than 35 mm Hg). The resulting pH usually reflects respiratory alkalosis. As ARDS becomes more severe, ABGs show respiratory acidosis (increasing PCO_2 [more than 45 mm Hg]) and metabolic acidosis (decreasing HCO_3 [less than 22 mEq/liter]) and a decreasing PO_2 despite oxygen therapy.

Other diagnostic tests include:

- *Pulmonary artery catheterization* helps identify the cause of pulmonary edema by evaluating capillary wedge pressure (PCWP); allows collection of pulmonary artery blood which shows decreased oxygen-saturation, reflecting tissue hypoxia; measures pulmonary artery pressure; and measures cardiac output by thermodilution techniques.
- *Serial chest X-rays* initially show bilateral infiltrates; in later stages, ground-glass appearance, and eventually (as hypoxemia becomes irreversible), "whiteouts" of both lung fields.

Differential diagnosis must rule out cardiogenic pulmonary edema, pulmonary vasculitis, and diffuse pulmonary hemorrhage. To establish etiology, laboratory work should include sputum Gram stain, culture and sensitivity, and blood cultures to detect infections; toxicology screen for drug ingestion; and, when pancreatitis is a consideration, a serum amylase determination.

Treatment

When possible, treatment is designed to correct the underlying cause of ARDS and to prevent progression and potentially fatal complications of hypoxemia and respiratory acidosis. Supportive medical care consists of administering humidified oxygen by a tight-fitting mask, which allows for use of continuous positive airway pressure (CPAP). Hypoxemia that doesn't respond adequately to these measures requires ventilatory support with intubation, volume ventilation, and positive end-expiratory pressure (PEEP). Other supportive measures include fluid restriction, diuretics, and correction of electrolyte and acid-base abnormalities.

When ARDS requires mechanical ventilation, sedatives, narcotics, or neuromuscular blocking agents, such as tubocurarine or pancuronium bromide, may be ordered to minimize restlessness and thereby oxygen consumption and carbon dioxide production, and to facilitate ventilation. When ARDS results from fat emboli or chemical injuries to the lungs, a short course of high-dose steroids may help if given early. Treatment to reverse severe metabolic acidosis with sodium bicarbonate may be necessary, and use of fluids and vasopressors may be required to maintain blood pressure. Nonviral infections require antimicrobial drugs.

Special considerations

ARDS requires careful monitoring and supportive care.

- Frequently assess the patient's respiratory status. Be alert for retractions on inspiration. Note rate, rhythm, and depth of respirations, and watch for dyspnea and the use of accessory muscles of respiration. On auscultation, listen for adventitious or diminished breath sounds. Check for clear, frothy sputum that may indicate pulmonary edema.
- Observe and document the hypoxemic patient's neurologic status (level of consciousness, mental sluggishness).
- Maintain a patent airway by suctioning, using sterile, nontraumatic technique. When necessary, instill normal saline solution to help liquefy tenacious secretions.
- Closely monitor heart rate and blood pressure. Watch for dysrhythmias that may result from hypoxemia, acid-base disturbances, or electrolyte imbalance. With pulmonary artery catheterization, know the desired PCWP level; check readings often and watch for decreasing mixed venous oxygen saturation.
- Monitor serum electrolytes and correct imbalances. Measure intake and output, and weigh patient daily.
- Check ventilator settings frequently, and empty condensation from tubing promptly to assure maximum oxygen delivery. Monitor ABG studies; check for metabolic and respiratory acidosis and PO_2 changes. The patient with severe hypoxemia may need controlled mechanical ventilation with positive airway pressure. Give sedatives, as needed, to reduce restlessness. Since PEEP may decrease cardiac output, check for hypotension, tachycardia, and decreased urinary output. Suction only as needed so that PEEP is maintained. Reposition often and record any increase in secretions, temperature, or hypotension that may indicate a deteriorating condition.
- Monitor nutrition, maintain joint mobility, and prevent skin breakdown. Accurately record calorie intake. Give tube feedings and hyperalimentation, as ordered. Perform passive range-of-motion exercises or help the patient perform active exercises, if possible. Provide meticulous skin care. Plan patient care to allow periods of uninterrupted sleep.
- Provide emotional support. Warn the patient who is recovering from ARDS that recovery will take some time and that he will feel weak for a while.
- Watch for and immediately report all respiratory changes in the patient who has suffered injuries that may adversely affect the lungs, especially during the 2- to 3-day period after the injury, when the patient may appear to be improving.

Pulmonary Edema

Pulmonary edema is the accumulation of fluid in the extravascular spaces of the lung. In cardiogenic pulmonary edema, fluid accumulation results from elevations in pulmonary venous and capillary hydrostatic pressures. A common complication of cardiac disorders, pulmonary edema can occur as a chronic condition or develop quickly and rapidly become fatal.

Causes

Pulmonary edema usually results from left ventricular failure due to arteriosclerotic, hypertensive, cardiomyopathic, or valvular cardiac disease. In such disorders, the compromised left ventricle requires increased filling pressures to maintain adequate output; these pressures are transmitted to the left atrium, pulmonary veins, and pulmonary capillary bed. This increased pulmonary capillary hydrostatic force promotes transudation of intravascular fluids into the pulmonary interstitium, decreasing lung compliance and interfering with gas exchange. Other factors that may predispose to pulmonary edema include:

- infusion of excessive volumes of I.V. fluids
- decreased serum colloid osmotic pressure as a result of nephrosis, protein-losing enteropathy, extensive burns, hepatic disease, or nutritional deficiency
- impaired lung lymphatic drainage from Hodgkin's disease or obliterative lymphangitis after radiation
- mitral stenosis and left atrial myxoma, which impair left atrial emptying
- pulmonary veno-occlusive disease.

Signs and symptoms

The early symptoms of pulmonary edema reflect interstitial fluid accumulation and diminished lung compliance: dyspnea on exertion, paroxysmal nocturnal dyspnea, orthopnea, and coughing. Clinical features include tachycardia, tachypnea, dependent rales, and a diastolic (S_3) gallop. With severe pulmonary edema, the alveoli and bronchioles may fill with fluid and intensify the early symptoms. Respiration becomes labored and rapid, with more diffuse crackles and coughing productive of frothy, bloody sputum. Tachycardia increases and dysrhythmias may occur. Skin becomes cold, clammy, diaphoretic, and cyanotic. Blood pressure falls and pulse becomes thready as cardiac output falls.

Symptoms of severe heart failure with pulmonary edema may also include depressed level of consciousness and confusion.

Diagnosis

Clinical features of pulmonary edema permit a working diagnosis. Arterial blood gases usually show hypoxia; P_{CO_2} is variable. Both profound respiratory alkalosis and acidosis may occur. Metabolic acidosis occurs when cardiac output is low. Chest X-ray shows diffuse haziness of the lung fields and, often, cardiomegaly and pleural effusions. Pulmonary artery catheterization helps identify left ventricular failure by showing elevated pulmonary wedge pressures. This helps to rule out adult respiratory distress syndrome—in which pulmonary wedge pressure is usually normal.

Treatment

Treatment of pulmonary edema is designed to reduce extravascular fluid, to improve gas exchange and myocardial function, and, if possible, to correct underlying pathology. Administration of high concentrations of oxygen by cannula, mask, and, if necessary, assisted ventilation improves oxygen delivery to the tissues and often improves acid-base disturbances. A bronchodilator, such as aminophylline, may decrease bronchospasm and enhance myocardial contractility. Diuretics, such as furosemide and ethacrynic acid, promote diuresis, thereby assisting in the mobilization of extravascular fluid.

Treatment of myocardial dysfunction includes digitalis or pressor agents to increase cardiac contractility, antiarrhythmics (particularly when dysrhythmias are associated with decreased cardiac output), and, occasionally, arterial vasodilators, such as nitroprusside, which decrease peripheral vascular resistance and thereby decrease left ventricular workload. Other treatment includes morphine to reduce anxiety and dyspnea and to dilate the systemic venous bed. Rotating tourniquets may be used as an emergency measure to reduce venous return to the heart from the extremities.

Special considerations

- Carefully monitor the vulnerable patient for early signs of pulmonary edema, especially tachypnea, tachycardia, and abnormal breath sounds. Report any ab-

normalities. Check for peripheral edema, which may also indicate that fluid is accumulating in pulmonary tissue.
- Administer oxygen, as ordered.
- Monitor vital signs every 15 to 30 minutes while administering nitroprusside in 5% dextrose in water by I.V. drip. Discard unused nitroprusside solution after 4 hours, and protect it from light by wrapping the bottle or bag with aluminum foil. Watch for dysrhythmias in patients receiving digitalis and for marked respiratory depression in those receiving morphine.
- Assess the patient's condition frequently, and record response to treatment. Monitor arterial blood gases, oral and I.V. fluid intake, urinary output, and, in the patient with a pulmonary artery catheter, pulmonary end diastolic and wedge pressures. Check cardiac monitor often. Report changes immediately.
- Record the sequence and time of rotating tourniquets.
- Reassure the patient, who will be frightened by decreased respiratory capability, in a calm voice and explain all procedures to him. Provide emotional support to his family as well.

Cor Pulmonale

The World Health Organization defines chronic cor pulmonale as "hypertrophy of the right ventricle resulting from diseases affecting the function and/or the structure of the lungs, except when these pulmonary alterations are the result of diseases that primarily affect the left side of the heart or of congenital heart disease." Invariably, cor pulmonale follows some disorder of the lungs, pulmonary vessels, chest wall, or respiratory control center. For instance, chronic obstructive pulmonary disease (COPD) produces pulmonary hypertension, which leads to right ventricular hypertrophy and failure. Since cor pulmonale generally occurs late during the course of COPD and other irreversible diseases, prognosis is generally poor.*

Causes and incidence

Approximately 85% of patients with cor pulmonale have COPD, and 25% of patients with bronchial COPD eventually develop cor pulmonale. Other respiratory disorders that produce cor pulmonale include:
- obstructive lung diseases such as emphysema
- restrictive lung diseases such as pneumoconiosis, cystic fibrosis, interstitial pneumonitis, bronchiectasis, scleroderma, and sarcoidosis
- loss of lung tissue after extensive lung surgery
- pulmonary vascular diseases such as recurrent thromboembolism, primary pulmonary hypertension, schistosomiasis, and pulmonary vasculitis
- respiratory insufficiency without pulmonary disease, as seen in chest wall disorders such as kyphoscoliosis, neuromuscular incompetence due to muscular dystrophy and amyotrophic lateral sclerosis, polymyositis, and spinal cord lesions above C6
- obesity hypoventilation syndrome (pickwickian syndrome) and upper airway obstruction
- living at high altitudes (chronic mountain sickness).

Pulmonary capillary destruction and pulmonary vasoconstriction (usually secondary to hypoxia) reduce the cross-sectional area of the pulmonary vascular bed, thus increasing pulmonary vascular resistance and causing pulmonary hypertension. To compensate for the extra work needed to force blood through the lungs, the right ventricle dilates and hypertrophies. In response to low oxygen content, the bone marrow produces more red blood cells, causing erythrocytosis. When the hematocrit exceeds

55%, blood viscosity increases, which further aggravates pulmonary hypertension and increases the hemodynamic load on the right ventricle. Right ventricular failure is the result.

Cor pulmonale accounts for about 25% of all types of heart failure. It's most common in areas of the world where the incidence of cigarette smoking and COPD is high; cor pulmonale affects middle-aged to elderly men more often than women, but incidence in women is increasing. In children, cor pulmonale may be a complication of cystic fibrosis, hemosiderosis, upper airway obstruction, scleroderma, extensive bronchiectasis, neurologic diseases affecting respiratory muscles, or abnormalities of the respiratory control center.

Signs and symptoms

As long as the heart can compensate for the increased pulmonary vascular resistance, clinical features reflect the underlying disorder and occur mostly in the respiratory system. They include chronic productive cough, exertional dyspnea, wheezing respirations, fatigue, and weakness. Progression of cor pulmonale is associated with dyspnea (even at rest) that worsens on exertion, tachypnea, orthopnea, edema, weakness, and right upper quadrant discomfort. Chest examination reveals findings characteristic of the underlying lung disease.

Signs of cor pulmonale and right ventricular failure include dependent edema; distended neck veins; enlarged, tender liver; prominent parasternal or epigastric cardiac impulse; hepatojugular reflux; and tachycardia. Decreased cardiac output may cause a weak pulse and hypotension. Chest examination yields various findings, depending on the underlying cause of cor pulmonale. In COPD, auscultation reveals rales, rhonchi, and diminished breath sounds. When the disease is secondary to upper airway obstruction or damage to central nervous system respiratory centers, chest examination may be normal except for a right ventricular lift, gallop rhythm, and loud pulmonic component of S_2. Tricuspid insufficiency produces a pansystolic murmur heard at the lower left sternal border; its intensity increases on inspiration, distinguishing it from a murmur due to mitral valve disease. A right ventricular early murmur that increases on inspiration can be heard at the left sternal border or over the epigastrium. A systolic pulmonic ejection click may also be heard. Drowsiness and alterations in consciousness may also occur.

Diagnosis

Pulmonary artery pressure measurements (by pulmonary artery catheter) show increased right ventricular and pulmonary artery pressures as a result of increased pulmonary vascular resistance. Both right ventricular systolic and pulmonary artery systolic pressures will be more than 30 mm Hg. Pulmonary artery diastolic pressure will be greater than 15 mm Hg.

- *Echocardiography* or *angiography* indicates right ventricular enlargement.
- *Chest X-ray* shows large central pulmonary arteries and suggests right ventricular enlargement by rightward enlargement of cardiac silhouette on an anterior chest film.
- *Arterial blood gases* show decreased PO_2 (often less than 70 mm Hg and never more than 90 mm Hg).
- *EKG* frequently shows dysrhythmias such as premature atrial and ventricular contractions and atrial fibrillation during severe hypoxia; it may also show right bundle branch block, right axis deviation, prominent P waves and inverted T wave in right precordial leads, and right ventricular hypertrophy.
- *Pulmonary function tests* show results consistent with the underlying pulmonary disease.
- *Hematocrit* is often greater than 50%.

Treatment

Treatment of cor pulmonale is designed to reduce hypoxemia, increase the patient's exercise tolerance, and, when possible, correct the underlying condition. In addition to bed rest, treatment may include administration of:

- *digitalis glycoside* (digoxin).
- *antibiotics* when respiratory infection is present; culture and sensitivity of sputum specimen aid in selection of antibiotics.
- *potent pulmonary artery vasodilators* (such as diazoxide, nitroprusside, or hydralazine) in primary pulmonary hypertension.
- *oxygen* by mask or cannula in concentrations ranging from 24% to 40%, depending on arterial PO_2, as necessary; in acute cases, therapy may also include mechanical ventilation; patients with underlying COPD generally shouldn't receive high concentrations of oxygen because of possible subsequent respiratory depression.
- *low-salt diet, restricted fluid intake,* and *diuretics* such as furosemide to reduce edema. Occasionally, cor pulmonale may require phlebotomy to reduce red cell mass.
- *anticoagulation* with small doses of heparin, since there may be increased risk of thromboembolism.

Depending on the underlying cause, some variations in treatment may be indicated. For example, a tracheotomy may be necessary if the patient has an upper airway obstruction, and steroids may be used in patients with a vasculitis or autoimmune phenomenon.

Special considerations

- Plan diet carefully with the patient and the staff dietitian. Since the patient may lack energy and tire easily when eating, provide small, frequent feedings rather than three heavy meals.
- Prevent fluid retention by limiting the patient's fluid intake to 1,000 to 2,000 ml/day and providing a low-sodium diet. Make sure the patient with cor pulmonale understands the need for this restriction, since patients with COPD probably have been encouraged to drink up to 10 glasses of water a day.
- Monitor serum potassium levels closely if the patient is receiving diuretics. Low serum potassium levels can potentiate the risk of dysrthythmias associated with digitalis.
- Watch the patient for signs of digitalis toxicity, such as complaints of anorexia, nausea, vomiting, and yellow halos around visual images; monitor for cardiac dysrhythmias. Teach the patient to check his radial pulse before taking digoxin or any digitalis glycoside and to notify the doctor if he detects changes in pulse rate.
- Reposition bedridden patients often to prevent atelectasis.
- Provide meticulous respiratory care, including oxygen therapy and, for COPD patients, pursed-lip breathing exercises. Periodically measure arterial blood gases and watch for signs of respiratory failure: change in pulse rate; deep, labored respirations; and increased fatigue produced by exertion.

Before discharge:

- Make sure the patient understands the importance of maintaining a low-salt diet, weighing himself daily, and watching for and immediately reporting edema. Teach him to detect edema by pressing the skin over his shins with one finger, holding it for a second or two, then checking for a finger impression.
- Instruct the patient to allow himself frequent rest periods and to do his breathing exercises regularly.
- If the patient needs suctioning or supplemental oxygen therapy at home, refer him to a social service agency that can help him obtain the necessary equipment, and, as necessary, arrange for follow-up examinations.
- Since pulmonary infection often exacerbates COPD and cor pulmonale, tell the patient to watch for and immediately report early signs of infection, such as increased sputum production, change in sputum color, increased coughing or wheezing, chest pain, fever, and tightness in the chest. Tell the patient to avoid crowds and persons known to have pulmonary infections, especially during the flu season.
- Warn the patient to avoid nonprescribed medications, such as sedatives, that may depress the ventilatory drive.

Legionnaires' Disease

Legionnaires' disease is an acute bronchopneumonia produced by a fastidious, gram-negative bacillus. It derives its name and notoriety from the peculiar, highly publicized disease that struck 182 people (29 of whom died) at an American Legion convention in Philadelphia in July 1976. This disease may occur epidemically or sporadically, usually in late summer or early fall. Its severity ranges from a mild illness, with or without pneumonitis, to multilobar pneumonia, with a mortality as high as 15%. A milder, self-limiting form (Pontiac syndrome) subsides within a few days but leaves the patient fatigued for several weeks; this form mimics Legionnaires' disease but produces few or no respiratory symptoms, no pneumonia, and no fatalities.

Causes and incidence

Legionnaires' disease bacterium (LDB), recently named *Legionella pneumophila,* is an aerobic, gram-negative bacillus that probably is transmitted by an airborne route. In past epidemics, it has spread through cooling towers or evaporation condensers in air-conditioning systems. However, LDB also flourishes in soil and excavation sites. It does not spread from person to person.

Legionnaires' disease occurs more often in men than in women and is most likely to affect:

- persons in the middle-aged to elderly age-group.
- immunocompromised patients (particularly those receiving corticosteroids, for example, after a transplant), or those with lymphoma or other disorders associated with delayed hypersensitivity.
- patients with a chronic underlying disease, such as diabetes, chronic renal failure, or chronic obstructive pulmonary disease (COPD).
- alcoholics.
- cigarette smokers (three to four times more likely to develop Legionnaires' disease than nonsmokers).

Signs and symptoms

The multisystem clinical features of Legionnaires' disease follow a predictable sequence, although onset of the disease may be gradual or sudden. After a 2- to 10-day incubation period, nonspecific, prodromal signs and symptoms appear, including diarrhea, anorexia, malaise, diffuse myalgias and generalized weakness, headache, recurrent chills, and an unremitting fever, which develops within 12 to 48 hours with a temperature that may reach 105° F. (40.5° C.). A cough then develops that, initially, is nonproductive but eventually may produce grayish, nonpurulent, and occasionally, blood-streaked sputum.

Other characteristic features of LDB are nausea, vomiting, disorientation, mental sluggishness, confusion, mild temporary amnesia, pleuritic chest pain, tachypnea, dyspnea, fine rales, and in 50% of patients, bradycardia. Patients who develop pneumonia may also experience hypoxia. Other complications include hypotension, delirium, congestive heart failure, arrhythmias, acute respiratory failure, renal failure, and shock (usually fatal).

Diagnosis

Patient history focuses on possible sources of infection and predisposing conditions. In addition:

- *Chest X-ray* shows patchy, localized infiltration, which progresses to multilobar consolidation (usually involving the lower lobes), pleural effusion, and in fulminant disease, opacification of the entire lung.
- *Auscultation* reveals fine rales, progressing to coarse rales as the disease advances.
- *Abnormal test results* include leuko-

cytosis, increased erythrocyte sedimentation rate, moderate increase in liver enzymes (SGOT, SGPT, alkaline phosphatase), decreased PO_2, and, initially, decreased PCO_2. Bronchial washings, blood and pleural fluid cultures, and transtracheal aspirates rule out other pulmonary infections.

Definitive tests include direct immunofluorescence of respiratory tract secretions and tissue, culture of *L. pneumophila,* and indirect fluorescent antibody testing of serum comparing acute samples with convalescent samples drawn at least 3 weeks later. A convalescent serum showing a fourfold or greater rise in antibody titer for LDB confirms this diagnosis.

Treatment

Antibiotic treatment begins as soon as Legionnaires' disease is suspected and diagnostic material is collected and shouldn't await laboratory confirmation. Erythromycin is the drug of choice, but if it's not effective alone, rifampin can be added to the regimen. If erythromycin is contraindicated, rifampin or rifampin with tetracycline may be used. Supportive therapy includes administration of antipyretics, fluid replacement, circulatory support with pressor drugs, if necessary, and oxygen administration by mask or cannula or by mechanical ventilation with positive end-expiratory pressure (PEEP).

Special considerations

- Closely monitor respiratory status. Evaluate chest wall expansion, depth and pattern of respirations, cough, and chest pain. Watch for restlessness, which may indicate the patient is hypoxemic, requiring suctioning, repositioning, or more aggressive oxygen therapy.
- Continually monitor vital signs, arterial blood gases, level of consciousness, and dryness and color of lips and mucous membranes. Watch for signs of shock (decreased blood pressure, thready pulse, diaphoresis, clammy skin).
- Keep the patient comfortable; avoid chills and exposure to drafts. Provide mouth care frequently. If necessary, apply soothing cream to the nostrils.
- Replace fluid and electrolytes, as needed. The patient with renal failure may require dialysis.
- Provide mechanical ventilation and other respiratory therapy, as needed. Teach the patient how to cough effectively, and encourage deep breathing exercises. Stress the need to continue these until recovery is complete.
- Give antibiotic therapy, as ordered, and observe carefully for side effects.

Atelectasis

Atelectasis is incomplete expansion of lobules (clusters of alveoli) or lung segments, which may result in partial or complete lung collapse. This causes the loss of regions of the lung for gas exchange; unoxygenated blood passes through these areas unchanged, thereby producing hypoxia. Atelectasis may be chronic or acute and occurs to some degree in many patients undergoing upper abdominal or thoracic surgery. Prognosis depends on prompt removal of any airway obstruction, relief of hypoxia, and reexpansion of collapsed lung.

Causes

Atelectasis often results from bronchial occlusion by mucous plugs (a special problem in persons with chronic obstructive pulmonary disease), bronchiectasis, cystic fibrosis, and in those who smoke heavily (smoking increases mucus production and damages cilia). Atelectasis may also result from occlusion by foreign bodies, bronchogenic carcinoma, and inflammatory lung disease.

Other causes include idiopathic respiratory distress syndrome of the newborn (hyaline membrane disease), oxygen toxicity, and pulmonary edema, in which alveolar surfactant changes increase surface tension and permit complete alveolar deflation.

External compression, which inhibits full lung expansion, or any condition that makes deep breathing painful may also cause atelectasis. Such compression or pain may result from upper abdominal surgical incisions, rib fractures, pleuritic chest pain, tight dressings around the chest, or obesity (which elevates the diaphragm and reduces tidal volume). Atelectasis may also result from prolonged immobility, since this causes preferential ventilation of one area of the lung over another, or mechanical ventilation using constant small tidal volumes without intermittent deep breaths. Central nervous system depression (as in drug overdose) eliminates periodic sighing and is a predisposing factor of progressive atelectasis.

Signs and symptoms

Clinical effects vary with the cause of collapse, the degree of hypoxia, and any underlying disease but generally include some dyspnea. Atelectasis of a small area of the lung may produce only minimal symptoms that subside without specific treatment. However, massive collapse can produce severe dyspnea, anxiety, cyanosis, diaphoresis, peripheral circulatory collapse, tachycardia, and substernal or intercostal retraction. Also, atelectasis may result in compensatory hyperinflation of unaffected areas of the lung, mediastinal shift to the affected side, and elevation of the ipsilateral hemidiaphragm.

Diagnosis

Diagnosis requires an accurate patient history, physical examination, and most importantly, a chest X-ray. Auscultation reveals decreased breath sounds. When a large portion of the lung is collapsed, percussion is dull. However, extensive areas of "microatelectasis" may exist without abnormalities on chest X-ray. In widespread atelectasis, chest X-ray shows characteristic horizontal lines in the lower lung zones and, with segmental or lobar collapse, characteristic dense shadows often associated with hyperinflation of neighboring lung zones. If the cause is unknown, diagnostic procedures may include bronchoscopy to rule out an obstructing neoplasm or a foreign body.

Treatment

Treatment includes incentive spirometry, chest percussion, postural drainage, and frequent coughing and deep breathing exercises. If these measures fail, bronchoscopy may be helpful in removing secretions. Humidity and bronchodilators can improve mucociliary clearance and dilate airways; they are sometimes used with a nebulizer.

Atelectasis secondary to an obstructing neoplasm may require surgery or radiation therapy. Postoperative thoracic and abdominal surgery patients require analgesics to facilitate deep breathing, which minimizes the risk of atelectasis.

Special considerations

- To prevent atelectasis, encourage postoperative and other high-risk patients to cough and deep breathe every 1 to 2 hours. To minimize pain during coughing exercises in postoperative patients, hold a pillow tightly over the incision; teach the patient this technique as well. *Gently* reposition these patients often and help them walk as soon as possible. Administer adequate analgesics to control pain.
- During mechanical ventilation, tidal volume should be maintained at 10 to 15 ml/kg of the patient's body weight to ensure adequate expansion of lungs. Use the sigh mechanism on the ventilator, if appropriate, to intermittently increase tidal volume at the rate of three to four sighs per hour.
- Use an incentive spirometer to encourage deep inspiration through posi-

tive reinforcement. Teach the patient how to use the spirometer and encourage him to use it every 1 to 2 hours.

- Humidify inspired air and encourage adequate fluid intake to mobilize secretions. To promote loosening and clearance of secretions, use postural drainage and chest percussion.
- If the patient is intubated or uncooperative, provide suctioning, as needed. Use sedatives with discretion, since they depress respirations and the cough reflex and suppress sighing. But remember that the patient will not cooperate with treatment if he is in pain.
- Assess breath sounds and ventilatory status frequently and report any changes immediately.
- Teach the patient about respiratory care, including postural drainage, coughing, and deep breathing.
- Encourage the patient to stop smoking, to lose weight, or both, as needed. Refer him to appropriate support groups for help.
- Provide reassurance and emotional support, since the patient will undoubtedly be frightened by his limited breathing capacity.

Respiratory Acidosis

An acid-base disturbance characterized by reduced alveolar ventilation and manifested by hypercapnia (P_{CO_2} greater than 45 mm Hg), respiratory acidosis can be acute (due to a sudden failure in ventilation) or chronic (as in long-term pulmonary disease). Prognosis depends on severity of the underlying disturbance, as well as the patient's general clinical condition.

Causes

Some predisposing factors in respiratory acidosis:

- *Drugs:* Narcotics, anesthetics, hypnotics, and sedatives decrease the sensitivity of the respiratory center.
- *Central nervous system (CNS) trauma:* Medullary injury may impair ventilatory drive.
- *Chronic metabolic alkalosis:* Respiratory compensatory mechanisms attempt to normalize pH by decreasing alveolar ventilation.
- *Neuromuscular disease* (such as myasthenia gravis, Guillain-Barré syndrome, and poliomyelitis): Failure of respiratory muscles to respond properly to respiratory drive reduces alveolar ventilation.

In addition, respiratory acidosis can result from airway obstruction or parenchymal lung disease which interferes with alveolar ventilation; chronic obstructive pulmonary disease (COPD); asthma; severe adult respiratory distress syndrome (ARDS); chronic bronchitis; large pneumothorax; extensive pneumonia; and pulmonary edema.

Hypoventilation compromises excretion of CO_2 produced through metabolism. The retained CO_2 then combines with H_2O to form an excess of carbonic acid (H_2CO_3), decreasing the blood pH. As a result, concentration of hydrogen ions in body fluids, which directly reflects acidity, increases.

Signs and symptoms

Acute respiratory acidosis produces CNS disturbances that reflect changes in the pH of CSF rather than increased CO_2 levels in cerebral circulation. Effects range from restlessness, confusion, and apprehension to somnolence, with a fine or flapping tremor (asterixis), or coma. The patient may complain of headaches and exhibit dyspnea and tachypnea with papilledema and depressed reflexes. Unless the patient is receiving oxygen, hypoxemia accompanies respiratory acidosis. This disorder may also cause cardiovascular abnormalities, such as tachycardia, hypertension, atrial and ventricular arrhythmias, and in severe acidosis, hypotension with vasodilation (bounding pulses and warm periphery).

Diagnosis

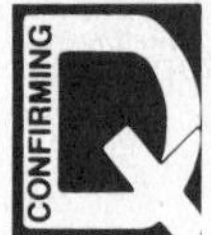

Arterial blood gases confirm respiratory acidosis: P_{CO_2} over the normal 45 mmHg; pH usually below the normal range of 7.35 to 7.45; and HCO_3 normal in the acute stage, but elevated in the chronic stage.

Treatment

Effective treatment for respiratory acidosis is designed to correct the underlying source of alveolar hypoventilation.

Significantly reduced alveolar ventilation may require mechanical ventilation until the underlying condition can be effectively treated. In COPD this includes bronchodilators, oxygen, and antibiotics; drug therapy for conditions such as myasthenia gravis; removal of foreign bodies from the airway; antibiotics for pneumonia; dialysis to remove toxic drugs; and correction of metabolic alkalosis.

Dangerously low blood pH levels (less than 7.15) can produce profound CNS and cardiovascular deterioration and may require administration of sodium bicarbonate I.V. In chronic lung disease, elevated CO_2 may persist despite optimal treatment.

Special considerataions

• Be alert for critical changes in the patient's respiratory, CNS, and cardiovascular functions. Report any such changes immediately, as well as any variations in arterial blood gases and electrolyte status. Maintain adequate hydration.

• Maintain a patent airway and provide adequate humidification if acidosis requires mechanical ventilation. Perform tracheal suctioning regularly and vigorous chest physiotherapy, if ordered. Continuously monitor ventilator settings and respiratory status.

• To prevent respiratory acidosis, closely monitor patients with COPD and chronic CO_2 retention for signs of acidosis. Also, administer oxygen at low flow rates and closely monitor all patients who receive narcotics and sedatives. Instruct the patient who has received a general anesthetic to turn, cough, and perform deep-breathing exercises frequently to prevent the onset of respiratory acidosis.

Respiratory Alkalosis

Respiratory alkalosis is a condition marked by a decrease in P_{CO_2} less than 35 mmHg, which is due to alveolar hyperventilation. Uncomplicated respiratory alkalosis leads to a decrease in hydrogen ion concentration, which causes elevated blood pH. Hypocapnia occurs when the elimination of CO_2 by the lungs exceeds the production of CO_2 at the cellular level.

Causes

Causes of respiratory alkalosis fall into two categories:

• *pulmonary*—pneumonia, interstitial lung disease, pulmonary vascular disease, and acute asthma

• *nonpulmonary*—anxiety, fever, aspirin toxicity, metabolic acidosis, CNS disease (inflammation or tumor), gram-negative septicemia, and hepatic failure.

Signs and symptoms

The cardinal sign of respiratory alkalosis is deep, rapid breathing, possibly above 40 respirations a minute and much like the Kussmaul breathing of diabetic acidosis. Such hyperventilation usually leads to CNS and neuromuscular disturbances, causing light-headedness or dizziness (subnormal CO_2 levels decrease cerebral blood flow), agitation, circumoral and peripheral paresthesias, carpopedal spasms, twitching (possibly progressing to tetany), and muscle weakness. Characteristic effects of severe respiratory alkalosis include hyperpnea and cardiac arrhythmias (that may fail to respond to conventional treatment).

Diagnosis

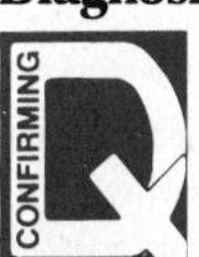

Arterial blood gases confirm respiratory alkalosis and rule out respiratory compensation for metabolic acidosis: PCO_2 below 35 mmHg; pH elevated in proportion to fall in PCO_2 in the acute stage, but falling toward normal in the chronic stage; HCO_3 normal in the acute stage, but below normal in the chronic stage.

Treatment

Treatment is designed to eradicate the underlying condition—for example, removal of ingested toxins, treatment of fever or sepsis, and treatment of CNS disease. In severe respiratory alkalosis, the patient may be instructed to breathe into a paper bag, which helps relieve acute anxiety and increases CO_2 levels.

Prevention of hyperventilation in patients receiving mechanical ventilation requires monitoring arterial blood gases and adjusting dead space or minute ventilation volume.

Special considerations

- Watch for and report any changes in neurologic, neuromuscular, or cardiovascular functions.
- Remember that twitching and cardiac arrhythmias may be associated with alkalemia and electrolyte imbalances. Monitor arterial blood gases and serum electrolytes closely, reporting any variations immediately.
- Explain all diagnostic tests and procedures to reduce anxiety.

Pneumothorax

Pneumothorax is an accumulation of air or gas between the parietal and visceral pleurae. The amount of air or gas trapped in the intrapleural space determines the degree of lung collapse. In a tension pneumothorax, the air in the pleural space is under higher pressure than air in adjacent lung and vascular structures. Without prompt treatment, a tension or a large pneumothorax results in fatal pulmonary and circulatory impairment.

Causes and incidence

Spontaneous pneumothorax usually occurs in otherwise healthy adults aged 20 to 40. Air leakage from ruptured congenital blebs adjacent to the visceral pleural surface, near the apex of the lung, causes this form of pneumothorax. Less often, it results from underlying pulmonary disease—for instance, an emphysematous bulla that ruptures during exercise or coughing, or tubercular or malignant lesions that erode into the pleural space. Spontaneous pneumothorax may also occur in interstitial lung disease, such as eosinophilic granuloma.

Traumatic pneumothorax may result from insertion of a central venous pressure line, thoracic surgery, or a penetrating chest injury, such as a gunshot or knife wound, or it may follow a transbronchial biopsy. It may also occur during thoracentesis or a closed pleural biopsy. When traumatic pneumothorax follows a penetrating chest injury, it often coexists with hemothorax (blood in pleural space).

In *tension pneumothorax*, positive pleural pressure develops as a result of any of the causes of traumatic pneumothorax. When air enters the pleural space through a tear in lung tissue and is unable to leave by the same vent, each inspiration traps air in the pleural space, resulting in positive pleural pressure. This in turn causes collapse of the ipsilateral lung and marked impairment of venous return, which can severely compromise cardiac output, and may cause a mediastinal shift. Decreased filling of the great veins of the chest results in diminished cardiac output and lowered blood pressure.

Pneumothorax can also be classified as open or closed. In *open pneumothorax* (usually the result of trauma), air flows between the pleural space and the outside of the body. In *closed pneumothorax,* air reaches the pleural space directly from the lung.

Signs and symptoms

The cardinal features of pneumothorax are sudden, sharp, pleuritic pain (exacerbated by movement of the chest, breathing, and coughing); asymmetric chest wall movement; shortness of breath; and cyanosis. In moderate to severe pneumothorax, profound respiratory distress may develop, with signs of tension pneumothorax: weak and rapid pulse, pallor, neck vein distention, anxiety. Tension pneumothorax produces the most severe respiratory symptoms; a spontaneous pneumothorax that releases only a small amount of air into the pleural space may cause no symptoms.

Diagnosis

Sudden, sharp chest pain and shortness of breath suggest pneumothorax.

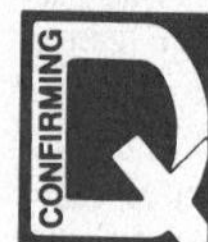

Chest X-ray showing air in the pleural space and, possibly, mediastinal shift confirms this diagnosis. In the absence of a definitive chest X-ray, physical examination occasionally reveals:

- *on inspection:* overexpansion and rigidity of the affected chest side; in tension pneumothorax, neck vein distention with hypotension and tachycardia.
- *on palpation:* crackling beneath the skin, indicating subcutaneous emphysema (air in tissue) and decreased vocal fremitus.
- *on percussion:* hyperresonance on the affected side.
- *on auscultation:* decreased or absent breath sounds over the collapsed lung.

If the pneumothorax is significant, arterial blood gas findings include pH less than 7.35, P_{O_2} less than 80 mmHg, and P_{CO_2} above 45 mmHg.

Treatment

Treatment is conservative for spontaneous pneumothorax in which no signs of increased pleural pressure (indicating tension pneumothorax) appear, lung collapse is less than 30%, and the patient shows no signs of dyspnea or other indications of physiologic compromise. Such treatment consists of bed rest; careful monitoring of blood pressure, pulse rate, and respirations; oxygen administration; and possibly, needle aspiration of air with a large-bore needle attached to a syringe. If more than 30% of lung is collapsed, treatment to reexpand the lung includes placing a thoracostomy tube in the second or third intercostal space in the midclavicular line, connected to an underwater seal or low suction pressures.

Recurring spontaneous pneumothorax requires thoracotomy and pleurectomy; these procedures prevent recurrence by causing the lung to adhere to the parietal pleura. Traumatic and tension pneumothoraces require chest tube drainage; traumatic pneumothorax may also require surgical repair.

Special considerations

- Watch for pallor, gasping respirations, and sudden chest pain. Carefully monitor vital signs at least every hour for indications of shock, increasing respiratory distress, or mediastinal shift. Listen for breath sounds over both lungs. Falling blood pressure, and rising pulse and respiration rates may indicate tension pneumothorax, which could be fatal without prompt treatment.
- Urge the patient to control coughing and gasping during thoracotomy. How-

ever, after the chest tube is in place, encourage him to cough and breathe deeply (at least once an hour) to facilitate lung expansion.

• In the patient undergoing chest tube drainage, watch for continuing air leakage (bubbling), indicating the lung defect has failed to close; this may require surgery. Also, watch for increasing subcutaneous emphysema by checking around the neck or at the tube insertion site for crackling beneath the skin. If the patient is on a ventilator, watch for difficulty in breathing in time with the ventilator, as well as pressure changes on ventilator gauges.

• Change dressings around the chest tube insertion site, as necessary. Be careful not to reposition or dislodge the tube. If the tube dislodges, place a petrolatum gauze dressing over the opening immediately to prevent rapid lung collapse.

• Monitor vital signs frequently after thoracotomy. Also, for the first 24 hours, assess respiratory status by checking breath sounds hourly. Observe the chest tube site for leakage, and note the amount and color of drainage. Walk the patient, as ordered (usually on the first postoperative day), to facilitate deep inspiration and lung expansion.

• Reassure the patient, and explain what pneumothorax is, what causes it, and all diagnostic tests and procedures. Make him as comfortable as possible. (The patient with pneumothorax is usually most comfortable sitting upright.)

Pneumonia

Pneumonia is an acute infection of the lung parenchyma which often impairs gas exchange. Prognosis is generally good for people who have normal lungs and adequate host defenses before the onset of pneumonia; however, bacterial pneumonia is the fifth leading cause of death in debilitated patients.

Causes

Pneumonia can be classified in several ways:

• *Microbiologic etiology*—Pneumonia can be viral, bacterial, fungal, protozoal, mycobacterial, mycoplasmal, or rickettsial in origin.

• *Location*—Bronchopneumonia involves distal airways and alveoli; lobular pneumonia, part of a lobe; and lobar pneumonia, an entire lobe.

• *Type*—Primary pneumonia results from inhalation or aspiration of a pathogen; it includes pneumococcal and viral pneumonia. Secondary pneumonia may follow initial lung damage from a noxious chemical or other insult (superinfection), or may result from hematogenous spread of bacteria from a distant focus.

Predisposing factors to bacterial and viral pneumonia include chronic illness and debilitation, cancer (particularly lung cancer), abdominal and thoracic surgery, atelectasis, common colds or other viral respiratory infections, chronic respiratory disease (COPD, asthma, bronchiectasis, cystic fibrosis), influenza, smoking, malnutrition, alcoholism, sickle cell disease, tracheostomy, exposure to noxious gases, aspiration, and immunosuppressive therapy. Predisposing factors to aspiration pneumonia include old age, debilitation, nasogastric tube feedings, impaired gag reflex, poor oral hygiene, and decreased level of consciousness.

Signs and symptoms

The five cardinal symptoms of early bacterial pneumonia are coughing, sputum production, pleuritic chest pain, shaking chills, and fever. Physical signs vary widely, ranging from diffuse, fine rales to signs of localized or extensive consolidation and pleural effusion.

Complications include hypoxemia,

TYPES OF PNEUMONIA

TYPE	SIGNS AND SYMPTOMS
VIRAL	
Influenza (prognosis poor even with treatment; 50% mortality)	• Cough (initially nonproductive; later, purulent sputum), marked cyanosis, dyspnea, high fever, chills, substernal pain and discomfort, moist rales, frontal headache, myalgia • Death results from cardiopulmonary collapse.
Adenovirus (insidious onset; generally affects young adults)	• Sore throat, fever, cough, chills, malaise, small amounts of mucoid sputum, retrosternal chest pain, anorexia, rhinitis, adenopathy, scattered rales, and rhonchi
Respiratory syncytial virus/RSV (most prevalent in infants and children)	• Listlessness, irritability, tachypnea with retraction of intercostal muscles, slight sputum production, fine moist rales, fever, severe malaise, and possibly, cough or croup
Measles/rubeola	• Fever, dyspnea, cough, small amounts of sputum, coryza, skin rash, and cervical adenopathy
Chicken pox/varicella (uncommon in children, but present in 30% of adults with varicella)	• Cough, dyspnea, cyanosis, tachypnea, pleuritic chest pain, hemoptysis and rhonchi 1 to 6 days after onset of rash
Cytomegalovirus/CMV	• Difficult to distinguish from other nonbacterial pneumonias • Fever, cough, shaking chills, dyspnea, cyanosis, weakness, and diffuse rales • Occurs in neonates as devastating multisystemic infection; in normal adults resembles mononucleosis; in immunocompromised hosts, varies from clinically inapparent to devastating infection
BACTERIAL	
Streptococcus (*Diplococcus pneumoniae*)	• Sudden onset of a single, shaking chill, and sustained temperature of 102° to 104° F. (38.9° to 40° C.); often preceded by upper respiratory tract infection
Klebsiella	• Fever and recurrent chills; cough producing rusty, bloody, viscous sputum (currant jelly); cyanosis of lips and nail beds due to hypoxemia; shallow, grunting respirations • Likely in patients with chronic alcoholism, pulmonary disease, and diabetes
Staphylococcus	• Temperature of 102° to 104° F. (38.9° to 40° C.), recurrent shaking chills, bloody sputum, dyspnea, tachypnea, and hypoxemia • Should be suspected with viral illness, such as influenza or measles, and in patients with cystic fibrosis
ASPIRATION	
Results from vomiting and aspiration of gastric or oropharyngeal contents into trachea and lungs	• Noncardiogenic pulmonary edema may follow damage to respiratory epithelium from contact with stomach acid. • Rales, dyspnea, cyanosis, hypotension, and tachycardia • May be subacute pneumonia with cavity formation, or lung abscess may occur if foreign body is present

DIAGNOSIS	TREATMENT
• *Chest X-ray:* diffuse bilateral bronchopneumonia radiating from hilus • *WBC:* normal to slightly elevated • *Sputum smears:* no specific organisms	*Supportive:* for respiratory failure, endotracheal intubation and ventilator assistance; for fever, hypothermia blanket or antipyretics; for influenza A; amantadine
• *Chest X-ray:* patchy distribution of pneumonia, more severe than indicated by physical examination • *WBC:* normal to slightly elevated	• Treat symptoms only. • Mortality low; usually clears with no residual effects
• *Chest X-ray:* patchy bilateral consolidation • *WBC:* normal to slightly elevated	• *Supportive:* humidified air, oxygen, antimicrobials often given until viral etiology confirmed • Complete recovery in 1 to 3 weeks
• *Chest X-ray:* reticular infiltrates, sometimes with hilar lymph node enlargement • *Lung tissue specimen:* characteristic giant cells	• *Supportive:* bed rest, adequate hydration, antimicrobials; assisted ventilation, if necessary
• *Chest X-ray:* shows more extensive pneumonia than indicated by physical examination, and bilateral, patchy, diffuse, nodular infiltrates • *Sputum analysis:* predominant mononuclear cells and characteristic intranuclear inclusion bodies, with characteristic skin rash confirm diagnosis	• *Supportive:* adequate hydration, oxygen therapy in critically ill patients
• *Chest X-ray:* in early stages, variable patchy infiltrates; later, bilateral, nodular, and more predominant in lower lobes • *Percutaneous aspiration of lung tissue, transbronchial biopsy or open lung biopsy:* microscopic examination shows typical intranuclear and cytoplasmic inclusions; the virus can be cultured from lung tissue	• Generally, benign and self-limiting in mononucleosis-like form • *Supportive:* adequate hydration and nutrition, oxygen therapy, bed rest • In immunosuppressed patients, disease is more severe and may be fatal
• *Chest X-ray:* areas of consolidation, often lobar • *WBC:* elevated • *Sputum culture:* may show gram-positive *S. pneumoniae;* this organism not always recovered	• *Antimicrobial therapy:* penicillin G (or erythromycin, if patient's allergic to penicillin) for 7 to 10 days. Such therapy begins after obtaining culture specimen but without waiting for results.
• *Chest X-ray:* typically, but not always, consolidation in the upper lobe that causes bulging of fissures • *WBC:* elevated • *Sputum culture and Gram stain:* may show gram-negative cocci *Klebsiella*	• *Antimicrobial therapy:* aminoglycoside plus, in serious infections, a cephalosporin
• *Chest X-ray:* multiple abscesses and infiltrates; high incidence of empyema • *WBC:* elevated • *Sputum culture and Gram stain:* may show gram-positive staphylococci	• *Antimicrobial therapy:* nafcillin or oxacillin for 14 days if staphylococci are penicillinase producing • Chest tube drainage of empyema
• *Chest X-ray:* locates areas of infiltrates, which suggest diagnosis	• *Antimicrobial therapy:* penicillin G or clindamycin • *Supportive:* oxygen therapy, suctioning, coughing, deep breathing, adequate hydration, and I.V. steroids

respiratory failure, pleural effusion, empyema, lung abscess, and bacteremia, with spread of infection to other parts of the body resulting in meningitis, endocarditis, and pericarditis.

Diagnosis

Clinical features, chest X-ray showing infiltrates, and sputum smear demonstrating acute inflammatory cells support this diagnosis. Positive blood cultures in patients with pulmonary infiltrates strongly suggest pneumonia produced by the organisms isolated from the blood cultures. Pleural effusions, if present, should be tapped and fluid analyzed for evidence of infection in the pleural space. Occasionally, a transtracheal aspirate of tracheobronchial secretions or bronchoscopy with brushings may be done to obtain material for smear and culture. The patient's response to antimicrobial therapy also provides important evidence of the presence of pneumonia.

Treatment

Antimicrobial therapy varies with the causative agent. Therapy should be reevaluated early in the course of treatment. Supportive measures include humidified oxygen therapy for hypoxia, mechanical ventilation for respiratory failure, a high-calorie diet and adequate fluid intake, bed rest, and an analgesic to relieve pleuritic chest pain. Patients with severe pneumonia on mechanical ventilation may require positive end-expiratory pressure to facilitate adequate oxygenation.

Special considerations

Correct supportive care can increase patient comfort, avoid complications, and speed recovery.

Throughout the illness:

- Maintain patent airway and adequate oxygenation. Measure arterial blood gases, especially in hypoxic patients. Administer supplemental oxygen if PO_2 is less than 55 to 60 mm Hg. Patients with underlying chronic lung disease should be given oxygen cautiously.
- Teach the patient how to cough and perform deep breathing exercises to clear secretions, and encourage him to do so often. In severe pneumonia that requires endotracheal intubation or tracheostomy with or without mechanical ventilation, provide thorough respiratory care and suction often, using sterile technique, to remove secretions.
- Obtain sputum specimens as needed, by suction if the patient can't produce specimens independently. Collect specimens in a sterile container and deliver them promptly to the microbiology laboratory.
- Administer antibiotics, as ordered, and pain medication, as needed; record the patient's response to medications. Fever and dehydration may require I.V. fluids and electrolyte replacement.
- Maintain adequate nutrition to offset high caloric utilization secondary to infection. Ask the dietary department to provide a high-calorie, high-protein diet consisting of soft, easy-to-eat foods. Encourage the patient to eat. As necessary, supplement oral feedings with nasogastric tube feedings or parenteral nutrition. Monitor fluid intake and output.
- Provide a quiet, calm environment for the patient, with frequent rest periods.
- Give emotional support by explaining all procedures (especially intubation and suctioning) to the patient and his family. Encourage family visits. Provide diversionary activities appropriate to the patient's age.
- To control the spread of infection, dispose of secretions properly. Tell the patient to sneeze and cough into a disposable tissue; tape a waxed bag to the side of the bed for used tissues.

To prevent pneumonia:

- Advise the patient to avoid using antibiotics indiscriminately during minor viral infections, since this may result in upper airway colonization with antibiotic-resistant bacteria. If the patient then develops pneumonia, the organisms producing the pneumonia may require treatment with more toxic antibiotics.
- Encourage annual influenza vacci-

nation and Pneumovax for high-risk patients such as those with COPD, chronic heart disease, and sickle cell disease.
• Urge all bedridden and postoperative patients to perform deep breathing and coughing exercises frequently. Position such patients properly to promote full aeration and drainage of secretions.
• To prevent aspiration during nasogastric tube feedings, elevate the patient's head, check the position of the tube, and administer feeding slowly. Don't give large volumes at one time, since this could cause vomiting. If the patient has an endotracheal tube, inflate the tube cuff. Keep his head elevated for at least ½ hour after feeding.

Pulmonary Embolism and Infarction

The most common pulmonary complication in hospitalized patients, pulmonary embolism is an obstruction of the pulmonary arterial bed by a dislodged thrombus or foreign substance. It strikes an estimated 6 million adults each year in the United States, resulting in 100,000 deaths. Although pulmonary infarction may be so mild as to be asymptomatic, massive embolism (more than 50% obstruction of pulmonary arterial circulation) and infarction can be rapidly fatal.

Causes

Pulmonary embolism generally results from dislodged thrombi originating in the leg veins. More than half of such thrombi arise in the deep veins of the legs and are usually multiple. Other less common sources of thrombi are the pelvic veins, renal veins, hepatic vein, right heart, and upper extremities. Such thrombus formation results directly from vascular wall damage, venostasis, or hypercoagulability of the blood.

Rarely, the emboli contain air, fat, amniotic fluid, talc (from drugs intended for oral administration which are injected intravenously by addicts), or tumor cells. Thrombi may embolize spontaneously during clot dissolution or may be dislodged during trauma, sudden muscular action, or a change in peripheral blood flow.

Rarely, pulmonary infarction (tissue death) may evolve from pulmonary embolism. Pulmonary infarction develops more frequently when pulmonary embolism occurs in patients with chronic cardiac or pulmonary disease. However if the embolus obstructs a large vessel, bronchial circulation may provide an adequate oxygen supply to the lung supplied by the occluded vessel.

Predisposing factors to pulmonary embolism include long-term immobility, chronic pulmonary disease, congestive heart failure or atrial fibrillation, thrombophlebitis, polycythemia vera, thrombocytosis, autoimmune hemolytic anemia, sickle cell disease, varicose veins, recent surgery, advanced age, pregnancy, lower extremity fractures or surgery, burns, obesity, vascular injury, malignancy, or oral contraceptives.

Signs and symptoms

Total occlusion of the main pulmonary artery is rapidly fatal; smaller or fragmented emboli produce symptoms that vary with the size, number, and location of the emboli. Usually, the first symptom of pulmonary embolism is dyspnea, which may be accompanied by anginal or pleuritic chest pain. Other clinical features include tachycardia, productive cough (sputum may be blood-tinged), low-grade fever, and pleural effusion. Less common signs include massive hemoptysis, splinting of the chest, leg edema, and, with a large embolus, cyanosis, syncope, and distended neck veins.

In addition, pulmonary embolism may cause pleural friction rub and signs of circulatory collapse (weak, rapid pulse; hypotension) and signs of hypoxia (restlessness).

Diagnosis

History reveals any predisposing conditions for pulmonary embolism.

- *Chest X-ray* helps to rule out other pulmonary diseases; shows areas of atelectasis, elevated diaphragm and pleural effusion, prominent pulmonary artery, and, occasionally, the characteristic wedge-shaped infiltrate suggestive of pulmonary embolism.
- *Lung scan* shows perfusion defects in areas beyond occluded vessels; normal lung scan rules out pulmonary embolism.
- *Pulmonary angiography* is the most definitive test but requires a skilled angiographer and radiologic equipment; it also poses some risk to the patient. Its use depends on the uncertainty of the diagnosis and the need to avoid unnecessary anticoagulant therapy in high-risk patients.
- *EKG* is inconclusive but helps distinguish pulmonary embolism from myocardial infarction. In extensive embolism, EKG may show right axis deviation, right bundle branch block, tall peaked P waves, depression of S-T segments and T-wave inversions (indicative of right heart strain), and supraventricular tachydysrhythmias.
- *Auscultation* occasionally reveals a right ventricular S_3 gallop and increased intensity of a pulmonic component of S_2. Also, crackles and a pleural rub may be heard at the site of embolism.
- *Arterial blood gas measurements* showing decreased P_{O_2} and P_{CO_2} are characteristic but do not always occur.

If pleural effusion is present, thoracentesis may rule out empyema, which indicates pneumonia.

Treatment

Treatment is designed to maintain adequate cardiovascular and pulmonary functions during resolution of the obstruction and to prevent recurrence of embolic episodes. Since most emboli largely resolve within 10 to 14 days, treatment consists of oxygen therapy, as needed, and anticoagulation with heparin to inhibit new thrombus formation. Heparin therapy is monitored by daily coagulation studies (partial thromboplastin time [PTT]). Patients with massive pulmonary embolism and shock may require fibrinolytic therapy with urokinase or streptokinase to enhance fibrinolysis of the pulmonary emboli and remaining thrombi. Emboli that cause hypotension may require the use of vasopressors. Treatment for septic emboli requires antibiotic therapy, not anticoagulants, and evaluation for the infection's source, particularly endocarditis.

Surgery to interrupt the inferior vena cava is reserved for patients who can't take anticoagulants or who have recurrent emboli during anticoagulant therapy. It should not be done without angiographic demonstration of pulmonary embolism. Surgery consists of vena caval ligation, plication, or insertion of a device (umbrella filter) to filter blood returning to the heart and lungs.

To prevent postoperative venous thromboembolism, a combination of heparin and dihydroergotamine (Embolex) may be administered. Embolex is more effective than heparin alone.

Special considerations

- Give oxygen by nasal cannula or mask. Check arterial blood gases in the event of fresh emboli or worsening dyspnea. Be prepared to provide endotracheal intubation with assisted ventilation if breathing is severely compromised.
- Administer heparin, as ordered, through I.V. push or continuous drip. Monitor coagulation studies daily. Effective heparin therapy raises PTT to approximately 24 times normal. Watch closely for nosebleed, petechiae, and other signs of abnormal bleeding; check stools for occult blood. Tell the patient to prevent bleeding by using an electric razor instead of a safety razor and to brush his teeth with a soft toothbrush.
- After the patient is stable, encourage him to move about often, and assist with

isometric and range-of-motion exercises. Check pedal pulses, temperature, and color of feet to detect venostasis. *Never* vigorously massage the patient's legs. Offer diversional activities to promote rest and relieve restlessness.
• Walk the patient as soon as possible after surgery to prevent venostasis.
• Maintain adequate nutrition and fluid balance to promote healing.
• Report frequent pleuritic chest pain, so analgesics can be prescribed. Also, incentive spirometry can assist in deep breathing. Provide tissues and a bag, for easy disposal of expectorations.
• Warn the patient not to cross his legs; this promotes thombus formation.
• To relieve anxiety, explain procedures and treatments. Encourage the patient's family to participate in his care.
• Most patients need treatment with an oral anticoagulant (warfarin) for 4 to 6 months after a pulmonary embolism. Advise these patients to watch for signs of bleeding (bloody stools, blood in urine, large ecchymoses), to take the prescribed medication exactly as ordered, and to avoid taking any additional medication (even for headaches or colds) or changing doses of medication without consulting their doctors. Stress the importance of follow-up laboratory tests (prothrombin time [PT]) to monitor anticoagulant therapy.
• To prevent pulmonary emboli, encourage early ambulation in patients predisposed to this condition. With close medical supervision, low-dose heparin may be useful prophylactically.

Sarcoidosis

Sarcoidosis is a multisystemic, granulomatous disorder that characteristically produces lymphadenopathy, pulmonary infiltration, and skeletal, liver, eye, or skin lesions. It occurs most often in young adults (aged 20 to 40). In the United States, sarcoidosis occurs predominantly among Blacks, affecting twice as many women as men. Acute sarcoidosis usually resolves within 2 years. Chronic, progressive sarcoidosis, which is uncommon, is associated with pulmonary fibrosis and progressive pulmonary disability.

Causes and incidence

The cause of sarcoidosis is unknown, but the following possible causes have been considered:
• *hypersensitivity response* (possibly from T cell imbalance) to such agents as atypical mycobacteria, fungi, and pine pollen
• *genetic predisposition* (suggested by a slightly higher incidence of sarcoidosis within the same family)
• *chemicals* such as zirconium or beryllium can lead to illnesses resembling sarcoidosis, suggesting an extrinsic cause for this disease.

Signs and symptoms

Initial symptoms of sarcoidosis include arthralgia (in the wrists, ankles, and elbows), fatigue, malaise, and weight loss. Other clinical features vary according to the extent and location of the fibrosis:
• *respiratory*—breathlessness, cough (usually nonproductive), substernal pain; complications in advanced pulmonary disease include pulmonary hypertension and cor pulmonale
• *cutaneous*—erythema nodosum, subcutaneous skin nodules with maculopapular eruptions, extensive nasal mucosal lesions.
• *ophthalmic*—anterior uveitis (common); glaucoma, blindness (rare)
• *lymphatic*—bilateral hilar and right paratracheal lymphadenopathy, and splenomegaly
• *musculoskeletal*—muscle weakness,

polyarthralgia, pain, punched-out lesions on phalanges
• *hepatic*—granulomatous hepatitis, usually asymptomatic
• *genitourinary*—hypercalciuria
• *cardiovascular*—arrhythmias (premature beats, bundle branch or, complete heart block) and, rarely, cardiomyopathy
• *CNS*—cranial or peripheral nerve palsies, basilar meningitis, convulsions, pituitary and hypothalamic lesions producing diabetes insipidus.

Diagnosis

Typical clinical features with appropriate laboratory data and X-ray findings suggest sarcoidosis. A positive Kveim-Siltzbach skin test supports the diagnosis. In this test, the patient receives an intradermal injection of an antigen prepared from human sarcoidal spleen or lymph nodes from patients with sarcoidosis. If the patient has active sarcoidosis, granuloma develops at the injection site in 2 to 6 weeks. This reaction is considered positive when a biopsy of the skin at the injection site shows discrete epitheloid cell granuloma. Other relevant findings include:
• *chest X-ray*—bilateral hilar and right paratracheal adenopathy with or without diffuse interstitial infiltrates; occasionally large nodular lesions are present in lung parenchyma
• *lymph node, skin, or lung biopsy*—noncaseating granulomas with negative cultures for mycobacteria and fungi
• *other laboratory data*—rarely, increased serum calcium, mild anemia, leukocytosis, hyperglobulinemia
• *pulmonary function tests*—decreased total lung capacity and compliance, and decreased diffusing capacity
• *arterial blood gases*—decreased arterial oxygen tension.

Negative tuberculin skin test, fungal serologies, and sputum cultures for mycobacteria and fungi, as well as negative biopsy cultures, help rule out infection.

Treatment

Asymptomatic sarcoidosis requires no treatment. However, sarcoidosis that causes ocular, respiratory, CNS, cardiac, or systemic symptoms (such as fever and weight loss) requires treatment with systemic or topical steroids; as does sarcoidosis that produces hypercalcemia or destructive skin lesions. Such therapy is usually continued for 1 to 2 years, but some patients may need lifelong therapy. Other treatment includes a low-calcium diet and avoidance of direct exposure to sunlight in patients with hypercalcemia.

Special considerations

• Watch for and report any complications. Be aware of any abnormal lab results (anemia, for example) which could alter patient care.
• For the patient with arthralgia, administer analgesics, as ordered. Record signs of progressive muscle weakness.
• Provide a nutritious, high-calorie diet and plenty of fluids. If the patient has hypercalcemia, suggest a low-calcium diet. Weigh the patient regularly to detect weight loss.
• Monitor respiratory function. Check chest X-rays for extent of lung involvement; note and record any bloody sputum or increase in sputum. If the patient has pulmonary hypertension or end-stage cor pulmonale, check arterial blood gases, watch for arrhythmias, and administer oxygen, as needed.
• Since steroids may induce or worsen diabetes mellitus, test urine for glucose and acetone at least every 12 hours at the beginning of steroid therapy. Also, watch for other steroid side effects, such as fluid retention, electrolyte imbalance (especially hypokalemia), moonface, hypertension, and personality change. During or after steroid withdrawal (particularly in association with infection or other stress), watch for and report vomiting, orthostatic hypotension, hypoglycemia, restlessness, anorexia, malaise, and fatigue. Remember that the patient on long-term or high-dose steroid therapy is vulnerable to infection.
• When preparing the patient for discharge, stress the need for compliance with prescribed steroid therapy and reg-

ular, careful follow-up examinations and treatment. Refer the patient with failing vision to community support and resource groups and the American Foundation for the Blind, if necessary.

Lung Abscess

Lung abscess is a lung infection accompanied by pus accumulation and tissue destruction. The abscess may be putrid (due to anaerobic bacteria) or nonputrid (due to anaerobes or aerobes), and often has a well-defined border. The availability of effective antibiotics has made lung abscess much less common than it was in the past.

Causes

Lung abscess is a manifestation of necrotizing pneumonia, often the result of aspiration of oropharyngeal contents. Poor oral hygiene with dental or gingival (gum) disease is strongly associated with putrid lung abscess. Septic pulmonary emboli commonly produce cavitary lesions. Infected cystic lung lesions and cavitating bronchial carcinoma must be distinguished from lung abscesses.

Signs and symptoms

The clinical effects of lung abscess include a cough that may produce bloody, purulent, or foul-smelling sputum, pleuritic chest pain, dyspnea, excessive sweating, chills, fever, headache, malaise, diaphoresis, and weight loss. Complications include rupture into the pleural space, which results in empyema and, rarely, massive hemorrhage. Chronic lung abscess may cause localized bronchiectasis. Failure of an abscess to improve with antibiotic treatment suggests possible underlying neoplasm or other causes of obstruction.

Diagnosis

- Auscultation of the chest may reveal rales and decreased breath sounds.
- Chest X-ray shows a localized infiltrate with one or more clear spaces, usually containing air-fluid levels.
- Percutaneous aspiration of an abscess may be attempted or bronchoscopy used to obtain cultures to identify the causative organism. Bronchoscopy is only used if abscess resolution is eventful and the patient's condition permits it.
- Blood cultures, Gram stain, and culture of sputum are also used to detect the causative organism; leukocytosis (WBC count greater than $10,000/mm^3$) is commonly present.

Treatment

Treatment consists of prolonged antibiotic therapy, often lasting for months, until radiographic resolution or definite stability occurs. Symptoms usually disappear in a few weeks. Postural drainage may facilitate discharge of necrotic material into upper airways where expectoration is possible; oxygen therapy may relieve hypoxemia. Poor response to therapy requires resection of the lesion or removal of the diseased section of the lung. All patients need rigorous follow-up and serial chest X-rays.

Special considerations

Care emphasizes aiding the patient with chest physiotherapy (including coughing and deep breathing), increasing fluid intake to loosen secretions, and providing a quiet, restful atmosphere.

To prevent lung abscess in the unconscious patient and the patient with seizures, first prevent aspiration of secretions. Do this by suctioning the patient and by positioning him to promote drainage of secretions. Give good mouth care and encourage patients to practice good oral hygiene.

Hemothorax

In hemothorax, blood from damaged intercostal, pleural, mediastinal, and (infrequently) lung parenchymal vessels enters the pleural cavity. Depending on the amount of bleeding and the underlying cause, hemothorax may be associated with varying degrees of lung collapse and mediastinal shift. Pneumothorax—air in the pleural cavity—often accompanies hemothorax.

Causes

Hemothorax usually results from blunt or penetrating chest trauma; in fact, about 25% of patients with such trauma have hemothorax. Less often, it results from thoracic surgery, pulmonary infarction, neoplasm, dissecting thoracic aneurysm, or anticoagulant therapy.

Signs and symptoms

The patient with hemothorax may experience chest pain, tachypnea, and mild to severe dyspnea, depending on the amount of blood in the pleural cavity and associated pathology. If respiratory failure results, the patient may appear anxious, restless, possibly stuporous, and cyanotic; marked blood loss produces hypotension and shock. The affected side of the chest expands and stiffens, while the unaffected side rises and falls with the patient's gasping respirations.

Diagnosis

Characteristic clinical signs with a history of trauma strongly suggest hemothorax. Percussion reveals dullness and, on auscultation, decreased to absent breath sounds over the affected side. Thoracentesis yields blood or serosanguineous fluid; chest X-rays show pleural fluid with or without mediastinal shift. Blood gases may document respiratory failure; hemoglobin may be decreased, depending on blood loss.

Treatment

Treatment is designed to stabilize the patient's condition, stop the bleeding, evacuate blood from the pleural space, and re-expand the underlying lung. Mild hemothorax usually clears rapidly in 10 to 14 days, requiring only observation for further bleeding. In severe hemothorax, thoracentesis serves not only as a diagnostic tool, but also to remove fluid from the pleural cavity.

After diagnosis is confirmed, a chest tube is inserted quickly into the sixth intercostal space in the posterior axillary line. Suction may be used; a large-bore tube is used to prevent clot blockage. If the chest tube doesn't improve the patient's condition, he may need thoracotomy to evacuate blood and clots and control bleeding.

Special considerations

- Give oxygen by face mask or nasal cannula.
- Give I.V. fluids and blood transfusions (monitored by a central venous pressure [CVP] line), as needed, to treat shock. Monitor blood gases often.
- Explain all procedures to the patient to allay his fears. Assist with thoracentesis. Warn the patient not to cough during this procedure.
- Observe chest tube drainage carefully and record volume drained (at least every hour). Milk the chest tube every hour to keep it open and free of clots. If the tube is warm and full of blood, and the bloody fluid level in the water-seal bottle is rising rapidly, report this immediately. The patient may need immediate surgery.
- Watch the patient closely for pallor and gasping respirations. Monitor his vital signs diligently. Falling blood pressure, rising pulse rate, and rising respiration rate may indicate shock or massive bleeding.

Pulmonary Hypertension

In adults, pulmonary hypertension is indicated by a resting systolic pulmonary artery pressure above 30mmHg and a mean pulmonary artery pressure above 18mmHg. It may be primary (rare) or secondary (far more common). Primary, *or* idiopathic, pulmonary hypertension *occurs most often in women between ages 20 and 40, usually is fatal within 3 to 4 years, and shows the highest mortality among pregnant women.* Secondary pulmonary hypertension *results from existing cardiac and/or pulmonary disease. Prognosis depends on the severity of the underlying disorder.*

Causes

Primary pulmonary hypertension begins as hypertrophy of the small pulmonary arteries. The medial and intimal muscle layers of these vessels thicken, decreasing distensibility and increasing resistance. This disorder then progresses to vascular sclerosis and obliteration of small vessels. Because this form of pulmonary hypertension occurs in association with collagen diseases, it is thought to result from altered immune mechanisms.

Usually, pulmonary hypertension is secondary to hypoxemia from an underlying disease process, including:

- *alveolar hypoventilation* from chronic obstructive pulmonary disease (most common cause in the United States), sarcoidosis, diffuse interstitial pneumonia, malignant metastases, and certain diseases, such as scleroderma. These diseases may cause pulmonary hypertension through alveolar destruction and increased pulmonary vascular resistance. Other disorders that cause alveolar hypoventilation without lung tissue damage include obesity and kyphoscoliosis.
- *vascular obstruction* from pulmonary embolism, vasculitis, and disorders that cause obstructions of small or large pulmonary veins, such as left atrial myxoma, idiopathic veno-occlusive disease, fibrosing mediastinitis, and mediastinal neoplasm.
- *primary cardiac disease,* which may be congenital or acquired. Congenital defects that cause left-to-right shunting of blood—such as patent ductus arteriosus, or atrial or ventricular septal defect—increase blood flow into the lungs and, consequently, raise pulmonary vascular pressure. Acquired cardiac disease, such as rheumatic valvular disease and mitral stenosis, increases pulmonary venous pressure by restricting blood flow returning to the heart.

Signs and symptoms

Most patients complain of increasing dyspnea on exertion, weakness, syncope, and fatigability. Many also show signs of right heart failure, including peripheral edema, ascites, neck vein distention, and hepatomegaly. Other clinical effects vary according to the underlying disorder.

Diagnosis

Characteristic diagnostic findings in patients with pulmonary hypertension include the following:

- *auscultation:* abnormalities associated with the underlying disorder
- *arterial blood gases:* hypoxemia (decreased Po_2)
- *EKG:* in right ventricular hypertrophy, shows right axis deviation and tall or peaked P waves in inferior leads
- *cardiac catheterization:* increased pulmonary artery pressures (PAP)—pulmonary systolic pressure above 30 mmHg; pulmonary capillary wedge pressure (PCWP) increases if the underlying cause is left atrial myxoma, mitral stenosis, or left ventricular failure—otherwise, PCWP is normal

- *pulmonary angiography:* detects filling defects in pulmonary vasculature, such as those that develop in patients with pulmonary emboli
- *pulmonary function tests:* in underlying obstructive disease, may show decreased flow rates and increased residual volume; in underlying restrictive disease, total lung capacity may decrease.

Treatment

Treatment usually includes oxygen therapy to decrease hypoxemia and resulting pulmonary vascular resistance. For patients with right ventricular failure, treatment also includes fluid restriction, digitalis to increase cardiac output, and diuretics to decrease intravascular volume and extravascular fluid accumulation. Of course, an important goal of treatment is correction of the underlying cause.

Special considerations

Pulmonary hypertension requires keen observation and careful monitoring, as well as skilled supportive care.

- Administer oxygen therapy, as ordered, and observe the response. Report any signs of increasing dyspnea so the doctor can adjust treatment accordingly.
- Monitor arterial blood gases for acidosis and hypoxemia. Report any change in level of consciousness immediately.
- When caring for a patient with right heart failure, especially one receiving diuretics, record weight daily, carefully measure intake and output, and explain all medications and diet restrictions. Check for increasing neck vein distention, which may indicate fluid overload.
- Monitor vital signs, especially blood pressure and heart rate. Watch for hypotension and tachycardia. If the patient has a pulmonary artery catheter, check PAP and PCWP, as ordered, and report any changes.
- Before discharge, help the patient adjust to the limitations imposed by this disorder. Advise against overexertion and suggest frequent rest periods between activities. Refer the patient to the social services department if special equipment, such as oxygen equipment, is needed for home use. Make sure he understands the prescribed diet and medications.

Pleural Effusion and Empyema

Pleural effusion is an excess of fluid in the pleural space. Normally, this space contains a small amount of extracellular fluid that lubricates the pleural surfaces. Increased production or inadequate removal of this fluid results in pleural effusion. Empyema is the accumulation of pus and necrotic tissue in the pleural space. Blood (hemothorax) and chyle (chylothorax) may also collect in this space.

Causes

The balance of osmotic and hydrostatic pressures in parietal pleural capillaries normally results in fluid movement into the pleural space. Balanced pressures in visceral pleural capillaries promote reabsorption of this fluid. Excessive hydrostatic pressure or decreased osmotic pressure can cause excessive amounts of fluid to pass across intact capillaries. The result is a transudative pleural effusion, an ultrafiltrate of plasma containing low concentrations of protein. Such effusions frequently result from congestive heart failure, hepatic disease with ascites, peritoneal dialysis, hypoalbuminemia, and disorders resulting in overexpanded intravascular volume.

Exudative pleural effusions result when capillaries exhibit increased permeability with or without changes in hydrostatic and colloid osmotic pressures, allowing protein-rich fluid to leak into the pleural space. Exudative pleural effusions occur with tuberculosis, subphrenic abscess, pancreatitis, bacterial or fungal pneumonitis or empyema, malignancy, pulmonary embolism with or without infarction, collagen disease (lupus erythematosus and rheumatoid arthritis), myxedema, and chest trauma.

Empyema is usually associated with infection in the pleural space. Such infection may be idiopathic, or may be related to pneumonitis, carcinoma, perforation, or esophageal rupture.

Signs and symptoms

Patients with pleural effusion characteristically display symptoms relating to the underlying pathology. Most patients with large effusions, particularly those with underlying pulmonary disease, complain of dyspnea. Those with effusions associated with pleurisy complain of pleuritic chest pain. Other clinical features depend on the cause of the effusion. Patients with empyema also develop fever and malaise.

Diagnosis

Chest X-ray shows radiopaque fluid in dependent regions. Auscultation of the chest reveals decreased breath sounds; percussion detects dullness over the effused area, which doesn't change with respiration. These tests verify pleural effusion. However, diagnosis also requires other tests to distinguish transudative from exudative effusions and to help pinpoint the underlying disorder. The most useful test is thoracentesis, in which analysis of aspirated pleural fluid shows:

- *transudative effusions:* specific gravity usually <1.015 and protein <3 g/dl
- *exudative effusions:* ratio of protein in pleural fluid to serum ≥ 0.5, pleural fluid lactic dehydrogenase (LDH) $\geq$ 200 IU, and ratio of LDH in pleural fluid to LDH in serum ≥ 0.6
- *empyema:* acute inflammatory WBCs and microorganisms
- *empyema or rheumatoid arthritis:* extremely decreased pleural fluid glucose levels.

In addition, if a pleural effusion results from esophageal rupture or pancreatitis, fluid amylase levels are usually higher than serum levels. Aspirated fluid may be tested for LE cells, antinuclear antibodies, and neoplastic cells. It may also be analyzed for color and consistency; acid-fast bacillus, fungal, and bacterial cultures; and triglycerides (in chylothorax). Cell analysis shows leukocytosis in empyema. Negative tuberculin skin test strongly rules against tuberculosis as the cause. In exudative pleural effusions in which thoracentesis is not definitive, pleural biopsy may be done; it is particularly useful for confirming tuberculosis or malignancy.

Treatment

Depending on the amount of fluid present, symptomatic effusion may require thoracentesis to remove fluid, or careful monitoring of the patient's own reabsorption of the fluid. Hemothorax requires drainage to prevent fibrothorax formation. Treatment of empyema requires insertion of one or more chest tubes after thoracentesis, to allow drainage of purulent material, and possibly, decortication (surgical removal of the thick coating over the lung) or rib resection to allow open drainage and lung expansion. Empyema also requires parenteral antibiotics. Associated hypoxia requires oxygen administration.

Special considerations

- Explain thoracentesis to the patient. Before the procedure, tell the patient to expect a stinging sensation from the local anesthetic and a feeling of pressure when the needle is inserted. Instruct him to tell you immediately if he feels uncomfortable or has trouble breathing during the procedure.
- Give reassurance during thoracentesis. Remind the patient to breathe normally and avoid sudden movements, such as coughing or sighing. Monitor vital signs, and watch for syncope. If fluid is removed too quickly, the patient may suffer bradycardia, hypotension, pain, pulmonary edema, or even cardiac arrest. Watch for respiratory distress or pneu-

mothorax (sudden onset of dyspnea, cyanosis) after thoracentesis.
• Administer oxygen and, in empyema, antibiotics, as ordered.
• Encourage the patient to do deep breathing exercises to promote lung expansion. Use an incentive spirometer to promote deep breathing.
• Provide meticulous chest tube care, and use aseptic technique for changing dressings around the tube insertion site in empyema. Ensure tube patency by watching for bubbles in the underwater seal chamber. Record the amount, color, and consistency of any tube drainage.
• If the patient has open drainage through a rib resection or intercostal tube, use hand and dressing precautions. Since weeks of such drainage are usually necessary to obliterate the space, make visiting nurse referrals for patients who will be discharged with the tube in place.
• If pleural effusion was a complication of pneumonia or influenza, advise prompt medical attention for chest colds.

Pleurisy
(Pleuritis)

Pleurisy is inflammation of the visceral and parietal pleurae that line the inside of the thoracic cage and envelop the lungs.

Causes
Pleurisy develops as a complication of pneumonia, tuberculosis, viruses, systemic lupus erythematosus, rheumatoid arthritis, uremia, Dressler's syndrome, malignancy, pulmonary infarction, and chest trauma. Pleuritic pain is caused by the inflammation or irritation of sensory nerve endings in the parietal pleura. As the lungs inflate and deflate, the visceral pleura covering the lungs moves against the fixed parietal pleura lining the pleural space, causing pain. This disorder usually begins suddenly.

Signs and symptoms
Sharp, stabbing pain that increases with respiration may be so severe that it limits movement on the affected side during breathing. Dyspnea also occurs. Other symptoms vary according to the underlying pathologic process.

Diagnosis
Auscultation of the chest reveals a characteristic *pleural friction rub*—a coarse, creaky sound heard during late inspiration and early expiration, directly over the area of pleural inflammation. Palpation over the affected area may reveal coarse vibration.

Treatment
Treatment is generally symptomatic and includes anti-inflammatory agents, analgesics, and bed rest. Severe pain may require an intercostal nerve block of two or three intercostal nerves. Pleurisy with pleural effusion calls for thoracentesis as both a therapeutic and a diagnostic measure.

Special considerations
• Stress the importance of bed rest and plan your care to allow the patient as much uninterrupted rest as possible.
• Administer antitussives and pain medication, as ordered, but be careful not to overmedicate. If the pain requires a narcotic analgesic, warn the patient about to be discharged to avoid overuse because such medication depresses coughing and respiration.
• Encourage the patient to cough. To minimize pain, apply firm pressure at the site of the pain during coughing exercises.

CHRONIC DISORDERS

Chronic Obstructive Pulmonary Disease

(Chronic obstructive lung disease [COLD])

Chronic obstructive pulmonary disease (COPD) is chronic airway obstruction that results from emphysema, chronic bronchitis, asthma, or any combination of these disorders. Usually, more than one of these underlying conditions coexist; most often, bronchitis and emphysema occur together. The most common chronic lung disease, COPD affects an estimated 17 million Americans, and its incidence is rising. It affects males more often than females, probably because until recently men were more likely to smoke heavily. It doesn't always produce symptoms and causes only minimal disability in many patients. However, COPD tends to worsen with time.

Causes

Predisposing factors to COPD include cigarette smoking, recurrent or chronic respiratory infections, and allergies. Smoking is by far the most important of these factors; it impairs ciliary action and macrophage function, and causes inflammation in airways, increased mucus production, destruction of alveolar septae, and peribronchiolar fibrosis. Early inflammatory changes may reverse if the patient stops smoking before lung destruction is extensive. Familial and hereditary factors (such as deficiency of alpha$_1$-antitrypsin) may also predispose to the development of COPD.

Signs and symptoms

The typical patient, a long-term cigarette smoker, has no symptoms until middle age, when his ability to exercise or do strenuous work gradually starts to decline, and he begins to develop a productive cough. While subtle at first, these signs become more pronounced as the patient gets older and the disease progresses. Eventually the patient develops dyspnea on minimal exertion, frequent respiratory infections, intermittent or continuous hypoxemia, and grossly abnormal pulmonary function studies. In its advanced form, COPD may cause thoracic deformities, overwhelming disability, cor pulmonale, severe respiratory failure, and death.

Treatment and special considerations

Treatment is designed to relieve symptoms and prevent complications. Because most COPD patients receive outpatient treatment, they need comprehensive patient teaching to help them comply with therapy and understand the nature of this chronic, progressive disease. If programs in pulmonary rehabilitation are available, encourage the patient to enroll.

- Urge the patient to stop smoking and avoid other respiratory irritants. Suggest that he install an air conditioner with an air filter in his home; it may prove helpful.
- Explain that bronchodilators alleviate bronchospasm and enhance mucociliary clearance of secretions. Familiarize the patient with his prescribed bronchodilators.
- Administer antibiotics, as ordered, to treat respiratory infections. Stress the need to complete the prescribed course of antibiotic therapy. Teach the patient and his family how to recognize early signs of infection; warn the patient to avoid contact with persons with respiratory infections. Encourage good oral hygiene to help prevent infection. Pneumococcal vaccination every 3 years and annual influenza vaccinations are important preventive measures.
- To strengthen the muscles of respira-

CHRONIC OBSTRUCTIVE PULMONARY DISEASE

DISEASE	CAUSES AND PATHOPHYSIOLOGY	CLINICAL FEATURES
Emphysema • Abnormal irreversible enlargement of air spaces distal to terminal bronchioles due to destruction of alveolar walls, resulting in decreased elastic recoil properties of lungs • Most common cause of death from respiratory disease in the United States	• Cigarette smoking, deficiency of alpha-antitrypsin • Recurrent inflammation associated with release of proteolytic enzymes from cells in lungs causes bronchiolar and alveolar wall damage and, ultimately, destruction. Loss of lung supporting structure results in decreased elastic recoil and airway collapse on expiration. Destruction of alveolar walls decreases surface area for gas exchange.	• Insidious onset, with dyspnea the predominant symptom • *Other signs and symptoms of* long-term disease: chronic cough, anorexia, weight loss, malaise, "barrel chest," use of accessory muscles of respiration, prolonged expiratory period with grunting, pursed-lip breathing and tachypnea, peripheral cyanosis, and clubbing digital • *Complications* include recurrent respiratory tract infections, cor pulmonale, and respiratory failure.
Chronic bronchitis • Excessive mucus production with productive cough for at least 3 months a year for 2 successive years • Only a minority of patients with the clinical syndrome of chronic bronchitis develop significant airway obstruction.	• Severity of disease related to amount and duration of smoking; respiratory infection exacerbates symptoms • Hypertrophy and hyperplasia of bronchial mucous glands, increased goblet cells, damage to cilia, squamous metaplasia of columnar epithelium, and chronic leukocytic and lymphocytic infiltration of bronchial walls; widespread inflammation, distortion, narrowing of airways, and mucus within the airways produce resistance in small airways and cause severe ventilation-perfusion imbalance	• Insidious onset, with productive cough and exertional dyspnea predominant symptoms • *Other signs and symptoms:* colds associated with increased sputum production and worsening dyspnea which take progressively longer to resolve; copious sputum (gray, white, or yellow); weight gain due to edema; cyanosis; tachypnea; wheezing; prolonged expiratory time, use of accessory muscles of respiration
Asthma • Increased bronchial reactivity to a variety of stimuli, which produces episodic bronchospasm and airway obstruction • Asthma with onset in adulthood: often without distinct allergies; asthma with onset in childhood: often associated with definite allergens. Status asthmaticus is an acute asthma attack with severe bronchospasm that fails to clear with bronchodilator therapy. • *Prognosis:* More than half of asthmatic children become asymptomatic as adults; more than half of asthmatics with onset after age 15 have persistent disease, with occasional severe attacks.	• Possible mechanisms include allergy (family tendency, seasonal occurrence); allergic reaction results in release of mast cell vasoactive and bronchospastic mediators • Upper airway infection, exercise, anxiety, and rarely, coughing or laughing can precipitate an asthma attack. • Paroxysmal airway obstruction associated with nasal polyps may be seen in response to aspirin or indomethacin ingestion. • Airway obstruction from spasm of bronchial smooth muscle narrows airways; inflammatory edema of the bronchial wall and inspissation of tenacious mucoid secretions are also important, particularly in status asthmaticus.	• History of intermittent attacks of dyspnea and wheezing • Mild wheezing progresses to severe dyspnea, audible wheezing, chest tightness (a feeling of not being able to breathe), and cough productive of thick mucus. • *Other signs:* prolonged expiration, intercostal and supraclavicular retraction on inspiration, use of accessory muscles of respiration, flaring nostrils, tachypnea, tachycardia, perspiration, and flushing; patients often have symptoms of eczema and allergic rhinitis ("hay fever"). • Status asthmaticus, unless treated promptly, can progress to respiratory failure.

CONFIRMING DIAGNOSTIC MEASURES	MANAGEMENT
• *Physical examination:* hyperresonance on percussion, decreased breath sounds, expiratory prolongation, quiet heart sounds • *Chest X-ray:* in advanced disease, flattened diaphragm, reduced vascular markings at lung periphery, overaeration of lungs, vertical heart, enlarged anteroposterior chest diameter, large retrosternal air space • *Pulmonary function tests:* increased residual volume, total lung capacity, and compliance; decreased vital capacity, diffusing capacity, and expiratory volumes • *Arterial blood gases:* reduced Po_2 with normal Pco_2 until late in disease • *EKG:* tall, symmetric P waves in leads II, III, and AVF; vertical QRS axis; signs of right ventricular hypertrophy late in disease • *RBC:* increased hemoglobin late in disease when persistent severe hypoxia is present	• Bronchodilators, such as aminophylline, to reverse bronchospasm and promote mucociliary clearance • Antibiotics to treat respiratory infection; flu vaccine to prevent influenza; and Pneumovax to prevent pneumococcal pneumonia • Adequate fluid intake and, in selected patients, chest physiotherapy to mobilize secretions • O_2 at low-flow settings to treat hypoxia • Avoidance of smoking and air pollutants
• *Physical examination:* rhonchi and wheezes on auscultation, expiratory elongation; neck vein distention, pedal edema • *Chest X-ray:* may show hyperinflation and increased bronchovascular markings • *Pulmonary function tests:* increased residual volume, decreased vital capacity and forced expiratory volumes, normal static compliance and diffusing capacity • *Arterial blood gases:* decreased Po_2; normal or increased Pco_2 • *Sputum:* contains many organisms and neutrophils • *EKG:* may show atrial arrhythmias; peaked P waves in leads II, III, and AVF; and occasionally, right ventricular hypertrophy	• Antibiotics for infections • Avoidance of smoking and air pollutants • Bronchodilators to relieve bronchospasm and facilitate mucociliary clearance • Adequate fluid intake and chest physiotherapy to mobilize secretions • Ultrasonic or mechanical nebulizer treatments to loosen secretions and aid in mobilization • Occasionally, patients respond to corticosteroids. • Diuretics for edema • Oxygen for hypoxia
• *Physical examination:* usually normal between attacks; auscultation shows rhonchi and wheezing throughout lung fields on expiration and, at times, inspiration; absent or diminished breath sounds during severe obstruction. Loud bilateral wheezes may be grossly audible; chest is hyperinflated. • *Chest X-ray:* hyperinflated lungs with air trapping during attack; normal during remission • *Sputum:* presence of Curschmann's spirals (casts of airways), Charcot-Leyden crystals, and eosinophils • *Pulmonary function tests:* during attacks, decreased forced expiratory volumes which improve significantly after inhaled bronchodilator; increased residual volume and, occasionally, total lung capacity; may be normal between attacks • *Arterial blood gases:* decreased Po_2; decreased, normal, or increased Pco_2 (in severe attack) • *EKG:* sinus tachycardia during an attack; severe attack may produce signs of cor pulmonale (right axis deviation, peaked P wave) which resolve after the attack. • *Skin tests:* may identify allergens	• Aerosol containing beta-adrenergic agents such as metaproterenol or albuterol; also, oral beta-adrenergic agents (terbutaline) and oral methylxanthines (aminophylline). Occasionally, patients require inhaled, oral, or I.V. corticosteroids. • *Emergency treatment:* O_2 therapy, corticosteroids, and bronchodilators such as subcutaneous epinephrine, intravenous aminophylline, and inhaled agents such as metaproterenol. • Monitor for deteriorating respiratory status and note sputum characteristics; provide adequate fluid intake and oxygen, as ordered. • *Prevention:* Tell the patient to avoid possible allergens and to use antihistamines, decongestants, inhalation of cromolyn powder, and oral or aerosol bronchodilators, as ordered. Explain the influence of stress and anxiety on asthma and frequent association with exercise (particularly running) and cold air.

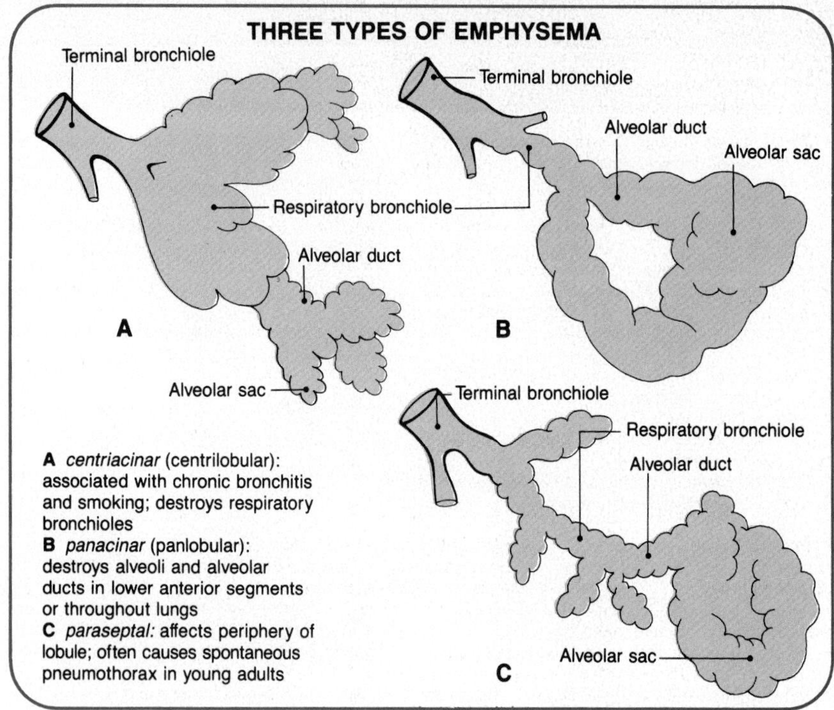
THREE TYPES OF EMPHYSEMA
Terminal bronchiole
Respiratory bronchiole
Alveolar duct
Alveolar sac
A
Terminal bronchiole
Alveolar duct
Alveolar sac
B
Terminal bronchiole
Respiratory bronchiole
Alveolar duct
Alveolar sac
C
A *centriacinar* (centrilobular): associated with chronic bronchitis and smoking; destroys respiratory bronchioles
B *panacinar* (panlobular): destroys alveoli and alveolar ducts in lower anterior segments or throughout lungs
C *paraseptal:* affects periphery of lobule; often causes spontaneous pneumothorax in young adults

tion, teach the patient to take slow, deep breaths and exhale through pursed lips.

• To help mobilize secretions, teach the patient how to cough effectively. If the patient with copious secretions has difficulty mobilizing secretions, teach his family how to perform postural drainage and chest physiotherapy. If secretions are thick, urge the patient to drink 12 to 15 glasses of fluid a day. A home humidifier may be beneficial, particularly in the winter.

• Administer low concentrations of oxygen, as ordered. Perform blood gas analysis to determine O_2 need and to avoid CO_2 narcosis. If the patient is to continue O_2 therapy at home, teach him how to use the equipment correctly. Patients with COPD rarely require more than 2 to 3 liters per minute to maintain adequate oxygenation. Higher flow rates will further increase PO_2, but patients whose ventilatory drive is largely based on hypoxemia will often develop markedly increased PCO_2 tensions. In these patients, chemoreceptors in the brain are relatively insensitive to the increase in CO_2. Teach patients and family that excessive O_2 therapy may eliminate the hypoxic respiratory drive, causing confusion and drowsiness, signs of CO_2 narcosis.

• Emphasize the importance of a balanced diet. Since the patient may tire easily when eating, suggest frequent, small meals and consider using oxygen, administered by nasal cannula, during meals.

• Help the patient and his family adjust their life-styles to accommodate the limitations imposed by this debilitating chronic disease. Instruct the patient to allow for daily rest periods and to exercise daily as his doctor directs.

• As COPD progresses, encourage the patient to discuss his fears.

• To help prevent COPD, advise all people, especially those with a family history of COPD or those in its early stages, not to smoke.

• Assist in the early detection of COPD by urging persons to have periodic physical examinations, including spirometry and medical evaluation of a chronic cough, and to seek treatment for recurring respiratory infections promptly.
• Set a good example by not smoking.

Bronchiectasis

A condition marked by chronic abnormal dilation of bronchi and destruction of bronchial walls, bronchiectasis can occur throughout the tracheobronchial tree or can be confined to one segment or lobe. However, it is usually bilateral and involves the basilar segments of the lower lobes. This disease has three forms: cylindrical (fusiform), varicose, and saccular (cystic). It affects people of both sexes and all ages. Because of the availability of antibiotics to treat acute respiratory tract infections, the incidence of bronchiectasis has dramatically decreased in the past 20 years. Its incidence is highest among Eskimos and the Maoris of New Zealand. Bronchiectasis is irreversible.

Causes

The different forms of bronchiectasis may occur separately or simultaneously. In *cylindrical bronchiectasis*, the bronchi expand unevenly, with little change in diameter, and end suddenly in a squared-off fashion. In *varicose bronchiectasis*, abnormal, irregular dilation and narrowing of the bronchi give the appearance of varicose veins. In *saccular bronchiectasis*, many large dilations end in sacs.

This disease results from conditions associated with repeated damage to bronchial walls, and abnormal mucociliary clearance, which cause a breakdown of supporting tissue adjacent to airways. Such conditions include:

• mucoviscidosis (cystic fibrosis of the pancreas)
• immunologic disorder (agammaglobulinemia, for example)
• recurrent, inadequately treated bacterial respiratory tract infections, such as tuberculosis, and as a complication of measles, pneumonia, pertussis, or influenza
• obstruction (by a foreign body, tumor, or stenosis) in association with recurrent infection
• inhalation of corrosive gas or repeated aspiration of gastric juices into the lungs
• congenital anomalies (uncommon), such as bronchomalacia, congenital bronchiectasis, and Kartagener's syndrome (bronchiectasis, sinusitis, and dextrocardia), and a variety of rare disorders, such as immotile-cilia syndrome.

In bronchiectasis, hyperplastic squamous epithelium denuded of cilia replaces ulcerated columnar epithelium. Abscess formation involving all layers of the bronchial wall produces inflammatory cells and fibrous tissue, resulting in both dilation and narrowing of the airways. Mucous plugs or fibrous tissue obliterates smaller bronchioles, while peribronchial lymphoid tissue becomes hyperplastic. Extensive vascular proliferation of bronchial circulation occurs and produces frequent hemoptysis.

Signs and symptoms

Initially, bronchiectasis may be asymptomatic. When symptoms do arise, they're often attributed to other illnesses. The patient usually complains of frequent bouts of pneumonia or hemoptysis. The classic symptom, however, is a chronic cough that produces copious, foul-smelling, mucopurulent secretions, possibly totaling several cupfuls daily. Characteristic findings include coarse rales during inspiration over involved lobes or segments, occasional wheezes, dyspnea, sinusitis, weight loss, anemia,

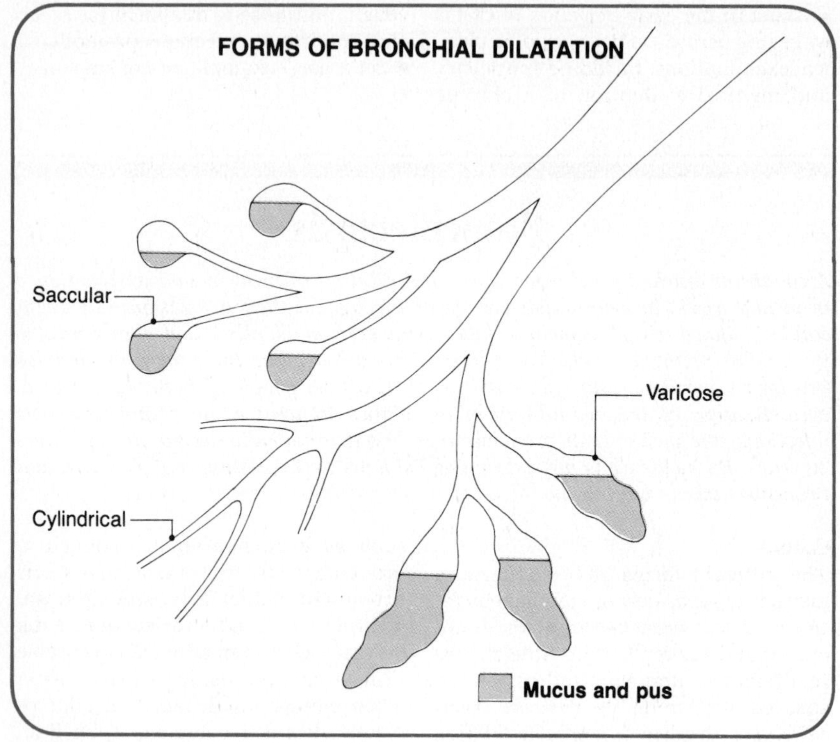

malaise, clubbing, recurrent fever, chills, and other signs of infection.

Advanced bronchiectasis may produce chronic malnutrition and amyloidosis, as well as right heart failure and cor pulmonale due to hypoxic pulmonary vasoconstriction.

Diagnosis

History of recurrent bronchial infections, pneumonia, and hemoptysis in a patient whose chest X-rays show peribronchial thickening, areas of atelectasis, and scattered cystic changes suggests bronchiectasis. Bronchography, however, is the most reliable diagnostic tool. Although this test is not done routinely, it should be considered for patients being evaluated for possible surgery or those with recurrent or severe hemoptysis. In bronchography, a radiopaque dye outlines the bronchial walls, revealing the location and extent of the disease. Bronchoscopy does not establish this diagnosis, but helps identify the source of secretions or the site of bleeding in hemoptysis.

Other helpful laboratory tests include:

- *sputum culture and Gram's stain* to identify predominant organisms
- *blood count* for possible anemia and leukocytosis
- *pulmonary function studies* to detect decreased vital capacity, expiratory flow, and hypoxemia; these tests also help determine the physiologic severity of the disease and the effects of therapy, and help evaluate patients for surgery. If symptoms warrant, evaluation may include urinalysis and EKG (the latter is normal unless cor pulmonale develops). When cystic fibrosis is suspected as the underlying cause of bronchiectasis, a sweat electrolyte test is useful.

Treatment

Treatment includes antibiotics, given P.O. or I.V., for 7 to 10 days or until sputum production decreases. Bronchodilators, with postural drainage and chest percussion, help remove secretions if the patient has bronchospasm and thick, tenacious sputum. Bronchoscopy may occasionally be used to aid mobilization of secretions. Hypoxia requires oxygen therapy; severe hemoptysis often requires lobectomy or segmental resection.

Special considerations

Throughout this illness, provide supportive care and help the patient adjust to the permanent changes in life-style that irreversible lung damage necessitates. Thorough teaching is vital.

- Administer antibiotics, as ordered, and explain all diagnostic tests. Perform chest physiotherapy, including postural drainage and chest percussion designed for involved lobes, several times a day. The best times to do this are early morning and just before bedtime. Instruct the patient to maintain each position for 10 minutes, then perform percussion and tell him to cough. Show family members how to do postural drainage and percussion. Also, teach the patient coughing and deep breathing techniques to promote good ventilation and the removal of secretions.
- Advise the patient to stop smoking, since it stimulates secretions and irritates the airways. Refer the patient to a local self-help group.
- Provide a warm, quiet, comfortable environment, and urge the patient to rest as much as possible. Encourage balanced, high-protein meals to promote good health and tissue healing, and plenty of fluids to aid expectoration. Give frequent mouth care to remove foul-smelling sputum. Teach the patient to dispose of all secretions properly.
- Tell the patient to avoid air pollutants and people with upper respiratory infections. Instruct him to take medications (especially antibiotics) exactly as ordered.
- To help prevent this disease, vigorously treat bacterial pneumonia and stress the need for immunization to prevent childhood diseases.

Tuberculosis

An acute or chronic infection caused by Mycobacterium tuberculosis *and, sometimes, other strains of* Mycobacteria, *tuberculosis (TB) is characterized by pulmonary infiltrates, formation of granulomas with caseation, fibrosis, and cavitation. The American Lung Association estimates that active disease afflicts nearly 14 out of every 100,000 people. Those living in crowded, poorly-ventilated conditions are most likely to become infected. Prognosis is excellent with correct treatment.*

Causes

After exposure to *M. tuberculosis*, roughly 5% of infected persons develop active tuberculosis within 1 year; in the remainder, microorganisms cause a latent infection. The host's immunologic defense system usually controls the tubercle bacillus by killing it or walling it up in a tiny nodule (tubercle). However, the bacillus may lie dormant within the tubercle for years and later reactivate and spread, causing active infection.

Although the primary focus of infection is in the lungs, mycobacteria commonly exist in other parts of the body, such as the kidneys and the lymph nodes. A number of factors increase the likelihood of reactivation of infection: gastrectomy, uncontrolled diabetes mellitus, Hodgkin's disease, leukemia, treatment with corticosteroids and immunosuppressives, and silicosis.

Transmission is by droplet nuclei produced when infected persons cough or sneeze. After inhalation, if a tubercle bacillus settles in an alveolus, infection occurs, with alveolar capillary dilation and endothelial cell swelling. Alveolitis results, with replication of tubercle bacilli and influx of polymorphonuclear leukocytes. These organisms disseminate through the lymph system to the circulatory system and then throughout the body. Cell-mediated immunity to the mycobacteria, which develops about 3 to 6 weeks later, usually contains the infection and arrests the disease. If the infection reactivates, the body's response characteristically leads to caseation—the conversion of necrotic tissue to a cheese-like material. The caseum may localize, undergo fibrosis, or excavate and form cavities, the walls of which are studded with multiplying tubercle bacilli. If this happens, infected caseous debris may spread throughout the lungs by the tracheobronchial tree. Sites of extrapulmonary TB include pleura, meninges, joints, lymph nodes, peritoneum, genitourinary tract, and bowel.

Signs and symptoms

In primary infection, after an incubation period of from 4 to 8 weeks, TB is usually asymptomatic but may produce nonspecific symptoms, such as fatigue, weakness, anorexia, weight loss, night sweats, and low-grade fever. In reactivation, symptoms may include a cough that produces mucopurulent sputum, occasional hemoptysis, and chest pains.

Diagnosis

Diagnostic tests include physical examination, chest X-ray, tuberculin skin test, and sputum smears and cultures to identify tubercle bacilli. Diagnosis must be precise, since several other diseases (lung carcinoma, lung abscess, pneumoconiosis, bronchiectasis) may mimic tuberculosis. The following procedures permit diagnosis:

- *Auscultation* detects crepitant rales, bronchial breath sounds, wheezes, and whispered pectoriloquy.
- *Chest percussion* detects a dullness over the affected area, indicating consolidation or pleural fluid.
- *Chest X-ray* shows nodular lesions, patchy infiltrates (mainly in upper lobes), cavity formation, scar tissue, and calcium deposits; however, it may not be able to distinguish active from inactive TB.
- *Tuberculin skin test* detects infection with tuberculosis but doesn't distinguish the disease from uncomplicated infection. In this test, intermediate-strength purified protein derivative (PPD) or 5 tuberculin units (0.1 ml) are injected intracutaneously on the forearm and read in 48 to 72 hours; a positive reaction (equal to or more than 10 mm induration) develops within 2 to 10 weeks after infection with the tubercle bacillus in both active and inactive TB.

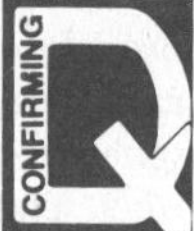

- *Stains and cultures* (of sputum, CSF, urine, drainage from abscess, or pleural fluid) show heat-sensitive, nonmotile, aerobic, acid-fast bacilli.

Treatment

Antitubercular therapy with daily oral doses of isoniazid or rifampin (with ethambutol added in some cases) for at least 9 months usually cures tuberculosis. After 2 to 4 weeks the disease generally is no longer infectious, and the patient can resume his normal life-style while continuing to take medication. Patients with atypical mycobacterial disease or drug-resistant TB may require second-line drugs, such as capreomycin, streptomycin, para-aminosalicylic acid, pyrazinamide, and cycloserine.

Special considerations

- Isolate the infectious patient in a quiet, well-ventilated room until he's no longer contagious. Teach the patient to cough and sneeze into tissues and to dispose of all secretions properly. Place a covered trash can nearby or tape a waxed bag to the side of the bed for used tissues. Instruct the patient to wear a mask when outside of his room. Visitors and hospital personnel should also wear masks when they are in the patient's room.
- Remind the patient to get plenty of rest. Stress the importance of eating balanced meals to promote recovery. If the patient is anorexic, urge him to eat small meals

throughout the day. Record weight weekly.

• Be alert for side effects of medications. Since isoniazid sometimes leads to hepatitis or peripheral neuritis, monitor SGOT and SGPT levels. To prevent or treat peripheral neuritis, give pyridoxine (vitamin B_6) as ordered. If the patient receives ethambutol, watch for optic neuritis; if it develops, discontinue the drug. If he receives rifampin, watch for hepatitis and purpura. Observe the patient for other complications, such as hemoptysis.

• Before discharge, teach the patient to watch for side effects from medication and warn him to report them immediately. Emphasize the importance of regular follow-up examinations, and instruct the patient and his family concerning the signs and symptoms of recurring tuberculosis. Stress the need to follow long-term treatment faithfully.

• Advise persons who have been exposed to infected patients to receive tuberculin tests and, if ordered, chest X-rays and prophylactic isoniazid.

PNEUMOCONIOSES

Silicosis

Silicosis is a progressive disease characterized by nodular lesions, which frequently progress to fibrosis. It is the most common form of pneumoconiosis. Silicosis can be classified according to the severity of pulmonary disease and the rapidity of its onset and progression; it usually occurs as a simple asymptomatic illness. Acute silicosis develops after 1 to 3 years in workers (sand blasters, tunnel workers) exposed to very high concentrations of respirable silica. Accelerated silicosis appears after an average of 10 years of exposure to lower concentrations of free silica. Chronic silicosis develops after 20 or more years of exposure to lower concentrations of free silica. Prognosis is good, unless the disease progresses into the complicated fibrotic form, which causes respiratory insufficiency and cor pulmonale, and is associated with pulmonary tuberculosis.

Causes

Silicosis results from the inhalation and pulmonary deposition of respirable crystalline silica dust, mostly from quartz. The danger to the worker depends on the concentration of dust in the atmosphere, the percentage of respirable free silica particles in the dust, and the duration of exposure. Respirable particles are less than 10 microns in diameter, but the disease-causing particles deposited in the alveolar space are usually 1 to 3 microns in diameter.

Industrial sources of silica in its pure form include the manufacture of ceramics (flint) and building materials (sandstone). It occurs in mixed form in the production of construction materials (cement); it's found in powder form (silica flour) in paints, porcelain, scouring soaps, and wood fillers, and in the mining of gold, coal, lead, zinc, and iron. Foundry workers, boiler scalers, and stonecutters are all exposed to silica dust and, therefore, are at high risk of developing silicosis.

Nodules result when alveolar macrophages ingest silica particles, which they are unable to process. As a result, the macrophages die and release proteolytic enzymes into the surrounding tissue. The subsequent inflammation attracts other macrophages and fibroblasts into the region to produce fibrous tissue and wall off the reaction. The resulting nodule has an onionskin appearance when viewed under a microscope. Nodules develop adjacent to terminal and respiratory bronchioles, concentrate in the upper lobes, and are frequently accompanied by bullous changes in both lobes. If the disease process does not progress, minimal physiologic disturbances and no disability occur. Occasionally, however, the fibrotic response accelerates, engulfing and destroying large areas of the lung (progressive massive fibrosis [PMF] or conglomerate lesions). Fibrosis may continue despite termination of exposure to dust.

Signs and symptoms

Silicosis initially may be asymptomatic, or it may produce dyspnea on exertion, often attributed to being "out of shape" or "slowing down." If the disease progresses to the chronic and complicated stage, dyspnea on exertion worsens, and other symptoms—usually tachypnea and an insidious dry cough, which is most pronounced in the morning—appear. Progression to the advanced stage causes dyspnea on minimal exertion, worsening cough, and pulmonary hypertension, which in turn leads to right ventricular failure and cor pulmonale. Patients with silicosis have a high incidence of active tuberculosis, which should be considered when evaluating a patient with this disease. CNS changes—confusion, lethargy, decrease in the rate and depth of respiration as P_{CO_2} increases—also occur in advanced silicosis. Other clinical features include malaise, disturbed sleep, and hoarseness. (*Note:* The severity of these symptoms may not correlate with chest X-ray findings or the results of pulmonary function studies.)

Diagnosis

Patient history reveals occupational exposure to silica dust. Physical examination is normal in *simple silicosis;* in *chronic silicosis* with conglomerate lesions, it may reveal decreased chest expansion, diminished intensity of breath sounds, areas of hypo- and hyperresonance, fine to medium rales, and tachypnea. In *simple silicosis,* chest X-rays show small, discrete, nodular lesions distributed throughout both lung fields but typically concentrated in the upper lung zones; the hilar lung nodes may be enlarged and exhibit "eggshell" calcification. In *complicated silicosis,* X-rays show one or more conglomerate masses of dense tissue.

Pulmonary function studies yield the following results:

- *FVC:* reduced in complicated silicosis
- *FEV_1:* reduced in obstructive disease (emphysematous areas of silicosis); reduced in complicated silicosis, but ratio of FEV_1 to FVC is normal or high
- *MVV:* reduced in both restrictive and obstructive diseases
- *DL_{CO}*: reduced when fibrosis destroys alveolar walls and obliterates pulmonary capillaries, or when fibrosis thickens alveolar capillary membrane.

In addition, arterial blood gas studies show:

- P_{O_2}: normal in simple silicosis; may be significantly decreased in the late stages of chronic or complicated disease, when the patient breathes room air
- P_{CO_2}: normal in early stages but may decrease due to hyperventilation; may increase as restrictive pattern develops, particularly if the patient is hypoxic and has severe impairment of alveolar ventilation.

Treatment and special considerations

The goal of treatment is to relieve respiratory symptoms, to manage hypoxia and cor pulmonale, and to prevent respiratory tract irritation and infections. Treatment also includes careful observation for the development of tuberculosis. Respiratory symptoms may be relieved through daily use of bronchodilating aerosols and increased fluid intake (at least 3 liters daily). Steam inhalation and chest physical therapy techniques, such as controlled coughing and segmental bronchial drainage, with chest percussion and vibration, help clear secretions. In severe cases, it may be necessary to administer oxygen by cannula or mask (1 to 2 liters/min) for the patient with chronic hypoxia, or by mechanical ventilation if arterial oxygen cannot be maintained above 40 mmHg. Respiratory infections require prompt administration of antibiotics.

• Teach the patient to prevent infections by avoiding crowds and persons with respiratory infections, and by receiving influenza and pneumococcal vaccines.

• Increase exercise tolerance by encouraging regular activity. Advise the patient to plan his daily activities to decrease the work of breathing; he should pace himself, rest often, and generally move slowly through his daily routine.

Asbestosis

Asbestosis is a form of pneumoconiosis characterized by diffuse interstitial fibrosis. It can develop as long as 15 to 20 years after regular exposure to asbestos has ended. Asbestos also causes pleural plaques and mesotheliomas of pleura and the peritoneum; a potent co-carcinogen, it aggravates the risk of lung cancer in cigarette smokers.

Causes

Asbestosis results from the inhalation of respirable asbestos fibers (50 microns or more in length, 0.5 microns or less in diameter), which assume a longitudinal orientation in the airway, move in the direction of airflow, and penetrate respiratory bronchioles and alveolar walls. Sources include the mining and milling of asbestos, the construction industry (where asbestos is used in a prefabricated form), and the fireproofing and textile industries; asbestos is also used in the production of paints, plastics, and brake and clutch linings.

Asbestos-related diseases develop in families of asbestos workers as a result of exposure to fibrous dust shaken off workers' clothing at home. Such diseases develop in the general public as a result of exposure to fibrous dust or waste piles from nearby asbestos plants.

Inhaled fibers become encased in a brown, proteinlike sheath rich in iron (ferruginous bodies or asbestos bodies), found in sputum and lung tissue. Interstitial fibrosis develops in lower lung zones, causing obliterative changes in lung parenchyma and pleurae. Raised hyaline plaques may form in parietal pleura, diaphragm, and pleura contiguous with the pericardium.

Signs and symptoms

Clinical features may appear before chest X-ray changes. The first symptom is usually dyspnea on exertion, typically after 10 years' exposure. As fibrosis extends, dyspnea on exertion increases, until eventually, dyspnea occurs even at rest; advanced disease also causes a dry cough (may be productive in smokers), chest pain (often pleuritic), recurrent respiratory infections, and tachypnea.

Cardiovascular complications include pulmonary hypertension, right ventricular hypertrophy, and cor pulmonale. Finger clubbing commonly occurs.

Diagnosis

Patient history reveals occupational, family, or neighborhood exposure to asbestos fibers. Physical examination reveals characteristic dry, crackling rales at bases of the lungs. Chest X-rays show fine, irregular, and linear diffuse infiltrates; extensive fibrosis results in a "honeycomb" or "ground glass" appearance. X-rays may also show pleural thickening and pleural calcification, with bilateral obliteration of costophrenic angles and, in later stages, an enlarged heart with a classic "shaggy" heart border.

Pulmonary function studies show:

- *VC, FVC, and TLC:* decreased
- *FEV_1:* decreased or normal
- *DL*CO: reduced when fibrosis destroys alveolar walls and thickens alveolar capillary membrane.

Arterial blood gas analysis reveals:

- *PO_2*: decreased
- *PCO_2*: low due to hyperventilation.

Treatment and special considerations

The goal of treatment is to relieve respiratory symptoms and, in advanced disease, manage hypoxia and cor pulmonale. Respiratory symptoms may be relieved by chest physical therapy techniques, such as controlled coughing and segmental bronchial drainage, with chest percussion and vibration. Aerosol therapy, inhaled mucolytics, and increased fluid intake (at least 3 liters daily) may also help relieve respiratory symptoms. Diuretics, digitalis preparations, and salt restriction may be indicated for patients with cor pulmonale. Hypoxia requires oxygen administration by cannula or mask (1 to 2 liters/min), or by mechanical ventilation if arterial oxygen cannot be maintained above 40 mmHg. Respiratory infections require prompt administration of antibiotics.

- Teach the patient to prevent infections by avoiding crowds and persons with infections and by receiving influenza and pneumococcal vaccines.
- Improve the patient's ventilatory efficiency by encouraging physical reconditioning, energy conservation in daily activities, and relaxation techniques.

Berylliosis

(Beryllium poisoning, beryllium disease)

Berylliosis, a form of pneumoconiosis, is a systemic granulomatous disorder with dominant pulmonary manifestations. It occurs in two forms: acute nonspecific pneumonitis and chronic noncaseating granulomatous disease with interstitial fibrosis, which may cause death from respiratory failure and cor pulmonale. Most patients with chronic interstitial disease become only slightly to moderately disabled by impaired lung function and other symptoms, but with each acute exacerbation the prognosis worsens.

Causes

Berylliosis is caused by the inhalation of beryllium dusts, fumes, and mists, with the pattern of disease related to the "dose" inhaled. Beryllium may also be absorbed through the skin. This disease occurs among beryllium alloy workers, cathode ray tube makers, gas mantle makers, missile technicians, and nuclear reactor workers; it's generally associated with the milling and use of beryllium, not with the mining of beryl ore. Berylliosis may also affect the families of workers as a result of dust shaken off workers' clothing at home and people who live near plants where beryllium alloy is used. The mechanism by which beryllium exerts its toxic effect is unknown.

Signs and symptoms

Absorption of beryllium through broken skin produces an itchy rash, which usually subsides within 2 weeks after exposure. A "beryllium ulcer" results from accidental implantation of beryllium metal in the skin.

Respiratory signs and symptoms of acute berylliosis include swelling and ulceration of nasal mucosa, which may progress to septal perforation, tracheitis, and bronchitis (dry cough). Acute pulmonary disease may develop rapidly (within 3 days) or weeks later, producing a progressive dry cough, tightness in the chest, substernal pain, tachycardia, and signs of bronchitis. This form of the disease has a significant mortality related to respiratory failure.

About 10% of patients with acute berylliosis develop chronic disease 10 to 15 years after exposure. The chronic form causes increasing dyspnea that becomes progressively unremitting, along with mild chest pain, dry unproductive cough, and tachypnea. Pneumothorax may occur, with pulmonary scarring and bleb formation.

Cardiovascular complications include pulmonary hypertension, right ventricular hypertrophy, and cor pulmonale. Other clinical features include hepatosplenomegaly, renal calculi, lymphadenopathy, anorexia, and fatigue.

Diagnosis

Patient history reveals occupational, family, or neighborhood exposure to beryllium dust, fumes, or mists. In *acute berylliosis,* chest X-rays may be suggestive of pulmonary edema, showing acute miliary process or a patchy acinous filling, and diffuse infiltrates with prominent peribronchial markings. In *chronic berylliosis,* X-rays show reticulonodular infiltrates and hilar adenopathy, and large coalescent infiltrates in both lungs.

Pulmonary function studies show decreased VC, FVC, RV/TLC, and DLCO, and compliance as lungs stiffen from fibrosis. Arterial blood gas analysis shows decreased P_{O_2} and P_{CO_2}.

The in vitro lymphocyte transformation test diagnoses berylliosis and monitors workers for occupational exposure to beryllium. Positive beryllium patch test establishes only hypersensitivity to beryllium, not the presence of disease. Tissue biopsy and spectrographic analysis are positive for most exposed workers but not absolutely diagnostic. In addition, urinalysis may show beryllium in urine, but this only indicates exposure. Differential diagnosis must rule out sarcoidosis and granulomatous infections.

Treatment and special considerations

Beryllium ulcer requires excision or curettage. Acute berylliosis requires prompt corticosteroid therapy. Hypoxia may require oxygen administration by nasal cannula or mask (1 to 2 liters/min). Severe respiratory failure requires mechanical ventilation if arterial oxygen cannot be maintained above 40 mmHg.

Chronic berylliosis is usually treated with corticosteroids, although it's not certain that steroids alter the progression of the disease. A lifelong maintenance dose may be necessary.

Respiratory symptoms may be treated with bronchodilators, increased fluid intake (at least 3 liters daily), and chest physical therapy techniques. Diuretics, digitalis preparations, and salt restriction may be useful in patients with cor pulmonale.

- Teach the patient to prevent infection by avoiding crowds and persons with infection, and by receiving influenza and pneumococcal vaccines.
- Encourage the patient to practice physical reconditioning, energy conservation in daily activities, and relaxation techniques.

Coal Worker's Pneumoconiosis

(Black lung disease, coal miner's disease, miner's asthma, anthracosis, anthracosilicosis)

A progressive nodular pulmonary disease, coal worker's pneumoconiosis (CWP) occurs in two forms. Simple CWP is characterized by small lung opacities; in complicated CWP, also known as progressive massive fibrosis (PMF), masses of fibrous tissue occasionally develop in the lungs of patients with simple CWP. The risk of developing CWP depends upon the duration of exposure to coal dust (usually

15 years or longer), intensity of exposure (dust count, particle size), location of the mine, silica content of the coal (anthracite coal has the highest silica content), and the worker's susceptibility. Incidence of CWP is highest among anthracite coal miners in the eastern United States. Prognosis varies. Simple asymptomatic disease is self-limiting, although progression to complicated CWP is more likely if CWP begins after a relatively short period of exposure. Complicated CWP may be disabling, resulting in severe ventilatory failure and right heart failure secondary to pulmonary hypertension.

Causes

CWP is caused by the inhalation and prolonged retention of respirable coal dust particles (less than 5 microns in diameter). *Simple CWP* results in the formation of macules (accumulations of macrophages laden with coal dust) around the terminal and respiratory bronchioles, surrounded by a halo of dilated alveoli. Macule formation leads to atrophy of supporting tissue, causing permanent dilation of small airways (focal emphysema). Simple disease may progress to *complicated CWP*, involving one or both lungs. In this form of the disease, fibrous tissue masses enlarge and coalesce, causing gross distortion of pulmonary structures (destruction of vasculature, alveoli, and airways).

Signs and symptoms

Simple CWP is asymptomatic, especially in nonsmokers. Symptoms appear if PMF develops and include exertional dyspnea and a cough that is occasionally productive of inky-black sputum, when fibrotic changes undergo avascular necrosis and their centers cavitate. Other clinical features of CWP include increasing dyspnea and a cough that produces milky, gray, clear, or coal-flecked sputum. Recurrent bronchial and pulmonary infections produce yellow, green, or thick sputum.

Complications include pulmonary hypertension, right ventricular hypertrophy and cor pulmonale, and pulmonary tuberculosis. In cigarette smokers, chronic bronchitis and emphysema may also complicate the disease.

Diagnosis

Patient history reveals exposure to coal dust. Physical examination shows barrel chest, hyperresonant lungs with areas of dullness, diminished breath sounds, rales, rhonchi, and wheezes. In *simple CWP*, chest X-rays show small opacities (less than 10 mm in diameter), which may be present in all lung zones but are more prominent in the upper lung zones; in *complicated CWP*, one or more large opacities (1 to 5 cm in diameter), possibly exhibiting cavitation, are seen.

The results of pulmonary function studies include:

- *VC:* normal in simple CWP, but decreased with PMF
- *FEV_1:* decreased in complicated disease
- *RV/TLC:* normal in simple CWP; decreased in PMF
- *DLCO*: significantly decreased in complicated CWP as alveolar septae are destroyed and pulmonary capillaries obliterated.

In addition, arterial blood gas studies show:

- PO_2: normal in simple CWP, but decreased in complicated disease
- PCO_2: normal in simple CWP, but may decrease due to hyperventilation; may also increase if the patient is hypoxic and has severe impairment of alveolar ventilation.

Treatment and special considerations

The goal of treatment is to relieve respiratory symptoms, to manage hypoxia and cor pulmonale, and to avoid respiratory tract irritants and infections. Treatment also includes careful observation for the development of tuberculosis. Respiratory symptoms may be relieved through bronchodilator therapy with theophylline or aminophylline (if bronchospasm is reversible), oral or inhaled sympathomimetic amines (metaproterenol), corticosteroids (oral prednisone or an aerosol form of beclomethasone), or cromolyn sodium aerosol. Chest physical therapy techniques, such as controlled coughing and segmental bronchial drainage, with chest percussion and vibration, help remove secretions.

Other measures include increased fluid intake (at least 3 liters daily) and respiratory therapy techniques, such as aerosol therapy, inhaled mucolytics, and intermittent positive pressure breathing (IPPB). Diuretics, digitalis preparations, and salt restriction may be indicated in cor pulmonale. In severe cases, it may be necessary to administer oxygen for hypoxia by cannula or mask (1 to 2 liters/min) if the patient has chronic hypoxia, or by mechanical ventilation if arterial oxygen cannot be maintained above 40 mmHg. Respiratory infections require prompt administration of antibiotics.

- Teach the patient to prevent infections by avoiding crowds and persons with respiratory infections, and by receiving influenza and pneumococcal vaccines.
- Encourage the patient to stay active to avoid a deterioration in his physical condition, but to pace his activities and practice relaxation techniques.

Selected References

Bell, C. William. *Home Care and Rehabilitation in Respiratory Medicine*. Philadelphia: J.B. Lippincott, Co., 1984.

Boyda, Ellen K., *Respiratory Problems*, vol. 5. Oradell, N.J.: Medical Economics, 1983.

Burton, George G., and Hodgkin, John E., eds. *Respiratory Care: A Guide to Clinical Practice*, 2nd ed. Philadelphia: J.B. Lippincott Co., 1984.

Harper, Rosalind W. *A Guide to Respiratory Care: Physiology and Clinical Applications*. Philadelphia: J.B. Lippincott Co., 1982.

Hinshaw, H. Corwin, et al. *Diseases of the Chest*, 4th ed. Philadelphia: J.B. Lippincott Co., 1980.

Moser, Kenneth M., and Spragg, Robert G. *Respiratory Emergencies*, 2nd ed. St. Louis: C.V. Mosby Co., 1982.

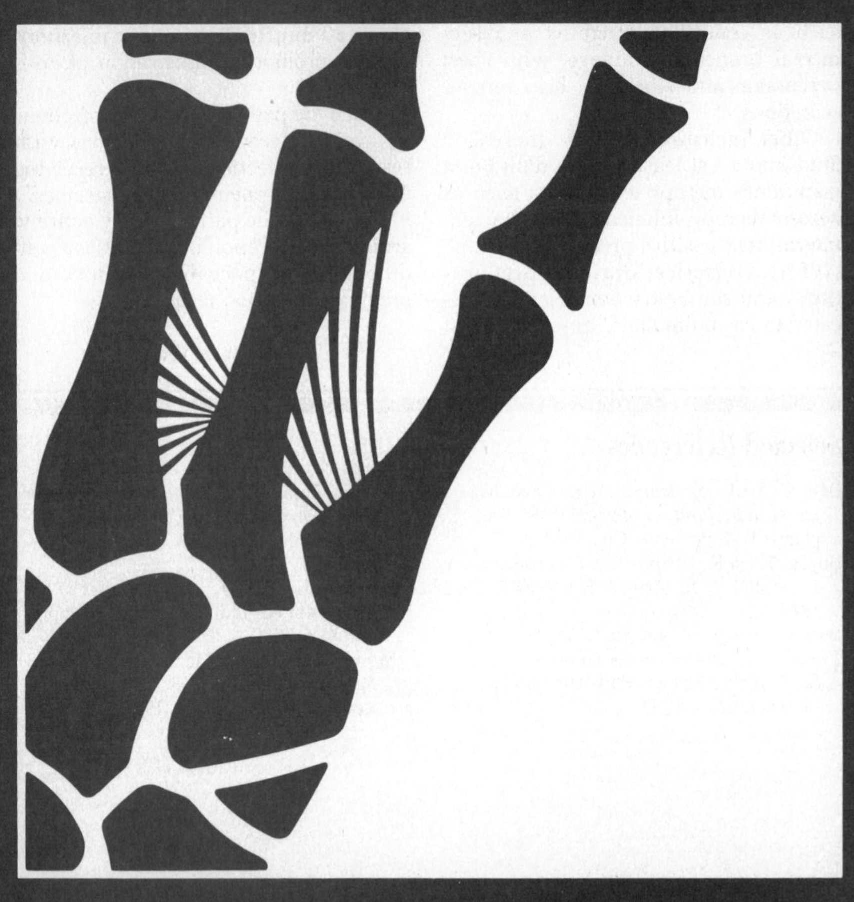

8 Musculoskeletal Disorders

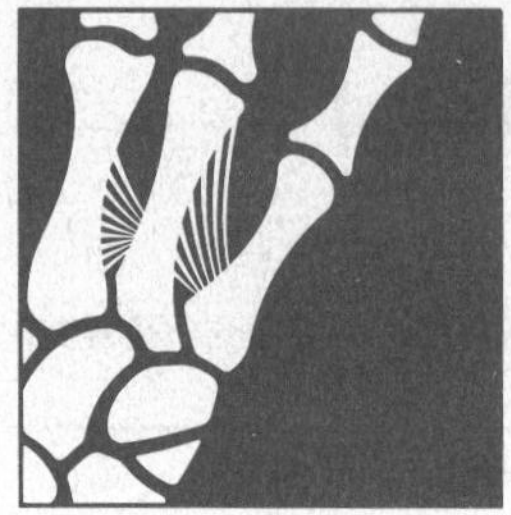

Musculoskeletal Disorders

Introduction

A complex system of bones, muscles, ligaments, tendons, and other connective tissue, the musculoskeletal system gives the body form and shape. It also protects vital organs, makes movement possible, stores calcium and other minerals, and provides the site for hematopoiesis.

The human skeleton contains 206 bones, which are composed of inorganic salts, such as calcium and phosphate, imbedded in a framework of collagen fibers. Bones are classified by shape: long, short, flat, or irregular.

Long bones

Long bones are found in the extremities, and include the humerus, radius, and ulna of the arm; the femur, tibia, and fibula of the leg; the phalanges, metacarpals, and metatarsals. These bones have a long shaft, or diaphysis, and widened, bulbous ends, called epiphyses. A long bone is made up mainly of compact bone, which surrounds the medullary cavity (also called the yellow marrow), a storage site for fat. The lining of the medullary cavity (the endosteum) is a thin layer of connective tissue. The outer layer is the periosteum.

In children and young adults, epiphyseal cartilage separates the diaphysis and epiphysis, allowing the bone to grow longer. In adults, in whom bone growth is complete, this cartilage is ossified and forms the epiphyseal line. The epiphysis also has a surface layer made up of compact bone, but its center is made of spongy or cancellous bone. Cancellous bone contains open spaces between thin threads of bone, called trabeculae, which are arranged in various directions to correspond with the lines of maximum stress or pressure. This gives the bone added structural strength.

Unlike cancellous bone, adult compact bone is composed of numerous orderly networks of interconnecting canals. Each of these networks is called a haversian system and consists of a central haversian canal surrounded by layers (lamellae) of bone. Between adjacent lamellae are small openings called lacunae, which contain bone cells or osteocytes. All lacunae are joined by an interconnecting network of tiny canals called canaliculi, each of which contains one or more capillaries and provides a route for tissue fluids. The haversian system runs parallel to the bone's long axis and is responsible for carrying blood to the bone through blood vessels that enter the system through Volkmann's canal.

Short, flat, or irregular bones

Short bones include the tarsal and carpal bones; flat bones, the frontal and parietal bones of the cranium, ribs, sternum, scapulae, ilium, and pubis; and irregular bones, the bones of the spine (vertebrae, sacrum, coccyx) and certain bones of the skull—the sphenoid, ethmoid, and mandible.

A short, flat, or irregular bone has an outer layer of compact bone and an inner portion of spongy bone, which in some bones—the sternum and certain areas in the flat bones of the skull—contain red marrow.

All bones are covered by a fibrous layer called the periosteum except at joints, where they're covered by articular cartilage.

Joints

The tissues connecting two bones comprise a joint, which allows for motion between the bones and provides stability. Joints, like bones, have varying forms.

• *Fibrous joints,* called synarthroses, have only minute motion and provide stability when tight union is necessary, as in the sutures that join the cranial bones.

• *Cartilaginous joints,* called amphiarthroses, allow limited motion, as between vertebrae.

• *Synovial joints,* called diarthroses, are the most common and allow the greatest degree of movement. Such joints include the elbows and knees. Synovial joints have special characteristics: the bones' two articulating surfaces have a smooth hyaline covering (articular cartilage), which is resilient to pressure; their opposing surfaces are congruous and glide smoothly on each other; a fibrous (articular) capsule holds them together. Beneath the capsule, lining the joint cavity, is the synovial membrane, which secretes a clear viscous fluid called synovial fluid. This fluid lubricates the two opposing surfaces during motion and also nourishes the articular cartilage. Surrounding a synovial joint are ligaments, muscles, and tendons, which strengthen and stabilize the joint but allow free movement.

In some synovial joints, the synovial membrane forms two additional structures—bursae and tendon sheaths—which reduce friction that normally accompanies movement. Bursae are small, cushionlike sacs lined with synovial membranes and filled with synovial fluid; most are located between tendons and bones. Tendon sheaths wrap around the tendon and cushion it as it crosses the joint.

There are two types of synovial joint movements: angular and circular. Angular movements include *flexion* (decrease in joint angle), *extension* (increase in the joint angle), and *hyperextension* (increase in the angle of extension beyond the usual arc). Joints of the knees, elbows, and phalanges permit such movement. Other angular movements are *abduction* (movement away from the body's midline) and *adduction* (movement toward the body's midline).

Circular movements include *rotation* (motion around a central axis), as in the ball and socket joints of the hips and shoulders; *pronation* (wrist motion to place palmar surface of the hand down, with the thumb toward the body); *supination* (begging position, with palm up). Other kinds of movement are *inversion* (movement facing inward), *eversion* (movement facing outward), *protraction* (as in forward motion of mandible), and *retraction* (returning protracted part into place).

Muscles make motion possible

Muscle tissues' most specialized feature—contractility—makes movement of bones and joints possible. Muscles also pump blood through the body, move food through the intestines, and make breathing possible. Muscular activity produces heat, making it an important component in temperature regulation. Muscles maintain body positions, such as sitting and standing. Muscle mass accounts for about 40% of a man's weight.

Muscles are classified in many ways. *Skeletal* muscles are attached to bone; *visceral* muscles permit function of internal organs; and *cardiac* muscles comprise the heart wall. Also, muscles may be striated or nonstriated (smooth), depending on their cellular configuration.

When muscles are classified according to activity, they are voluntary or involuntary. *Voluntary* muscles can be controlled at will and are under the influence of the somatic nervous system; these are the skeletal muscles. *Involuntary* muscles, controlled by the autonomic nervous system, include the cardiac and visceral muscles.

Each skeletal muscle is composed of many elongated muscle cells, called *muscle fibers,* through which run slender threads of protein, called myofibrils. Muscle fibers are held together in bundles by sheaths of fibrous tissue, called fascia. Blood vessels and nerves pass into muscles through the fascia to reach the individual muscle fibers.

Skeletal muscles are attached to bone directly or indirectly by fibrous cords known as tendons. The least movable end of the muscle attachment (generally proximal) is called the point of origin; the most movable end (generally distal) is the point of insertion.

Mechanism of contraction

To stimulate muscle contraction and movement, the brain sends motor impulses by the peripheral motor nerves to the voluntary muscle, which contains motor nerve fibers. These fibers reach membranes of skeletal muscle cells at neuromuscular (myoneural) junctions. When an impulse reaches the myoneural junction, the neurochemical acetylcholine is released. This triggers the transient release of calcium from the sarcoplasmic reticulum, a membranous network in the muscle fiber, which, in turn, triggers muscle contraction. The energy source for such contraction is adenosine triphosphate (ATP). ATP release is also triggered by the impulse at the myoneural junction. Relaxation of a muscle is believed to take place by reversal of the above mechanisms.

Musculoskeletal assessment

Patients with musculoskeletal disorders are often elderly, have other concurrent medical conditions, or are victims of trauma. Generally, they face prolonged immobilization. These factors make thorough assessment essential. Your assessment should include a complete history and a careful physical examination.

Interview the patient carefully to obtain a complete medical, social, and personal history. Ask about general activity (does he jog daily, or is he sedentary?), which may be significantly altered by musculoskeletal disease or trauma. Obtain information about occupation, diet, sexual activity, and elimination habits, and try to assess how the problem will affect body image. Also, ask how he functions at home. Can he perform daily activities? Does he have trouble getting around? Are there stairs where he lives? Where are the bathroom and bedroom? Does he use any prosthetic devices? Ask

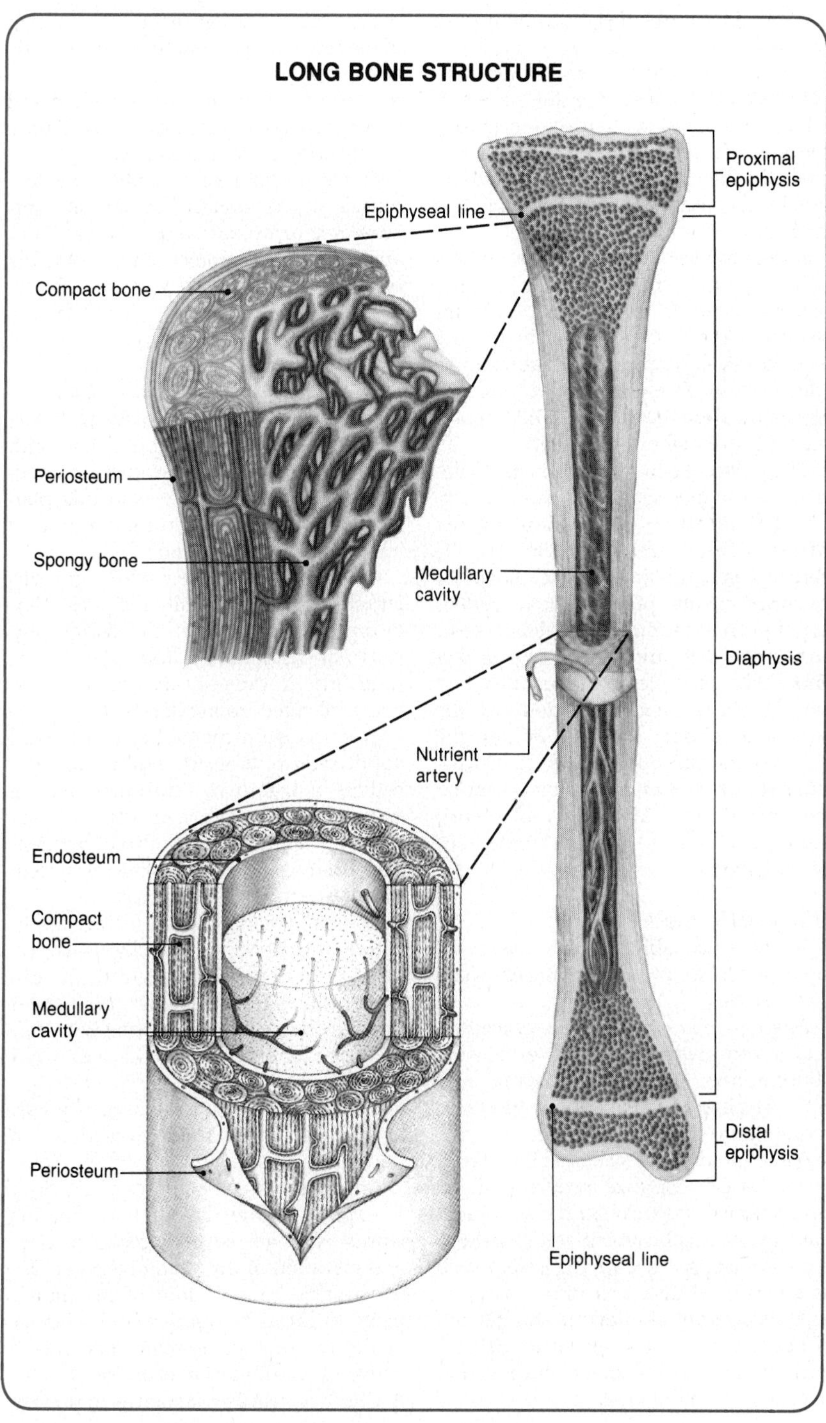
LONG BONE STRUCTURE
Proximal epiphysis
Epiphyseal line
Compact bone
Periosteum
Spongy bone
Medullary cavity
Diaphysis
Nutrient artery
Endosteum
Compact bone
Medullary cavity
Periosteum
Distal epiphysis
Epiphyseal line

if other family members can help with his care.

Get an accurate account of the musculoskeletal problem. Ask the patient if it has caused him to change his everyday routine. When did symptoms begin and how did they progress? Has the patient previously received treatment for this problem?

Assess the level of pain. Is the patient in pain at the moment? Evaluate past and present response to treatment. For instance, if the patient has arthritis and uses corticosteroids, ask him about their effectiveness. Does he require more or less medication than before? Did he comply with prescribed treatment?

The physical examination helps to determine diagnosis and records any existing disabilities for evaluating the effects of future treatment. Observe the patient's general appearance. Look for localized edema, pigmentation, reddening of pressure points, point tenderness, and other deformities (atrophy or kyphosis, for example). Note mobility and gait. To check range of motion, ask the patient to abduct, adduct, or flex the muscles in question. Check neurovascular status, including motion sensation and circulation. Measure and record discrepancies in muscle circumference or leg length.

Diagnostic tools

• *X-ray* is probably the most useful diagnostic tool for evaluating musculoskeletal diseases.
• *Myelography* is an invasive procedure that is especially helpful for evaluating abnormalities of the spinal canal and cord. Myelography entails injection of a radiopaque contrast medium into the subarachnoid space of the spine. Then, serial X-rays visualize progress of the contrast medium through the subarachnoid space. Displacement of the medium indicates a space-occupying lesion, such as a herniated disk or a tumor.
• *Arthrography* similarly is an injection of opaque contrast material to give information regarding shape, outline, and integrity of a joint capsule.
• *Arthroscopy* is the visual examination of the interior of a joint with a fiberoptic endoscope.
• *Bone scan* identifies areas of increased bone activity or active bone formation by injection of radioisotopes.

Other useful tests include bone and muscle biopsies, electromyography, microscopic examination of synovial fluid, and multiple laboratory studies of urine and blood to identify systemic abnormalities.

Patient care

Each patient with musculoskeletal disease needs an individual care plan formulated early in his hospital stay, with the doctor, physical therapist, and occupational therapist. Develop this plan with short- and long-term goals, during and after hospitalization.

Caring for the patient with a musculoskeletal disease usually includes managing at least one of the following: traction, casts, braces, splints, crutches, intermittent range-of-motion devices, and prolonged immobilization.

Traction is the manual or mechanical application of a steady pulling force to reduce a fracture, minimize muscle spasms, or immobilize or align a joint.
• *Skin traction* is the indirect application of traction to the skeletal system through skin and soft tissues.
• *Skeletal traction* is the direct application of traction to bones by transversing the affected bone with a pin (Steinmann's pin) or wire (Kirschner wire) or by gripping the bone with calipers or a tonglike device (Gardner-Wells tongs).
• *Manual traction,* for emergency use, is the direct application of traction to a body part by hand.

During the use of all types of traction:
• Explain to the patient how traction works, and advise how much activity and elevation of the head of the bed are permissible. Inform him of the anticipated duration of traction and whether or not the traction is removable. Teach active range-of-motion exercises.
• Check neurovascular status to prevent

nerve damage. Also, make sure the mattress is firm, that the traction ropes aren't frayed, that they're on the center track of the pulley, and that traction weights are hanging free. Thoroughly investigate any complaint the patient makes.

- Check for signs of infection (odor, local inflammation and drainage, fever) at pin sites if the patient is in skeletal traction. Also, check with the doctor regarding pin site care, such as use of peroxide or povidone-iodine.

Ideally, a cast immobilizes without adding too much weight. It's snug-fitting but doesn't constrict, and has a smooth inner surface and smooth edges to prevent pressure or skin irritation. Casts require comprehensive patient teaching.

- A wet cast takes 24 to 48 hours to dry. To prevent indentations, tell the patient not to squeeze the cast with his fingers; not to cover or walk on the cast until it has dried; not to bump a damp cast on hard surfaces, since dents can cause pressure areas. Warn the patient that while the cast is drying he'll feel a transient sensation of heat under the cast.
- Emphasize the need to keep the cast above heart level for *24 hours* following its application, to reduce swelling in the extremity.
- While the cast is drying and after drying is complete, the patient should watch for and immediately report persistent pain in the extremity inside or distal to the cast, as well as edema, changes in skin color, coldness, or tingling or numbness in this area. If any of these signs occur, tell the patient to position the casted body part above heart level and notify his doctor.
- The patient should also report drainage through the cast, or an odor that may indicate infection. Warn against inserting foreign objects under the cast, getting it wet, pulling out its padding, or scratching inside it. Tell the patient to seek immediate attention for a broken cast.
- Instruct the patient to exercise the joints above and below the cast to prevent stiffness and contracture.

Braces, splints, and slings also provide alignment, immobilization, and pain relief for musculoskeletal diseases. Slings and splints are usually used for short-term immobilization. Explain to the patient and his family why these appliances are necessary, and show them how to properly apply the sling, splint, or brace for optimal benefit. Tell the patient how long the appliance will have to be worn, and advise him of any activity limitations that must be observed. If the patient has a brace, check with his orthotist about proper care. Encourage the patient to refer additional questions to his doctor. Teach proper crutch-walking.

Coping with immobility

Immobilized patients require meticulous care to prevent complications. Without constant care, the bedridden patient becomes susceptible to decubitus ulcers, caused by the increased pressure on tissue over bony prominences, and is especially vulnerable to cardiopulmonary complications.

- To prevent decubitus ulcers, turn the patient regularly, massage areas over bony prominences, and place a flotation pad, a sheepskin pad, or an alternating-air-current, egg crate, or foam mattress under bony prominences. Show the patient how to use a Balkan frame with a trapeze to move about in bed.
- Increase fluid intake to minimize risk of renal calculi.
- Perform passive range-of-motion exercises on the affected side, as ordered, to prevent contractures, and instruct the patient in active range-of-motion exercises on the unaffected side. Apply footboards or high-topped sneakers to prevent footdrop.
- Since most bedridden patients involuntarily perform a Valsalva maneuver when using the upper arms and trunk to move, instruct the patient to exhale (instead of holding his breath) as he turns. This will prevent possible cardiac complications that result from increased intrathoracic pressure.
- Emphasize the importance of coughing and deep breathing, and teach the

patient how to use the incentive spirometer, if ordered.

• Because constipation is a common problem in bedridden patients, establish a bowel program (fluids, roughage, laxatives, stool softeners), as needed.

Rehabilitation
Restoring the patient to his former state of health is not always possible. When it is not, help the patient adjust to a modified life-style. During hospitalization, promote independence by letting him finish difficult tasks by himself. If necessary, refer the patient to a community facility for continued rehabilitation.

CONGENITAL DISORDERS

Clubfoot

(Talipes)

Clubfoot, the most common congenital disorder of the lower extremities, is marked primarily by a deformed talus and shortened Achilles tendon, which give the foot a characteristic clublike appearance. In talipes equinovarus, the foot points downward (equinus) and turns inward (varus), while the front of the foot curls toward the heel (forefoot adduction).

Clubfoot, which has an incidence of approximately 1 per 1,000 live births, usually occurs bilaterally and is twice as common in boys as in girls. It may be associated with other birth defects, such as myelomeningocele, spina bifida, and arthrogryposis. Clubfoot is correctable with prompt treatment.

Causes
A combination of genetic and environmental factors in utero appears to cause clubfoot. Heredity is a definite factor in some cases, although the mechanism of transmission is undetermined. If a child is born with clubfoot, his sibling has a 1 in 35 chance of being born with the same anomaly. Children of a parent with clubfoot have 1 chance in 10. In children without a family history of clubfoot, this anomaly seems linked to arrested development during the ninth and tenth weeks of embryonic life, when the feet are formed. Researchers also suspect muscle abnormalities, leading to variations in length and tendon insertions, as possible causes of clubfoot.

Signs and symptoms
Talipes equinovarus varies greatly in severity. Deformity may be so extreme that the toes touch the inside of the ankle, or it may be only vaguely apparent. In every case, the talus is deformed, the Achilles tendon shortened, and the calcaneus somewhat shortened and flattened. Depending on the degree of the varus deformity, the calf muscles are shortened and underdeveloped, with soft-tissue contractures at the site of the deformity. The foot is tight in its deformed position and resists manual efforts to push it back into normal position. Clubfoot is painless, except in elderly, arthritic patients. In older children, clubfoot may be secondary to paralysis, poliomyelitis, or cerebral palsy, in which case treatment must include management of the underlying disease.

Diagnosis
Early diagnosis of clubfoot is usually no problem, because the deformity is ob-

vious. In subtle deformity, however, true clubfoot must be distinguished from apparent clubfoot (metatarsus varus or pigeon toe). Apparent clubfoot results when a fetus maintains a position in utero that gives his feet a clubfoot appearance at birth. This can usually be corrected manually. Another form of apparent clubfoot is inversion of the feet, resulting from the peroneal type of progressive muscular atrophy and progressive muscular dystrophy. In true clubfoot, X-rays show superimposition of the talus and the calcaneus and a ladderlike appearance of the metatarsals.

Treatment

Treatment for clubfoot is administered in three stages: correcting the deformity, maintaining the correction until the foot regains normal muscle balance, and observing the foot closely for several years to prevent the deformity from recurring. In newborns, corrective treatment for true clubfoot should begin *at once*. An infant's foot contains large amounts of cartilage; the muscles, ligaments, and tendons are supple. The ideal time to begin treatment is during the first few days and weeks of life—when the foot is most malleable.

Clubfoot deformities are usually corrected in sequential order: forefoot adduction first, then varus (or inversion), then equinus (or plantar flexion). Trying to correct all three deformities at once only results in a misshapen, rocker-bottomed foot. Forefoot adduction is corrected by uncurling the front of the foot away from the heel (forefoot abduction); the varus deformity is corrected by turning the foot so the sole faces outward (eversion); and finally, equinus is corrected by casting the foot with the toes pointing up (dorsiflexion). This last correction may have to be supplemented with a subcutaneous tenotomy of the Achilles tendon and posterior capsulotomy of the ankle joint.

Several therapeutic methods have been tested and found effective in correcting clubfoot. The first is simple manipulation and casting, whereby the foot is gently manipulated into a partially corrected position, then held there in a cast for several days or weeks. (The skin should be painted with a nonirritating adhesive liquid beforehand to prevent the cast from slipping.) After the cast is removed, the foot is manipulated into an even better position and casted again. This procedure is repeated as many times as necessary. In some cases, the shape of the cast can be transformed through a series of wedging maneuvers (Kite method), instead of changing the cast each time.

After correction of clubfoot, proper foot alignment should be maintained through exercise, night splints, and orthopedic shoes. With manipulating and casting, correction usually takes about 3 months. The Denis Browne splint, a device that consists of two padded, metal footplates connected by a flat, horizontal bar, is sometimes used as a follow-up measure to help promote bilateral correction and strengthen the foot muscles.

Resistant clubfoot may require surgery. Older children, for example, with recurrent or neglected clubfoot usually need surgery. Tenotomy, tendon transfer, stripping of the plantar fascia, and capsulotomy are some of the surgical procedures that may be used. In severe cases, bone surgery (wedge resections, osteotomy, or astragalectomy) may be appropriate. After surgery, a cast is applied to preserve the correction. Whenever clubfoot is severe enough to require surgery, it's rarely totally correctable; however, surgery can usually ameliorate the deformity.

Special considerations

The primary concern is recognition of clubfoot as early as possible, preferably in newborn infants.

- Look for any exaggerated attitudes in an infant's feet. Make sure you can recognize the difference between true clubfoot and apparent clubfoot. Don't use excessive force in trying to manipulate a clubfoot. The foot with apparent clubfoot moves easily.
- Stress the importance of prompt treat-

ment to parents. Make sure they understand that clubfoot demands immediate therapy and orthopedic supervision until growth is completed.

• After casting, elevate the child's feet with pillows. Check the toes every 1 to 2 hours for temperature, color, sensation, motion, and capillary refill time; watch for edema. Before a child in a clubfoot cast is discharged, teach parents to recognize circulatory impairment.

• Insert plastic petals over the top edges of a new cast while it's still wet, to keep urine from soaking and softening the cast. When the cast is dry, "petal" the edges with adhesive tape to keep out plaster crumbs and prevent skin irritation. Perform good skin care under the cast edges every 4 hours. After washing and drying the skin, rub it with alcohol. (Don't use oils or powders; they tend to macerate the skin.)

• Warn parents of an older child not to let the foot part of the cast get soft and thin from wear. If it does, much of the correction may be lost.

• When the Kite method is being used, check circulatory status frequently; it may be impaired because of increased pressure on tissues and blood vessels. The equinus correction especially places considerable strain on ligaments, blood vessels, and tendons.

• After surgery, elevate the child's feet with pillows to decrease swelling and pain. Report any signs of discomfort or pain immediately. Try to locate the source of pain—it may result from cast pressure, not the incision. If bleeding occurs under the cast, circle the location and mark the time on the cast. If bleeding spreads, report it.

• Explain to the older child and his parents that in older children, surgery can improve clubfoot but can't totally correct it.

• Emphasize the need for long-term orthopedic care to maintain correction. Teach parents the prescribed exercises that the child can do at home. Urge them to make the child wear the corrective shoes ordered and the splints during naps and at night. Make sure they understand that treatment for clubfoot continues during the entire growth period. Correcting this defect permanently takes time and patience.

Congenital Hip Dysplasia

Congenital dysplasia, an abnormality of the hip joint present from birth, is the most common disorder that affects the hip joints of children under age 3. It can be unilateral or bilateral. This abnormality occurs in three forms of varying severity: unstable hip dysplasia, *in which the hip is positioned normally but can be dislocated by manipulation;* subluxation or incomplete dislocation, *in which the femoral head rides on the edge of the acetabulum; and* complete dislocation, *in which the femoral head is totally outside the acetabulum.*

Congenital hip subluxation or dislocation can cause abnormal acetabular development and permanent disability. About 85% of affected infants are females.

Causes

Unproven theories exist concerning the cause of congenital hip dysplasia.

• Hormones that relax maternal ligaments in preparation for labor may also cause laxity of infant ligaments around the capsule of the hip joint.

• Dislocation is 10 times more common after breech delivery (malpositioning in utero) than after cephalic delivery.

Signs and symptoms

Clinical effects of hip dysplasia vary with age. In newborns, dysplasia produces no gross deformity or pain. However, in complete dysplasia, the hip rides above the acetabulum, causing the leg on the affected side to appear shorter or the affected hip more prominent. As the child grows older and begins to walk, uncorrected bilateral dysplasia may cause him to sway from side to side, a condition known as "duck waddle"; unilateral dysplasia may produce a limp. If corrective treatment isn't begun until after age 2, congenital hip dysplasia may cause degenerative hip changes, lordosis, joint malformation, and soft-tissue damage.

Diagnosis

Several observations during physical examination of the relaxed child strongly suggest congenital hip dysplasia. First, place the child on his back, and inspect the folds of skin over his thighs. Usually, a child in this position has an equal number of thigh folds on each side, but a child with subluxation or dislocation may have an extra fold on the affected side (this extra fold is also apparent when the child lies prone). Next, with the child lying prone, check for alignment of the buttock fold. In a child with dysplasia, the buttock fold on the affected side is higher. In addition, abduction of the affected hip is restricted.

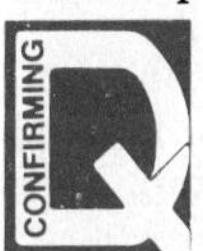

A positive Ortolani's or Trendelenburg's sign confirms congenital hip dysplasia. To test for the Ortolani sign, place the infant on his back, with his hip flexed and in abduction. Adduct the hip while pressing the femur downward. This will dislocate the hip. Then, abduct the hip while moving the femur upward. If you hear a click or feel a jerk (produced by the femoral head moving over the acetabular rim) this indicates subluxation in an infant younger than 1 month; this sign indicates subluxation or complete dislocation in an older infant.

To elicit Trendelenburg's sign, have the child rest his weight on the side of the dislocation and lift his other knee. His pelvis drops on the normal side because of weak abductor muscles in the affected hip. However, when the child stands with his weight on the normal side and lifts the other knee, the pelvis remains horizontal; these phenomena make up a positive Trendelenburg's sign.

X-rays show the location of the femur head and a shallow acetabulum; X-rays can also monitor the progress of the disease or treatment.

Treatment

The earlier the infant receives treatment, the better his chances are for normal development. Treatment varies with the patient's age. In infants younger than 3 months, treatment includes *gentle* manipulation to reduce the dislocation, followed by holding the hips in a flexed and abducted position with a splint-brace or harness, to maintain the reduction. The infant must wear this apparatus continuously for 2 to 3 months and then use a night splint for another month, so the joint capsule can tighten and stabilize in correct alignment.

If treatment doesn't begin until after age 3 months, it may include bilateral skin traction (in infants) or skeletal traction (in children who have started walking) in an attempt to reduce the dislocation by gradually abducting the hips. If traction fails, gentle closed reduction under general anesthetic can further abduct the hips; the child is then placed in a spica cast for 4 to 6 months. If closed treatment fails, open reduction, followed by immobilization in a spica cast for an average of 6 months, or osteotomy may be considered.

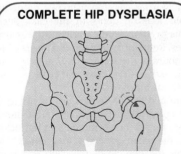

COMPLETE HIP DYSPLASIA

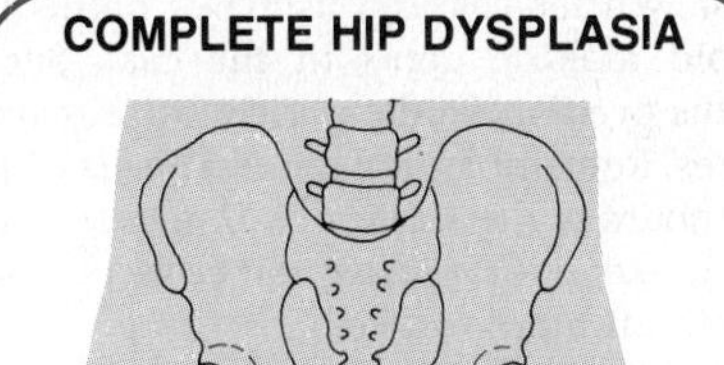

In complete dislocation, the femoral head (right) is totally displaced outside the acetabulum.

In the child aged 2 to 5 years, treatment is difficult and includes skeletal traction and subcutaneous adductor tenotomy. Treatment begun after age 5 rarely restores satisfactory hip function.

Special considerations

The child who must wear a splint, brace, or body cast needs special personal care, requiring parent teaching.

- Teach parents how to correctly splint or brace the hips, as ordered. Stress the need for frequent checkups.
- Listen sympathetically to the parents' expressions of anxiety and fear. Explain possible causes of congenital hip dislocation, and give reasssurance that early, prompt treatment will probably result in complete correction.
- During the child's first few days in a cast or splint-brace, encourage his parents to stay with him as much as possible to calm and reassure him, since restricted movement will make him irritable.
- Assure parents that the child will adjust to this restriction and return to normal sleeping, eating, and playing behavior in a few days.
- Instruct parents to remove braces and splints while bathing the infant but to replace them immediately afterward. Stress good hygiene; parents should bathe and change the child frequently and wash his perineum with warm water and soap at each diaper change.

If treatment requires a spica cast:

- When transferring the child immediately after casting, use your palms to avoid making dents in the cast. Such dents predispose the patient to pressure sores. Remember that the cast needs 24 to 48 hours to dry naturally. Don't use heat to make it dry faster, since heat also makes it more fragile.
- Immediately after the cast is applied, use a plastic sheet to protect it from moisture around the perineum and buttocks. Cut the sheet in strips long enough to cover the outside of the cast, and tuck them about a finger length beneath the cast edges. Using overlapping strips of tape, tack the corner of each petal to the outside of the cast. Remove the plastic under the cast every 4 hours; then wash, dry, and retuck it. Disposable diapers folded lengthwise over the perineum may also be used.
- Position the child either on a Bradford frame elevated on blocks, with a bedpan under the frame, or on pillows to support the child's legs. Be sure to keep the cast dry, and change diapers often.
- Wash and dry the skin under the cast edges every 2 to 4 hours, and rub it with alcohol. Don't use oils or powders; they can macerate skin.
- Turn the child every 2 hours during the day, and every 4 hours at night. Check color, sensation, and motion of the infant's legs and feet. Be sure to examine all his toes. Notify the doctor of dusky, cool, or numb toes.
- Shine a flashlight under the cast every 4 hours to check for objects and crumbs. Check the cast daily for odors, which may herald infection. Record temperature daily.
- If the child complains of itching, he may benefit from diphenhydramine. Or you may aim a hair dryer set on cool at the cast edges to relieve itching. Don't scratch or probe under the cast. Investigate any persistent itching.
- Provide adequate nutrition, and maintain adequate fluid intake to avoid renal calculi and constipation, both complications of inactivity.
- If the child is very restless, apply a jacket restraint to keep him from falling out of bed or off the frame.
- Provide adequate stimuli to promote growth and development. If the child's hips are abducted in a froglike position, tell parents that he may be able to fit on a kiddy car. Encourage parents to let the child sit at a table by seating him on pillows on a chair, to put him on the floor for short periods of play and to let him play with other children his age.
- Tell parents to watch for signs that the child is outgrowing the cast (cyanosis, cool extremities, pain).
- Tell the parents that treatment may be prolonged and requires patience.

Muscular Dystrophy

Muscular dystrophy is actually a group of congenital disorders characterized by progressive symmetric wasting of skeletal muscles without neural or sensory defects. Paradoxically, these wasted muscles tend to enlarge because of connective tissue and fat deposits, giving an erroneous impression of muscle strength. Four main types of muscular dystrophy occur: pseudohypertrophic *(Duchenne's)* muscular dystrophy, *which accounts for 50% of all cases;* facioscapulohumeral *(Landouzy-Dejerine)* dystrophy; limb-girdle *(Erb's)* dystrophy; *and a* mixed *type.*

Prognosis varies. Duchenne's muscular dystrophy generally strikes during early childhood and results in death within 10 to 15 years of onset. Facioscapulohumeral and limb-girdle dystrophies usually don't shorten life expectancy. The mixed type progresses rapidly and is usually fatal within 5 years after onset.

Causes and incidence

Duchenne's muscular dystrophy is an X-linked recessive disorder, affecting males most often; incidence is approximately 4 per 100,000. Facioscapulohumeral dystrophy is an autosomal dominant disorder that is transmitted to both sexes. Limb-girdle muscular dystrophy may be inherited in several ways but is usually an autosomal recessive disorder that affects both sexes. The mixed type doesn't appear to be inherited and strikes both sexes.

Exactly how these inherited and acquired defects cause progressive muscle weakness isn't clear. They may cause an abnormality in muscle fiber intracellular metabolism, possibly related to an enzyme deficiency or dysfunction, or to an inability to synthesize, absorb, or metabolize some unknown substance vital to muscle function. Vitamin E deficiency has been suggested as a possible cause, but this hypothesis has not been confirmed.

Signs and symptoms

Although four types of muscular dystrophy cause progressive muscular deterioration, degree of severity and age of onset vary.

Duchenne's muscular dystrophy begins insidiously, between ages 3 and 5. Initially, it affects leg and pelvic muscles but eventually spreads to the involuntary muscles. Muscle weakness produces a waddling gait, toe-walking, and lordosis. Children with this disorder have difficulty climbing stairs, fall down often, can't run properly, and their scapulae flare out (or "wing") when they raise their arms. Calf muscles especially become enlarged and firm. Muscle deterioration progresses rapidly, and contractures develop. Usually, these children are confined to wheelchairs by ages 9 to 12. Late in the disease, progressive weakening of cardiac muscle causes tachycardia, electrocardiogram abnormalities, and pulmonary complications. Death commonly results from sudden heart failure, respiratory failure, or infection.

Facioscapulohumeral dystrophy is a slowly progressive and relatively benign form of muscular dystrophy that usually occurs before age 10 but may develop during adolescence. Initially, it weakens the muscles of the face, shoulders, and upper arms but eventually spreads to all voluntary muscles, producing a pendulous lower lip and absence of the nasolabial fold. Early symptoms include inability to pucker the mouth or whistle, abnormal facial movements, and absence of facial movements when laughing or crying. Other signs consist of diffuse facial flattening that leads to a masklike expression, winging of the scapulae, inability to raise the arms above the head, and, in infants, inability to suckle.

Limb-girdle dystrophy follows a similarly slow course and often causes only slight disability. Usually, it begins between ages 6 and 10; less often, in early adulthood. Muscle weakness first appears in the upper arm and pelvic muscles. Other symptoms include winging of the scapulae, lordosis with abdominal protrusion, waddling gait, poor balance, and inability to raise the arms.

Mixed dystrophy generally begins between ages 30 and 50, affects all voluntary muscles, and causes rapidly progressive deterioration.

Diagnosis

Characteristic abnormalities of gait and other voluntary movements, with a typical medical and family history, suggest this diagnosis.

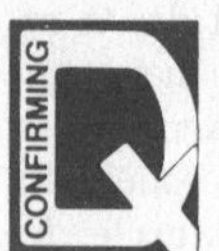

A muscle biopsy showing fat and connective tissue deposits confirms it. Electromyography often shows short, weak bursts of electrical activity in affected muscles, but this isn't conclusive. However, with a positive muscle biopsy, electromyography can help rule out neurogenic muscle atrophy by showing intact muscle innervation.

Other relevant laboratory results in Duchenne's muscular dystrophy include increased urinary creatinine excretion and elevated serum levels of creatinine phosphokinase (CPK), lactate dehydrogenase, and transaminase. Usually, CPK level rises before muscle weakness becomes severe and is a good early indicator of Duchenne's muscular dystrophy. These diagnostic tests are also useful for genetic screening, since unaffected carriers of Duchenne's muscular dystrophy also show elevated CPK and other enzyme levels.

Treatment

No treatment can stop the progressive muscle impairment of muscular dystrophy, but orthopedic appliances, exercise, physical therapy, and surgery to correct contractures can help preserve mobility and independence. Family members who are carriers of muscular dystrophy should receive genetic counseling regarding the risk of transmitting this disease. Amniocentesis can't detect muscular dystrophy, but it can reveal the fetus' sex, so it's often recommended for known carriers of Duchenne's muscular dystrophy who are pregnant.

Special considerations

Comprehensive long-term care and follow-up, patient and family teaching, and psychological support can help the patient and family deal with this disorder.

- When respiratory involvement occurs in Duchenne's muscular dystrophy, encourage coughing, deep breathing exercises, and diaphragmatic breathing. Teach parents how to recognize early signs of respiratory complications.
- Encourage and assist with active and passive range-of-motion exercises to preserve joint mobility and prevent muscle atrophy. Advise the patient to avoid long periods of bed rest and inactivity; if necessary, limit TV viewing and other sedentary activities. Refer the patient for physical therapy. Splints, braces, surgery to correct contractures, grab bars, overhead slings, and a wheelchair can help preserve mobility. A footboard or high-topped sneakers and a foot cradle increase comfort and prevent footdrop.
- Because inactivity may cause constipation, encourage adequate fluid intake, increase dietary bulk, and obtain an order for a stool softener. Since such a patient is prone to obesity because of reduced physical activity, help him and his family plan a low-calorie, high-protein, high-fiber diet.
- Always allow the patient plenty of time to perform even simple physical tasks, since he's apt to be slow and awkward.
- Encourage communication between family members to help them deal with the emotional strain this disorder produces. Provide emotional support to help the patient cope with continual changes in body image.
- Help the child with Duchenne's muscular dystrophy maintain peer relationships and realize his intellectual potential by encouraging his parents to keep him in a regular school as long as possible.
- If necessary, refer adult patients for

sexual counseling. Refer those who must learn new job skills for vocational rehabilitation. (Contact your state's Department of Labor and Industry for more information.) For information on social services and financial assistance, refer these patients and their families to Muscular Dystrophy Association, Inc.

JOINTS

Septic Arthritis

(Infectious arthritis)

A medical emergency, septic arthritis is caused by bacterial invasion of a joint, resulting in inflammation of the synovial lining. If the organisms enter the joint cavity, effusion and pyogenesis follow, with eventual destruction of bone and cartilage. Septic arthritis can lead to ankylosis and even fatal septicemia. However, prompt antibiotic therapy and joint aspiration or drainage cures most patients.

Causes

In most cases of septic arthritis, bacteria spread from a primary site of infection, usually in adjacent bone or soft tissue, through the bloodstream to the joint. Common infecting organisms include four strains of gram-positive cocci: *Staphylococcus aureus, Streptococcus pyogenes, Streptococcus pneumoniae,* and *Streptococcus viridans;* two strains of gram-negative cocci: *Neisseria gonorrhoeae* and *Hemophilus influenzae;* and various gram-negative bacilli: *Escherichia coli, Salmonella,* and *Pseudomonas,* for example. Anaerobic organisms such as gram-positive cocci usually infect adults, and children over age 2. *H. influenzae* most often infects children under age 2.

Various factors can predispose a person to septic arthritis. Any concurrent bacterial infection (of the genitourinary or the upper respiratory tract, for example) or serious chronic illness (such as malignancy, renal failure, rheumatoid arthritis, systemic lupus erythematosus, diabetes, or cirrhosis) heightens susceptibility. Consequently, alcoholics and elderly persons run a higher risk of developing septic arthritis. Of course, susceptibility increases with diseases that depress the autoimmune system or with prior immunosuppressive therapy. Intravenous drug abuse (by heroin addicts, for example) can also cause septic arthritis. Other predisposing factors include recent articular trauma, joint surgery, intraarticular injections, and local joint abnormalities.

Signs and symptoms

Acute septic arthritis begins abruptly, causing intense pain, inflammation, and swelling of the affected joint, with low-grade fever. It usually affects a single joint. It most often develops in the large joints but can strike any joint, including the spine and small peripheral joints. Systemic signs of inflammation may not appear in some patients. Migratory polyarthritis sometimes precedes localization of the infection. If the bacteria invade the hip, pain may occur in the groin, upper thigh, or buttock, or may be referred to the knee.

Diagnosis

Identifying the causative organism in a Gram stain or culture of synovial fluid or a biopsy of synovial membrane confirms septic arthritis. Joint fluid analysis shows gross pus or watery, cloudy fluid

OTHER TYPES OF ARTHRITIS

• *Intermittent hydrarthrosis*—a rare, benign, condition characterized by regular, recurrent joint effusions—most commonly affects the knee. The patient may have difficulty moving the affected joint but have no other arthritic symptoms. The cause of intermittent hydrarthrosis is unknown; onset is usually at or soon after puberty and may be linked to familial tendencies, allergies, or menstruation. No effective treatment exists.

• *Traumatic arthritis* results from blunt, penetrating, or repeated trauma or from forced inappropriate motion of a joint or ligament. Clinical effects may include swelling, pain, tenderness, joint instability, and internal bleeding. Treatment includes analgesics, anti-inflammatories, application of cold followed by heat, and, if needed, compression dressings, splinting, joint aspiration, casting, or possibly surgery.

• *Schönlein-Henoch purpura,* a vasculitic syndrome, is marked by palpable purpura, abdominal pain, and arthralgia that most commonly affects the knees and ankles, producing swollen, warm, and tender joints without joint erosion or deformity. Most patients have microscopic hematuria and proteinuria 4 to 8 weeks after onset. Renal involvement is also common. Incidence is highest in children and young adults, occurring most often in the spring after a respiratory infection. Treatment may include corticosteroids.

• *Hemophilic arthrosis* produces transient or permanent joint changes. Often precipitated by trauma, hemophilic arthrosis usually arises between ages 1 and 5 and tends to recur until about age 10. It usually affects only one joint at a time—most commonly the knee, elbow, or ankle—and tends to recur in the same joint. Initially, the patient may feel only mild discomfort; later, he may experience warmth, swelling, tenderness, and severe pain with adjacent muscle spasm that leads to flexion of the extremity. Mild hemophilic arthrosis may cause only limited stiffness that subsides within a few days. In prolonged bleeding, however, symptoms may subside after weeks or months or not at all. Severe hemophilic arthrosis may be accompanied by fever and leukocytosis; severe, prolonged, or repeated bleeding may lead to chronic hemophilic joint disease. Effective treatment includes I.V. infusion of the deficient clotting factor, bed rest with the affected extremity elevated, application of ice packs, analgesics, and joint aspiration. Physical therapy includes progressive range-of-motion and muscle-strengthening exercises, to restore motion and to prevent contractures and muscle atrophy.

of decreased viscosity usually with 50,000/mm^3 or more white cells, containing primarily neutrophils. When synovial fluid culture is negative, positive blood culture may confirm the diagnosis. Synovial fluid glucose is often low as compared to a simultaneous 6-hour postprandial blood sugar.

Other diagnostic measures:

• *X-rays* can show typical changes as early as 1 week after initial infection—distention of joint capsules, for example, followed by narrowing of joint space (indicating cartilage damage) and erosions of bone (joint destruction).

• *Radioisotope joint scan* for less accessible joints (such as spinal articulations) may help detect infection or inflammation but isn't itself diagnostic.

• *WBC count* may be elevated, with many polymorphonuclear cells; erythrocyte sedimentation rate is increased.

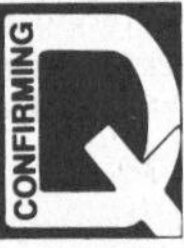

• *Two sets of positive culture* and *Gram stain smears* of skin exudates, sputum, urethral discharge, stools, urine, or nasopharyngeal smear confirm septic arthritis.

• *Lactic assay* can distinguish septic from nonseptic arthritis.

Treatment

Antibiotic therapy should begin promptly; it may be modified when sensitivity results become available. Penicillin G is effective against infections caused by *S. aureus*, *S. pyogenes*, *S. pneumoniae*, *S. viridans*, and *N. gonorrhoeae*. A penicillinase-resistant penicillin, such as nafcillin, is recommended for penicillin G–resistant strains of *S. aureus;* ampicillin, for *H. influenzae;* gentamicin, for gram-negative bacilli. Medication selection requires drug sensitivity studies of the infecting organism. Bioassays or bactericidal assays of synovial fluid and bioassays of blood may confirm clearing of the infection.

Treatment of septic arthritis requires monitoring of progress through frequent analysis of joint fluid cultures, synovial fluid leukocyte counts, and glucose determinations. Codeine or propoxyphene can be given for pain, if needed. (Aspirin causes a misleading reduction in swelling, hindering accurate monitoring of progress.) The affected joint can be immobilized with a splint or put into traction until movement can be tolerated.

Needle aspiration (arthrocentesis) to remove grossly purulent joint fluid should be repeated daily until fluid appears normal. If excessive fluid is aspirated or the leukocyte count remains elevated, open surgical drainage (usually arthrotomy with lavage of the joint) may be necessary for resistant infection or chronic septic arthritis.

Late reconstructive surgery is warranted only for severe joint damage and only after all signs of active infection have disappeared, which usually takes several months. In some cases, the recommended procedure may be arthroplasty or joint fusion. Prosthetic replacement remains controversial since it may exacerbate the infection, but has helped patients with damaged femoral heads or acetabula.

Special considerations

Management of septic arthritis demands meticulous supportive care, close observation, and control of infection.

- Practice strict aseptic technique with all procedures. Wash hands carefully before and after giving care. Dispose of soiled linens and dressings properly. Prevent contact between immunosuppressed patients and infected patients.
- Watch for signs of joint inflammation: heat, redness, swelling, pain, or drainage. Monitor vital signs and fever pattern. Remember that corticosteroids mask signs of infection.
- Check splints or traction regularly. Keep the joint in proper alignment, but avoid prolonged immobilization. Start passive range-of-motion exercises immediately, and progress to active exercises as soon as the patient can move the affected joint and put weight on it.
- Monitor pain levels and medicate accordingly, especially before exercise, remembering that the pain of septic arthritis is easy to underestimate. Administer analgesics and narcotics for acute pain, and heat or ice packs for moderate pain.
- Carefully evaluate the patient's condition after joint aspiration. Provide emotional support throughout the diagnostic tests and procedures, which should be previously explained to the patient. Warn the patient before the first aspiration that it will be *extremely* painful.
- Discuss all prescribed medications with the patient. Explain why therapy must be carefully monitored.

Gout

(Gouty arthritis)

Gout is a metabolic disease marked by urate deposits, which cause painfully arthritic joints. It can strike any joint but favors those in the feet and legs. Primary gout *usually occurs in men older than age 30 and in postmenopausal women;* secondary gout *occurs in the elderly. Gout follows an intermittent course and often leaves patients totally free of symptoms for years between attacks. Gout can lead to chronic disability or incapacitation and, rarely, severe hypertension and progressive renal disease. Prognosis is good with treatment.*

SYDENHAM'S DESCRIPTION OF GOUT

For clarity and vividness, few passages in medical literature can rival the following classic description of an acute gout attack written by Thomas Sydenham, the famous 17th-century British doctor who suffered from gout for 34 years:

"The victim goes to bed and sleeps in good health. About two o'clock in the morning he is awakened by a severe pain in the great toe; more rarely in the heel, ankle, or instep. This pain is like that of a dislocation, and yet the parts feel as if cold water were poured over them. Then follow chills and shivers, and a little fever. The pain, which was at first moderate, becomes more intense. With its intensity the chills and shivers increase. After a time this comes to its height, accommodating itself to the bones and ligaments of the tarsus and metatarsus. Now it is a violent stretching and tearing of the ligaments—now it is a gnawing pain and now a pressure and tightening. So exquisite and lively meanwhile is the feeling of the part affected, that it cannot bear the weight of bedclothes nor the jar of a person walking in the room. The night is passed in torture, sleeplessness, turning of the part affected, and perpetual change of posture; the tossing about of the body being as incessant as the pain of the tortured joint, and being worse as the fit comes on. Hence the vain effort by change of posture, both in the body and the limb affected, to obtain an abatement of the pain."*

* THE WORKS OF THOMAS SYDENHAM, translated by R.G. Latham (London: Sydenham Society 1850), Vol. II, p. 214.

Causes

Although the exact cause of primary gout remains unknown, it seems linked to a genetic defect in purine metabolism, which causes overproduction of uric acid (hyperuricemia), retention of uric acid, or both. In secondary gout, which develops during the course of another disease (such as obesity, diabetes mellitis, hypertension, sickle cell anemia, and renal disease), hyperuricemia results from the breakdown of nucleic acid. Secondary gout can also follow drug therapy, especially after hydrochlorothiazide or pyrazinamide, which interferes with urate excretion. Increased concentration of uric acid leads to urate deposits, called *tophi,* in joints or tissues, causing local necrosis or fibrosis.

Signs and symptoms

Gout develops in four stages: asymptomatic, acute, intercritical, and chronic. In asymptomatic gout, serum urate levels rise but produce no symptoms. As the disease progresses, it may cause hypertension or nephrolithiasis, with severe back pain. The first acute attack strikes suddenly and peaks quickly. Although it generally involves only one or a few joints, this initial attack is extremely painful. Affected joints appear hot, tender, inflamed, dusky-red, or cyanotic. The metatarsophalangeal joint of the great toe usually becomes inflamed first (podagra), then the instep, ankle, heel, knee, or wrist joints. Sometimes a low-grade fever is present. Mild acute attacks often subside quickly but tend to recur at irregular intervals. Severe attacks may persist for days or weeks.

Intercritical periods are the symptom-free intervals between gout attacks. Most patients have a second attack within 6 months to 2 years, but in some the second attack is delayed for 5 to 10 years. Delayed attacks are more common in those who are untreated and tend to be longer and more severe than initial attacks. Such attacks are also polyarticular, invariably affecting joints in the feet and legs, and are sometimes accompanied by fever. A migratory attack sequentially strikes various joints and the Achilles tendon, and is associated with either subdeltoid or olecranon bursitis.

Eventually, chronic polyarticular gout sets in. This final, unremitting stage of the disease (chronic or tophaceous gout) is marked by persistent painful polyarthritis, with large, subcutaneous tophi in cartilage, synovial membranes, tendons, and soft tissue. Tophi form in fingers, hands, knees, feet, ulnar sides of the forearms, helix of the ear, Achilles tendons, and, rarely, in internal organs, such as the kidneys and myocardium. The skin over the tophus may ulcerate and release a chalky, white exudate or pus. Chronic inflammation and tophaceous deposits precipitate secondary joint degeneration, with eventual erosions, deformity, and disability. Kidney involvement, with associated tubular damage, leads to chronic renal dysfunction. Hypertension and albuminuria occur in some patients; urolithiasis is common.

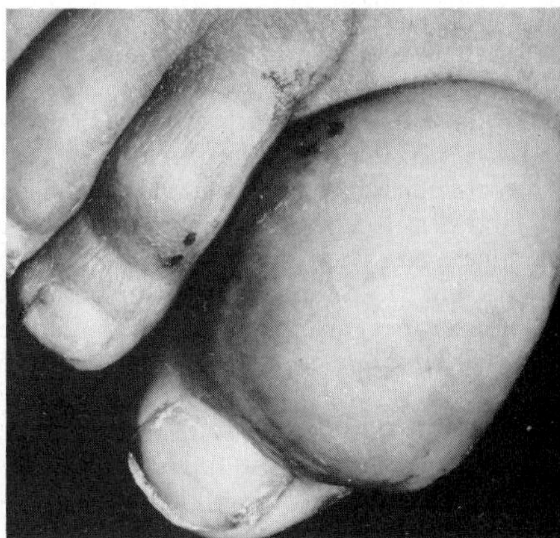

The final stage of gouty arthritis (chronic or tophaceous gout) is marked by painful polyarthritis, with large, subcutaneous, tophaceous deposits in cartilage, synovial membranes, tendons, and soft tissue. The skin over the tophus is shiny, thin, and taut.

Diagnosis

The presence of monosodium urate monohydrate crystals in synovial fluid taken from an inflamed joint or tophous establishes the diagnosis. Aspiration of synovial fluid (arthrocentesis) or of tophaceous material reveals needlelike intracellular crystals of sodium urate.

Although hyperuricemia isn't specifically diagnostic of gout, serum uric acid is above normal. Urinary uric acid is usually higher in secondary gout than in primary gout.

Initially, X-ray examinations are normal. However, in chronic gout, X-rays show damage of the articular cartilage and subchondral bone. Outward displacement of the overhanging margin from the bone contour characterizes gout.

Treatment

Correct management seeks to terminate an acute attack, reduce hyperuricemia, and prevent recurrence, complications, and the formation of kidney stones. Treatment for the patient with acute gout consists of bed rest; immobilization and protection of the inflamed, painful joints; and local application of heat or cold. Analgesics, such as acetaminophen, relieve the pain associated with mild attacks, but acute inflammation requires concomitant treatment with colchicine (P.O. or I.V.) every hour for 8 hours, until the pain subsides or nausea, vomiting, cramping, or diarrhea develops. Phenylbutazone or indomethacin in therapeutic doses may be used instead but is less specific. Resistant inflammation may require corticosteroids or corticotropin (I.V. drip or I.M.), or joint aspiration and an intraarticular corticosteroid injection.

Treatment for chronic gout aims to decrease serum uric acid level. Continuing maintenance dosage of allopurinol is often given to suppress uric acid formation or control uric acid levels, preventing further attacks. However, this powerful drug should be used cautiously in patients with renal failure. Colchicine prevents recurrent acute attacks until uric acid returns to its normal level, but doesn't affect the acid level. Uricosuric agents—probenecid and sulfinpyrazone—promote uric acid excretion and inhibit accumulation of uric acid, but their value is limited in patients with renal impairment. These medications should not be given to patients with urinary stones.

Adjunctive therapy emphasizes a few dietary restrictions, primarily the avoidance of alcohol and purine-rich foods.

Obese patients should try to lose weight, because obesity puts additional stress on painful joints.

In some cases, surgery may be necessary to improve joint function or correct deformities. Tophi must be excised and drained if they become infected or ulcerated. They can also be excised to prevent ulceration, improve the patient's appearance, or make it easier for him to wear shoes or gloves.

Special considerations

- Encourage bed rest, but use a bed cradle to keep bedcovers off extremely sensitive, inflamed joints.
- Give pain medication, as needed, especially during acute attacks. Apply hot or cold packs to inflamed joints. Administer anti-inflammatory medication and other drugs, as ordered. Watch for side effects. Be alert for gastrointestinal disturbances with colchicine.
- Urge the patient to drink plenty of fluids (up to 2 liters a day) to prevent formation of kidney stones. When forcing fluids, record intake and output accurately. Be sure to monitor serum uric acid levels regularly. Alkalinize urine with sodium bicarbonate or other agent, if ordered.
- Watch for acute gout attacks 24 to 96 hours after surgery. Even minor surgery can precipitate an attack. Before and after surgery, administer colchinine to help prevent gout attacks, as ordered.
- Make sure the patient understands the importance of checking serum uric acid levels periodically. Tell him to avoid high-purine foods, such as anchovies, liver, sardines, kidneys, sweetbreads, lentils, and alcoholic beverages—especially beer and wine—which raise the urate level. Explain the principles of a gradual weight reduction diet to obese patients. Such a diet features foods containing moderate amounts of protein and very little fat.
- Advise the patient receiving allopurinol, probenecid, and other drugs to report any side effects immediately. (Side effects may include such things as drowsiness, dizziness, nausea, vomiting, urinary frequency, and dermatitis.) Warn the patient taking probenecid or sulfinpyrazone to avoid aspirin or any other salicylate. Their combined effect causes urate retention.
- Inform the patient that long-term colchicine therapy is essential during the first 3 to 6 months of treatment with uricosuric drugs or allopurinol.

PSEUDOGOUT

Pseudogout, or calcium pyrophosphate disease, results when calcium pyrophosphate crystals collect in periarticular joint structures. Without treatment, it leads to permanent joint damage in about half of the patients it affects, most of whom are elderly.

Like gout, pseudogout causes abrupt joint pain and swelling—most commonly affecting the knee, wrist, ankle, and other peripheral joints. These recurrent, self-limiting attacks may be triggered by stress, trauma, surgery, severe dieting, thiazide therapy, and alcohol abuse. Associated symptoms are similar to those of rheumatoid arthritis.

Diagnosis of pseudogout depends on joint aspirations and synovial biopsy to detect calcium pyrophosphate crystals. X-rays reveal calcific densities in the fibrocartilage and linear markings along bone ends. Blood tests may detect an underlying endocrine or metabolic disorder.

Effective treatment of pseudogout may include joint aspiration to relieve fluid pressure; instillation of steroids; administration of analgesics, phenylbutazone, salicylates, or other nonsteroidal anti-inflammatories; and, if appropriate, treatment of the underlying endocrine or metabolic disorder.

Neurogenic Arthropathy

(Charcot's arthropathy)

Neurogenic arthropathy, most common in men over age 40, is a progressively degenerative disease of peripheral and axial joints, resulting from impaired sensory innervation. The loss of sensation in the joints causes progressive deterioration, resulting from trauma or primary disease, which leads to laxity of supporting ligaments and eventual disintegration of the affected joints.

Causes and incidence

In adults, the most common cause of neurogenic arthropathy is diabetes mellitus. Other causes include tabes dorsalis (especially among patients aged 40 to 60), syringomyelia (progresses to neurogenic arthropathy in about 25% of patients), myelopathy of pernicious anemia, spinal cord trauma, paraplegia, hereditary sensory neuropathy, Charcot-Marie-Tooth disease. Rarely, amyloidosis, peripheral nerve injury, myelomeningocele (in children), leprosy, and alcoholism cause neurogenic arthropathy.

Frequent intraarticular injection of corticosteroids has also been linked to neurogenic arthropathy. The analgesic effect of the corticosteroids may mask symptoms and allow continuous damaging stress to accelerate joint destruction.

Signs and symptoms

Neurogenic arthropathy begins insidiously with swelling, warmth, increased mobility, and instability in a single joint or in many joints. It can progress to deformity. The first clue to vertebral neuroarthropathy, which progresses to gross spinal deformity, may be nothing more than a mild, persistent backache. Characteristically, pain is minimal despite obvious deformity.

The specific joint affected varies. Diabetes usually attacks the joints and bones of the feet; tabes dorsalis attacks the large weight-bearing joints, such as the knee, hip, ankle, or lumbar and dorsal vertebrae (Charcot spine); syringomyelia, the shoulder, elbow, or cervical intervertebral joint. Neurogenic arthropathy related to intraarticular injection of corticosteroids usually develops in the hip or knee joint.

Diagnosis

Patient history of painless joint deformity and underlying primary disease suggests neurogenic arthropathy. Physical examination may reveal bone fragmentation in advanced disease. X-rays confirm diagnosis and assess severity of joint damage. In the early stage of the disease, soft-tissue swelling or effusion may be the only overt effect; in the advanced stage, articular fracture, subluxation, erosion of articular cartilage, periosteal new bone formation, and excessive growth of marginal loose bodies (osteophytosis) or resorption may be seen.

Other diagnostic measures include:

- *vertebral examination:* narrowing of disk spaces, deterioration of vertebrae, and osteophyte formation, leading to ankylosis and deforming kyphoscoliosis
- *synovial biopsy:* bony fragments and bits of calcified cartilage.

Treatment

Effective management relieves associated pain with analgesics and immobilization, using crutches, splints, braces, and restriction of weight-bearing.

In severe disease, surgery may include arthrodesis or, in severe diabetic neuropathy, amputation. However, surgery risks further damage through nonunion and infection.

Special considerations

Assess the pattern of pain and give analgesics, as needed. Check sensory perception, range of motion, alignment, joint swelling, and the status of underlying disease.

- Teach the patient joint protection techniques; to avoid physically stressful actions that may cause pathologic fractures; and to take safety precautions, such as removing throw rugs and clutter that may cause falls.
- Advise the patient to report severe joint pain, swelling, or instability. Warm compresses may be applied to relieve local pain and tenderness.
- Instruct the patient in the proper technique for crutches or other orthopedic devices. Stress the importance of proper fitting and regular professional readjustment of such devices. Warn that impaired sensation might allow damage from these aids without discomfort.
- Emphasize the need to continue regular treatment of the underlying disease.

Osteoarthritis

The most common form of arthritis, osteoarthritis is chronic, causing deterioration of the joint cartilage and formation of reactive new bone at the margins and subchondral areas of the joints. This degeneration results from a breakdown of chondrocytes, most often in the hips and knees.

Osteoarthritis is widespread, occurring equally in both sexes. Incidence is after age 40; its earliest symptoms generally begin in middle age and may progress with advancing age.

Disability depends on the site and severity of involvement, and can range from minor limitation of the fingers to severe disability in persons with hip or knee involvement. Rate of progression varies, and joints may remain stable for years in an early stage of deterioration.

Causes

Primary osteoarthritis, a normal part of aging, results from many things, including metabolic, genetic, chemical, and mechanical factors. Secondary osteoarthritis usually follows an identifiable predisposing event—most commonly trauma or congenital deformity—and leads to degenerative changes.

Signs and symptoms

The most common symptom of osteoarthritis is joint pain, particularly after exercise or weight bearing, that is usually relieved by rest. Other common symptoms include: stiffness in the morning and after exercise (relieved by rest), aching during changes in weather, "grating" of the joint during motion, and limited movement. The severity of these effects increases with poor posture, obesity, and occupational stress.

Osteoarthritis of the interphalangeal joints produces irreversible changes in the distal joints (Heberden's nodes) and proximal joints (Bouchard's nodes). These nodes may be painless at first but eventually become red, swollen, and tender, causing numbness and loss of dexterity.

Diagnosis

A thorough physical examination confirms typical symptoms, and lack of systemic symptoms rules out an inflammatory joint disorder, such as rheumatoid arthritis. X-rays of the affected joint help confirm diagnosis of osteoarthritis. X-rays may require posterior, anterior, lateral, and oblique views (with spinal involvement), and typically show:

- narrowing of joint space or margin
- cystlike bony deposits in joint space and margins
- joint deformity due to degeneration or articular damage

• bony growths at weight-bearing areas (hips, knees).

No laboratory test is specific for osteoarthritis.

Treatment

Treatment is primarily palliative, through medication and surgery. Medications for relief of pain and joint inflammation include aspirin (or other nonnarcotic analgesics), phenylbutazone, indomethacin, fenoprofen, ibuprofen, propoxyphene, and, in some cases, intraarticular injections of corticosteroids. Such injections may delay the development of nodes in the hands.

Effective treatment also reduces stress by supporting or stabilizing the joint with crutches, braces, cane, walker, cervical collar, or traction. Other supportive measures include massage, moist heat, paraffin dips for hands, protective techniques for preventing undue stress on the joints, adequate rest, particularly after activity, and, occasionally, exercise when the knees are affected.

The following surgical procedures are reserved for patients who have severe osteoarthritis with disability or uncontrollable pain:

• *arthroplasty* (partial or total): replacement of deteriorated part of joint with prosthetic appliance
• *arthrodesis:* surgical fusion of bones; used primarily in spine (laminectomy)
• *osteoplasty:* scraping of deteriorated bone from joint
• *osteotomy:* change in alignment of bone to relieve stress by excision of wedge of bone or cutting of bone.

Special considerations

• Promote adequate rest, particularly after activity. Plan rest periods during the day, and provide for adequate sleep at night. Moderation is the key—teach the patient to "pace" daily activities.
• Assist with physical therapy, and encourage the patient to perform gentle range-of-motion exercises.
• If the patient needs surgery, provide appropriate preoperative and postoperative care.

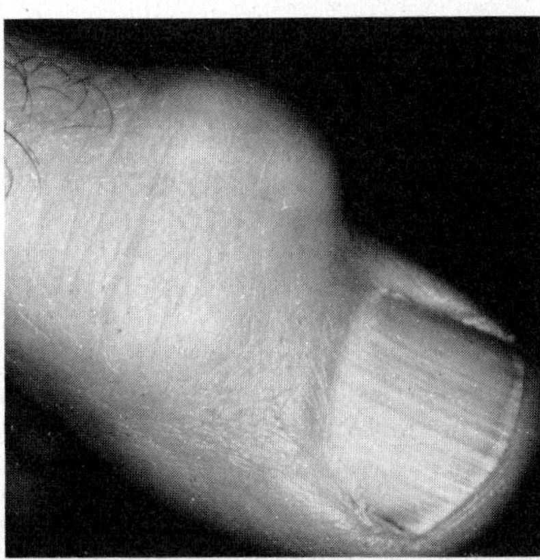

Osteoarthritis of the interphalangeal joints produces irreversible changes in the distal joints (Heberden's nodes). These nodes can be initially painless, with gradual progression or sudden flare-up of redness, swelling, tenderness, and impairment of sensation and dexterity.

• Provide emotional support and reassurance to help the patient cope with limited mobility. Explain that osteoarthritis is *not* a systemic disease.

Specific patient care depends on the affected joint:

• *Hand:* Apply hot soaks and paraffin dips to relieve pain, as ordered.
• *Spine (lumbar and sacral):* Recommend firm mattress (or bed board) to decrease morning pain.
• *Spine (cervical):* Check cervical collar for constriction; watch for redness with prolonged use.
• *Hip:* Use moist heat pads to relieve pain and administer antispasmodic drugs, as ordered. Assist with range-of-motion and strengthening exercises, always making sure the patient gets the proper rest afterward. Check crutches, cane, braces, and walker for proper fit, and teach the patient to use them correctly. For example, the patient with unilateral joint involvement should use an orthopedic appliance (such as a cane or walker) on the normal side. Advise use of cushions when sitting, as well as use of an elevated toilet seat.
• *Knee:* Twice daily, assist with prescribed range-of-motion exercises, ex-

ercises to maintain muscle tone, and progressive resistance exercises to increase muscle strength. Provide elastic supports or braces if needed.

To minimize the long-term effects of osteoarthritis, teach the patient to:

• plan for adequate rest during the day, after exertion, and at night.
• take medication exactly as prescribed, and report side effects immediately.
• avoid overexertion. The patient should take care to stand and walk correctly, to minimize weight-bearing activities, and to be especially careful when stooping or picking up objects.
• always wear well-fitting supportive shoes; don't allow the heels to become too worn down.
• install safety devices at home, such as guard rails in the bathroom.
• do range-of-motion exercises as gently as possible.
• maintain proper body weight to lessen strain on joints.

BONES

Osteomyelitis

Osteomyelitis is a pyogenic bone infection that may be chronic or acute. It commonly results from a combination of local trauma—usually quite trivial but resulting in hematoma formation—and an acute infection originating elsewhere in the body. Although osteomyelitis often remains localized, it can spread through the bone to the marrow, cortex, and periosteum. Acute osteomyelitis is usually a blood-borne disease, which most often affects rapidly growing children. Chronic osteomyelitis (rare) is characterized by multiple draining sinus tracts and metastatic lesions.

Causes and incidence

Osteomyelitis occurs more often in children than in adults—and particularly in boys—usually as a complication of an acute localized infection. The most common sites in children are the lower end of the femur and the upper end of the tibia, humerus, and radius. In adults, the most common sites are the pelvis and vertebrae, generally the result of contamination associated with surgery or trauma. The incidence of both chronic and acute osteomyelitis is declining, except in drug abusers. With prompt treatment, prognosis for acute osteomyelitis is very good; for chronic osteomyelitis, which is more prevalent in adults, prognosis is still poor.

The most common pyogenic organism in osteomyelitis is *Staphylococcus aureus;* others include *Streptococcus pyogenes, Pneumococcus, Pseudomonas aeruginosa, Escherichia coli,* and *Proteus vulgaris.* Typically, these organisms find a culture site in a hematoma from recent trauma or in a weakened area, such as the site of local infection (for example, furunculosis), and spread directly to bone. As the organisms grow and form pus within the bone, tension builds within the rigid medullary cavity, forcing pus through the haversian canals. This forms a subperiosteal abscess that deprives the bone of its blood supply and eventually may cause necrosis. In turn, necrosis stimulates the periosteum to create new bone (involucrum); the old bone (sequestrum) detaches and works its way out through an abscess or the sinuses. By the time sequestrum forms, osteomyelitis is chronic.

Signs and symptoms

Onset of *acute* osteomyelitis is usually rapid, with sudden pain in the affected bone, and tenderness, heat, swelling, and restricted movement over it. Associated systemic symptoms may include tachycardia, sudden fever, nausea, and malaise. Generally, the clinical features of both chronic and acute osteomyelitis are the same, except that chronic infection can persist intermittently for years, flaring up spontaneously after minor trauma. Sometimes, however, the only symptom of chronic infection is the persistent drainage of pus from an old pocket in a sinus tract.

Diagnosis

Patient history, physical examination, and blood tests help to confirm osteomyelitis:

- *White blood cell count* shows leukocytosis.
- *Erythrocyte sedimentation rate* is elevated.
- *Blood cultures* identify causative organism.

X-rays may not show bone involvement until the disease has been active for some time, usually 2 to 3 weeks. Bone scans can detect early infection. Diagnosis must rule out poliomyelitis, rheumatic fever, myositis, and bone fractures.

Treatment

To prevent further bone damage, treatment for acute osteomyelitis should begin before definitive diagnosis. Treatment includes administration of large doses of antibiotics I.V. (usually a penicillinase-resistant penicillin, such as nafcillin or oxacillin) after blood cultures are taken; early surgical drainage to relieve pressure buildup and sequestrum formation; immobilization of the affected bone by plaster cast, traction, or bed rest; and supportive measures, such as analgesics and I.V. fluids.

If an abscess forms, treatment includes incision and drainage, followed by a culture of the drainage. Antibiotic therapy to control infection may include administration of systemic antibiotics; intracavitary instillation of antibiotics through closed-system continuous irrigation with low intermittent suction; limited irrigation with blood drainage system with suction (Hemovac); or local application of packed, wet, antibiotic-soaked dressings.

In addition to antibiotics and immobilization, chronic osteomyelitis usually requires surgery to remove dead bone (sequestrectomy) and to promote drainage (saucerization). Prognosis is poor even after surgery. Patients are often in great pain and require prolonged hospitalization. Resistant chronic osteomyelitis in an arm or leg may necessitate amputation.

Special considerations

Your major concerns are to control infection, protect the bone from injury, and offer meticulous supportive care.

- Use strict aseptic technique when changing dressings and irrigating wounds. Wash your hands before and after giving care. If the patient is in skeletal traction for compound fractures, cover insertion points of pin tracks with small, dry dressings, and tell him not to touch the skin around the pins and wires. When cleaning the wound, always start at the center and work out.
- Administer I.V. fluids to maintain adequate hydration, as necessary. Provide a diet high in protein and vitamin C.
- Assess vital signs, wound appearance, and new pain, which may indicate secondary infection, daily.
- Carefully monitor suctioning equipment. Don't let containers of solution being instilled become empty, allowing air into the system. Monitor the amount of solution instilled and suctioned.
- Support the affected limb with firm pillows. Keep the limb level with the body; *don't* let it sag. Provide good skin care. Turn him gently every 2 hours and watch for signs of developing decubitus ulcers.
- Provide good cast care. Support the cast with firm pillows and "petal" the edges with pieces of adhesive tape or moleskin to smooth rough edges. Check circulation and drainage: if a wet spot appears on the cast, circle it with a marking pen and note the time of appearance (on the cast). Be aware of how

much drainage is expected. Check the circled spot at least every 4 hours. Report any enlargement immediately.

- Protect the patient from mishaps, such as jerky movements and falls, which may threaten bone integrity. Report sudden pain, crepitus, or deformity immediately. Watch for any sudden malposition of the limb, which may indicate fracture.
- Provide emotional support and appropriate diversions. Before discharge, teach the patient how to protect and clean the wound and, most importantly, how to recognize signs of recurring infection (increased temperature, redness, localized heat, and swelling). Stress the need for follow-up examinations. Instruct the patient to seek prompt treatment for possible sources of recurrence—blisters, boils, styes, and impetigo.

Osteoporosis

Osteoporosis is a metabolic bone disorder in which the rate of bone resorption accelerates while the rate of bone formation slows down, causing a loss of bone mass. Bones affected by this disease lose calcium and phosphate salts and thus become porous, brittle, and abnormally vulnerable to fracture. Osteoporosis may be primary or secondary to an underlying disease. Primary osteoporosis is often called senile or postmenopausal osteoporosis because it most commonly develops in elderly, postmenopausal women.

Causes

The cause of primary osteoporosis is unknown; however, a mild but prolonged negative calcium balance, resulting from an inadequate dietary intake of calcium, may be an important contributing factor—so may declining gonadal adrenal function, faulty protein metabolism due to estrogen deficiency, and sedentary lifestyle. Causes of secondary osteoporosis are many: prolonged therapy with steroids or heparin, total immobilization or disuse of a bone (as with hemiplegia, for example), alcoholism, malnutrition, malabsorption, scurvy, lactose intolerance, hyperthyroidism, osteogenesis imperfecta, and Sudeck's atrophy (localized to hands and feet, with recurring attacks).

Signs and symptoms

Osteoporosis is usually discovered when an elderly person bends to lift something, hears a snapping sound, then feels a sudden pain in the lower back. Vertebral collapse, producing a backache with pain that radiates around the trunk, is the most common presenting feature. Any movement or jarring aggravates the backache.

In another common pattern, osteoporosis can develop insidiously, with increasing deformity, kyphosis, loss of height, and a markedly aged appearance. As vertebral bodies weaken, spontaneous wedge fractures, pathologic fractures of the neck and femur, Colles' fractures following a minor fall, and hip fractures are all common.

Osteoporosis primarily affects the weight-bearing vertebrae. Only when the condition is advanced or severe, as in Cushing's syndrome or hyperthyroidism, do comparable changes occur in the skull, ribs, and long bones.

Diagnosis

Differential diagnosis must exclude other causes of rarefying bone disease, especially those affecting the spine, such as metastatic carcinoma and advanced multiple myeloma. Initial evaluation attempts to identify the specific cause of osteoporosis through patient history.

- *X-rays* show typical degeneration in the lower thoracic and lumbar vertebrae.

The vertebral bodies may appear flattened, with varying degrees of collapse and wedging, and may look denser than normal. Loss of bone mineral becomes evident in later stages.

- *Serum calcium, phosphorus,* and *alkaline phosphatase* are all within normal limits, but *parathyroid hormone* may be elevated.
- *Bone biopsy* shows thin, porous, but otherwise normal-looking bone.

Treatment

Treatment is basically symptomatic and aims to prevent additional fractures and control pain. A physical therapy program, emphasizing gentle exercise and activity, is an important part of the treatment. Estrogen may be given to decrease the rate of bone resorption; fluoride, to stimulate bone formation; and calcium and vitamin D, to support normal bone metabolism. However, drug therapy merely arrests osteoporosis and doesn't cure it. Weakened vertebrae should be supported, usually with a back brace. Surgery can correct pathologic fractures of the femur by open reduction and internal fixation. Colles' fracture requires reduction with plaster immobilization for 4 to 10 weeks.

The incidence of senile osteoporosis may be reduced through adequate intake of dietary calcium and regular exercise. Hormonal and fluoride treatments may also offer some preventive benefit and are sometimes used this way. Secondary osteoporosis can be prevented through effective treatment of the underlying disease, as well as through judicious use of steroid therapy, early mobilization after surgery or trauma, decreased alcohol consumption, careful observation for signs of malabsorption, and prompt treatment of hyperthyroidism.

Special considerations

Your care plan should focus on the patient's fragility, stressing careful positioning, ambulation, and prescribed exercises.

- Check the patient's skin daily for redness, warmth, and new sites of pain, which may indicate new fractures. Encourage activity; help the patient walk several times daily. As appropriate, perform passive range-of-motion exercises or encourage the patient to perform active exercises. Make sure the patient regularly attends scheduled physical therapy sessions.
- Impose safety precautions. Keep side rails up to prevent the patient from falling out of bed. Move the patient gently and carefully at all times. Explain to the patient's family and ancillary hospital personnel how easily an osteoporotic patient's bones can fracture.
- Provide a balanced diet, high in nutrients that support skeletal metabolism: vitamin D, calcium, and protein. Administer analgesics, as needed. Apply heat to relieve pain.
- Before discharge, make sure the patient and his family clearly understand the prescribed drug regimen. Tell them how to recognize significant side effects and to report them immediately. The patient should also report any new pain sites immediately, especially after trauma, no matter how slight. Advise the patient to sleep on a firm mattress and avoid excessive bed rest. Make sure he knows how to wear his back brace. If a female patient is taking estrogen, emphasize the need for routine gynecologic checkups, including Pap smears, and tell her to report any abnormal bleeding.
- Thoroughly explain osteoporosis to the patient and his family. If the patient and family don't understand the nature of this disease, they may feel the fractures could have been prevented if they had been more careful.
- Teach the patient good body mechanics—to stoop before lifting anything, and to avoid twisting movements and prolonged bending.
- Instruct the female patient taking estrogen in the proper technique for self-examination of the breasts. Tell her to perform this examination at least once a month and to report any lumps immediately.

Legg-Calvé-Perthes Disease

(Coxa plana)

Legg-Calvé-Perthes disease is ischemic necrosis leading to eventual flattening of the head of the femur due to vascular interruption. This usually unilateral condition occurs most frequently in boys aged 4 to 10 and tends to recur in families. Legg-Calvé-Perthes disease occurs bilaterally in 20% of patients.

Although this disease usually runs its course in 3 to 4 years, it may lead to premature osteoarthritis later in life from misalignment of the acetabulum and the flattened femoral head.

Causes

Vascular obstructive changes that initiate Legg-Calvé-Perthes disease are unknown. The disease occurs in four stages:

- Spontaneous vascular interruption causes necrosis of the femoral head: 1 to 3 weeks.
- New blood supply causes bone resorption and deposition of new bone cells; deformity may result from pressure on weakened area: 6 months to 1 year.
- New bone replaces necrotic bone: 2 to 3 years.
- Completion of healing or regeneration fixes shape of the joint: residual stage.

Signs and symptoms

The first indication of Legg-Calvé-Perthes disease is usually a persistent limp that becomes progressively severe. This symptom appears during the second stage, when bone resorption and deformity begin. Other effects may include mild pain (in the hip, thigh, or knee) that is aggravated by activity and relieved by rest, muscle spasm, atrophy of muscles in the upper thigh, slight shortening of the leg, and severely restricted abduction and rotation of the hip.

Diagnosis

A thorough physical examination and clinical history suggest Legg-Calvé-Perthes disease. Hip X-rays taken every 3 to 4 months confirm the diagnosis, with findings that vary according to the stage of the disease. Diagnostic evaluation must also differentiate between Legg-Calvé-Perthes disease (restriction of only the abduction and rotation of the hip) and infection or arthritis (restriction of all motion). Aspiration and culture of synovial fluid rule out joint sepsis.

Treatment

The aim of treatment is to protect the femoral head from further stress and damage by containing it within the acetabulum. After 3 months of bed rest, therapy may include reduced weight-bearing through bed rest in bilateral split counterpoised traction, then application of hip abduction splint or cast, or weight-bearing while a splint, cast, or brace holds the leg in abduction. Analgesics help relieve pain.

For a young child in the early stages of the disease, osteotomy and subtrochanteric derotation provide maximum confinement of the epiphysis within the acetabulum to allow return of the femoral head to normal shape and full range of motion. Proper placement of the epiphysis thus allows remolding with ambulation. Postoperatively, the patient requires a spica cast for about 2 months.

Special considerations

When caring for the hospitalized child:

- Monitor fluid intake and output. Maintain sufficient fluid balance. Provide a diet sufficient for growth but one that doesn't cause excessive weight gain, which might necessitate cast change with ultimate loss of the corrective position.
- Provide good cast care. Always turn a child in a wet cast with your palms,

since depressions in the plaster may lead to pressure sores. Turn the child every 2 to 3 hours to expose the cast to air. After the cast dries, "petal" it with pieces of adhesive tape or moleskin, changing them as they become soiled. Protect the cast with a plastic covering during each bowel movement.

• Watch for complications. Check toes for color, temperature, swelling, sensation, and motion; report dusky, cool, numb toes immediately. Check the skin under the cast with a flashlight every 4 hours while the patient is awake. Follow a consistent plan of washing, drying (alcohol may be used), and rubbing the skin under cast edges to improve circulation and prevent skin breakdown. *Never* use oils or powders under the cast, since they increase skin breakdown and soften the cast. Check under the cast daily for odors, particularly after surgery, to detect skin breakdown or wound problems. Report persistent soreness.

• Administer analgesics, as ordered.

• Relieve itching by using a hair dryer (set on cool) at the cast edges; this also decreases dampness from perspiration. If itching becomes excessive, get an order for an antipruritic. *Never* insert an object under the cast to scratch.

• Provide emotional support. Explain all procedures and the need for bed rest, cast, or braces to the child; encourage him to verbalize his fears and anxiety. Encourage parents to participate in their child's care. Teach them proper cast care and how to recognize signs of skin breakdown. Offer tips for making home management of the bedridden child easier. Tell them what special supplies are needed: pajamas and trousers a size larger (open the side seam, and attach Velcro fasteners to close it), bedpan, adhesive tape, moleskin, and, possibly, a hospital bed.

• After removal of the cast, debride dry, scaly skin *gradually* by applying lotion after bathing.

• Stress the need for follow-up care to monitor rehabilitation. Also stress home tutoring and socialization to promote normal growth and development.

Osgood-Schlatter Disease

(Osteochondrosis)

Osgood-Schlatter disease is a painful, incomplete separation of the epiphysis of the tibial tubercle from the tibial shaft. It's most common in active adolescent boys, frequently affecting one or both knees. Severe disease may cause permanent tubercle enlargement.

Causes

Osgood-Schlatter disease probably results from trauma, before the complete fusion of the epiphysis to the main bone has occurred (between ages 10 and 15). Such trauma may be a single violent action or repeated knee flexion against tight quadriceps muscle. Other causes include locally deficient blood supply and genetic factors.

Signs and symptoms

The patient complains of constant aching and pain and tenderness below the kneecap which worsens during any activity that causes forceful contraction of the patellar tendon on the tubercle, such as ascending or descending stairs. Such pain may be associated with some obvious soft-tissue swelling, localized heat, and local tenderness.

Diagnosis

Physical examination supports the diagnosis: the examiner forces the tibia into internal rotation while slowly extending the patient's knee from 90° of flexion; at about 30°, such flexion produces pain

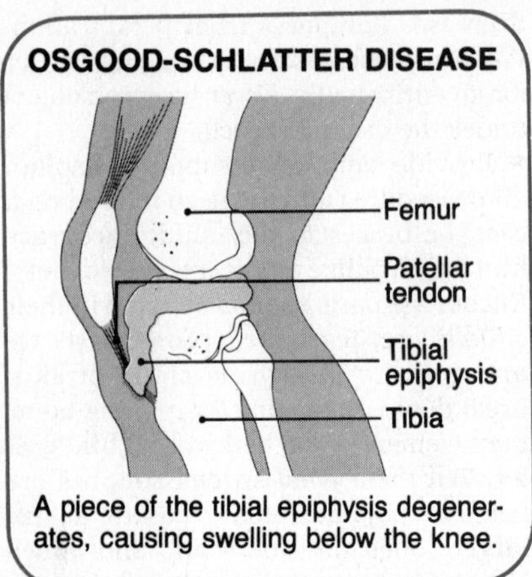

A piece of the tibial epiphysis degenerates, causing swelling below the knee.

that subsides immediately with external rotation of the tibia.

X-rays may be normal or show epiphyseal separation and soft-tissue swelling for up to 6 months after onset; eventually, they may show bone fragmentation.

Treatment

Treatment usually consists of immobilization for 6 to 8 weeks, and supportive measures. Leg immobilization through reinforced elastic knee support, plaster cast, or splint allows revascularization and reossification of the tubercle and minimizes the pull of the quadriceps. Supportive measures include activity restrictions and, possibly, cortisone injections into the joint to relieve tenderness. In very mild cases, simple restriction of predisposing activities (bicycling, running) may be adequate.

Rarely, conservative measures fail, and surgery may be necessary. Such surgery includes removal or fixation of the epiphysis or drilling holes through the tubercle to the main bone to form channels for rapid revascularization.

Special considerations

- Monitor the patient's circulation, sensation, and pain, and watch for excessive bleeding after surgery.
- Assess daily for limitation of motion. Administer analgesics, as needed.
- Make sure knee support or splint isn't too tight. Keep the cast dry and clean, and "petal" it around the top and bottom margins to avoid skin irritation. Teach proper use of crutches. Tell the patient to protect the injured knee with padding and to avoid trauma and repeated flexion (running, contact sports).
- Monitor for muscle atrophy.
- Give reassurance and emotional support, since disruption of normal activities is difficult for an active teenager. Emphasize that restrictions are temporary.

Paget's Disease

(Osteitis deformans)

Paget's disease is a slowly progressive metabolic bone disease characterized by an initial phase of excessive bone resorption (osteoclastic phase), followed by a reactive phase of excessive abnormal bone formation (osteoblastic phase). The new bone structure, which is chaotic, fragile, and weak, causes painful deformities of both external contour and internal structure. Paget's disease usually localizes in one or several areas of the skeleton (most frequently the lower torso), but occasionally, skeletal deformity is widely distributed. It can be fatal, particularly when it is associated with congestive heart failure (widespread disease creates a continuous need for high cardiac output), bone sarcoma, or giant cell tumors.

Causes and incidence

Paget's disease occurs worldwide but is extremely rare in Asia, the Middle East, Africa, and Scandinavia. In the United

States, it affects approximately 2.5 million people over age 40 (mostly men). Although its exact cause is unknown, one theory holds that early viral infection (possibly with mumps virus) causes a dormant skeletal infection that erupts many years later as Paget's disease.

Signs and symptoms

Clinical effects of Paget's disease vary. Early stages may be asymptomatic, but when pain does develop, it is usually severe and persistent and may coexist with impaired movement resulting from impingement of abnormal bone on the spinal cord or sensory nerve root. Such pain intensifies with weight-bearing.

The patient with skull involvement shows characteristic cranial enlargement over frontal and occipital areas (hat size may increase) and may complain of headaches. Other deformities include kyphosis (spinal curvature due to compression fractures of pagetic vertebrae), accompanied by a barrel-shaped chest and asymmetric bowing of the tibia and femur, which often reduces height. Pagetic sites are warm and tender and are susceptible to pathologic fractures after minor trauma. Pagetic fractures heal slowly and often incompletely.

Bony impingement on the cranial nerves may cause blindness and hearing loss with tinnitus and vertigo. Other complications include hypertension, renal calculi, hypercalcemia, gout, congestive heart failure, and a waddling gait (from softening of pelvic bones).

Diagnosis

X-rays taken before overt symptoms develop show increased bone expansion and density. A bone scan, which is more sensitive than X-rays, clearly shows early pagetic lesions (radioisotope concentrates in areas of active disease). Bone biopsy reveals characteristic mosaic pattern. Other laboratory findings include:

- anemia
- elevated serum alkaline phosphatase (an index of osteoblastic activity and bone formation)
- elevated 24-hour urine levels for hydroxyproline (amino acid excreted by kidneys and an index of osteoclastic hyperactivity). Increasing use of routine chemistry screens—which include serum alkaline phosphatase—is making early diagnosis more common.

Treatment

Primary treatment consists of drug therapy and includes one of the following:

- *calcitonin* (a hormone, given subcutaneously or I.M.) and *etidronate* (P.O.) to retard bone resorption (which relieves bone lesions) and reduce serum alkaline phosphate and urinary hydroxyproline secretion. Although calcitonin requires long-term maintenance therapy, there is noticeable improvement after the first few weeks of treatment; etidronate produces improvement after 1 to 3 months.
- *mithramycin,* a cytotoxic antibiotic, to decrease calcium, urinary hydroxyproline, and serum alkaline phosphatase. This medication produces remission of symptoms within 2 weeks and biochemical improvement in 1 to 2 months. However, mithramycin may destroy platelets or compromise renal function.

Self-administration of calcitonin and etidronate helps patients with Paget's disease lead near-normal lives. Nevertheless, these patients may need surgery to reduce or prevent pathologic fractures, correct secondary deformities, and relieve neurologic impairment. To decrease the risk of excessive bleeding due to hypervascular bone, drug therapy with calcitonin and etidronate or mithramycin must precede surgery. Joint replacement is difficult because bonding material (methyl methacrylate) doesn't set properly on pagetic bone.

Other treatment is symptomatic and supportive and varies according to symptoms. Aspirin, indomethacin, or ibuprofen usually controls pain.

Special considerations

- To evaluate the effectiveness of analgesics, assess level of pain daily. Watch for new areas of pain or restricted movements—which may indicate new fracture sites—and sensory or motor disturbances, such as difficulty in hearing, seeing, or walking.

- Monitor serum calcium and alkaline phosphatase levels.
- If the patient is confined to prolonged bed rest, prevent decubitus ulcers by providing good skin care. Reposition the patient frequently, and use a flotation mattress. Provide high-topped sneakers to prevent footdrop.
- Monitor intake and output. Encourage adequate fluid intake to minimize renal calculi formation.
- Demonstrate how to inject calcitonin properly and rotate injection sites. Warn the patient that side effects may occur (nausea, vomiting, local inflammatory reaction at injection site, facial flushing, itching of hands, and fever). Give reassurance that these side effects are usually mild and infrequent.
- To help the patient adjust to the changes in life-style imposed by this disease, teach him how to pace activities and, if necessary, how to use assistive devices. Encourage him to follow a recommended exercise program—avoiding both immobilization and excessive activity. Suggest a firm mattress or a bedboard to minimize spinal deformities. Warn against imprudent use of analgesics. To prevent falls at home, advise removal of throw rugs and other small obstacles.
- Emphasize the importance of regular checkups, including the eyes and ears.
- Tell the patient receiving etidronate to take this medication with fruit juice 2 hours before or after meals (milk or other high-calcium fluids impair absorption), to divide daily dosage to minimize side effects, and to watch for and report stomach cramps, diarrhea, fractures, and increasing or new bone pain.
- Tell the patient receiving mithramycin to watch for signs of infection, easy bruising, bleeding, and temperature elevation, and to report for regular follow-up laboratory tests.
- Help the patient and family make use of community support resources, such as a visiting nurse or home health agency. For more information, refer them to the Paget's Disease Foundation.

Hallux Valgus

Hallux valgus is a lateral deviation of the great toe at the metatarsophalangeal joint. It occurs with medial enlargement of the first metatarsal head and bunion formation (bursa and callus formation at the bony prominence).

Causes and incidence

Hallux valgus may be congenital or familial but is more often acquired from degenerative arthritis or prolonged pressure on the foot, especially from narrow-toed, high-heeled shoes that compress the forefoot. Consequently, hallux valgus is more common in women.

In congenital hallux valgus, abnormal bony alignment (increased space between first and second metatarsal [metatarsus primus varus]) causes bunion formation. In acquired hallux valgus, bony alignment is normal at the outset of the disorder.

Signs and symptoms

Hallux valgus characteristically begins as a tender bunion covered by deformed, hard, erythematous skin and palpable bursa, often distended with fluid. The first indication of hallux valgus may be pain over the bunion from shoe pressure. Pain can also stem from traumatic arthritis, bursitis, or abnormal stresses on the foot, since hallux valgus changes the body's weight-bearing pattern. In an advanced stage, a flat, splayed forefoot may occur, with severely curled toes (hammer toes) and formation of a small bunion on the fifth metatarsal.

Diagnosis

A red, tender bunion makes hallux valgus obvious. X-rays confirm diagnosis by showing medial deviation of first metatarsal and lateral deviation of the great toe.

Treatment

In the very early stages of acquired hallux valgus, good foot care and proper shoes may eliminate the need for further treatment. Other useful measures for early management include felt pads to protect the bunion, foam pads or other devices to separate the first and second toes at night, and a supportive pad and exercises to strengthen the metatarsal arch. Early treatment is vital in patients predisposed to foot problems, such as those with rheumatoid arthritis or diabetes mellitus. If the disease progresses to severe deformity with disabling pain, bunionectomy is necessary.

After surgery, the toe is immobilized in its corrected position one of two ways: with a soft compression dressing (which may cover the entire foot or just the great toe and the second toe, which serves as a splint) or with a short cast (such as a light slipper spica cast).

The patient may need crutches or controlled weight-bearing. Depending on the extent of their surgery, some patients walk on their heels a few days after surgery; others must wait 4 to 6 weeks to bear weight on the affected foot. Supportive treatment may include physical therapy, such as warm compresses, soaks, and exercises, and analgesics to relieve pain and stiffness.

Special considerations

Before surgery, obtain a patient history and assess the neurovascular status of the foot (temperature, color, sensation, blanching sign). If necessary, teach the patient how to walk with crutches.

After bunionectomy:

- Apply ice to reduce swelling. Increase negative venous pressure and reduce edema by supporting the foot with pillows, elevating the foot of the bed, or putting the bed in a Trendelenburg position.
- Record the neurovascular status of the toes, including the patient's ability to move the toes (dressing may inhibit movement), every hour for the first 24 hours, then every 4 hours. Report any change in neurovascular status to the surgeon immediately.
- Prepare the patient for walking by having him dangle his foot over the side of the bed for a short time before he gets up, allowing a gradual increase in venous pressure. If crutches are needed,

HAMMER TOE

In hammer toe, the toe assumes a clawlike pose from hyperextension of the metatarsophalangeal joint, flexion of the proximal interphalangeal joint, and hyperextension of the distal interphalangeal joint, usually under pressure from hallux valgus displacement. This causes a painful corn on the back of the interphalangeal joint and on the bone end, and a callus on the sole of the foot, both of which make walking painful. Hammer toe may be mild or severe, and can affect one toe or all five, as in clawfoot (which also causes a very high arch).

Hammer toe can be congenital (and familial) or acquired from constantly wearing short, narrow shoes, which put pressure on the end of the long toe. Acquired hammer toe is commonly bilateral and often develops in children who rapidly outgrow shoes and socks.

In young children, or adults with early deformity, repeated foot manipulation and splinting of the affected toe relieve discomfort and may correct the deformity. Other treatment includes protection of protruding joints with felt pads, corrective footwear (open-toed shoes and sandals, or special shoes that conform to the shape of the foot), the use of a metatarsal arch support, and exercises, such as passive manual stretching of the proximal interphalangeal joint. Severe deformity requires surgical fusion of the proximal interphalangeal joint in a straight position.

supervise the patient in using them, and make sure this skill is mastered before discharge. The patient should have a proper cast shoe or boot to protect the cast or dressing.

- Before discharge, instruct the patient to limit activities, to rest frequently with feet elevated, to elevate his feet whenever he feels pain or has edema, and to wear wide-toed shoes and sandals after the dressings are removed.
- Teach proper foot care, such as cleanliness, massages, and cutting toenails straight across to prevent ingrown nails and infection.
- Suggest exercises to do at home to strengthen foot muscles, such as standing at the edge of a step on the heel, then raising and inverting the top of the foot.
- Stress the importance of follow-up care and prompt medical attention for painful bunions, corns, and calluses.

Kyphosis

(Roundback)

Kyphosis is an anteroposterior curving of the spine that causes a bowing of the back, commonly at the thoracic, but sometimes at the thoracolumbar or sacral, level. Normally, the spine displays some convexity, but excessive thoracic kyphosis is pathologic. Kyphosis occurs in children and adults.

Causes and incidence

Congenital kyphosis is rare but usually severe, with resultant cosmetic deformity and reduced pulmonary function.

Adolescent kyphosis (Scheuermann's disease, juvenile kyphosis, vertebral epiphysitis), the most common form of this disorder, may result from growth retardation or a vascular disturbance in the vertebral epiphysis (usually at the thoracic level) during periods of rapid growth, or from congenital deficiency in the thickness of the vertebral plates. Other causes include infection, inflammation, aseptic necrosis, and disk degeneration. The subsequent stress of weight-bearing on the compromised vertebrae may result in the thoracic hump often seen in adolescents with kyphosis. Symptomatic adolescent kyphosis is more prevalent in girls than in boys and occurs most often between ages 12 and 16.

Adult kyphosis (adult roundback) may result from aging and associated degeneration of intervertebral disks, atrophy, and osteoporotic collapse of the vertebrae; from endocrine disorders such as hyperparathyroidism, and Cushing's disease; and from prolonged steroid therapy. Adult kyphosis may also result from conditions such as arthritis, Paget's disease, polio, compression fracture of the thoracic vertebrae, metastatic tumor, plasma cell myeloma, or tuberculosis. In both children and adults, kyphosis may also result from poor posture.

Disk lesions called Schmorl's nodes may develop in anteroposterior curving of the spine and are localized protrusions of nuclear material through the cartilage plates and into the spongy bone of the vertebral bodies. If the anterior portions of the cartilage are destroyed, bridges of new bone may transverse the intervertebral space, causing ankylosis.

Signs and symptoms

Development of adolescent kyphosis is usually insidious, often occurring after a history of excessive sports activity, and may be asymptomatic except for the obvious curving of the back (sometimes more than 90°). In some adolescents, kyphosis may produce mild pain at the apex of the curve (about 50% of patients), fatigue, tenderness or stiffness in the involved area or along the entire spine, and prominent vertebral spinous processes at the lower dorsal and upper lumbar levels, with compensatory increased lumbar lordosis, and hamstring tightness. Rarely, kyphosis may induce neurologic damage: spastic paraparesis secondary to spinal cord compression or herniated nucleus pulposus. In both adolescent and adult forms of kyphosis that are not due to poor posture alone, the spine will not straighten out when the patient assumes a recumbent position.

Adult kyphosis produces a characteristic roundback appearance, possibly associated with pain, weakness of the back, and generalized fatigue. Unlike the adolescent form, adult kyphosis rarely produces local tenderness, except in senile osteoporosis with recent compression fracture.

Diagnosis

Physical examination reveals curvature of the thoracic spine in varying degrees of severity. X-rays may show vertebral wedging, Schmorl's nodes, irregular end plates, and possibly mild scoliosis of 10° to 20°. Adolescent kyphosis must be distinguished from tuberculosis and other inflammatory or neoplastic diseases that cause vertebral collapse; the severe pain, bone destruction, or systemic symptoms associated with these diseases help to rule out a diagnosis of kyphosis. Other sites of bone disease, primary sites of malignancy, and infection must also be evaluated, possibly through vertebral biopsy.

Treatment

For kyphosis caused by poor posture alone, treatment may consist of therapeutic exercises, bed rest on a firm mattress (with or without traction), and a brace to straighten the kyphotic curve until spinal growth is complete. Corrective exercises include pelvic tilt to decrease lumbar lordosis, hamstring stretch to overcome muscle contractures, and thoracic hyperextension to flatten the kyphotic curve. These exercises may be performed in or out of the brace. Lateral X-rays taken every 4 months evaluate correction. Gradual weaning from the brace can begin after maximum correction of the kyphotic curve, vertebral wedging has decreased, and the spine has reached full skeletal maturity. Loss of correction indicates that weaning from the brace has been too rapid, and time out of the brace is decreased accordingly.

Treatment for both adolescent and adult kyphosis also includes appropriate measures for the underlying cause and, possibly, spinal arthrodesis for relief of symptoms. Although rarely necessary, surgery may be recommended when kyphosis causes neurologic damage, a spinal curve greater than 60°, or intractable and disabling back pain in a patient with full skeletal maturity. Preoperative measures may include halo-femoral traction. Corrective surgery includes a posterior spinal fusion with spinal instrumentation, iliac bone grafting, and plaster immobilization. Anterior spinal fusion followed by immobilization in plaster may be necessary when kyphosis produces a spinal curve greater than 70°.

Special considerations

Effective management of kyphosis necessitates first-rate supportive care for patients in traction or a brace, skillful patient teaching, and sensitive emotional support.

- Teach the patient with adolescent kyphosis caused by poor posture alone the prescribed therapeutic exercises and the fundamentals of good posture. Suggest bed rest when pain is severe. Encourage use of a firm mattress, preferably with a bed board. If the patient needs a brace, explain its purpose and teach him how and when to wear it. Teach good skin care. The patient should not use lotions, ointments, or powders where the brace contacts the skin. Warn that only the doctor or orthotist should adjust the brace.
- If corrective surgery is needed, explain all preoperative tests thoroughly, as well as the need for postoperative traction or casting, if applicable. After surgery, check neurovascular status every 2 to 4 hours for the first 48 hours, and report any changes immediately. Turn the patient often by logrolling him.

• Offer pain medication every 3 or 4 hours for the first 48 hours. Institute blood product replacement, if ordered. Accurately measure fluid intake and output, including urine specific gravity. Insert a nasogastric tube and a Foley catheter, if ordered; a rectal tube may also be necessary if paralytic ileus causes abdominal distention.
• Give meticulous skin care. Check the skin at the cast edges several times a day; use heel and elbow protectors to prevent skin breakdown. Remove antiembolism stockings, if ordered, at least three times a day for at least 30 minutes. Change dressings as ordered.
• Provide emotional support. The adolescent patient is likely to exhibit mood changes and periods of depression. Maintain communication, and offer frequent encouragement and reassurance.
• Assist during removal of sutures and application of a new cast (usually about 10 days after surgery). Encourage gradual ambulation (often with the use of a tilt-table in the physical therapy department). At discharge, provide detailed, written cast care instructions. Tell the patient to immediately report pain, burning, skin breakdown, loss of feeling, tingling, numbness, or cast odor. Advise the patient to drink plenty of liquids to avoid constipation, and to report any illness (especially abdominal pain or vomiting) immediately. Arrange for home visits by a social worker and a home care nurse.

Herniated Disk

(Ruptured or slipped disk, herniated nucleus pulposus)

Herniated disk occurs when all or part of the nucleus pulposus—the soft, gelatinous, central portion of an intervertebral disk (nucleus pulposus)—is forced through the disk's weakened or torn outer ring (anulus fibrosus). When this happens, the extruded disk may impinge on spinal nerve roots as they exit from the spinal canal or on the spinal cord itself, resulting in back pain and other signs of nerve root irritation. Herniated disk usually occurs in adults (mostly men) under age 45.

Causes

Herniated disks may result from severe trauma or strain or may be related to intervertebral joint degeneration. In the elderly, whose disks have begun to degenerate, minor trauma may cause herniation. Ninety percent of herniation usually occurs in the lumbar and lumbosacral regions; 8% occurs in the cervical area, and 1% to 2% in the thoracic area. Patients with a congenitally small lumbar spinal canal or with osteophyte formation along the vertebrae may be more susceptible to nerve root compression with a herniated disk and more likely to have neurologic symptoms.

Signs and symptoms

The overriding symptom of lumbar herniated disk is severe, low back pain, which radiates to the buttocks, legs, and feet, usually unilaterally. When herniation follows trauma, the pain may begin suddenly, subside in a few days, then recur at shorter intervals and with progressive intensity. Sciatic pain follows, beginning as a dull pain in the buttocks. Valsalva's maneuver, coughing, sneezing, or bending intensifies the pain, which is often accompanied by muscle spasms. Herniated disk may also cause sensory and motor loss in the area innervated by the compressed spinal nerve root and, in later stages, weakness and atrophy of leg muscles.

Diagnosis

Obtaining a careful patient history is vital, since the mechanisms that intensify disk pain are diagnostically significant.

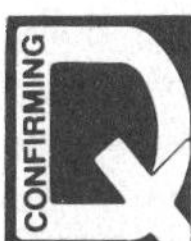

The straight-leg–raising test and its variants are perhaps the best tests for herniated disk. For the straight-leg–raising test, the patient lies in a supine position while the examiner places one hand on the patient's ilium, to stabilize the pelvis, and the other hand under the ankle, then slowly raises the patient's leg. The test is positive only if the patient complains of posterior leg (sciatic) pain, not back pain. In LeSegue's test, the patient lies flat while the thigh and knee are flexed to a 90° angle. Resistance and pain, as well as loss of ankle or knee-jerk reflex, indicate spinal root compression.

X-rays of the spine are essential to rule out other abnormalities, but may not diagnose herniated disk, since marked disk prolapse can be present despite a normal X-ray. A thorough check of the patient's peripheral vascular status—including posterior tibial and dorsalis pedis pulses, and skin temperature of extremities—helps rule out ischemic disease, another cause of leg pain or numbness. After physical examination and X-rays, myelography or computed tomography scan provides the most specific diagnostic information, showing spinal canal compression by herniated disk material.

Treatment

Unless neurologic impairment progresses rapidly, treatment is initially conservative and consists of several weeks of bed rest (possibly with pelvic traction), heat applications, and an exercise program. Aspirin reduces inflammation and edema at the site of injury; rarely, corticosteroids, such as dexamethasone, may be prescribed for the same purpose. Muscle relaxants, especially diazepam or methocarbamol, also may be beneficial.

A herniated disk that fails to respond to conservative treatment may necessitate surgery. The most common procedure, laminectomy, involves excision of a portion of the lamina and removal of the protruding disk (nucleus pulposus). If laminectomy doesn't alleviate pain and disability, a spinal fusion may be necessary to overcome segmental instability. Laminectomy and spinal fusion are sometimes performed concurrently to stabilize the spine.

Chemonucleolysis—injection of the enzyme chymopapain into the herniated disk to dissolve nucleus polposus—is a possible alternative to laminectomy. Microdiskectomy can also be used to remove fragments of nucleus polposus.

Special considerations

Herniated disk requires supportive care, careful patient teaching, and strong emotional support to help the patient cope with the discomfort and frustration of chronic low back pain.

- If the patient requires myelography, question him carefully about allergies to iodides, iodine-containing substances, or seafood, since such allergies may indicate sensitivity to the test's radiopaque dye. Reinforce previous explanations of the need for this test, and tell the patient to expect some pain. Assure him that he'll receive a sedative before the test, if needed, to keep him as calm and comfortable as possible. After the test, urge the patient to remain in bed with his head elevated (especially if metrizamide was used) and to drink plenty of fluids. Monitor intake and output. Watch for seizures and allergic reaction.
- During conservative treatment, watch for any deterioration in neurologic status (especially during the first 24 hours after admission), which may indicate an urgent need for surgery. Use antiembolism stockings, as prescribed, and encourage the patient to move his legs, as allowed. Provide high-topped sneakers to prevent footdrop. Work closely with the physical therapy department to ensure a consistent regimen of leg- and back-strengthening exercises. Give plenty of fluids to prevent renal stasis, and remind the patient to cough, deep breathe, and use blow bottles or an incentive spirometer to preclude pulmonary complications. Provide good skin care. Assess for bowel function. Use a fracture bedpan for the patient on complete bed rest.

• After laminectomy, microdiskectomy, or spinal fusion, enforce bed rest, as ordered. If a blood drainage system (Hemovac) is in use, check the tubing frequently for kinks and a secure vacuum. Empty the Hemovac at the end of each shift, as ordered, and record the amount and color of drainage. Report colorless moisture on dressings (possible cerebrospinal fluid leakage) or excessive drainage immediately. Observe neurovascular status of legs (color, motion, temperature, sensation).
• Monitor vital signs, check for bowel sounds and abdominal distention. Use logrolling technique to turn the patient. Administer analgesics, as ordered, especially 30 minutes before initial attempts at sitting or walking. Give the patient assistance during his first attempt to walk. Provide a straight-backed chair for limited sitting.
• Teach the patient who has undergone spinal fusion how to wear a brace. Assist with straight-leg–raising and toe-pointing exercises, as ordered. Before discharge, teach proper body mechanics—bending at the knees and hips (never at the waist), standing straight, carrying objects close to the body. Advise the patient to lie down when tired and to sleep on his side (never on his abdomen) on an extra-firm mattress or a bed board. Urge maintenance of proper weight to prevent lordosis caused by obesity.
• Before chemonucleolysis, make sure the patient is not allergic to meat tenderizers (chymopapain is a similar substance). Such an allergy contraindicates the use of this enzyme, which can produce severe anaphylaxis in a sensitive patient. After chemonucleolysis, enforce bed rest, as ordered. Administer analgesics and apply heat, as needed. Urge the patient to cough and deep breathe. Assist with special exercises, and tell the patient to continue these exercises after discharge.
• Tell the patient who must receive a muscle relaxant of possible side effects, especially drowsiness. Warn him to avoid activities that require alertness until he has built up a tolerance to the drug's sedative effects.
• Provide emotional support. Try to cheer the patient during periods of frustration and depression. Assure him of his progress, and offer encouragement.

Scoliosis

Scoliosis is a lateral curvature of the spine that may be found in the thoracic, lumbar, or thoracolumbar spinal segment. The curve may be convex to the right (more common in thoracic curves) or to the left (more common in lumbar curves). Rotation of the vertebral column around its axis occurs and may cause rib cage deformity. Scoliosis is often associated with kyphosis (humpback) and lordosis (swayback).

Causes

Scoliosis may be functional or structural. *Functional (postural) scoliosis* usually results from poor posture or a discrepancy in leg lengths, not fixed deformity of the spinal column. In *structural scoliosis,* curvature results from a deformity of the vertebral bodies. Structural scoliosis may be:
• *congenital:* usually related to a congenital defect, such as wedge vertebrae, fused ribs or vertebrae, or hemivertebrae
• *paralytic or musculoskeletal:* develops several months after asymmetric paralysis of the trunk muscles due to polio, cerebral palsy, or muscular dystrophy
• *idiopathic (the most common form):* may be transmitted as an autosomal dominant or multifactoral trait. This form appears in a previously straight spine during the growing years.

Idiopathic scoliosis can be classified

PARENT TEACHING AID

How to Detect Scoliosis

Dear Parents:
To check your child for scoliosis—abnormal curvature of the spine—perform this simple test. First, have your child remove her shirt and stand up straight. Then look at her back, and answer these questions:

- Is one shoulder higher than the other, or is one shoulder blade more prominent?
- When the child's arms hang loosely at her sides, does one arm swing away from the body more than the other?
- Is one hip higher or more prominent than the other?
- Does the child seem to tilt to one side?

Then, ask your child to bend forward, with arms hanging down and palms together at knee level. Can you see a hump on the back at the ribs or near the waist?

If your answer to any of these questions is "yes," notify your doctor. Your child needs careful evaluation for scoliosis.

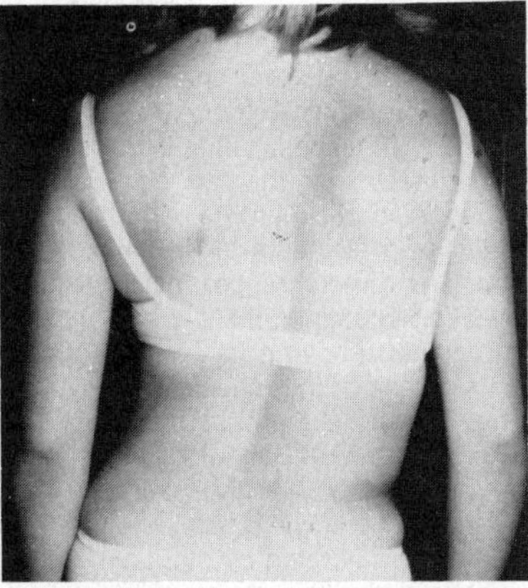

Patient shown above demonstrates the obvious effects of scoliosis. Notice this patient tilts to the right; her left hip is higher than her right hip; her right shoulder is higher than her left shoulder; and she holds her right arm further from her body than her left arm.

This parent teaching aid may be reproduced by office copier for distribution to parents.

as *infantile,* which affects mostly male infants between birth and age 3 and causes left thoracic and right lumbar curves; *juvenile,* which affects both sexes between ages 4 and 10 and causes varying types of curvature; or *adolescent,* which generally affects girls between age 10 and achievement of skeletal maturity and causes varying types of curvature.

Signs and symptoms

The most common curve in functional or structural scoliosis arises in the thoracic segment, with convexity to the right, and compensatory curves (S curves) in the cervical segment above and the lumbar segment below, both with convexity to the left. As the spine curves laterally, compensatory curves develop to maintain body balance and mark the deformity. Scoliosis rarely produces subjective symptoms until it's well established; when symptoms do occur, they include backache, fatigue, and dyspnea. Since many teenagers are shy about their bodies, their parents suspect that something is wrong only after they notice uneven hemlines, pantlegs that appear unequal in length, or subtle physical signs like one hip appearing higher than the other. Untreated scoliosis may result in pulmonary insufficiency (curvature may decrease lung capacity), back pain, degenerative arthritis of the spine, disk disease, and sciatica.

Diagnosis

Anterior, posterior, and lateral spinal X-rays, taken with the patient standing upright and bending, confirm scoliosis and determine the de-

CAST SYNDROME

Cast syndrome is a serious complication that sometimes follows spinal surgery and application of a body cast. Characterized by nausea, abdominal pressure, and vague abdominal pain, cast syndrome probably results from hyperextension of the spine. Hyperextension of the spine accentuates lumbar lordosis, with compression of the third portion of the duodenum between the superior mesenteric artery anteriorly, and the aorta and vertebral column posteriorly. High intestinal obstruction produces nausea, vomiting, and ischemic infarction of the mesentery.

After removal of the cast, treatment includes decompression and removal of gastric contents with a nasogastric tube and suction. The patient is given I.V. fluids and nothing by mouth. Antiemetics should be given sparingly, since they may mask symptoms of cast syndrome. Surgery may be required to release the ligament of Treitz, which attaches to the fourth portion of the duodenum. Untreated cast syndrome may be fatal.

Teach patients who are discharged in body jackets, localizer casts, or high hip spica casts how to recognize cast syndrome, which may develop as late as several weeks or months after application of the cast.

gree of curvature (Cobb method) and flexibility of the spine. Physical examination reveals unequal shoulder heights, elbow levels, and heights of the iliac crests. Muscles on the convex side of the curve may be rounded; those on the concave side, flattened, producing asymmetry of paraspinal muscles.

Treatment

The severity of the deformity and potential spine growth determine appropriate treatment, which may include close observation, exercise, a brace (for example, Milwaukee brace), surgery, or a combination of these. To be most effective, treatment should begin early, when spinal deformity is still subtle.

A curve of less than 25° is mild and monitored by X-rays and an examination every 3 months. An exercise program that includes sit-up pelvic tilts, spine hyperextension, push-ups, and breathing exercises may strengthen torso muscles and prevent curve progression. A heel lift may help.

A curve of 30° to 50° requires spinal exercises and a brace. (Transcutaneous electrical stimulation may be used as an alternative.) Usually, a brace halts progression in most patients but doesn't reverse established curvature. The Milwaukee brace consists of a leather or plastic pelvic girdle that holds one anterior and two posterior metal uprights connected to a neck ring. It can be adjusted as the patient grows and is worn until bone growth is complete.

A curve of 40° or more requires surgery (spinal fusion), since a lateral curve continues to progress at the rate of 1° a year even after skeletal maturity.

Some surgeons prescribe Cotrel dynamic traction for 7 to 10 days for preoperative preparation. This traction consists of a belt-pulley-weight system. While in traction, the patient should exercise for 10 minutes every hour, increasing muscle strength while keeping the vertebral column immobile.

Surgery corrects lateral curvature by posterior spinal fusion and internal stabilization with a Harrington rod. A distraction rod on the concave side of the curve "jacks" the spine into a straight position and provides an internal splint. An alternative procedure, anterior spinal fusion with Dwyer or Zielke instrumentation, corrects curvature with vertebral staples and an anterior stabilizing cable. Most spinal fusions require postoperative immobilization in a localizer cast (Risser cast) for 3 to 6 months. Postoperatively, periodic checkups are required for several months to monitor stability of the correction.

Special considerations

Scoliosis often affects adolescent girls, who are likely to find limitations on their activities and treatment with orthopedic appliances distressing. Therefore, provide emotional support, along with meticulous skin and cast care, and patient teaching.

If the patient needs a brace:

• Enlist the help of a physical therapist, a social worker, and an orthotist (orthopedic appliance specialist). Before the patient goes home, explain what the brace does and how to care for it (how to check the screws for tightness and pad the uprights to prevent excessive wear on clothing). Suggest that loose-fitting, oversized clothes be worn for greater comfort.

• Tell the patient to wear the brace 23 hours a day and to remove it only for bathing and exercise. While she's still adjusting to the brace, tell her to lie down and rest several times a day.

• Suggest a soft mattress if a firm one is uncomfortable.

• To prevent skin breakdown, advise the patient not to use lotions, ointments, or powders on areas where the brace contacts the skin. Instead, suggest she use rubbing alcohol or tincture of benzoin to toughen the skin. Tell her to keep the skin dry and clean and to wear a snug T-shirt under the brace.

• Advise the patient to increase activities gradually and avoid vigorous sports. Emphasize the importance of conscientiously performing prescribed exercises. Recommend swimming during the 1 hour out of the brace but strongly warn against diving.

• Instruct the patient to turn her whole body, instead of just her head, when looking to the side. To make reading easier, tell her to hold the book so she can look straight ahead at it instead of down. If she finds this difficult, help her to obtain prism glasses.

If the patient needs traction or a cast before surgery:

• Explain these procedures to the patient and family. Remember that application of a body cast can be traumatic, since it's done on a special frame and the patient's head and face are covered throughout the procedure.

• Check the skin around the cast edge

COBB METHOD FOR MEASURING ANGLE OF CURVATURE

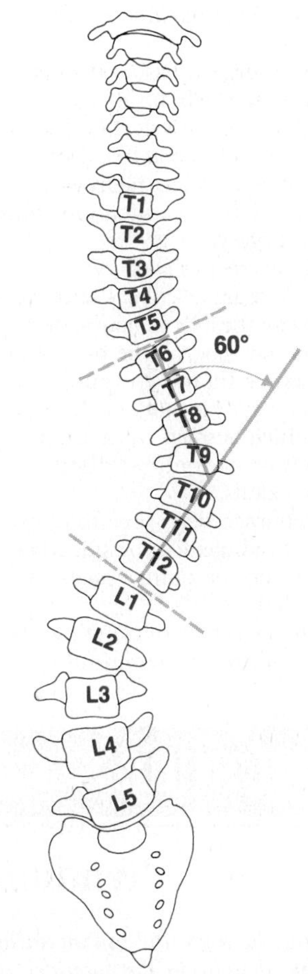

The Cobb method measures the angle of curvature in scoliosis. The top vertebra in the curve (T6 in the illustration) is the uppermost vertebra whose upper face tilts toward the curve's concave side. The bottom vertebra in the curve (T12) is the lowest vertebra whose lower face tilts toward the curve's concave side. The angle at which perpendicular lines drawn from the upper face of the top vertebra and the lower face of the bottom vertebra intersect is the angle of the curve.

daily. Keep the cast clean and dry, and edges of the cast "petaled" (padded). Warn the patient not to insert or let anything get under the cast and to immediately report cracks in the cast, pain, burning, skin breakdown, numbness, or odor.

- Before surgery, assure the patient and family that she'll have adequate pain control postoperatively. Check sensation, movement, color, and blood supply in all extremities to detect neurovascular deficit, a serious complication following spinal surgery.

After corrective surgery:

- Check neurovascular status every 2 to 4 hours for the first 48 hours; then several times a day. Logroll the patient often.
- Measure intake, output, and urine specific gravity to monitor effects of blood loss, which is often substantial.
- Monitor abdominal distention and bowel sounds.
- Encourage deep-breathing exercises to avoid pulmonary complications.
- Medicate for pain, especially before any activity.
- Promote active range-of-motion arm exercises to help maintain muscle strength. Remember that any exercise, even brushing the hair or teeth, is helpful. Encourage the patient to perform quadriceps-setting, calf-pumping, and active range-of-motion exercises of ankles and feet.
- Watch for skin breakdown and signs of cast syndrome. Teach the patient how to recognize these signs.
- Remove antiembolism stockings for at least 30 minutes daily.
- Offer emotional support to help prevent depression that may result from altered body image and immobility. Encourage the patient to wear her own clothes, wash her hair, and use makeup.
- If the patient is being discharged with a Harrington rod and cast and must have bed rest, arrange for a social worker and a visiting nurse to provide home care. Before discharge, check with the surgeon about activity limitations, and make sure the patient understands them.
- If you work in a school, screen children routinely for scoliosis during physical examinations.

MUSCLE & CONNECTIVE TISSUE

Tendinitis and Bursitis

Tendinitis *is a painful inflammation of tendons and of tendon-muscle attachments to bone, usually in the shoulder rotator cuff, hip, Achilles tendon, or hamstring.* Bursitis *is a painful inflammation of one or more of the bursae—closed sacs that are lubricated with small amounts of synovial fluid which facilitate the motion of muscles and tendons over bony prominences. Bursitis usually occurs in the subdeltoid, olecranon, trochanteric, calcaneal, or prepatellar bursae.*

Causes and incidence

Tendinitis commonly results from trauma (such as strain during sports activity), another musculoskeletal disorder (rheumatic diseases, congenital defects), postural misalignment, abnormal body development, or hypermobility.

Bursitis usually occurs in middle age from recurring trauma that stresses or pressures a joint or from an inflammatory joint disease (rheumatoid arthritis, gout). Chronic bursitis follows attacks of acute bursitis or repeated trauma and infection. Septic bursitis may result from wound infection or from bacterial invasion of skin over the bursa.

PATIENT TEACHING AID

Exercises for Shoulder Pain

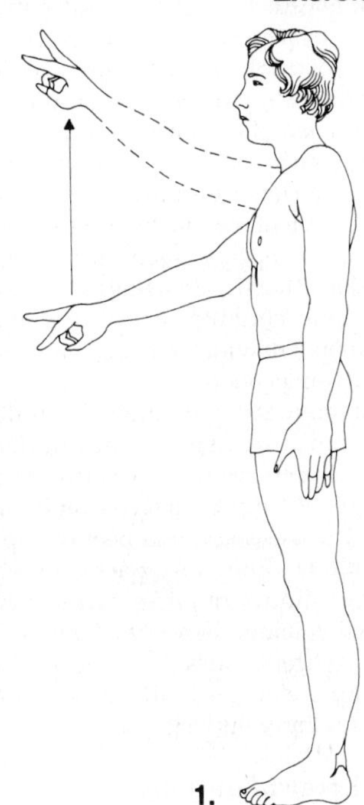

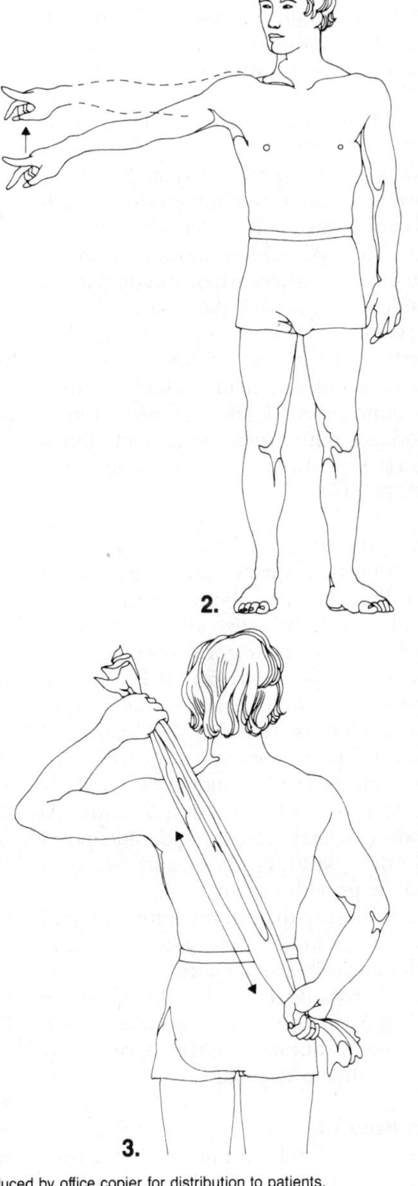

1. Stand facing a wall an arm's length away. Slowly, walk your fingers up the wall as high as you can. Then walk your fingers back down.

2. Then stand at a right angle to the wall and repeat the exercise. As your hand gets higher, step closer to the wall to allow your shoulder the maximum range of motion.

3. Grasp the ends of a large bath towel behind your back. Then simulate the motion of drying your back, reaching and pulling as far as possible. Reverse the position of your arms and repeat the exercise.

Signs and symptoms

The patient with tendinitis of the shoulder complains of restricted shoulder movement, especially abduction, and localized pain, which is most severe at night and often interferes with sleep. The pain extends from the acromion (the shoulder's highest point) to the deltoid muscle insertion, predominately in the so-called painful arc—that is, when the patient abducts his arm between 50° and 130°. Fluid accumulation causes swelling. In calcific tendinitis, calcium deposits in the tendon cause proximal weakness and, if calcium erodes into adjacent bursae, acute calcific bursitis.

In bursitis, fluid accumulation in the bursae causes irritation, inflammation, sudden or gradual pain, and limited movement. Other symptoms vary according to the affected site. Subdeltoid bursitis impairs arm abduction; prepatellar bursitis (housemaid's knee) produces pain when the patient climbs stairs; hip bursitis makes crossing the legs painful.

Diagnosis

In tendinitis, X-rays may be normal at first but later show bony fragments, osteophyte sclerosis, or calcium deposits. Arthrography is usually normal, with occasional small irregularities on the undersurface of the tendon. Diagnosis of tendinitis must rule out other causes of shoulder pain, such as myocardial infarction, cervical spondylosis, and tendon tear or rupture. Significantly, in tendinitis, heat aggravates shoulder pain; in other painful joint disorders, heat usually provides relief.

Localized pain and inflammation and a history of unusual strain or injury 2 to 3 days before onset of pain are the bases for diagnosing bursitis. During early stages, X-rays are usually normal, except in calcific bursitis, where X-rays may show calcium deposits.

Treatment

Treatment to relieve pain includes resting the joint (by immobilization with a sling, splint, or cast), systemic analgesics, application of cold or heat, ultrasound, or local injection of an anesthetic and corticosteroids to reduce inflammation. A mixture of a corticosteroid and an anesthetic, such as lidocaine, generally provides immediate pain relief. Extended-release injections of a corticosteroid, such as triamcinolone or prednisolone, offer longer pain relief. Until the patient is free of pain and able to perform range-of-motion exercises easily, treatment also includes oral anti-inflammatory agents, such as sulindac and indomethacin. Short-term analgesics include codeine, propoxyphene, acetaminophen with codeine, and, occasionally, oxycodone.

Supplementary treatment includes fluid removal by aspiration, physical therapy to preserve motion and prevent frozen joints (improvement usually follows in 1 to 4 weeks), and heat therapy; for calcific tendinitis, ice packs. Rarely, calcific tendinitis requires surgical removal of calcium deposits. Long-term control of chronic bursitis and tendinitis may require changes in life-style to prevent recurring joint irritation.

Special considerations

- Assess the severity of pain and the range of motion to determine effectiveness of the treatment.
- Before injecting corticosteroids or local anesthetics, ask the patient about his drug allergies.
- Assist with intraarticular injection. Scrub the patient's skin thoroughly with povidone-iodine or a comparable solution, and shave the injection site, if necessary. After the injection, massage the area to ensure penetration through the tissue and joint space. Apply ice intermittently for about 4 hours to minimize pain. Avoid applying heat to the area for 2 days.

Since patient teaching is essential, tell the patient to:

- take anti-inflammatory agents with milk to minimize gastrointestinal distress, and to report any signs of distress immediately.
- perform strengthening exercises and

to avoid activities that aggravate the joint.
• wear a triangular sling during the first few days of an attack of subdeltoid bursitis or tendinitis to support the arm and protect the shoulder, particularly at night. Demonstrate how to wear the sling so it won't put too much weight on the shoulder. Instruct the patient's family how to pin the sling or how to tie a square knot that will lie flat on the back of the patient's neck. To protect the shoulder during sleep, a splint may be worn instead of a sling. Instruct the patient to remove the splint during the day.
• maintain joint mobility and prevent muscle atrophy by performing exercises or physical therapy when he is free of pain.

Epicondylitis

(Tennis elbow, epitrochlear bursitis)

Epicondylitis is inflammation of the forearm extensor supinator tendon fibers at their common attachment to the lateral humeral epicondyle, which produces acute or subacute pain.

Causes and incidence

Epicondylitis probably begins as a partial tear and is common among tennis players or persons whose activities require a forceful grasp, wrist extension against resistance, or frequent rotation of the forearm. Untreated epicondylitis may become disabling.

Signs and symptoms

The patient's initial symptom is elbow pain that gradually worsens and often radiates to the forearm and back of the hand whenever he grasps an object or twists his elbow. Other associated signs and symptoms include tenderness over the involved lateral or medial epicondyle or over the head of the radius, and a weak grasp. In rare instances, epicondylitis may cause local heat, swelling, or restricted range of motion.

Diagnosis

Since X-rays are almost always negative, diagnosis typically depends on clinical signs and symptoms and a patient history of playing tennis or engaging in similar activities. The pain can be reproduced by wrist extension and supination with lateral involvement, or by flexion and pronation with medial epicondyle involvement.

Treatment

Treatment aims to relieve pain, usually by local injection of corticosteroid and a local anesthetic and by systemic anti-inflammatory therapy with aspirin or indomethacin. Supportive treatment includes an immobilizing splint from the distal forearm to the elbow, which generally relieves pain in 2 to 3 weeks; heat therapy, such as warm compresses, short wave diathermy, and ultrasound (alone or in combination with diathermy); and physical therapy, such as manipulation and massage to detach the tendon from the chronically inflamed periosteum. A "tennis elbow strap" has helped many patients. This strap, which is wrapped snugly around the forearm approximately 2.5 cm below the epicondyle, helps relieve the strain on affected forearm muscles and tendons. If these measures prove ineffective, surgical release of the tendon at the epicondyle may be necessary.

Special considerations

• Assess level of pain, range of motion, and sensory function. Monitor heat therapy to prevent burns.
• Advise the patient to take anti-inflammatory drugs with food to avoid gastrointestinal irritation.

• Instruct the patient to rest the elbow until inflammation subsides.
• Remove the support daily, and gently move the arm to prevent stiffness and contracture.
• Instruct the patient to follow the prescribed exercise program. For example, he may stretch his arm and flex his wrist to the maximum, then press the back of his hand against a wall until he can feel a pull in his forearm, and hold this position for 1 minute.
• Advise the patient to warm up for 15 to 20 minutes before beginning any sports activity.
• Urge the patient to wear an elastic support or splint during any activity that stresses the forearm or elbow.

Achilles Tendon Contracture

Achilles tendon contracture is a shortening of the Achilles tendon (tendo calcaneus or heel cord), which causes foot pain and strain, with limited ankle dorsiflexion.

Causes
Achilles tendon contracture may reflect a congenital structural anomaly or a muscular reaction to chronic poor posture, especially in women who wear high-heeled shoes or joggers who land on the balls of their feet instead of their heels. Other causes include paralytic conditions of the legs, such as poliomyelitis or cerebral palsy.

Signs and symptoms
Sharp, spasmodic pain during dorsiflexion of the foot characterizes the reflex type of Achilles tendon contracture. In footdrop (fixed equinus), contracture of the flexor foot muscle prevents placing the heel on the ground.

Diagnosis
Physical examination and patient history suggest Achilles tendon contracture.

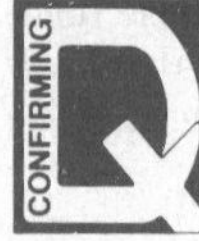

A simple test confirms achilles tendon contracture: while the patient keeps his knee flexed, the examiner places the foot in dorsiflexion; gradual knee extension forces the foot into plantar flexion.

Treatment
Conservative treatment aims to correct Achilles tendon contracture by raising the inside heel of the shoe in the reflex type; gradually lowering the heels of shoes (sudden lowering can aggravate the problem), and stretching exercises, if the cause is high heels; or using support braces or casting to prevent footdrop in a paralyzed patient. Alternative therapy includes using wedged plaster casts or stretching the tendon by manipulation. Analgesics may be given to relieve pain.

With fixed footdrop, treatment may include surgery (z-tenotomy), although this procedure may weaken the tendon. Z-tenotomy allows further stretching by cutting the tendon. After surgery, a short leg cast maintains the foot in 90° dorsiflexion for 6 weeks. Some surgeons allow partial weight-bearing on a walking cast after 2 weeks.

Special considerations
After surgery to lengthen the Achilles tendon:
• Elevate the casted foot to decrease venous pressure and edema by raising the foot of the bed or supporting the foot with pillows.
• Record the neurovascular status of the toes (temperature, color, sensation, capillary refill time, toe mobility) every hour for the first 24 hours, then every 4 hours. If any changes are detected, increase the elevation of the patient's legs and notify the surgeon immediately.

• Prepare the patient for ambulation by having him dangle his foot over the side of the bed for short periods (5 to 15 minutes) before he gets out of bed, allowing for gradual increase of venous pressure. Assist the patient in walking, as ordered (usually within 24 hours of surgery), using crutches and a non-weight-bearing or touch-down gait.
• Protect the patient's skin with moleskin or by "petaling" the edges of the cast. Before discharge, teach the patient how to care for the cast, and advise him to elevate his foot regularly when sitting or whenever the foot throbs or becomes edematous. Also, make sure the patient understands how much exercise and walking are recommended after discharge.
• To prevent Achilles tendon contracture in paralyzed patients, apply support braces, universal splints, casts, or high-topped sneakers. Make sure the weight of the sheets doesn't keep paralyzed feet in plantar flexion. For other patients, teach good foot care and urge them to seek immediate medical care for foot problems. Warn women against wearing high heels constantly, and suggest regular foot (dorsiflexion) exercises.

Carpal Tunnel Syndrome

The most common of the nerve entrapment syndromes, carpal tunnel syndrome results from compression of the median nerve at the wrist, within the carpal tunnel, through which it passes along with blood vessels, and flexor tendons to the fingers and thumb. This compression neuropathy causes sensory and motor changes in the median distribution of the hand. Carpal tunnel syndrome usually occurs in women between ages 30 and 60 and poses a serious occupational health problem. Assembly-line workers and packers and persons who repeatedly use poorly designed tools are most likely to develop this disorder. Any strenuous use of the hands—sustained grasping, twisting, or flexing—aggravates this condition.

Causes

The carpal tunnel is formed by the carpal bones and the transverse carpal ligament. Inflammation or fibrosis of the tendon sheaths that pass through the carpal tunnel often causes edema and compression of the median nerve. Many conditions can cause the contents or structure of the carpal tunnel to swell and press the median nerve against the transverse carpal ligament. Such conditions include rheumatoid arthrtitis, flexor tenosynovitis (often associated with rheumatic disease), nerve compression, pregnancy, renal failure, menopause, diabetes mellitus, acromegaly, edema following Colles' fracture, hypothyroidism, amyloidosis, myxedema, benign tumors, tuberculosis, and other granulomatous diseases. Another source of damage to the median nerve is dislocation or acute sprain of the wrist.

Signs and symptoms

The patient with carpal tunnel syndrome usually complains of weakness, pain, burning, numbness, or tingling in one or both hands. This paresthesia affects the thumb, forefinger, middle finger, and half of the fourth finger. The patient is unable to clench his hand into a fist; the nails may be atrophic, the skin dry and shiny.

Because of vasodilatation and venous stasis, symptoms are often worse at night and in the morning. The pain may spread to the forearm and, in severe cases, as far as the shoulder. The patient can usually relieve such pain by shaking his hands vigorously or dangling his arms at his side.

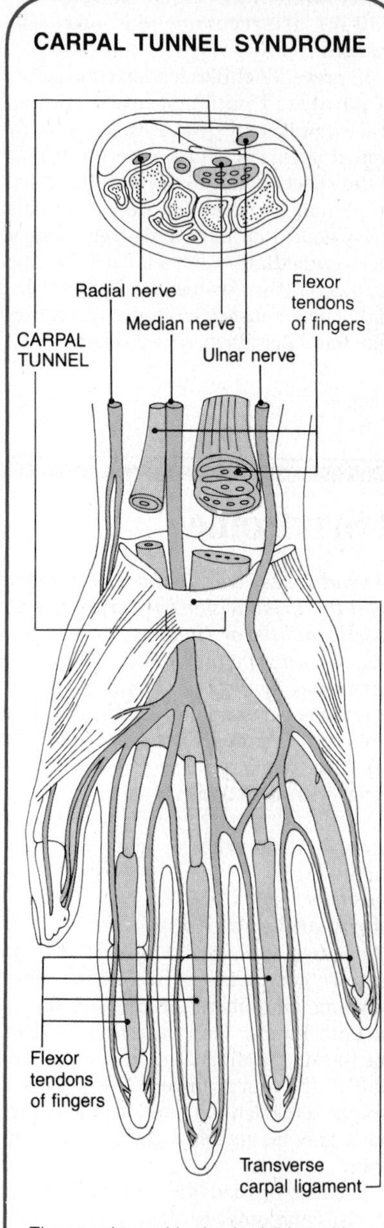

The carpal tunnel is clearly visible in this palmar view and cross-section of a right hand. Note the median nerve, flexor tendons of fingers, and blood vessels passing through the tunnel on their way from the forearm to the hand.

Diagnosis

Physical examination reveals decreased sensation to light touch or pinpricks in the affected fingers. Thenar muscle atrophy occurs in about half of all cases of carpal tunnel syndrome. The patient exhibits a positive Tinel's sign (tingling over the median nerve on light percussion) and responds positively to Phalen's wrist-flexion test (holding the forearms vertically and allowing both hands to drop into complete flexion at the wrists for 1 minute reproduces symptoms of carpal tunnel syndrome). A compression test supports this diagnosis: a blood pressure cuff inflated above systolic pressure on the forearm for 1 to 2 minutes provokes pain and paresthesia along the distribution of the median nerve.

Electromyography detects a median nerve motor conduction delay of more than 5 milliseconds. Other laboratory tests may identify underlying disease.

Treatment

Conservative treatment should be tried first, including resting the hands by splinting the wrist in neutral extension for 1 to 2 weeks. If a definite link has been established between the patient's occupation and the development of carpal tunnel syndrome, he may have to seek other work. Effective treatment may also require correction of an underlying disorder. When conservative treatment fails, the only alternative is surgical decompression of the nerve by sectioning the entire transverse carpal tunnel ligament. Neurolysis (freeing of the nerve fibers) may also be necessary.

Special considerations

- Administer mild analgesics, as needed. Encourage the patient to use his hands as much as possible; however, if the condition has impaired the dominant hand, you may have to help with eating and bathing.
- Teach the patient how to apply a splint. Tell him not to make it too tight. Show him how to remove the splint to perform gentle range-of-motion exercises, which should be done daily. Make sure the pa-

tient knows how to do these exercises before he's discharged.

• After surgery, monitor vital signs, and regularly check the color, sensation, and motion of the affected hand.

• Advise the patient who is about to be discharged to occasionally exercise his hands in warm water. If the arm is in a sling, tell him to remove the sling several times a day to do exercises for his elbow and shoulder.

• Suggest occupational counseling for the patient who has to change jobs because of carpal tunnel syndrome.

Torticollis

(Wryneck)

This neck deformity, in which the sternocleidomastoid neck muscles are spastic or shortened, causes bending of the head to the affected side and rotation of the chin to the opposite side. This disorder may be congenital or acquired. Incidence of congenital (muscular) torticollis is highest in infants after difficult delivery (breech presentation), in firstborn infants, and in girls. Acquired torticollis usually develops during the first 10 years of life or after age 40.

Causes

Possible causes of congenital torticollis include malposition of the head in utero, prenatal injury, fibroma, interruption of blood supply, or fibrotic rupture of the sternocleidomastoid muscle, with hematoma and scar formation.

The three types of acquired torticollis—acute, spasmodic, and hysterical—have differing causes. The acute form results from muscular damage caused by inflammatory diseases, such as myositis, lymphadenitis, and tuberculosis, and from cervical spinal injuries that produce scar tissue contracture. The spasmodic form results from rhythmic muscle spasms caused by an organic CNS disorder (probably due to irritation of the nerve root by arthritis or osteomyelitis). Hysterical torticollis is due to a psychogenic inability to control neck muscles.

Signs and symptoms

The first sign of congenital torticollis is often a firm, nontender, palpable enlargement of the sternocleidomastoid muscle that is visible at birth and for several weeks afterward. It slowly regresses during a period of 6 months, although incomplete regression can cause permanent contracture. If the deformity is severe, the infant's face and head flatten from sleeping on the affected side; this asymmetry gradually worsens. The infant's chin turns away from the side of the shortened muscle, and his head tilts to the shortened side. His shoulder may elevate on the affected side, restricting neck movement.

The first sign of acquired torticollis is usually recurring unilateral stiffness of neck muscles, followed by a drawing sensation and a momentary twitching or contraction that pulls the head to the affected side. This type of torticollis often produces severe neuralgic pain throughout the head and neck.

Diagnosis

A history of painless neck deformity from birth suggests congenital torticollis; gradual onset of painful neck deformity suggests acquired torticollis. However, diagnosis must rule out tuberculosis of the cervical spine, pharyngeal or tonsillar inflammations, spinal accessory nerve damage, ruptured transverse ligaments, subdural hematoma, dislocations and fractures, scoliosis, congenital abnormalities of the cervical spine, rheumatoid arthritis, and osteomyelitis.

TORTICOLLIS

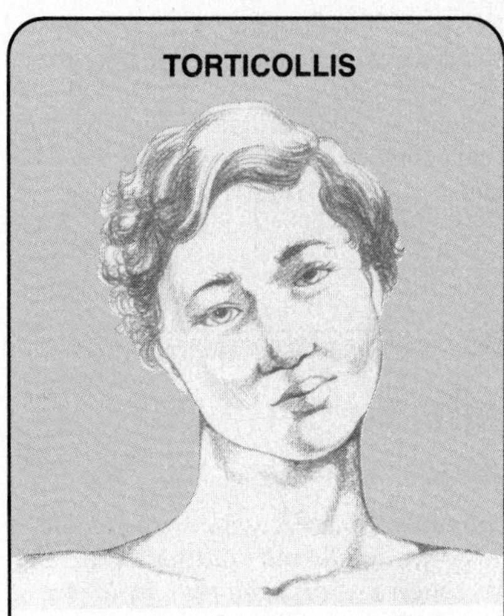

In torticollis, contraction of the sternocleidomastoid neck muscles produces a twisting of the neck and an unnatural position of the head.

In acquired torticollis, cervical spine X-rays are negative for bone or joint disease but may reveal an associated disorder (such as tuberculosis, scar tissue formation, or arthritis).

Treatment

Treatment of congenital torticollis aims to stretch the shortened muscle. Nonsurgical treatment includes passive neck stretching and proper positioning during sleep for an infant and active stretching exercises for an older child, for example, touching the ear opposite the affected side to the shoulder and touching the chin to the same shoulder.

Surgical correction involves sectioning the sternocleidomastoid muscle; this should be done during preschool years and only if other therapies fail.

Treatment of acquired torticollis aims to correct the underlying cause of the disease. In the acute form, application of heat, cervical traction, and gentle massage may help relieve pain. Stretching exercises and a neck brace may relieve symptoms of the spasmodic and hysterical forms. Treatment of elderly patients with acquired torticollis may include administration of levodopa-carbidopa, carbamazepine (Tegretol), and haloperidol (Haldol).

Special considerations

To aid early diagnosis of torticollis of the congenital type, observe the infant for limited neck movement, and thoroughly assess his degree of discomfort.

Teach the parents of an affected child how to perform stretching exercises with the child. Suggest that they place toys or hanging mobiles on the side of the crib opposite the affected side of the child's neck, to encourage the child to move his head and stretch his neck.

If surgery is necessary, prepare the patient by shaving the neck to the hairline on the affected side.

After corrective surgery, follow these guidelines:

- Monitor the patient closely for nausea or signs of respiratory complications, especially if he's in cervical traction. Keep suction equipment available to prevent aspiration.
- The patient may be in a cast or in traction day and night or at night only. Give meticulous cast care, including the monitoring of circulation, sensation, and color around the cast. Protect the cast around the patient's chin and mouth with waterproof material. Check for skin irritation, pressure areas, or softening of cast pad.
- Provide emotional support for the patient and family to relieve their anxiety due to fear, pain, limitations from the brace or traction, and an altered body image.
- Begin stretching exercises, such as those outlined above, as soon as the patient can tolerate them.
- Before discharge, explain to the patient or parents the importance of continuing daily heat applications, massages, and stretching exercises, as prescribed, and of keeping the cast clean and dry. Emphasize that physical therapy is essential for a successful rehabilitation after the cast is removed.

Selected References

Aegerter, Ernest E., and Kilpatrick, John A., Jr. *Orthopedic Diseases: Physiology, Pathology, Radiology,* 4th ed. Philadelphia: W.B. Saunders Co., 1975.

Calin, Andrei. *Diagnosis and Management of Rheumatoid Arthritis.* Reading, Mass.: Addison-Wesley Publishing Co., 1984.

Cassidy, James T. *Textbook of Pediatric Rheumatology.* New York: John Wiley & Sons, 1982.

Coventry, Mark B., ed. *Yearbook of Orthopedics, 1984.* Chicago: Year Book Medical Pubs., 1984.

Jahss, Melvin H. *Disorders of the Foot,* vol. I. Philadelphia: W.B. Saunders Co., 1982.

Karn, M.A., et al. "Postoperative Management of Patients Following Posterior Spinal Fusion," *Orthopedic Nursing* 3(2):21-25, March/April 1984.

Kelley, William N., et al. *Textbook of Rheumatology,* 2nd ed. Philadelphia: W.B. Saunders Co., 1985.

Klenerman, L. *The Foot and Its Disorders,* 2nd ed. St. Louis: C.V. Mosby Co., 1982.

McCarthy, Daniel J., ed. *Arthritis and Allied Conditions: A Textbook of Rheumatology,* 10th ed. Philadelphia: Lea & Febiger, 1985.

Rake, Robert F., ed. *Conn's Current Therapy.* Philadelphia: W.B. Saunders Co., 1984.

Riggs, Gail K., and Gall, Eric P., eds. *Rheumatic Diseases: Rehabilitation and Management.* Boston: Butterworth Publishers, 1984.

Rodnan, Gerald P., et al., eds. *Primer on Rheumatic Diseases.* Atlanta: Arthritis Foundation, 1983.

Scoles, Peter V. *Pediatric Orthopedics in Clinical Practice.* Chicago: Year Book Medical Pubs., 1982.

Tachdjian, Mihran O. *The Child's Foot.* Philadelphia: W.B. Saunders Co., 1984.

Utsinger, Peter D., et al. *Rheumatoid Arthritis: Etiology, Diagnosis, Management.* Philadelphia: J.B. Lippincott Co., 1985.

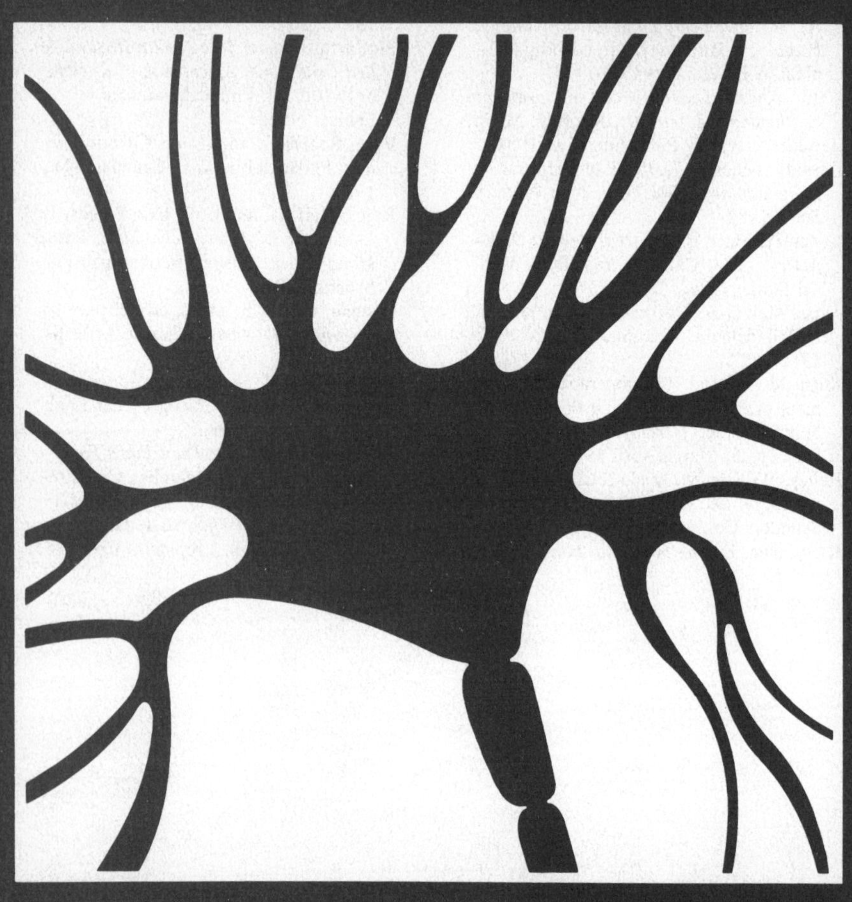

9 Neurologic Disorders

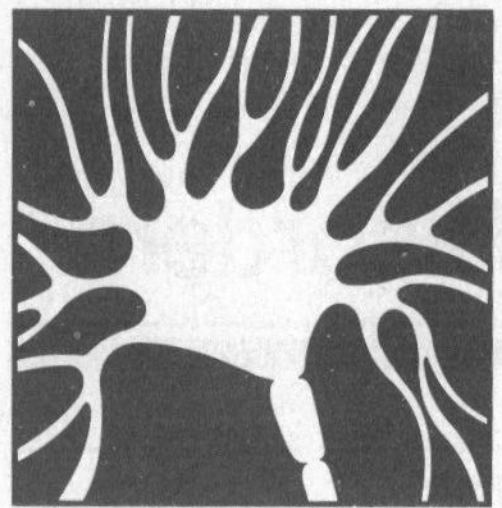

Neurologic Disorders

Introduction

The neurologic system, the body's communications network, coordinates and organizes the functions of all body systems. This intricate network has three main divisions:

• *central nervous system (CNS),* the control center, made up of the brain and the spinal cord

• *peripheral nervous system,* which includes nerves that connect the CNS to remote body parts and relay and receive messages from them

• *autonomic nervous system,* which regulates involuntary functioning of internal organs.

Fundamental unit

The fundamental unit of the nervous system is the neuron, a highly specialized conductor cell that receives and transmits electrochemical nerve impulses. It has a special, distinguishing structure. Delicate, threadlike nerve fibers extend from the central cell body and transmit signals: *axons* carry impulses away from the cell body; *dendrites* carry impulses to it. Most neurons have multiple dendrites but only one axon. *Sensory (afferent) neurons* transmit impulses from special receptors to the spinal cord or the brain; *motor (efferent) neurons* transmit impulses from the CNS to regulate activity of muscles or glands; and *interneurons (connecting or association neurons)* shuttle signals through complex pathways between sensory and motor neurons. Interneurons account for 99% of all the neurons in the nervous system and include most of the neurons in the brain itself.

Intricate control system

This intricate network of interlocking receptors and transmitters, with the brain and spinal cord, forms a dynamic control system—a living computer—that controls and regulates every mental and physical function. From birth to death, this astonishing system efficiently organizes the body's affairs—controlling the smallest action, thought, or feeling; monitoring communication and instinct for survival; and allowing introspection, wonder, abstract thought, and—unique to humans—awareness of one's own intelligence. The brain, the primary center of this central system, is the large soft mass of nervous tissue housed within the cranium, and protected and supported by the meninges.

The fragile brain and spinal cord are protected by bone (the skull and vertebrae), cushioning cerebrospinal fluid (CSF), and three membranes:

• The *dura mater,* or outer sheath, is made of tough white fibrous tissue.

• The *arachnoid membrane,* the middle layer, is delicate and lacelike.

• The *pia mater,* the inner meningeal layer, is made of fine blood vessels held together by connective tissue. It's thin and transparent, and clings to the brain and spinal cord surfaces, carrying branches of the cerebral arteries deep into the brain's fissures and sulci.

Between the dura mater and the arachnoid membrane is the *subdural space;* between the pia mater and the arachnoid membrane is the *subarachnoid space.* Within the subarachnoid space and the brain's four ventricles is *cerebrospinal fluid,* a liquid containing water and traces of organic materials (especially protein), glucose, and minerals.

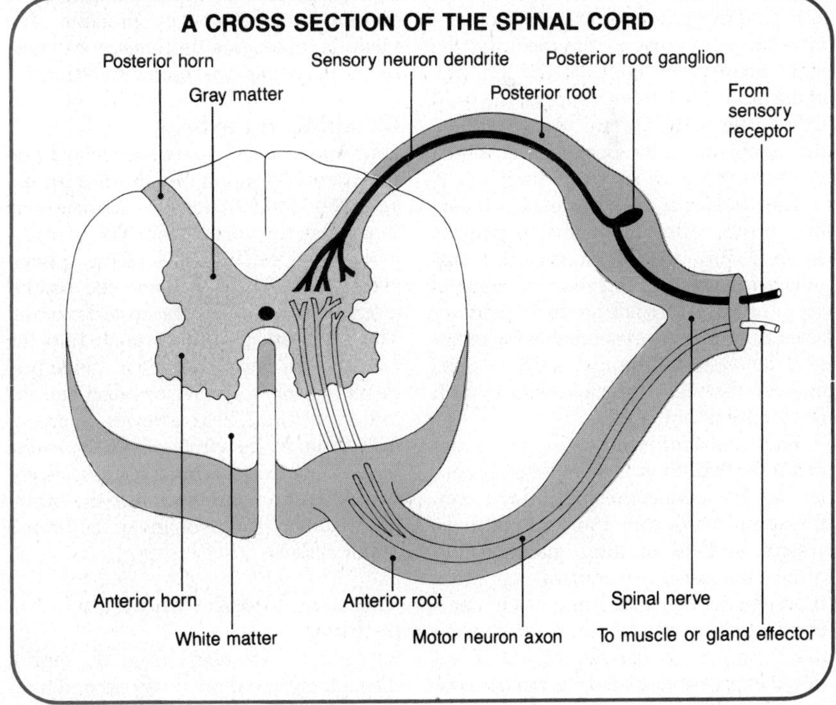

CSF is formed from blood in capillary networks called *choroid plexi,* which are located primarily in the brain's lateral ventricles. CSF is eventually reabsorbed into the venous blood through the *arachnoid villi,* in dural sinuses on the brain's surface.

The *cerebrum,* the largest portion of the brain, houses the nerve center that controls sensory and motor activities, and intelligence. The outer layer of the cerebrum, the *cerebral cortex,* consists of neuron cell bodies, or gray matter; the inner layers consist of axons, or white matter, plus basal ganglia, which control motor coordination and steadiness. The cerebral surface is deeply convoluted, furrowed with elevations (gyri) and depressions (sulci). The *longitudinal fissure* divides the cerebrum into two hemispheres connected by a wide band of nerve fibers called the *corpus callosum,* which allows the hemispheres to share learning and intellect. Both hemispheres don't share equally—one always dominates, giving one side control over the other. Because motor impulses descending from the brain through the pyramidal tract cross in the medulla, the right hemisphere controls the left side of the body; the left hemisphere, the right side of the body. Several fissures divide the cerebrum into lobes, each of which is associated with specific functions.

The *thalamus,* a relay center below the corpus callosum, further organizes cerebral function by transmitting impulses to and from appropriate areas of the cerebrum. In addition to its primary relay function, it's responsible for primitive emotional response, such as fear, and for distinguishing pleasant stimuli from unpleasant ones.

The *hypothalamus,* which lies beneath the thalamus, is an autonomic center that has connections with the brain, the spinal cord, the autonomic nervous system, and the pituitary gland. It regulates temperature control, appetite, blood pressure, breathing, sleep patterns, and peripheral nerve discharges that occur with behavioral and emotional expression. It also has partial control of pituitary gland secretion and stress reaction.

The base of the brain

Beneath the cerebrum, at the base of the brain, is the *cerebellum,* also called the hindbrain. It's responsible for smooth muscle movements, coordinating sensory impulses with muscle activity, and maintaining muscle tone and equilibrium.

The *brain stem* houses cell bodies for most of the cranial nerves and includes the *midbrain,* the *pons,* and the *medulla oblongata.* With the thalamus and the hypothalamus, it makes up a nerve network called the *reticular formation,* which acts as an arousal mechanism. It also relays nerve impulses between the spinal cord and other parts of the brain. The midbrain is the reflex center for the third and fourth cranial nerves, and mediates pupillary reflexes and eye movements. The pons helps regulate respirations. It's also the reflex center for the fifth through eighth cranial nerves, and mediates chewing, taste, saliva secretion, hearing, and equilibrium. The medulla oblongata influences cardiac, respiratory, and vasomotor functions.

Bloodline to the brain

Four major arteries—two *vertebral* and two *carotid*—supply the brain with oxygenated blood. These arteries originate in or near the aortic arch. The two vertebral arteries (branches of the subclavians) converge to become the basilar artery, which supplies the posterior brain. The common carotids branch into the two internal carotids, which divide further to supply the anterior brain and the middle brain. These arteries interconnect through the *circle of Willis,* at the base of the brain. This anastomosis ensures continual circulation to the brain, despite interruption of any of the brain's major vessels.

The spinal cord: Conductor pathway

Extending downward from the brain, through the vertebrae, to the second lumbar vertebra is the *spinal cord,* a two-way conductor pathway between the brain stem and the peripheral nervous system. The spinal cord is also the reflex center for activities that don't require brain control, such as a knee-jerk reaction to a reflex hammer.

A cross section of the spinal cord shows an internal H-shaped mass of gray matter divided into horns, which consist primarily of neuron cell bodies. Cell bodies in the *posterior,* or *dorsal, horn* primarily relay sensations; those in the *anterior,* or *ventral, horn* are needed for voluntary or reflex motor activity. The white matter surrounding the outer part of these horns consists of myelinated nerve fibers grouped functionally in vertical columns called *tracts.*

The *sensory,* or *ascending, tracts* carry sensory impulses up the spinal cord to the brain, while *motor,* or *descending, tracts* carry motor impulses down the spinal cord. The brain's motor impulses reach a descending tract and continue through the peripheral nervous system by *upper motor neurons.* These neurons originate in the brain and form two major systems:

• The *pyramidal system* (corticospinal tract) is responsible for fine, skilled movements of skeletal muscle. An impulse in this system originates in the frontal lobe's motor cortex, and travels downward to the pyramids of the medulla, where it crosses to the opposite side of the spinal cord.

• The *extrapyramidal system* (extracorticospinal tract) controls gross motor movements. An impulse traveling in this system originates in the frontal lobe's motor cortex, and is mediated by basal ganglia, the thalamus, cerebellum, and reticular formation before descending to the spinal cord.

Reaching outlying areas

Messages transmitted through the spinal cord reach outlying areas through the *peripheral nervous system,* which originates in 31 pairs of segmentally arranged spinal nerves attached to the spinal cord. Spinal nerves are numbered

A LOOK AT THE LOBES

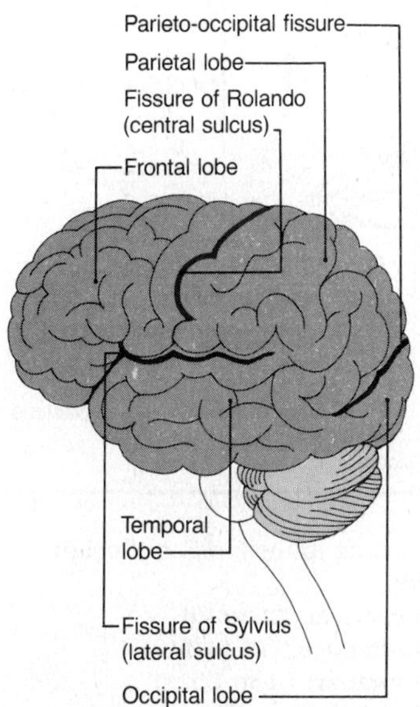

Several fissures divide the cerebrum into hemispheres and lobes; each lobe has a specific function. The *fissure of Sylvius* (lateral sulcus) separates the temporal lobe from the frontal and parietal lobes. The *fissure of Rolando* (central sulcus) separates the frontal lobes from the parietal lobe. The *parieto-occipital fissure* separates the occipital lobe from the two parietal lobes.

• The *frontal lobe* controls voluntary muscle movements and contains motor areas (including the motor area for speech, or Broca's area). It's the center for personality, behavioral, and intellectual functions, such as judgment, memory, and problem-solving; for autonomic functions; and for cardiac and emotional resonses.

• The *temporal lobe* is the center for taste, hearing, and smell, and in the brain's dominant hemisphere, interprets spoken language.

• The *parietal lobe* coordinates and interprets sensory information from the opposite side of the body.

• The *occipital lobe* interprets visual stimuli.

STRUCTURE OF THE NEURON

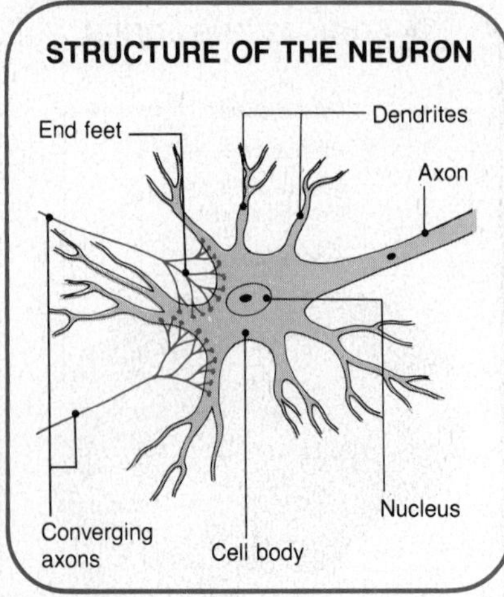

according to their point of origin in the cord:

- 8 cervical: C1 to C8
- 12 thoracic: T1 to T12
- 5 lumbar: L1 to L5
- 5 sacral: S1 to S5
- 1 coccygeal.

On the cross section of the spinal cord, you'll see that these spinal nerves are attached to the spinal cord by two roots:

- The *anterior,* or *ventral, root* consists of motor fibers that relay impulses from the cord to glands and muscles.
- The *posterior,* or *dorsal, root* consists of sensory fibers that relay sensory information from receptors to the cord. The posterior root has a swelling on it—the posterior root ganglion—which is made up of sensory neuron cell bodies.

After leaving the vertebral column, each spinal nerve separates into *rami* (branches), which distribute peripherally, with extensive but organized overlapping. This overlapping reduces the chance of lost sensory or motor function from interruption of a single spinal nerve.

Two functional systems

- The *somatic (voluntary) nervous system* is activated by will but can also function independently. It's responsible for all conscious and higher mental processes and for subconscious and reflex actions, such as shivering.
- The *autonomic (involuntary) nervous system* regulates functions of the unconscious level to control involuntary body functions, such as digestion, respiration, and cardiovascular function. It's usually divided into two antagonistic systems. The *sympathetic nervous system* controls energy expenditure, especially in stressful situations, by releasing the adrenergic catecholamine *norepinephrine.* The *parasympathetic nervous system* helps conserve energy by releasing the cholinergic neurohormone *acetylcholine.* These antagonistic systems balance each other to support homeostasis.

Assessing neurologic function

A complete neurologic assessment helps confirm the diagnosis in a suspected neurologic disorder. It establishes a clinical baseline and can offer lifesaving clues to rapid deterioration. Neurologic assessment includes:

- *Patient history:* In addition to the usual information, try to elicit the patient's and his family's perception of the disorder. Use the patient interview to make observations that help evaluate mental status and behavior.
- *Physical examination:* Pay particular attention to obvious abnormalities that may signal serious neurologic problems, for example, fluid draining from the nose or ears.
- *Neurologic examination:* Determine cerebral, cerebellar, motor, sensory, and cranial nerve function.

Obviously, there isn't always time for a complete neurologic examination during bedside assessment. Therefore, it is necessary to select priorities. For example, typical ongoing bedside assessment focuses on level of consciousness, pupillary response, motor function, reflexes, and vital signs. However, when time permits, a complete neurologic examination can provide valuable information regarding total neurologic function.

Mental status, intellect, and behavior

Mental status and behavior are good indicators of cerebral function, and they're easy to assess. Note the patient's appearance, mannerisms, posture, facial expression, grooming, and tone of voice. Check for orientation to time, place, and person, and for memory of recent and past events. To test intellect, ask the patient to count backward from 100 by 7s, to read aloud, or to interpret a common proverb, and see how well he understands and follows commands. But if you make such checks frequently, vary your questions to avoid a programmed response.

Level of consciousness

Level of consciousness is the single most valuable indicator of neurologic function. It can vary from alertness (response to verbal stimulus) to coma (failure to respond even to painful stimulus). It's best to document the patient's exact response to the stimulus: "patient pulled away in response to nail bed pressure" rather than just to write "stuporous."

The Glasgow Coma Scale (GCS), which assesses eye opening as well as verbal and motor responses, provides a quick standardized account of neurologic status and is becoming widely used. In this test, each response receives a numerical value. For instance, if the patient readily responds verbally, and is oriented to time, place, and person, he scores a 5; if he's totally unable to respond verbally, he scores a 1. A score of 15 for all three parts is normal; 7 or less indicates coma; 3—the lowest score possible—generally (but not always) points to brain death. Although the GCS is useful, it's not a substitute for a complete neurologic assessment.

Assessing motor function

Inability to perform the following simple tests, or observation of tics, tremors, or other abnormalities during such testing suggests cerebellar dysfunction.

- Ask the patient to touch his nose with each index finger, alternating hands. Repeat this test with his eyes closed.
- Instruct the patient to tap the index finger and thumb of each hand together rapidly.
- Have the patient draw a figure eight in the air with his foot.
- To test tandem walk, ask the patient to walk heel to toe in a straight line.
- To test balance, perform the Romberg test: Ask the patient to stand with feet together, eyes closed, and arms outstretched without losing balance.

Motor function is a good indicator of level of consciousness and can also point to central or peripheral nervous system damage. During all tests of motor function, watch for differences between right and left side functions.

- To check gait, ask the patient to walk while you observe posture, balance, and coordination of leg movement and arm swing.
- To check muscle tone, palpate muscles at rest and in response to passive flexion. Look for flaccidity, spasticity, and rigidity. Measure muscle size, and look for involuntary movements, such as rapid jerks, tremors, or contractions.
- To evaluate muscle strength, have the patient grip your hands and squeeze. Then, ask him to push against your palm with his foot. Compare muscle strength on each side, using a 5-point scale (5 is normal strength, 0 is complete paralysis). Also test the patient's ability to extend and flex the neck, elbows, wrists, fingers, toes (especially the great toe), hips, and knees; to extend the spine; to contract and relax the abdominal muscles; and to rotate the shoulders.
- Rate reflexes on a 4-point scale (4 is hyperactive reflex, 0 is absent reflex). Before testing reflexes, see that the patient is comfortable and relaxed. Then, to test superficial reflexes, stroke the skin of the abdominal, gluteal, plantar, and scrotal regions with a moderately sharp object (such as a key) that won't puncture the skin. A normal reflex is flexion in response to this stimulus. To test deep reflexes, use a reflex hammer to briskly tap the biceps, the triceps, and the brachioradialis (wrist), patellar (knee), and Achilles tendon regions. Normal response is rapid muscle extension and contraction.

Assessing sensory function

Impaired or absent sensation in the trunk or extremities can point to brain, spinal cord, or peripheral nerve damage. It's important to determine the extent of sensory dysfunction, since this helps locate neurologic damage. For instance, localized dysfunction indicates local peripheral nerve damage; dysfunction over a single dermatome (an area served by 1 of the 31 pairs of spinal nerves) indicates damage to the nerve's dorsal root; and dysfunction extending over more than one dermatome suggests brain or spinal cord damage.

In assessing sensory function, always test both sides of symmetric areas; for instance, both arms, not just one. Reassure the patient that the test won't be painful.

- *Superficial pain perception:* Lightly press the point of an open safety pin against the patient's skin. Don't press hard enough to scratch the skin.
- *Thermal sensitivity:* The patient tells what he feels when you place a test tube filled with hot water and one filled with cold water against his skin.
- *Tactile sensitivity:* Ask the patient to close his eyes and tell you what he feels when touched lightly on hands, wrists, arms, thighs, lower legs, feet, and trunk with a wisp of cotton.
- *Sensitivity to vibration:* Place the base of a vibrating tuning fork against the patient's wrists, elbows, knees, or other bony prominences. Hold it in place, and ask the patient to tell you when it stops vibrating.
- *Position sense:* Move the patient's toes or fingers up, down, and to the side. Ask the patient to tell you the direction of movement.
- *Discriminatory sensation:* Ask the patient to close his eyes and identify familiar textures (velvet, burlap) or objects placed in his hand, or numbers and letters traced on his palm.
- *Two-point discrimination:* Using calipers or other sharp objects, touch the patient in two different places simultaneously. Ask if he can feel one or two points.

Localize cranial nerve function

By using the simple tests that follow, you can reliably localize cranial nerve dysfunction.

- *Olfactory nerve (I):* Have the patient close his eyes and, using each nostril separately, try to identify common nonirritating smells, such as cinnamon, coffee, or peppermint.
- *Optic nerve (II):* Examine the patient's eyes with an ophthalmoscope, and have him read a Snellen eye chart or a newspaper. To test peripheral vision, ask him to cover one eye and fix his other eye on a point directly in front of him. Then, ask if he can see you wiggle your finger to his far right or left.
- *Oculomotor nerve (III):* Compare the size and shape of the patient's pupils, and the equality of pupillary response to a small light in a darkened room.
- *Trochlear nerve (IV) and abducens nerve (VI):* To assess for conjugate and lateral eye movement, ask the patient to follow your finger with his eyes, as you slowly move it from his far left to his far right.
- *Trigeminal nerve (V):* To test facial sensory response, stroke the patient's jaws, cheeks, and forehead with a cotton applicator, the point of a pin, or test tubes filled with hot or cold water. Since testing for a blink reflex is irritating to the patient, it's not commonly done. If you must test for this response (it may be decreased in patients who wear contact lenses), touch the cornea lightly with a wisp of cotton or tissue, and avoid repeating the test, if possible. To test for jaw jerk, ask the patient to hold his mouth slightly open, then tap the middle of his chin with a reflex hammer. The jaw should jerk closed.
- *Facial nerve (VII):* To test upper and lower facial motor function, ask the patient to raise his eyebrows, wrinkle his forehead, or show his teeth. To test sense of taste, ask him to identify the taste of well-known salty, sour, sweet, and bitter substances, which you have placed on his tongue.
- *Acoustic nerve (VIII):* Ask the patient to identify common sounds, such as a

GLASGOW COMA SCALE

To quickly assess a patient's level of consciousness and to uncover baseline changes, use the Glasgow Coma Scale. This assessment tool grades consciousness in relation to eye opening and motor and verbal responses. A decreased reaction score in one or more categories warns of impending neurologic crisis. A patient scoring 7 or less is comatose and probably has severe neurologic damage.

TEST	PATIENT'S REACTION	SCORE
Eye opening response	Open spontaneously	4
	Open to verbal command	3
	Open to pain	2
	No response	1
Best motor response	Obeys verbal command	6
	Localizes painful stimuli	5
	Flexion-withdrawal	4
	Flexion-abnormal (decorticate rigidity)	3
	Extension (decerebrate rigidity)	2
	No response	1
Best verbal response	Oriented and converses	5
	Disoriented and converses	4
	Inappropriate words	3
	Incomprehensible sounds	2
	No response	1
TOTAL		**3-15**

ticking clock. With a tuning fork, test for air and bone conduction.

• *Glossopharyngeal nerve (IX):* To test gag reflex, touch a tongue depressor to each side of the patient's pharynx.

• *Vagus nerve (X):* Observe ability to swallow, and watch for symmetric movements of soft palate when the patient says, "Ah."

• *Spinal accessory nerve (XI):* To test shoulder muscle strength, palpate the patient's shoulders, and ask him to shrug against a resistance.

• *Hypoglossal nerve (XII):* To test tongue movement, ask the patient to stick out his tongue. Inspect it for tremor, atrophy, or lateral deviation. To test for strength, ask the patient to move his tongue from side to side while you hold a tongue depressor against it.

Testing for a firm diagnosis

A firm diagnosis of many neurologic disorders often requires a wide range of relevant diagnostic tests. If possible, noninvasive tests are done first and may include the following:

- *A skull X-ray* identifies skull malformations, fractures, erosion, or thickening that may indicate tumors or increased intracranial pressure (ICP).
- *Computed tomography (CT) scan* is a series of X-rays of "slices" of the brain, which produces a three-dimensional effect. It's used to identify intracranial tumor, hemorrhage, or malformation, and cerebral atrophy, calcification, edema, and infarction. If a contrast medium is used, this is an invasive procedure.
- *Nuclear magnetic resonance imaging (NMR),* or magnetic resonance imaging (MRI), is a new diagnostic test that's similar to a CT scan but views the CNS in greater detail.
- *Electroencephalography* detects abnormal electrical activity in the brain, which may result from a seizure, a psychological or metabolic disorder, a tumor, mental retardation, or drug overdose.
- *Echoencephalography* determines if the midline structures in the brain have shifted, indicating a lesion.

Invasive tests may include:

- *Lumbar puncture:* A needle is inserted into the subarachnoid space of the spinal cord, usually between L3 and L4 (or L4 and L5), allowing aspiration of cerebrospinal fluid (CSF) for examination. This specimen is used to detect infection or hemorrhage; to determine cell count, and glucose, protein, and globulin levels; and to measure CSF pressure. Lumbar puncture is usually contraindicated in hydrocephalus and in known increased ICP, since quick reduction in pressure may cause brain herniation.
- *Myelography:* Following a lumbar puncture and CSF removal, a radiologic dye is instilled. X-rays determine spinal cord compression related to back pain or extremity weakness, and show spinal abnormalities.
- *Pneumoencephalography:* This test is seldom used now that CT scans are available. After lumbar puncture, a small amount of air is introduced into the subarachnoid space. A subsequent X-ray visualizes tumors and lesions in the brain stem and the ventricles.
- *Arteriography (cerebral angiography):* A catheter is inserted into an artery—usually the femoral artery—and is indirectly threaded up to the carotid artery. Then, a radiopaque dye is injected, which allows X-ray visualization of the cerebral vasculature. Sometimes the catheter is threaded directly into the brachial or carotid artery. This test can show cerebral vascular abnormalities and spasms, plus arterial changes due to tumor, arteriosclerosis, hemorrhage, aneurysm, or blockage from a cerebrovascular accident.
- *Ventriculography:* Air is introduced into the lateral ventricle through an opening in the skull, usually in the occipital region. X-rays are then taken and are used to identify tumors or anomalies that affect the ventricular system.
- *Brain scan:* A scanner measures gamma rays produced by a radioisotope injected I.V. Uptake and distribution of isotope in the brain can detect intracranial masses or vascular lesions.
- *Intracranial pressure (ICP) monitoring:* In this diagnostic test, a screw-type device with a sensor tip is inserted into a burr hole, usually in the parietal region. A transducer attached to the screw converts CSF pressure readings into electric impulses, which are visualized by an oscilloscope and recorded on a printout.

  An alternate method uses an intraventricular catheter with a three-way stopcock, flushing solution, and a manometer. ICP monitoring is done when even a slight rise in ICP is an emergency or when a precipitous rise may occur, as in a ruptured cerebral aneurysm or cerebral edema.
- *Electromyography:* A needle inserted into selected muscles at rest and during voluntary contraction picks up nerve impulses and measures nerve conduction time. This test is used to detect lower motor neuron disorders, neuromuscular disorders, and nerve damage.

CONGENITAL ANOMALIES

Cerebral Palsy

The most common cause of crippling in children, cerebral palsy comprises a group of neuromuscular disorders resulting from prenatal, perinatal, or postnatal CNS damage. Although nonprogressive, these disorders may become more obvious as an affected infant grows older. Three major types of cerebral palsy occur—spastic, athetoid, *and* ataxic—*sometimes in mixed forms. Motor impairment may be minimal (sometimes apparent only during physical activities such as running) or severely disabling. Associated defects, such as seizures, speech disorders, and mental retardation, are common. Prognosis varies. In mild impairment, proper treatment may make a near-normal life possible.*

Cerebral palsy occurs in an estimated 1.5 to 5:1,000 live births every year. Incidence is highest in premature infants (anoxia plays the greatest role in contributing to cerebral palsy) and in those who are small for their gestational age. Cerebral palsy is slightly more common in males than in females and occurs more often in whites.

Signs and symptoms

The *spastic* form of cerebral palsy predominates, affecting about 70% of patients. This form is characterized by hyperactive deep tendon reflexes, increased stretch reflexes, rapid alternating muscle contraction and relaxation, muscle weakness, underdevelopment of affected limbs, muscle contraction in response to manipulation, and a tendency toward contractures. Typically, a child with spastic cerebral palsy walks on his toes with a scissors gait, crossing one foot in front of the other.

In *athetoid cerebral palsy*, which affects about 20% of patients, involuntary movements—grimacing, wormlike writhing, dystonia, and sharp jerks—impair voluntary movement. Usually, these involuntary movements affect the arms more severely than the legs; involuntary facial movements may make speech difficult. These athetoid movements become more severe during stress, decrease with relaxation, and disappear entirely during sleep.

Ataxic cerebral palsy accounts for about 10% of patients. Its characteristics include disturbed balance, incoordination (especially of the arms), hypoactive reflexes, nystagmus, muscle weakness, tremor, lack of leg movement during infancy, and a wide gait as the child begins to walk. Ataxia makes sudden or fine movements almost impossible.

Some children with cerebral palsy display a combination of these clinical features. In most, impaired motor function makes eating, especially swallowing, difficult, and retards growth and development. Up to 40% of these children are mentally retarded, about 25% have seizure disorders, and about 80% have impaired speech. Many also have dental abnormalities, vision and hearing defects, and reading disabilities.

Diagnosis

Early diagnosis is essential for effective treatment and requires careful clinical observation during infancy and precise neurologic assessment. Suspect cerebral palsy whenever an infant:

- has difficulty sucking or keeping the nipple or food in his mouth
- seldom moves voluntarily, or has arm or leg tremors with voluntary movement
- crosses his legs when lifted from behind rather than pulling them up or "bicycling" like a normal infant

CAUSES OF CEREBRAL PALSY

Conditions that result in cerebral anoxia, hemorrhage, or other damage are probably responsible for cerebral palsy.

- *Prenatal causes:* maternal infection (especially rubella), radiation, anoxia, toxemia, maternal diabetes, abnormal placental attachment, malnutrition, and isoimmunization
- *Perinatal and birth difficulties:* forceps delivery, breech presentation, placenta previa, abruptio placentae, depressed maternal vital signs from general or spinal anesthetic, prolapsed cord with delay in delivery of head, premature birth, prolonged or unusually rapid labor, multiple birth (especially infants born last in a multiple birth)
- *Infection or trauma during infancy:* kernicterus resulting from erythroblastosis fetalis, brain infection, head trauma, prolonged anoxia, brain tumor, cerebral circulatory anomalies causing blood vessel rupture, and systemic disease resulting in cerebral thrombosis or embolus.

- has legs that are hard to separate, making diaper changing difficult
- persistently uses only one hand or, as he gets older, uses his hands well but not his legs.

Infants at particular risk include those with low birth weight, low Apgar scores at 5 minutes, seizures, and metabolic disturbances. However, all infants should have a screening test for cerebral palsy as a regular part of their 6-month checkup.

Treatment

Cerebral palsy can't be cured, but proper treatment can help affected children reach their full potential within the limits set by this disorder. Such treatment requires a comprehensive and cooperative effort involving doctors, nurses, teachers, psychologists, the child's family, and occupational, physical, and speech therapists. Home care is often possible. Treatment usually includes:

- braces or splints and special appliances, such as adapted eating utensils and a low toilet seat with arms, to help these children perform activities independently
- an artificial urinary sphincter for the incontinent child who can use the hand controls
- range-of-motion exercises to minimize contractures
- orthopedic surgery to correct contractures
- phenytoin, phenobarbital, or another anticonvulsant to control seizures
- sometimes muscle relaxants or neurosurgery to decrease spasticity.

Children with milder forms of cerebral palsy should attend a regular school; severely afflicted children need special education classes.

Special considerations

A child with cerebral palsy may be hospitalized for orthopedic surgery and for treatment of other complications.

- Speak slowly and distinctly. Encourage the child to ask for things he wants. Listen patiently and don't rush him.
- Plan an adequate diet to meet the child's high energy needs.
- During meals, maintain a quiet, unhurried atmosphere with as few distractions as possible. The child may need special utensils and a chair with a solid footrest. Teach him to place food far back in his mouth to facilitate swallowing.
- Encourage the child to chew food thoroughly, drink through a straw, and suck on lollipops, to develop the muscle control needed to minimize drooling.
- Allow the child to wash and dress independently, assisting only as needed. The child may need clothing modifications.
- Give all care in an unhurried manner; otherwise, muscle spasticity may increase.
- Encourage the child and his family to participate in the care plan so they can continue it at home.
- Care for associated hearing or visual disturbances, as necessary.
- Give frequent mouth care and dental

care, as necessary.
- Reduce muscle spasms that increase postoperative pain by moving and turning the child carefully after surgery.
- After orthopedic surgery, give good cast care. Wash and dry the skin at the edge of the cast frequently, and rub it with alcohol. Reposition the child often, check for foul odor, and ventilate under the cast with a blow-dryer. Use a flashlight to check for skin breakdown beneath the cast. Help the child relax, perhaps by giving a warm bath, before reapplying a bivalved cast.

Help parents deal with their child's handicap:
- A good understanding of normal growth and development will enable you to work with parents to set realistic goals.
- Assist in planning crafts and other activities.
- Stress the child's need to develop peer relationships; warn the parents against being overprotective.
- Identify and deal with family stress. Parents may feel unreasonable guilt about their child's handicap and may need psychological counseling.
- Make a referral to supportive community organizations. For more information, tell parents to contact the United Cerebral Palsy Association, Inc., or their local cerebral palsy agency.

Hydrocephalus

Hydrocephalus is an excessive accumulation of cerebrospinal fluid (CSF) within the ventricular spaces of the brain. It occurs most often in newborns, but it can also occur in adults as a result of injury or disease. In infants, hydrocephalus enlarges the head; and in both infants and adults, resulting compression can damage brain tissue. With early detection and surgical intervention, prognosis improves but remains guarded. Even after surgery, such complications as mental retardation, impaired motor function, and vision loss can persist. Without surgery, prognosis is poor: mortality may result from increased intracranial pressure in persons of all ages; infants may also die prematurely of infection and malnutrition.

Causes

Hydrocephalus may result from an obstruction in CSF flow (noncommunicating hydrocephalus) or from faulty absorption of CSF (communicating hydrocephalus).

In noncommunicating hydrocephalus, the obstruction occurs most frequently between the third and fourth ventricles, at the aqueduct of Sylvius, but it can also occur at the outlets of the fourth ventricle (foramina of Luschka and Magendie) or, rarely, at the foramen of Monro. This obstruction may result from faulty fetal development, infection (syphilis, granulomatous diseases, meningitis), a tumor, cerebral aneurysm, or a blood clot (after intracranial hemorrhage).

In communicating hydrocephalus, faulty absorption of CSF may result from

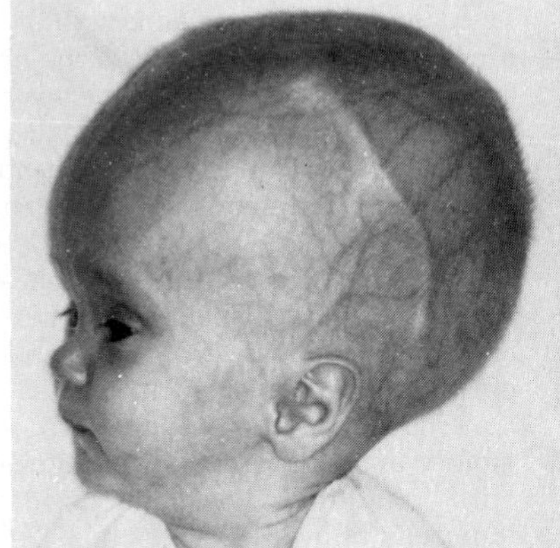

In infants, characteristic changes of hydrocephalus include marked enlargement of the head; distended scalp veins; thin, shiny, and fragile-looking scalp skin; and underdeveloped neck muscles.

NORMAL CIRCULATION OF CSF

CSF is produced from blood in a capillary network (choroid plexus) in the brain's lateral ventricles. From the lateral ventricles, CSF flows through the interventricular foramen (foramen of Monro) to the third ventricle. From there, it flows through the aqueduct of Sylvius to the fourth ventricle and through the foramina of Luschka and Magendie to the cisterna of the subarachnoid space.

Then, the fluid passes under the base of the brain, upward over the brain's upper surfaces, and down around the spinal cord. Eventually, CSF reaches the arachnoid villi, where it's reabsorbed into venous blood at the venous sinuses.

Normally, the amount of fluid produced (about 500 ml/day) equals the amount absorbed. The average amount circulated at one time is 150 to 175 ml.

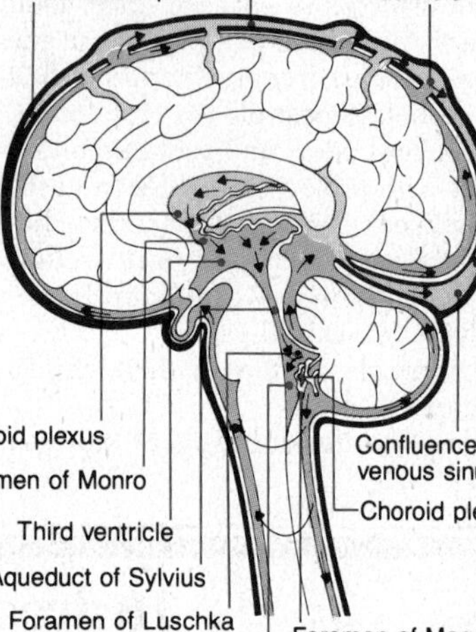

surgery to repair a myelomeningocele, adhesions between meninges at the base of the brain, or meningeal hemorrhage. Rarely, a tumor in the choroid plexus causes overproduction of CSF, producing hydrocephalus.

Signs and symptoms

In infants, the unmistakable sign of hydrocephalus is enlargement of the head clearly disproportionate to the infant's growth. Other characteristic changes in hydrocephalic infants include distended scalp veins; thin, fragile- and shiny-looking scalp skin; and underdeveloped neck muscles. In severe hydrocephalus, the roof of the orbit is depressed, the eyes are displaced downward, and the sclera are prominent. A high-pitched, shrill cry; abnormal muscle tone of the legs; irritability; anorexia; and vomiting often occur. In adults and older children, indicators of hydrocephalus include decreased level of consciousness, ataxia, incontinence, and impaired intellect.

Diagnosis

In infants, abnormally large head size for the patient's age strongly suggests this diagnosis. Skull X-rays show thinning of the skull with separation of sutures and widening of fontanelles; ventriculography shows enlargement of the brain's ventricles. Angiography, pneumoencephalography, CT scan, and magnetic resonance imaging can differentiate between hydrocephalus and intracranial lesions and can also demonstrate the Arnold-Chiari deformity, which occurs with hydrocephalus.

Treatment

Surgical correction is the only treatment for hydrocephalus. Usually, such surgery consists of insertion of a ventriculoperitoneal shunt, which transports excess fluid from the lateral ventricle into the peritoneal cavity. A less common procedure is insertion of a ventriculoatrial shunt, which drains fluid from the brain's lateral ventricle into the right atrium of the heart, where the fluid makes its way into the venous circulation.

Complications of surgery include shunt infection, septicemia (after ventriculoatrial shunt), adhesions and paralytic ileus, migration, peritonitis, and intestinal perforation (with peritoneal shunt).

Special considerations

On initial assessment, obtain a complete history from the patient or the family. Note general behavior, especially irritability, apathy, or decreased level of consciousness. Perform a neurologic assessment. Examine the eyes: pupils should be equal and reactive to light. In adults and older children, evaluate movements and motor strength in extremities. (Watch especially for ataxia.) Ask the patient if he has headaches, and watch for projectile vomiting; both are signs of increased intracranial pressure. Also watch for convulsions. Note changes in vital signs.

Before surgery to insert a shunt:

- Encourage maternal/infant bonding when possible. When caring for the infant yourself, hold him on your lap for feeding; stroke and cuddle him, and speak soothingly.
- Check fontanelles for tension or fullness, and measure and record head circumference. On the patient's chart, draw a picture showing where to measure the head so that other staff members measure it in the same place, or mark the forehead with ink.
- To prevent postfeeding aspiration and hypostatic pneumonia, place the infant on his side and reposition every 2 hours, or prop him up in an infant seat.
- To prevent skin breakdown, make sure his earlobe is flat, and place a sheepskin or rubber foam under his head.
- When turning the infant, move his head, neck, and shoulders with his body, to reduce strain on his neck.
- Feed the infant slowly. To lessen strain from the weight of the infant's head on your arm while holding him during feeding, place his head, neck, and shoulders on a pillow.

After surgery:

- Place the infant on the side opposite the operative site, with his head level with his body unless the doctor's orders specify otherwise.
- Check temperature, pulse rate, blood pressure, and level of consciousness. Also check fontanelles for fullness daily. Watch for vomiting, which may be an early sign of increased intracranial pressure and shunt malfunction.
- Watch for signs of infection, especially meningitis: fever, stiff neck, irritability, or tense fontanelles. Also watch for redness, swelling, or other signs of local infection over the shunt tract. Check dressing often for drainage.
- Listen for bowel sounds after ventriculoperitoneal shunt.
- Check the infant's growth and development periodically, and help the parents set goals consistent with ability and potential. Help parents focus on their child's strengths, not his weaknesses. Discuss special education programs, and emphasize the infant's need for sensory stimulation appropriate for his age. Teach parents to watch for signs of shunt malfunction, infection, and paralytic ileus. Tell them that shunt insertion requires periodic surgery to lengthen the shunt as the child grows older, to correct malfunctioning, or to treat infection.

ARNOLD-CHIARI SYNDROME

The Arnold-Chiari syndrome frequently accompanies hydrocephalus, especially when a myelomeningocele is also present. In this condition, an elongation or tonguelike downward projection of the cerebellum and medulla extends through the foramen magnum into the cervical portion of the spinal canal, impairing CSF drainage from the fourth ventricle.

In addition to signs and symptoms of hydrocephalus, infants with this syndrome have nuchal rigidity, noisy respirations, irritability, vomiting, weak sucking reflex, and a preference for hyperextension of neck.

Treatment requires surgery to insert a shunt like that used in hydrocephalus. Surgical decompression of the cerebellar tonsils at the foramen magnum is sometimes indicated.

Cerebral Aneurysm

Cerebral aneurysm is a localized dilation of a cerebral artery that results from a weakness in the arterial wall. Its most common form is the berry aneurysm, a saclike outpouching in a cerebral artery. Cerebral aneurysms usually arise at an arterial junction in the circle of Willis, the circular anastomosis forming the major cerebral arteries at the base of the brain. Cerebral aneurysms often rupture and cause subarachnoid hemorrhage.

Prognosis is guarded. Probably half the patients suffering subarachnoid hemorrhages die immediately; of those persons who survive untreated, 40% die from the effects of hemorrhage; another 20% die later from recurring hemorrhage. With new and better treatment, prognosis is improving.

Causes and incidence

Cerebral aneurysm may result from a congenital defect, a degenerative process, or a combination of both. For example, hypertension and atherosclerosis may disrupt blood flow and exert pressure against a congenitally weak arterial wall, stretching it like an overblown balloon and making it likely to rupture. After such rupture, blood spills into the space normally occupied by CSF (subarachnoid hemorrhage). Sometimes, it also spills into brain tissue and subsequently forms a clot. This may result in potentially fatal increased intracranial pressure (ICP) and brain tissue damage.

Incidence is slightly higher in women than in men, especially those in their late 40s or early to mid-50s, but cerebral aneurysm may occur at any age, in both women and men.

Signs and symptoms

Occasionally, rupture of a cerebral aneurysm causes premonitory symptoms that last several days, such as headache, nuchal rigidity, stiff back and legs, and intermittent nausea. Normally, however, onset is abrupt and without warning, causing a sudden severe headache, nausea, vomiting, and, depending on the severity and location of bleeding, altered consciousness (including deep coma).

Bleeding causes meningeal irritation, resulting in nuchal rigidity, back and leg pain, fever, restlessness, irritability, occasional seizures, and blurred vision. Bleeding into the brain tissues causes hemiparesis, hemisensory defects, dysphagia, and visual defects. If the aneurysm is near the internal carotid artery, it compresses the oculomotor nerve and causes diplopia, ptosis, dilated pupil, and inability to rotate the eye.

The severity of symptoms varies considerably from patient to patient, depending on the site and amount of bleeding. To better describe their conditions, patients with ruptured cerebral aneurysms are grouped as follows:

• *Grade I: Minimal bleed.* Patient is alert with no neurologic deficit; he may have a slight headache and nuchal rigidity.
• *Grade II: Mild bleed.* Patient is alert, with a mild to severe headache, nuchal rigidity, and, possibly, third-nerve palsy.
• *Grade III: Moderate bleed.* Patient is confused or drowsy, with nuchal rigidity and, possibly, a mild focal deficit.
• *Grade IV: Severe bleed.* Patient is stuporous, with nuchal rigidity and, possibly, mild to severe hemiparesis.
• *Grade V: Moribund (often fatal).* If nonfatal, patient is in deep coma or decerebrate.

Generally, cerebral aneurysm poses three major threats:

• *death from increased ICP:* increased ICP may push the brain downward, impair brain stem function, and cut off blood supply to the part of the brain that supports vital functions.
• *rebleed:* generally, after the initial bleeding episode, a clot forms and seals the rupture, which reinforces the wall of the aneurysm for 7 to 10 days. How-

MOST COMMON SITES OF CEREBRAL ANEURYSM

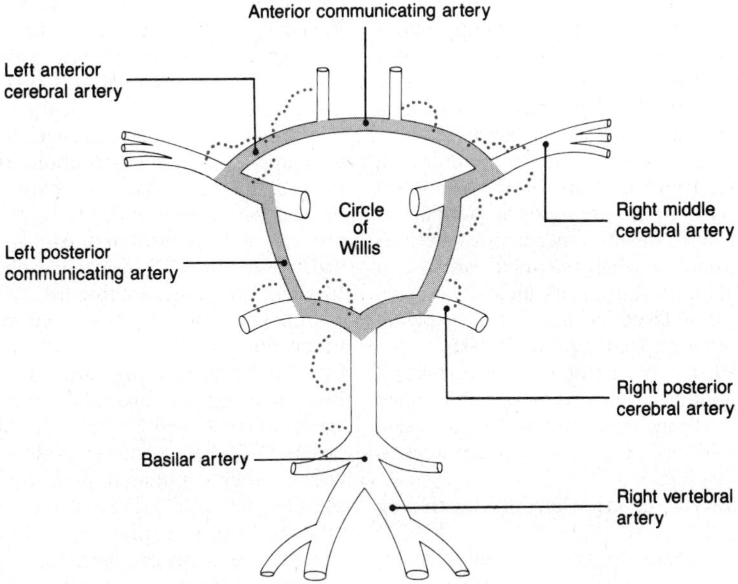

Anterior communicating artery
Left anterior cerebral artery
Right middle cerebral artery
Circle of Willis
Left posterior communicating artery
Right posterior cerebral artery
Basilar artery
Right vertebral artery

ever, after the seventh day, fibrinolysis begins to dissolve the clot and increases the risk of rebleeding. This rebleeding produces signs and symptoms similar to those accompanying the initial hemorrhage. Rebleeds during the first 48 to 72 hours following initial hemorrhage are not uncommon and contribute to the high mortality.

• *vasospasm:* why this occurs isn't clearly understood. Usually, vasospasm occurs in blood vessels adjacent to the aneurysm, but it may extend to major vessels of the brain, causing ischemia and altered brain function.

Other complications include acute hydrocephalus (a result of abnormal accumulation of CSF within the cranial cavity because of CSF blockage by blood or adhesions) and pulmonary embolism (a possible side effect of aneurysm treatment with aminocaproic acid or deep vein thrombosis).

Diagnosis

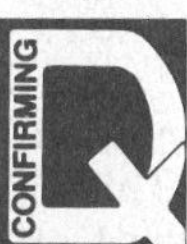

Angiography can pinpoint an unruptured cerebral aneurysm. Unfortunately, diagnosis of cerebral aneurysm usually follows its rupture. Then, diagnostic evaluation includes patient history, physical examination, and certain laboratory tests.

• *Lumbar puncture* can detect blood in CSF and increased ICP.

• *Skull X-ray* may show calcification in the walls of a large aneurysm.

• *EKG* often shows flattened or depressed T waves.

• *CT scan* locates the clot and identifies hydrocephalus, areas of infarction, and extent of blood spillage within the cisterns around the brain.

Other baseline laboratory studies include complete blood count, urinalysis, measurement of arterial blood gases, coagulation studies, serum osmolality, and electrolyte and glucose levels.

Treatment

Treatment aims to reduce the risk of rebleeding by repairing the aneurysm. Usually, surgical repair (by clipping, ligation, or wrapping the aneurysm neck with muscle) takes place 7 to 10 days after the initial bleed; however, surgery performed within 1 to 2 days after hemorrhage has also shown promise in grades I and II. When surgical correction is risky (in very elderly patients or those with heart, lung, or other serious diseases), or when the aneurysm is in a particularly dangerous location or surgery is delayed because of vasospasm, conservative treatment includes:

- bed rest in a quiet, darkened room; if immediate surgery isn't possible, such bed rest may continue for 4 to 6 weeks
- avoidance of coffee, other stimulants, and aspirin
- codeine or another analgesic, as needed
- hydralazine or another hypotensive agent if the patient is hypertensive
- corticosteroids to reduce edema
- phenobarbital or another sedative
- aminocaproic acid, a fibrinolytic inhibitor, to minimize the risk of rebleed by delaying blood clot lysis. However, this drug's effectiveness is controversial.

After surgical repair, the patient's condition depends on the extent of damage from the initial bleed and the degree of success of the treatment of the resulting complications. Surgery cannot improve the patient's neurologic condition unless it removes a hematoma or reduces the compression effect.

Special considerations

An accurate neurologic assessment, good patient care, patient and family teaching, and psychological support can speed recovery and reduce complications.

- During initial treatment after hemorrhage, establish and maintain a patent airway, since the patient may need supplementary oxygen. Position the patient to promote pulmonary drainage and prevent upper airway obstruction. If he's intubated, preoxygenation with 100% oxygen before suctioning to remove secretions will prevent hypoxia and vasodilation from CO_2 accumulation. Give frequent nose and mouth care.
- Impose aneurysm precautions to minimize the risk of rebleed and to avoid increased ICP. Such precautions include bed rest in a quiet, darkened room (keep the head of the bed flat or under 30°, as ordered); limited visitors; avoidance of coffee, other stimulants, and strenuous physical activity; and restricted fluid intake. Be sure to explain why these restrictive measures are necessary.

Along with these preventive measures, good patient care can minimize other complications:

- Turn the patient often. Encourage deep breathing and leg movement. Warn the patient to avoid all unnecessary physical activity. Assist with active range-of-motion exercises (unless the doctor has forbidden them); if the patient is paralyzed, perform regular passive range-of-motion exercises.
- Monitor arterial blood gases, level of consciousness, and vital signs often, and accurately measure intake and output. Avoid taking temperature rectally, since

ANEURYSM CLIP

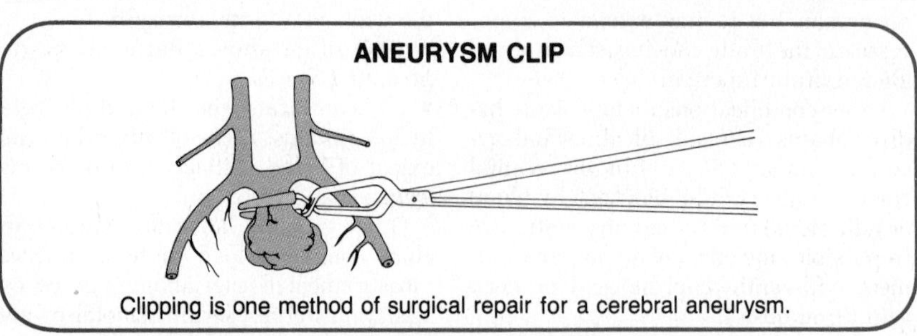

Clipping is one method of surgical repair for a cerebral aneurysm.

vagus nerve stimulation may cause cardiac arrest.

• Watch for these danger signals, which may indicate an enlarging aneurysm, rebleeding, intracranial clot, vasospasm, or other complication: decreased level of consciousness, unilateral enlarged pupil, onset or worsening of hemiparesis or motor deficit, increased blood pressure, slowed pulse, worsening of headache or sudden onset of a headache, renewed or worsened nuchal rigidity, renewed or persistent vomiting.

• Give fluids, as ordered, and monitor I.V. infusions to avoid increased ICP.

• If the patient has facial weakness, assist him during meals, placing food in the unaffected side of his mouth. If he can't swallow, insert a nasogastric tube, as ordered, and give all tube feedings slowly. Prevent skin breakdown by taping the tube so it doesn't press against the nostril. If the patient can eat, provide a high-bulk diet (bran, salads, and fruit) to prevent straining at stool, which can increase ICP. Get an order for a stool softener, such as dioctyl sodium sulfosuccinate, or a mild laxative, and administer, as ordered. *Don't* force fluids. Implement a bowel program based on previous habits. If the patient is receiving steroids, check the stool for blood.

• With third or facial nerve palsy, administer artificial tears to the affected eye, and tape the eye shut at night to prevent corneal damage.

• To minimize stress, give a sedative, as ordered. Watch for signs of oversedation, and report them immediately. If the patient is confused, raise the side rails to help protect him from injury. If possible, avoid using restraints, since these can cause agitation and raise ICP.

• Administer hydralazine or another hypotensive agent, as ordered. Carefully monitor blood pressure and report *any* significant change, but especially a rise in systolic pressure, immediately.

• Administer aminocaproic acid I.V. in dextrose 5% in water, P.O. or as ordered. Give it at least every 2 hours to maintain therapeutic blood levels. (Renal insufficiency may require dosage adjustment.) Monitor the patient for adverse reactions, such as nausea and diarrhea, which are most common with oral administration, and phlebitis, most common with I.V. administration. Reduce deep vein thrombosis by applying elastic stockings.

• If the patient can't speak, establish a simple means of communication, or use cards or a slate. Try to limit conversation to topics that won't further frustrate the patient. Encourage his family to speak to him in a normal tone, even if he doesn't seem to respond.

• Provide emotional support, and include the patient's family in his care as much as possible. Encourage family members to adopt a positive attitude, but discourage unrealistic goals.

• Before discharge, make a referral to a visiting nurse or a rehabilitation center when necessary.

Spinal Cord Defects

(Spina bifida, meningocele, myelomeningocele)

Defective embryonic neural tube closure during the first trimester of pregnancy results in various malformations of the spine. Generally, these defects occur in the lumbosacral area, but they are occasionally found in the sacral, thoracic, and cervical areas.

Spina bifida occulta is the most common and least severe spinal cord defect. It's characterized by incomplete closure of one or more vertebrae without protrusion of the spinal cord or meninges.

However, in more severe forms of spina bifida, incomplete closure of one or more vertebrae causes protrusion of the spinal contents in an external sac or cystic lesion. In spina bifida with meningocele, this sac contains meninges and CSF. In spina bifida with myelomeningocele (meningomyelocele), this sac contains meninges, CSF, and a portion of the spinal cord or nerve roots distal to the conus medullaris.

Prognosis varies with the degree of accompanying neurologic deficit. It's worst in patients with large open lesions, neurogenic bladders (which predispose to infection and renal failure), or total paralysis of the legs. Because such features are usually absent in spina bifida occulta and meningocele, prognosis is much better than in myelomeningocele, and many patients with these conditions can lead normal lives.

Causes and incidence

Normally, about 20 days after conception, the embryo develops a neural groove in the dorsal ectoderm. This groove rapidly deepens, and the two edges fuse to form the neural tube. By about day 23, this tube is completely closed except for an opening at each end. Theoretically, if the posterior portion of this neural tube fails to close by the fourth week of gestation, or if it closes but then splits open from a cause such as an abnormal increase in CSF later in the first trimester, a spinal defect results.

Viruses, radiation, and other environmental factors may be responsible for such defects. However, spinal cord defects occur more often in offspring of women who have previously had children with similar defects, so genetic factors may also be responsible.

Spina bifida is relatively common and affects about 5% of the population. In the United States, about 12,000 infants each year are born with some form of spina bifida; spina bifida with myelomeningocele is less common than spina bifida occulta and spina bifida with meningocele. Incidence is highest in persons of Welsh or Irish ancestry.

ENCEPHALOCELE

An encephalocele is a congenital saclike protrusion of the meninges and brain through a defective opening in the skull. Usually, it's in the occipital area, but it may also occur in the parietal, nasopharyngeal, or frontal area.

Clinical effects of encephalocele vary with the degree of tissue involvement and location of the defect. Paralysis and hydrocephalus are common.

Treatment includes surgery during infancy to place protruding tissues back in the skull, excise the sac, and correct associated craniofacial abnormalities. Always handle an infant with encephalocele carefully and avoid pressure on the sac. Both before and after surgery, watch for signs of increased intracranial pressure (bulging fontanelles). As the child grows older, teach his parents to watch for developmental deficiencies that may signal mental retardation.

Signs and symptoms

Spina bifida occulta is often accompanied by a depression or dimple, tuft of hair, soft fatty deposits, port wine nevi, or a combination of these abnormalities on the skin over the spinal defect; however, such signs may be absent. Spina bifida occulta doesn't usually cause neurologic dysfunction but occasionally is associated with foot weakness or bowel and bladder disturbances. Such disturbances are especially likely during rapid growth phases, when the spinal cord's ascent within the vertebral column may be impaired by its abnormal adherence to other tissues.

In both meningocele and myelomeningocele, a saclike structure protrudes over the spine. Like spina bifida occulta, meningocele rarely causes neurologic deficit. But myelomeningocele, depending on the level of the defect, causes permanent neurologic dysfunction, such as flaccid or spastic paralysis and bowel and blad-

TYPES OF SPINAL CORD DEFECTS

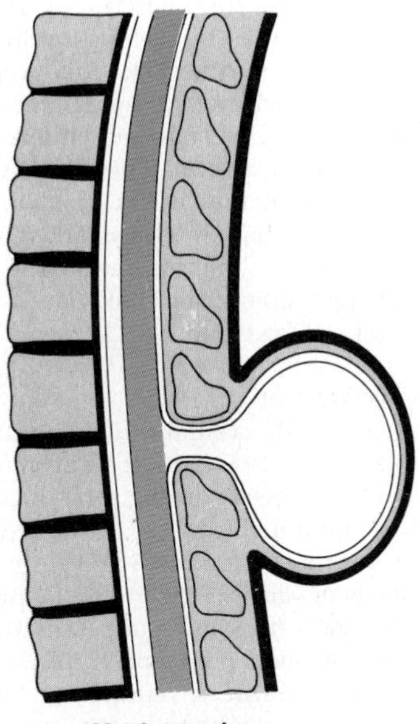
Meningocele

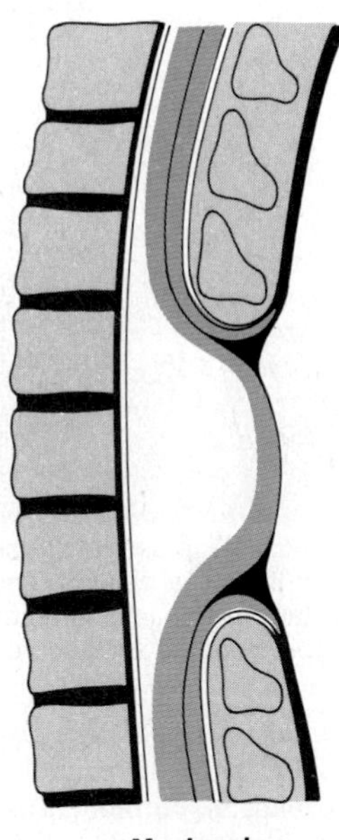
Myelocele

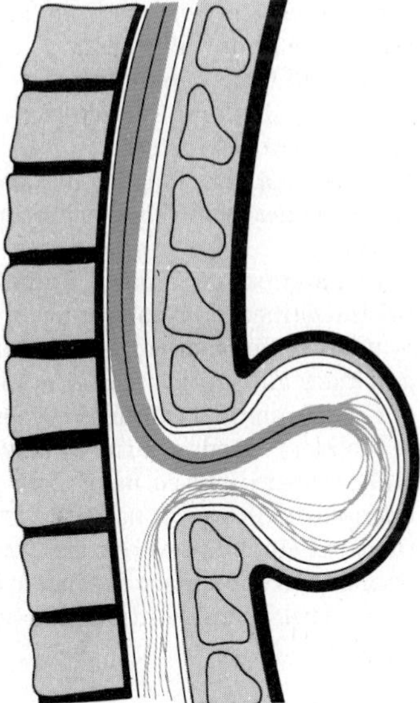
Myelomeningocele

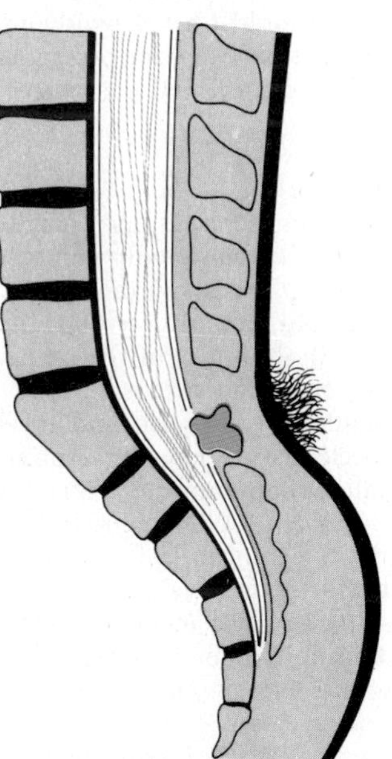
Spina Bifida Occulta

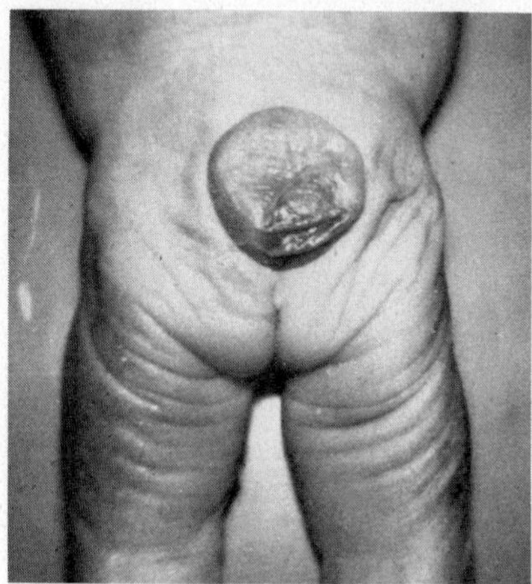

In myelomeningocele, a saclike structure protrudes over the spinal column. This structure contains meninges, cerebrospinal fluid, and a portion of the spinal cord.

der incontinence. Associated disorders include trophic skin disturbances (ulcerations, cyanosis), clubfoot, knee contractures, hydrocephalus (in about 90% of patients), and possibly mental retardation, Arnold-Chiari syndrome (in which part of the brain protrudes into the spinal canal), and curvature of the spine.

Diagnosis

Spina bifida occulta is often overlooked, although it's occasionally palpable and spinal X-ray can show the bone defect. Myelography can differentiate it from other spinal abnormalities, especially spinal cord tumors.

Usually, meningocele and myelomeningocele are obvious on examination; transillumination of the protruding sac can sometimes distinguish between them. (In meningocele, it typically transilluminates; in myelomeningocele, it doesn't.) In myelomeningocele, a pinprick examination of the legs and trunk shows the level of sensory and motor involvement; skull X-rays, cephalic measurements, and CT scan demonstrate associated hydrocephalus. Other appropriate laboratory tests in patients with myelomeningocele include urinalysis, urine cultures, and tests for renal function in older children and adults with urinary incontinence.

Although amniocentesis can detect only open defects, such as myelomeningocele and meningocele, this procedure is recommended for all pregnant women who have previously had children with spinal cord defects, since these women are at an increased risk of having children with similar defects. If these defects are present, amniocentesis shows increased alpha-fetoprotein levels by 14 weeks of gestation.

Treatment

Spina bifida occulta usually requires no treatment. However, if neuromuscular problems occur during growth, surgery may be indicated.

Treatment for meningocele consists solely of surgical closure of the protruding sac and continual assessment of growth and development. Treatment of myelomeningocele requires surgical repair of the sac and supportive measures to promote independence and prevent further complications. Unfortunately, surgery can't reverse neurologic deficit. Usually, a shunt is necessary to relieve associated hydrocephalus.

In older children or adults, rehabilitation measures include:

- waist supports, long leg braces, walkers, crutches, and other orthopedic appliances
- diet and bowel training to manage fecal incontinence or colostomy
- neurogenic bladder management with a urinary antiseptic, regular application of Credé's method (manual compression of bladder) to reduce urinary stasis, possibly intermittent catheterization, and antispasmodics such as bethanechol or propantheline. In severe cases, insertion of an artificial urinary sphincter is often successful; urinary diversion may be helpful.

Special considerations

Care of the patient with a severe spinal defect requires a team approach, with the neurosurgeon, orthopedist, urologist, nurse, social worker, occupational and physical therapists, and parents. Obviously, care is most complex when the neurologic deficit is severe. Immediate goals include psychological support to help parents accept the diagnosis, and pre- and postoperative care. Long-term goals include patient and family teaching, and measures to prevent contractures, decubitus ulcers, urinary tract infections, and other complications.

Before surgery for meningocele or myelomeningocele:

- Prevent local infection by cleansing the defect gently with sterile saline solution or other solutions, as ordered. Inspect the defect often for signs of infection, and cover it with sterile dressings moistened with sterile saline solution. Don't use ointments on the defect, since they may cause skin maceration. Prevent skin breakdown by placing sheepskin or a foam pad under the infant. Keep skin clean, and apply lotion to knees, elbows, chin, and other pressure areas. Give antibiotics, as ordered.
- Handle the infant carefully, and don't apply pressure to the defect. Usually, he can't wear a diaper or a shirt until after surgical correction, because it will irritate the sac, so keep him warm in an infant incubator (Isolette). Position him on his abdomen to prevent contamination of the sac with urine or feces. Hold and cuddle the infant, but avoid placing pressure on the sac. When holding him on your lap, position him on his abdomen, and teach parents to do the same.
- Measure head circumference daily, and watch for signs of hydrocephalus and meningeal irritation, such as fever or nuchal rigidity.
- Contractures can be minimized by passive range-of-motion exercises and casting. To prevent hip dislocation, moderately abduct hips with a pad between the knees, or with sandbags and ankle rolls.
- Monitor intake and output. Watch for decreased skin turgor, dryness, or other signs of dehydration. To prevent urinary tract infection, Credé the bladder every 2 hours during the day and once during the night. Provide meticulous skin care to genitals and buttocks to prevent infection.
- Ensure adequate nutrition.

After surgical repair of the defect:

- Watch for hydrocephalus, which often follows such surgery. Measure the child's head circumference, as ordered.
- Monitor vital signs often. Watch for signs of shock, infection, and increased intracranial pressure (projectile vomiting). Remember that before age 2, infants don't show typical signs of increased intracranial pressure, since suture lines aren't fully closed. In infants, the most telling sign is bulging fontanelles.
- Change the dressing regularly, as ordered, and check for drainage, wound rupture, and infection.
- If leg casts have been applied to prevent deformities, watch for signs that the child is outgrowing the cast. Petal its edges with plastic to prevent softening and skin irritation. Use a blow-dryer to dry skin under the cast. Periodically check for foul odor and other indications of skin breakdown.

Teach parents how to cope with the infant's physical problems and successfully meet long-range treatment goals. For example, teach them how to:

- recognize early signs of complications, such as hydrocephalus, decubitus ulcers, and urinary tract infection.
- provide psychological support and encourage a positive attitude.
- Credé the bladder regularly. Encourage parents to begin training their child in a bladder routine by age 3. Emphasize the need for increased fluid intake to prevent urinary tract infection. Teach intermittent catheterization and conduit hygiene, as ordered. If the child has an artificial urinary sphincter, teach him how to use it.
- prevent bowel obstruction. Stress the need for increased fluid intake, a high-bulk diet, exercise, and use of a stool softener, as ordered. Teach parents to empty their child's bowel by exerting slight pressure on his abdomen, telling him to bear down, and giving a glycerin suppository, as needed.

• recognize developmental lags early (a possible result of hydrocephalus). If present, stress the importance of follow-up IQ assessment to help plan realistic educational goals. The child may need to attend a school with special facilities. Also, stress the need for stimulation to ensure maximum mental development. Help parents plan activities appropriate to their child's age and abilities.

Refer parents for genetic counseling, and suggest that amniocentesis be performed in future pregnancies. For more information and names of support groups, refer parents to the Spina Bifida Association of America.

PAROXYSMAL DISORDERS

Headache

The most common patient complaint, headache usually occurs as a symptom of an underlying disorder. Ninety percent of all headaches are vascular, muscle contraction, or a combination; 10% are due to underlying intracranial, systemic, or psychological disorders. Migraine headaches, probably the most intensively studied, are throbbing, vascular headaches that usually begin to appear in childhood or adolescence and recur throughout adulthood. Affecting up to 10% of Americans, they're more common in females and have a strong familial incidence.

Causes

Most chronic headaches result from tension—muscle contraction—which may be caused by emotional stress, fatigue, menstruation, or environmental stimuli (noise, crowds, bright lights). Other possible causes include glaucoma; inflammation of the eyes or mucosa of the nasal or paranasal sinuses; diseases of the scalp, teeth, extracranial arteries, or external or middle ear; and muscle spasms of the face, neck, or shoulders. In addition, headaches may be caused by vasodilators (nitrates, alcohol, histamine), systemic disease, hypoxia, hypertension, head trauma and tumor, intracranial bleeding, abscess, or aneurysm.

The cause of migraine headache is unknown, but it is associated with constriction and dilation of intracranial and extracranial arteries. Certain biochemical abnormalities are thought to occur during a migraine attack. These include local leakage of a vasodilator polypeptide called neurokinin through the dilated arteries and a decrease in the plasma level of serotonin.

Headache pain may emanate from the pain-sensitive structures of the skin, scalp, muscles, arteries, veins; cranial nerves V, VII, IX, and X; and cervical nerves 1, 2, and 3. Intracranial mechanisms of headache include traction or displacement of arteries, venous sinuses, or venous tributaries, and inflammation or direct pressure on the cranial nerves with afferent pain fibers.

Signs and symptoms

Initially, migraine headache usually produces unilateral, pulsating pain, which later becomes more generalized. The headache is often preceded by a scintillating scotoma, hemianopsia, unilateral paresthesias, or speech disorders. The patient may experience irritability, anorexia, nausea, vomiting, and photophobia.

Both muscle contraction and traction-

CLINICAL FEATURES OF MIGRAINE HEADACHES

TYPE	SIGNS AND SYMPTOMS
Common migraine (*most prevalent*) Usually occurs on weekends and holidays	• Prodromal symptoms (fatigue, nausea and vomiting, and fluid imbalance) precede headache by about a day. • Sensitivity to light and noise (most prominent feature) • Headache pain (unilateral or bilateral, aching or throbbing)
Classic migraine Usually occurs in compulsive personalities and within families	• Prodromal symptoms include visual disturbances, such as zigzag lines and bright lights (most common), sensory disturbances (tingling of face, lips, and hands), or motor disturbances (staggering gait). • Recurrent and periodic headaches
Hemiplegic and ophthalmoplegic migraine (*rare*) Usually occurs in young adults	• Severe, unilateral pain • Extraocular muscle palsies (involving third cranial nerve) and ptosis • With repeated headaches, possible permanent third cranial nerve injury • In hemiplegic migraine, neurologic deficits (hemiparesis, hemiplegia) may persist after headache subsides.
Basilar artery migraine Occurs in young women before their menstrual periods	• Prodromal symptoms usually include partial vision loss followed by vertigo; ataxia; dysarthria; tinnitus; and sometimes, tingling of fingers and toes, lasting from several minutes to almost an hour. • Headache pain, severe occipital throbbing, vomiting

inflammatory vascular headaches produce a dull, persistent ache, tender spots on the head and neck, and a feeling of tightness around the head, with a characteristic "hatband" distribution. The pain is often severe and unrelenting. If caused by intracranial bleeding, these headaches may result in neurologic deficits, such as paresthesias and muscle weakness; narcotics fail to relieve pain in these cases. If caused by a tumor, pain is most severe when the patient awakens.

Diagnosis

Diagnosis requires a history of recurrent headaches and physical examination of the head and neck. Such examination includes percussion, auscultation for bruits, inspection for signs of infection, and palpation for defects, crepitus, or tender spots (especially after trauma). Firm diagnosis also requires a complete neurologic examination, assessment for other systemic diseases—such as hypertension—and a psychosocial evaluation, when such factors are suspected. Diagnostic tests include skull X-rays (including cervical spine and sinus), EEG, CT scan, brain scan, and lumbar puncture.

Treatment

Depending on the type of headache, analgesics—ranging from aspirin to codeine or meperidine—may provide symptomatic relief. A tranquilizer, such as diazepam, may help during acute attacks. Other measures include identification and elimination of causative factors and, possibly, psychotherapy for headaches caused by emotional stress. Chronic tension headaches may also require muscle relaxants.

For migraine headache, ergotamine alone or with caffeine is the most effective treatment. These drugs and other analgesics work best when taken early in the course of an attack. If nausea and vomiting make oral administration impossible, these drugs may be given as rectal suppositories. Drugs that can help prevent migraine headache include propranolol and calcium channel blockers, such as verapamil and diltiazem.

Special considerations

Headaches rarely necessitate hospitalization unless they're caused by a serious underlying disorder. If this is the case, direct your patient's care to the primary problem.

- Obtain a complete patient history: duration and location of the headache; time of day it usually begins; nature of the pain (intermittent or throbbing); concurrence with other symptoms, such as blurred vision; precipitating factors, such as tension, menstruation, loud noises, menopause, or alcohol; medications being taken, such as oral contraceptives; or prolonged fasting.
- Using the history as a guide, help the patient understand the reason for headaches so he can avoid exacerbating factors. Advise him to lie down in a dark, quiet room during an attack and to place ice packs on his forehead or a cold cloth over his eyes.
- Instruct the patient to take the prescribed medication at the onset of migraine symptoms, to prevent dehydration by drinking plenty of fluids after nausea and vomiting subside, and to use other headache relief measures.
- The patient with migraine usually needs to be hospitalized only if nausea and vomiting are severe enough to induce dehydration and possible shock.

Epilepsy

(Seizure disorder)

Epilepsy is a condition of the brain characterized by a susceptibility to recurrent seizures (paroxysmal events associated with abnormal electrical discharges of neurons in the brain). Epilepsy probably affects 1% to 2% of the population. However, the prognosis is good if the patient with epilepsy adheres strictly to his prescribed treatment.

Causes

In about half the cases of epilepsy the cause is unknown. However, some possible causes of epilepsy include:

- birth trauma (inadequate oxygen supply to the brain, blood incompatibility, or hemorrhage)
- perinatal infection
- anoxia
- infectious diseases (meningitis, encephalitis, or brain abscess)
- ingestion of toxins (mercury, lead, or carbon monoxide)
- tumors of the brain
- inherited disorders or degenerative disease, such as phenylketonuria or tuberous sclerosis
- head injury or trauma
- metabolic disorders, such as hypoglycemia or hypoparathyroidism
- cerebrovascular accident (hemorrhage, thrombosis, or embolism).

Signs and symptoms

The hallmarks of epilepsy are recurring seizures, which can be classified as partial or generalized (some patients may be affected by more than one type).

Partial seizures arise from a localized area of the brain, causing specific symptoms. In some patients, partial seizure activity may spread to the entire brain, causing a generalized seizure. Partial seizures include jacksonian and complex partial seizures (psychomotor or temporal lobe).

A jacksonian seizure begins as a localized motor seizure characterized by a spread of abnormal activity to adjacent areas of the brain. It typically produces a stiffening or jerking in one extremity, accompanied by a tingling sensation in the same area. For example, it may start in the thumb and spread to the entire hand and arm. The patient seldom loses consciousness. A jacksonian seizure may progress to a generalized tonic-clonic seizure.

The symptoms of a complex partial seizure are variable but usually include purposeless behavior. This seizure may begin with an aura, a sensation the patient feels immediately before a seizure. An aura represents the beginning of abnormal electrical discharges within a focal area of the brain and may include a pungent smell, gastrointestinal distress (nausea or indigestion), a rising or sinking feeling in the stomach, a dreamy feeling, an unusual taste, or a visual disturbance. Overt signs of a complex partial seizure include a glassy stare, picking at one's clothes, aimless wandering, lip-smacking or chewing motions, and unintelligible speech. Mental confusion may last several minutes after the seizure; as a result, an observer may mistakenly suspect intoxication with alcohol or drugs, or psychosis.

Generalized seizures, as the term suggests, cause a generalized electrical abnormality within the brain and include several distinct types:

Absence (petit mal) seizures occur most often in children, although they may affect adults as well. They usually begin with a brief change in level of consciousness, indicated by blinking or rolling of the eyes, a blank stare, and slight mouth movements. The patient retains his posture and continues preseizure activity without difficulty. Typically, each seizure lasts from 1 to 10 seconds. If not properly treated, seizures can recur as often as 100 times a day. An absence seizure may progress to generalized tonic-clonic seizures.

The *myoclonic (bilateral massive epileptic myoclonus) seizure* is characterized by brief, involuntary muscular jerks of the body or extremities, which may occur in a rhythmic fashion.

A *generalized tonic-clonic (grand mal) seizure* typically begins with a loud cry, precipitated by air rushing from the lungs through the vocal cords. The patient then falls to the ground, losing consciousness. The body stiffens (tonic phase), then alternates between episodes of muscular spasm and relaxation (clonic phase). Tongue-biting, incontinence, labored breathing, apnea, and subsequent cyanosis may also occur. The seizure stops in 2 to 5 minutes, when abnormal electrical conduction of the neurons is completed. The patient then regains consciousness but is somewhat confused and may have difficulty talking. If he can talk, he may complain of drowsiness, fatigue, headache, muscle soreness, and arm or leg weakness. He may fall into deep sleep following the seizure.

An *akinetic seizure* is characterized by a general loss of postural tone and a temporary loss of consciousness. It occurs in young children. It's sometimes called a "drop attack" because it causes the child to fall.

Status epilepticus is a continuous seizure state, which can occur in all seizure types. The most life-threatening example is generalized tonic-clonic status epilepticus, a continuous generalized tonic-clonic seizure without intervening return of consciousness. Status epilepticus is accompanied by respiratory distress. It can result from abrupt withdrawal of antiepileptic medications, hypoxic encephalopathy, acute head trauma, metabolic encephalopathy, or septicemia secondary to encephalitis or meningitis.

Diagnosis

Clinically, the diagnosis of epilepsy is based on the occurrence of one or more seizures and proof or the assumption that the condition which led to them is still present.

Important diagnostic information is

obtained from the patient's history and description of seizure activity and from family history, thorough physical and neurologic examinations, and computed tomography (CT) scan. This scan offers density readings of the brain and may indicate abnormalities in internal structures. Paroxysmal abnormalities on the EEG confirm the diagnosis of epilepsy by providing evidence of the continuing tendency to have seizures. A negative EEG does not rule out epilepsy, since the paroxysmal abnormalities occur intermittently. Other helpful tests may include serum glucose and calcium studies, skull X-rays, lumbar puncture, brain scan, and cerebral angiography.

Treatment

Generally, treatment for epilepsy consists of drug therapy specific to the type of seizure. The most commonly prescribed drugs include phenytoin, carbamazepine, phenobarbital, or primidone administered individually for generalized tonic-clonic seizures and complex partial seizures. Valproic acid, clonazepam, and ethosuximide are commonly prescribed for absence seizures.

A patient taking antiepileptic medications requires constant monitoring for toxic signs, such as nystagmus, ataxia, lethargy, dizziness, drowsiness, slurred speech, irritability, nausea, and vomiting.

If drug therapy fails, treatment may include surgical removal of a demonstrated focal lesion to attempt to bring an end to seizures. Emergency treatment for status epilepticus usually consists of diazepam, phenytoin, or phenobarbital; 50% dextrose I.V. (when seizures are secondary to hypoglycemia); and thiamine I.V. (in the presence of chronic alcoholism or withdrawal).

Special considerations

A key to support is a true understanding of the nature of epilepsy and of the myths and misconceptions that surround this disorder.

- Encourage the patient and family to express their feelings about the patient's condition. Answer their questions, and help them cope by dispelling some of the myths about epilepsy; for example, the myth that epilepsy is contagious. Assure them that epilepsy is controllable for most patients who follow a prescribed regimen of medication, and that most patients maintain a normal life-style.

Since drug therapy is the treatment of choice for most persons with epilepsy, information about the medications is invaluable.

- Stress the need for compliance with the prescribed drug schedule. Assure the patient that antiepileptic drugs are safe *when taken as ordered*. Reinforce dosage instructions, and find methods to help the patient remember to take medications. Caution him to monitor the amount of medication left so he doesn't run out of it.
- Warn against possible side effects—drowsiness, lethargy, hyperactivity, confusion, visual and sleep disturbances—all of which indicate the need for dosage adjustment. Phenytoin therapy may lead to hyperplasia of the gums, which may be relieved by conscientious oral hygiene. Instruct the patient to report side effects immediately.
- When administering phenytoin intravenously, use a large vein, and monitor vital signs frequently. Avoid I.M. administration and mixing with dextrose solutions.
- Emphasize the importance of having antiepileptic drug blood levels checked at regular intervals, even if the seizures are under control.
- Warn the patient against drinking alcoholic beverages.
- Know which social agencies in your community can help epileptic patients. Refer the patient to the Epilepsy Foundation of America for general information and to the state motor vehicle department for information about a driver's license.

Generalized tonic-clonic seizures may necessitate first aid. So be sure to instruct the patient's family how to give such aid correctly:

- Avoid restraining the patient during a

seizure. Help the patient to a lying position, loosen any tight clothing, and place something flat and soft, such as a pillow, jacket, or hand, under his head. Clear the area of hard objects. *Don't* force anything into the patient's mouth if his teeth are clenched—a tongue blade or spoon could lacerate mouth and lips or displace teeth, precipitating respiratory distress. However, if the patient's mouth is open, protect his tongue by placing a soft object (such as folded cloth) between his teeth. Turn his head to provide an open airway. After the seizure subsides, reassure the patient that he's all right, orient him to time and place, and inform him that he's had a seizure.

- If the patient has a complex partial seizure, *don't* restrain him during the seizure. Clear the area of any hard objects. Protect him from injury by gently calling his name and directing him away from the source of danger. After the seizure passes, reassure him and tell him that he's just had a seizure.

BRAIN & SPINAL CORD DISORDERS

Cerebrovascular Accident

(Stroke)

A cerebrovascular accident (CVA) is a sudden impairment of cerebral circulation in one or more of the blood vessels supplying the brain. CVA interrupts or diminishes oxygen supply and often causes serious damage or necrosis in brain tissues. The sooner circulation returns to normal after CVA, the better chances are for complete recovery. However, about half of those who survive a CVA remain permanently disabled and experience a recurrence within weeks, months, or years.

Causes and incidence

CVA is the third most common cause of death in the United States today and the most common cause of neurologic disability. It strikes 500,000 people each year; half of them die as a result.

Factors that increase the risk of CVA include history of transient ischemic attacks, atherosclerosis, hypertension, dysrhythmias, EKG changes, rheumatic heart disease, diabetes mellitus, gout, postural hypotension, cardiac or myocardial enlargement, high serum triglyceride levels, lack of exercise, use of oral contraceptives, cigarette smoking, and family history of CVA.

The major causes of CVA are thrombosis, embolism, and hemorrhage. *Thrombosis* is the most common cause of CVA in middle-aged and elderly persons, among whom there is a higher incidence of atherosclerosis, diabetes, and hypertension. CVA results from obstruction of a blood vessel. Typically, the main site of the obstruction is in extracerebral vessels, but sometimes it is intracerebral. Thrombosis causes ischemia in brain tissue supplied by the affected vessel, as well as congestion and edema; the latter may produce more clinical effects than thrombosis itself, but these symptoms subside with the edema. Thrombosis tends to develop while the patient is asleep or shortly after he awakens; however, it can also occur during surgery or following a myocardial infarction. The risk of thrombosis increases with obesity, smoking, or the use of oral contraceptives.

Embolism, the second most common cause of CVA, is an occlusion of a blood vessel caused by a fragmented clot, a tumor, fat, bacteria, or air. It can occur at any age, especially among patients with

TRANSIENT ISCHEMIC ATTACK (TIA)

A TIA is a recurrent episode of neurologic deficit, lasting from seconds to hours, that clears within 12 to 24 hours. It's usually considered a warning sign of an impending thrombotic CVA. In fact, TIAs have been reported in 50% to 80% of patients who have had a cerebral infarction from such thrombosis. The age of onset varies. Incidence rises dramatically after age 50 and is highest among blacks and men.

In TIA, microemboli released from a thrombus probably temporarily interrupt blood flow, especially in the small distal branches of the arterial tree in the brain. Small spasms in those arterioles may impair blood flow and also precede TIA. Predisposing factors are the same as for thrombotic CVAs. The most distinctive characteristics of TIAs are the transient duration of neurologic deficits and complete return of normal function. The symptoms of TIA easily correlate with the location of the affected artery. These symptoms include double vision, speech deficits (slurring or thickness), unilateral blindness, staggering or uncoordinated gait, unilateral weakness or numbness, falling because of weakness in the legs, and dizziness.

During an active TIA, the aim of treatment is to prevent a completed stroke and consists of aspirin or anticoagulants to minimize the risk of thrombosis. After or between attacks, preventive treatment includes carotid endartectomy or cerebral microvascular bypass.

a history of rheumatic heart disease, endocarditis, posttraumatic valvular disease, myocardial fibrillation and other cardiac dysrhythmias, or following open-heart surgery. It usually develops rapidly—in 10 to 20 seconds—and without warning. When an embolus reaches the cerebral vasculature, it cuts off circulation by lodging in a narrow portion of an artery, most often the middle cerebral artery, causing necrosis and edema. If the embolus is septic and infection extends beyond the vessel wall, an abscess or encephalitis may develop. If the infection is within the vessel wall, an aneurysm may form, which could lead to cerebral hemorrhage.

Hemorrhage, the third most common cause of CVA, like embolism, may occur suddenly, at any age. Such hemorrhage results from chronic hypertension or aneurysms, which cause sudden rupture of a cerebral artery. The rupture diminishes blood supply to the area served by this artery. In addition, blood accumulates deep within the brain, further compressing neural tissue and causing even greater damage.

CVAs are classified according to their course of progression. The least severe is the transient ischemic attack (TIA), or "little stroke," which results from a temporary interruption of blood flow, most often in the carotid and vertebrobasilar arteries. A progressive stroke, or stroke-in-evolution (thrombus-in-evolution), begins with slight neurologic deficit, and worsens in a day or two. In a completed stroke, neurologic deficits are maximal right at onset.

Signs and symptoms

Clinical features of CVA vary with the artery affected (and, consequently, the portion of the brain it supplies), the severity of damage, and the extent of collateral circulation that develops to help the brain compensate for decreased blood supply. If the CVA occurs in the left hemisphere, it produces symptoms on the right side; if in the right hemisphere, symptoms are on the left side. However, a CVA that causes cranial nerve damage produces signs of cranial nerve dysfunction on the same side as the hemorrhage. Symptoms are usually classified according to the artery affected:

- *middle cerebral artery:* aphasia, dysphasia, visual field cuts, and hemiparesis on affected side (more severe in the face and arm than in the leg)
- *carotid artery:* weakness, paralysis, numbness, sensory changes, and visual disturbances on affected side; altered level of consciousness, bruits, head-

aches, aphasia, ptosis
• *vertebrobasilar artery:* weakness on affected side, numbness around lips and mouth, visual field cuts, diplopia, poor coordination, dysphagia, slurred speech, dizziness, amnesia, ataxia
• *anterior cerebral artery:* confusion, weakness and numbness (especially in the leg) on affected side, incontinence, loss of coordination, impaired motor and sensory functions, personality changes
• *posterior cerebral arteries:* visual field cuts, sensory impairment, dyslexia, coma, cortical blindness. Usually, paralysis is absent.

Symptoms can also be classified as premonitory, generalized, and focal. Premonitory symptoms, such as drowsiness, dizziness, headache, and mental confusion, are rare. Generalized symptoms, such as headache, vomiting, mental impairment, convulsions, coma, nuchal rigidity, fever, and disorientation, are typical. Focal symptoms, such as sensory and reflex changes, reflect the site of hemorrhage or infarct and may worsen.

Diagnosis

Diagnosis of CVA is based on observation of clinical features, a history of risk factors, and the results of diagnostic tests. Definitive tests for CVA victims are:
• *computed tomography scan*—shows evidence of thrombotic or hemorrhagic stroke, tumor, or hydrocephalus
• *brain scan*—shows ischemic areas but may not be positive for up to 2 weeks after the CVA.

Other supporting tests include:
• *lumbar puncture*—in hemorrhagic stroke, CSF may be bloody
• *ophthalmoscopy*—may show signs of hypertension and atherosclerotic changes in retinal arteries
• *angiography*—outlines blood vessels and pinpoints the site of occlusion or rupture
• *EEG*—may help to localize the area of damage.

Other baseline laboratory studies include urinalysis; coagulation studies; CBC; serum osmolality; and electrolyte, glucose, triglyceride, creatinine, and blood urea nitrogen levels.

Treatment

Surgery to improve cerebral circulation for patients with thrombotic or embolic CVA includes endarterectomy (removal of atherosclerotic plaques from inner arterial wall) or microvascular bypass (extracranial vessel is surgically anastomosed to an intracranial vessel).

Medications useful in CVA include:
• anticonvulsants, such as phenytoin or phenobarbital, to treat or prevent seizures
• stool softeners, such as dioctyl sodium sulfosuccinate, to avoid straining, which increases intracranial pressure (ICP)
• corticosteroids, such as dexamethasone, to minimize associated cerebral edema
• analgesics, such as codeine, to relieve headache that may follow hemorrhagic CVA. Usually, aspirin is contraindicated in hemorrhagic CVA since it increases bleeding tendencies, but it may be useful in preventing TIAs.

Special considerations

Effective care of patients with CVA is complex and demands careful application of technical skills, keen observation, precise assessment, and supportive care. During the acute phase, such care emphasizes continuing neurologic assessment, support of respiration, continuous monitoring of vital signs, careful positioning to prevent aspiration and contractures, management of GI problems, and careful monitoring of fluid, electrolyte, and nutritional intake. Patient care must also prevent complications, such as infection.
• Maintain patent airway and oxygenation. Loosen constricting clothes. Watch for ballooning of the cheek with respiration. The side that balloons is the side affected by the stroke. If the patient is unconscious, he could aspirate saliva, so keep him in a lateral position to allow secretions to drain naturally or suction secretions, as needed. Insert an artificial airway, and start mechanical ventilation

or supplemental oxygen, if necessary.

• Check vital signs and neurologic status, record observations, and report any significant changes to the doctor. Monitor blood pressure, level of consciousness, pupillary changes, motor function (voluntary and involuntary movements), sensory function, speech, skin color, temperature, signs of increased ICP, and nuchal rigidity or flaccidity. Remember, if CVA is impending, blood pressure rises suddenly, pulse is rapid and bounding, and the patient may complain of headache. Also, watch for signs of pulmonary emboli, such as chest pains, shortness of breath, dusky color, tachycardia, fever, and changed sensorium. If the patient is unresponsive, monitor his blood gases often and alert the doctor to increased PCO_2 or decreased PO_2 levels.

• Maintain fluid and electrolyte balance. If the patient can take liquids P.O., offer them as often as fluid limitations permit. Administer I.V. fluids, as ordered; never give too much too fast, since this can increase ICP. Offer the urinal or bedpan every 2 hours. If the patient is incontinent, he may need a Foley catheter but this should be avoided, if possible, because of the risk of infection.

• Ensure adequate nutrition. Check for gag reflex before offering small oral feedings of semisolid foods. Place the food tray within the patient's visual field. If oral feedings aren't possible, insert a nasogastric tube.

• Manage gastrointestinal problems. Be alert for signs that the patient is straining at stool, since this increases ICP. Modify diet, administer stool softeners, as ordered, and give laxatives, if necessary. If the patient vomits (usually during the first few days), keep him positioned on his side to prevent aspiration.

• Give careful mouth care. Clean and irrigate the patient's mouth to remove food particles. Care for his dentures, as needed.

• Provide meticulous eye care. Remove secretions with a cotton ball and sterile normal saline solution. Instill eyedrops, as ordered. Patch the patient's affected eye if he can't close the lid.

• Position the patient, and align his extremities correctly. Use high-topped sneakers to prevent footdrop and contracture; and egg crate, flotation, or pulsating mattresses, or sheepskin to prevent decubitus ulcers. To prevent pneumonia, turn the patient at least every 2 hours. Elevate the affected hand to control dependent edema, and place it in a functional position.

• Assist the patient with exercise. Perform range-of-motion exercises for both the affected and unaffected sides. Teach and encourage the patient to use his unaffected side to exercise his affected side.

• Give medications, as ordered, and watch for and report side effects.

• Establish and maintain communication with the patient. If he is aphasic, set up a simple method of communicating basic needs. Then, remember to phrase your questions so he'll be able to answer using this system. Repeat yourself quietly and calmly (remember, he isn't deaf!) and use gestures if necessary to help him understand. Even the unresponsive patient can hear, so don't say anything in his presence you wouldn't want him to hear and remember.

• Provide psychological support. Set realistic short-term goals. Involve the patient's family in his care when possible, and explain his deficits and strengths.

Begin your rehabilitation of the patient with CVA on admission. The amount of teaching you'll have to do depends on the extent of neurologic deficit.

• Establish rapport with the patient. Spend time with him, and provide a means of communication. Simplify your language, asking yes-or-no questions whenever possible. Don't correct his speech or treat him like a child. Remember that building rapport may be difficult because of the mood changes that may result from brain damage or as a reaction to being dependent.

• If necessary, teach the patient to comb his hair, dress, and wash. With the aid of a physical and an occupational therapist, obtain appliances, such as walking frames, hand bars by the toilet, and ramps, as needed. If speech therapy is indicated, encourage the patient to begin as soon as possible and follow through with the speech pathologist's suggestions. To reinforce teaching, involve the patient's family in all aspects of rehabilitation. With their cooperation and support, devise a realistic discharge plan, and let them help decide when the patient can return home.

- Before discharge, warn the patient or his family to report any premonitory signs of a CVA, such as severe headache, drowsiness, confusion, and dizziness. Emphasize the importance of regular follow-up visits.
- If aspirin has been prescribed to minimize the risk of embolic stroke, tell the patient to watch for possible gastrointestinal bleeding related to ulcer formation. Make sure the patient realizes that he cannot substitute acetaminophen for aspirin.

To help prevent CVA:

Stress the need to control diseases such as diabetes or hypertension. Teach all patients (especially those at high risk) the importance of following a low-cholesterol, low-salt diet; watching their weight; increasing activity; avoiding smoking and prolonged bed rest; and minimizing stress.

Meningitis

In meningitis, the brain and the spinal cord meninges become inflamed, usually as a result of bacterial infection. Such inflammation may involve all three meningeal membranes—the dura mater, the arachnoid, and the pia mater. Prognosis is good and complications are rare, especially if the disease is recognized early and the infecting organism responds to antibiotics. However, mortality in untreated meningitis is 70% to 100%. Prognosis is poorer for infants and the elderly.

Causes

Meningitis is almost always a complication of another bacterial infection—bacteremia (especially from pneumonia, empyema, osteomyelitis, and endocarditis), sinusitis, otitis media, encephalitis, myelitis, or brain abscess—usually caused by *Neisseria meningitidis, Hemophilus influenzae, Streptococcus (Diplococcus) pneumoniae,* and *Escherichia coli.* Meningitis may also follow skull fracture, a penetrating head wound, lumbar puncture, or ventricular shunting procedures. Aseptic meningitis may result from a virus or other organism. Sometimes, no causative organism can be found.

Meningitis often begins as an inflammation of the pia-arachnoid, which may progress to congestion of adjacent tissues and destroy some nerve cells.

Signs and symptoms

The cardinal signs of meningitis are those of infection (fever, chills, malaise) and of increased intracranial pressure (headache, vomiting, and, rarely, papilledema). Signs of meningeal irritation include nuchal rigidity, positive Brudzinski's and Kernig's signs, exaggerated and symmetrical deep tendon reflexes, and opisthotonos (a spasm in which the back and extremities arch backward so that the body rests on the head and heels). Other manifestations of meningitis are sinus arrhythmias; irritability; photophobia, diplopia, and other visual problems; and delirium, deep stupor, and coma. An infant may show signs of infection but often is simply fretful and refuses to eat. Such an infant may vomit a great deal, leading to dehydration; this prevents a bulging fontanelle and thus masks this important sign of increased intracranial pressure (ICP). As this illness progresses, twitching, seizures (in 30% of infants), or coma may develop. Most older children have the same symp-

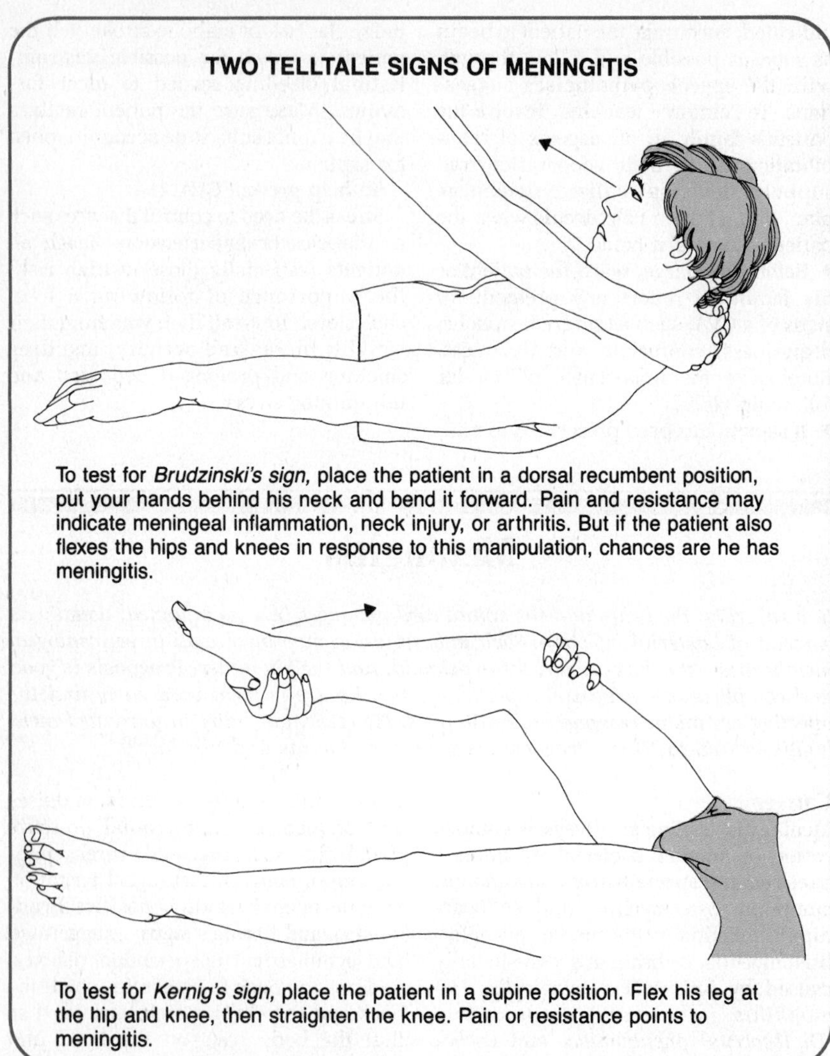

To test for *Brudzinski's sign,* place the patient in a dorsal recumbent position, put your hands behind his neck and bend it forward. Pain and resistance may indicate meningeal inflammation, neck injury, or arthritis. But if the patient also flexes the hips and knees in response to this manipulation, chances are he has meningitis.

To test for *Kernig's sign,* place the patient in a supine position. Flex his leg at the hip and knee, then straighten the knee. Pain or resistance points to meningitis.

toms as adults. In subacute meningitis, onset may be insidious.

Diagnosis

A lumbar puncture showing typical CSF findings and positive Brudzinski's and Kernig's signs usually establish this diagnosis. The following tests can uncover the primary sites of infection: cultures of blood, urine, and nose and throat secretions; a chest X-ray; an EKG; and a complete physical examination, with special attention to skin, ears, and sinuses. CSF pressure is elevated, resulting from obstruction of CSF outflow at the arachnoid villi. The fluid may appear cloudy or milky white, depending on the number of white blood cells present. CSF protein levels tend to be high; glucose levels may be low. (However, in subacute meningitis, CSF findings may vary.) CSF culture and sensitivity tests usually identify the infecting organism, unless it's a virus. Leukocytosis and serum electrolyte abnormalities are also common. CT scan can rule out cerebral hematoma, hemorrhage, or tumor.

Treatment

Treatment of meningitis includes appropriate antibiotic therapy and vigorous supportive care. Usually, I.V. antibiotics are given for at least 2 weeks and are followed by oral antibiotics. Such antibiotics include penicillin G, ampicillin, or nafcillin. However, if the patient is allergic to penicillin, anti-infective therapy includes tetracycline, chloramphenicol, or kanamycin. Other drugs include a cardiac glycoside, such as digoxin, to control dysrhythmias, mannitol to decrease cerebral edema, an anticonvulsant (usually given I.V.) or a sedative to reduce restlessness, and aspirin or acetaminophen to relieve headache and fever. Supportive measures include bed rest, hypothermia, and measures to prevent dehydration. Isolation is necessary if nasal cultures are positive. Of course, treatment includes appropriate therapy for any coexisting conditions, such as endocarditis or pneumonia.

To prevent meningitis, prophylactic antibiotics are sometimes used after ventricular shunting procedures, skull fracture, or penetrating head wounds, but this use is controversial.

ASEPTIC MENINGITIS

Aseptic meningitis is a benign syndrome characterized by headache, fever, vomiting, and meningeal symptoms. It results from some form of virus infection including enteroviruses (most common), arboviruses, herpes simplex virus, mumps virus, or lymphocytic choriomeningitis virus.

Aseptic meningitis begins suddenly with a fever up to 104° F. (40.0° C.), alterations in consciousness (drowsiness, confusion, stupor), and neck or spine stiffness, which is slight at first. (The patient experiences such stiffness when bending forward.) Other signs and symptoms include headaches, nausea, vomiting, abdominal pain, poorly defined chest pain, and sore throat.

Patient history of recent illness and knowledge of seasonal epidemics are essential in differentiating among the many forms of aseptic meningitis. Negative bacteriologic cultures and CSF analysis showing pleocytosis and increased protein suggest the diagnosis. Isolation of the virus from CSF confirms it.

Treatment is supportive, including bed rest, maintenance of fluid and electrolyte balance, analgesics for pain, and exercises to combat residual weakness. Isolation is not necessary. Careful handling of excretions and good handwashing technique prevent spreading the disease.

Special considerations

• Assess neurologic function often. Observe level of consciousness and signs of increased ICP (plucking at the bedcovers, vomiting, convulsions, a change in motor function and vital signs). Also watch for signs of cranial nerve involvement (ptosis, strabismus, diplopia).

• Watch for deterioration. Be especially alert for a temperature increase up to 102° F. (38.9° C.), deteriorating level of consciousness, onset of seizures, and altered respirations, all of which may signal an impending crisis.

• Monitor fluid balance. Maintain adequate fluid intake to avoid dehydration, but avoid fluid overload because of the danger of cerebral edema. Measure central venous pressure, and intake and output accurately.

• Watch for side effects of I.V. antibiotics and other drugs. To avoid infiltration and phlebitis, check the I.V. site often, and change the site according to hospital policy.

• Position the patient carefully to prevent joint stiffness and neck pain. Turn him often, according to a planned positioning schedule. Assist with range-of-motion exercises.

• Maintain adequate nutrition and elimination. It may be necessary to provide small, frequent meals or supplement these meals with nasogastric tube or parenteral feedings. To prevent constipation and minimize the risk of increased ICP resulting from straining at stool, give the patient a mild laxative or stool softener.

• Ensure the patient's comfort. Provide mouth care regularly. Maintain a quiet environment. Darkening the room may decrease photophobia. Relieve headache with a nonnarcotic analgesic, such as aspirin or acetaminophen, as ordered. (Narcotics interfere with accurate neurologic assessment.)

• Provide reassurance and support. The patient may be frightened by his illness and frequent lumbar punctures. If he's delirious or confused, attempt to reorient him often. Reassure the family that the delirium and behavior changes caused by meningitis usually disappear. However, if a severe neurologic deficit appears permanent, refer the patient to a rehabilitation program as soon as the acute phase of this illness has passed.

• To help prevent development of meningitis, teach patients with chronic sinusitis or other chronic infections the importance of proper medical treatment. Follow strict aseptic technique when treating patients with head wounds or skull fractures.

Encephalitis

Encephalitis is a severe inflammation of the brain, usually caused by a mosquito-borne or, in some areas, a tickborne virus. However, transmission by means other than arthropod bites may occur through ingestion of infected goat's milk and accidental injection or inhalation of the virus. Eastern equine encephalitis may produce permanent neurologic damage and is often fatal.

In encephalitis, intense lymphocytic infiltration of brain tissues and the leptomeninges causes cerebral edema, degeneration of the brain's ganglion cells, and diffuse nerve cell destruction.

Causes

Encephalitis generally results from infection with arboviruses specific to rural areas. However, in urban areas, encephalitis is most frequently caused by enteroviruses (coxsackievirus, poliovirus, and echovirus). Other causes include herpesvirus, mumps virus, adenoviruses, and demyelinating diseases following measles, varicella, rubella, or vaccination.

Between World War I and the Depression, a type of encephalitis known as lethargic encephalitis, von Economo's disease, or sleeping sickness occurred with some regularity. The causative virus was never clearly identified, and the disease is rare today. Even so, the term sleeping sickness persists and is often mistakenly used to describe other types of encephalitis as well.

Signs and symptoms

All viral forms of encephalitis have similar clinical features, although certain differences do occur. Usually, the acute illness begins with sudden onset of fever, headache, and vomiting, and progresses to include signs and symptoms of meningeal irritation (stiff neck and back) and neuronal damage (drowsiness, coma, paralysis, convulsions, ataxia, organic psychoses). After the acute phase of the illness, coma may persist for days or weeks.

The severity of arbovirus encephalitis may range from subclinical to rapidly fatal necrotizing disease. Herpes encephalitis also produces signs and symptoms that vary from subclinical to acute and often fatal fulminating disease. Associated effects include disturbances of taste or smell.

Diagnosis

During an encephalitis epidemic, diagnosis is readily made on clinical findings and patient history. However, sporadic cases are difficult to distinguish from other febrile illnesses, such as gastroenteritis or meningitis. When possible, identification of the virus in CSF or blood confirms this diagnosis. The common viruses that also cause herpes, measles, and mumps are easier to identify than arboviruses. Arboviruses and herpesviruses can be isolated by inoculating young mice with a specimen taken from the patient. In herpes encephalitis, serologic studies may show rising titers of complement-fixing antibodies.

In all forms of encephalitis, CSF pressure is elevated, and despite inflammation, the fluid is often clear. WBC and protein levels in CSF are slightly elevated, but the glucose level remains normal. An EEG reveals abnormalities. Occasionally, a CT scan may be ordered to rule out cerebral hematoma.

Treatment

The antiviral agent vidarabine is effective only against herpes encephalitis. Treatment of all other forms of encephalitis is entirely supportive. Drug therapy includes phenytoin or another anticonvulsant, usually given I.V.; glucocorticoids to reduce cerebral inflammation and resulting edema; sedatives for restlessness; and aspirin or acetaminophen to relieve headache and reduce fever. Other supportive measures include adequate fluid and electrolyte intake to prevent dehydration, and appropriate antibiotics for associated infections, such as pneumonia or sinusitis. Isolation is unnecessary.

Special considerations

During the acute phase of the illness:

- Assess neurologic function often. Observe level of consciousness and signs of increased intracranial pressure (increasing restlessness, plucking at the bedcovers, vomiting, convulsions, and changes in pupil size, motor function, and vital signs). Also watch for cranial nerve involvement (ptosis, strabismus, diplopia), abnormal sleep patterns, and behavior changes.
- Maintain adequate fluid intake to prevent dehydration, but avoid fluid overload, which may increase cerebral edema. Measure and record intake and output accurately.
- Give vidarabine by slow I.V. infusion only. Watch for side effects, such as tremor, dizziness, hallucinations, anorexia, nausea, vomiting, diarrhea, pruritus, rash, and anemia; also watch for side effects of other drugs. Check the infusion site often to avoid infiltration and phlebitis.
- Carefully position the patient to prevent joint stiffness and neck pain, and turn him often. Assist with range-of-motion exercises.
- Maintain adequate nutrition. It may be necessary to give the patient small, frequent meals or to supplement these meals with nasogastric tube or parenteral feedings.
- To prevent constipation and minimize the risk of increased intracranial pressure resulting from straining at stool, give a mild laxative or stool softener.
- Provide good mouth care.
- Maintain a quiet environment. Darkening the room may decrease photophobia and headache. If the patient naps during the day and is restless at night, plan daytime activities to minimize napping and promote sleep at night.
- Provide emotional support and reassurance, since the patient is apt to be frightened by the illness and frequent diagnostic tests.
- If the patient is delirious or confused, attempt to reorient him often. Providing a calendar or a clock in the patient's room may be helpful.
- Reassure the patient and his family that behavior changes caused by encephalitis usually disappear. If a neurologic deficit is severe and appears permanent, refer the patient to a rehabilitation program as soon as the acute phase has passed.

Brain Abscess

(Intracranial abscess)

Brain abscess is a free or encapsulated collection of pus usually found in the temporal lobe, cerebellum, or frontal lobes. It can vary in size and may occur singly or multilocularly. Brain abscess has a relatively low incidence. Although it can occur at any age, it is most common in persons between ages 10 and 35 and is rare in the elderly.

Untreated brain abscess is usually fatal; with treatment, prognosis is only fair, and about 30% of patients develop focal seizures. Multiple metastatic abscesses secondary to systemic or other infections have the poorest prognosis.

Causes

Brain abscess is usually secondary to some other infection, especially otitis media, sinusitis, dental abscess, and mastoiditis. Other causes include subdural empyema; bacterial endocarditis; bacteremia; pulmonary or pleural infection; pelvic, abdominal, and skin infections; and cranial trauma, such as a penetrating head wound or compound skull fracture. Brain abscess also occurs in about 2% of children with congenital heart disease, possibly because the hypoxic brain is a good culture medium for bacteria. The most common infecting organisms are pyogenic bacteria, such as *Staphylococcus aureus, Streptococcus viridans,* and *Streptococcus hemolyticus.* Penetrating head trauma or bacteremia usually leads to staphylococcal infection; pulmonary disease, to streptococcal infection.

Brain abscess usually begins with localized inflammatory necrosis and edema, septic thrombosis of vessels, and suppurative encephalitis. This is followed by thick encapsulation of accumulated pus, and adjacent meningeal infiltration by neutrophils, lymphocytes, and plasma cells.

Signs and symptoms

Onset varies according to cause, but generally, brain abscess produces clinical effects similar to those of a brain tumor. Early symptoms result from increased intracranial pressure (ICP) and include constant intractable headache, worsened by straining; nausea; vomiting; and focal or generalized seizures. Typical later symptoms include ocular disturbances, such as nystagmus, decreased vision, and inequality of pupils. Other features differ with the site of the abscess:

- *temporal lobe abscess:* auditory-receptive dysphasia, central facial weakness, hemiparesis
- *cerebellar abscess:* dizziness, coarse nystagmus, gaze weakness on lesion side, tremor, ataxia
- *frontal lobe abscess:* expressive dysphasia, hemiparesis with unilateral motor seizure, drowsiness, inattention, mental function impairment.

Signs of infection, such as fever, pallor, and bradycardia, are absent until late stages unless they result from the predisposing condition. If the abscess is encapsulated, they may never appear. Depending on abscess size and location, level of consciousness varies from drowsiness to deep stupor.

Diagnosis

A history of infection—especially of the middle ear, mastoid, nasal sinuses, heart, or lungs—or a history of congenital heart disease, along with a physical examination showing such characteristic clinical features as increased ICP, point to brain abscess. An EEG, computed tomography (CT) scan, and, occasionally, arteriography (which highlights abscess by a halo) help locate the site.

Examination of CSF can help confirm infection, but most doctors agree that lumbar puncture is usually too risky, because it can release the increased ICP and provoke cerebral herniation. Other tests include culture and sensitivity of drainage to identify the causative organism, skull X-rays, radioisotope scan, and, rarely, ventriculography.

Treatment

Therapy consists of antibiotics to combat the underlying infection, and surgical aspiration or drainage of the abscess. However, surgery is delayed until the abscess becomes encapsulated (CT scan helps determine this) and is contraindicated in patients with congenital heart disease or another debilitating cardiac condition. Administration of a penicillinase-resistant antibiotic, such as nafcillin or methicillin, for at least 2 to 3 weeks before surgery can reduce the risk of spreading infection. Other treatment during the acute phase is palliative and supportive and includes mechanical ventilation, administration of I.V. fluids with diuretics (urea, mannitol) and glucocorticoids (dexamethasone) to combat increased ICP and cerebral edema. Anticonvulsants, such as phenytoin and phenobarbital, help prevent seizures.

Special considerations

The patient with an acute brain abscess requires intensive care monitoring.

- Frequently assess neurologic status, especially the level of consciousness, speech, and motor, sensory, and cranial nerve functions. Watch for signs of increased ICP (decreased level of consciousness, vomiting, abnormal pupil response, and depressed respirations), which may lead to cerebral herniation with signs such as fixed and dilated pupils, widened pulse pressure, tachycardia, and absent respirations.
- Record vital signs at least every 1 to 2 hours.
- Monitor fluid intake and output carefully, since fluid overload could contribute to cerebral edema.

If surgery is necessary, explain the procedure to the patient and answer his questions.

After surgery:

- Continue frequent neurologic assessment. Monitor vital signs, and intake and output.
- Watch for signs of meningitis (nuchal rigidity, headaches, chills, sweats), an ever-present threat.
- Be sure to change a damp dressing often, using aseptic technique and noting amount of drainage. *Never allow bandages to remain damp.* To promote drainage and prevent reaccumulation of the abscess, position the patient on the operative side.
- If the patient remains stuporous or comatose for an extended period, give meticulous skin care to prevent decubitus ulcers, and position him to preserve function and prevent contractures.
- If the patient requires isolation because of postoperative drainage, make sure he and his family understand why.
- Ambulate the patient as soon as possible to prevent immobility and encourage independence.
- To prevent brain abscess, stress the need for treatment of otitis media, mastoiditis, dental abscess, and other infections. Give prophylactic antibiotics, as ordered, after compound skull fracture or penetrating head wound.

Huntington's Disease

(Huntington's chorea, hereditary chorea, chronic progressive chorea, adult chorea)

Huntington's disease is a hereditary disease in which degeneration in the cerebral cortex and basal ganglia causes chronic progressive chorea and mental deterioration, ending in dementia. Huntington's disease usually strikes persons between ages 25 and 55 (the average age is 35); however, 2% of cases occur in children, and 5%, as late as age 60. Death usually results 10 to 15 years after onset, from suicide, congestive heart failure, or pneumonia.

Causes and incidence

The cause of Huntington's disease is unknown. Because this disease is transmitted as an autosomal dominant trait, either sex can transmit and inherit it. Each child of a parent with this disease has a 50% chance of inheriting it; however, the child who doesn't inherit it can't pass it on to his own children. Because of hereditary transmission, Huntington's disease is prevalent in areas where affected families have lived for several generations. A study is being made of children in families with Huntington's disease in order to develop ways of identifying this disease before onset of symptoms.

Signs and symptoms

Onset is insidious. The patient eventually becomes totally dependent—emotionally and physically—through loss of musculoskeletal control. Gradually, he develops progressively severe choreic movements. Such movements are rapid, often violent, and purposeless. Initially, they are unilateral and more prominent in the face and arms than in the legs, progressing from mild fidgeting to grimacing, tongue smacking, dysarthria (indistinct speech), athetoid movements (especially of the hands) related to emotional state, and torticollis.

Ultimately, the patient with Huntington's disease develops dementia, although the dementia doesn't always progress at the same rate as the chorea. Dementia can be mild at first but eventually severely disrupts the personality. Such personality changes include obstinacy, carelessness, untidiness, moodiness, apathy, inappropriate behavior, loss of memory and concentration, and sometimes paranoia.

Diagnosis

There is no reliable confirming test for Huntington's disease. Diagnosis is based on a characteristic clinical history: progressive chorea and dementia, onset in early middle age (35 to 40), and confirmation of a genetic link. Helpful tests include pneumoencephalography, which shows characteristic butterfly dilation of the brain's lateral ventricles, and CT scan, which shows brain atrophy.

Treatment and special considerations

Since Huntington's disease has no known cure, treatment is supportive, protective, and symptomatic. Tranquilizers, as well as chlorpromazine, haloperidol, or imipramine, help control choreic movements, but they can't stop mental deterioration. They also alleviate discomfort and depression, making the patient easier to manage. However, tranquilizers increase patient rigidity. To control choreic movements without rigidity, choline may be prescribed. Institutionalization is often necessary because of mental deterioration.

- Provide physical support by attending to the patient's basic needs, such as hygiene, skin care, bowel and bladder care, and nutrition. Increase this support as mental and physical deterioration makes him increasingly immobile.
- Offer emotional support to the patient and family. Teach them about the disease, and listen to their concerns and special problems. Keep in mind the patient's dysarthria, and allow him extra time to express himself, thereby decreasing frustration. Teach the family to participate in the patient's care.
- Stay alert for possible suicide attempts. Control the patient's environment to protect him from suicide or other self-inflicted injury. Pad the side rails of the bed, but avoid restraints, which may cause the patient to injure himself with violent, uncontrolled movements.
- Make sure affected families receive genetic counseling. All affected family members should realize that each of their offspring has a 50% chance of inheriting

this disease.

- Refer the patient and family to appropriate community organizations: visiting nurse services, social services, psychiatric counseling, and long-term care facility.
- For more information about this degenerative disease, refer the patient and family to the Committee to Combat Huntington's Disease or the National Huntington's Disease Association.

Parkinson's Disease

(Parkinsonism, paralysis agitans, shaking palsy)

Named for James Parkinson, the English doctor who wrote the first accurate description of the disease in 1817, Parkinson's disease characteristically produces progressive muscle rigidity, akinesia, and involuntary tremor. Deterioration progresses for an average of 10 years, at which time death usually results from aspiration pneumonia or some other infection. Parkinson's disease, one of the most common crippling diseases in the United States, affects men more often than women. According to current statistics, Parkinson's strikes 1 in every 100 people over age 60. Because of increased longevity, this amounts to roughly 60,000 new cases diagnosed annually in the United States alone.

Causes

Although the cause of Parkinson's disease is unknown, study of the extrapyramidal brain nuclei (corpus striatum, globus pallidus, substantia nigra) has established that a dopamine deficiency prevents affected brain cells from performing their normal inhibitory function within the central nervous system.

Signs and symptoms

The cardinal symptoms of Parkinson's disease are muscle rigidity and akinesia, and an insidious tremor that begins in the fingers (unilateral pill-roll tremor), increases during stress or anxiety, and decreases with purposeful movement and sleep. Muscle rigidity results in resistance to passive muscle stretching, which may be uniform (lead-pipe rigidity) or jerky (cogwheel rigidity). Akinesia causes the patient to walk with difficulty (gait lacks normal parallel motion and may be retropulsive or propulsive). It also produces a high-pitched, monotone voice; drooling; a masklike facial expression; loss of posture control (the patient walks with body bent forward); and dysarthria, dysphagia, or both. Occasionally, akinesia may also cause oculogyric crises (eyes are fixed upward, with involuntary tonic movements) or blepharospasm (eyelids are completely closed). Parkinson's disease itself doesn't impair the intellect, but a coexisting disorder, such as arteriosclerosis, may.

Diagnosis

Generally, laboratory data are of little value in identifying Parkinson's disease; consequently, diagnosis is based on the patient's age and history, and the characteristic clinical picture. However, urinalysis may support the diagnosis by revealing decreased dopamine levels. Conclusive diagnosis is possible only after ruling out other causes of tremor, involutional depression, cerebral arteriosclerosis, and, in patients under age 30, intracranial tumors, Wilson's disease, or phenothiazine or other drug toxicity.

Treatment

Since there's no cure for Parkinson's disease, the primary aim of treatment is to relieve symptoms and keep the patient functional as long as possible. Treatment consists of drugs, physical therapy, and, in severe disease states unresponsive to drugs, stereotactic neurosurgery.

Drug therapy usually includes levodopa, a dopamine replacement that is most effective during early stages. This drug is given in increasing doses until symptoms are relieved or side effects appear. Because these side effects can be serious, levodopa is now frequently given in combination with carbidopa to halt peripheral dopamine synthesis. When levodopa proves ineffective or too toxic, alternative drug therapy includes anticholinergics, such as trihexyphenidyl; antihistamines, such as diphenhydramine; and amantadine, an antiviral agent.

When drug therapy fails, stereotactic neurosurgery is sometimes an effective alternative. In this procedure, electrical coagulation, freezing, radioactivity, or ultrasound destroys the ventrolateral nucleus of the thalamus to prevent involuntary movement. Such neurosurgery is most effective in comparatively young, otherwise healthy persons with unilateral tremor or muscle rigidity. Like drug therapy, neurosurgery is a palliative measure that can only *relieve* symptoms.

Individually planned physical therapy complements drug treatment and neurosurgery to maintain normal muscle tone and function. Appropriate physical therapy includes both active and passive range-of-motion exercises, routine daily activities, walking, and baths and massage to help relax muscles.

Special considerations

Effectively caring for the patient with Parkinson's disease requires careful monitoring of drug treatment, emphasis on teaching self-reliance, and generous psychological support.

- Monitor drug treatment so dosage can be adjusted to minimize side effects.
- If the patient has surgery, watch for signs of hemorrhage and increased intracranial pressure by frequently checking level of consciousness and vital signs.
- Encourage independence. The patient with excessive tremor may achieve partial control of his body by sitting on a chair and using its arms to steady himself. Remember that fatigue may cause him to depend more on others.
- Help the patient overcome problems related to eating and elimination. For example, if he has difficulty eating, offer supplementary or small, frequent meals to increase caloric intake. Help establish a regular bowel routine by encouraging him to drink at least 2,000 ml of liquids daily and eat high-bulk foods. He may need an elevated toilet seat to assist him from a standing to a sitting position.
- Give the patient and family emotional support. Teach them about the disease, its progressive stages, and drug side effects. Show the family how to prevent decubitus ulcers and contractures by proper positioning. Inform them of the dietary restrictions levodopa imposes, and explain household safety measures to prevent accidents. Help the patient and family express their feelings and frustrations about the progressively debilitating effects of the disease. Establish long- and short-term treatment goals, and be aware of the patient's need for intellectual stimulation and diversion.

To obtain more information, refer the patient and family to the National Parkinson Foundation or the United Parkinson Foundation.

Myelitis and Acute Transverse Myelitis

Myelitis, or inflammation of the spinal cord, can result from several diseases. Poliomyelitis affects the cord's gray matter and produces motor dysfunction; leukomyelitis affects only the white matter and produces sensory dysfunction. These types of myelitis can attack any level of the spinal cord, causing partial destruction or scattered lesions. Acute transverse myelitis, which affects the entire thickness of the spinal cord, produces both motor and sensory dysfunctions. This form of myelitis, which has a rapid onset, is the most devastating.

The prognosis depends on the severity of cord damage and prevention of complications. If spinal cord necrosis occurs, prognosis for complete recovery is poor. Even without necrosis, residual neurologic deficits usually persist after recovery. Patients who develop spastic reflexes early in the course of the illness are more likely to recover than those who don't.

Causes

Acute transverse myelitis has a variety of causes. It often follows acute infectious diseases, such as measles or pneumonia (the inflammation occurs after the infection has subsided), and primary infections of the spinal cord itself, such as syphilis or acute disseminated encephalomyelitis. Acute transverse myelitis can accompany demyelinating diseases, such as acute multiple sclerosis, and inflammatory and necrotizing disorders of the spinal cord, such as hematomyelia.

Certain toxic agents (carbon monoxide, lead, and arsenic) can cause a type of myelitis in which acute inflammation (followed by hemorrhage and possible necrosis) destroys the entire circumference (myelin, axis cylinders, and neurons) of the spinal cord. Other forms of myelitis may result from poliovirus, herpes zoster, herpesvirus B, or rabies virus; disorders that cause meningeal inflammation, such as syphilis, abscesses and other suppurative conditions, and tuberculosis; smallpox or polio vaccination; parasitic and fungal infections; and chronic adhesive arachnoiditis.

Signs and symptoms

In acute transverse myelitis, onset is rapid, with motor and sensory dysfunctions below the level of spinal cord damage appearing in 1 to 2 days.

Patients with acute transverse myelitis develop flaccid paralysis of the legs (sometimes beginning in just one leg) with loss of sensory and sphincter functions. Such sensory loss may follow pain in the legs or trunk. Reflexes disappear in the early stages but may reappear later. The extent of damage depends on the level of the spinal cord affected; transverse myelitis rarely involves the arms. If spinal cord damage is severe, it may cause shock (hypotension and hypothermia).

Diagnosis

Paraplegia of rapid onset usually points to acute transverse myelitis. In such patients, neurologic examination confirms paraplegia or neurologic deficit below the level of the spinal cord lesion and absent or, later, hyperactive reflexes. CSF may be normal or show increased lymphocytes or elevated protein levels.

Diagnostic evaluation must rule out spinal cord tumor and identify the cause of any underlying infection.

Treatment

No effective treatment exists for acute transverse myelitis. However, this condition requires appropriate treatment of any underlying infection. Some patients with postinfectious or multiple sclerosis-induced myelitis have received steroid therapy, but its benefits aren't clear.

Special considerations

- Frequently assess vital signs. Watch carefully for signs of spinal shock (hypotension and excessive sweating).
- Prevent contractures with range-of-motion exercises and proper alignment.
- Watch for signs of urinary tract infections from Foley catheters.
- Prevent skin infections and decubitus ulcers with meticulous skin care. Check pressure points often and keep skin clean and dry; use a water bed or other pressure-relieving device.
- Initiate rehabilitation immediately. Assist the patient with physical therapy, bowel and bladder training, and lifestyle changes his condition requires.

Primary Degenerative Dementia

(Alzheimer's Disease)

Primary degenerative dementia accounts for over half of all dementias. An estimated 5% of persons over the age of 65 have a severe form of this disease, and 12% suffer from mild to moderate dementia. Because this is a primary progressive dementia, the prognosis for a patient with this disease is poor.

Causes

The cause of primary degenerative dementia is unknown. However, several factors are thought to be implicated in this disease. These include *neurochemical factors,* such as deficiencies in neurotransmitter substances of acetylcholine, somatostatin, substance P, and norepinephrine; *environmental factors,* such as aluminum and manganese; *viral factors,* such as slow-growing central nervous system viruses; *trauma;* and *genetic immunologic factors.* The brain tissue of patients with primary degenerative dementia has three hallmark features: neurofibrillary tangles, neuritic plaques, and granulovascular degeneration.

Signs and symptoms

Onset is insidious. Initially, the patient experiences almost imperceptible changes, such as forgetfulness, recent memory loss, difficulty learning and remembering new information, deterioration in personal hygiene and appearance, and an inability to concentrate. Gradually, tasks that require abstract thinking and activities that require judgment become more difficult. Progressive difficulty in communication and severe deterioration in memory, language, and motor function results in a loss of coordination and an inability to write or speak. Personality changes (restlessness, irritability) and nocturnal awakenings are common. Eventually, the patient becomes disoriented, and emotional lability and physical and intellectual disability progress. The patient becomes very susceptible to infection and accidents. Usually, death results from infection.

Diagnosis

Early diagnosis of primary degenerative dementia is difficult because of the subtlety of the patient's signs and symptoms. Diagnosis relies on an accurate history from a reliable family member, mental status and neurologic examinations, and psychometric testing. A positron emission transaxial tomography scan measures the metabolic activity of the cerebral cortex and may help confirm early diagnosis. An electroencephalogram and a computed tomography (CT) scan may help diagnose later stages of primary degenerative dementia. Currently, primary degenerative dementia is diagnosed by exclusion; a variety of tests are performed to rule out other disorders. A true diagnosis of this disease cannot be confirmed until death, when pathologic findings are found at autopsy.

Treatment

Therapy consists of cerebral vasodilators, such as ergoloid mesylates (Hydergine), isoxsuprine (Vasodilan), and cyclandelate (Cyclospasmol) to enhance the brain's circulation; hyperbaric oxygen to increase oxygenation to the brain; psychostimulators, such as methylphenidate (Ritalin), to enhance the patient's mood; and antidepressants if depression seems to exacerbate the patient's dementia. Most drug therapies currently being used are experimental. These include choline salts, lecithin, physostigmine, deanol, enkephalins, and naloxone, which may slow the disease process. Another approach to treatment includes avoiding antacids, use of aluminum cooking utensils, and aluminum-containing deodorants to help decrease aluminum intake.

ORGANIC BRAIN SYNDROME

Although many behavioral disturbances are clearly linked to organic brain dysfunction, the clinical syndromes associated with this type of impairment are sometimes hard to detect. Why? Because these clinical syndromes aren't always determined by the affected area of the brain or even by the extent of tissue damage. Instead, the way in which the patient's personality interacts with the brain injury determines the specific clinical effects that develop. General symptoms often include impairment of orientation, memory, and intellectual and emotional function. These primary cognitive deficits help to distinguish organic brain syndromes from neurosis and depression.

Diagnosis of an organic brain syndrome depends on a detailed history of the onset of cognitive and behavioral disturbances; a complete neurologic assessment; and such tests as electroencephalograms, computed tomography scans, brain X-rays, cerebrospinal fluid analysis, and psychological studies. Organic brain syndromes are classified by etiology and specific clinical effects. Causes include infection, brain trauma, nutritional deficiency, cerebrovascular disease, degenerative disease, tumor, toxins, and metabolic or endocrine disorders.

Effective treatment requires correction of the underlying cause. Special considerations may include reality orientation, emotional support for the patient and family, providing a safe environment, mat therapy for an agitated or aggressive patient, and referral for psychological counseling.

Special considerations

Overall care is focused on supporting the patient's abilities and compensating for those abilities he has lost.

- Establish an effective communication system with the patient and family to help them adjust to the patient's altered cognitive abilities.
- Offer emotional support to the patient and family. Teach them about the disease, and listen to their concerns.
- Protect the patient from injury by providing a safe, structured environment.
- Encourage the patient to exercise, as ordered, to help maintain mobility.

Reye's Syndrome

Reye's syndrome is an acute childhood illness that causes fatty infiltration of the liver with concurrent hyperammonemia, encephalopathy, and increased intracranial pressure (ICP). In addition, fatty infiltration of the kidneys, brain, and myocardium may occur. Reye's syndrome affects children from infancy to adolescence and occurs equally in boys and girls. It affects whites over age 1 more often than blacks.

Prognosis depends on the severity of CNS depression. Previously, mortality was as high as 90%. Today, though, ICP monitoring and, consequently, early treatment of increased ICP, along with other treatment measures, have cut mortality to about 20%. Death is usually a result of cerebral edema or respiratory arrest. Comatose patients who survive may have residual brain damage.

Causes and incidence

Reye's syndrome almost always follows within 1 to 3 days of an acute viral infection, such as an upper respiratory infection, type B influenza, or varicella (chicken pox). Incidence often rises during influenza outbreaks and may be linked to aspirin use.

STAGES OF TREATMENT FOR REYE'S SYNDROME

SIGNS AND SYMPTOMS	BASELINE TREATMENT	BASELINE INTERVENTION
Stage I: vomiting, lethargy, hepatic dysfunction	• To decrease intracranial pressure and brain edema, give I.V. fluids at ⅔ maintenance. Also give an osmotic diuretic or furosemide. • To treat hypoprothrombinemia, give vitamin K; if vitamin K is unsuccessful, give fresh frozen plasma. • Monitor serum ammonia, blood glucose, plasma osmolality every 4 to 8 hours to check progress.	• Monitor vital signs and check level of consciousness for increasing lethargy. Take vital signs more often as the patient's condition deteriorates. • Monitor fluid intake and output to prevent fluid overload. Maintain urine output at 1.0 ml/kg/hr; plasma osmolality, 290 mOsm; and blood glucose, 150 mg/ml. (*Goal:* Keep glucose high, osmolality normal to high, and ammonia low.) Also, restrict protein.
Stage II: hyperventilation, delirium, hepatic dysfunction, hyperactive reflexes	• Continue baseline treatment.	• Maintain seizure precautions. • Immediately report any signs of coma that require invasive, supportive therapy, such as intubation. • Keep head of bed at 30° angle.
Stage III: coma, hyperventilation, decorticate rigidity, hepatic dysfunction	• Continue baseline and seizure treatment. • Monitor ICP with a subarachnoid screw or other invasive device. • Provide endotracheal intubation and mechanical ventilation to control P_{CO_2} levels. A paralyzing agent, such as pancuronium I.V., may help maintain ventilation. • Give mannitol I.V. or glycerol by nasogastric tube.	• Monitor ICP (should be <20 before suctioning) or give thiopental I.V., as ordered; as necessary, hyperventilate the patient. • When ventilating the patient, maintain P_{CO_2} between 20 and 30 torr and P_{O_2} between 80 and 100 torr. • Closely monitor cardiovascular status with a pulmonary artery catheter or central venous pressure line. • Give good skin and mouth care, and range-of-motion exercises.
Stage IV: deepening coma; decerebrate rigidity; large, fixed pupils; minimal hepatic dysfunction	• Continue baseline and supportive care. • If all previous measures fail, some pediatric centers use barbiturate coma, decompressive craniotomy, hypothermia, or exchange transfusion.	• Check patient for loss of reflexes and signs of flaccidity. • Give the family the extra support they need, considering their child's poor prognosis.
Stage V: seizures, loss of deep tendon reflexes, flaccidity, respiratory arrest, ammonia level above 300 mg/100 ml	• Continue baseline and supportive care.	• Help the family to face the patient's impending death.

In Reye's syndrome, damaged hepatic mitochondria disrupt the urea cycle, which normally changes ammonia to urea for its excretion from the body. This results in hyperammonemia, hypoglycemia, and an increase in serum short-chain fatty acids, leading to encephalopathy. Simultaneously, fatty infiltration is found in renal tubular cells, neuronal tissue, and muscle tissue, including the heart.

Signs and symptoms

The severity of the child's signs and symptoms varies with the degree of encephalopathy and cerebral edema. In any case, Reye's syndrome develops in five stages: After the initial viral infection, a brief recovery period follows when the child doesn't seem seriously ill. A few days later, he develops intractable vomiting; lethargy; rapidly changing mental status (mild to severe agitation, confusion, irritability, delirium); rising blood pressure, respiratory rate, and pulse rate; and hyperactive reflexes.

Reye's syndrome often progresses to coma. As coma deepens, seizures develop, followed by decreased tendon reflexes and, frequently, respiratory failure.

Increased ICP, a serious complication, results from cerebral edema. Such edema may develop as a result of acidosis, increased cerebral metabolic rate, and an impaired autoregulatory mechanism.

Diagnosis

A history of a recent viral disorder with typical clinical features strongly suggests Reye's syndrome. An increased serum ammonia level, abnormal clotting studies, and hepatic dysfunction confirm it. Testing serum salicylate level rules out aspirin overdose. Absence of jaundice despite increased liver transaminase levels rules out acute hepatic failure and hepatic encephalopathy.

Abnormal test results may include:

- *liver function studies:* SGOT and SGPT elevated to twice normal levels; bilirubin usually normal
- *liver biopsy:* fatty droplets uniformly distributed throughout cells
- *CSF analysis:* WBC less than 10/mm^3; with coma, increased CSF pressure
- *coagulation studies:* PT and PTT prolonged
- *blood values:* serum ammonia levels elevated; serum glucose levels normal or, in 15% of cases, low; serum fatty acid and lactate levels increased.

For more information, refer parents to the National Reye's Syndrome Foundation. Advise parents to give nonsalicylate analgesics and antipyretics, such as acetaminophen (Tylenol).

Guillain-Barré Syndrome

(Infectious polyneuritis, Landry-Guillain-Barré syndrome, acute idiopathic polyneuritis)

Guillain-Barré syndrome is an acute, rapidly progressive and potentially fatal form of polyneuritis that causes muscle weakness and mild distal sensory loss. This syndrome can occur at any age but is most common between ages 30 and 50; it affects both sexes equally. Recovery is spontaneous and complete in about 95% of patients, although mild motor or reflex deficits in the feet and legs may persist. Prognosis is best when symptoms clear between 15 and 20 days after onset.

Causes and incidence

Precisely what causes Guillain-Barré syndrome is unknown, but it may be a cell-mediated immunologic attack on peripheral nerves in response to a virus. The major pathologic effect is segmental demyelination of the peripheral nerves. Since this syndrome causes inflammation and degenerative changes in both the posterior (sensory) and anterior (motor) nerve roots, signs of sensory and motor losses occur simultaneously.

Signs and symptoms

About 50% of patients with Guillain-Barré syndrome have a history of minor febrile illness, usually an upper respiratory tract infection or, less often, gastroenteritis. When infection precedes onset of Guillain-Barré syndrome, signs of infection subside before neurologic features appear. Other possible precipitating factors include surgery, rabies or swine influenza vaccination, viral illness, Hodgkin's or some other malignant disease, and lupus erythematosus.

Muscle weakness, the major neurologic sign, usually appears in the legs first (ascending type), then extends to the arms and facial nerves in 24 to 72 hours. Sometimes, muscle weakness develops in the arms first (descending type), or in the arms and legs simultaneously. In milder forms of this disease, muscle weakness may affect only the cranial nerves or may not occur at all.

Another common neurologic sign is paresthesia, which sometimes precedes muscle weakness but tends to vanish quickly. However, some patients with this disorder never develop this symptom. Other clinical features may include facial diplegia (possibly with ophthalmoplegia [ocular paralysis]), dysphagia or dysarthria, and, less often, weakness of the muscles supplied by the 11th cranial (spinal accessory) nerve. Muscle weakness develops so quickly that muscle atrophy doesn't occur, but hypotonia and areflexia do. Stiffness and pain in the form of a severe "charley horse" often occur.

The clinical course of Guillain-Barré syndrome is divided into three phases. The *initial phase* begins when the first definitive symptom develops; it ends 1 to 3 weeks later, when no further deterioration is noted. The *plateau phase* lasts several days to 2 weeks and is followed by the *recovery phase*, which is believed to coincide with remyelination and axonal process regrowth. The recovery phase extends over a period of 4 to 6 months; patients with severe disease may take up to 2 years to recover, and recovery may not be complete.

Significant complications of Guillain-Barré syndrome include mechanical ventilatory failure, aspiration, pneumonia, sepsis, joint contractures, and deep vein thrombosis. Unexplained autonomic nervous system involvement may cause sinus tachycardia or bradycardia, hypertension, postural hypotension, or loss of bladder and bowel sphincter control.

Diagnosis

A history of preceding febrile illness (usually a respiratory tract infection) and typical clinical features suggest Guillain-Barré syndrome.

Several days after onset of signs and symptoms, CSF protein level begins to rise, peaking in 4 to 6 weeks, probably as a result of widespread inflammatory disease of the nerve roots. CSF white blood cell count remains normal, but in severe disease CSF pressure may rise above normal. Probably because of predisposing infection, complete blood count shows leukocytosis and a shift to immature forms early in the illness, but blood studies soon return to normal. Electromyography may show repeated firing of the same motor unit, instead of widespread sectional stimulation. Nerve conduction velocities are slowed soon after paralysis develops. Diagnosis must rule out similar diseases, such as acute poliomyelitis.

Treatment

Treatment is primarily supportive, consisting of endotracheal intubation or tracheotomy if the patient has difficulty clearing secretions.

A trial dose of prednisone may be tried if the course of the disease is relentlessly progressive. If prednisone produces no noticeable improvement after 7 days, the drug is discontinued. Plasma exchange treatment for patients with Guillain-Barré syndrome is currently under investigation.

Special considerations

- Watch for ascending sensory loss, which precedes motor loss. Also, monitor vital signs and level of consciousness.
- Assess and treat respiratory dysfunction. If respiratory muscles are weak, take serial vital capacity recordings. Use a respirometer with a mouthpiece or a face mask for bedside testing.
- Obtain arterial blood gas measurements. Since neuromuscular disease results in primary hypoventilation with hypoxemia and hypercapnia, watch for PO_2 below 70 mm Hg, which signals respiratory failure. Be alert for signs of rising PCO_2 (confusion, tachypnea).
- Auscultate breath sounds, turn and position the patient, and encourage coughing and deep breathing. Begin respiratory support at the first sign of dyspnea (in adults, vital capacity less than 800 ml; in children, less than 12 ml/kg body weight) or decreasing PO_2.
- If respiratory failure becomes imminent, establish an emergency airway with an endotracheal tube.
- Give meticulous skin care to prevent skin breakdown and contractures. Establish a strict turning schedule; inspect the skin (especially sacrum, heels, and ankles) for breakdown, and reposition the patient every 2 hours. After each position change, stimulate circulation by carefully massaging pressure points. Also, use foam, gel, or alternating pressure pads at points of contact.
- Perform passive range-of-motion exercises within the patient's pain limits, perhaps using a Hubbard tank. (Although this disease doesn't produce pain, exercising little-used muscles will.) Remember that the proximal muscle group of the thighs, shoulders, and trunk will be the most tender and will cause the most pain on passive movement and turning. When the patient's condition stabilizes, change to gentle stretching and active assistance exercises.
- To prevent aspiration, test the gag reflex, and elevate the head of the bed before giving the patient anything to eat. If the gag reflex is absent, give nasogastric feedings until this reflex returns.

TESTING FOR THORACIC SENSATION

When Guillain-Barré syndrome progresses rapidly, test for ascending sensory loss by touching the patient or pressing his skin lightly with a pin every hour. Move systematically from the iliac crest (T12) to the scapula, occasionally substituting the blunt end of the pin to test the patient's ability to discriminate between sharp and dull. Mark the level of diminished sensation to measure any change. If diminished sensation ascends to T8 or higher, the patient's intercostal muscle function (and consequently respiratory function) will probably be impaired. As Guillain-Barré syndrome subsides, sensory and motor weakness descends to the lower thoracic segments, heralding a return of intercostal and extremity muscle function.

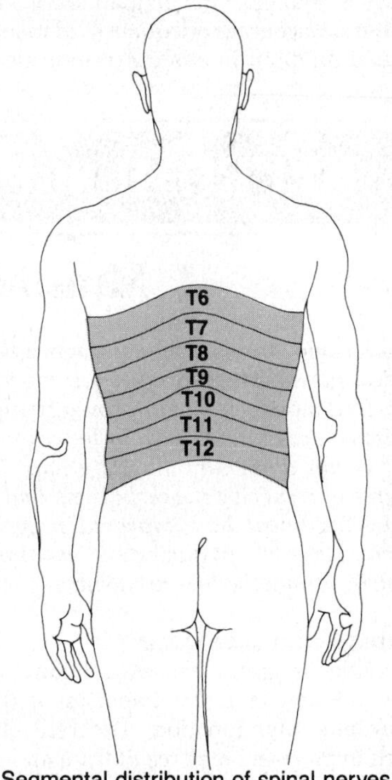

Segmental distribution of spinal nerves to back of the body

KEY

T = thoracic segments

- As the patient regains strength and can tolerate a vertical position, be alert for postural hypotension. Monitor blood pressure and pulse during tilting periods and, if necessary, apply toe-to-groin elastic bandages or an abdominal binder to prevent postural hypotension.
- Inspect the patient's legs regularly for signs of thrombophlebitis (localized pain, tenderness, erythema, edema, positive Homans' sign), a common complication of Guillain-Barré syndrome. To prevent thrombophlebitis, apply antiembolism stockings and give prophylactic anticoagulants, as ordered.
- If the patient has facial paralysis, give eye and mouth care every 4 hours. Protect the corneas with isotonic eyedrops and conical eye shields.
- Watch for urinary retention. Measure and record intake and output every 8 hours, and offer the bedpan every 3 to 4 hours. Encourage adequate fluid intake (2,000 ml/day), unless contraindicated. If urinary retention develops, begin intermittent catheterization, as ordered. Since the abdominal muscles are weak, the patient may need manual pressure on the bladder (Credé's method) before he can urinate.
- To prevent and relieve constipation, offer prune juice and a high-bulk diet. If necessary, give daily or alternate-day suppositories (glycerin or bisacodyl), or Fleet enemas, as ordered.
- Before discharge, prepare a home care plan. Teach the patient how to transfer from bed to wheelchair, from wheelchair to toilet or to tub, and how to walk short distances with a walker or a cane. Teach the family how to help him eat, compensating for facial weakness, and how to help him avoid skin breakdown. Stress the need for a regular bowel and bladder routine. Refer the patient for physical therapy, as needed.

NEUROMUSCULAR DISORDERS

Myasthenia Gravis

Myasthenia gravis produces sporadic but progressive weakness and abnormal fatigability of striated (skeletal) muscles, which are exacerbated by exercise and repeated movement but improved by anticholinesterase drugs. Usually, this disorder affects muscles innervated by the cranial nerves (face, lips, tongue, neck, and throat), but it can affect any muscle group. Myasthenia gravis follows an unpredictable course of recurring exacerbations and periodic remissions. There's no known cure. Drug treatment has improved prognosis and allows patients to lead relatively normal lives except during exacerbations. When the disease involves the respiratory system, it may be life-threatening.

Causes and incidence

Myasthenia gravis causes a failure in transmission of nerve impulses at the neuromuscular junction. Theoretically, such impairment may result from an autoimmune response, ineffective acetylcholine release, or inadequate muscle fiber response to acetylcholine.

Myasthenia gravis affects 1 in 25,000 persons. It occurs at any age, but incidence is highest between ages 20 and 40. It is three times more common in women than in men. About 20% of infants born to myasthenic mothers have transient (or occasionally persistent) myasthenia. Frequently, myasthenia gravis coexists with immunologic and thyroid disorders. In fact, 15% of myasthenic patients have thymomas. Spontaneous remissions occur in about 25% of patients.

Signs and symptoms

The dominant symptoms of myasthenia gravis are skeletal muscle weakness and fatigability. In the early stages, easy fatigability of certain muscles may appear with no other findings. Later, it may be severe enough to cause paralysis. Typically, myasthenic muscles are strongest in the morning but weaken throughout the day, especially after exercise. Short rest periods temporarily restore muscle function. Muscle weakness is progressive; more and more muscles become weak, and eventually some muscles may lose function entirely. Resulting symptoms depend on the muscle group affected; they become more intense during menses and after emotional stress, prolonged exposure to sunlight or cold, or infections.

Onset may be sudden or insidious. In many patients, weak eye closure, ptosis, and diplopia are the first signs that something is wrong. Myasthenic patients usually have blank and expressionless faces and nasal vocal tones. They experience frequent nasal regurgitation of fluids and have difficulty chewing and swallowing. Because of this, they often worry about choking. Their eyelids droop, and they may have to tilt their heads back to see. Their neck muscles may become too weak to support their heads without bobbing.

In patients with weakened respiratory muscles, decreased tidal volume and vital capacity make breathing difficult and predispose to pneumonia and other respiratory tract infections. Respiratory muscle weakness (myasthenic crisis) may be severe enough to require an emergency airway and mechanical ventilation.

Diagnosis

Muscle fatigability that improves with rest strongly suggests a diagnosis of myasthenia gravis. Tests for this neurologic condition record the effect of exercise and subsequent rest on muscle weakness. Electromyography, with repeated neural stimulation, may help confirm this diagnosis.

But the classic proof of myasthenia gravis is improved muscle function after an I.V. injection of edrophonium or neostigmine. In myasthenic patients, muscle function improves within 30 to 60 seconds and lasts up to 30 minutes. However, long-standing ocular muscle dysfunction often fails to respond to such testing. This same test can differentiate a myasthenic crisis from a cholinergic crisis (caused by acetylcholine overactivity at the neuromuscular junction, possibly due to anticholinesterase overdose). Diagnostic evaluation should rule out thyroid disease and, in all adults, thymoma (by mediastinal X-ray).

Treatment

Treatment is symptomatic. Anticholinesterase drugs, such as neostigmine and pyridostigmine, counteract fatigue and muscle weakness and allow about 80% of normal muscle function. However, these drugs become less effective as the disease worsens. Corticosteroids may be beneficial in relieving symptoms.

Patients with thymomas require thymectomy, which may cause remission in some cases of adult-onset myasthenia. Acute exacerbations that cause severe respiratory distress necessitate emergency treatment. Tracheotomy, ventilation with a positive-pressure ventilator, and vigorous suctioning to remove secretions usually bring improvement in a few days. Because anticholinesterase drugs aren't effective in myasthenic crisis, they're discontinued until respiratory function begins to improve. Such crisis requires immediate hospitalization and vigorous respiratory support.

Special considerations

Careful baseline assessment, early recognition and treatment of potential crises, supportive measures, and thorough patient teaching can minimize exacerbations and complications. Continuity of care is essential.

- Establish an accurate neurologic and respiratory baseline. Thereafter, monitor tidal volume and vital capacity regularly. The patient may need a ventilator and frequent suctioning to remove accumulating secretions.

- Be alert for signs of an impending crisis (increased muscle weakness, respiratory distress, difficulty in talking or chewing).
- Evenly space administration of drugs, and give them on time, as ordered, to prevent relapses. Be prepared to give atropine for anticholinesterase overdose or toxicity.
- Plan exercise, meals, patient care, and activities to make the most of energy peaks. For example, give medication 20 to 30 minutes before meals to facilitate chewing or swallowing. Allow the patient to participate in his care.
- When swallowing is difficult, give soft, solid foods instead of liquids to lessen the risk of choking.
- After a severe exacerbation, try to increase social activity as soon as possible.
- Patient teaching is essential, since myasthenia gravis is usually a lifelong condition. Help the patient plan daily activities to coincide with energy peaks. Stress the need for frequent rest periods throughout the day. Emphasize that periodic remissions, exacerbations, and day-to-day fluctuations are common.
- Teach the patient how to recognize side effects and signs of toxicity of anticholinesterase drugs (headaches, weakness, sweating, abdominal cramps, nausea, vomiting, diarrhea, excessive salivation, and bronchospasm) and corticosteroids.
- Warn the patient to avoid strenuous exercise, stress, infection, and needless exposure to the sun or cold weather. All of these things may worsen signs and symptoms. Wearing an eye patch or glasses with one frosted lens may help the patient with diplopia.
- For more information and an opportunity to meet myasthenics who lead full, productive lives, refer the patient to the Myasthenia Gravis Foundation.

Amyotrophic Lateral Sclerosis

(Lou Gehrig's disease)

Amyotrophic lateral sclerosis (ALS) is the most common motor neuron disease of muscular atrophy. Other motor neuron diseases include progressive muscular atrophy and progressive bulbar palsy. Generally, onset occurs between ages 40 and 70. ALS is fatal within 3 to 10 years after onset, usually a result of aspiration pneumonia or respiratory failure.

Causes and incidence

ALS occurs in 2 to 7 of every 100,000 persons. Generally, it affects men four times more often than women and is more common in whites than in blacks. In about 10% of cases, ALS is inherited as an autosomal dominant trait and affects men and women equally. In noninherited ALS, incidence is highest among persons whose occupations require strenuous physical labor.

ALS and other motor neuron diseases may result from several causes:

- nutritional deficiency of motor neurons related to a disturbance in enzyme metabolism
- metabolic interference in nucleic acid production by the nerve fibers
- autoimmune disorders that affect immune complexes in the renal glomerulus and basement membrane.

Precipitating factors for acute deterioration include trauma, viral infections, and physical exhaustion. Disorders that must be differentiated from ALS include central nervous system syphilis, multiple sclerosis, spinal cord tumors, and syringomyelia.

Signs and symptoms

Patients with ALS develop fasciculations, accompanied by atrophy and weakness, especially in the muscles of the forearms and the hands. Other signs include impaired speech; difficulty chewing, swallowing, and breathing, particularly if the brain stem is affected; and, occasionally, choking and excessive drooling. Mental deterioration doesn't usually occur, but patients may become depressed as a reaction to the disease. Progressive bulbar palsy may cause crying spells or inappropriate laughter.

Diagnosis

Characteristic clinical features indicate a combination of upper and lower motor neuron involvement without sensory impairment. Electromyography and muscle biopsy help show nerve, rather than muscle, disease. Protein content of CSF is increased in one third of patients, but this finding alone doesn't confirm ALS. Diagnosis must rule out multiple sclerosis, spinal cord neoplasm, polyarteritis, syringomyelia, myasthenia gravis, and progressive muscular dystrophy.

Treatment

No effective treatment exists for ALS. Management aims to control symptoms and provide emotional, psychological, and physical support.

Special considerations

This cruel, demeaning neurologic disease challenges the patient's and his care givers' ability to cope. Since mental status remains intact while progressive physical degeneration takes place, the patient acutely perceives every change.

Care begins with a complete neurologic assessment, a baseline for future evaluations of progressing disease.

- Implement a rehabilitation program designed to maintain independence as long as possible.
- Help the patient obtain equipment, such as a walker and a wheelchair. Arrange for a visiting nurse to oversee the patient's status, to provide support, and to teach the family about the illness.
- Depending on the patient's muscular capacity, assist with bathing, personal hygiene, and transfers from wheelchair to bed. Help establish a regular bowel and bladder routine.
- To help the patient handle increased accumulation of secretions and dysphagia, teach him to suction himself. He should have a suction machine handy at home to reduce fear of choking.
- To prevent skin breakdown, provide good skin care when the patient is bedridden. Turn him often, keep his skin clean and dry, and use sheepskins or pressure-relieving devices.
- If the patient has trouble swallowing, give him soft, solid foods and position him upright during meals. Gastrostomy and nasogastric tube feedings may be necessary if he can no longer swallow. Teach the patient (if he's still able to feed himself) or family how to administer gastrostomy feedings.
- Provide emotional support. Prepare the patient and family for his eventual death, and encourage the start of the grieving process. Patients with ALS may benefit from a hospice program.

MOTOR NEURON DISEASE

In its final stages, motor neuron disease affects both upper and lower motor neuron cells. However, the site of initial cell damage varies:

- *progressive bulbar palsy:* degeneration of upper motor neurons in the medulla oblongata
- *progressive muscular atrophy:* degeneration of lower motor neurons in the spinal cord
- *amyotrophic lateral sclerosis:* degeneration of upper motor neurons in the medulla oblongata and lower motor neurons in the spinal cord

Multiple Sclerosis

Multiple sclerosis (MS) is characterized by exacerbations and remissions caused by progressive demyelination of the white matter of the brain and the spinal cord. It's a major cause of chronic disability in young adults. Sporadic patches of demyelination in various parts of the central nervous system induce widely disseminated and varied neurologic dysfunction.

Prognosis is variable. MS may progress rapidly, disabling the patient by early adulthood or causing death within months of onset. However, 70% of patients lead active, productive lives with prolonged remissions.

Incidence

Onset occurs between ages 20 and 40 (average age is 27). The disease affects women to men in a ratio of 3:2; whites to blacks, 5:1. Incidence is low in Japan; it is generally higher among urban populations and upper socioeconomic groups. Family history of MS and living in a cold, damp climate increase the risk.

Causes

The exact cause of MS is unknown, but current theories suggest a slow-acting viral infection, an autoimmune response of the nervous system, or an allergic response to an infectious agent. Other theoretical causes include trauma, anoxia, toxins, nutritional deficiencies, vascular lesions, and anorexia, all of which may contribute to destruction of axons and the myelin sheath. Emotional stress, overwork, fatigue, pregnancy, and acute respiratory infections all have been known to precede onset of this illness. Endogenous, constitutional, and genetic factors may also contribute.

Signs and symptoms

Clinical findings in MS correspond to the extent and site of myelin destruction, the extent of remyelination, and the adequacy of subsequent restored synaptic transmission. Symptoms may be transient or may last for hours or weeks; they may wax and wane with no predictable pattern, vary from day to day, and be bizarre and difficult for the patient to describe.

In most patients, visual problems and sensory impairment, such as numbness and tingling sensations (paresthesia), are the first signs that anything is wrong. Other characteristic changes include:

- *ocular disturbances:* optic neuritis, diplopia, ophthalmoplegia, blurred vision, and nystagmus
- *muscle dysfunction:* weakness, paralysis ranging from monoplegia to quadriplegia, spasticity, hyperreflexia, intention tremor, gait ataxia
- *urinary disturbances:* incontinence, frequency, urgency, and frequent infections
- *emotional lability:* mood swings, irritability, euphoria, or depression.

Associated signs and symptoms include poorly articulated or scanning speech, and dysphagia. Clinical effects may be so mild that the patient may be unaware of them, or so bizarre that he appears hysterical.

Diagnosis

Because early symptoms may be mild, years may elapse between onset of the first signs and the diagnosis. Diagnosis requires evidence of multiple neurologic attacks and characteristic remissions and exacerbations. Since diagnosis is so difficult, periodic testing and close observation are necessary, perhaps for years, depending on the course of the disease.

Abnormal EEG occurs in one third of patients. Lumbar puncture shows elevated gamma globulin fraction of IgG but normal total CSF protein levels. Such elevated CSF gamma globulin is significant only when serum gamma globulin levels are normal, and it reflects hyperactivity of the immune system because of chronic demyelination. Oligoclonal bands of immunoglobulin can be detected when CSF gamma globulin is examined by electrophoresis. These are present in most patients and can be found even when the percentage of CSF gamma globulin is normal. In addition, CSF white blood cell count is slightly increased. Diagnosis also may include a psychological evaluation.

Differential diagnosis must rule out spinal cord compression, foramen magnum tumor (often, such a tumor exactly mimics the exacerbations and remissions of MS), multiple small strokes, syphilis or other infection, and psychological disturbances.

Treatment

The aim of treatment is to shorten exacerbations and, if possible, relieve neurologic deficits, so the patient can resume a normal life-style. Because MS is thought to have allergic and inflammatory causes, ACTH, prednisone, or dexamethasone is used to reduce the associated edema of the myelin sheath during exacerbations. ACTH and corticosteroids seem to relieve symptoms and hasten remission but don't prevent future exacerbations.

Other drugs used with ACTH and corticosteroids include chlordiazepoxide to mitigate mood swings, baclofen or dantrolene to relieve spasticity, and bethanechol or oxybutynin to relieve urinary retention and minimize frequency and urgency. During acute exacerbation, supportive measures include bed rest, comfort measures such as massages, prevention of fatigue, prevention of decubitus ulcers, bowel and bladder training (if necessary), treatment of bladder infections with antibiotics, physical therapy, and counseling.

Special considerations

Appropriate care depends on the severity of the disease and the symptoms.

- Assist with physical therapy. Increase patient comfort with massages and relaxing baths. Make sure the bathwater isn't too hot, since it may temporarily intensify otherwise subtle symptoms. Assist with active, resistive, and stretching exercises to maintain muscle tone and joint mobility, decrease spasticity, improve coordination, and boost morale.
- Educate the patient and family concerning the chronic course of multiple sclerosis. Emphasize the need to avoid stress, infections, and fatigue and to maintain independence by developing

DEMYELINATION IN MULTIPLE SCLEROSIS

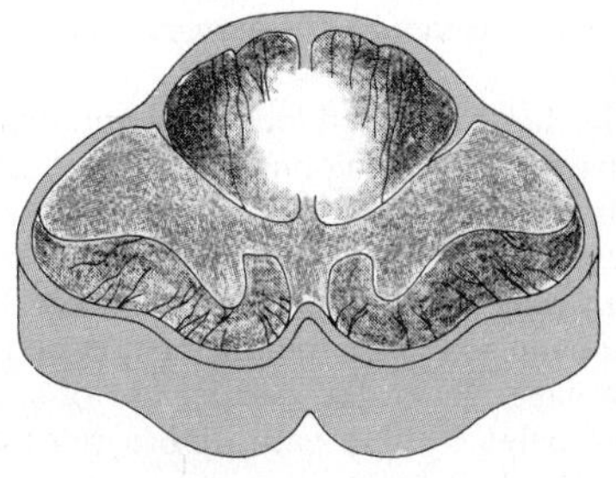

Transverse section of cervical spine shows partial loss of myelin, characteristic of multiple sclerosis. This degenerative process is called demyelination.

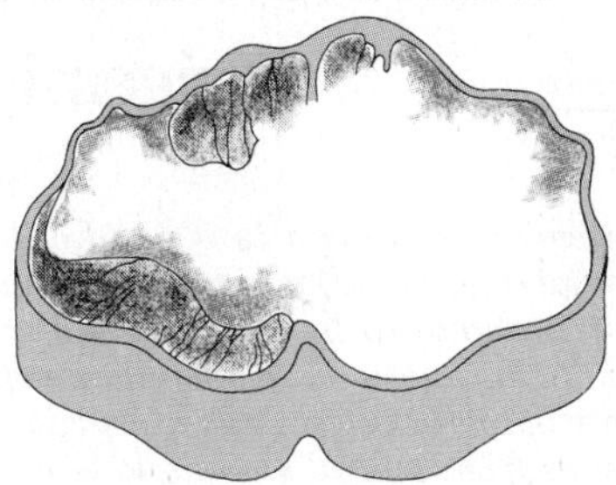

In this illustration, the loss of myelin is nearly complete. Clinical features of multiple sclerosis depend on the extent of demyelination.

new ways of performing daily activities. Be sure to tell the patient to avoid exposure to infections.
• Stress the importance of eating a nutritious, well-balanced diet that contains sufficient roughage to prevent constipation.
• Evaluate the need for bowel and bladder training during hospitalization. Encourage adequate fluid intake and regular urination. Eventually, the patient may require urinary drainage by self-catheterization or, in men, condom drainage. Teach the correct use of suppositories to help establish a regular bowel schedule.
• Watch for drug side effects. For instance, dantrolene may cause muscle weakness and decreased muscle tone.
• Promote emotional stability. Help the patient establish a daily routine to maintain optimal functioning. Activity level is regulated by tolerance level. Encourage regular rest periods to prevent fatigue, and daily physical exercise.
• Inform the patient that exacerbations are unpredictable, necessitating physical and emotional adjustments in life-style.
• For more information, refer him to the National Multiple Sclerosis Society.

PERIPHERAL NERVE DISORDERS

Trigeminal Neuralgia

(Tic douloureux)

Trigeminal neuralgia is a painful disorder of one or more branches of the fifth cranial (trigeminal) nerve that produces paroxysmal attacks of excruciating facial pain precipitated by stimulation of a trigger zone. It occurs mostly in people over age 40, in women more often than men, and on the right side of the face more often than the left. Trigeminal neuralgia can subside spontaneously, with remissions lasting from several months to years.

Causes

Although the cause remains undetermined, trigeminal neuralgia may reflect an afferent reflex phenomenon located centrally in the brain stem or more peripherally in the sensory root of the trigeminal nerve. Such neuralgia may also be related to compression of the nerve root by posterior fossa tumors, middle fossa tumors, or vascular lesions (subclinical aneurysm), although such lesions usually produce simultaneous loss of sensation. Occasionally, trigeminal neuralgia is a manifestation of multiple sclerosis or herpes zoster.

Whatever the cause, the pain of trigeminal neuralgia is probably produced by an interaction or short-circuiting of touch and pain fibers.

Signs and symptoms

Typically, the patient reports a searing or burning pain that occurs in lightninglike jabs and lasts from 1 to 15 minutes (usually 1 to 2 minutes) in an area innervated by one of the divisions of the trigeminal nerve, primarily the superior mandibular or maxillary division. The pain rarely affects more than one division, and seldom the first division (ophthalmic) or both sides of the face. It affects the second (maxillary) and third (mandibular) divisions of the trigeminal nerve equally.

These attacks characteristically follow stimulation of a trigger zone, usually by a light touch to a hypersensitive area, such as the tip of the nose, the cheeks, or the gums. Although attacks can occur at any time, they may follow a draft of air, exposure to heat or cold, eating, smiling, talking, or drinking hot or cold beverages. The frequency of attacks varies greatly, from many times a day to several times a month or year.

Between attacks, most patients are free of pain, although some have a constant, dull ache. No patient is ever free of the fear of the next attack.

Diagnosis

The patient's pain history is the basis for diagnosis, since trigeminal neuralgia produces no objective clinical or pathologic changes. Physical examination shows no impairment of sensory or motor function; indeed, sensory impairment implies a space-occupying lesion as the cause of pain.

Observation during the examination shows the patient favoring (splinting) the affected area. To ward off a painful attack, the patient often holds his face immobile when talking. He may also leave the affected side of his face unwashed and unshaven, or protect it with a coat or shawl. When asked where the pain occurs, he points to—but never touches—the affected area. Witnessing a typical attack helps to confirm diagnosis. Rarely, a tumor in the posterior fossa can produce pain that is clinically indistinguishable from trigeminal neuralgia. Skull X-rays, tomography, and computed tomography scan rule out sinus or tooth infections, and tumors.

Treatment

Oral administration of carbamazepine or phenytoin may temporarily relieve or prevent pain. Narcotics may be helpful during the pain episode.

When these medical measures fail or attacks become increasingly frequent or severe, neurosurgical procedures may provide permanent relief. The preferred procedure is percutaneous electrocoa-

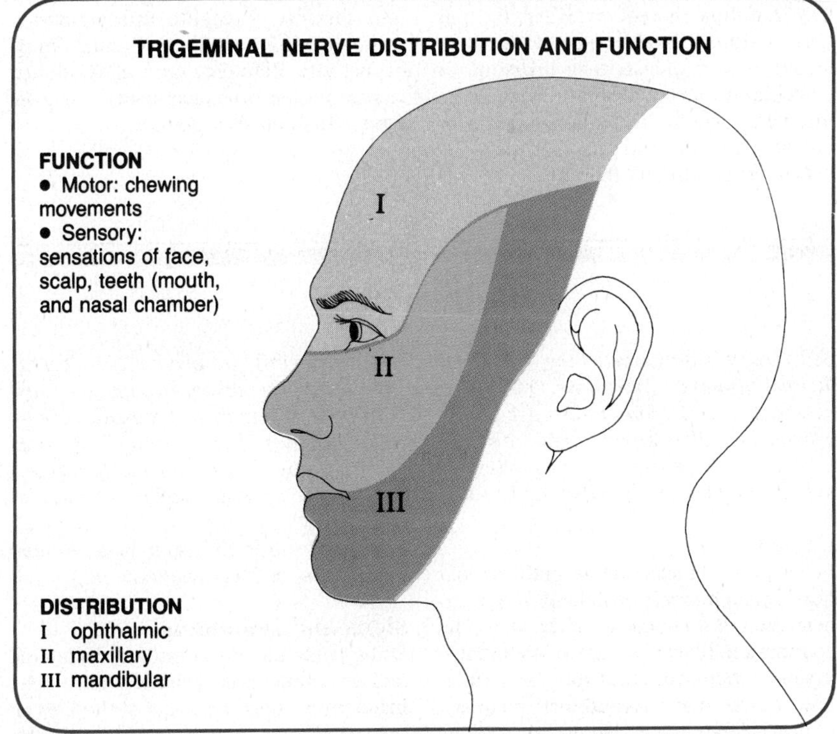

gulation of nerve rootlets, under local anesthetic. New treatments include a percutaneous radio frequency procedure, which causes partial root destruction and relieves pain, and microsurgery for vascular decompression of the trigeminal nerve.

Special considerations

- Observe and record the characteristics of each attack, including the patient's protective mechanisms.
- Provide adequate nutrition in small, frequent meals at room temperature.
- If the patient is receiving carbamazepine, watch for cutaneous and hematologic reactions (erythematous and pruritic rashes, urticaria, photosensitivity, exfoliative dermatitis, leukopenia, agranulocytosis, eosinophilia, aplastic anemia, thrombocytopenia) and, possibly, urinary retention and transient drowsiness. For the first 3 months of carbamazepine therapy, CBC and liver function should be monitored weekly, then monthly thereafter. Warn the patient to immediately report fever, sore throat, mouth ulcers, easy bruising, or petechial or purpuric hemorrhage, since these may signal thrombocytopenia or aplastic anemia and may require discontinuation of drug therapy.
- If the patient is receiving phenytoin, also watch for side effects, including ataxia, skin eruptions, gingival hyperplasia, and nystagmus.
- After resection of the first branch of the trigeminal nerve, tell the patient to avoid rubbing his eyes and using aerosol spray. Advise him to wear glasses or goggles outdoors and to blink often.
- After surgery to sever the second or third branch, tell the patient to avoid hot foods and drinks, which could burn his mouth, and to chew carefully to avoid biting his mouth. Advise him to place food in the unaffected side of his mouth when chewing, to brush his teeth and rinse his mouth often, and to see the dentist twice a year to detect cavities. (Cavities in the area of the severed nerve won't cause pain.)
- After surgical decompression of the root or partial nerve dissection, check neurologic and vital signs often.
- Provide emotional support, and encourage the patient to express his fear and anxiety. Promote independence through self-care and maximum physical activity. Reinforce natural avoidance of stimulation (air, heat, cold) of trigger zones (lips, cheeks, gums).

Bell's Palsy

Bell's palsy is a disease of the seventh cranial nerve (facial) that produces unilateral facial weakness or paralysis. Onset is rapid. While it affects all age-groups, it occurs most often in persons under age 60. In 80% to 90% of patients, it subsides spontaneously, with complete recovery in 1 to 8 weeks; however, recovery may be delayed in the elderly. If recovery is partial, contractures may develop on the paralyzed side of the face. Bell's palsy may recur on the same or opposite side of the face.

Causes

Bell's palsy blocks the seventh cranial nerve, which is responsible for motor innervation of the muscles of the face. The conduction block is due to an inflammatory reaction around the nerve (usually at the internal auditory meatus), which is often associated with infections and can result from hemorrhage, tumor, meningitis, or local trauma.

Signs and symptoms

Bell's palsy usually produces unilateral facial weakness, occasionally with aching pain around the angle of the jaw or behind the ear. On the weak side, the

BELL'S PALSY

Bell's palsy causes unilateral facial paralysis, producing a distorted appearance with an inability to wrinkle the forehead, close the eyelid, smile, show the teeth, or puff out the cheek.

Distorted appearance

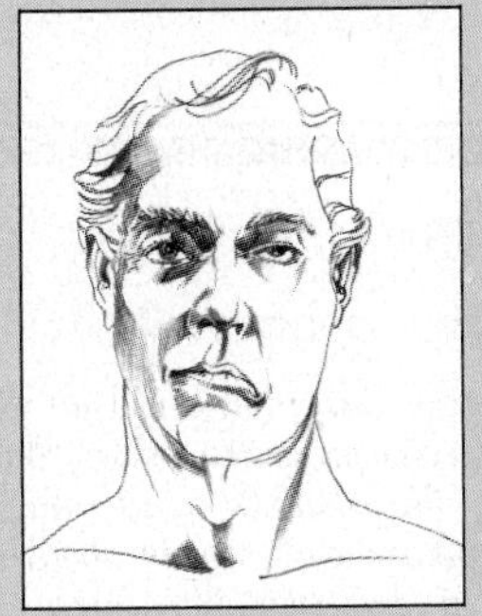

Wrinkling the forehead

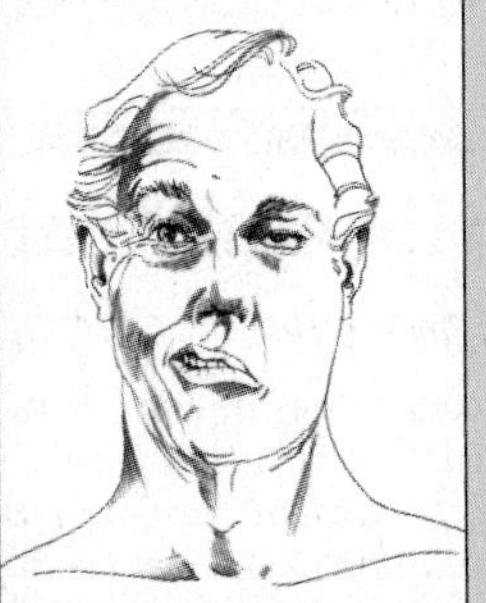

Smiling

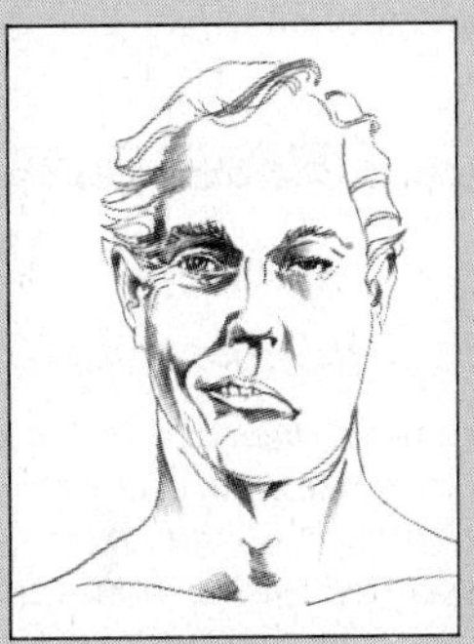

mouth droops (causing the patient to drool saliva from the corner of his mouth), and taste perception is distorted over the affected anterior portion of the tongue. In addition, the forehead appears smooth, and the patient's ability to close his eye on the weak side is markedly impaired. When he tries to close this eye, it rolls upward (Bell's phenomenon) and shows excessive tearing. Although Bell's phenomenon occurs in normal persons, it's not apparent, since the eye closes completely and covers this eye motion. In Bell's palsy, incomplete eye closure makes this upward motion obvious.

Diagnosis

Diagnosis is based on clinical presentation: distorted facial appearance and inability to raise the eyebrow, close the eyelid, smile, show the teeth, or puff out the cheek. After 10 days, electromyography helps predict the level of expected recovery by distinguishing temporary conduction defects from a pathologic interruption of nerve fibers.

Treatment and special considerations

Treatment consists of prednisone, an oral corticosteroid that reduces facial nerve edema and improves nerve conduction and blood flow. After the 14th day of prednisone therapy, electrotherapy may help prevent atrophy of facial muscles.

- During treatment with prednisone, watch for steroid side effects, especially gastrointestinal distress and fluid retention. If gastrointestinal distress is troublesome, a concomitant antacid usually provides relief. If the patient has diabetes, prednisone must be used with caution and necessitates frequent monitoring of serum glucose levels.
- To reduce pain, apply moist heat to the affected side of the face, taking care not to burn the skin.
- To help maintain muscle tone, massage the patient's face with a gentle upward motion two to three times daily for 5 to 10 minutes, or have him massage his face himself. When he's ready for active exercises, teach him to exercise by grimacing in front of a mirror.
- Advise the patient to protect his eye by covering it with an eyepatch, especially when outdoors. Tell him to keep warm and avoid exposure to dust and wind. When exposure is unavoidable, instruct him to cover his face.

• To prevent excessive weight loss, help the patient cope with difficulty in eating and drinking. Instruct him to chew on the unaffected side of his mouth. Provide a soft, nutritionally balanced diet, eliminating hot foods and fluids. Arrange for privacy at mealtimes to reduce embarrassment. Apply a facial sling to improve lip alignment. Also, give the patient frequent and complete mouth care, being particularly careful to remove residual food that collects between the cheeks and gums.
• Offer psychological support. Give reassurance that recovery is likely within 1 to 8 weeks.

Peripheral Neuritis

(Multiple neuritis, peripheral neuropathy, polyneuritis)

Peripheral neuritis is the degeneration of peripheral nerves supplying mainly the distal muscles of the extremities. It results in muscle weakness with sensory loss and atrophy, and decreased or absent deep tendon reflexes. This syndrome is associated with a noninflammatory degeneration of the axon and myelin sheaths, chiefly affecting the distal muscles of the extremities. Although peripheral neuritis can occur at any age, incidence is highest in men between ages 30 and 50. Because onset is usually insidious, patients may compensate by overusing unaffected muscles; however, onset is rapid with severe infection and chronic alcohol intoxication. If the cause can be identified and eliminated, prognosis is good.

Causes

Causes of peripheral neuritis include:
• chronic intoxication (ethyl alcohol, arsenic, lead, carbon disulfide, benzene, phosphorus, and sulfonamides)
• infectious diseases (meningitis, diphtheria, syphilis, tuberculosis, pneumonia, mumps, and Guillain-Barré syndrome)
• metabolic and inflammatory disorders (gout, diabetes mellitus, rheumatoid arthritis, polyarteritis nodosa, systemic lupus erythematosus)
• nutritive diseases (beriberi and other vitamin deficiencies, and cachectic states).

Signs and symptoms

The clinical effects of peripheral neuritis develop slowly, and the disease usually affects the motor and sensory nerve fibers. Neuritis typically produces flaccid paralysis, wasting, loss of reflexes, pain of varying intensity, loss of ability to perceive vibratory sensations, and paresthesia, hyperesthesia, or anesthesia in the hands and feet. Deep tendon reflexes are diminished or absent, and atrophied muscles are tender or hypersensitive to pressure or palpation. Footdrop may also be present. Cutaneous manifestations include glossy red skin and decreased sweating. Patients often have a history of clumsiness and may complain of frequent vague sensations.

Diagnosis

Patient history and physical examination delineate characteristic distribution of motor and sensory deficits. Electromyography may show a delayed action potential if this condition impairs motor nerve function.

Treatment

Effective treatment of peripheral neuritis consists of supportive measures to relieve pain, adequate bed rest, and physical therapy, as needed. Most important, however, the underlying cause must be identified and corrected. For instance, it's essential to identify and remove the toxic agent, correct nutritional and vitamin deficiencies (the patient needs a high-calorie diet rich in vitamins, especially B complex), or counsel the patient to avoid alcohol.

Special considerations

- Relieve pain with correct positioning, analgesics, or possibly phenytoin, which has been used experimentally for neuritic pain, especially if associated with diabetic neuropathy.
- Instruct the patient to rest and refrain from using the affected extremity. To prevent pressure sores, apply a foot cradle. To prevent contractures, arrange for the patient to obtain splints, boards, braces, or other orthopedic appliances.
- After the pain subsides, passive range-of-motion exercises or massage may be beneficial. Electrotherapy is advocated for nerve and muscle stimulation.

Selected References

Adams, R.D., and Victor, M. *Principles of Neurology*, 3rd ed. New York: McGraw-Hill Book Co., 1981.

Conway-Rutkowski, Barbara L. *Carini and Owen's Neurological and Neurosurgical Nursing*, 8th ed. St. Louis: C.V. Mosby Co., 1982.

Gilroy, John, and Holliday, Patti. *Basic Neurology*. New York: MacMillan Publishing Co., 1982.

Green, Barth, et al. *Intensive Care for Neurologic Trauma and Disease*. Orlando, Fla.: Academic Press, 1982.

Hickey, Joanne V.X. *The Clinical Practice of Neurological and Neurosurgical Nursing*. Philadelphia: J.B. Lippincott Co., 1981.

Nikas, Diana L. *Critically Ill Neurosurgical Patient*. New York: Churchill Livingstone, 1982.

Weisburg, Leon A., and Strub, Richard L. *Essentials of Clinical Neurology*. Baltimore: University Park Press, 1983.

Weller, R.O., et al. *Clinical Neuropathology*. New York: Springer-Verlag New York, 1983.

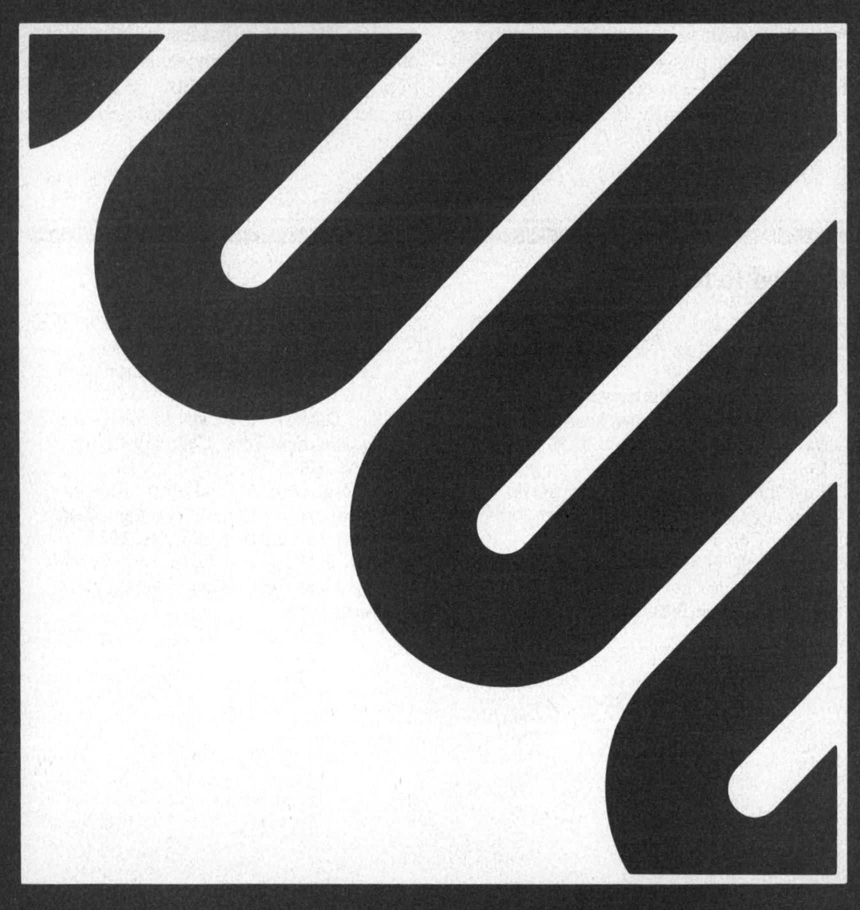

10 Gastrointestinal Disorders

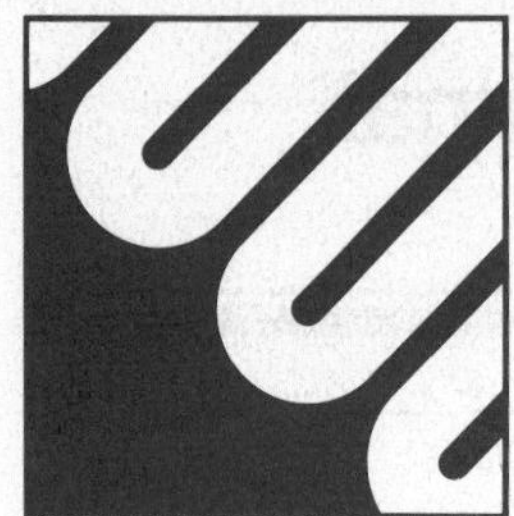

Gastrointestinal Disorders

Introduction

The gastrointestinal (GI) tract, also known as the alimentary canal, is a long hollow tube with glands and accessory organs (salivary glands, liver, gallbladder, and pancreas). The GI tract breaks down food—carbohydrates, fats, and proteins—into molecules small enough to permeate cell membranes, thus providing cells with the necessary energy to function properly; it prepares food for cellular absorption by altering its physical and chemical composition. Consequently, a malfunction along the GI tract can produce far-reaching metabolic effects, eventually threatening life itself. The GI tract is an unsterile system filled with bacteria and other flora; these organisms can cause superinfection from antibiotic therapy, or they can infect other systems when a GI organ ruptures. A common indication of GI problems is referred pain, which makes diagnosis especially difficult.

Accurate assessment vital

Your assessment of the patient with suspected GI disease must begin with a careful history that includes occupation, family history, and recent travel. Medical history should include previous hospital admissions; any surgery (including recent tooth extraction); family history of ulcers, colitis, or cancer; and any current medications, such as aspirin, steroids, or anticoagulants.

Next, have the patient describe his chief complaint in his own words. Does he have abdominal pain, indigestion, heartburn, or rectal bleeding? How long has he had it? What relieves these symptoms or makes them worse? Has he experienced nosebleeds or difficulty in swallowing recently? Has he had any recent weight loss or gain? Is he on a special diet? Does he drink alcoholic beverages or smoke? How much and how often? Ask about bowel habits. Does he regularly use laxatives or enemas? If he experiences nausea and vomiting, what does the vomitus look like? Does changing his position relieve nausea?

Next, try to define and locate any pain. Ask the patient to describe the pain. Is it dull, sharp, burning, aching, spasmodic, intermittent? Where is it located? How long does it last? When does it occur? Does it radiate? What relieves it?

Visual assessment

Observe how the patient looks and note appropriateness of behavior. Changes in fluid and electrolyte balance, severe infection, drug toxicity, and hepatic disease may cause abnormal behavior. Your visual examination should carefully check:

- *skin:* loss of turgor, jaundice, cyanosis, pallor, diaphoresis, petechiae, bruises, edema, texture (dry or oily)
- *head*—color of sclerae, sunken eyes,

dentures, caries, lesions, tongue (color, swelling, dryness), breath odor
- *chest*—shape
- *lungs*—rate, rhythm, and quality of respirations
- *abdomen*—size and shape (distention, contour, visible masses, protrusions), abdominal scars or fistulae, excessive skin folds (may indicate wasting), abnormal respiratory movements (inflammation of diaphragm).

Auscultation, palpation, and percussion

Auscultation provides helpful clues to GI abnormalities. For example, absence of bowel sounds over the area to the lower right of the umbilicus may indicate peritonitis. High-pitched sounds that coincide with colicky pain may indicate small bowel obstruction. Less intense, low-pitched rumbling noises may accompany minor irritation.

Palpating the abdomen after auscultation helps detect tenderness, muscle guarding, and abdominal masses. Watch for muscle tone (boardlike rigidity points to peritonitis; transient rigidity suggests severe pain) and tenderness (rebound tenderness may indicate peritoneal inflammation).

Percussion helps detect air, fluid, and solid matter in the abdomen.

Diagnostic tests

After physical assessment, several tests can identify GI malfunction.
- *Barium swallow* primarily examines the esophagus.
- In an *upper GI (UGI) series,* swal-

HISTOLOGY OF THE GI TRACT

The GI tract consists of four tissue layers whose structure varies in different organs:
- *mucous membrane:* innermost layer; secretes gastric juice and protects the tract
- *submucosa:* connective tissue that contains the major blood vessels
- *external muscle coat (muscularis externa):* double layer of smooth-muscle fibers; inner circular and outer longitudinal layers propel gastric contents downward by peristalsis
- *fibroserous coat (serosa):* outermost protective layer of connective tissue; forms the largest serous membrane of the body—the peritoneum. The peritoneum's parietal layer covers the walls of the abdominal cavity; the visceral layer drapes most of the abdominal organs, covering the upper surface of the pelvic organs.

PRIMARY SOURCE OF DIGESTIVE HORMONES

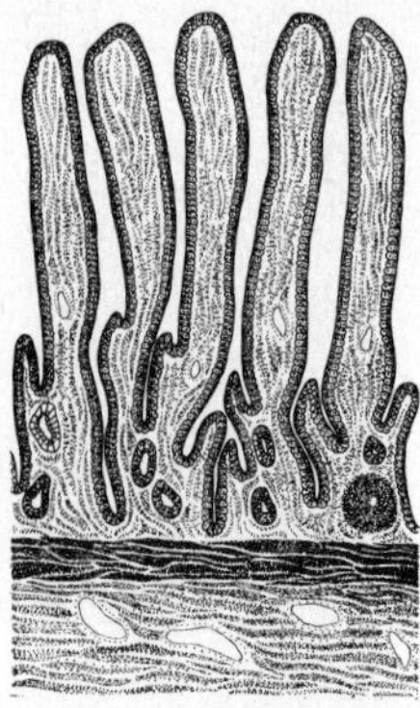

PYLORIC MUCOSA

Gastrin, which originates in the G cells of the pyloric antral mucosa (also from the duodenal and jejunal mucosa), stimulates secretion of HCl by parietal cells, and pepsinogen by chief cells.

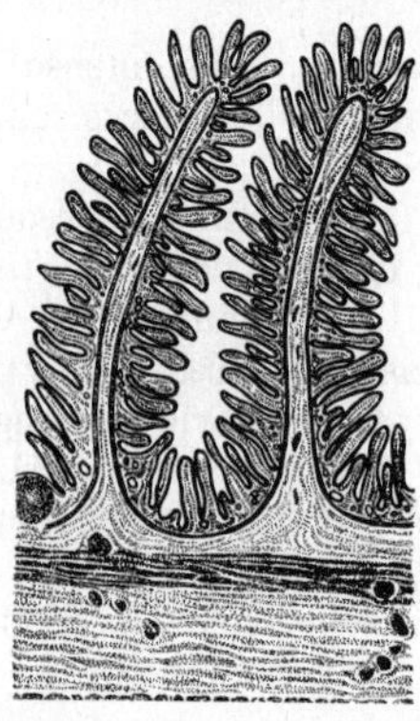

JEJUNAL MUCOSA

Gastric inhibitory peptide (GIP), which originates in the jejunal mucosa (also from duodenal mucosa), stimulates secretion of intestinal juice and insulin, and inhibits gastric acid secretion and motility.

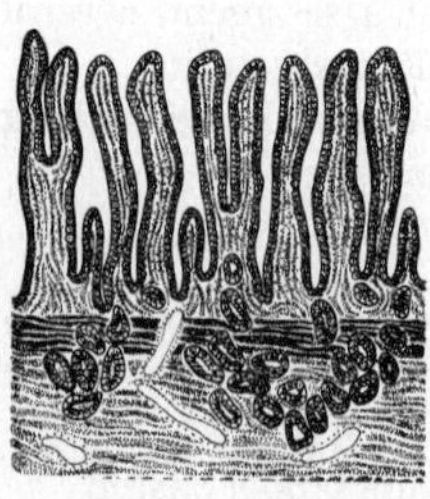

DUODENAL MUCOSA

Secretin, which originates in the duodenal mucosa, stimulates the pancreas to secrete alkaline fluid (water and HCO_3^-) into the duodenum, which neutralizes acid from the stomach.

Cholecystokinin-pancreozymin, which originates in the duodenal mucosa, stimulates pancreatic enzyme secretion, and contraction and evacuation of the gallbladder.

Motilin, which originates in the duodenal mucosa, slows gastric emptying and stimulates gastric acid and pepsin secretion.

Other digestive hormones
Three other digestive hormone-like substances are thought to originate in the hypothalamus, gastrointestinal tract, and neurons of the brain. These substances include substance P, which increases small bowel motility; bombesin, which increases gastrin secretion and small bowel motility; and somatosin, which inhibits secretion of gastrin, vasoactive intestinal polypeptide, GIP, secretin, and motilin. Other possible digestive hormones include enterogastrone, enteroglucagon, and somatostatin. More research is needed to confirm and clarify the existence and function of these hormones.

REVIEW OF ANATOMY AND PHYSIOLOGY

The GI tract includes the mouth, pharynx, esophagus, stomach (fundus, body, antrum), small intestine (duodenum, jejunum, ileum), and large intestine (cecum, colon, rectum, anal canal).

Digestion begins in the mouth through chewing and through the action of an enzyme, ptyalin (amylase), secreted in saliva, which breaks down starch. Digestion continues in the stomach, where the lining secretes gastric juice that contains hydrochloric acid and the enzymes pepsin (begins protein digestion), lipase (speeds hydrolysis of emulsified fats), and in infants, rennin (curdles milk). Through a churning motion, the stomach breaks food into tiny particles, mixes them with gastric juice, and pushes the mass toward the pylorus. The liquid portion (chyme) enters the duodenum in small amounts; any solid material remains in the stomach until it liquefies (usually from 1 to 6 hours). The stomach also produces an intrinsic factor necessary for the absorption of vitamin B_{12}. Although limited amounts of water, alcohol, and some drugs are absorbed in the stomach, chyme passes unabsorbed into the duodenum. Most digestion and absorption occur in the small intestine, where the surface area is increased by millions of villi in the mucous membrane lining. For digestion, the small intestine relies on a vast array of enzymes produced by the pancreas or by the intestinal lining itself. Pancreatic enzymes include tryspin, which digests protein to amino acids; lipase, which digests fat to fatty acids and glycerol; and amylase, which digests starches to sugars. Intestinal enzymes include erepsin, which digests protein to amino acids; lactase, maltase, and sucrase, which digest complex sugars like glucose, fructose, and galactose; and enterokinase, which activates trypsin.

In addition, bile, secreted by the liver, helps neutralize stomach acid and aids the small intestine to emulsify and absorb fats and fat-soluble vitamins.

By the time ingested material reaches the ileocecal valve (where the small intestine joins the large intestine), all its nutritional value has been absorbed.

The large intestine, so named because it's larger in diameter than the small intestine, absorbs water from the digestive material before passing it on for elimination. Rectal distention by feces stimulates the defecation reflex, which, when assisted by voluntary sphincter relaxation, permits defecation.

Throughout the GI tract, peristalsis propels ingested material along; sphincters prevent its reflux.

lowed barium sulfate proceeds into the esophagus, stomach, and small intestine, to reveal abnormalities. The barium outlines stomach walls and delineates ulcer craters and filling defects.

- A *small bowel series*, an extension of UGI, visualizes barium flowing through the small intestine to the ileocecal valve.
- A *barium enema (lower GI)* allows X-ray visualization of the colon.
- A *stool specimen* is useful with suspected GI bleeding, infection, or malabsorption. Guaiac test for occult blood, microscopic stool examination for ova and parasites, and tests for fat require several specimens.
- In *upper GI endoscopy,* insertion of a fiberoptic scope allows direct visual inspection of the esophagus, stomach, and, sometimes, duodenum; proctosigmoidoscopy permits inspection of the rectum and distal sigmoid colon; colonoscopy, inspection of descending, transverse, and ascending colon.
- *Gastric analysis* examines gastric secretions.
- *Endoscopic retrograde cholangiopancreatography (ERCP)* allows direct visualization of the esophagus, stomach, proximal duodenum, and pancreatic, hepatic, and biliary ducts.

Intubation

Certain GI disorders require intubation to empty the stomach and intestine, to aid diagnosis and treatment, to decompress obstructed areas, to detect and treat GI bleeding, and to administer medications or feedings. Tubes generally inserted through the nose are the short nasogastric tubes (the Levin, the Salem Sump, and the specialized Sengstaken-Blakemore) and the long intestinal tubes (Cantor and Miller-Abbott). The larger Ewald tube is usually inserted orally.

When caring for patients with tubes:

- Explain the procedure before intubation.
- Maintain accurate intake and output records. Measure gastric drainage every 8 hours; record amount, color, odor, and consistency. When irrigating the tube, note the amount of saline solution instilled and aspirated. Check for fluid and electrolyte imbalances.
- Provide good oral and nasal care. Brush the patient's teeth frequently; also provide mouthwash and lemon and glycerine swabs. Make sure the tube is secure but isn't causing too much pressure on the nostrils. Gently wash the area around the tube, and apply a water-soluble lubricant to soften crusts. These measures help prevent sore throat and nose, dry lips, nasal excoriation, and parotitis.
- Ensure maximum patient comfort. After insertion of a long intestinal tube, instruct the patient to turn from side to side to facilitate its passage through the GI tract. Note the tube's progress.
- To support the short tube's weight, anchor it to the patient's clothing.
- With both types of tubes, tell the patient to expect a feeling of dryness or a lump in the throat; if he is allowed, suggest he chew gum or eat hard candy to relieve these discomforts.
- Always keep a pair of scissors taped to the wall near the bed when the patient has a Sengstaken-Blakemore tube in place. If the tube should dislodge and obstruct the bronchus, cut the lumen to the balloons immediately. Sometimes the tube is taped to the face piece of a football-helmet worn by the patient to prevent the tube from dislodging and to put traction on the tube.
- After removing the tube from a patient with GI bleeding, watch for signs of recurrent bleeding, such as hematemesis, decreased hemoglobin, pallor, chills, and clamminess.
- Provide emotional support. Many people panic at the sight of a tube. Your calm, reassuring manner can help minimize their fear.

MOUTH & ESOPHAGUS

Stomatitis and Other Oral Infections

Stomatitis, inflammation of the oral mucosa, which may also extend to the buccal mucosa, lips, and palate, is a common infection. It may occur alone or as part of a systemic disease. There are two main types: acute herpetic stomatitis *and* aphthous stomatitis. *Acute herpetic stomatitis is usually self-limiting; however, it may be severe and, in newborns, may be generalized and potentially fatal. Aphthous stomatitis usually heals spontaneously, without a scar, in 10 to 14 days. Other oral infections include gingivitis, periodontitis, and Vincent's angina.*

Causes and incidence

Acute herpetic stomatitis results from herpes simplex virus. It's a common cause of stomatitis in children between ages 1 and 3.

Aphthous stomatitis is common in girls and female adolescents. Its predisposing factors include stress, fatigue, anxiety, febrile states, trauma, and solar overexposure.

ORAL INFECTIONS

DISEASE AND CAUSES	SIGNS AND SYMPTOMS	TREATMENT
Gingivitis (inflammation of the gingiva) • Early sign of hypovitaminosis, diabetes, blood dyscrasias • Occasionally related to use of oral contraceptives	• Inflammation with painless swelling, redness, change of normal contours, bleeding, and periodontal pocket (gum detachment from teeth)	• Removal of irritating factors (calculus, faulty dentures) • Good oral hygiene; regular dental check-ups; vigorous chewing • Oral or topical corticosteroids
Periodontitis (progression of gingivitis; inflammation of the oral mucosa) • Early sign of hypovitaminosis, diabetes, blood dyscrasias • Occasionally related to use of oral contraceptives • Dental factors: calculus, poor oral hygiene, malocclusion. Major cause of tooth loss after middle-age	• Acute onset of bright red gum inflammation, painless swelling of interdental papillae, easy bleeding • Loosening of teeth, typically without inflammatory symptoms, progressing to loss of teeth and alveolar bone • Acute systemic infection (fever, chills)	• Scaling, root planing, and curettage for infection control • Periodontal surgery to prevent recurrence • Good oral hygiene, regular dental checkups, vigorous chewing
Vincent's angina (trench mouth, necrotizing ulcerative gingivitis) • Fusiform bacillus or spirochete infection • Predisposing factors: stress, poor oral hygiene, insufficient rest, nutritional deficiency, smoking	• Sudden onset: painful, superficial bleeding gingival ulcers (rarely, on buccal mucosa) covered with a gray-white membrane • Ulcers become punched out lesions after slight pressure or irritation. • Malaise, mild fever, excessive salivation, bad breath, pain on swallowing or talking, enlarged submaxillary lymph nodes	• Removal of devitalized tissue with ultrasonic cavitron • Antibiotics (penicillin or erythromycin P.O.) for infection • Analgesics, as needed • Hourly mouth rinses (with equal amounts of hydrogen peroxide and warm water) • Soft, nonirritating diet; rest; no smoking • With treatment, improvement common within 24 hours
Glossitis (inflammation of the tongue) • Streptococcal infection • Irritation or injury; jagged teeth; ill-fitting dentures; biting during convulsions; alcohol; spicy foods; smoking; sensitivity to toothpaste or mouthwash • Vitamin B deficiency; anemia • Skin conditions: lichen planus, erythema multiforme, pemphigus vulgaris	• Reddened ulcerated or swollen tongue (may obstruct airway) • Painful chewing and swallowing • Speech difficulty • Painful tongue without inflammation	• Treatment of underlying cause • Topical anesthetic mouthwash or systemic analgesics (aspirin and acetaminophen) for painful lesions • Good oral hygiene; regular dental checkups; vigorous chewing • Avoidance of hot, cold, or spicy foods, and alcohol.

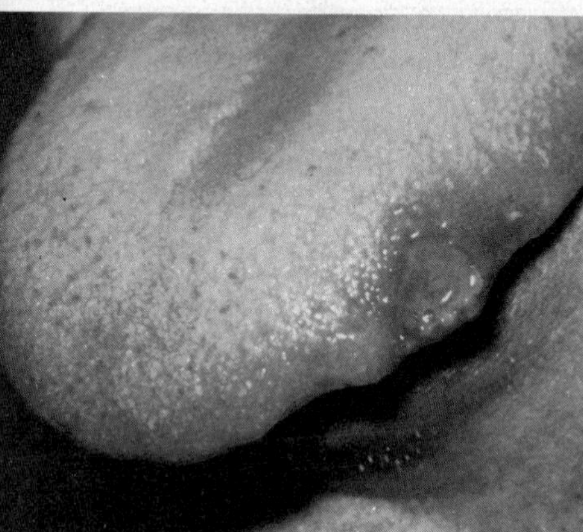

In aphthous stomatitis, numerous small round vesicles appear, soon breaking and leaving shallow ulcers with red areolae.

Signs and symptoms

Acute herpetic stomatitis begins suddenly with mouth pain, malaise, lethargy, anorexia, irritability, and fever, which may persist for 1 to 2 weeks. Gums are swollen and bleed easily, and the mucous membrane is extremely tender. Papulovesicular ulcers appear in the mouth and throat, and eventually become punched-out lesions with reddened areolae. Submaxillary lymphadenitis is common. Pain usually disappears from 2 to 4 days before healing of ulcers is complete. If the child with stomatitis sucks his thumb, these lesions spread to the hand.

A patient with aphthous stomatitis will typically report burning, tingling, and slight swelling of the mucous membrane. Single or multiple shallow ulcers with whitish centers and red borders appear and heal at one site but then appear at another.

Diagnosis

Diagnosis depends on physical examination, and, in Vincent's angina, a smear of ulcer exudate allows identification of the causative organism.

Treatment and special considerations

For acute herpetic stomatitis, treatment is conservative. For local symptoms, management includes warm-water mouth rinses (antiseptic mouthwashes are contraindicated because they are irritating) and a topical anesthetic to relieve mouth ulcer pain. Supplementary treatment includes bland or liquid diet and, in severe cases, I.V. fluids and bed rest.

For aphthous stomatitis, primary treatment is application of a topical anesthetic. Effective long-term treatment requires alleviation or prevention of precipitating factors.

Gastroesophageal Reflux

Gastroesophageal reflux is the backflow of gastric or duodenal contents, or both, into the esophagus and past the lower esophageal sphincter (LES), without associated belching or vomiting. Reflux may or may not cause symptoms or pathologic changes. Persistent reflux may cause reflux esophagitis (inflammation of the esophageal mucosa). Prognosis varies with the underlying cause.

Causes

The function of the LES—a high-pressure area in the lower esophagus, just above the stomach—is to prevent gastric contents from backing up into the esophagus. Normally, the LES creates pressure, closing the lower end of the esophagus, but relaxes after each swallow to allow food into the stomach. Reflux occurs when LES pressure is deficient or when pressure within the stomach exceeds LES pressure.

Studies have shown that a person with symptomatic reflux can't swallow often

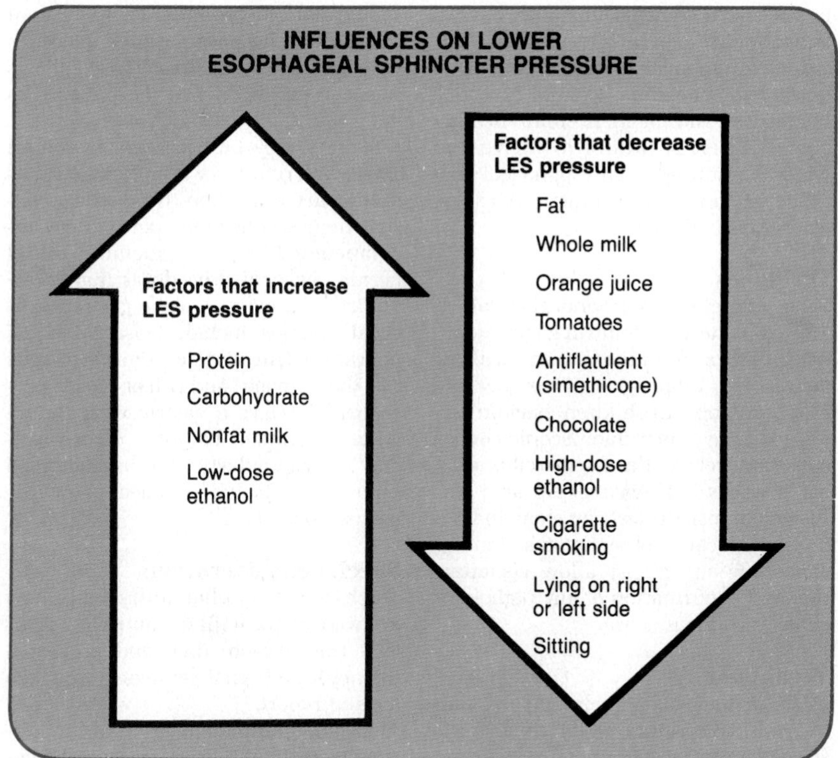

enough to create sufficient peristaltic amplitude to clear gastric acid from the lower esophagus. This results in prolonged periods of acidity in the esophagus when reflux occurs.

Predisposing factors include:

• pyloric surgery (alteration or removal of the pylorus), which allows reflux of bile or pancreatic juice.
• long-term nasogastric intubation (more than 4 or 5 days).
• any agent that lowers LES pressure: food, alcohol, cigarettes, anticholinergics (atropine, belladonna, propantheline), other drugs (morphine, diazepam, and meperidine).
• hiatal hernia (especially in children).
• any condition or position that increases intra-abdominal pressure.

Signs and symptoms

Gastroesophageal reflux doesn't always cause symptoms, and in patients showing clinical effects, physiologic reflux is not always confirmable. The most common feature of gastroesophageal reflux is heartburn, which may become more severe with vigorous exercise, bending, or lying down, and may be relieved by antacids or sitting upright. The pain of esophageal spasm resulting from reflux esophagitis tends to be chronic and may mimic angina pectoris, radiating to the neck, jaws, and arms. Other symptoms include odynophagia, which may be followed by a dull substernal ache from severe, long-term reflux; dysphagia from esophageal spasm, stricture, or esophagitis; and bleeding (bright red or dark brown). Rarely, nocturnal regurgitation wakens the patient with coughing, choking, and a mouthful of saliva. Reflux may be associated with hiatal hernia. Direct hiatal hernia becomes clinically significant *only* when reflux is confirmed.

Pulmonary symptoms result from reflux of gastric contents into the throat and subsequent aspiration and include chronic pulmonary disease or nocturnal wheezing, bronchitis, asthma, morning hoarseness, and cough. In children, other signs consist of failure to thrive and forceful vomiting from esophageal irritation. Such vomiting sometimes causes aspiration pneumonia.

Diagnosis

After a careful history and physical examination, tests to confirm gastroesophageal reflux include barium swallow fluoroscopy, esophageal pH probe, and esophagoscopy. In children, barium esophagography under fluoroscopic control can show reflux. Recurrent reflux after age 6 weeks is abnormal. An acid perfusion (Bernstein) test can show that reflux is the cause of symptoms. Finally, endoscopy and biopsy allow visualization and confirmation of any pathologic changes in the mucosa.

Treatment

Effective management relieves symptoms by reducing reflux through gravity, strengthening the LES with drug therapy, neutralizing gastric contents, and reducing intraabdominal pressure. To reduce intraabdominal pressure, the patient should sleep in a reverse Trendelenburg position (with the head of the bed elevated) and should avoid lying down after meals and late-night snacks. In uncomplicated cases, positional therapy is especially useful in infants and children. Antacids given 1 hour and 3 hours after meals and at bedtime are effective for intermittent reflux. Hourly administration is necessary for intensive therapy. A nondiarrheal, nonmagnesium antacid (aluminum carbonate, aluminum hydroxide) may be preferred, depending on the patient's bowel status. Bethanechol, a drug to increase LES pressure, stimulates smooth-muscle contraction and decreases esophageal acidity after meals (proven with pH probe). Metoclopramide and cimetidine have also been used with beneficial results. If possible, nasogastric intubation should not be continued for more than 4 or 5 days, because the tube interferes with sphincter integrity and itself allows reflux, especially when the patient lies flat.

Surgery may be necessary to control severe and refractory symptoms, such as pulmonary aspiration, hemorrhage, obstruction, severe pain, perforation, incompetent LES, or associated hiatal hernia. Surgical procedures that create an artificial closure at the gastroesophageal junction include Belsey Mark IV operation (invaginates the esophagus into the stomach) and Hill or Nissen procedures (creates a gastric wraparound with or without fixation). Also, vagotomy or pyloroplasty may be combined with an antireflux regimen to modify gastric contents.

Special considerations

Teach the patient what causes reflux, how to avoid reflux with an antireflux regimen (medication, diet, and positional therapy), and what symptoms to watch for and report.

- Instruct the patient to avoid any circumstance that increases intraabdominal pressure (such as bending, coughing, vigorous exercise, tight clothing, constipation, and obesity) or any substance that reduces sphincter control (cigarettes, alcohol, fatty foods, and certain drugs).
- Advise the patient to sit upright, particularly after meals, and to eat small, frequent meals. Tell him to avoid highly seasoned food, acidic juices, alcoholic drinks, bedtime snacks, and foods high in fat or carbohydrates, which reduce LES pressure. He should eat meals at least 2 to 3 hours before lying down.
- Tell patient to take antacids, as ordered (usually 1 hour and 3 hours after meals and at bedtime).
- Teach patient correct preparation for diagnostic testing. For example, he should not eat for 6 to 8 hours before barium X-ray or endoscopy.

After surgery using a thoracic approach, carefully watch and record chest tube drainage and respiratory status. If needed, give chest physiotherapy and oxygen. Position the patient with a nasogastric tube in semi-Fowler's position to help prevent reflux. Offer reassurance and emotional support.

Tracheoesophageal Fistula and Esophageal Atresia

Tracheoesophageal fistula is a developmental anomaly characterized by an abnormal connection between the trachea and the esophagus. It usually accompanies esophageal atresia, in which the esophagus is closed off at some point. Although these malformations have numerous anatomic variations, the most common, by far, is esophageal atresia with fistula to the distal segment.

These disorders, two of the most serious surgical emergencies in newborns, require immediate diagnosis and correction. They may coexist with other serious anomalies, such as congenital heart disease, imperforate anus, genitourinary abnormalities, and intestinal atresia. Esophageal atresia occurs in about 1 of every 4,000 live births; about one third of these infants are born prematurely.

Causes

Tracheoesophageal fistula and esophageal atresia result from failure of the embryonic esophagus and trachea to develop and separate correctly. The most common abnormality is type C tracheoesophageal fistula with esophageal atresia. In this type, the upper section of the esophagus terminates in a blind pouch, and the lower section ascends from the stomach and connects with the trachea by a short fistulous tract.

In type A atresia, both esophageal segments are blind pouches, and neither is connected to the airway. In type E (or H-type)—tracheoesophageal fistula without atresia—the fistula may occur anywhere between the level of the cricoid cartilage and the midesophagus but is usually higher in the trachea than in the esophagus. Such a fistula may be as small as a pinpoint. In types B and D, the upper portion of the esophagus opens into the trachea; infants with this anomaly may experience life-threatening aspiration of saliva or food.

Signs and symptoms

A newborn with type C tracheoesophageal fistula with esophageal atresia appears to swallow normally, but soon after swallowing coughs, struggles, becomes cyanotic, and stops breathing, as he aspirates fluids returning from the blind pouch of the esophagus through his nose and mouth. In such an infant, stomach distention may cause respiratory distress; air and gastric contents (bile and gastric secretions) may reflux through the fistula into the trachea, resulting in chemical pneumonitis.

An infant with type A esophageal atresia appears normal at birth. The infant swallows normally, but as secretions fill the esophageal sac and overflow into the oropharynx, he develops mucus in the oropharynx and drools excessively. When the infant is fed, regurgitation and respiratory distress follow aspiration. Suctioning the mucus and secretions temporarily relieves these symptoms. Excessive secretions and drooling in the newborn strongly suggest esophageal atresia.

Repeated episodes of pneumonitis, pulmonary infection, and abdominal distention may signal type E (or H-type) tracheoesophageal fistula. When a child with this disorder drinks, he coughs, chokes, and becomes cyanotic. Excessive mucus builds up in the oropharynx. Crying forces air from the trachea into

TYPES OF TRACHEOESOPHAGEAL ANOMALIES

Congenital malformations of the esophagus occur in about 1 in 4,000 live births. The American Academy of Pediatrics classification of the anatomic variations of tracheoesophageal anomalies is:

- **Type A** (7.7%): esophageal atresia without fistula
- **Type B** (0.8%): esophageal atresia with tracheoesophageal fistula to the proximal segment
- **Type C** (86.5%): esophageal atresia with fistula to the distal segment
- **Type D** (0.7%): esophageal atresia with fistula to both segments
- **Type E (or H-Type)** (4.2%): tracheoesophageal fistula without atresia

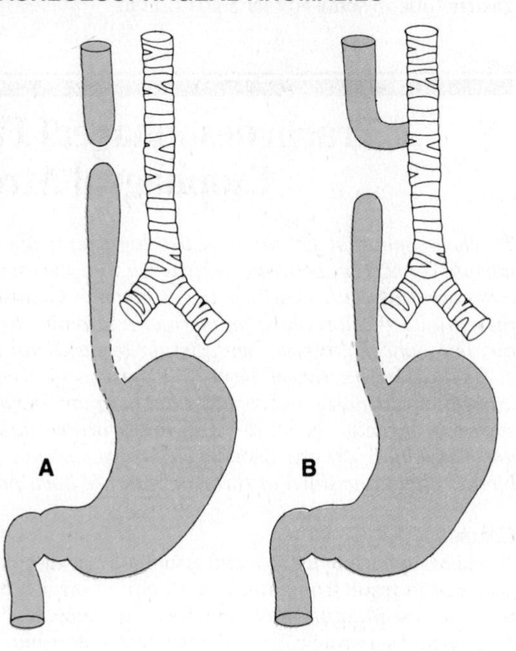

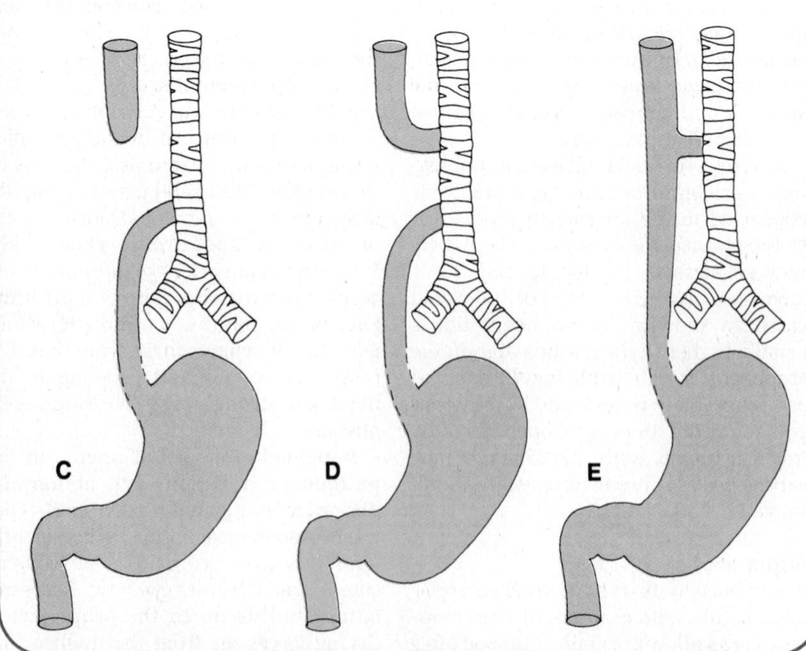

the esophagus, producing abdominal distention. Since such a child may appear normal at birth, this type of tracheoesophageal fistula may be overlooked, and diagnosis may be delayed as long as a year.

Both type B (proximal fistula) and type D (fistula to both segments) cause immediate aspiration of saliva into the airway, and bacterial pneumonitis.

Diagnosis

Respiratory distress and drooling in a newborn suggest tracheoesophageal fistula and esophageal atresia. The following procedures confirm it:

- *A size 10 or 12 French catheter passed through the nose* meets an obstruction (esophageal atresia) approximately 4″ to 5″ (10 to 13 cm) distal from the nostrils. Aspirate of gastric contents is less acidic than normal.
- *Chest X-ray* demonstrates the position of the catheter and can also show a dilated, air-filled upper esophageal pouch; pneumonia in the right upper lobe; or bilateral pneumonitis. Both pneumonia and pneumonitis suggest aspiration.
- *Abdominal X-ray* shows gas in the bowel in a distal fistula (type C) but none in a proximal fistula (type B) or in atresia without fistula (type A).
- *Cinefluorography* allows visualization on a fluoroscopic screen. After a size 10 or 12 French catheter is passed through the patient's nostril into the esophagus, a small amount of contrast medium is instilled to define the tip of the upper pouch and to differentiate between overflow aspiration from a blind end (atresia) and aspiration due to passage of liquids through a tracheoesophageal fistula.

Treatment

Tracheoesophageal fistula and esophageal atresia require surgical correction and are usually surgical emergencies. The type of surgical procedure and when it's performed depend on the nature of the anomaly, the patient's general condition, and the presence of coexisting congenital defects. For example, in a premature infant, a poor surgical risk, correction of combined tracheoesophageal fistula and esophageal atresia is done in two stages: first, gastrostomy (for gastric decompression, prevention of reflux, and feeding) and closure of the fistula; then 1 to 2 months later, anastomosis of the esophagus.

Both before and after surgery, positioning varies with the doctor's philosophy and the child's anatomy; the child may be placed supine, with his head low to facilitate drainage, or with his head elevated to prevent aspiration.

The child should receive I.V. fluids, as necessary, and appropriate antibiotics for superimposed infection.

Postoperative complications after correction of tracheoesophageal fistula include recurrent fistulas, esophageal motility dysfunction, esophageal stricture, recurrent bronchitis, pneumothorax, and failure to thrive. Esophageal motility dysfunction or hiatal hernia may develop after surgical correction of esophageal atresia.

Correction of esophageal atresia alone requires anastomosis of the proximal and distal esophageal segments in one or two stages. End-to-end anastomosis often produces postoperative stricture; end-to-side anastomosis is less likely to do so. If the esophageal ends are widely separated, treatment may include a colonic interposition (grafting a piece of the colon) or elongation of the proximal segment of the esophagus by bougienage. About 10 days after surgery, and again 1 month and 3 months later, X-rays are required to evaluate the effectiveness of surgical repair.

Postoperative treatment includes placement of a suction catheter in the upper esophageal pouch to control secretions and prevent aspiration; maintaining the infant in an upright position to avoid reflux of gastric juices into the trachea; I.V. fluids and nothing by mouth; gastrostomy to prevent reflux and allow feeding; and appropriate antibiotics for pneumonia.

Postoperative complications may include impaired esophageal motility (in one third of patients), hiatal hernia, and reflux esophagitis.

Special considerations

- Monitor respiratory status. Administer oxygen and perform pulmonary physiotherapy and suctioning, as needed. Provide a humid environment.
- Administer antibiotics and parenteral fluids, as ordered. Keep accurate intake and output records.
- If the patient has chest tubes postoperatively, check them frequently for patency. Maintain proper suction, measure and mark drainage periodically, and milk tubing, as necessary.
- Observe carefully for signs of complications, such as abnormal esophageal motility, recurrent fistulas, pneumothorax, and esophageal stricture.
- Maintain gastrostomy tube feedings, as ordered. Such feedings initially consist of dextrose and water (not more than 5% solution); later, add a proprietary formula (first diluted and then full strength). If the infant develops gastric atony, use an isoosmolar formula. Oral feedings can usually resume 8 to 10 days postoperatively. If gastrostomy feedings and oral feedings are impossible due to intolerance to them or decreased intestinal motility, the infant requires total parenteral nutrition.
- Give the infant a pacifier to satisfy his sucking needs but *only* when he can safely handle secretions, since sucking stimulates secretion of saliva.
- Offer the parents support and guidance in dealing with their infant's acute illness. Encourage them to participate in the infant's care and to hold and touch him as much as possible to facilitate bonding.

Corrosive Esophagitis and Stricture

Corrosive esophagitis is inflammation and damage to the esophagus after ingestion of a caustic chemical. Similar to a burn, this injury may be temporary or may lead to permanent stricture (narrowing or stenosis) of the esophagus that is correctable only through surgery. Severe injury can quickly lead to esophageal perforation, mediastinitis, and death from infection, shock, and massive hemorrhage (due to aortic perforation).

Causes

The most common chemical injury to the esophagus follows the ingestion of lye or other strong alkalies; less often, the ingestion of strong acids. The type and amount of chemical ingested determine the severity and location of the damage. In children, household chemical ingestion is accidental; in adults, it's usually a suicide attempt or gesture. The chemical may damage only the mucosa or submucosa, or may damage all layers of the esophagus.

Esophageal tissue damage occurs in three phases: the acute phase, edema and inflammation; the latent phase, ulceration, exudation, and tissue sloughing; and the chronic phase, diffuse scarring.

Signs and symptoms

Effects vary from none at all to intense pain in the mouth and anterior chest, marked salivation, inability to swallow, and tachypnea. Bloody vomitus containing pieces of esophageal tissue signals severe damage. Signs of esophageal perforation and mediastinitis, especially crepitation, indicate destruction of the entire esophagus. Inability to speak implies laryngeal damage.

The acute phase subsides in 3 to 4 days, enabling the patient to eat again. Fever suggests secondary infection. Symptoms of dysphagia return if stricture develops, usually within weeks; rarely, stricture is delayed and develops several years after the injury.

Diagnosis

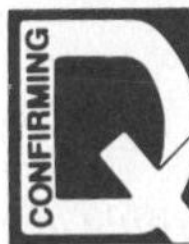

A history of chemical ingestion and physical examination revealing oropharyngeal burns (including white membranes and edema of the soft palate and uvula) usually confirm the diagnosis. The type and amount of the chemical ingested must be identified; this may sometimes be done by examining empty containers of the ingested material or by calling the poison control center.

Two procedures are helpful in evaluating the severity of the injury:

• *Endoscopy* (in the first 24 hours after ingestion) delineates the extent and location of the esophageal injury and assesses depth of the burn. This procedure may also be performed a week after ingestion to assess stricture development.

• *Barium swallow* (1 week after ingestion and every 3 weeks thereafter) may identify segmental spasm or fistula but doesn't always show mucosal injury.

Treatment

Conservative treatment for corrosive esophagitis and stricture includes monitoring the victim's condition; administering corticosteroids, such as prednisone and hydrocortisone, to control inflammation and inhibit fibrosis; and administering a broad-spectrum antibiotic, such as ampicillin, to protect the corticosteroid-immunosuppressed patient against infection by his own mouth flora.

Current treatment includes administering corticosteroids and antibiotics and performing endoscopy early. It may also include bougienage. This procedure involves passing a slender, flexible, cylindrical instrument called a bougie into the esophagus to dilate it and minimize stricture. Some doctors begin bougienage immediately and continue it regularly to maintain a patent lumen and prevent stricture; others delay it for a week to avoid the risk of esophageal perforation.

Surgery is necessary immediately for esophageal perforation or later to correct stricture untreatable with bougienage. Corrective surgery may involve transplanting a piece of the colon to the damaged esophagus. However, even after surgery, stricture may recur at the site of the anastomosis.

Supportive treatment includes I.V. therapy to replace fluids or total parenteral nutrition while the patient can't swallow, gradually progressing to clear liquids and a soft diet.

Special considerations

If you're the first health-care professional to see the person who has ingested a corrosive chemical, the quality of your emergency care will be critical. To meet this challenge, follow these important guidelines:

• *Do not induce vomiting or lavage,* as this will expose the esophagus and oropharynx to injury a second time.

• *Do not perform gastric lavage,* as the corrosive chemical may cause further damage to the mucous membrane of the GI lining.

• Provide vigorous support of vital functions, as needed, such as oxygen, mechanical ventilation, I.V. fluids, and treatment for shock depending on severity of injury.

• Carefully observe and record intake and output.

• Before X-rays and endoscopy, explain the procedure to the patient to lessen anxiety during the tests and to obtain cooperation.

• Since the adult who has ingested a corrosive agent has usually done so with suicidal intent, encourage and assist him and his family to seek psychological counseling.

• Provide emotional support for parents whose child has ingested a chemical. They'll be distraught and may feel guilty about the accident. After the emergency and without emphasizing blame, teach appropriate preventive measures, such as locking accessible cabinets and keeping all corrosive agents out of a child's reach.

Mallory-Weiss Syndrome

The Mallory-Weiss syndrome is mild to massive and usually painless bleeding due to a tear in the mucosa or submucosa of the cardia or lower esophagus. Such a tear, usually singular and longitudinal, results from prolonged or forceful vomiting. Sixty percent of these tears involve the cardia; 15%, the terminal esophagus; and 25%, the region across the esophagogastric junction. Mallory-Weiss syndrome is most common in men over age 40, especially alcoholics.

Causes

The direct cause of a tear in Mallory-Weiss syndrome is forceful or prolonged vomiting, probably when the upper esophageal sphincter fails to relax during vomiting; this lack of sphincter coordination seems more common after excessive intake of alcohol. Other factors and conditions that may also increase intra-abdominal pressure and predispose to esophageal tearing include coughing, straining during bowel movements, trauma, convulsions, childbirth, hiatal hernia, esophagitis, gastritis, and atrophic gastric mucosa.

Signs and symptoms

Typically, Mallory-Weiss syndrome begins with vomiting of blood or passing large amounts of blood rectally a few hours to several days after normal vomiting. This bleeding, which may be accompanied by epigastric or back pain, may range from mild to massive but is generally more profuse than in esophageal rupture. In Mallory-Weiss syndrome, the blood vessels are only partially severed, preventing retraction and closure of the lumen. Massive bleeding—most likely when the tear is on the gastric side, near the cardia—may quickly lead to fatal shock.

Diagnosis

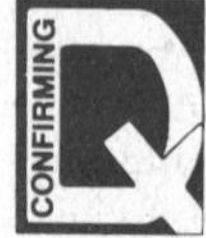

Identifying esophageal tears by fiberoptic endoscopy confirms Mallory-Weiss syndrome. These lesions, which usually occur near the gastroesophageal junction, appear as erythematous longitudinal cracks in the mucosa when recently produced and as raised, white streaks surrounded by erythema in older tears. Other helpful diagnostic measures include the following:
- *Angiography* (selective celiac arteriography) can determine the bleeding site but not the cause; this is used when endoscopy is not available
- *Gastrotomy* may be performed at the time of surgery.
- *Hematocrit* helps quantify blood loss.

Treatment

Treatment varies with the severity of bleeding. Usually, gastrointestinal bleeding stops spontaneously, and requires supportive measures and careful observation but no definitive treatment. However, if bleeding continues, treatment may include:
- angiography, with infusion of a vasoconstrictor (vasopressin) into the superior mesenteric artery or direct infusion into a vessel that leads to the bleeding artery.
- transcatheter embolization or thrombus formation with an autologous blood clot or other hemostatic material (insertion of artificial material, such as shredded absorbable gelatin sponge, or, less often, the patient's own clotted blood through a catheter into the bleeding vessel to aid thrombus formation).
- surgery to suture each laceration (for massive recurrent or uncontrollable bleeding).

Special considerations

- Evaluate respiratory status, monitor arterial blood gas measurements, and administer oxygen, as necessary.

• Assess the amount of blood loss, and record related symptoms, such as hematemesis and melena (including color, amount, consistency, and frequency). Monitor hematologic status (hemoglobin, hematocrit, red blood cells). Draw blood for coagulation studies (prothrombin time, partial thromboplastin time, and platelet count), and type and cross match. Try to keep three units of matched whole blood on hand at all times. Until blood is available, insert a large-bore (14- to 18-gauge) I.V. line, and start a temporary infusion of normal saline solution.
• Monitor vital signs, central venous pressure, urinary output, and overall clinical status.
• Explain diagnostic procedures carefully to facilitate the patient's cooperation and to promote his psychological well-being.
• Keep the patient warm.
• Obtain a history of recent medications taken, dietary habits, and use of alcohol.
• Avoid giving the patient medications that may cause nausea or vomiting. Administer antiemetics, as ordered, to prevent postoperative retching and vomiting.
• Reassure the patient that bleeding will subside.
• Advise the patient to avoid alcohol, aspirin, and other irritating substances.

Esophageal Diverticula

Esophageal diverticula are hollow outpouchings of one or more layers of the esophageal wall. They occur in three main areas: just above the upper esophageal sphincter (Zenker's, or pulsion, diverticulum, the most common type), near the midpoint of the esophagus (traction), and just above the lower esophageal sphincter (epiphrenic). Generally, esophageal diverticula occur later in life—although they can affect infants and children—and are three times more common in men than in women. Epiphrenic diverticula usually occur in middle-aged men; Zenker's, in men over age 60.

Causes

Esophageal diverticula are due either to primary muscular abnormalities that may be congenital or to inflammatory processes adjacent to the esophagus. Zenker's diverticulum occurs when the pouch results from increased intraesophageal pressure; traction diverticulum, when the pouch is pulled out by adjacent inflamed tissue. However, some authorities classify all diverticula as traction diverticula.

Zenker's diverticulum results from developmental muscular weakness of the posterior pharynx above the border of the cricopharyngeal muscle. The pressure of swallowing aggravates this weakness, as does contraction of the pharynx before relaxation of the sphincter. A midesophageal (traction) diverticulum is a response to scarring and pulling on esophageal walls by an external inflammatory process, such as tuberculosis. An epiphrenic diverticulum (rare) is generally right-sided and usually accompanies an esophageal motor disturbance, such as esophageal spasm or achalasia. It's thought to be caused by traction and pulsation.

Signs and symptoms

Both midesophageal and epiphrenic diverticula with an associated motor disturbance (achalasia or spasm) seldom produce symptoms but may cause dysphagia and heartburn. However, Zenker's diverticulum produces distinctly staged symptoms: initially, throat irritation and, later, dysphagia and near-complete obstruction. In early stages, regurgitation occurs soon after eating; in later stages, regurgitation after eating is delayed and may even occur during sleep, leading to food aspiration and pulmonary infection. Other symptoms include noise when liquids are swallowed, chronic cough, hoarseness, a bad taste in the mouth or foul breath, and, rarely, bleeding.

Diagnosis

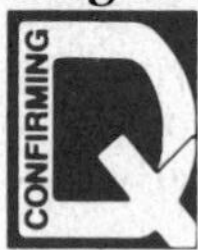

X-rays taken following a barium swallow usually confirm diagnosis by showing characteristic outpouching. Esophagoscopy can rule out another lesion; however, the procedure risks rupturing the diverticulum by passing the scope into it rather than into the lumen of the esophagus, a special danger with Zenker's diverticulum.

Treatment

Treatment of Zenker's diverticulum is usually palliative and includes a bland diet, thorough chewing, and drinking water after eating to flush out the sac. However, severe symptoms or a large diverticulum necessitates surgery to remove the sac or facilitate drainage. An esophagomyotomy may be necessary to prevent recurrence.

A midesophageal diverticulum seldom requires therapy except when esophagitis aggravates the risk of rupture. Then, treatment includes antacids and an antireflux regimen: keeping the head elevated, maintaining an upright position for 2 hours after eating, eating small meals, controlling chronic coughing, and avoiding constrictive clothing.

Epiphrenic diverticulum requires treatment of accompanying motor disorders, such as achalasia, by repeated dilations of the esophagus; of acute spasm by anticholinergic administration and diverticulum excision; and of dysphagia or severe pain by surgical excision or suspending the diverticulum to promote drainage. Depending on the patient's nutritional status, treatment may also include insertion of a nasogastric tube (passed carefully to prevent perforation) and tube feedings to prepare for the stress of surgery.

Special considerations

- Carefully observe and document symptoms.
- Regularly assess nutritional status (weight, caloric intake, appearance).
- If the patient regurgitates food and mucus, protect against aspiration by positioning carefully (head elevated or turned to one side). To prevent aspiration, tell the patient to empty any visible outpouching in the neck by massage or postural drainage before retiring.
- If the patient has dysphagia, record well-tolerated foods and what circumstances ease swallowing. Provide a "blenderized" diet, with vitamin or protein supplements, and encourage thorough chewing.
- Teach the patient about this disorder. Explain treatment instructions and diagnostic procedures.

Hiatal Hernia

(Hiatus hernia)

Hiatal hernia is a defect in the diaphragm that permits a portion of the stomach to pass through the diaphragmatic opening into the chest. Three types of hiatal hernia can occur: sliding hernia, paraesophageal *("rolling")* hernia, *or* mixed hernias, *which include features of both. In a sliding hernia, both the stomach and the gastroesophageal junction slip up into the chest, so the gastroesophageal junction is above the diaphragmatic hiatus. In paraesophageal hernia, a part of the greater curvature of the stomach rolls through the diaphragmatic defect. Treatment can prevent complications, such as strangulation of the herniated intrathoracic portion of the stomach.*

Causes and incidence

A sliding hernia is three to ten times more common than paraesophageal and mixed hernias combined. The incidence of hiatal hernia increases with age, and prevalence is higher in women than in men (especially the paraesophageal type).

Usually, hiatal hernia results from muscle weakening that's common with aging and may be secondary to esophageal carcinoma, kyphoscoliosis, trauma, or certain surgical procedures. It may also result from certain diaphragmatic malformations that may cause congenital weakness.

In hiatal hernia, the muscular collar around the esophageal and diaphragmatic junction loosens, permitting the lower portion of the esophagus and the stomach to rise into the chest when intra-abdominal pressure increases (possibly causing gastroesophageal reflux). Such increased intra-abdominal pressure may result from ascites, pregnancy, obesity, constrictive clothing, bending, straining, coughing, Valsalva's maneuver, or extreme physical exertion.

Signs and symptoms

Typically, a paraesophageal hernia produces no symptoms; it's usually an incidental finding on barium swallow. Since this type of hernia leaves the closing mechanism of the cardiac sphincter unchanged, it rarely causes acid reflux and reflux esophagitis. Symptoms result from displacement or stretching of the stomach and may include a feeling of fullness in the chest or pain resembling angina pectoris. Even if it produces no symptoms, this type of hernia needs surgical treatment because of the high risk of strangulation.

A sliding hernia without an incompetent sphincter produces no reflux or symptoms and, consequently, doesn't require treatment. When a sliding hernia causes symptoms, they are typical of gastric reflux, resulting from the incompetent lower esophageal sphincter, and may include the following:

- *Pyrosis* (heartburn) occurs from 1 to 4 hours after eating and is aggravated

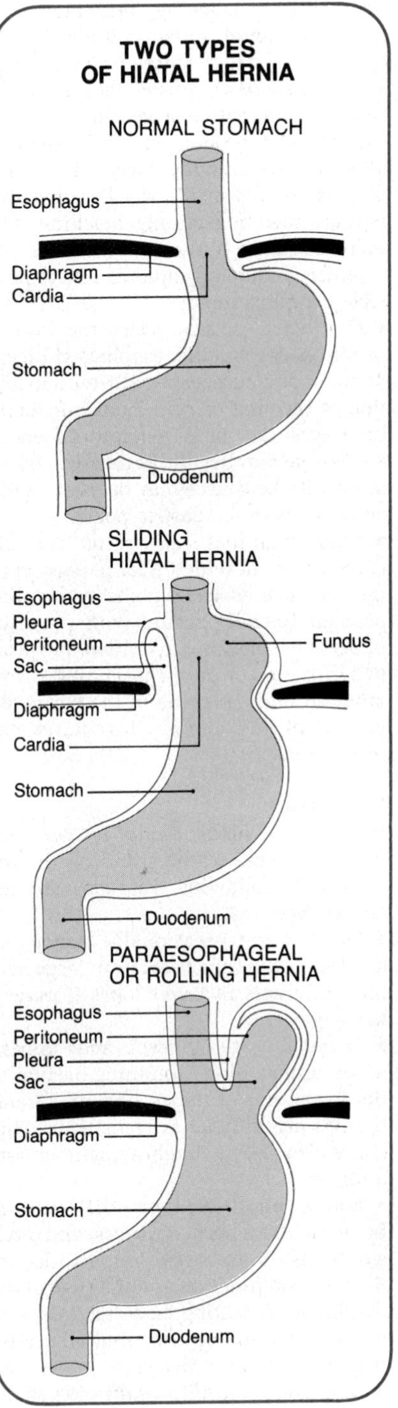

by reclining, belching, and increased intra-abdominal pressure. It may be accompanied by regurgitation or vomiting.
• *Retrosternal or substernal chest pain* results from reflux of gastric contents, distention of the stomach, and spasm or altered motor activity. Chest pain occurs most often after meals or at bedtime and is aggravated by reclining, belching, and increased intra-abdominal pressure.

Other common symptoms reflect possible complications:
• *Dysphagia* occurs when the hernia produces esophagitis, esophageal ulceration, or stricture, especially with ingestion of very hot or cold foods, alcoholic beverages, or a large amount of food.
• *Bleeding* may be mild or massive, frank or occult; the source may be esophagitis or erosions of the gastric pouch.
• *Severe pain and shock* result from incarceration, in which a large portion of the stomach is caught above the diaphragm (usually occurs with paraesophageal hernia). Incarceration may lead to perforation of gastric ulcer, and strangulation and gangrene of the herniated portion of the stomach. It requires immediate surgery.

Diagnosis

Diagnosis of hiatal hernia is based on typical clinical features and on the results of the following laboratory studies and procedures:
• *Chest X-ray* occasionally shows air shadow behind the heart with large hernia; infiltrates in lower lobes if patient has aspirated.
• In *barium study,* hernia may appear as an outpouching containing barium at the lower end of the esophagus. (Small hernias are difficult to recognize.) This study also shows diaphragmatic abnormalities.
• *Endoscopy and biopsy* differentiate between hiatal hernia, varices, and other small gastroesophageal lesions; identify the mucosal junction and the edge of the diaphragm indenting the esophagus; and can rule out malignancy that otherwise may be difficult to detect.
• *Esophageal motility studies* assess the presence of esophageal motor abnormalities before surgical repair of the hernia.
• *pH studies* assess for reflux of gastric contents.
• *Acid perfusion (Bernstein) test* indicates that heartburn results from esophageal reflux when perfusion of HCl through the nasogastric tube provokes this symptom.

Laboratory tests may indicate gastrointestinal bleeding as a complication of hiatal hernia:
• *CBC* may show hypochromic microcytic anemia when bleeding from esophageal ulceration occurs.
• *Stool guaiac test* may be positive.
• *Analysis of gastric contents* may reveal blood.

Treatment

The primary goals of treatment are to relieve symptoms by minimizing or correcting the incompetent cardia and to manage and prevent complications. Medical therapy is used first, because symptoms usually respond to it and because hiatal hernia tends to recur after surgery. Such therapy attempts to modify or reduce reflux by changing the quantity or quality of refluxed gastric contents; by strengthening the lower esophageal sphincter muscle pharmacologically; or by decreasing the amount of reflux through gravity. Such measures include restricting any activity that increases intra-abdominal pressure (coughing, straining, bending), giving antiemetics and cough suppressants, avoiding constrictive clothing, modifying diet, giving stool softeners or laxatives to prevent straining at stool, and discouraging smoking, because it stimulates gastric acid production. Modifying the diet means eating small, frequent, bland meals at least 2 hours before lying down (no bedtime snack); eating slowly; and avoiding spicy foods, fruit juices, alcoholic beverages, and coffee. Antacids also modify the fluid refluxed into the esophagus and are probably the best treatment for intermittent reflux. Intensive antacid therapy may call for hourly administration; however, the choice of antacid should take into consideration the patient's bowel function. Cimetidine also modifies the fluid refluxed into the esophagus.

To reduce the amount of reflux, the overweight patient should lose weight to decrease intraabdominal pressure. Elevating the head of the bed 6″ (15 cm) reduces gastric reflux by gravity.

Drug therapy to strengthen cardiac sphincter tone may include a cholinergic agent, such as bethanechol. Metoclopramide has also been used to stimulate smooth-muscle contraction, increase cardiac sphincter tone, and decrease reflux after eating.

Failure to control symptoms by medical means, or onset of complications, such as stricture, significant bleeding, pulmonary aspiration, strangulation, or incarceration, requires surgical repair. Techniques vary greatly, but most create an artificial closing mechanism at the gastroesophageal junction to strengthen the lower esophageal sphincter's barrier function. The surgeon may use an abdominal or a thoracic approach.

Special considerations

- To enhance compliance with treatment, teach the patient about this disorder. Explain treatment and diagnostic measures, and significant symptoms.
- Prepare the patient for diagnostic tests, as needed. After endoscopy, watch for signs of perforation (falling blood pressure, rapid pulse, shock, sudden pain).
- If surgery is scheduled, reinforce the explanation of the procedure and any preoperative and postoperative considerations. Tell him he probably won't be allowed to eat or drink and will have a nasogastric tube in place, with low suction, for 2 to 3 days postoperatively.
- After surgery, carefully record intake and output, including nasogastric or wound drainage.
- While the nasogastric tube is in place, provide meticulous mouth and nose care. Give ice chips to moisten oral mucous membranes. (Remember to include this ice in your intake and output record.)
- If the surgeon used a thoracic approach, the patient will have chest tubes in place. Carefully observe chest tube drainage and respiratory status, and perform pulmonary physiotherapy.
- Before discharge, tell the patient what foods he can eat (he may require a bland diet), and recommend small, frequent meals. Warn against activities that cause increased intraabdominal pressure, and advise slow return to normal functions. Tell him he'll probably be able to resume regular activity in 6 to 8 weeks.

STOMACH, INTESTINE & PANCREAS

Gastritis

Gastritis, an inflammation of the gastric mucosa, may be acute or chronic. Acute gastritis, the most common stomach disorder, produces mucosal reddening, edema, hemorrhage, and erosion. Gastritis is common in persons with pernicious anemia (as chronic atrophic gastritis). Although gastritis can occur at any age, it is more prevalent in the elderly.

Causes

Acute gastritis usually results from chronic ingestion of irritating foods, such as hot peppers (or an allergic reaction to them); alcoholic beverages; drugs, such as aspirin; or poisons, especially DDT, ammonia, mercury, and carbon tetrachloride. It can be part of hepatic disorders, such as portal hypertension; GI disorders, such as sprue; or infectious diseases, such as viruses, influenza, and typhoid fever. Other causes include Curling's ulcer (after a burn), Cushing's ulcer (from a CNS disorder), and GI injury that may be thermal (ingestion of hot fluids) or mechanical (swallowing a foreign object).

Corrosive gastritis results from the ingestion of strong acids or alkalies. Acute phlegmonous gastritis results from a rare bacterial (usually streptococcal) infection of the stomach wall.

Signs and symptoms

Typical effects of acute gastritis are GI bleeding (most common) and mild epigastric discomfort (postprandial distress). Epigastric discomfort may be the only symptom. Other possible signs: upper abdominal pain, belching, fever, malaise, nausea, vomiting, and hematemesis. Abdominal tenderness is rare.

> **CHRONIC GASTRITIS**
>
> Chronic gastritis results from recurring ingestion of an irritating substance or from pernicious anemia. The main types of chronic gastritis are fundal gland gastritis and chronic antral gastritis (pyloric gland gastritis). Fundal gland gastritis includes:
>
> - superficial gastritis—reddened edematous mucosa, with hemorrhages and small erosions
> - atrophic gastritis—inflammation in all stomach layers, with decreased number of parietal and chief cells
> - gastric atrophy—dull and nodular mucosa, with irregular, thickened, or nodular rugae.
>
> Many patients with chronic gastritis, particularly those with chronic antral gastritis, have no symptoms. When symptoms develop, they are typically indistinct and may include loss of appetite, feeling of fullness, belching, vague epigastric pain, nausea, and vomiting. Diagnosis requires biopsy.
>
> Usually no treatment is necessary, except for avoiding aspirin and spicy or irritating foods, and taking antacids if symptoms persist. If pernicious anemia is the underlying cause, then vitamin B_{12} should be administered. Chronic gastritis often progresses to acute gastritis.

Diagnosis

Patient history suggesting exposure to a GI irritant in a person with epigastric

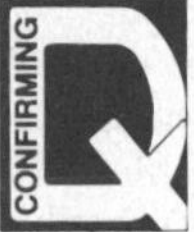

discomfort or other GI symptoms (particularly bleeding) suggest gastritis. A gastroscopy (often with biopsy) confirms it, when done before lesions heal (usually within 24 hours). However, gastroscopy is contraindicated after ingestion of a corrosive agent. X-rays rule out other diseases.

Treatment

Symptoms are usually relieved by eliminating the gastric irritant or other cause. For instance, the treatment for corrosive gastritis is neutralization with the appropriate antidote (emetics are contraindicated). Treatment for gastritis caused by other poisons includes emetics. Anticholinergics, such as methantheline bromide, histamine-antagonists, such as cimetidine, and antacids relieve GI distress. When gastritis causes massive bleeding, treatment includes blood replacement; iced saline lavage, possibly with norepinephrine; angiography, with vasopressin infused in normal saline solution; and surgery. Treatment for bacterial gastritis includes antibiotics, bland diet, and an antiemetic. Treatment for acute phlegmonous gastritis is vigorous antibiotic therapy, followed by surgical repair.

Special considerations

- Give antacids, anticholinergics, histamine-antagonists, and antibiotics, as ordered.
- Explain all diagnostic procedures to the patient.
- If the patient is vomiting, give antiemetics and, as ordered, replace I.V. fluids. Monitor fluid intake and output, and watch electrolyte balance.
- Watch for signs of GI bleeding (hema-

temesis, melena, drop in hematocrit, bloody nasogastric drainage) or hemorrhagic shock (hypotension, tachycardia, or restlessness). In corrosive gastritis, watch for signs of obstruction, perforation, or peritonitis, such as nausea, vomiting, diarrhea, abdominal pain, or fever.

- Urge the patient to seek immediate attention for recurring symptoms (hematemesis, nausea, or vomiting).

To prevent recurrence of gastritis, stress the importance of taking prescribed prophylactic medication exactly as ordered. Advise patients to prevent gastric irritation by taking steroids with milk, food, or antacids; by taking antacids between meals and at bedtime; by avoiding aspirin-containing compounds; and by avoiding spicy foods, hot fluids, alcohol, caffeine, and tobacco.

Gastroenteritis

(Intestinal flu, traveler's diarrhea, viral enteritis, food poisoning)

A self-limiting disorder, gastroenteritis is characterized by diarrhea, nausea, vomiting, and abdominal cramping. It occurs in persons of all ages and is a major cause of morbidity and mortality in underdeveloped nations. In the United States, gastroenteritis ranks second to the common cold as a cause of lost work time, and fifth as the cause of death among young children. It also can be life-threatening in the elderly and the debilitated.

Causes

Gastroenteritis has many possible causes:

- bacteria (responsible for acute food poisoning): *Staphylococcus aureus, Salmonella, Shigella, Clostridium botulinum, Escherichia coli, Clostridium perfringens*
- amebae: especially *Entamoeba histolytica*
- parasites: *Ascaris, Enterobius,* and *Trichinella spiralis*
- viruses (may be responsible for traveler's diarrhea): adeno-, echo-, or coxsackieviruses
- ingestion of toxins: plants or toadstools
- drug reactions: antibiotics
- enzyme deficiencies
- food allergens.

The bowel reacts to any of these enterotoxins with hypermotility, producing severe diarrhea and secondary depletion of intracellular fluid.

Signs and symptoms

Clinical manifestations vary depending on the pathologic organism and on the level of GI tract involved. However, gastroenteritis in adults is usually a self-limiting, nonfatal disease producing diarrhea, abdominal discomfort (ranging from cramping to pain), nausea, and vomiting. Other possible symptoms include fever, malaise, and borborygmi. In children, the elderly, and the debilitated, gastroenteritis produces the same symptoms, but these patients' intolerance to electrolyte and fluid losses leads to a higher mortality.

Diagnosis

Patient history can aid diagnosis of gastroenteritis. Stool culture (by direct rectal swab) or blood culture identifies causative bacteria or parasites.

Treatment

Treatment is usually supportive and consists of bed rest, nutritional support, and increased fluid intake. When gastroenteritis is severe or affects a young child or an elderly or debilitated person, treatment may necessitate hospitalization; specific antimicrobials; I.V. fluid and electrolyte replacement; bismuth-containing compounds, such as Pepto-Bismol; and antiemetics (P.O., I.M., or rectal suppository), such as prochlorperazine or trimethobenzamide.

Special considerations

Administer medications, as ordered; correlate dosages, routes, and times appropriately with the patient's meals and activities (for example, give antiemetics 30 to 60 minutes before meals).

- If the patient can eat, replace lost fluids and electrolytes with broth, ginger ale, and lemonade, as tolerated. Vary the diet to make it more enjoyable, and allow some choice of foods. Warn the patient to avoid milk and milk products, which may provoke recurrence.
- Record intake and output carefully. Watch for signs of dehydration, such as dry skin and mucous membranes, fever, and sunken eyes.
- Wash hands thoroughly after giving care to avoid spreading infection.
- To ease anal irritation, provide warm sitz baths or apply witch hazel compresses.
- If food poisoning is probable, contact public health authorities so they can interview patients and food handlers, and take samples of the suspected contaminated food.
- Teach good hygiene to prevent recurrence. Instruct patients to thoroughly cook foods, especially pork; refrigerate perishable foods, such as milk, mayonnaise, potato salad, and cream-filled pastry; always wash hands with warm water and soap before handling food, especially after using the bathroom; to clean utensils thoroughly; avoid drinking water or eating raw fruit or vegetables when visiting a foreign country; eliminate flies and roaches in the home.

Peptic Ulcers

Peptic ulcers—circumscribed lesions in the gastric mucosal membrane—can develop in the lower esophagus, stomach, pylorus, duodenum, or jejunum from contact with gastric juice (especially hydrochloric acid and pepsin). About 80% of all peptic ulcers are duodenal ulcers, which affect the proximal part of the small intestine and occur most often in men between ages 20 and 50. Gastric ulcers, which affect the stomach mucosa, are most common in both middle-aged and elderly men, especially among the poor and undernourished, and in chronic users of aspirin or alcohol. Benign gastric ulcers tend to recur. Duodenal ulcers often follow a chronic course, with remissions and exacerbations; 5% to 10% of patients develop complications that necessitate surgery.

Causes

Decreased mucosal resistance, inadequate mucosal blood flow, and defective mucus have all been associated with the development of peptic ulcers, but a precise cause has not been determined. Psychogenic factors may stimulate long-term overproduction of gastric secretions that can erode the stomach, duodenum, or esophagus. Normally, tightly packed epithelial cells protect the stomach against irritation. Back diffusion of acid through mucosa damaged by chronic gastritis or irritants, such as aspirin or alcohol, is a likely cause of gastric ulcers. In the elderly, the pylorus begins to wear down, permitting the reflux of bile into the stomach, a common cause of gastric ulcers in this age-group. For unknown reasons, these ulcers often strike people with type A blood and may become malignant more often than duodenal ulcers.

Acid hypersecretion, possibly caused by an overactive vagus nerve, contributes to the formation of duodenal ulcers. These ulcers tend to afflict people with type O blood, perhaps because such people don't secrete blood group antigens (mucopolysaccharides, which may serve to protect the mucosa) in their saliva and other body fluids. Duodenal ulcers may persist for life; when they do heal, they usually leave scars that can later break down and ulcerate again under hyperacidic conditions.

Signs and symptoms

Heartburn and indigestion usually signal the start of a gastric ulcer attack. Eating a large meal stretches the gastric wall, causing pain in the left epigastrium and a feeling of fullness and distention. Other typical effects include weight loss and repeated episodes of massive GI bleeding.

Duodenal ulcers produce heartburn, well-localized midepigastric pain (relieved by food), weight gain (since the patient eats to relieve discomfort), and a peculiar sensation of hot water bubbling in the back of the throat. Attacks usually occur about 2 hours after meals, whenever the stomach is empty, or after consumption of orange juice, coffee, aspirin, or alcohol. Exacerbations tend to recur several times a year, then fade into remission. Vomiting and other digestive disturbances are rare.

Both kinds of ulcers may be asymptomatic or may penetrate the pancreas and cause severe back pain. Other complications of peptic ulcers include perforation, hemorrhage, and pyloric obstruction.

Diagnosis

Upper GI tract X-rays show abnormalities in mucosa; gastric secretory studies show hyperchlorhydria.

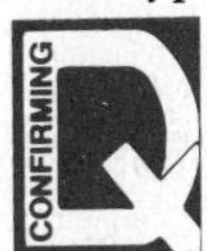

The presence of an ulcer is confirmed by upper GI endoscopy or esophagogastroduodenoscopy. Biopsy rules out malignancy. Stools may test positive for occult blood.

Treatment

Treatment is essentially symptomatic and emphasizes drug therapy and rest:

- antacids to reduce gastric acidity.
- cimetidine or ranitidine, histamine-receptor antagonists, to reduce gastric secretion; for short-term therapy (up to 8 weeks).
- anticholinergics, such as propantheline, to inhibit the vagus nerve effect on the parietal cells and to reduce gastrin production and excessive gastric activity in *duodenal ulcers;* these drugs are usually contraindicated in gastric ulcers, since they prolong gastric emptying and can aggravate the ulcer.
- physical rest and, for gastric ulcers only, sedatives and tranquilizers, such as chlordiazepoxide and phenobarbital.

If GI bleeding occurs, emergency treatment begins with passage of a nasogastric tube to allow for iced saline lavage, possibly containing norepinephrine. Angiography facilitates placement of an intraarterial catheter, followed by infusion of vasopressin to constrict blood vessels and control bleeding. This type of therapy allows postponement of surgery until the patient's condition stabilizes. Surgery is indicated for perforation, unresponsiveness to conservative treatment, and suspected malignancy. Surgical procedures for peptic ulcers include:

- *vagotomy and pyloroplasty:* severing one or more branches of the vagus nerve to reduce hydrochloric acid secretion and refashioning the pylorus to create a larger lumen and facilitate gastric emptying
- *distal subtotal gastrectomy* (with or without vagotomy): excising the antrum of the stomach, thereby removing the hormonal stimulus of the parietal cells, followed by anastomosis of the rest of the stomach to the duodenum or the jejunum.

Special considerations

Management of peptic ulcers requires careful administration of medications, thorough patient teaching, and skillful postoperative care.

- Administer medications, as ordered, and watch for cimetidine and anticholinergic side effects: dizziness, rash, mild diarrhea, muscle pain, leukopenia, and gynecomastia; and dry mouth, blurred vision, headache, constipation, and urinary retention, respectively. Anticholinergics are usually most effective when given 30 minutes before meals. Give sedatives and tranquilizers, as needed.

• Instruct the patient to take antacids 1 hour after meals. Advise the patient with a history of cardiac disease or on a sodium-restricted diet to take only low-sodium antacids. Warn that antacids may cause changes in bowel habits (diarrhea with magnesium-containing antacids, constipation with aluminum-containing antacids).

• Warn the patient to avoid aspirin-containing drugs, reserpine, indomethacin, and phenylbutazone, because they irritate the gastric mucosa. For the same reason, warn against excessive use of coffee, stressful situations, and alcoholic beverages during exacerbations (although alcohol may be consumed in moderation during remission). Advise the patient to stop smoking, because it stimulates gastric secretion.

After gastric surgery:

• Keep nasogastric tube patent. If the tube isn't functioning, don't reposition it; you may damage the suture line or anastomosis. Notify the surgeon promptly.

• Monitor intake and output, including nasogastric tube drainage. Check bowel sounds, and allow the patient nothing by mouth until peristalsis resumes and the nasogastric tube is removed or clamped.

• Replace fluids and electrolytes. Assess for signs of dehydration, sodium deficiency, and metabolic alkalosis, which may occur secondary to gastric suction.

• Control postoperative pain with narcotics and analgesics, as ordered.

• Watch for complications: hemorrhage; shock; iron, folate, or vitamin B_{12} deficiency anemia (from malabsorption or continued blood loss); and dumping syndrome (weakness, nausea, flatulence, diarrhea, distention, and palpitations within 30 minutes after a meal).

• To avoid dumping syndrome, advise the patient to lie down after meals; to drink fluids *between* meals rather than with meals; to avoid eating large amounts of carbohydrates; and to eat four to six small, high-protein, low-carbohydrate meals during the day.

Ulcerative Colitis

Ulcerative colitis is an inflammatory, often chronic disease that affects the mucosa and submucosa of the colon. It usually begins in the rectum and sigmoid colon, and often extends upward into the entire colon; it rarely affects the small intestine, except for the terminal ileum. Ulcerative colitis produces congestion, edema (leading to mucosal friability), and ulcerations that eventually develop into abscesses. Severity ranges from a mild, localized disorder to a fulminant disease that may cause a perforated colon, progressing to potentially fatal peritonitis and toxemia.

Causes and incidence

Ulcerative colitis occurs primarily in young adults, especially women; it is also more prevalent among Jews and in higher socioeconomic groups. Overall, incidence is rising.

Although the etiology of ulcerative colitis is unknown, possible predisposing factors include:

• family history of the disease
• bacterial infection
• allergic reaction to food, milk, or other substances that release inflammatory histamine in the bowel
• overproduction of enzymes that break down the mucous membranes
• emotional stress
• autoimmune reactions, such as arthritis, hemolytic anemia, erythema nodosum, and uveitis.

Signs and symptoms

The hallmark of ulcerative colitis is recurrent bloody diarrhea, often containing pus and mucus, interspersed with asymptomatic remissions. The intensity of these attacks varies with the extent of inflammation. Other symptoms include spastic rectum and anus, abdominal pain, irritability, weight loss, weakness, anorexia, nausea, and vomiting.

Ulcerative colitis may lead to complications affecting many body systems.

- *Blood:* anemia from iron deficiency, coagulation defects due to vitamin K deficiency
- *Skin:* erythema nodosum on the face and arms; pyoderma gangrenosum on the legs and ankles
- *Eye:* uveitis
- *Liver:* pericholangitis, sclerosing cholangitis, cirrhosis, possible cholangiocarcinoma
- *Musculoskeletal:* arthritis, ankylosing spondylitis, loss of muscle mass
- *Gastrointestinal:* strictures, pseudopolyps, stenosis, and perforated colon, leading to peritonitis and toxemia.

Patients with ulcerative colitis run a greater-than-normal risk of developing colorectal cancer, especially if onset of the disease occurs before age 15 or if it has persisted for longer than 10 years.

Diagnosis

Sigmoidoscopy showing increased mucosal friability, decreased mucosal detail, and thick inflammatory exudate suggests this diagnosis. Biopsy can help confirm it. Colonoscopy may be required to determine the extent of the disease and also to evaluate strictured areas and pseudopolyps. (Biopsy would then be done during colonoscopy.) Barium enema can assess the extent of the disease and detect complications, such as strictures and carcinoma.

Stool specimen should be cultured and analyzed for leukocytes, ova and parasites. Other supportive laboratory values include decreased serum levels of potassium, magnesium, hemoglobin, and albumin, as well as leukocytosis and increased prothrombin time. Elevated erythrocyte sedimentation rate correlates with the severity of the attack.

Treatment

The goals of treatment are to control inflammation, replace nutritional losses and blood volume, and prevent complications. Supportive treatment includes bed rest, I.V. fluid replacement, and a clear-liquid diet. For patients awaiting surgery or showing signs of dehydration and debilitation from excessive diarrhea, I.V. hyperalimentation rests the intestinal tract, decreases stool volume, and restores positive nitrogen balance. Blood transfusions or iron supplements may be needed to correct anemia.

Drug therapy to control inflammation includes adrenocorticotropic hormone and adrenal corticosteroids, such as prednisone, prednisolone, and hydrocortisone; sulfasalazine, which has anti-inflammatory and antimicrobial properties, may also be used. Antispasmodics, such as tincture of belladonna, and antidiarrheals, such as diphenoxylate compound, are used only for patients with frequent, troublesome diarrheal stools whose ulcerative colitis is under control. These drugs may precipitate massive dilation of the colon (toxic megacolon) and are generally contraindicated.

Surgery is the treatment of last resort if the patient has toxic megacolon, fails to respond to drugs and supportive measures, or finds symptoms unbearable. The most common surgical technique is proctocolectomy with ileostomy. Total colectomy and ileorectal anastomosis is done less often because of its mortality (2% to 5%). This procedure removes the entire colon and anastomoses the rectum and the terminal ileum; it requires observation of the remaining rectal stump for any signs of malignancy or colitis.

Pouch ileostomy, in which a pouch is created from a small loop of the terminal ileum and a nipple valve formed from the distal ileum, is gaining popularity in some areas. The resulting stoma opens just above the pubic hairline; the pouch empties through a catheter inserted in the stoma several times a day. In ulcerative colitis, colectomy to prevent colon cancer is controversial.

Special considerations

- Accurately record intake and output, particularly the frequency and volume of stools. Watch for signs of dehydration (poor skin turgor, furrowed tongue) and electrolyte imbalances, especially signs of hypokalemia (muscle weakness, paresthesia) and hypernatremia (tachycardia, flushed skin, fever, dry tongue). Monitor hemoglobin and hematocrit, and give blood transfusions, as ordered. Provide good mouth care for the patient who is allowed nothing by mouth.
- After each bowel movement, thoroughly clean the skin around the rectum. Provide an air mattress or sheepskin to help prevent skin breakdown.
- Administer medication, as ordered. Watch for side effects of prolonged corticosteroid therapy (moonface, hirsutism, edema, gastric irritation). Be aware that such therapy may mask infection.
- If the patient needs hyperalimentation, change dressings, as ordered, assess for inflammation at the insertion site, and check urine every 6 hours for sugar and acetone.
- Take precautionary measures if the patient is prone to bleeding. Watch closely for signs of complications, such as a perforated colon and peritonitis (fever, severe abdominal pain, abdominal rigidity and tenderness, cool clammy skin), and toxic megacolon (abdominal distention, decreased bowel sounds).

Carefully prepare the patient for surgery, especially by informing him about ileostomy.

- Explain what a stoma is, what it looks like, and how it differs from normal anatomy. Provide information (available from the United Ostomy Association), and arrange for the patient to be visited by an enterostomal therapist and a recovered ileostomate, if possible.
- Encourage the patient to verbalize his feelings. Provide emotional support and a quiet environment.
- Do a bowel preparation, as ordered. This usually involves keeping the patient on a clear-liquid diet, using cleansing enemas, and administering antimicrobials, such as neomycin.

After surgery, give meticulous supportive care and continue teaching correct stoma care.

- Keep the nasogastric tube patent. After removal of the tube, provide a clear-liquid diet, and gradually advance to a low-residue diet, as tolerated.
- After a proctocolectomy and ileostomy, teach good stoma care. Wash the skin around the stoma with soapy water and dry thoroughly. Apply karaya gum around the stoma's base to avoid irritation and make a watertight seal. Attach the pouch over the karaya ring. Cut an opening in the ring to fit over the stoma, and secure the pouch to the skin. Empty the pouch when it's one-third full. Encourage the patient to take over this care.
- After a pouch ileostomy, uncork the catheter every hour to allow contents to drain. After 10 to 14 days, gradually increase the length of time the catheter is left corked until it can be opened every 3 hours. Then, remove the catheter and reinsert it every 3 to 4 hours for drainage. Teach the patient how to insert the catheter and how to take care of the stoma.
- Encourage the patient to have regular physical examinations, since he risks developing colorectal cancer.

Necrotizing Enterocolitis

Necrotizing enterocolitis (NEC) is characterized by diffuse or patchy intestinal necrosis, accompanied by sepsis in about one third of cases. Sepsis usually involves Escherichia coli, Clostridia, Salmonella, Pseudomonas, *or* Klebsiella. *Initially, ne-*

crosis is localized, occurring anywhere along the intestine, but most often it is right-sided (in the ileum, ascending colon, or rectosigmoid). With early detection, the survival rate is 60% to 80%. If diffuse bleeding occurs, NEC usually results in disseminated intravascular coagulation (DIC).

Causes and incidence

NEC occurs most often among premature infants (less than 34 weeks gestation) and those of low birth weight (less than 5 lb [2.26 kg]). NEC is occurring more frequently in some areas, possibly due to the higher incidence and survival of premature infants and to newborns who have low birth weights. One in ten infants who develops NEC is full-term. Among premature and low-birth-weight infants in intensive care nurseries, incidence varies from 1% to 12%. NEC is related to 2% of all infant deaths.

The exact cause of NEC is unknown. Suggested predisposing factors include birth asphyxia, postnatal hypotension, respiratory distress, hypothermia, umbilical vessel catheterization, or patent ductus arteriosus. NEC may also be a response to significant prenatal stress, such as premature rupture of membranes, placenta previa, maternal sepsis, toxemia of pregnancy, or breech or cesarean birth.

According to current theory, NEC develops when the infant suffers perinatal hypoxemia due to shunting of blood from the gut to more vital organs. Subsequent mucosal ischemia provides an ideal medium for bacterial growth. Hypertonic formula may increase bacterial activity because—unlike maternal breast milk—it doesn't provide protective immunologic activity and because it contributes to the production of hydrogen gas. As the bowel swells and breaks down, gas-forming bacteria invade damaged areas, producing free air in the intestinal wall. This may result in fatal perforation and peritonitis.

Signs and symptoms

Any infant who has suffered from perinatal hypoxemia has the potential for developing NEC. A distended (especially tense or rigid) abdomen, with gastric retention, is the earliest and most common sign of oncoming NEC, usually appearing from 1 to 10 days after birth. Other clinical features are increasing residual gastric contents (which may contain bile), bile-stained vomitus, and occult blood in the stool. One fourth of patients have bloody diarrhea. A red or shiny, taut abdomen may indicate peritonitis.

Nonspecific signs and symptoms include thermal instability, lethargy, metabolic acidosis, jaundice, and DIC. The major complication is perforation, which requires surgery. Recurrence of NEC and mechanical and functional abnormalities of the intestine, especially stricture, are the usual cause of residual intestinal malfunction in any infant who survives acute NEC and may develop as late as 3 months postoperatively.

Diagnosis

Successful treatment of NEC relies on early recognition. Anteroposterior and

lateral abdominal X-rays confirm the diagnosis. These X-rays show nonspecific intestinal dilation and, in later stages of NEC, pneumatosis cystoides intestinalis (gas or air in the intestinal wall).

Blood studies show several abnormalities. Platelet count may fall below 50,000/mm³. Serum sodium levels are decreased, and arterial blood gases show metabolic acidosis (a result of sepsis). Infection-induced red blood cell breakdown elevates bilirubin levels. Blood and stool cultures identify the infecting organism; clotting studies and hemoglobin levels, associated DIC; guaiac test detects occult blood in the stool.

Treatment

The first signs of NEC necessitate removal of the umbilical catheter (arterial or venous) and discontinuation of oral intake for 7 to 10 days to rest the injured bowel. I.V. fluids, including hyperalimentation, maintain fluid and electrolyte balance and nutrition during this time; passage of a nasogastric (NG) tube aids bowel decompression. If coagulation studies indicate a need for transfusion, the infant usually receives dextran to promote hemodilution, increase mesenteric blood flow, and reduce platelet aggregation. Antibiotic therapy consists of parenteral administration of an aminoglycoside or ampicillin to suppress bacterial flora and prevent bowel perforation. (These drugs can also be administered through an NG tube, if necessary.) Anteroposterior and lateral X-rays every 4 to 6 hours monitor disease progression.

Surgery is indicated if the patient shows any of the following symptoms: signs of perforation (free intraperitoneal air on X-ray or symptoms of peritonitis), respiratory insufficiency (caused by severe abdominal distention), progressive and intractable acidosis, or DIC. Surgery removes all necrotic and acutely inflamed bowel and creates a temporary colostomy or ileostomy. Such surgery must leave at least 12" (30.48 cm) of bowel, or the infant may suffer from malabsorption or chronic vitamin B_{12} deficiency.

Special considerations

- Be alert for signs of gastric distention and perforation: apnea, cardiovascular shock, sudden drop in temperature, bradycardia, sudden listlessness, rag-doll limpness, increasing abdominal tenderness, edema, erythema, or involuntary rigidity of the abdomen. Take axillary temperatures to avoid perforating the bowel.
- Prevent cross-contamination by disposing of soiled diapers properly and washing hands with povidone-iodine after diaper changes.
- Try to prepare parents for potential deterioration in their infant's condition. Be honest and explain all treatments, including why feedings are withheld.
- After surgery, the infant needs mechanical ventilation. Gently suction secretions, and assess respiration often.
- Replace fluids (lost through NG tube and stoma drainage). Include drainage losses in output records. Weigh the infant daily. Daily weight gain of 0.35 to 0.7 oz (9.9 to 19.8 g) indicates a good response to therapy.

An infant with a temporary colostomy or ileostomy needs special care. Explain to the parents what a colostomy or ileostomy is and why it's necessary. Encourage them to participate in their infant's physical care after his condition is no longer critical.

- Because of the infant's small abdomen, the suture line is near the stoma; therefore, keeping the suture line clean can be a problem. Good skin care is essential, since the immature infant's skin is fragile and vulnerable to excoriation and the active enzymes in bowel secretions are corrosive. Improvise premature-sized colostomy bags from urine collection bags, medicine cups, or condoms. Karaya gum is helpful in making a seal. Watch for wound disruption, infection, and excoriation—potential dangers because of severe catabolism.
- Watch for intestinal malfunction from stricture or short-gut syndrome. Such complications usually develop 1 month after the infant resumes normal feedings.
- You may develop surrogate attachment to infants who require intensive care, but avoid unconscious exclusion of the parents. Encourage parental visits.

To help prevent NEC, encourage mothers to breast-feed, since breast milk contains live macrophages that fight infection and has a low pH that inhibits the growth of many organisms. Also, colostrum—fluid secreted before the milk—contains high concentrations of IgA, which directly protects the gut from infection and which the newborn lacks for several days postpartum. Tell mothers that they may refrigerate their milk for 48 hours but shouldn't freeze or heat it, since this destroys antibodies. Tell them to use plastic—not glass—containers, because leukocytes adhere to glass.

Crohn's Disease

(Regional enteritis, granulomatous colitis)

Crohn's disease is an inflammation of any part of the GI tract (usually the terminal ileum), which extends through all layers of the intestinal wall. It may also involve regional lymph nodes and the mesentery. Crohn's disease is most prevalent in adults aged 20 to 40. It is two to three times more common in Jews and least common in blacks.

Causes

Although the exact cause of Crohn's disease is unknown, possible causes include allergies and other immune disorders, lymphatic obstruction, and infection. However, no infecting organism has been isolated. Several factors also implicate a genetic cause: Crohn's disease sometimes occurs in monozygotic twins, and up to 5% of patients with Crohn's disease have one or more affected relatives. However, no simple pattern of Mendelian inheritance has been identified.

Whatever the cause of Crohn's disease, lacteal blockage in the intestinal wall leads to edema and, eventually, to inflammation, ulceration, stenosis, and abscess and fistula formation.

Signs and symptoms

Clinical effects vary according to the location and extent of the lesion, and at first may be mild and nonspecific. However, acute inflammatory signs and symptoms mimic appendicitis and include right lower quadrant pain, cramping, tenderness, flatulence, nausea, fever, and diarrhea. Bleeding may occur and, although usually mild, may be massive. Bloody stools may also occur.

Chronic symptoms, which are more typical of the disease, are more persistent and less severe; they include diarrhea (four to six stools a day) with right lower quadrant pain, steatorrhea, marked weight loss, and, rarely, clubbing of fingers. The patient may complain of weakness, lack of ambition, and inability to cope with everyday stress. Complications include intestinal obstruction, fistula formation between the small bowel and the bladder, perianal and perirectal abscesses and fistulas, intraabdominal abscesses, and perforation.

Diagnosis

Laboratory findings often indicate increased white blood cell count and erythrocyte sedimentation rate, hypokalemia, hypocalcemia, hypomagnesemia, and decreased hemoglobin. Barium enema showing the string sign (segments of stricture separated by normal bowel) supports this diagnosis. Sigmoidoscopy and colonoscopy may show patchy areas of inflammation, thus helping to rule out ulcerative colitis. However, definitive diagnosis is possible only after biopsy.

Treatment

Treatment is symptomatic. In debilitated patients, therapy includes intravenous hyperalimentation to maintain nutrition while resting the bowel. Drug therapy may include anti-inflammatory corticosteroids, immunosuppressive agents, such as azathioprine, and antibacterial agents, such as sulfasalazine. Metronidazole has proved to be effective in some patients. Opium tincture and diphenoxylate may help combat diarrhea but are contraindicated in patients with significant intestinal obstruction. Effective treatment requires important changes in life-style: physical rest, restricted fiber diet (no fruit or vegetables), and elimination of dairy products for lactose intolerance.

Surgery may be necessary to correct

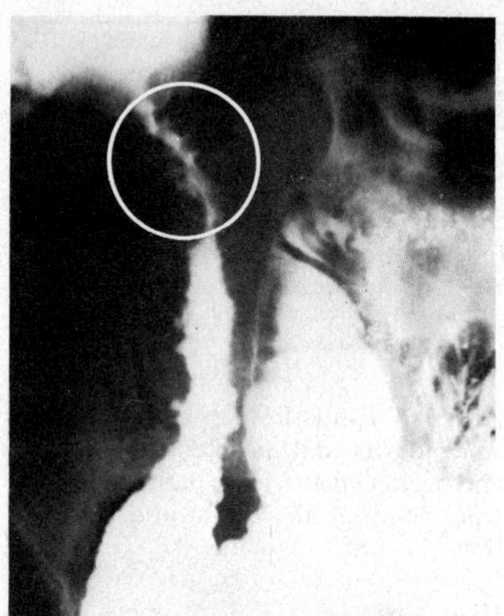

In Crohn's disease, the characteristic "string sign" (marked narrowing of the bowel), from inflammatory disease and scarring, strengthens the diagnosis.

bowel perforation, massive hemorrhage, fistulas, or acute intestinal obstruction. Colectomy with ileostomy is often necessary in patients with extensive disease of the large intestine and rectum.

Special considerations

- Record fluid intake and output (including the amount of stool), and weigh the patient daily. Watch for dehydration and maintain fluid and electrolyte balance. Be alert for signs of intestinal bleeding (bloody stools); check stools daily for occult blood.
- If the patient is receiving steroids, watch for side effects, such as GI bleeding. Remember that steroids can mask signs of infection.
- Check hemoglobin and hematocrit regularly. Give iron supplements and blood transfusions, as ordered.
- Give analgesics, as ordered.
- Provide good patient hygiene and meticulous mouth care if the patient is restricted to nothing by mouth. After each bowel movement, give good skin care. Always keep a clean, covered bedpan within the patient's reach. Ventilate the room to eliminate odors.
- Watch for fever and pain on urination, which may signal bladder fistula. Abdominal pain, fever, and hard, distended abdomen may indicate intestinal obstruction.
- Before ileostomy, arrange for a visit by an enterostomal therapist.
- After surgery, frequently check the patient's I.V. and nasogastric tube for proper functioning. Monitor vital signs, and fluid intake and output. Watch for wound infection. Provide meticulous stoma care, and teach it to the patient and family. Realize that ileostomy changes the patient's body image, so offer reassurance and emotional support.
- Stress the need for a severely restricted diet and bed rest, which may be trying, particularly for the young patient. Encourage him to try to reduce tension. If stress is clearly an aggravating factor, refer him for counseling.

Pseudomembranous Enterocolitis

Pseudomembranous enterocolitis is an acute inflammation and necrosis of the small and large intestines, which usually affects the mucosa but may extend into submucosa and, rarely, other layers. Marked by severe diarrhea, this rare condition is generally fatal in 1 to 7 days from severe dehydration and from toxicity, peritonitis, or perforation.

Causes

The exact cause of pseudomembranous enterocolitis is unknown; however, *Clostridium difficile* is thought to produce a toxin that may play a role in its development. Pseudomembranous enterocolitis has occurred postoperatively in debilitated patients who undergo abdominal surgery or patients who have been treated with broad-spectrum antibiotics. Whatever the cause, necrosed mucosa is replaced by a pseudomembrane filled with staphylococci, leukocytes, mucus, fibrin, and inflammatory cells.

Signs and symptoms
Pseudomembranous enterocolitis begins suddenly with copious watery or bloody diarrhea, abdominal pain, and fever. Serious complications may be associated with this disorder. They include such things as severe dehydration, electrolyte imbalance, hypotension, shock, and colonic perforation.

Diagnosis
Diagnosis is often difficult because of the abrupt onset of enterocolitis and the emergency situation it creates, so consideration of patient history is essential. A rectal biopsy through sigmoidoscopy confirms pseudomembranous enterocolitis. Stool cultures can identify *C. difficile.*

Treatment
A patient who is receiving broad-spectrum antibiotic therapy requires immediate discontinuation of the antibiotics. Effective treatment includes antibiotics such as vancomycin, metronidazole, or bacitracin. A patient with mild pseudomembranous enterocolitis may receive anion exchange resins, such as cholestyramine, to bind the toxin produced by *C. difficile.* Supportive treatment must maintain fluid and electrolyte balance and combat hypotension and shock with pressors, such as dopamine and levarterenol.

Special considerations
- Monitor vital signs, skin color, and level of consciousness. Immediately report signs of shock.
- Record fluid intake and output, including fluid lost in stools. Watch for dehydration (poor skin turgor, sunken eyes, and decreased urine output).
- Check serum electrolytes daily, and watch for clinical signs of hypokalemia, especially malaise, and weak, rapid, irregular pulse.

Irritable Bowel Syndrome

(Spastic colon, spastic colitis)

Irritable bowel syndrome is a common condition marked by chronic or periodic diarrhea, alternating with constipation, and accompanied by straining and abdominal cramps. Prognosis is good. Supportive treatment or avoidance of a known irritant often relieves symptoms.

Causes
This functional disorder is generally associated with psychological stress; however, it may result from physical factors, such as diverticular disease, ingestion of irritants (coffee, raw fruits or vegetables), lactose intolerance, abuse of laxatives, food poisoning, or colon cancer.

Signs and symptoms
Irritable bowel syndrome characteristically produces lower abdominal pain (usually relieved by defecation or passage of gas) and diarrhea that typically occurs during the day. These symptoms alternate with constipation or normal bowel function. Stools are often small and contain visible mucus. Dyspepsia and abdominal distention may occur.

Diagnosis
Diagnosis of irritable bowel syndrome requires a careful history to determine contributing psychological factors, such

as a recent stressful life change. Diagnosis must also rule out other disorders, such as amebiasis, diverticulitis, colon cancer, and lactose intolerance. Appropriate diagnostic procedures include sigmoidoscopy, colonoscopy, barium enema, rectal biopsy, and stool examination for blood, parasites, and bacteria.

Treatment

Therapy aims to relieve symptoms and includes counseling to help the patient understand the relationship between stress and his illness. Strict dietary restrictions aren't beneficial, but food irritants should be investigated and the patient instructed to avoid them. Rest and heat applied to the abdomen are helpful, as is judicious use of sedatives (phenobarbital) and antispasmodics (propantheline, diphenoxylate with atropine sulfate). However, with chronic use, the patient may become dependent on these drugs. If the cause of irritable bowel syndrome is chronic laxative abuse, bowel training may help correct the condition.

Special considerations

Since the patient with irritable bowel syndrome isn't hospitalized, focus your care on patient teaching.

- Tell the patient to avoid irritating foods, and encourage development of regular bowel habits.
- Help the patient deal with stress, and warn against dependence on sedatives or antispasmodics.
- Encourage regular checkups, since irritable bowel syndrome is associated with a higher-than-normal incidence of diverticulitis and colon cancer. For patients over age 40, emphasize the need for an annual sigmoidoscopy and rectal examination.

Celiac Disease

(Idiopathic steatorrhea, nontropical sprue, gluten enteropathy, celiac sprue)

Celiac disease is characterized by poor food absorption and intolerance of gluten, a protein in wheat and wheat products. Such malabsorption in the small bowel results from atrophy of the villi and a decrease in the activity and amount of enzymes in the surface epithelium. With treatment (eliminating gluten from the patient's diet), prognosis is good, but residual bowel changes may persist in adults.

Causes and incidence

This relatively uncommon disorder probably results from environmental factors and a genetic predisposition, but the exact mechanism is unknown. Two theories prevail: The first suggests that the disease involves an abnormal immune response. (The presence of HLA-B8 antigen in such a person may be the primary determinant of celiac disease, according to recent studies.)

The second theory proposes that an intramucosal enzyme defect produces an inability to digest gluten. Resulting tissue toxicity produces rapid cell turnover, increases epithelial lymphocytes, and damages surface epithelium of the small bowel.

Celiac disease affects twice as many females as males and occurs more often among relatives, especially siblings. Incidence in the general population is approximately 1 in 3,000. This disease primarily affects whites of northwestern European ancestry; it's rare among blacks, Jews, Orientals, and people of Mediterranean ancestry. It usually affects children but may occur in adults.

Signs and symptoms

This disorder produces clinical effects in many body systems.

- *Gastrointestinal:* recurrent attacks of diarrhea, steatorrhea, abdominal distention due to flatulence, stomach cramps, weakness, anorexia, and, occasionally, increased appetite without weight gain. Atrophy of intestinal villi leads to malabsorption of fat, carbohydrates, and protein. It also causes loss of calories, fat-soluble vitamins (A, D, and K), calcium, and essential minerals and electrolytes. In adults, celiac disease produces multiple, nonspecific ulcers in the small bowel, which may perforate or bleed.
- *Hematologic:* normochromic, hypochromic, or macrocytic anemia due to poor absorption of folate, iron, and vitamin B_{12} and to hypoprothrombinemia from jejunal loss of vitamin K
- *Musculoskeletal:* osteomalacia, osteoporosis, tetany, and bone pain (especially in the lower back, rib cage, and pelvis). These symptoms are due to calcium loss and vitamin D deficiency, which weakens the skeleton, causing rickets in children and compression fractures in adults.
- *Neurologic:* peripheral neuropathy, convulsions, or paresthesia
- *Dermatologic:* dry skin, eczema, psoriasis, dermatitis herpetiformis, and acne rosacea. Deficiency of sulfur-containing amino acids may cause generalized fine, sparse, prematurely gray hair; brittle nails; and localized hyperpigmentation on the face, lips, or mucosa.
- *Endocrine:* amenorrhea, hypometabolism, and possibly, with severe malabsorption, adrenocortical insufficiency
- *Psychosocial:* mood changes and irritability.

Symptoms may develop during the first year of life, when gluten is introduced into the child's diet as cereal. Clinical effects may disappear during adolescence and reappear in adulthood. One theory proposes that the age at which symptoms first appear depends on the strength of the genetic factor: a strong factor produces symptoms during the child's first 4 years; a weak factor, in late childhood or adulthood.

Diagnosis

Histologic changes seen on small-bowel biopsy specimens confirm the diagnosis: a mosaic pattern of alternating flat and bumpy areas on the bowel surface due to an almost total absence of villi and an irregular, blunt, and disorganized network of blood vessels. These changes appear most prominently in the jejunum.

Malabsorption and tolerance studies support the diagnosis. A glucose tolerance test shows poor absorption of glucose. A D-xylose tolerance test shows low urine and blood levels of xylose (less than 3 g over a 5-hour period); however, the presence of renal disease may cause a false-positive result. Serum carotene levels measure absorption. (The patient ingests carotene for several days before the test; since the body neither stores nor manufactures carotene, low serum levels indicate malabsorption.) Analyses of stool specimens (after a 72-hour stool collection) show excess fat.

Barium X-rays of the small bowel show protracted barium passage. The barium shows up in a segmented, coarse, scattered, and clumped pattern; the jejunum shows generalized dilation.

The following lab findings also support the diagnosis:
- low hemoglobin, hematocrit, leukocyte, and platelet counts
- reduced albumin, sodium, potassium, cholesterol, and phospholipid levels
- reduced prothrombin time.

Treatment

Treatment requires elimination of gluten from the patient's diet for life. Even with this exclusion, full return to normal absorption and bowel histology may not occur for months or at all.

Supportive treatment may include supplemental iron, vitamin B_{12}, and folic acid, reversal of electrolyte imbalance (by I.V. infusion, if necessary), I.V. fluid replacement for dehydration, corticosteroids (prednisone, hydrocortisone) to treat accompanying adrenal insufficiency, and vitamin K for hypoprothrombinemia.

Special considerations

- Explain necessity of a gluten-free diet to the patient (and to his parents, if the patient is a child). Advise elimination of wheat, barley, rye, and oats and foods made from them, such as breads and baked goods; suggest substitution of corn or rice. Advise the patient to consult a dietitian for a gluten-free diet, which is high in protein but low in carbohydrates and fats. Depending on individual tolerance, the diet initially consists of proteins and gradually expands to include other foods. Assess the patient's acceptance and understanding of the disease, and encourage regular reevaluation.
- Observe nutritional status and progress by daily calorie counts and weight checks. Also, evaluate tolerance to new foods. In the early stages, offer small, frequent meals to counteract anorexia.
- Assess fluid status: record intake, urine output, and number of stools (may exceed 10 per day). Watch for signs of dehydration, such as dry skin and mucous membranes, and poor skin turgor.
- Check serum electrolyte levels. Watch for signs of hypokalemia (weakness, lethargy, rapid pulse, nausea, and diarrhea) and of low calcium levels (impaired blood clotting, muscle twitching, and tetany).
- Monitor prothrombin time, hemoglobin, and hematocrit. Protect the patient from bleeding and bruising. Administer vitamin K, iron, folic acid, and vitamin B_{12}, as ordered. Early in treatment, give hematinic supplements I.M., using a separate syringe for each. Use the Z-track method to give iron I.M. If the patient can tolerate oral iron, give it between meals, when absorption is best. Dilute oral iron preparations, and give them through a straw to prevent staining teeth.
- Protect patients with osteomalacia from injury by keeping the side rails up and assisting with ambulation, as necessary.
- Give steroids, as ordered, and assess regularly for cushingoid side effects, such as hirsutism and muscle weakness.

Diverticular Disease

In diverticular disease, bulging pouches (diverticula) in the GI wall push the mucosal lining through the surrounding muscle. The most common site for diverticula is in the sigmoid colon, but they may develop anywhere, from the proximal end of the pharynx to the anus. Other typical sites are the duodenum, near the pancreatic border or the ampulla of Vater, and the jejunum. Diverticular disease of the stomach is rare and is often a precursor of peptic or neoplastic disease. Diverticular disease of the ileum (Meckel's diverticulum) is the most common congenital anomaly of the GI tract.

Diverticular disease has two clinical forms. In diverticulosis, *diverticula are present but do not cause symptoms. In* diverticulitis, *diverticula are inflamed and may cause potentially fatal obstruction, infection, or hemorrhage.*

Causes

Diverticular disease is most prevalent in men over age 40. Diverticula probably result from high intraluminal pressure on areas of weakness in the GI wall, where blood vessels enter.

Diet may also be a contributing factor, since lack of roughage reduces fecal residue, narrows the bowel lumen, and leads to higher intraabdominal pressure during defecation. The fact that diverticulosis is most prevalent in Western industrialized nations, where processing removes much of the roughage from foods, supports this theory. Diverticulosis is less common in nations where the diet contains more natural bulk and fiber.

In diverticulitis, retained undigested food mixed with bacteria accumulates in the diverticular sac, forming a hard mass (fecalith). This substance cuts off the blood supply to the thin walls of the sac, making them more susceptible to attack by colonic bacteria. Inflammation follows, possibly leading to perforation, abscess, peritonitis, obstruction, or hemorrhage. Occasionally, the inflamed colon segment may produce a fistula by adhering to the bladder or other organs.

MECKEL'S DIVERTICULUM

In Meckel's diverticulum, a congenital abnormality, a blind tube, like the appendix, opens into the distal ileum near the ileocecal valve. This disorder results from failure of the intra-abdominal portion of the yolk sac to close completely during fetal development. It occurs in 2% of the population, mostly in males.

Uncomplicated Meckel's diverticulum produces no symptoms, but complications cause abdominal pain, especially around the umbilicus, and dark red melena. The lining of the diverticulum may be either gastric mucosa or pancreatic tissue. This disorder may lead to peptic ulceration, perforation, and peritonitis, and may resemble acute appendicitis.

Meckel's diverticulum may also cause bowel obstruction when a fibrous band that connects the diverticulum to the abdominal wall, the mesentery, or other structures snares a loop of the intestine. This may cause intussusception into the diverticulum, or volvulus near the diverticular attachment to the back of the umbilicus or another intra-abdominal structure. Meckel's diverticulum should be considered in cases of gastrointestinal obstruction or hemorrhage, especially when routine gastrointestinal X-rays are negative.

Treatment is surgical resection of the inflamed bowel, and antibiotic therapy if infection is present.

Signs and symptoms

Diverticulosis usually produces no symptoms but may cause recurrent left lower quadrant pain. Such pain, often accompanied by alternating constipation and diarrhea, is relieved by defecation or the passage of flatus. Symptoms resemble irritable bowel syndrome and suggest that both disorders may coexist.

In elderly patients, a rare complication of diverticulosis (without diverticulitis) is hemorrhage from colonic diverticula, usually in the right colon. Such hemorrhage is usually mild to moderate and easily controlled but may occasionally be massive and life-threatening.

Mild diverticulitis produces moderate left lower abdominal pain, mild nausea, gas, irregular bowel habits, low-grade fever, and leukocytosis. In severe diverticulitis, the diverticula can rupture and produce abscesses or peritonitis. Such rupture occurs in up to 20% of such patients; its symptoms include abdominal rigidity and left lower quadrant pain. Peritonitis follows release of fecal material from the rupture site and causes signs of sepsis and shock (high fever, chills, hypotension). Rupture of diverticulum near a vessel may cause microscopic or massive hemorrhage, depending on the vessel's size.

Chronic diverticulitis may cause fibrosis and adhesions that narrow the bowel's lumen and lead to bowel obstruction. Symptoms of incomplete obstruction are constipation, ribbonlike stools, intermittent diarrhea, and abdominal distention. Increasing obstruction causes abdominal rigidity and pain, diminishing or absent bowel sounds, nausea, and vomiting.

Diagnosis

Diverticular disease frequently produces no symptoms, and is often found incidental to an upper GI barium X-ray series. Upper GI series confirms or rules out diverticulosis of the esophagus and upper bowel; a barium enema confirms or rules out diverticulosis of the lower bowel. Barium-filled diverticula can be single, multiple, or clustered like grapes, and may have a wide or narrow mouth. Barium outlines but does not fill diverticula blocked by impacted feces. In patients with acute diverticulitis, a barium enema may rupture the bowel, so this procedure requires caution. If irritable bowel syndrome accompanies diverticular disease, X-rays may reveal colonic spasm.

Biopsy rules out cancer; however, a colonoscopic biopsy is not recommended during acute diverticular disease because of the strenuous bowel preparation it requires. Blood studies may show elevated ESR in diverticulitis, especially if the diverticula are infected.

Treatment

Asymptomatic diverticulosis generally doesn't necessitate treatment. Intestinal diverticulosis with pain, mild GI distress, constipation, or difficult defecation may respond to a liquid or bland diet, stool softeners, and occasional doses of mineral oil. These measures relieve symptoms, minimize irritation, and lessen the risk of progression to diverticulitis. After pain subsides, patients also benefit from a high-residue diet and bulk medication, such as psyllium.

Treatment of mild diverticulitis without signs of perforation must prevent constipation and combat infection. It may include bed rest, a liquid diet, stool softeners, a broad-spectrum antibiotic, meperidine to control pain and relax smooth muscle, and an antispasmodic, such as propantheline, to control muscle spasms.

Diverticulitis that is refractory to medical treatment requires a colon resection to remove the involved segment. Perforation, peritonitis, obstruction, or fistula that accompanies diverticulitis may require a temporary colostomy to drain abscesses and rest the colon, followed by later anastomosis.

Patients who hemorrhage need blood replacement and careful monitoring of fluid and electrolyte balance. Such bleeding usually stops spontaneously. If it continues, angiography for catheter placement and infusion of vasopressin into the bleeding vessel is effective. Rarely, surgery may be required.

Special considerations

Management of uncomplicated diverticulosis chiefly involves thorough patient teaching about bowel and dietary habits.

- Explain what diverticula are and how they form.
- Make sure the patient understands the importance of dietary roughage and the harmful effects of constipation and straining at stool. Encourage increased intake of foods high in undigestible fiber, including fresh fruits and vegetables, whole grain bread, and wheat or bran cereals. Warn that a high-fiber diet may temporarily cause flatulence and discomfort. Advise the patient to relieve constipation with stool softeners or bulk-forming cathartics. But caution against taking bulk-forming cathartics without plenty of water; if swallowed dry, they may absorb enough moisture in the mouth and throat to swell and obstruct the esophagus or trachea.
- If the patient with diverticulosis is hospitalized, administer medication, as ordered; observe his stools carefully for frequency, color, and consistency; and keep accurate pulse and temperature charts, since they may signal developing inflammation or complications.

Management of diverticulitis depends on severity of symptoms:

- In mild disease, administer medications, as ordered; explain diagnostic tests and preparations for such tests; observe stools carefully; and maintain accurate records of temperature, pulse, respirations, and intake and output.
- Monitor carefully if the patient requires angiography and catheter placement for vasopressin infusion. Inspect the insertion site frequently for bleeding, check pedal pulses often, and keep the patient from flexing his legs at the groin.
- Watch for vasopressin-induced fluid retention (apprehension, abdominal cramps, convulsions, oliguria, or anuria) and severe hyponatremia (hypo-

tension; rapid, thready pulse; cold, clammy skin; and cyanosis.)

After surgery to resect the colon:

- Watch for signs of infection. Provide meticulous wound care, since perforation may have already infected the area. Check drain sites frequently for signs of infection (pus on dressing, foul odor) or fecal drainage. Change dressings, as necessary.
- Encourage coughing and deep breathing to prevent atelectasis.
- Watch for signs of postoperative bleeding (hypotension, and decreased hemoglobin and hematocrit).
- Record intake and output accurately.
- Keep the nasogastric tube patent. If it becomes dislodged, notify the surgeon immediately; don't attempt to reposition it yourself.
- As needed, teach colostomy care, and arrange for a visit by an enterostomal therapist.

Appendicitis

The most common major surgical disease, appendicitis is inflammation of the vermiform appendix due to an obstruction. Appendicitis may occur at any age and affects both sexes equally; however, between puberty and age 25, it's more prevalent in men. Since the advent of antibiotics, the incidence and the death rate of appendicitis have declined; if untreated, this disease is invariably fatal.

Causes

Appendicitis probably results from an obstruction of the intestinal lumen caused by a fecal mass, stricture, barium ingestion, or viral infection. This obstruction sets off an inflammatory process that can lead to infection, thrombosis, necrosis, and perforation. If the appendix ruptures or perforates, the infected contents spill into the abdominal cavity, causing peritonitis, the most common and most perilous complication of appendicitis.

Signs and symptoms

Typically, appendicitis begins with generalized or localized abdominal pain in the upper right abdomen, followed by anorexia, nausea, and vomiting (rarely profuse). Pain eventually localizes in the lower right abdomen (McBurney's point) with abdominal "boardlike" rigidity, retractive respirations, increasing tenderness, increasingly severe abdominal spasms, and almost invariably, rebound tenderness. (Rebound tenderness on the opposite side of the abdomen suggests peritoneal inflammation.)

Later symptoms include constipation (although diarrhea is also possible), slight fever, and tachycardia. Sudden cessation of abdominal pain indicates perforation or infarction of the appendix.

Diagnosis

Diagnosis of appendicitis is based on physical findings and characteristic clinical symptoms. Findings that support this diagnosis include a temperature of 99° to 102° F. (37.2° to 38.9° C.) and a moderately elevated WBC (12,000 to 15,000/mm^3), with increased immature cells. Diagnosis must rule out illnesses with similar symptoms: gastritis, gastroenteritis, ileitis, colitis, diverticulitis, pancreatitis, renal colic, bladder infection, ovarian cyst, and uterine disease.

Treatment

Appendectomy is the only effective treatment. If peritonitis develops, treatment involves gastrointestinal intubation, parenteral replacement of fluids and electrolytes, and administration of antibiotics.

Special considerations

If appendicitis is suspected, or during preparation for appendectomy:

• Administer I.V. fluids to prevent dehydration. *Never* administer cathartics or enemas, as they may rupture the appendix. Give the patient nothing by mouth, and administer analgesics judiciously, since they may mask symptoms.
• To lessen pain, place the patient in Fowler's position. (This is also helpful postoperatively.) *Never* apply heat to the lower right abdomen; this may cause the appendix to rupture.

After appendectomy:
• Monitor vital signs, and intake and output. Give analgesics, as ordered.
• Encourage the patient to cough, deep breathe, and turn frequently to prevent pulmonary complications.
• Document bowel sounds, passing of flatus, or bowel movements—signs of the return of peristalsis. These signs in a patient whose nausea and abdominal rigidity have subsided indicate readiness to resume oral fluids.
• Watch closely for possible surgical complications. Continuing pain and fever may signal an abscess. The complaint that "something gave way" may mean wound dehiscence. If an abscess or peritonitis develops, incision and drainage may be necessary. Frequently assess the dressing for wound drainage.
• Assist the patient to ambulate as soon as possible after surgery—usually within 12 hours.
• If peritonitis complicated appendicitis, a nasogastric tube may be needed to decompress the stomach and reduce nausea and vomiting. If so, record drainage, and give good mouth and nose care.

Peritonitis

Peritonitis is an acute or chronic inflammation of the peritoneum, the membrane that lines the abdominal cavity and covers the visceral organs. Such inflammation may extend throughout the peritoneum or may be localized as an abscess. Peritonitis commonly decreases intestinal motility and causes intestinal distention with gas. Mortality is 10%, with death usually a result of bowel obstruction; this mortality rate was much higher before the introduction of antibiotics.

Causes and incidence

Although the GI tract normally contains bacteria, the peritoneum is sterile. In peritonitis, however, bacteria invade the peritoneum. Generally, such infection results from inflammation and perforation of the GI tract, allowing bacterial invasion. Usually, this is a result of appendicitis, diverticulitis, peptic ulcer, ulcerative colitis, volvulus, strangulated obstruction, abdominal neoplasm, or a stab wound. Peritonitis may also result from chemical inflammation, as in rupture of the fallopian or an ovarian tube, or the bladder; perforation of a gastric ulcer; or released pancreatic enzymes.

In both chemical and bacterial inflammation, accumulated fluids containing protein and electrolytes make the transparent peritoneum opaque, red, inflamed, and edematous. Because the peritoneal cavity is so resistant to contamination, such infection is often localized as an abscess instead of disseminated as a generalized infection.

Signs and symptoms

The key symptom of peritonitis is sudden, severe, and diffuse abdominal pain that tends to intensify and localize in the area of the underlying disorder. For instance, if appendicitis causes the rupture, pain eventually localizes in the lower right quadrant. The patient often displays weakness, pallor, excessive sweating, and cold skin as a result of excessive loss of fluid, electrolytes, and protein into the abdominal cavity. Decreased intestinal motility and paralytic ileus result from the effect of bacterial toxins on the intestinal muscles. Intestinal obstruction causes nausea, vomiting, and abdominal rigidity.

Other clinical characteristics include hypotension, tachycardia, signs of dehydration (oliguria, thirst, dry swollen tongue, pinched skin), acutely tender abdomen associated with rebound tenderness, temperature of 103° F. (39.4° C.) or higher, and hypokalemia. Inflammation of the diaphragmatic peritoneum may cause shoulder pain and hiccups. Abdominal distention and resulting upward displacement of the diaphragm may decrease respiratory capacity. Typically, the patient with peritonitis tends to breathe shallowly and move as little as possible to minimize pain.

Diagnosis

Severe abdominal pain in a person with direct or rebound tenderness suggests peritonitis. Abdominal X-rays showing edematous and gaseous distention of the small and large bowel support the diagnosis. In the case of perforation of a visceral organ, the X-ray shows air in the abdominal cavity. Other appropriate tests include:

- *chest X-ray:* may show elevation of the diaphragm
- *blood studies:* leukocytosis (more than 20,000/mm^3)
- *paracentesis:* reveals bacteria, exudate, blood, pus, or urine
- *laparotomy:* may be necessary to identify the underlying cause.

Treatment

Early treatment of GI inflammatory conditions and preoperative and postoperative antibiotic therapy help prevent peritonitis. After peritonitis develops, emergency treatment must combat infection, restore intestinal motility, and replace fluids and electrolytes.

Massive antibiotic therapy usually includes administration of cefoxitin with an aminoglycoside or penicillin G and clindamycin with an aminoglycoside, depending on the infecting organisms. To decrease peristalsis and prevent perforation, the patient should receive nothing by mouth; he should receive supportive fluids and electrolytes parenterally.

Other supplementary treatment measures include preoperative and postoperative administration of an analgesic, such as meperidine; nasogastric intubation to decompress the bowel; and possible use of a rectal tube to facilitate passage of flatus.

When peritonitis results from perforation, surgery is necessary as soon as the patient's condition is stable enough to tolerate it. The aim of surgery is to eliminate the source of infection by evacuating the spilled contents and inserting drains. Occasionally, abdominocentesis may be necessary to remove accumulated fluid. Irrigation of the abdominal cavity with antibiotic solutions during surgery may be appropriate.

Special considerations

- Regularly monitor vital signs, fluid intake and output, and amount of nasogastric drainage or vomitus.
- Place the patient in semi-Fowler's position to help him deep breathe with less pain and thus prevent pulmonary complications.
- Counteract mouth and nose dryness due to fever and nasogastric intubation with regular cleansing and lubrication.

After surgery to evacuate the peritoneum:

- Maintain parenteral fluid and electrolyte administration, as ordered. Accurately record fluid intake and output, including nasogastric and incisional drainage.
- Place the patient in Fowler's position to promote drainage (through drainage tube) by gravity. Move him carefully, since the slightest movement will intensify the pain.
- Keep the side rails up and implement other safety measures, if fever and pain disorient the patient.
- Encourage and assist ambulation, as ordered, usually on the first postoperative day.
- Watch for signs of dehiscence (the patient may complain that "something gave

way") and abscess formation (continued abdominal tenderness and fever).

• Frequently assess for peristaltic activity by listening for bowel sounds and checking for gas, bowel movements, and soft abdomen. When peristalsis returns, and temperature and pulse rate are normal, gradually decrease parenteral fluids and increase oral fluids. If the patient has a nasogastric tube in place, clamp it for short intervals. If nausea or vomiting does not result, begin oral fluids, as ordered and tolerated.

Intestinal Obstruction

Intestinal obstruction is the partial or complete blockage of the lumen in the small or large bowel. Small bowel obstruction is far more common (90% of patients) and usually more serious. Complete obstruction in any part of the bowel, if untreated, can cause death within hours from shock and vascular collapse. Intestinal obstruction is most likely to occur after abdominal surgery or in persons with congenital bowel deformities.

Causes

Adhesions and strangulated hernias usually cause small bowel obstruction; carcinomas, large bowel obstruction. Mechanical intestinal obstruction results from foreign bodies (fruit pits, gallstones, worms) or compression of the bowel wall due to stenosis, intussusception, volvulus of the sigmoid or cecum, tumors, or atresia. Nonmechanical obstruction results from physiologic disturbances, such as paralytic ileus, electrolyte imbalances, toxicity (uremia, generalized infection), neurogenic abnormalities (spinal cord lesions), and thrombosis or embolism of mesenteric vessels.

Intestinal obstruction develops in three forms:

• *Simple:* Blockage prevents intestinal contents from passing, with no other complications.

• *Strangulated:* Blood supply to part or all of the obstructed section is cut off, in addition to blockage of the lumen.

• *Close-looped:* Both ends of a bowel section are occluded, isolating it from the rest of the intestine.

In all three forms, the physiologic effects are similar: When intestinal obstruction occurs, fluid, air, and gas collect near the site. Peristalsis increases temporarily, as the bowel tries to force its contents through the obstruction, injuring intestinal mucosa and causing distention at and above the site of the obstruction. This distention blocks the flow of venous blood and halts normal absorptive processes. As a result, the bowel begins to secrete water, sodium, and potassium into the fluid pooled in the lumen. Obstruction in the upper intestine results in metabolic alkalosis from dehydration and loss of gastric hydrochloric acid; lower obstruction causes slower dehydration and loss of intestinal alkaline fluids, resulting in metabolic acidosis. Ultimately, intestinal obstruction may lead to ischemia, necrosis, and death.

Signs and symptoms

Colicky pain, nausea, vomiting, constipation, and abdominal distention characterize small bowel obstruction. It may also cause drowsiness, intense thirst, malaise, and aching, and may dry up oral mucous membranes and the tongue. Auscultation reveals bowel sounds, borborygmi, and rushes; occasionally, these are loud enough to be heard without a stethoscope. Palpation elicits abdominal tenderness, with moderate distention; rebound tenderness occurs when obstruction has caused strangulation with ischemia. In late stages, signs of hypovolemic shock result from progressive dehydration and plasma loss.

In complete upper intestinal (small bowel) obstruction, vigorous peristaltic waves propel bowel contents toward the mouth instead of the rectum. Spasms may occur every 3 to 5 minutes and last about 1 minute each, with persistent epigastric or periumbilical pain. Passage of small amounts of mucus and blood may occur. The higher the obstruction, the earlier and more severe the vomiting. Vomitus initially contains gastric juice, then bile, and finally fecal contents of the ileum.

Symptoms of large bowel obstruction develop more slowly, because the colon can absorb fluid from its contents and distend well beyond its normal size. Constipation may be the only clinical effect for days. Colicky abdominal pain may then appear suddenly, producing spasms that last less than 1 minute each and recur every few minutes. Continuous hypogastric pain, and nausea may develop, but vomiting is usually absent at first. Large bowel obstruction can cause dramatic abdominal distention: loops of large bowel may become visible on the abdomen. Eventually, complete large bowel obstruction may cause fecal vomiting, continuous pain, or localized peritonitis.

Patients with partial obstruction may display any of the above symptoms in a milder form. However, leakage of liquid stool around the obstruction is common in partial obstruction.

Diagnosis

Progressive, colicky, abdominal pain and distention, with or without nausea and vomiting, suggest bowel obstruction; X-rays confirm it. Abdominal films show the presence and location of intestinal gas or fluid. In small bowel obstruction, a typical "stepladder" pattern emerges, with alternating fluid and gas levels apparent in 3 to 4 hours. In large bowel obstruction, barium enema reveals a distended, air-filled colon or a closed loop of sigmoid with extreme distention (in sigmoid volvulus).

PARALYTIC (ADYNAMIC) ILEUS

Paralytic ileus is a physiologic form of intestinal obstruction that usually develops in the small bowel after abdominal surgery. It causes decreased or absent intestinal motility that usually disappears spontaneously after 2 to 3 days. This condition can develop as a response to trauma, toxemia, or peritonitis, or as a result of electrolyte deficiencies (especially hypokalemia) and the use of certain drugs, such as ganglionic blocking agents and anticholinergics. It can also result from vascular causes, such as thrombosis or embolism. Excessive air swallowing may contribute to it, but paralytic ileus brought on by this factor alone seldom lasts more than 24 hours.

Clinical effects of paralytic ileus include severe abdominal distention, extreme distress, and possibly, vomiting. The patient may be severely constipated or may pass flatus and small, liquid stools. Paralytic ileus lasting longer than 48 hours necessitates intubation for decompression and nasogastric suctioning. Because of the absence of peristaltic activity, a weighted Cantor tube may be necessary in the patient with extraordinary abdominal distention. However, such procedures must be used with extreme caution, because any additional trauma to the bowel can aggravate ileus. When paralytic ileus results from surgical manipulation of the bowel, treatment may also include cholinergic agents, such as neostigmine or bethanechol.

When caring for patients with paralytic ileus, warn those receiving cholinergic agents to expect certain paradoxical side effects, such as intestinal cramps and diarrhea. Remember that neostigmine produces cardiovascular side effects, usually bradycardia and hypotension. Check frequently for returning bowel sounds.

Laboratory results supporting this diagnosis include:

- decreased sodium, chloride, and potassium levels (due to vomiting)
- slightly elevated WBC (with necrosis, peritonitis, or strangulation)

• increased serum amylase level (possibly from irritation of pancreas by bowel loop).

Treatment

Preoperative therapy consists of correction of fluid and electrolyte imbalances, decompression of the bowel to relieve vomiting and distention, and treatment of shock and peritonitis. Strangulated obstruction usually necessitates blood replacement as well as I.V. fluid administration. Passage of a Levin tube, followed by use of the longer and weighted Miller-Abbott tube, usually accomplishes decompression, especially in small bowel obstruction. Close monitoring of the patient's condition determines duration of treatment; if the patient fails to improve or his condition deteriorates, surgery is necessary. In large bowel obstruction, surgical resection with anastomosis, colostomy, or ileostomy commonly follows decompression with a Levin tube.

Hyperalimentation may be appropriate if the patient suffers a protein deficit from chronic obstruction, postoperative or paralytic ileus, or infection. Drug therapy includes analgesics or sedatives, such as meperidine or phenobarbital (but not opiates, since they inhibit GI motility), and antibiotics for peritonitis caused by strangulation or infarction of the bowel.

Special considerations

Effective management of intestinal obstruction, a life-threatening condition that often causes overwhelming pain and distress, requires skillful supportive care and keen observation.

• Monitor vital signs frequently. A drop in blood pressure may indicate reduced circulating blood volume due to blood loss from a strangulated hernia. Remember, as much as 10 liters of fluid can collect in the small bowel, drastically reducing plasma volume. Observe closely for signs of shock (pallor, rapid pulse, and hypotension).

• Stay alert for signs of metabolic alkalosis (changes in sensorium; slow, shallow respirations; hypertonic muscles; tetany) or acidosis (shortness of breath on exertion; disorientation; and, later, deep, rapid breathing, weakness, and malaise). Watch for signs and symptoms of secondary infection, such as fever and chills.

• Monitor urinary output carefully to assess renal function, circulating blood volume, and possible urinary retention due to bladder compression by the distended intestine. If you suspect bladder compression, catheterize the patient for residual urine immediately after he has voided. Also measure abdominal girth frequently to detect progressive distention.

• Provide fastidious mouth and nose care if the patient has undergone decompression by intubation or vomited. Look for signs of dehydration (thick, swollen tongue; dry, cracked lips; dry oral mucous membranes). Record amount and color of drainage from the decompression tube. Irrigate the tube, if necessary, with normal saline solution to maintain patency. If a weighted tube has been inserted, check periodically to make sure it's advancing. Help the patient turn from side to side (or walk around, if he can) to facilitate passage of the tube.

• Keep the patient in Fowler's position as much as possible to promote pulmonary ventilation and ease respiratory distress from abdominal distention. Listen for bowel sounds, and watch for signs of returning peristalsis (passage of flatus and mucus through the rectum).

• Explain all diagnostic and therapeutic procedures to the patient and answer any questions he may have. Make sure he understands that these procedures are necessary to relieve the obstruction and reduce pain. Tell the patient to lie on his left side for about a half hour before X-rays are taken. Prepare him and his family for the possibility of surgery, and provide emotional support and positive reinforcement afterward. Arrange for an enterostomal therapist to visit the patient who has had a colostomy.

Inguinal Hernia

(Rupture)

A hernia occurs when part of an internal organ protrudes through an abnormal opening in the containing wall of its cavity. Most hernias occur in the abdominal cavity. Although many kinds of abdominal hernias are possible, inguinal hernias are most common. In an inguinal hernia, the large or small intestine, omentum, or bladder protrudes into the inguinal canal. Hernias can be reducible (if the hernia can be manipulated back into place with relative ease), incarcerated (if the hernia can't be reduced because adhesions have formed in the hernial sac), or strangulated (part of the herniated intestine becomes twisted or edematous, seriously interfering with normal blood flow and peristalsis, and possibly leading to intestinal obstruction and necrosis).

Causes and incidence

An inguinal hernia may be indirect or direct. An indirect inguinal hernia, the more common form, results from weakness in the fascial margin of the internal inguinal ring. In an indirect hernia, abdominal viscera leave the abdomen through the inguinal ring and follow the spermatic cord (in males) or round ligament (in females); they emerge at the external ring and extend down the inguinal canal, often into the scrotum or labia. An indirect inguinal hernia may develop at any age, is three times more common in males, and is especially prevalent in infants under age 1.

Direct inguinal hernia results from a weakness in the fascial floor of the inguinal canal. Instead of entering the canal through the internal ring, the hernia passes through the posterior inguinal wall, protrudes directly through the transverse fascia of the canal (in an area known as Hesselbach's triangle), and comes out at the external ring.

In males, during the seventh month of gestation, the testicle normally descends into the scrotum, preceded by the peritoneal sac. If the sac closes improperly, it leaves an opening through which the intestine can slip. In either sex, a hernia can result from weak abdominal muscles (caused by congenital malformation, trauma, or aging) or increased intra-abdominal pressure (due to heavy lifting, pregnancy, obesity, or straining).

Signs and symptoms

Inguinal hernia usually causes a lump to appear over the herniated area when the patient stands or strains. The lump disappears when the patient is supine. Tension on the herniated contents may cause a sharp, steady pain in the groin, which fades when the hernia is reduced. Strangulation produces severe pain, and may lead to partial or complete bowel obstruction and even intestinal necrosis. Partial bowel obstruction may cause anorexia, vomiting, pain and tenderness in the groin, an irreducible mass, and diminished bowel sounds. Complete obstruction may cause shock, high fever, absent bowel sounds, and bloody stools. In an infant, an inguinal hernia often coexists with an undescended testicle or a hydrocele.

Diagnosis

In a patient with a large hernia, physical examination reveals an obvious swelling or lump in the inguinal area. In the patient with a small hernia, the affected area may simply appear full. Palpation of the inguinal area while the patient is performing Valsalva's maneuver confirms the diagnosis. To detect a hernia in a male patient, the patient is asked to stand with his ipsilateral leg slightly flexed and his weight resting on the other leg. The examiner inserts an index finger into the lower part of the scrotum and invaginates the scrotal skin so the finger

COMMON SITES OF HERNIA

• *Umbilical hernia* results from abnormal muscular structures around the umbilical cord. This hernia is quite common in newborns but also occurs in women who are obese or who have had several pregnancies. Since most umbilical hernias in infants close spontaneously, surgery is warranted only if the hernia persists for more than 4 or 5 years. Taping or binding the affected area or supporting it with a truss may relieve symptoms until the hernia closes. Severe congenital umbilical hernia allows the abdominal viscera to protrude outside the body. This condition necessitates immediate repair.

• *Incisional (ventral) hernia* develops at the site of previous surgery, usually along vertical incisions. This hernia may result from a weakness in the abdominal wall, perhaps as a result of an infection or impaired wound healing. Inadequate nutrition, extreme abdominal distention, or obesity also predispose to incisional hernia. Palpation of an incisional hernia may reveal several defects in the surgical scar. Effective repair requires pulling the layers of the abdominal wall together without creating tension. If this isn't possible, surgical reconstruction uses Teflon, Marlex mesh, or tantalum mesh to close the opening.

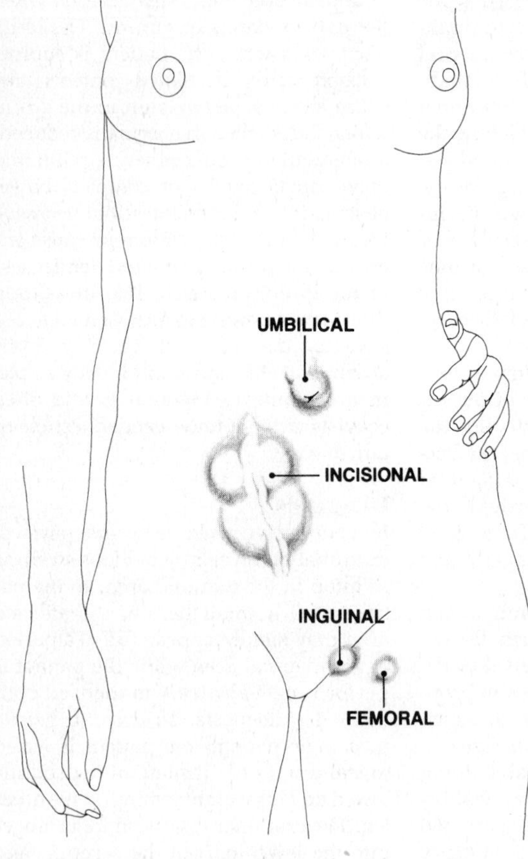

• *Inguinal hernia* can be direct or indirect. Indirect inguinal hernia causes the abdominal viscera to protrude through the inguinal ring and follow the spermatic cord (in males); or round ligament (in females). Direct inguinal hernia results from a weakness in the fascial floor of the inguinal canal.

• *Femoral hernia* occurs where the femoral artery passes into the femoral canal. Typically, a fatty deposit within the femoral canal enlarges and eventually creates a hole big enough to accommodate part of the peritoneum and bladder. A femoral hernia appears as a swelling or bulge at the pulse point of the large femoral artery. It's usually a soft, pliable, reducible, nontender mass, but often becomes incarcerated or strangulated.

advances through the external inguinal ring to the internal ring (about 1½" to 2" [4 to 5 cm] through the inguinal canal). The patient is then told to cough. If the examiner feels pressure against the fingertip, an indirect hernia exists; if pressure is felt against the side of the finger, a direct hernia exists.

Patient history of sharp or "catching" pain when lifting or straining may help confirm the diagnosis. Suspected bowel obstruction requires X-rays and a WBC count (may be elevated).

Treatment

If the hernia is reducible, the pain may be temporarily relieved by pushing the hernia back into place. A truss may keep the abdominal contents from protruding into the hernial sac, although it won't cure the hernia. This device is especially beneficial for an elderly or debilitated patient, since any surgery is potentially hazardous to him.

For infants, adults, and otherwise healthy elderly patients, herniorrhaphy is the treatment of choice. Herniorrhaphy replaces the contents of the hernial sac into the abdominal cavity and closes the opening. This procedure is often performed under local anesthetic in a short-term unit, or as a single-day admission. Another effective surgical procedure for repairing hernia is hernioplasty, which reinforces the weakened area with steel mesh, fascia, or wire.

A strangulated or necrotic hernia necessitates bowel resection. Rarely, an extensive resection may require temporary colostomy. In either case, bowel resection lengthens postoperative recovery and requires massive doses of antibiotics, parenteral fluids, and electrolyte replacements.

Special considerations

- Apply a truss only after a hernia has been reduced. For best results, apply it in the morning, before the patient gets out of bed.
- To prevent skin irritation, tell the patient to bathe daily and apply liberal amounts of cornstarch or baby powder. Warn against applying the truss over clothing, since this reduces the effectiveness of the truss and may make it slip.
- Watch for and immediately report signs of incarceration and strangulation. Don't try to reduce an incarcerated hernia, since this may perforate the bowel. If severe intestinal obstruction arises because of hernial strangulation, inform the doctor immediately. A nasogastric tube may be inserted promptly to empty the stomach and relieve pressure on the hernial sac.
- Before surgery, closely monitor vital signs. Administer I.V. fluids, and analgesics for pain, as ordered. Control fever with acetaminophen or tepid sponge baths, as ordered. Place the patient in Trendelenburg position to reduce pressure on the hernia site.
- Give special reassurance and support to a child scheduled for hernia repair. Encourage him to ask questions, and answer them as simply as possible. Offer appropriate diversions to distract him from the impending surgery.
- After surgery, make sure the patient voids within 8 to 12 hours. Check the incision and dressing at least three times a day for drainage, inflammation, or swelling. Check for normal bowel sounds and watch for fever.
- Observe carefully for postoperative scrotal swelling. To reduce such swelling, support the scrotum with a rolled towel and apply an ice bag.
- Encourage fluid intake to maintain hydration and prevent constipation. Teach deep-breathing exercises, and show the patient how to splint the incision before coughing.
- Before discharge, warn the patient against lifting or straining. In addition, tell him to watch for signs of infection (oozing, tenderness, warmth, redness) at the incision site, and to keep the incision clean and covered until the sutures are removed.
- Advise the patient not to resume normal activity or return to work without the surgeon's permission.

Intussusception

Intussusception is a telescoping (invagination) of a portion of the bowel into an adjacent distal portion. Intussusception may be fatal, especially if treatment is delayed more than 24 hours.

Causes and incidence

Intussusception is most common in infants and occurs three times more often in males than in females; 87% of children with intussusception are under age 2; 70% of these children are between ages 4 and 11 months.

Studies suggest that intussusception may be linked to viral infections, since seasonal peaks are noted—in the spring-summer, coinciding with peak incidence of enteritis, and in the midwinter, coinciding with peak incidence of respiratory tract infections.

The cause of most cases of intussusception in infants is unknown. In older children, polyps, alterations in intestinal motility, hemangioma, lymphosarcoma, lymphoid hyperplasia, or Meckel's diverticulum may trigger the process. In adults, intussusception usually results from benign or malignant tumors (65% of patients). It may also result from polyps, Meckel's diverticulum, gastroenterostomy with herniation, or an appendiceal stump.

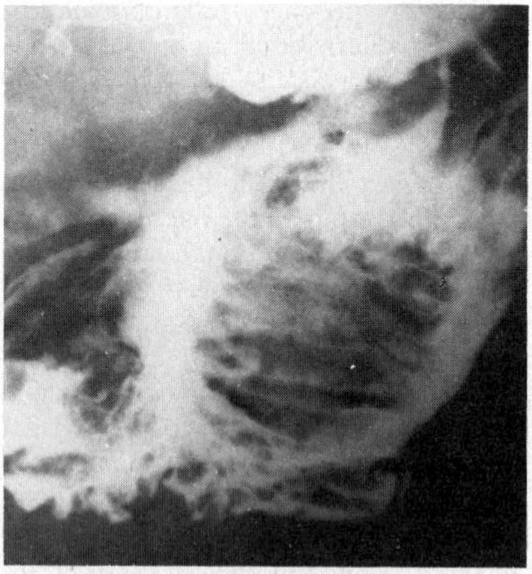

This barium study confirms retrograde intussusception following gastrojejunostomy by showing the characteristic "coiled spring" appearance caused by barium coating on the outer layers of the jejunum. Barium also outlines the stomach pouch.

When a bowel segment (the intussusceptum) invaginates, peristalsis propels it along the bowel, pulling more bowel along with it; the receiving segment is the intussuscipiens. This invagination produces edema, hemorrhage from venous engorgement, incarceration, and obstruction. If treatment is delayed for longer than 24 hours, strangulation of the intestine usually occurs, with gangrene, shock, and perforation.

Signs and symptoms

In an infant or child, intussusception produces four cardinal clinical effects:

- *intermittent attacks of colicky pain,* which cause the child to scream, draw his legs up to his abdomen, turn pale and diaphoretic, and possibly, display grunting respirations
- initially, *vomiting of stomach contents;* later, of bile-stained or fecal material
- *"currant jelly" stools,* which contain a mixture of blood and mucus
- *tender, distended abdomen, with a palpable, sausage-shaped abdominal mass;* often, the viscera are absent from the lower right quadrant.

In adults, intussusception produces nonspecific, chronic, and intermittent symptoms, including colicky abdominal pain and tenderness, vomiting, diarrhea (occasionally constipation), bloody stools, and weight loss. Abdominal pain usually localizes in the lower right quadrant, radiates to the back, and increases with eating. Adults with severe intussusception may develop strangulation with excruciating pain, abdominal distention, and tachycardia.

Diagnosis

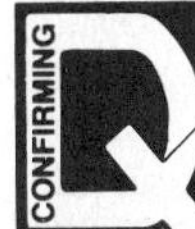

Barium enema confirms colonic intussusception when it shows the characteristic coiled spring sign; it also delineates the extent of intussusception. Upright abdominal X-rays may show a soft-tissue mass and signs of complete or partial obstruction, with dilated loops of bowel. WBC up to 15,000/mm³ indicates obstruction; greater than 15,000/mm³, strangulation; more than 20,000/mm³, bowel infarction should be considered.

Treatment

In children, therapy may include hydrostatic reduction or surgery. Surgery is indicated for children with recurrent intussusception, for those who show signs of shock or peritonitis, and for those in whom symptoms have been present longer than 24 hours. In adults, surgery is always the treatment of choice.

During hydrostatic reduction, the radiologist drips a barium solution into the rectum from a height of not more than 3′ (0.9 m); fluoroscopy traces the progress of the barium. If the procedure is successful, the barium backwashes into the ileum, and the mass disappears. If not, the procedure is stopped, and the patient is prepared for surgery.

During surgery, manual reduction is attempted first. After compressing the bowel above the intussusception, the doctor attempts to milk the intussusception back through the bowel. However, if manual reduction fails, or if the bowel is gangrenous or strangulated, the doctor will perform a resection of the affected bowel segment. In addition, he'll probably perform a prophylactic appendectomy at this time.

Special considerations

- Monitor vital signs before and after surgery. A change in temperature may indicate sepsis; infants may become hypothermic at onset of infection. Rising pulse rate and falling blood pressure may be signs of peritonitis.
- Check intake and output. Watch for signs of dehydration and bleeding. If the patient is in shock, give blood or plasma, as ordered.
- A nasogastric tube is inserted to decompress the intestine and minimize vomiting. Monitor tube drainage, and replace volume lost, as ordered.
- After surgery, administer broad-spectrum antibiotics, as ordered, and give meticulous wound care. Most incisions heal without complications. However, closely check the incision for inflammation, drainage, or suture separation.
- Encourage the patient to cough productively by turning him from side to side. Take care to splint the incision when he coughs, or teach him to do so himself. In addition, make sure he takes 10 deep breaths an hour.
- Oral fluids may be resumed postoperatively when bowel sounds and peristalsis return, nasogastric tube drainage is minimal, the abdomen remains soft, and vomiting does not occur when the nasogastric tube is clamped briefly for a trial period. When the patient tolerates oral fluids well, the tube can be removed and the patient's diet gradually returned to normal, as tolerated.
- Check for abdominal distention after the patient resumes a normal diet, and monitor his general condition.
- Offer special reassurance and emotional support to the child and parents. This condition is considered a pediatric emergency, and parents are often unprepared for their child's hospitalization and possible surgery; they may feel guilty for not seeking medical aid when their child first began exhibiting symptoms. Similarly, the child is unprepared for an abrupt separation from his parents and familiar environment.

To minimize the stress of hospitalization, encourage parents to participate in their child's care as much as possible. Be flexible about visiting hours.

Volvulus

Volvulus is a twisting of the intestine at least 180° on its mesentery, which results in blood vessel compression.

Causes and incidence

In volvulus, twisting may result from an anomaly of rotation, an ingested foreign body, or an adhesion; in some cases, however, the cause is unknown. Volvulus usually occurs in a bowel segment with a mesentery long enough to twist. The most common area, particularly in adults, is the sigmoid; the small bowel is a common site in children. Other common sites include the stomach and cecum. Volvulus secondary to meconium ileus may occur in patients with cystic fibrosis.

Signs and symptoms

Vomiting and rapid, marked abdominal distention follow sudden onset of severe abdominal pain. Without immediate treatment, volvulus can lead to strangulation of the twisted bowel loop, ischemia, infarction, perforation, and fatal peritonitis.

Diagnosis

Sudden onset of severe abdominal pain and physical examination that may reveal a palpable mass suggest volvulus. Appropriate special tests include:

- *X-rays:* Abdominal X-rays may show obstruction and abnormal air-fluid levels in the sigmoid and cecum; in midgut volvulus, abdominal X-rays may be normal.
- *Barium enema:* In cecal volvulus, barium fills the colon distal to the section of cecum; in sigmoid volvulus in children, barium may twist to a point, and, in adults, barium may take on an "ace of spades" configuration.
- *Upper GI series:* In midgut volvulus, obstruction and possibly a twisted contour show in a narrow area near the duodenojejunal junction, where barium will not pass.
- *White blood cell count:* In strangulation, the count is greater than 15,000/mm^3; in bowel infarction, greater than 20,000/mm^3.

Treatment and special considerations

Treatment varies according to the severity and location of the volvulus. For children with midgut volvulus, treatment is surgical. For adults with sigmoid volvulus, nonsurgical treatment includes proctoscopy to check for infarction, and reduction by careful insertion of a sigmoidoscope or a long rectal tube to deflate the bowel. Success of nonsurgical reduction is indicated by expulsion of gas and immediate relief of abdominal pain. If the bowel is distended but viable, surgery consists of detorsion (untwisting); if the bowel is necrotic, surgery includes resection and anastomosis. Prolonged hyperalimentation and I.V. antibiotics are usually necessary. Occasionally, sedatives are needed.

After surgical correction of volvulus:

- Monitor vital signs, watching for temperature changes (a sign of sepsis), and a rapid pulse rate and falling blood pressure (signs of shock and peritonitis). Carefully monitor fluid intake and output (including stool), electrolytes, and complete blood count. Be sure to measure and record drainage from nasogastric tube and drains.
- Encourage frequent coughing and deep breathing. Reposition the patient often, and suction him, as needed.
- Keep dressings clean and dry. Record any excessive or unusual drainage. Later, check for incisional inflammation and separation of sutures.
- When bowel sounds and peristalsis return, begin oral feedings with clear liquids, as ordered. Before removing the

nasogastric tube, clamp it for a trial period, and watch for abdominal distention. When solid food can be tolerated, gradually expand the diet. Reassure the patient and family, and explain all diagnostic procedures. If the patient is a child, encourage parents to participate in their child's care to minimize the stress of hospitalization.

Hirschsprung's Disease

(Congenital megacolon, congenital aganglionic megacolon)

Hirschsprung's disease is a congenital disorder of the large intestine, characterized by absence or marked reduction of parasympathetic ganglion cells in the colorectal wall. This disorder impairs intestinal motility and causes severe, intractable constipation. Without prompt treatment, an infant with colonic obstruction may die within 24 hours from enterocolitis that leads to severe diarrhea and hypovolemic shock. With prompt treatment, prognosis is good.

Causes and incidence

In Hirschsprung's disease, the aganglionic bowel segment contracts without the reciprocal relaxation needed to propel feces forward. In 90% of patients, this aganglionic segment is in the rectosigmoid area, but it occasionally extends to the entire colon and parts of the small intestine.

Hirschsprung's disease is believed to be a familial, congenital defect, and occurs in 1 in 2,000 to 1 in 5,000 live births. It's up to seven times more common in males than in females (although the aganglionic segment is usually shorter in males than in females) and is more prevalent in whites. Total aganglionosis affects both sexes equally. Females with Hirschsprung's disease are at higher risk of having affected children.

This disease often coexists with other congenital anomalies, particularly trisomy 21 and anomalies of the urinary tract, such as megaloureter.

Signs and symptoms

Clinical effects usually appear shortly after birth, but mild symptoms may not be recognized until later in childhood or during adolescence (usually) or adulthood (rarely). The newborn with Hirschsprung's disease commonly fails to pass meconium within 24 to 48 hours, shows signs of obstruction (bile-stained or fecal vomiting, abdominal distention), irritability, feeding difficulties (poor sucking, refusal to take feedings), failure to thrive, dehydration (pallor, loss of skin turgor, dry mucous membranes, sunken eyes), and overflow diarrhea. The infant may also exhibit abdominal distention that causes rapid breathing and grunting. Rectal examination reveals a rectum empty of stool and, when the examining finger is withdrawn, an explosive gush of malodorous gas and liquid stool. Such examination may temporarily relieve GI symptoms. In infants, the main cause of death is enterocolitis, caused by fecal stagnation that leads to bacterial overgrowth, production of bacterial toxins, intestinal irritation, profuse diarrhea, hypovolemic shock, and perforation.

The older child has intractable constipation (usually requiring laxatives and enemas), abdominal distention, and easily palpated fecal masses. In severe cases, failure to grow is characterized by wasted extremities and loss of subcutaneous tissue, with a large protuberant abdomen.

Adult megacolon, although rare, usually affects men. The patient has abdominal distention, rectal bleeding (rare), and a history of chronic intermittent constipation. He is generally in poor physical condition.

Diagnosis

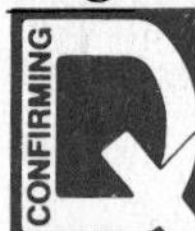

Rectal biopsy provides definitive diagnosis by showing absence of ganglion cells. Suction aspiration using a small tube inserted into the rectum may be performed initially. If findings of suction aspiration are inconclusive, diagnosis requires full-thickness surgical biopsy under general anesthetic. In older infants, barium enema showing a narrowed segment of distal colon with a sawtooth appearance and a funnel-shaped segment above it confirms the diagnosis and assesses the extent of intestinal involvement. Significantly, infants with Hirschsprung's disease retain barium longer than the usual 12 to 24 hours, so delayed films are often helpful when other characteristic signs are absent. Other tests include rectal manometry, which detects failure of the internal anal sphincter to relax and contract, and upright plain films of the abdomen, which show marked colonic distention.

Treatment

Surgical treatment involves pulling the normal ganglionic segment through to the anus. However, such corrective surgery is usually delayed until the infant is at least 10 months old and better able to withstand it. Management of an infant until the time of surgery consists of daily colonic lavage to empty the bowel. If total obstruction is present in the newborn, a temporary colostomy or ileostomy is necessary to decompress the colon. A preliminary bowel prep with an antibiotic, such as neomycin or nystatin, is necessary before surgery. The surgical technique used is based on the three main corrective procedures: the Duhamel, Soave, or Swenson pull-through procedure.

Special considerations

Before emergency decompression surgery:

- Maintain fluid and electrolyte balance, and prevent shock. Provide adequate nutrition, and hydrate with I.V. fluids, as needed. Transfusions may be necessary to correct shock or dehydration. Relieve respiratory distress by keeping the patient in an upright position (place an infant in an infant seat).

After colostomy or ileostomy:

- Place the infant in a heated incubator, with the temperature set at 98° to 99° F. (36.6° to 37.2° C.), or in a radiant warmer. Monitor vital signs, watching for sepsis and enterocolitis (increased respiratory rate with abdominal distention).
- Carefully monitor and record fluid intake and output (including drainage from ileostomy or colostomy) and electrolytes. Ileostomy is especially likely to cause excessive electrolyte loss. Also, measure and record nasogastric drainage, and replace fluids and electrolytes, as ordered. Check stools carefully for excess water—a sign of fluid loss.
- Check urine for specific gravity, glucose (hyperalimentation may lead to osmotic diuresis), and blood.
- To prevent aspiration pneumonia and skin breakdown, turn and reposition the patient often. Also, suction the nasopharynx frequently.
- Keep the area around the stoma clean and dry, and cover it with dressings or a colostomy or ileostomy appliance to absorb drainage. Use aseptic technique until the wound heals. Watch for prolapse, discoloration, or excessive bleeding. (Slight bleeding is common.) To prevent excoriation, use a powder such as karaya gum or a protective stoma disk.
- Oral feeding can begin when bowel sounds return. An infant may tolerate predigested formulas best.
- Teach parents to recognize the signs of fluid loss and dehydration (decreased urinary output, sunken eyes, poor skin turgor) and of enterocolitis (sudden marked abdominal distention, vomiting, diarrhea, fever, lethargy).
- Before discharge, if possible, make sure the parents consult with an enterostomal therapist, for valuable tips for colostomy and ileostomy care.

Before corrective surgery:

- At least once a day, colonic lavage with

normal saline solution is necessary to evacuate the colon, since ordinary enemas and laxatives won't clean it adequately. Keep accurate records of how much lavage solution is instilled. Repeat lavage until the return solution is completely free of fecal particles.

• Administer antibiotics for bowel preparation, as ordered.

After corrective surgery:

• Keep the wound clean and dry, and check for significant inflammation (some inflammation is normal). Do not use a rectal thermometer or suppository until the wound has healed. After 3 to 4 days, the infant will have a first bowel movement, a liquid stool, which will probably create discomfort. Record the number of stools.

• Check urine for blood, especially in a boy; extensive surgical manipulation may cause bladder trauma.

• Watch for signs of possible anastomic leaks (sudden development of abdominal distention unrelieved by gastric aspiration, temperature spike, extreme irritability), which may lead to pelvic abscess.

• Begin oral feedings when active bowel sounds begin and nasogastric drainage decreases. As an additional check, clamp the nasogastric tube for brief, intermittent periods, as ordered. If abdominal distention develops, the patient isn't ready to begin oral feedings. Begin oral feedings with clear fluids, increasing bulk as tolerated.

• Instruct parents to watch for foods that increase the number of stools and to avoid offering these foods. Reassure them that their child will probably gain sphincter control and be able to eat a normal diet. But warn that complete continence may take several years to develop and constipation may recur at times.

• Because an infant with Hirschsprung's disease needs surgery and hospitalization so early in life, parents have difficulty establishing an emotional bond with their child. To promote bonding, encourage them to participate in their child's care as much as possible.

Inactive Colon

(Lazy colon, colonic stasis, atonic constipation)

Inactive colon is a state of chronic constipation that, if untreated, may lead to fecal impaction. It's common in elderly persons and invalids because of their inactivity and is often relieved with diet and exercise.

Causes

Inactive colon usually results from some deficiency in the three elements necessary for normal bowel activity: dietary bulk, fluid intake, and exercise. Other possible causes can include habitual disregard of the impulse to defecate, emotional conflicts, chronic use of laxatives, or prolonged dependence on enemas, which dull rectal sensitivity to the presence of feces.

Signs and symptoms

The primary symptom of inactive colon is chronic constipation. The patient often strains to produce hard, dry, stools accompanied by mild abdominal discomfort. Straining can aggravate other rectal conditions, such as hemorrhoids.

Diagnosis

A patient history of dry, hard, infrequent stools suggests inactive colon. A digital rectal examination reveals stool in the lower portion of the rectum and a palpable colon. Proctoscopy may show an unusually small colon lumen, prominent veins, and an abnormal amount of mucus. Diagnostic tests to rule out other causes include upper GI series, barium enema, and examination of stool for occult blood from neoplasms.

Treatment

Treatment varies according to the patient's age and condition. A higher bulk diet, sufficient exercise, and increased fluid intake often relieve constipation. Treatment for severe constipation may include bulk-forming laxatives, such as psyllium, or well-lubricated glycerin suppositories; for fecal impaction, manual removal of feces is necessary. Administration of an oil-retention enema usually precedes feces removal; an enema is also necessary afterward. For lasting relief of constipation, the patient with inactive colon must modify bowel habits.

Special considerations

Patient education can often help break the constipation habit. Advise the patient to follow these guidelines:

- Drink at least eight to ten glasses (at least 2 liters) of liquid every day, since fluids help keep the intestinal contents in a semisolid state for easier passage. This is particularly important for an older patient. Tell the patient to stimulate the bowel with a drink of hot coffee, warm lemonade, iced liquids—plain or with lemon—or prune juice before breakfast or in the evening.
- Add fiber to the diet with foods such as whole grain cereals (rolled oats, bran, shredded wheat, brown rice, whole wheat bread, oatmeal) to contribute bulk and induce peristalsis. However, warn that too much bran can create an irritable bowel, so the patient should check labels on foods for fiber content (low fiber—0.3 to 1 g; moderate fiber—1.1 to 2 g; high fiber—2.1 to 4.2 g). Increase bulk content of the diet slowly to prevent flatulence, which is sometimes a transient effect of a high-bulk diet. Include fresh fruits, with skins, in the diet for additional bulk. Also include raw and coarse vegetables (broccoli, Brussels sprouts, cabbage, cauliflower, cucumbers, lettuce, and turnips).
- Consume fat-containing foods, such as bacon, butter, cream, and oil, in moderation, since these things will help to soften intestinal contents but sometimes cause diarrhea.
- Avoid highly refined foods, such as white rice, cream of wheat, farina, white pastries, pie or cake, macaroni, spaghetti, noodles, candy, cookies, and ice cream.
- Rest at least 6 hours every night.
- Incorporate moderate exercise, such as walking, into the daily routine.
- Avoid overuse of laxatives, and maintain a regular time for bowel movements (usually after breakfast). Autosuggestion, relaxation, and use of a small footstool to promote thigh flexion while sitting on the toilet may be helpful. To help him relax, suggest that he bring pleasant reading material. Tell the patient to respond promptly to the urge to defecate. If he worries about constipation, assure him that a 2- to 3-day interval between bowel movements can be normal.
- Take bulk-forming laxatives, such as psyllium, with at least 8 oz (240 ml) of liquid. Juices, soft drinks, or other pleasant-tasting liquids help mask this drug's grittiness.

If the patient with inactive colon is hospitalized:

- Assist the elderly patient with inactive colon during a bowel movement to a bedside commode, since using a bedpan causes additional strain. However, if the patient must use a bedpan, have him sit in Fowler's position, or have him sit on the pan at the side of his bed, to facilitate elimination. Occasional digital rectal stimulation or abdominal massage near the sigmoid area may help stimulate a bowel movement. *Caution:* If the patient has a history of arteriosclerosis, congestive heart failure, or hypertension, constipation and straining may induce a "bathroom coronary" or a cerebrovascular accident.
- If the patient requires enemas, avoid using a sodium biphosphate enema too often. Its hypertonic solution can absorb as much as 10% of the colon's sodium content or draw intestinal fluids into the colon, causing dehydration. Also, don't overuse other types of enemas.

Pancreatitis

Pancreatitis, inflammation of the pancreas, occurs in acute and chronic forms and may be due to edema, necrosis, or hemorrhage. In men, this disease is commonly associated with alcoholism, trauma, or peptic ulcer; in women, with biliary tract disease. Prognosis is good when pancreatitis follows biliary tract disease but poor when it follows alcoholism. Mortality rises as high as 60% when pancreatitis is associated with necrosis and hemorrhage.

Causes

The most common causes of pancreatitis are biliary tract disease and alcoholism, but it can also result from pancreatic carcinoma, trauma, or certain drugs, such as glucocorticoids, sulfonamides, chlorothiazide, and azathioprine. This disease also may develop as a complication of peptic ulcer, mumps, or hypothermia. Rarer causes are stenosis or obstruction of the sphincter of Oddi, hyperlipemia, metabolic endocrine disorders (hyperparathyroidism, hemochromatosis), vasculitis or vascular disease, viral infections, mycoplasmal pneumonia, and pregnancy.

Afro-Asian syndrome (diabetes, pancreatic insufficiency and calcification) occurs in young persons, probably from malnutrition and alcoholism, and leads to pancreatic atrophy. Regardless of the cause, pancreatitis involves autodigestion: the enzymes normally excreted by the pancreas digest pancreatic tissue.

Signs and symptoms

In many patients, the first and only symptom of mild pancreatitis is steady epigastric pain centered close to the umbilicus, radiating between the tenth thoracic and sixth lumbar vertebrae, and unrelieved by vomiting. However, a severe attack causes extreme pain, persistent vomiting, abdominal rigidity, diminished bowel activity (suggesting peritonitis), crackles at lung bases, and left pleural effusion. Severe pancreatitis may produce extreme malaise and restlessness, with mottled skin, tachycardia, low-grade fever (100° to 102° F. [37.7° to 38.8° C.]), and cold, sweaty extremities. Proximity of the inflamed pancreas to the bowel may cause ileus.

If pancreatitis damages the islets of Langerhans, complications may include diabetes mellitus. Fulminant pancreatitis causes massive hemorrhage and total destruction of the pancreas, resulting in diabetic acidosis, shock, or coma.

CHRONIC PANCREATITIS

Chronic pancreatitis is usually associated with alcoholism (in over half of all patients), but can also follow hyperparathyroidism, hyperlipemia, or infrequently, gallstones, trauma, or peptic ulcer. Inflammation and fibrosis cause progressive pancreatic insufficiency and eventually destroy the pancreas. Symptoms of chronic pancreatitis include constant dull pain with occasional exacerbations, malabsorption, severe weight loss, and hyperglycemia (leading to diabetic symptoms). Relevant diagnostic measures include patient history, X-rays showing pancreatic calcification, elevated ESR, and examination of stool for steatorrhea.

The severe pain of chronic pancreatitis often requires large doses of analgesics or narcotics, making addiction a serious problem. Treatment also includes a low-fat diet and oral administration of pancreatic enzymes, such as pancreatin or pancrelipase to control steatorrhea, insulin or oral hypoglycemics to curb hyperglycemia, and occasionally, surgical repair of biliary or pancreatic ducts, or the sphincter of Oddi to reduce pressure and promote the flow of pancreatic juice. Prognosis is good if the patient can avoid alcohol; poor if he can't.

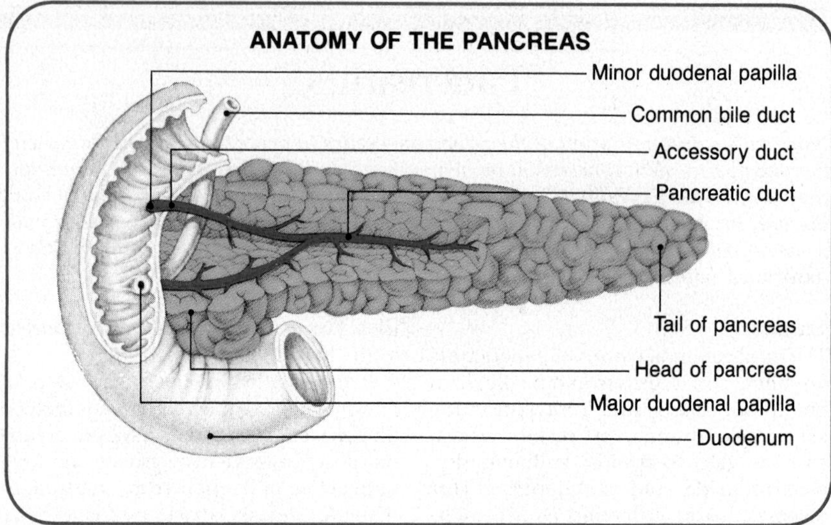

Diagnosis

A careful patient history (especially for alcoholism) and physical examination are the first steps in diagnosis, but the retroperitoneal position of the pancreas makes physical assessment difficult.

Dramatically elevated serum amylase levels—frequently over 500 units—confirm pancreatitis and rule out perforated peptic ulcer, acute cholecystitis, appendicitis, and bowel infarction or obstruction. Similarly dramatic elevations of amylase also occur in urine, ascites, or pleural fluid. Characteristically, amylase levels return to normal 48 hours after onset of pancreatitis, despite continuing symptoms. Supportive laboratory values include:

- increased serum lipase levels, which rise more slowly than serum amylase
- low serum calcium (hypocalcemia) from fat necrosis and formation of calcium soaps
- White blood cell counts range from 8,000 to 20,000/mm^3, with increased polymorphonuclear leukocytes
- elevated glucose levels—as high as 500 to 900 mg/dl, indicating hyperglycemia
- hematocrit occasionally exceeding 50% concentrations.

Results of other tests may include:

- EKG changes (prolonged Q-T segment but normal T wave), which help diagnose hypocalcemia
- abdominal X-rays that show dilation of the small or large bowel or calcification of the pancreas
- GI series, indicating extrinsic pressure on the duodenum or stomach due to edema of the pancreas head
- chest X-rays showing left-sided pleural effusion
- I.V. cholangiography to help distinguish acute cholecystitis from acute pancreatitis
- analysis of abdominal fluid to detect amylase levels as high as 7,000 units. In the patient with a perforated bowel, it may also detect bacteria or bile.

Treatment

Treatment must maintain circulation and fluid volume, relieve pain, and decrease pancreatic secretions. Emergency treatment for shock (the most common cause of death in early-stage pancreatitis) consists of vigorous I.V. replacement of electrolytes and proteins. Metabolic acidosis secondary to hypovolemia and impaired cellular perfusion requires vigorous fluid volume replacement.

Treatment may also include meperidine for pain (although it may cause spasm of the sphincter of Oddi); diazepam for restlessness and agitation; and antibiotics, such as gentamicin, clindamycin, or chloramphenicol, for bacterial infections. Hypocalcemia requires infusion of 10% calcium gluconate; serum glucose levels greater than 300 to 350 mg/dl require insulin therapy.

After the emergency phase, continuing I.V. therapy should provide adequate electrolytes and protein solutions that don't stimulate the pancreas (glucose or free amino acids) for 5 to 7 days. If the patient is not ready to resume oral feedings by then, hyperalimentation may be necessary. Nonstimulating elemental gavage feedings may be safer because of the decreased risk of infection and overinfusion. In extreme cases, laparotomy to drain the pancreatic bed, 95% pancreatectomy, or a combination of cholecystostomy-gastrostomy, feeding jejunostomy, and drainage may be necessary.

Special considerations

Acute pancreatitis is a life-threatening emergency. Design your care plan to provide meticulous supportive care and continuous monitoring of vital systems.

- Monitor vital signs and pulmonary artery pressure closely. If the patient has a central venous pressure line instead of a pulmonary artery catheter, monitor it closely for volume expansion (it shouldn't rise above 10 cmH_2O). Give plasma or albumin, if ordered, to maintain blood pressure. Record fluid intake and output; check urine output hourly, and monitor electrolyte levels. Assess for crackles, rhonchi, or decreased breath sounds.
- For bowel decompression, maintain constant nasogastric suctioning, and give nothing by mouth. Perform good mouth and nose care.
- Watch for signs of calcium deficiency—tetany, cramps, carpopedal spasm, and convulsions. If you suspect hypocalcemia, keep airway and suction apparatus handy and pad side rails.
- Administer analgesics, as needed, to relieve the patient's pain and anxiety. Remember that anticholinergics reduce salivary and sweat gland secretions. Warn the patient that he may experience dry mouth and facial flushing. *Caution:* Narrow-angle glaucoma contraindicates the use of atropine or its derivatives.
- Watch for adverse reactions to antibiotics: nephrotoxicity with aminoglycosides; pseudomembranous enterocolitis with clindamycin; and blood dyscrasias with chloramphenicol.
- Don't confuse thirst due to hyperglycemia (indicated by serum glucose levels up to 350 mg/dl and sugar and acetone in urine) with dry mouth due to nasogastric intubation and anticholinergics.
- Watch for complications due to hyperalimentation, such as sepsis, hypokalemia, overhydration, and metabolic acidosis. Watch for fever, cardiac irregularities, changes in arterial blood gas measurements, and deep respirations. Use strict aseptic technique when caring for the catheter insertion site.

ANORECTUM

Hemorrhoids

Hemorrhoids are varicosities in the superior or inferior hemorrhoidal venous plexus. Dilation and enlargement of the superior plexus produce internal hemorrhoids; dilation and enlargement of the inferior plexus produce external hemorrhoids that may protrude from the rectum. Generally, incidence is highest between ages 20 and 50 and includes both sexes.

Causes

Hemorrhoids probably result from increased intravenous pressure in the hemorrhoidal plexus. Predisposing factors include occupations that require prolonged standing or sitting; straining due to constipation, diarrhea, coughing, sneezing, or vomiting; heart failure; hepatic disease, such as cirrhosis, amebic abscesses, or hepatitis; alcoholism; anorectal infections; loss of muscle tone due to old age, rectal surgery, or episiotomy; anal intercourse; and pregnancy.

Signs and symptoms

Although hemorrhoids may be asymptomatic, they characteristically cause painless, intermittent bleeding, which occurs on defecation. Bright-red blood appears on stool or on toilet paper due to injury of the fragile mucosa covering the hemorrhoid. These first-degree hemorrhoids may itch due to poor anal hygiene. When second-degree hemorrhoids prolapse, they're usually painless and spontaneously return to the anal canal following defecation. Third-degree hemorrhoids cause constant discomfort and prolapse in response to any increase in intraabdominal pressure. They must be manually reduced. Thrombosis of external hemorrhoids produces sudden rectal pain and a subcutaneous, large, firm lump that the patient can feel. If hemorrhoids cause severe or recurrent bleeding, they may lead to secondary anemia with significant pallor, fatigue, and weakness. However, such systemic complications are rare.

Diagnosis

Physical examination confirms external hemorrhoids. Proctoscopy confirms internal hemorrhoids and rules out rectal polyps.

Treatment

Treatment depends on the type and severity of the hemorrhoid and on the patient's overall condition. Generally, treatment includes measures to ease pain, combat swelling and congestion,

TYPES OF HEMORRHOIDS

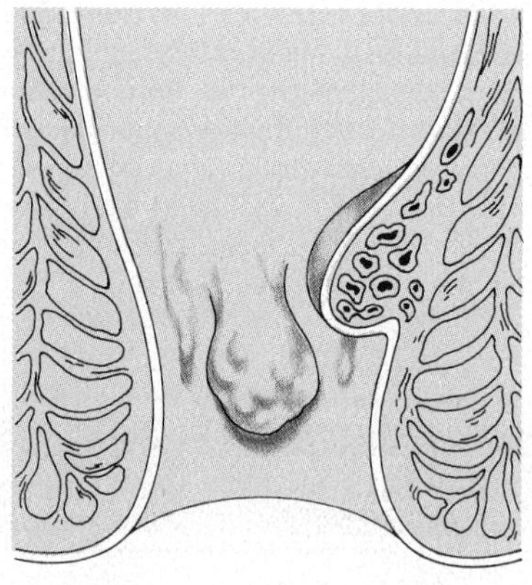

Frontal and cross section view of internal hemorrhoids.

Covered by mucosa, internal hemorrhoids bulge into the rectal lumen and may prolapse during defecation.

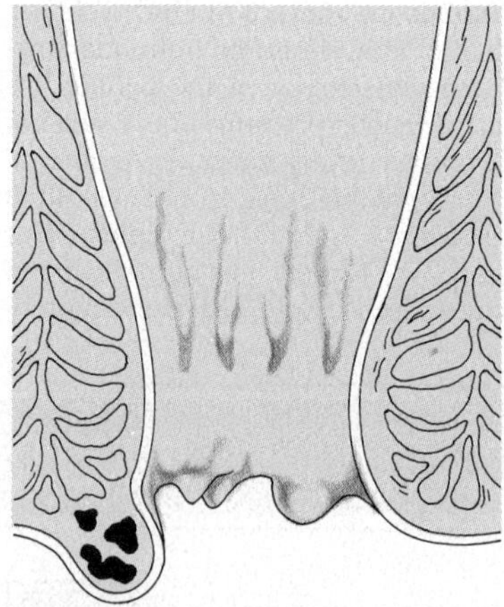

Frontal and cross section view of external hemorrhoids.

Covered by skin, external hemorrhoids protrude from the rectum and are more likely to thrombose than internal hemorroids.

and regulate bowel habits. Patients can relieve constipation by increasing the amount of raw vegetables, fruit, and whole grain cereal in the diet or by using stool softeners. Venous congestion can be prevented by avoiding prolonged sitting on the toilet; and local swelling and pain decreased with local anesthetic agents (lotions, creams, or suppositories), astringents, or cold compresses, followed by warm sitz baths or thermal packs. Rarely, the patient with chronic, profuse bleeding may require blood transfusion.

Other nonsurgical treatments are: injection of a sclerosing solution to produce scar tissue that decreases prolapse, manual reduction, and hemorrhoid ligation or freezing.

Hemorrhoidectomy, the most effective treatment, is necessary for patients with severe bleeding, intolerable pain and pruritus, and large prolapse. This procedure is contraindicated in patients with blood dyscrasias (acute leukemia, aplastic anemia, or hemophilia) or gastrointestinal carcinoma, and during the first trimester of pregnancy.

Special considerations

- To prepare the patient for hemorrhoidectomy, administer an enema, as ordered (usually 2 to 4 hours before surgery), and record the results. Shave the perianal area, and clean the anus and surrounding skin.
- Postoperatively, check for signs of prolonged rectal bleeding, administer adequate analgesics (usually morphine or meperidine), and provide sitz baths, as ordered.
- As soon as the patient can resume oral feedings, administer a bulk medication, such as psyllium, about 1 hour after the evening meal, to ensure a daily stool. Warn against using stool-softening medications soon after hemorrhoidectomy, since a firm stool acts as a natural dilator to prevent anal stricture from the scar tissue. (Some patients may need repeated digital dilation to prevent such narrowing.)
- Keep the wound site clean to prevent infection and irritation.
- Before discharge, stress the importance of regular bowel habits and good anal hygiene. Warn against too vigorous wiping with washcloths and using harsh soaps. Encourage the use of medicated astringent pads and white toilet paper (the fixative in colored paper can irritate the skin).

Anorectal Abscess and Fistula

Anorectal abscess is a localized collection of pus due to inflammation of the soft tissue near the rectum or anus. Such inflammation may produce an anal fistula—an abnormal opening in the anal skin—that may communicate with the rectum. Such disorders develop four times as often in men as in women, possibly because men wear rougher clothing that produces friction on the perianal skin and interferes with air circulation.

Causes

The inflammatory process that leads to abscess may begin with an abrasion or tear in the lining of the anal canal, rectum, or perianal skin, and subsequent infection by *Escherichia coli,* staphylococci, or streptococci. Such trauma may result from injections for treatment of internal hemorrhoids, enema-tip abrasions, puncture wounds from ingested eggshells or fishbones, or insertion of foreign objects. Other preexisting lesions include infected anal fissure, infections from the anal crypt through the anal gland, ruptured anal hematoma, prolapsed thrombosed internal hemorrhoids, and septic lesions in the pelvis, such as acute appendicitis, acute salpingitis, and diverticulitis. Systemic illnesses that may cause abscesses include ulcerative colitis and Crohn's disease. However, many abscesses develop without preexisting lesions.

As the abscess produces more pus, a fistula may form in the soft tissue beneath the muscle fibers of the sphincters (especially the external sphincter), usually extending into the perianal skin. The internal (primary) opening of the abscess/fistula is usually near the anal glands and crypts; the external (secondary) opening, in the perianal skin.

Signs and symptoms

Characteristics are throbbing pain and tenderness at the site of the abscess. A hard, painful lump develops on one side, preventing comfortable sitting.

Diagnosis

Anorectal abscess is detectable on physical examination:

- *Perianal abscess* (80% of patients) is a red, tender, localized, oval swelling close to the anus. Sitting or coughing increases pain, and pus may drain from the abscess. Digital examination reveals no abnormalities.
- *Ischiorectal abscess* (15% of patients) involves the entire perianal region on the affected side of the anus. It's tender but may not produce drainage. Digital examination reveals a tender induration bulging into the anal canal.
- *Submucous or high intermuscular abscess* (5% of patients) may produce a dull, aching pain in the rectum, tenderness and, occasionally, induration. Digital examination reveals a smooth swelling of the upper part of the anal canal or lower rectum.
- *Pelvirectal abscess* (rare) produces fever, malaise, and myalgia but no local anal or external rectal signs or pain. Digital examination reveals a tender mass high in the pelvis, perhaps extending into one of the ischiorectal fossae.

If the abscess drains by forming a fistula, the pain usually subsides and the major signs become pruritic drainage and subsequent perianal irritation. The external opening of a fistula generally appears as a pink or red, elevated, discharging sinus or ulcer on the skin near the anus. Depending on the infection's severity, the patient may have chills, fever, nausea, vomiting, and malaise. Digital examination may reveal a palpable indurated tract and a drop or two of pus on palpation. The internal opening may be palpated as a depression or ulcer in the midline anteriorly or at the dentate line posteriorly. Examination with a probe may require an anesthetic.

Sigmoidoscopy, barium studies, and colonoscopy may be done to rule out other conditions.

Treatment

Anorectal abscesses require surgical incision under caudal anesthesia to promote drainage. Fistulas require a fistulotomy—removal of the fistula and associated granulation tissue—under caudal anesthesia. If the fistula tract is epithelialized, treatment requires fistulectomy—removal of the fistulous tract—followed by insertion of drains, which remain in place for 48 hours.

Special considerations

After incision to drain anorectal abscess:

- provide adequate medication for pain relief, as ordered.
- examine the wound frequently to assess proper healing, which should progress from the inside out. Healing should be complete in 4 to 5 weeks for perianal fistulas; in 12 to 16 weeks, for deeper wounds.
- inform the patient that complete recovery takes time. Offer encouragement.
- stress the importance of perianal cleanliness.
- dispose of soiled dressings properly.
- be alert for the first postoperative bowel movement. The patient may suppress the urge to defecate because of anticipated pain; the resulting constipation increases pressure at the wound site. Such a patient benefits from a stool-softening laxative, Hydrocil, or Metamucil.

Rectal Polyps

Rectal polyps are masses of tissue that rise above the mucosal membrane and protrude into the gastrointestinal tract. Types of polyps include common polypoid adenomas, villous adenomas, hereditary polyposis, focal polypoid hyperplasia, and juvenile polyps (hamartomas). Most rectal polyps are benign. However, villous and hereditary polyps show a marked inclination to become malignant. Indeed, a striking feature of familial polyposis is its frequent association with rectosigmoid adenocarcinoma.

Causes and incidence

Villous adenomas are most prevalent in men over age 55; common polypoid adenomas, in Caucasian women between ages 45 and 60. Incidence in both sexes rises after age 70. Juvenile polyps occur most frequently among children under age 10 and are characterized by rectal bleeding. Predisposing factors include heredity, age, infection, and diet. Formation of polyps results from unrestrained cell growth in the upper epithelium.

Signs and symptoms

Because rectal polyps don't generally cause symptoms, they are usually discovered incidentally during a digital examination or rectosigmoidoscopy. Their most common sign is rectal bleeding: high rectal polyps leave a streak of blood on the stool; low rectal polyps bleed freely.

Rectal polyps vary in appearance:

- *Common polypoid adenomas* are small (usually less than 1 cm), multiple lesions (typically two to five) that are redder than normal mucosa. These lesions are frequently pedunculated—attached to rectal mucosa by a long, thin stalk—and granular, with a red, lobular, or eroded surface.
- *Villous adenomas* are sessile—attached to the mucosa by a wide base—and vary in size from 0.5 to 12 cm. They are soft, friable, and finely lobulated. They may grow large and cause painful defecation; however, because adenomas are soft, they rarely cause bowel obstruction. Sometimes adenomas prolapse outside the anus, expelling parts of the adenoma with the feces. These polyps may cause diarrhea, bloody stools, and subsequent fluid and electrolyte depletion, with hypotension and oliguria.
- In *hereditary polyposis,* rectal polyps resemble benign adenomas but occur in hundreds of small (0.5 cm) lesions, filling the entire mucosal surface. Accompanying signs include diarrhea, bloody stools, and secondary anemia. In a patient with hereditary polyposis, a change in bowel habits with abdominal pain usually signals rectosigmoid cancer.
- *Juvenile polyps* are large, inflammatory lesions, often without an epithelial covering. Mucus-filled cysts cover their usually smooth surface.
- *Focal polypoid hyperplasia* produces small (less than 3 mm), granular, sessile lesions, similar to the colon in color, or gray or translucent. They usually occur at the rectosigmoid junction.

Diagnosis

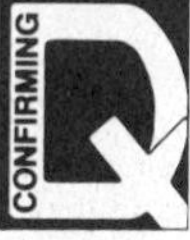

Firm diagnosis of rectal polyps requires identification of the polyps through proctosigmoidoscopy or colonoscopy, and rectal biopsy. Barium enema can help identify polyps that are located high in the colon. Supportive laboratory findings include occult blood in the stool, low hemoglobin and hematocrit (with anemia), and possibly, serum electrolyte imbalances.

Treatment

Treatment varies according to the type and size of polyps, and their location within the colon. Common polypoid adenomas less than 1 cm in size require polypectomy, frequently by fulguration (destruction by high-frequency electricity) during endoscopy. For common polypoid adenomas over 4 cm and all invasive villous adenomas, treatment usually consists of abdominoperineal resection. Focal polypoid hyperplasia requires local fulguration. Depending on gastrointestinal involvement, hereditary polyps necessitate total abdominoperineal resection with a permanent ileostomy, subtotal colectomy with ileoproctostomy, or ileal anal anastomosis. Juvenile polyps are prone to autoamputation; if this doesn't occur, snare removal during colonoscopy is the treatment of choice.

Special considerations

During diagnostic evaluation:

- Check sodium, potassium, and chloride levels daily in the patient with fluid imbalance; adjust fluid and electrolytes, as necessary. Administer normal saline solution with potassium I.V., as ordered. Weigh the patient daily, and record the amount of diarrhea. Watch for signs of dehydration (decreased urine, increased BUN levels).
- Tell the patient to watch for and report evidence of rectal bleeding.

After biopsy and fulguration:

- Check for signs of perforation and hemorrhage, such as sudden hypotension, decrease in hemoglobin or hematocrit, shock, abdominal pain, and passage of red blood through the rectum.
- Watch for and record the first bowel movement, which may not occur for 2 to 3 days.
- Ambulate the patient within 24 hours of the procedure.
- Provide sitz baths for 3 days.
- If the patient has benign polyps, stress the need for routine follow-up studies to check the polypoid growth rate.
- Prepare the patient with precancerous or familial lesions for abdominoperineal resection. Provide emotional support and preoperative instruction.
- After ileostomy or subtotal colectomy with ileoproctostomy, properly care for abdominal dressings, I.V. lines, and Foley catheter. Record intake and output, and check vital signs for hypotension and surgical complications. Administer pain medication, as ordered. To prevent embolism, ambulate the patient as soon as possible, and apply antiembolism stockings; encourage range-of-motion exercises. Provide enterostomal therapy and teach stoma care.

Anorectal Stricture, Stenosis, or Contracture

In anorectal stricture, anorectal lumen size decreases; stenosis prevents dilation of the sphincter.

Causes

Anorectal stricture results from scarring after anorectal surgery or inflammation, inadequate postoperative care, or laxative abuse.

Signs and symptoms

The patient with anorectal stricture strains excessively when defecating and is unable to completely evacuate his bowel. Other clinical effects include pain, bleeding, and pruritus ani.

Diagnosis

Visual inspection reveals narrowing of the anal canal. Digital examination reveals tenderness and tightness.

Treatment and special considerations

Surgical removal of scar tissue is the most effective treatment. Digital or instrumental dilation may be beneficial but may cause additional tears and splits. If the cause of stricture is inflammation,

correction of the underlying inflammatory process is necessary.
• Prepare the patient for the digital examination and testing by explaining procedures thoroughly.
• After surgery, check vital signs often until the patient is stable. Watch for signs of hemorrhage (excessive bleeding on rectal dressing).
• If surgery was performed under spinal anesthetic, record first leg motion, and keep the patient lying flat for 6 to 8 hours after surgery.
• When the patient's condition is stable, resume normal diet, and record time of first bowel movement. Administer stool softeners, as ordered. Give analgesics, provide sitz baths, and change perianal dressing, as ordered.

Pilonidal Disease

In pilonidal disease, a coccygeal cyst—which usually contains hair—becomes infected and produces an abscess, a draining sinus, or a fistula. Incidence is highest among hirsute, Caucasian men aged 18 to 30.

Causes
Pilonidal disease may develop congenitally from a tendency to hirsutism, or it may be acquired from stretching or irritation of the sacrococcygeal area (intergluteal fold) from prolonged rough exercise (such as horseback riding), heat, excessive perspiration, or constricting clothing.

Signs and symptoms
Generally, a pilonidal cyst produces no symptoms until it becomes infected, causing local pain, tenderness, swelling, or heat. Other clinical features include continuous or intermittent purulent drainage, chills, fever, headache, and malaise.

Diagnosis
Physical examination confirms the diagnosis and may reveal a series of openings along the midline, with thin, brown, foul-smelling drainage or a protruding tuft of hair. Pressure on the sinus tract may produce a purulent drainage. Passing a probe back through the sinus tract toward the sacrum should not reveal a perforation between the anterior sinus and anal canal. Cultures of discharge from the infected sinus may show staphylococci or skin bacteria but do not usually contain bowel bacteria.

Treatment
Conservative treatment of pilonidal disease consists of incision and drainage of abscesses, regular extraction of protruding hairs, and sitz baths (four to six times daily). However, persistent infections may necessitate surgical excision of the entire affected area. After excision of a pilonidal abscess, the patient requires regular follow-up care to monitor wound healing. The surgeon may periodically palpate the wound during healing with a cotton-tipped applicator, curette excess granulation tissue, and extract loose hairs to promote wound healing from the inside out and to prevent dead cells from collecting in the wound. Complete healing may take several months.

Special considerations
• Before incision and drainage of pilonidal abscess, assure the patient he'll receive adequate pain relief.
• After surgery, check the compression dressing for signs of excessive bleeding; change the dressing, as directed. Encourage the patient to walk within 24 hours.
• Tell the patient to wear a gauze sponge over the wound site after the dressing is removed, to allow ventilation and prevent friction from clothing. Recommend

the continued use of sitz baths, followed by air-drying instead of rubbing or patting dry with a towel.
- After healing, the patient should briskly wash the area daily with a washcloth to remove loose hairs. Encourage obese patients to lose weight.

Rectal Prolapse

Rectal prolapse is the circumferential protrusion of one or more layers of the mucous membrane through the anus. Prolapse may be complete (with displacement of the anal sphincter or bowel herniation) or partial (mucosal layer).

Causes and incidence

Rectal prolapse usually occurs in men under age 40, in women around age 45 (three times more often than men), and in children aged 1 to 3 (especially those with cystic fibrosis). Predisposing factors include increased intra-abdominal pressure, especially from straining at stool; conditions that affect the pelvic floor or rectum, such as weak sphincters; or weak longitudinal, rectal, or levator ani muscles due to neurologic disorders, injury, tumors, aging, and chronic wasting diseases, such as tuberculosis, cystic fibrosis, or whooping cough; and nutritional disorders.

RECTAL PROLAPSE

Partial rectal prolapse (involves rectal mucosa only)

Complete prolapse (involves all layers of rectum)

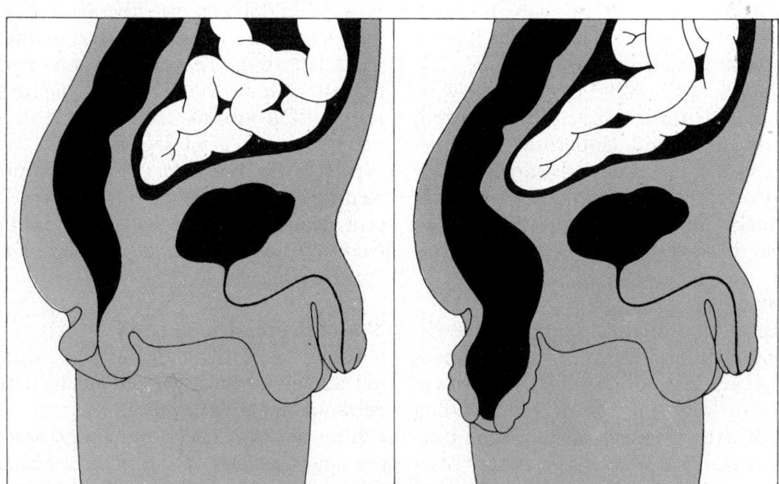

Partial rectal prolapse involves only the mucosa and a small mass of radial mucosal folds. However, in complete rectal prolapse (also known as procidentia), the full rectal wall, sphincter muscle, and a large mass of concentric mucosal folds protrude. Ulceration is possible after complete prolapse.

Signs and symptoms

In rectal prolapse, protrusion of tissue from the rectum may occur during defecation or walking. Other symptoms include a persistent sensation of rectal fullness, bloody diarrhea, and pain in the lower abdomen due to ulceration. Hemorrhoids or rectal polyps may coexist with a prolapse.

Diagnosis

Typical clinical features and visual examination confirm diagnosis. In complete prolapse, examination reveals the full thickness of the bowel wall and, possibly, the sphincter muscle protruding, and mucosa falling into bulky, concentric folds. In partial prolapse, examination reveals only partially protruding mucosa and a smaller mass of radial mucosal folds. Straining during examination may disclose the full extent of prolapse.

Treatment and special considerations

Treatment varies according to the underlying cause. Sometimes eliminating this cause (straining, coughing, nutritional disorders) is the only treatment necessary. In a child, prolapsed tissue usually diminishes as the child grows. In an older patient, injection of a sclerosing agent to cause a fibrotic reaction fixes the rectum in place. Severe or chronic prolapse requires surgical repair by strengthening or tightening the sphincters with wire or by anterior or rectal resection of prolapsed tissue.

- Help the patient prevent constipation by teaching correct diet and stool-softening regimen. Advise the patient with severe prolapse and incontinence to wear a perineal pad.
- Before surgery, explain possible complications, including permanent rectal incontinence.
- After surgery, watch for immediate complications (hemorrhage) and later ones (pelvic abscess, fever, pus drainage, pain, rectal stenosis, constipation, or pain on defecation). Teach perineal strengthening exercises: have the patient lie down, with his back flat on the mattress; then ask him to pull in his abdomen and squeeze while taking a deep breath; or have the patient repeatedly squeeze and relax his buttocks while sitting on a chair.

Anal Fissure

Anal fissure is a laceration or crack in the lining of the anus that extends to the circular muscle. Posterior fissure, the most common, is equally prevalent in males and females. Anterior fissure, the rarer type, is 10 times more common in females. Prognosis is very good, especially with fissurectomy and good anal hygiene.

Causes and incidence

Posterior fissure results from passage of large, hard stools that stretch the lining beyond its limits. Anterior fissure usually results from strain on the perineum during childbirth and, rarely, from scar stenosis. Occasionally, anal fissure is secondary to proctitis, anal tuberculosis, or carcinoma.

Signs and symptoms

Onset of an acute anal fissure is characterized by tearing, cutting, or burning pain during or immediately after bowel movement. A few drops of blood may streak toilet paper or underclothes. Painful anal sphincter spasms result from ulceration of a "sentinel pile" (swelling at the lower end of the fissure). A fissure may heal spontaneously and completely, or it may partially heal and break open again. Chronic fissure produces scar tissue that hampers normal bowel evacuation.

Diagnosis

Anoscopy showing longitudinal tear and typical clinical features help establish diagnosis. Digital examination that elicits pain and bleeding supports this diagnosis. Also, gentle traction on perianal skin can create sufficient eversion to visualize the fistula directly.

Treatment and special considerations

Treatment varies according to severity of the tear. For superficial fissures without hemorrhoids, forcible digital dilation of anal sphincters under local anesthetic stretches the lower portion of the anal sphincter. For complicated fissures, treatment includes surgical excision of tissue, adjacent skin, and mucosal tags, and division of internal sphincter muscle from external.

- Prepare the patient for rectal examination; explain the necessity for the procedure.
- Provide hot sitz baths, warm soaks, and local anesthetic ointment to relieve pain. A low–residue diet, adequate fluid intake, and stool softeners prevent straining during defecation.
- Control diarrhea with diphenoxylate or other antidiarrheals.

Pruritus Ani

Pruritus ani is perianal itching, irritation, or superficial burning. This disorder is more common in men than in women and is rare in children.

Causes and incidence

Factors that contribute to pruritus ani include overcleaning of perianal area (harsh soap, vigorous rubbing with washcloth or toilet paper); minor trauma caused by straining to defecate; poor hygiene; sensitivity to spicy foods, coffee, alcohol, food preservatives, perfumed or colored toilet paper, detergents, or certain fabrics; specific medications (antibiotics, antihypertensives, or antacids that cause diarrhea); excessive sweating (in occupations associated with physical labor or high stress levels); anal skin tags; systemic disease, especially diabetes; certain skin lesions, such as squamous cell carcinoma, basal cell carcinoma, Bowen's disease, Paget's disease, melanoma, syphilis, and tuberculosis; fungus or parasite infection; and local anorectal disease (fissure, hemorrhoids, fistula).

Signs and symptoms

The key symptom of pruritus ani is perianal itching or burning after a bowel movement, during stress, or at night. In acute pruritus ani, scratching produces reddened skin, with weeping excoriations; in chronic pruritus ani, skin becomes thick and leathery, with excessive pigmentation.

Diagnosis

Detailed patient history is essential. Rectal examination rules out fissures and fistulas; biopsy rules out carcinoma. Allergy testing may also be helpful.

Treatment and special considerations

After elimination of the underlying cause, treatment is symptomatic.

- Make sure the patient understands his condition and the causes.
- Advise the patient to avoid self-prescribed creams or powders, perfumed soaps, and colored toilet paper, because they may be irritating. Teach him to keep the perianal area clean and dry. Suggest witch hazel pads for wiping, and cotton balls tucked between buttocks to absorb moisture.

Proctitis

Proctitis is acute or chronic inflammation of the rectal mucosa. Prognosis is good unless massive bleeding occurs.

Causes and incidence

Contributing factors include chronic constipation, habitual laxative use, emotional upset, radiation (especially for cancer of the cervix and of the uterus), endocrine dysfunction, rectal injury, rectal medications, bacterial infections, allergies (especially to milk), vasomotor disturbance that interferes with normal muscle control, and food poisoning.

Signs and symptoms

Key symptoms include tenesmus, constipation, a feeling of rectal fullness, and left abdominal cramps. The patient feels an intense urge to defecate, which produces a small amount of stool that may contain blood and mucus.

Diagnosis

In acute proctitis, sigmoidoscopy shows edematous, bright-red or pink rectal mucosa that's thick, shiny, friable, and possibly ulcerated. In chronic proctitis, sigmoidoscopy shows thickened mucosa, loss of vascular pattern, and stricture of the rectal lumen. Other supportive tests include biopsy to rule out carcinoma and a bacteriologic examination. Detailed patient history is essential.

Treatment and special considerations

Primary treatment eliminates the underlying cause (fecal impaction, laxatives, or other medications). Soothing enemas, or steroid (hydrocortisone) suppositories or enemas may be helpful if proctitis is due to radiation. Tranquilizers may be appropriate for the patient with emotional stress.

Tell the patient to watch for and report bleeding and other persistent symptoms. Fully explain proctitis and its treatment to help him understand the disorder and prevent its recurrence. As appropriate, offer emotional support and reassurance during rectal examinations and treatment.

Selected References

Bolinger, Jeanne, et al. "Gastric Bypass For Morbid Obesity," *Nursing81* 11(1):54-59, January 1981.

Gannon, R.B., and Pickett, K. "Jaundice," *American Journal of Nursing* 83(3): 404-07, March 1983.

Grant, Allan Kerr, and Skyring, A.P., eds. *The Clinical Diagnosis of Gastrointestinal Disease*. Boston: Blackwell Scientific Pubns., 1981.

Greenberger, Norton J. *Gastrointestinal Disorders*. Chicago: Year Book Medical Pubs., 1980.

Kosel, K., et al. "Total Pancreatectomy and Islet Cell Autotransplantation," *American Journal of Nursing* 82:568-71, April 1982.

Sleisinger, Marvin H., and Fordtran, John S. *Gastrointestinal Disease: Pathophysiology, Diagnosis, Management*, 3rd ed., vols. 1 and 2. Philadelphia: W.B. Saunders Co., 1983.

Spiro, Howard M. *Clinical Gastroenterology*, 2nd ed. New York: Macmillan Publishing Co., 1983.

Sugar, E.C. "Hirschsprung's Disease," *American Journal of Nursing* 81:2065-67, November 1981.

Taylor, P.D. "Liver Transplantation," *American Journal of Nursing* 8:1672-73, September 1981.

Thompson, Marie Ann. "Managing the Patient with Liver Dysfunction," *Nursing81* 11(11):100-07, November 1981.

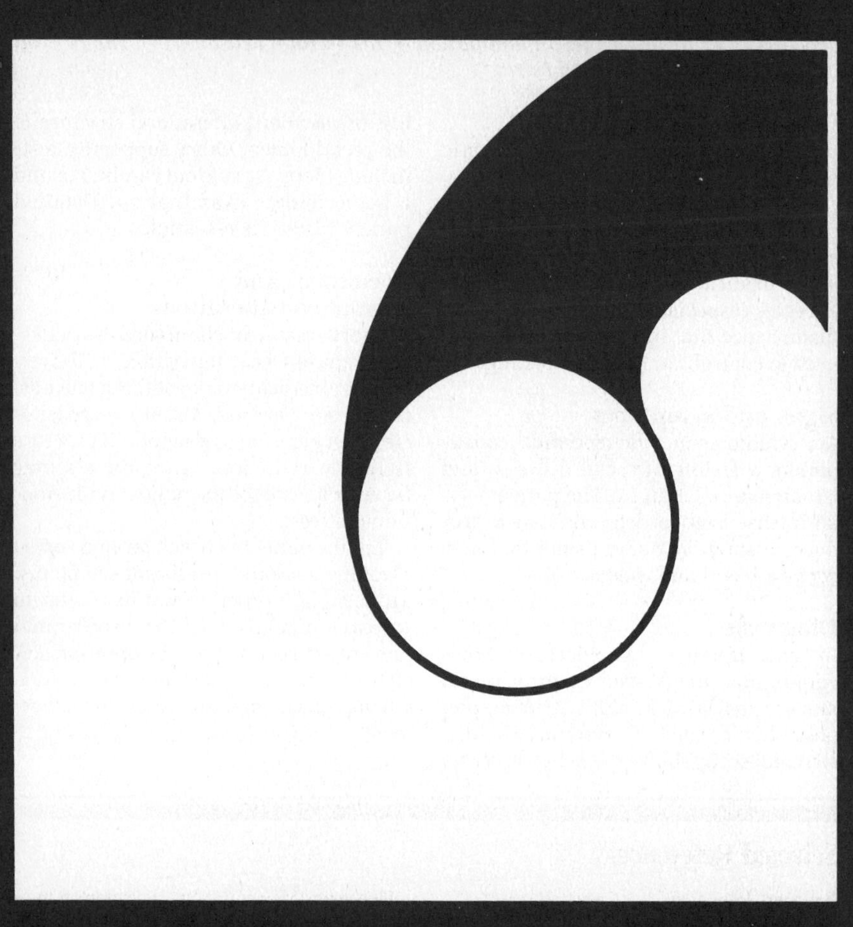

11 Hepatobiliary Disorders

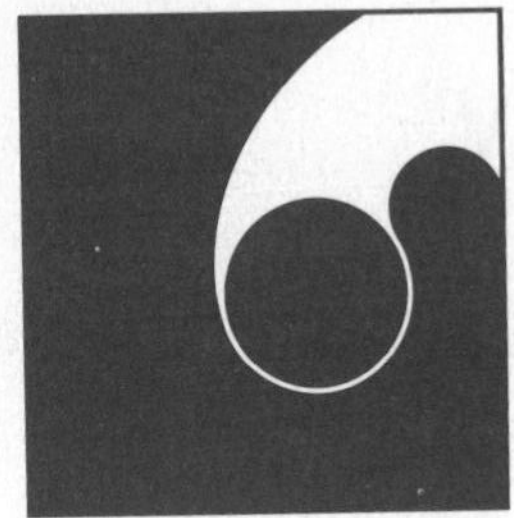

Hepatobiliary Disorders

Introduction

The liver is the largest internal organ in the human body, weighing slightly more than 3 lb (1,200 to 1,600 g) in the average adult. It's also one of the busiest, performing well over 100 separate functions. The most important of these are the formation and secretion of bile, detoxification of harmful substances, storage of vitamins, and metabolism of carbohydrates, fats, and proteins. This remarkably resilient organ serves as the body's warehouse and is absolutely essential to life.

Lobular structure

Located above the right kidney, stomach, pancreas, and intestines, and immediately below the diaphragm, the liver divides into a left and a right lobe (the right lobe is six times larger than the left), which are separated by the falciform ligament. Glisson's capsule, a network of connective tissue, covers the entire organ and extends into the parenchyma along blood vessels and bile ducts. Within the parenchyma, cylindrical lobules comprise the basic functional units of the liver, consisting of cellular plates that radiate from a central vein—like spokes in a wheel. Small bile canaliculi fit between the cells in the plates and empty into terminal bile ducts. These ducts join two larger ones, which merge into a single hepatic duct upon leaving the liver. The hepatic duct then joins the cystic duct to form the common bile duct.

The liver receives blood from two major sources: the hepatic artery and the portal vein. These two vessels carry approximately 1,500 ml of blood per minute to the liver, nearly 75% of which is supplied by the portal vein. Sinusoids—offshoots of both the hepatic artery and portal vein—run between each row of hepatic cells. Phagocytic Kupffer's cells, part of the reticuloendothelial system, line the sinusoids, destroying old or defective red blood cells and detoxifying harmful substances. The liver has a large lymphatic supply, and consequently, cancer frequently metastasizes there.

One of the liver's most important functions is the conversion of bilirubin, a breakdown product of hemoglobin, into bile. Liberated by the spleen into plasma and bound loosely to albumin, bilirubin reaches the liver in an unconjugated (water-insoluble) state. The liver then conjugates or dissociates it, converting it to a water-soluble derivative before excreting it as bile. All hepatic cells continually form bile.

The liver also detoxifies many substances through inactivation as well as through conjugation. Inactivation involves reduction, oxidation, and hydroxylation. To inactivate gonadal and adrenocortical hormones, for example, the liver reduces them to their derivatives, making them more soluble so they can be excreted in bile and urine. Another important liver function is the inactivation of many drugs. All the barbiturates (except phenobarbital and barbital), for example, are metabolized primarily in the liver. Such drugs must be used with caution in hepatic disease, since their effects may be markedly prolonged. As still another example of its amazing versatility, the liver forms vitamin A from certain vegetables and stores vitamins K, D, and B_{12}. It also stores iron in the form of ferritin.

Metabolic functions

Finally, the liver figures indispensably in the metabolism of the three major food groups: carbohydrates, fats, and proteins. In carbohydrate metabolism, the liver plays one of its most vital roles by extracting excess glucose from the blood and reserving it for times when blood glucose levels fall below normal; at such times, the liver releases glucose into the circulation, and then replenishes the supply by a process called glyconeogenesis (gluconeogenesis). To prevent dangerously low blood glucose levels, the liver can also convert galactose or amino acids into glucose. The liver also forms many critical chemical compounds from the intermediate products of carbohydrate metabolism.

Liver cells metabolize fats more quickly and efficiently than do any other body cells, breaking them down into glycerol and fatty acids, then converting the fatty acids into small molecules that can be oxidized. The liver performs more than half the body's preliminary breakdown of fats. This remarkable organ also produces great quantities of cholesterol and phospholipids, manufactures lipoproteins, and synthesizes fat from carbohydrates and proteins, to be transported in lipoproteins for eventual storage in adipose tissue.

Like so many of its functions, the liver's role in protein metabolism is essential to life. The liver deaminates amino acids so they can be used for energy or converted into fats or carbohydrates. It forms urea to remove ammonia from body fluids and all plasma proteins (as much as 50 to 100 g/day) except gamma globulin. The liver is such an effective synthesizer of protein that it can replenish as much as half its plasma proteins in 4 to 7 days. The liver also synthesizes nonessential amino acids and forms other important chemical compounds from amino acids.

Assessing for liver disease

A careful physical examination and patient history can often detect telltale signs of hepatic disease. Watch especially for its cardinal signs: jaundice (a result of increased serum bilirubin levels), ascites (often accompanied by hemodilution, edema, and oliguria), and hepatomegaly. Its symptoms may include right upper quadrant abdominal pain, lassitude, anorexia, nausea, and vomiting. To detect hepatomegaly, palpate the liver's left lobe, in the epigastrium between the xiphoid process and the umbilicus. Another primary sign is portal hypertension, or portal vein pressure greater than 6 to 12 cmH_2O. Auscultating a venous hum over the patient's abdomen suggests portal hypertension. Another test for portal hypertension is surgical insertion of a catheter into the portal vein to measure hepatic vein pressure.

Carefully assess the patient's neurologic status, since neurologic symptoms such as those associated with hepatic encephalopathy (confusion, muscle tremors, and asterixis) may signal onset of life-threatening hepatic failure.

Other common manifestations of hepatic disease include pallor (often linked to cirrhosis or carcinoma), parotid gland enlargement (in alcoholism-induced liver damage), Dupuytren's contracture, gynecomastia, testicular atrophy, decreased axillary or pubic hair, bleeding disorders (ecchymosis, purpura), spider angiomas, and palmar erythema. Careful abdominal palpation and auscultation can also detect hepatoma or metastasis (either turns the liver rock-hard and causes abdominal bruits) and postnecrotic cirrhosis. In hepatitis, palpation may elicit tenderness at the liver's edge. In neoplastic disease or hepatic abscess, auscultation may detect a pleural friction rub.

Comprehensive history essential

Ask if the patient has ever had jaundice, anemia, or a splenectomy. Ask about occupation and possible contact with rodents or exposure to toxins (carbon tetrachloride, beryllium, or vinyl chloride); all may predispose to hepatic disease. Don't overlook recent trips to other countries, especially to areas where hepatic disease is endemic.

Be sure to ask about alcohol consumption, which holds paramount significance in suspected hepatic disease. Remember, the alcoholic often deliberately underestimates how much he drinks, so interview friends and relatives as well. Ask about recent contact with a jaundiced person and about any recent blood or plasma transfusions, blood tests, tattoos, or dental work. Find out if the patient takes any drugs (especially parenteral narcotics, hallucinogens, or stimulants). Also, inquire if onset of symptoms was abrupt or insidious, or followed a recent abdominal injury that could have damaged the liver. Ask if the patient bruises or bleeds easily. Check color of stools and urine, and ask about any change in bowel habits. Ask if the patient's weight has fluctuated recently.

Liver function studies

The numerous tests that are available to detect hepatic disease reflect the liver's multiple functions. Perhaps the most useful tests are the so-called liver function studies, which measure serum enzymes and other substances. The following results are typical in hepatic disease:

- increased serum and urine bilirubin
- increased alkaline phosphatase and 5′-nucleotidase
- elevated transaminase levels (aminotransferases)—serum glutamic-oxaloacetic transaminase (SGOT) and serum glutamic-pyruvic transaminase (SGPT)—these enzymes are particularly useful in detecting hepatocellular damage, viral hepatitis, and acute hepatic necrosis.
- elevated gamma glutamyl transpeptidase (GGT)—this test is especially helpful, because this enzyme level rises even while hepatic damage is still minimal.
- hypoalbuminemia—suggests subacute or massive hepatic necrosis, cirrhosis
- hyperglobulinemia—suggests chronic inflammatory disorders
- prolonged prothrombin (PT) or partial thromboplastin time (PTT)—suggests hepatitis or cirrhosis
- elevated serum ammonia
- decreased serum total cholesterol
- positive lupus erythematosus (LE) cell

test in chronic active hepatitis and presence of hepatitis B antigen.

After liver trauma, liver function studies are less reliable. For instance, tests done long after the injury might miss an initial rise in serum transaminase levels. Less specific, and therefore less useful tests include elevated urine urobilinogen, lactic dehydrogenase (LDH), and ornithine carbamyl transferase (OCT).

Other useful diagnostic tests include:
• *abdominal X-rays*—may indicate gross hepatomegaly and hepatic masses by elevation or distortion of the diaphragm, and may show calcification in the gallbladder, biliary tree, pancreas, and liver
• *barium studies*—may indicate an elevated left hepatic lobe by displacing the barium-filled stomach laterally and posteriorly
• *oral cholecystography*—useful because parenchymal dysfunction and impaired bile excretion decrease excretion of contrast material and prevent visualization of the gallbladder
• *I.V. cholangiography*—visualizes the intrahepatic and extrahepatic bile ducts and localizes obstructing lesions in the major ducts
• *percutaneous transhepatic cholangiography*—distinguishes between mechanical biliary obstruction and intrahepatic cholestasis
• *angiography*—demonstrates hepatic arterial circulation (deranged in cirrhosis) and helps diagnose primary or secondary hepatic tumor masses
• *radioisotope liver scans (scintiscans)*—may show an area of decreased uptake (a "hole") using colloidal or bengal scan, or an area of increased uptake (a "hot spot") using gallium scan in hepatoma or hepatic abscess
• *portal and hepatic vein manometry*—localizes obstructions in the extrahepatic portion of the portal vein, portal inflow system, or pressure in the presinusoidal vessels
• *percutaneous liver biopsy*—can determine the cause of unexplained hepatomegaly, hepatosplenomegaly, cholestasis, or persistent abnormal liver function tests; also useful in suspected systemic infiltrative disease (sarcoidosis, for example) and suspected primary or metastatic hepatic tumors
• *peritoneoscopy*—visualizes the serosal lining, liver, gallbladder, spleen, and other organs; useful in unexplained hepatomegaly, ascites, or abdominal mass
• *laparotomy*—used only when thorough clinical, laboratory, and biopsy studies fail to identify hepatic disease.

Gallbladder anatomy

The gallbladder is a pear-shaped organ that lies in the fossa on the underside of the liver, and is capable of holding 50 ml of bile. Attached to the large organ above by connective tissue, the peritoneum, and blood vessels, the gallbladder is divided into four parts: the fundus, or broad inferior end; the body, which is funnel-shaped and bound to the duodenum; the neck, which empties into the cystic duct; and the infundibulum, which lies between the body and the neck, and sags to form Hartmann's pouch. The hepatic artery supplies both the cystic and hepatic ducts with blood, which drains out of the gallbladder through the cystic vein. Rich lymph vessels in the submucosal layer also drain the gallbladder, as well as the head of the pancreas.

The biliary duct system provides a passage for bile from the liver to the intestine and regulates bile flow. The gallbladder itself collects, concentrates, and stores bile. The normally functioning gallbladder also removes water and electrolytes from hepatic bile, increases the concentration of the larger solutes, and lowers its pH below 7. In gallbladder disease, bile becomes more alkaline, altering bile salts and cholesterol, and predisposing the organ to stone formation.

Mechanisms of contraction

The gallbladder responds to both sympathetic and parasympathetic innervation. Sympathetic stimulation inhibits muscle contraction; mild vagal stimulation causes the gallbladder to contract and the sphincter of Oddi to relax; stronger stimulation causes the sphincter to contract. The gallbladder also responds to substances released by the intestine. For instance, after chyme (semiliquid, partially digested food) enters the duodenum from the stomach, the duodenum releases cholecystokinin (CCK) and pancreozymin (PCZ) into the bloodstream, and stimulates the gallbladder to contract. The gallbladder also produces secretin, which stimulates the liver to secrete bile and CCK-PCZ. The gallbladder may also respond to some type of hormonal control, a theory based in part on the fact that the gallbladder empties more slowly during pregnancy.

Assessing for gallbladder disease

During your physical examination of a patient with suspected gallbladder disease, look for its telltale signs: pain, jaundice (a result of blockage of the common bile duct), fever, chills, indigestion, nausea, and intolerance of fatty foods. Pain may range from vague discomfort (as when pressure within the common bile duct gradually increases) to deep visceral pain (as when the gallbladder suddenly distends). Abrupt onset of pain with epigastric distress indicates gallbladder inflammation or obstruction of bile outflow by a stone or spasm.

Onset of jaundice also varies. If the gallbladder is healthy, jaundice may be delayed several days after bile duct blockage; if the gallbladder is absent or diseased, jaundice may appear within 24 hours after the blockage. Other effects of obstruction—pruritus, steatorrhea, and bleeding tendencies—may accompany jaundice. Gallbladder disorders rarely cause internal bleeding, but when they do—as in cholecystitis or obstructive clots in the biliary tree from gastrointestinal bleeding—they can be fatal.

Diagnostic tests

After a thorough patient history and careful assessment of clinical features, accurate diagnosis of gallbladder disease begins with oral *cholecystography*, which visualizes the gallbladder after the patient has ingested radiopaque dye. However, visualization depends on absorption of the dye from the small intestine, the liver's capacity to remove the dye from the blood and excrete it in bile, the patency of the ductal system, and the ability of the gallbladder to concentrate and store the dye. (This test may be repeated to rule out inadequate preparation.) Normally, the gallbladder fills about 13 hours after ingestion of the dye. Presence of stones or failure to visualize the gallbladder is significant.

Other diagnostic tests for gallbladder disease include:

- *percutaneous transhepatic cholangiography*—differentiates obstructive from intrahepatic types of jaundice, and detects hepatic dysfunction and calculi. Needle insertion in a bile duct permits withdrawal of bile and injection of dye. Fluoroscopic tests evaluate the filling of the hepatic and biliary trees.
- *duodenal drainage*—diagnoses cholelithiasis, choledocholithiasis, biliary obstruction, hepatic cirrhosis, and pancreatic disease, and differentiates types of jaundice. This test is especially useful when gallbladder function is poor or absent; when cholecystography fails to visualize the gallbladder or yields negative results despite continuing symptoms; or when cholecystography is contraindicated because of the patient's condition. In this test, a tube is passed through the gastrointestinal tract into the duodenum and CCK-PCZ is given to stimulate the gallbladder. This permits measurement of bile flow and also specimen collection, which is examined for mucus, blood, cholesterol crystals, pancreatic enzymes, cancer cells, bacteria, or calcium bilirubinate.
- *endoscopic retrograde cholangiopancreatography*—duodenal endoscopy dye injection and fluoroscopy are used to visualize and cannulate Vater's papilla. This test is particularly useful in locating obstruction, stones, carcinoma, or stricture.

Other appropriate tests for biliary disease are the same as those for hepatic disease, since their symptoms are similar and diagnosis often must distinguish between them.

LIVER DISEASES

Viral Hepatitis

A fairly common systemic disease, viral hepatitis is marked by liver cell destruction, necrosis, and autolysis, leading to anorexia, jaundice, and hepatomegaly. More than 70,000 cases are reported annually in the United States. This disease has three forms: type A (infectious or short-incubation hepatitis), type B (serum or long-incubation hepatitis), and type non-A, non-B hepatitis. All three types are found worldwide. Type B hepatitis rarely occurs in epidemics but has a higher mortality than type A hepatitis, which tends to be benign and self-limiting. Type non-A, non-B hepatitis is similar to type B, but less severe.

Causes and incidence

Type A hepatitis is highly contagious and is usually transmitted by the fecal-oral route, although occasionally it's transmitted parenterally. The most common cause is ingestion of contaminated food, water, or milk. Outbreaks of type A hepatitis often occur after people have eaten seafood that came from polluted water. Type B hepatitis, which is generally transmitted parenterally, can also be spread through contact with human secretions and feces. Nurses, doctors, laboratory technicians, blood bank workers, and dentists are frequent victims of type B hepatitis, often as a result of wearing defective gloves while working. In addition, the incidence of both type A and type B hepatitides appears to be rising among homosexuals, presumably because of oral and anal sexual contact. Type non-A, non-B hepatitis accounts

COMPARING TYPES OF HEPATITIS

	TYPE A (infectious)	TYPE B (serum)	TYPE NON-A, NON-B
Age incidence	Children, young adults	Any age	Adults
Seasonal incidence	Fall, winter	Anytime	Anytime
Transmission	Food, water, semen, tears, stools, and possibly urine	Serum, blood and blood products, and semen	Serum, blood and blood products, and possibly food
Incubation	15 to 45 days	40 to 180 days	15 to 160 days
Onset	Sudden	Insidious	Insidious
Serum markers	Anti-HAV	HBsAg + anti-HBs	
Prognosis	Good	Worsens with age	Moderate
Carrier state	No	Yes	Unknown

for 10% of posttransfusion hepatitis in the United States, and transmission usually results from commercial blood donations.

In most patients with hepatitis, liver cells eventually regenerate with little or no residual damage. Patients usually recover readily, with a lifelong immunity to type A hepatitis (but not to type B). Old age and serious underlying disorders make complications more likely. Prognosis is poor if edema and hepatic encephalopathy develop.

Signs and symptoms

The preicteric phase of viral hepatitis begins with fatigue, malaise, arthralgia, myalgia, headache, anorexia, photophobia, pharyngitis, cough, and coryza. This disease also causes nausea and vomiting, often with alterations in the senses of taste and smell. Fever, with temperature of 100° to 101° F. (37.7° to 38.3° C.), may be associated with liver and lymph node enlargement. Symptoms begin suddenly in type A hepatitis and insidiously in type B; they disappear with the onset of jaundice. Type non-A, non-B hepatitis has a clinical course similar to type B hepatitis but is milder.

Mild weight loss, dark urine, clay-colored stools, and yellow scleras and skin signal the start of the icteric phase of hepatitis. In this second phase, anorexia may continue, the liver remains enlarged and tender, and the patient complains of discomfort and pain in the right upper abdominal quadrant. Splenomegaly, cervical adenopathy, bile obstruction, irritability, and severe pruritus may develop.

Jaundice may last from 1 to 2 weeks. It results from the damaged liver cells' inability to remove bilirubin from the blood but doesn't indicate the disease's severity. Occasionally, hepatitis occurs without jaundice. After jaundice disappears, the patient continues to experience fatigue, flatulence, abdominal pain or tenderness, and indigestion, although appetite usually returns and liver enlargement subsides. The posticteric, or convalescent, phase generally lasts from 2 to 12 weeks; this phase often lasts longer in patients with acute type B or non-A, non-B hepatitis.

Complications include chronic hepatitis, which may be benign (chronic persistent hepatitis) or active (chronic aggressive hepatitis). About 25% of patients with chronic aggressive hepatitis die from hepatic failure. Life-threatening fulminant hepatitis develops in about 1% of patients, causing unremitting hepatic failure with encephalopathy. It progresses to coma and commonly leads to death within 2 weeks.

Diagnosis

Patient history revealing recent exposure to drugs, chemicals, or jaundiced persons or recent blood transfusions or injections, in the presence of typical clinical features, strongly suggests viral hepatitis. Recently pierced ears may also be significant, since contaminated instruments can cause hepatitis.

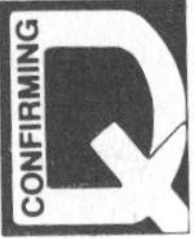

The presence of hepatitis B surface antigens (HBsAg) and hepatitis B antibodies (anti-HBs) confirms a diagnosis of type B hepatitis. HBsAg—sometimes called Australia antigen because it was originally discovered in the serum of an Australian aborigine—appears early in the disease, but blood levels may be negative later, giving a false-negative reading if drawn too late. Detection of an antibody to type A hepatitis (anti-HAV) confirms diagnosis.

In the presence of HBsAg, anti-HBs, and anti-HAV, other laboratory results, such as atypical lymphocytes and hypoglycemia, support a diagnosis of viral hepatitis, type A or type B; in their absence, these tests confirm type non-A, non-B hepatitis:

- prolonged prothrombin time (more than 3 seconds longer than normal indicates severe liver damage)
- elevated serum glutamic-oxaloacetic transaminase and serum glutamic-pyruvic transaminase levels and slightly elevated serum alkaline phosphatase, reflecting the presence of enzymes in the blood

- elevated serum and urine bilirubin (with jaundice)
- low serum albumin and high serum globulin
- increased cephalin flocculation and thymol turbidity levels
- liver biopsy and scan showing patchy necrosis.

Hepatitis may be mistaken for infectious mononucleosis. During the preicteric phase of acute type B hepatitis, a serum sickness–like syndrome sometimes occurs, causing arthralgia, arthritis, rash, angioedema, and sometimes hematuria and proteinuria, which may be misdiagnosed as rheumatoid arthritis or lupus erythematosus.

About 10% of patients with type B hepatitis remain HBsAg-positive for 6 months. With anti-HBs and chronic HBsAg, the patient may be a carrier or have chronic low-grade active hepatitis.

Treatment

No specific treatment exists for hepatitis. The patient should rest in the early stages of the illness and combat anorexia by eating small meals high in calories and protein. (Protein intake should be reduced if signs of precoma—lethargy, confusion, mental changes—develop.) Large meals are usually better tolerated in the morning. Antiemetics (trimethobenzamide or benzquinamide) may be given ½ hour before meals to relieve nausea and prevent vomiting; phenothiazines have a cholestatic effect and should be avoided. If vomiting persists, the patient will require I.V. infusions.

In severe hepatitis, corticosteroids may give the patient a sense of well-being and may stimulate appetite, while decreasing itching and inflammation. Give corticosteroids sparingly, however, since their use in hepatitis is controversial.

Report all cases of hepatitis to health officials. Ask the patient to name anyone he came in contact with recently.

Special considerations

Base your care plan on supportive care, observation, and emotional support.

- Wear gloves when handling fluids and feces from a patient with type A hepatitis and when drawing blood from a patient with type B hepatitis.
- Inform visitors about isolation precautions.
- Encourage the patient to eat. Don't overload his meal tray; too much food

PREVENTION OF VIRAL HEPATITIS

Immune globulin (IG)—or gamma globulin—is 80% to 90% effective in preventing type A hepatitis in contacts. In confirmed type A cases, IG should be given to high-risk contacts as soon as possible after exposure, but within 2 weeks after jaundice appears in the patients. Type A hepatitis is transmitted through the fecal-oral route; household, intimate, sexual, and institutional contacts are at high risk.

Most IG made in the United States contains low titers of antibody against type B hepatitis, which probably transmits some passive protection. However, a combination of hepatitis B vaccine (HB vaccine) and hepatitis B immune globulin (HBIG) currently offers the best protection after exposure to type B hepatitis. HB vaccine and HBIG should be given prophylactically to newborn infants whose mothers are HBsAg-positive. HBIG should be given I.M. after the infant has stabilized, preferably within 12 hours after birth; HB vaccine may be given I.M. at the same time in a different site, or within 7 days after birth. Infants of HBeAg-positive mothers need extra HBIG with the vaccine. HB vaccine and HBIG should be given prophylactically within 24 hours to persons who have had significant oral or percutaneous contact with an HBsAg-positive fluid. Sexual contact with an HBsAg-positive patient may require a single dose of HBIG if it can be given within 14 days of the last contact. If the patient remains HBsAg-positive 3 months after detection, the contact may need a second dose. If he becomes a chronic carrier, the contact may need HB vaccine. Homosexual men may need a dose of HBIG and the HB vaccine series.

on the tray will only diminish his appetite. And don't overmedicate; this too will diminish his appetite. Force fluids (at least 4,000 ml/day). Encourage the anorectic patient to drink fruit juices. Also offer chipped ice and effervescent soft drinks, to maintain adequate hydration without inducing vomiting.

- Record weight daily, and keep accurate intake and output records. Observe feces for color, consistency, frequency, and amount.
- Watch for signs of hepatic coma, dehydration, pneumonia, vascular problems, and decubitus ulcers.
- With fulminant hepatitis, maintain electrolyte balance and a patent airway, and control bleeding. Be sure to correct hypoglycemia and any other complications while awaiting liver regeneration and repair.
- Before discharge, emphasize the importance of having regular medical checkups for at least 1 year. Be sure to warn the patient not to drink any alcohol during this time period, and teach him how to recognize signs of a recurrence. Refer the patient for follow-up, as needed.

Nonviral Hepatitis

Nonviral inflammation of the liver (toxic or drug-induced hepatitis) is a form of hepatitis that usually results from exposure to certain chemicals or drugs. Most patients recover from this illness, although a few develop fulminating hepatitis or cirrhosis.

Causes

Various hepatotoxins—carbon tetrachloride, acetaminophen, trichloroethylene, poisonous mushrooms, vinyl chloride—can cause the toxic form of this disease. Following exposure to these agents, liver damage (diffuse fatty infiltration of liver cells and necrosis) usually occurs within 24 to 48 hours, depending on the size of the dose. Alcohol, anoxia, and preexisting liver disease exacerbate the toxic effects of some of these agents.

Drug-induced (idiosyncratic) hepatitis may stem from a hypersensitivity reaction unique to the affected individual, unlike toxic hepatitis, which appears to affect all persons indiscriminately. Among the drugs that may cause this type of hepatitis are halothane, sulfonamides, isoniazid, methyldopa, and phenothiazines (cholestasis-induced hepatitis). In hypersensitive persons, symptoms of hepatic dysfunction may appear at any time during or after exposure to these drugs but usually emerge after 2 to 5 weeks of therapy. Not all adverse drug reactions are toxic. Oral contraceptives, for example, may impair liver function and produce jaundice without causing necrosis, fatty infiltration of liver cells, or a hypersensitive reaction.

Signs and symptoms

Clinical features of toxic and drug-induced hepatitis vary with the severity of the liver damage and the causative agent. In most patients, symptoms resemble those of viral hepatitis: anorexia, nausea, vomiting, jaundice, dark urine, hepatomegaly, possible abdominal pain (with acute onset and massive necrosis), and clay-colored stools or pruritus with the cholestatic form of hepatitis. Carbon tetrachloride poisoning also produces headache, dizziness, drowsiness, and vasomotor collapse; halothane-related hepatitis produces fever, moderate leukocytosis, and eosinophilia; chlorpromazine produces abrupt fever, rash, arthralgias, lymphadenopathy, and epigastric or right upper quadrant pain.

Diagnosis

Diagnostic findings include elevations in

serum transaminase (SGOT, SGPT), both total and direct bilirubin (with cholestasis), alkaline phosphatase, white blood cell (WBC) count, and eosinophils (possible in drug-induced type). Liver biopsy may help identify the underlying pathology, especially infiltration with WBCs and eosinophils. Liver function tests have limited value in distinguishing between nonviral and viral hepatitis.

Treatment and special considerations

Effective treatment must remove the causative agent by lavage, catharsis, or hyperventilation, depending on the route of exposure. Dimercaprol may serve as an antidote for toxic hepatitis caused by gold or arsenic poisoning but doesn't prevent drug-induced hepatitis caused by other substances. Corticosteroids may be ordered for patients with the drug-induced type. Thioctic acid, an investigational drug, may be successful with mushroom poisoning. Preventive measures should include instructing the patient about the proper use of drugs and the proper handling of cleaning agents and solvents.

Cirrhosis and Fibrosis

Cirrhosis is a chronic hepatic disease characterized by diffuse destruction and fibrotic regeneration of hepatic cells. As necrotic tissue yields to fibrosis, this disease alters liver structure and normal vasculature, impairs blood and lymph flow, and ultimately causes hepatic insufficiency. It's twice as common in men as in women and is especially prevalent among malnourished chronic alcoholics over age 50. Mortality is high: many patients die within 5 years of onset. Prognosis is better in noncirrhotic forms of hepatic fibrosis, which cause minimal hepatic dysfunction and don't destroy liver cells.

Causes

The following clinical types of cirrhosis reflect its diverse etiology:

- *Portal, nutritional, or alcoholic cirrhosis* (Laennec's), the most common type, occurs in 30% to 50% of cirrhotic patients, up to 90% of whom have a history of alcoholism. Liver damage results from malnutrition, especially of dietary protein, and chronic alcohol ingestion. Fibrous tissue forms in portal areas and around central veins.
- *Biliary cirrhosis* (15% to 20% of patients) results from bile duct diseases, which suppress bile flow.
- *Postnecrotic (posthepatitic) cirrhosis* (10% to 30% of patients) stems from various types of hepatitis.
- *Pigment cirrhosis* (5% to 10% of patients) may stem from disorders such as hemochromatosis.
- *Cardiac cirrhosis* (rare) refers to liver damage caused by right heart failure.
- *Idiopathic cirrhosis* (about 10% of patients) has no known cause.

Noncirrhotic fibrosis may result from schistosomiasis or congenital hepatic fibrosis, or may be idiopathic.

Signs and symptoms

Clinical manifestations of cirrhosis and fibrosis are similar for all types, regardless of cause. Early indications are vague but usually include gastrointestinal symptoms (anorexia, indigestion, nausea, vomiting, constipation, or diarrhea) and dull abdominal ache. Major and late symptoms develop as a result of hepatic insufficiency and portal hypertension, and include the following:

- *respiratory*—pleural effusion, limited thoracic expansion due to abdominal ascites, interfering with efficient gas exchange and leading to hypoxia
- *CNS*—progressive symptoms of hepatic encephalopathy: lethargy, mental

PORTAL HYPERTENSION AND ESOPHAGEAL VARICES

Portal hypertension—elevated pressure in the portal vein—occurs when blood flow meets increased resistance. The disorder is a common result of cirrhosis but may also stem from mechanical obstruction and occlusion of the hepatic veins (Budd-Chiari syndrome). As portal pressure rises, blood backs up into the spleen and flows through collateral channels to the venous system, bypassing the liver. Consequently, portal hypertension produces splenomegaly with thrombocytopenia, dilated collateral veins (esophageal varices, hemorrhoids, or prominent abdominal veins), and ascites. Nevertheless, in many patients the first sign of portal hypertension is bleeding from esophageal varices—dilated tortuous veins in the submucosa of the lower esophagus. Such varices often cause massive hematemesis, requiring emergency treatment to control hemorrhage and prevent hypovolemic shock.

- *Endoscopy* identifies the ruptured varix as the bleeding site and excludes other potential sources in the upper gastrointestinal tract.
- *Angiography* may aid diagnosis but is less precise than endoscopy.
- *Vasopressin* infused into the superior mesenteric artery may temporarily stop bleeding; when angiography is unavailable, vasopressin may be infused by I.V. drip, diluted with 5% dextrose in water (except in patients with coronary vascular disease), but this route is usually less effective.
- *A Minnesota* or *Sengstaken-Blakemore tube* may also help control hemorrhage by applying pressure on bleeding site. Iced saline lavage through the tube may help control bleeding.

The use of vasopressin or a Minnesota or Sengstaken-Blakemore tube is a temporary measure, especially in the patient with a severely deteriorated liver. Fresh blood and fresh frozen plasma, if available, are preferred for blood transfusions, to replace clotting factors. Treatment with lactulose promotes elimination of old blood from the gastrointestinal tract and combats excessive production and accumulation of ammonia.

Appropriate surgical bypass procedures include portosystemic anastomosis, splenorenal shunt, and mesocaval shunt. A portacaval or a mesocaval shunt decreases pressure within the liver, as well as reduces ascites, plasma loss, and risk of hemorrhage by directing blood from the liver into collateral vessels. Emergency shunts carry a mortality of 25% to 50%. Clinical evidence suggests that the portosystemic bypass does not prolong the patient's survival time; however, he will eventually die of hepatic coma rather than of hemorrhage.

Care for the patient who has portal hypertension with esophageal varices focuses on careful monitoring for signs and symptoms of hemorrhage and subsequent hypotension, compromised oxygen supply, and altered level of consciousness.

- Monitor vital signs, urinary output, and central venous pressure to determine fluid volume status.
- Assess level of consciousness often.
- Provide emotional support and reassurance in the wake of massive gastrointestinal bleeding, which is always a frightening experience.
- Keep the patient as quiet and comfortable as possible, but remember that tolerance for sedatives and tranquilizers may be decreased because of liver damage.
- Clean the patient's mouth, which may be dry and flecked with dried blood.
- Carefully monitor the patient with a Minnesota or Sengstaken-Blakemore tube in place for persistent bleeding in gastric drainage, signs of asphyxiation from tube displacement, proper inflation of balloons, and correct traction to maintain tube placement.

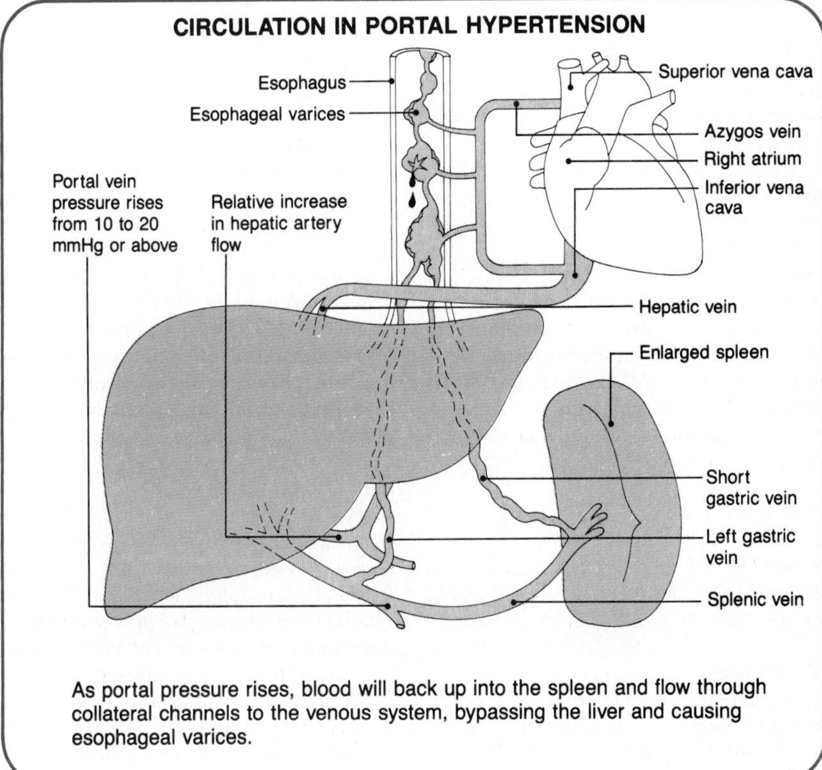

As portal pressure rises, blood will back up into the spleen and flow through collateral channels to the venous system, bypassing the liver and causing esophageal varices.

changes, slurred speech, asterixis (flapping tremor), peripheral neuritis, paranoia, hallucinations, extreme obtundation, and coma

- *hematologic*—bleeding tendencies (nosebleeds, easy bruising, bleeding gums), anemia
- *endocrine*—testicular atrophy, menstrual irregularities, gynecomastia, and loss of chest and axillary hair
- *skin*—severe pruritus, extreme dryness, poor tissue turgor, abnormal pigmentation, spider angiomas, palmar erythema, and possibly jaundice
- *hepatic*—jaundice, hepatomegaly, ascites, edema of the legs, hepatic encephalopathy, and hepatorenal syndrome comprise the other major effects of full-fledged cirrhosis
- *miscellaneous*—musty breath, enlarged superficial abdominal veins, muscle atrophy, pain in the upper right abdominal quadrant that worsens when the patient sits up or leans forward, palpable liver or spleen, and temperature of 101° to 103° F. (38.3° to 39.4° C.). Bleeding from esophageal varices results from portal hypertension.

Diagnosis

Liver biopsy, the definitive test for cirrhosis, detects destruction and fibrosis of hepatic tissue; liver scan shows abnormal thickening and a liver mass. Cholecystography and cholangiography visualize the gallbladder and the biliary duct system, respectively; splenoportal venography visualizes the portal venous system. Percutaneous transhepatic cholangiography differentiates extrahepatic from intrahepatic obstructive jaundice and discloses hepatic pathology and presence of gallstones.

The following laboratory findings are

characteristic of cirrhosis:

- decreased white blood cell count, hemoglobin and hematocrit, albumin, serum electrolytes (sodium, potassium, chlorides, and magnesium), and cholinesterase
- elevated globulin, serum ammonia, total bilirubin, alkaline phosphatase, serum transaminase (SGOT and SGPT), lactate dehydrogenase, and thymol turbidity
- anemia, neutropenia, and thrombocytopenia, with prolonged prothrombin and partial thromboplastin times
- deficiencies of vitamins A, B_{12}, C, and K; folic acid; and iron
- abnormal Bromsulphalein (BSP) excretion and glucose tolerance test (possible)
- positive tests for galactose tolerance and urine bilirubin
- fecal urobilinogen greater than 40 to 280/mg in 24 hours, urine urobilinogen greater than 0 to 1.16/mg in 24 hours.

Treatment

Treatment is designed to remove or alleviate the underlying cause of cirrhosis or fibrosis, prevent further liver damage, and prevent or treat complications. The patient may benefit from a high-calorie and moderate- to high-protein diet, but developing hepatic encephalopathy mandates restricted protein intake. In addition, sodium is usually restricted to 200 to 500 mg/day, fluids to 1,000 to 1,500 ml/day.

If the patient's condition continues to deteriorate, he may need tube feedings or hyperalimentation. Other supportive measures include supplemental vitamins—A, B complex, D, and K—to compensate for the liver's inability to store them, and vitamin B_{12}, folic acid, and thiamine for deficiency anemia. Rest, moderate exercise, and avoidance of exposure to infections and toxic agents are essential.

Drug therapy requires special caution, since the cirrhotic liver can't detoxify harmful substances efficiently. Alcohol is prohibited; sedatives should be avoided or prescribed with great care. When absolutely necessary, antiemetics, such as trimethobenzamide or benzquinamide, may be given for nausea; vasopressin, for esophageal varices; and diuretics, such as furosemide or spironolactone, for edema. However, diuretics require careful monitoring, since fluid and electrolyte imbalance may precipitate hepatic encephalopathy.

Paracentesis and infusions of salt-poor albumin may alleviate ascites. Surgical procedures include ligation of varices, splenectomy, esophagogastric resection, and splenorenal or portacaval anastomosis to relieve portal hypertension. Programs for prevention of cirrhosis usually emphasize avoidance of alcohol.

Special considerations

Cirrhotic patients need close observation, first-rate supportive care, and sound nutritional counseling.

- Check skin, gums, stools, and emesis regularly for bleeding. Apply pressure to injection sites to prevent bleeding. Warn the patient against taking aspirin, straining at stool, and blowing his nose or sneezing too vigorously. Suggest using an electric razor and soft toothbrush.
- Observe closely for signs of behavioral or personality changes. Report increasing stupor, lethargy, hallucinations, or neuromuscular dysfunction. Arouse the patient periodically to determine level of consciousness. Watch for asterixis, a sign of developing hepatic encephalopathy.
- To assess fluid retention, weigh the patient and measure abdominal girth daily, inspect ankles and sacrum for dependent edema, and accurately record intake and output. Carefully evaluate the patient before, during, and after paracentesis; this drastic loss of fluid may induce shock.
- To prevent skin breakdown associated with edema and pruritus, avoid using soap when you bathe the patient; instead, use lubricating lotion or moisturizing agents. Handle the patient gently, and turn and reposition him often to keep skin intact.
- Tell the patient that rest and good nutrition will conserve energy and decrease

metabolic demands on the liver. Urge him to eat frequent small meals. Stress the need to avoid infections and abstain from alcohol. Refer the patient to Alcoholics Anonymous, if necessary.

Liver Abscess

A liver abscess occurs when bacteria or protozoa destroy hepatic tissue, producing a cavity, which fills with infectious organisms, liquefied liver cells, and leukocytes. Necrotic tissue then walls off the cavity from the rest of the liver.

While a liver abscess is relatively uncommon, it carries a mortality of 30% to 50%. This rate soars to more than 80% with multiple abscesses and to more than 90% with complications, such as rupture into the peritoneum, pleura, or pericardium. About 70% of pyogenic liver abscesses occur among men, usually between ages 20 and 30.

Causes

In pyogenic liver abscesses, the common infecting organisms are *Escherichia coli, Klebsiella, Enterobacter* species, *Salmonella, Staphylococcus,* and enterococcus. Such organisms may invade the liver directly after a liver wound, or they may spread from the lungs, skin, or other organs by the hepatic artery, portal vein, or biliary tract. Pyogenic abscesses are generally multiple and often follow cholecystitis, peritonitis, pneumonia, and bacterial endocarditis.

An amebic abscess results from infection with the protozoa *Entamoeba histolytica,* the organism that causes amebic dysentery. Amebic liver abscesses usually occur singly, in the right lobe.

Signs and symptoms

The clinical manifestations of a liver abscess depend on the degree of involvement. Some patients are acutely ill; in others, the abscess is recognized only at autopsy, after death from another illness. Onset of symptoms of a pyogenic abscess is usually sudden; in an amebic abscess, onset is more insidious. Common signs include right abdominal and shoulder pain, weight loss, fever, chills, diaphoresis, nausea, vomiting, and anemia. Signs of right pleural effusion, such as dyspnea and pleural pain, develop if the abscess extends through the diaphragm. Liver damage may cause jaundice.

Diagnosis

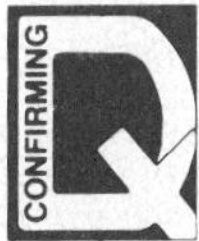

A liver scan showing filling defects at the area of the abscess more than ¾" (1.9 cm), together with characteristic clinical features, confirms this diagnosis. A liver ultrasound may indicate defects caused by the abscess but is less definitive than a liver scan. In a chest X-ray, the diaphragm on the affected side appears raised and fixed. A computed tomography scan verifies diagnosis after liver scan or ultrasound. Relevant laboratory values include elevated serum transaminase (SGOT, SGPT), alkaline phosphatase, bilirubin, and white blood cell count (usually more elevated in pyogenic abscess than in amebic), and decreased serum albumin. In pyogenic abscess, a blood culture can identify the bacterial agent; in amebic abscess, a stool culture and serologic and hemagglutination tests can isolate *Entamoeba histolytica.*

Treatment

If the organism causing the liver abscess is unknown, long-term antibiotic therapy begins immediately with aminoglycosides, cephalosporins, clindamycin, or chloramphenicol. If cultures demonstrate that the infectious organism is *Escherichia coli,* treatment includes ampicillin; if *Entamoeba histolytica,* it includes emetine, chloroquine, or metronidazole. The therapy continues for 2 to 4 months. Surgery is usually avoided, but it may be done for a single pyogenic abscess or for an amebic abscess that fails to respond to antibiotics.

Special considerations

• Provide supportive care, monitor vital signs (especially temperature), and maintain fluid and nutritional intake.

• Administer anti-infectives and antibiotics, as ordered, and watch for possible side effects. Stress the importance of compliance with therapy.

• Explain diagnostic and surgical procedures.

• Watch carefully for complications of abdominal surgery, such as hemorrhage or infection.

Fatty Liver

(Steatosis)

A common clinical finding, fatty liver is the accumulation of triglycerides and other fats in liver cells. In severe fatty liver, fat comprises as much as 40% of the liver's weight (as opposed to 5% in a normal liver) and the weight of the liver may increase from 3.31 lb (1.5 kg) to as much as 11 lb (4.9 kg). Minimal fatty changes are temporary and asymptomatic; severe or persistent changes may cause liver dysfunction. Fatty liver is usually reversible by simply eliminating the cause; however, this disorder may result in recurrent infection or sudden death from fat emboli in the lungs.

Causes

The most common cause of fatty liver in the United States and in Europe is chronic alcoholism, with the severity of hepatic disease directly related to the amount of alcohol consumed. Other causes include malnutrition (especially protein deficiency), obesity, diabetes mellitus, jejunoileal bypass surgery, Cushing's syndrome, Reye's syndrome, pregnancy, large doses of hepatotoxins—such as I.V. tetracycline—carbon tetrachloride intoxication, prolonged I.V. hyperalimentation, and DDT poisoning. Whatever the cause, fatty infiltration of the liver probably results from mobilization of fatty acids from adipose tissues or altered fat metabolism.

Signs and symptoms

Clinical features of fatty liver vary with the degree of lipid infiltration, and many patients are asymptomatic. The most typical sign is a large, tender liver (hepatomegaly). Common symptoms include upper right quadrant pain (with massive or rapid infiltration), ascites, edema, jaundice, and fever (all with hepatic necrosis or biliary stasis). Nausea, vomiting, and anorexia are less common. Splenomegaly usually accompanies cirrhosis. Rarer changes are spider angiomas, varices, transient gynecomastia, and menstrual disorders.

Diagnosis

Typical clinical features—especially in patients with chronic alcoholism, malnutrition, poorly controlled diabetes mellitus, or obesity—suggest fatty liver.

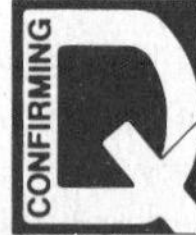

A liver biopsy confirms excessive fat in the liver. The following liver function tests support this diagnosis:

• *albumin*—somewhat low
• *globulin*—usually elevated
• *cholesterol*—usually elevated
• *total bilirubin*—elevated
• *alkaline phosphatase*—elevated
• *transaminase*—usually low (less than 300 units)
• *prothrombin time*—possibly prolonged.

Other findings may include anemia, leukocytosis, elevated white blood cell count, albuminuria, hyperglycemia or hypoglycemia, and deficiencies of iron, folic acid, and vitamin B_{12}.

Treatment

Treatment for fatty liver is essentially supportive and consists of correcting the underlying condition or eliminating its cause. For instance, when fatty liver results from I.V. hyperalimentation, decreasing the rate of carbohydrate infusion may correct the disease. In alcoholic fatty liver, abstinence from alcohol and a proper diet can begin to correct liver changes within 4 to 8 weeks. Such correction requires comprehensive patient teaching.

Special considerations

- Suggest counseling for alcoholics. Provide emotional support for their families as well.
- Teach diabetics and their families about proper care, such as the purpose of insulin injections, diet, and exercise. Refer them to public health nurses or to group classes, as necessary, to promote compliance with treatment. Emphasize the need for long-term medical supervision, and urge them to report any changes in their health immediately.
- Instruct obese patients and their families about proper diet. Warn against fad diets, since they may be nutritionally inadequate. Recommend medical supervision for those more than 20% overweight. Encourage attendance at group diet and exercise programs, and, if necessary, suggest behavior modification programs to correct eating habits. Be sure to follow up on your patient's progress, and provide positive reinforcement for any weight loss.
- Assess for malnutrition, especially protein deficiency, in those with chronic illness. Suggest an adequate diet.
- Advise patients receiving hepatotoxins and those who risk occupational exposure to DDT to watch for and immediately report signs of toxicity.
- Inform all patients that fatty liver is reversible *only* if they strictly follow the therapeutic program; otherwise, they risk permanent liver damage.

MASSIVE ASCITES IN FATTY LIVER

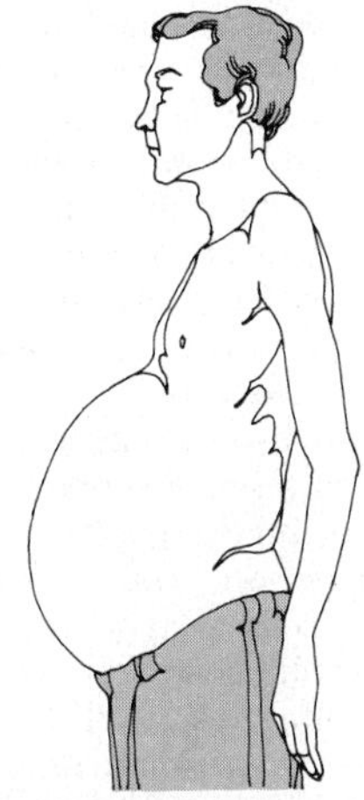

A possible effect of fatty liver is massive ascites. Emaciated extremities and upper thorax are also typical of ascites.

Wilson's Disease

(Hepatolenticular degeneration)

Wilson's disease is a rare, inherited metabolic disorder characterized by retention of excessive amounts of copper in the liver, brain, kidneys, and corneas. These deposits produce the characteristic Kayser-Fleischer rings and eventually lead to tissue necrosis and fibrosis, causing a variety of clinical effects, especially hepatic disease and neurologic changes. Wilson's disease is progressive and, if untreated, leads to fatal hepatic failure.

Causes and incidence

Wilson's disease is inherited as an autosomal recessive trait only when *both* parents carry the abnormal gene. There is a 25% chance that carrier parents will transmit Wilson's disease (and a 50% chance they will transmit the carrier state) to each of their offspring. The disease occurs most often among eastern European Jews, Sicilians, and southern Italians, probably as a result of consanguineous marriages.

This genetic disorder causes excessive intestinal absorption of copper and subsequent decreased excretion of copper in the stool. Copper accumulates first in the liver. As liver cells necrose, they release copper into the bloodstream, which then carries it to other tissues. For example, in the kidneys, excretion of excessive amounts of unbound copper in the urine (hypercupriuria) results from deficiency of ceruloplasmin, a serum enzyme normally bound to copper. The deposit of copper in the tissue decreases serum copper (hypocupremia).

Signs and symptoms

Clinical manifestations of Wilson's disease usually appear between ages 6 and 20, although signs and symptoms can occur as late as age 40. They result from damage to the body tissues caused by progressive copper deposition and vary according to the patient and the state of his disease.

KAYSER-FLEISCHER RING

Wilson's disease produces a characteristic rust-colored ring around the cornea (Kayser-Fleischer ring), caused by copper deposits.

The most characteristic symptom of Wilson's disease is Kayser-Fleischer ring—a rusty brown ring of pigment at the periphery of the corneas. Fever may also occur in acute disease or with intercurrent infection. Other clinical features depend on the area affected:

- *liver* (including spleen): hepatomegaly, splenomegaly, ascites, jaundice, hematemesis, spider angiomas, and thrombocytopenia, eventually leading to cirrhosis or subacute necrosis of the liver
- *blood*: anemia and leukopenia
- *CNS*: "wing-flapping" tremors in arms, "pill-rolling" tremors in hands, facial and muscular rigidity, dysarthria, unsteady gait, and emotional and behavioral changes
- *genitourinary tract*: aminoaciduria, proteinuria, uricosuria, glycosuria, and phosphaturia
- *musculoskeletal system* (in severe disease): muscle-wasting, contractures, deformities, osteomalacia, and pathologic fractures.

Diagnosis

Several tests suggest Wilson's disease:

- *serum ceruloplasmin:* less than 20 mg/100 ml
- *serum copper:* less than 80 mcg/100 ml
- *urine copper:* more than 100 mcg/24 hours (may be as high as 1,000 mcg)
- *liver biopsy:* excessive copper deposits (250 mcg/g dry weight), tissue changes indicative of chronic active hepatitis, fatty liver, or cirrhosis.

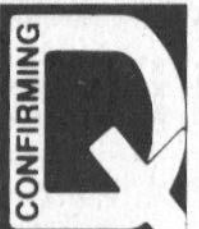

Revelation of Kayser-Fleischer rings during slit-lamp ophthalmic examination confirms diagnosis. However, rings are present only when the disease has progressed beyond the liver.

Treatment

Treatment aims to reduce the amount of copper in the tissues, prevent additional accumulation, and manage hepatic disease. The most effective treatment for Wilson's disease consists of lifetime therapy using pyridoxine (vitamin B_6) in conjunction with D-penicillamine, a copper-chelating agent that mobilizes copper from the tissues and promotes its excretion in the urine. However, about one third of patients are sensitive to penicillamine, necessitating dosage adjustment or discontinuation. If an adverse reaction recurs after penicillamine therapy is resumed, the patient may require treatment with corticosteroids, such as prednisone. Treatment also includes potassium and sodium supplements before meals, to prevent gastrointestinal absorption of copper.

Special considerations

- Since penicillamine is chemically related to penicillin, ask if the patient is allergic to penicillin before administering the first dose. Watch closely for allergic reactions, such as fever, skin rash, adenopathy, severe leukopenia, and thrombocytopenia. Always give penicillamine on an empty stomach. If gastrointestinal irritation develops, provide enteric-coated tablets.
- Tell the patient and his family what foods to avoid on a low-copper diet (mushrooms, nuts, chocolate, dried fruit, liver, and shellfish). Suggest the use of distilled water, since most tap water flows through copper pipes.
- Be sure to emphasize the necessity of lifetime therapy. Assist the patient and his family with arrangements for continuing education, physical or vocational rehabilitation, and community nursing services, as needed.
- Provide emotional support. The neurologic changes Wilson's disease produces often lead to its misdiagnosis as a psychiatric disorder. Reassure the patient that his condition has a treatable physical basis.
- For a patient in an advanced stage of the disease, encourage as much self-care as possible to prevent further mental and physical deterioration. Plan an exercise schedule. Avoid sensory deprivation or overload. Prevent accidents and injuries that could occur as a result of neurologic deficits.
- If the patient is in a terminal stage, support the family in their grief.
- Suggest genetic counseling for couples who are blood relatives or who have a relative with Wilson's disease. Explain that the chance of their having a child with Wilson's disease is 25% with *each* pregnancy. Teach parents the disease's early symptoms, so they can seek prompt treatment for their child; stress regular pediatric examinations.

Hepatic Encephalopathy

(Hepatic coma)

Hepatic encephalopathy is a neurologic syndrome that develops as a complication of chronic liver disease. Most common in patients with cirrhosis, this syndrome is due primarily to ammonia intoxication of the brain. It may be acute and self-limiting, or chronic and progressive. Treatment requires correction of the precipitating cause and reduction of blood ammonia levels. In advanced stages, prognosis is extremely poor despite vigorous treatment.

Causes

Hepatic encephalopathy follows rising blood ammonia levels. Normally, the ammonia produced by protein breakdown in the bowel is metabolized to urea in the liver. When portal blood shunts past the liver, ammonia directly enters the systemic circulation and is carried to the brain. Such shunting may result from the collateral venous circulation that develops in portal hypertension or from surgically created portal-systemic shunts. Cirrhosis further compounds this problem, because impaired hepatocellular function prevents conversion of ammonia that reaches the liver.

Other factors that predispose rising ammonia levels include excessive protein intake, sepsis, excessive accumulation of nitrogenous body wastes (from constipation or gastrointestinal hemorrhage), and bacterial action on protein and urea to form ammonia. Certain other factors heighten the brain's sensitivity to ammonia intoxication: fluid and electrolyte imbalance (especially metabolic alkalosis), hypoxia, azotemia, impaired glucose metabolism, infection, and administration of sedatives, narcotics, and general anesthetics.

Signs and symptoms

Clinical manifestations of hepatic encephalopathy vary (depending on the severity of neurologic involvement) and develop in four stages:

- *prodromal stage*—early symptoms are often overlooked because they're so subtle: slight personality changes (disorientation, forgetfulness, slurred speech) and a slight tremor
- *impending stage*—tremor progresses into asterixis (liver flap, flapping tremor), the hallmark of hepatic encephalopathy. Asterixis is characterized by quick, irregular extensions and flexions of the wrists and fingers, when the wrists are held out straight and the hands flexed upward. Lethargy, aberrant behavior, and apraxia also occur.
- *stuporous stage*—hyperventilation; patient stuporous but noisy and abusive when aroused
- *comatose stage*—hyperactive reflexes, a positive Babinski's sign, fetor hepaticus (musty, sweet odor to the breath), and coma.

Diagnosis

Clinical features, a positive history of liver disease, and elevated serum ammonia levels in venous and arterial samples confirm hepatic encephalopathy. Other supportive lab values include an electroencephalogram that slows as the disease progresses, elevated bilirubin, and prolonged prothrombin time.

Treatment

Effective treatment stops progression of encephalopathy by reducing blood ammonia levels. Such treatment eliminates ammonia-producing substances from the gastrointestinal tract by administration of neomycin to suppress bacterial flora (preventing them from converting amino acids into ammonia), sorbitol-induced catharsis to produce osmotic diarrhea, continuous aspiration of blood from the stomach, reduction of dietary protein intake, and administration of lactulose to reduce the blood ammonia levels. Lactulose traps ammonia in the bowel and promotes its excretion. It's effective because bacterial enzymes change lactulose to lactic acid, thereby rendering the colon too acidic for bacterial growth. At the same time, the resulting increase in free hydrogen ions prevents diffusion of ammonia through the mucosa; lactulose promotes conversion of systemically absorbable NH_3 to NH_4, which is poorly absorbed and can be excreted. Lactulose syrup may be given 30 to 45 ml P.O. three or four times daily. For acute hepatic coma, 300 ml diluted with 700 ml water may be administered by retention enema. Lactulose therapy requires careful monitoring of fluid and electrolyte balance. The usual dose of neomycin is 3 to 4 g/day P.O. or by retention enema. Although neomycin is nonabsorbable at recommended dosages, an amount that exceeds 4 g/day may produce irreversible hearing loss and nephrotoxicity.

Treatment may also include potassium supplements (80 to 120 mEq/day, P.O. or I.V.) to correct alkalosis (from increased ammonia levels), especially if the patient is taking diuretics. Sometimes, hemodialysis can temporarily clear toxic blood. Exchange transfusions may provide dramatic but temporary improvement; however, these require a particularly large amount of blood. Salt-poor albumin may be used to maintain fluid and electrolyte balance, replace depleted albumin levels, and restore plasma.

Special considerations

- Frequently assess and record the patient's level of consciousness. Continually orient him to place and time. Remember to keep a daily record of the patient's handwriting to monitor progression of neurologic involvement.
- Monitor intake, output, and fluid and electrolyte balance. Check daily weight and measure abdominal girth. Watch for, and immediately report, signs of anemia (decreased hemoglobin), infection, alkalosis (increased serum bicarbonate), and gastrointestinal bleeding (melena, hematemesis).
- Give drugs, as ordered, and watch for side effects.
- Ask the dietary department to provide the specified low-protein diet, with carbohydrates supplying most of the calories. Provide good mouth care.
- Promote rest, comfort, and a quiet atmosphere. Discourage stressful exercise.
- Use restraints, if necessary, but avoid sedatives. Protect the comatose patient's eyes from corneal injury by using artificial tears or eye patches.
- Provide emotional support for the patient's family in the terminal stage of encephalopathy.

GALLBLADDER & DUCT DISEASES

Cholelithiasis, Choledocholithiasis, Cholangitis, Cholecystitis, Cholesterolosis, Biliary Cirrhosis, and Gallstone Ileus

Diseases of the gallbladder and biliary tract are common and often painful conditions that usually require surgery and may be life-threatening. They are often associated with deposition of calculi and inflammation.

Causes and incidence

Cholelithiasis, stones or calculi (gallstones) in the gallbladder, results from changes in bile components. Gallstones are made of cholesterol, calcium bilirubinate, or a mixture of cholesterol and bilirubin pigment. They arise during periods of sluggishness in the gallbladder due to pregnancy, oral contraceptives, diabetes mellitus, celiac disease, cirrhosis of the liver, and pancreatitis. Cholelithiasis is the fifth leading cause of hospitalization among adults, and accounts for 90% of all gallbladder and duct diseases. Prognosis is usually good with treatment unless infection occurs, in which case prognosis depends on its severity and response to antibiotics.

One out of every ten patients with gallstones develops *choledocholithiasis* or gallstones in the common bile duct (sometimes called "common duct stones"). This occurs when stones passed out of the gallbladder lodge in the hepatic and common bile ducts and obstruct the flow of bile into the duodenum. Prognosis is good unless infection occurs.

Cholangitis, infection of the bile duct, is often associated with choledocholithiasis and may follow percutaneous transhepatic cholangiography. Predisposing factors may include bacterial or metabolic alteration of bile acids. Widespread inflammation may cause fibrosis and stenosis of the common bile duct.

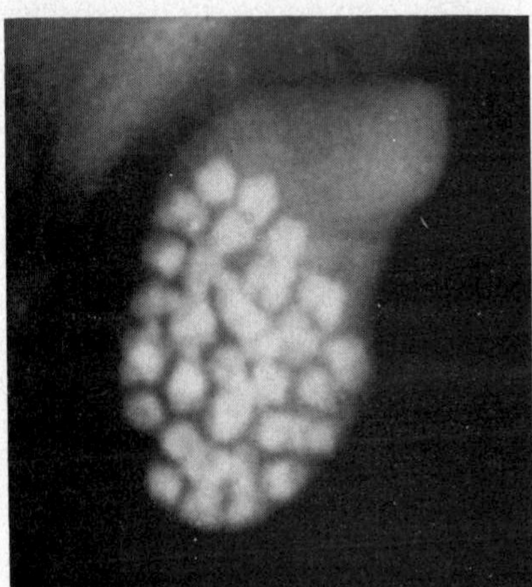
Oral cholecystography shows stones in the gallbladder.

Prognosis for this rare condition is poor—stenosing or primary sclerosing cholangitis is almost always fatal.

Cholecystitis, acute or chronic inflammation of the gallbladder, is usually associated with a gallstone impacted in the cystic duct, causing painful distention of the gallbladder. Cholecystitis accounts for 10% to 25% of all patients requiring gallbladder surgery. The acute form is most common during middle age; the chronic form, among the elderly. Prognosis is good with treatment.

Cholesterolosis, cholesterol polyps or deposits of cholesterol crystals in the submucosa of the gallbladder, may result from bile secretions containing high concentrations of cholesterol and insufficient bile salts. These polyps may be localized or speckle the entire gallbladder with yellow spots. Cholesterolosis, the most common pseudotumor, is not related to widespread inflammation of the mucosa or lining of the gallbladder. Prognosis is good with surgery.

Biliary cirrhosis, ascending infection of the biliary system, sometimes follows viral destruction of liver and duct cells, but the primary cause is unknown. This condition usually leads to obstructive jaundice and involves the portal and periportal spaces of the liver. It strikes women aged 40 to 60 nine times more often than men. Prognosis is poor.

Gallstone ileus results from a gallstone lodging at the terminal ileum. This condition is more common in the elderly. Prognosis is good with surgery.

Postcholecystectomy syndrome (PCS) commonly results from residual gallstones or stricture of the common bile duct. It occurs in 1% to 5% of all patients whose gallbladders have been surgically removed and may produce right upper quadrant abdominal pain, biliary colic, fatty food intolerance, dyspepsia, and indigestion. Prognosis is good with surgery or treatment.

Generally, gallbladder and duct diseases occur during middle age. Between ages 20 and 50, they're six times more common in women, but incidence between men and women becomes equal after age 50. Incidence rises with each succeeding decade.

Signs and symptoms

Although gallbladder disease may be asymptomatic (even when X-rays reveal gallstones), acute cholelithiasis, acute cholecystitis, choledocholithiasis, and cholesterolosis produce the symptoms of a classic gallbladder attack. Such an attack often follows meals rich in fats (such as fried food, cream, and chocolate) or may occur in the middle of the night, suddenly awakening the patient. It begins with acute abdominal pain in the right upper quadrant. This pain may radiate to the back, between the shoulders, or to the front of the chest; the pain may be so severe that the patient seeks emergency room care. Other features may include recurring fat intolerance, biliary colic, belching that leaves a sour taste in the mouth, flatulence, indigestion, diaphoresis, nausea, vomiting, chills, and low-grade fever. Jaundice may occur if a stone obstructs the common bile duct (small stones are more likely to do this than larger ones). Clay-colored stools may also occur with choledocholithiasis.

Clinical features of cholangitis include a rise in eosinophils, jaundice, abdominal pain, high fever, and chills; biliary cirrhosis may produce jaundice, related itching, weakness, fatigue, slight weight loss, and abdominal pain. Gallstone ileus produces signs of small bowel obstruction—nausea, vomiting, abdominal distention, and absent bowel sounds if the bowel is completely obstructed. Its most telling sign is intermittent recurrence of colicky pain over several days.

Diagnosis

Echography and X-rays detect gallstones. Specific procedures include:

- *ultrasound:* reflects stones in the gallbladder with 96% accuracy
- *percutaneous transhepatic cholangiography:* imaging done under fluoroscopic control, distinguishes between gallbladder disease and cancer of the pancreatic head in patients with jaundice
- *endoscopic retrograde cholangiopancreatography:* visualizes the biliary tree after insertion of an endoscope down the esophagus into the duodenum, cannulation of the common bile and pancreatic ducts, and injection of contrast medium
- *hida scan* (of the gallbladder): detects obstruction of the cystic duct
- *computed tomography scan:* although not used routinely, helps distinguish between obstructive and nonobstructive jaundice
- *flat plate of the abdomen:* identifies calcified, but not cholesterol, stones with 15% accuracy
- *oral cholecystography:* shows stones in the gallbladder and biliary duct obstruction
- *intravenous cholangiography:* visualizes the ductal system; rarely used.

Elevated icteric index, total bilirubin, urine bilirubin, and alkaline phosphatase support the diagnosis. White blood cell count is slightly elevated during a cholecystitis attack. Differential diagnosis is essential, because gallbladder

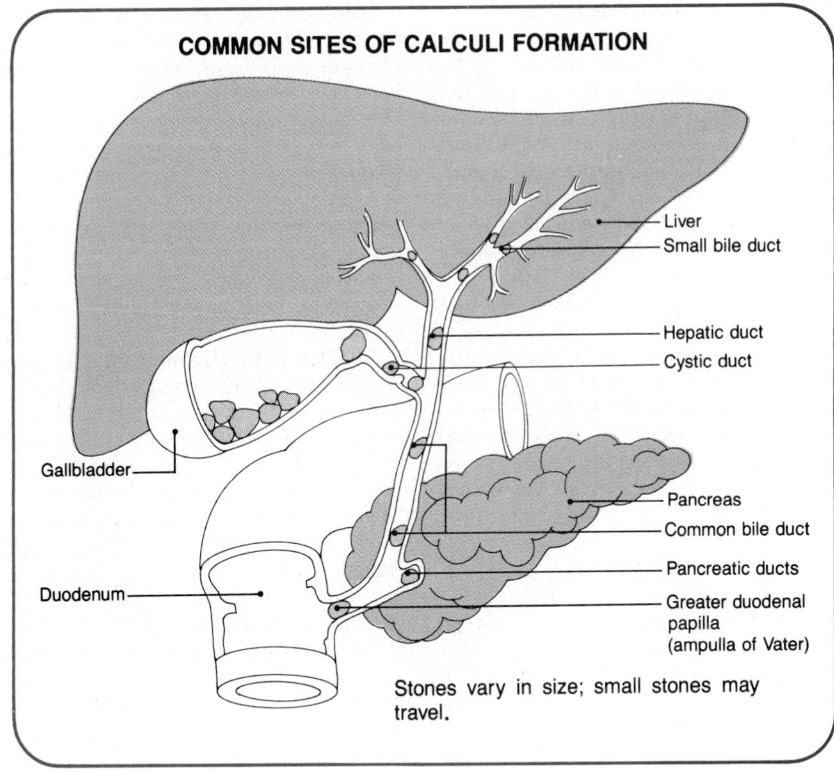

disease can mimic other diseases (myocardial infarction, angina, pancreatitis, pancreatic head cancer, pneumonia, peptic ulcer, hiatal hernia, esophagitis, and gastritis). Serum amylase distinguishes gallbladder disease from pancreatitis. With suspected heart disease, serial enzyme tests and electrocardiogram should precede gallbladder and upper GI diagnostic tests.

Treatment

Surgery, usually elective, is the treatment of choice for gallbladder and duct disease. Surgery may include cholecystectomy, cholecystectomy with operative cholangiography, and possibly exploration of the common bile duct. Other treatment includes a low-fat diet to prevent attacks, and vitamin K for itching, jaundice, and bleeding tendencies due to vitamin K deficiency. Treatment during an acute attack may include insertion of a nasogastric tube and an I.V., and possibly antibiotic administration.

A recently developed nonsurgical treatment for choledocholithiasis involves insertion of a flexible catheter, formed around a T tube, through a sinus tract into the common bile duct. Guided by fluoroscopy, the catheter is directed toward the stone. A Dormia basket is threaded through the catheter, opened, twirled to entrap the stone, closed, and withdrawn.

Chenodiol, a newly available drug that dissolves radiolucent stones, provides an alternative for patients who are poor surgical risks or who refuse surgery. However, use of chenodiol is limited by the need for prolonged treatment, the high incidence of adverse effects, and the frequency of stone reformation after treatment is stopped.

Special considerations

Patient care for gallbladder and duct disease focuses on supportive care and close postoperative observation.

- Before surgery, teach the patient to deep-breathe, cough, expectorate, and perform leg exercises that are necessary after surgery. Also teach splinting, repositioning, and ambulation techniques. Explain the procedures that will be performed before, during, and after surgery, to help ease the patient's anxiety and to help ensure his cooperation.
- After surgery, monitor vital signs for signs of bleeding, infection, or atelectasis. Evaluate the incision site for bleeding. Serosanguineous and bile drainage is common during the first 24 to 48 hours if the patient has a wound drain such as a Jackson-Pratt or Penrose drain. If, after a choledochostomy, a T-tube drain is placed in the duct and attached to a drainage bag, make sure there is no kink in the drainage tube. Also check for adequate connecting tubing from the T tube that's well secured to the patient to prevent dislodgment. Measure and record drainage daily (200 to 300 ml is normal). Teach patients who will be discharged with a T tube how to empty it, change the dressing, and provide proper skin care.
- Monitor intake and output. Allow the patient nothing by mouth for 24 to 48 hours or until bowel sounds return and nausea and vomiting cease (postoperative nausea may indicate a full urinary bladder). If the patient doesn't void within 8 hours (or if the amount voided is inadequate based on I.V. fluid intake), percuss over the symphysis pubis for bladder distention. (This is especially important in patients receiving anticholinergics.) Avoid catheterization if possible.
- Encourage deep breathing and leg exercises every hour. The patient should ambulate in the evening or morning after surgery. Discourage sitting in a chair, and provide elastic stockings to support leg muscles and promote venous blood flow, thus preventing stasis and possible clot formation. Check daily for a positive Homans' sign (pain on dorsiflexion of the foot or calf tenderness, both signs of phlebitis and thrombophlebitis). Have the patient rest in slight Fowler's position as much as possible to direct any abdominal drainage into the pelvic cavity rather than allowing it to accumulate under the diaphragm.

• Evaluate the location, duration, and character of any pain. Report sudden pain that the patient describes as a tearing of the incision (possible wound dehiscence) and chest or back pain. Administer adequate medication to relieve pain, especially before such activities as deep-breathing and ambulation, which increase pain. Abdominal distention is common sometime during the second and third postoperative days and may aggravate pain. Abdominal distention resolves spontaneously as bowel function returns.

• At discharge (usually 4 to 10 days after surgery), advise the patient against heavy lifting or straining for 6 weeks. Urge him to walk daily. Tell him that food restrictions are unnecessary unless he has an intolerance to a specific food or some underlying condition (diabetes, atherosclerosis, obesity) that requires such restriction.

Selected References

Bates, Robin. "The Elusive Illness," *Nova*. WGBH Educational Foundation, 1980.

Bockus, Henry, ed. *Gastroenterology*, 4th ed. Philadelphia: W.B. Saunders Co, 1984.

Given, Barbara A., and Simmons, Sandra J. *Gastroenterology in Clinical Nursing*, 4th ed. St. Louis: C.V. Mosby Co., 1983.

Greenberger, Norton J. *Gastrointestinal Disorders*. Chicago: Year Book Medical Pubs., 1980.

Hoofnagle, J.H., et al. "Transmission of Non-A, Non-B Hepatitis," *Annals of Internal Medicine* 87(1):14-20, July 1977.

Immunization Practices Advisory Committee. "Postexposure Prophylaxis of Hepatitis B," *Annals of Internal Medicine* 101(3):351-54, September 1984.

Schiff, Leon, ed. *Diseases of the Liver*, 5th ed. Philadelphia: J.B. Lippincott Co., 1982.

Schoenfield, Leslie J. "Gallstones and Other Biliary Diseases," *Clinical Symposia (CIBA)* 34(4):2-32, 1982.

Thorpe, Constance J., and Caprini, Joseph A. "Gallbladder Disease: Current Trends and Treatments," *American Journal of Nursing* 80(12):2181-85, December 1980.

Zimmerman, Hyman J. *Hepatotoxicity: The Adverse Effects of Drugs and Other Chemicals in the Liver*. East Norwalk, Conn.: Appleton-Century-Crofts, 1978.

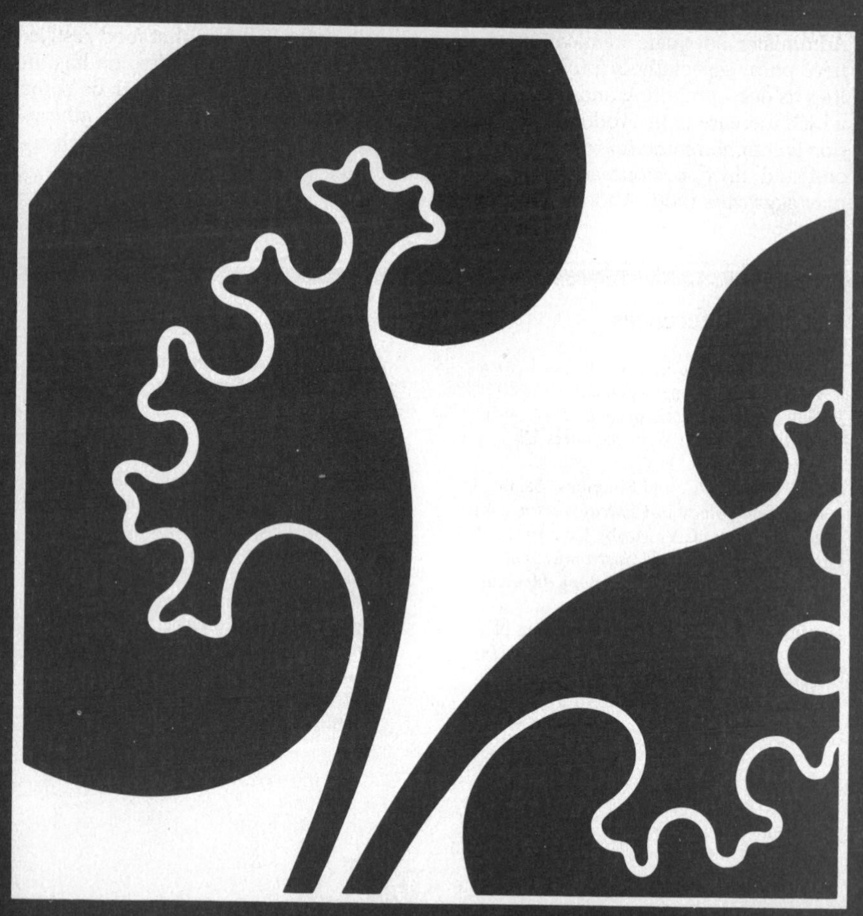

12 Renal and Urologic Disorders

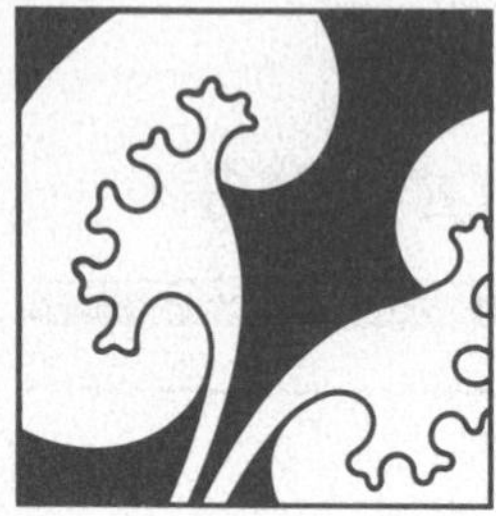

Renal and Urologic Disorders

Introduction

Renal-related diseases currently affect more than 8 million Americans—a fact that suggests you'll probably deal with renal patients often. To give such patients the best possible care, you need to know normal anatomy and physiology, specific pathophysiologic conditions, assessment, and treatment.

Kidneys and homeostasis

Through the production and elimination of urine, the kidneys maintain homeostasis. These vital organs regulate the volume, electrolyte concentration, and acid-base balance of body fluids; detoxify the blood and eliminate wastes; regulate blood pressure; and aid in erythropoiesis. The kidneys eliminate wastes from the body through urine formation (by glomerular filtration, tubular reabsorption, and tubular secretion) and excretion. Glomerular filtration, the process of filtering the blood flowing through the kidneys, depends on the permeability of the capillary walls, vascular pressure, and filtration pressure. The normal glomerular filtration rate (GFR) is about 120 ml/minute.

Clearance measures function

Clearance, the volume of plasma that can be cleared of a substance per unit of time, depends on how renal tubular cells handle the substance that has been filtered by the glomerulus:

- If the tubules don't reabsorb or secrete the substance, clearance equals the GFR.
- If the tubules reabsorb it, clearance is less than the GFR.
- If the tubules secrete it, clearance is greater than the GFR.
- If the tubules reabsorb and secrete it, clearance is less than, equal to, or greater than the GFR.

The most accurate measure of glomerular function is creatinine clearance, since this substance is only filtered by the glomerulus and is not reabsorbed by the tubules.

The transport of filtered substances in tubular reabsorption or secretion may be active (requiring the expenditure of energy) or passive (requiring none). For example, energy is required to move sodium across tubular cells (active transport), but none is required to move urea (passive transport). The amount of reabsorption or secretion of a substance depends on the maximum tubular transport capacity (Tm) for that substance—that is, the greatest amount of a substance that can be reabsorbed or secreted per minute without saturating the system.

Water regulation

Hormones partially control water regulation by the kidneys. Hormonal control depends on the response of osmoreceptors to changes in osmolality. The two hormones involved are antidiuretic hormone (ADH), produced by the pituitary gland, and aldosterone, produced by the adrenal cortex. ADH alters the collecting tubules' permeability to water. When plasma concentration of ADH is high, the tubules are very permeable to water, so a greater amount of water is reabsorbed, creating a high concentration but small volume of urine. The reverse is true if ADH concentration is low.

Aldosterone, however, regulates sodium and water reabsorption from the distal tubules. High plasma aldosterone

ASSESSMENT OF SERUM AND URINE VALUES IN RENAL DISEASE

	NORMAL SERUM VALUE	DEVIATION	NORMAL URINE VALUE	DEVIATION
Sodium	136-146 mEq/L	↑ or N	50-130 mEq/L	V
Potassium	3.5-5.5 mEq/L	↑	20-70 mEq/L	↓
Chloride	96-106 mEq/L	↑	50-130 mEq/L	↓
Calcium	8.5-10.5 mg/ 100 ml	↓	5-12 mEq/L	↓
Phosphorus	2-4.5 mg/100 ml	↑	1 g/24 hr	V
Magnesium	1.6-2.2 mEq/L	↑ or N	2-18 mEq/L	↓
CO_2 combining power	24 mEq/L	↓		
Specific gravity			1.003-1.030	↓
pH			5.0-8.0	↑
BUN/Urea	9-18 mg/100 ml	↑	10-20 g/L	↓
Creatinine	0.7-1.5 mg/100 ml	↑	1.0-1.6 g/24 hr	↓
Osmolality	280-295 mOsm/kg	V	500-1,200 mOsm/ kg	↓
Uric acid	3-7 mg/100 ml	↑		
Glucose	70-100 mg/100 ml	N	0	N
Protein	6-8 g/100 ml	↓ or N	0	V
Hematocrit	40%-50%	↓		
Hemoglobin	12-16 g/100 ml	↓		
WBC	4,000-10,000/mm^3	V	<2,000,000/24 hr	V
RBC			<1,000,000/24 hr	V
Casts			<100,000/24 hr	V
Bacteria			<100,000 organisms/ml	V
Alkaline phosphatase	5-13 K-A-U	↑		

KEYS: ↑ = increased, ↓ = decreased, N = normal, V = varies

STRUCTURE OF THE KIDNEYS

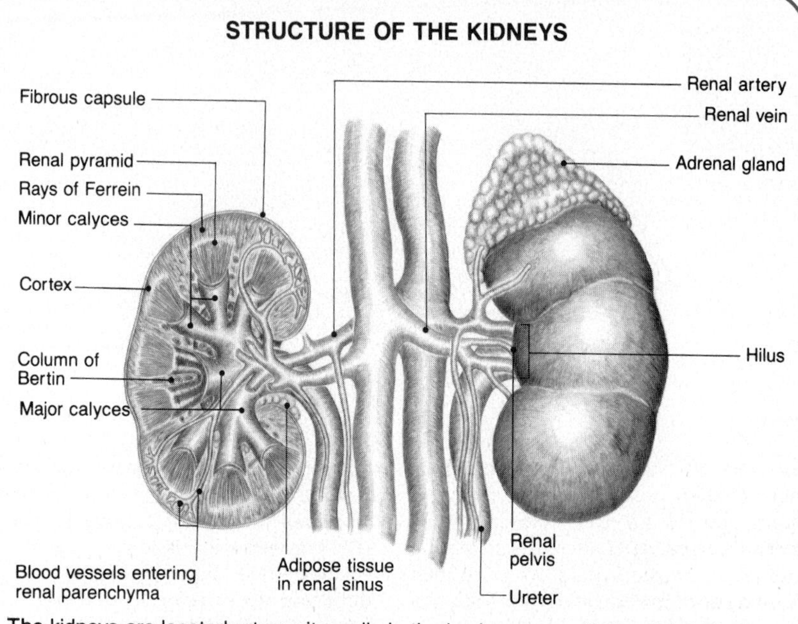

The kidneys are located retroperitoneally in the lumbar area, with the right kidney a little lower than the left because of the liver mass above it. The left kidney is slightly longer than the right and closer to the midline. The kidneys assume different locations with changes in body position. The coverings of the kidneys consist of the true or fibrous capsule, perirenal fat, renal fascia, and pararenal fat.

Renal arteries branch into five segmental arteries that supply different areas of the kidneys. The segmental arteries then branch into several divisions from which the afferent arterioles and vasa recta arise. Renal veins follow a similar branching pattern, characterized by stellate vessels and segmental branches, and empty into the inferior vena cava. The tubular system receives its blood supply from a peritubular capillary network of vessels.

concentration promotes sodium and water reabsorption from the tubules and decreases sodium and water excretion in the urine; low plasma aldosterone concentration promotes sodium and water excretion.

Aldosterone also helps control the distal tubular secretion of potassium. Other factors that determine potassium secretion include the amount of potassium ingested, number of hydrogen ions secreted, level of intracellular potassium, amount of sodium in the distal tubule, and the GFR.

The countercurrent mechanism is the method by which the kidneys concentrate urine; this mechanism is composed of a multiplication system and an exchange system, which occur in the renal medulla via the limbs of the loop of Henle and the vasa recta. It achieves active transport of sodium and chloride between the loop of Henle and the medullary interstitial fluid. Failure of this mechanism produces polyuria and nocturia.

To regulate acid-base balance, the kidneys secrete hydrogen ions, reabsorb sodium and bicarbonate ions, acidify phosphate salts, and synthesize ammonia—all of which keep the blood at its normal pH of 7.37 to 7.43.

The kidneys assist in regulating blood pressure by synthesizing and secreting

REVIEW OF RENAL AND UROLOGIC ANATOMY

The gross structure of each kidney includes the lateral and medial margins, the hilus, the renal sinus, and renal parenchyma. The hilus, located at the medial margin, is the indentation where the blood and lymph vessels enter the kidney and the ureter emerges. The hilus leads to the renal sinus, which is a spacious cavity filled with adipose tissue, branches of the renal vessels, calyces, the renal pelvis, and the ureter. The renal sinus is surrounded by parenchyma, which consists of a cortex and a medulla. The cortex (outermost layer of the kidney) contains glomeruli (parts of the nephron), cortical arches (areas that separate the medullary pyramids from the renal surface), columns of Bertin (areas that separate the pyramids from one another), and medullary rays of Ferrein (long, delicate processes from the bases of the pyramids that mix with the cortex).

The medulla contains pyramids (cone-shaped structures of parenchymal tissue), papillae (apical ends of the pyramids through which urine oozes into the minor calyces), and papillary ducts of Bellini (collecting ducts in the pyramids that empty into the papillae).

The ureters are a pair of retroperitoneally located, mucosa-lined, fibromuscular tubes that transport urine from the renal pelvis to the urinary bladder. Although the ureters have no sphincters, their oblique entrance into the bladder creates a mucosal fold that may produce a sphincterlike action.

The adult urinary bladder is a spherical, hollow muscular sac, with a normal capacity of 300 to 500 ml. It is located anterior and inferior to the peritoneal cavity, and posterior to the pubic bones. The gross structure of the bladder includes the fundus (large central, posterosuperior portion of the bladder), the apex (anterosuperior region), the body (posteroinferior region containing the ureteral orifices), and the urethral orifice, or neck (most inferior portion of the bladder). The three orifices comprise a triangular area called the trigone.

Functional units

The functional units of each kidney are its 1 to 3 million nephrons. Each nephron is composed of the renal corpuscle and the tubular system. The renal corpuscle includes the glomerulus (a network of minute blood vessels) and Bowman's capsule (an epithelial sac surrounding the glomerulus that is part of the tubular system). The renal corpuscle has a vascular pole, where the afferent arteriole enters and the efferent arteriole emerges, and a urinary pole that narrows to form the beginning of the tubular system. The tubular system includes the proximal convoluted tubule, the loop of Henle, and the distal convoluted tubule. The last portion of the nephron consists of the collecting duct.

Innervation and vasculature

The kidneys are innervated by sympathetic branches from the celiac plexus, upper lumbar splanchnic and thoracic nerves, and the intermesenteric and superior hypogastric plexuses, which form a plexus around the kidneys. Similar numbers of sympathetic and parasympathetic nerves from the renal plexus, superior hypogastric plexus, and intermesenteric plexus innervate the ureters. Nerves that arise from the inferior hypogastric plexuses innervate the bladder. The parasympathetic nerve supply to the bladder controls micturition.

The ureters receive their blood supply from the renal, vesical, gonadal, and iliac arteries, and the abdominal aorta. The ureteral veins follow the arteries and drain into the renal vein. The bladder receives blood through vesical arteries. Vesical veins unite to form the pudendal plexus, which empties into the iliac veins. A rich lymphatic system drains the renal cortex, the kidneys, the ureters, and the bladder.

renin in response to an actual, or perceived, decrease in the volume of extracellular fluid. Renin, in turn, acts on a substrate to form angiotensin I, which is converted to angiotensin II. Angiotensin II increases arterial blood pressure by peripheral vasoconstriction and stimulation of aldosterone secretion. The resulting increase in the aldosterone level promotes the reabsorption of sodium and water to correct the fluid deficit and renal ischemia.

The kidneys secrete erythropoietin in response to decreased oxygen tension in the renal blood supply. Erythropoietin then acts on the bone marrow to increase the production of RBCs.

Renal tubular cells synthesize active vitamin D and help regulate calcium balance and bone metabolism.

Clinical assessment

Assessment of the renal and urologic systems begins with an accurate patient history; assessment also requires a thorough physical examination and certain laboratory data and test results from invasive and noninvasive procedures. When obtaining a patient history, ask about symptoms that pertain specifically to the pathology of the renal and urologic systems, such as frequency or urgency; and about the presence of any systemic diseases that can produce renal or urologic dysfunction, such as hypertension, diabetes mellitus, or bladder infections. Family history may also suggest a genetic predisposition to certain renal diseases, such as glomerulonephritis or polycystic kidney disease. Also, ask what medications the patient has been taking; abuse of analgesics or antibiotics may cause nephrotoxicity.

Physical examination for renal disease

The first step in physical examination is careful observation of the patient's overall appearance, since renal disease affects all body systems. Examine the patient's skin for color, turgor, intactness, texture; mucous membranes for color, secretions, odor, and intactness; eyes for periorbital edema and vision; general activity for motion, gait, and posture; muscle movement for motor function and general strength; and mental status for level of consciousness, orientation, and response to stimuli.

Renal disease causes distinctive changes in vital signs: hypertension due to fluid and electrolyte imbalances and hyperactivity of the renin-angiotensin system; a strong, fast, irregular pulse due to fluid and electrolyte imbalances; hyperventilation to compensate for metabolic acidosis; and an increased susceptibility to infection due to overall decreased resistance. Palpation and percussion may reveal little, since the kidneys and bladder are difficult to palpate unless they are enlarged or distended.

Relevant laboratory data

Laboratory tests analyze serum levels of chemical substances, such as uric acid, creatinine, and BUN; tests also determine urine characteristics, including the presence of RBCs, WBCs, casts, or bacteria; specific gravity and pH; and physical properties, such as clarity, color, and odor.

Noninvasive monitoring includes the following:

• *Intake and output assessment:* Intake and output measurement helps assess the patient's hydration status but is not a valid evaluation of renal function, since urine output varies with different types of renal pathology. However, to provide the most useful and accurate information, use calibrated containers, establish baseline values for each patient, compare measurement patterns, and validate intake and output measurements by weighing the patient daily. Also, monitor all fluid losses—including blood, emesis, diarrhea, and wound and stoma drainage.

• *Specimen collection:* Meticulous collection is vital for valid laboratory data. If the patient is collecting the specimen, explain the importance of cleaning the meatal area thoroughly. The culture specimen should be caught midstream, in a sterile container; a specimen for urinalysis, in a clean container, preferably

INVASIVE DIAGNOSTIC TESTS FOR ASSESSING THE RENAL AND UROLOGIC SYSTEM

PROCEDURE AND PURPOSE	SPECIAL CONSIDERATIONS
Cystoscopy: Visualizes the inside of the bladder with a fiberoptic scope	*Before:* Give sedatives, as ordered. *After:* Offer increased fluids; administer analgesics; watch for hematuria and signs of perforation, hemorrhage, and infection (chills, fever, increased pulse rate, shock).
Cystourethrography: Determines size and shape of bladder and urethra through X-rays and instilled contrast medium	*During:* Catheterize the patient. *After:* Offer increased fluids; observe for hypersensitivity reaction (chills, fever, increased pulse rate, itching, hives).
Cystometry: Evaluates bladder pressure, sensation, and capacity	*Before:* Observe voiding; catheterize for residual urine. *After:* Remove catheter; watch for stress incontinence when patient coughs; watch voiding; catheterize for residual urine.
Intravenous pyelography (IVP): Visualizes renal parenchyma, calyces, pelves, ureters, and bladder with X-rays and contrast medium	*After:* Observe for hypersensitivity reaction (chills, fever, increased pulse rate, itching, hives); watch for hematomas at injection site.
Nephrotomography: Visualizes parenchyma, calyces, and pelves in layers after I.V. injection of contrast medium, followed by tomography	*After:* Observe for hypersensitivity reaction (chills, fever, increased pulse rate, itching, hives).
Renal angiography: Visualizes arterial tree, capillaries, and venous drainage of the kidney, using contrast medium injected into a catheter in the femoral artery or vein	*After:* Observe for hypersensitivity reaction (chills, fever, increased pulse rate, itching, hives), hematomas and hemorrhage at injection site, and nephrotoxicity. Offer increased fluids.
Renal scan: Determines renal function by visualizing the appearance and disappearance of radioisotopes within the kidney	*After:* Observe for hypersensitivity reaction (chills, fever, increased pulse rate, itching, hives).
Renal biopsy: Obtains specimen for developing histologic diagnosis and determines therapy and prognosis	*Before:* Make sure patient's clotting times, prothrombin times, and platelet count are recorded on his chart and that the patient has had IVP. Place patient in prone position with his side slightly elevated on a towel or pillow, and clean the skin over the area to be biopsied. *During:* Help the patient maintain proper position. Tell him to lie still and hold his breath if the biopsy is done at the bedside. Often, however, it's done in the operating room. *After:* Instruct the patient to breathe normally. Apply gentle pressure to the bandage site. Watch for hemorrhage and hematoma at the biopsy site and for hematuria. Enforce bed rest for 24 hours postprocedure. Offer increased fluids.

COMMON RENAL SYMPTOMS

SYMPTOM	POSSIBLE CAUSE
Frequency	Infection, diabetes
Nocturia	Infection
Urgency	Infection, prostatic disease
Hesitancy	Prostatic enlargement
Oliguria	Failure, insufficiency, neoplasms
Dysuria	Infection
Dribbling	Prostatic enlargement, strictures
Hematuria	Glomerular diseases, trauma, neoplasms
Pyuria	Infection
Edema	Nephrotic syndrome, failure
Incontinence	Infection, neoplasms, prolapsed uterus
Renal colic	Calculi
Proteinuria	Glomerular diseases, infection

at the first voiding of the day. Begin a 24-hour specimen collection after discarding the first voiding; such specimens often necessitate special handling or preservatives. When obtaining a urine specimen from a catheterized patient, don't take the specimen from the collection bag; instead, aspirate a sample through the collection port in the catheter, with a sterile needle and a syringe.

• *X-ray:* A plain film of the abdomen (kidney-ureter-bladder) assesses the size, shape, position, and possible areas of calcification.

If the patient needs invasive diagnostic procedures such as cystoscopy, intravenous pyelography, and renal angiography, explain each procedure carefully to allay anxiety and encourage cooperation. Prepare the patient for the procedure, as appropriate; afterward, observe for complications, such as hypersensitivity and hemorrhage, by monitoring vital signs, intake and output, and general status. Document the patient's response to the procedure.

Treatment methods

Treatment of intractable renal or urinary system dysfunction may require urinary diversion, dialysis, or renal transplantation. Urinary diversion is the creation of an abnormal outlet for excreting urine. Several methods of urinary diversion may be performed: ileal conduit, cutaneous ureterostomy, ureterosigmoidostomy, or the creation of a rectal bladder.

In dialysis, a semipermeable membrane, osmosis, and diffusion imitate normal kidney function by eliminating excess body fluids, maintaining or restoring plasma electrolyte and acid-base balances, and removing waste products and dialyzable poisons from the blood. Dialysis is most often used for patients with acute or chronic renal failure. The two most common types are peritoneal dialysis and hemodialysis.

In peritoneal dialysis, a dialysate solution is infused into the peritoneal cavity. Substances then diffuse through the peritoneal membrane. Waste products remain in the solution and are removed.

Hemodialysis separates solutes by differential diffusion through a cellophane membrane placed between the blood and the dialysate solution, in an external receptacle. Since the blood must actually pass out of the body into a dialysis machine, hemodialysis requires an access route to the blood supply by an arteriovenous fistula or cannula or by a bovine or synthetic graft. When caring for a patient with such vascular access routes, monitor the patency of the access, prevent infection, and promote safety and adequate function. After dialysis, watch for complications, which may include headache, vomiting, agitation, and twitching.

Patients with end-stage renal disease may benefit from renal transplantation, despite its limitations: a shortage of donor kidneys, the chance of transplant rejection, and the need for medications and lifelong follow-up care. After renal transplantation, maintain fluid and electrolyte balance, prevent infection, monitor for rejection, and promote psychological well-being.

CONGENITAL ANOMALIES

Medullary Sponge Kidney

In medullary sponge kidney, the collecting ducts in the renal pyramids dilate, and cavities, clefts, and cysts form in the medulla. This disease may affect only a single pyramid in one kidney or all pyramids in both kidneys. The kidneys are usually somewhat enlarged but may be of normal size; they appear spongy.

Since this disorder is usually asymptomatic and benign, it's often overlooked until the patient reaches adulthood. Although medullary sponge kidney may be found in both sexes and in all age-groups, it primarily affects men aged 40 to 70. It occurs in about 1 in every 5,000 to 20,000 persons. Prognosis is generally very good. Medullary sponge kidney is unrelated to medullary cystic disease; these conditions are similar only in the presence and location of the cysts.

Causes

Medullary sponge kidney may be transmitted as an autosomal dominant trait, but this remains unproven. Most nephrologists still consider it a congenital abnormality.

Signs and symptoms

Symptoms usually appear only as a result of complications and are seldom present before adulthood. Such complications include formation of calcium phosphate stones, which lodge in the dilated cystic collecting ducts or pass through a ureter, and infection secondary to dilation of the ducts. These complications, which occur in about 30% of patients, are likely to produce severe colic, hematuria, lower urinary tract infection (burning on urination, urgency, frequency), and pyelonephritis.

Secondary impairment of renal function from obstruction and infection occurs in only about 10% of patients.

Diagnosis

Intravenous pyelography is usually the key to diagnosis, often showing a characteristic flowerlike appearance of the pyramidal cavities when they fill with contrast material. Retrograde pyelography or excretory urography may show renal calculi, but these tests are usually avoided because of the risk of infection.

Urinalysis is generally normal unless complications develop; however, it may show a slight reduction in concentrating ability or hypercalciuria.

Diagnosis must distinguish medullary sponge kidney from renal tuberculosis, renal tubular acidosis, and papillary necrosis.

Treatment

Treatment focuses on preventing or treating complications caused by stones and infection. Specific measures include increasing fluid intake and monitoring renal function and urine. New symptoms necessitate immediate evaluation.

Since medullary sponge kidney is a benign condition, surgery is seldom necessary, except to remove stones during acute obstruction. Only serious, uncontrollable infection or hemorrhage requires nephrectomy.

Special considerations

- Explain the disease to the patient and his family. Stress that the condition is benign and the prognosis good.
- To prevent infection, instruct the patient to bathe often and use proper toilet hygiene. Such hygiene is especially important for a female patient, since the proximity of the urinary meatus and the anus increases the risk of infection.
- If infection occurs, stress the impor-

tance of completing the prescribed course of antibiotic therapy.
- Emphasize the need for fluids.
- Explain all diagnostic procedures, and provide emotional support. Demonstrate how to collect a clean-catch urine specimen for culture. Check for allergy to intravenous pyelography dye.
- When the patient is hospitalized for a stone, strain all urine, administer analgesics freely, and force fluids. Before discharge, tell the patient to watch for and report any signs of stone passage and urinary tract infection.

Polycystic Kidney Disease

An inherited disorder, polycystic kidney disease is characterized by multiple, bilateral, grapelike clusters of fluid-filled cysts that grossly enlarge the kidneys, compressing and eventually replacing functioning renal tissue. This disease appears in two distinct forms. The infantile form causes stillbirth or early neonatal death. A few infants with this disease survive for 2 years and then develop fatal renal, congestive heart, or respiratory failure. Onset of the adult form is insidious but usually becomes obvious between ages 30 and 50; rarely, it may not cause symptoms until the patient is in his seventies. In the adult form, renal deterioration is more gradual but, like the infantile form, progresses relentlessly to fatal uremia.

Prognosis in adults is extremely variable. Progression may be slow, even after symptoms of renal insufficiency appear. However, after uremic symptoms develop, polycystic disease is usually fatal within 4 years, unless the patient receives treatment with dialysis.

Causes and incidence

While both types of polycystic kidney disease are genetically transmitted, the incidence in two distinct age-groups and different inheritance patterns suggest two unrelated disorders. The infantile type appears to be inherited as an autosomal recessive trait; the adult type, as an autosomal dominant trait. Both types affect males and females equally.

Signs and symptoms

The newborn with infantile polycystic disease often has pronounced epicanthal folds, a pointed nose, a small chin, and floppy, low-set ears (Potter facies). At birth, he has huge bilateral masses on the flanks that are symmetrical, tense, and cannot be transilluminated. He characteristically shows signs of respiratory distress and congestive heart failure. Eventually, he develops uremia and renal failure. Accompanying hepatic fibrosis may cause portal hypertension and bleeding varices to develop as well.

Adult polycystic kidney disease is often asymptomatic while the patient's in his thirties and forties, but may induce nonspecific symptoms, such as hypertension, polyuria, and urinary tract infection. Later, the patient develops overt symptoms related to the enlarging kidney mass, such as lumbar pain, widening girth, and swollen or tender abdomen. Such abdominal pain is usually worsened by exertion and relieved by lying down. In advanced stages, this disease may cause recurrent hematuria; life-threatening retroperitoneal bleeding resulting from cyst rupture; proteinuria; and colicky abdominal pain from the ureteral passage of clots or calculi. Generally, about 10 years after symptoms appear, progressive compression of kidney structures by the enlarging mass produces renal failure and uremia.

Diagnosis

A family history and a physical examination revealing large bilateral, irregular masses in the flanks strongly suggest polycystic kidney disease. In advanced stages, grossly enlarged and palpable kidneys make the diagnosis obvious. In patients with these findings, the following laboratory results are typical:

- *Intravenous or retrograde pyelography* reveals enlarged kidneys, with elongation of pelvis, flattening of the calyces, and indentations caused by cysts. Excretory urography of the newborn shows poor excretion of contrast medium.
- *Ultrasound* and *tomography* show kidney enlargement and presence of cysts; tomography demonstrates multiple areas of cystic damage.
- *Urinalysis* and *creatinine clearance tests*—nonspecific tests that evaluate renal function—indicate abnormalities.

Diagnosis must rule out the presence of renal tumors.

Treatment

Polycystic kidney disease can't be cured, but careful management of associated urinary tract infections and secondary hypertension may prolong life. Progressive renal failure requires treatment similar to that for other types of renal disease, including dialysis or, rarely, kidney transplant.

When adult polycystic kidney disease is discovered in the asymptomatic stage, careful monitoring is required, including urine cultures and creatinine clearance tests repeated at 6-month intervals. When urine culture detects infection, prompt and vigorous antibiotic treatment is necessary even for asymptomatic infection. As renal impairment progresses, selected patients may undergo dialysis, transplantation, or both. Cystic abscess or retroperitoneal bleeding may require surgical drainage; intractable pain (a rare symptom) may also require surgery. However, since this disease is bilateral, nephrectomy usually isn't recommended, because it aggravates the risk of infection in the remaining kidney.

Special considerations

Since polycystic kidney disease is usually relentlessly progressive, comprehensive patient teaching and emotional support are essential.

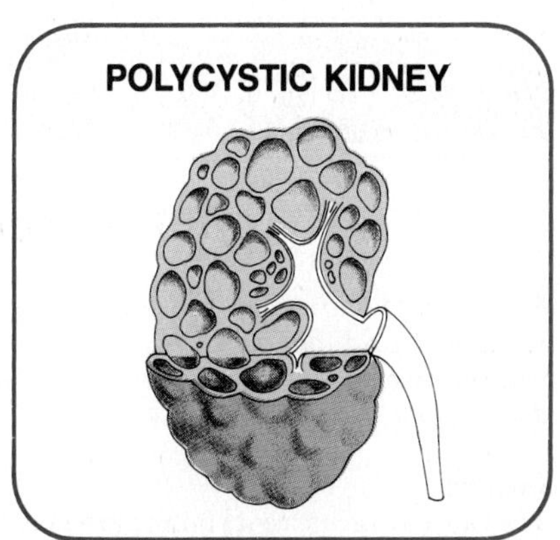

- Refer the young adult patient or parents of infants with polycystic kidney disease for genetic counseling. Such parents will probably have many questions about the risk to other offspring.
- Provide supportive care to minimize any associated symptoms. Carefully assess the patient's life-style and his physical and mental state; determine how rapidly the disease is progressing. Use this information to plan individualized patient care.
- Acquaint yourself with all aspects of end-stage renal disease, including dialysis and transplantation, so you can provide appropriate care and patient teaching as the disease progresses.
- Explain all diagnostic procedures to the patient or to his family, if the patient's an infant. Before beginning intravenous pyelography and other procedures that use an iodine-based contrast medium, determine whether the patient has ever had an allergic reaction to iodine or shellfish. Even if the patient has no history of allergy, watch for a possible allergic reaction after performing the procedures.
- Administer antibiotics, as ordered, for urinary tract infection. Stress to the patient the need to take medication exactly as prescribed, even if symptoms are minimal or absent.

ACUTE RENAL DISORDERS

Acute Renal Failure

Acute renal failure is the sudden interruption of kidney function due to obstruction, reduced circulation, or renal parenchymal disease. It's usually reversible with medical treatment; otherwise, it may progress to end-stage renal disease, uremic syndrome, and death.

Causes

The causes of acute renal failure are classified as prerenal, intrinsic (or parenchymal), and postrenal. Prerenal failure is associated with diminished blood flow to the kidneys. Such decreased flow may result from hypovolemia, shock, embolism, blood loss, sepsis, pooling of fluid in ascites or burns, and cardiovascular disorders, such as congestive heart failure, dysrhythmias, and tamponade.

Intrinsic renal failure results from damage to the kidneys themselves, usually due to acute tubular necrosis. Such damage may also result from acute poststreptococcal glomerulonephritis, systemic lupus erythematosus, periarteritis nodosa, vasculitis, sickle-cell disease, bilateral renal vein thrombosis, nephrotoxins, ischemia, renal myeloma, and acute pyelonephritis.

Postrenal failure results from bilateral obstruction of urinary outflow. Its multiple causes include kidney stones, blood clots, papillae from papillary necrosis, tumors, benign prostatic hypertrophy, strictures, and urethral edema from catheterization.

Signs and symptoms

Acute renal failure is a critical illness. Its early signs are oliguria, azotemia, and, rarely, anuria. Electrolyte imbalance, metabolic acidosis, and other severe effects follow, as the patient becomes increasingly uremic and renal dysfunction disrupts other body systems.

- *Gastrointestinal:* anorexia, nausea, vomiting, diarrhea or constipation, stomatitis, bleeding, hematemesis, dry mucous membranes, uremic breath
- *Central nervous system:* headache, drowsiness, irritability, confusion, peripheral neuropathy, convulsions, coma
- *Cutaneous:* dryness, pruritus, pallor, purpura, and, rarely, uremic frost
- *Cardiovascular:* early in the disease, hypotension; later, hypertension, dysrhythmias, fluid overload, congestive heart failure, systemic edema, anemia, altered clotting mechanisms
- *Respiratory:* pulmonary edema, Kussmaul's respirations.

Fever and chills indicate infection, a common complication.

Diagnosis

A patient history of renal disease suggests possible causes.

Blood test results indicating intrinsic acute renal failure include elevated BUN, serum creatinine, and potassium; and low blood pH, bicarbonate, hematocrit, and hemoglobin. Urine samples show casts, cellular debris, decreased specific gravity, and, in glomerular diseases, proteinuria and urine osmolality close to serum osmolality. Urine sodium level is < 20 mEq/liter if oliguria results from decreased perfusion; > 40 mEq/liter if it results from an intrinsic problem.

Other studies include ultrasound of the kidneys, plain films of the abdomen and the kidney-ureter-bladder, intravenous pyelography, renal scan, retrograde pyelography, and nephrotomography.

Treatment

Supportive measures include a diet high in calories and low in protein, sodium, and potassium, with supplemental vitamins and restricted fluids. Meticulous electrolyte monitoring is essential to detect hyperkalemia. If hyperkalemia occurs, acute therapy may include dialysis, hypertonic glucose and insulin infusions, and sodium bicarbonate—all administered I.V.—and sodium polystyrene sulfonate, P.O. or by enema, to remove potassium from the body.

If measures fail to control uremic symptoms, hemodialysis or peritoneal dialysis may be necessary.

Special considerations

- Measure and record intake and output, including all body fluids, such as wound drainage, nasogastric output, and diarrhea. Weigh the patient daily.
- Assess hematocrit and hemoglobin levels and replace blood components, as ordered. *Don't* use whole blood if the patient is prone to congestive heart failure and can't tolerate extra fluid volume.
- Monitor vital signs. Watch for and report any signs of pericarditis (pleuritic chest pain, tachycardia, pericardial friction rub), inadequate renal perfusion (hypotension), and acidosis.
- Maintain proper electrolyte balance. Strictly monitor potassium levels. Watch for symptoms of hyperkalemia (malaise, anorexia, paresthesia, or muscle weakness) and EKG changes (tall peaked T waves, widening QRS segment, and disappearing P waves), and report them immediately. Avoid administering medications containing potassium.
- Assess the patient frequently, especially during emergency treatment to lower potassium levels. If the patient receives hypertonic glucose and insulin infusions, monitor potassium levels. If you give sodium polystyrene sulfonate rectally, make sure the patient doesn't retain it and become constipated, to prevent bowel perforation.
- Maintain nutritional status. Provide a high-calorie, low-protein, low-sodium, and low-potassium diet, with vitamin supplements. Give the anorectic patient small, frequent meals.
- Use aseptic technique, since the patient with acute renal failure is highly susceptible to infection. Don't allow personnel with upper respiratory tract infections to care for the patient.
- Prevent complications of immobility by encouraging frequent coughing and deep breathing and by performing passive range-of-motion exercises. Help the patient walk as soon as possible. Add lubricating lotion to the patient's bathwater to combat skin dryness.
- Provide good mouth care frequently, since mucous membranes are dry. If stomatitis occurs, an antibiotic solution may be ordered. Have the patient swish the solution around in his mouth before swallowing.
- Monitor for gastrointestinal bleeding by guaiac-testing all stools for blood. Administer medications carefully, especially antacids and stool softeners.
- Use appropriate safety measures, such as side rails and restraints, since the patient with CNS involvement may be dizzy or confused.
- Provide emotional support to the patient and his family. Reassure them by clearly and fully explaining all procedures.
- During peritoneal dialysis, position the patient carefully. Elevate the head of the bed to reduce pressure on the diaphragm and aid respiration. Be alert for signs of infection (cloudy drainage, elevated temperature) and, rarely, bleeding. If pain occurs, reduce the amount of dialysate. Monitor the diabetic patient's blood glucose periodically, and administer insulin, as ordered. Watch for complications, such as peritonitis, atelectasis, hypokalemia, pneumonia, and shock.
- If the patient requires hemodialysis, check the site of the arteriovenous shunt or fistula every 2 hours for patency and signs of clotting. Don't use the arm with the shunt or fistula for taking blood pressures or drawing blood. Keep two bulldog clips attached to the dressing over the shunt; use them to clamp off the shunt if it becomes disconnected. During dialysis, monitor vital signs, clotting times, blood flow, the function of the vascular

access site, and arterial and venous pressures. Watch for complications, such as septicemia, embolism, hepatitis, and rapid fluid and electrolyte loss. After dialysis, monitor vital signs and the vascular access site; watch for signs of fluid and electrolyte imbalances.

Acute Pyelonephritis

(Acute infective tubulointerstitial nephritis)

One of the most common renal diseases, acute pyelonephritis is a sudden inflammation caused by bacteria that primarily affects the interstitial area and the renal pelvis or, less often, the renal tubules. With treatment and continued follow-up, prognosis is good, and extensive permanent damage is rare.

Causes and incidence

Acute pyelonephritis results from bacterial infection of the kidneys. Infecting bacteria usually are normal intestinal and fecal flora that grow readily in urine. The most common causative organism is *Escherichia coli,* but *Proteus, Pseudomonas, Staphylococcus aureus,* and *Streptococcus faecalis* (enterococcus) may also cause such infections.

Typically, the infection spreads from the bladder to the ureters, then to the kidneys, as in vesicoureteral reflux. Vesicoureteral reflux may result from congenital weakness at the junction of the ureter and the bladder. Bacteria refluxed to intrarenal tissues may create colonies of infection within 24 to 48 hours. Infection may also result from instrumentation (such as catheterization, cystoscopy, or urologic surgery), from a hematogenic infection (as in septicemia or endocarditis), or possibly from lymphatic infection.

Pyelonephritis may also result from an inability to empty the bladder (for example, in patients with neurogenic bladder), urinary stasis, or urinary obstruction due to tumors, strictures, or benign prostatic hypertrophy.

Pyelonephritis occurs more often in females, probably because of a shorter urethra and the proximity of the urinary meatus to the vagina and the rectum—both conditions allow bacteria to reach the bladder more easily—and a lack of the antibacterial prostatic secretions produced in the male.

Incidence increases with age and is higher in the following groups:

- *Sexually active women:* Intercourse in-

CHRONIC PYELONEPHRITIS

Chronic pyelonephritis is a persistent kidney inflammation that can scar the kidneys and may lead to chronic renal failure. Its etiology may be bacterial, metastatic, or urogenous. This disease is most common in patients who are predisposed to recurrent acute pyelonephritis, such as those with urinary obstructions or vesicoureteral reflux.

Patients with chronic pyelonephritis may have a childhood history of unexplained fevers or bed-wetting. Clinical effects may include flank pain, anemia, low urine specific gravity, proteinuria, leukocytes in urine, and especially in late stages, hypertension. Uremia rarely develops from chronic pyelonephritis unless structural abnormalities exist in the excretory system. Bacteriuria may be intermittent. When no bacteria are found in the urine, diagnosis depends on intravenous pyelography (renal pelvis may appear small and flattened) and renal biopsy.

Effective treatment of chronic pyelonephritis requires control of hypertension, elimination of the existing obstruction (when possible), and long-term antimicrobial therapy.

creases the risk of bacterial contamination.

- *Pregnant women:* About 5% develop asymptomatic bacteriuria; if untreated, about 40% develop pyelonephritis.
- *Diabetics:* Neurogenic bladder causes incomplete emptying and urinary stasis; glycosuria may support bacterial growth in the urine.
- *Persons with other renal diseases:* Compromised renal function aggravates susceptibility.

Signs and symptoms

Typical clinical features include urgency, frequency, burning during urination, dysuria, nocturia, and hematuria (usually microscopic but may be gross). Urine may appear cloudy and have an ammoniacal or fishy odor. Other common symptoms include a temperature of 102° F. (38.9° C.) or higher, shaking chills, flank pain, anorexia, and general fatigue.

These symptoms characteristically develop rapidly over a few hours or a few days. Although these symptoms may disappear within days, even without treatment, residual bacterial infection is likely and may cause later recurrence of symptoms.

Diagnosis

Diagnosis requires urinalysis and culture. Typical findings include:

- *Pyuria* (pus in urine): Urine sediment reveals the presence of leukocytes singly, in clumps, and in casts; and, possibly, a few RBCs.
- *Significant bacteriuria:* Urine culture reveals more than 100,000 organisms/mm^3 of urine.
- *Low specific gravity and osmolality:* These findings result from a temporarily decreased ability to concentrate urine.
- *Slightly alkaline urine pH.*
- *Proteinuria, glycosuria, and ketonuria:* These conditions are less common.

X-rays also help in the evaluation of acute pyelonephritis. A plain film of the kidneys-ureters-bladder may reveal calculi, tumors, or cysts in the kidneys and the urinary tract. Intravenous pyelography may show asymmetrical kidneys.

Treatment

Treatment centers on antibiotic therapy appropriate to the specific infecting organism after identification by urine culture and sensitivity studies. For example, enterococcus requires treatment with ampicillin, penicillin G, or vancomycin. *Staphylococcus* requires penicillin G or, if resistance develops, a semisynthetic penicillin, such as nafcillin, or a cephalosporin. *Escherichia coli* may be treated with sulfisoxazole, nalidixic acid, and nitrofurantoin; *Proteus,* with ampicillin, sulfisoxazole, nalidixic acid, and a cephalosporin; and *Pseudomonas,* with gentamicin, tobramycin, and carbenicillin. When the infecting organism cannot be identified, therapy usually consists of a broad-spectrum antibiotic, such as ampicillin or cephalexin. If the patient is pregnant, antibiotics must be prescribed cautiously. Urinary analgesics, such as phenazopyridine, are also appropriate.

Symptoms may disappear after several days of antibiotic therapy. Although urine usually becomes sterile within 48 to 72 hours, the course of such therapy is 10 to 14 days. Follow-up treatment includes reculturing urine 1 week after drug therapy stops, then periodically for the next year to detect residual or recurring infection. Most patients with uncomplicated infections respond well to therapy and don't suffer reinfection.

In infection from obstruction or vesicoureteral reflux, antibiotics may be less effective; treatment may then necessitate surgery to relieve the obstruction or correct the anomaly. Patients at high risk of recurring urinary tract and kidney infections—such as those with prolonged use of an indwelling catheter or maintenance antibiotic therapy—require long-term follow-up.

Special considerations

- Administer antipyretics for fever.
- Force fluids to achieve urinary output of more than 2,000 ml/day. This helps to empty the bladder of contaminated

urine. Don't encourage intake of more than 2 to 3 liters, because this may decrease the effectiveness of the antibiotics.

- Provide an acid-ash diet to prevent stone formation.
- Teach proper technique for collecting a clean-catch urine specimen. Be sure to refrigerate or culture a urine specimen within 30 minutes of collection to prevent overgrowth of bacteria.
- Stress the need to complete prescribed antibiotic therapy, even after symptoms subside. Encourage long-term follow-up care for high-risk patients.

To prevent acute pyelonephritis:

- Observe strict sterile technique during catheter insertion and care.
- Instruct females to prevent bacterial contamination by wiping the perineum from front to back after defecation.
- Advise routine checkups for patients with a history of urinary tract infections. Teach them to recognize signs of infection, such as cloudy urine, burning on urination, urgency, and frequency, especially when accompanied by a low-grade fever.

Acute Poststreptococcal Glomerulonephritis

(Acute glomerulonephritis)

Acute poststreptococcal glomerulonephritis (APSGN) is a relatively common bilateral inflammation of the glomeruli. It follows a streptococcal infection of the respiratory tract or, less often, a skin infection, such as impetigo. APSGN is most common in boys aged 3 to 7, but can occur at any age. Up to 95% of children and up to 70% of adults with APSGN recover fully; the rest may progress to chronic renal failure within months.

Causes

APSGN results from the entrapment and collection of antigen-antibody (produced as an immunologic mechanism in response to streptococcus) in the glomerular capillary membranes, inducing inflammatory damage and impeding glomerular function. Sometimes, the immune complement further damages the glomerular membrane. The damaged and inflamed glomerulus loses the ability to be selectively permeable, and allows RBCs and proteins to filter through as the glomerular filtration rate falls. Uremic poisoning may result.

Signs and symptoms

Generally, APSGN begins within 1 to 3 weeks after untreated pharyngitis. The most common symptoms are mild to moderate edema, proteinuria, azotemia, hematuria (smoky or coffee-colored urine), oliguria (less than 400 ml/24 hours), and fatigue. Mild to severe hypertension may result from either sodium or water retention (caused by decreased glomerular filtration rate), or inappropriate renin release. Congestive heart failure from hypervolemia leads to symptoms of pulmonary edema: shortness of breath, dyspnea, and orthopnea.

Diagnosis

Diagnosis requires a detailed patient history, and assessment of clinical symptoms and laboratory tests. Blood values (elevated electrolytes, BUN, and creatinine) and urine values (RBCs, WBCs, mixed cell casts, and protein) indicate renal failure. In addition, elevated antistreptolysin-O titers (in 80% of patients), elevated streptozyme and anti-DNase B titers, and low-serum complement levels verify recent streptococcal infection. A throat culture may also show group A beta-hemolytic streptococcus. Kidney-ureter-bladder X-rays show bilateral kidney enlargement. A renal biopsy may be necessary to confirm diagnosis or assess renal tissue status.

Treatment

The goals of treatment are relief of symptoms and prevention of complications. Vigorous supportive care includes bed rest, fluid and dietary sodium restrictions, and correction of electrolyte imbalances (possibly with dialysis, although this is rarely necessary). Therapy may include diuretics, such as metolazone or furosemide, to reduce extracellular fluid overload, and an antihypertensive, such as hydralazine. The use of antibiotics to prevent secondary infection or transmission to others is controversial.

Special considerations

APSGN usually resolves within 2 weeks, so patient care is primarily supportive:

- Check vital signs and electrolyte values. Monitor intake and output and daily weight. Assess renal function daily through serum creatinine, BUN, and urine creatinine clearance. Watch for and immediately report signs of acute renal failure (oliguria, azotemia, and acidosis).
- Consult the dietitian to provide a diet high in calories and low in protein, sodium, potassium, and fluids.
- Protect the debilitated patient against secondary infection by providing good nutrition, using good hygienic technique, and preventing contact with infected persons.
- Bed rest is necessary during the acute phase. Allow the patient to *gradually* resume normal activities as symptoms subside.
- Provide emotional support for the patient and family. If the patient's on dialysis, explain the procedure fully.
- Advise the patient with a history of chronic upper respiratory tract infections to immediately report signs of infection (fever, sore throat).
- Tell the patient that follow-up examinations are necessary to detect chronic renal failure. Stress the need for regular blood pressure, urinary protein, and renal function assessments during the convalescent months to detect recurrence. After APSGN, gross hematuria may recur during nonspecific viral infections; abnormal urinary findings may persist for years.
- Encourage pregnant women with histories of APSGN to have frequent medical evaluations, since pregnancy further stresses the kidneys and increases the risk of chronic renal failure.

Acute Tubular Necrosis

(Acute tubulointerstitial nephritis)

Acute tubular necrosis (ATN) accounts for about 75% of all cases of acute renal failure and is the most common cause of acute renal failure in critically ill patients. ATN injures the tubular segment of the nephron, causing renal failure and uremic syndrome. Mortality ranges from 40% to 70%, depending on complications from underlying diseases. Nonoliguric forms of ATN have a better prognosis.

Causes

ATN results from ischemic or nephrotoxic injury, most commonly in debilitated patients, such as the critically ill or those who have undergone extensive surgery. In ischemic injury, disruption of blood flow to the kidneys may result from circulatory collapse, severe hypotension, trauma, hemorrhage, dehydration, cardiogenic or septic shock, surgery, anesthetics, or reactions to transfusions. Nephrotoxic injury may follow ingestion of certain chemical agents or result from a hypersensitive reaction of the kidneys. Since nephrotoxic ATN doesn't damage the basement membrane of the nephron, it's potentially reversible. However, ischemic ATN can damage the epithelial and

NEPHROTOXIC INJURY INCREASING

Incidence of acute tubular necrosis (ATN) from ingestion or inhalation of toxic substances is rising. This exposure may occur in the hospital, to an already debilitated patient, from such toxic agents as antibiotics (aminoglycosides, for example) and contrast media. Other nephrotoxic agents include pesticides, fungicides, heavy metals (mercury, arsenic, lead, bismuth, uranium), and organic solvents containing carbon tetrachloride or ethylene glycol (cleaning fluids or industrial solvents). Ingestion of these substances may be accidental or intentional.

Nephrotoxic injury causes multiple symptoms similar to those of renal failure, particularly azotemia, anemia, acidosis, overhydration, and hypertension; and, less often, fever, skin rash, and eosinophilia.

Treatment consists of identifying the nephrotoxic substance, eliminating its use, and removing it from the body by any means available, such as hemodialysis in extreme cases. Treatment is supportive during the course of acute renal failure.

basement membranes and can cause lesions in the renal interstitium.

ATN may result from:

- diseased tubular epithelium that allows leakage of glomerular filtrate across the membranes and reabsorption of filtrate into the blood.
- obstruction of urine flow by the collection of damaged cells, casts, RBCs, and other cellular debris within the tubular walls.
- ischemic injury to glomerular epithelial cells, resulting in cellular collapse and decreased glomerular capillary permeability.
- ischemic injury to vascular endothelium, eventually resulting in cellular swelling and obstruction.

Signs and symptoms

ATN is usually difficult to recognize in its early stages, because effects of the critically ill patient's primary disease may mask the symptoms of ATN. The first recognizable effect may be decreased urine output. Generally, hyperkalemia and the characteristic uremic syndrome soon follow, with oliguria (or, rarely, anuria) and confusion, which may progress to uremic coma. Other possible complications may include congestive heart failure, uremic pericarditis, pulmonary edema, uremic lung, anemia, anorexia, intractable vomiting, and poor wound healing due to debilitation.

Fever and chills may signify the onset of infection, the leading cause of death in ATN.

Diagnosis

Diagnosis is usually delayed until the condition has progressed to an advanced stage. The most significant laboratory clues are urinary sediment containing RBCs and casts, and dilute urine of a low specific gravity (1.010), low osmolality (less than 400 mOsm/kg), and high sodium level (40 to 60 mEq/liter). Blood studies reveal elevated BUN and serum creatinine levels, anemia, defects in platelet adherence, metabolic acidosis, and hyperkalemia. EKG may show dysrhythmias (from electrolyte imbalances) and, with hyperkalemia, widening QRS segment, disappearing P waves, and tall, peaked T waves.

Treatment

Treatment for patients with ATN consists of vigorous supportive measures during the acute phase until normal kidney function resumes.

Initial treatment may include administration of diuretics and infusion of a large volume of fluids to flush tubules of cellular casts and debris and to replace fluid loss. However, this treatment carries a risk of fluid overload. Long-term fluid management requires daily replacement of projected and calculated losses (including insensible loss).

Other appropriate measures to control complications include transfusion of packed RBCs for anemia and administration of antibiotics for infection. Hyperkalemia may require emergency I.V. administration of 50% glucose, regular insulin, and sodium bicarbonate. Sodium polystyrene sulfonate with sorbitol may be given P.O. or by enema to reduce extracellular potassium levels. Peritoneal dialysis or hemodialysis may be needed if the patient is catabolic.

Special considerations

- Maintain fluid balance. Watch for fluid overload, a common complication of therapy. Accurately record intake and output, including wound drainage, nasogastric output, and peritoneal dialysis and hemodialysis balances. Weigh the patient daily.
- Monitor hemoglobin and hematocrit, and administer blood products, as needed. Use fresh packed cells instead of whole blood to prevent fluid overload and congestive heart failure.
- Maintain electrolyte balance. Monitor laboratory results, and report imbalances. Enforce dietary restriction of foods containing sodium and potassium, such as bananas, orange juice, and baked potatoes. Check for potassium content in prescribed medications (for example, potassium penicillin). Provide adequate calories and essential amino acids, while restricting protein intake to maintain an anabolic state. Total parenteral nutrition may be indicated in the severely debilitated or catabolic patient.
- Use aseptic technique, particularly when handling catheters, since the debilitated patient is vulnerable to infection. Immediately report fever, chills, delayed wound healing, or flank pain if the patient has a Foley catheter in place.
- Watch for complications. If anemia worsens (pallor, weakness, lethargy with decreased hemoglobin), administer RBCs, as ordered. For acidosis, give sodium bicarbonate or assist with dialysis in severe cases, as ordered. Watch for signs of diminishing renal perfusion (hypotension and decreased urinary output). Encourage coughing and deep breathing to prevent pulmonary complications.
- Perform passive range-of-motion exercises. Provide good skin care; apply lotion or bath oil for dry skin. Help the patient to walk as soon as possible, but guard against exhaustion.
- Provide reassurance and emotional support. Encourage the patient and family to express their fears. Fully explain each procedure; repeat the explanation each time the procedure is done. Help the patient and family set realistic goals according to individual prognosis.
- To prevent ATN, make sure all patients are well hydrated before surgery or after X-rays that use a contrast medium. Administer mannitol, as ordered, to high-risk patients before and during these procedures. Carefully monitor patients receiving blood transfusions to detect early signs of transfusion reaction (fever, rash, chills), and discontinue such transfusion immediately.

Renal Infarction

Renal infarction is the formation of a coagulated, necrotic area in one or both kidneys that results from renal blood vessel occlusion. The location and size of the infarction depend on the site of vascular occlusion. Most often, infarction affects the renal cortex, but it can extend into the medulla. Residual renal function after infarction depends on the extent of the damage from the infarction.

Causes

In 75% of patients, renal infarction results from renal artery embolism secondary to mitral stenosis, infective endocarditis, atrial fibrillation, microthrombi in the left ventricle, rheumatic

SITES OF RENAL INFARCTION

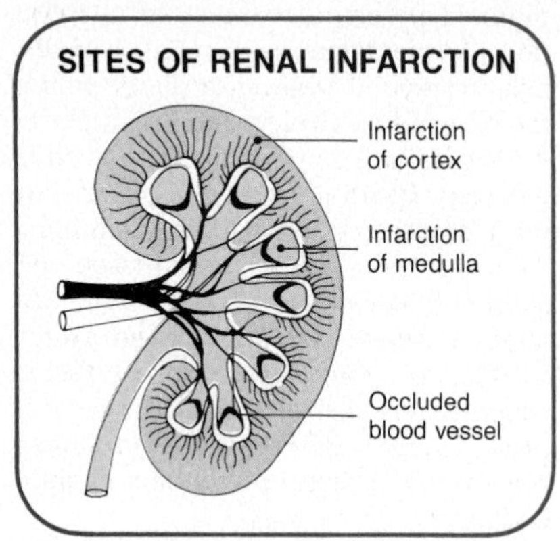

valvular disease, or recent myocardial infarction. The embolism reduces the rate of blood flow to renal tissue and leads to ischemia. The rate and degree of blood flow reduction determine whether or not the insult will be acute or chronic as arterial narrowing progresses.

Less common causes of renal infarction are atherosclerosis, with or without thrombus formation; and thrombus from flank trauma, sickle-cell anemia, scleroderma, and arterionephrosclerosis.

Signs and symptoms

Although renal infarction may be asymptomatic, typical symptoms include severe upper abdominal pain or gnawing flank pain and tenderness, costovertebral tenderness, fever, anorexia, nausea, and vomiting. When arterial occlusion causes infarction, the affected kidney is small and not palpable. Renovascular hypertension, a frequent complication that may occur several days after infarction, results from reduced blood flow, which stimulates the renin-angiotensin mechanism.

Diagnosis

A history of predisposing cardiovascular disease or other factors in a patient with typical clinical features strongly suggests renal infarction. Firm diagnosis requires appropriate laboratory tests:

• *Urinalysis* reveals proteinuria and microscopic hematuria.

• *Urine enzyme levels,* especially lactate dehydrogenase (LDH) and alkaline phosphatase, are often elevated as a result of tissue destruction.

• *Serum enzyme levels,* especially SGOT, alkaline phosphatase, and LDH, are elevated. Blood studies may also reveal leukocytosis and increased ESR.

• *Intravenous pyelography (IVP)* shows diminished or absent excretion of contrast dye, indicating vascular occlusion or urethral obstruction.

• *Isotopic renal scan,* a benign, noninvasive technique, demonstrates absent or reduced blood flow to the kidneys.

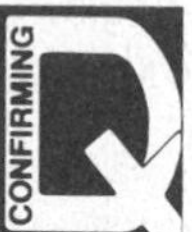

• *Renal arteriography* provides absolute proof of existing infarction but is used as a last resort, since it is a high-risk procedure.

Treatment

Infection in the infarcted area or significant hypertension may require surgical repair of the occlusion or nephrectomy. Surgery to establish collateral circulation to the area can relieve renovascular hypertension. Persistent hypertension may respond to antihypertensives and a low-sodium diet. Additional treatments may include administration of intraarterial streptokinase, to lyse blood clots, and catheter embolectomy.

Special considerations

Assess the degree of renal function and offer supportive care to maintain homeostasis.

• Monitor intake and output, vital signs (particularly blood pressure), electrolytes, and daily weight. Watch for signs of fluid overload, such as dyspnea, tachycardia, pulmonary edema, and electrolyte imbalances.

• Carefully explain all diagnostic procedures.

• Provide reassurance and emotional support for the patient and family.

• Encourage the patient to return for follow-up examination, which usually includes IVP or a renal scan to assess regained renal function.

Renal Calculi

(Kidney stones)

Renal calculi may form anywhere in the urinary tract but usually develop in the renal pelvis or the calyces of the kidneys. Such formation follows precipitation of substances normally dissolved in the urine (calcium oxalate, calcium phosphate, magnesium ammonium phosphate, or occasionally, urate or cystine). Renal calculi vary in size and may be solitary or multiple. They may remain in the renal pelvis or enter the ureter and may damage renal parenchyma; large calculi cause pressure necrosis. In certain locations, calculi cause obstruction, with resultant hydronephrosis, and tend to recur.

Causes

Among Americans, renal calculi develop in 1 in 1,000 persons, are more common in men (especially those aged 30 to 50) than in women, and are rare in Blacks and children. They're particularly prevalent in certain geographic areas, such as southeastern United States (stone belt), possibly because a hot climate promotes dehydration or because of regional dietary habits. Although the exact cause of renal calculi is unknown, predisposing factors include the following:

- *Dehydration:* Decreased urine production concentrates calculus-forming substances.
- *Infection:* Infected, damaged tissue serves as a site for calculus development; pH changes provide a favorable medium for calculus formation (especially for magnesium ammonium phosphate or calcium phosphate calculi); or infected calculi (usually magnesium ammonium phosphate or staghorn calculi) may develop if bacteria serve as the nucleus in calculus formation. Such infections may promote destruction of renal parenchyma.
- *Obstruction:* Urinary stasis (as in immobility from spinal cord injury) allows calculus constituents to collect and adhere, forming calculi. Obstruction also promotes infection, which, in turn, compounds the obstruction.
- *Metabolic factors:* These factors may predispose to renal calculi: hyperparathyroidism, renal tubular acidosis, elevated uric acid (usually with gout), defective metabolism of oxalate, genetic defect in metabolism of cystine, and excessive intake of vitamin D or dietary calcium.

Signs and symptoms

Clinical effects vary with size, location, and etiology of the calculi. Pain, the key symptom, usually results from obstruction; large, rough calculi occlude the opening to the ureter and increase the frequency and force of peristaltic contractions. The pain of classic renal colic travels from the costovertebral angle to the flank, to the suprapubic region and external genitalia. The intensity of this pain fluctuates and may be excruciating at its peak. If calculi are in the renal pelvis and calyces, pain may be more constant and dull. Back pain (from calculi that produce an obstruction within a kidney) and severe abdominal pain (from calculi traveling down a ureter) may also occur. Nausea and vomiting usually accompany severe pain.

Other associated signs include fever, chills, hematuria (when calculi abrade a ureter), abdominal distention, pyuria, and rarely, anuria (from bilateral obstruction, or unilateral obstruction in the patient with one kidney).

Diagnosis

Diagnosis is based on the clinical picture and the following tests:

- *Kidney-ureter-bladder X-rays* reveal most renal calculi.
- *Stone analysis* shows mineral content.

TYPES OF RENAL CALCULI

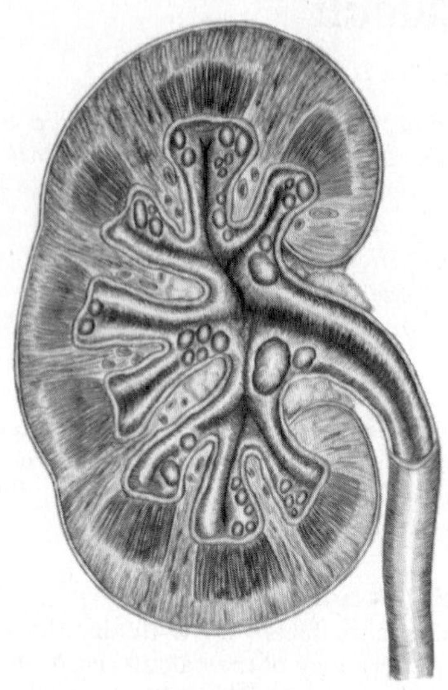

Multiple small calculi may vary in size; they may remain in the renal pelvis or pass down the ureter.

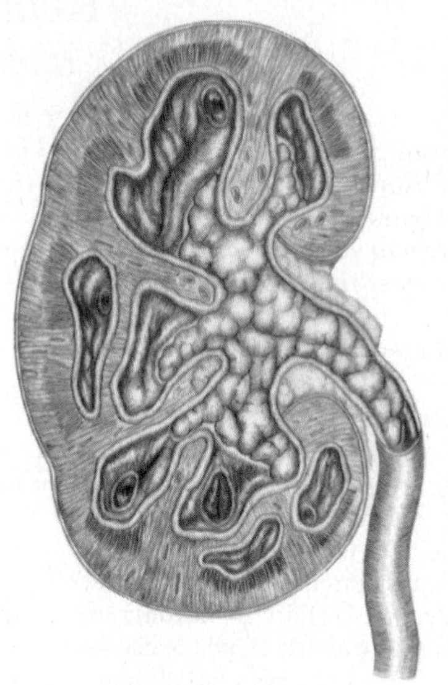

A staghorn calculus (a cast of the calyceal and pelvic collecting system) may form from a stone that stays in the kidney.

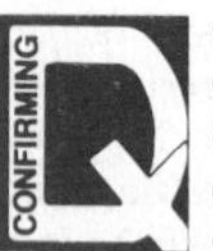

- *Intravenous pyelography* confirms the diagnosis and determines size and location of calculi.
- *Kidney ultrasonography* is an easily performed noninvasive, nontoxic test to detect obstructive changes, such as hydronephrosis.
- *Urine culture* of midstream sample may indicate urinary tract infection.
- *Urinalysis* may be normal, or may show increased specific gravity and acid or alkaline pH suitable for different types of stone formation. Other urinalysis findings include hematuria (gross or microscopic), crystals (urate, calcium, or cystine), casts, and pyuria with or without bacteria and WBCs.
- A *24-hour urine collection* is evaluated for calcium oxalate, phosphorus, and uric acid excretion levels.

Other laboratory results support this diagnosis:

- *Serial blood calcium and phosphorus levels* detect hyperparathyroidism and show increased calcium level in proportion to normal serum protein.
- *Blood protein level* determines level of free calcium unbound to protein.
- *Blood chloride and bicarbonate levels* may show renal tubular acidosis.
- *Increased blood uric acid levels* may indicate gout as the cause.

Diagnosis must rule out appendicitis, cholecystitis, peptic ulcer, and pancreatitis as potential sources of pain.

Treatment

Since 90% of renal calculi are smaller than 5 mm in diameter, treatment usually consists of measures to promote their natural passage. Along with vigorous hydration, such treatment includes antimicrobial therapy (varying with the cultured organism) for infection; analgesics, such as meperidine, for pain; and diuretics to prevent urinary stasis and further calculus formation (thiazides decrease calcium excretion into the urine). Prophylaxis to prevent calculus formation includes a low-calcium diet for absorptive hypercalciuria, parathyroidectomy for hyperparathyroidism, allopurinol for uric acid calculi, and daily administration of ascorbic acid P.O. to acidify the urine.

Calculi too large for natural passage may require surgical removal. When a calculus is in the ureter, a cystoscope may be inserted through the urethra and the calculus manipulated with catheters or retrieval instruments. Extraction of calculi from other areas (kidney calyx, renal pelvis) may necessitate a flank or lower abdominal approach. Percutaneous ultrasonic lithotripsy and extracorporeal shock wave lithotripsy shatter the calculus into fragments for removal by suction or natural passage.

Special considerations

- To aid diagnosis, maintain a 24- to 48-hour record of urine pH, with nitrazine pH paper; strain all urine through gauze or a tea strainer, and save all solid material recovered for analysis.
- To facilitate spontaneous passage, encourage the patient to walk, if possible. Also promote sufficient intake of fluids to maintain a urinary output of 3 to 4 liters/day (urine should be very dilute and colorless). To help acidify urine, offer fruit juices, particularly cranberry juice. If the patient can't drink the required amount of fluid, supplemental I.V. fluids may be given. Record intake and output and daily weight to assess fluid status and renal function.
- Stress the importance of proper diet and compliance with drug therapy. For example, if the patient's stone is caused by a hyperuricemic condition, advise the patient or whoever prepares his meals which foods are high in purine.
- If surgery is necessary, give reassurance by supplementing and reinforcing what the surgeon has told the patient about the procedure. The patient is apt to be fearful, especially if surgery includes removal of a kidney, so emphasize the fact that the body can adapt well to one kidney. If he is to have an abdominal or flank incision, teach deep breathing and coughing exercises.
- After surgery, the patient will probably have an indwelling catheter or a nephrostomy tube. Unless one of his kidneys was removed, expect bloody drainage

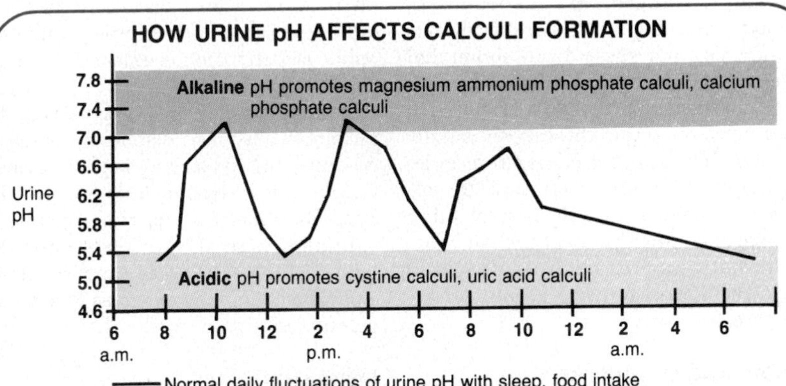

Normally, the pH of urine fluctuates from slightly acidic to slightly alkaline over a 24-hour period. This fluctuation has the periodicity shown above. If urine pH is consistently acidic or alkaline, the urine provides a medium suitable for calculi formation: acidic urine promotes formation of cystine and uric acid calculi; alkaline urine promotes formation of calcium phosphate and magnesium ammonium phosphate calculi. Calcium oxalate calculi can form in urine of varying pH.

from the catheter. Never irrigate the catheter without a doctor's order. Check dressings regularly for bloody drainage, and know how much drainage to expect. Immediately report suspected hemorrhage (excessive drainage, rising pulse rate). Use sterile technique when changing dressings or providing catheter care.

• Watch for signs of infection (rising fever, chills), and give antibiotics, as ordered. To prevent pneumonia, encourage frequent position changes, and ambulate the patient as soon as possible. Have him hold a small pillow over the operative site to splint the incision and thereby facilitate deep breathing and coughing exercises.

• Before discharge, teach the patient and family the importance of following the prescribed dietary and medication regimens to prevent recurrence of calculi. Encourage increased fluid intake. If appropriate, show the patient how to check his urine pH, and instruct him to keep a daily record. Tell him to immediately report symptoms of acute obstruction (pain, inability to void).

Renal Vein Thrombosis

Renal vein thrombosis, clotting in the renal vein, results in renal congestion, engorgement, and possibly, infarction. Such thrombosis may affect both kidneys and may occur in an acute or a chronic form. Chronic thrombosis usually impairs renal function, causing nephrotic syndrome. Abrupt onset of thrombosis that causes extensive damage may precipitate rapidly fatal renal infarction. If thrombosis affects both kidneys, prognosis is poor. However, less severe thrombosis that affects only one kidney, or gradual progression that allows development of collateral circulation may preserve partial renal function.

Causes

Renal vein thrombosis often results from a tumor that obstructs the renal vein (usually hypernephroma). Other causes include thrombophlebitis of the inferior vena cava (may result from abdominal trauma) or blood vessels of the legs, congestive heart failure, and periarteritis. In infants, renal vein thrombosis usually follows diarrhea that causes severe dehydration. Chronic renal vein thrombosis is often a complication of other glomerulopathic diseases, such as amyloidosis, diabetic nephropathy, and membranoproliferative glomerulonephritis.

Signs and symptoms

Clinical features of renal vein thrombosis vary with speed of onset. Rapid onset of venous obstruction produces severe lumbar pain, and tenderness in the epigastric region and the costovertebral angle. Other characteristic features include fever, leukocytosis, pallor, hematuria, proteinuria, peripheral edema, and when the obstruction is bilateral, oliguria and other uremic signs. The kidneys enlarge and become easily palpable. Hypertension is unusual, but may develop.

Gradual onset causes symptoms of nephrotic syndrome. Peripheral edema is possible, but pain is generally absent. Other clinical signs include proteinuria, hypoalbuminemia, and hyperlipemia.

Infants with this disease have enlarged kidneys, oliguria, and renal insufficiency that may progress to acute or chronic renal failure.

Diagnosis

• *Intravenous pyelography* provides reliable diagnostic evidence. In acute renal vein thrombosis, the kidneys appear enlarged and excretory function diminishes. Contrast medium seems to "smudge" necrotic renal tissue. In chronic thrombosis, it may show ureteral indentations that result from collateral venous channels. Renal arteriography and biopsy may also confirm the diagnosis.

• *Urinalysis* reveals gross or microscopic hematuria, proteinuria (more than 2 g/day in chronic disease), casts, and oliguria.

• *Blood studies* show leukocytosis, hypoalbuminemia, and hyperlipemia.

Treatment

Treatment is most effective for gradual thrombosis that affects only one kidney. Anticoagulant therapy (heparin or warfarin) may prove helpful, particularly if long-term. Effective surgery must be performed within 24 hours of thrombosis but even then has limited success, since thrombi often extend into the small veins. Extensive intrarenal bleeding may necessitate nephrectomy.

Patients who survive abrupt thrombosis with extensive renal damage develop nephrotic syndrome and require treatment for renal failure, such as dialysis and, possibly, transplantation. Some infants with renal vein thrombosis recover completely following heparin therapy or surgery; others suffer irreversible kidney damage.

Special considerations

• Assess renal function regularly. Monitor vital signs, intake and output, daily weight, and electrolytes.

• Administer diuretics for edema, as ordered, and enforce dietary restrictions, such as limited sodium and potassium intake.

• Monitor closely for signs of pulmonary emboli (chest pain, dyspnea).

• If heparin is given by constant I.V. infusion, frequently monitor partial thromboplastin time to determine the patient's response to it. Dilute the drug; administer it by infusion pump or controller, so the patient receives the least amount necessary.

• During anticoagulant therapy, watch for and report signs of bleeding, such as tachycardia, hypotension, hematuria, bleeding from nose or gums, ecchymoses, petechiae, and tarry stools. Instruct the patient on maintenance warfarin therapy to use an electric razor and a soft toothbrush and to avoid trauma. Suggest that he wear a medical identification bracelet, and tell him to avoid aspirin, which aggravates bleeding tendencies. Stress the need for close medical follow-up.

CHRONIC RENAL DISORDERS

Nephrotic Syndrome

Nephrotic syndrome (NS) is a condition characterized by marked proteinuria, hypoalbuminemia, hyperlipemia, and edema. Although NS is not a disease itself, it results from a specific glomerular defect and indicates renal damage. Prognosis is highly variable, depending on the underlying cause. Some forms may progress to end-stage renal failure.

Causes and incidence

About 75% of NS results from primary (idiopathic) glomerulonephritis. Classifications include the following:

• In *lipid nephrosis (nil lesions)*—main cause of NS in children—glomerulus appears normal by light microscopy. Some tubules may contain increased lipid deposits.

• *Membranous glomerulonephritis*—most common lesion in adult idiopathic NS—is characterized by uniform thickening of the glomerular basement membrane containing dense deposits and

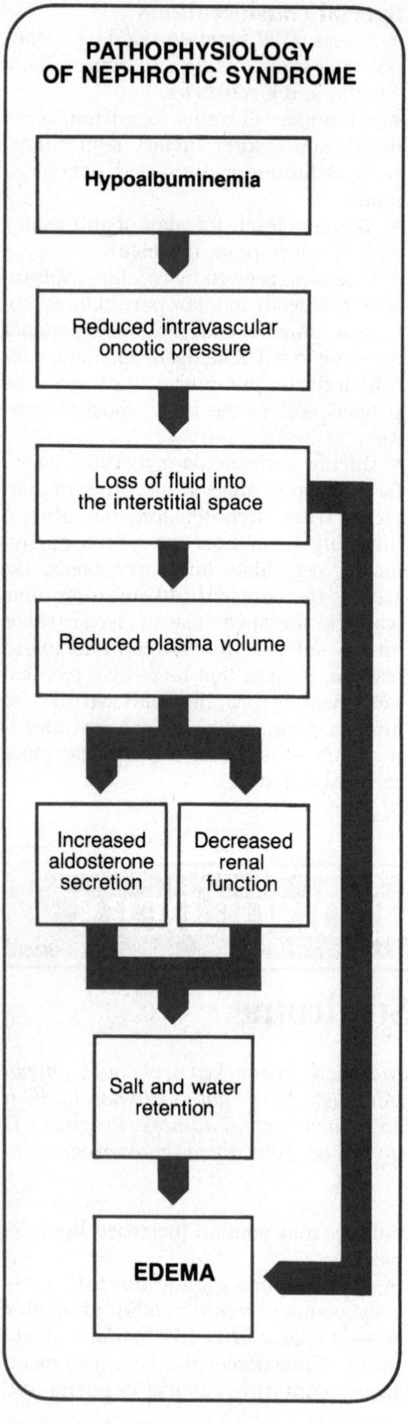

PATHOPHYSIOLOGY OF NEPHROTIC SYNDROME

Hypoalbuminemia → Reduced intravascular oncotic pressure → Loss of fluid into the interstitial space → Reduced plasma volume → Increased aldosterone secretion / Decreased renal function → Salt and water retention → EDEMA

(Loss of fluid into the interstitial space → EDEMA)

eventually progresses to renal failure.

- *Focal glomerulosclerosis* can develop spontaneously at any age, follow renal transplantation, or result from heroin abuse. Reported incidence of this condition is 10% in children with NS and up to 20% in adults. Lesions initially affect the deeper glomeruli, causing hyaline sclerosis, with later involvement of the superficial glomeruli. These lesions generally cause slowly progressive deterioration in renal function. Remissions occur occasionally.
- In *membranoproliferative glomerulonephritis*, slowly progressive lesions develop in the subendothelial region of the basement membrane. These lesions may follow infection, particularly streptococcal infection. This disease occurs primarily in children and young adults.

Other causes of NS include metabolic diseases, such as diabetes mellitus; collagen-vascular disorders, such as systemic lupus erythematosus and periarteritis nodosa; circulatory diseases, such as congestive heart failure, sickle-cell anemia, and renal vein thrombosis; nephrotoxins, such as mercury, gold, and bismuth; allergic reactions; and infections, such as tuberculosis or enteritis. Other possible causes are pregnancy, hereditary nephritis, multiple myeloma, and other neoplastic diseases.

These diseases increase glomerular protein permeability, leading to increased urinary excretion of protein, especially albumin, and subsequent hypoalbuminemia.

Signs and symptoms

The dominant clinical feature of nephrotic syndrome is mild to severe dependent edema of the ankles or sacrum, or periorbital edema, especially in children. Such edema may lead to ascites, pleural effusion, and swollen external genitalia. Accompanying symptoms may include orthostatic hypotension, lethargy, anorexia, depression, and pallor. Major complications are malnutrition, infection, coagulation disorders, thromboembolic vascular occlusion, and accelerated atherosclerosis.

Diagnosis

Consistent proteinuria in excess of 3.5 g/24 hours strongly suggests NS; examination of urine also reveals increased number of hyaline, granular, and waxy, fatty casts, and oval fat bodies. Serum values that support the diagnosis are increased cholesterol, phospholipids, and triglycerides and decreased albumin levels. Histologic identification of the lesion requires kidney biopsy.

Treatment

Effective treatment of NS necessitates correction of the underlying cause, if possible. Supportive treatment consists of protein replacement with a nutritional diet of 1.5 g protein/kg of body weight, with restricted sodium intake; diuretics for edema; and antibiotics for infection.

Some patients respond to an 8-week course of corticosteroid therapy (such as prednisone), followed by a maintenance dose. Others respond better to a combination course of prednisone and azathioprine (Imuran) or cyclophosphamide (Cytoxan).

Special considerations

- Frequently check urine protein. (Urine containing protein appears frothy.)
- Measure blood pressure while patient is supine and also while he's standing; immediately report a drop in blood pressure that exceeds 20 mm Hg.
- After kidney biopsy, watch for bleeding and shock.
- Monitor intake and output and check weight at the same time each morning—after the patient voids and before he eats—and while he's wearing the same kind of clothing. Ask the dietitian to plan a high-protein, low-sodium diet.
- Give good skin care, since the patient with NS usually has edema.
- To avoid thrombophlebitis, encourage activity and exercise, and provide antiembolism stockings, as ordered.
- Watch for and teach the patient and family how to recognize drug therapy side effects, such as bone marrow toxicity from cytotoxic immunosuppressives and cushingoid symptoms (muscle weakness, mental changes, acne, moon face, hirsutism, girdle obesity, purple striae, amenorrhea) from long-term steroid therapy. Other steroid complications include masked infections, increased susceptibility to infections, ulcers, GI bleeding, and steroid-induced diabetes; a steroid crisis may occur if the drug is discontinued abruptly. To prevent GI complications, administer steroids with an antacid or with cimetidine or ranitidine. Explain that steroid side effects will subside when therapy stops.
- Offer the patient and family reassurance and support, especially during the acute phase, when edema is severe and the patient's body image changes.

Chronic Glomerulonephritis

A slowly progressive disease, chronic glomerulonephritis is characterized by inflammation of the glomeruli, which results in sclerosis, scarring, and eventual renal failure. This condition usually remains subclinical until the progressive phase begins, marked by proteinuria, cylindruria (presence of granular tube casts), and hematuria. By the time it produces symptoms, chronic glomerulonephritis is usually irreversible.

Causes

Common causes of chronic glomerulonephritis include primary renal disorders, such as membranoproliferative glomerulonephritis, membranous glomerulopathy, focal glomerulosclerosis, rapidly progressive glomerulonephritis, and, less often, poststreptococcal glomerulonephritis. Systemic disorders that may cause chronic glomerulonephritis include lupus erythematosus, Goodpasture's syndrome, or hemolytic-uremic syndrome.

Signs and symptoms

Chronic glomerulonephritis usually develops insidiously and asymptomatically, often over many years. At any time, however, it may suddenly become progressive, producing nephrotic syndrome, hypertension, proteinuria, and hematuria. In late stages of progressive chronic glomerulonephritis, it may accelerate to uremic symptoms, such as azotemia, nausea, vomiting, pruritus, dyspnea, malaise, and fatigability. Mild to severe edema and anemia may accompany these symptoms. Severe hypertension may cause cardiac hypertrophy, leading to congestive heart failure, and may accelerate the development of advanced renal failure, eventually necessitating dialysis or transplantation.

Diagnosis

Patient history and physical assessment seldom suggest glomerulonephritis. Suspicion develops from urinalysis revealing proteinuria, hematuria, cylindruria, and RBC casts. Rising BUN and serum creatinine levels indicate advanced renal insufficiency. X-ray or ultrasound shows smaller kidneys. Kidney biopsy identifies underlying disease and provides data needed to guide therapy.

Treatment

Treatment is essentially nonspecific and symptomatic, with its goals to control hypertension with antihypertensives and a sodium-restricted diet; to correct fluid and electrolyte imbalances through restrictions and replacement; to reduce edema with diuretics, such as furosemide; and to prevent congestive heart failure. Treatment may also include antibiotics (for symptomatic urinary tract infections), dialysis, or transplantation.

Special considerations

Patient care is primarily supportive, focusing on continual observation and sound patient teaching.

- Accurately monitor vital signs, intake and output, and daily weight to evaluate fluid retention. Observe for signs of fluid, electrolyte, and acid-base imbalances.
- Ask the dietitian to plan low-sodium, high-calorie meals with adequate protein.
- Administer medications, as ordered, and provide good skin care (because of pruritus and edema) and oral hygiene. Instruct the patient to continue taking prescribed antihypertensives as scheduled, even if he's feeling better, and to report any side effects. Advise him to take diuretics in the morning, so he won't have to disrupt his sleep to void, and teach him how to assess ankle edema.
- Warn the patient to report signs of infection, particularly urinary tract infection, and to avoid contact with persons who have infections. Urge follow-up examinations to assess renal function.
- Help the patient adjust to this illness by encouraging him to express his feelings. Explain all necessary procedures beforehand, and answer the patient's questions about them.

Cystinuria

An autosomal recessive disorder, cystinuria is an inborn error of amino acid transport in the kidneys and intestine that allows excessive urinary excretion of cystine and other dibasic amino acids and results in recurrent cystine renal calculi. It is the most common defect of amino acid transport, but with proper treatment, prognosis is good.

Causes and incidence

Cystinuria is inherited as an autosomal recessive defect, and occurs in approximately 1 in 15,000 live births. It is more prevalent in persons of short stature; the reason for this is unknown. Although this disorder affects both sexes, it is more severe in males.

Impaired renal tubular reabsorption of dibasic amino acids (cystine, lysine, arginine, and ornithine) results in excessive amino acid concentration and excretion in the urine. When cystine concentration exceeds its solubility, it precipitates and forms crystals, precursors of cystine calculi. Excessive excretion of the other three amino acids produces no ill effects.

Signs and symptoms

The clinical effects of cystinuria result from cystine or mixed cystine calculi, which develop most frequently between ages 10 and 30. Typically, such calculi may cause dull flank pain from renal parenchymal and capsular distention, nausea, vomiting, abdominal distention from acute renal colic (due to smooth-muscle spasm and hyperperistalsis), hematuria, and tenderness in the costovertebral angle or over the kidneys.

Renal calculi may also cause urinary tract obstruction, with resultant secondary infection (chills; fever; burning, itching, or pain on urination; frequency; and foul-smelling urine) and, with prolonged ureteral obstruction, marked hydronephrosis and a visible or palpable flank mass.

Diagnosis

Typical clinical features and a positive family history of renal disease or kidney stones suggest cystinuria, but the following laboratory data confirm it:

- *Chemical analysis of calculi* shows cystine crystals, with a variable amount of calcium. Pure cystine stones are radiolucent on X-ray, but most contain some calcium. These stones are light yellow or brownish-yellow, and granular; they may be large.
- *Blood studies* may show elevated serum WBC, especially with a urinary tract infection, and elevated clearance of cystine, lysine, arginine, and ornithine.
- *Urinalysis* with amino acid chromatography indicates aminoaciduria, consisting of cystine, lysine, arginine, and ornithine. Urine pH is usually less than 5.
- *Microscopic examination of urine* shows hexagonal, flat cystine crystals. When glacial acetic acid is added to chilled urine, cystine crystals resemble benzene rings.
- *Cyanide-nitroprusside test* is positive. In cystinuria, a urine specimen made alkaline by adding ammonia turns magenta when nitroprusside is added to it.

Confirming tests also include excretory urography to determine renal function, and kidney-ureter-bladder X-rays to determine size and location of calculi.

Treatment

No effective treatment exists to decrease cystine excretion. Increasing fluid intake to maintain a minimum 24-hour urine volume of 3,000 ml and reduce urine cystine concentration is the primary means of dissolving excess cystine and preventing cystine stones. Sodium bicarbonate and an alkaline-ash diet (high in vegetables and fruit, low in protein) alkalinize urine, increasing cystine solubility. However, this therapy may provide a favorable environment for formation of calcium phosphate stones. Penicillamine can also increase cystine solubility but should be used with caution because of its toxic side effects and high incidence of allergic reaction. Treatment may also include surgical removal of renal calculi, when necessary, and appropriate measures to prevent and treat urinary tract infection.

Special considerations

In addition to general supportive care, management of cystinuria focuses on careful patient teaching to promote compliance with the treatment regimen.

- Emphasize the need to maintain increased, evenly spaced fluid intake, even through the night.
- Teach the patient how to recognize

signs of renal calculi and urinary tract infection, and tell him to report any symptoms immediately.
• Teach the patient to check urine pH and record the results.
• Carefully monitor sodium bicarbonate administration, since metabolic alkalosis may develop. Arterial bicarbonate level can be estimated by subtracting 2 from the serum CO_2 level.
• Explain to the patient receiving penicillamine that it may cause an allergic or serum sickness–type reaction. Other side effects may include severe proteinuria, neutropenia, tinnitus, and taste impairment.

Renovascular Hypertension

Renovascular hypertension is a rise in systemic blood pressure resulting from stenosis of the major renal arteries or their branches or from intrarenal atherosclerosis. This narrowing or sclerosis may be partial or complete, and the resulting blood pressure elevation, benign or malignant. Approximately 5% to 10% of patients with high blood pressure display renovascular hypertension; it is most common in persons under age 30 or over age 50.

Causes

Atherosclerosis (especially in older men) and fibromuscular diseases of the renal artery wall layers—such as medial fibroplasia and, less commonly, intimal and subadventitial fibroplasia—are the primary causes in 95% of all patients with renovascular hypertension. Other causes include arteritis, anomalies of the renal arteries, embolism, trauma, tumor, and dissecting aneurysm.

Stenosis or occlusion of the renal artery stimulates the affected kidney to release the enzyme renin, which converts angiotensinogen—a plasma protein—to angiotensin I. As angiotensin I circulates through the lungs and liver, it converts to angiotensin II, which causes peripheral vasoconstriction, increased arterial pressure and aldosterone secretion, and, eventually, hypertension.

Signs and symptoms

In addition to elevated systemic blood pressure, renovascular hypertension usually produces symptoms common to hypertensive states, such as headache, palpitations, tachycardia, anxiety, lightheadedness, decreased tolerance of temperature extremes, retinopathy, and mental sluggishness. Significant complications include congestive heart failure, myocardial infarction, cerebrovascular accident, and, occasionally, renal failure.

Diagnosis

In addition to thorough patient and family histories, diagnosis requires isotopic renal blood flow scan and rapid-sequence intravenous pyelography to identify abnormalities of renal blood flow and discrepancies of kidney size and shape. Renal arteriography reveals the actual arterial stenosis or obstruction; samples from both the right and left renal veins are obtained for comparison of plasma renin levels with those in the inferior vena cava. Increased renin level implicates the affected kidney and determines whether surgical correction can reverse hypertension.

Treatment

Surgery, the treatment of choice, is performed to restore adequate circulation and to control severe hypertension or severely impaired renal function by renal artery bypass, endarterectomy, arterioplasty, or, as a last resort, nephrectomy. Balloon catheter renal artery dilation is used in selected cases to correct renal artery stenosis without the risks and morbidity of surgery. Symptomatic measures include antihypertensives, diuretics, and a sodium-restricted diet.

Special considerations

The care plan must emphasize helping the patient and family understand renovascular hypertension and the importance of following prescribed treatment.

- Accurately monitor intake and output and daily weight. Check blood pressure in both arms regularly, with the patient lying down and standing. A drop of 20 mm Hg or more on arising may necessitate an adjustment in antihypertensive medications. Assess renal function daily.
- Administer drugs, as ordered. Maintain fluid and sodium restrictions. Explain the purpose of a low-sodium diet.
- Explain the diagnostic tests, and prepare the patient appropriately; for example, adequately hydrate the patient before tests that use contrast media. Make sure the patient is not allergic to the dye used in diagnostic tests. After intravenous pyelography or arteriography, watch for complications.
- If a nephrectomy is necessary, reassure the patient that the remaining kidney is adequate for renal function.
- Postoperatively, watch for bleeding and hypotension. If the sutures around the renal vessels slip, the patient can quickly go into shock, since kidneys receive 25% of cardiac output.
- Provide a quiet, stress-free environment, if possible. Urge the patient and family members to have regular blood pressure screenings.

Hydronephrosis

Hydronephrosis is an abnormal dilation of the renal pelvis and the calyces of one or both kidneys, caused by an obstruction of urine flow in the genitourinary tract. Although partial obstruction and hydronephrosis may not produce symptoms initially, the pressure built up behind the area of obstruction eventually results in symptomatic renal dysfunction.

Causes

Almost any type of obstructive uropathy can result in hydronephrosis. The most common causes are benign prostatic hypertrophy, urethral strictures, and calculi; less common causes include strictures or stenosis of the ureter or bladder outlet, congenital abnormalities, abdominal tumors, blood clots, and neurogenic bladder. If obstruction is in the urethra or bladder, hydronephrosis is usually bilateral; if obstruction is in a ureter, it's usually unilateral. Obstructions distal to the bladder cause the bladder to dilate and act as a buffer zone, delaying hydronephrosis. Total obstruction of urine flow with dilation of the collecting system ultimately causes complete cortical atrophy and cessation of glomerular filtration.

Signs and symptoms

Clinical features of hydronephrosis vary with the cause of the obstruction. In some patients, hydronephrosis produces no symptoms or only mild pain and slightly decreased urinary flow; in others, it may produce severe, colicky renal pain or dull flank pain that may radiate to the groin, and gross urinary abnormalities, such as hematuria, pyuria, dysuria, alternating oliguria and polyuria, or complete anuria. Other symptoms of hydronephrosis include nausea, vomiting, abdominal fullness, pain on urination, dribbling, or hesitancy. Unilateral obstruction may cause pain on only one side, usually in the flank area.

The most common complication of an obstructed kidney is infection (pyelonephritis), due to stasis that exacerbates renal damage and may create a life-threatening crisis. Paralytic ileus frequently accompanies acute obstructive uropathy.

Diagnosis

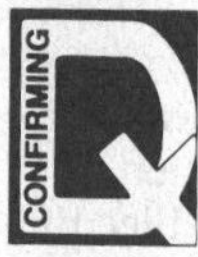

While the patient's clinical features may suggest hydronephrosis, intravenous pyelography, retrograde pyelography, renal ultrasound, and renal function studies are necessary to confirm it.

Treatment

The goals of treatment are to preserve renal function and prevent infection through surgical removal of the obstruction, such as dilation for stricture of the urethra or prostatectomy for benign prostatic hypertrophy.

If renal function has already been affected, therapy may include a diet low in protein, sodium, and potassium. This diet is designed to stop the progression of renal failure before surgery. Inoperable obstructions may necessitate decompression and drainage of the kidney using a nephrostomy tube emplaced temporarily or permanently in the renal pelvis. Concurrent infection requires appropriate antibiotic therapy.

Special considerations

- Explain hydronephrosis, as well as the purpose of intravenous pyelography and other diagnostic procedures. Check the patient for allergy to intravenous pyelography dye.
- Administer medication for pain, as needed and prescribed.
- Postoperatively, closely monitor intake and output, vital signs, and fluid and electrolyte status. Watch for a rising pulse rate and cold, clammy skin, which indicate possible impending hemorrhage and shock. Monitor renal function studies daily.
- If a nephrostomy tube has been inserted, check it frequently for bleeding and patency. Irrigate the tube only as ordered, and don't clamp it.
- If the patient is to be discharged with a nephrostomy tube in place, teach him how to care for it properly.
- To prevent progression of hydronephrosis to irreversible renal disease, urge older men (especially those with family histories of benign prostatic hypertrophy or prostatitis) to have routine medical checkups. Teach them to recognize and report symptoms of hydronephrosis (colicky pain, hematuria) or urinary tract infection.

Renal Tubular Acidosis

Renal tubular acidosis (RTA)—a syndrome of persistent dehydration, hyperchloremia, hypokalemia, metabolic acidosis, and nephrocalcinosis—results from the kidneys' inability to conserve bicarbonate. This disorder occurs as distal RTA (Type I, or classic RTA) or proximal RTA (Type II). Prognosis is usually good but depends on the severity of renal damage that precedes treatment.

Causes and incidence

Metabolic acidosis usually results from renal excretion of bicarbonate. However, metabolic acidosis associated with RTA results from a defect in the kidneys' normal tubular acidification of urine.

Distal RTA results from an inability of the distal tubule to secrete hydrogen ions against established gradients across the tubular membrane. This results in decreased excretion of titratable acids and ammonium, increased loss of potassium and bicarbonate in the urine, and systemic acidosis. Prolonged acidosis causes mobilization of calcium from bone and, eventually, hypercalciuria, predisposing to the formation of renal calculi.

Distal RTA may be classified as primary or secondary.

• *Primary distal RTA* may occur sporadically or through a hereditary defect and is most prevalent in females, older children, adolescents, and young adults.

• *Secondary distal RTA* has been linked to many renal or systemic conditions, such as starvation, malnutrition, hepatic cirrhosis, and several genetically transmitted disorders.

Proximal RTA results from defective reabsorption of bicarbonate in the proximal tubule. This causes bicarbonate to flood the distal tubule, which normally secretes hydrogen ions, and leads to impaired formation of titratable acids and ammonium for excretion. Ultimately, metabolic acidosis results.

Proximal RTA occurs in two forms:

• In *primary proximal RTA,* the reabsorptive defect is idiopathic and is the only disorder present.

• In *secondary proximal RTA,* the reabsorptive defect may be one of several defects and is due to proximal tubular cell damage from a disease, such as Fanconi's syndrome.

Signs and symptoms

In infants, RTA produces anorexia, vomiting, occasional fever, polyuria, dehydration, growth retardation, apathy, weakness, tissue wasting, constipation, nephrocalcinosis, and rickets.

In children and adults, RTA may lead to urinary tract infection, rickets, and growth problems. Possible complications of RTA include nephrocalcinosis and pyelonephritis.

Diagnosis

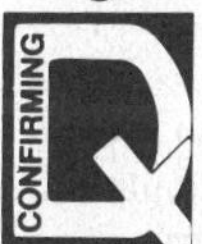

Demonstration of impaired acidification of urine with systemic metabolic acidosis confirms distal RTA. Demonstration of bicarbonate wasting due to impaired reabsorption confirms proximal RTA.

Other relevant laboratory results show:

• decreased serum bicarbonate, pH, potassium, and phosphorus

• increased serum chloride and alkaline phosphatase

• alkaline pH, with low titratable acids and ammonium content in urine; increased urinary bicarbonate and potassium, low specific gravity.

In later stages, X-rays may show nephrocalcinosis.

Treatment

Supportive treatment for patients with RTA requires replacement of those substances being abnormally excreted, especially bicarbonate, and may include sodium bicarbonate tablets or Shohl's solution to control acidosis, potassium P.O. for dangerously low potassium levels, and vitamin D for bone disease. If pyelonephritis occurs, treatment may include antibiotics as well.

Treatment for renal calculi secondary to nephrocalcinosis varies and may include supportive therapy until the calculi pass or until surgery for severe obstruction is performed.

Special considerations

• Urge compliance with all medication instructions. Inform the patient and his family that the prognosis for RTA and bone lesion healing is directly related to the adequacy of treatment.

• Monitor laboratory values, especially potassium, for hypokalemia.

• Test urine for pH, and strain it for calculi.

• If rickets develops, explain the condition and its treatment to the patient and his family.

• Teach the patient how to recognize signs and symptoms of calculi (hematuria, low abdominal or flank pain). Advise him to immediately report any such signs and symptoms.

• Instruct the patient with low potassium levels to eat foods with a high potassium content, such as bananas and baked potatoes. Orange juice is also high in potassium.

• Since RTA may be caused by a genetic defect, encourage family members to seek genetic counseling or screening for this disorder.

Fanconi's Syndrome

(de Toni-Fanconi syndrome)

Fanconi's syndrome is a renal disorder that produces malfunctions of the proximal renal tubules, leading to hyperkalemia, hypernatremia, glycosuria, phosphaturia, aminoaciduria, uricosuria, bicarbonate wasting, and eventually, retarded growth and development, and rickets. Since treatment of Fanconi's syndrome is usually unsuccessful, it commonly leads to end-stage renal failure, and the patient may survive only a few years after its onset.

Causes and incidence

Idiopathic congenital Fanconi's syndrome is most prevalent in children and affects both sexes equally. Onset of the hereditary form usually occurs during the first 6 months of life, although another hereditary form also occurs in adults. The more serious adult form of this disease is acquired Fanconi's syndrome; it is secondary to Wilson's disease, cystinosis, galactosemia, or exposure to a toxic substance (heavy metal poisoning).

Fanconi's syndrome produces characteristic changes in the proximal renal tubules, such as shortening of the connection to glomeruli by an abnormally narrow segment (swan's neck)—a result of the atrophy of epithelial cells and loss of proximal tubular mass volume.

Signs and symptoms

Changes in the proximal renal tubules result in decreased tubular reabsorption of glucose, phosphate, amino acid, bicarbonate, potassium, and occasionally, water. An infant with Fanconi's syndrome appears normal at birth, although birth weight may be low. At about age 6 months, the infant shows failure to thrive, weakness, dehydration (associated with polyuria, vomiting, and anorexia), constipation, acidosis, cystine crystals in the corneas and conjunctivas, and peripheral retinal pigment degeneration. Typically, the skin is yellow and has little pigmentation, even in summer. Refractory rickets or osteomalacia may be severe, and linear growth is slow. Bicarbonate loss causes acidosis; potassium loss, weakness; water loss, dehydration. Renal calculi rarely occur.

In adults, symptoms of Fanconi's syndrome are secondary to hypophosphatemia, hypokalemia, and glycosuria. Their clinical effects include osteomalacia, muscle weakness and paralysis, and metabolic acidosis.

Diagnosis

Diagnosis requires evidence of excessive 24-hour urinary excretion of glucose, phosphate, amino acids, bicarbonate, and potassium (generally, serum values correspond to the decrease in these components). Other results include elevated phosphorus and nitrogen levels with increased renal dysfunction, and increased alkaline phosphatase with rickets. Hyperchloremic acidosis and hypokalemia support the diagnosis. (*Caution:* Glucose tolerance test is contraindicated for these patients, because it may cause a fatal shocklike reaction.) In a child with refractory rickets, growth retardation is evident; serum sample shows increased alkaline phosphatase and, with renal dysfunction, decreased calcium.

Treatment

Treatment is symptomatic, with replacement therapy appropriate to the patient's specific deficiencies. For example, a patient with rickets receives large doses of vitamin D; with acidosis and hypokalemia, supplements containing a flavored mixture of sodium and potassium citrate; and with hypocalcemia, calcium supplements (close monitoring is necessary to prevent hypercalcemia). When diminishing renal function causes hyperphosphatemia, treatment includes aluminum hydroxide antacids to bind phosphate in the intestine and prevent its absorption. Acquired Fanconi's syndrome requires treatment of the underlying cause. End-stage Fanconi's syndrome occasionally requires dialysis. Other treatment is symptomatic.

Special considerations

- Help the patient with acquired Fanconi's syndrome or the parents of an infant with inherited Fanconi's syndrome understand the seriousness of this disease (including the possibility of dialysis) and the need to comply with drug and dietary therapy. If the patient has rickets, help him accept the changes in his body image.
- Because the prognosis for acquired Franconi's syndrome is poor, the patient with this disorder may be apathetic about taking medication. Encourage compliance with therapy.
- Monitor renal function closely. Make sure 24-hour urine specimens are collected accurately. Watch for fluid and electrolyte imbalances, particularly hypokalemia and hyponatremia; disturbed regulatory function characterized by anemia and hypertension; and uremic symptoms characteristic of renal failure (oliguria, anorexia, vomiting, muscle twitching, and pruritus).
- Instruct the patient with acquired Fanconi's sydrome to follow a diet for chronic renal failure, as ordered.

Chronic Renal Failure

Chronic renal failure is usually the end result of a gradually progressive loss of renal function; occasionally, it's the result of a rapidly progressive disease of sudden onset. Few symptoms develop until after more than 75% of glomerular filtration is lost; then the remaining normal parenchyma deteriorates progressively, and symptoms worsen as renal function decreases.

If this condition continues unchecked, uremic toxins accumulate and produce potentially fatal physiologic changes in all major organ systems. If the patient can tolerate it, maintenance dialysis or kidney transplant can sustain life.

Causes

Chronic renal failure may result from:

- *chronic glomerular disease,* such as glomerulonephritis
- *chronic infections,* such as chronic pyelonephritis or tuberculosis
- *congenital anomalies,* such as polycystic kidneys
- *vascular diseases,* such as renal nephrosclerosis or hypertension
- *obstructive processes,* such as calculi
- *collagen diseases,* such as systemic lupus erythematosus
- *nephrotoxic agents,* such as long-term aminoglycoside therapy
- *endocrine diseases,* such as diabetic neuropathy.

Such conditions gradually destroy the nephrons and eventually cause irreversible renal failure. Similarly, acute renal failure that fails to respond to treatment becomes chronic renal failure.

This syndrome may progress through the following stages:

- reduced renal reserve (creatinine clearance glomerular filtration rate [GFR] is 40 to 70 ml/minute)
- renal insufficiency (GFR 20 to 40 ml/minute)
- renal failure (GFR 10 to 20 ml/minute)
- end-stage renal disease (GFR less than 10 ml/minute).

Signs and symptoms

Chronic renal failure produces major changes in all body systems:

• *Renal* and *urologic:* Initially, salt-wasting and consequent hyponatremia produce hypotension, dry mouth, loss of skin turgor, listlessness, fatigue, and nausea; later, somnolence and confusion develop. As the number of functioning nephrons decreases, so does the kidneys' capacity to excrete sodium, resulting in salt retention and overload. Accumulation of potassium causes muscle irritability, then muscle weakness as the potassium level continues to rise. Fluid overload and metabolic acidosis also occur. Urinary output decreases; urine is very dilute and contains casts and crystals.

• *Cardiovascular:* Renal failure leads to hypertension, dysrhythmias (including life-threatening ventricular tachycardia or fibrillation), cardiomyopathy, uremic pericarditis, pericardial effusion with possible cardiac tamponade, congestive heart failure, and peripheral edema.

• *Respiratory:* Pulmonary changes include reduced pulmonary macrophage activity with increased susceptibility to infection, pulmonary edema, pleuritic pain, pleural friction rub and effusions, uremic pleuritis and uremic lung (or uremic pneumonitis), dyspnea due to congestive heart failure, and Kussmaul's respirations as a result of acidosis.

• *Gastrointestinal:* Inflammation and ulceration of gastrointestinal mucosa cause stomatitis, gum ulceration and bleeding, and, possibly, parotitis, esophagitis, gastritis, duodenal ulcers, lesions on the small and large bowel, uremic colitis, pancreatitis, and proctitis. Other gastrointestinal symptoms include a metallic taste in the mouth, uremic fetor (ammonia smell to breath), anorexia, nausea, and vomiting.

• *Cutaneous:* Typically, the skin is pallid, yellowish bronze, dry, and scaly. Other cutaneous symptoms include severe itching, purpura, ecchymoses, petechiae, uremic frost (most often in critically ill or terminal patients), thin brittle fingernails with characteristic lines, and dry, brittle hair that may change color and fall out easily.

• *Neurologic:* Restless leg syndrome, one of the first signs of peripheral neuropathy, causes pain, burning, and itching in the legs and feet, which may be relieved by voluntarily shaking, moving, or rocking them. Eventually, this condition progresses to paresthesia and motor nerve dysfunction (usually bilateral footdrop) unless dialysis is initiated. Other signs and symptoms include muscle cramping and twitching, shortened memory and attention span, apathy, drowsiness, irritability, confusion, coma, and convulsions. EEG changes indicate metabolic encephalopathy.

• *Endocrine:* Common endocrine abnormalities include stunted growth patterns in children (even with elevated growth hormone levels), infertility and decreased libido in both sexes, amenorrhea and cessation of menses in women, impotence and decreased sperm production in men, increased aldosterone secretion (related to increased renin production), and impaired carbohydrate metabolism (increased blood glucose levels similar to diabetes mellitus).

• *Hematopoietic:* Anemia, decreased RBC survival time, blood loss from dialysis and gastrointestinal bleeding, mild thrombocytopenia, and platelet defects occur. Other problems include increased bleeding and clotting disorders, demonstrated by purpura, hemorrhage from body orifices, easy bruising, ecchymoses, and petechiae.

• *Skeletal:* Calcium-phosphorus imbalance and consequent parathyroid hormone imbalances cause muscle and bone pain, skeletal demineralization, pathologic fractures, and calcifications in the brain, eyes, gums, joints, myocardium, and blood vessels. Arterial calcification may produce coronary artery disease. In children, renal osteodystrophy (renal rickets) may develop.

Diagnosis

Diagnosis of chronic renal failure is based on clinical assessment, a history of chronic progressive debilitation, and gradual deterioration of renal function as determined by creatinine clearance tests. The following laboratory findings

CONTINUOUS AMBULATORY PERITONEAL DIALYSIS

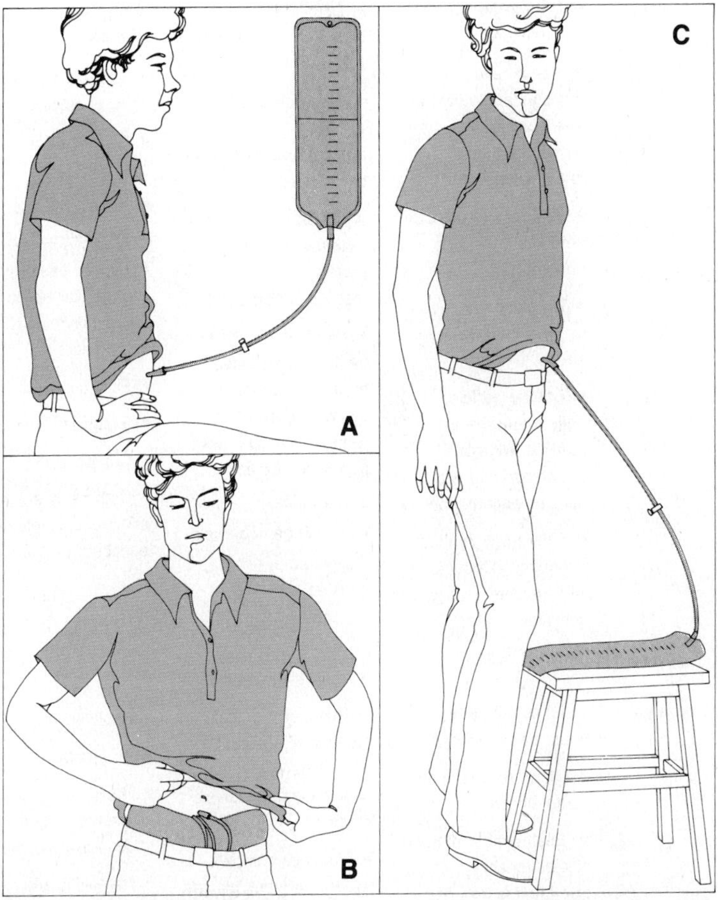

Continuous ambulatory peritoneal dialysis (CAPD) is a relatively new, increasingly useful alternative to hemodialysis in patients with renal failure. Using the peritoneum as a dialysis membrane, it allows almost uninterrupted exchange of dialysis solution. With this method, four to six exchanges of fresh dialysis solution are infused each day. The approximate dwell-time for the daytime exchanges is 5 hours; for the overnight exchange, the dwell-time is 8 to 10 hours. After each dwell-time, the patient removes the dialyzing solution by gravity drainage. This form of dialysis offers the unique advantages of a simple, easily taught procedure and patient independence from a special treatment center.

A. In this procedure, a Tenchkoff catheter is surgically implanted in the abdomen, just below the umbilicus. A bag of dialysis solution is aseptically attached to the tube, and the fluid allowed to flow into the peritoneal cavity (this takes about 10 minutes).

B. The dialyzing fluid remains in the peritoneal cavity for about 4 to 6 hours. During this time, the bag may be rolled up and placed under a shirt or blouse, and the patient can go about normal activities while dialysis takes place.

C. The fluid is then drained out of the peritoneal cavity through gravity flow by unrolling the bag and suspending it below the pelvis (drainage takes about 20 minutes). After it drains, the patient aseptically connects a new bag of dialyzing solution and fills the peritoneal cavity again. He repeats this procedure four to six times a day.

COMPARISON OF PERITONEAL DIALYSIS AND HEMODIALYSIS

TYPE	ADVANTAGES	DISADVANTAGES	POSSIBLE COMPLICATIONS
Peritoneal dialysis	• Can be performed immediately • Requires less complex equipment and less specialized personnel than hemodialysis • Requires small amounts of heparin or none at all • No blood loss; minimal cardiovascular stress • Can be performed by patient anywhere (CAPD), without assistance and with minimal patient teaching • Allows patient independence without long interruptions in daily activities • Lower cost	• Contraindicated within 72 hours of abdominal surgery • Requires 48 to 72 hours for significant response to treatment • Severe protein loss necessitates high-protein diet (up to 100 g/day) • High risk of peritonitis; repeated bouts may cause scarring, preventing further treatments with peritoneal dialysis • Urea clearance less than with hemodialysis (60%)	• Bacterial or chemical peritonitis • Pain (abdominal, low back, shoulder) • Shortness of breath, or dyspnea • Atelectasis and pneumonia • Severe loss of protein into the dialysis solution in the abdominal cavity (10 to 20 g/day) • Fluid overload • Excessive fluid loss • Constipation • Catheter site inflammation, infection, or leakage
Hemodialysis	• Takes only 3 to 5 hours per treatment • Faster results in an acute situation • Total number of hours of maintenance treatment is only half that of peritoneal dialysis • In an acute situation, can use an I.V. route without a surgical access route	• Requires surgical creation of a vascular access between circulation and dialysis machine • Requires complex water treatment, dialysis equipment, and highly trained personnel • Requires administration of larger amounts of heparin • Confines patient to special treatment unit	• Septicemia • Air emboli • Rapid fluid and electrolyte imbalance (disequilibrium syndrome) • Hemolytic anemia • Metastatic calcification • Increased risk of hepatitis • Hypo- or hypertension • Itching • Pain (generalized or in chest) • Heparin overdose, possibly causing hemorrhage • Leg cramps • Nausea and vomiting • Headache

also aid in diagnosis:

• *Blood studies* show elevated BUN, serum creatinine, and potassium levels; decreased arterial pH and bicarbonate; and low hemoglobin and hematocrit.
• *Urine specific gravity* becomes fixed at 1.010; urinalysis may show proteinuria, glycosuria, erythrocytes, leukocytes, and casts, depending on the etiology.
• *X-ray studies* include kidney-ureter-bladder films, intravenous pyelography, nephrotomography, renal scan, and renal arteriography.
• *Kidney biopsy* allows histologic identification of underlying pathology.

Treatment

Hemodialysis or peritoneal dialysis (particularly newer techniques—continuous ambulatory peritoneal dialysis [CAPD] and continuous cyclic peritoneal dialysis [CCPD]) can help control most manifestations of end-stage renal disease; altering dialyzing bath fluids can correct fluid and electrolyte disturbances. However, anemia, peripheral neuropathy, cardiopulmonary and GI complications, sexual dysfunction, and skeletal defects may persist. In addition, maintenance dialysis itself may produce complications, including serum hepatitis (hepatitis B) due to numerous blood transfusions, protein-wasting, refractory ascites, and dialysis dementia.

Conservative treatment aims to correct specific symptoms. A low-protein diet reduces the production of end-products of protein metabolism that the kidneys can't excrete. (A patient receiving continuous peritoneal dialysis should have a high-protein diet.) A high-calorie diet prevents ketoacidosis and the negative nitrogen balance that results in catabolism and tissue atrophy. Such a diet also restricts sodium and potassium.

Maintaining fluid balance requires careful monitoring of vital signs, weight changes, and urine volume (if present). Loop diuretics, such as Lasix (if some renal function remains), and fluid restriction can reduce fluid retention. Digitalis may be used to mobilize edema fluids; antihypertensives, to control blood pressure and associated edema. Antiemetics taken before meals may relieve nausea and vomiting; cimetidine or ranitidine may decrease gastric irritation. Methylcellulose or docusate can help prevent constipation.

Treatment may also include regular stool analysis (guaiac test) to detect occult blood and, as needed, cleansing enemas to remove blood from the gastrointestinal tract. Anemia necessitates iron and folate supplements; severe anemia requires infusion of fresh frozen packed cells or washed packed cells. However, transfusions relieve anemia only temporarily. Androgen therapy (testosterone or nandrolone) may increase RBC production.

Drug therapy often relieves associated symptoms: an antipruritic, such as trimeprazine or diphenhydramine, for itching and aluminum hydroxide gel to lower serum phosphate levels. The patient may also benefit from supplementary vitamins (particularly B vitamins and vitamin D) and essential amino acids.

Careful monitoring of serum potassium levels is necessary to detect hyperkalemia. Emergency treatment for severe hyperkalemia includes dialysis therapy, and administration of 50% hypertonic glucose I.V., regular insulin, calcium gluconate I.V., sodium bicarbonate I.V., and cation exchange resins, such as sodium polystyrene sulfonate. Cardiac tamponade resulting from pericardial effusion may require emergency pericardial tap or surgery.

Blood gas measurements may indicate acidosis; intensive dialysis and thoracentesis can relieve pulmonary edema and pleural effusions.

Special considerations

Since chronic renal failure has such widespread clinical effects, it requires meticulous and carefully coordinated supportive care.

• Good skin care is important. Bathe the patient daily, using superfatted soaps, oatmeal baths, and skin lotion to ease pruritus. Give good perineal care, using mild soap and water. Pad the side rails to guard against ecchymoses. Turn the patient often, and use an egg-crate mattress to prevent skin breakdown.

- Provide good oral hygiene. Brush the patient's teeth often with a soft brush or sponge tip to reduce breath odor. Hard candy and mouthwash minimize bad taste in the mouth and alleviate thirst.
- Offer small, palatable meals that are also nutritious; try to provide favorite foods within dietary restrictions. Encourage intake of high-calorie foods. Instruct the outpatient to avoid high-sodium foods and high-potassium foods. Encourage adherence to fluid and protein restrictions. To prevent constipation, stress the need for exercise and sufficient dietary bulk.
- Watch for hyperkalemia. Observe for cramping of the legs and abdomen, and diarrhea. As potassium levels rise, watch for muscle irritability and a weak pulse rate. Monitor EKG for tall, peaked T waves, widening QRS segment, prolonged PR interval, and disappearance of P waves, indicating hyperkalemia.
- Assess hydration status carefully. Check for jugular vein distention, and auscultate the lungs for rales. Measure daily intake and output carefully, including all drainage, emesis, diarrhea, and blood loss. Record daily weight, presence or absence of thirst, axillary sweat, dryness of tongue, hypertension, and peripheral edema.
- Monitor for bone or joint complications. Prevent pathologic fractures by turning the patient carefully and ensuring his safety. Provide passive range-of-motion exercises for the bedridden patient.
- Encourage deep breathing and coughing to prevent pulmonary congestion. Listen often for rales, rhonchi, and decreased lung sounds. Be alert for clinical effects of pulmonary edema (dyspnea, restlessness, rales). Administer diuretics and other medications, as ordered.
- Maintain strict aseptic technique. Use a micropore filter during I.V. therapy. Watch for signs of infection (listlessness, high fever, leukocytosis). Urge the outpatient to avoid contact with infected persons during the cold and flu season.
- Carefully observe and document seizure activity. Infuse sodium bicarbonate for acidosis, and sedatives or anticonvulsants for seizures, as ordered. Pad the side rails and keep an oral airway and suction setup at bedside. Assess neurologic status periodically, and check for Chvostek's and Trousseau's signs, indicators of low serum calcium levels.
- Observe for signs of bleeding. Watch for prolonged bleeding at puncture sites and at the vascular access site used for hemodialysis. Monitor hemoglobin and hematocrit, and check stool, urine, and vomitus for blood.
- Report signs of pericarditis, such as a pericardial friction rub and chest pain.

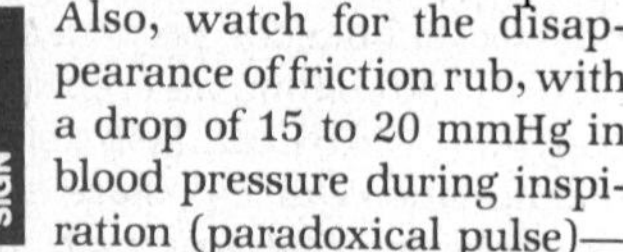

Also, watch for the disappearance of friction rub, with a drop of 15 to 20 mmHg in blood pressure during inspiration (paradoxical pulse)—an early sign of pericardial tamponade.

- Schedule medications carefully. Give iron before meals, aluminum hydroxide gels after meals, and antiemetics, as necessary, a half hour before meals. Administer antihypertensives at appropriate intervals. If the patient requires a rectal infusion of sodium polystyrene sulfonate for dangerously high potassium levels, apply an emollient to soothe the perianal area. Be sure the sodium polystyrene sulfonate enema is expelled; otherwise, it will cause constipation and won't lower potassium levels. Recommend antacid cookies as an alternative to aluminum hydroxide gels needed to bind gastrointestinal phosphate.

If the patient requires dialysis:

- Prepare the patient by fully explaining the procedure. Be sure that he understands how to protect and care for the arteriovenous shunt, fistula, or other vascular access. Check the vascular access site every 2 hours for patency and the extremity for adequate blood supply and intact nervous function (temperature, pulse rate, capillary refill, and sensation). If the patient has a shunt, look for bright red blood pulsating in the tube, and listen for a bruit on auscultation. If a fistula is present, feel for a thrill and listen for a bruit. Report signs of possible clotting. Don't use the arm with the vascular access site to take blood pressure readings, draw blood, or give injections. Keep two bulldog clamps or hemostats attached to the shunt dressing in case the shunt becomes disconnected.

- Withhold the 6 a.m. (or morning) dose of antihypertensive on the morning of dialysis, and instruct the outpatient to do the same.
- Check the patient's hepatitis antigen status. If it's positive, he is a carrier of hepatitis B and requires stool, needle, blood, and excretion precautions.
- Monitor hemoglobin and hematocrit. Instruct the anemic patient to conserve energy and to rest frequently.
- After dialysis, check for disequilibrium syndrome, a result of sudden correction of blood chemistry abnormalities. Symptoms range from a headache to seizures. Also, check for excessive bleeding from the dialysis site. Apply pressure dressing or absorbable gelatin sponge, as indicated. Monitor blood pressure carefully after dialysis.
- A patient undergoing dialysis is under a great deal of stress, as is his family. Refer them to appropriate counseling agencies for assistance in coping with chronic renal failure.

Alport's Syndrome

Alport's syndrome is a hereditary nephritis characterized by recurrent gross or microscopic hematuria. It's associated with deafness, albuminuria, and variably progressive azotemia.

Cause and incidence

Alport's syndrome is transmitted as an X-linked, autosomal trait and affects males more often and more severely than females. Men with hematuria and proteinuria often develop end-stage renal disease in their thirties or forties. Respiratory infection often precipitates recurrent bouts of hematuria; however, streptococcal infection isn't linked to Alport's syndrome.

Signs and symptoms

The primary clinical feature of Alport's syndrome is recurrent gross or microscopic hematuria, which typically appears during early childhood. The next most common symptom is deafness (especially to high-frequency sounds). Other signs and symptoms that may be associated with Alport's syndrome include proteinuria, pyuria, red cell casts in urine, and, possibly, flank pain or other abdominal symptoms, although many patients are initially asymptomatic. Ocular features may include cataracts, and, less commonly, keratoconus, microspherophakia, myopia, retinitis pigmentosa, and nystagmus. Hypertension is often associated with progressive renal failure.

Diagnosis

A family history of recurrent hematuria, deafness, and renal failure (especially in males) suggests Alport's syndrome. Laboratory tests include urinalysis of all family members; blood studies to detect immunoglobulins and complement components; and audiometry testing. Renal biopsy confirms diagnosis.

Treatment and special considerations

Effective treatment is supportive and symptomatic. It may include antibiotic therapy for associated respiratory or urinary tract infection; a hearing aid for hearing loss; eyeglasses or contact lenses to improve vision; antihypertensive therapy for associated hypertension; and dialysis or renal transplantation for end-stage renal failure.

Refer the patient and family for genetic counseling as appropriate.

LOWER URINARY TRACT DISORDERS

Lower Urinary Tract Infection

Cystitis and urethritis, the two forms of lower urinary tract infection (UTI), are nearly 10 times more common in women than in men and affect approximately 10% to 20% of all women at least once. Lower UTI is also a prevalent bacterial disease in children, with girls also most commonly affected. In men and children, lower UTIs are frequently related to anatomic or physiologic abnormalities and therefore require extremely close evaluation. UTIs often respond readily to treatment, but recurrence and resistant bacterial flare-up during therapy are possible.

Causes

Most lower UTIs result from ascending infection by a single gram-negative enteric bacteria, such as *Escherichia coli, Klebsiella, Proteus, Enterobacter, Pseudomonas,* or *Serratia.* However, in a patient with neurogenic bladder, an indwelling catheter, or a fistula between the intestine and bladder, lower UTI may result from simultaneous infection with multiple pathogens. Recent studies suggest that infection results from a breakdown in local defense mechanisms in the bladder that allow bacteria to invade the bladder mucosa and multiply. These bacteria cannot be readily eliminated by normal micturition.

Bacterial flare-up during treatment is generally caused by the pathogenic organism's resistance to the prescribed antimicrobial therapy. The presence of even a small number (less than 10,000/ml) of bacteria in a midstream urine sample obtained during treatment casts doubt on the effectiveness of treatment.

In 99% of patients, recurrent lower UTI results from reinfection by the same organism or from some new pathogen; in the remaining 1%, recurrence reflects persistent infection, usually from renal calculi, chronic bacterial prostatitis, or a structural anomaly that may become a source of infection.

The high incidence of lower UTI among women may result from the shortness of the female urethra (1¼" to 2" [3 to 5 cm]), which predisposes women to infection caused by bacteria from the vagina, perineum, rectum, or a sexual partner. Men are less vulnerable because their urethras are longer (7¾" [19.68 cm]) and their prostatic fluid serves as an antibacterial shield. In both men and women, infection usually ascends from the urethra to the bladder.

Signs and symptoms

Lower UTI usually produces urgency, frequency, dysuria, cramps or spasms of the bladder, itching, a feeling of warmth during urination, nocturia, and possibly urethral discharge in males. Inflammation of the bladder wall also causes hematuria and fever. Other common features include low back pain, malaise, nausea, vomiting, abdominal pain or tenderness over the bladder area, chills, and flank pain.

Diagnosis

Characteristic clinical features and a microscopic urinalysis showing RBCs and WBCs greater than 10/high-power field suggest lower UTI.

A clean, midstream urine specimen revealing a bacterial count of more than 100,000/ml confirms the diagnosis. Lower counts do not necessarily rule out infection, especially if the patient is voiding frequently, since bacteria require 30 to 45 minutes to reproduce in urine. Careful midstream, clean-catch collection is preferred to catheterization, which can reinfect the bladder with urethral bacteria.

Sensitivity testing determines the appropriate therapeutic antimicrobial agent. If patient history and physical examination warrant, a blood test or a stained smear of the discharge rules out venereal disease. Voiding cystoureterography or intravenous pyelography may detect congenital anomalies that predispose the patient to recurrent UTIs.

Treatment

Appropriate antimicrobials are the treatment of choice for most initial lower UTIs. A 7- to 10-day course of antibiotic therapy is standard, but recent studies suggest that a single dose of an antibiotic or a 3- to 5-day antibiotic regimen may be sufficient to render the urine sterile. After 3 days of antibiotic therapy, urine culture should show no organisms. If the urine is not sterile, bacterial resistance has probably occurred, making the use of a different antimicrobial necessary. Single-dose antibiotic therapy with amoxicillin or co-trimoxazole may be effective in women with acute noncomplicated UTI. A urine culture taken 1 to 2 weeks later indicates whether or not the infection has been eradicated.

Recurrent infections due to infected renal calculi, chronic prostatitis, or structural abnormality may necessitate surgery; prostatitis also requires long-term antibiotic therapy. In patients without these predisposing conditions, long-term, low-dosage antibiotic therapy is the treatment of choice.

Special considerations

The care plan should include careful patient teaching, supportive measures, and proper specimen collection.

- Explain the nature and purpose of antimicrobial therapy. Emphasize the importance of completing the prescribed course of therapy or, with long-term prophylaxis, of adhering strictly to ordered dosage. Urge the patient to drink plenty of water (at least eight glasses a day). Stress the need to maintain a consistent fluid intake of about 2,000 ml/day. More or less than this amount may alter the effect of the prescribed antimicrobial. Fruit juices, especially cranberry juice, and oral doses of vitamin C may help acidify the urine and enhance the action of the medication.
- Watch for gastrointestinal disturbances from antimicrobial therapy. Nitrofurantoin macrocrystals, taken with milk or a meal, prevent such distress. If therapy includes phenazopyridine, warn the patient that this drug may turn urine red-orange.
- Suggest warm sitz baths for relief of perineal discomfort. If baths are not effective, apply heat sparingly to the perineum, but be careful not to burn the patient. Apply topical antiseptics, such as povidone-iodine ointment, on the urethral meatus, as necessary.
- Collect all urine samples for culture and sensitivity testing carefully and promptly. Teach the female patient how to clean the perineum properly and keep the labia separated during voiding. A noncontaminated midstream specimen is essential for accurate diagnosis.
- To prevent recurrent lower UTIs, teach the female patient to carefully wipe the perineum from front to back and to clean it thoroughly with soap and water after defecation. Advise an infection-prone woman to void immediately after sexual intercourse. Stress the need to drink plenty of fluids routinely and to avoid postponing urination. Recommend frequent comfort stops during long car trips. Also stress the need to completely empty the bladder. To prevent recurrent infections in men, urge prompt treatment of predisposing conditions such as chronic prostatitis.

Vesicoureteral Reflux

In vesicoureteral reflux, urine flows from the bladder back into the ureters and eventually into the renal pelvis or the parenchyma. Because the bladder empties poorly, urinary tract infection may result, possibly leading to acute or chronic pyelonephritis with renal damage.

Vesicoureteral reflux is most common during infancy in boys and during early childhood (ages 3 to 7) in girls. Primary vesicoureteral reflux that results from congenital anomalies is most prevalent in females and is rare in blacks. Up to 25% of asymptomatic siblings of children with diagnosed primary vesicoureteral reflux also show reflux.

Causes and incidence

In patients with vesicoureteral reflux, incompetence of the ureterovesical junction allows backflow of urine into the ureter when the bladder contracts during voiding. Such incompetence may result from congenital anomalies of the ureters or bladder, including short or absent intravesical ureter, ureteral ectopia lateralis (greater-than-normal lateral placement of ureters), and gaping or golf-hole ureteral orifice. It also may be caused by inadequate detrusor muscle buttress in the bladder, stemming from congenital paraureteral bladder diverticulum, acquired diverticulum (from outlet obstruction), flaccid neurogenic bladder, and high intravesical pressure from outlet obstruction or an unknown cause. Vesicoureteral reflux may also result from cystitis, with inflammation of the intravesical ureter, which causes edema and fixation of the intramural ureter and usually leads to reflux in persons with congenital ureteral or bladder anomalies or other predisposing conditions.

Signs and symptoms

Vesicoureteral reflux typically manifests itself as the signs and symptoms of urinary tract infection: frequency, urgency, burning on urination, hematuria, foul-smelling urine, and, in infants, dark, concentrated urine. With upper urinary tract involvement, signs and symptoms usually include high fever, chills, flank pain, vomiting, and malaise. In children, fever, nonspecific abdominal pain, and diarrhea may be the only clinical effects. Rarely, children with minimal symptoms remain undiagnosed until puberty or adulthood, when they begin to exhibit clear signs of renal impairment—anemia, hypertension, and lethargy.

Diagnosis

Symptoms of urinary tract infection provide the first clues to diagnosis of vesicoureteral reflux. In infants, hematuria or strong-smelling urine may be the first indication; palpation may reveal a hard, thickened bladder (hard mass deep in the pelvis) if posterior urethral valves are causing an obstruction in male infants.

Cystoscopy, with instillation of a solution containing methylene blue or indigo carmine dye, may confirm the diagnosis. After the bladder is emptied and refilled with clear sterile water, color-tinged efflux from either ureter positively confirms reflux.

Other pertinent laboratory studies include the following:

- *Clean-catch urinalysis* shows bacterial count greater than 100,000/mm³. Microscopic examination may reveal WBCs, RBCs, and an increased urine pH in the presence of infection. Specific gravity less than 1.010 demonstrates inability to concentrate urine.
- *Elevated creatinine* (greater than 1.2 mg/dl) and *elevated BUN* (greater than 18 mg/dl) demonstrate advanced renal dysfunction.
- *Intravenous pyelography* may show

dilated lower ureter, ureter visible for its entire length, hydronephrosis, calyceal distortion, and renal scarring.
- *Voiding cystourethrography* identifies and determines the degree of reflux and shows when reflux occurs. It may also pinpoint the causative anomaly. In this procedure, contrast material is instilled into the bladder, and X-rays are taken before, during, and after voiding. Radioisotope scanning and renal ultrasound may also be used to detect reflux.
- *Catheterization of the bladder* after the patient voids determines the amount of residual urine.

Treatment

The goal of treatment in a patient with vesicoureteral reflux is to prevent pyelonephritis and renal dysfunction with antibiotic therapy and, when necessary, vesicoureteral reimplantation. Appropriate surgical procedures create a normal valve effect at the junction by reimplanting the ureter into the bladder wall at a more oblique angle.

Antimicrobial therapy is usually effective for reflux that is secondary to infection, reflux related to neurogenic bladder, and, in children, reflux related to a short intravesical ureter (which abates spontaneously with growth). Reflux related to infection generally subsides after the infection is cured. However, 80% of girls with vesicoureteral reflux will have recurrent urinary tract infections within a year. Recurrent infection requires long-term prophylactic antibiotic therapy and careful patient follow-up (cystoscopy and intravenous pyelography every 4 to 6 months) to track the degree of reflux.

Urinary tract infection that recurs despite adequate prophylactic antibiotic therapy necessitates vesicoureteral reimplantation. Bladder outlet obstruction in neurogenic bladder requires surgery only if renal dysfunction is present. After surgery, as after antibiotic therapy, close medical follow-up is necessary (pyelography every 2 to 3 years and urinalysis once a month for a year), even if symptoms have not recurred.

Special considerations

- To ensure complete emptying of the bladder, teach the patient with vesicoureteral reflux to double void (void once and then try to void again in a few minutes). Also, since his natural urge to urinate may be impaired, advise him to void every 2 to 3 hours whether or not he feels the urge.
- Since the diagnostic tests may frighten the child, encourage one of his parents to stay with him during all procedures. Explain the procedures to the parents and to the child, if he's old enough to understand.
- If surgery is necessary, explain postoperative care: suprapubic catheter in the male, Foley catheter in the female; and, in both, one or two ureteral catheters or splints brought out of the bladder through a small abdominal incision. The suprapubic or Foley catheter keeps the bladder empty and prevents pressure from stressing the surgical wound; ureteral catheters drain urine directly from the renal pelvis. After complicated reimplantations, all catheters remain in place for 7 to 10 days. Explain that the child will be able to move and walk with the catheters but must be very careful not to dislodge them.
- Postoperatively, closely monitor fluid intake and output. Give analgesics and antibiotics, as ordered. Make sure the catheters are patent and draining well. Maintain sterile technique during catheter care. Watch for fever, chills, and flank pain, which suggest a blocked catheter.
- Before discharging the patient, stress the importance of close follow-up care and adequate fluid intake throughout childhood.
- Instruct parents to watch for and report recurring signs of urinary tract infection (painful, frequent, burning urination; foul-smelling urine).
- If the child is taking antimicrobial drugs, make sure his parents understand the importance of completing the prescribed therapy or maintaining low-dose prophylaxis.

Neurogenic Bladder

(Neuromuscular dysfunction of the lower urinary tract, neurologic bladder dysfunction, neuropathic bladder)

Neurogenic bladder refers to all types of bladder dysfunction caused by an interruption of normal bladder innervation. Subsequent complications include incontinence, residual urine retention, urinary infection, stone formation, and renal failure. A neurogenic bladder can be spastic (hypertonic, reflex, or automatic) or flaccid (hypotonic, atonic, nonreflex, or autonomous).

Causes

At one time, neurogenic bladder was thought to result primarily from spinal cord injury; now, it appears to stem from a host of underlying conditions:

- *cerebral disorders,* such as cerebrovascular accident, brain tumor (meningioma and glioma), Parkinson's disease, multiple sclerosis, dementia, and incontinence caused by aging
- *spinal cord disease or trauma,* such as spinal stenosis (causing cord compression) or arachnoiditis (causing adhesions between the membranes covering the cord), cervical spondylosis, myelopathies from hereditary or nutritional deficiencies, and, rarely, tabes dorsalis
- *disorders of peripheral innervation,* including autonomic neuropathies resulting from endocrine disturbances, such as diabetes mellitus (most common)
- *metabolic disturbances,* such as hypothyroidism, porphyria, or uremia (infrequent)
- *acute infectious diseases,* such as Guillain-Barré syndrome
- *heavy metal toxicity*
- *chronic alcoholism*
- *collagen diseases,* such as systemic lupus erythematosus
- *vascular diseases,* such as atherosclerosis
- *distant effects of cancer,* such as primary oat cell carcinoma of the lung
- *herpes zoster*
- *sacral agenesis.*

An upper motor neuron lesion (above S2 to S4) causes spastic neurogenic bladder, with spontaneous contractions of detrusor muscles, elevated intravesical voiding pressure, bladder wall hypertrophy with trabeculation, and urinary sphincter spasms. A lower motor neuron lesion (below S2 to S4) causes flaccid neurogenic bladder, with decreased intravesical pressure, increased bladder capacity and large residual urine retention, and poor detrusor contraction.

Signs and symptoms

Neurogenic bladder produces a wide range of clinical effects, depending on the underlying cause and its effect on the structural integrity of the bladder. Usually, this disorder causes some degree of incontinence, changes in initiation or interruption of micturition, and inability to empty the bladder completely. Other effects of neurogenic bladder include vesicoureteral reflux, deterioration or infection in the upper urinary tract, and hydroureteral nephrosis.

Depending on the site and extent of the spinal cord lesion, *spastic neurogenic bladder* may produce involuntary or frequent scanty urination, without a feeling of bladder fullness, and possibly spontaneous spasms of the arms and legs. Anal sphincter tone may be increased. Tactile stimulation of the abdomen, thighs, or genitalia may precipitate voiding and spontaneous contractions of the arms and legs. With cord lesions in the upper thoracic (cervical) level, bladder distention can trigger hyperactive autonomic reflexes, resulting in severe hypertension, bradycardia, and headaches.

Flaccid neurogenic bladder may be associated with overflow incontinence, diminished anal sphincter tone, and a greatly distended bladder (evident on percussion or palpation), but without the accompanying feeling of bladder fullness due to sensory impairment.

Diagnosis

Since the causes of neurogenic bladder are so varied, diagnosis must begin with a meticulous patient history, including a thorough neurologic history (especially for injury to the spinal cord) and a history of bowel, urologic, and sexual function. Physical examination includes a complete assessment for overt neurologic disease and the following tests:

- *Spinal fluid analysis* showing increased protein level may indicate cord tumor; increased gamma globulin may indicate multiple sclerosis.
- *Skull and vertebral column X-rays* show fracture, dislocation, congenital anomalies, or metastasis.
- *Myelography* shows spinal cord compression (from tumor, spondylosis, or arachnoiditis).
- *EEG* may be abnormal in the presence of a brain tumor.
- *Electromyelography* confirms presence of peripheral neuropathy.
- *Brain and computed tomography scans* localize and identify brain masses.

Other tests assess bladder function:

- *Cystometry* evaluates bladder nerve supply and detrusor muscle tone.
- *Urethral pressure profile* determines urethral function.
- *Urinary flow study (uroflow)* shows diminished or impaired urinary flow.
- *Retrograde urethrography* reveals presence of strictures and diverticula.
- *Voiding cystography* evaluates bladder neck function and continence.

Treatment

The goals of treatment are to maintain the integrity of the upper urinary tract, control infection, and prevent urinary incontinence through evacuation of the bladder, drug therapy, surgery, or, less often, neural blocks and electrical stimulation. Techniques of bladder evacuation include Credé's method, Valsalva's maneuver, and intermittent self-catheterization. Credé's method—application of manual pressure over the lower abdomen—promotes complete emptying of the bladder. After appropriate instruction, most patients can perform this maneuver themselves. Even when performed properly, however, Credé's method isn't always successful and doesn't always eliminate the need for catheterization.

Intermittent self-catheterization—more effective than either Credé's method or Valsalva's maneuver—has proven a major advance in the treatment of neurogenic bladder, since it allows complete emptying of the bladder without the risks of a Foley catheter. Generally, a male can perform this procedure more easily, but a female can learn self-catheterization with the help of a mirror. Intermittent self-catheterization, in conjunction with a bladder-retraining program, is especially useful in patients with flaccid neurogenic bladder.

Drug therapy for neurogenic bladder may include bethanechol and phenoxybenzamine to facilitate bladder emptying and propantheline, methantheline, flavoxate, dicyclomine, and imipramine to facilitate urine storage. When conservative treatment fails, surgery may correct the structural impairment through transurethral resection of the bladder neck, a Y-V plasty, urethral dilation, external sphincterotomy, or urinary diversion procedures. Implantation of an artificial urinary sphincter may be necessary if permanent incontinence follows surgery.

Special considerations

Care for patients with neurogenic bladder varies according to the underlying cause and the method of treatment.

- Explain all diagnostic tests clearly so the patient understands the procedure, the time involved, and the possible results. Assure the patient that the lengthy diagnostic process is necessary to identify the most effective treatment plan. After the treatment plan is chosen, explain it to the patient in detail.

- Use strict aseptic technique during insertion of a Foley catheter (a temporary measure to drain the incontinent patient's bladder). Don't interrupt the closed drainage system for any reason. Obtain urine specimens with a syringe and small-bore needle inserted through the aspirating port of the catheter itself (below the junction of the balloon instillation site). Irrigate in the same manner, if ordered.
- Clean the catheter insertion site with soap and water at least twice a day. Don't allow the catheter to become encrusted. Use a sterile applicator to apply antibiotic ointment around the meatus after catheter care. Keep the drainage bag below the tubing, and don't raise the bag above the level of the bladder. Clamp the tubing, or empty the bag before transferring the patient to a wheelchair or stretcher to prevent accidental urine reflux. If urinary output is considerable, empty the bag more frequently than once every 8 hours, since bacteria can multiply in standing urine and migrate up the catheter and into the bladder.
- Watch for signs of infection (fever, cloudy or foul-smelling urine). Encourage the patient to drink plenty of fluids to prevent calculus formation and infection from urinary stasis. Try to keep the patient as mobile as possible. Perform passive range-of-motion exercises, if necessary.
- If urinary diversion procedure is to be performed, arrange for consultation with an enterostomal therapist, and coordinate the care plans.
- Before discharge, teach the patient and his family evacuation techniques, as necessary (Credé's method, intermittent catheterization). Counsel him regarding sexual activities. Remember, the incontinent patient feels embarrassed and distressed. Provide emotional support.

Congenital Anomalies of the Ureter, Bladder, and Urethra

Congenital anomalies of the ureter, bladder, and urethra are among the most common birth defects, occurring in about 5% of all births. Some of these abnormalities are obvious at birth; others are not apparent and are recognized only after they produce symptoms.

Causes

The most common malformations include duplicated ureter, retrocaval ureter, ectopic orifice of the ureter, stricture or stenosis of the ureter, ureterocele, exstrophy of the bladder, congenital bladder diverticulum, hypospadias, and epispadias. Their causes are unknown; diagnosis and treatment vary.

Special considerations

- Since these anomalies aren't always obvious at birth, carefully evaluate the newborn's urogenital function. Document the amount and color of urine, voiding pattern, strength of stream, and any indications of infection, such as fever and urine odor. Tell parents to watch for these signs at home.
- In all children, watch for signs of obstruction, such as dribbling, oliguria or anuria, abdominal mass, hypertension, fever, bacteriuria, or pyuria.
- Monitor renal function daily; record intake and output accurately.
- Follow strict aseptic technique in handling cystostomy tubes or Foley catheters.
- Make sure that ureteral, suprapubic, or urethral catheters remain in place and don't become contaminated. Document type, color, and amount of drainage.

CONGENITAL ANOMALIES OF THE URETER AND BLADDER

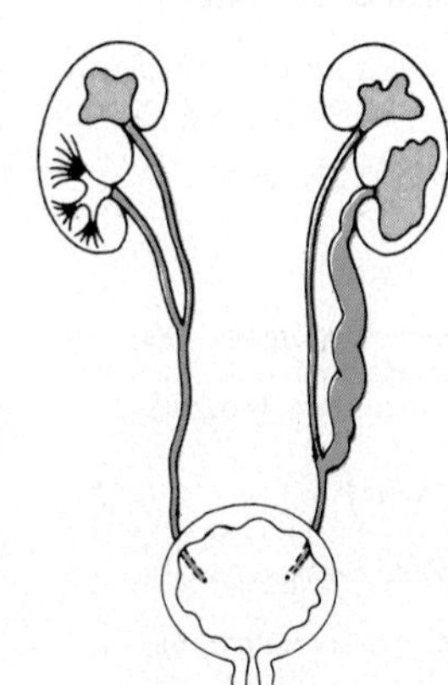

DUPLICATED URETER

PATHOPHYSIOLOGY

- Most common ureteral anomaly
- *Complete,* a double collecting system with two separate pelves, each with its own ureter and orifice
- *Incomplete* (y type), two separate ureters join before entering bladder

CLINICAL FEATURES

- Persistent or recurrent infection
- Frequency, urgency, or burning on urination
- Diminished urinary output
- Flank pain, fever, and chills

DIAGNOSIS AND TREATMENT

- Intravenous pyelography
- Voiding cystoscopy
- Cystoureterography
- Retrograde pyelography
- Surgery for obstruction, reflux, or severe renal damage

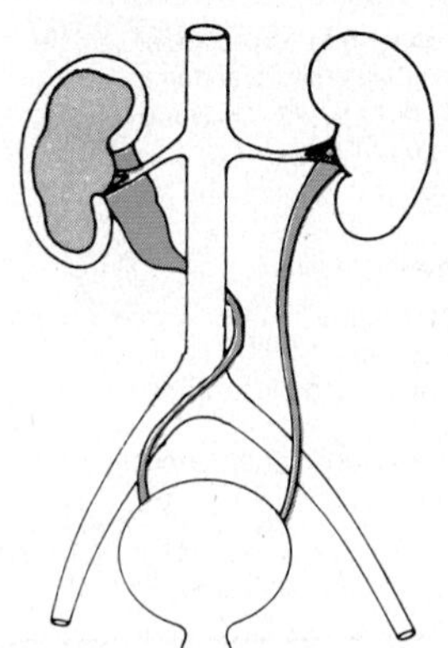

RETROCAVAL URETER (PREURETERAL VENA CAVA)

PATHOPHYSIOLOGY

- Right ureter passes behind the inferior vena cava before entering the bladder. Compression of the ureter between the vena cava and the spine causes dilation and elongation of the pelvis; hydroureter, hydronephrosis; fibrosis and stenosis of ureter in the compressed area.
- Relatively uncommon; higher incidence in males

CLINICAL FEATURES

- Right flank pain
- Recurrent urinary tract infection
- Renal calculi
- Hematuria

DIAGNOSIS AND TREATMENT

- Intravenous or retrograde pyelography demonstrates superior ureteral enlargement with spiral appearance.
- Surgical resection and anastomosis of ureter with renal pelvis, or reimplantation into bladder

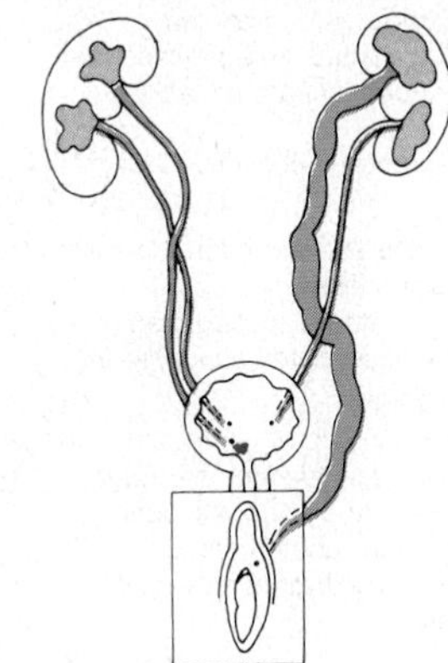

ECTOPIC ORIFICE OF URETER

PATHOPHYSIOLOGY

- Ureters single or duplicated. In females, ureteral orifice usually inserts in urethra or vaginal vestibule, beyond external urethral sphincter; in males, in prostatic urethra, or in seminal vesicles or vas deferens

CLINICAL FEATURES

- Symptoms rare when ureteral orifice opens between trigone and bladder neck
- Obstruction, reflux, and incontinence (dribbling) in 50% of females
- In males, flank pain, frequency, urgency

DIAGNOSIS AND TREATMENT

- Intravenous pyelography
- Urethroscopy, vaginoscopy
- Voiding cystourethrography
- Resection and ureteral reimplantation into bladder for incontinence

CONGENITAL ANOMALIES OF THE URETER AND BLADDER (continued)

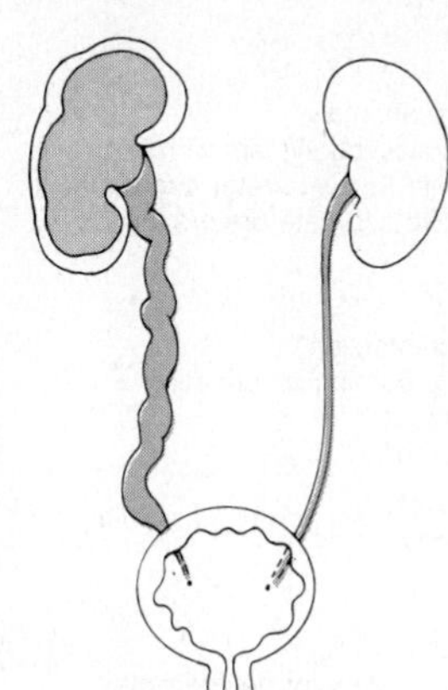

STRICTURE OR STENOSIS OF URETER

PATHOPHYSIOLOGY

- Most common site, the distal ureter above ureterovesical junction; less common, ureteropelvic junction; rare, the midureter
- Discovered during infancy in 25% of patients; before puberty in most
- More common in males

CLINICAL FEATURES

- Megaloureter or hydroureter (enlarged ureter), with hydronephrosis when stenosis occurs in distal ureter
- Hydronephrosis alone when stenosis occurs at ureteropelvic junction

DIAGNOSIS AND TREATMENT

- Ultrasound
- Intravenous and retrograde pyelography
- Voiding cystography
- Surgical repair of stricture. Nephrectomy for severe renal damage

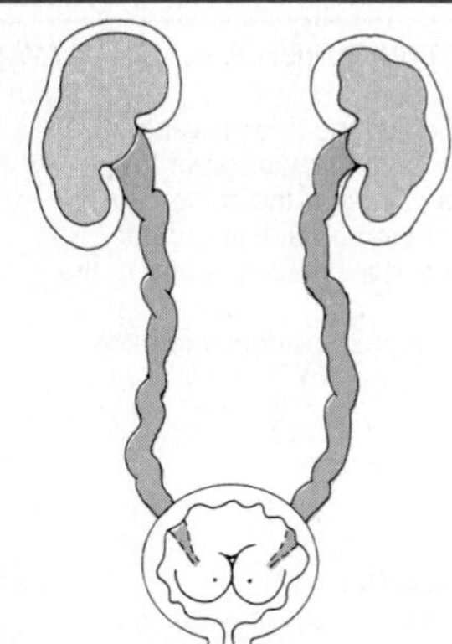

URETEROCELE

PATHOPHYSIOLOGY

- Bulging of submucosal ureter into bladder can be 1 or 2 cm, or can almost fill entire bladder
- Unilateral, bilateral, ectopic with resulting hydroureter, and hydronephrosis

CLINICAL FEATURES

- Obstruction
- Persistent or recurrent infection

DIAGNOSIS AND TREATMENT

- Voiding cystourethrography
- Intravenous pyelography and cystoscopy show thin, translucent mass.
- Surgical excision or resection of ureterocele, with reimplantation of ureter

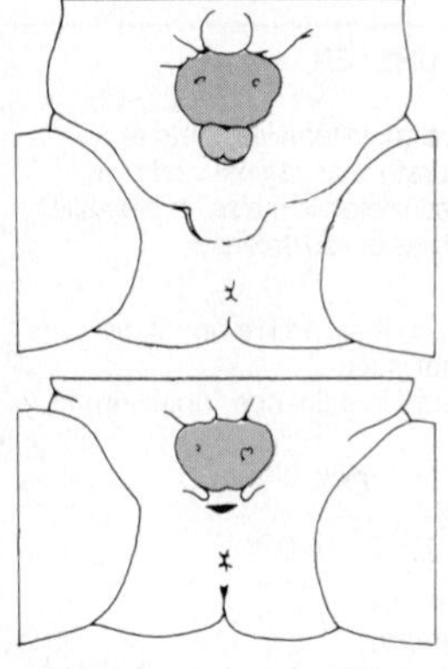

EXSTROPHY OF BLADDER

PATHOPHYSIOLOGY

- Absence of anterior abdominal and bladder wall allows the bladder to protrude onto abdomen.
- In males, associated epispadias and undescended testes; in females, cleft clitoris, separated labia, or absent vagina
- Skeletal or intestinal anomalies possible

CLINICAL FEATURES

- Obvious at birth, with urine seeping onto abdominal wall from abnormal ureteral orifices
- Surrounding skin is excoriated; exposed bladder mucosa ulcerated; infection; associated abnormalities

DIAGNOSIS AND TREATMENT

- Intravenous pyelography
- Surgical closure of defect, and bladder and urethra reconstruction during infancy to allow pubic bone fusion; alternative treatment includes protective dressing and diapering; urinary diversion eventually necessary for most patients

CONGENITAL ANOMALIES OF THE URETER AND BLADDER (continued)

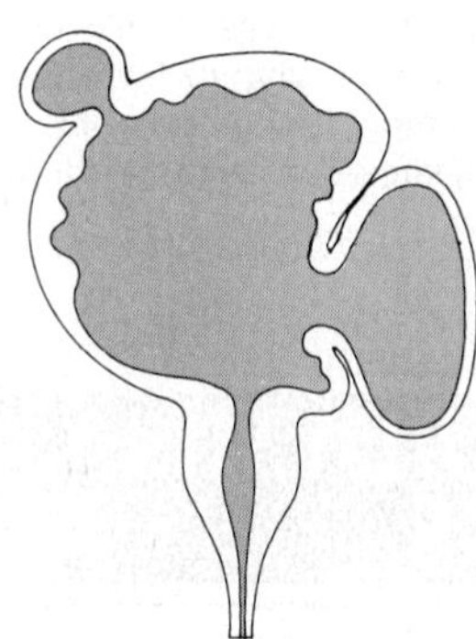

CONGENITAL BLADDER DIVERTICULUM

PATHOPHYSIOLOGY

- Circumscribed pouch or sac (diverticulum) of bladder wall
- Can occur anywhere in bladder, usually lateral to ureteral orifice. Large diverticulum at orifice can cause reflux.

CLINICAL FEATURES

- Fever, frequency, and painful urination
- Urinary tract infection
- Cystitis, particularly in males

DIAGNOSIS AND TREATMENT

- Intravenous pyelography shows diverticulum.
- Retrograde cystography shows vesicoureteral reflux in ureter.
- Surgical correction for reflux

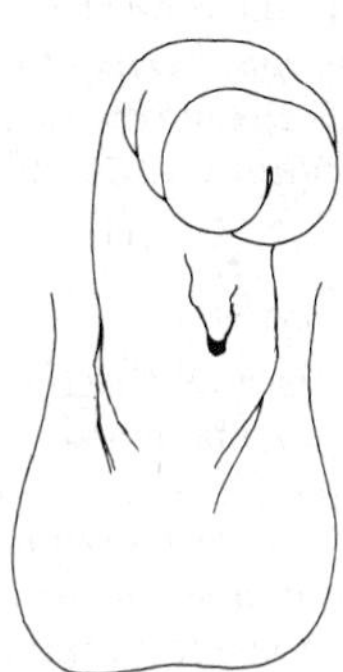

HYPOSPADIAS

PATHOPHYSIOLOGY

- Urethral opening is on ventral surface of penis or, in females (rare), within the vagina.
- Occurs in 1 of 300 live male births. Genetic factor suspected in less severe cases.

CLINICAL FEATURES

- Usually associated with chordee, making normal urination with penis elevated impossible
- Absence of ventral prepuce
- Vaginal discharge in females

DIAGNOSIS AND TREATMENT

- Mild disorder requires no treatment.
- Surgical repair of severe anomaly usually necessary before child reaches school age

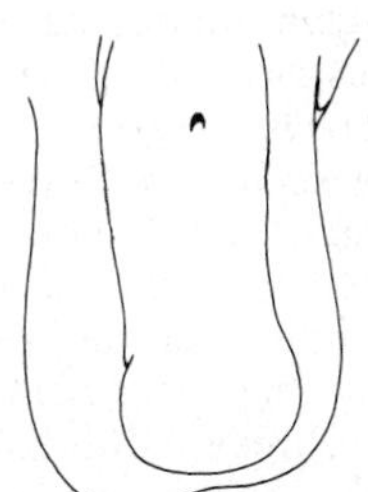

EPISPADIAS

PATHOPHYSIOLOGY

- Urethral opening on dorsal surface of penis; in females, a fissure of the upper wall of urethra
- A rare anomaly; usually develops in males; often accompanies bladder exstrophy.

CLINICAL FEATURES

- In mild cases, orifice appears along dorsum of glans; in severe cases, along dorsum of penis.
- In females, bifid clitoris and short, wide urethra

DIAGNOSIS AND TREATMENT

- Surgical repair, in several stages, almost always necessary

• Apply sterile saline pads to protect the exposed mucosa of the newborn with bladder exstrophy. Don't use heavy clamps on the umbilical cord, and avoid dressing or diapering the infant. Place the infant in an incubator, and direct a stream of saline mist onto the bladder to keep it moist. Use warm water and mild soap to keep the surrounding skin clean. Rinse well, and keep the area as dry as possible to prevent excoriation.

• Provide reassurance and emotional support to the parents. When possible, allow them to participate in their child's care to promote normal bonding. As appropriate, suggest or arrange for genetic counseling.

PROSTATE & EPIDIDYMIS DISORDERS

Prostatitis

Prostatitis, inflammation of the prostate gland, may be acute or chronic. Acute prostatitis *most often results from gram-negative bacteria and is easy to recognize and treat. However,* chronic prostatitis, *the most common cause of recurrent urinary tract infection (UTI) in men, is less easy to recognize. As many as 35% of men over age 50 have chronic prostatitis.*

Causes

About 80% of bacterial prostatitis results from infection by *Escherichia coli;* the rest, from infection by *Klebsiella, Enterobacter, Proteus, Pseudomonas, Streptococcus,* or *Staphylococcus.* Such infection probably spreads to the prostate gland by the hematogenous route or from ascending urethral infection, invasion of rectal bacteria by way of lymphatics, reflux of infected bladder urine into prostate ducts, or, less commonly, infrequent or excessive sexual intercourse or urethral instrumentation, such as cystoscopy or catheterization. Chronic prostatitis usually develops as a result of bacterial invasion from the urethra.

Signs and symptoms

Acute prostatitis begins with sudden fever, chills, low back pain, a feeling of myalgia, perineal fullness, and arthralgia. Urination becomes more frequent and more urgent. Dysuria, nocturia, and some degree of urinary obstruction may also occur. The urine may appear cloudy. When palpated rectally, the prostate is markedly tender, indurated, swollen, firm, and warm.

Clinical features of chronic bacterial prostatitis vary. Although some patients are asymptomatic, this condition usually elicits the same urinary symptoms as the acute form but to a lesser degree. Other possible signs include painful ejaculation, hemospermia, persistent urethral discharge, and sexual dysfunction. UTI is a common complication.

Diagnosis

Although a urine culture can often identify the causative infectious organism, and characteristic rectal examination findings suggest prostatitis (especially in the acute phase), firm diagnosis depends

on the comparison of urine cultures of samples obtained by the Meares and Stamey technique. This test requires four specimens: one collected when the patient starts voiding (voided bladder one—VB1); another midstream (VB2); another after the patient stops voiding and the doctor massages the prostate to produce secretions (expressed prostate secretions—EPS); and a final voided specimen (VB3). A significant increase in colony count of the prostatic specimens (EPS and VB3) confirms prostatitis.

Treatment

Systemic antibiotic therapy, using the best antibiotics available based on sensitivity studies, is the treatment of choice for acute prostatitis. Aminoglycosides, such as gentamicin or tobramycin, may be the most effective drugs for severe cases. Co-trimoxazole is widely used to treat chronic prostatitis, which usually requires a long-term course of treatment (at least 6 weeks).

Supportive therapy includes bed rest, adequate hydration, and administration of analgesics, antipyretics, and stool softeners, as necessary.

If drug therapy is unsuccessful in treating chronic prostatitis, treatment may include transurethral resection of the prostate. To be effective, this procedure requires removal of all infected tissue. The procedure is usually not performed on young adults, because it usually leads to retrograde ejaculation and sterility. Total prostatectomy is curative but may cause sexual impotence and incontinence.

Special considerations

- Ensure bed rest and adequate hydration. Provide stool softeners and administer sitz baths, as ordered.
- As necessary, prepare to assist with suprapubic needle aspiration of the bladder or a suprapubic cystostomy.
- Administer prescribed medications, as ordered. Emphasize to the patient the need for strict adherence to the prescribed drug treatment regimen. Instruct the patient to drink at least eight glasses of water a day. Tell him to immediately report signs of possible adverse drug reactions, such as rash, nausea, vomiting, fever, chills, and gastrointestinal irritation.

Epididymitis

This infection of the epididymis, the testicle's cordlike excretory duct, is one of the most common infections of the male reproductive tract. It usually affects adults and is rare before puberty. Epididymitis may spread to the testicle itself, causing orchitis; bilateral epididymitis may cause sterility.

Causes

Epididymitis usually results from pyogenic organisms, such as staphylococci, *Escherichia coli,* and streptococci. Generally, such organisms result from established urinary tract infection or prostatitis and reach the epididymis through the lumen of the vas deferens. Rarely, epididymitis is secondary to a distant infection, such as pharyngitis or tuberculosis, that spreads through the lymphatics or, less commonly, the bloodstream. Other causes include trauma, gonorrhea, syphilis, or a chlamydial infection. Trauma may reactivate a dormant infection or initiate a new one. Epididymitis is a complication of prostatectomy and may also result from chemical irritation by extravasation of urine through the vas deferens.

Signs and symptoms

The key symptoms are pain, extreme tenderness, and swelling in the groin and scrotum. Other clinical effects include high fever, malaise, and a characteristic waddle—an attempt to protect the groin and scrotum during walking. An acute hydrocele may also occur as a reaction to the inflammatory process.

Diagnosis

Clinical features suggest epididymitis, but diagnosis requires laboratory tests:

ORCHITIS

Orchitis, infection of the testicles, is a serious complication of epididymitis. This infection may also result from mumps, which may lead to sterility, and, less often, from another systemic infection, testicular torsion, or severe trauma. Its typical effects include unilateral or bilateral tenderness, gradual onset of pain, and swelling of the scrotum and testicles. The affected testicle may be red and hot. Nausea and vomiting also occur. Sudden cessation of pain indicates testicular ischemia, which may result in permanent damage to one or both testicles.

Treatment consists of immediate antibiotic therapy or, in mumps orchitis, diethylstilbestrol (DES), which may relieve pain, swelling, and fever. Corticosteroids are still experimental. Severe orchitis may require surgery to incise and drain the hydrocele and to improve testicular circulation. Other treatment is similar to that for epididymitis. To prevent mumps orchitis, stress the need for prepubertal males to receive mumps vaccine (or gamma globulin injection after contracting mumps).

- *Urinalysis:* Increased WBC count indicates infection.
- *Urine culture and sensitivity:* Findings may identify causative organism.
- *Serum WBC count:* > 10,000/mm³ in infection.

However, in epididymitis accompanied by orchitis, diagnosis must be made cautiously, since symptoms mimic those of testicular torsion, a condition requiring urgent surgical intervention.

Treatment

The goal of treatment is to reduce pain and swelling and combat infection. Therapy must begin immediately, particularly in the patient with bilateral epididymitis, since sterility is always a threat. During the acute phase, treatment consists of bed rest, scrotal elevation with towel rolls or adhesive strapping, broad-spectrum antibiotics, and analgesics. An ice bag applied to the area may reduce swelling and relieve pain (heat is contraindicated, since it may damage germinal cells, which are viable only at or below normal body temperature). When pain and swelling subside and allow walking, an athletic supporter may prevent pain. Occasionally, corticosteroids may be prescribed to help counteract inflammation, but their use is controversial.

In the older patient undergoing open prostatectomy, bilateral vasectomy may be necessary to prevent epididymitis as a postoperative complication; however, antibiotic therapy alone may prevent it. When epididymitis is refractory to antibiotic therapy, epididymectomy under local anesthetic is necessary.

Special considerations

- Watch closely for abscess formation (localized, hot, red, tender area) or extension of infection into the testes. Closely monitor temperature, and ensure adequate fluid intake.
- Since the patient is usually very uncomfortable, administer analgesics, as necessary. During bed rest, check often for proper scrotum elevation.
- Before discharge, emphasize the importance of completing the prescribed antibiotic therapy, even after symptoms subside.
- If the patient faces the possibility of sterility, suggest supportive counseling, as necessary.

Benign Prostatic Hypertrophy

Although most men over age 50 have some prostatic enlargement, in benign prostatic hypertrophy or hyperplasia (BPH), the prostate gland enlarges sufficiently to com-

press the urethra and cause some overt urinary obstruction. Depending on the size of the enlarged prostate, the age and health of the patient, and the extent of obstruction, BPH is treated symptomatically or surgically.

Causes

Recent evidence suggests a link between BPH and hormonal activity. As men age, production of androgenic hormones decreases, causing an imbalance in androgen and estrogen levels, and high levels of dihydrotestosterone, the main prostatic intracellular androgen. Other theoretical causes include neoplasm, arteriosclerosis, inflammation, and metabolic or nutritional disturbances.

Whatever the cause, BPH begins with changes in periurethral glandular tissue. As the prostate enlarges, it may extend into the bladder and obstruct urinary outflow by compressing or distorting the prostatic urethra. BPH may also cause a pouch to form in the bladder that retains urine when the rest of the bladder empties. This retained urine may lead to calculus formation or cystitis.

Signs and symptoms

Clinical features of BPH depend on the extent of prostatic enlargement and the lobes affected. Characteristically, the condition starts with a group of symptoms known as "prostatism": reduced urinary stream caliber and force, difficulty starting micturition (straining), feeling of incomplete voiding, and, occasionally, urinary retention. As obstruction increases, urination becomes more frequent, with nocturia, incontinence, and possibly hematuria. Physical examination indicates a visible midline mass (distended bladder) that represents an incompletely emptied bladder; rectal palpation discloses an enlarged prostate. Examination may detect secondary anemia and, possibly, renal insufficiency secondary to obstruction.

As BPH worsens, complete urinary obstruction may follow infection or ingestion of decongestants, tranquilizers, alcohol, antidepressants, or anticholinergics. Possible complications include infection, renal insufficiency, hemorrhage, and shock.

Diagnosis

Clinical features and a rectal examination are usually sufficient for diagnosis. Other findings help to confirm this diagnosis:

- *Intravenous pyelography* may indicate urinary tract obstruction, calculi or tumors, and filling and emptying defects in the bladder.
- *Elevated BUN and creatinine levels* suggest impaired renal function.
- *Urinalysis and urine culture* show hematuria, pyuria, and, when bacterial count is more than 100,000/mm^3, urinary tract infection.

When symptoms are severe, a cystourethroscopy is the definitive diagnostic measure, but this examination is performed only immediately before surgery, to help determine the best operative procedure. It can show prostate enlargement, bladder wall changes, and a raised bladder.

Treatment

Conservative therapy includes prostatic massages, sitz baths, short-term fluid restriction (to prevent bladder distention), and, if infection develops, antimicrobials. Regular sexual intercourse may help relieve prostatic congestion.

Surgery is the only effective therapy for relief of acute urinary retention, hydronephrosis, severe hematuria, and recurrent urinary tract infection or for palliative relief of intolerable symptoms. A transurethral resection may be performed if the prostate weighs less than 2 oz (56.7 g). (Weight is approximated by digital examination.) In this procedure, a resectoscope removes tissue with a wire loop and electric current. For patients who are at high risk, continuous drainage with a Foley catheter alleviates urinary retention.

Other appropriate procedures involve open surgical removal:

- *suprapubic* (transvesical): most common and especially useful when pros-

tatic enlargement remains within the bladder
- *perineal:* for a large gland in an older patient; usually results in impotence and incontinence
- *retropubic* (extravesical): allows direct visualization; potency and continence are usually maintained.

Special considerations

Prepare the patient for diagnostic tests and surgery, as appropriate.
- Monitor and record the patient's vital signs, intake and output, and daily weight. Watch closely for signs of postobstructive diuresis (such as increased urine output and hypotension), which may lead to serious dehydration, lowered blood volume, shock, electrolyte loss, and anuria.
- Administer antibiotics, as ordered, for urinary tract infection, urethral instrumentation, and cystoscopy.
- If urinary retention is present, insert a Foley catheter (although this is usually difficult in a patient with BPH). If the catheter can't be passed transurethrally, assist with suprapubic cystostomy (under local anesthetic). Watch for rapid bladder decompression.

After prostatic surgery:
- Maintain patient comfort, and watch for and prevent postoperative complications. Observe for immediate dangers—shock and hemorrhage—of prostatic bleeding. Check the catheter frequently (every 15 minutes for the first 2 to 3 hours) for patency and urine color; check the dressings for bleeding.
- Postoperatively, many urologists insert a three-way catheter and establish continuous bladder irrigation. Keep the catheter open at a rate sufficient to maintain returns that are clear and light pink. Watch for fluid overload from absorption of the irrigating fluid into systemic circulation. If a regular catheter is used, observe it closely. If drainage stops because of clots, irrigate the catheter, as ordered, usually with 80 to 100 ml normal saline solution, while maintaining *strict* aseptic technique.
- Also watch for septic shock, the most serious complication of prostatic surgery. Immediately report severe chills, sudden fever, tachycardia, hypotension, or other signs of shock. Start rapid infusion of antibiotics I.V., as ordered. Watch for pulmonary embolus, heart failure, and renal shutdown. Monitor vital signs, central venous pressure, and arterial pressure continuously. The patient may need intensive supportive care in the intensive care unit.
- Administer belladonna and opium suppositories or other anticholinergics, as ordered, to relieve painful bladder spasms that often occur after transurethral resection.
- Take patient comfort measures after an open procedure: provide suppositories (except after perineal prostatectomy), analgesic medication to control incisional pain, and frequent dressing changes.
- Continue infusing I.V. fluids until the patient can drink sufficient fluids (2,000 to 3,000 ml/day) to maintain adequate hydration.
- Administer stool softeners and laxatives, as ordered, to prevent straining. *Don't* check for fecal impaction, since a rectal examination may precipitate bleeding.
- After the catheter is removed, the patient may experience frequency, dribbling, and occasional hematuria. Reassure him that he will gradually regain urinary control. Explain this to the patient's family so they can reinforce this reassurance.
- Reinforce prescribed limits on activity. Warn the patient against lifting, strenuous exercise, and long automobile rides, since these increase bleeding tendency. Also caution the patient to restrict sexual activity for at least several weeks after discharge.
- Instruct the patient to follow the prescribed oral antibiotic drug regimen, and tell him the indications for using gentle laxatives. Urge him to seek medical care immediately if he can't void, if he passes bloody urine, or if he develops a fever.

MEDIAL VIEW OF THE BRAIN

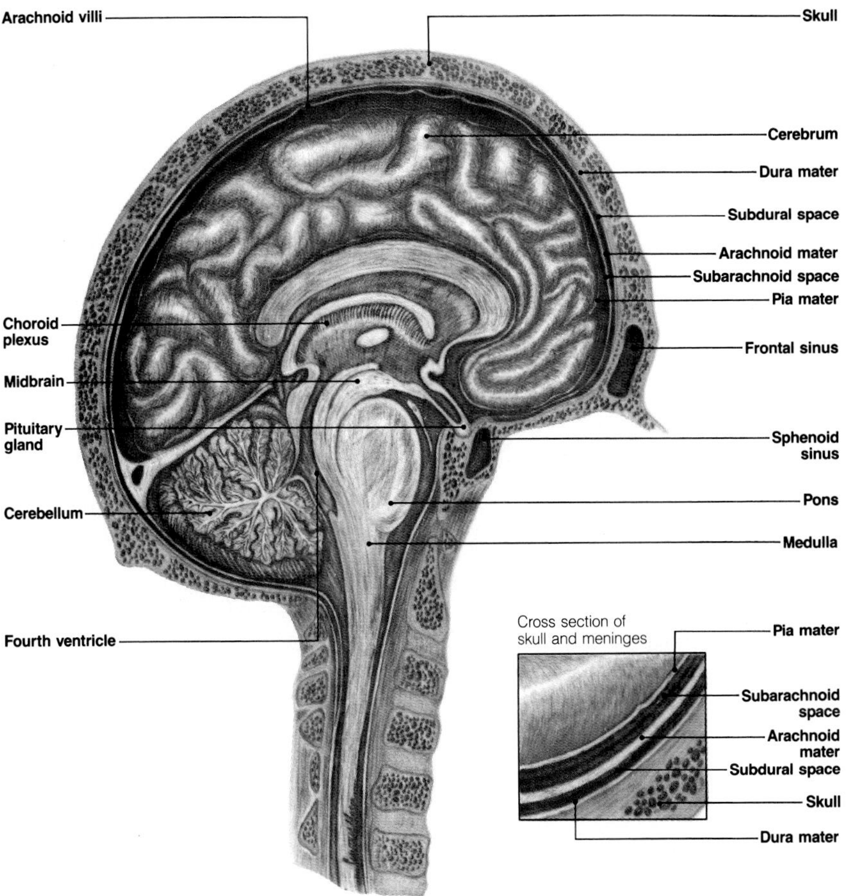
Arachnoid villi
Skull
Cerebrum
Dura mater
Subdural space
Arachnoid mater
Subarachnoid space
Pia mater
Choroid plexus
Frontal sinus
Midbrain
Pituitary gland
Sphenoid sinus
Pons
Cerebellum
Medulla
Fourth ventricle
Cross section of skull and meninges
Pia mater
Subarachnoid space
Arachnoid mater
Subdural space
Skull
Dura mater

Nerve origin

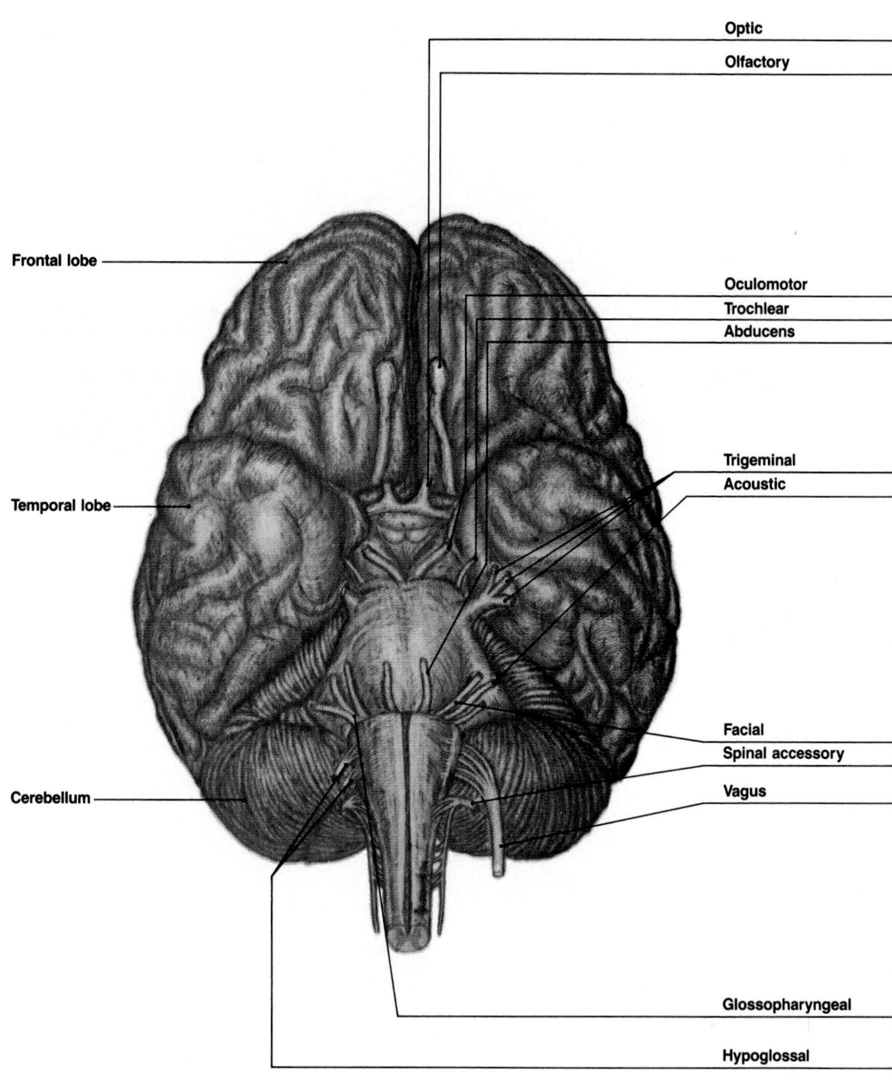

Optic
Olfactory
Frontal lobe
Oculomotor
Trochlear
Abducens
Trigeminal
Acoustic
Temporal lobe
Facial
Spinal accessory
Vagus
Cerebellum
Glossopharyngeal
Hypoglossal

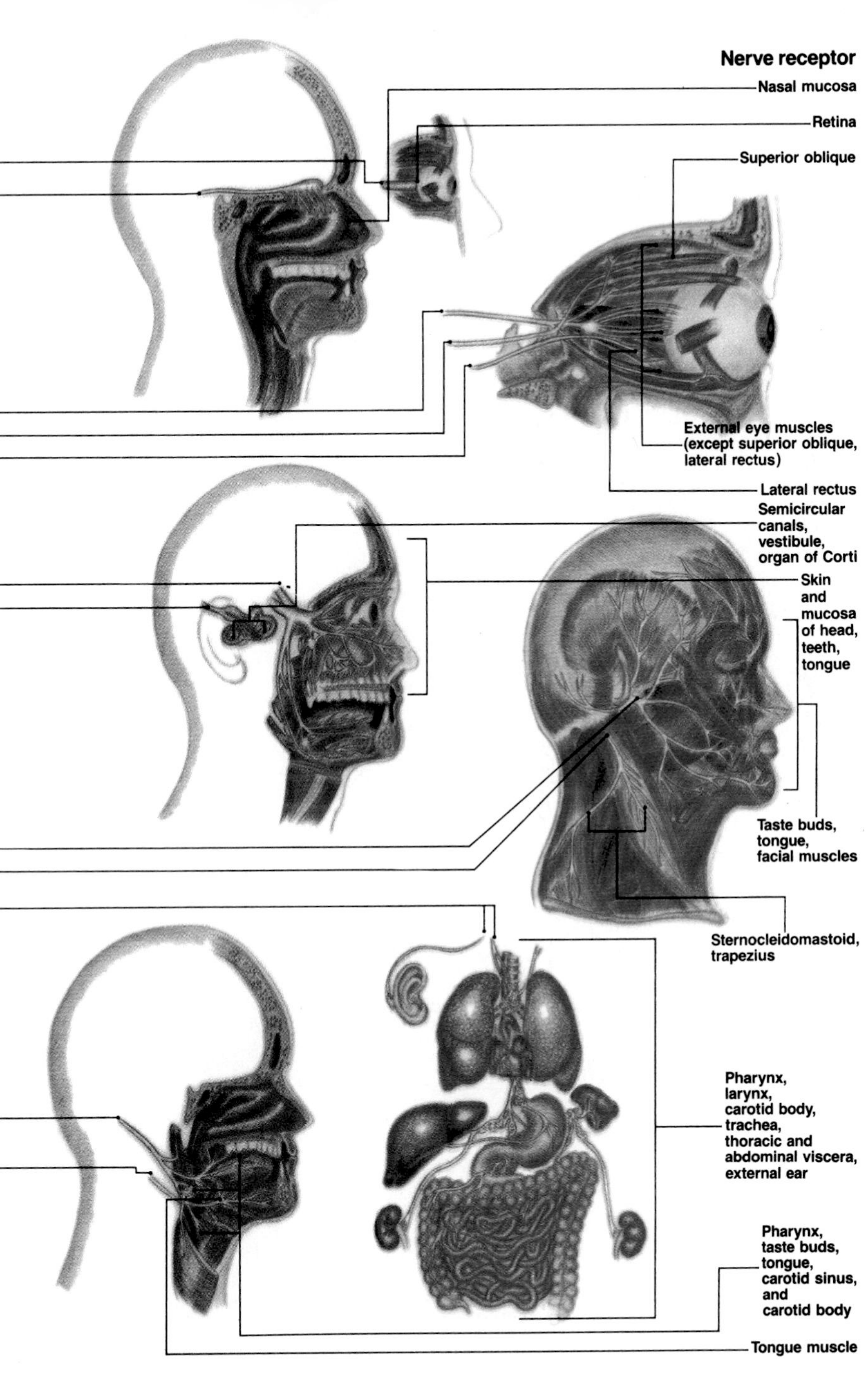
Nerve receptor
Nasal mucosa
Retina
Superior oblique
External eye muscles (except superior oblique, lateral rectus)
Lateral rectus
Semicircular canals, vestibule, organ of Corti
Skin and mucosa of head, teeth, tongue
Taste buds, tongue, facial muscles
Sternocleidomastoid, trapezius
Pharynx, larynx, carotid body, trachea, thoracic and abdominal viscera, external ear
Pharynx, taste buds, tongue, carotid sinus, and carotid body
Tongue muscle

AUTONOMIC NERVOUS SYSTEM

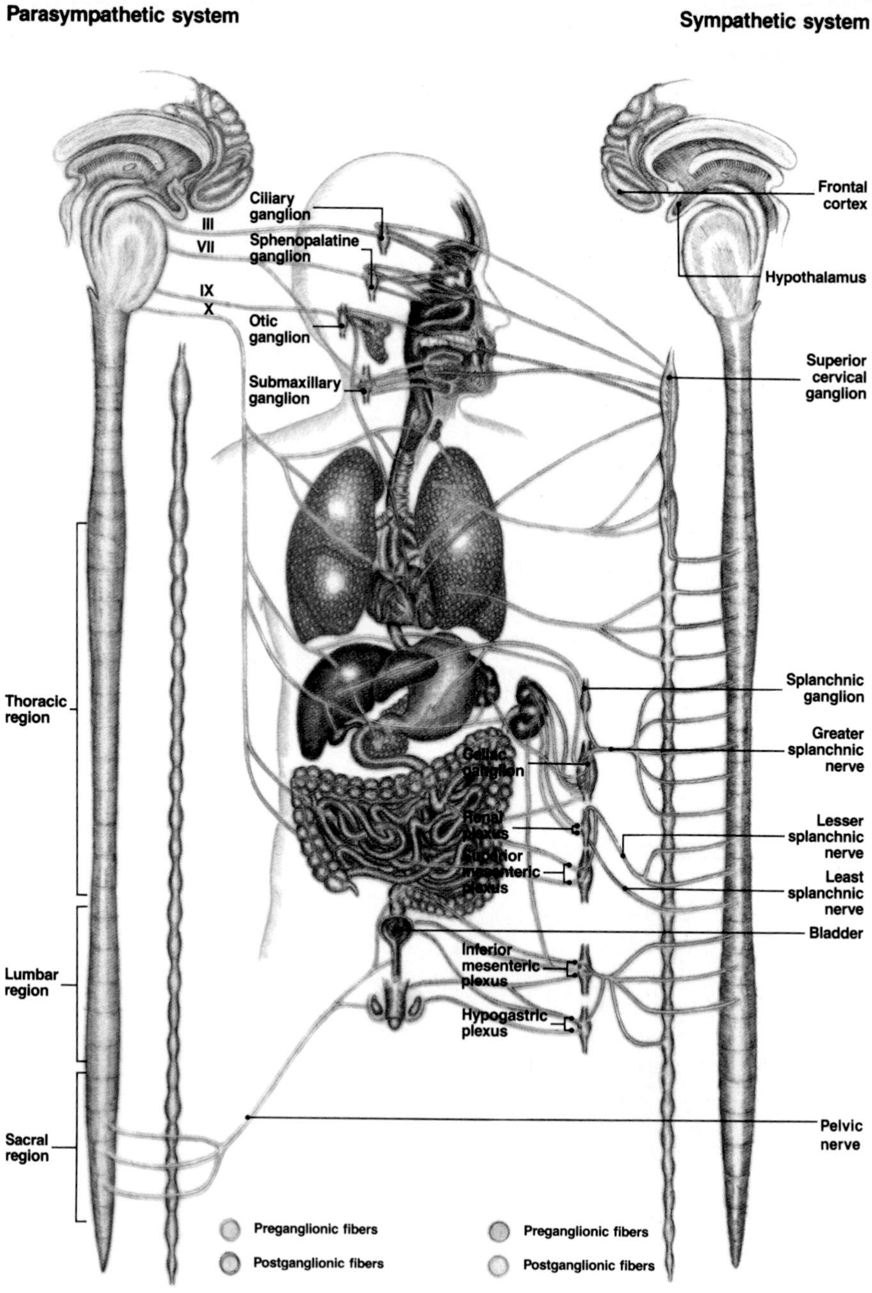

Parasympathetic system

Sympathetic system

Ciliary ganglion
III
VII
Sphenopalatine ganglion
IX
X
Otic ganglion
Submaxillary ganglion
Thoracic region
Lumbar region
Sacral region
Celiac ganglion
Renal plexus
Superior mesenteric plexus
Inferior mesenteric plexus
Hypogastric plexus
Frontal cortex
Hypothalamus
Superior cervical ganglion
Splanchnic ganglion
Greater splanchnic nerve
Lesser splanchnic nerve
Least splanchnic nerve
Bladder
Pelvic nerve

Preganglionic fibers
Postganglionic fibers

Preganglionic fibers
Postganglionic fibers

NORMAL HEART

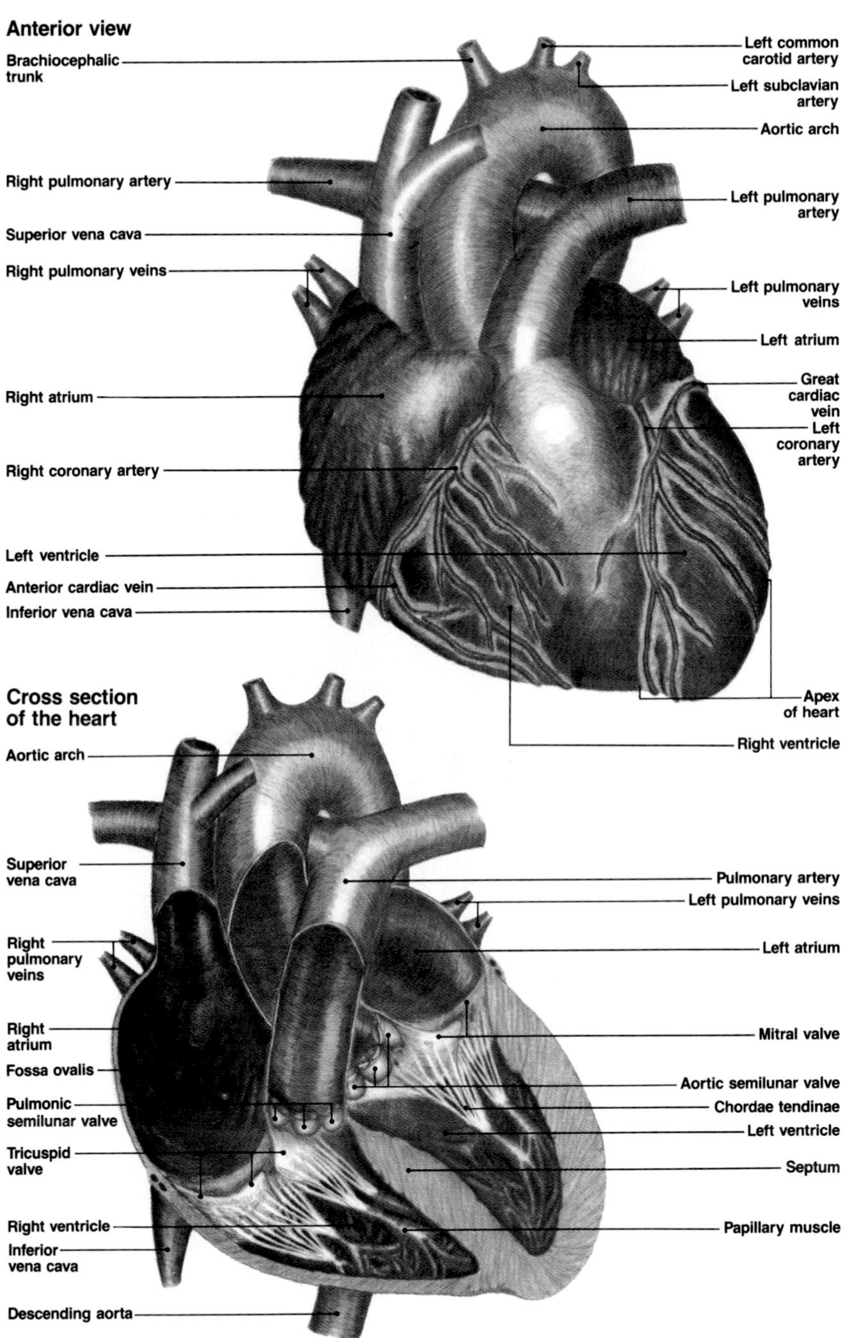
Anterior view
Brachiocephalic trunk
Left common carotid artery
Left subclavian artery
Aortic arch
Right pulmonary artery
Left pulmonary artery
Superior vena cava
Right pulmonary veins
Left pulmonary veins
Left atrium
Great cardiac vein
Right atrium
Left coronary artery
Right coronary artery
Left ventricle
Anterior cardiac vein
Inferior vena cava
Apex of heart
Right ventricle
Cross section of the heart
Aortic arch
Superior vena cava
Pulmonary artery
Left pulmonary veins
Right pulmonary veins
Left atrium
Right atrium
Mitral valve
Fossa ovalis
Aortic semilunar valve
Pulmonic semilunar valve
Chordae tendinae
Left ventricle
Tricuspid valve
Septum
Right ventricle
Papillary muscle
Inferior vena cava
Descending aorta

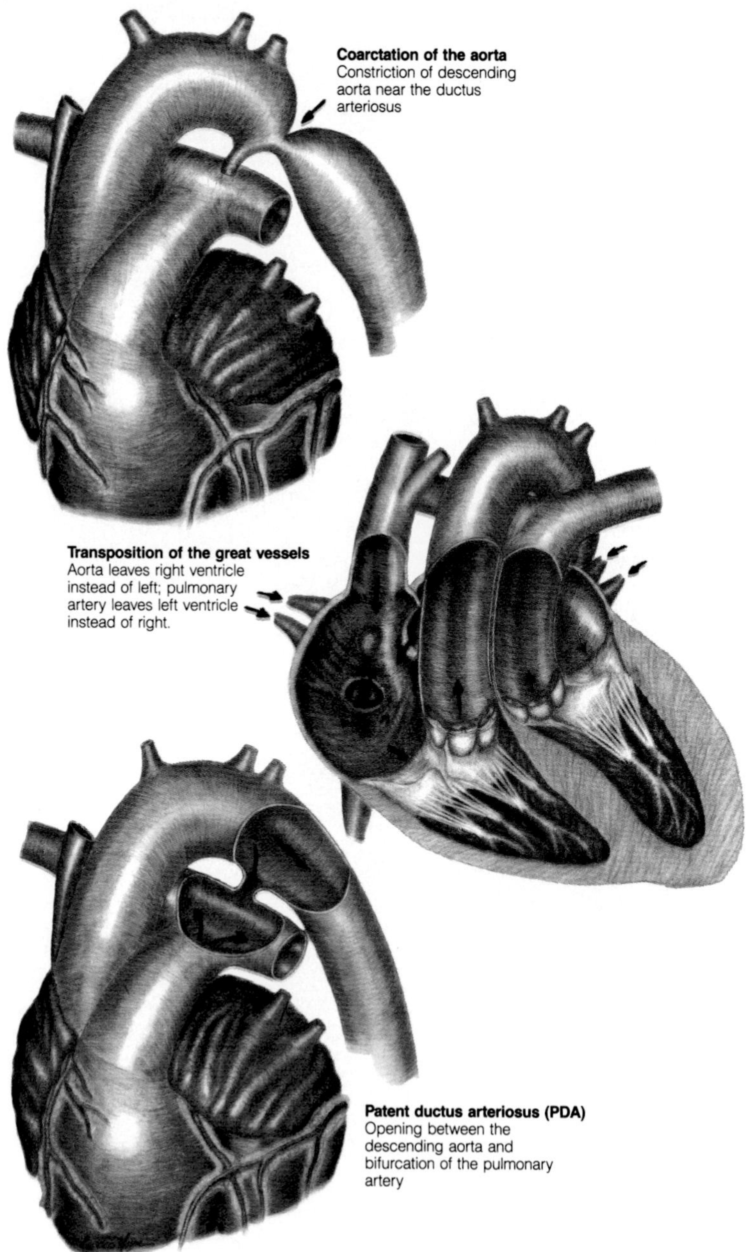
Coarctation of the aorta
Constriction of descending aorta near the ductus arteriosus
Transposition of the great vessels
Aorta leaves right ventricle instead of left; pulmonary artery leaves left ventricle instead of right.
Patent ductus arteriosus (PDA)
Opening between the descending aorta and bifurcation of the pulmonary artery

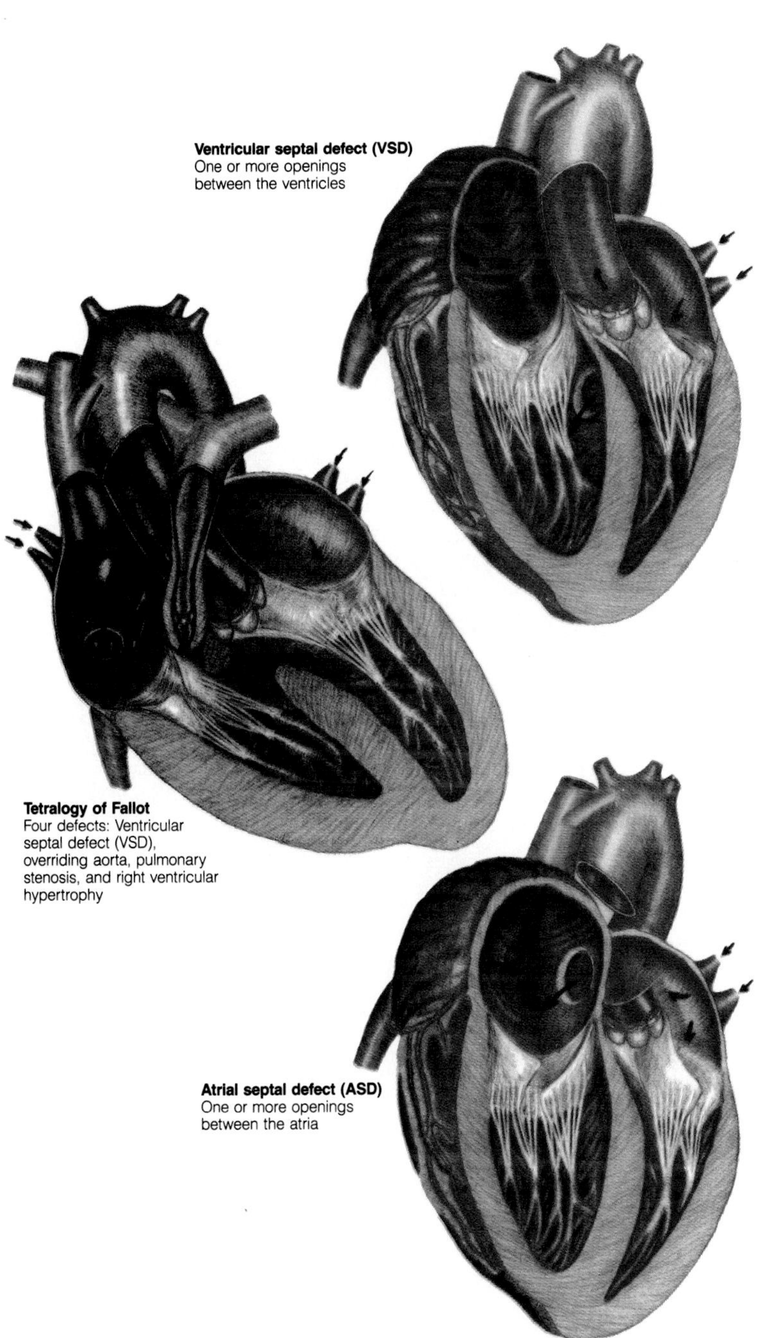
Ventricular septal defect (VSD)
One or more openings
between the ventricles
Tetralogy of Fallot
Four defects: Ventricular
septal defect (VSD),
overriding aorta, pulmonary
stenosis, and right ventricular
hypertrophy
Atrial septal defect (ASD)
One or more openings
between the atria

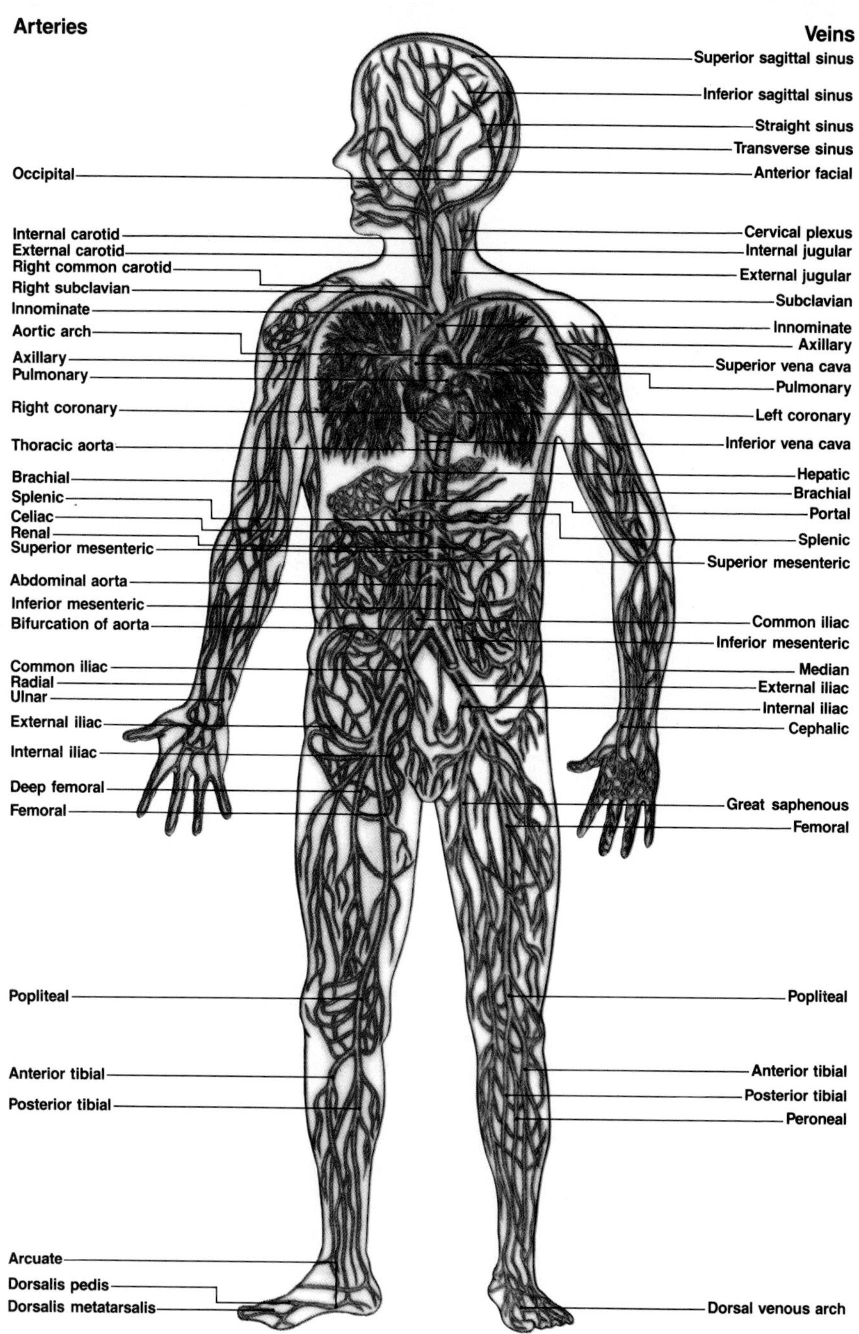

Arteries
Veins
Superior sagittal sinus
Inferior sagittal sinus
Straight sinus
Transverse sinus
Occipital
Anterior facial
Internal carotid
External carotid
Right common carotid
Right subclavian
Innominate
Aortic arch
Axillary
Pulmonary
Right coronary
Thoracic aorta
Brachial
Splenic
Celiac
Renal
Superior mesenteric
Abdominal aorta
Inferior mesenteric
Bifurcation of aorta
Common iliac
Radial
Ulnar
External iliac
Internal iliac
Deep femoral
Femoral
Popliteal
Anterior tibial
Posterior tibial
Arcuate
Dorsalis pedis
Dorsalis metatarsalis
Cervical plexus
Internal jugular
External jugular
Subclavian
Innominate
Axillary
Superior vena cava
Pulmonary
Left coronary
Inferior vena cava
Hepatic
Brachial
Portal
Splenic
Superior mesenteric
Common iliac
Inferior mesenteric
Median
External iliac
Internal iliac
Cephalic
Great saphenous
Femoral
Popliteal
Anterior tibial
Posterior tibial
Peroneal
Dorsal venous arch

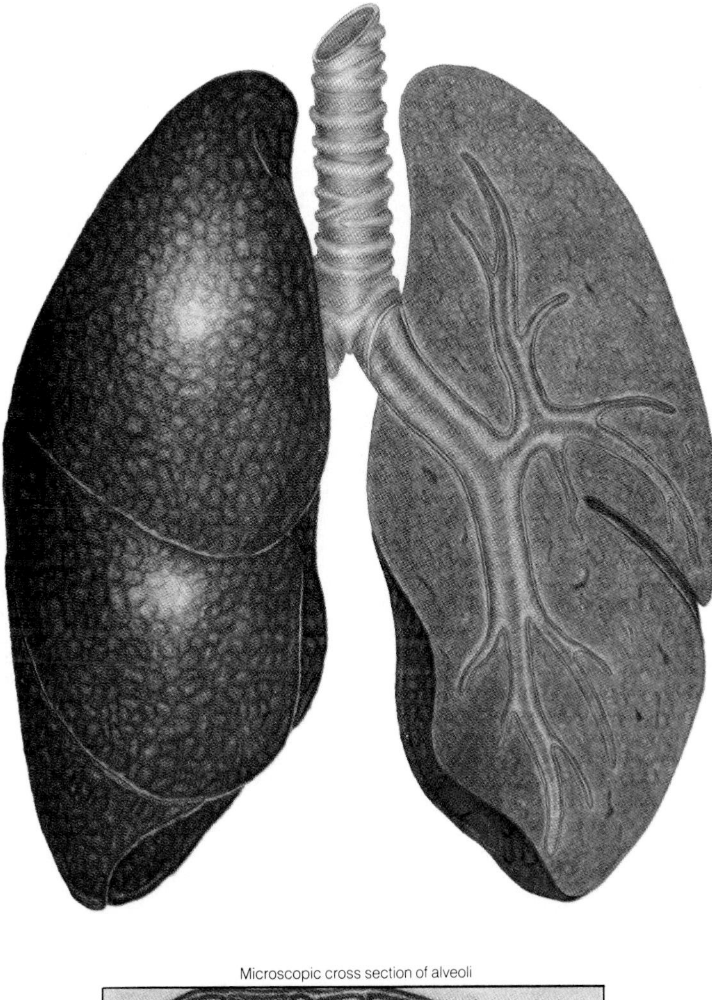

Microscopic cross section of alveoli

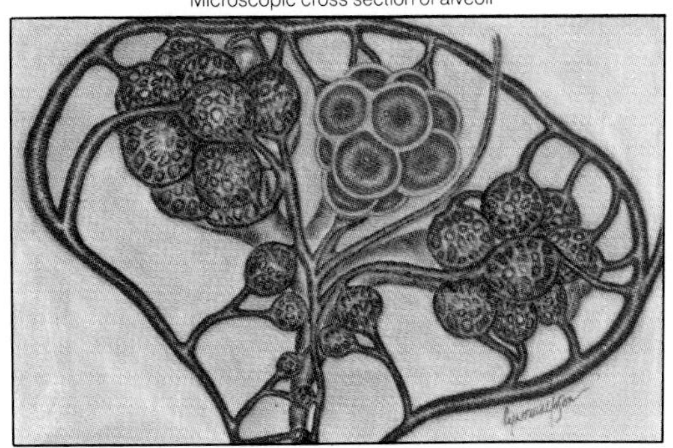

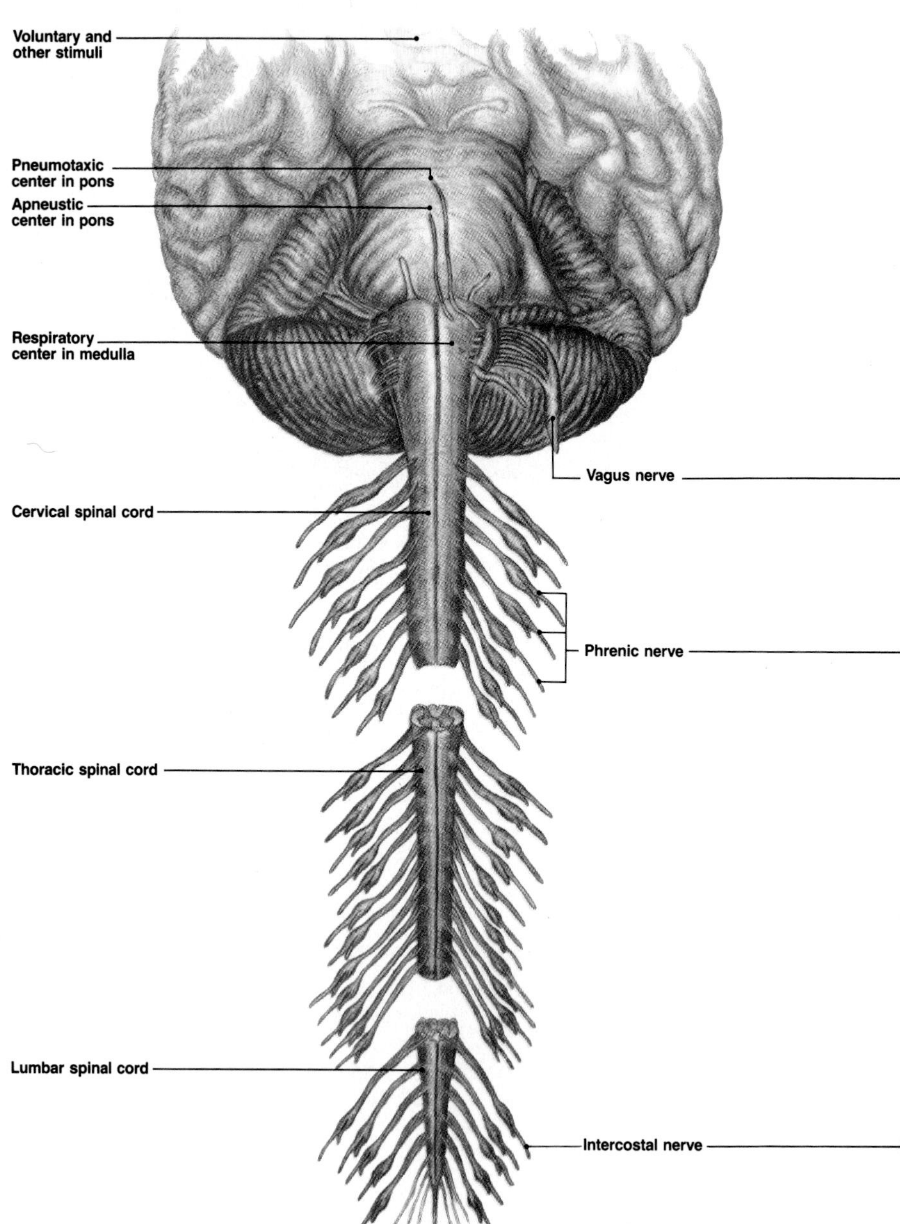
Voluntary and
other stimuli
Pneumotaxic
center in pons
Apneustic
center in pons
Respiratory
center in medulla
Vagus nerve
Cervical spinal cord
Phrenic nerve
Thoracic spinal cord
Lumbar spinal cord
Intercostal nerve

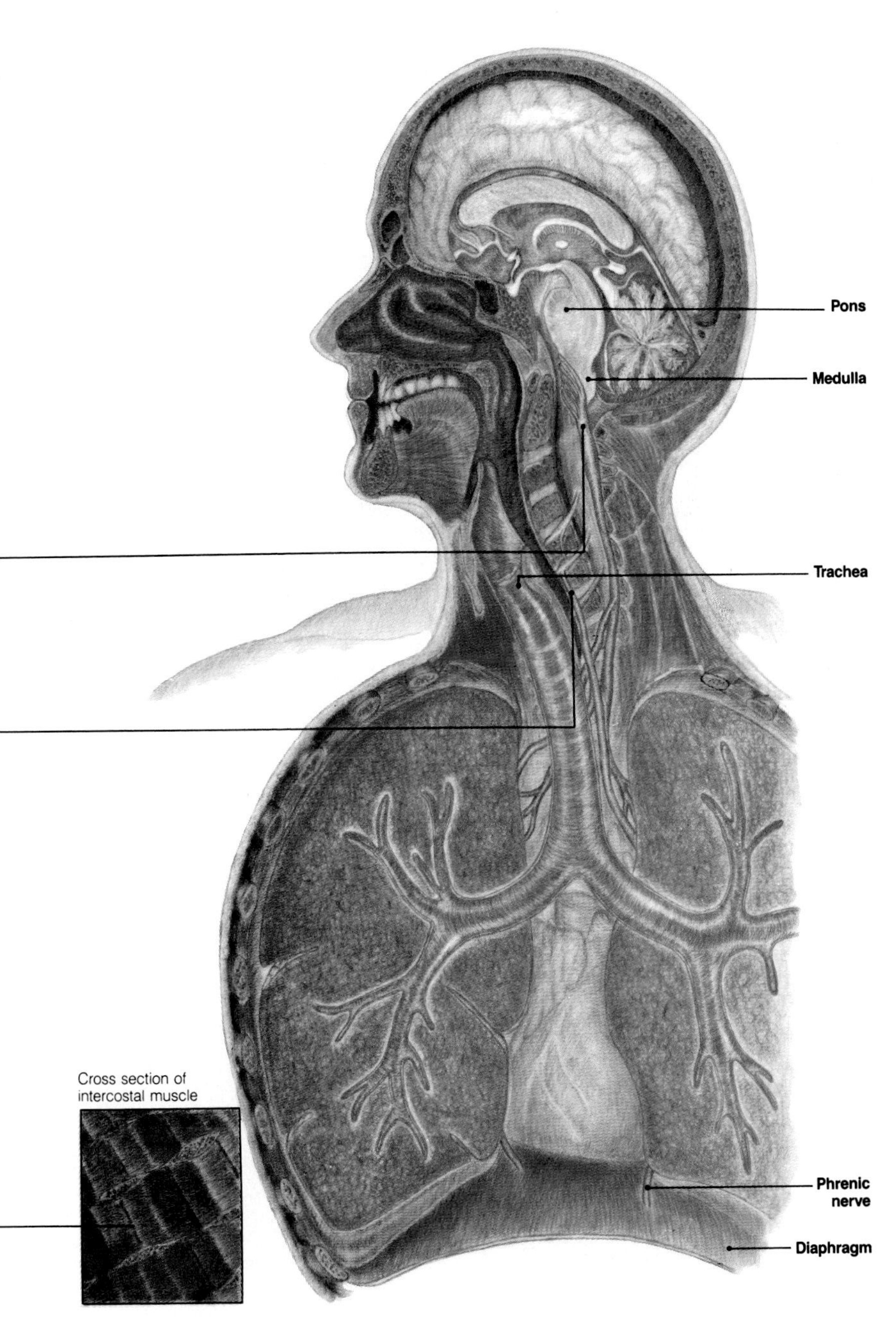
Pons
Medulla
Trachea
Phrenic nerve
Diaphragm
Cross section of intercostal muscle

PATHOLOGY IN FOUR COMMON LUNG DISEASES

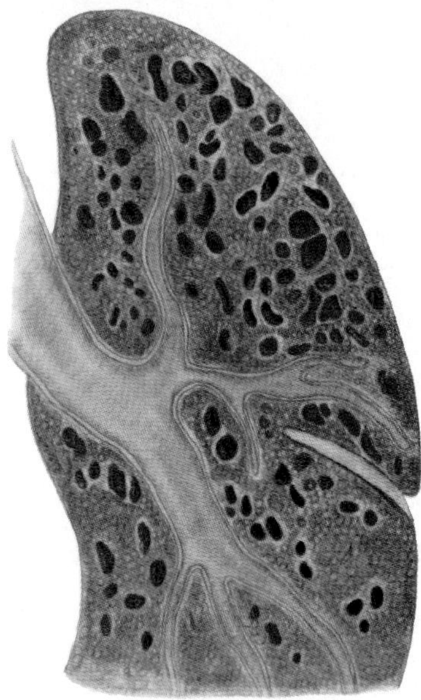

Emphysema

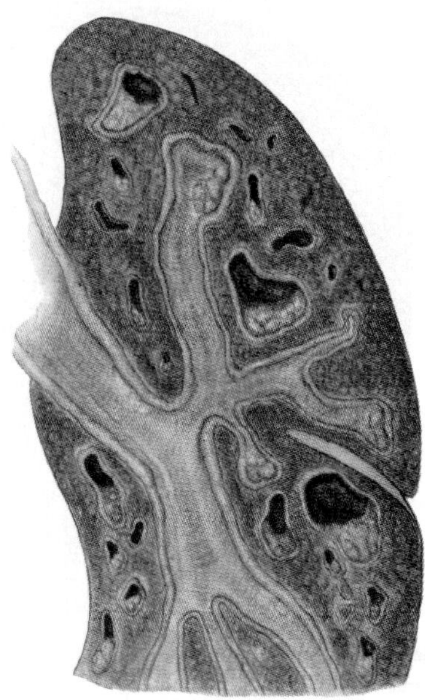

Bronchiectasis

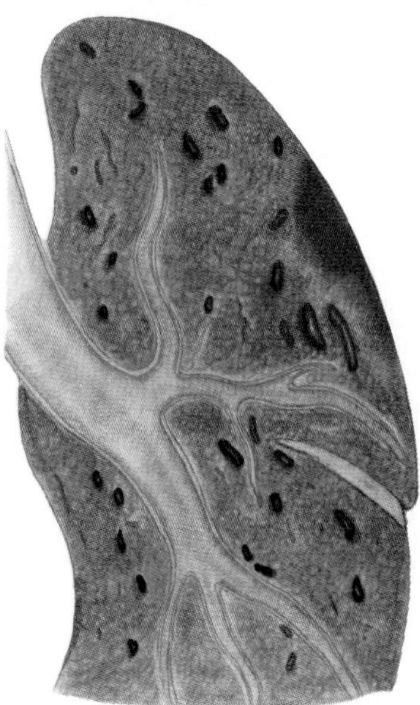

Pulmonary emboli and infarction

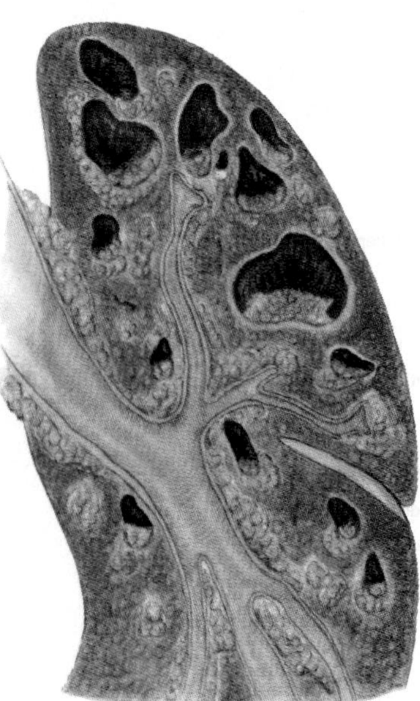

Tuberculosis

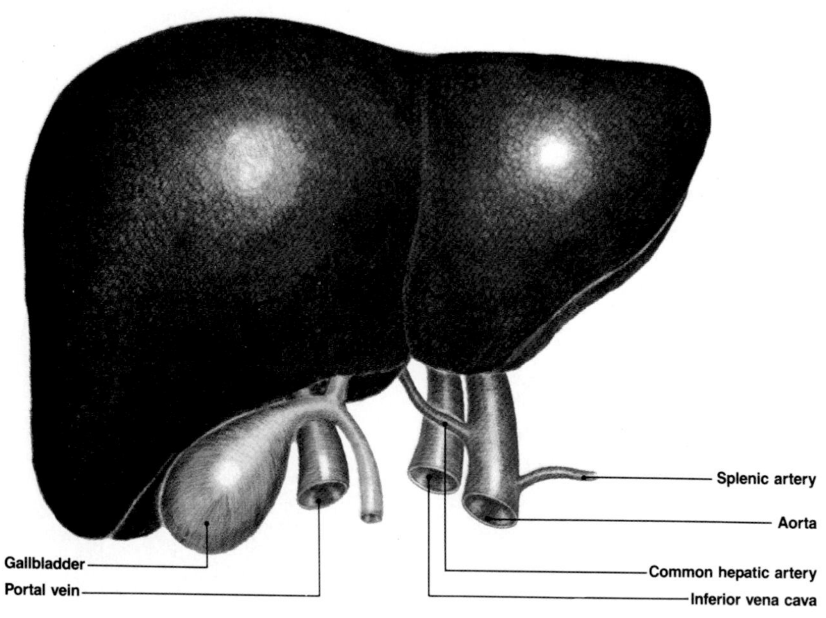

Microscopic view of liver lobule

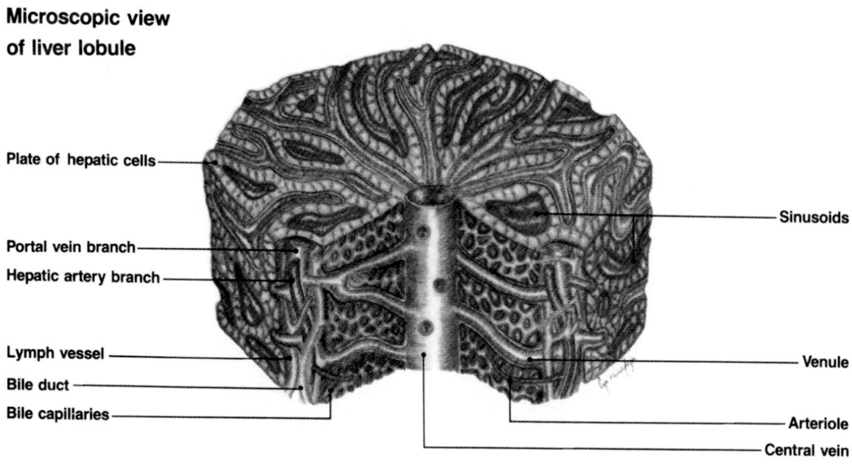

Hypothalamus and pituitary

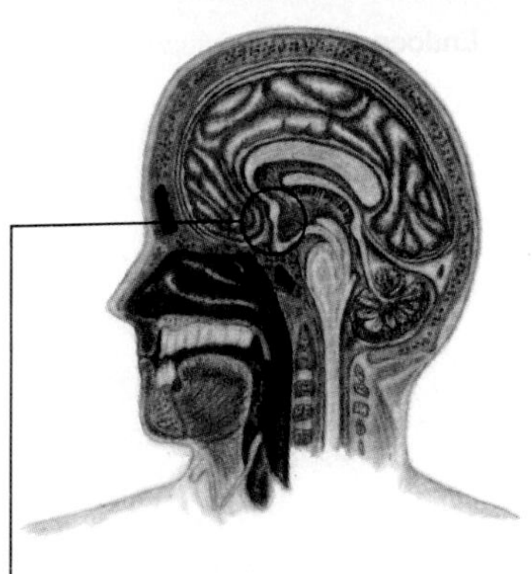

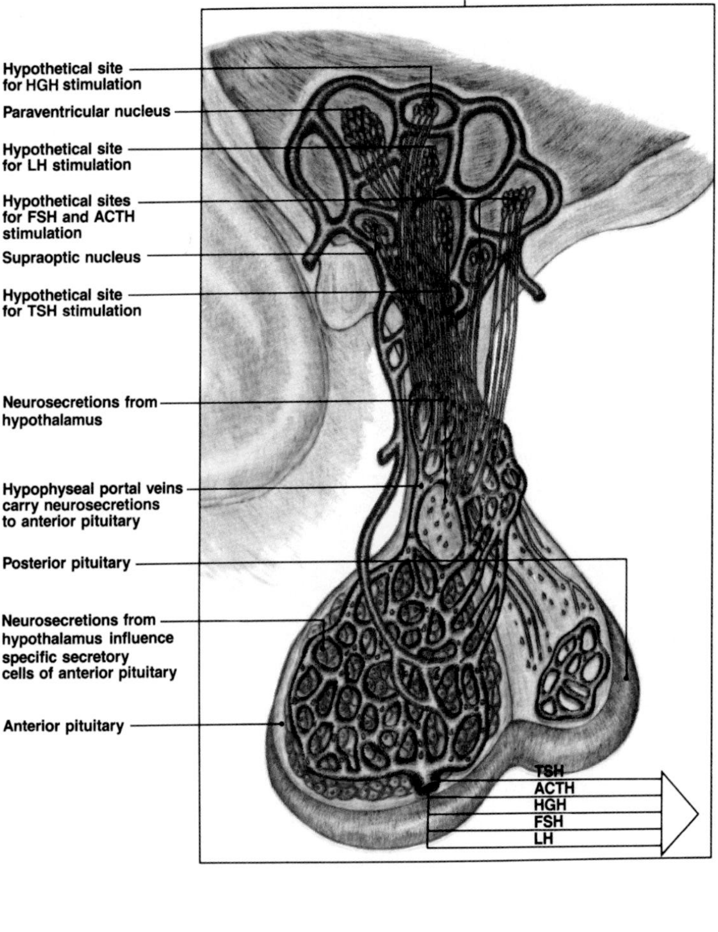

Hypothetical site for HGH stimulation

Paraventricular nucleus

Hypothetical site for LH stimulation

Hypothetical sites for FSH and ACTH stimulation

Supraoptic nucleus

Hypothetical site for TSH stimulation

Neurosecretions from hypothalamus

Hypophyseal portal veins carry neurosecretions to anterior pituitary

Posterior pituitary

Neurosecretions from hypothalamus influence specific secretory cells of anterior pituitary

Anterior pituitary

TSH
ACTH
HGH
FSH
LH

Endocrine target organs

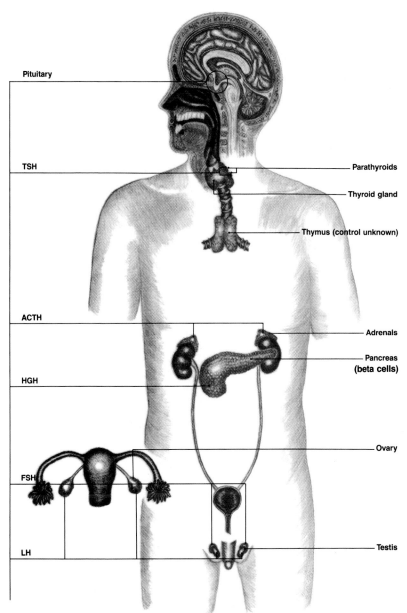

Pituitary

TSH

Parathyroids

Thyroid gland

Thymus (control unknown)

ACTH

Adrenals

Pancreas
(beta cells)

HGH

Ovary

FSH

Testis

LH

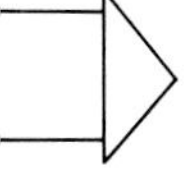

GASTROINTESTINAL TRACT

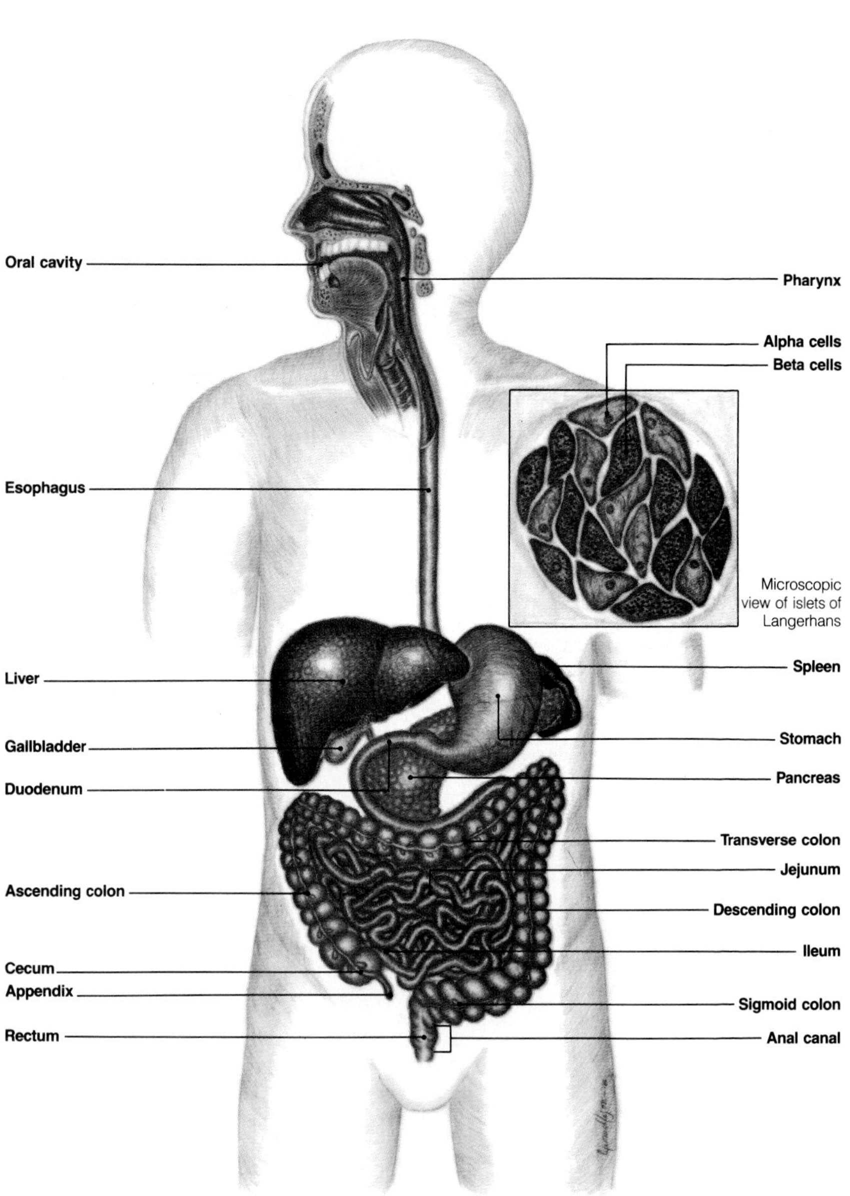
Oral cavity
Pharynx
Alpha cells
Beta cells
Esophagus
Microscopic view of islets of Langerhans
Liver
Spleen
Stomach
Gallbladder
Pancreas
Duodenum
Transverse colon
Jejunum
Ascending colon
Descending colon
Ileum
Cecum
Appendix
Sigmoid colon
Rectum
Anal canal

Selected References

Brenner, Barry M., and Stein, Jay H. "Acute Renal Failure," in *Contemporary Issues in Nephrology,* vol 6. New York: Churchill Livingstone, 1982.

Bricker, Neal S., and Kirschenbaum, Michael A. *The Kidney: Diagnosis and Management*. New York: John Wiley & Sons, 1984.

Brown, R.B. *Clinical Urology Illustrated.* Baltimore: Williams & Wilkins Co., 1982.

Brundage, Dorothy J. *Nursing Management of Renal Problems,* 2nd ed. St. Louis: C.V. Mosby Co., 1980.

Cheigh, Jhoong S., et al. *Manual of Clinical Nephrology*. Boston: Martinus Nijhoff Publishers, 1981.

Dalton, John R. *Basic Clinical Urology*. Philadelphia: J.B. Lippincott Co., 1982.

First, Martin Roy. *Chronic Renal Failure: Pathophysiology, Clinical Manifestations, and Management*. New Hyde Park, N.Y.: Medical Examination Pub. Co., 1982.

Flamenbaum, Walter. *Nephrology: An Approach to the Patient with Renal Disease*. Philadelphia: J.B. Lippincott Co., 1982.

Franklin, Stanley S., ed. *Practical Nephrology*. New York: John Wiley & Sons, 1981.

Gonick, Harvey C., ed. *Current Nephrology*. New York: John Wiley & Sons, 1983.

Hamburger, Jean, et al., eds. *Renal Transplantation: Theory and Practice,* 2nd ed. Baltimore: Williams & Wilkins Co., 1981.

Kaufman, Joseph J. *Current Urologic Therapy*. Philadelphia: W.B. Saunders Co., 1980.

Leaf, Alexander, et al., eds. *Renal Pathophysiology—Recent Advances.* New York: Raven Press Pubs., 1980.

Lerner, Judith, and Khan, Zafar. *Mosby's Manual of Urologic Nursing*. St. Louis: C.V. Mosby Co., 1982.

Schrier, Robert W., ed. *Renal and Electrolyte Disorders,* 2nd ed. Boston: Little, Brown & Co., 1980.

Smith, Donald R. *General Urology,* 11th ed. Los Altos, Calif.: Lange Medical Pubns., 1984.

Stein, Jay H. *Nephrology,* New York: Grune & Stratton, 1980.

Stone, William J., and Rabin, Pauline L., eds. *End-Stage Renal Disease*. Orlando, Fla.: Academic Press, 1983.

"Symposium on Endurology," *Urologic Clinics of North America* 9(1):1-205, February 1982.

"Symposium on Surgery of Stone Disease," *Urologic Clinics of North America* 10(1):583-766, November 1983.

Valtin, Heinz. *Renal Function: Mechanisms Preserving Fluid and Solute Balance in Health,* 2nd ed. Boston: Little, Brown & Co., 1983.

Wright, Lucius F. *Maintenance Hemodialysis*. Boston: G.K. Hall & Co., 1981.

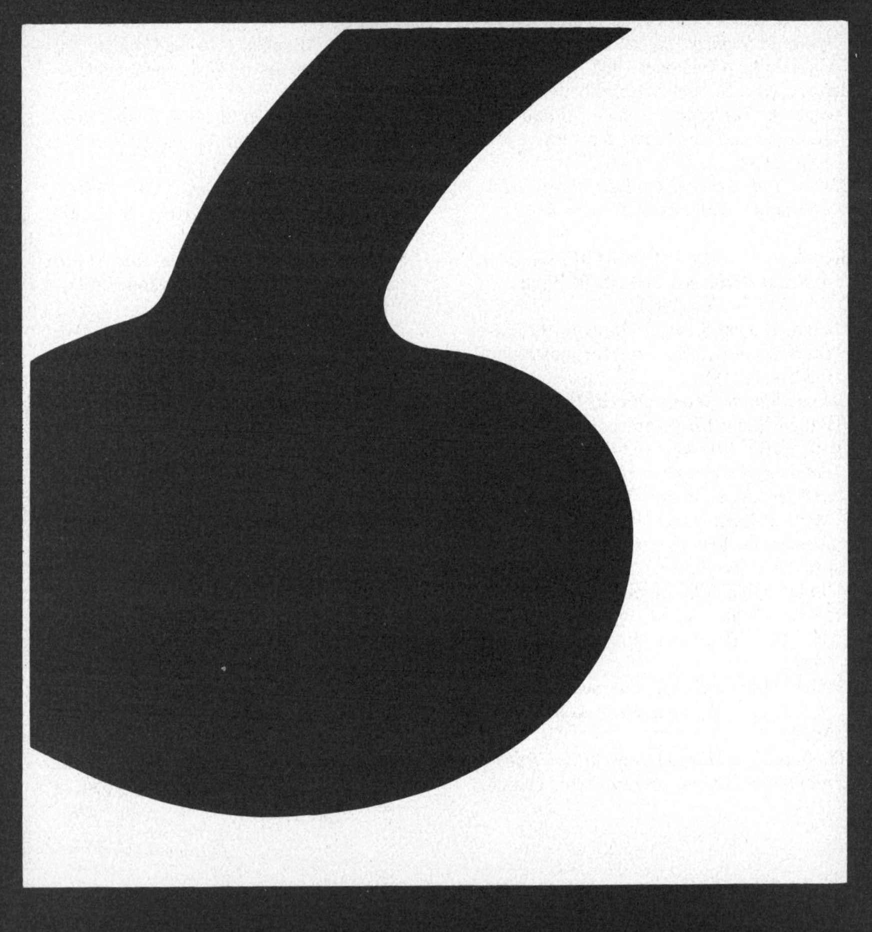

13 Endocrine Disorders

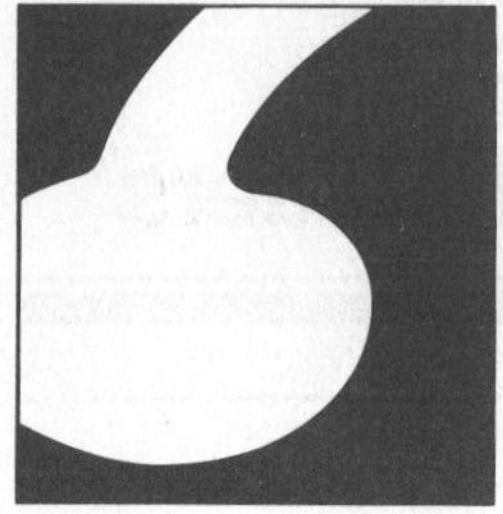

Endocrine Disorders

Introduction

Together with the nervous system, the endocrine system regulates and integrates the body's metabolic activities. The endocrine system meets the nervous system at the hypothalamus. The hypothalamus, the highest integrative center for the endocrine and autonomic nervous systems, controls endocrine organs by neural and hormonal pathways. A hormone is a chemical transmitter released from specialized cells into the bloodstream, which carries it to specialized organ-receptor cells that respond to it.

Neural pathways connect the hypothalamus to the posterior pituitary, or neurohypophysis. Neural stimulation to the posterior pituitary provokes the secretion of two effector hormones: antidiuretic hormone (ADH) and oxytocin.

Hypothalamic control

The hypothalamus also exerts hormonal control at the anterior pituitary through releasing and inhibiting factors, which arrive by a portal system. Hypothalamic hormones stimulate the pituitary to release trophic hormones, such as adrenocorticotropic hormone (ACTH), thyroid-stimulating hormone (TSH), luteinizing hormone (LH), and follicle-stimulating hormone (FSH), and to release or inhibit effector hormones, such as the growth hormone (GH) and prolactin (PRL). In turn, secretion of trophic hormones stimulates the adrenal cortex, thyroid, and gonads. In a patient whose clinical condition suggests endocrine pathology, this complex hormonal sequence requires careful evaluation at each level to identify the dysfunction; dysfunction may result from defects of releasing, trophic, or effector hormones, or of the target tissue. Hyperthyroidism, for example, may result from an excess of thyrotropin-releasing hormone (TRH), of TSH, or of thyroid hormone.

In addition to hormonal and neural controls, a negative feedback system regulates the endocrine system. The mechanism of feedback may be simple or complex. Simple feedback occurs when the level of one substance regulates secretion of a hormone. For example, low serum calcium stimulates parathyroid hormone (PTH) secretion; high serum calcium inhibits it. Complex feedback occurs through the hypothalamic-pituitary-target organ axis. For example, secretion of the hypothalamic corticotropin-releasing hormone (CRH) releases pituitary ACTH, which, in turn, stimulates adrenal cortisol secretion. Subsequently, a rise in serum cortisol inhibits ACTH by decreasing CRH secretion. Steroid therapy disrupts the hypothalamic-pituitary-adrenal (HPA) axis by suppressing hypothalamic-pituitary secretion. Because abrupt withdrawal of steroids doesn't allow time for recovery of the HPA axis to stimulate cortisol secretion, it can induce life-threatening adrenal crisis.

Endocrine pathology

Common dysfunctions of the endocrine system are classified as hypofunction and hyperfunction, inflammation, and tumor. The source of hypofunction and hyperfunction may originate in the hypothalamus or in the pituitary or effector glands. Inflammation may be acute or subacute, as in thyroiditis, but is usually chronic, often resulting in glandular hypofunction. Tumors can occur within a gland—as in thyroid carcinoma or pheochromocytoma—or in other areas, resulting in ectopic hormone production. Certain lung tumors, for example, secrete ADH or PTH.

The study of endocrine function focuses on measuring the level or the effect of a hormone. Radioimmunoassay, for example, measures insulin levels; a fasting blood glucose test measures insulin's effects. Sophisticated techniques of hormone measurement have improved diagnosis of endocrine disorders.

While diagnostic tests are needed to confirm endocrine disorders, clinical data usually provide the first clues to these disorders. Nursing assessment can reveal common signs and symptoms of endocrine dysfunction, such as excessive or delayed growth, wasting, weakness, polydipsia, polyuria, and mental changes. The quality and distribution of hair, skin pigmentation, and distribution of body fat are also significant.

Aside from assessment, nurses have the additional responsibilities of patient preparation, including instruction and support during testing, and proper specimen collection, particularly of 12- or 24-hour urine specimens.

Hormonal effects

In response to the hypothalamus, the *posterior pituitary* secretes oxytocin and ADH. Oxytocin stimulates contraction of the uterus and is responsible for the milk let-down reflex in lactating women. ADH controls the concentration of body fluids by altering the permeability of the distal convoluted tubules and collecting ducts of the kidneys, to conserve water. The secretion of ADH depends on the plasma osmolality as monitored by hypothalamic neurons. Circulatory shock and severe hemorrhage are the most powerful stimulators of ADH; other stimulators include pain, emotional stress, trauma, morphine, tranquilizers, certain anesthetics, and positive-pressure breathing.

The syndrome of inappropriate ADH secretion (SIADH) is a heterogamous disorder with four separate types of osmoregulatory defects. Generally, however, overhydration suppresses ADH

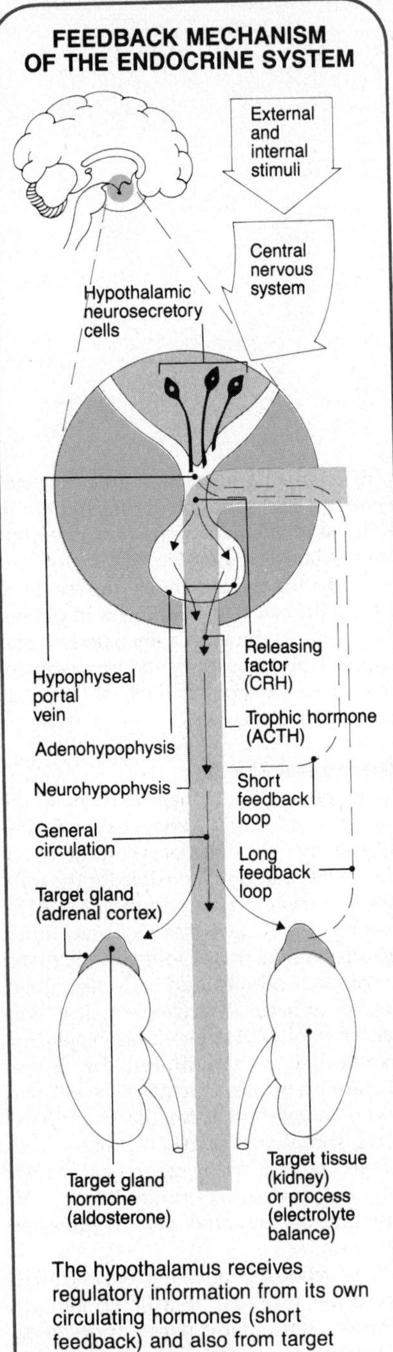

The hypothalamus receives regulatory information from its own circulating hormones (short feedback) and also from target glands (long feedback).

secretion (so, incidentally, does alcohol). Deficiency of ADH causes a condition of high urinary output known as diabetes insipidus.

The *anterior pituitary* secretes prolactin, which stimulates milk secretion, and human growth hormone (HGH), which affects most body tissues. HGH stimulates growth by increasing protein synthesis and fat mobilization and by decreasing carbohydrate utilization. Hyposecretion of HGH results in dwarfism; hypersecretion causes gigantism in children and acromegaly in adults.

The *thyroid gland* secretes the iodinated hormones thyroxine (T_4) and triiodothyronine (T_3). Thyroid hormones are necessary for normal growth and development and act on many tissues to increase metabolic activity and protein synthesis. Deficiency of thyroid hormone causes varying degrees of hypothyroidism, from a mild, clinically insignificant form to the life-threatening extreme, myxedema coma. Congenital hypothyroidism causes cretinism. Hypersecretion causes hyperthyroidism and, in extreme cases, thyrotoxic crisis. Excessive secretion of TSH causes hyperplasia of the thyroid gland and results in goiter.

The *parathyroid glands* secrete PTH, which regulates calcium and phosphate metabolism. PTH elevates serum calcium levels by stimulating resorption of calcium and phosphate from bone, reabsorption of calcium and excretion of phosphate by the kidneys, and by combined action with vitamin D, absorption of calcium and phosphate from the gastrointestinal tract. Thyrocalcitonin, a secretion from the thyroid, opposes the effect of PTH and therefore decreases serum calcium. Hyperparathyroidism causes hypercalcemia; hypoparathyroidism causes hypocalcemia. Altered calcium levels may also result from nonendocrine causes, such as metastatic bone disease.

The *endocrine pancreas* produces glucagon from the alpha cells and insulin from the beta cells. Glucagon, the hormone of the fasting state, releases stored glucose to raise the blood glucose level. Insulin, the hormone of the nourished state, facilitates glucose transport, promotes glucose storage, stimulates protein synthesis, and enhances free fatty acid uptake and storage. Insulin deficiency causes diabetes mellitus. Insulin excess can result from an insulinoma.

The *adrenal cortex* secretes mineralocorticoids, glucocorticoids, and sex steroids. Aldosterone, a mineralocorticoid, regulates the reabsorption of sodium and the excretion of potassium by the kidneys. Although affected by ACTH, aldosterone is also regulated by angiotensin II, which, in turn, is regulated by renin. Together, aldosterone, angiotensin, and renin may be implicated in the pathogenesis of hypertension. An excess of aldosterone (aldosteronism) can result primarily from hyperplasia or from adrenal adenoma or secondarily from many conditions, including congestive heart failure and cirrhosis.

Cortisol, a glucocorticoid, stimulates gluconeogenesis, increases protein breakdown and free fatty acid mobilization, suppresses the immune response, and provides for an appropriate response to stress. Hyperactivity of the adrenal cortex results in Cushing's syndrome; hypoactivity of the adrenal cortex causes Addison's disease and, in extreme cases, adrenal crisis. Adrenogenital syndromes may result from overproduction of sex steroids.

The *adrenal medulla* is an aggregate of nervous tissue that produces the catecholamines epinephrine and norepinephrine, both of which cause vasoconstriction. Epinephrine also causes the "fight or flight" response—dilation of bronchioles and increased blood pressure, blood sugar, and heart rate. Pheochromocytoma, a tumor of the adrenal medulla, causes hypersecretion of catecholamines and results in characteristic sustained or paroxysmal hypertension.

The *testes* synthesize and secrete testosterone in response to gonadotropic hormones, especially LH, from the anterior pituitary gland; spermatogenesis occurs in response to FSH. The *ovaries* produce sex steroid hormones (primarily estrogen and progesterone) in response to anterior pituitary trophic hormones.

Chronic endocrine abnormalities are common health problems. For example, deficiencies of cortisol, thyroid hormone, or insulin require lifelong replacement of these hormones for survival. Consequently, these conditions make special demands on your skills during ongoing patient assessment, situations of acute illness, and patient teaching.

PITUITARY DISORDERS

Hypopituitarism

(Panhypopituitarism and dwarfism)

Hypopituitarism is a complex syndrome marked by metabolic dysfunction, sexual immaturity, and growth retardation (when it occurs in childhood), resulting from a deficiency of the hormones secreted by the anterior pituitary gland. Panhypopituitarism refers to a generalized condition caused by partial or total failure of all six of this gland's vital hormones—ACTH, TSH, LH, FSH, HGH, and prolactin. Partial hypopituitarism and complete hypopituitarism (panhypopituitarism) occur in adults and children; in children, these diseases may cause dwarfism and pubertal delay. Prognosis may be good with adequate replacement therapy and correction of the underlying causes.

Causes

The most common cause of primary hypopituitarism is tumor. Other causes include congenital defects (hypoplasia or aplasia of the pituitary gland); pituitary infarction (most often from postpartum hemorrhage); or partial or total hypophysectomy by surgery, irradiation, or chemical agents; and, rarely, granulomatous disease (tuberculosis, for example). Occasionally, hypopituitarism may have no identifiable cause. Secondary hypopituitarism stems from a deficiency of releasing hormones produced by the hypothalamus—either ideopathic or a possible result of infection, trauma, or tumor.

Primary hypopituitarism usually develops in a predictable pattern of hormonal failures. It generally starts with hypogonadism or gonadotropin failure (decreased FSH and LH). In adults, it causes cessation of menses in women and impotence in men. Growth hormone deficiency follows; in children, this causes short stature, delayed growth, and possibly delayed puberty. Subsequent failure of thyrotropin (decreased TSH) causes hypothyroidism; finally, adrenocorticotropic failure (decreased ACTH) results in adrenal insufficiency. However, when hypopituitarism follows surgical ablation or trauma, the pattern of hormonal events may not necessarily follow this sequence.

Occasionally, damage to the neurohypophysis from one of the above causes is extensive enough to cause diabetes insipidus.

Signs and symptoms

Clinical features of hypopituitarism usually develop slowly and vary greatly with the severity of the disorder and the number of deficient hormones. Signs and symptoms of hypopituitarism in adults may include gonadal failure (secondary amenorrhea, impotence, infertility, decreased libido), diabetes insipidus, hypothyroidism (tiredness, lethargy, sensitivity to cold, menstrual disturbances), and adrenocortical insufficiency (hypoglycemia, anorexia, nausea, abdominal pain, hypotension).

Postpartum necrosis of the pituitary (Sheehan's syndrome) characteristically causes failure of lactation, menstruation, and growth of pubic and axillary hair; and symptoms of thyroid and adrenocortical failure.

In children, hypopituitarism causes retarded growth or delayed puberty. Dwarfism usually isn't apparent at birth, but early signs begin to appear during the first few months of life; by age 6 months, growth retardation is obvious. Although these children generally enjoy good health, pituitary dwarfism may cause chubbiness due to fat deposits in the lower trunk, delayed secondary tooth eruption, and, possibly, hypoglycemia. Growth continues at less than half the normal rate—sometimes extending into the patient's twenties or thirties—to an average height of 4′ (122 cm), with normal proportions.

When hypopituitarism strikes before puberty, it totally prevents development of secondary sexual characteristics (including facial and body hair). In males, it produces undersized testes, penis, and prostate gland; absent or minimal libido; and inability to initiate and maintain an erection. In females, it usually causes immature development of the breasts, sparse or absent pubic and axillary hair, and primary amenorrhea.

Panhypopituitarism may induce a host of mental and physiologic abnormalities, including lethargy, psychosis, orthostatic hypotension, bradycardia, anemia, and anorexia. However, clinical manifestations of hormonal deficiencies resulting from pituitary destruction don't become apparent until 75% of the gland is destroyed. Total loss of all hormones released by the anterior pituitary invariably proves fatal unless treated.

Neurologic signs associated with hypopituitarism and produced by pituitary tumors include headache, bilateral temporal hemianopia, loss of visual acuity, and, possibly, blindness. Acute hypopituitarism resulting from surgery or infection is often associated with fever, hypotension, vomiting, and hypoglycemia—all characteristic of adrenal insufficiency.

Diagnosis

In suspected hypopituitarism, evaluation must confirm hormonal deficiency due to impairment or destruction of the anterior pituitary gland and rule out disease of the target organs (adrenals, gonads, and thyroid) or the hypothalamus. Low serum levels of thyroxine (T_4), for example, indicate diminished thyroid gland function, but further tests are necessary to identify the source of this dysfunction as the thyroid, pituitary, or hypothalamus.

Radioimmunoassay showing decreased plasma levels of some or all pituitary hormones (except ACTH, which requires more sophisticated testing), accompanied by end-organ hypofunction, suggests pituitary failure and eliminates target gland disease. Failure of TRH administration to increase TSH or prolactin concentrations rules out hypothalamic dysfunction as the cause of hormonal deficiency.

Provocative tests are helpful. To pinpoint the source of low hydroxycorticosteroid levels, P.O. administration of metyrapone blocks cortisol synthesis, which should stimulate pituitary secretion of ACTH. Insulin-induced hypoglycemia also stimulates ACTH secretion. Persistently low levels of ACTH indicate pituitary or hypothalamic failure. These tests require careful medical supervision, because they may precipitate an adrenal crisis.

Diagnosis of dwarfism requires measurement of growth hormone levels in the blood after administration of regular insulin (inducing hypoglycemia) or levodopa (causing hypotension). These drugs should provoke increased secretion of growth hormone. Persistently low growth hormone levels, despite provocative testing, confirm growth hormone deficiency. Computed tomography scan, pneumoencephalography, or cerebral angiography confirms the presence of intrasellar or extrasellar tumors.

Treatment

Replacement of hormones secreted by the target glands is the most effective treatment for hypopituitarism and panhypopituitarism. Hormonal replacement includes cortisol, thyroxine, and androgen or cyclic estrogen. Prolactin need not be replaced. The patient of reproductive age may benefit from administration of FSH and human chorionic gonadotropin (HCG) to boost fertility.

HGH, obtained from cadaver pituitaries, is effective for treating dwarfism and stimulates growth increases as great as 4″ to 6″ (10 to 15 cm) in the first year of treatment. Growth rate tapers off in later years. After pubertal changes have occurred, the effects of HGH therapy are limited. (The National Pituitary Agency, which supplies HGH, currently withdraws treatment after the patient attains a height of 5′ [152 cm].) Occasionally, a child becomes unresponsive to HGH therapy, even with larger doses, perhaps because of antibody formation against the hormone. In such refractory patients, small doses of androgen may again stimulate growth, but extreme caution is necessary to prevent premature closure of the epiphyses. Children with hypopituitarism may also need replacement of adrenal and thyroid hormones and, as they approach puberty, sex hormones.

Special considerations

Caring for patients with hypopituitarism and panhypopituitarism requires an understanding of hormonal effects and strong skills in offering physical and psychological support.

- Keep track of the results of all laboratory tests for hormonal deficiencies, and know what they mean. Until replacement therapy is complete, check for signs of thyroid deficiency (increasing lethargy), adrenal deficiency (weakness, orthostatic hypotension, hypoglycemia, fatigue, and weight loss), and gonadotropin deficiency (decreased libido, lethargy, and apathy).
- Watch for anorexia in the patient with panhypopituitarism. Help plan a menu containing favorite foods—ideally, high-

calorie foods. Monitor for weight loss or gain.
• If the patient has trouble sleeping, encourage exercise during the day.
• Record temperature, blood pressure, and heart rate every 4 to 8 hours. Check eyelids, nailbeds, and skin for pallor, which indicates anemia.
• Prevent infection by giving meticulous skin care. Since the patient's skin is probably dry, use oil or lotion instead of soap. If body temperature is low, provide additional clothing and covers, as needed, to keep the patient warm.
• Darken the room if the patient has a tumor that is causing headaches and visual disturbances. Help with any activity that requires good vision, such as reading the menu. The patient with bilateral hemianopia may be able to see only out of the corners of the eyes, so be sure to stand where he can see you, and advise the family to do the same.
• During insulin testing, monitor closely for signs of hypoglycemia (initially, slow cerebration, tachycardia, and nervousness, progressing to convulsions). Keep 50% dextrose in water available for I.V. administration to correct hypoglycemia rapidly.
• To prevent postural hypotension, be sure to keep the patient supine during levodopa testing.
• Instruct the patient to wear a medical identification bracelet. Teach him to administer steroids parenterally in case of an emergency.
• Refer the family of a child with dwarfism to appropriate community resources for psychological counseling, since the emotional stress caused by this disorder increases as the child becomes more aware of his condition.

Hyperpituitarism

(Acromegaly and gigantism)

A chronic, progressive disease marked by hormonal dysfunction and startling skeletal overgrowth, hyperpituitarism appears in two forms: acromegaly occurs after epiphyseal closure, causing bone thickening, and transverse growth and visceromegaly; gigantism begins before epiphyseal closure and causes proportional overgrowth of all body tissues. Although prognosis depends on the causative factor, this disease usually reduces life expectancy.

Causes and incidence

In hyperpituitarism, oversecretion of HGH produces changes throughout the body, resulting in acromegaly and, when such oversecretion occurs before puberty, gigantism. Eosinophilic or mixed-cell adenomas of the anterior pituitary gland may cause this oversecretion, but the etiology of the tumors themselves remains unclear. Occasionally, hyperpituitarism occurs in more than one family member, suggesting a possible genetic cause.

In acromegaly, signs and symptoms develop slowly. Early effects include soft-tissue swelling and hypertrophy of the extremities and face. This rare form of hyperpituitarism occurs equally among men and women, usually between ages 30 and 50.

In gigantism, proportional overgrowth of all body tissues starts before epiphyseal closure. This causes remarkable height increases of as much as 6″ (15 cm) a year. Gigantism affects infants and children, causing them to attain as much as three times the normal height for their age. As adults, they may ultimately reach a height of more than 80″ (203 cm).

Signs and symptoms

Acromegaly develops slowly and typically produces diaphoresis, oily skin, hypermetabolism, and hypertrichosis. Severe headache, central and peripheral nervous system impairment, bitemporal hemianopia, loss of visual acuity, and blindness may result from the underlying intrasellar tumor.

Hypersecretion of HGH produces cartilaginous and connective tissue overgrowth, resulting in a characteristic hulking appearance, with an enlarged supraorbital ridge and thickened ears and nose. Prognathism becomes marked and may interfere with chewing. Laryngeal hypertrophy, paranasal sinus enlargement, and thickening of the tongue cause the voice to sound deep and hollow. Distal phalanges display an arrowhead appearance on X-rays, and the fingers are thickened. Irritability, hostility, and various psychological disturbances may occur.

Prolonged effects of excessive HGH secretion include bowed legs, barrel chest, arthritis, osteoporosis, kyphosis, hypertension, and arteriosclerosis. Both gigantism and acromegaly may also cause signs of glucose intolerance and clinically apparent diabetes mellitus, due to the insulin-antagonistic character of HGH.

Gigantism develops abruptly, producing some of the same skeletal abnormalities seen in acromegaly. In infants, it may cause a highly arched palate, muscular hypotonia, slanting eyes, and exophthalmos. As the disease progresses, the pituitary tumor enlarges and invades normal tissue, resulting in the loss of other trophic hormones such as TSH, LH, FSH, and ACTH, which causes the target organ to stop functioning.

Diagnosis

Radioimmunoassay shows increased plasma HGH levels. However, since HGH is not secreted at a steady rate, a random sampling may be misleading. The glucose suppression test offers more reliable information. Glucose normally suppresses HGH secretion; therefore, a glucose infusion that fails to suppress the hormone level to below the accepted normal value of 5 ng, when combined with characteristic clinical features, strongly suggests hyperpituitarism.

In addition, skull X-rays, CT scan, arteriography, and pneumoencephalography determine the presence and extent of the pituitary lesion. Bone X-rays showing a thickening of the cranium (especially of frontal, occipital, and parietal bones) and of the long bones, as well as osteoarthritis in the spine, support this diagnosis.

Treatment

The aim of treatment is to curb overproduction of HGH through removal of the underlying tumor by cranial or transsphenoidal hypophysectomy or pituitary radiation therapy. In acromegaly, surgery is mandatory when a tumor causes blindness or other severe neurologic disturbances. Postoperative therapy often requires replacement of thyroid, cortisone, and gonadal hormones. Adjunctive treatment may include bromocriptine, which inhibits HGH synthesis.

Special considerations

- Grotesque body changes characteristic of this disorder can cause severe psychological stress. Provide emotional support to help the patient cope with an altered body image.
- Assess for skeletal manifestations, such as arthritis of the hands and osteoarthritis of the spine. Administer medications, as ordered. To promote maximum joint mobility, perform or assist with range-of-motion exercises.
- Evaluate muscular weakness, especially in the patient with late-stage acromegaly. Check the strength of his handclasp. If it's very weak, help with tasks such as cutting food.
- Keep the skin dry. Avoid using an oily lotion, since the skin is already oily.
- Test urine for glucose. Check for signs of hyperglycemia (sweating, fatigue, polyuria, polydipsia).
- Be aware that the tumor may cause visual problems. If the patient has hemianopia, stand where he can see you. Remember, this disease can also cause inexplicable mood changes. Reassure the

family that these mood changes result from the disease and can be modified with treatment.

- Before surgery, reinforce what the surgeon has told the patient, and try to allay the patient's fear with a clear and honest explanation of the scheduled operation. If the patient is a child, explain to parents that such surgery prevents permanent soft-tissue deformities but won't correct bone changes that have already taken place. Arrange for counseling, if necessary, to help the child and parents cope with these permanent defects.
- After surgery, diligently monitor vital signs and neurologic status. Immediately report any alteration in level of consciousness, pupil equality, or visual acuity, as well as vomiting, falling pulse rate, or rising blood pressure. These changes may signal an increase in intracranial pressure due to intracranial bleeding.
- Check blood glucose often. Remember, HGH levels usually fall rapidly after surgery, removing an insulin-antagonist effect in many patients and possibly precipitating hypoglycemia. Measure intake and output hourly, and report large increases. Transient diabetes insipidus, which sometimes occurs after surgery for hyperpituitarism, can cause such increases in urine output.
- If the transsphenoidal approach is used, a large nasal packing is kept in place for several days. Since the patient must breathe through his mouth, give good mouth care. Pay special attention to the mucous membranes—which usually become very dry—and the incision site under the upper lip, at the top of the gum line. The surgical site is packed with a piece of tissue generally taken from a midthigh donor site. Watch for cerebrospinal fluid (CSF) leaks from the packed site. Look for increased external nasal drainage or drainage into the nasopharynx. CSF leaks may necessitate additional surgery to repair the leak.
- Encourage the patient to ambulate on the first or second day after surgery.
- Before discharge, emphasize the importance of continuing hormone replacement therapy, if ordered. Make sure the patient and family understand which hormones are to be taken and why, as well as the correct times and dosages. Warn against stopping the hormones suddenly.
- Advise the patient to wear a medical identification bracelet at all times and to bring his hormone replacement schedule with him whenever he returns to the hospital.
- Instruct the patient to have follow-up examinations at least once a year for the rest of his life, since a slight chance exists that the tumor which caused his hyperpituitarism may recur.

Diabetes Insipidus

(Pituitary diabetes insipidus)

Diabetes insipidus results from a deficiency of circulating vasopressin (also called antidiuretic hormone [ADH]). This uncommon condition occurs equally among both sexes, usually between ages 10 and 20. Incidence is slightly higher today than in the past because of the increased use of hypophysectomy to treat breast cancer and other disorders. In uncomplicated diabetes insipidus, prognosis is good and patients usually lead normal lives, with adequate water replacement. In cases complicated by an underlying disorder, such as breast cancer, prognosis varies.

Causes

Primary diabetes insipidus (50% of patients) is familial or idiopathic in origin. Secondary diabetes insipidus results from intracranial neoplastic or metastatic lesions, hypophysectomy or other neurosurgery, or head trauma—which damages the neurohypophyseal structures. It can also result from infection, granulomatous disease, and vascular lesions. (*Note:* Pituitary diabetes insipidus should not be confused with nephrogenic diabetes insipidus, a rare congenital disturbance of water metabolism that results from renal tubular resistance to vasopressin.)

Normally, the hypothalamus synthesizes vasopressin. The posterior pituitary gland (or neurohypophysis) stores vasopressin and releases it into general circulation, where it causes the kidneys to reabsorb water by making the distal and collecting tubule cells water-permeable. The absence of vasopressin in diabetes insipidus allows the filtered water to be excreted in the urine instead of being reabsorbed.

Signs and symptoms

Diabetes insipidus typically produces extreme polyuria (usually 4 to 16 liters/day of dilute urine, but sometimes as much as 30 liters/day). As a result, the patient is extremely thirsty and drinks great quantities of water to compensate for the body's water loss. This disorder may also result in slight to moderate nocturia and, in severe cases, extreme fatigue from inadequate rest caused by frequent voiding and excessive thirst. Other characteristic features of diabetes insipidus include signs and symptoms of dehydration (poor tissue turgor, dry mucous membranes, constipation, muscle weakness, dizziness, and hypotension). These symptoms usually begin abruptly, commonly appearing within 1 to 2 days after basal skull fracture, cerebrovascular accident, or surgery. Relief of cerebral edema or of increased intracranial pressure may cause all of these symptoms to subside just as rapidly as they began.

Diagnosis

Urinalysis reveals almost colorless urine of low osmolality (50 to 200 mOsm/kg, less than that of plasma) and low specific gravity (less than 1.005).

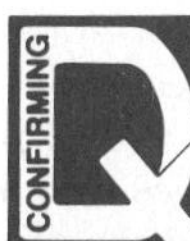

However, diagnosis requires evidence of vasopressin deficiency, resulting in renal inability to concentrate urine during a water restriction test: After baseline vital signs, weight, and urine and plasma osmolalities are obtained, the patient is deprived of fluids and observed to make sure he doesn't drink anything surreptitiously. Hourly measurements then record the total volume of urine output, body weight, urine osmolality or specific gravity, and plasma osmolality. Throughout the test, blood pressure and pulse rate must be monitored for signs of postural hypotension. Fluid deprivation continues until the patient loses 3% of his body weight (indicating severe dehydration) or until severe postural hypotension occurs. This test may end sooner if no further rise in urine osmolality appears in three consecutive urine samples and if plasma osmolality is greater than normal (usually after 8 to 16 hours).

Hourly measurements of urine volume and specific gravity are continued after subcutaneous injection of 5 units of aqueous vasopressin. Patients with pituitary diabetes insipidus respond to vasopressin with decreased urine output and increased specific gravity. (Patients with nephrogenic diabetes insipidus show no response to vasopressin.)

Treatment

Until the cause of diabetes insipidus can be identified and eliminated, administration of various forms of vasopressin or of a vasopressin stimulant can control fluid balance and prevent dehydration:

- *vasopressin tannate:* an oil preparation administered I.M.; effective for 48 to 96 hours
- *vasopressin injection:* an aqueous preparation administered subcutaneously or I.M. several times a day, since effectiveness lasts only for 2 to 6 hours; often used in acute disease
- *desmopressin:* nasal spray absorbed through the mucous membranes, or injectable form given subcutaneously or I.V.; effective up to 20 hours

• *lypressin:* short-acting nasal spray with significant disadvantages—variable dosage, nasal congestion and irritation, ulcerated nasal passages (with repeated use), substernal chest tightness, coughing, and dyspnea (after accidental inhalation of large doses)
• *chlorpropamide:* reduces the polyuria of diabetes insipidus by possibly releasing ADH or potentiating its effects.

Special considerations

• Record fluid intake and output carefully. Maintain fluid intake to prevent severe dehydration. Watch for signs of hypovolemic shock, and monitor blood pressure and heart and respiratory rates regularly, especially during the water deprivation test. Check weight daily. If the patient is dizzy or has muscle weakness, keep the side rails up and assist with walking.
• Monitor urine specific gravity between doses. Watch for a decrease in specific gravity, with increasing urinary output, indicating the return of polyuria and necessitating administration of the next dose or a dosage increase.
• Observe the patient receiving chlorpropamide for signs of hypoglycemia. Tell the patient about possible drug side effects. Make sure calorie intake is adequate; keep orange juice or another carbohydrate handy to treat hypoglycemic attacks. Watch for decreasing urinary output and increasing specific gravity between doses. Check laboratory values for hyponatremia and hypoglycemia.
• If constipation develops, add more bulk foods and fruit juices to the diet. If necessary, obtain an order for a mild laxative, such as milk of magnesia. Provide meticulous skin and mouth care; apply petrolatum, as needed, to cracked or sore lips.
• Before discharge, teach the patient how to monitor intake and output. Instruct him to administer vasopressin I.M. or by nasal insufflation only after onset of polyuria—not before—to prevent excess fluid retention and water intoxication. Tell him to report weight gain; it may mean dosage is too high. Recurrence of polyuria, as reflected on the intake and output sheet, indicates dosage is too low. Because of its viscosity, warn the patient never to administer vasopressin tannate while the suspension is cold. Show him how to warm the vial in his hands and to rotate it gently to disperse the active particles throughout the oil.
• Identify all patients with coronary artery disease; they need special periodic evaluations, since vasopressin constricts the arteries.
• Advise the patient to wear a medical identification bracelet and to carry his medication with him at all times.

THYROID DISORDERS

Hypothyroidism in Adults

Hypothyroidism, a state of low serum thyroid hormone, results from hypothalamic, pituitary, or thyroid insufficiency. The disorder can progress to life-threatening myxedema coma. Hypothyroidism is most prevalent in women; in the United States, incidence is rising significantly in persons aged 40 to 50.

Causes

Hypothyroidism results from inadequate production of thyroid hormone—usually because of dysfunction of the thyroid gland due to surgery (thyroidectomy), irradiation therapy (particularly with ^{131}I), inflammation, chronic autoimmune thyroiditis (Hashimoto's disease), or inflammatory conditions, such as amyloidosis and sarcoidosis. It may also result from pituitary failure to produce thyroid-stimulating hormone (TSH), hypothalamic failure to produce thyrotropin-releasing hormone (TRH), inborn errors of thyroid hormone synthesis, inability to synthesize thyroid hormone because of iodine deficiency (usually dietary), or the use of antithyroid medications, such as propylthiouracil.

In patients with hypothyroidism, infection, exposure to cold, and sedatives may precipitate myxedema coma.

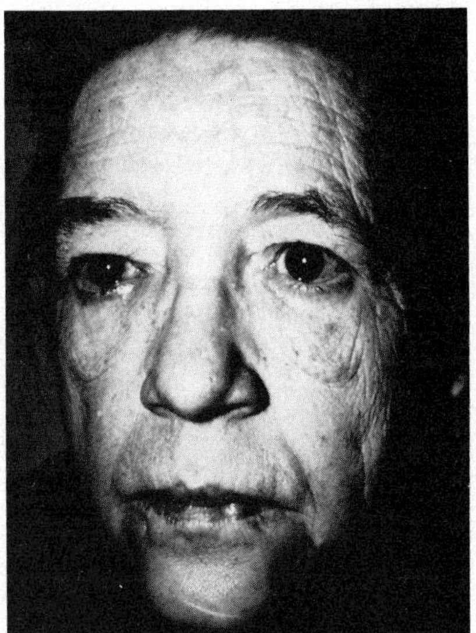

Characteristic myxedematous symptoms in adults include dry, flaky, inelastic skin; puffy face; and upper eyelid droop.

Signs and symptoms

Typically, the early clinical features of hypothyroidism are vague: fatigue, forgetfulness, sensitivity to cold, unexplained weight gain, and constipation. As the disorder progresses, characteristic myxedematous symptoms appear: decreasing mental stability; dry, flaky, inelastic skin; puffy face, hands, and feet; hoarseness; periorbital edema; upper eyelid droop; dry, sparse hair; and thick, brittle nails. Cardiovascular involvement leads to decreased cardiac output, slow pulse rate, signs of poor peripheral circulation, and, occasionally, arteriosclerosis and cardiac enlargement. Other common effects include anorexia, abdominal distention, menorrhagia, decreased libido, infertility, ataxia, intention tremor, and nystagmus. Reflexes show delayed relaxation time (especially in the Achilles tendon).

Progression to myxedema coma is usually gradual, but when stress aggravates severe or prolonged hypothyroidism, coma may develop abruptly. Clinical effects include progressive stupor, hypoventilation, hypoglycemia, hyponatremia, hypotension, and hypothermia.

Diagnosis

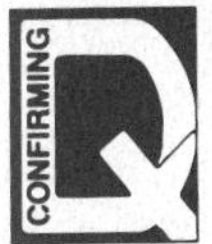

Radioimmunoassay confirms hypothyroidism with low T_3 and T_4 levels. Supportive laboratory findings include:

- increased TSH level with hypothyroidism due to thyroid insufficiency; decreased TSH level with hypothyroidism due to hypothalamic or pituitary insufficiency.
- elevated levels of serum cholesterol, carotene, alkaline phosphatase, and triglycerides.
- normocytic normochromic anemia.

In myxedema coma, laboratory tests may also show low serum sodium, and decreased pH and increased PCO_2 in arterial blood gases, indicating respiratory acidosis.

Treatment

Therapy for hypothyroidism consists of gradual thyroid replacement with levothyroxine (T_4), liothyronine (T_3), liotrix, or thyroid USP (desiccated). During myxedema coma, effective treatment supports vital functions while restoring euthyroidism. To support blood pressure and pulse rate, treatment includes I.V. administration of levothyroxine and hydrocortisone to correct possible pituitary or adrenal insufficiency. Hypoventilation necessitates oxygenation and vigorous respiratory support. Other supportive measures include careful fluid replacement and antibiotics for infection.

Special considerations

To manage the hypothyroid patient:

- Provide a high-bulk, low-calorie diet and encourage activity to combat constipation and promote weight loss. Administer cathartics and stool softeners, as needed.
- After thyroid replacement therapy begins, watch for symptoms of hyperthyroidism, such as restlessness, sweating, and excessive weight loss.
- Tell the patient to report any signs of aggravated cardiovascular disease, such as chest pain and tachycardia.
- To prevent myxedema coma, tell the patient to continue his course of antithyroid medication even if his symptoms subside.
- Warn the patient to report infection immediately and to make sure any doctor who prescribes drugs for him knows about the underlying hypothyroidism.

Treatment of myxedema coma requires supportive care:

- Check frequently for signs of decreasing cardiac output (such as falling urinary output).
- Monitor temperature until stable. Provide extra blankets and clothing and a warm room to compensate for hypothermia. Rapid rewarming may cause vasodilation and vascular collapse.
- Record intake and output and daily weight. As treatment begins, urinary output should increase and body weight decrease; if not, report this immediately.
- Turn the edematous bedridden patient every 2 hours, and provide skin care, particularly around bony prominences, at least once a shift.
- Avoid sedation when possible or reduce dosage, since hypothyroidism delays metabolism of many drugs.
- Maintain patent I.V. line. Monitor serum electrolytes carefully when administering I.V. fluids.
- Monitor vital signs carefully when administering levothyroxine, since rapid correction of hypothyroidism can cause adverse cardiac effects. Report chest pain or tachycardia immediately. Watch for hypertension and congestive heart failure in the elderly patient.
- Check arterial blood gases for indications of hypoxia and respiratory acidosis to determine whether the patient needs ventilatory assistance.
- Since myxedema coma may have been precipitated by an infection, check possible sources of infection, such as blood or urine, and obtain sputum cultures.

Hypothyroidism in Children

(Cretinism)

Deficiency of thyroid hormone secretion during fetal development or early infancy results in infantile cretinism (congenital hypothyroidism). Untreated hypothyroidism is characterized in infants by respiratory difficulties, persistent jaundice, and hoarse crying; in older children, by stunted growth (dwarfism), bone and muscle dystrophy, and mental deficiency. Cretinism occurs three times more often in girls than in boys. Early diagnosis and treatment allow the best prognosis; infants treated before age 3 months usually grow and develop normally. However, athyroid children who remain untreated beyond age 3 months and children with acquired hypothyroidism who remain untreated beyond age 2 suffer irreversible mental retardation; their skeletal abnormalities are reversible with treatment.

Causes

In infants, cretinism usually results from defective embryonic development that causes congenital absence or underdevelopment of the thyroid gland. The next most common cause can be traced to an inherited enzymatic defect in the synthesis of thyroxine, caused by an autosomal recessive gene. Less frequently, antithyroid drugs taken during pregnancy produce cretinism in infants. In children older than age 2, cretinism usually results from chronic autoimmune thyroiditis.

Signs and symptoms

At birth, the weight and length of an infant with infantile cretinism appear normal, but characteristic signs of hypothyroidism develop by the time he's 3 to 6 months old. An exception to this is the breast-fed infant, in whom onset of most symptoms may be delayed until weaning, because breast milk contains small amounts of thyroid hormone.

Typically, an infant with cretinism sleeps excessively, seldom cries (except for occasional hoarse crying), and is generally inactive. Because of this, his parents may describe him as a "good baby—no trouble at all." However, such behavior actually results from lowered metabolism and progressive mental impairment. The infant with cretinism also exhibits abnormal deep tendon reflexes, hypotonic abdominal muscles, a protruding abdomen, and slow, awkward movements. He has feeding difficulties, develops constipation, and, because his immature liver can't conjugate bilirubin, becomes jaundiced.

His large, protruding tongue obstructs respiration, making breathing loud and noisy and forcing him to open his mouth to breathe. He may have dyspnea on exertion, anemia, abnormal facial features—such as a short forehead; puffy, wide-set eyes (periorbital edema); wrinkled eyelids; a broad, short, upturned nose—and a dull expression, resulting from mental retardation. His skin is cold and mottled because of poor circulation, and his hair is dry, brittle, and dull. Teeth erupt late and tend to decay early; body temperature is below normal; and pulse rate is slow.

In the child who acquires hypothyroidism after age 2, appropriate treatment is likely to prevent mental retardation. However, growth retardation becomes apparent in short stature (due to delayed epiphyseal maturation, particularly in the legs), obesity, and a head that appears abnormally large because the arms and legs are stunted. An older child may show delayed or accelerated sexual development.

Diagnosis

A high serum level of TSH, associated with low T_3 and T_4 levels, points to cretinism. Since early detection and treatment can minimize the effects of cretinism, many states require measurement of infant thyroid hormone levels at birth.

Thyroid scan (^{131}I uptake test) shows decreased uptake levels and confirms the absence of thyroid tissue in athyroid children. Increased gonadotropin levels are compatible with sexual precocity in older children and may coexist with hypothyroidism. EKG shows bradycardia and flat or inverted T waves in untreated infants. Hip, knee, and thigh X-rays reveal absence of the femoral or tibial epiphyseal line and delayed skeletal development that is markedly inappropriate for the child's chronologic age. A low T_4 level associated with a normal TSH level suggests hypothyroidism secondary to hypothalamic or pituitary disease, a rare condition.

Treatment

Early detection is mandatory to prevent irreversible mental retardation and permit normal physical development.

Treatment in infants younger than age 1 consists of replacement therapy with levothyroxine P.O., beginning with moderate doses. Dosage gradually increases to levels sufficient for lifelong maintenance. (Rapid increase in dosage may precipitate thyrotoxicity.) Doses are proportionately higher in children than in adults, because children metabolize thyroid hormone more quickly. Therapy in older children includes levothyroxine.

Special considerations

Prevention, early detection, comprehensive parent teaching, and psychological support are essential. Know the early signs. Be especially wary if parents emphasize how good and how quiet their new baby is.

After cretinism is diagnosed, provide supportive care during hormonal replacement:

- During early management of infantile cretinism, monitor blood pressure and pulse rate; report hypertension and tachycardia immediately. But remember—normal infant heart rate is approximately 120 beats per minute. If the infant's tongue is unusually large, position him on his side and observe him frequently to prevent airway obstruction. Check rectal temperature every 2 to 4 hours. Keep the infant warm and his skin moist.
- Inform parents that the child will require lifelong treatment with thyroid supplements. Teach them to recognize signs of overdose: rapid pulse rate, irritability, insomnia, fever, sweating, and weight loss. Stress the need to comply with treatment to prevent further mental impairment.
- Provide support to help parents deal with a child who may be mentally retarded. Help them adopt a positive but realistic attitude and focus on their child's strengths rather than his weaknesses. Encourage them to provide stimulating activities to help the child reach maximum potential. Refer them to supportive community resources.
- To prevent infantile cretinism, emphasize the importance of adequate nutrition during pregnancy, including iodine-rich foods and the use of iodized salt or, in case of sodium restriction, an iodine supplement.

Thyroiditis

Inflammation of the thyroid gland occurs as autoimmune thyroiditis (long-term inflammatory disease), subacute granulomatous thyroiditis (self-limiting inflammation), Riedel's thyroiditis (rare, invasive fibrotic process), and miscellaneous thyroiditis (acute suppurative, chronic infective, and chronic noninfective). Thyroiditis is more common in women than in men.

Causes

Although the causes of the four types of thyroiditis vary, all seem related to bacterial or viral infection, or the body's immune response to it.

Autoimmune thyroiditis is due to antibodies to thyroid antigens in the blood. It may cause inflammation and lymphocytic infiltration (Hashimoto's thyroiditis). Glandular atrophy (myxedema) and Graves' disease are linked to autoimmune thyroiditis.

Subacute granulomatous thyroiditis usually follows mumps, influenza, or coxsackievirus or adenovirus infection. *Riedel's thyroiditis* may be the result of an autoimmune or subacute process.

Miscellaneous thyroiditis results from bacterial invasion of the gland in suppurative thyroiditis; tuberculosis, syphilis, or actinomycosis in the chronic infective form; and sarcoidosis and amyloidosis in chronic noninfective thyroiditis.

Signs and symptoms

Autoimmune thyroiditis is usually asymptomatic and commonly occurs in women, with peak incidence in middle age. It's the most prevalent cause of spontaneous hypothyroidism.

In subacute granulomatous thyroiditis, moderate thyroid enlargement may follow an upper respiratory tract infection or a sore throat. The thyroid may be painful and tender, and dysphagia may occur.

In Riedel's thyroiditis, the gland enlarges slowly as it is replaced by hard, fibrous tissues. This fibrosis may compress the trachea or the esophagus. The thyroid feels firm.

Clinical effects of miscellaneous thyroiditis are characteristic of pyogenic infection: fever, pain, tenderness, and reddened skin over the gland.

Diagnosis

Precise diagnosis depends on the type of thyroiditis:

- *autoimmune:* positive precipitin test, high titers of thyroglobulin, microsomal antibodies present in serum
- *subacute granulomatous:* elevated erythrocyte sedimentation rate (ESR), increased thyroid hormone levels, decreased thyroidal radioiodine uptake
- *chronic infective and noninfective:* variance in findings, depending on underlying infection or other disease.

Treatment

Treatment varies with the type of thyroiditis. Drug therapy includes levothyroxine for accompanying hypothyroidism, analgesics and anti-inflammatory drugs for mild subacute granulomatous thyroiditis, propranolol for transient hyperthyroidism, and steroids for severe episodes of acute illness. Suppurative thyroiditis requires antibiotic therapy. A partial thyroidectomy may be necessary to relieve tracheal or esophageal compression in Riedel's thyroiditis.

Special considerations

- Before treatment, obtain a patient history to identify underlying diseases that may cause thyroiditis, such as tuberculosis or a recent viral infection.
- Check vital signs, and examine the patient's neck for unusual swelling, enlargement, or redness. Provide a liquid diet if the patient has difficulty swallowing, especially when due to fibrosis. If the neck is swollen, measure and record the circumference daily to monitor progressive enlargement.
- Administer antibiotics, as ordered, and report and record elevations in temperature, which may indicate developing resistance to the antibiotic.
- Instruct the patient to watch for and report signs of hypothyroidism (lethargy, restlessness, sensitivity to cold, forgetfulness, or dry skin)—especially if he has Hashimoto's thyroiditis, which often causes hypothyroidism; check for signs of hyperthyroidism (nervousness, tremor, weakness), which often occur in subacute thyroiditis.
- After thyroidectomy, check vital signs every 15 to 30 minutes until the patient's condition stabilizes. Stay alert for signs of tetany secondary to accidental parathyroid injury during surgery. Keep 10% calcium gluconate available for I.V. use, if needed. Assess dressings frequently for excessive bleeding. Watch for signs of airway obstruction, such as difficulty in talking or increased swallowing; keep tracheotomy equipment handy.
- Explain to the patient that lifelong thyroid hormone replacement therapy is necessary. Tell him to watch for signs of overdosage, such as nervousness and palpitations.

Simple Goiter

(Nontoxic goiter)

Simple goiter, thyroid gland enlargement not caused by inflammation or a neoplasm, is commonly classified as endemic or sporadic. Endemic goiter usually results from geographically related nutritional factors, such as iodine-depleted soil or iodine deficiency that accompanies malnutrition. Areas in the United States where this deficiency is most common are called "goiter belts" and include the midwest, the northwest, and the Great Lakes region. Sporadic goiter follows ingestion of certain drugs or foods and affects no particular segment of the population.

Simple goiter is found most frequently in females, especially during adolescence, pregnancy, and menopause. With treatment, prognosis is good.

Causes

Simple goiter occurs when the thyroid gland can't secrete enough thyroid hormone to meet metabolic requirements; as a result, the thyroid mass increases to compensate for inadequate hormone synthesis. Such compensation usually overcomes mild to moderate hormonal impairment. Since TSH levels are generally within normal limits in patients with simple goiter, goitrogenesis probably results from impaired intrathyroidal hormone synthesis and depletion of glandular iodine that increases the thyroid gland's sensitivity to TSH. However, increased levels of TSH may be transient and therefore missed. Endemic goiter is usually due to inadequate dietary intake of iodine, which leads to inadequate secretion of thyroid hormone. Iodized salt prevents this deficiency.

Sporadic goiter commonly results from ingestion of large amounts of goitrogenic foods or use of goitrogenic drugs. Goitrogenic foods contain agents that decrease thyroxine production, and include rutabagas, cabbage, soybeans, peanuts, peaches, peas, strawberries, spinach, and radishes. Goitrogenic drugs include propylthiouracil, iodides, phenylbutazone, para-aminosalicylic acid, cobalt, and lithium. In a pregnant woman, such substances may cross the placenta and affect the fetus.

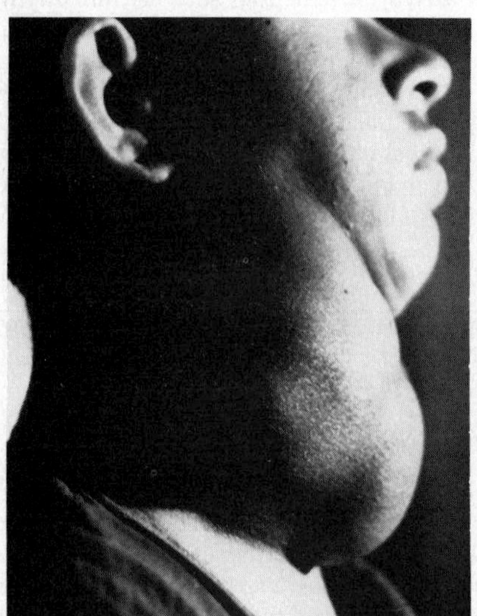

Massive multinodular goiter causes gross distention and swelling of the neck.

Inherited defects may cause insufficient thyroxine synthesis or impaired iodine metabolism. Since families tend to congregate in one geographic area, this familial factor may contribute to endemic and sporadic goiters.

Signs and symptoms

Thyroid enlargement may range from a single, small nodule to massive, multinodular goiter. Because simple goiter doesn't alter the patient's metabolic state, clinical features arise solely from thyroid enlargement, and include respiratory distress and dysphagia from compression of the trachea and esophagus, and swelling and distention of the neck. In addition, large goiters may obstruct venous return, produce venous engorgement, and rarely, induce development of collateral venous circulation of the chest. Such obstruction may cause dizziness or syncope (Pemberton's sign) when the patient raises his arms above his head.

Diagnosis

Detailed patient history may reveal goitrogenic medications or foods, or endemic influence. Diagnostic laboratory tests include:

- *TSH or T_3 serum concentration:* high or normal
- *T_4 serum concentrations:* low-normal or normal
- *^{131}I uptake:* normal or increased (50% of the dose at 24 hours)
- *protein-bound iodine:* low-normal or normal
- *urinary excretion of iodine:* low.

Diagnosis must rule out disorders with similar clinical effects: Graves' disease, Hashimoto's thyroiditis, and thyroid carcinoma.

Treatment

The goal of treatment is to reduce thyroid hyperplasia. Exogenous thyroid hormone replacement (with levothyroxine, desiccated thyroid, or liothyronine) is the treatment of choice; it inhibits TSH secretion and allows the gland to rest. Small doses of iodide (Lugol's or potassium iodide solution) often relieve goiter that results from iodine deficiency. Sporadic goiter requires avoidance of known goitrogenic drugs or food. A large goiter unresponsive to treatment may require subtotal thyroidectomy.

Special considerations

- Watch for progressive thyroid gland enlargement and for the development of hard nodules in the gland, which may indicate malignancy.
- To maintain constant hormone levels, instruct the patient to take prescribed thyroid hormone preparations at the same time each day. Also, tell him to watch for and immediately report signs of thyrotoxicosis: increased pulse rate, palpitations, nausea, vomiting, diarrhea, sweating, tremors, agitation, and shortness of breath.
- Instruct the patient with endemic goiter to use iodized salt to supply the daily 150 to 300 mcg iodine necessary to prevent goiter.
- Monitor the patient taking goitrogenic drugs for signs of sporadic goiter.

Hyperthyroidism

(Graves' disease, Basedow's disease, Parry's disease, thyrotoxicosis)

Hyperthyroidism is a metabolic imbalance that results from thyroid hormone overproduction. The most common form of hyperthyroidism is Graves' disease, which increases thyroxine production, enlarges the thyroid gland (goiter), and causes multiple system changes. Incidence of Graves' disease is highest between ages 30 and 40, especially in persons with family histories of thyroid abnormalities; only 5% of hyperthyroid patients are younger than age 15. With treatment, most patients can lead normal lives. However, thyroid storm—an acute exacerbation of hyperthyroidism—is a medical emergency that may lead to life-threatening cardiac, hepatic, or renal failure.

Causes

Graves' disease may result from genetic and immunologic factors. Increased incidence in monozygotic twins, for example, points to an inherited factor, probably an autosomal recessive gene. This disease occasionally coexists with abnormal iodine metabolism and other endocrine abnormalities, such as diabetes mellitus, thyroiditis, and hyperparathyroidism. Graves' disease is also associated with production of autoantibodies (long-acting thyroid stimulator [LATS], LATS-protector, and human thyroid adenyl cyclase stimulator), possibly caused by a defect in suppressor-T-lymphocyte function that allows the formation of these autoantibodies.

In a person with latent hyperthyroidism, excessive dietary intake of iodine and, possibly, stress can precipitate clinical hyperthyroidism. Similarly, in a person with inadequately treated hyperthyroidism, stressful conditions—including surgery, infection, toxemia of pregnancy, and diabetic ketoacidosis—can precipitate thyroid storm.

Signs and symptoms

The classic symptoms of Graves' disease are an enlarged thyroid (goiter), nervousness, heat intolerance, weight loss despite increased appetite, sweating, diarrhea, tremor, and palpitations. Ex-

OTHER FORMS OF HYPERTHYROIDISM

Toxic adenoma—a small, benign nodule in the thyroid gland that secretes thyroid hormone—is the second most common cause of hyperthyroidism. The cause of toxic adenoma is unknown; incidence is highest in the elderly. Clinical effects are essentially similar to those of Graves' disease, except that toxic adenoma doesn't induce ophthalmopathy, pretibial myxedema, or acropachy. Presence of adenoma is confirmed by radioactive iodine (^{131}I) uptake and thyroid scan, which show a single hyperfunctioning nodule suppressing the rest of the gland. Treatment includes ^{131}I therapy, or surgery to remove adenoma after antithyroid drugs achieve a euthyroid state.

- *Thyrotoxicosis factitia* results from chronic ingestion of thyroid hormone for thyrotropin suppression in patients with thyroid carcinoma, or from thyroid hormone abuse by persons who are trying to lose weight.
- *Functioning metastatic thyroid carcinoma* is a rare disease that causes excess production of thyroid hormone.
- *TSH-secreting pituitary tumor* causes overproduction of thyroid hormone.
- *Subacute thyroiditis* is a virus-induced granulomatous inflammation of the thyroid, producing transient hyperthyroidism associated with fever, pain, pharyngitis, and tenderness in the thyroid gland.
- *Silent thyroiditis* is a self-limiting, transient form of hyperthyroidism, with histologic thyroiditis but no inflammatory symptoms.

ophthalmos is considered most characteristic but is absent in many patients with hyperthyroidism. Many other symptoms are common, as hyperthyroidism profoundly affects virtually every body system:

- *CNS:* difficulty in concentrating because increased thyroxine secretion accelerates cerebral function; excitability or nervousness due to increased basal metabolic rate (BMR); fine tremor, shaky handwriting, and clumsiness from increased activity in the spinal cord area that controls muscle tone; emotional instability and mood swings, ranging from occasional outbursts to overt psychosis
- *Skin, hair, and nails:* smooth, warm, flushed skin (patient sleeps with minimal covers and little clothing); fine, soft hair; premature graying and increased hair loss in both sexes; friable nails and onycholysis (distal nail separated from the bed); pretibial myxedema (dermopathy), producing thickened skin, accentuated hair follicles, raised red patches of skin that are itchy and sometimes painful, with occasional nodule formation. Microscopic examination shows increased mucin deposits.
- *Cardiovascular system:* tachycardia; full, bounding pulse; wide pulse pressure; cardiomegaly; increased cardiac output and blood volume; visible point of maximal impulse (PMI); paroxysmal supraventricular tachycardia and atrial fibrillation (especially in the elderly); and occasionally, systolic murmur at the left sternal border
- *Respiratory system:* dyspnea on exertion and at rest, possibly from cardiac decompensation and increased cellular oxygen utilization
- *Gastrointestinal system:* possible anorexia; nausea and vomiting due to increased gastrointestinal mobility and peristalsis; increased defecation; soft stools or, with severe disease, diarrhea; and liver enlargement
- *Musculoskeletal system:* weakness, fatigue, and muscle atrophy; rare coexistence with myasthenia gravis; generalized or localized paralysis associated with hypokalemia may occur; and occasional acropachy—soft-tissue swelling, accompanied by underlying bone changes where new bone formation occurs.
- *Reproductive system:* in females, oligomenorrhea or amenorrhea, decreased fertility, higher incidence of spontaneous abortions; in males, gynecomastia due to increased estrogen levels; in both sexes, diminished libido
- *Eyes:* exophthalmos (produced by the combined effects of accumulation of mucopolysaccharides and fluids in the

retroorbital tissues that force the eyeball outward, and of lid retraction that produces the characteristic staring gaze); occasional inflammation of conjunctivae, corneas, or eye muscles; diplopia; and increased tearing.

When hyperthyroidism escalates to thyroid storm, these symptoms can be accompanied by extreme irritability, hypertension, tachycardia, vomiting, temperature up to 106° F. (41.1° C.), delirium, and coma.

Diagnosis

Patient history and physical examination suggest hyperthyroidism. The following laboratory tests confirm it:

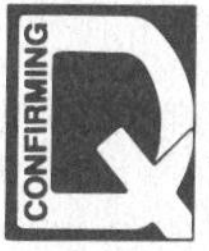

- *Radioimmunoassay* showing increased serum T_4 and T_3 concentrations confirms the diagnosis. (This test is contraindicated if the patient is pregnant.)
- *Thyroid scan* reveals increased uptake of ^{131}I.
- *Thyroid-releasing hormone (TRH) stimulation test* indicates hyperthyroidism if thyroid-stimulating hormone (TSH) level fails to rise within 30 minutes after administration of TRH.
- *BMR* is elevated in hyperthyroidism, but this test has largely been superseded by the more reliable and efficient measurements of T_3 and T_4.

Other supportive test results show increased serum protein-bound iodine (PBI) and decreased serum cholesterol and total lipids. Ultrasonography confirms subclinical ophthalmopathy.

Treatment

The primary forms of treatment for hyperthyroidism are antithyroid drugs, ^{131}I, and surgery. Appropriate treatment depends on the size of the goiter, the causes, the patient's age and parity, and how long surgery will be delayed (if the patient is a candidate for it).

Antithyroid drug therapy is used for children, young adults, pregnant women, and patients who refuse surgery or ^{131}I treatment. Thyroid hormone antagonists include propylthiouracil (PTU) and methimazole, which block thyroid hormone synthesis. Although hypermetabolic symptoms subside from 4 to 8 weeks after such therapy begins, the patient must continue taking the medication for 6 months to 2 years. In many patients, concomitant propranolol is used to manage tachycardia and other peripheral effects of excessive hypersympathetic activity. In pregnant women, moderate doses of propranolol have been administered without ill effects.

During pregnancy, antithyroid medication should be kept at the minimum dosage required to keep maternal thyroid function normal until delivery and to minimize the risk of fetal hypothyroidism—even though most infants of hyperthyroid mothers are born with mild and transient hyperthyroidism. (Neonatal hyperthyroidism may even necessitate treatment with antithyroid drugs and propranolol for 2 to 3 months.) Because exacerbation of hyperthyroidism sometimes occurs in the puerperium, continuous control of maternal thyroid function is essential. Approximately 3 to 6 months postpartum, antithyroid drugs can be gradually tapered down and thyroid function reassessed (drugs may be discontinued at that time). Throughout antithyroid treatment, the mother should not breast-feed, as this may cause neonatal hypothyroidism.

Another major form of therapy for hyperthyroidism is a single P.O. dose of ^{131}I—the treatment of choice for patients not planning to have children. (Patients of reproductive age must give informed consent for this treatment, since small amounts of ^{131}I concentrate in the gonads.) During treatment with ^{131}I, the thyroid gland picks up the radioactive element as it would regular iodine. Subsequently, the radioactivity destroys some of the cells that normally concentrate iodine and produce thyroxine, thus decreasing thyroid hormone production and normalizing thyroid size and function. In most patients, hypermetabolic symptoms diminish from 6 to 8 weeks after such treatment. However, some patients may require a second dose.

Subtotal (partial) thyroidectomy is indicated for the patient younger than age 40 who has a very large goiter and whose hyperthyroidism has repeatedly relapsed after drug therapy. Thyroidectomy removes part of the thyroid gland, thus decreasing its size and capacity for hormone production. Preoperatively, the patient may receive iodides (Lugol's solution or saturated solution of potassium iodide), antithyroid drugs, or high doses of propranolol, to help prevent thyroid storm. If euthyroidism is not achieved, surgery should be delayed and propranolol administered to decrease the systemic effects (cardiac dysrhythmias) caused by hyperthyroidism.

After ablative treatment with ^{131}I or surgery, patients require regular, frequent medical supervision for the rest of their lives, because they usually develop hypothyroidism, sometimes as long as several years after treatment.

Therapy for hyperthyroid ophthalmopathy includes local applications of topical medications but may require high doses of corticosteroids, given systemically or, in severe cases, injected into the retrobulbar area. A patient with severe exophthalmos that causes pressure on the optic nerve may require surgical decompression to lessen pressure on the orbital contents.

Treatment of thyroid storm includes administration of an antithyroid drug such as PTU, propranolol I.V. to block sympathetic effects, a corticosteroid to inhibit the conversion of T_4 to T_3 and to replace depleted cortisol, and an iodide to block release of thyroid hormone. Supportive measures include nutrients, vitamins, fluid administration, and sedation, as necessary.

Special considerations

Patients with hyperthyroidism require vigilant care to prevent acute exacerbations and complications.

- Record vital signs and weight. Monitor serum electrolytes, and check periodically for hyperglycemia and glycosuria. Carefully monitor cardiac function if the patient is elderly or has coronary artery disease. If the cardiac rate is more than 100 beats per minute, check blood pressure and pulse rate often. Check level of consciousness and urinary output. If the patient is pregnant, tell her to watch closely during the first trimester for signs of spontaneous abortion (spotting, occasional mild cramps) and report such signs immediately.
- Encourage bed rest, and keep the room cool, quiet, and dark. The patient with dyspnea will be most comfortable sitting upright or in high Fowler's position.
- Remember, extreme nervousness may produce bizarre behavior. Reassure the patient and family that such behavior subsides with treatment. Provide sedatives, as necessary.
- To promote weight gain, provide a balanced diet, with six meals a day. If the patient has edema, suggest a low-sodium diet.
- If iodide is part of the treatment, mix it with milk to prevent gastrointestinal distress, and administer it through a straw to prevent tooth discoloration.
- Watch for signs of thyroid storm (tachycardia, hyperkinesis, fever, vomiting, hypertension). Check intake and output carefully to ensure adequate hydration and fluid balance. Closely monitor blood pressure, cardiac rate and rhythm, and temperature. If the patient has a high fever, reduce it with appropriate hypothermic measures (sponging, hypothermia blankets, and acetaminophen; avoid aspirin because it raises thyroxine levels). Maintain an I.V. line and give drugs, as ordered.
- If the patient has exophthalmos or other ophthalmopathy, suggest sunglasses or eyepatches to protect his eyes from light. Moisten the conjunctivae often with isotonic eyedrops. Warn the patient with severe lid retraction to avoid sudden physical movements that might cause the lid to slip behind the eyeball.

Thyroidectomy necessitates meticulous postoperative care to prevent complications:

- Check often for respiratory distress, and keep a tracheotomy tray at bedside.
- Watch for evidence of hemorrhage into

the neck, such as a tight dressing with no blood on it. Change dressings and perform wound care, as ordered; check the *back* of the dressing for drainage. Keep the patient in semi-Fowler's position, and support his head and neck with sandbags to ease tension on the incision.

- Check for dysphagia or hoarseness from possible laryngeal nerve injury.
- Watch for signs of hypoparathyroidism (tetany, numbness), a complication that results from accidental removal of the parathyroid glands during surgery.
- Stress the importance of regular medical follow-up after discharge, since hypothyroidism may develop from 2 to 4 weeks postoperatively.

Drug therapy and ^{131}I therapy require careful monitoring and comprehensive patient teaching:

- After ^{131}I therapy, tell the patient not to expectorate or cough freely, because his saliva is radioactive for 24 hours. Stress the need for repeated measurement of serum thyroxine levels. Be sure the patient understands he must not resume antithyroid drug therapy.
- In the patient taking PTU and methimazole, monitor CBC periodically to detect leukopenia, thrombocytopenia, and agranulocytosis. Instruct him to take these medications with meals to minimize GI distress, and to avoid over-the-counter cough preparations because many contain iodine. Tell him to report fever, enlarged cervical lymph nodes, sore throat, mouth sores, and other signs of blood dyscrasia and any rash or skin eruptions—signs of hypersensitivity.
- Watch the patient taking propranolol for signs of hypotension (dizziness, decreased urinary output). Tell him to rise slowly after sitting or lying down to prevent orthostatic syncope.
- Instruct the patient taking antithyroid drugs or ^{131}I therapy to report any symptoms of hypothyroidism.

PARATHYROID DISORDERS

Hypoparathyroidism

Hypoparathyroidism is a deficiency of parathyroid hormone (PTH) caused by disease, injury, or congenital malfunction of the parathyroid glands. Since the parathyroid glands primarily regulate calcium balance, hypoparathyroidism causes hypocalcemia, producing neuromuscular symptoms ranging from paresthesia to tetany. The clinical effects of hypoparathyroidism are usually correctable with replacement therapy. However, some complications of this disorder, such as cataracts and basal ganglion calcifications, are irreversible.

Causes and incidence

Hypoparathyroidism may be acute or chronic and is classified as idiopathic, acquired, or reversible.

Idiopathic hypoparathyroidism may result from an autoimmune genetic disorder or the congenital absence of the parathyroid glands. *Acquired hypoparathyroidism* often results from accidental removal of or injury to one or more parathyroid glands during thyroidectomy or other neck surgery or, rarely, from massive thyroid irradiation. It may also result from ischemic infarction of the parathyroids during surgery, or from hemochromatosis, sarcoidosis, amyloidosis, tuberculosis, neoplasms, or trauma. An *acquired, reversible hypoparathyroidism* may result from hypomagnesemia-induced impairment of hormone synthesis, from suppression of normal gland function due to hypercalcemia, or from delayed maturation of parathyroid function.

PTH normally maintains blood calcium levels by increasing bone resorption and gastrointestinal absorption of calcium. It also maintains an inverse relationship between serum calcium and phosphate levels by inhibiting phosphate reabsorption in the renal tubules. Abnormal PTH production in hypoparathyroidism disrupts this delicate balance.

Incidence of the idiopathic and reversible forms is highest in children; that of the irreversible acquired form, in older patients who have undergone surgery for hyperthyroidism.

Signs and symptoms

Although mild hypoparathyroidism may be asymptomatic, it usually produces hypocalcemia and high serum phosphate levels that affect the central nervous system as well as other body systems. Chronic hypoparathyroidism typically causes neuromuscular irritability, increased deep tendon reflexes, Chvostek's sign (hyperirritability of the facial nerve, producing a characteristic spasm when it's tapped), dysphagia, organic brain syndrome, psychosis, mental deficiency in children, and tetany.

Acute (overt) tetany begins with a tingling in the fingertips, around the mouth, and, occasionally, in the feet. This tingling spreads and becomes more severe, producing muscle tension and spasms and consequent adduction of the thumbs, wrists, and elbows. Pain varies with the degree of muscle tension but rarely affects the face, legs, and feet. Chronic tetany is usually unilateral and less severe; it may cause difficulty in walking and a tendency to fall. Both forms of tetany can lead to laryngospasm, stridor, and, eventually, cyanosis. They may also cause elementary partial, absence, or tonoclonic seizures. These CNS abnormalities tend to be exaggerated during hyperventilation, pregnancy, infection, withdrawal of thyroid hormone, and administration of diuretics and before menstruation.

Other clinical effects include abdominal pain; dry, lusterless hair; spontaneous hair loss; brittle fingernails that develop ridges or fall out; dry, scaly skin; cataracts; and weakened tooth enamel, which causes teeth to stain, crack, and decay easily. Hypocalcemia may induce cardiac dysrhythmias and may eventually lead to congestive heart failure.

Diagnosis

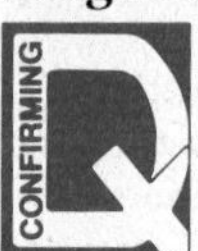

The following test results confirm the presence of hypoparathyroidism:

- *radioimmunoassay for parathyroid hormone:* decreased PTH concentration
- *serum calcium:* decreased level
- *serum phosphorus:* increased level (more than 5.4 mg/1 dl)
- *X-rays:* increased bone density
- *EKG:* increased QT and ST intervals due to hypocalcemia.

The following test helps provoke clinical evidence of hypoparathyroidism: inflating a blood pressure cuff on the upper arm to above systolic blood pressure elicits Trousseau's sign (carpal spasm).

Treatment

Treatment initially includes vitamin D, with or without supplemental calcium. Such therapy is usually lifelong, except in patients with the reversible form of the disease. If the patient can't tolerate the pure form of vitamin D, alternatives include dihydrotachysterol, if renal function is adequate, and calcitriol, if renal function is severely compromised.

Acute life-threatening tetany calls for immediate I.V. administration of calcium gluconate to raise serum calcium levels. If the patient is awake and able to cooperate, he can help raise ionized serum calcium levels by breathing into a paper bag and then inhaling his own CO_2; this produces hypoventilation and mild respiratory acidosis. Sedatives and anticonvulsants may control spasms until calcium levels rise. Chronic tetany calls for maintenance of serum calcium levels with oral calcium supplements.

Special considerations

- While awaiting diagnosis of hypoparathyroidism in a patient with a history of tetany, maintain a patent I.V. line and keep calcium I.V. available. Because the patient is vulnerable to convulsions, maintain seizure precautions. Also, keep a tracheotomy tray and endotracheal tube at bedside, since laryngospasm may result from hypocalcemia.

• For the patient with tetany, administer 10% calcium gluconate slow I.V. (1 mg/minute), and maintain a patent airway. Such a patient may also require intubation, and sedation with diazepam I.V. Monitor vital signs often after administration of diazepam I.V. to make certain blood pressure and heart rate return to normal.

• Advise the patient to follow a high-calcium, low-phosphorus diet, and tell him which foods are permitted.

• When caring for the patient with chronic disease, particularly a child, stay alert for minor muscle twitching (especially in the hands) and for signs of laryngospasm (respiratory stridor or dysphagia), since these effects may signal onset of tetany.

• For the patient on drug therapy, emphasize the importance of checking serum calcium levels at least three times a year. Instruct the patient to watch for signs of hypercalcemia and to keep medications away from light.

• Because the patient with chronic disease has prolonged QT intervals on EKG, watch for heart block and signs of decreasing cardiac output. Closely monitor the patient receiving both digitalis and calcium, since calcium potentiates the effect of digitalis. Stay alert for signs of digitalis toxicity (dysrhythmias, nausea, fatigue, visual changes).

• Instruct the patient with scaly skin to use creams to soften his skin. Also, tell him to keep his nails trimmed to prevent them from splitting.

Hyperparathyroidism

Hyperparathyroidism is characterized by overactivity of one or more of the four parathyroid glands, resulting in excessive secretion of parathyroid hormone (PTH). Such hypersecretion of PTH promotes bone resorption and leads to hypercalcemia and hypophosphatemia. In turn, increased renal and gastrointestinal absorption of calcium occurs.

Causes

Hyperparathyroidism may be primary or secondary. In primary hyperparathyroidism, one or more of the parathyroid glands enlarges, increasing PTH secretion and elevating serum calcium levels. The most common cause is a single adenoma. Other causes include a genetic disorder or multiple endocrine neoplasia. Primary hyperparathyroidism usually occurs between ages 30 and 50 but can also occur in children and the elderly. It affects women two to three times more frequently than men.

In secondary hyperparathyroidism, excessive compensatory production of PTH stems from a hypocalcemia-producing abnormality outside the parathyroid gland, which causes a resistance to the metabolic action of PTH. Some hypocalcemia-producing abnormalities are rickets, vitamin D deficiency, chronic renal failure, or osteomalacia due to phenytoin or laxative abuse.

Signs and symptoms

Clinical effects of primary hyperparathyroidism result from hypercalcemia and are typically present in several body systems:

• *Renal:* nephrocalcinosis due to elevated levels of calcium and phosphorus; possibly, recurring nephrolithiasis, which may lead to renal insufficiency. Renal manifestations are the most common effects of hyperparathyroidism.

• *Skeletal and articular:* chronic low back pain and easy fracturing due to bone degeneration; bone tenderness; chondrocalcinosis; occasional severe osteopenia, especially on the vertebrae; erosions of the juxtaarticular surface; subchondrial fractures; traumatic synovitis; and pseudogout
• *Gastrointestinal:* pancreatitis, causing constant, severe epigastric pain radiating to the back; peptic ulcers, causing abdominal pain, hematemesis, nausea, and vomiting
• *Neuromuscular:* marked muscle weakness and atrophy, particularly in the legs
• *Central nervous system:* psychomotor and personality disturbances, depression, overt psychosis, stupor, and, possibly, coma
• *Other:* skin necrosis, cataracts, calcium microthrombi to lungs and pancreas, polyuria, anemia, and subcutaneous calcification.

Similarly, in secondary hyperparathyroidism, decreased serum calcium levels may produce the same features of calcium imbalance, with skeletal deformities of the long bones (rickets, for example), as well as symptoms of the underlying disease.

Diagnosis

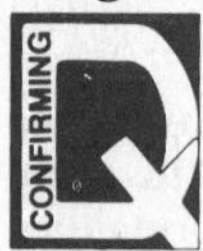

In primary disease, a high concentration of serum PTH on radioimmunoassay, with accompanying hypercalcemia, confirms the diagnosis. In addition, X-rays show diffuse demineralization of bones, bone cysts, outer cortical bone absorption, and subperiosteal erosion of the radial aspect of the middle fingers. Microscopic examination of the bone with tests such as X-ray spectrophotometry typically demonstrates increased bone turnover. Laboratory tests reveal elevated urine and serum calcium, chloride, and alkaline phosphatase levels, and decreased serum phosphorus level.

Hyperparathyroidism may also raise uric acid and creatinine levels and increase basal acid secretion and serum immunoreactive gastrin. Increased serum amylase levels may indicate acute pancreatitis.

Laboratory findings in secondary hyperparathyroidism show normal or slightly decreased serum calcium levels and variable serum phosphorus levels, especially when hyperparathyroidism is due to rickets, osteomalacia, or renal disease. Patient history may reveal familial renal disease, convulsive disorders, or drug ingestion. Other laboratory values and physical examination findings identify the cause of secondary hyperparathyroidism.

Treatment

Treatment varies, depending on the cause of the disease. Treatment for primary hyperparathyroidism may include surgery to remove the adenoma or, depending on the extent of hyperplasia, all but half of one gland (the remaining part of the gland is necessary to maintain normal PTH levels). Such surgery may relieve bone pain within 3 days. However, renal damage may be irreversible.

Preoperatively—or if surgery isn't feasible or necessary—other treatments can decrease calcium levels. Such treatments include: forcing fluids; limiting dietary intake of calcium; promoting sodium and calcium excretion through forced diuresis using normal saline solution (up to 6 liters in life-threatening circumstances), furosemide, or ethacrynic acid; and administering oral sodium or potassium phosphate, calcitonin, or mithramycin.

Therapy for potential postoperative magnesium and phosphate deficiencies includes I.V. administration of magnesium and phosphate, or sodium phosphate solution given P.O. or by retention enema. In addition, during the first 4 or 5 days after surgery, when serum calcium falls to low normal levels, supplemental calcium may be necessary; vitamin D or calcitriol may also be used to raise the serum calcium level.

Treatment of secondary hyperparathyroidism must correct the underlying cause of parathyroid hypertrophy, and includes vitamin D therapy or, in the patient with renal disease, aluminum hydroxide for hyperphosphatemia. In the patient with renal failure, peritoneal dialysis therapy is necessary to lower calcium levels and may have to continue for life. In the patient with chronic secondary hyperparathyroidism, the enlarged glands may not revert to normal size and function even after calcium levels have been controlled.

Special considerations

Care emphasizes prevention of complications from the underlying disease and its treatment.

- Obtain pretreatment baseline serum potassium, calcium, phosphate, and magnesium levels, since these values may change abruptly during treatment.
- During hydration to reduce serum calcium level, record intake and output accurately. Strain urine to check for stones. Provide at least 3 liters of fluid a day, including cranberry or prune juice. As ordered, obtain blood and urine samples to measure sodium, potassium, and magnesium levels, especially for the patient taking furosemide.
- Auscultate for lung sounds often. Listen for signs of pulmonary edema in the patient receiving large amounts of saline solution I.V., especially if he has pulmonary or cardiac disease. Monitor the patient on digitalis carefully, since elevated calcium levels can rapidly produce toxic effects.
- Since the patient is predisposed to pathologic fractures, assist with walking, keep the bed at its lowest position, and raise the side rails. Lift the immobilized patient carefully to minimize bone stress, and check X-rays so you know which bones are weakest. Schedule care to allow the patient with muscle weakness as much rest as possible.
- Watch for signs of peptic ulcer and administer antacids, as appropriate.

After parathyroidectomy:

- Check frequently for respiratory distress, and keep a tracheotomy tray at bedside. Watch for postoperative complications, such as renal colic, acute psychosis, laryngeal nerve damage, or, rarely, hemorrhage. Monitor intake and output carefully.

BONE RESORPTION IN PRIMARY HYPERPARATHYROIDISM

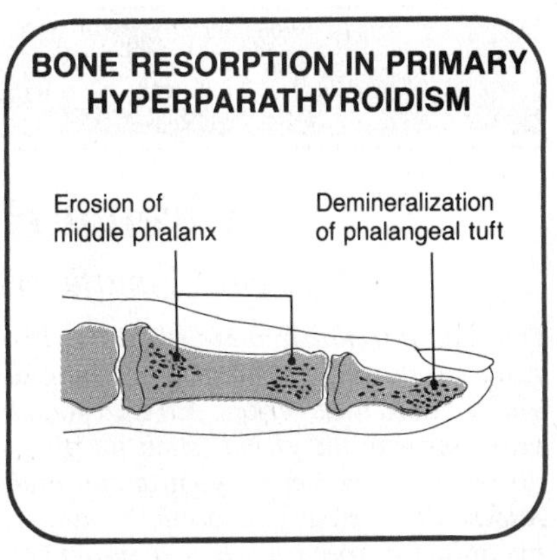

- Check for swelling at the operative site. Place the patient in semi-Fowler's position, and support his head and neck with sandbags to decrease edema, which may cause pressure on the trachea.
- Watch for signs of mild tetany, such as complaints of tingling in the hands and around the mouth. These symptoms should subside quickly but may be prodromal signs of tetany, so keep calcium gluconate I.V. available for emergency administration. Watch for increased neuromuscular irritability and other signs of severe tetany, and report them immediately. Ambulate the patient as soon as possible postoperatively, even though he may find this uncomfortable, since pressure on bones speeds up bone recalcification.
- Check laboratory results for low serum calcium and magnesium levels.
- Monitor mental status and watch for listlessness. In the patient with persistent hypercalcemia, check for muscle weakness and signs of psychosis.
- Before discharge, advise the patient of the possible side effects of drug therapy. Emphasize the need for periodic follow-up through laboratory blood tests. If hyperparathyroidism was not corrected surgically, warn the patient to avoid calcium-containing antacids and thiazide diuretics.

ADRENAL DISORDERS

Adrenal Hypofunction

(Adrenal insufficiency, Addison's disease)

Primary adrenal hypofunction (Addison's disease) originates within the adrenal gland itself and is characterized by decreased mineralocorticoid, glucocorticoid, and androgen secretion. Adrenal hypofunction can also occur secondary to a disorder outside the gland (such as pituitary tumor, with ACTH deficiency), but aldosterone secretion frequently continues intact. A relatively uncommon disorder, Addison's disease can occur at any age and in both sexes. Secondary adrenal hypofunction occurs when a patient abruptly stops taking long-term exogenous steroid therapy. With early diagnosis and adequate replacement therapy, prognosis for adrenal hypofunction is good.

Adrenal crisis (addisonian crisis), a critical deficiency of mineralocorticoids and glucocorticoids, generally follows acute stress, sepsis, trauma, or surgery in patients who have chronic adrenal insufficiency. A medical emergency, adrenal crisis necessitates immediate, vigorous treatment.

Causes

Addison's disease occurs when more than 90% of the adrenal gland is destroyed. Such massive destruction usually results from an autoimmune process in which circulating antibodies react specifically against the adrenal tissue. Other causes include tuberculosis (once the chief cause but now accounting for less than 30% of cases), bilateral adrenalectomy, hemorrhage into the adrenal gland, neoplasms, and fungal infections, such as histoplasmosis. Rarely, a familial tendency to autoimmune disease predisposes to Addison's disease as well as to other endocrinopathies.

Secondary adrenal hypofunction that results in glucocorticoid deficiency can stem from hypopituitarism (causing decreased ACTH secretion), abrupt withdrawal of long-term corticosteroid therapy, or removal of a nonendocrine, ACTH-secreting tumor (long-term exogenous corticosteroid stimulation suppresses pituitary ACTH secretion and results in adrenal gland atrophy). Adrenal crisis follows when trauma, surgery, or other physiologic stress exhausts the body's stores of glucocorticoids in a person with adrenal hypofunction.

Signs and symptoms

Addison's disease typically produces such effects as weakness, fatigue, weight loss, and various gastrointestinal disturbances, such as nausea, vomiting, anorexia, and chronic diarrhea. The disorder also usually causes a conspicuous bronze coloration of the skin. The patient appears to be deeply suntanned, especially in the creases of the hands and over the metacarpophalangeal joints, the elbows, and the knees. He also may exhibit a darkening of scars, areas of vitiligo (absence of pigmentation), and increased pigmentation of the mucous membranes, especially the buccal mucosa. Such abnormal skin and mucous membrane coloration results from decreased secretion of cortisol (one of the glucocorticoids), which causes the pituitary gland to simultaneously secrete excessive amounts of ACTH and melanocyte-stimulating hormone (MSH).

Associated cardiovascular abnormalities in Addison's disease include postural hypotension, decreased cardiac size and output, and a weak, irregular pulse. Other clinical effects include decreased tolerance for even minor stress, poor coordination, fasting hypoglycemia (due to decreased glyconeogenesis), and a craving for salty food. Addison's disease may also retard axillary and pubic hair growth in females, decrease libido (due to decreased androgen production), and in severe cases, cause amenorrhea.

Secondary adrenal hypofunction produces similar clinical effects but without hyperpigmentation, since ACTH and MSH levels are low. Because aldosterone secretion may continue at fairly normal levels in secondary adrenal hypofunction, this condition does not necessarily cause accompanying hypotension and electrolyte abnormalities.

Adrenal crisis produces profound weakness, fatigue, nausea, vomiting, hypotension, dehydration, and occasionally, high fever followed by hypothermia. If untreated, this condition can ultimately cause vascular collapse, renal shutdown, coma, and death.

Diagnosis

Diagnosis requires the demonstration of decreased concentrations of corticosteroids in the plasma or urine, and an accurate determination as to whether adrenal hypofunction is primary or secondary. After baseline plasma and urine steroid testing (24-hour urine collection for 17-ketosteroids [17-KS] and 17-hydroxycorticosteroids [17-OHCS]), special provocative tests are necessary.

The *metyrapone test* requires P.O. or I.V. administration of metyrapone, which blocks cortisol production and should stimulate the release of ACTH from the hypothalamic-pituitary system. In Addison's disease, the hypothalamic-pituitary system responds normally, and plasma reveals high levels of ACTH; however, plasma levels of compound S (cortisol precursor) and urinary concentration of 17-OHCS don't rise. This test is followed by the *ACTH stimulation test,* which involves I.V. administration of ACTH over 6 to 8 hours, after samples have been obtained to determine baseline plasma cortisol and 24-hour urine cortisol levels. In Addison's disease, plasma and urine cortisol levels fail to rise normally in response to ACTH; in secondary disease, repeated doses of ACTH over successive days produce a gradual increase in cortisol levels, until normal values are reached.

In a patient with typical symptoms, the following laboratory findings strongly suggest acute adrenal insufficiency:

- decreased cortisol levels in plasma (less than 10 mcg/dl in the morning, with lower levels in the evening). However, this test is time-consuming, and therapy shouldn't be delayed for results.
- decreased serum sodium and fasting blood sugar
- increased serum potassium and BUN
- elevated hematocrit, and lymphocyte and eosinophil counts
- X-rays showing a small heart, and adrenal calcification.

Treatment

For all patients with primary or secondary adrenal hypofunction, corticosteroid replacement, usually with cortisone or hydrocortisone (both also have mineralocorticoid effect), is the primary treatment and must continue for life. Addison's disease may also necessitate desoxycorticosterone I.M., a pure mineralocorticoid, or fludrocortisone P.O., a synthetic that acts as a mineralocorticoid; both prevent dangerous dehydration and hypotension. Women with Addison's disease who have muscle weakness and decreased libido may benefit from testosterone injections but risk unfortunate masculinizing effects.

Adrenal crisis requires prompt I.V. bolus administration of 100 mg hydrocortisone. Later, 50 to 100 mg doses are given I.M., or are diluted with dextrose in saline solution and given I.V. until the patient's condition stabilizes; up to 300 mg/day of hydrocortisone and 3 to 5 liters of I.V. saline solution may be required during the acute stage. With proper treatment, the crisis usually subsides quickly; blood pressure should stabilize, and water and sodium levels return to normal. After the crisis, maintenance doses of hydrocortisone preserve physiologic stability.

Special considerations

- In adrenal crisis, monitor vital signs carefully, especially for hypotension, volume depletion, and other signs of shock (decreased level of consciousness and urinary output). Watch for hyperkalemia before treatment and for hypokalemia after treatment (from excessive mineralocorticoid effect).
- If the patient also has diabetes, check blood glucose periodically, since steroid replacement may necessitate adjustment of insulin dosage.
- Record weight and intake and output carefully, since the patient may have volume depletion. Until onset of mineralocorticoid effect, force fluids to replace excessive fluid loss.

To manage the patient receiving maintenance therapy:

- Arrange for a diet that maintains sodium and potassium balances.
- If the patient is anorectic, suggest six small meals a day to increase calorie intake. Ask the dietitian to provide a diet high in protein and carbohydrates. Keep a late-morning snack available in case the patient becomes hypoglycemic.
- Observe the patient receiving steroids for cushingoid signs, such as fluid retention around the eyes and face. Watch for fluid and electrolyte imbalance, especially if the patient is receiving mineralocorticoids. Monitor weight and check blood pressure to assess body fluid status. Remember, steroids administered in the late afternoon or evening may cause stimulation of the CNS and insomnia in some patients. Check for petechiae, since the patient bruises easily.
- In women receiving testosterone injections, watch for and report facial hair growth and other signs of masculinization. A dosage adjustment may be necessary.
- If the patient receives glucocorticoids alone, observe for orthostatic hypotension or electrolyte abnormalities, which may indicate a need for mineralocorticoid therapy.
- Explain that lifelong steroid therapy is necessary. Advise him of symptoms of overdosage and underdosage. Tell him that dosage may need to be increased during times of stress (when he has a cold, for example). Warn that infection, injury, or profuse sweating in hot weather may precipitate adrenal crisis.
- Instruct the patient to always carry a medical identification card stating that he takes a steroid and giving the name of the drug and the dosage. Teach the patient how to give himself an injection of hydrocortisone. Tell him to keep an emergency kit available containing hydrocortisone in a prepared syringe for use in times of stress. Warn that any stress may necessitate additional cortisone to prevent a crisis.

Cushing's Syndrome

Cushing's syndrome is a cluster of clinical abnormalities due to excessive levels of adrenocortical hormones (particularly cortisol) or related corticosteroids and, to a lesser extent, androgens and aldosterone. Its unmistakable signs include rapidly developing adiposity of the face (moon face), neck, and trunk, and purple striae on the skin. Cushing's syndrome is most common in females. Prognosis depends on the underlying cause; it is poor in untreated persons and in those with untreatable ectopic ACTH-producing carcinoma or metastatic adrenal carcinoma.

Causes

In approximately 70% of patients, Cushing's syndrome results from excess production of ACTH and consequent hyperplasia of the adrenal cortex. Overproduction of ACTH may stem from pituitary hypersecretion (Cushing's disease), an ACTH-producing tumor in another organ (particularly bronchogenic or pancreatic carcinoma), or administration of synthetic glucocorticoids or ACTH.

In the remaining 30% of patients, Cushing's syndrome results from a cortisol-secreting adrenal tumor, which is usually benign. In infants, the usual cause of Cushing's syndrome is adrenal carcinoma.

Signs and symptoms

Like other endocrine disorders, Cushing's syndrome induces changes in multiple body systems, depending on the adrenocortical hormone involved. Clinical effects may include the following signs and symptoms:

- *Endocrine and metabolic systems:* steroid diabetes, with decreased glucose tolerance, fasting hyperglycemia, and glucosuria
- *Musculoskeletal system:* muscle weakness due to hypokalemia or to loss of muscle mass from increased catabolism, pathologic fractures due to decreased bone mineral, and skeletal growth retardation in children
- *Skin:* purplish striae; fat pads above the clavicles, over the upper back (buffalo hump), on the face (moon face), and throughout the trunk, with slender arms and legs; little or no scar formation; poor wound healing; acne and hirsutism in women
- *Gastrointestinal system:* peptic ulcer, resulting from increased gastric secretions and pepsin production, and decreased gastric mucus
- *Central nervous system (CNS):* irritability and emotional lability, ranging from euphoric behavior to depression or psychosis; insomnia
- *Cardiovascular system:* hypertension due to sodium and water retention; left ventricular hypertrophy; capillary weakness due to protein loss, which leads to bleeding, petechiae, and ecchymosis
- *Immunologic system:* increased susceptibility to infection due to decreased lymphocyte production and suppressed antibody formation; decreased resistance to stress. Suppressed inflammatory response may mask even a severe infection.
- *Renal and urologic systems:* sodium and secondary fluid retention; increased potassium excretion; inhibited ADH secretion; ureteral calculi from increased bone demineralization, with hypercalciuria
- *Reproductive system:* increased androgen production, causing gynecomastia in males and clitoral hypertrophy, mild virilism, and amenorrhea or oligomenorrhea in females.

Diagnosis

Initially, diagnosis of Cushing's syndrome requires determination of plasma and urine steroid levels. In normal persons, plasma cortisol levels are higher in the morning and decrease gradually through the day (diurnal variation). In patients with Cushing's syndrome, cortisol levels do not fluctuate and remain consistently elevated; 24-hour urine sample demonstrates elevated free cortisol levels.

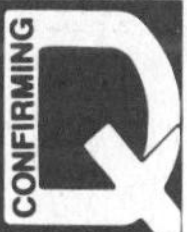

A low-dose dexamethasone suppression test confirms the diagnosis of Cushing's syndrome. A high-dose dexamethasone suppression test can determine if Cushing's syndrome results from pituitary dysfunction (Cushing's disease). In this test, dexamethasone suppresses plasma cortisol levels, and urinary 17-OHCS and 17-KGS fall to 50% or less of basal levels. Failure to suppress these levels indicates that the syndrome results from an adrenal tumor or a nonendocrine, ACTH-secreting tumor. This test can produce false-positive results.

In a stimulation test, administration of metyrapone, which blocks cortisol production by the adrenal glands, tests the ability of the pituitary gland and the hypothalamus to detect and correct low levels of plasma cortisol by increasing ACTH production. The patient with Cushing's disease reacts to this stimulus by secreting an excess of plasma ACTH as measured by levels of urinary com-

SYMPTOMS OF CUSHINGOID SYNDROME

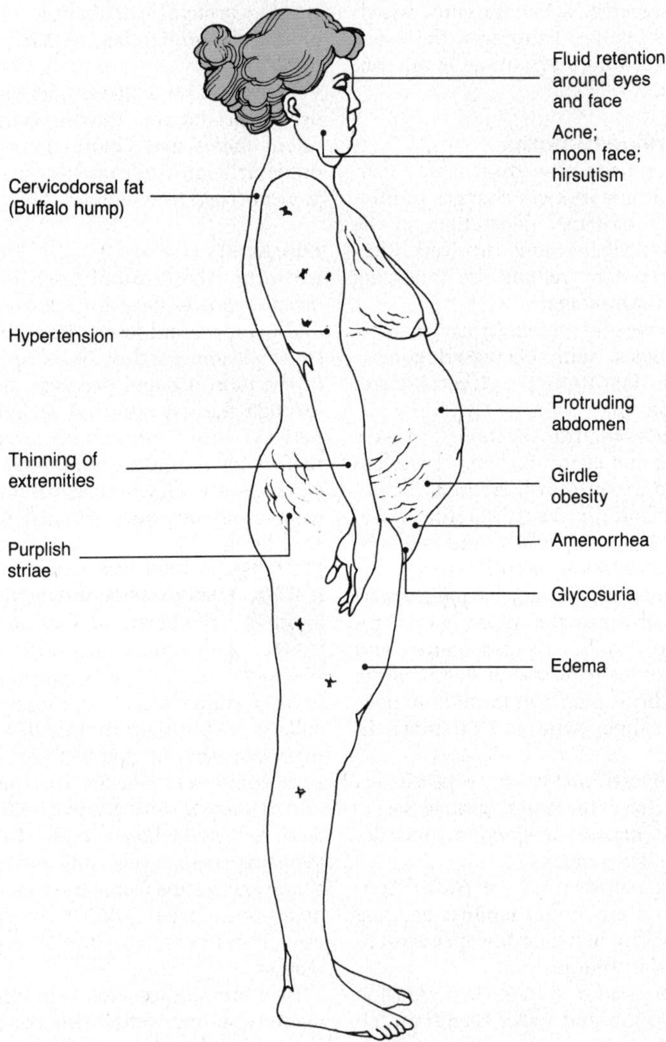

Long-term treatment with corticosteroids may produce a side effect called cushingoid syndrome—a condition marked by obvious fat deposits between the shoulders and around the waist, and widespread systemic abnormalities.

In addition to the symptoms shown in the illustration, observe for renal disorders, hyperglycemia, tissue wasting, muscular weakness, and labile emotional state.

pound S or 17-OHCS. If the patient has an adrenal or a nonendocrine ACTH-secreting tumor, the pituitary gland—which is suppressed by the high cortisol levels—cannot respond normally, so steroid levels remain stable or fall.

Ultrasound, computed tomography (CT) scan, or angiography localize adrenal tumors; CT scan of the head identifies pituitary tumors.

Treatment

Management to restore hormone balance and reverse Cushing's syndrome may necessitate radiation or drug therapy or surgery. For example, pituitary-dependent Cushing's syndrome with adrenal hyperplasia and severe cushingoid symptoms—such as psychosis, poorly controlled steroid diabetes, osteoporosis, and severe pathologic fractures—may require bilateral adrenalectomy, hypophysectomy, or pituitary irradiation. Nonendocrine ACTH-producing tumors require excision of the tumor, followed by drug therapy (mitotane, metyrapone, or aminoglutethimide) to decrease cortisol levels if symptoms persist.

Aminoglutethimide and cyproheptadine decrease cortisol levels and have been beneficial for many cushingoid patients. Aminoglutethimide alone, or in combination with metyrapone, may also be useful in metastatic adrenal carcinoma.

Before surgery, the patient with cushingoid symptoms needs special management to control hypertension, edema, diabetes, and cardiovascular manifestations and to prevent infection. Glucocorticoid administration on the morning of surgery can help prevent acute adrenal insufficiency during surgery.

Cortisol therapy is essential during and after surgery, to help the patient tolerate the physiologic stress imposed by removal of the pituitary or adrenals. If normal cortisol production resumes, steroid therapy may be gradually tapered and eventually discontinued. However, bilateral adrenalectomy or total hypophysectomy mandates lifelong steroid replacement therapy to correct hormonal deficiencies. Patients with pituitary-dependent Cushing's disease may develop Nelson's syndrome (pituitary chromophobe adenoma) after bilateral adrenalectomy.

Special considerations

Patients with Cushing's syndrome require painstaking assessment and vigorous supportive care.

- Frequently monitor vital signs, especially blood pressure. Carefully observe the hypertensive patient who also has cardiac disease.
- Check laboratory reports for hypernatremia, hypokalemia, hyperglycemia, and glycosuria.
- Because the cushingoid patient is likely to retain sodium and water, check for edema, and monitor daily weight and intake and output carefully. To minimize weight gain, edema, and hypertension, ask the dietary department to provide a diet that is high in protein and potassium but low in calories, carbohydrates, and sodium.
- Watch for infection—a particular problem in Cushing's syndrome.
- If the patient has osteoporosis and is bedridden, carefully perform passive range-of-motion exercises.
- Remember, Cushing's syndrome produces emotional lability. Record incidents that upset the patient, and try to prevent such situations from occurring, if possible. Help him get the physical and mental rest he needs—by sedation, if necessary. Offer support to the emotionally labile patient throughout the difficult testing period.

After bilateral adrenalectomy and pituitary surgery, give meticulous postoperative care:

- Report wound drainage or temperature elevation immediately. Use strict aseptic technique in changing the patient's dressings.
- Administer analgesics and replacement steroids, as ordered.
- Monitor urinary output, and check vital signs carefully, watching for signs of shock (decreased blood pressure, increased pulse rate, pallor, and cold,

clammy skin). To counteract shock, give vasopressors and increase the rate of I.V. fluids, as ordered. Because mitotane, aminoglutethimide, and metyrapone decrease mental alertness and produce physical weakness, assess neurologic and behavioral status, and warn the patient of CNS side effects. Also watch for severe nausea, vomiting, and diarrhea.

- Check laboratory reports for hypoglycemia due to removal of the source of cortisol, a hormone that maintains blood glucose levels.
- Check for abdominal distention and return of bowel sounds following adrenalectomy.
- Check regularly for signs of adrenal hypofunction—orthostatic hypotension, apathy, weakness, fatigue—indicators that steroid replacement is inadequate.
- In the patient undergoing pituitary surgery, check for and immediately report signs of increased intracranial pressure (confusion, agitation, changes in level of consciousness, nausea, and vomiting). Watch for hypopituitarism.

Provide comprehensive teaching to help the patient cope with lifelong treatment:

- Advise the patient to take replacement steroids with antacids or meals, to minimize gastric irritation. (Usually, it's helpful to take two thirds of the dosage in the morning and the remaining third in the early afternoon to mimic diurnal adrenal secretion.)
- Tell the patient to carry a medical identification card and to immediately report physiologically stressful situations, such as infections, which necessitate increased dosage.
- Instruct the patient to watch closely for signs of inadequate steroid dosage (fatigue, weakness, dizziness) and of overdosage (severe edema, weight gain). Emphatically warn against discontinuing steroid dosage, because this may produce a fatal adrenal crisis.

Hyperaldosteronism

In hyperaldosteronism, hypersecretion of the mineralocorticoid aldosterone by the adrenal cortex causes excessive reabsorption of sodium and water, and excessive renal excretion of potassium.

Causes and incidence

Hyperaldosteronism may be primary or secondary. Primary hyperaldosteronism (Conn's syndrome) is uncommon; in 70% of patients, it results from a benign aldosterone-producing adrenal adenoma. Incidence is three times higher in women than in men, and is highest between ages 30 and 50. In 15% to 30% of patients with primary hyperaldosteronism, the cause is unknown; rarely, the cause is adrenocortical hyperplasia (in children) or carcinoma.

In primary hyperaldosteronism, chronic aldosterone excess is independent of the renin-angiotensin system and, in fact, it suppresses plasma renin activity. This aldosterone excess enhances sodium reabsorption by the kidneys, which leads to hypernatremia and, simultaneously, hypokalemia and increased extracellular fluid volume. Expansion of intravascular fluid volume also occurs and results in volume-dependent hypertension and increased cardiac output.

Ingestion of an excessive amount of licorice or licoricelike substances can produce a syndrome similar to primary hyperaldosteronism, due to the mineralocorticoid activity of glycyrrhizic acid.

Secondary hyperaldosteronism results from extra-adrenal pathology, which stimulates the adrenal gland to increase production of aldosterone. For example, conditions that reduce renal blood flow (renal artery stenosis) and extracellular fluid volume or produce a sodium deficit activate the renin-angiotensin system and, subsequently, increase aldosterone secretion. Thus, secondary hyperaldosteronism may result from conditions that induce hypertension through increased renin production (such as Wilms' tumor), ingestion of oral contraceptives, and pregnancy.

However, secondary hyperaldosteronism may also result from disorders unrelated to hypertension. Such disorders may or may not cause edema. For example, nephrotic syndrome, hepatic cirrhosis with ascites, and congestive heart failure commonly induce edema; Bartter's syndrome and salt-losing nephritis do not.

Signs and symptoms

Most clinical effects of hyperaldosteronism result from hypokalemia, which increases neuromuscular irritability and produces muscular weakness; intermittent, flaccid paralysis; fatigue; headaches; paresthesia; and possibly, tetany, as a result of metabolic alkalosis, which can lead to hypocalcemia. Diabetes mellitus is common, perhaps because hypokalemia interferes with normal insulin secretion. Hypertension and its accompanying complications are also common. Other characteristic signs include visual disturbances and loss of renal concentrating ability, producing nocturnal polyuria and polydipsia. Azotemia and bacilluria indicate chronic potassium depletion nephropathy.

Diagnosis

Persistently low serum potassium levels in a nonedematous patient who isn't taking diuretics, doesn't have obvious gastrointestinal losses (from vomiting or diarrhea), and has a normal sodium intake suggest hyperaldosteronism. If hypokalemia develops in a hypertensive patient shortly after starting treatment with potassium-wasting diuretics (such as thiazides), and it persists after the diuretic has been discontinued and potassium replacement therapy has been instituted, evaluation for hyperaldosteronism is necessary.

Low plasma renin level after volume depletion by diuretic administration and upright posture, and a high plasma aldosterone level after volume expansion by salt loading confirm primary (Conn's) hyperaldosteronism in a hypertensive patient without edema.

Serum bicarbonate level is often elevated, with ensuing alkalosis due to hydrogen and potassium ion loss in the distal renal tubules. Other tests show markedly increased urinary aldosterone levels, increased plasma aldosterone levels, and in secondary hyperaldosteronism, increased plasma renin levels.

A suppression test is useful to differentiate between primary and secondary hyperaldosteronism. During this test, the patient receives desoxycorticosterone P.O. for 3 days, while plasma aldosterone levels and urinary metabolites are continuously measured. These levels decrease in secondary hyperaldosteronism but remain the same in primary (Conn's). Simultaneously, renin levels are low in primary hyperaldosteronism and high in secondary hyperaldosteronism.

Other helpful diagnostic evidence includes an increase in plasma volume of 30% to 50% above normal, EKG signs of hypokalemia (ST segment depression and U waves), chest X-ray showing left ventricular hypertrophy from chronic hypertension, and localization of tumor by adrenal angiography or CAT scan.

Treatment

Although treatment for primary hyperaldosteronism may include unilateral adrenalectomy, administration of a potassium-sparing diuretic—spironolactone—and sodium restriction may control hyperaldosteronism without surgery. Bilateral adrenalectomy reduces blood pressure for most patients with idiopathic primary hyperaldosteronism. However, some degree of hypertension persists in most patients, even after surgery, necessitating treatment with spironolactone or other antihypertensive therapy. Such patients also require lifelong adrenal hormone replacement.

Treatment of secondary hyperaldosteronism must include correction of the underlying cause.

Special considerations

- Monitor and record urinary output, blood pressure, weight, and serum potassium levels.
- Watch for signs of tetany (muscle twitching, Chvostek's sign) and for hypokalemia-induced cardiac dysrhythmias, paresthesia, or weakness. Give potassium replacement, as ordered, and keep calcium gluconate I.V. available.
- Ask the dietitian to provide a low-sodium, high-potassium diet.
- After adrenalectomy, watch for weakness, hyponatremia, rising serum potassium levels, and signs of adrenal insufficiency, especially hypotension.
- If the patient is taking spironolactone, advise him to watch for signs of hyperkalemia. Tell him that impotence and gynecomastia may follow long-term use.
- Tell the patient who must take steroid hormone replacement to wear a medical alert bracelet.

Adrenogenital Syndrome

Adrenogenital syndrome results from disorders of adrenocortical steroid biosynthesis. This syndrome may be inherited (congenital adrenal hyperplasia [CAH]) or acquired, usually as a result of an adrenal tumor (adrenal virilism). Salt-losing CAH may cause fatal adrenal crisis in newborns.

Causes and incidence

CAH is the most prevalent adrenal disorder in infants and children; simple virilizing CAH and salt-losing CAH are the most common forms. Acquired adrenal virilism is rare and affects females twice as often as males.

CAH is transmitted as an autosomal recessive trait that causes deficiencies in the enzymes needed for adrenocortical secretion of cortisol and, possibly, aldosterone. Compensatory secretion of ACTH produces varying degrees of adrenal hyperplasia. In simple virilizing CAH, deficiency of the enzyme 21-hydroxylase results in underproduction of cortisol. In turn, this cortisol deficiency stimulates increased secretion of ACTH, producing large amounts of cortisol precursors and androgens that do not require 21-hydroxylase for synthesis.

In salt-losing CAH, 21-hydroxylase is almost completely absent. ACTH secretion increases, causing excessive production of cortisol precursors, including salt-wasting compounds. However, plasma cortisol levels and aldosterone—both dependent on 21-hydroxylase—fall precipitously and, in combination with the excessive production of salt-wasting compounds, precipitate acute adrenal crisis. ACTH hypersecretion stimulates adrenal androgens, possibly even more than in simple virilizing CAH, and produces masculinization.

Other rare CAH enzyme deficiencies exist and lead to increased or decreased production of affected hormones.

Signs and symptoms

The newborn female with simple virilizing CAH has ambiguous genitalia (enlarged clitoris, with urethral opening at the base; some labioscrotal fusion) but normal genital tract and gonads. As she grows older, signs of progressive virilization develop: early appearance of pubic and axillary hair, deep voice, acne, and facial hair. The newborn male with this condition has no obvious abnormality; however, at prepuberty he shows accentuated masculine characteristics, such as deepened voice and an enlarged phallus, with frequent erections. At puberty, females fail to begin menstruation, and males have small testes. Both males and females with this condition may be taller than other children their age due to rapid bone and muscle growth, but since excessive androgen levels hasten epiphyseal closure, abnormally short adult stature results.

Salt-losing CAH in females causes more complete virilization than the simple form and results in development of male external genitalia without testes. Since males with this condition have no external genital abnormalities, immediate neonatal diagnosis is difficult, and is commonly delayed until the infant develops severe systemic symptoms. Characteristically, such an infant is apathetic, fails to eat, and has diarrhea; he develops symptoms of adrenal crisis in the first week of life (vomiting, dehydration from hyponatremia, hyperkalemia). Unless this condition is treated promptly, dehydration and hyperkalemia may lead to cardiovascular collapse and cardiac arrest.

Diagnosis

Physical examination revealing pseudohermaphroditism in females, or precocious puberty in both sexes strongly suggests CAH.

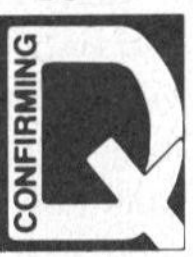

The following laboratory findings confirm the diagnosis: elevated urinary 17-ketosteroids (17-KS), which can be suppressed by administering dexamethasone P.O.; elevated urinary metabolites of hormones, particularly pregnanetriol; elevated plasma 17-hydroxyprogesterone; and normal or decreased urinary levels of 17-hydroxycorticosteroids.

Symptoms of adrenal hypofunction or adrenal crisis in the first week of life strongly suggest salt-losing CAH. Hyperkalemia, hyponatremia, and hypochloremia in the presence of excessive urinary 17-KS and pregnanetriol, and decreased urinary aldosterone confirm it.

Treatment

Simple virilizing CAH requires correction of the cortisol deficiency and inhibition of excessive pituitary ACTH production by daily administration of

ACQUIRED ADRENAL VIRILISM

Acquired adrenal virilism results from virilizing adrenal tumors, carcinomas, or adenomas. This rare disorder is twice as common in females as it is in males. Although acquired adrenal virilism can develop at any age, its clinical effects vary with the patient's age at onset:

- *prepubescent girls:* pubic hair, clitoral enlargement; at puberty, no breast development, menses delayed or absent
- *prepubescent boys:* hirsutism, macrogenitosomia precox (excessive body development, with marked enlargement of genitalia). Occasionally, the penis and prostate equal those of an adult male in size; however, testicular maturation fails to occur.
- *women (especially middle-aged):* dark hair on legs, arms, chest, back, and face; pubic hair extending toward navel; oily skin, sometimes with acne; menstrual irregularities; muscular hypertrophy (masculine resemblance); male pattern balding; and atrophy of breasts and uterus
- *men:* no overt signs; discovery of tumor usually accidental
- *all patients:* good muscular development; taller than average during childhood and adolescence; short stature as adults due to early closure of epiphyses.

Diagnostic tests:

- *urinary total 17-ketosteroids (17-KS):* greatly elevated, but levels vary daily; dexamethasone P.O. doesn't suppress 17-KS.
- *plasma levels of dehydroepiandrosterone (DHA):* greatly elevated
- *serum electrolytes:* normal
- *X-ray of kidneys:* may show downward displacement of kidneys by tumor.

Treatment requires surgical excision of tumor and metastases (if present), when possible, or radiation therapy and chemotherapy. Preoperative treatment may include glucocorticoids. With treatment, prognosis is very good in patients with slow-growing and nonrecurring tumors. Periodic follow-up urine testing (for increased 17-KS) to check for possible tumor recurrence is essential.

HERMAPHRODITISM

True hermaphroditism (hermaphrodism, intersexuality) is a rare condition characterized by both ovarian and testicular tissues. External genitalia are usually ambiguous but may be completely male or female, and thus can mask hermaphroditism until puberty. The hermaphrodite almost always has a uterus (fertility is rare) and ambiguous gonads distributed:

- *bilaterally:* testis and ovary on both sides, ovatestes
- *unilaterally:* ovary or testis on one side; an ovatestis on the other
- *asymmetrically or laterally:* an ovary and a testis on opposite sides.

Since the Y chromosome is needed to develop testicular tissue, hermaphroditism in infants with XX karyotypes is particularly perplexing but may possibly result from mosaicism (XX/XY, XX/XXY), hidden mosaicism, or hidden gene alterations. In patients with XX karyotype, ovaries are usually better developed than in those with XY karyotype. Fifty percent of hermaphrodites have 46,XX karyotype, 20% have XY, and 30% are mosaics.

Although ambiguous external genitalia suggest hermaphroditism, chromosomal studies (particularly a buccal smear for Barr bodies, indicating an XX karyotype), a 24-hour urine specimen for 17-ketosteroids to rule out congenital adrenal hyperplasia, and gonadal biopsy are necessary to confirm it.

Sexual assignment, based on the anatomy of the external genitalia, and prognosis for most successful plastic reconstruction should be made as early as possible to prevent physical and psychologic consequences of delayed reassignment. During such surgery, inappropriate reproductive organs are removed to prevent incongruous secondary sex characteristics at puberty. Hormonal replacement may be necessary.

Nursing intervention emphasizes psychologic support of the parents and reinforcement of their choice about sexual assignment.

cortisone or hydrocortisone. Such treatment returns androgen production to normal levels. Measurement of urinary 17-KS determines the initial dose of cortisone or hydrocortisone; this dose is usually large and is given I.M. Later dosage is modified according to decreasing urinary 17-KS levels. Infants must continue to receive cortisone or hydrocortisone I.M. until age 18 months; after that, they may take it P.O.

The infant with salt-losing CAH in adrenal crisis requires immediate I.V. sodium chloride and glucose infusion to maintain fluid and electrolyte balance and to stabilize vital signs. If saline and glucose infusion doesn't control symptoms while diagnosis is being established, desoxycorticosterone I.M. and, occasionally, hydrocortisone I.V. are necessary. Later, maintenance includes mineralocorticoid (desoxycorticosterone) and glucocorticoid (cortisone or hydrocortisone) replacement.

Sex chromatin and karyotype studies determine the genetic sex of patients with ambiguous external genitalia. Females with masculine external genitalia require reconstructive surgery, such as correction of the labial fusion and of the urogenital sinus. Such surgery is usually scheduled between ages 1 and 3, after the effect of cortisone therapy has been assessed.

Special considerations

- Suspect CAH in infants hospitalized for failure to thrive, dehydration, or diarrhea, as well as in tall, sturdy-looking children with a record of numerous episodic illnesses.
- When caring for an infant with adrenal crisis, keep the I.V. line patent, infuse fluids, and give steroids, as ordered. Monitor body weight, blood pressure, and serum electrolytes carefully, especially sodium and potassium levels. Watch for cyanosis, hypotension, tachycardia, tachypnea, and signs of shock. Keep external stress to a minimum.
- If the child is receiving maintenance therapy with steroid injections, rotate I.M. injection sites to prevent atrophy;

tell parents to do the same. Teach them the possible side effects (cushingoid symptoms) of long-term therapy. Explain that maintenance therapy with hydrocortisone, cortisone, or implanted desoxycorticosterone pellets is essential for life. Warn parents not to withdraw these drugs suddenly, since potentially fatal adrenal insufficiency will result. Instruct parents to report stress and infection, which require increased steroid dosages.

- Monitor the patient receiving desoxycorticosterone for edema, weakness, and hypertension. Be alert for significant weight gain and rapid changes in height, since normal growth is an important indicator of adequate therapy.
- Instruct the patient to wear a medical identification bracelet indicating that he's on prolonged steroid therapy and providing information about dosage.
- Help parents of a female infant with male genitalia to understand that she is physiologically a female and that this abnormality can be surgically corrected. Arrange for counseling, if necessary.

Pheochromocytoma

A pheochromocytoma is a chromaffin-cell tumor of the adrenal medulla that secretes an excess of the catecholamines epinephrine and norepinephrine, which results in severe hypertension, increased metabolism, and hyperglycemia. This disorder is potentially fatal, but prognosis is generally good with treatment. However, pheochromocytoma-induced kidney damage is irreversible.

Causes and incidence

A pheochromocytoma may result from an inherited autosomal dominant trait. According to some estimates, about 0.5% of newly diagnosed patients with hypertension have pheochromocytoma. While this tumor is usually benign, it may be malignant in as many as 10% of these patients. It affects all races and both sexes, occurring primarily between ages 30 and 40.

Signs and symptoms

The cardinal sign of pheochromocytoma is persistent or paroxysmal hypertension. Common clinical effects include palpitations, tachycardia, headache, diaphoresis, pallor, warmth or flushing, paresthesia, tremor, excitation, fright, nervousness, feelings of impending doom, abdominal pain, tachypnea, nausea, and vomiting. Postural hypotension and paradoxical response to antihypertensive drugs are common, as are associated glycosuria, hyperglycemia, and hypermetabolism. Patients with hypermetabolism may show marked weight loss, but some patients with pheochromocytomas are obese. Symptomatic episodes may recur as seldom as once every 2 months or as often as 25 times a day. They may occur spontaneously or may follow certain precipitating events, such as postural change, exercise, laughing, smoking, induction of anesthesia, urination, or a change in environmental or body temperature.

Often, pheochromocytoma is diagnosed during pregnancy, when uterine pressure on the tumor induces more frequent attacks; such attacks can prove fatal for both mother and fetus as a result of cerebrovascular accident, acute pulmonary edema, cardiac arrhythmias, or hypoxia. In such patients, the risk of spontaneous abortion is high, but most fetal deaths occur during labor or immediately after birth.

Diagnosis

A history of acute episodes of hypertension, headache, sweating, and tachycardia—particularly in a patient with hyperglycemia, glycosuria, and hypermetabolism—strongly suggests pheochromocytoma. A patient who experiences intermittent attacks may show no abnormality during a latent phase. The tumor is rarely palpable; however, when it is, palpation of the surrounding area may induce a typical acute attack and help confirm the diagnosis. Generally, diagnosis depends on laboratory findings.

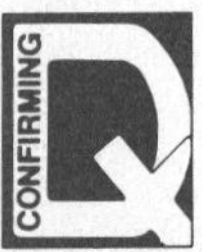

Increased urinary excretion of total free catecholamine and its metabolites, vanillylmandelic acid (VMA) and metanephrine, as measured by an analysis of a 2- to 4-hour or a 24-hour urine collection, confirms pheochromocytoma. Labile blood pressure necessitates urine collection during a hypertensive episode and comparison of this specimen to a baseline specimen. Direct assay of total plasma catecholamines may show levels 10 to 50 times higher than normal.

Provocative tests with tyramine or glucagon and depressor tests (phentolamine) suggest the diagnosis. However, because they may precipitate a hypertensive crisis or result in a false positive or negative, they're rarely used.

Angiography demonstrates an adrenal medullary tumor; intravenous pyelography with nephrotomography, adrenal venography, or computed tomography (CT) scan helps localize the tumor.

Treatment

Surgical removal of the tumor is the treatment of choice. To decrease blood pressure, alpha-adrenergic blocking agents (phentolamine or phenoxybenzamine) or, more recently, metyrosine (blocks catecholamine synthesis) is administered from 1 day to 2 weeks before surgery. A beta-adrenergic blocking agent (propranolol) may also be used after achieving alpha blockade. Postoperatively, I.V. fluids, plasma volume expanders, vasopressors, and, possibly, transfusions may be required if marked hypotension occurs. However, persistent hypertension in the immediate postoperative period is more common.

If surgery isn't feasible, alpha- and beta-adrenergic blocking agents—such as phenoxybenzamine and propranolol, respectively—are beneficial in controlling catecholamine effects and preventing attacks.

Acute attack or hypertensive crisis requires I.V. administration of phentolamine (push or drip) or nitroprusside to normalize blood pressure.

Special considerations

- To ensure the reliability of urine catecholamine measurements, make sure the patient avoids foods high in vanillin (such as coffee, nuts, chocolate, and bananas) for 2 days before urine collection of VMA. Also, be aware of possible drug therapy that may interfere with the accurate determination of VMA (such as guaifenesin and salicylates). Collect the urine in a special container, with hydrochloric acid, that has been prepared by the laboratory.
- Obtain blood pressure readings often, since transient hypertensive attacks are possible. Tell the patient to report headaches, palpitations, nervousness, or other symptoms of an acute attack. If hypertensive crisis develops, monitor blood pressure and heart rate every 2 to 5 minutes until blood pressure stabilizes at an acceptable level.
- Check urine for glucose, and watch for weight loss from hypermetabolism.
- After surgery, blood pressure may rise or fall sharply. Keep the patient quiet; provide a private room, if possible, since excitement may trigger a hypertensive episode. Postoperative hypertension is common, because the stress of surgery and manipulation of the adrenal gland stimulate secretion of catecholamines. Since this excess secretion causes profuse sweating, keep the room cool, and change the patient's clothing and bedding often. If the patient receives phentolamine, monitor blood pressure closely. Observe and record side effects: dizziness, hypotension, tachycardia. The first 24 to 48 hours immediately after surgery are the most critical, since blood pressure can drop drastically.

• If the patient is receiving vasopressors I.V., check blood pressure every 3 to 5 minutes, and regulate the drip to maintain a safe pressure. Arterial pressure lines facilitate constant monitoring.
• Watch for abdominal distention and return of bowel sounds.
• Check dressings and vital signs for indications of hemorrhage (increased pulse rate, decreased blood pressure, cold and clammy skin, pallor, unresponsiveness).
• Give analgesics for pain, as ordered, but monitor blood pressure carefully, since many analgesics, especially meperidine, can cause hypotension.
• If autosomal dominant transmission of pheochromocytoma is suspected, the patient's family should also be evaluated for this condition.

PANCREATIC & MULTIPLE DISORDERS

Multiple Endocrine Neoplasia

(Wermer's syndrome, Sipple's syndrome)

Multiple endocrine neoplasia (MEN) is a hereditary disorder in which two or more endocrine glands develop hyperplasia, adenoma, or carcinoma, concurrently or consecutively. Two of the types that occur are well documented; a third may exist. MEN I (Wermer's syndrome) involves hyperplasia and adenomatosis of the parathyroids, islet cells of the pancreas, pituitary, and, rarely, adrenals and thyroid gland; and MEN II (Sipple's syndrome) involves medullary carcinoma of the thyroid, with hyperplasia and adenomatosis of the adrenal medulla (pheochromocytoma) and parathyroids. MEN I is the most common form.

Causes and incidence

MEN usually results from autosomal dominant inheritance, affects both males and females, and may occur at any time from adolescence to old age.

Signs and symptoms

Clinical effects of MEN may develop in various combinations and orders, depending on the glands involved. The most common symptom of MEN I is peptic ulceration, perhaps associated with the Zollinger-Ellison syndrome (marked by increased gastrin production from nonbeta islet cell tumors of the pancreas). Hypoglycemia may result from pancreatic beta islet cell tumors, with increased insulin production. When MEN I affects the parathyroids, it produces signs of hyperparathyroidism, including hypercalcemia (since the parathyroids are primarily responsible for the regulation of calcium and phosphorus levels). When MEN causes pituitary tumor, it usually triggers pituitary hypofunction but can also result in hyperfunction. MEN I rarely produces renal and skeletal complications.

Characteristic features of MEN II with medullary carcinoma of the thyroid include enlarged thyroid mass, with resultant increased calcitonin, and, occasionally, ectopic ACTH, causing Cushing's syndrome. With tumors of the adrenal medulla, symptoms include headache, tachydysrhythmias, and hypertension; with adenomatosis or hyperplasia of the parathyroids, symptoms result from renal calculi.

Diagnosis

Investigating symptoms of pituitary tumor, hypoglycemia, hypercalcemia, or gastrointestinal hemorrhage may lead to a diagnosis of MEN. Diagnostic tests must be used to carefully evaluate each affected endocrine gland. For example, radioimmunoassay showing increased levels of gastrin in patients with peptic ulceration and Zollinger-Ellison syndrome suggests the need for follow-up studies for MEN I, since 50% of patients with Zollinger-Ellison syndrome have MEN. After confirmation of MEN, family members must also be assessed for this inherited syndrome.

Treatment

Treatment must eradicate the tumors. Subsequent therapy controls residual symptoms. In MEN I, peptic ulceration is usually the most urgent clinical feature, so primary treatment emphasizes control of bleeding or resection of necrotic tissue. In hypoglycemia caused by insulinoma, P.O. administration of diazoxide or glucose can keep blood glucose within acceptable limits. However, subtotal (partial) pancreatectomy is frequently required. Because all parathyroid glands have the potential for neoplastic enlargement, subtotal parathyroidectomy may also be required, along with transphenoidal hypophysectomy. In MEN II, treatment for adrenal medullary tumor includes antihypertensives and resection of the tumor.

Special considerations

Supportive care depends on the body system involved.
- If MEN involves the pancreas, monitor blood and urine glucose levels frequently. If it affects the adrenal glands, monitor blood pressure closely, especially during drug therapy.
- Manage peptic ulcers, hypoglycemia, and other complications, as needed.
- If pituitary tumor is suspected, watch for signs of pituitary trophic hormone dysfunction, which may affect any of the endocrine glands. Also, be aware that pituitary apoplexy (sudden severe headache, altered level of consciousness, visual disturbances) may occur.

Diabetes Mellitus

A chronic disease of insulin deficiency or resistance, diabetes mellitus is characterized by disturbances in carbohydrate, protein, and fat metabolism. A leading cause of death by disease in the United States, this syndrome contributes to about 50% of myocardial infarctions and about 75% of strokes, as well as to renal failure and peripheral vascular disease. It's also the leading cause of new blindness.

This condition occurs in two forms: insulin-dependent diabetes mellitus *(IDDM, ketosis-prone, or juvenile diabetes) and the more prevalent* noninsulin-dependent diabetes mellitus *(NIDDM, ketosis-resistant, or maturity-onset diabetes). IDDM usually occurs before age 30 (although it may occur at any age); the patient is usually thin and requires exogenous insulin and dietary management to achieve control. Conversely, NIDDM usually occurs in obese adults after age 40 and is most often treated with diet and exercise (possibly in combination with hypoglycemic drugs), although treatment may include insulin therapy.*

Causes and incidence

Diabetes mellitus affects an estimated 5% of the population of the United States (10 to 12 million persons), about half of whom are undiagnosed. Incidence is equal in males and females and rises with age.

Although recent studies show that certain cases of IDDM are viral in origin, heredity strongly influences most diabetes. Precipitating factors include:
- obesity: causes resistance to endogenous insulin
- physiologic or emotional stress: causes prolonged elevation of stress hormone levels (cortisol, epinephrine, glucagon, and growth hormone), which raises blood glucose, in turn placing increased

demands on the pancreas

- pregnancy and oral contraceptives: increase levels of estrogen and placental hormones, which antagonize insulin
- other medications that are known insulin antagonists: thiazide diuretics, adrenal corticosteroids, phenytoin.

Insulin transports glucose into the cell for use as energy and storage as glycogen. It also stimulates protein synthesis and free fatty acid storage in the fat depots. Insulin deficiency compromises the body tissues' access to essential nutrients for fuel and storage.

Signs and symptoms

Diabetes may begin dramatically with ketoacidosis or insidiously as in mild diabetes, which is often asymptomatic. Its most common symptom is fatigue, from energy deficiency and a catabolic state. Insulin deficiency causes hyperglycemia, which pulls fluid from body tissues, causing osmotic diuresis, polyuria, and dehydration. Other signs include polydipsia, dry mucous membranes, and poor skin turgor. Edema and sugar deposits cause changes in the lens, which result in visual disturbances. In ketoacidosis or hyperglycemic hyperosmolar nonketotic coma, dehydration may cause hypovolemia and shock. Wasting of glucose in the urine usually produces weight loss and hunger in IDDM, even if the patient eats voraciously.

Long-term effects of diabetes may include retinopathy, nephropathy, atherosclerosis, peripheral and autonomic neuropathy. Peripheral neuropathy usually affects the feet and may cause numbness or pain. Autonomic neuropathy may manifest itself in several ways, including gastroparesis (leading to delayed gastric emptying and a feeling of nausea and fullness after meals), nocturnal diarrhea, and postural hypotension.

Because hyperglycemia impairs resistance to infection, diabetes may result in skin and urinary tract infections, vaginitis, and anal pruritus. Glucose content of the epidermis and urine encourages bacterial growth.

Diagnosis

Symptoms of uncontrolled diabetes and random elevated blood glucose or glucosuria suggest diabetes. Confirmation

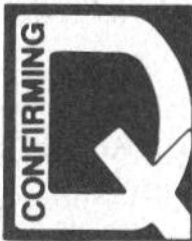

requires a fasting plasma glucose above 140 mg/dl; or, with normal fasting glucose, a blood glucose level above 200 mg/dl during the first 2 hours of a glucose tolerance test (GTT). An ophthalmologic examination may show diabetic retinopathy. Other diagnostic and monitoring tests include the cortisone GTT to elicit stress-induced diabetes, blood insulin level determination, urine testing for glucose and acetone, and glycosylated hemoglobin (hemoglobin A_{1c}) determination, which reflects recent glucose control.

Treatment

Effective treatment normalizes blood glucose and prevents complications. In IDDM, these goals are achieved with insulin replacement that mimics normal pancreatic function. Current means of insulin replacement include mixed, split doses of regular insulin and NPH injected twice a day; premeal injections of short-acting regular insulin with intermediate NPH injections at bedtime; and continuous subcutaneous insulin infusion (insulin pump). An additional treatment, pancreas transplantation, is still experimental. Diabetic treatment also requires a strict diet carefully planned to meet nutritional needs, to control blood glucose levels, and to reach and maintain appropriate body weight. For the obese diabetic, weight reduction is a dietary goal. In IDDM, the calorie allotment may be high, depending on growth stage and activity level. However, to be successful, the diet must be followed consistently and meals eaten at regular times.

Patients with NIDDM may require oral hypoglycemics. These medications stimulate endogenous insulin production and may also increase insulin sensitivity at the cellular level.

Treatment for long-term diabetic complications may include transplantation

PATIENT TEACHING AID

Mixing Regular and Long-acting Insulins

Dear Patient:
Your doctor has prescribed regular and long-acting insulins to control your diabetes. To avoid separate injections, you can mix these two types and administer them together. Here are the steps you must follow:

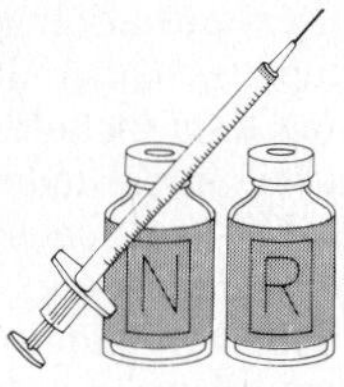

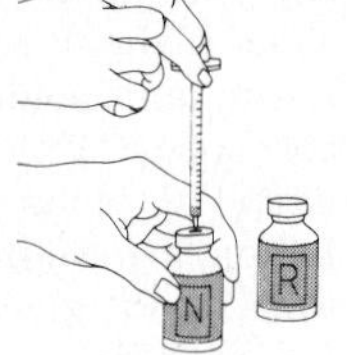

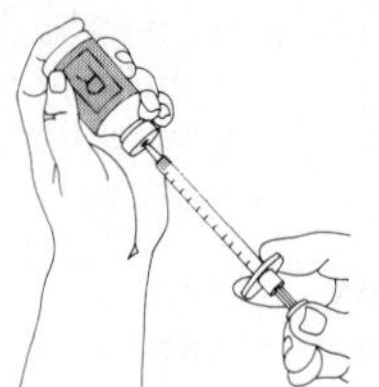

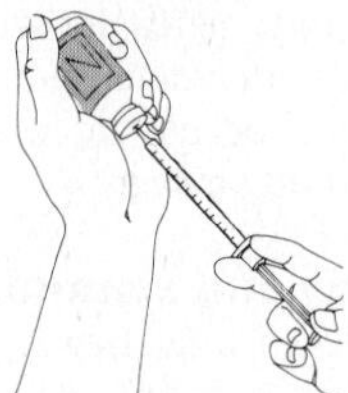

1. *Check your equipment.* Always wash your hands first, and prepare the mixture in a clean area. Make sure you have alcohol swabs, both types of insulin, and the proper syringe for the insulin concentration. Then, warm each vial by rolling it gently between your palms.

2. *Put air into the vial of long-acting insulin.* Clean the rubber stopper of the vial with an alcohol swab. To put air into the syringe, pull the plunger back to the appropriate number of units of long-acting insulin. Then, insert the needle into the top of the vial, making sure the point doesn't touch the insulin. Push in the plunger, and withdraw the syringe.

3. *Withdraw your dose of regular insulin.* Clean the rubber stopper of the regular insulin vial with an alcohol swab. Next, pull back the plunger to the necessary number of units of regular insulin, and inject air into the bottle. With the needle still in the bottle, turn the bottle upside down, and withdraw the proper dose of regular insulin.

4. *Withdraw your dose of long-acting insulin.* Clean the top of the long-acting insulin vial, and insert the needle into it, without pushing down the plunger. Then, invert the bottle, and withdraw the appropriate number of units. (Remember to pull the plunger back to the number of units needed for the *total* dose. For instance, if you have 10 units of regular insulin in the syringe and you need 20 units of long-acting insulin, pull the plunger back to 30 units.)

or dialysis for renal failure, photocoagulation for retinopathy, and vascular surgery for large vessel disease. Meticulous blood glucose control is essential.

Special considerations

Management of diabetes focuses on comprehensive teaching, recognition and care of the patient in crisis, and prevention of complications.

- Stress that compliance with the prescribed program is essential. Tailor your teaching to the patient's needs, abilities, and developmental stage. Include diet; purpose, administration, and possible side effects of medication; exercise; monitoring techniques; hygiene; and the prevention and recognition of hypoglycemia and hyperglycemia. To motivate the patient's adherence to required life-style changes, emphasize the significance of the effect of blood glucose control on long-term health.
- Watch for acute complications of diabetes and diabetic therapy, especially hypoglycemia (vagueness, slow cerebra-

tion, dizziness, weakness, pallor, tachycardia, diaphoresis, seizures, and coma); immediately give carbohydrates in the form of fruit juice, hard candy, honey, or, if the patient is unconscious, glucagon or dextrose I.V. Also be alert for signs of ketoacidosis (acetone breath, dehydration, weak and rapid pulse, Kussmaul's respirations) and hyperosmolar coma (polyuria, thirst, neurologic abnormalities, stupor). These hyperglycemic crises require I.V. fluids, insulin, and, possibly, potassium replacement.

• Monitor diabetic control by testing urine for glucose and acetone and obtaining blood glucose levels. (Urine glucose tests should be reported in mg% glucose instead of plus values.) A patient with NIDDM may test once daily using the glucose oxidase method (such as Tes-Tape); a patient with IDDM may test four times a day using the two-drop copper sulfate reduction method (such as Clinitest) and an acetone test; a patient with renal disease (in whom urine testing is unreliable) should monitor control of blood glucose using a home glucose-monitoring device.

• Watch for diabetic effects on the cardiovascular system, such as cerebral vascular, coronary artery, and peripheral vascular disease. Treat all injuries, cuts, and blisters (particularly on the lower extremities) meticulously. Stay alert for signs of urinary tract infection, renal failure, and Kimmelstiel-Wilson syndrome (protein and RBCs in urine, edema); the latter results from vascular deterioration in the kidneys and is a leading cause of death in young adult diabetics. Urge regular ophthalmologic examinations for early detection of diabetic retinopathy.

• Assess the patient for signs of diabetic neuropathy (numbness or pain in arms and legs, footdrop, neurogenic bladder). Emphasize the need for personal safety, since decreased sensation can mask injuries. Minimize complications by maintaining strict blood glucose control.

• To prevent diabetes, teach persons at high risk to avoid precipitative factors; for example, females with family histories of diabetes should have thorough medical counseling about the use of contraceptives and the risks of pregnancy. Advise genetic counseling for young adult diabetics who are planning families.

• Further information about diabetes and patient-teaching aids may be obtained from the Juvenile Diabetes Foundation, the American Diabetes Association, the American Association of Diabetes Educators, and the manufacturers of products used by diabetics.

Selected References

Camuñas, C. "Transsphenoidal Hypophysectomy," *American Journal of Nursing* 80(10):1820-23, October 1980.

Collu, Robert, et al., eds., *Pediatric Endocrinology*. Comprehensive Endocrinology Series. New York: Raven Press Pubs., 1981.

DeGroot, Leslie J., et al., *The Thyroid and Its Diseases*, 5th ed. New York: John Wiley & Sons, 1984.

Felig, Philip, et al., *Endocrinology and Metabolism*. New York: McGraw-Hill Book Co., 1981.

Guthrie, Diana W., and Guthrie, Richard A., eds. *Nursing Management of Diabetes Mellitus*, 2nd ed. St. Louis: C.V. Mosby Co., 1982.

Hershman, J.M. *Endocrine Pathophysiology: A Patient-Oriented Approach*, 2nd ed. Philadelphia: Lea & Febiger, 1982.

Kempe, C. Henry, et al., eds. *Current Pediatric Diagnosis and Treatment*, 8th ed. Los Altos, Calif.: Lange Medical Pubns., 1984.

Krieger, Dorothy T., and Bardin, C. Wayne. *Current Therapy in Endocrinology, 1983-1984*. St. Louis: C.V. Mosby Co., 1983.

Pillitteri, Adele. *Child Health Nursing: Care of the Growing Family*, 2nd ed. Boston: Little, Brown & Co., 1981.

Williams, Robert H. *Textbook of Endocrinology*, 6th ed. Philadelphia: W.B. Saunders Co., 1981.

14 Metabolic and Nutritional Disorders

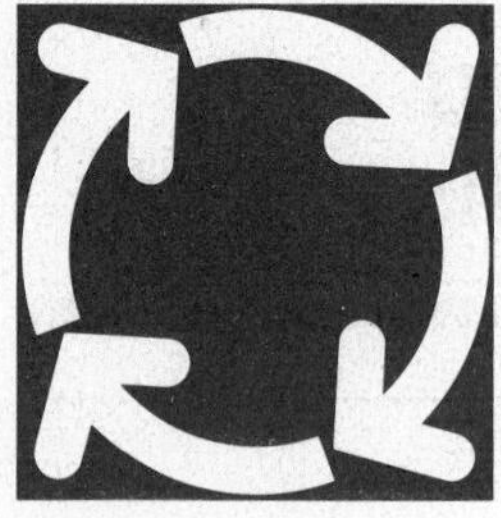

Metabolic and Nutritional Disorders

Introduction

Metabolism is the physiologic process that absorbs nutrients and converts them into forms that produce energy and continually rebuild body cells. Metabolism has two phases: catabolism and anabolism. In catabolism, the energy-producing phase of metabolism, the body breaks down large food molecules into smaller ones; in anabolism, the tissue-building phase, the body converts small molecules into larger ones (such as antibodies to keep the body capable of fighting infection). Both phases are accomplished by means of a chemical process using energy.

Carbohydrates: Primary energy source

The body gets most of its energy by metabolizing carbohydrates, especially glucose. Glucose catabolism proceeds in three phases:

- *Glycolysis,* a series of chemical reactions, converts glucose molecules into pyruvic or lactic acid.
- The *citric acid cycle* removes ionized hydrogen atoms from pyruvic acid and produces carbon dioxide.
- *Oxidative phosphorylation* traps energy from the hydrogen electrons and combines the hydrogen ions and electrons with oxygen to form water and the common form of biologic energy, adenosine triphosphate (ATP).

Other essential processes in carbohydrate metabolism include glycogenesis—the formation of glycogen, a storage form of glucose—which occurs when cells become saturated with glucose 6-phosphate (an intermediate product of glycolysis); glycogenolysis, the reverse process, which converts glycogen into glucose 6-phosphate in muscle cells and liberates free glucose in the liver; and gluconeogenesis, or "new" glucose formation from protein amino acids or fat glycerols.

A complex interplay of hormonal and neural controls regulates the homeostasis of glucose metabolism. Hormone secretions of five endocrine glands dominate this regulatory function:

- Beta cells of the islets of Langerhans secrete the glucose-regulating hormone *insulin,* which decreases blood sugar levels.
- Alpha cells of the islets of Langerhans secrete *glucagon,* which increases the blood glucose level by stimulating phosphorylase activity to accelerate liver glycogenolysis.
- The adrenal medulla, as a response to stress, secretes *epinephrine,* which stimulates liver and muscle glycogenolysis to increase the blood glucose level.
- *Adrenocorticotropic hormone (ACTH)* and *glucocorticoids* also increase blood glucose levels. Glucocorticoids accelerate gluconeogenesis by promoting the flow of amino acids to the liver, where

they are synthesized into glucose.

• *Growth hormone (GH)* limits the storage of fat and favors fat catabolism; consequently, it inhibits carbohydrate catabolism and thus raises blood glucose levels.

• *Thyroid-stimulating hormone (TSH)* and *thyroid hormone* have mixed effects on carbohydrate metabolism and may raise or lower blood glucose levels.

Fats: Catabolism and anabolism

The breaking up of triglycerides—lipolysis—yields fatty acids and glycerol. Beta-oxidation breaks down fatty acids into acetyl coenzyme A, which can then enter the citric acid cycle phase; glycerol can also undergo gluconeogenesis or enter the glycolytic pathways to produce energy. Conversely, lipogenesis is the chemical formation of fat from excess

ESSENTIAL NUTRIENTS AND THEIR FUNCTIONS

NUTRIENTS	FUNCTIONS
Carbohydrates	• Energy source
Fats and essential fatty acids	• Energy source; essential for growth, normal skin, and membranes
Proteins and amino acids	• Synthesis of all body proteins, growth, and tissue maintenance
Water-soluble vitamins:	
• Ascorbic acid (C)	• Collagen synthesis, wound healing, antioxidation
• Thiamine (B_1)	• Coenzyme in carbohydrate (CHO) metabolism
• Riboflavin (B_2)	• Coenzyme in energy metabolism
• Niacin	• Coenzyme in CHO, fat, energy metabolism, and tissue metabolism
• Vitamin B_{12}	• DNA and RNA synthesis; erythrocyte formation
• Folic acid	• Coenzyme in amino acid metabolism; heme and hemoglobin formation
Fat-soluble vitamins:	
• Vitamin A	• Vision in dim light, mucosal epithelium integrity, tooth development, endocrine function
• Vitamin D	• Regulation of calcium and phosphate absorption and metabolism; renal phosphate clearance
• Vitamin E	• Antioxidation; essential for muscle, liver, and RBC integrity
• Vitamin K	• Blood clotting (catalyzes synthesis of prothrombin by liver)

carbohydrates and proteins or from the fatty acids and glycerol products of lipolysis. Adipose tissue is the primary storage site for excess fat and thus is the greatest source of energy reserve. Certain unsaturated fatty acids are necessary for synthesis of vital body compounds. Because the body cannot produce these essential fatty acids, they must be provided through diet. Insulin, GH, catecholamines, ACTH, and glucocorticoids control fat metabolism in an inverse relationship with carbohydrate metabolism; large amounts of carbohydrates promote fat storage, and deficiency of available carbohydrates promotes fat breakdown for energy needs.

Proteins: Anabolism

The primary process in protein metabolism is anabolism. Catabolism is relegated to a supporting role in protein metabolism—a reversal of the roles played by these two processes in carbohydrate and fat metabolisms. By synthesizing proteins—the tissue-building foods—the body derives substances essential for life, such as plasma proteins, and can reproduce, control cell growth, and repair itself. However, when carbohydrates or fats are unavailable as energy sources, or when energy demands are exceedingly high, protein catabolism converts protein into an available energy source. Protein metabolism consists of many processes, including:

- Deamination: a catabolic and energy-producing process occurring in the liver with the splitting off of the amino acid to form ammonia and a keto acid
- Transamination: anabolic conversion of keto acids to amino acids
- Urea formation: a catabolic process occurring in the liver, producing urea, the end product of protein catabolism.

GH and the male hormone testosterone stimulate protein anabolism; ACTH prompts secretion of glucocorticoids, which, in turn, facilitate protein catabolism. Normally, the rate of protein anabolism equals the rate of protein catabolism—a condition known as nitrogen balance (because ingested nitrogen equals nitrogen waste excreted in urine, feces, and sweat). When excessive catabolism causes the amount of nitrogen excreted to exceed the amount ingested, a state of *negative nitrogen balance* exists—usually the result of starvation and cachexia.

Fluid and electrolyte balance

A critical component of metabolism is fluid and electrolyte balance. Water is an essential body substance and constitutes almost 60% of an adult's body weight and more than 75% of a newborn's body weight. In both older and obese adults, the ratio of water to body weight drops; children and lean people have a higher proportion of water in their bodies.

Body fluids can be classified as intracellular (or cellular) and extracellular. Intracellular fluid constitutes about 50% of total body weight and 60% of all body fluid and contains large quantities of potassium and phosphates but very little sodium and chloride. Conversely, extracellular fluid contains mostly sodium and chloride but very little potassium and phosphates. Divided into interstitial, cerebrospinal, intraocular, and gastrointestinal fluids and plasma, extracellular fluid supplies cells with nutrients and other substances needed for cellular function. The many components of body fluids have the important function of preserving osmotic pressure and acid-base and anion-cation balance.

Homeostasis is a stable state—the equilibrium of chemical and physical properties of body fluid. Body fluids contain two kinds of dissolved substances: those that dissociate in solution (electrolytes) and those that do not. For example, glucose, when dissolved in water, does not break down into smaller particles; but sodium chloride dissociates in solution into sodium cations (+) and chloride anions (−). The composition of these electrolytes in body fluids is electrically balanced so the positively charged ions (cations: sodium, potassium, calcium, and magnesium) equal the negatively charged ions (anions: chloride, bicarbonate, sulfate, phos-

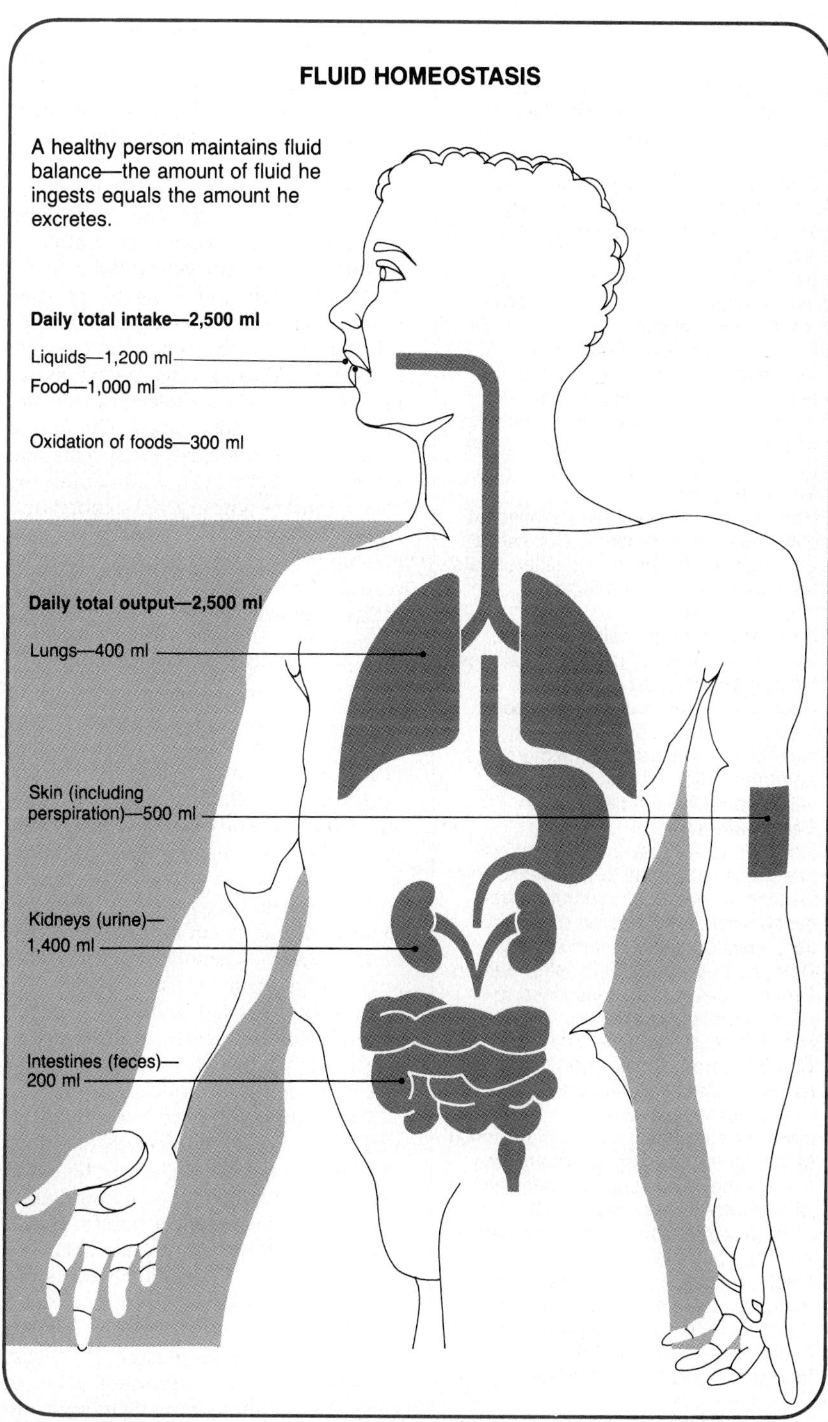
FLUID HOMEOSTASIS
A healthy person maintains fluid balance—the amount of fluid he ingests equals the amount he excretes.
Daily total intake—2,500 ml
Liquids—1,200 ml
Food—1,000 ml
Oxidation of foods—300 ml
Daily total output—2,500 ml
Lungs—400 ml
Skin (including perspiration)—500 ml
Kidneys (urine)—1,400 ml
Intestines (feces)—200 ml

LABORATORY TESTS: ASSESSING NUTRITIONAL STATUS

Blood and urine tests provide the most precise data about nutritional status. In fact, they often reveal nutritional problems before they're clinically apparent. The list below explains some common laboratory tests and what their results may indicate.

Serum vitamins and minerals
Vitamins commonly screened for deficiency include A, B, B_{12}, folic acid, ascorbic acid, beta carotene, riboflavin, and, sometimes, zinc, calcium, magnesium, and other minerals.

Serum nutrients
Glucose levels help assess suspected diabetes or hypoglycemia. Cholesterol and triglyceride levels help differentiate the type of hyperlipoproteinemia.

Nitrogen balance
A negative nitrogen balance indicates inadequate intake of protein or calories.

Hemoglobin and hematocrit
Decreased levels can occur in protein-calorie malnutrition, but they can also reflect overhydration, hemorrhage, and hemolytic disease. Elevated values may occur in dehydration.

Serum albumin
Reduced levels may indicate visceral protein depletion due to GI disease, liver disease, or nephrotic syndrome. Reduced levels also occur in overhydration, elevated levels in dehydration.

Delayed hypersensitivity skin testing
One or more positive responses, in 24 to 48 hours, to intradermally injected common recall antigens (mumps virus, *Candida,* streptokinase-streptodornase) indicates intact cell-mediated immunity. Negative, delayed, or absent response may indicate protein-calorie malnutrition (although trauma, sepsis, and chemotherapy may also suppress immunity).

Creatinine-height index (CHI)
This calculated value, based on creatinine clearance and the patient's height, reflects muscle mass and estimates muscle protein depletion. Reduced CHI may indicate protein-calorie malnutrition; however, it may also indicate impaired renal function.

phate, proteinate, and carbonic and other organic acids). Although these particles are present in relatively low concentrations, any deviation from their normal levels can have profound physiologic effects.

In homeostasis—an ever-changing but balanced state—water and electrolytes and other solutes move continually between cellular and extracellular compartments. Such motion is made possible by semipermeable membranes that allow diffusion, filtration, and active transport. Diffusion refers to the movement of particles or molecules from an area of greater concentration to one of lesser concentration. Normally, particles move randomly and constantly until the concentrations within given solutions are equal. Diffusion also depends on permeability, electrical gradient, and pressure gradient. Particles, however, cannot diffuse against any of these gradients without energy and a carrier substance (active transport). ATP is released from cells to aid particles needing energy to pass through the cell membrane.

The diffusion of water from a solution of low concentration to one of high concentration is called osmosis. The pressure that develops when a selectively permeable cell membrane separates solutions of different strengths of concentrations is known as osmotic pressure, expressed in terms of osmols or milliosmols (mOsm). Osmotic activity is described in terms of osmolality—the osmotic pull exerted by all particles per unit of water, expressed in mOsm/kg of water—or osmolarity, when expressed in mOsm/liter of solution.

The normal range of body fluid osmolality is 285 to 295 mOsm. Solutions of 50 mOsm above or below the high and low points of this normal range exert little or no osmotic effect (isosmolality). A solution below 240 mOsm contains a lower particle concentration than plasma (hypo-osmolar), while a solution over 340 mOsm has a higher particle concentration than plasma (hyperosmolar). Rapid I.V. administration of isosmolar solutions to patients who are debilitated, are very old or very young, or have cardiac or renal insufficiency could lead to extracellular fluid volume overload and induce pulmonary edema and congestive heart failure.

Continuous I.V. administration of hypo-osmolar solutions decreases serum osmolality and leads to excess intracellular fluid volume (water intoxication). Continuous I.V. administration of hyperosmolar solutions results in intracellular dehydration, increased serum osmolality, and, eventually, extracellular fluid volume deficit due to excessive urinary excretion.

Regulation of pH

Primarily through the complex chemical regulation of carbonic acid by the lungs and of base bicarbonate by the kidneys, the body maintains the hydrogen ion concentration to keep the extracellular fluid pH between 7.35 and 7.45. Nutritional deficiency or excess, disease, injury, or metabolic disturbance can interfere with normal homeostatic mechanisms and cause a lowering of pH (acidosis) or a rise in pH (alkalosis).

Assessing homeostasis

The goal of metabolism and homeostasis is to maintain the complex environment of extracellular fluid—the plasma—which nourishes and supports every body cell. This special environment is subject to multiple interlocking influences and readily reflects any disturbance in nutrition, chemical or fluid content, and osmotic pressure. Such disturbances are detectable by various laboratory determinations. For example, measurements of albumin-transferrin and other blood proteins, electrolyte concentration, enzyme and antibody levels, and urine and blood chemistry levels (lipoproteins, glucose, BUN, creatinine, and creatinine-height index) accurately reflect the state of metabolism, homeostasis, and nutrition throughout the body. Results of such laboratory tests, of course, supplement the information obtained from dietary history and physical examination—which offer gross clinical information about the quality, quantity, and efficiency of metabolic processes. To support such clinical information, anthropometry, height-weight ratio, and skin-fold thickness determinations offer specific determination of tissue nutritional status.

The following measures can help you maintain your patient's homeostasis:

- Obtain a complete dietary history to determine if carbohydrate, fat, protein, vitamin, mineral, and water intake is adequate to meet the body's needs for energy production and for tissue repair and growth. Remember that during periods of rapid tissue synthesis (growth, pregnancy, healing), protein needs increase.
- Consult a dietitian about any patient who may be malnourished (malabsorption syndromes, renal or hepatic disease, clear-liquid diets). Carefully planned meals that provide adequate amounts of carbohydrates, fats, and protein are necessary for convalescence. Supplementary carbohydrate snacks are often needed to spare protein and achieve a positive nitrogen balance.
- Accurately record intake and output to assess fluid balance (this includes intake of oral liquids or I.V. solutions, and urine, gastric, and stool ouput).
- Weigh the patient daily—at the same time, with the same-type clothing, and on the same scale. Remember, a weight loss of 2.2 lb (1 kg) is equivalent to the loss of 1 liter of fluid.
- Observe the patient closely for insensible water or unmeasured fluid losses (such as through diaphoresis). Remember, fluid loss from the skin and lungs (normally 900 ml/day) can reach as high as 2,000 ml/day from diaphoresis and hyperventilation.
- Recognize I.V. solutions that are hypo-osmolar, such as 0.45% NaCl (half–normal saline solution). Isosmolar solutions include normal saline solution (0.9% NaCl), 5% dextrose in 0.2% NaCl, Ringer's solutions, and 5% dextrose in water. Examples of hyperosmolar solutions are 5% dextrose in normal saline solution, 10% dextrose in water, and 5% dextrose in Ringer's lactate solution.

• When continuously administering hypo-osmolar solutions, watch for signs of water intoxication: headaches, behavior changes (confusion or disorientation), nausea, vomiting, rising blood pressure, and falling pulse rate.
• When continuously administering hyperosmolar solutions, be alert for signs of hypovolemia: thirst, dry mucous membranes, slightly falling blood pressure, rising pulse rate and respirations, low-grade fever (99° F. [37.2° C.]), and elevated hematocrit, hemoglobin, and BUN.
• Administer fluid cautiously, especially to the patient with cardiopulmonary disease, and watch for signs of overhydration: constant and irritating cough, dyspnea, moist rales, rising central venous pressure, and pitting edema (late sign). When the patient is in an upright position, neck and hand vein engorgement is a common sign of fluid overload, possibly from administration of hyperosmolar solutions.
• Teach elderly patients and others vulnerable to fluid imbalances, and parents of newborns, the importance of maintaining adequate fluid intake.

NUTRITIONAL IMBALANCE

Vitamin A Deficiency

A fat-soluble vitamin absorbed in the gastrointestinal tract, vitamin A maintains epithelial tissue and retinal function. Consequently, deficiency of this vitamin may result in night blindness, decreased color adjustment, keratinization of epithelial tissue, and poor bone growth. Healthy adults have adequate vitamin A reserves to last up to a year; children often do not. Each year, more than 80,000 persons worldwide—mostly children in underdeveloped countries—lose their sight from severe vitamin A deficiency. This condition is rare in the United States, although many disadvantaged children have substandard levels of vitamin A. With therapy, the chance of reversing symptoms of night blindness and milder conjunctival changes is excellent. When corneal damage is present, emergency treatment is necessary.

Causes

Vitamin A deficiency usually results from inadequate dietary intake of foods high in vitamin A (liver, kidney, butter, milk, cream, cheese, and fortified margarine) or carotene, a precursor of vitamin A found in dark green leafy vegetables, and yellow or orange fruits and vegetables.

Less common causes include:
• *malabsorption* due to celiac disease, sprue, obstructive jaundice, cystic fibrosis, giardiasis, or habitual use of mineral oil as a laxative.
• *massive urinary excretion* caused by cancer, tuberculosis, pneumonia, nephritis, or urinary tract infection.
• *decreased storage and transport* of vitamin A due to hepatic disease.

Signs and symptoms

Typically, the first symptom of vitamin A deficiency is night blindness (nyctalopia), which usually becomes apparent when the patient enters a dark place or is caught in the glare of oncoming headlights while driving at night. This condition can progress to xerophthalmia, or drying of the conjunctivas, with development of gray plaques (Bitot's spots); if unchecked, perforation, scarring, and blindness may result. Keratinization of epithelial tissue causes dry, scaly skin; follicular hyperkeratosis; and shrinking and hardening of the mucous membranes, possibly leading to infections of the eyes and the respiratory or genitourinary tract. An infant with severe vitamin A deficiency shows signs of failure to thrive and apathy, along with dry skin and corneal changes, which can lead to ulceration and rapid destruction of the cornea.

Diagnosis

Dietary history and characteristic ocular lesions suggest vitamin A deficiency.

Decreased carotene levels (less than 40 mcg/dl) also suggest vitamin A deficiency, but they fluctuate with seasonal ingestion of fruits and vegetables. Serum levels of vitamin A that fall below 20 mcg/dl confirm vitamin A deficiency.

Treatment

Mild conjunctival changes or night blindness requires vitamin A replacement in the form of cod liver oil or halibut liver oil. Acute deficiency requires aqueous vitamin A solution I.M., especially when corneal changes have occurred. Therapy for underlying biliary obstruction consists of administration of bile salts; for pancreatic insufficiency, pancreatin. Dry skin responds well to cream- or petrolatum-based products.

In patients with chronic malabsorption of fat-soluble vitamins, and in those with low dietary intake, prevention of vitamin A deficiency requires aqueous I.V. supplements or a water-miscible preparation P.O.

Special considerations

- Administer oral vitamin A supplements with or after meals or parenterally, as ordered. Watch for signs of hypercarotenemia (orange coloration of the skin and eyes) and hypervitaminosis A (rash, hair loss, anorexia, transient hydrocephalus, and vomiting in children; bone pain, hepatosplenomegaly, diplopia, and irritability in adults). If these signs occur, discontinue supplements, and notify the doctor immediately. (Hypercarotenemia is relatively harmless; hypervitaminosis A may be toxic.)
- Since vitamin A deficiency usually results from dietary insufficiency, provide nutritional counseling and, if necessary, referral to an appropriate community agency.

Vitamin B Deficiencies

Vitamin B complex is a group of water-soluble vitamins essential to normal metabolism, cell growth, and blood formation. The most common deficiencies involve thiamine (B_1), riboflavin (B_2), niacin, pyridoxine (B_6), and cobalamin (B_{12}).

Causes and incidence

Thiamine deficiency results from malabsorption or inadequate dietary intake of vitamin B_1. Beriberi, a serious thiamine-deficiency disease, is most prevalent in Orientals, who subsist mainly on diets of unenriched rice and wheat. Although this disease is uncommon in the United States, alcoholics may develop cardiac (wet) beriberi with high-output congestive heart failure, neuropathy, and cerebral disturbances. In times of stress (pregnancy, for example), malnourished young adults may develop beriberi; infantile beriberi may appear in infants on low-protein diets or in those breast-fed by thiamine-deficient mothers.

Riboflavin deficiency (ariboflavinosis) results from a diet deficient in milk, meat, fish, green leafy vegetables, and legumes. Chronic alcoholism or prolonged diarrhea may also induce deficiency of riboflavin (or of any of the other water-soluble B-complex vitamins). Exposure of milk to sunlight or treatment of legumes with baking soda can destroy riboflavin.

Niacin deficiency, in its advanced form,

produces pellagra, which affects the skin, central nervous system, and gastrointestinal tract. Although this deficiency is now rarely found in the United States, it was once common among Southerners who subsisted mainly on corn and consumed minimal animal protein. (Corn is low in niacin and in available tryptophan, the amino acid from which the body synthesizes niacin.) Niacin deficiency is still common in parts of Egypt, Yugoslavia, Romania, and Africa, where corn is the dominant staple food. Niacin deficiency can also occur secondary to carcinoid syndrome or Hartnup disease.

Pyridoxine deficiency usually results from destruction of pyridoxine by autoclaving infant formulas. A frank deficiency is uncommon in adults, except in patients taking pyridoxine antagonists, such as isoniazid and penicillamine.

Cobalamin deficiency most commonly results from an absence of intrinsic factor in gastric secretions, or an absence of receptor sites after ileal resection. Other causes include malabsorption syndromes associated with diverticulosis, sprue, intestinal infestation, regional ileitis, and gluten enteropathy, and a diet low in animal protein.

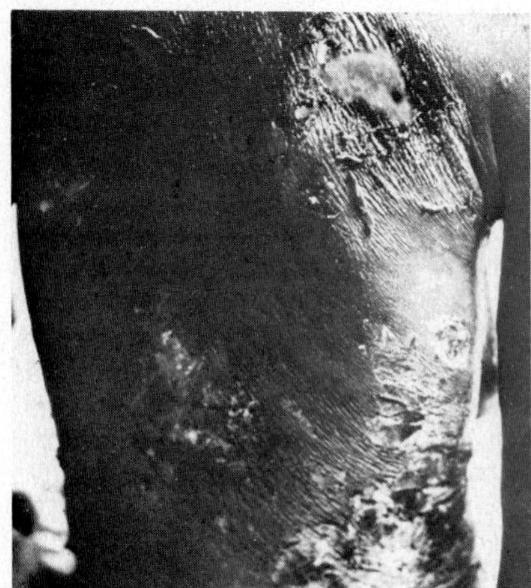

This patient with pellagra shows dark, scaly, advanced dermatitis. Such dermatitis usually occurs on areas exposed to the sun.

Signs and symptoms

Thiamine deficiency causes polyneuritis and, possibly, Wernicke's encephalopathy and Korsakoff's psychosis. In infants (infantile beriberi), this deficiency produces edema, irritability, abdominal pain, pallor, vomiting, loss of voice, and possibly convulsions. In wet beriberi, severe edema starts in the legs and moves up through the body; dry beriberi causes multiple neurologic symptoms and an emaciated appearance. Thiamine deficiency may also cause cardiomegaly, palpitations, tachycardia, dyspnea, and circulatory collapse. Constipation and indigestion are common; ataxia, nystagmus, and ophthalmoplegia are also possible.

Riboflavin deficiency characteristically causes cheilosis (cracking of the lips and corners of the mouth), sore throat, and glossitis. It may also cause seborrheic dermatitis in the nasolabial folds, scrotum, and vulva, and possibly, generalized dermatitis involving the arms, legs, and trunk. This deficiency can also affect the eyes, producing burning, itching, light sensitivity, tearing, and vascularization of the corneas. Late-stage riboflavin deficiency causes neuropathy, mild anemia, and in children, growth retardation.

Niacin deficiency in its early stages produces fatigue, anorexia, muscle weakness, headache, indigestion, mild skin eruptions, weight loss, and backache. In advanced stages (pellagra), it produces dark, scaly dermatitis, especially on exposed parts of the body, that makes the patient appear to be severely sunburned. The mouth, tongue, and lips become red and sore, which may interfere with eating. Common GI symptoms include nausea, vomiting, and diarrhea. Associated CNS aberrations—confusion, disorientation, and neuritis—may become severe enough to induce hallucinations and paranoia. Because of this triad of symptoms, pellagra is sometimes called a "3-D" syndrome—dementia, dermatitis, and diarrhea. If not reversed by therapeutic doses of niacin, pellagra can be fatal.

RECOMMENDED DAILY ALLOWANCE OF B-COMPLEX VITAMINS

VITAMIN	MEN (23-50)	WOMEN (23-50)	INFANTS	CHILDREN (1-10)
B_1*	1.4 mg	1.0 mg	0.4 mg	0.7 to 1.2 mg
B_2*	1.6 mg	1.2 mg	0.5 mg	0.8 to 1.4 mg
niacin*	18 mg	13 mg	5 to 8 mg	9 to 16 mg
B_6	2.2 mg	2.0 mg	0.4 mg	0.9 to 1.6 mg
B_{12}	3 mcg	3 mcg	0.3 mcg	2.0 to 3.0 mg

requirements per 1,000 kilocalories of dietary intake

Pyridoxine deficiency in infants causes a wide range of distressing symptoms: dermatitis, occasional cheilosis or glossitis that does not respond to riboflavin therapy, abdominal pain, vomiting, ataxia, and convulsions. This deficiency can also lead to CNS disturbances, particularly in infants.

Cobalamin deficiency causes pernicious anemia, which produces various GI symptoms (anorexia, weight loss, abdominal discomfort, constipation, diarrhea, and glossitis); peripheral neuropathy; and, possibly, spinal cord involvement (ataxia, spasticity, and hyperactive reflexes).

Diagnosis

The following values confirm vitamin B deficiency:

- *Thiamine deficiency:* serum thiamine levels less than 2 mcg/dl; elevated levels of serum pyruvate and alpha-ketoglutarate, especially after exercise and glucose administration; low thiamine concentration in urine
- *Riboflavin deficiency:* serum riboflavin level less than 15 mcg/dl
- *Niacin deficiency:* serum niacin levels less than 30 mcg/dl; diminished or absent metabolites (N-methyl niacinamide and N-methylpyridone) in urine
- *Pyridoxine deficiency:* xanthurenic acid more than 50 mg/day in 24-hour urine collection after administration of 10 g L-tryptophan; decreased levels of serum and RBC transaminases; reduced excretion of pyridoxic acid in urine
- *Cobalamin deficiency:* cobalamin serum levels less than 150 pg/ml. Tests to discover the cause of the deficiency include gastric analysis and hemoglobin studies. In addition, Schilling test measures absorption of radioactive cobalamin with and without intrinsic factor; X-rays must rule out gastric cancer, which is common among patients with pernicious anemia.

Prevention and treatment

Appropriate dietary adjustments and supplementary vitamins can prevent or correct vitamin B deficiencies:

- *Thiamine deficiency:* a high-protein diet, with adequate calorie intake, possibly supplemented by B-complex vitamins for early symptoms. Thiamine-rich foods include pork, peas, wheat bran, oatmeal, and liver. Alcoholic beriberi may require thiamine supplements or administration of thiamine hydrochloride as part of a B-complex concentrate.
- *Riboflavin deficiency*: supplemental riboflavin in patients with intractable diarrhea or increased demand for riboflavin as a result of growth, pregnancy, lactation, or wound healing. Good sources of riboflavin are meats, enriched flour, milk and dairy foods, green leafy vegetables, eggs, and cereal. Acute riboflavin deficiency requires daily oral doses of riboflavin alone or in combination with other B-complex vitamins. Riboflavin supplements can also be administered I.V. or I.M. as the sodium salt of riboflavin phosphate.
- *Niacin deficiency*: supplemental B-complex vitamins and dietary enrichment in patients at risk due to marginal diets or alcoholism. Meats, fish, peanuts, brewer's yeast, enriched breads, and cereals are rich in niacin; milk and eggs, in tryptophan. Confirmed niacin deficiency requires daily doses of niacin-

amide P.O. or I.V.

• *Pyridoxine deficiency*: prophylactic pyridoxine therapy in infants and epileptic children; supplemental B-complex vitamins in patients with anorexia, malabsorption, or those taking isoniazid or penicillamine. Some women who take oral contraceptives may have to supplement their diets with pyridoxine. Confirmed pyridoxine deficiencies require oral or parenteral pyridoxine. Children with convulsive seizures stemming from metabolic dysfunction may require daily doses of 200 to 600 mg pyridoxine.

• *Cobalamin deficiency*: parenteral cyanocobalamin in patients with reduced gastric secretion of hydrochloric acid, lack of intrinsic factor, some malabsorption syndromes, or ileum resections. Strict vegetarians may have to supplement their diets with oral vitamin B_{12}. Depending on the severity of the deficiency, supplementary cyanocobalamin is usually given parenterally for 5 to 10 days, followed by monthly or daily vitamin B_{12} supplements.

Special considerations

An accurate dietary history provides a baseline for effective dietary counseling.

• Identify and observe patients who risk vitamin B deficiencies—alcoholics, the elderly, pregnant women, and persons on limited diets.

• Administer prescribed supplements. Make sure patients understand how important it is that they adhere strictly to their prescribed treatment for the rest of their lives. Watch for side effects from large doses of niacinamide, in patients with niacin deficiency. Remember, prolonged intake of niacin can cause hepatic dysfunction. Caution patients with Parkinson's disease receiving pyridoxine that this drug can impair response to levodopa therapy.

• Explain all tests and procedures. Reassure patients that, with treatment, prognosis is good. Refer patients to appropriate assistance agencies if their diets are inadequate due to socioeconomic conditions.

Vitamin C Deficiency

(Scurvy)

Vitamin C (ascorbic acid) deficiency leads to scurvy or inadequate production of collagen, an extracellular substance that binds the cells of the teeth, bones, and capillaries. Historically common among sailors and others deprived of fresh fruits and vegetables for long periods of time, vitamin C deficiency is uncommon today in the United States, except in alcoholics, persons on restricted-residue diets, and infants weaned from breast milk to cow's milk without a vitamin C supplement.

Causes

The primary cause of this deficiency is a diet lacking foods rich in vitamin C, such as citrus fruits, tomatoes, cabbage, broccoli, spinach, and berries. Since the body can't store this water-soluble vitamin in large amounts, the supply needs to be replenished daily. Other causes include:

• destruction of vitamin C in foods by overexposure to air or by overcooking.

• excessive ingestion of vitamin C during pregnancy, which causes the newborn to require large amounts of the vitamin after birth.

• marginal intake of vitamin C during periods of physiologic stress—caused by infectious disease, for example—which can deplete tissue saturation of vitamin C.

Signs and symptoms

Clinical features of vitamin C deficiency appear as capillaries become increasingly fragile. In an adult, it produces petechiae, ecchymoses, follicular hyperkeratosis (especially on the buttocks and legs), anemia, anorexia, limb and joint pain (especially in the knees), pallor, weakness, swollen or bleeding gums, loose teeth, lethargy, insomnia, poor wound healing, and ocular hemorrhages in the bulbar conjunctivae. Vitamin C deficiency can also cause beading, fractures of the costochondral junctions of the ribs or epiphysis, and psychological disturbances—irritability, depression, hysteria, and hypochondriasis.

In a child, vitamin C deficiency produces tender, painful swelling in the legs, causing the child to lie with his legs partially flexed. Other symptoms include fever, diarrhea, and vomiting.

Diagnosis

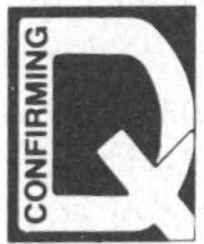

Dietary history revealing an inadequate intake of ascorbic acid suggests vitamin C deficiency; serum ascorbic acid levels less than 0.4 mg/dl and WBC ascorbic acid levels less than 25 mg/dl help confirm it.

Treatment

Since scurvy is potentially fatal, treatment begins immediately to restore adequate vitamin C intake by daily doses of 100 to 200 mg vitamin C in synthetic form or in orange juice in mild disease and by doses as high as 500 mg/day in severe disease. Symptoms usually subside in 2 to 3 days; hemorrhages and bone disorders, in 2 to 3 weeks.

To prevent vitamin C deficiency, patients unable or unwilling to consume foods rich in vitamin C or those facing surgery should take daily supplements of ascorbic acid. Vitamin C supplement may also prevent this deficiency in recently weaned infants or those drinking formula not fortified with vitamin C.

Special considerations

- Administer ascorbic acid P.O. or by slow I.V. infusion, as ordered. Avoid moving the patient unnecessarily to prevent irritation of painful joints and muscles. Encourage him to drink orange juice.

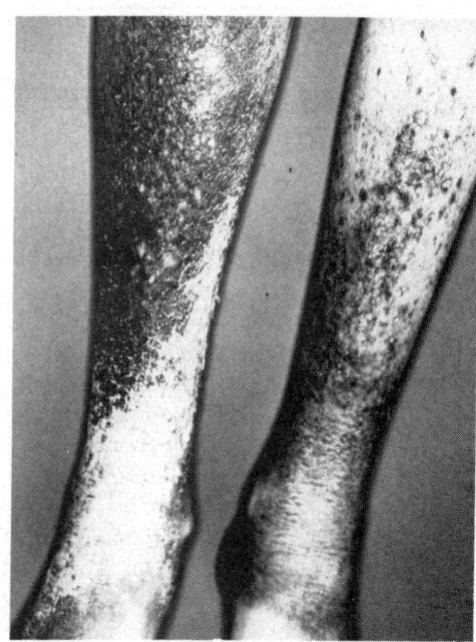

Follicular hyperkeratosis from scurvy usually occurs on the legs.

- Explain the importance of supplemental ascorbic acid. Counsel the patient and his family about good dietary sources of vitamin C.
- However, discourage the patient from taking too much vitamin C. Explain that excessive doses of ascorbic acid may cause nausea, diarrhea, and renal calculi formation and may also interfere with anticoagulant therapy.

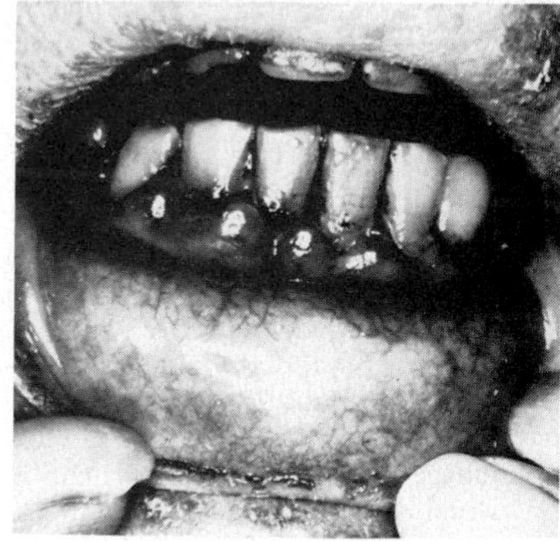

In adults, scurvy causes swollen or bleeding gums and loose teeth.

Vitamin D Deficiency

(Rickets)

Vitamin D deficiency causes failure of normal bone calcification, which results in rickets in infants and young children, and osteomalacia in adults. With treatment, prognosis is good. However, in rickets, bone deformities usually persist, while in osteomalacia, deformities may disappear.

Causes and incidence

Vitamin D deficiency results from inadequate dietary intake of preformed vitamin D, malabsorption of vitamin D, or too little exposure to sunlight.

Once a common childhood disease, rickets is now rare in the United States but occasionally appears in breast-fed infants who do not receive a vitamin D supplement or in infants receiving a formula with a nonfortified milk base. This deficiency may also occur in overcrowded, urban areas where smog limits sunlight penetration; incidence is highest in Black children who, because of their pigmentation, absorb less sunlight. (Solar ultraviolet rays irradiate 7-dehydrocholesterol, a precursor of vitamin D, to form calciferol.)

Osteomalacia, also uncommon in the United States, is most prevalent in the Orient, among young multiparas who eat a cereal diet and have minimal exposure to sunlight. Other causes include:

- *vitamin D–resistant rickets* (refractory rickets, familial hypophosphatemia) from an inherited impairment of renal tubular reabsorption of phosphate (from vitamin D insensitivity).
- *conditions that lower absorption of fat-soluble vitamin D,* such as chronic pancreatitis, celiac disease, Crohn's disease, cystic fibrosis, gastric or small bowel resections, fistulas, colitis, and biliary obstruction.
- *hepatic or renal disease,* which interferes with the formation of hydroxylated calciferol, necessary to initiate the formation of a calcium-binding protein in intestinal absorption sites.
- *malfunctioning parathyroid gland* (decreased secretion of parathyroid hormone), which contributes to calcium deficiency (normally, vitamin D controls absorption of calcium and phosphorus through the intestine) and interferes with activation of vitamin D in the kidneys.

Signs and symptoms

Early indications of vitamin D deficiency are profuse sweating, restlessness, and irritability. Chronic deficiency induces numerous bone malformations due to softening of the bones: bowlegs, knock-knees, rachitic rosary (beading of ends of ribs), enlargement of wrists and ankles, pigeon breast, delayed closing of the fontanelles, softening of the skull, and bulging of the forehead. Other rachitic features are poorly developed muscles (potbelly) and infantile tetany. These bone deformities may also produce difficulty in walking and in climbing stairs, spontaneous multiple fractures, and pain in the legs and lower back.

Diagnosis

Physical examination, dietary history, and laboratory tests establish diagnosis. Test results include plasma calcium serum levels <7.5 mg/100 ml, inorganic phosphorus serum levels <3 mg/100 ml, serum citrate levels <2.5 mg/100 ml, and alkaline phosphatase <4 Bodansky units/100 ml—all of which suggest vitamin D deficiency.

X-rays confirm diagnosis by showing characteristic bone deformities and abnormalities, such as Looser's zones.

Treatment and special considerations

For osteomalacia and rickets—except

when due to malabsorption—treatment consists of massive P.O. doses of vitamin D or cod liver oil. For rickets refractory to vitamin D or in rickets accompanied by hepatic or renal disease, treatment includes 25-hydroxycholecalciferol, 1,25-dihydroxycholecalciferol, or a synthetic analog of active vitamin D.

- Obtain a dietary history to assess the patient's current vitamin D intake. Encourage him to eat foods high in vitamin D—fortified milk, fish liver oils, herring, liver, and egg yolks—and get sufficient sun exposure. If deficiency is due to socioeconomic conditions, refer the patient to an appropriate community agency.
- If the patient must take vitamin D for a prolonged period, tell him to watch for signs of vitamin D toxicity (headache, nausea, constipation, and, after prolonged use, renal calculi).
- To prevent rickets, administer supplementary aqueous preparations of vitamin D for chronic fat malabsorption, hydroxylated cholecalciferol for refractory rickets, and supplemental vitamin D for breast-fed infants.

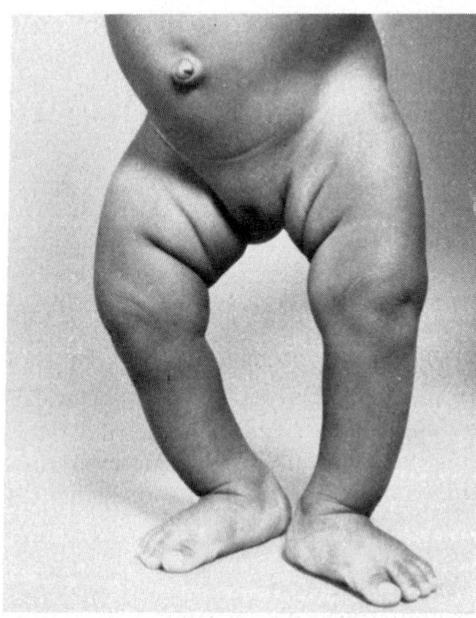

This infant with rickets shows characteristic bowing of the legs.

Vitamin E Deficiency

In humans, vitamin E (tocopherol) appears to act primarily as an antioxidant, preventing intracellular oxidation of polyunsaturated fatty acids and other lipids. Deficiency of vitamin E usually manifests as hemolytic anemia in low–birth-weight or premature infants. With treatment, prognosis is good.

Causes and incidence

Vitamin E deficiency in infants usually results from formulas high in polyunsaturated fatty acids that are fortified with iron but not vitamin E. Such formulas increase the need for antioxidant vitamin E, because the iron supplement catalyzes the oxidation of RBC lipids. A newborn has low tissue concentrations of vitamin E to begin with, since only a small amount passes through the placenta; the mother retains most of it. Since vitamin E is a fat-soluble vitamin, deficiency develops in conditions associated with fat malabsorption, such as kwashiorkor, celiac disease, or cystic fibrosis. These conditions may induce megaloblastic or hemolytic anemia, and creatinuria, all of which are reversible with vitamin E administration.

Vitamin E deficiency is uncommon in adults but is possible in persons whose diets are high in polyunsaturated fatty acids, which increase vitamin E requirements, and in persons with vitamin E malabsorption, which impairs red blood cell survival.

Signs and symptoms

Vitamin E deficiency is difficult to recognize, but its early symptoms include edema and skin lesions in infants and muscle weakness or intermittent claudication in adults. In premature infants, vitamin E deficiency produces hemolytic anemia, thrombocythemia, and erythematous papular skin eruption, followed by desquamation.

Diagnosis

Dietary and medical histories suggest vitamin E deficiency.

Serum alpha-tocopherol levels below 0.5 mg/dl in adults and below 0.2 mg/dl in infants confirm it. Creatinuria, increased creatine phosphokinase, hemolytic anemia, and elevated platelet count generally support the diagnosis.

Treatment and special considerations

Replacement of vitamin E with a water-soluble supplement, either P.O. or parenteral, is the only appropriate treatment.

- As ordered, prevent deficiency by providing vitamin E supplements for low-birth-weight infants receiving formulas not fortified with vitamin E and for adults with vitamin E malabsorption. Many commercial multivitamin supplements are easily absorbed by patients with vitamin E malabsorption.
- Inform new mothers who plan to breast-feed that human milk provides adequate vitamin E.
- Encourage adult patients to eat foods high in vitamin E; good sources include vegetable oils (corn, safflower, soybean, cottonseed), whole grains, dark green leafy vegetables, nuts, and legumes. Tell them that heavy consumption of polyunsaturated fatty acids increases the need for vitamin E.
- If vitamin E deficiency is related to socioeconomic conditions, refer the patient to appropriate community agencies.

Vitamin K Deficiency

Deficiency of vitamin K, an element necessary for formation of prothrombin and other clotting factors in the liver, produces abnormal bleeding. If the deficiency is corrected, prognosis is excellent.

Causes and incidence

Vitamin K deficiency is common among newborns in the first few days postpartum due to poor placental transfer of vitamin K and inadequate production of vitamin K–producing intestinal flora. Its other causes include prolonged use of drugs, such as the anticoagulant dicumarol and antibiotics that destroy normal intestinal bacteria; decreased flow of bile to the small intestine from obstruction of the bile duct or bile fistula; malabsorption of vitamin K due to sprue, pellagra, bowel resection, ileitis, or ulcerative colitis; chronic hepatic disease, with impaired response of hepatic ribosomes to vitamin K; and cystic fibrosis, with fat malabsorption. Vitamin K deficiency rarely results from insufficient dietary intake of this vitamin.

Signs and symptoms

The cardinal sign of vitamin K deficiency is an abnormal bleeding tendency, accompanied by prolonged prothrombin time; these signs disappear with administration of vitamin K. Without treatment, such bleeding may be severe and possibly fatal.

Diagnosis

A prothrombin time 25% longer than the normal range of 10 to 20 seconds, measured by the Quick method, confirms the diagnosis of vitamin K deficiency after other causes of prolonged prothrombin time (such as anticoagulant therapy or hepatic disease) have been ruled out. Repetition of this test in 24 hours (and regularly during treatment) monitors success of therapy.

Treatment and special considerations

Administration of vitamin K corrects abnormal bleeding tendencies. To prevent vitamin K deficiency:

- Administer vitamin K to newborns and patients with fat malabsorption or with prolonged diarrhea resulting from colitis, ileitis, or long-term antibiotic drug therapy.
- Warn against self-medication with or overuse of antibiotics, because these drugs destroy the intestinal bacteria necessary to generate significant amounts of vitamin K.
- If the deficiency has a dietary cause, help the patient and family plan a diet that includes important sources of vitamin K, such as green leafy vegetables, cauliflower, tomatoes, cheese, egg yolks, and liver.

Hypervitaminoses A and D

Hypervitaminosis A is excessive accumulation of vitamin A; hypervitaminosis D, of vitamin D. Although these are toxic conditions, they usually respond well to treatment. They are most prevalent in infants and children, usually as a result of accidental or misguided overdosage by parents. A related, benign condition called hypercarotenemia results from excessive consumption of carotene, a chemical precursor of vitamin A.

Causes and incidences

Vitamins A and D are fat-soluble vitamins that accumulate in the body because they aren't dissolved and excreted in the urine. Generally, hypervitaminoses A and D result from ingestion of excessive amounts of supplemental vitamin preparations. A single dose of more than 1 million units of vitamin A can cause acute toxicity; daily doses of 15,000 to 25,000 units taken over weeks or months have proven toxic in infants and children. For the same dose to produce toxicity in adults, ingestion over years is necessary. Ingestion of only 1,600 to 2,000 units of vitamin D is sufficient to cause toxicity.

Hypervitaminosis A may occur in patients receiving pharmacologic doses of vitamin A for dermatologic disorders. Hypervitaminosis D may occur in patients receiving high doses of the vitamin as treatment for hypoparathyroidism, rickets, and the osteodystrophy of chronic renal failure and in infants who consume fortified milk and cereals, plus

IMPORTANT FACTS ABOUT VITAMINS A AND D

VITAMIN	SOURCES	RECOMMENDED DIETARY ALLOWANCE (RDA)	ACTION
Vitamin A	• Carrots, sweet potatoes, dark leafy green vegetables, butter, margarine, liver, egg yolk	• Children: 1,400 IU • Adults: 4,000 to 5,000 IU • Lactating women: 6,000 IU	• Produces retinal pigment and maintains epithelial tissue
Vitamin D	• Ultraviolet light, fortified foods (especially milk)	• 400 IU daily	• Promotes absorption and regulates metabolism of calcium and phosphorus

a vitamin supplement. Concentrations of vitamin A in common foods are generally low enough not to pose a danger of excessive intake. However, a benign condition called hypercarotenemia results from excessive consumption of vegetables high in carotene (a protovitamin that the body converts into vitamin A), such as carrots, sweet potatoes, and dark green leafy vegetables.

Signs and symptoms

Chronic hypervitaminosis A produces anorexia, irritability, headache, hair loss, malaise, itching, vertigo, bone pain, bone fragility, and dry, peeling skin. It may also cause hepatosplenomegaly and emotional lability. Acute toxicity may also produce transient hydrocephalus and vomiting. (Hypercarotenemia manifests yellow or orange skin coloration.)

Hypervitaminosis D causes anorexia, headache, nausea, vomiting, weight loss, polyuria, and polydipsia. Since vitamin D promotes calcium absorption, severe toxicity can lead to hypercalcemia, including calcification of soft tissues, as in the heart, aorta, and renal tubules. Lethargy, confusion, and coma may accompany severe hypercalcemia.

Diagnosis

A thorough patient history suggests hypervitaminosis A; elevated serum vitamin A level (over 90 mcg/dl) confirms it. Patient history and elevated serum calcium level (over 10.1 mg/dl) suggest hypervitaminosis D; elevated serum vitamin D level confirms it. In children, X-rays showing calcification of tendons, ligaments, and subperiosteal tissues support this diagnosis. Elevated serum carotene level (over 250 mcg/dl) confirms hypercarotenemia.

Treatment

Withholding vitamin supplements usually corrects hypervitaminosis A quickly and hypervitaminosis D gradually. Hypercalcemia may persist for weeks or months after the patient stops taking vitamin D. Treatment for severe hypervitaminosis D may include glucocorticoids to control hypercalcemia and prevent renal damage. In the acute stage, diuretics or other emergency measures for severe hypercalcemia may be necessary. Hypercarotenemia responds well to dietary exclusion of foods high in carotene.

Special considerations

- Keep the patient comfortable, and reassure him that symptoms will subside after he stops taking the vitamin.
- Make sure the patient or the parents of a child with these conditions understand that vitamins aren't innocuous. Explain the hazards associated with excessive vitamin intake. Point out that vitamin A and D requirements can easily be met with a diet containing dark green leafy vegetables, fruits, and fortified milk or milk products.
- To prevent hypervitaminosis A or D, monitor serum vitamin A levels in patients receiving doses above the recommended daily dietary allowance and serum calcium levels in patients receiving pharmacologic doses of vitamin D.

Iodine Deficiency

Iodine deficiency is the absence of sufficient levels of iodine to satisfy daily metabolic requirements. Because the thyroid gland uses most of the body's iodine stores, iodine deficiency is apt to cause hypothyroidism and thyroid gland hypertrophy (endemic goiter). Other effects of deficiency range from dental caries to cretinism in infants born to iodine-deficient mothers. Iodine deficiency is most common in pregnant or lactating women due to their exaggerated metabolic need for this element. Iodine deficiency is readily responsive to treatment with iodine supplements.

Causes

Iodine deficiency usually results from insufficient ingestion of dietary sources of iodine, mostly iodized table salt, seafood, and dark green leafy vegetables. (Normal iodine requirements range from 35 mcg/day for infants to 150 mcg/day for lactating women; the average adult needs 1 mcg/kg of body weight.)

Iodine deficiency may also result from an increase in metabolic demands during pregnancy, lactation, and adolescence.

Signs and symptoms

Clinical features of iodine deficiency depend on the degree of hypothyroidism that develops (in addition to the development of a goiter). Mild deficiency may produce only mild, nonspecific symptoms such as lassitude, fatigue, and loss of motivation. Severe deficiency usually generates the typically overt and unmistakable features of hypothyroidism: bradycardia; decreased pulse pressure and cardiac output; weakness; hoarseness; dry, flaky, inelastic skin; puffy face; thick tongue; delayed relaxation phase in deep tendon reflexes; poor memory; hearing loss; chills; anorexia; and nystagmus. In women, iodine deficiency may also cause menorrhagia and amenorrhea.

Cretinism—hypothyroidism that develops in utero or in early infancy—is characterized by failure to thrive, neonatal jaundice, and hypothermia. By age 3 to 6 months, the infant may display spastic diplegia and signs and symptoms similar to those seen in infants with Down's syndrome.

Diagnosis

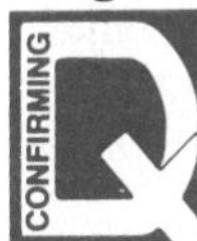

Abnormal laboratory test results include low T_4 with high ^{131}I uptake, low 24-hour urine iodine, and high TSH. Radioiodine uptake test traces ^{131}I in the thyroid 24 hours after administration; T_3- or T_4-resin uptake test shows values 25% below normal.

Treatment and special considerations

Severe iodine deficiency necessitates administration of iodine supplements (potassium iodide [SSKI]). Mild deficiency may be corrected by increasing iodine intake through the use of iodized table salt and consumption of iodine-rich foods (seafood and green leafy vegetables).

- Administer SSKI preparation in milk or juice to reduce gastric irritation and mask its metallic taste. Tell the patient to drink the solution through a straw, to prevent tooth discoloration. Store the solution in a light-resistant container.
- To prevent iodine deficiency, recommend use of iodized salt and consumption of iodine-rich foods for high-risk patients—especially adolescents and pregnant or lactating women.
- Advise pregnant women that severe iodine deficiency may produce cretinism in newborns, and instruct them to watch for early signs of iodine deficiency, such as fatigue, lassitude, weakness, and decreased mental function.

Zinc Deficiency

Zinc, an essential trace element that is present in the bones, teeth, hair, skin, testes, liver, and muscles, is also a vital component of many enzymes. Zinc promotes synthesis of DNA, RNA, and, ultimately, protein and maintains normal blood concentrations of vitamin A by mobilizing it from the liver.

Zinc deficiency is most common in persons from underdeveloped countries, especially in the Middle East. Children are most susceptible to this deficiency during periods of rapid growth. Prognosis is good with correction of the deficiency.

Causes

Zinc deficiency usually results from excessive intake of foods (containing iron, calcium, vitamin D, and the fiber and phytates in cereals) that bind zinc to form insoluble chelates that prevent its absorption. Occasionally, it results from blood loss due to parasitism and low dietary intake of foods containing zinc. Alcohol and corticosteroids increase renal excretion of zinc.

Signs and symptoms

Zinc deficiency produces hepatosplenomegaly, sparse hair growth, soft and misshapen nails, poor wound healing, anorexia, hypogeusesthesia (decreased taste acuity), dysgeusia (unpleasant taste), hyposmia (decreased odor acuity), dysosmia (unpleasant odor in nasopharynx), severe iron deficiency anemia, bone deformities, and, when chronic, hypogonadism, dwarfism, and hyperpigmentation.

Diagnosis

Serum zinc levels below 121 (± 19) mcg/dl confirm zinc deficiency and indicate altered phosphate metabolism, imbalance between aerobic and anaerobic metabolisms, and decreased pancreatic enzymes.

Treatment and special considerations

Treatment consists of correcting the underlying cause of the deficiency and administering zinc supplements, as necessary. Prevention requires a balanced diet including seafood, oatmeal, bran, meat, eggs, nuts, and dry yeast and correct use of calcium and iron supplements. Advise the patient to take zinc supplements with milk or meals to prevent gastric distress and vomiting.

Obesity

Obesity is an excess of body fat, generally 20% above ideal body weight. Prognosis for correction of obesity is poor: fewer than 30% of patients succeed in losing 20 lb (9 kg), and only half of these maintain the loss over a prolonged period.

Causes and incidence

Obesity results from excessive calorie intake and inadequate expenditure of energy. Theories to explain this condition include hypothalamic dysfunction of hunger and satiety centers, genetic predisposition, abnormal absorption of nutrients, and impaired action of gastrointestinal and growth hormones and of hormonal regulators, such as insulin. An inverse relationship between socioeconomic status and the prevalence of obesity has been documented, especially in women. Obesity in parents increases the probability of obesity in children, from genetic or environmental factors, such as activity levels and learned patterns of eating. Psychological factors may also contribute to obesity.

Diagnosis

Observation and comparison of height and weight to a standard table indicate obesity. Measurement of the thickness of subcutaneous fat folds with calipers provides an approximation of total body fat. Although this measurement is reliable and isn't subject to daily fluctuations, it has little meaning for the patient in monitoring subsequent weight loss. Obesity may lead to serious complications, such as respiratory difficulties, hypertension, cardiovascular disease, diabetes mellitus, renal disease, gallbladder disease, and psychosocial difficulties.

Treatment

Successful management of obesity must decrease the patient's daily calorie intake, while increasing his activity level. Effective treatment must be based on a balanced, low-calorie diet that eliminates foods high in fat or sugar. To achieve long-term benefits, lifelong maintenance of these improved eating and exercise patterns is necessary.

The popular low-carbohydrate diets offer no long-term advantage; rapid early weight reduction is due to loss of water, not fat. These and other crash or fad diets have the overwhelming drawback that they don't teach the patient long-term modification of eating patterns and often lead to the "yo-yo syndrome"—episodes of repeated weight loss followed by weight gain.

Total fasting is an effective method of rapid weight reduction but requires close monitoring and supervision to minimize risks of ketonemia, electrolyte imbalance, hypotension, and loss of lean body mass. Prolonged fasting or very low-calorie diets have been associated with sudden death, possibly resulting from cardiac dysrhythmias caused by electrolyte abnormalities. These methods also neglect patient reeducation, which is necessary for long-term weight maintenance.

Treatment may also include hypnosis and behavior modification techniques, which promote fundamental changes in eating habits and activity patterns. In addition, psychotherapy may be beneficial for some patients, since weight reduction may lead to depression or even psychosis.

Amphetamines and amphetamine congeners have been used to enhance compliance with a prescribed diet by temporarily suppressing the appetite and creating a feeling of well-being. However, because their value in long-term weight control is questionable, and they have a significant potential for dependence and abuse, their use is generally avoided. If these drugs are used at all, they should be prescribed only for short-term therapy and should be monitored carefully.

As a last resort, *morbid* obesity (body weight $\geqslant$ 200% of standard) may be treated surgically with gastroplasty (gastric stapling). Gastroplasty decreases the volume of food that the stomach can hold and thus produces satiety with small intake. This technique causes fewer complications than jejunoileal bypass, which induces a permanent malabsorption syndrome.

Special considerations

- Obtain an accurate diet history to identify the patient's eating patterns and the importance of food to his life-style. Ask the patient to keep a careful record of what, where, and when he eats to help identify situations that normally provoke overeating.
- Explain the prescribed diet carefully, and encourage compliance to improve health status.
- To increase calorie expenditure, promote increased physical activity, including an exercise program. Recommended activity levels vary according to the patient's general condition and cardiovascular status.
- If the patient is taking appetite-suppressing drugs, watch carefully for signs of dependence or abuse and for side effects, such as insomnia, excitability, dry mouth, and gastrointestinal disturbances.
- Teach the patient who is grossly obese the importance of good skin care to prevent breakdown in moist skin folds. Regular use of powder to keep skin dry is recommended.
- To help prevent obesity in children, teach parents to avoid overfeeding their infants and to familiarize themselves with actual nutritional needs and optimum growth rates. Discourage parents from using food to reward or console their children, from emphasizing the importance of "clean plates," and from allowing eating to prevent hunger rather than to satisfy it.
- Encourage physical activity and exercise, especially in children and young adults, to establish lifelong patterns. Suggest low-calorie snacks, such as raw vegetables.

Protein-calorie Malnutrition

One of the most prevalent and serious depletion disorders, protein-calorie malnutrition (PCM) occurs as marasmus (protein-calorie deficiency), characterized by growth failure and wasting, and as kwashiorkor (protein deficiency), characterized by tissue edema and damage. Both forms vary from mild to severe and may be fatal, depending on accompanying stress (particularly sepsis or injury) and duration of deprivation. PCM increases the risk of death from pneumonia, chickenpox, or measles.

Causes and incidence

Both marasmus (nonedematous PCM) and kwashiorkor (edematous PCM) are common in underdeveloped countries and in areas where dietary amino acid content is insufficient to satisfy growth requirements. Kwashiorkor typically occurs at about age 1, after infants are weaned from breast milk to a protein-deficient diet of starchy gruels or sugar water, but it can develop at any time during the formative years. Marasmus affects infants aged 6 to 18 months as a result of breast-feeding failure or a debilitating condition, such as chronic diarrhea.

In industrialized countries, PCM may occur secondary to chronic metabolic disease that decreases protein and calorie intake or absorption, or trauma that increases protein and calorie requirements. In the United States, PCM is estimated to occur to some extent in 50% of surgical and 48% of medical patients. Those who are not allowed anything by mouth for an extended period are at high risk of developing PCM. Conditions that increase protein-calorie requirements include severe burns and injuries, systemic infections, and cancer (accounts for the largest group of hospitalized patients with PCM). Conditions that cause defective utilization of nutrients include malabsorption syndrome, short-bowel syndrome, and Crohn's disease.

Signs and symptoms

Children with chronic PCM are small for their chronologic age and tend to be physically inactive, mentally apathetic, and susceptible to frequent infections. Anorexia and diarrhea are common. In acute PCM, children are small, gaunt, and emaciated, with no adipose tissue. Skin is dry and "baggy," and hair is sparse and dull brown or reddish yellow. Temperature is low; pulse rate and respirations, slowed. Such children are weak, irritable, and usually hungry, although they may have anorexia, with nausea and vomiting.

Unlike marasmus, chronic kwashiorkor allows the patient to grow in height, but adipose tissue diminishes as fat metabolizes to meet energy demands. Edema often masks severe muscle wasting; dry, peeling skin and hepatomegaly are common. Patients with secondary PCM show signs similar to marasmus, primarily loss of adipose tissue and lean body mass, lethargy, and edema. Severe secondary PCM may cause loss of immunocompetence.

Diagnosis

Clinical appearance, dietary history, and anthropometry confirm PCM. If the patient does not suffer from fluid retention, weight change over time is the best index of nutritional status. Other factors support the diagnosis:

- height and weight less than 80% of standard for the patient's age and sex, and below standard arm circumference and triceps skinfold
- serum albumin less than 2.8 g/100 ml (normal 3.3 to 4.3 g/100 ml)
- urinary creatinine (24-hour), which shows lean body mass status by relating

CLINICAL FEATURES OF MALNUTRITION

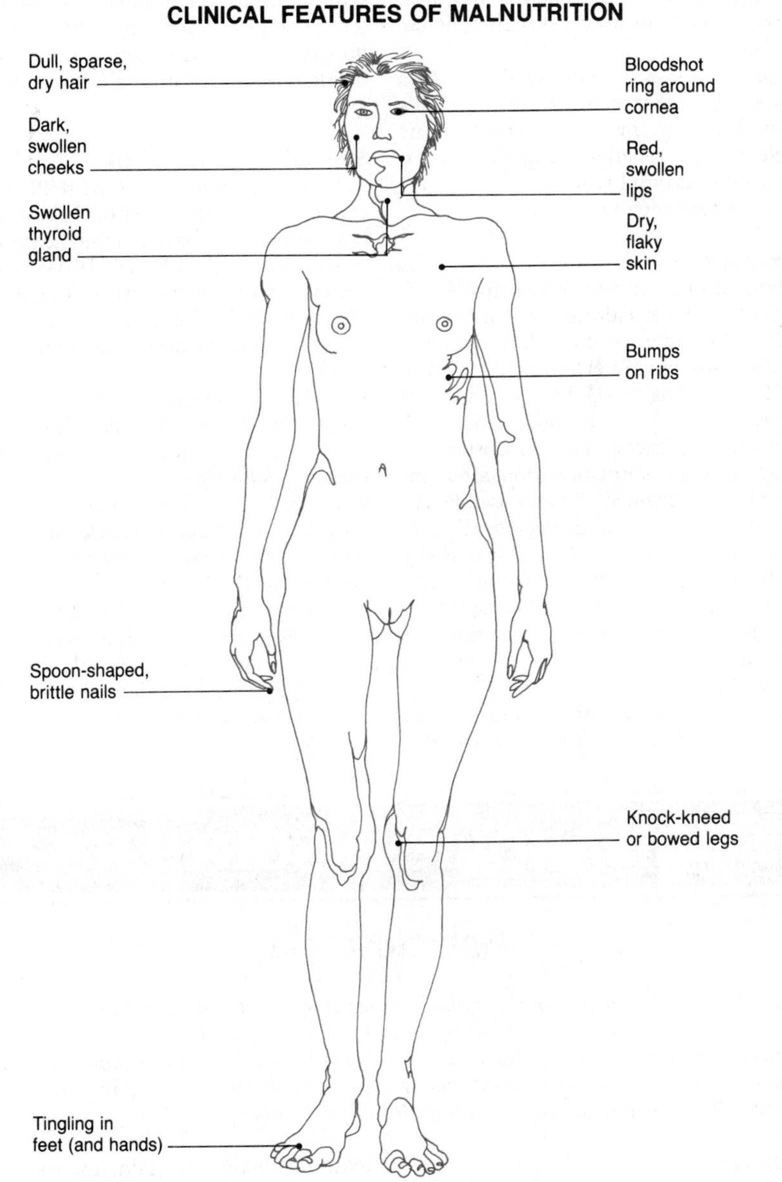

The generalized body reaction to prolonged states of malnourishment produces a characteristic clinical picture of reduced body mass and abnormalities in rapidly regenerating body tissues. In addition, CNS effects cause behavioral modifications: mental apathy; anorexia; lethargy; and in order to preserve the delicate energy balance, chronically limited energy expenditure. Immunologic competence is severely compromised, and mortality from common infectious diseases is abnormally high.

creatinine excretion to height and ideal body weight, to yield creatinine-height index
• skin tests with standard antigens (streptokinase-streptodornase) to indicate degree of immune compromise by determining reactivity expressed as a percent of normal reaction
• moderate anemia.

Treatment
The aim of treatment is to provide sufficient proteins, calories, and other nutrients for nutritional rehabilitation and maintenance. When treating severe PCM, restoring fluid and electrolyte balance parentally is the initial concern. A patient who shows normal absorption may receive enteral nutrition after anorexia has subsided. When possible, the preferred treatment is oral feeding of high-quality protein foods, especially milk, and protein-calorie supplements. A patient who is unwilling or unable to eat may require supplementary feedings through a nasogastric tube or total parenteral nutrition (TPN) through a central venous catheter. Accompanying infection must also be treated, preferably with antibiotics that do not inhibit protein synthesis. Cautious realimentation is essential to prevent complications from overloading the compromised metabolic system.

Special considerations
• Encourage the patient with PCM to consume as much nutritious food and beverage as possible (it's often helpful to "cheer him on" as he eats). Assist the patient to eat, if necessary. Cooperate closely with the dietitian to monitor intake, and provide acceptable meals and snacks.
• If TPN is necessary, observe strict aseptic technique when handling catheters, tubes, and solutions and during dressing changes.
• Watch for PCM in patients who've been hospitalized for a prolonged period, have had no oral intake for several days, or have cachectic disease.
• To help eradicate PCM in developing countries, encourage prolonged breast feeding, educate mothers about their children's needs, and provide supplementary foods, as needed.

METABOLIC DISORDERS

Galactosemia

Galactosemia is any disorder of galactose metabolism. It produces symptoms ranging from cataracts and liver damage to mental retardation and occurs in two forms: classic galactosemia and galactokinase-deficiency galactosemia. Although a galactose-free diet relieves most symptoms, galactosemia-induced mental impairment is irreversible; some residual vision impairment may also persist.

Causes
Both forms of galactosemia are inherited as autosomal recessive defects and occur in about 1 in 60,000 births in the United States. Up to 1.25% of the population is heterozygous for the classic galactosemia gene. Classic galactosemia results from a defect in the enzyme galactose-1-phosphate uridyl transferase. Galactokinase-deficiency galactosemia, the rarer form of this disorder, stems from a deficiency of the enzyme galactokinase. In both forms of galactosemia, the inability to normally metabolize the sugar galactose (which is mainly formed by digestion of the disaccharide lactose that's present in milk) causes galactose accumulation.

Signs and symptoms

In children who are homozygous for the classic galactosemia gene, signs are evident at birth or begin within a few days after milk ingestion, and include failure to thrive, vomiting, and diarrhea. Other clinical effects include liver damage (which causes jaundice, hepatomegaly, cirrhosis, ascites), splenomegaly, galactosuria, proteinuria, and aminoaciduria. Cataracts may also be present at birth or develop later. Pseudotumor cerebri may occur.

Continued ingestion of galactose or lactose-containing foods may cause mental retardation, malnourishment, progressive hepatic failure, and death—from the still unknown process of galactose metabolites accumulating in body tissues. Although treatment may prevent mental impairment, galactosemia can produce a short attention span, difficulty with spatial and mathematical relationships, and apathetic, withdrawn behavior. Cataracts may be the only sign of galactokinase deficiency, resulting from the accumulation of galactitol, a metabolic by-product of galactose, in the lens.

Diagnosis

Deficiency of the enzyme galactose-1-phosphate uridyl transferase in RBCs confirms classic galactosemia; decreased RBC levels of galactokinase confirm galactokinase deficiency. Other related laboratory results include increased galactose levels in blood (normal value in children is less than 20 mg/dl) and urine (must use galactose oxidase to avoid confusion with other reducing sugars). Galactose measurements in blood and urine must be interpreted carefully, because some children who consume large amounts of milk have elevated plasma galactose concentrations and galactosuria but are not galactosemic. Also, newborns excrete galactose in their urine for about a week after birth; premature infants, even longer. Other test results include:

- *liver biopsy:* typical acinar formation
- *liver enzymes (SGOT, SGPT):* elevated
- *urinalysis:* albumin in urine
- *ophthalmoscopy:* punctate lesions in the fetal lens nucleus (with treatment, cataracts regress)
- *amniocentesis:* prenatal diagnosis of galactosemia (recommended for heterozygous and homozygous parents).

Treatment and special considerations

Elimination of galactose and lactose from the diet causes most effects to subside. The infant gains weight; liver anomalies, nausea, vomiting, galactosemia, proteinuria, and aminoaciduria disappear; and cataracts regress. To eliminate galactose and lactose from an infant's diet, replace cow's milk formula or breast

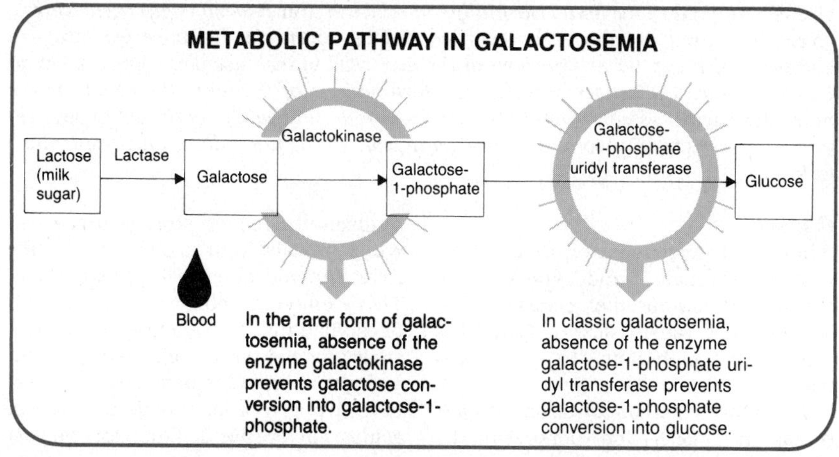
METABOLIC PATHWAY IN GALACTOSEMIA
Lactose (milk sugar)
Lactase
Galactose
Galactokinase
Galactose-1-phosphate
Galactose-1-phosphate uridyl transferase
Glucose
Blood
In the rarer form of galactosemia, absence of the enzyme galactokinase prevents galactose conversion into galactose-1-phosphate.
In classic galactosemia, absence of the enzyme galactose-1-phosphate uridyl transferase prevents galactose-1-phosphate conversion into glucose.

PARENT TEACHING AID

Diet for Galactosemia

Dear Parent:
If your child has galactosemia, make sure he follows a diet free of lactose. He may eat:
- fish and animal products (except brains and mussels)
- fresh fruits and vegetables (except peas and lima beans)
- only bread and rolls made from cracked wheat.

He should avoid:
- dairy products
- puddings, cookies, cakes, pies
- food coloring
- instant potatoes
- canned and frozen foods (if lactose is listed as an ingredient).

milk with a meat-base or soybean formula. As the child grows, a balanced, galactose-free diet must be maintained. A pregnant woman who is heterozygous or homozygous for galactosemia should also follow a galactose-restricted diet. Such a diet supports normal growth and development and may delay symptoms in the newborn.
- Teach the parents about dietary restrictions and stress the importance of compliance. Warn them to read medication labels carefully and avoid giving any that contain lactose fillers.
- If the child has a learning disability, help parents secure educational assistance. Refer parents who want to have other children for genetic counseling. In some states, screening of all newborns for galactosemia is required by law.

Glycogen Storage Diseases

Glycogen storage diseases consist of at least eight distinct errors of metabolism, all inherited, that alter the synthesis or degradation of glycogen, the form in which glucose is stored in the body. Normally, muscle and liver cells store glycogen. Muscle glycogen is used in muscle contraction; liver glycogen can be converted into free glucose, which can then diffuse out of the liver cells to increase blood glucose levels. Glycogen storage diseases manifest as dysfunctions of the liver, the heart, or the musculoskeletal system. Symptoms vary from mild and easily controlled hypoglycemia to severe organ involvement that may lead to cardiac failure and respiratory failure.

Causes

Almost all glycogen storage diseases (Types I through V and Type VII) are transmitted as autosomal recessive traits. The mode of transmission of Type VI is unknown; Type VIII may be an X-linked trait.

The most common glycogen storage disease is Type I—von Gierke's, or hepatorenal glycogen storage disease—which results from a deficiency of the liver enzyme glucose-6-phosphatase. This enzyme converts glucose-6-phosphate into free glucose and is necessary for the release of stored glycogen and glucose into the bloodstream, to relieve hypoglycemia. Infants may die of acidosis before age 2; if they survive past

RARE FORMS OF GLYCOGEN STORAGE DISEASE

TYPE	CLINICAL FEATURES	DIAGNOSTIC TEST RESULTS
II *(Pompe's)* Absence of alpha-1,4-glucosidase (acid maltase)	• *Infants:* cardiomegaly, profound hypotonia, and, occasionally, endocardial fibroelastosis (usually fatal before age 1 due to cardiac or respiratory failure) • *Some infants and young children:* muscular weakness and wasting, variable organ involvement (slower progression, usually fatal by age 19) • *Adults:* muscle weakness without organomegaly (slowly progressive but not fatal)	• *Muscle biopsy:* increased concentration of glycogen with normal structure; alpha 1,4-glucosidase deficiency • *EKG* (in infants): large QRS complexes in all leads; inverted T waves; shortened PR interval • *Electromyography* (in adults): muscle fiber irritability; myotonic discharges • *Amniocentesis:* alpha-1,4-glucosidase deficiency • *Placenta or umbilical cord examination:* alpha-1,4-glucosidase deficiency
III *(Cori's)* Absence of debranching enzyme (amylo-1,6-glucosidase) (*Note:* predominant cause of glycogen storage disease in Israel)	• *Young children:* massive hepatomegaly, which may disappear by puberty; growth retardation; moderate splenomegaly; hypoglycemia • *Adults:* progressive myopathy • Occasionally, moderate cardiomegaly, cirrhosis, muscle wasting, hypoglycemia	• *Liver biopsy:* deficient debranching activity; increased glycogen concentration • *Lab tests* (in children only): elevated SGOT or SGPT; increased erythrocyte glycogen
IV *(Andersen's)* Deficiency of branching enzyme (amylo-1,4-1,6-transglucosidase) (*Note:* extremely rare)	• *Infants:* hepatosplenomegaly, ascites, muscle hypotonia; usually fatal before age 2 from progressive cirrhosis	• *Liver biopsy:* deficient branching enzyme activity; glycogen molecule has longer outer branches.
V *(McArdle's)* Deficiency of muscle phosphorylase	• *Children:* mild or no symptoms • *Adults:* muscle cramps and pain during strenuous exercise, possibly resulting in myoglobinuria and renal failure • *Older patients:* significant muscle weakness and wasting	• *Serum lactate:* no increase in venous levels in sample drawn from extremity after ischemic exercise • *Muscle biopsy:* lack of phosphorylase activity; increased glycogen content
VI *(Hers')* Possible deficiency of hepatic phosphorylase	• Mild symptoms (similar to those of Type I), requiring no treatment	• *Liver biopsy:* decreased phosphorylase *b* activity, increased glycogen concentration
VII Deficiency of muscle phosphofructokinase	• Muscle cramps during strenuous exercise, resulting in myoglobinuria and possible renal failure • Reticulocytosis	• *Serum lactate:* no increase in venous levels in sample drawn from extremity after ischemic exercise • *Muscle biopsy:* deficient phosphofructokinase; marked rise in glycogen concentration • *Blood studies:* low erythrocyte phosphofructokinase activity; reduced half-life of RBCs
VIII Deficiency of hepatic phosphorylase kinase	• Mild hepatomegaly • Mild hypoglycemia	• *Liver biopsy:* deficient phosphorylase *b* kinase activity; increased liver glycogen • *Blood study:* deficient phosphorylase *b* kinase in leukocytes

this age, with proper treatment, they may grow normally and live to adulthood, with only minimal hepatomegaly. However, there is a danger of adenomatous liver nodules, which may be premalignant.

Signs and symptoms

Primary clinical features of the liver glycogen storage diseases (Types I, III, IV, VI, and VIII) are hepatomegaly and rapid onset of hypoglycemia and ketosis when food is withheld. Symptoms of the muscle glycogen storage diseases (Types II, V, and VII) include poor muscle tone; Type II may result in death from heart failure.

In addition, Type I may produce the following symptoms:

- *infants:* acidosis, hyperlipidemia, gastrointestinal bleeding, coma
- *children:* low resistance to infection and, without proper treatment, short stature
- *adolescents:* gouty arthritis and nephropathy; chronic tophaceous gout; bleeding (especially epistaxis); small superficial vessels visible in skin, due to impaired platelet function; fat deposits in cheeks, buttocks, and subcutaneous tissues; poor muscle tone; enlarged kidneys; xanthomas over extensor surfaces of arms and legs; steatorrhea; multiple, bilateral, yellow lesions in fundi; and osteoporosis, probably secondary to negative calcium balance. Correct treatment of glycogen storage disease should prevent all of these effects.

Diagnosis

Liver and muscle biopsies are the key tests in diagnosing Type I glycogen storage disease:

- *Liver biopsy* confirms diagnosis by showing normal glycogen synthetase and phosphorylase enzyme activities but reduced or absent glucose-6-phosphatase activity. Glycogen structure is normal, but amounts are elevated.

- *Laboratory studies* of plasma demonstrate low glucose levels but high levels of free fatty acids, triglycerides, cholesterol, and uric acid. Serum analysis reveals high pyruvic acid levels and high lactic acid levels. Prenatal diagnoses are available for Types II, III, and IV.
- *Injection of glucagon or epinephrine* increases pyruvic and lactic acid levels but does not increase blood glucose levels. Glucose tolerance test curve typically shows depletional hypoglycemia and reduced insulin output. Intrauterine diagnosis is possible.

Treatment

For Type I, the aims of treatment are to maintain glucose homeostasis and prevent secondary consequences of hypoglycemia through frequent feedings and constant nocturnal nasogastric drip with Polycose, dextrose, or Vivonex. Treatment includes a low-fat diet, with normal amounts of protein and calories; carbohydrates should contain glucose or glucose polymers only.

Therapy for Type III includes frequent feedings and a high-protein diet. Type IV requires a high-protein, high-calorie diet; bed rest; diuretics; sodium restriction; and paracentesis, if necessary, to relieve ascites. Types V and VII require no treatment except avoidance of strenuous exercise. No treatment is necessary for Types VI and VIII, and no effective treatment exists for Type II.

Special considerations

When managing Type I disease:

- Advise the patient or parents to include carbohydrate foods containing mainly starch in his diet and to sweeten foods with glucose only.
- Before discharge, teach the patient or family member how to pass a nasogastric tube, use a pump with alarm capacity, monitor blood glucose with Dextrostix, and recognize symptoms of hypoglycemia.
- Watch for and report signs of infection (fever, chills, myalgia) and of hepatic encephalopathy (mental confusion, stupor, asterixis, coma) due to increased blood ammonia levels.

When managing other types:

- *Type II:* Explain test procedures, such as electromyography and electroencephalography, thoroughly.
- *Type III:* Instruct the patient to eat a high-protein diet (eggs, nuts, fish, meat, poultry, and cheese).
- *Type IV:* Watch for signs of hepatic failure (nausea, vomiting, irregular bowel function, clay-colored stools, right upper quadrant pain, jaundice, dehydration, electrolyte imbalance, edema, and changes in mental status, progressing to coma).

When caring for patients with Types II, III, and IV glycogen storage disease, offer parents reassurance and emotional support. Recommend and arrange for genetic counseling, if appropriate.

- *Types V through VIII:* Care for these patients is minimal. Explain the disorder to the patient and his family, and help them accept the limitations imposed by his particular type of glycogen storage disease.

Hypoglycemia

Hypoglycemia is an abnormally low glucose level in the bloodstream. It occurs when glucose burns up too rapidly, when the glucose release rate falls behind tissue demands, or when excessive insulin enters the bloodstream. Hypoglycemia is classified as reactive or fasting. Reactive hypoglycemia *results from the reaction to the disposition of meals or the administration of excessive insulin.* Fasting hypoglycemia *causes discomfort during long periods of abstinence from food—for example, in the early morning hours before breakfast. Although hypoglycemia is a specific endocrine imbalance, its symptoms are often vague and depend on how quickly the patient's glucose levels drop. If not corrected, severe hypoglycemia may result in coma and irreversible brain damage.*

Causes

Reactive hypoglycemia may take several forms. In a diabetic patient, it may result from administration of too much insulin or—less commonly—too much oral hypoglycemia medication. In a mildly diabetic patient (or one in the early stages of diabetes mellitus), reactive hypoglycemia may result from delayed and excessive insulin production after carbohydrate ingestion. Similarly, a nondiabetic patient may suffer reactive hypoglycemia from a sharp increase in insulin output after a meal. Sometimes called *postprandial hypoglycemia,* this type of reactive hypoglycemia usually disappears when the patient eats something sweet. In some patients, reactive hypoglycemia may have no known cause (idiopathic reactive) or may result from hyperalimentation due to gastric dumping syndrome and from impaired glucose tolerance.

Fasting hypoglycemia usually results from an excess of insulin or insulin-like substance or from a decrease in counterregulatory hormones. It can be *exogenous,* resulting from such external factors as alcohol or drug ingestion, or *endogenous,* resulting from organic problems.

Endogenous hypoglycemia may result from tumors or liver disease. Insulinomas, small islet cell tumors in the pancreas, secrete excessive amounts of insulin, which inhibits hepatic glucose production. They are generally benign (in 90% of patients). Extrapancreatic tumors, though uncommon, can also cause hypoglycemia by increasing glucose utilization and inhibiting glucose output. Such tumors occur primarily in the mesenchyma, liver, adrenal cortex, gastrointestinal system, and lymphatic system. They may be benign or malignant. Among nonendocrine causes of fasting hypoglycemia are severe liver diseases, including hepatitis, cancer, cirrhosis, and liver congestion associated with congestive heart failure. All of these conditions reduce the uptake and release of glycogen from the liver. Some endocrine causes include destruction of pancreatic islet cells; adrenocortical insufficiency, which contributes to hypoglycemia by reducing the production of cortisol and cortisone needed for gluconeogenesis; and pituitary insufficiency, which reduces ACTH and GH levels.

Hypoglycemia is at least as common in newborns and children as it is in adults. Usually, infants develop hypoglycemia because of an increased number of cells per unit of body weight and because of increased demands on stored liver glycogen to support respirations, thermoregulation, and muscular activity. In full-term infants, hypoglycemia may occur 24 to 72 hours after birth and is usually transient. In infants who are premature or small for gestational age, onset of hypoglycemia is much more rapid—it can occur as soon as 6 hours after birth—due to their small, immature livers, which produce much less glycogen. Maternal disorders that can produce hypoglycemia in infants within 24 hours after birth include diabetes mellitus, toxemia, erythroblastosis, and glycogen storage disease.

Signs and symptoms

Signs and symptoms of reactive hypoglycemia include fatigue and malaise, nervousness, irritability, trembling, tension, headache, hunger, cold sweats, and rapid heart rate. These same clinical effects usually characterize fasting hypoglycemia. In addition, fasting hypoglycemia may also cause central nervous system (CNS) disturbances; for example, blurry or double vision, confusion, motor weakness, hemiplegia, convulsions, or coma.

In infants and children, signs and symptoms of hypoglycemia are vague. A newborn's refusal to feed may be the primary clue to underlying hypoglycemia. Associated CNS effects include tremors, twitching, weak or high-pitched cry, sweating, limpness, convulsions, and coma.

Diagnosis

Dextrostix or Chemstrips provide quick screening methods for determining blood glucose level. A color change that corresponds to < 45 mg/dl indicates the need for a venous blood sample.

Laboratory testing confirms diagnosis by showing decreased blood glucose values. The following values indicate hypoglycemia:

- *Full-term infants:*
  < 30 mg/dl before feeding
  < 40 mg/dl after feeding
- *Pre-term infants:*
  < 20 mg/dl before feeding
  < 30 mg/dl after feeding
- *Children and adults:*
  < 40 mg/dl before meal
  < 50 mg/dl after meal

In addition, a 5-hour glucose tolerance test may be administered to provoke reactive hypoglycemia. Following a 12-hour fast, laboratory testing to detect plasma insulin and plasma glucose levels may identify fasting hypoglycemia.

Treatment

Effective treatment of reactive hypoglycemia requires dietary modification to help delay glucose absorption and gastric emptying. Usually, this includes small, frequent meals; ingestion of complex carbohydrates, fiber, and fat; and avoidance of simple sugars, alcohol, and fruit drinks. The patient may also receive anticholinergic drugs to slow gastric emptying and intestinal motility and to inhibit vagal stimulation of insulin release.

For fasting hypoglycemia, surgery and drug therapy are usually required. In patients with insulinoma, removal of the tumor is the treatment of choice. Drug therapy may include nondiuretic thiazides, such as diazoxide, to inhibit insulin secretion; streptozocin; and hormones, such as glucocorticoids and long-acting glycogen.

Therapy for newborn infants who have hypoglycemia or risk developing it includes preventive measures. A hypertonic solution of 10% to 25% dextrose, calculated at 2 to 4 ml/kg of body weight and administered I.V., should correct a severe hypoglycemic state in newborns. To reduce the chance of hypoglycemia developing in high-risk infants, such infants should receive feedings—either breast milk or a solution of 5% to 10% glucose and water—as soon after birth as possible.

Special considerations

- Watch for and report signs of hypoglycemia (such as poor feeding) in high-risk infants.
- Monitor infusion of hypertonic glucose in the newborn to avoid hyperglycemia, circulatory overload, and cellular dehydration. Terminate glucose solutions gradually, to prevent hypoglycemia caused by hyperinsulinemia.
- Explain the purpose and procedure for any diagnositc tests. Collect blood samples at the appropriate times, as ordered.
- Monitor the effects of drug therapy, and watch for the development of any side effects.
- Teach the patient which foods to include in his diet (complex carbohydrates, fiber, fat) and which foods to avoid (simple sugars, alcohol). Refer the patient and family for dietary counseling, as appropriate.

Hereditary Fructose Intolerance

Hereditary fructose intolerance is an inability to metabolize fructose. After eliminating fructose from the diet, symptoms subside within weeks. Older children and adults with hereditary fructose intolerance have normal intelligence and apparently normal liver and kidney function.

Causes

Transmitted as an autosomal recessive trait, hereditary fructose intolerance results from a deficiency in the enzyme fructose-1-phosphate aldolase. The enzyme operates at only 1% to 10% of its normal biological activity, thus preventing rapid uptake of fructose by the liver after ingestion of fruit or foods containing cane sugar.

Signs and symptoms

Typically, clinical features of hereditary fructose intolerance appear shortly after dietary introduction of foods containing fructose or sucrose. Symptoms are more severe in infants than in older persons and include hypoglycemia, nausea, vomiting, pallor, excessive sweating, cyanosis, and tremor. In newborns and young children, continuous ingestion of foods containing fructose may result in failure to thrive, hypoglycemia, jaundice, hyperbilirubinemia, ascites, hepatomegaly, vomiting, dehydration, hypophosphatemia, albuminuria, aminoaciduria, seizures, convulsions, coma, febrile episodes, substernal pain, and anemia.

Diagnosis

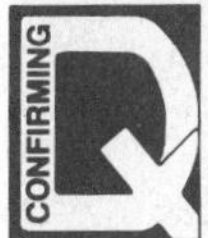

Although a dietary history often suggests hereditary fructose intolerance, a fructose tolerance test (using glucose oxidase or paper chromatography to measure glucose levels) usually confirms it. However, liver biopsy showing a deficiency in fructose-1-phosphate aldolase may be necessary for definitive diagnosis. Supportive values may include decreased serum inorganic phosphorus levels. Urine studies may show fructosuria and albuminuria.

Treatment and special considerations

Treatment of hereditary fructose intolerance consists of exclusion of fructose and sucrose (cane sugar or table sugar) from the diet. Tell the patient to avoid fruits containing fructose and vegetables containing sucrose (sugar beets, sweet potatoes, and peas), because sucrose is digested to glucose and fructose in the intestine.

Refer the patient and family for genetic and dietary counseling, as appropriate.

Hyperlipoproteinemia

Hyperlipoproteinemia occurs as five distinct metabolic disorders, all of which may be inherited. Types I and III are transmitted as autosomal recessive traits; Types II, IV, and V are transmitted as autosomal dominant traits. About one in five persons with elevated plasma lipids and lipoproteins has hyperlipoproteinemia. It is marked by increased plasma concentrations of one or more lipoproteins. Hyperlipoproteinemia may also occur secondary to other conditions, such as diabetes, pancreatitis, hypothyroidism, or renal disease. This disorder affects lipid transport in serum and produces varied clinical changes, from relatively mild symptoms that can be corrected by dietary management to potentially fatal pancreatitis.

Signs and symptoms

- *Type I:* recurrent attacks of severe abdominal pain similar to pancreatitis, usually preceded by fat intake; abdominal spasm, rigidity, or rebound tenderness; hepatosplenomegaly, with liver or spleen tenderness; papular or eruptive xanthomas (pinkish-yellow cutaneous deposits of fat) over pressure points and extensor surfaces; lipemia retinalis (reddish-white retinal vessels); malaise; anorexia; and fever

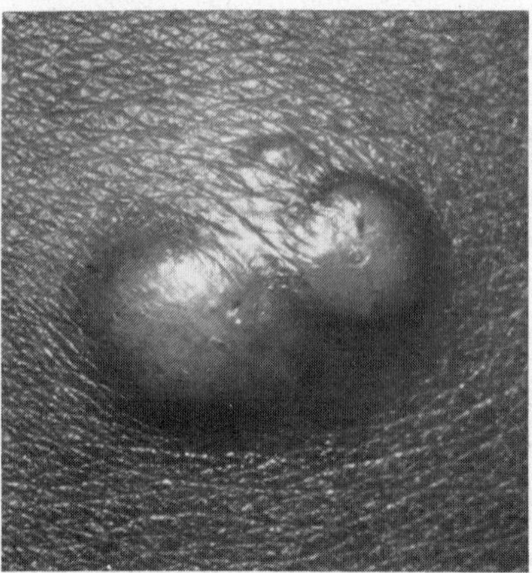

Papular xanthomas, cutaneous deposits of fat, are characteristic of Type I hyperlipoproteinemia.

- *Type II:* tendinous xanthomas (firm masses) on the Achilles tendons and tendons of the hands and feet, tuberous xanthomas, xanthelasma, juvenile corneal arcus (opaque ring surrounding the corneal periphery), accelerated atherosclerosis and premature coronary artery disease, and recurrent polyarthritis and tenosynovitis
- *Type III:* peripheral vascular disease manifested by claudication or tuboeruptive xanthomas (soft, inflamed, pedunculated lesions) over the elbows and knees; palmar xanthomas on the hands, particularly fingertips; premature atherosclerosis
- *Type IV:* predisposition to atherosclerosis and early coronary artery disease, exacerbated by excessive calorie intake, obesity, diabetes, and hypertension
- *Type V:* abdominal pain (most common), pancreatitis, peripheral neurop-

TYPES OF HYPERLIPOPROTEINEMIA

TYPE	CAUSES AND INCIDENCE	DIAGNOSTIC FINDINGS
I (Frederickson's hyperlipoproteinemia, fat-induced hyperlipemia, idiopathic familial)	• Deficient or abnormal lipoprotein lipase, resulting in decreased or absent post-heparin lipolytic activity • Relatively rare • Present at birth	• Chylomicrons (very-low-density lipoprotein [VLDL], low-density lipoprotein [LDL], high-density lipoprotein [HDL]), in plasma 14 hours or more after last meal • High elevated serum chylomicrons and triglycerides; slightly elevated serum cholesterol • Lower serum lipoprotein lipase • Leukocytosis
II (familial hyperbetalipoproteinemia, essential familial hypercholesterolemia)	• Deficient cell surface receptor that regulates LDL degradation and cholesterol synthesis, resulting in increased levels of plasma LDL over joints and pressure points • Onset between ages 10 and 30	• Increased plasma concentrations of LDL • Increased serum LDL and cholesterol • Amniocentesis shows increased LDL.
III (familial broad-beta disease, xanthoma tuberosum)	• Unknown underlying defect results in deficient conversion of triglyceride-rich VLDL to LDL. • Uncommon; usually occurs after age 20 but can occur earlier in men	• Abnormal serum beta-lipoprotein • Elevated cholesterol and triglycerides • Slightly elevated glucose tolerance • Hyperuricemia
IV (endogenous hypertriglyceridemia, hyperbetalipoproteinemia)	• Usually occurs secondary to obesity, alcoholism, diabetes, or emotional disorders • Relatively common, especially in middle-aged men	• Elevated VLDL • Abnormal levels of triglycerides in plasma; variable increase in serum • Normal or slightly elevated serum cholesterol • Mildly abnormal glucose tolerance • Family history • Early coronary artery disease
V (mixed hypertriglyceridemia, mixed hyperlipidemia)	• Defective triglyceride clearance causes pancreatitis; usually secondary to another disorder, such as obesity or nephrosis • Uncommon; onset usually occurs in late adolescence or early adulthood.	• Chylomicrons in plasma • Elevated plasma VLDL • Elevated serum cholesterol and triglycerides

athy, eruptive xanthomas on extensor surfaces of the arms and legs, lipemia retinalis, and hepatosplenomegaly.

Treatment and prognosis

The first goal is to identify and treat any underlying problem, such as diabetes. If no underlying problem exists, then primary treatment for Types II, III, and IV is dietary management, especially restriction of cholesterol intake, possibly supplemented by drug therapy (cholestyramine, clofibrate, niacin) to lower plasma triglyceride or cholesterol level when diet alone is ineffective.

Type I hyperlipoproteinemia requires long-term weight reduction, with fat intake restricted to less than 40 to 60 g/day. A 20- to 40-g/day medium-chain triglyceride diet may be ordered to supplement calorie intake. The patient should also avoid alcoholic beverages, to decrease plasma triglycerides. Prognosis is good with treatment; without treatment, death can result from pancreatitis.

For Type II, dietary management to restore normal lipid levels and decrease the risk of atherosclerosis includes restriction of cholesterol intake to less than 300 mg/day for adults and less than 150 mg/day for children; triglycerides must be restricted to less than 100 mg/day for children and adults. Diet should also be high in polyunsaturated fats. In familial hypercholesterolemia, nicotinic acid with a bile acid usually normalizes low-density lipoprotein levels. For severely affected children, portacaval shunt is a last resort to reduce plasma cholesterol levels. Prognosis remains poor regardless of treatment; in homozygotes, myocardial infarction usually causes death before age 30.

For Type III, dietary management includes restriction of cholesterol intake to less than 300 mg/day; carbohydrates must also be restricted, while polyunsaturated fats are increased. Clofibrate and niacin help lower blood lipid levels. Weight reduction is helpful. With strict adherence to prescribed diet, prognosis is good.

For Type IV, weight reduction may normalize blood lipid levels without additional treatment. Long-term dietary management includes restricted cholesterol intake, increased polyunsaturated fats, and avoidance of alcoholic beverages. Clofibrate and niacin may lower plasma lipid levels. Prognosis remains uncertain, however, because of predisposition to premature coronary artery disease.

The most effective treatment for Type V is weight reduction and long-term maintenance of a low-fat diet. Alcoholic beverages must be avoided. Niacin, clofibrate, gemfibrozil, and a 20- to 40-g/day medium-chain triglyceride diet may prove helpful. Prognosis is uncertain because of the risk of pancreatitis. Increased fat intake may cause recurrent bouts of illness, possibly leading to pseudocyst formation, hemorrhage, and death.

Special considerations

Nursing care for hyperlipoproteinemia emphasizes careful monitoring for drug side effects and teaching the importance of long-term dietary management.

- Administer cholestyramine before meals or before bedtime. This drug must not be given with other medications. Watch for side effects, such as nausea, vomiting, constipation, steatorrhea, rashes, and hyperchloremic acidosis. Also watch for malabsorption of other medications and fat-soluble vitamins.
- Give clofibrate, as ordered. Watch for side effects, such as cholelithiasis, cardiac dysrhythmias, intermittent claudication, thromboembolism, nausea, weight gain (from fluid retention), and myositis.
- *Don't* administer niacin to patients with active peptic ulcers or hepatic disease. Use with caution in patients with diabetes. In other patients, watch for side effects, such as flushing, pruritus, hyperpigmentation, and exacerbation of inactive peptic ulcers.
- Urge the patient to adhere to his diet (usually 1,000 to 1,500 calories/day) and to avoid excess sugar and alcoholic beverages, to minimize intake of saturated fats (higher in meats, coconut oil), and to increase intake of polyunsaturated fats (vegetable oils).
- Instruct the patient, for the 2 weeks preceding serum cholesterol and serum triglyceride tests, to maintain a steady weight and to adhere strictly to the prescribed diet. He should also fast for 12 hours preceding the test.
- Instruct women with elevated serum lipids to avoid oral contraceptives or drugs that contain estrogen.

Gaucher's Disease

Gaucher's disease, the most common lipidosis, causes an abnormal accumulation of glucocerebrosides in reticuloendothelial cells. It occurs in three forms: Type I (adult); Type II (infantile); and Type III (juvenile). Type II can prove fatal within 9 months of onset, usually from pulmonary involvement.

Causes and incidence

Gaucher's disease results from an autosomal recessive inheritance, which causes decreased activity of the enzyme glucocerebrosidase. Type I is 30 times more prevalent in Eastern Europeans of Jewish ancestry. Types II and III are less common.

Signs and symptoms

Key signs of all types of Gaucher's disease are hepatosplenomegaly and bone lesions. In Type I, bone lesions lead to thinning of cortices, pathologic fractures, collapsed hip joints, and, eventually, vertebral compression. Severe episodic pain may develop in the legs, arms, and back but usually not until adolescence. (The adult form of Gaucher's disease is generally diagnosed while the patient is in his teens; the word adult is used loosely here.) Other clinical effects of Type I are fever, abdominal distention (from hypotonicity of the large bowel), respiratory problems (pneumonia or, rarely, cor pulmonale), easy bruising and bleeding, anemia, and, rarely, pancytopenia. Older patients may develop a yellow pallor and brown-yellow pigmentation on the face and legs.

In Type II, motor dysfunction and spasticity occur at age 6 to 7 months. Other signs of the infantile form of Gaucher's disease include abdominal distention, strabismus, muscular hypertonicity, retroflexion of the head, neck rigidity, dysphagia, laryngeal stridor, hyperreflexia, seizures, respiratory distress, and easy bruising and bleeding.

Clinical effects of Type III after infancy include convulsions, hypertonicity, strabismus, poor coordination and mental ability, and, possibly, easy bruising and bleeding.

Diagnosis

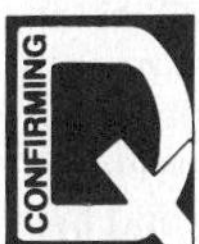

Bone marrow aspiration showing Gaucher's cells and direct assay of glucocerebrosidase activity, which can be performed on venous blood, confirm this diagnosis. Supportive laboratory results include increased serum acid phosphatase level, decreased platelets and serum iron level, and, in Type III, abnormal EEG after infancy.

Treatment and special considerations

Treatment is mainly supportive and consists of vitamins, supplemental iron or liver extract to prevent anemia caused by iron deficiency and to alleviate other hematologic problems, blood transfusions for anemia, splenectomy for thrombocytopenia, and strong analgesics for bone pain. Enzyme replacement therapy is still experimental but looks promising.

- In the patient confined to bed, prevent pathologic fractures by turning him carefully. If he is ambulatory, see that he is assisted when getting out of bed or walking.
- Observe closely for changes in pulmonary status.
- Explain all diagnostic tests and procedures to the patient and/or his parents. Help the patient accept the limitations imposed by this disorder.
- Recommend genetic counseling for parents who want to have another child.

Amyloidosis

Amyloidosis is a rare, chronic disease resulting in the accumulation of an abnormal fibrillar scleroprotein (amyloid), which infiltrates body organs and soft tissues. Amyloidosis is classified in two ways, based on histologic findings: perireticular type, *which affects the inner coats of blood vessels, and* pericollagen type, *which affects the outer coats of blood vessels and also involves the parenchyma.*

Although prognosis varies with type and with the site and extent of involvement, amyloidosis sometimes results in permanent—usually even life-threatening—organ damage.

Causes and incidence

Amyloidosis is sometimes familial, especially in persons of Portuguese ancestry. It may occur in conjunction with tuberculosis, chronic infection, rheumatoid arthritis, multiple myeloma, Hodgkin's disease, paraplegia, and brucellosis. It may also accompany the aging process.

In amyloidosis, accumulation and infiltration of amyloid produces pressure and causes atrophy of nearby cells. Reticuloendothelial cell dysfunction and abnormal immunoglobulin synthesis occur in some types of amyloidosis. In the United States, evidence of amyloidosis on autopsy is 0.5%, but true incidence is difficult to determine.

Signs and symptoms

Amyloidosis produces dysfunction of the kidneys, heart, GI tract, peripheral nerves, and, rarely, the liver.

• *Kidneys:* The primary sign of renal involvement is proteinuria, leading to nephrotic syndrome and eventual renal failure.

• *Heart:* Amyloidosis often causes intractable congestive heart failure, due to amyloid deposits in the subendocardium, endocardium, and myocardium.

• *GI tract:* GI amyloidosis may produce stiffness and enlargement of the tongue, hindering enunciation. In addition, it may decrease intestinal motility and produce malabsorption, bleeding, infiltration of blood vessel walls, abdominal pain, constipation, and diarrhea. Tumorlike amyloid deposits may occur in all portions of this system. Chronic malabsorption may lead to malnutrition and predispose to infection.

• *Peripheral nervous system:* The appearance of peripheral neuropathy indicates peripheral nerve involvement.

• *Liver:* Hepatic amyloidosis is rare and usually coexists with other forms of this disease. It generally produces liver enlargement, often with azotemia, anemia, albuminuria, and mild jaundice.

Diagnosis

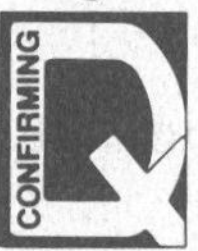

Diagnosis depends on histologic examination of a tissue biopsy specimen, using a polarizing or electron microscope. Rectal mucosa biopsy is the best screening test, since it's less hazardous than kidney or liver biopsy. Depending on the location of amyloid deposits, other biopsy sites include the gingiva, skin, and nerves.

In cardiac amyloidosis, other findings include faint heart sounds and an EKG showing low voltage and conduction or rhythm abnormalities resembling those of myocardial infarction. In hepatic amyloidosis, liver function studies are generally normal, except for slightly elevated serum alkaline phosphatase.

Treatment

Treatment is mainly supportive but may include corticosteroids and other immunosuppressives to minimize inflammation. Transplantation may be useful for amyloidosis-induced renal failure. Patients with cardiac amyloidosis require conservative treatment; digitalis must be given with caution to prevent dangerous dysrhythmias. Malnutrition caused by malabsorption in end-stage GI involvement may require total parenteral nutrition.

Special considerations

• Maintain nutrition and fluid balance; give analgesics to relieve intestinal pain; control constipation or diarrhea; and manage infection and fever.

• Provide good mouth care for the patient with tongue involvement. Refer him for speech therapy, if needed; provide an alternate method of communication if he can't talk.

• Assess airway patency when the tongue is involved, and prevent respiratory tract compromise by gentle and adequate suctioning, when indicated. Keep a tracheostomy tray at bedside.

• When long-term bed rest is necessary,

properly position the patient, and turn him often to prevent decubitus ulcers. Perform range-of-motion exercises to prevent contractures.

• Provide psychological support. Exercise patience and understanding to help the patient cope with this chronic illness.

Porphyrias

Porphyrias are metabolic disorders that affect the biosynthesis of heme (a component of hemoglobin) and cause excessive production and excretion of porphyrins or their precursors. Porphyrins, which are present in all protoplasm, figure prominently in energy storage and utilization. Classification of porphyrias depends on the site of excessive porphyrin production; they may be erythropoietic (erythroid cells in bone marrow), hepatic (in the liver), or erythrohepatic (in bone marrow and liver). An acute episode of intermittent hepatic porphyria may cause fatal respiratory paralysis. In the other forms of porphyrias, prognosis is good with proper treatment.

Causes

Porphyrias are inherited as autosomal dominant traits, except for Günther's disease (autosomal recessive trait) and toxic-acquired porphyria (usually from ingestion of or exposure to lead). Menstruation often precipitates acute porphyria in premenopausal women.

Signs and symptoms

Porphyrias are generally marked by photosensitivity, acute abdominal pain, and neuropathy.

Hepatic porphyrias may produce a complex syndrome marked by distinct neurologic and hepatic dysfunction:

• Neurologic symptoms include chronic brain syndrome, peripheral neuropathy and autonomic effects, tachycardia, labile hypertension, severe colicky lower abdominal pain, and constipation.

• During an acute attack, fever, leukocytosis, and fluid and electrolyte imbalance may occur.

• Structural hepatic effects include fatty infiltration of the liver, hepatic siderosis, and focal hepatocellular necrosis.

• Skin lesions may cause itching and burning, erythema, and altered pigmentation and edema in areas exposed to light. Some chronic skin changes include milia (white papules on the dorsal aspects of the hands) and hirsutism on the upper cheeks and periorbital areas.

Diagnosis

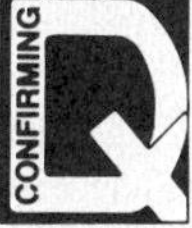

Generally, diagnosis requires screening tests for porphyrins or their precursors (such as aminolevulinic acid [ALA] and porphobilinogen [PBG]) in urine, stool, or blood or, occasionally, skin biopsy. Urinary lead level of 0.2 mg/liter confirms toxic-acquired porphyria.

Other laboratory values may include increased serum iron levels in porphyria cutanea tarda; leukocytosis, SIADH, and elevated bilirubin and alkaline phosphatase in acute intermittent porphyria.

Treatment and special considerations

• Warn the patient against excessive sun exposure. Administer beta-carotene to reduce photosensitivity.

• Administer hemin (an enzyme-inhibitor derived from processed red blood cells) to control recurrent attacks of acute intermittent porphyria, Günther's disease, variegate porphyria, and hereditary coproporphyria.

• Encourage a high-carbohydrate diet to decrease urinary excretion of ALA and PBG, with restricted fluid intake to inhibit release of ADH.

• Warn the patient to avoid precipitating factors, especially alcohol, barbiturates, estrogens, and fasting.

CLINICAL VARIANTS OF PORPHYRIA

PORPHYRIA	SIGNS AND SYMPTOMS	TREATMENT
ERYTHROPOIETIC PORPHYRIA		
Günther's disease • Usual onset before age 5	• Red urine (earliest, most characteristic sign); severe cutaneous photosensitivity, leading to vesicular or bullous eruptions on exposed areas, and eventual scarring and ulceration • Hypertrichosis • Brown or red-stained teeth • Splenomegaly, hemolytic anemia	• Anti-inflammatory ointments, such as 1% hydrocortisone, for dermatitis • Prednisone to reverse anemia • Transfusion of packed red cells to inhibit erythropoiesis and reduce level of excreted porphyrins • Hemin for recurrent attacks • Splenectomy for hemolytic anemia
ERYTHROHEPATIC PORPHYRIA		
Protoporphyria • Usually affects children • Occurs most often in males	• Photosensitive dermatitis • Hemolytic anemia • Chronic hepatic disease	• Avoidance of causative factors • Beta-carotene to reduce photosensitivity
Toxic-acquired porphyria • Usually affects children • Significant mortality	• Acute colicky pain • Anorexia, nausea, vomiting • Neuromuscular weakness • Behavioral changes • Convulsions, coma	• Chlorpromazine I.V. (25 mg every 4 to 6 hours during an acute attack) to relieve pain and GI symptoms • Avoidance of lead exposure
HEPATIC PORPHYRIA		
Acute intermittent porphyria • Most common form • Affects females most often, usually between ages 15 and 40	• Colicky abdominal pain with fever, general malaise, and hypertension • Peripheral neuritis, behavioral changes, possibly leading to frank psychosis • Respiratory paralysis can occur	• Chlorpromazine I.V. (25 mg every 4 to 6 hours) to relieve abdominal pain and control psychic abnormalities • Avoidance of barbiturates, infections, alcohol, and fasting • Hemin for recurrent attacks
Variegate porphyria • Usual onset between ages 30 and 50 • Occurs almost exclusively among South African whites • Affects males and females equally	• Skin lesions, extremely fragile skin in exposed areas • Hypertrichosis • Hyperpigmentation • Abdominal pain during acute attack • Neuropsychiatric manifestations	• High-carbohydrate diet • Avoidance of sunlight, or wearing protective clothing when avoidance isn't possible • Hemin for recurrent attacks
Porphyria cutanea tarda • Most frequent in men aged 40 to 60 • Highest incidence in South Africans	• Facial pigmentation • Red-brown urine • Photosensitive dermatitis • Hypertrichosis	• Avoidance of precipitating factors, such as alcohol and estrogens • Phlebotomy at 2-week intervals to lower serum iron level
Hereditary coproporphyria • Rare • Affects males and females equally	• Asymptomatic or mild neurologic, abdominal, or psychiatric symptoms	• High-carbohydrate diet • Avoidance of barbiturates • Hemin for recurrent attacks

HOMEOSTATIC IMBALANCE

Potassium Imbalance

Potassium, a cation that is the dominant cellular electrolyte, facilitates contraction of both skeletal and smooth muscles—including myocardial contraction—and figures prominently in nerve impulse conduction, acid-base balance, enzyme action, and cell membrane function. Because serum potassium level has such a narrow range (3.5 to 5 mEq/liter), a slight deviation in either direction can produce profound clinical consequences. Paradoxically, both hypokalemia (potassium deficiency) and hyperkalemia (potassium excess) can lead to muscle weakness and flaccid paralysis, because both create an ionic imbalance in neuromuscular tissue excitability. Both conditions also diminish excitability and conduction rate of the heart muscle, which may lead to cardiac arrest.

Causes

Since many foods contain potassium, hypokalemia rarely results from a dietary deficiency. Instead, potassium loss results from:

- *excessive gastrointestinal or urinary losses,* such as vomiting, gastric suction, diarrhea, dehydration, anorexia, or chronic laxative abuse.
- *trauma* (injury, burns, or surgery), in which damaged cells release potassium, which enters serum or extracellular fluid, to be excreted in the urine.
- *chronic renal disease,* with tubular potassium wasting.
- *certain drugs,* especially potassium-wasting diuretics, steroids, and certain sodium-containing antibiotics (carbenicillin).
- *acid-base imbalances,* which cause potassium shifting into cells without true depletion in alkalosis.
- *prolonged potassium-free I.V. therapy.*
- *hyperglycemia,* causing osmotic diuresis and glycosuria.
- *Cushing's syndrome, primary hyperaldosteronism, excessive ingestion of licorice,* and *severe serum magnesium deficiency.*

Hyperkalemia results from the kidneys' inability to excrete excessive amounts of potassium infused intravenously or administered orally; from decreased urine output, renal dysfunction or failure; or the use of potassium-sparing diuretics, such as triamterene, by patients with renal disease. It may also result from any injuries or conditions that release cellular potassium or favor its retention, such as burns, crushing injuries, failing renal function, adrenal gland insufficiency, dehydration, or diabetic acidosis.

Diagnosis

- *Hypokalemia:* serum potassium levels < 3.5 mEq/liter.
- *Hyperkalemia:* serum potassium levels > 5 mEq/liter.

Additional tests may be necessary to determine the underlying cause of the imbalance.

Treatment

For hypokalemia, replacement therapy with potassium chloride (I.V. or P.O.) is the primary treatment. When diuresis is necessary, spironolactone, a potassium-sparing diuretic, may be administered concurrently with a potassium-wasting diuretic to minimize potassium loss. Hypokalemia can be prevented by giving a maintenance dose of potassium I.V. to patients who may not take anything by mouth and to others predisposed to potassium loss.

For hyperkalemia, rapid infusion of

10% calcium gluconate decreases myocardial irritability and temporarily prevents cardiac arrest but doesn't correct serum potassium excess; it's also contraindicated in patients receiving digitalis. As an emergency measure, sodium bicarbonate I.V. increases pH and causes potassium to shift back into the cells. Insulin and 10% to 50% glucose I.V. also move potassium back into cells, but their effect lasts only 6 hours; repeated use is less effective. Sodium polystyrene sulfonate (Kayexalate) with 70% sorbitol produces exchange of sodium ions for potassium ions in the intestine. Hemodialysis or peritoneal dialysis also aids in removal of excess potassium.

Special considerations

For the patient with hypokalemia:

- Check serum potassium and other electrolyte levels often in patients apt to develop potassium imbalance and in those requiring potassium replacement; they are vulnerable to overcorrection to hyperkalemia.
- Assess intake and output carefully. Remember, the kidneys excrete 80% to 90% of ingested potassium. Never give supplementary potassium to a patient whose urinary output is below 600 ml/day. Also, measure gastrointestinal loss from suctioning or vomiting.
- Administer slow-release potassium or dilute oral potassium supplements in 4 oz (120 ml) or more of water or fluid to reduce irritation of gastric and small-bowel mucosa. Determine the patient's chloride level. If the level is low, give a potassium chloride supplement, as ordered; if it's normal, administer potassium gluconate, as ordered.
- Give potassium I.V. only after it is diluted in solution; potassium is very irritating to vascular, subcutaneous, and fatty tissues and may cause phlebitis or tissue necrosis if it infiltrates. Infuse slowly (no more than 20 mEq/liter/hour) to prevent hyperkalemia. *Never* administer by I.V. push or bolus; it may cause cardiac arrest.
- Carefully monitor patients receiving

CLINICAL FEATURES OF POTASSIUM IMBALANCE

DYSFUNCTION	HYPOKALEMIA	HYPERKALEMIA
Cardiovascular	• Dizziness, hypotension, arrhythmias, EKG changes (flattened T waves, elevated U waves, depressed ST segment), cardiac arrest (with serum potassium levels $<$ 2.5 mEq/liter)	• Tachycardia and later bradycardia, EKG changes (tented and elevated T waves, widened QRS, prolonged PR interval, flattened or absent P waves, depressed ST segment), cardiac arrest (with levels $>$ 7.0 mEq/liter)
Gastrointestinal	• Nausea and vomiting, anorexia, diarrhea, abdominal distention, paralytic ileus or decreased peristalsis	• Nausea, diarrhea, abdominal cramps
Musculoskeletal	• Muscle weakness and fatigue, leg cramps	• Muscle weakness, flaccid paralysis
Genitourinary	• Polyuria	• Oliguria, anuria
CNS	• Malaise, irritability, confusion, mental depression, speech changes, decreased reflexes, respiratory paralysis	• Hyperreflexia progressing to weakness, numbness, tingling, and flaccid paralysis
Acid-base balance	• Metabolic alkalosis	• Metabolic acidosis

EKG CHANGES IN POTASSIUM IMBALANCE

HYPOKALEMIA

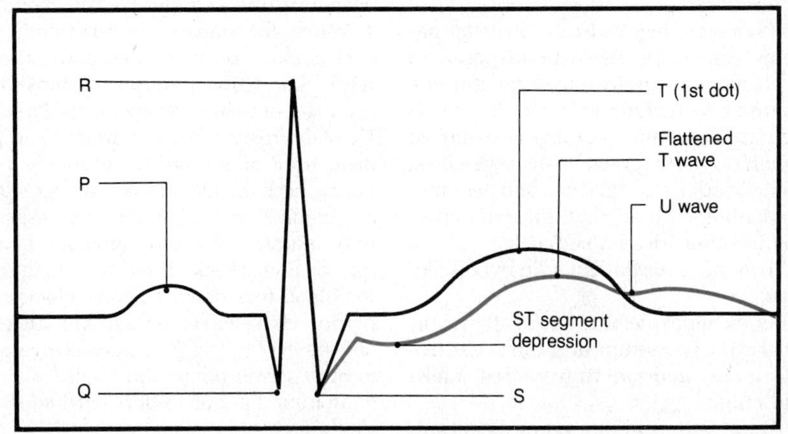

KEY

EKG tracing in hypo- and hyperkalemia

EKG tracing in normal potassium balance

HYPERKALEMIA

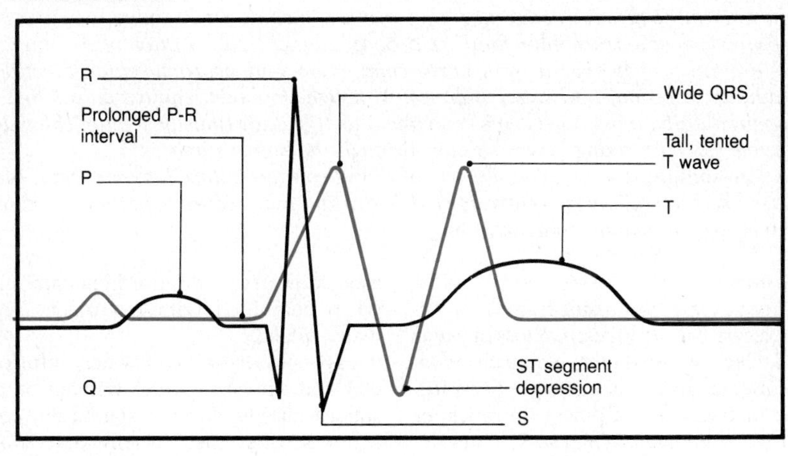

digitalis, since hypokalemia enhances the action of digitalis and may produce signs of digitalis toxicity (anorexia, nausea, vomiting, blurred vision, and dysrhythmias).

- To prevent hypokalemia, instruct patients (especially those predisposed to hypokalemia due to long-term diuretic therapy) to include in their diet foods rich in potassium—oranges, bananas, tomatoes, dark green leafy vegetables, milk, dried fruits, apricots, and peanuts.
- Monitor cardiac rhythm, and report any irregularities immediately.

To manage the patient with hyperkalemia:

- As in hypokalemia, frequently monitor serum potassium and other electrolyte levels, and carefully record intake and output.
- Administer sodium polystyrene sulfonate orally or rectally (by retention enema). Watch for signs of hypokalemia with prolonged use and for clinical effects of hypoglycemia (muscle weakness, syncope, hunger, diaphoresis) with repeated insulin and glucose treatment.
- Watch for signs of hyperkalemia in predisposed patients, especially those with poor urinary output or those receiving potassium supplements P.O. or I.V. Administer no more than 10 to 20 mEq/liter of potassium chloride per hour; check the I.V. infusion site for signs of phlebitis or infiltration of potassium into tissues. Also, before giving a blood transfusion, check to see how long ago the blood was donated; older blood cell hemolysis releases potassium. Infuse only *fresh* blood for patients with average to high serum potassium levels.
- Monitor for and report cardiac dysrhythmias.

Sodium Imbalance

Sodium is the major cation (90%) in extracellular fluid; potassium, the major cation in intracellular fluid. During repolarization, the sodium-potassium pump continually shifts sodium into the cells and potassium out of the cells; during depolarization, it does the reverse. Sodium cation functions include maintaining tonicity and concentration of extracellular fluid, acid-base balance (reabsorption of sodium ion and excretion of hydrogen ion), nerve conduction and neuromuscular function, glandular secretion, and water balance. Although the body requires only 2 to 4 g of sodium daily, most Americans consume 6 to 10 g daily (mostly sodium chloride, as table salt), excreting excess sodium through the kidneys and skin.

A low-sodium diet or excessive use of diuretics may induce hyponatremia (decreased serum sodium concentration); dehydration may induce hypernatremia (increased serum sodium concentration).

Causes

Hyponatremia can result from:

- excessive gastrointestinal loss of water and electrolytes due to vomiting, suctioning, or diarrhea; excessive perspiration or fever; use of potent diuretics; or tap-water enemas. When such losses decrease circulating fluid volume, increased secretion of antidiuretic hormone (ADH) promotes maximum water reabsorption, which further dilutes serum sodium. These factors are especially likely to cause hyponatremia when combined with too much free-water intake.
- excessive drinking of water, infusion of I.V. dextrose in water without other solutes, malnutrition or starvation, and a low-sodium diet, usually in combination with one of the other causes.
- trauma, surgery (wound drainage), or burns, which cause sodium to shift into damaged cells.
- adrenal gland insufficiency (Addi-

CLINICAL EFFECTS OF SODIUM IMBALANCE

DYSFUNCTION	HYPONATREMIA	HYPERNATREMIA
CNS	• Anxiety, headaches, muscle twitching and weakness, convulsions	• Fever, agitation, restlessness, convulsions
Cardiovascular	• Hypotension; tachycardia; with severe deficit, vasomotor collapse, thready pulse	• Hypertension, tachycardia, pitting edema, excessive weight gain
Gastrointestinal	• Nausea, vomiting, abdominal cramps	• Rough, dry tongue; intense thirst
Genitourinary	• Oliguria or anuria	• Oliguria
Respiratory	• Cyanosis with severe deficiency	• Dyspnea, respiratory arrest, and death (from dramatic rise in osmotic pressure)
Cutaneous	• Cold clammy skin, decreased skin turgor	• Flushed skin; dry, sticky mucous membranes

son's disease) or hypoaldosteronism.

- cirrhosis of the liver with ascites.
- syndrome of inappropriate antidiuretic hormone secretion (SIADH), resulting from brain tumor, cerebrovascular accident, pulmonary disease, or neoplasm with ectopic ADH production. Certain drugs, such as chlorpropamide and clofibrate, may produce an SIADH-like syndrome.

Causes of hypernatremia include:

- decreased water intake. When severe vomiting and diarrhea cause water loss that exceeds sodium loss, serum sodium levels rise, but overall extracellular fluid volume decreases.
- excess adrenocortical hormones, as in Cushing's syndrome.
- ADH deficiency (diabetes insipidus).
- salt intoxication (less common), which may be produced by excessive ingestion of table salt.

Signs and symptoms

Sodium imbalance has profound physiologic effects and can induce severe central nervous system, cardiovascular, and gastrointestinal abnormalities. For example, hyponatremia may cause renal dysfunction or, if serum sodium loss is abrupt or severe, may result in seizures; hypernatremia may produce pulmonary edema, circulatory disorders, and decreased level of consciousness.

Diagnosis

Hyponatremia is defined as serum sodium level less than 135 mEq/liter; hypernatremia, as serum sodium level greater than 145 mEq/liter. However, additional laboratory studies are necessary to determine etiology and differentiate between a true deficit and an apparent deficit due to sodium shift or to hypervolemia or hypovolemia. In true hyponatremia, supportive values include urine sodium greater than 100 mEq/24 hours, with low serum osmolality; in true hypernatremia, urine sodium is less than 40 mEq/24 hours, with high serum osmolality.

Treatment

Therapy for mild hyponatremia usually consists of restricted free-water intake when it is due to hemodilution, SIADH, or conditions such as congestive heart failure, cirrhosis of the liver, and renal failure. If fluid restriction alone fails to normalize serum sodium levels, demeclocycline or lithium, which blocks ADH action in the renal tubules, can be used to promote water excretion. In extremely rare instances of severe symptomatic hyponatremia, when serum sodium levels fall below 110 mEq/liter, treatment may include infusion of 3% or 5% saline solution.

Treatment with saline infusion requires

careful monitoring of venous pressure to prevent potentially fatal circulatory overload. The aim of treatment of secondary hyponatremia is to correct the underlying disorder.

Primary treatment of hypernatremia is administration of salt-free solutions (such as dextrose in water) to return serum sodium levels to normal, followed by infusion of 0.45% sodium chloride to prevent hyponatremia. Other measures include a sodium-restricted diet and discontinuation of drugs that promote sodium retention.

Special considerations

When managing the patient with hyponatremia:

- Watch for and report extremely low serum sodium and accompanying serum chloride levels. Monitor urine specific gravity and other laboratory results. Record fluid intake and output accurately, and weigh the patient daily.
- During administration of isosmolar or hyperosmolar saline solution, watch closely for signs of hypervolemia (dyspnea, rales, engorged neck or hand veins). Report conditions that may cause excessive sodium loss—diaphoresis or prolonged diarrhea or vomiting, and severe burns.
- Refer the patient on maintenance dosage of diuretics to a dietitian for instruction about dietary sodium intake.
- To prevent hyponatremia, administer isosmolar solutions.

When managing the patient with hypernatremia:

- Measure serum sodium levels every 6 hours or at least daily. Monitor vital signs for changes, especially for rising pulse rate. Watch for signs of hypervolemia, especially in the patient receiving I.V. fluids.
- Record fluid intake and output accurately, checking for body fluid loss. Weigh the patient daily.
- Obtain a drug history to check for drugs that promote sodium retention.
- Explain the importance of sodium restriction, and teach the patient how to plan a low-sodium diet. Closely monitor the serum sodium levels of high-risk patients.

Calcium Imbalance

Calcium plays an indispensable role in cell permeability, formation of bones and teeth, blood coagulation, transmission of nerve impulses, and normal muscle contraction. Nearly all (99%) of the body's calcium is found in the bones. The remaining 1% exists in ionized form in serum, and it is the maintenance of the 1% of ionized calcium in the serum that is critical to healthy neurologic function. The parathyroid glands regulate ionized calcium and determine its resorption into bone, absorption from the gastrointestinal mucosa, and excretion in urine and feces. Severe calcium imbalance requires emergency treatment, since a deficiency (hypocalcemia) can lead to tetany and convulsions; excess (hypercalcemia), to cardiac arrhythmias.

Causes

Common causes of hypocalcemia include:

- *inadequate intake of calcium and vitamin D,* in which inadequate levels of vitamin D inhibit intestinal absorption of calcium.
- *hypoparathyroidism* as a result of injury, disease, or surgery that decreases or eliminates secretion of parathyroid hormone (PTH), which is necessary for calcium absorption and normal serum calcium levels.
- *malabsorption or loss of calcium from the gastrointestinal tract,* caused by increased intestinal motility from severe diarrhea or laxative abuse. Malabsorption of calcium from the gastrointestinal

tract can also result from inadequate levels of vitamin D or PTH, or a reduction in gastric acidity, decreasing the solubility of calcium salts.

- *severe infections or burns,* in which diseased and burned tissue traps calcium from the extracellular fluid.
- *overcorrection of acidosis,* resulting in alkalosis, which causes decreased ionized calcium and induces symptoms of hypocalcemia.
- *pancreatic insufficiency,* which may cause malabsorption of calcium and subsequent calcium loss in feces. In pancreatitis, participation of calcium ions in saponification contributes to calcium loss.
- *renal failure,* resulting in excessive excretion of calcium secondary to increased retention of phosphate.
- *hypomagnesemia,* which causes decreased PTH secretion and blocks the peripheral action of that hormone.

Causes of hypercalcemia include:

- *Hyperparathyroidism* increases serum calcium levels by promoting calcium absorption from the intestine, resorption from bone, and reabsorption from the kidneys.
- *Hypervitaminosis D* can promote increased absorption of calcium from the intestine.
- *Tumors* raise serum calcium levels by destroying bone or by releasing PTH or a PTH-like substance, osteoclast-activating factor, prostaglandins, and perhaps, a vitamin D–like sterol.
- *Multiple fractures and prolonged immobilization* release bone calcium and raise the serum calcium level.
- *Multiple myeloma* promotes loss of calcium from bone.

Other causes include milk-alkali syndrome, sarcoidosis, hyperthyroidism, adrenal insufficiency, thiazide diuretics, and loss of serum albumin secondary to renal disease.

Signs and symptoms

Calcium deficit causes nerve fiber irritability and repetitive muscle spasms. Consequently, characteristic symptoms of hypocalcemia include perioral paresthesia, twitching, carpopedal spasm, tetany, seizures, and possibly, cardiac arrhythmias. Chvostek's sign and Trousseau's sign are reliable indicators of hypocalcemia.

SYMPTOMS OF CALCIUM IMBALANCE

DYSFUNCTION	HYPOCALCEMIA	HYPERCALCEMIA
CNS	• Anxiety, irritability, twitching around mouth, laryngospasm, convulsions, Chvostek's sign, Trousseau's sign	• Drowsiness, lethargy, headaches, depression or apathy, irritability, confusion
Musculoskeletal	• Paresthesia (tingling and numbness of the fingers), tetany or painful tonic muscle spasms, facial spasms, abdominal cramps, muscle cramps, spasmodic contractions	• Weakness, muscle flaccidity, bone pain, pathologic fractures
Cardiovascular	• Arrhythmias, hypotension	• Signs of heart block, cardiac arrest in systole, hypertension
Gastrointestinal	• Increased GI motility, diarrhea	• Anorexia, nausea, vomiting, constipation, dehydration, polydipsia
Other	• Blood-clotting abnormalities	• Renal polyuria, flank pain, and eventually, azotemia

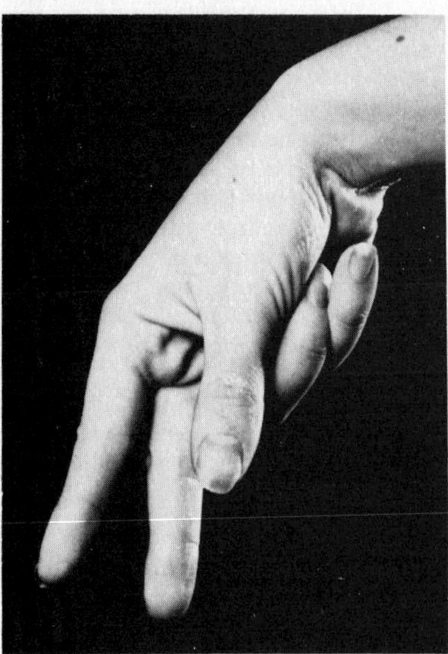

To check for Trousseau's sign, apply a blood pressure cuff to the patient's arm. A carpopedal spasm that causes thumb adduction and phalangeal extension, as shown, confirms tetany.

Clinical effects of hypercalcemia include muscle weakness, decreased muscle tone, lethargy, anorexia, constipation, nausea, vomiting, dehydration, polydipsia, and polyuria. Severe hypercalcemia (serum levels that exceed 5.7 mEq/liter) may produce cardiac dysrhythmias and, eventually, coma.

Diagnosis

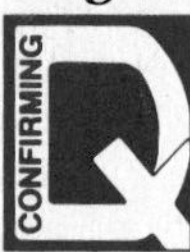

A serum calcium level less than 4.5 mEq/liter confirms hypocalcemia; a level above 5.5 mEq/liter confirms hypercalcemia. (However, since approximately one half of serum calcium is bound to albumin, changes in serum protein must be considered when interpreting serum calcium levels.) The Sulkowitch urine test shows increased calcium precipitation in hypercalcemia. In hypocalcemia, EKG reveals lengthened QT interval, prolonged ST segment, and dysrhythmias; in hypercalcemia, shortened QT interval and heart block.

Treatment

Treatment varies and requires correction of the acute imbalance, followed by maintenance therapy and correction of the underlying cause. Mild hypocalcemia may require nothing more than an adjustment in diet to allow adequate intake of calcium, vitamin D, and protein, possibly with oral calcium supplements. Acute hypocalcemia is an emergency that needs immediate correction by I.V. administration of calcium gluconate or calcium chloride. Chronic hypocalcemia also requires vitamin D supplements to facilitate gastrointestinal absorption of calcium. To correct mild deficiency states, the amounts of vitamin D in most multivitamin preparations are adequate. For severe deficiency, vitamin D is used in four forms: ergocalciferol (vitamin D_2), cholecalciferol (vitamin D_3), calcitriol, and dihydrotachysterol, a synthetic form of vitamin D_2.

Treatment of hypercalcemia primarily eliminates excess serum calcium through hydration with normal saline solution, which promotes calcium excretion in urine. Loop diuretics, such as ethacrynic acid and furosemide, also promote calcium excretion. (Thiazide diuretics are contraindicated in hypercalcemia, because they inhibit calcium excretion.) Corticosteroids, such as prednisone and hydrocortisone, are helpful in treating sarcoidosis, hypervitaminosis D, and certain tumors. Mithramycin can also lower serum calcium level and is especially effective against hypercalcemia secondary to certain tumors. Calcitonin may also be helpful in certain instances. Sodium phosphate solution administered P.O. or by retention enema promotes deposition of calcium in bone and inhibits its absorption from the gastrointestinal tract.

Special considerations

Watch for hypocalcemia in patients receiving massive transfusions of citrated blood and in those with chronic diarrhea, severe infections, and insufficient dietary intake of calcium and protein (especially the elderly).

• Monitor serum calcium levels every 12 to 24 hours, and report a calcium deficit less than 4.5 mEq/liter immediately. When giving calcium supplements, frequently check pH level, since an alkalotic state that exceeds 7.45 pH inhibits calcium ionization. Check for Trousseau's and Chvostek's signs.
• Administer calcium gluconate slow I.V. in 5% dextrose in water (*never* in saline solution, which encourages renal calcium loss). Don't add calcium gluconate I.V. to solutions containing bicarbonate; it will precipitate. When administering calcium solutions, watch for anorexia, nausea, and vomiting—possible signs of overcorrection to hypercalcemia.
• If the patient is receiving calcium chloride, watch for abdominal discomfort.
• Monitor the patient closely for a possible drug interaction if he's receiving digitalis with large doses of oral calcium supplements; watch for signs of digitalis toxicity (anorexia, nausea, vomiting, yellow vision, and cardiac arrhythmias). Administer oral calcium supplements 1 to 1½ hours after meals or with milk.
• Provide a quiet, stress-free environment for the patient with tetany. Observe seizure precautions for patients with severe hypocalcemia that may lead to convulsions.
• To prevent hypocalcemia, advise all patients—especially the elderly—to eat foods rich in calcium, vitamin D, and protein, such as fortified milk and cheese. Explain how important calcium is for normal bone formation and blood coagulation. Discourage chronic use of laxatives. Also, warn hypocalcemic patients not to overuse antacids, since these may aggravate the condition.

If the patient has hypercalcemia:
• Monitor serum calcium levels frequently. Watch for cardiac arrhythmias if serum calcium level exceeds 5.7 mEq/liter. Increase fluid intake to dilute calcium in serum and urine, and to prevent renal damage and dehydration. Watch for signs of congestive heart failure in patients receiving normal saline solution diuresis therapy.
• Administer loop diuretics (not thiazide diuretics), as ordered. Monitor intake and output, and check urine for renal calculi and acidity. Provide acid-ash drinks, such as cranberry or prune juice, since calcium salts are more soluble in acid than in alkali.
• Check EKG and vital signs frequently. In the patient receiving digitalis, watch for signs of toxicity, such as anorexia, nausea, vomiting, and bradycardia (often with arrhythmia).
• Ambulate the patient as soon as possible. Handle the patient with chronic hypercalcemia *gently* to prevent pathologic fractures. If the patient is bedridden, reposition him frequently, and encourage range-of-motion exercises to promote circulation and prevent urinary stasis and calcium loss from bone.
• To prevent recurrence, suggest a low-calcium diet, with increased fluid intake.

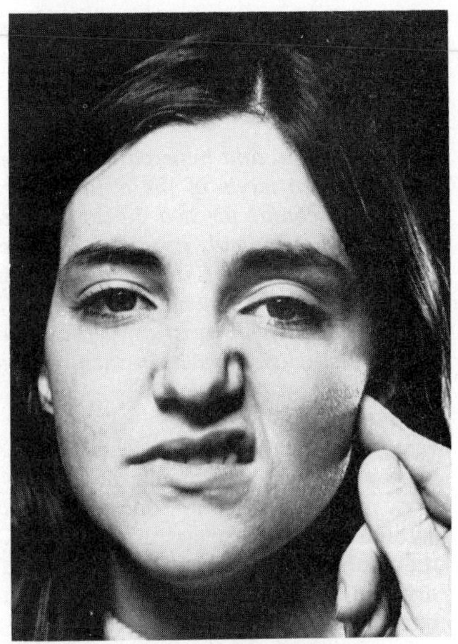
To check for Chvostek's sign, tap the facial nerve above the mandibular angle, adjacent to the ear lobe. A facial muscle spasm that causes the patient's upper lip to twitch, as shown, confirms tetany.

Chloride Imbalance

Hypochloremia and hyperchloremia are, respectively, conditions of deficient or excessive serum levels of the anion chloride. A predominantly extracellular anion, chloride accounts for two thirds of all serum anions. Secreted by stomach mucosa as hydrochloric acid, it provides an acid medium conducive to digestion and activation of enzymes. Chloride also participates in maintaining acid-base and body water balances, influences the osmolality or tonicity of extracellular fluid, plays a role in the exchange of oxygen and carbon dioxide in RBCs, and helps activate salivary amylase (which, in turn, activates the digestive process).

Causes

Hypochloremia may result from:

- decreased chloride intake or absorption, as in low dietary sodium intake, sodium deficiency, potassium deficiency, metabolic alkalosis; prolonged use of mercurial diuretics; or administration of dextrose I.V. without electrolytes.
- excessive chloride loss, resulting from prolonged diarrhea or diaphoresis; loss of hydrochloric acid in gastric secretions, due to vomiting, gastric suctioning, or gastric surgery.

Hyperchloremia may result from:

- excessive chloride intake or absorption—as in hyperingestion of ammonium chloride, or ureterointestinal anastomosis—allowing reabsorption of chloride by the bowel.
- hemoconcentration, caused by dehydration.
- compensatory mechanisms for other metabolic abnormalities, as in metabolic acidosis, brain stem injury causing neurogenic hyperventilation, and hyperparathyroidism.

Signs and symptoms

Hypochloremia is usually associated with hyponatremia and its characteristic muscular weakness and twitching, since renal chloride loss always accompanies sodium loss, and sodium reabsorption is not possible without chloride. However, if chloride depletion results from metabolic alkalosis secondary to loss of gastric secretions, chloride is lost independently from sodium; typical symptoms are muscle hypertonicity, tetany, and shallow, depressed breathing.

Because of the natural affinity of sodium and chloride ions, hyperchloremia usually produces clinical effects associated with hypernatremia and resulting extracellular fluid volume excess (agitation, tachycardia, hypertension, pitting edema, dyspnea). Hyperchloremia associated with metabolic acidosis is due to excretion of base bicarbonate by the kidneys, and induces deep, rapid breathing; weakness; diminished cognitive ability; and ultimately, coma.

Diagnosis

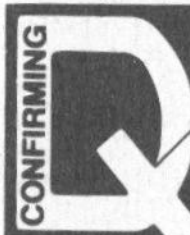

Serum chloride level < 98 mEq/liter confirms hypochloremia; supportive values with metabolic alkalosis include serum pH > 7.45 and serum CO_2 > 32 mEq/liter.

Serum chloride level > 108 mEq/liter confirms hyperchloremia; with metabolic acidosis, serum pH is < 7.35 and serum CO_2 is < 22 mEq/liter.

Treatment

The aims of treatment for hypochloremia are to correct the condition that causes excessive chloride loss and to give oral replacement, such as salty broth. When oral therapy is not possible or when emergency measures are necessary, treatment may include normal saline solution I.V. (if hypovolemia is present) or chloride-containing drugs, such as ammonium chloride, to increase serum chloride levels, and potassium chloride for metabolic alkalosis. For severe hyperchloremic acidosis, treatment consists of sodium bicarbonate I.V. to raise serum bicarbonate level and permit renal excretion of the chloride anion, since bicarbonate and chloride compete for combination with sodium. For mild hyperchloremia, Ringer's lactate solution is administered; it converts to bicarbonate in the liver, thus increasing base bicarbonate to correct acidosis.

In either kind of chloride imbalance, treatment must correct the underlying disorder.

Special considerations

When managing the patient with hypochloremia:

- Monitor serum chloride levels frequently, particularly during I.V. therapy.
- Watch for signs of hyperchloremia or hypochloremia. Be alert for respiratory difficulty.
- To prevent hypochloremia, monitor laboratory results (serum electrolytes and blood gases) and fluid intake and output of patients who are vulnerable to chloride imbalance, particularly those recovering from gastric surgery. Record and report excessive or continuous loss of gastric secretions. Also report prolonged infusion of dextrose in water without saline.

When managing the patient with hyperchloremia:

- Check serum electrolyte levels every 3 to 6 hours. If the patient is receiving high doses of sodium bicarbonate, watch for signs of overcorrection (metabolic alkalosis, respiratory depression) or lingering signs of hyperchloremia, which indicate inadequate treatment.
- To prevent hyperchloremia, check laboratory results for elevated serum chloride or potassium imbalance if the patient is receiving I.V. solutions containing sodium chloride, and monitor fluid intake and output. Also, watch for signs of metabolic acidosis. When administering I.V. fluids containing Ringer's lactate solution, monitor flow rate according to the patient's age, physical condition, and bicarbonate level. Report any irregularities promptly.

Magnesium Imbalance

Magnesium is the second most common cation in intracellular fluid. Although its major function is to enhance neuromuscular integration, it also stimulates parathyroid hormone (PTH) secretion, thus regulating intracellular fluid calcium levels. Therefore, magnesium deficiency (hypomagnesemia) may result in transient hypoparathyroidism and/or interference with the peripheral action of PTH. Magnesium may also regulate skeletal muscles through its influence on calcium utilization by depressing acetylcholine release at synaptic junctions. In addition, magnesium activates many enzymes for proper carbohydrate and protein metabolism, aids in cell metabolism and the transport of sodium and potassium across cell membranes, and influences sodium, potassium, calcium, and protein levels.

Approximately one third of magnesium taken into the body is absorbed through the small intestine and is eventually excreted in urine; the remaining unabsorbed magnesium is excreted in stool.

Since many common foods contain magnesium, a dietary deficiency is rare. Hypomagnesemia generally follows impaired absorption or too-rapid excretion of magnesium. It frequently coexists with other electrolyte imbalances, especially low calcium and potassium levels. Magnesium excess (hypermagnesemia) is common in patients with renal failure and excessive intake of magnesium-containing antacids.

Causes

Hypomagnesemia usually results from impaired absorption of magnesium in intestines or excessive excretion in urine or stool. Possible causes include:

- decreased magnesium intake or absorption, as in malabsorption syndrome, chronic diarrhea, or postoperative complications after bowel resection; chronic alcoholism; prolonged diuretic therapy, nasogastric suctioning, or administration of parenteral fluids without magnesium salts; starvation or malnutrition.
- excessive loss of magnesium, as in severe dehydration and diabetic acidosis; hyperaldosteronism and hypoparathyroidism, which result in hypokalemia and hypocalcemia; hyperparathyroidism and hypercalcemia; excessive release of adrenocortical hormones; diuretic therapy.

Hypermagnesemia results from the kidneys' inability to excrete magnesium that was either absorbed from the intestines or infused. Common causes of hypermagnesemia include:

- chronic renal insufficiency.
- use of laxatives (magnesium sulfate, milk of magnesia, and magnesium citrate solutions), especially with renal insufficiency.
- overuse of magnesium-containing antacids.
- severe dehydration (resulting oliguria can cause magnesium retention).
- overcorrection of hypomagnesemia.

Signs and symptoms

Hypomagnesemia causes neuromuscular irritability and cardiac arrythmias. Hypermagnesemia causes CNS and respiratory depression, in addition to neuromuscular and cardiac effects.

Diagnosis

Decreased serum magnesium levels (less than 1.5 mEq/liter) confirm hypomagnesemia; increased levels (greater than 2.5 mEq/liter), hypermagnesemia. Low levels of other serum electrolytes (especially potassium and calcium) often coexist with hypomagnesemia. In fact, unresponsiveness to correct treatment for hypokalemia strongly suggests hypomagnesemia. Similarly, elevated levels of other serum electrolytes are associated with hypermagnesemia.

Treatment

The aim of therapy for magnesium imbalance is identification and correction of the underlying cause.

Treatment of mild hypomagnesemia consists of daily magnesium supplements I.M. or P.O.; of severe hypomagnesemia, magnesium sulfate I.V. (10 to 40 mEq/liter diluted in I.V. fluid). Magnesium intoxication (a possible side ef-

SIGNS AND SYMPTOMS OF MAGNESIUM IMBALANCE

DYSFUNCTION	HYPOMAGNESEMIA	HYPERMAGNESEMIA
Neuromuscular	• Hyperirritability, tetany, leg and foot cramps, Chvostek's sign (facial muscle spasms induced by tapping the branches of the facial nerve)	• Diminished reflexes, muscle weakness, flaccid paralysis, respiratory muscle paralysis that may cause respiratory embarrassment
CNS	• Confusion, delusions, hallucinations, convulsions	• Drowsiness, flushing, lethargy, confusion, diminished sensorium
Cardiovascular	• Arrhythmias, vasomotor changes (vasodilation and hypotension), occasionally, hypertension	• Bradycardia, weak pulse, hypotension, heart block, cardiac arrest (common with serum levels of 25 mEq/liter)

fect) requires calcium gluconate I.V.

Therapy for hypermagnesemia includes increased fluid intake and loop diuretics, such as furosemide, with impaired renal function; calcium gluconate (10%), a magnesium antagonist, for temporary relief of symptoms in an emergency; and peritoneal dialysis or hemodialysis if renal function fails or if excess magnesium can't be eliminated.

Special considerations

For patients with hypomagnesemia:

- Monitor serum electrolytes (including magnesium, calcium, and potassium) daily for mild deficits and every 6 to 12 hours during replacement therapy.
- Measure intake and output frequently (urinary output shouldn't fall below 25 ml/hour or 600 ml/day). Remember, the kidneys excrete excess magnesium, and hypermagnesemia could occur with renal insufficiency.
- Monitor vital signs during I.V. therapy. Infuse magnesium replacement slowly, and watch for bradycardia, heart block, and decreased respirations. Have calcium gluconate I.V. available to reverse hypermagnesemia from overcorrection.
- Advise patients to eat foods high in magnesium, such as fish and green vegetables.
- Watch for and report signs of hypomagnesemia in patients with predisposing diseases or conditions, especially those not permitted anything by mouth or who receive I.V. fluids without magnesium.

For patients with hypermagnesemia:

- Frequently assess level of consciousness, muscle activity, and vital signs.
- Keep accurate intake and output records. Provide sufficient fluids for adequate hydration and maintenance of renal function.
- Report abnormal serum electrolyte levels immediately.
- Monitor and report EKG changes (peaked T waves, increased PR intervals, widened QRS complex).
- Watch patients receiving digitalis and calcium gluconate simultaneously, since calcium excess enhances digitalis action, predisposing the patient to digitalis intoxication.
- Advise patients not to abuse laxatives and antacids containing magnesium, particularly the elderly or those patients with compromised renal function.
- Watch for signs of hypermagnesemia in predisposed patients. Observe closely for respiratory distress if magnesium serum levels rise above 10 mEq/liter.

Phosphorus Imbalance

Phosphorus exists primarily in inorganic combination with calcium in teeth and bones. In extracellular fluid, the phosphate ion supports several metabolic functions: utilization of B vitamins, acid-base homeostasis, bone formation, nerve and muscle activity, cell division, transmission of hereditary traits, and metabolism of carbohydrates, proteins, and fats. Renal tubular reabsorption of phosphate is inversely regulated by calcium levels—an increase in phosphorus causes a decrease in calcium. An imbalance causes hypophosphatemia or hyperphosphatemia. Incidence of hypophosphatemia varies with the underlying cause; hyperphosphatemia occurs most often in children, who tend to consume more phosphorus-rich foods and beverages than adults, and in children and adults with renal insufficiency. Prognosis for both conditions depends on the underlying cause.

Causes

Hypophosphatemia is usually the result of inadequate dietary intake; it is often related to malnutrition resulting from a prolonged catabolic state or chronic alcoholism. It may also stem from intes-

FOODS HIGH IN PHOSPHORUS (P)

FOOD	PORTION	P (mg)
Almonds	⅔ cup	475
Beef liver (fried)	3½ oz	476
Broccoli (cooked)	⅔ cup	62
Carbonated beverage	12 oz	up to 500
Milk (whole)	8 oz	93
Turkey (roasted)	3½ oz	251

tinal malabsorption, chronic diarrhea, hyperparathyroidism with resultant hypercalcemia, hypomagnesemia, or deficiency of vitamin D, which is necessary for intestinal phosphorus absorption. Other important causes include chronic use of antacids containing aluminum hydroxide, use of hyperalimentation solution with inadequate phosphate content, renal tubular defects, tissue damage in which phosphorus is released by injured cells, and diabetic acidosis.

Hyperphosphatemia is generally secondary to hypocalcemia, hypervitaminosis D, hypoparathyroidism, or renal failure (often due to stress or injury). It may also result from overuse of laxatives with phosphates or phosphate enemas.

Signs and symptoms

Hypophosphatemia produces anorexia, muscle weakness, tremor, paresthesia, and, when persistent, osteomalacia, causing bone pain. Impaired red blood cell functions may occur in hypophosphatemia due to alterations in oxyhemoglobin dissociation, which may result in peripheral hypoxia. Hyperphosphatemia usually remains asymptomatic unless it results in hypocalcemia, with tetany and convulsions.

Diagnosis

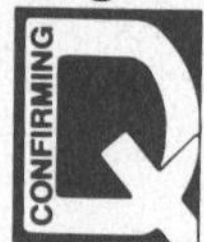

Serum phosphorus level less than 1.7 mEq/liter or 2.5 mg/dl confirms hypophosphatemia. Urine phosphorus level more than 1.3 g/24 hours supports this diagnosis.

Serum phosphorus level over 2.6 mEq/liter or 4.5 mg/dl confirms hyperphosphatemia. Supportive values include decreased levels of serum calcium (less than 9 mg/dl) and urine phosphorus (less than 0.9 g/24 hours).

Treatment

The treatment goal is to correct the underlying cause of phosphorus imbalance. Until this is done, management of hypophosphatemia consists of phosphorus replacement, with a high-phosphorus diet and P.O. administration of phosphate salt tablets or capsules. Severe hypophosphatemia requires I.V. infusion of potassium phosphate. Severe hyperphosphatemia may require peritoneal dialysis or hemodialysis to lower the serum phosphorus level.

Special considerations

- Carefully monitor serum electrolyte, calcium, magnesium, and phosphorus levels. Report any changes immediately.

To manage hypophosphatemia:

- Record intake and output accurately. Administer potassium phosphate slow I.V. to prevent overcorrection to hyperphosphatemia. Assess renal function, and be alert for hypocalcemia when giving phosphate supplements. If phosphate salt tablets cause nausea, use capsules instead.
- To prevent recurrence, advise the patient to follow a high-phosphorus diet containing milk and milk products, kidney, liver, turkey, and dried fruits.

To manage hyperphosphatemia:

- Monitor intake and output. If urinary output falls below 25 ml/hour or 600 ml/day, notify the doctor immediately, since decreased output can seriously affect renal clearance of excess serum phosphorus.
- Watch for signs of hypocalcemia, such as muscle twitching and tetany, which often accompany hyperphosphatemia.
- To prevent recurrence, advise the patient to eat foods with low phosphorus content, such as vegetables. Obtain dietary consultation if the condition results from chronic renal insufficiency.

Syndrome of Inappropriate Antidiuretic Hormone Secretion

Syndrome of inappropriate antidiuretic hormone secretion (SIADH) is marked by excessive release of ADH, which disturbs fluid and electrolyte balance. Such disturbances result from inability to excrete dilute urine, retention of free water, expansion of extracellular fluid volume, and hyponatremia. SIADH occurs secondary to diseases that affect the osmoreceptors (supraoptic nucleus) of the hypothalamus. Prognosis depends on the underlying disorder and response to treatment.

Causes

The most common cause of SIADH (80% of patients) is oat cell carcinoma of the lung, which secretes excessive ADH or vasopressor-like substances. Other neoplastic diseases—such as pancreatic and prostatic cancer, Hodgkin's disease, and thymoma—may also trigger SIADH. Less common causes include:

- *Central nervous system disorders:* brain tumor or abscess, cerebrovascular accident, head injury, Guillain-Barré syndrome, and lupus erythematosus
- *pulmonary disorders:* pneumonia, tuberculosis, lung abscess, and positive-pressure ventilation
- *drugs:* chlorpropamide, vincristine, cyclophosphamide, carbamazepine, clofibrate, and morphine
- *miscellaneous conditions:* myxedema and psychosis.

Signs and symptoms

SIADH may produce weight gain despite anorexia, nausea, and vomiting; muscle weakness; restlessness; and possibly coma and convulsions. Edema is rare unless water overload exceeds 4 liters, since much of the free water excess is within cellular boundaries.

Diagnosis

Complete medical history revealing positive water balance may suggest SIADH.

Serum osmolality less than 280 mOsm/kg of water and serum sodium less than 123 mEq/liter confirm it (normal urine osmolality is one and a half serum values). Supportive laboratory values include high urine sodium secretion (more than 20 mEq/liter) without diuretics. In addition, diagnostic studies show normal renal function and no evidence of dehydration.

Treatment

Treatment for SIADH is symptomatic and begins with restricted water intake (500 to 1,000 ml/day). With severe water intoxication, administration of 200 to 300 ml of 5% saline may be necessary to raise serum sodium level. When possible, treatment should include correction of the underlying cause of SIADH. If SIADH is due to malignancy, success in alleviating water retention may be obtained by surgical resection, irradiation, or chemotherapy. If fluid restriction is ineffective, demeclocycline or lithium may be helpful by blocking the renal response to ADH.

Special considerations

- Closely monitor and record intake and output, vital signs, and daily weight. Watch for hyponatremia.
- Observe for restlessness, irritability, convulsions, congestive heart failure, and unresponsiveness due to hyponatremia and water intoxication.
- To prevent water intoxication, explain to the patient and his family why he *must* restrict his intake.

Metabolic Acidosis

Metabolic acidosis is a physiologic state of excess acid accumulation and deficient base bicarbonate produced by an underlying pathologic disorder. Symptoms result from the body's attempts to correct the acidotic condition through compensatory mechanisms in the lungs, kidneys, and cells. Metabolic acidosis is more prevalent among children, who are vulnerable to acid-base imbalance because their metabolic rates are faster and their ratios of water to total-body weight are lower. Severe or untreated metabolic acidosis can be fatal.

Causes

Metabolic acidosis usually results from excessive burning of fats in the absence of usable carbohydrates. This can be caused by diabetic ketoacidosis, chronic alcoholism, malnutrition, or a low-carbohydrate, high-fat diet—all of which produce more keto acids than the metabolic process can handle. Other causes include:

- *anaerobic carbohydrate metabolism:* a decrease in tissue oxygenation or perfusion, as occurs with pump failure after myocardial infarction, or with pulmonary or hepatic disease, shock, or anemia forces a shift from aerobic to anaerobic metabolism, causing a corresponding rise in lactic acid level.
- *renal insufficiency and failure (renal acidosis):* underexcretion of metabolized acids or inability to conserve base.
- *diarrhea and intestinal malabsorption:* loss of sodium bicarbonate from the intestines, causing the bicarbonate buffer system to shift to the acidic side. For example, ureteroenterostomy and Crohn's disease can also induce metabolic acidosis.

Less frequently, metabolic acidosis results from salicylate intoxication (overuse of aspirin), exogenous poisoning, or Addison's disease (due to increased excretion of sodium and chloride, and retention of potassium ions).

ANION GAP (THE DELTA)

The anion gap is the difference between concentrations of serum cations and anions—determined by measuring one cation (sodium) and two anions (chloride and bicarbonate). The normal concentration of sodium is 140 mEq/liter; of chloride, 102 mEq/liter; and of bicarbonate, 26 mEq/liter. Thus, the anion gap between *measured* cations (actually sodium alone) and *measured* anions is about 12 mEq/liter (140 minus 128).

Concentrations of potassium, calcium, and magnesium (*unmeasured* cations), or proteins, phosphate, sulfate, and organic acids (*unmeasured* anions) are not needed to measure the anion gap. Added together, the concentration of unmeasured cations would be about 11 mEq/liter; of unmeasured anions, about 23 mEq/liter. Thus, the normal anion gap between unmeasured cations and anions is about 12 mEq/liter (23 minus 11)—give or take 2 mEq/liter for normal variation. An anion gap over 14 mEq/liter indicates *metabolic acidosis.* It may result from accumulation of excess organic acids or from retention of hydrogen ions, which chemically bond with bicarbonate and decrease bicarbonate levels.

Signs and symptoms

In mild acidosis, symptoms of the underlying disease may obscure any direct clinical evidence. Metabolic acidosis typically begins with headache and lethargy, progressing to drowsiness, CNS depression, Kussmaul's respirations (as the lungs attempt to compensate by "blowing off" CO_2), stupor, and if the condition is severe and goes untreated, coma and death. Associated gastrointestinal distress usually produces anorexia, nausea, vomiting, and diarrhea, and may lead to dehydration. Underlying diabetes mellitus may cause fruity breath from catabolism of fats and excretion of accumulated acetone through the lungs.

Diagnosis

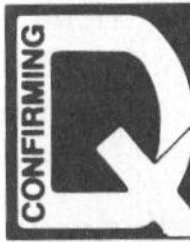

Arterial pH below 7.35 confirms metabolic acidosis. In severe acidotic states, pH may fall to 7.10 and arterial blood gas P_{CO_2} may be normal or < 34 mm Hg as compensatory mechanisms take hold. HCO_3 may be < 22 mEq/liter. Supportive findings include:

- *urine pH:* < 4.5 in the absence of renal disease
- *serum potassium levels:* > 5.5 mEq/liter from chemical buffering
- *glucose:* > 150 mg/dl in diabetes
- *serum ketone bodies:* elevated in diabetes mellitus
- *plasma lactic acid:* elevated in lactic acidosis
- *anion gap:* > 14 mEq/liter indicates metabolic acidosis (diabetic ketoacidosis, aspirin overdose, alcohol poisoning).

Treatment

Treatment for metabolic acidosis includes sodium bicarbonate I.V. to neutralize blood acidity, careful evaluation and correction of electrolyte imbalances, and, ultimately, correction of the underlying cause. For example, in diabetic ketoacidosis, low-dose continuous I.V. insulin infusion is recommended.

Special considerations

- Keep sodium bicarbonate ampules handy for emergency administration. Frequently monitor vital signs, laboratory results, and level of consciousness, since changes can occur rapidly.
- In diabetic acidosis, watch for secondary changes due to hypovolemia, such as decreasing blood pressure.
- Record intake and output accurately to monitor renal function. Watch for signs of excessive serum potassium—weakness, flaccid paralysis, and dysrhythmias, possibly leading to cardiac arrest. After treatment, check for overcorrection to hypokalemia.
- Because metabolic acidosis commonly causes vomiting, position the patient to prevent aspiration. Prepare for possible convulsions with seizure precautions.
- Provide good oral hygiene. Use sodium bicarbonate washes to neutralize mouth acids, and lubricate the patient's lips with lemon and glycerine swabs.
- To prevent metabolic acidosis, carefully observe patients receiving I.V. therapy or who have intestinal tubes in place, as well as those suffering from shock, hyperthyroidism, hepatic disease, and circulatory failure, or dehydration. Teach the patient with diabetes how to routinely test urine for sugar and acetone, and encourage strict adherence to insulin or oral hypoglycemic therapy.

Metabolic Alkalosis

A clinical state marked by decreased amounts of acid or increased amounts of base bicarbonate, metabolic alkalosis causes metabolic, respiratory, and renal responses, producing characteristic symptoms—most notably, hypoventilation. This condition is always secondary to an underlying cause. With early diagnosis and prompt treatment, prognosis is good; however, untreated metabolic alkalosis may lead to coma and death.

Causes

Metabolic alkalosis results from loss of acid, retention of base, or renal mechanisms associated with decreased serum levels of potassium and chloride.

Causes of critical acid loss include

vomiting, nasogastric tube drainage or lavage without adequate electrolyte replacement, fistulas, and the use of steroids and certain diuretics (furosemide, thiazides, and ethacrynic acid). Hyperadrenocorticism is another cause of severe acid loss. Cushing's disease, primary hyperaldosteronism, and Bartter's syndrome, for example, all lead to retention of sodium and chloride, and urinary loss of potassium and hydrogen.

Excessive retention of base can result from excessive intake of bicarbonate of soda or other antacids (usually for treatment of gastritis or peptic ulcer), excessive intake of absorbable alkali (as in milk-alkali syndrome, often seen in patients with peptic ulcers), administration of excessive amounts of I.V. fluids with high concentrations of bicarbonate or lactate, or respiratory insufficiency—all of which cause chronic hypercapnia, from high levels of plasma bicarbonate.

Signs and symptoms

Clinical features of metabolic alkalosis result from the body's attempt to correct the acid-base imbalance, primarily through hypoventilation. Other manifestations include irritability, picking at bedclothes (carphology), twitching, confusion, nausea, vomiting, and diarrhea (which aggravates alkalosis). Cardiovascular abnormalities—such as atrial tachycardia—and respiratory disturbances—such as cyanosis and apnea—also occur. In the alkalotic patient, diminished peripheral blood flow during repeated blood pressure checks may provoke carpopedal spasm in the hand—a possible sign of impending tetany (Trousseau's sign). Uncorrected metabolic alkalosis may progress to convulsions and coma.

Diagnosis

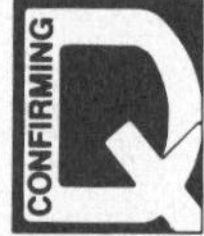

Blood pH level > 7.45 and HCO_3 > 29 mEq/liter confirm diagnosis. A PCO_2 > 45 mmHg indicates attempts at respiratory compensation. Serum electrolyte levels show potassium 3.5 mEq/liter and chloride 98 mEq/liter. Other characteristic findings include:

- *Urine pH* is usually about 7.
- *Urinalysis* reveals alkalinity after the renal compensatory mechanism begins to excrete bicarbonate.
- *EKG* may show low T wave, merging with a P wave, and atrial tachycardia.

Treatment

The goal of treatment is to correct the underlying cause of metabolic alkalosis. Therapy for severe alkalosis may include cautious administration of ammonium chloride I.V. to release hydrogen chloride and restore concentration of extracellular fluid and chloride levels. Potassium chloride and normal saline solution (except in the presence of congestive heart failure) are usually sufficient to replace losses from gastric drainage. Electrolyte replacement with potassium chloride and discontinuing diuretics correct metabolic alkalosis resulting from potent diuretic therapy.

Special considerations

Structure the care plan around cautious I.V. therapy, keen observation, and strict monitoring of the patient's status.

- Dilute potassium when giving I.V. containing potassium salts. Monitor the infusion rate to prevent damage to blood vessels; watch for signs of phlebitis. When administering ammonium chloride 0.9%, limit the infusion rate to 1 liter in 4 hours; faster administration may cause hemolysis of RBCs. Avoid overdosage, since it may cause overcorrection to metabolic acidosis. Don't give ammonium chloride with signs of hepatic or renal disease.
- Watch closely for signs of muscle weakness, tetany, or decreased activity. Monitor vital signs frequently, and record intake and output to evaluate respiratory, fluid, and electrolyte status. Remember, respiratory rate usually decreases in an effort to compensate for alkalosis. Hypotension and tachycardia may indicate electrolyte imbalance, especially hypokalemia.
- Observe seizure precautions.
- To prevent metabolic alkalosis, warn

patients against overusing alkaline agents. Irrigate nasogastric tubes with isotonic saline solution instead of plain water to prevent loss of gastric electrolytes. Monitor I.V. fluid concentrations of bicarbonate or lactate. Teach patients with ulcers to recognize signs of milk-alkali syndrome: a distaste for milk, anorexia, weakness, and lethargy.

Selected References

Bondy, Philip K., and Rosenberg, Leon E. *Metabolic Control of Disease,* 8th ed. Philadelphia: W.B. Saunders Co., 1980.

Cohn, Robert M., and Roth, Karl. *Metabolic Disease: A Guide to Early Recognition.* Philadelphia: W.B. Saunders Co., 1983.

Kee, Joyce L. *Fluids and Electrolytes with Clinical Applications: A Programmed Approach,* 3rd ed. New York: John Wiley & Sons, 1982.

Metheny, Norma, and Snively, W.D., Jr. *Nurses' Handbook of Fluid Balance,* 4th ed. Philadelphia: J.B. Lippincott Co., 1983.

Robinson, Corinne H., and Lawler, Marilyn R. *Normal and Therapeutic Nutrition,* 16th ed. New York: Macmillan Publishing Co., 1982.

Stanbury, John B., et al., eds. *The Metabolic Basis of Inherited Disease,* 5th ed. New York: McGraw-Hill Book Co., 1983.

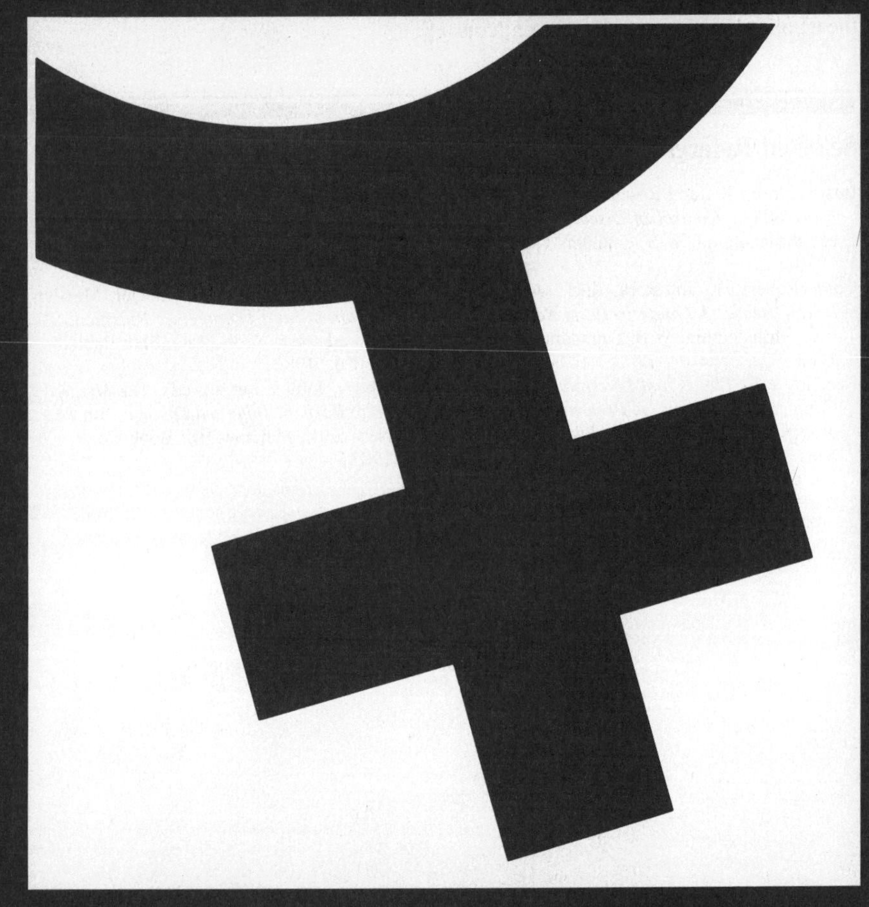

15 Obstetric and Gynecologic Disorders

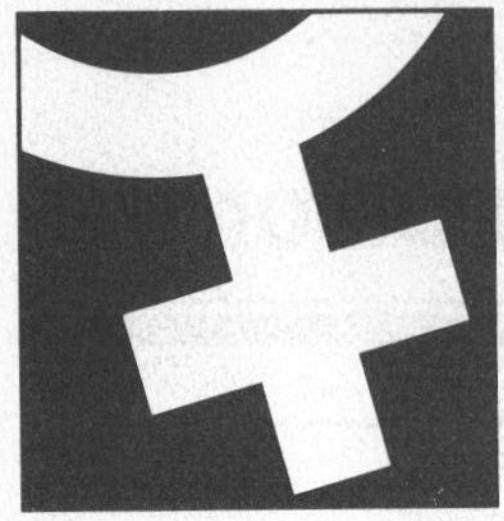

Obstetric and Gynecologic Disorders

Introduction

Medical care of the obstetric or gynecologic patient reflects a growing interest in improving the quality of health care for females. Today, you must be able to assess, counsel, teach, and refer these patients, while weighing such relevant factors as the desire to have children, problems of sexual adjustment, and self-image. Frequently, the situation is further complicated by the fact that multiple obstetric and gynecologic abnormalities often occur simultaneously. For example, a patient with dysmenorrhea may also have trichomonal vaginitis, dysuria, and unsuspected infertility. Her condition may be further complicated by associated urologic disorders, due to the proximity of the urinary and reproductive systems. This tendency to multiple and complex disorders is readily understandable upon review of the anatomic structure of the female genitalia.

External structures

Female genitalia include the following external structures, collectively known as the *vulva:* mons pubis (or mons veneris), labia majora, labia minora, clitoris, vestibule, urethral meatus, hymen, Bartholin's glands and Skene's glands (paraurethral glands), fourchette, and perineum. The size, shape, and color of these structures—as well as pubic hair distribution, and skin texture and pigmentation—vary from person to person and race to race. Furthermore, these external structures undergo distinct changes during the life cycle.

The *mons pubis* is the pad of fat over the symphysis pubis (pubic bone), which is usually covered by the base of the inverted triangular patch of pubic hair that grows over the vulva after puberty.

The *labia majora* are the two thick, longitudinal folds of fatty tissue that extend from the mons pubis to the perineum. The labia majora protect the perineum and contain large sebaceous glands that help maintain lubrication. Virtually absent in the young child, their development is a characteristic sign of onset of puberty. The skin of the more prominent parts of the labia majora is pigmented, and darkens after puberty.

The *labia minora* are the two thin, longitudinal folds of skin that border the vestibule. Firmer than the labia majora, they extend from the clitoris to the fourchette.

The *clitoris* is the small, protuberant organ located just beneath the arch of the mons pubis. The clitoris contains erectile tissue, venous cavernous spaces, and specialized sensory corpuscles that are stimulated during coitus.

The *vestibule* is the oval space bordered by the clitoris, labia minora, and fourchette. The *urethral meatus* is located in the anterior portion of the vestibule; the *vaginal meatus,* in the posterior portion. The *hymen* is the elastic membrane that partially obstructs the vaginal meatus in virgins.

Several glands lubricate the vestibule. *Skene's glands* open on both sides of the urethral meatus; *Bartholin's glands,* on both sides of the vaginal meatus.

The *fourchette* is the posterior junction of the labia majora and labia minora. The *perineum,* which includes the underlying muscles and fascia, is the external surface of the floor of the pelvis,

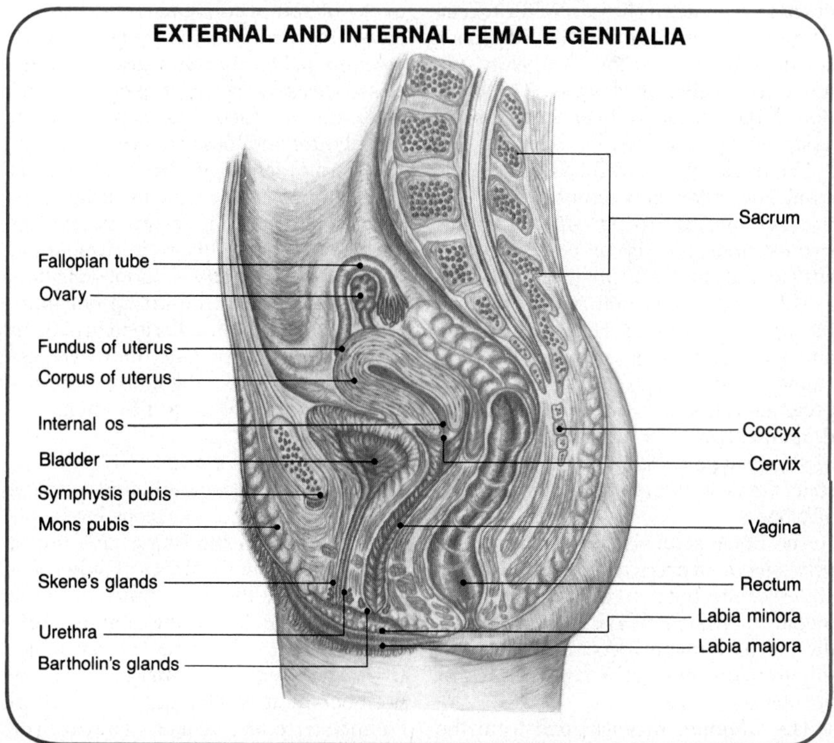

extending from the fourchette to the anus.

Internal structures

The following internal structures are included in the female genitalia: vagina, cervix, uterus, fallopian tubes (or oviducts), and ovaries.

The *vagina* occupies the space between the bladder and the rectum. A muscular, membranous tube approximately 3″ (7.5 cm) long, the vagina connects the uterus and the vestibule of the external genitalia. It serves as a passageway for sperm to the fallopian tubes, for the discharge of menstrual fluid, and for childbirth.

The *cervix,* or neck of the uterus, protrudes at least ¾″ (2 cm) into the proximal end of the vagina. A rounded, conical structure, the cervix joins the uterus and the vagina at a 45° to 90° angle.

The *uterus* is the hollow, pear-shaped organ in which the conceptus grows during pregnancy. The part of the uterus above the junction of the fallopian tubes is called the *fundus;* the part below this junction is called the *corpus.* The junction of the corpus and cervix forms the *lower uterine segment.*

The thick uterine wall consists of mucosal, muscular, and serous layers. The inner mucosal lining—the *endometrium*—undergoes cyclic changes to facilitate and maintain pregnancy.

The smooth muscular middle layer—the *myometrium*—interlaces the uterine and ovarian arteries and veins that circulate blood through the uterus. During pregnancy, this vascular system expands dramatically. After abortion or childbirth, the myometrium contracts to constrict the vasculature and control the loss of blood.

The outer serous layer—the *parietal peritoneum*—covers all the fundus, part of the corpus, but none of the cervix. This incompleteness allows surgical entry into the uterus without incision of the peritoneum, thereby reducing the risk of peritonitis.

The *fallopian tubes* extend from the sides of the fundus and terminate near the ovaries. Through ciliary and muscular action, these small tubes (3¼″ to 5½″ [8 to 14 cm] long) carry ova from the ovaries to the uterus and facilitate the movement of sperm from the uterus toward the ovaries. Fertilization of the ovum normally occurs in a fallopian tube. The same ciliary and muscular action helps move a *zygote* (fertilized ovum) down to the uterus, where it implants in the blood-rich inner uterine lining, the *endometrium.*

The *ovaries* are two almond-shaped organs, one on either side of the fundus, situated behind and below the fallopian tubes. The ovaries produce ova and two primary hormones—estrogen and progesterone—in addition to small amounts of androgen. These hormones, in turn, produce and maintain secondary sex characteristics, prepare the uterus for pregnancy, and stimulate mammary gland development.

The ovaries are connected to the uterus by the uteroovarian ligament and are divided into two parts: the *cortex,* which contains primordial and graafian follicles in various stages of development, and the *medulla,* which consists primarily of vasculature and loose connective tissue.

A normal female is born with at least 400,000 primordial follicles in her ovaries. At puberty, these ova precursors become graafian follicles, in response to the effects of pituitary gonadotropic hormones—follicle-stimulating hormone (FSH) and luteinizing hormone (LH). In the life cycle of a female, however, less than 500 ova eventually mature and develop the potential for fertilization.

The menstrual cycle

Maturation of the hypothalamus and the resultant increase in hormone levels initiate puberty. In the young girl, breast development—the first sign of puberty—is followed by the appearance of pubic and axillary hair and the characteristic adolescent growth spurt. The reproductive system begins to undergo a series of hormone-induced changes that result in *menarche,* onset of menstruation (or

PATIENT TEACHING AID

Menstrual Cycle

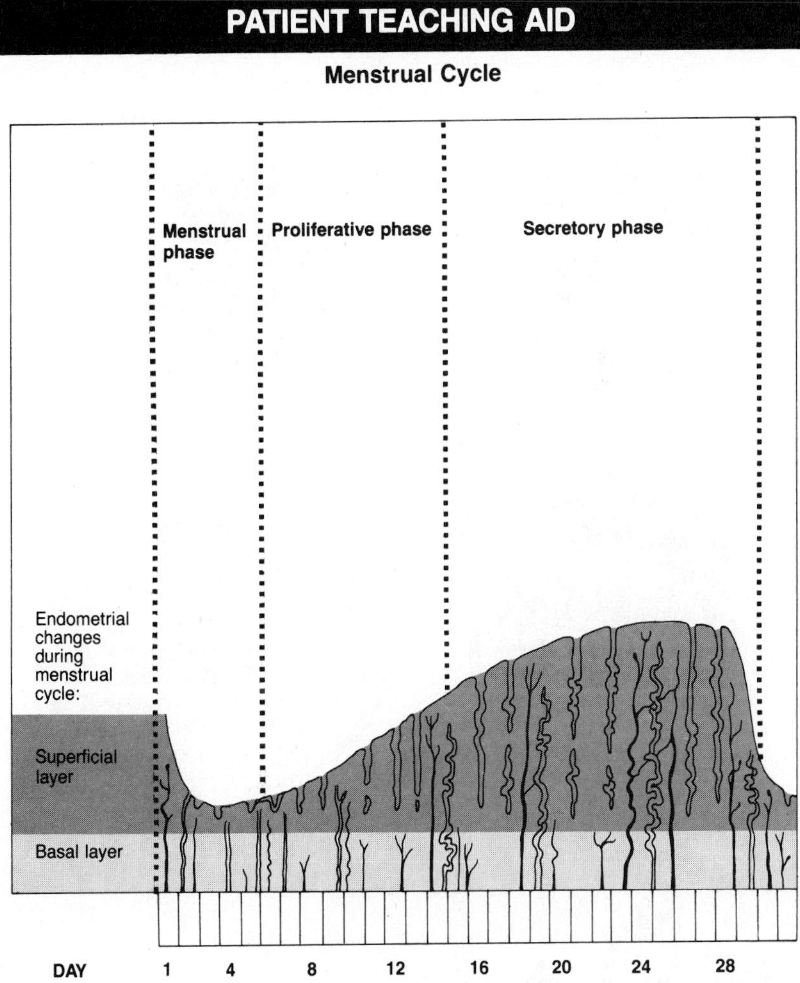

Dear Patient:

Your menstrual cycle is divided into three distinct phases:

- The menstrual phase starts on the first day of menstruation. The top layer of the endometrium (the material lining the uterus) breaks down and flows out of the body. This flow, called the menses, consists of blood, mucus, and unneeded tissue.
- During the proliferative phase, the endometrium begins to thicken, and the level of estrogen in the blood rises.
- In the secretory phase, the endometrium continues to thicken to nourish an embryo should fertilization occur. Without fertilization, the top layer of the endometrium breaks down, and the menstrual phase of the cycle begins again.

FOLLICULAR CYCLE
(Corresponding to days of the menstrual cycle)

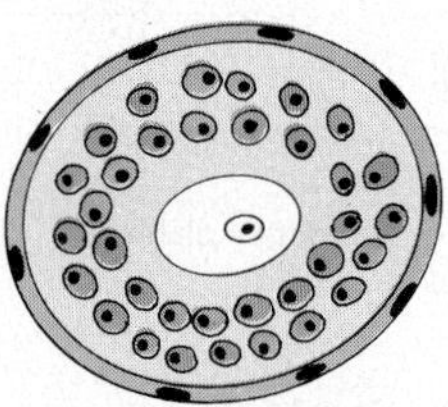

1. Early follicular phase
Days 1 to 5

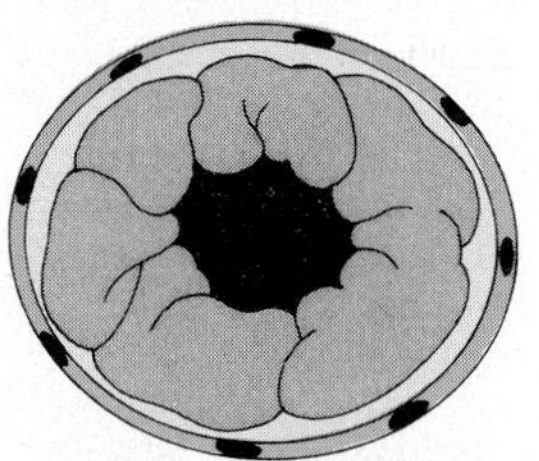

4. Early luteal phase
Days 16 to 20

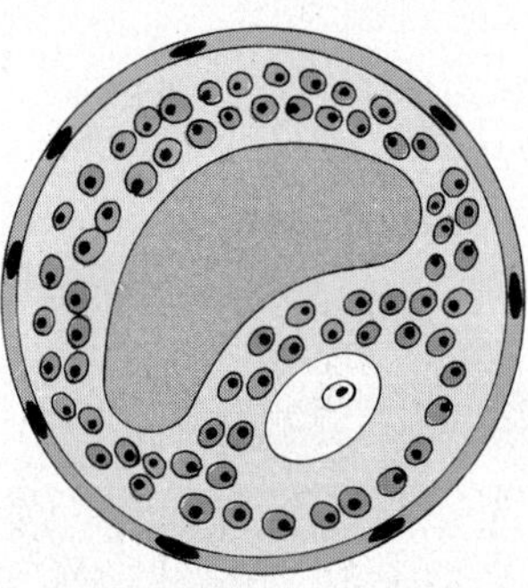

2. Late follicular phase
Days 6 to 10

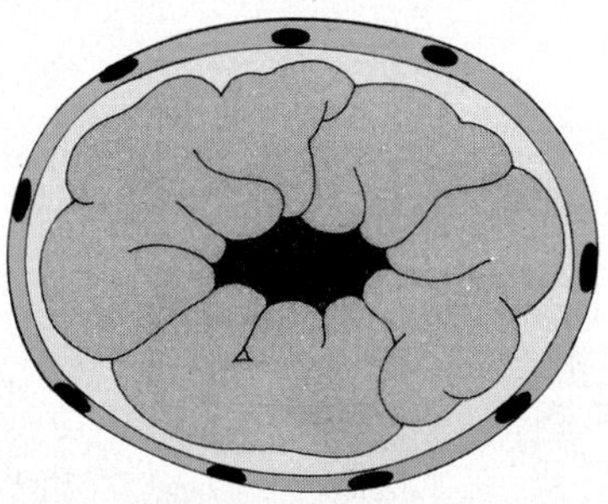

5. Midluteal phase
Days 21 to 25

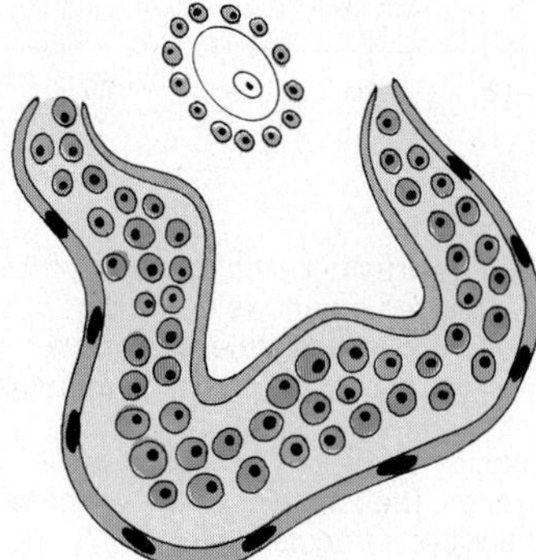

3. Ovulatory phase
Days 11 to 15

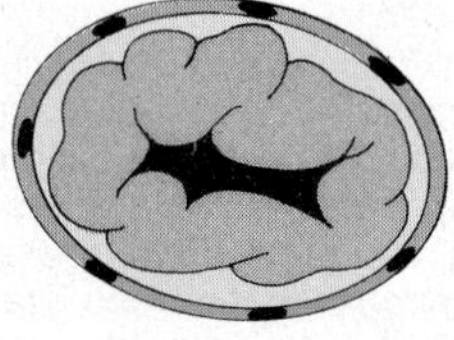

6. Late luteal phase
Days 26 to 28

menses). In North American females, menarche usually occurs at about age 13 but may occur anytime between ages 9 and 18. Usually, initial menstrual periods are irregular and anovulatory, but after a year or so, periods generally are more regular.

The menstrual cycle is made up of three different phases: menstrual, proliferative (estrogen-dominated), and secretory (progesterone-dominated). These phases correspond to the phases of ovarian function. The menstrual and proliferative phases correspond to the follicular ovarian phase; the secretory phase, to the luteal ovarian phase.

The *menstrual phase* begins with day 1 of menstruation. During this phase, decreased estrogen and progesterone levels provoke shedding of most of the endometrium. When these hormone levels are low, positive feedback causes the hypothalamus to produce LH-releasing factor and FSH-releasing factor. These two factors, in turn, stimulate pituitary secretion of FSH and LH. FSH stimulates the growth of ovarian follicles; LH stimulates these follicles to secrete estrogen.

The *proliferative phase* begins with the cessation of the menstrual period and ends with ovulation. During this phase, the increased amount of estrogen secreted by the developing ovarian follicles causes the endometrium to proliferate in preparation for possible pregnancy. Around day 14 of a 28-day menstrual cycle (the average length), these high estrogen levels trigger ovulation—the rupture of one of the developing follicles and subsequent release of an ovum.

The *secretory phase* extends from the day of ovulation to about 3 days before the next menstrual period (premenstrual phase). In most women, this final phase of the menstrual cycle lasts 13 to 15 days (its length varies less than those of the menstrual and proliferative phases). After ovulation, the ruptured follicle that released the ovum remains under the influence of LH. It then becomes the *corpus luteum* and starts secreting progesterone, in addition to estrogen.

In the nonpregnant female, LH controls the secretions of the corpus luteum; in the pregnant female, human chorionic gonadotropin (HCG) controls them. At the end of the secretory phase, the uterine lining is ready to receive and nourish a zygote. If fertilization doesn't occur, increasing estrogen and progesterone levels decrease LH and FSH production. Since LH is necessary to maintain the corpus luteum, a decrease in LH production causes the corpus luteum to atrophy and stop secreting estrogen and progesterone. The thickened uterine lining then begins to slough off, and menstruation begins again, renewing the cycle.

However, if fertilization and pregnancy do occur, the endometrium grows even thicker. After implantation of the zygote (about 5 or 6 days after fertilization), the endometrium becomes the *decidua.* Chorionic villi produce HCG soon after implantation, stimulating the corpus luteum to continue secreting estrogen and progesterone, a process that prevents further ovulation and menstruation.

HCG continues to stimulate the corpus luteum until the placenta—the vascular organ that develops to transport materials to and from the fetus—forms and starts producing its own estrogen and progesterone. After the placenta takes over hormonal production, secretions of the corpus luteum are no longer needed to maintain the pregnancy, and the corpus luteum gradually decreases its function and begins to degenerate.

Pregnancy

Cell multiplication and differentiation begin in the zygote at the moment of conception. By about 17 days after conception, the placenta has established circulation to what is now an *embryo* (the term used for the conceptus between the 2nd and 7th weeks of pregnancy). By the end of the embryonic stage, fetal structures are formed. Further development now consists primarily of growth and maturation of already formed structures. From this point until birth, the conceptus is called a *fetus.*

First trimester

The length of a normal pregnancy ranges from 240 to 300 days. Although pregnancies vary in duration, they're conveniently divided into three trimesters.

During the first trimester, a female usually experiences physical changes, such as amenorrhea, urinary frequency, nausea and vomiting (more severe in the morning or when the stomach is empty), breast swelling and tenderness, fatigue, increased vaginal secretions, and constipation.

Within 7 to 10 days after conception, pregnancy tests, which detect HCG in the urine and serum, are usually positive. Although such positive tests strongly suggest pregnancy, a pelvic examination helps confirm it by showing Hegar's sign (cervical and uterine softening), Chadwick's sign (a bluish coloration of the vagina and cervix resulting from increased venous blood circulation), and an enlarged uterus.

The first trimester is a critical time during pregnancy. Rapid cell differentiation makes the developing embryo or fetus highly susceptible to the teratogenetic effects of viruses, alcohol, cigarettes, caffeine, and other drugs.

Second trimester

From the 13th to the 26th week of pregnancy, uterine and fetal size increase substantially, causing weight gain, a thickening waistline, abdominal enlargement, and, possibly, reddish streaks as abdominal skin stretches (striation). In addition, pigment changes may cause skin alterations, such as linea nigra, melasma (mask of pregnancy), and a darkening of the areolae of the nipples.

Other physical changes may include diaphoresis, increased salivation, indigestion, continuing constipation, hemorrhoids, nosebleeds, and some dependent edema. The breasts become larger and heavier, and approximately 19 weeks after the last menstrual period, they may secrete colostrum. By about the 16th to 18th week of pregnancy, the fetus is large enough for the mother to feel it move (quickening).

Third trimester

During this period, the mother feels Braxton Hicks contractions—sporadic episodes of painless uterine tightening—which help strengthen uterine muscles in preparation for labor. Increasing uterine size may displace pelvic and intestinal structures, causing indigestion, protrusion of the umbilicus, shortness of breath, and insomnia. The mother may experience backaches because she walks with a swaybacked posture to counteract her frontal weight. By lying down, she can help minimize the development of varicose veins, hemorrhoids, and ankle edema.

Labor and delivery

About 2 to 4 weeks before birth, lightening—the descent of the fetal head into the pelvis—shifts the uterine position. This relieves pressure on the diaphragm and enables the mother to breathe more easily.

Onset of labor characteristically produces low back pain and passage of a small amount of bloody "show," a brownish or blood-tinged plug of cervical mucus. As labor progresses, the cervix becomes soft, then effaces and dilates; the amniotic membranes may rupture spontaneously, causing a gush or leakage of amniotic fluid. Uterine contractions become increasingly regular, frequent, intense, and longer.

Labor is usually divided into four stages:

- *Stage I,* the longest stage, lasts from onset of regular contractions until full cervical dilation (4" [10 cm]). Average duration of this stage is about 12 hours for a primigravida and 6 hours for a multigravida.
- *Stage II* lasts from full cervical dilation until delivery of the infant—about 1 to 2 hours for a primigravida, 30 minutes for a multigravida.
- *Stage III,* the time between delivery and expulsion of the placenta, usually lasts 3 to 4 minutes for a primigravida and 4 to 5 minutes for a multigravida, but may last up to 1 hour.
- *Stage IV* constitutes a period of re-

STAGES OF LABOR

LIGHTENING

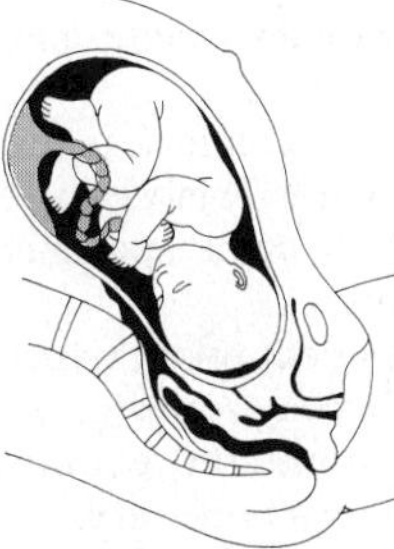

Descent of the fetal head into the pelvis

STAGE I

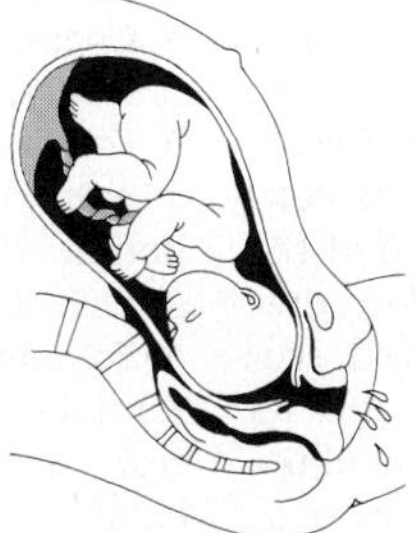

Onset of regular contractions and breaking of the amniotic sac

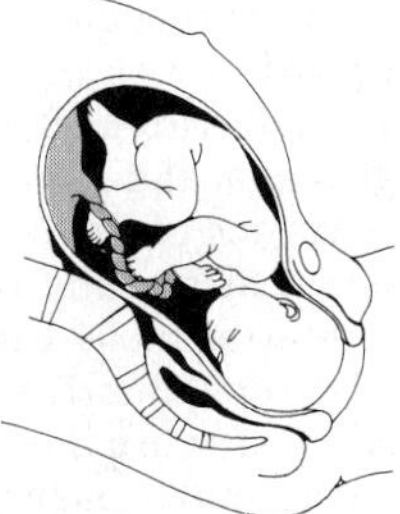

Full cervical dilation

STAGE II

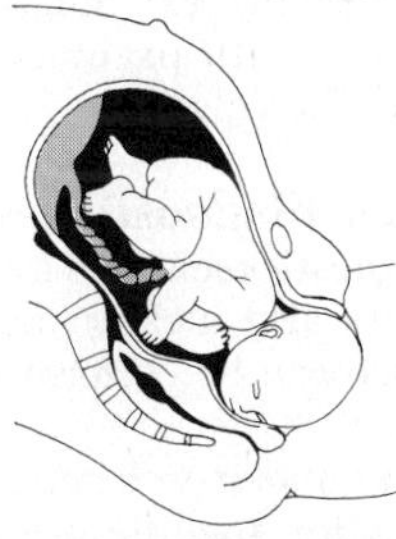

Delivering the head

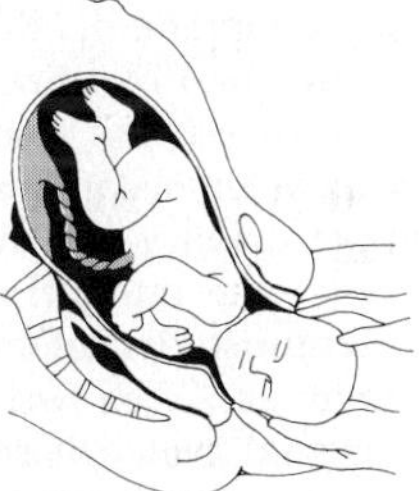

Rotating the head

STAGE III

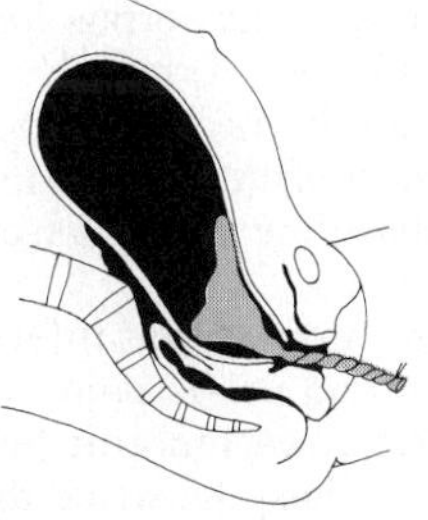

Uterine contractions

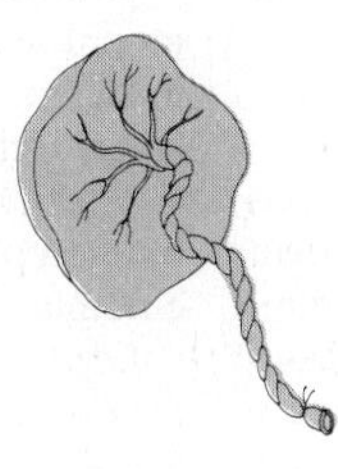

Expulsion of the placenta

STAGE IV

Reestablishment of homeostasis during this stage includes recuperation from anesthetic (if used), normalization of vital signs, cessation of bleeding, and return of muscle tone.

covery during which homeostasis is reestablished. This final stage lasts 1 to 4 hours after expulsion of the placenta.

Sources of pathology

In no other part of the body do so many interrelated physiologic functions occur in such proximity as in the area of the female reproductive tract. Besides the internal genitalia, the female pelvis contains the organs of the urinary and the gastrointestinal systems (bladder, ureters, urethra, sigmoid colon, and rectum). The reproductive tract and its surrounding area are thus the site of urination, defecation, menstruation, ovulation, copulation, impregnation, and parturition. It's easy to understand how an abnormality in one pelvic organ can readily induce abnormality in another.

When conducting a pelvic examination, therefore, you must consider all possible sources of pathology. Remember that some serious abnormalities of the pelvic organs can be asymptomatic. Remember, too, that some abnormal findings in the pelvic area may result from pathologic changes in other organ systems, such as the upper urinary and the gastrointestinal tracts, the endocrine glands, and the neuromusculoskeletal system. Pain symptoms are often associated with the menstrual cycle; therefore, in many common diseases of the female reproductive tract, such pain follows a cyclic pattern. A patient with pelvic inflammatory disease, for example, may complain of increasing premenstrual pain that is relieved by onset of menstruation.

Pelvic examination

A pelvic examination and a thorough patient history are essential for any patient with symptoms related to the reproductive tract or adjacent body systems. Document any history of pregnancy, miscarriage, and abortion. Ask her if she has experienced any recent changes in her urinary habits or menstrual cycle. If she practices birth control, find out what method she uses and whether she has experienced any side effects.

Then, prepare the patient for the pelvic examination as follows:

- Ask the patient if she's douched within the last 24 hours. Explain that douching washes away cells or organisms that the examination is designed to evaluate.
- Check the patient's weight and blood pressure.
- For the patient's comfort, instruct her to empty her bladder before the examination. Provide a urine specimen container, if needed.
- To help the patient relax, which is essential for a thorough pelvic examination, explain what the examination entails and why it's necessary.
- If the patient is scheduled for a Papanicolaou (Pap) smear, inform her that another smear may have to be taken later. To reduce her anxiety, reassure her that this is done to confirm the results of the first test. If she has never had a Pap smear before, tell her it is painless.
- After the examination, provide the patient with premoistened tissues to clean the vulva.

Other diagnostic tests

Diagnostic measures for gynecologic disorders also include the following tests, which can be performed in the doctor's office:

- *wet smear* to examine vaginal secretions for specific organisms, such as *Trichomonas vaginalis, Candida albicans,* or *Hemophilus vaginalis,* or to evaluate semen specimens in rape or infertility cases
- *endometrial biopsy* to assess hormonal secretions of the corpus luteum, to determine whether normal ovulation is occurring, and to check for neoplasia
- *dilation and curettage (D & C)* to evaluate atypical bleeding and to detect carcinoma.

Laparoscopy to evaluate infertility, dysmenorrhea, and pelvic pain, and as a means of sterilization can be performed only in a hospital while the patient is under anesthesia.

GYNECOLOGIC DISORDERS

Premenstrual Syndrome

Premenstrual syndrome (PMS) is characterized by a varying syndrome that appears 7 to 14 days before menses and usually subsides with its onset. The effects of PMS range from minimal discomfort to severe, disruptive symptoms and can include nervousness, irritability, depression, and multiple somatic complaints. This disorder occurs in 30% of women, usually striking those between ages 20 and 40. Incidence seems to rise with age and parity.

Causes

Although the direct cause of PMS is unknown, it is believed to result from a progesterone deficiency in the luteal phase of the menstrual cycle or from an increased estrogen-progesterone ratio. About 10% of patients with PMS have elevated prolactin levels.

Other conditions that may possibly contribute to PMS include abnormal carbohydrate metabolism, imbalance of salt and water, mental and emotional disorders, and tubal ligation. There also seems to be a relationship between PMS and changes in endorphin levels.

Signs and symptoms

Clinical effects vary widely among patients and may include any combination of the following:

- *behavioral*—mild to severe personality changes, nervousness, hostility, irritability, agitation, sleep disturbances, fatigue, lethargy, and depression
- *somatic*—breast tenderness or swelling, abdominal tenderness or bloating, joint pain, headache, edema, diarrhea or constipation, and exacerbations of skin problems (such as acne or skin rash), respiratory problems (such as asthma), or neurologic problems (such as seizures).

Diagnosis

Patient history shows typical menstrually related symptoms. To help ensure an accurate history, the patient may be asked to record menstrual symptoms and body temperature on a calendar for 2 to 3 months prior to diagnosis. Estrogen and progesterone blood levels may be evaluated to help rule out hormonal imbalance. Psychological evaluation is also recommended to rule out or detect an underlying psychiatric disorder.

Treatment

Treatment is primarily symptomatic and may include tranquilizers, sedatives, antidepressants, vitamins, and progestins. Effective treatment may require a diet that's low in simple sugars, caffeine, and salt, with adequate amounts of protein and complex carbohydrates and, possibly, vitamin supplements. (Salt restriction or the use of diuretics may be unnecessary.)

Special considerations

- Inform the patient that self-help groups exist for women with PMS; if appropriate, help her contact such a group.
- Obtain a complete patient history to help identify any emotional problems that may contribute to PMS. If necessary, refer the patient for psychological counseling.
- If possible, discuss life-style changes—such as avoiding stimulants, for example—that might help alleviate symptoms by reducing stress and anxiety.
- Advise further medical consultation if severe symptoms disrupt the patient's normal life-style.

Dysmenorrhea

Dysmenorrhea—painful menstruation—is the most common gynecologic complaint and a leading cause of absenteeism from school (affects 10% of high school girls each month) and work (estimated 140 million work hours lost annually). Dysmenorrhea can occur as a primary disorder or secondary to an underlying disease. Since primary dysmenorrhea is self-limiting, prognosis is generally good. Prognosis for secondary dysmenorrhea depends on the underlying disorder.

Causes and incidence

Although primary dysmenorrhea is unrelated to any identifiable cause, possible contributing factors include hormonal imbalances and psychogenic factors. The pain of dysmenorrhea probably results from increased prostaglandin secretion, which intensifies normal uterine contractions. Dysmenorrhea may also be secondary to such gynecologic disorders as endometriosis, cervical stenosis, uterine leiomyomas, uterine malposition, pelvic inflammatory disease, pelvic tumors, or adenomyosis.

Since dysmenorrhea almost always follows an ovulatory cycle, both the primary and secondary forms are rare during the first 2 years of menses, which are usually anovulatory. After age 20, dysmenorrhea is generally secondary.

CAUSES OF PELVIC PAIN

The characteristic pelvic pain of dysmenorrhea must be distinguished from the acute pain caused by many other disorders, such as:

- *gastrointestinal disorders:* appendicitis, acute diverticulitis, acute or chronic cholecystitis, chronic cholelithiasis, acute pancreatitis, peptic ulcer perforation, intestinal obstruction
- *urinary tract disorders:* cystitis, renal calculi
- *reproductive disorders:* acute salpingitis, chronic inflammation, degenerating fibroid, ovarian cyst torsion
- *pregnancy disorders:* impending abortion (pain and bleeding early in pregnancy), ectopic pregnancy, abruptio placentae, uterine rupture, leiomyoma degeneration, toxemia
- *emotional conflicts:* psychogenic (functional) pain.

Other conditions that may mimic dysmenorrhea include ovulation and normal uterine contractions experienced in pregnancy.

Signs and symptoms

Dysmenorrhea produces sharp, intermittent, cramping, lower abdominal pain, which usually radiates to the back, thighs, groin, and vulva. Such pain—sometimes compared to labor pains—typically starts with or immediately before menstrual flow and peaks within 24 hours. Dysmenorrhea may also be associated with the characteristic signs and symptoms of premenstrual syndrome (urinary frequency, nausea, vomiting, diarrhea, headache, chills, abdominal bloating, painful breasts, depression, and irritability).

Diagnosis

Pelvic examination, a detailed patient history, and, if necessary, psychiatric evaluation may suggest the cause of dysmenorrhea.

Primary dysmenorrhea is diagnosed when secondary causes are ruled out. Appropriate tests (such as laparoscopy, dilation and curettage, and X-rays) are used to diagnose underlying disorders in secondary dysmenorrhea.

Treatment

Initial treatment aims to relieve pain. Pain-relief measures may include:

- *analgesics,* such as aspirin, for mild to moderate pain (most effective when

taken 24 to 48 hours before onset of menses). Aspirin is especially effective for treating dysmenorrhea because it also inhibits prostaglandin synthesis.
• *narcotics* if pain is severe (infrequently used).
• *prostaglandin inhibitors* (such as mefenamic acid and ibuprofen) to relieve pain by decreasing the severity of uterine contractions.
• *heat* applied locally to the lower abdomen (may relieve discomfort in women but is not recommended in young girls because appendicitis may mimic dysmenorrhea).

For *primary dysmenorrhea,* sex steroid therapy is an alternative to treatment with antiprostaglandins or analgesics. Such therapy usually consists of oral contraceptives to relieve pain by suppressing ovulation. (Patients who are attempting pregnancy should rely on antiprostaglandin therapy instead of oral contraceptives for relief from primary dysmenorrhea.)

Because persistently severe dysmenorrhea may have a psychogenic cause, psychological evaluation and treatment may be helpful.

In *secondary dysmenorrhea,* treatment is designed to identify and correct the underlying cause. This may include surgical treatment of underlying disorders, such as endometriosis or uterine leiomyomas, but only after conservative therapy fails.

Rarely, severe and disabling dysmenorrhea may require insertion of a stem pessary into the cervical os, transection of the uterosacral ligaments (Doyce operation), or presacral neurectomy (Cotte's operation).

Special considerations

Effective patient management focuses on relief of symptoms, emotional support, and patient teaching, especially for the adolescent.
• Obtain a complete patient history focusing on gynecologic complaints, including information on symptoms of pelvic disease such as excessive bleeding, changes in bleeding pattern, vaginal discharge, and dyspareunia.
• Provide patient teaching. Explain normal anatomy and physiology to the patient, as well as the nature of dysmenorrhea. This may be a good opportunity, if warranted, to provide the adolescent patient with information on pregnancy and contraception.
• Encourage the patient to keep a record of menstrual symptoms and to seek medical care if her symptoms persist.

Vulvovaginitis

Vulvovaginitis is inflammation of the vulva (vulvitis) and vagina (vaginitis). Because of the proximity of these two structures, inflammation of one usually precipitates inflammation of the other. Vulvovaginitis may occur at any age and affects most females at some time. Prognosis is good with treatment.

Causes

Common causes of vaginitis (with or without consequent vulvitis) include:
• infection with *Trichomonas vaginalis,* a protozoan flagellate, usually transmitted through sexual intercourse.
• infection with *Candida albicans (Monilia),* a fungus that requires glucose for growth. Incidence rises during the secretory phase of the menstrual cycle. Such infection occurs twice as often in pregnant females as in nonpregnant females. It also commonly affects users of oral contraceptives, diabetics, and patients receiving systemic therapy with broad-spectrum antibiotics (incidence may reach 75%).
• infection with *Hemophilus vaginalis,*

a gram-negative bacillus.

- venereal infection with *Neisseria gonorrhoeae* (gonorrhea), a gram-negative diplococcus.
- viral infection with venereal warts (condylomata acuminata) or herpesvirus Type II, usually transmitted by sexual intercourse.
- vaginal mucosa atrophy in menopausal women due to decreasing levels of estrogen, which predisposes to bacterial invasion.

Common causes of vulvitis include:

- parasitic infection (*Phthirus pubis* [crab louse]).
- trauma (skin breakdown may lead to secondary infection).
- poor personal hygiene, especially from contamination with urine, feces, or vaginal secretions.
- chemical irritations, or allergic reactions to feminine hygiene sprays, douches, detergents, clothing, or toilet paper.
- vulval atrophy in menopausal women due to decreasing estrogen levels.

Signs and symptoms

In trichomonal vaginitis, vaginal discharge is thin, bubbly, green-tinged, and malodorous. This infection causes marked irritation and itching, and urinary symptoms, such as burning and frequency. Monilia vaginitis produces a thick, white, cottage-cheese–like discharge and red, edematous mucous membranes, with white flecks adhering to the vaginal wall, and is often accompanied by intense itching. Hemophilus vaginitis produces a gray, foul-smelling discharge. Gonorrhea may produce no symptoms at all, or a profuse, purulent discharge and dysuria.

Acute vulvitis causes a mild to severe inflammatory reaction, including edema, erythema, burning, and pruritus. Severe pain on urination and dyspareunia may necessitate immediate treatment. Herpes infection may cause painful ulceration or vesicle formation during the active phase. Chronic vulvitis generally causes relatively mild inflammation, possibly associated with severe edema that may involve the entire perineum.

Diagnosis

Diagnosis of vaginitis requires identification of the infectious organism during microscopic examination of vaginal exudate on a wet slide preparation (a drop of vaginal exudate placed in normal saline solution).

- In trichomonal infections, the presence of motile, flagellated trichomonads confirms the diagnosis.
- In monilia vaginitis, 10% potassium hydroxide is added to the slide, and microscopic examination seeks "clue cells" (granular epithelial cells); however, diagnosis requires identification of *C. albicans* fungi.
- Gonorrhea necessitates culture of vaginal exudate on Thayer-Martin or Transgrow medium to confirm diagnosis.

Diagnosis of vulvitis or suspected venereal disease may require CBC, urinalysis, cytology screening, biopsy of chronic lesions to rule out malignancy, and culture of exudate from acute lesions.

Treatment

Common therapeutic measures include the following:

- metronidazole P.O. for the patient with trichomonal vaginitis, and all sexual partners (if possible), since recurrence often results from reinfection by an asymptomatic male.
- vaginal ointments and suppositories, such as nystatin, for monilia vaginitis.
- local antibiotic therapy for hemophilus vaginitis.
- systemic antibiotic therapy (penicillin and probenicid) for the patient with gonorrhea, and all sexual partners.

Cold compresses or cool sitz baths may provide relief from pruritus in acute vulvitis; severe inflammation may require warm compresses. Other therapy includes avoiding drying soaps, wearing loose clothing to promote air circulation, and applying topical corticosteroids to reduce inflammation. Chronic vulvitis may respond to topical hydrocortisone or antipruritics and good hygiene (especially in elderly or incontinent patients). Topical estrogen ointments may be used to treat atrophic vulvovaginitis. No cure currently exists for herpesvirus infections; however, oral and topical acyclovir (Zovirax) decreases the duration and symptoms of active lesions.

Special considerations

• Ask the patient if she has any drug allergies. Stress the importance of taking the medication for the length of time prescribed, even if symptoms subside.

• Teach the patient how to insert vaginal ointments and suppositories. Tell her to remain prone for at least 30 minutes after insertion to promote absorption (insertion at bedtime is ideal). Suggest she wear a pad to prevent staining her underclothing.

• Encourage good hygiene. Advise the patient with a history of recurrent vulvovaginitis to wear all-cotton underpants. Advise her to avoid wearing tight-fitting pants and panty hose, which favors the growth of the infecting organisms.

• Report cases of venereal disease to the local public health authorities.

• Advise the patient of the correlation between sexual contact and the spread of vaginal infections.

Ovarian Cysts

Ovarian cysts are usually nonneoplastic sacs on an ovary that contain fluid or semisolid material. Although these cysts are usually small and produce no symptoms, they require thorough investigation as possible sites of malignant change. Common ovarian cysts include follicular cysts, lutein cysts (granulosa-lutein [corpus luteum] and theca-lutein cysts), and polycystic (or sclerocystic) ovarian disease. Ovarian cysts can develop any time between puberty and menopause, including during pregnancy. Granulosa-lutein cysts occur infrequently, usually during early pregnancy. Prognosis for nonneoplastic ovarian cysts is excellent.

Causes

Follicular cysts are generally very small and arise from follicles that overdistend instead of going through the atretic stage of the menstrual cycle. When such cysts persist into menopause, they secrete excessive amounts of estrogen in response to the hypersecretion of follicle-stimulating hormone and luteinizing hormone that normally occurs during menopause.

Granulosa-lutein cysts, which occur within the corpus luteum, are functional, nonneoplastic enlargements of the ovaries, caused by excessive accumulation of blood during the hemorrhagic phase of the menstrual cycle. *Theca-lutein cysts* are commonly bilateral and filled with clear, straw-colored fluid; they are often associated with hydatidiform mole, choriocarcinoma, or hormone therapy (with human chorionic gonadotropin [HCG] or clomiphene citrate).

Polycystic ovarian disease is part of

FOLLICULAR CYST

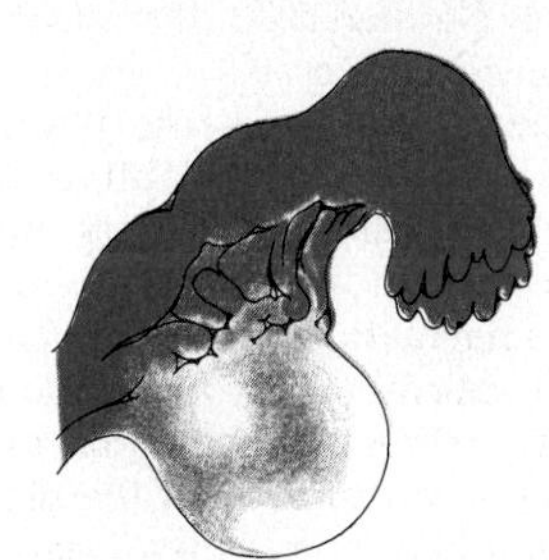

A common type of ovarian cyst, a follicular cyst is usually semi-transparent and overdistended with watery fluid that is visible through its thin walls.

the Stein-Leventhal syndrome and stems from endocrine abnormalities.

Signs and symptoms

Small ovarian cysts (such as follicular cysts) usually don't produce symptoms unless torsion or rupture causes signs of an acute abdomen (abdominal tenderness, distention, and rigidity). Large or multiple cysts may induce mild pelvic discomfort, low back pain, dyspareunia, or abnormal uterine bleeding secondary to a disturbed ovulatory pattern. Ovarian cysts with torsion induce acute abdominal pain similar to that of appendicitis.

Granulosa-lutein cysts that appear early in pregnancy may grow as large as 2″ to 2½″ (5 to 6 cm) in diameter and produce unilateral pelvic discomfort and, if rupture occurs, massive intraperitoneal hemorrhage. In nonpregnant women, these cysts may cause delayed menses, followed by prolonged or irregular bleeding. Polycystic ovarian disease may also produce secondary amenorrhea, oligomenorrhea, or infertility.

Diagnosis

Generally, characteristic clinical features suggest ovarian cysts.

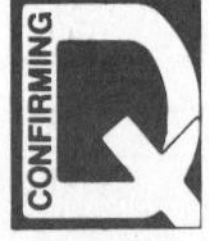

Visualization of the ovary through ultrasound, laparoscopy, or surgery (often for another condition) confirms ovarian cysts.

Extremely elevated HCG titers strongly suggest theca-lutein cysts.

In polycystic ovarian disease, physical examination demonstrates bilaterally enlarged polycystic ovaries. Tests reveal slight elevation of urinary 17-ketosteroids and anovulation (shown by basal body temperature graphs and endometrial biopsy). Direct visualization must rule out paraovarian cysts of the broad ligament, salpingitis, endometriosis, and neoplastic cysts.

Treatment

Follicular cysts generally don't require treatment, since they tend to disappear spontaneously within 60 days. However, if they interfere with daily activities, clomiphene citrate P.O. for 5 days or progesterone I.M. (also for 5 days) reestablishes the ovarian hormonal cycle and induces ovulation. Oral contraceptives may also accelerate involution of functional cysts (including both types of lutein cysts and follicular cysts).

Treatment for granulosa-lutein cysts that occur during pregnancy is symptomatic, since these cysts diminish during the third trimester and rarely require surgery. Theca-lutein cysts disappear spontaneously after elimination of the hydatidiform mole, destruction of choriocarcinoma, or discontinuation of HCG or clomiphene citrate therapy.

Treatment for polycystic ovarian disease may include drugs, such as hydrocortisone or clomiphene citrate, to induce ovulation or, if drug therapy fails to induce ovulation, surgical wedge resection of one half to one third of the ovary.

Surgery frequently becomes necessary for both diagnosis and treatment. For example, a cyst that remains after one menstrual period should be removed; pathologic studies confirm diagnosis.

Special considerations

Thorough patient teaching is a primary consideration. Carefully explain the nature of the particular cyst, the type of discomfort—if any—the patient is apt to experience, and how long the condition is expected to last.

- Preoperatively, watch for signs of cyst rupture, such as increasing abdominal pain, distention, and rigidity. Monitor vital signs for fever, tachypnea, or hypotension, a sign of possible peritonitis or intraperitoneal hemorrhage. Administer sedatives, as ordered, to assure adequate preoperative rest.
- Postoperatively, encourage frequent movement in bed and early ambulation, as ordered. Early ambulation effectively prevents pulmonary embolism.
- Provide emotional support. Offer appropriate reassurance if the patient fears cancer or infertility.
- The patient may be worried about the possibility of recurrence, but you can as-

sure her that recurrence is unlikely.

- Before discharge, advise the patient to increase her at-home activity gradually—preferably over 4 to 6 weeks. Tell her to abstain from intercourse, using tampons, and douching during this time.

Endometriosis

Endometriosis is the presence of endometrial tissue outside the lining of the uterine cavity. Such ectopic tissue is generally confined to the pelvic area, most commonly around the ovaries, uterovesical peritoneum, uterosacral ligaments, and the cul-de-sac, but it can appear anywhere in the body. Active endometriosis usually occurs between ages 30 and 40, especially in women who postpone childbearing; it's uncommon before age 20. Severe symptoms of endometriosis may have an abrupt onset or may develop over many years. Generally, this disorder becomes progressively severe during the menstrual years; after menopause, it tends to subside.

Causes

The direct cause is unknown, but familial susceptibility or recent surgery that necessitated opening the uterus (such as a cesarean section) may predispose a woman to endometriosis. Although neither of these possible predisposing factors explains all the lesions in endometriosis or their location, research focuses on the following possible causes:

- *Transportation:* During menstruation, the fallopian tubes expel endometrial fragments that implant on the ovaries or pelvic peritoneum.
- *Formation in situ:* Inflammation or a hormonal change triggers metaplasia (differentiation of coelomic epithelium to endometrial epithelium).
- *Induction* (a combination of transportation and of formation in situ): The endometrium chemically induces undifferentiated mesenchyma to form endometrial epithelium. (This is the most likely cause.)

Signs and symptoms

The classic symptom of endometriosis is acquired dysmenorrhea, which may produce constant pain in the lower abdomen and in the vagina, posterior pelvis, and back. This pain usually begins from 5 to 7 days before menses reaches its peak and lasts for 2 to 3 days. It differs from primary dysmenorrheal pain, which is more cramplike and concentrated in the abdominal midline. However, the severity of pain doesn't necessarily indicate the extent of the disease.

Other clinical features depend on the location of the ectopic tissue:

- *ovaries* and *oviducts:* infertility and profuse menses
- *ovaries* or *cul-de-sac:* deep-thrust dyspareunia
- *bladder:* suprapubic pain, dysuria, hematuria
- *rectovaginal septum* and *colon:* painful defecation, rectal bleeding with menses, pain in the coccyx or sacrum
- *small bowel* and *appendix:* nausea and vomiting, which worsen before menses, and abdominal cramps
- *cervix, vagina,* and *perineum:* bleeding from endometrial deposits in these areas during menses.

The primary complication of endometriosis is infertility. It can also cause spontaneous abortion.

Diagnosis

Pelvic examination suggests endometriosis. Palpation may detect multiple tender nodules on uterosacral ligaments or in the rectovaginal septum. These nodules enlarge and become more tender during menses. Palpation may also uncover ovarian enlargement in the pres-

STAGING ENDOMETRIOSIS

A point system created by the American Fertility Society (AFS) grades endometrial implants or adhesions according to size, character, and location. To determine the stage of endometrial involvement, compare the total number of assigned points to the staging scale below. A score of 1 to 5 indicates minimal involvement (Stage I endometriosis), whereas a score of more than 40 indicates severe involvement (Stage IV endometriosis).

AFS Point System

		Endometriosis	<1 cm	1.3 cm	>3 cm
Peritoneum		Superficial	1	2	4
		Deep	2	4	6
Ovary	R	Superficial	1	2	4
	R	Deep	4	16	20
	L	Superficial	1	2	4
	L	Deep	4	16	20

Posterior Cul-de-sac Obliteration	Partial	Complete
	4	40

		Adhesions	<1.3 Enclosure	1.3-2.3 Enclosure	>2.3 Enclosure
Ovary	R	Filmy	1	2	4
	R	Dense	4	8	16
	L	Filmy	1	2	4
	L	Dense	4	8	16
Tube	R	Filmy	1	2	4
	R	Dense	4*	8*	16
	L	Filmy	1	2	4
	L	Dense	4*	8*	16

*If the fimbriated end of the fallopian tube is completely enclosed, change the point assignment to 16.

Staging Scale: Stage I (Minimal)—1-5, Stage II (Mild)—6-15
Stage III (Moderate)—16-40, Stage IV (Severe)—> 40

ence of endometrial cysts on the ovaries or thickened, nodular adnexa (as in pelvic inflammatory disease). Laparoscopy may confirm diagnosis and determine the stage of the disease. Barium enema rules out malignant or inflammatory bowel disease.

Treatment

Treatment varies according to the stage of the disease and the patient's age and desire to have children. Conservative therapy for young women who want to have children includes androgens, such as danazol, which produce a temporary remission in Stages I and II. Progestins and oral contraceptives also relieve symptoms.

When ovarian masses are present (Stages III and IV), surgery must rule out malignancy. Conservative surgery is possible; but treatment of choice for women who don't want to bear children or for extensive disease (Stages III and IV) is a total abdominal hysterectomy with bilateral salpingo-oophorectomy.

Special considerations

- Minor gynecologic procedures are contraindicated immediately before and during menstruation.
- Advise adolescents to use sanitary napkins instead of tampons; this can help prevent retrograde flow in girls with a narrow vagina or small introitus.
- Since infertility is a possible complication, advise the patient who wants children not to postpone childbearing.
- Recommend an annual pelvic examination and Pap smear to all patients.

Uterine Leiomyomas

(Myomas, fibromyomas, fibroids)

The most common benign tumors in women, uterine leiomyomas are smooth-muscle tumors. They are usually multiple and generally occur in the uterine corpus, although they may appear on the cervix or on the round or broad ligament. Uterine leiomyomas are often called fibroids, but this term is misleading, since these tumors consist of muscle cells and not fibrous tissue. Uterine leiomyomas occur in approximately 20% of all women over age 35 and affect blacks three times more often than whites. Malignancy (leiomyosarcoma) develops in only 0.1% of patients.

Causes

The cause of uterine leiomyomas is unknown, but excessive levels of estrogen and human growth hormone (HGH) may influence tumor formation by stimulating susceptible fibromuscular elements. Large doses of estrogen and the later stages of pregnancy increase both tumor size and HGH levels. Conversely, uterine leiomyomas usually shrink or disappear after menopause, when estrogen production decreases.

Signs and symptoms

Usually, submucosal hypermenorrhea is the cardinal sign of uterine leiomyomas, although other forms of abnormal endometrial bleeding, as well as dysmenorrhea, are possible. Pain may occur if the tumors twist or degenerate after circulatory occlusion or infection or if the uterus contracts in an attempt to expel a pedunculated submucous leiomyoma. Large tumors may produce a feeling of heaviness in the abdomen; pressure on surrounding organs may cause secondary pain, intestinal obstruction, constipation, and urinary frequency or urgency. Irregular uterine enlargement may occur, often asymptomatically.

Diagnosis

Clinical findings and patient history suggest uterine leiomyomas. Blood studies showing anemia from abnormal bleeding support the diagnosis; palpation of the tumor, revealing a round or irregular mass, helps to confirm it. Other diagnostic procedures include dilation and curettage or submucosal hysterosalpingography to detect submucosal leiomyomas, or laparoscopy to visualize subserous leiomyomas on the uterine surface.

Treatment

Treatment depends on the severity of symptoms, size and location of the tumors, and the patient's age, parity, pregnancy status, desire to have children, and general health.

If they have caused problems in the past, or if they are likely to threaten a future pregnancy, small leiomyomas may be surgically removed. This is the treatment of choice for a young woman who wants to have children.

Tumors that twist or grow large enough to cause intestinal obstruction require a hysterectomy, with preservation of the ovaries, if possible.

If the patient is pregnant, but her uterus is no larger than a 6-month normal uterus by the 16th week of pregnancy, the outcome for the pregnancy is favorable, and surgery is usually unnecessary. However, if a pregnant woman has a leiomyomatous uterus the size of a 5- to 6-month normal uterus by the 9th week of pregnancy, spontaneous abortion will probably occur, especially with a cervical leiomyoma. If surgery is necessary, a hysterectomy is usually performed 5 to 6 months after delivery (when involution is complete), with preservation of the ovaries, if possible.

Special considerations

- Tell the patient to report any abnormal bleeding or pelvic pain immediately.
- If a hysterectomy or oophorectomy is indicated, explain the effects of the operation on menstruation, menopause, and sexual activity to the patient.
- Reassure the patient that she won't experience premature menopause if her ovaries are left intact.
- If it is necessary for the patient to have a multiple myomectomy, make sure she understands pregnancy is still possible. However, if the uterine cavity is entered during surgery, explain that a cesarean delivery may be necessary.
- In a patient with severe anemia due to excessive bleeding, administer iron and blood transfusions, as ordered.

Precocious Puberty

In females, precocious puberty is onset of pubertal changes (breast development, pubic and axillary hair, and menarche) before age 9 (normally, the mean age for menarche is 13). In true precocious puberty, the ovaries mature and pubertal changes progress in an orderly manner. In pseudoprecocious puberty, pubertal changes occur without corresponding ovarian maturation.

Causes

About 85% of all true precocious puberty in females is constitutional, resulting from early development and activation of the endocrine glands without corresponding abnormality. Other causes of true precocious puberty are pathologic and include CNS disorders resulting from tumors, trauma, infection, or other lesions. These CNS disorders include hypothalamic tumors, intracranial tumors (pinealoma, granuloma, hamartoma), hydrocephaly, degenerative encephalopathy, tuberous sclerosis, neurofibromatosis, encephalitis, skull injuries, meningitis, and peptic arachnoiditis. Albright's syndrome, Silver's syndrome, and juvenile hypothyroidism are conditions often associated with female precocity.

Pseudoprecocious puberty may result from increased levels of sex hormones due to ovarian and adrenocortical tumors, adrenal cortical virilizing hyperplasia, and ingestion of estrogens or androgens. It may also result from increased end-organ sensitivity to low levels of circulating sex hormones, whereby estrogens promote premature breast development and androgens promote premature pubic and axillary hair growth.

Signs and symptoms

The usual pattern of precocious puberty in females is a rapid growth spurt, thelarche (breast development), pubarche (pubic hair development), and menarche—all before age 9. These changes may occur independently or simultaneously.

Diagnosis

Diagnosis requires a complete patient history, a thorough physical examination, and special tests to differentiate between true and pseudoprecocious puberty and to indicate what treatment may be necessary. X-rays of hands, wrists, knees, and hips determine bone age and possible premature epiphyseal closure. Other tests detect abnormally high hormonal levels for the patient's age: vaginal smear for estrogen secretion, urinary tests for gonadotropic activity and excretion of 17-ketosteroids, and radioimmunoassay for both luteinizing and follicle-stimulating hormones.

As indicated, laparoscopy or exploratory laparotomy may verify a suspected abdominal lesion; electroencephalography, ventriculography, pneumoencephalography, CAT scan, or angiography can detect CNS disorders.

Treatment

Although still controversial, treatment of constitutional true precocious puberty may include medroxyprogesterone to reduce secretion of gonadotropins and prevent menstruation. Other therapy depends on the cause of precocious puberty and its stage of development:

- *Adrenogenital syndrome* necessitates cortical or adrenocortical steroid replacement.
- *Abdominal tumors* necessitate surgery to remove ovarian and adrenal tumors. Regression of secondary sex characteristics may follow such surgery, especially in young children.
- *Choriocarcinomas* require surgery and chemotherapy.
- *Hypothyroidism* requires thyroid extract or levothyroxine to decrease gonadotropic secretions.
- *Drug ingestion* requires that the medication be discontinued.

In precocious thelarche and pubarche, no treatment is necessary.

Special considerations

The dramatic physical changes produced by precocious puberty can be upsetting and alarming for the child and her family. Provide a calm, supportive atmosphere, and encourage the patient and family to express their feelings about these changes. Explain all diagnostic procedures, and tell the patient and family that surgery may be necessary.

- To prevent psychological damage, explain her condition to the child in terms she can understand, to prevent feelings of shame and loss of self-esteem. Provide appropriate sex education, including information on menstruation and related hygiene.
- Tell parents that although their daughter seems physically mature, she is not psychologically mature, and the discrepancy between physical appearance and psychological and psychosexual maturation may create problems. Warn them against expecting more of her than they'd expect of other children her age.
- Suggest that parents continue to dress their daughter in clothes that are appropriate for her age and styles that don't call attention to her physical development.
- Reassure parents that precocious puberty *doesn't* usually precipitate precocious sexual behavior.

Menopause

Menopause is the gradual decline and eventual cessation of menstruation and of the physiologic mechanisms that cause it. Menopause includes a complex syndrome of physiologic and psychosocial changes—the climacteric—caused by declining ovarian function.

Causes and incidence

Menopause occurs in three forms:

• *Physiologic menopause,* the normal decline in ovarian function due to aging, begins in most women between ages 40 and 50, and results in infrequent ovulation, decreased menstrual function, and eventually, cessation of menstruation (usually between ages 45 and 55).

• *Pathologic menopause* (premature menopause), the gradual or abrupt cessation of menstruation before age 40, occurs idiopathically in about 5% of women in the United States. However, certain diseases, especially severe infections and reproductive tract tumors, may cause pathologic menopause by seriously impairing ovarian function. Other factors that may precipitate pathologic menopause include malnutrition, debilitation, extreme emotional stress, excessive radiation exposure, and surgical procedures that impair ovarian blood supply.

• *Artificial menopause* is the cessation of ovarian function following radiation therapy or surgical procedures, such as oophorectomy.

Signs and symptoms

The decline in ovarian function and consequent decreased estrogen level that characterize all forms of menopause produce various menstrual cycle irregularities: a decrease in the amount and duration of menstrual flow, spotting, and episodes of amenorrhea and polymenorrhea (possibly with hypermenorrhea). These irregularities may last only a few months or may persist for several years before menstruation ceases permanently.

The following changes may occur in the body's systems but usually not until after the permanent cessation of menstruation:

• *reproductive system:* shrinkage of vulval structures and loss of subcutaneous fat, possibly leading to atrophic vulvitis; atrophy of vaginal mucosa and flattening of vaginal rugae, possibly causing bleeding after coitus or douching; vaginal itching, and discharge from bacterial invasion; and loss of capillaries in the atrophying vaginal wall, causing the pink, rugal lining to become smooth and white. Menopause may also produce excessive vaginal dryness and dyspareunia due to decreased lubrication from the vaginal walls and decreased secretion from Bartholin's glands; a reduction in the size of the ovaries and oviducts; and progressive pelvic relaxation, as the supporting structures of the reproductive tract lose their tone due to the absence of estrogen.

• *urinary system:* atrophic cystitis due to the deleterious effects of decreased estrogen levels on bladder mucosa and related structures, causing pyuria, dysuria, urinary frequency, urgency, and incontinence. Urethral carbuncles from loss of urethral tone and thinning of the mucosa may cause dysuria, meatal tenderness, and occasionally, hematuria.

• *mammary system:* reduction in breast size

• *integumentary system:* loss of skin elasticity and turgor due to estrogen deprivation, loss of pubic and axillary hair, and occasionally, slight alopecia

• *autonomic nervous system:* hot flashes and night sweats (in 60% of women), vertigo, syncope, tachycardia, dyspnea, tinnitus, emotional disturbances (such as irritability, nervousness, crying spells, fits of anger), and exacerbation of preexisting neurotic disorders (such as depression, anxiety, and compulsive, manic, or schizoid behavior).

Menopause may also induce atherosclerosis and osteoporosis. The role of estrogen deficiency in causing atherosclerosis is unclear. However, a decrease in estrogen level is known to contribute to osteoporosis, or bone loss caused by increased bone resorption and decreased bone formation, which may lead to long-bone fractures. Maximum bone loss occurs in weight-bearing bones, commonly producing kyphosis and, possibly, severe pain.

Artificial menopause, without estrogen replacement, produces symptoms within 2 to 5 years in 95% of women. Since the cessation of menstruation in both pathologic and artificial menopause is often abrupt, severe vasomotor and emotional disturbances may result. Menstrual bleeding after 1 year of amenorrhea may indicate organic disease.

Diagnosis

Patient history and typical clinical features suggest menopause. A Pap smear may support the diagnosis by showing the influence of estrogen deficiency on vaginal mucosa. In addition, radioimmunoassay reveals the following blood hormone levels:

- estrogen: 0 to 14 ng/dl
- plasma estradiol: 15 to 40 pg/ml
- estrone: 25 to 50 pg/ml.

Radioimmunoassay also shows the following urine values:

- estrogen: 6 to 28 mcg/24 hours
- pregnanediol (urinary secretion of progesterone): 0.3 to 0.9 mg/24 hours.

The most striking endocrine change occurs in the secretion of pituitary gonadotropins. Follicle-stimulating hormone production may increase as much as 15 times its normal level; luteinizing hormone production, as much as 5 times.

X-rays of the spine, femurs, or metacarpals may show osteopenia or osteoporosis. Pelvic examination, endometrial biopsy, and dilation and curettage may be performed to rule out suspected organic disease in the presence of abnormal menstrual bleeding.

THE ESTROGEN CONTROVERSY

Estrogen replacement therapy (ERT) to counteract decreasing estrogen levels during menopause persists as a controversial issue. Those in favor of ERT claim that it successfully controls the physical and emotional symptoms of menopause; opponents argue that ERT produces undesirable side effects, such as vaginal bleeding, breast tenderness, nausea, vomiting, abdominal bloating, and uterine cramps. At the heart of the controversy, however, is the increased risk of endometrial cancer in women who take supplemental estrogen.

According to recent studies, these are the facts concerning estrogen use:

- ERT has proven to be an effective treatment for two complaints associated with menopause—hot flashes and atrophic vaginitis. It also prevents osteoporosis by reducing bone resorption and halts postmenopausal bone loss.
- The increased risk of cancer is directly linked to the duration of ERT. Use of supplemental estrogen for more than 5 years multiplies the risk by as much as 15 times in the general population; its use for less than 1 year only doubles the risk.
- The risk of cancer does not significantly decrease with the use of cyclic therapy or of progestins for 7 days each month.
- To minimize the risk of cancer, estrogen should be prescribed in the lowest possible dosage.
- Women who experience menopause prematurely or as a result of surgery may need ERT to prevent osteoporosis.
- Smoking increases the risk of thromboembolic disease in users of ERT.
- Women with family histories of gynecologic cancer should not use ERT.

Treatment

Since physiologic menopause is a normal process, it may not require treatment. Atypical or adenomatous hyperplasia necessitates the administration of drugs such as medroxyprogesterone or norethindrone, which cause the endometrium to "shed," followed by methyltestosterone to suppress endometrial growth. Cystic endometrial hyperplasia does not require treatment. If osteoporosis occurs, estrogen therapy may be necessary.

Controversy continues over the efficacy of estrogen replacement therapy (ERT). However, recent evidence supports use of ERT in menopausal and postmenopausal women. Women who take estrogen must be monitored regularly to detect possible cancer early.

Special considerations

- Provide the patient who is considering ERT with all the facts about this controversial therapy so she can make an informed decision. Make sure she realizes the need for regular monitoring.
- Advise the patient not to discontinue contraceptive measures until confirmation that menstruation has ceased.
- Reassure the patient experiencing physiologic menopause that current body changes are normal and predictable.
- If the patient considers menopause a threat to her femininity, reassure her that she is still capable of enjoying an active sex life. If the patient is unusually distressed, suggest psychological counseling.
- Tell the patient to immediately report vaginal bleeding or spotting after cessation of menstruation.

Female Infertility

Infertility, the inability to conceive after regular intercourse for at least 1 year without contraception, affects approximately 10% to 15% of all couples in the United States. About 40% to 50% of all infertility is attributed to the female. (See also MALE INFERTILITY, *pages 980 to 982.) Following extensive investigation and treatment, approximately 50% of these infertile couples achieve pregnancy. Of the 50% who do not, 10% have no pathologic basis for infertility; the prognosis in this group becomes extremely poor if pregnancy is not achieved after 3 years.*

Causes

The causes of female infertility may be functional, anatomic, or psychologic:

- *Functional:* complex hormonal interactions determine the normal function of the female reproductive tract and require an intact hypothalamic-pituitary-ovarian axis, a system that stimulates and regulates the production of hormones necessary for normal sexual development and function. Any defect or malfunction of this system axis can cause infertility, due to insufficient gonadotropin secretions (both luteinizing and follicle-stimulating hormones). The ovary controls, and is controlled by, the hypothalamus through a system of negative and positive feedback mediated by estrogen production. Insufficient gonadotropin levels may result from infections, tumors, or neurologic disease of the hypothalamus or pituitary gland. Hypothyroidism also impairs fertility.
- *Anatomic causes are the following:*

—*Ovarian factors* are related to anovulation and oligoovulation (infrequent ovulation) and are a major cause of infertility. Pregnancy or direct visualization provides irrefutable evidence of ovulation. Presumptive signs of ovulation include regular menses, cyclic changes reflected in basal body temperature readings, postovulatory progesterone levels, and endometrial changes due to the presence of progesterone. Absence of presumptive signs suggests anovulation. Ovarian failure, in which no ova are produced by the ovaries, may result from ovarian dysgenesis or premature menopause. Amenorrhea is often associated with ovarian failure. Oligo-ovulation may be due to a mild hormonal imbalance in gonadotropin production and regulation and may be caused by polycystic disease of the ovary or abnormalities in the adrenal or thyroid gland that adversely affect hypothalamic-pituitary functioning.

—*Uterine abnormalities* may include congenitally absent uterus, bicornuate or double uterus, leiomyomas, or Asherman's syndrome, in which the anterior and posterior uterine walls adhere because of scar tissue formation.

—*Tubal and peritoneal factors* are due to faulty tubal transport mechanisms and unfavorable environmental influences affecting the sperm, ova, or recently fertilized ovum. Tubal loss or impairment may occur secondary to ectopic pregnancy.

Frequently, tubal and peritoneal factors result from anatomic abnormalities: bilateral occlusion of the tubes due to salpingitis (resulting from gonorrhea, tuberculosis, or puerperal sepsis), peritubal adhesions (resulting from endometriosis, pelvic inflammatory disease, use of an intrauterine device for contraception, diverticulosis, or childhood rupture of the appendix), and uterotubal obstruction due to tubal spasm.

—*Cervical factors* may include malfunctioning cervix that produces deficient or excessively viscous mucus and is impervious to sperm, preventing entry into the uterus. In cervical infection, viscous mucus may contain spermicidal macrophages. The possible existence of cervical antibodies that immobilize sperm is also under investigation.

- *Psychological problems* probably account for relatively few cases of infertility. Occasionally, ovulation may stop under stress due to failure of LH release. Marital discord may affect the frequency of intercourse. More often, however, psychological problems result from, rather than cause, infertility.

Symptoms and diagnosis

The inability to achieve pregnancy after having regular intercourse without contraception for at least 1 year suggests infertility.

Diagnosis requires a complete physical examination and health history, including specific questions on the patient's reproductive and sexual function, past diseases, mental state, previous surgery, types of contraception used in the past, and family history. Irregular, painless menses may indicate anovulation. A history of pelvic inflammatory disease may suggest fallopian tube blockage.

The following tests assess ovulation:

- *Basal body temperature graph* shows a sustained elevation in body temperature postovulation until just before onset of menses, indicating the approximate time of ovulation.
- *Endometrial biopsy,* done on or about day 5 after the basal body temperature elevates, provides histologic evidence that ovulation has occurred.
- *Progesterone blood levels,* measured when they should be highest, can show a luteal phase deficiency.

The following procedures assess structural integrity of the fallopian tubes, the ovaries, and the uterus:

- *Hysterosalpingography* provides radiologic evidence of tubal obstruction and abnormalities of the uterine cavity by injecting radiopaque contrast fluid through the cervix.
- *Endoscopy* confirms the results of hysterosalpingography and visualizes the endometrial cavity by hysteroscopy or explores the posterior surface of the uterus, fallopian tubes, and ovaries by culdoscopy. Laparoscopy allows visualization of the abdominal and pelvic areas.

Male-female interaction studies include the following:

- *Postcoital test* (Sims-Huhner test) examines the cervical mucus for motile sperm cells following intercourse that takes place at midcycle (as close to ovulation as possible).
- *Immunologic or antibody testing* detects spermicidal antibodies in the sera of the female. Further research is being conducted in this area.

Treatment

Treatment depends on identifying the underlying abnormality or dysfunction within the hypothalamic-pituitary-ovarian complex. In hyperactivity or hypoactivity of the adrenal or thyroid gland, hormone therapy is necessary; progesterone deficiency requires progesterone replacement. Anovulation necessitates treatment with clomiphene, human menopausal gonadotropins, or human chorionic gonadotropin; ovulation usually occurs several days after such administration. If mucus production decreases (a side effect of clomiphene), small doses of estrogen to improve the quality of cervical mucus may be given concomitantly.

Surgical restoration may correct certain anatomic causes of infertility, such as fallopian tube obstruction. Surgery may also be necessary to remove tumors located within or near the hypothalamus or pituitary gland. Endometriosis requires drug therapy (danazol or medroxyprogesterone, or noncyclic administration of oral contraceptives), surgical removal of areas of endometriosis, or a combination of both.

Artifical insemination has proven to be an effective treatment for infertility problems. In vitro (test tube) fertilization has also been successful.

Special considerations

Management includes providing the infertile couple with emotional support and information about diagnostic and treatment techniques.

An infertile couple may suffer loss of self-esteem; they may feel angry, guilty, or inadequate, and the diagnostic procedures for this disorder may intensify their fear and anxiety. You can help by explaining these procedures thoroughly. Above all, encourage the patient and her partner to talk about their feelings, and listen to what they have to say with a nonjudgmental attitude.

If the patient requires surgery, tell her what to expect postoperatively; this, of course, depends on which procedure is to be performed.

Pelvic Inflammatory Disease

Pelvic inflammatory disease (PID) is any acute, subacute, recurrent, or chronic infection of the oviducts and ovaries, with adjacent tissue involvement. It includes inflammation of the cervix (cervicitis), uterus (endometritis), fallopian tubes (salpingitis), and ovaries (oophoritis), which can extend to the connective tissue lying between the broad ligaments (parametritis). Early diagnosis and treatment prevents damage to the reproductive system. Untreated PID may cause infertility and may lead to potentially fatal septicemia, pulmonary emboli, and shock.

Causes

PID can result from infection with aerobic or anaerobic organisms. The aerobic organism *Neisseria gonorrhoeae* is its most common cause, because it most readily penetrates the bacteriostatic barrier of cervical mucus.

Normally, cervical secretions have a protective and defensive function. Therefore, conditions or procedures that alter or destroy cervical mucus impair this bacteriostatic mechanism and allow bacteria present in the cervix or vagina to ascend into the uterine cavity; such procedures include conization or cauterization of the cervix.

Uterine infection can also follow the transfer of contaminated cervical mucus into the endometrial cavity by instrumentation. Consequently, PID can follow insertion of an intrauterine device, use of a biopsy curet or of an irrigation catheter, or tubal insufflation. Other predisposing factors include abortion, pelvic

FORMS OF PELVIC INFLAMMATORY DISEASE

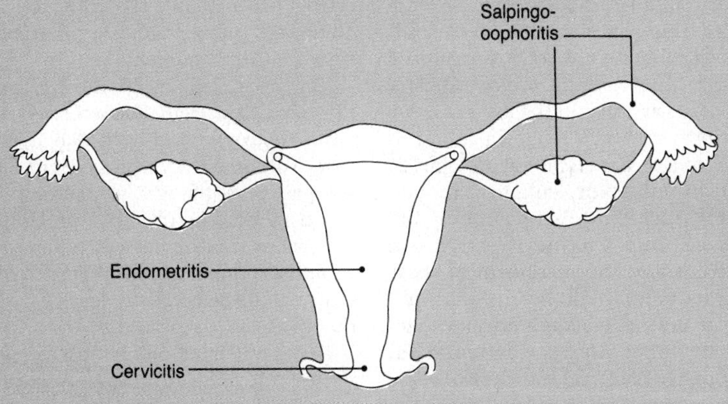

CLINICAL FEATURES	DIAGNOSTIC FINDINGS
Salpingo-oophoritis • *Acute:* sudden onset of lower abdominal and pelvic pain, usually following menses; increased vaginal discharge; fever; malaise; lower abdominal pressure and tenderness; tachycardia; pelvic peritonitis • *Chronic:* recurring acute episodes	• Blood studies show leukocytosis or normal WBC. • X-ray may show ileus. • Pelvic exam reveals extreme tenderness. • Smear of cervical or periurethral gland exudate shows gram-negative intracellular diplococci.
Cervicitis • *Acute:* purulent, foul-smelling vaginal discharge; vulvovaginitis, with itching or burning; red, edematous cervix; pelvic discomfort; sexual dysfunction; metrorrhagia; infertility; spontaneous abortion • *Chronic:* cervical dystocia, laceration or eversion of the cervix, ulcerative vesicular lesion (when cervicitis results from herpes simplex virus II)	• Cultures for *N. gonorrhoeae* are positive (> 90% of patients). • Cytologic smears may reveal severe inflammation. • If cervicitis is not complicated by salpingitis, WBC normal or slightly elevated; ESR elevated. • In *acute cervicitis,* cervical palpation reveals tenderness. • In *chronic cervicitis,* causative organisms are usually staphylococcus or streptococcus.
Endometritis (generally postpartum or postabortion) • *Acute:* mucopurulent or purulent vaginal discharge oozing from the cervix; edematous, hyperemic endometrium, possibly leading to ulceration and necrosis (with virulent organisms); lower abdominal pain and tenderness; fever; rebound pain; abdominal muscle spasm; thrombophlebitis of uterine and pelvic vessels (in severe forms) • *Chronic:* recurring acute episodes (increasingly common because of widespread use of IUDs)	• In severe infection, palpation may reveal boggy uterus. • Uterine and blood samples positive for causative organism, usually staphylococcus. • WBC and ESR are elevated.

surgery, and infection during or after pregnancy.

Bacteria may also enter the uterine cavity through the bloodstream or from drainage from a chronically infected fallopian tube, a pelvic abscess, a ruptured appendix, diverticulitis of the sigmoid colon, or other infectious foci.

The most common bacteria found in cervical mucus are staphylococci, streptococci, diphtheroids, chlamydiae, and coliforms, including *Pseudomonas* and *Escherichia coli.* Uterine infection can result from any one or several of these organisms or may follow the multiplication of normally nonpathogenic bacteria in an altered endometrial environment. Bacterial multiplication is most common during parturition, because the endometrium is atrophic, quiescent, and not stimulated by estrogen.

Signs and symptoms

Clinical features of PID vary with the affected area but generally include a profuse, purulent vaginal discharge, sometimes accompanied by low-grade fever and malaise (particularly if gonorrhea is the cause). The patient experiences lower abdomen pain; movement of the cervix or palpation of the adnexa may be extremely painful.

Diagnosis

Diagnostic tests generally include:

- *Gram stain* of secretions from the endocervix or cul-de-sac. Culture and sensitivity testing aids selection of the appropriate antibiotic. Urethral and rectal secretions may also be cultured.
- *ultrasonography* to identify an adnexal or uterine mass. (X-rays seldom identify pelvic masses.)
- *culdocentesis* to obtain peritoneal fluid or pus for culture and sensitivity testing.

In addition, patient history is significant. In general, PID is associated with recent sexual intercourse, IUD insertion, childbirth, or abortion.

Treatment

To prevent progression of PID, antibiotic therapy begins immediately after culture specimens are obtained. Such therapy can be reevaluated as soon as laboratory results are available (usually after 24 to 48 hours). Infection may become chronic if treated inadequately.

The preferred antibiotic therapy for PID resulting from gonorrhea is penicillin G procaine I.M. in two injection sites, combined with probenecid P.O. If the patient is allergic to penicillin, tetracycline may be used. (A patient with gonorrhea may also require therapy for syphilis.) Supplemental treatment of PID may include bed rest, analgesics, and I.V. therapy.

Development of pelvic abscess necessitates adequate drainage. A ruptured pelvic abscess is a life-threatening condition. If this complication develops, the patient may need a total abdominal hysterectomy, with bilateral salpingo-oophorectomy.

Special considerations

- After establishing that the patient has no drug allergies, administer antibiotics and analgesics, as ordered.
- Check for elevated temperature. If fever persists, carefully monitor fluid intake and output for signs of dehydration.
- Watch for abdominal rigidity and distention, possible signs of developing peritonitis. Provide frequent perineal care if vaginal drainage occurs.
- To prevent recurrence, encourage compliance with treatment, and explain the nature and seriousness of PID.
- Stress the need for the patient's sexual partner to be examined and, if necessary, treated for infection.
- Since PID may cause painful intercourse, advise the patient to consult with her doctor about sexual activity.
- To prevent infection after minor gynecologic procedures, such as dilation and curettage, tell the patient to immediately report any fever, increased vaginal discharge, or pain. After such procedures, instruct her to avoid douching or intercourse for at least 7 days.

UTERINE BLEEDING DISORDERS

Amenorrhea

Amenorrhea is the abnormal absence or suppression of menstruation. Primary amenorrhea is the absence of menarche in an adolescent (by age 18). Secondary amenorrhea is the failure of menstruation for at least 3 months after normal onset of menarche.

Causes

Amenorrhea is normal before puberty, after menopause, or during pregnancy and lactation; it is pathologic at any other time. As a disorder, it usually results from anovulation due to hormonal abnormalities, such as decreased secretion of estrogen, gonadotropins, luteinizing hormone, and follicle-stimulating hormone; lack of ovarian response to gonadotropins; or constant presence of progesterone or other endocrine abnormalities.

Amenorrhea may also result from the absence of a uterus, endometrial damage, or from ovarian, adrenal, or pituitary tumors. It is also linked to emotional disorders, and is common in patients with severe disorders such as depression and anorexia nervosa. Mild emotional disturbances tend merely to distort the ovulatory cycle, while severe psychic trauma may abruptly change the bleeding pattern or may completely suppress one or more full ovulatory cycles. Amenorrhea may also result from malnutrition and, occasionally, from prolonged use of oral contraceptives.

Symptoms and diagnosis

A history of failure to menstruate in a female over age 18 confirms primary amenorrhea. Secondary amenorrhea can be diagnosed when a change is noted in a previously established menstrual pattern (absence of menstruation for 3 months). A thorough physical and pelvic examination rules out pregnancy, as well as anatomic abnormalities (such as cervical stenosis) that may cause false amenorrhea (cryptomenorrhea), in which menstruation occurs without external bleeding.

Onset of menstruation within 1 week after administration of pure progestational agents, such as medroxyprogesterone and progesterone, indicates a functioning uterus. If menstruation does not occur, special diagnostic studies are appropriate.

Blood and urine studies may reveal hormonal imbalances—such as lack of ovarian response to gonadotropins (elevated pituitary gonadotropins) and failure of gonadotropin secretion (low pituitary gonadotropin levels). Tests for identification of dominant or missing hormones include cervical mucus ferning, vaginal cytologic examinations, basal body temperature, endometrial biopsy (during dilation and curettage), urinary 17-ketosteroids, and plasma progesterone, testosterone, and androgen levels. A complete medical workup, including appropriate X-rays, laparoscopy, and a biopsy, may determine ovarian, adrenal, and pituitary tumors.

Treatment

Generally, appropriate hormone replacement reestablishes menstruation. Treatment of amenorrhea not related to hormone deficiency depends on the underlying cause. For example, amenorrhea that results from a tumor usually requires surgery.

Special considerations

- Explain all diagnostic procedures.

- Provide reassurance and emotional support. Psychiatric counseling may be necessary if amenorrhea results from emotional disturbances.
- After treatment, teach the patient how to keep an accurate record of her menstrual cycles to aid early detection of recurrent amenorrhea.

Abnormal Premenopausal Bleeding

Abnormal premenopausal bleeding refers to any bleeding that deviates from the normal menstrual cycle before menopause. These deviations include menstrual bleeding that is abnormally infrequent (oligomenorrhea), abnormally frequent (polymenorrhea), excessive (menorrhagia or hypermenorrhea), deficient (hypomenorrhea), or irregular (metrorrhagia [uterine bleeding between menses]). Rarely, symptoms of menstruation are not accompanied by external bleeding (cryptomenorrhea). Premenopausal bleeding may merely be troublesome or can result in severe hemorrhage; however, prognosis depends on the underlying cause. Abnormal patterns of bleeding often respond to hormonal or other therapy.

Causes and incidence

Causes of abnormal premenopausal bleeding vary with the type of bleeding.

- *Oligomenorrhea* and *polymenorrhea* usually result from anovulation due to an endocrine or systemic disorder.
- *Menorrhagia* usually results from local lesions, such as uterine leiomyomas, endometrial polyps, and endometrial hyperplasia. It may also result from endometritis, salpingitis, and anovulation.
- *Hypomenorrhea* results from local, endocrine, or systemic disorders, or from blockage due to partial obstruction by the hymen or to cervical obstruction.
- *Cryptomenorrhea* may result from an imperforate hymen or cervical stenosis.
- *Metrorrhagia* usually results from slight physiologic bleeding from the endometrium during ovulation but may also result from local disorders, such as uterine malignancy, cervical erosions, polyps (which tend to bleed after intercourse), or inappropriate estrogen therapy. Complications of pregnancy can also cause premenopausal bleeding. Such bleeding may be as mild as spotting or as severe as menorrhagia.

Signs and symptoms

Bleeding not associated with abnormal pregnancy is usually painless, but it may be severely painful. When bleeding is associated with abnormal pregnancy, other symptoms include nausea, breast tenderness, bloating, and fluid retention. Severe or prolonged bleeding causes anemia, especially in patients with underlying disease (such as blood dyscrasias) and in patients receiving anticoagulants.

Diagnosis

The typical clinical picture confirms abnormal premenopausal bleeding. Special tests identify the underlying cause:

- *Serum hormone levels* reflect adrenal, pituitary, or thyroid dysfunction.
- *Urinary 17-ketosteroids* reveal adrenal hyperplasia, hypopituitarism, or polycystic ovarian disease.
- *Endometrial sampling* rules out malignancy and should be performed in all patients that experience premenopausal bleeding.
- *Pelvic examination, Pap smear, and history* rule out local or malignant causes.
- *CBC* rules out anemia.

If testing rules out pelvic and hormonal causes of abnormal bleeding, a complete hematologic survey (including platelet count and bleeding time) is appropriate to determine clotting abnormalities.

Treatment

Treatment depends on the type of bleeding abnormality and its cause. Menstrual irregularity alone may not require therapy unless it interferes with the patient's attempt to achieve or avoid conception or leads to anemia. When it does require treatment, clomiphene induces ovulation. Electrocautery, chemical cautery, or cryosurgery can remove cervical polyps; dilation and curettage, uterine polyps. Organic disorders—such as cervical or uterine malignancy—may necessitate hysterectomy, radium or X-ray therapy, or both of these treatments, depending on the site and extent of the disease. And, of course, anemia and infections require appropriate treatment.

CAUSES OF ABNORMAL PREMENOPAUSAL BLEEDING

	HYPOMENORRHEA	OLIGOMENORRHEA	METRORRHAGIA	POLYMENORRHEA	MENORRHAGIA
Malnutrition	•	•			
Hyperthyroidism	•	•			
Hypothyroidism				•	•
Severe psychic trauma	•	•			•
Blood dyscrasias			•	•	•
Severe infections	•	•			
Endometritis			•		
Drugs (such as digitalis, corticosteroids, anticoagulants)				•	
Uterine tumors			•		•

Special considerations

- If a patient complains of abnormal bleeding, tell her to record the dates of the bleeding and the number of tampons or pads she uses per day. This helps to assess the cyclic pattern and the amount of bleeding.
- Instruct the patient to report abnormal bleeding immediately to help rule out major hemorrhagic disorders, such as occur in abnormal pregnancy.
- To prevent abnormal bleeding due to organic causes, and for early detection of malignancy, encourage the patient to have a Pap smear and a pelvic examination annually.
- Offer reassurance and support. The patient may be particularly anxious about excessive or frequent blood loss and the passage of clots. Suggest that she minimize blood flow by avoiding strenuous activity and occasionally lying down with her feet elevated.

Dysfunctional Uterine Bleeding

Dysfunctional uterine bleeding (DUB) refers to abnormal endometrial bleeding without recognizable organic lesions. Prognosis varies with the cause. DUB is the indication for almost 25% of gynecologic surgery.

Causes

DUB usually results from an imbalance in the hormonal-endometrial relationship, where persistent and unopposed stimulation of the endometrium by estrogen occurs. Disorders that cause sustained high estrogen levels are polycystic ovary syndrome, obesity, immaturity of the hypothalamic-pituitary-ovarian mechanism (in postpubertal teenagers), and anovulation (in women in their late 30s or early 40s).

In most cases of DUB, the endometrium shows no pathologic changes. However, in chronic unopposed estrogen stimulation (as from a hormone-producing ovarian tumor), the endometrium may show hyperplastic or malignant changes.

Signs and symptoms

DUB usually occurs as metrorrhagia (episodes of vaginal bleeding between menses); it may also occur as hypermenorrhea (heavy or prolonged menses, longer than 8 days) or chronic polymenorrhea (menstrual cycle of less than 18 days). Such bleeding is unpredictable and can cause anemia.

Diagnosis

Diagnostic studies must rule out other causes of excessive vaginal bleeding, such as organic, systemic, psychogenic, and endocrine causes, including malignancy, polyps, incomplete abortion, pregnancy, and infection.

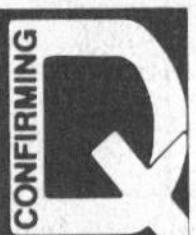

Dilation and curettage (D & C), and biopsy results confirm the diagnosis by revealing endometrial hyperplasia. Hematocrit and hemoglobin levels determine the need for blood or iron replacement.

Treatment

High-dose estrogen-progestogen combination therapy (oral contraceptives), the primary treatment, is designed to control endometrial growth and reestablish a normal cyclic pattern of menstruation. These drugs are usually administered four times daily for 5 to 7 days, even though bleeding usually stops in 12 to 24 hours. (The patient's age and the cause of bleeding help determine the drug choice and dosage.) In patients over age 35, endometrial biopsy is necessary before the start of estrogen therapy to rule out endometrial adenocarcinoma. Progestogen therapy is a necessary alternative in some women, such as those susceptible to the adverse effects of estrogen (thrombophlebitis, for example).

If drug therapy is ineffective, a D & C serves as a supplementary treatment, through removal of a large portion of the bleeding endometrium. Also, a D & C can help determine the original cause of hormonal imbalance and can aid in planning further therapy. Regardless of the primary treatment, the patient may need iron replacement or transfusions of packed cells or whole blood, as indicated, because of anemia caused by recurrent bleeding.

Special considerations

- Explain the importance of adhering to the prescribed hormonal therapy. If a D & C is ordered, explain this procedure and its purpose.
- Stress the need for regular checkups to assess treatment.

Postmenopausal Bleeding

Postmenopausal bleeding is defined as bleeding from the reproductive tract that occurs 1 year or more after cessation of menses. Sites of bleeding include the vulva, vagina, cervix, and endometrium. Prognosis varies with the cause.

Causes

Postmenopausal bleeding may result from:

- *exogenous estrogen,* when administration is excessive or prolonged or when small amounts are given in the presence of a hypersensitive endometrium.
- *endogenous estrogen production,* especially when levels are high, as in persons with estrogen-producing ovarian

tumor; however, in some persons, even slight fluctuation in estrogen levels may cause bleeding.
• *atrophic endometrium* due to low estrogen levels.
• *atrophic vaginitis,* usually triggered by trauma during coitus in the absence of estrogen production.
• *aging,* which increases vascular vulnerability by thinning epithelial surfaces, increasing vascular fragility, producing degenerative tissue changes, and decreasing resistance to infections.
• *cervical or endometrial cancer* (more common after age 60).
• *adenomatous hyperplasia* or *atypical adenomatous hyperplasia* (usually considered a premalignant lesion).

Signs and symptoms
Vaginal bleeding, the predominant symptom, ranges from spotting to outright hemorrhage; its duration also varies. Other symptoms depend on the cause. Excessive estrogen stimulation, for example, may also produce copious cervical mucus; estrogen deficiency may cause vaginal mucosa to atrophy.

Diagnosis
Diagnostic evaluation of the patient with postmenopausal bleeding should include physical examination (especially pelvic examination), a detailed history, standard laboratory tests (such as CBC), and cytologic examination of smears from the cervix and the endocervical canal. Dilation and curettage (D & C) shows pathologic findings in the endometrium.

Diagnosis must rule out underlying degenerative or systemic disease. For instance, evidence of elevated levels of endogenous estrogen may suggest an ovarian tumor. Before testing for estrogen levels, the patient must stop all sources of exogenous estrogen intake—including face and body creams that contain estrogen—to rule out excessive exogenous estrogen as a cause.

Treatment
Emergency treatment to control massive hemorrhage is rarely necessary, except in advanced malignancy. Treatment may include D & C to relieve bleeding. Other therapy varies according to the underlying cause. Estrogen creams and suppositories are usually very effective in correcting estrogen deficiency, since they are rapidly absorbed. Hysterectomy is indicated for repeated episodes of postmenopausal bleeding from the endometrial cavity. Such bleeding may indicate endometrial cancer.

Special considerations
• Obtain a detailed patient history to rule out excessive exogenous estrogen as a cause of bleeding. Ask the patient about use of cosmetics (especially face and body creams), drugs, and other products that may contain estrogen. Discuss the risks and benefits of estrogen replacement therapy with her.
• Provide emotional support. The patient will probably be afraid that the bleeding indicates cancer.
• To prevent disorders that cause postmenopausal bleeding, stress the fact that periodic gynecologic examinations are as important after menopause as they were before.

DISORDERS OF PREGNANCY

Abortion

Abortion is the spontaneous or induced (therapeutic) expulsion of the products of conception from the uterus before fetal viability (fetal weight of less than 17½ oz

[500 g] and gestation of less than 20 weeks). Up to 15% of all pregnancies and approximately 30% of first pregnancies end in spontaneous abortion (miscarriage). At least 75% of miscarriages occur during the first trimester. Incidence of legal therapeutic abortions is rising in the United States. Roughly 25% of all pregnancies end in elective abortions, usually during the first trimester.

Causes

Spontaneous abortion may result from fetal, placental, or maternal factors. Fetal factors usually cause such abortions at 9 to 12 weeks of gestation and include:

- defective embryologic development due to abnormal chromosome division (most common cause of fetal death)
- faulty implantation of fertilized ovum
- failure of the endometrium to accept the fertilized ovum.

Placental factors usually cause abortion around the 14th week of gestation, when the placenta takes over the hormone production necessary to maintain the pregnancy, and include:

- premature separation of the normally implanted placenta
- abnormal placental implantation
- abnormal platelet function.

Maternal factors usually cause abortion between 11 and 19 weeks of gestation and include:

- maternal infection, severe malnutrition, abnormalities of the reproductive organs (especially incompetent cervix, in which the cervix dilates painlessly and bloodlessly in the second trimester)
- endocrine problems, such as thyroid dysfunction or lowered estriol secretion
- trauma, including any type of surgery that necessitates manipulation of the pelvic organs
- blood group incompatibility and Rh isoimmunization (still under investigation as a possible cause)
- drug ingestion.

The goal of *therapeutic abortion* is to preserve the mother's mental or physical health in cases of rape, unplanned pregnancy, or medical conditions, such as moderate or severe cardiac dysfunction.

Signs and symptoms

Prodromal symptoms of spontaneous abortion may include a pink discharge for several days or a scant brown discharge for several weeks before onset of cramps and increased vaginal bleeding. For a few hours the cramps intensify and occur more frequently; then the cervix dilates for expulsion of uterine contents. If the entire contents are expelled, cramps and bleeding subside. However, if any contents remain, cramps and bleeding continue.

Diagnosis

Diagnosis of spontaneous abortion is based on clinical evidence of expulsion of uterine contents, pelvic examination, and laboratory studies. Human chorionic gonadotropin (HCG) in the blood or urine confirms pregnancy; decreased HCG levels suggest spontaneous abortion. Pelvic examination determines the size of the uterus and whether this size is consistent with the length of the pregnancy. Tissue cytology indicates evidence of products of conception. Laboratory tests reflect decreased hematocrit and hemoglobin levels due to blood loss.

Treatment

An accurate evaluation of uterine contents is necessary before planning treatment. The progression of spontaneous abortion cannot be prevented, except in those cases caused by an incompetent cervix. Hospitalization is necessary to control severe hemorrhage. Severe bleeding requires transfusion with packed RBCs or whole blood. Initially, I.V. administration of oxytocin stimulates uterine contractions. If remnants remain in the uterus, dilation and curettage (D & C) or dilation and evacuation (D & E) should be performed.

A D & E is also used in first-trimester therapeutic abortions. In second-trimester therapeutic abortions, an injection of hypertonic saline solution or of prostaglandin into the amniotic sac or insertion of a prostaglandin vaginal suppository induces labor and expulsion of uterine contents.

After an abortion, spontaneous or induced, an Rh-negative female with a negative indirect Coombs' test should receive Rh_o (D) immune globulin (human) to prevent future Rh isoimmunization.

In a habitual aborter, spontaneous abortion can result from an incompetent cervix. Treatment, therefore, involves surgical reinforcement of the cervix (Shirodkar-Barter procedure) about 14 to 16 weeks after the last menstrual period. A few weeks before the estimated delivery date, the sutures are removed, and the patient awaits the onset of labor. An alternative procedure, especially for the woman who wants to have more children, is to leave the sutures in place, and to deliver the infant by cesarean section.

Special considerations

Before possible abortion:

- Explain all procedures thoroughly.
- The patient should *not* have bathroom privileges, because she may expel uterine contents without knowing it. After she uses the bedpan, inspect the contents carefully for intrauterine material.

After spontaneous or elective abortion:

- Note the amount, color, and odor of vaginal bleeding. Save all the pads the patient uses, for evaluation.
- Administer analgesics and oxytocin, as ordered.
- Give good perineal care.
- Obtain vital signs every 4 hours for 24 hours.
- Monitor urinary output.

Care of the patient who has had a spontaneous abortion includes emotional support and counseling during the grieving process. Encourage the patient and her partner to express their feelings. Some couples may want to talk to a member of the clergy or, depending on their religion, may wish to have the fetus baptized.

The patient who has had a therapeutic abortion also benefits from support. Encourage her to verbalize her feelings. Remember, she may feel ambivalent about the procedure; intellectual and emotional acceptance of abortion are not the same. Refer her for counseling, if necessary.

To prepare the patient for discharge:

- Tell the patient to expect vaginal bleeding or spotting and to report bleed-

TYPES OF SPONTANEOUS ABORTION

- *Threatened abortion:* Bloody vaginal discharge occurs during the first half of pregnancy. Approximately 20% of pregnant women have vaginal spotting or actual bleeding early in pregnancy; of these, about 50% abort.
- *Inevitable abortion:* Membranes rupture and the cervix dilates. As labor continues, the uterus expels the products of conception.
- *Incomplete abortion:* Uterus retains part or all of the placenta. Before the 10th week of gestation, the fetus and placenta usually are expelled together; after the 10th week, separately. Because part of the placenta may adhere to the uterine wall, bleeding continues. Hemorrhage is possible because the uterus doesn't contract and seal the large vessels that fed the placenta.
- *Complete abortion:* Uterus passes all the products of conception. Minimal bleeding usually accompanies complete abortion because the uterus contracts and compresses the maternal blood vessels that fed the placenta.
- *Missed abortion:* Uterus retains the products of conception for 2 months or more after the death of the fetus. Uterine growth ceases; uterine size may even seem to decrease. Prolonged retention of the dead products of conception may cause coagulation defects, such as disseminated intravascular coagulation (DIC).
- *Habitual abortion:* Spontaneous loss of three or more consecutive pregnancies constitutes habitual abortion.
- *Septic abortion:* Infection accompanies abortion. This may occur with spontaneous abortion but usually results from an illegal abortion.

ing that lasts longer than 8 to 10 days or excessive, bright-red blood immediately.

- Advise the patient to watch for signs of infection, such as a temperature higher than 100° F. (37.8° C.) and foul-smelling vaginal discharge.
- Encourage the gradual increase of daily activities to include whatever tasks the patient feels comfortable doing (cooking, sewing, cleaning, for example), as long as these activities don't increase vaginal bleeding or cause fatigue. Most patients return to work within 1 to 4 weeks.
- Urge 2 to 3 weeks' abstinence from intercourse, and encourage use of a contraceptive when intercourse is resumed.
- Instruct the patient to avoid using tampons for 2 to 4 weeks.
- Be sure to inform the patient who desires an elective abortion of all the available alternatives. She needs to know what the procedure involves, what the risks are, and what to expect during and after the procedure, both emotionally and physically. Be sure to ascertain whether the patient is comfortable with her decision to have an elective abortion. Encourage her to verbalize her thoughts both when the procedure is performed and at a follow-up visit, usually 2 weeks later. If you identify an inappropriate coping response, refer the patient for professional counseling.
- To help prevent elective abortion, medical and nursing personnel need to make contraceptive information available. An educated population motivated to utilize contraception would have little need for elective abortion.
- Tell the patient to see her doctor in 2 to 4 weeks for a follow-up examination.

To minimize the risk of future spontaneous abortions, emphasize to the pregnant woman the importance of good nutrition and the need to exclude alcohol, cigarettes, and drugs. Most clinicians recommend that the couple wait two or three normal menstrual cycles after a spontaneous abortion has occurred before attempting conception. If the patient has a history of habitual spontaneous abortions, suggest that she and her partner have thorough examinations. For the woman, this includes premenstrual endometrial biopsy, a hormone assessment (estrogen, progesterone, and thyroid, follicle-stimulating, and luteinizing hormones), and hysterosalpingography and laparoscopy to detect anatomic abnormalities. Genetic counseling may also be indicated.

Ectopic Pregnancy

Ectopic pregnancy is the implantation of the fertilized ovum outside the uterine cavity. The most common site is the fallopian tube (more than 90% of ectopic implantations occur in the fimbria, ampulla, or isthmus), but other possible sites may include the interstitium, tubo-ovarian ligament, ovary, abdominal viscera, and internal cervical os. In whites, ectopic pregnancy occurs in 1 in 200 pregnancies; in nonwhites, in 1 in 120. Prognosis is good with prompt diagnosis, appropriate surgical intervention, and control of bleeding; rarely, in cases of abdominal implantation, the fetus may survive to term. Usually, subsequent intrauterine pregnancy is achieved.

Causes

Conditions that prevent or retard the passage of the fertilized ovum through the fallopian tube and into the uterine cavity include:

- *endosalpingitis,* an inflammatory reaction that causes folds of the tubal mucosa to agglutinate, narrowing the tube.
- *diverticula,* the formation of blind pouches that cause tubal abnormalities.

IMPLANTATION SITES OF ECTOPIC PREGNANCY

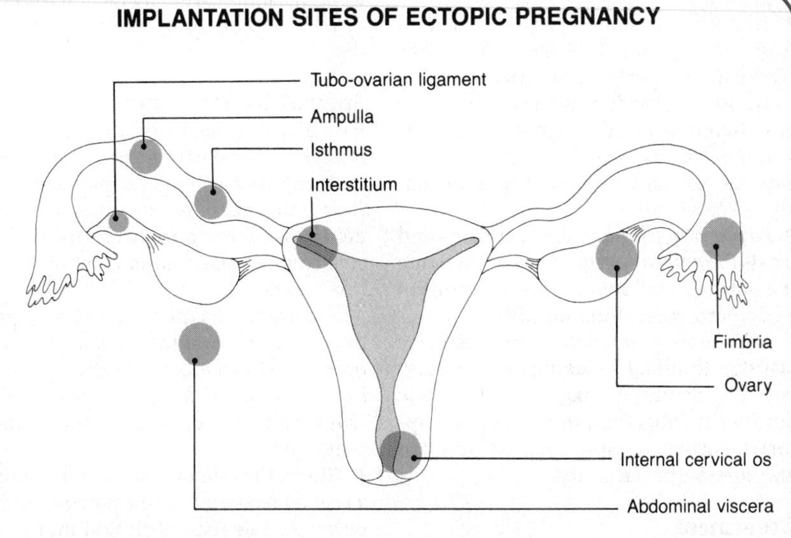

In 90% of patients with ectopic pregnancy, the ovum implants in the fallopian tube, either in the fimbria, ampulla, or isthmus. Other possible sites of implantation include the interstitium, tubo-ovarian ligament, ovary, abdominal viscera, and internal cervical os.

- *tumors* pressing against the tube.
- *previous surgery* (tubal ligation or resection, or adhesions from previous abdominal or pelvic surgery).
- *transmigration of the ovum* (from one ovary to the opposite tube), resulting in delayed implantation.

Rarely, ectopic pregnancy may result from congenital defects in the reproductive tract or ectopic endometrial implants in the tubal mucosa. Ectopic pregnancy may also be related to use of an intrauterine device (IUD). Such use may exaggerate the risk of ectopic pregnancy, because an IUD causes localized action on the cellular lining of the uterus, extending into the fallopian tubes.

Signs and symptoms

Ectopic pregnancy sometimes produces symptoms of normal pregnancy or no symptoms other than mild abdominal pain (the latter is especially likely in abdominal pregnancy), making diagnosis difficult. Characteristic clinical effects after fallopian tube implantation include amenorrhea or abnormal menses, followed by slight vaginal bleeding, and unilateral pelvic pain over the mass. Rupture of the tube causes life-threatening complications, including hemorrhage, shock, and peritonitis. The patient experiences sharp lower abdominal pain, possibly radiating to the shoulders and neck, often precipitated by activities that increase abdominal pressure, such as a bowel movement; she feels extreme pain upon motion of the cervix and palpation of the adnexa during a pelvic examination. She has a tender, boggy uterus.

Diagnosis

Clinical features, patient history, and the results of a pelvic examination suggest ectopic pregnancy. The following tests confirm it:

- *Serum pregnancy test* shows presence of human chorionic gonadotropin.
- *Real time ultrasonography* determines intrauterine pregnancy or ovarian cyst (performed if serum pregnancy test

is positive).
• In *culdocentesis,* fluid is aspirated from the vaginal cul-de-sac to detect free blood in the peritoneum (performed if ultrasonography detects the absence of a gestational sac in the uterus).
• *Laparoscopy* reveals pregnancy outside the uterus (performed if culdocentesis is positive).
• *Exploratory laparotomy* confirms and treats the ectopic pregnancy by removing the affected fallopian tube (salpingectomy) and controlling bleeding.

Decreased hemoglobin and hematocrit due to blood loss support the diagnosis. Differential diagnosis must rule out uterine abortion, appendicitis, ruptured corpus luteum cyst, salpingitis, and torsion of the ovary.

Treatment

If culdocentesis is positive for blood in the peritoneum, laparotomy and salpingectomy are indicated, possibly preceded by laparoscopy. Patients who wish to have children can undergo microsurgical repair of the fallopian tube. The ovary is saved, if possible; however, ovarian pregnancy necessitates oophorectomy. Interstitial pregnancy may require hysterectomy; abdominal pregnancy requires a laparotomy to remove the fetus, except in rare cases, when the fetus survives to term or calcifies undetected in the abdominal cavity.

Supportive treatment includes transfusion with whole blood or packed red cells to replace excessive blood loss, administration of broad-spectrum antibiotics I.V. for septic infection, administration of supplemental iron P.O. or I.M., and institution of a high-protein diet.

Special considerations

Patient care measures include careful monitoring and assessment of vital signs and vaginal bleeding, preparing the patient with excessive blood loss for emergency surgery, and providing blood replacement and emotional support and reassurance.
• Record the location and character of the pain, and administer analgesics, as ordered. (Remember, however, that analgesics may mask the symptoms of intraperitoneal rupture of the ectopic pregnancy.)
• Check the amount, color, and odor of vaginal bleeding. Ask the patient the date of her last menstrual period and to describe the character of this period.
• Observe for signs of pregnancy (enlarged breasts, soft cervix).
• Provide a quiet, relaxing environment, and encourage the patient to freely express her feelings of fear, loss, and grief.

To prevent ectopic pregnancy:
• Advise prompt treatment of pelvic infections to prevent diseases of the fallopian tube. Inform patients who have undergone surgery involving the fallopian tubes or those with confirmed pelvic inflammatory disease that they are at increased risk of ectopic pregnancy.
• Tell the patient who is vulnerable to ectopic pregnancy to delay using an IUD until after she has completed her family.

Hyperemesis Gravidarum

Unlike the transient nausea and vomiting normally experienced between the sixth and twelfth weeks of pregnancy, hyperemesis gravidarum is severe and unremitting nausea and vomiting that persists after the first trimester. If untreated, it produces substantial weight loss; starvation; dehydration, with subsequent fluid and electrolyte imbalance (hypokalemia); and acid-base disturbances (acidosis and alkalosis). This syndrome occurs in approximately 1 in 200 pregnancies. Prognosis is good with appropriate treatment.

Causes
Although its cause is unknown, hyperemesis gravidarum often affects pregnant females with conditions that produce high levels of human chorionic gonadotropin, such as hydatidiform mole or multiple pregnancy. Its other possible causes include pancreatitis (elevated serum amylase levels are common), biliary tract disease, drug toxicity, inflammatory obstructive bowel disease, and vitamin deficiency (especially of B_6). In some patients, it may be related to psychological factors, such as ambivalence toward pregnancy.

Signs and symptoms
The cardinal symptoms of hyperemesis gravidarum are unremitting nausea and vomiting. The vomitus initially contains undigested food, mucus, and small amounts of bile; later, it contains only bile and mucus; and finally, blood and material that resembles coffee grounds. Persistent vomiting causes substantial weight loss and eventual emaciation. Associated effects may include pale, dry, waxy, and possibly jaundiced skin; subnormal or elevated temperature; rapid pulse; a fetid, fruity breath odor from acidosis; and CNS symptoms such as confusion, delirium, headache, lassitude, stupor, and possibly coma.

Diagnosis
Diagnosis depends on a history of uncontrolled nausea and vomiting that persists beyond the first trimester, evidence of substantial weight loss, and other characteristic clinical features. Serum analysis shows decreased protein, chloride, sodium, and potassium levels and increased BUN levels. Other laboratory tests reveal ketonuria, slight proteinuria, and elevated hemoglobin and WBC levels. Diagnosis must rule out other conditions with similar clinical effects.

Treatment
Hyperemesis gravidarum may necessitate hospitalization to correct electrolyte imbalance and prevent starvation. I.V. infusions maintain nutrition until the patient can tolerate oral feedings. She progresses slowly to a clear liquid diet, then a full liquid diet, and finally, small, frequent meals of high-protein solid foods. A midnight snack helps stabilize blood glucose levels; vitamin B supplements help correct vitamin deficiency.

When vomiting stops and electrolyte balance has been restored, the pregnancy usually continues without recurrence of hyperemesis gravidarum. Most patients feel better as they begin to regain normal weight, but some continue to vomit throughout the pregnancy, requiring extended treatment. If appropriate, some patients may benefit from consultations with clinical nurse specialists, psychologists, or psychiatrists.

Special considerations
- Encourage the patient to eat. Suggest dry foods and decreased liquid intake during meals. Company and diversionary conversation at mealtime may be beneficial.
- Instruct the patient to remain upright for 45 minutes after eating to decrease reflux.
- Provide reassurance and a calm, restful atmosphere. Encourage the patient to discuss her feelings regarding her pregnancy.
- Before discharge, provide good nutritional counseling.

Pregnancy-Induced Hypertension

(Toxemia of pregnancy)

Pregnancy-induced hypertension, a potentially life-threatening disorder, usually develops late in the second trimester or in the third trimester. Preeclampsia, *the nonconvulsive form of toxemia, develops in about 7% of pregnancies. It is mild or severe, and the incidence is significantly higher in low socioeconomic groups.* Eclampsia *is the convulsive form of toxemia. About 5% of females with preeclampsia develop eclampsia; of these, about 15% die from toxemia itself or its complications. Fetal mortality is high due to the increased incidence of premature delivery.*

Causes

The cause of pregnancy-induced hypertension is unknown, but it appears to be related to inadequate prenatal care (especially poor nutrition), parity (more prevalent in primigravidas), multiple pregnancies, preexisting diabetes mellitus or hypertension, hydramnios, or hydatidiform mole. Other theories postulate a long list of potential toxic sources, such as autolysis of placental infarcts, autointoxication, uremia, maternal sensitization to total proteins, and pyelonephritis.

Signs and symptoms

Mild preeclampsia generally produces the following clinical effects: hypertension, proteinuria, generalized edema (especially of the hands, face, and feet), and sudden weight gain of more than 3 lb (1.36 kg) a week during the second trimester or more than 1 lb (0.45 kg) a week during the third trimester.

Severe preeclampsia is marked by increased hypertension and proteinuria, eventually leading to the development of oliguria. Other symptoms that may indicate worsening preeclampsia include blurred vision due to retinal arteriolar spasms, epigastric pain or heartburn, irritability, emotional tension, and severe frontal headache.

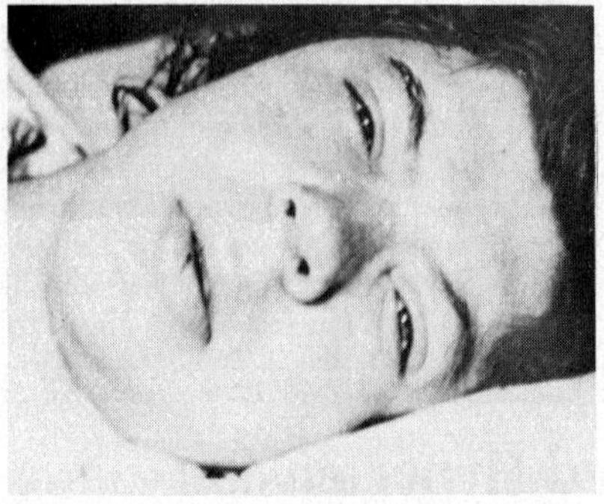

This woman's face shows some of the classic symptoms of preeclampsia—edema of the face and eyelids, and coarsening of the features.

In eclampsia, all the clinical manifestations of preeclampsia are magnified and are associated with convulsions and, possibly, coma. Complications of persistent convulsions include cerebral hemorrhage, blindness, abruptio placentae, premature labor, stillbirth, renal failure, and hepatic damage.

Diagnosis

The following findings suggest mild preeclampsia:

- *elevated blood pressure readings:* 140 systolic, or a rise of 30 mm Hg or greater above the patient's normal systolic pressure, measured on two occasions, 6 hours apart; 90 diastolic, or a rise of 15 mm Hg or greater above the patient's normal diastolic pressure, measured on two occasions, 6 hours apart
- *proteinuria:* more than 500 mg/24 hours.

These findings suggest severe preeclampsia:

- *higher blood pressure readings:* 160/110 mm Hg or higher on two occasions, 6 hours apart, at bed rest
- *increased proteinuria:* 5 g/24 hours or more
- *oliguria:* urine output less than or equal to 400 ml/24 hours
- *deep tendon reflexes:* possibly hyperactive as CNS irritability increases.

Typical clinical features—especially convulsions—with typical findings for severe preeclampsia strongly suggest eclampsia. In addition, ophthalmoscopic examination may reveal vascular spasm, papilledema, retinal edema or detachment, and arteriovenous nicking or hemorrhage.

Real time ultrasonography and stress and nonstress tests evaluate fetal well-being. In the stress test, oxytocin stimulates contractions; fetal heart tones are then monitored electronically. In the nonstress test, fetal heart tones are monitored electronically during periods of fetal activity, without oxytocin stimulation. Electronic monitoring reveals stable or increased fetal heart tones during periods of fetal activity.

Treatment

Therapy for preeclampsia is designed to halt the disorder's progress—specifically, the early effects of eclampsia, such as convulsions, residual hypertension, and renal shutdown—and to ensure fetal survival. Some doctors advocate the prompt induction of labor, especially if the patient is near term; others follow a more conservative approach. Therapy may include sedatives, such as phenobarbital, along with complete bed rest, to relieve anxiety, reduce hypertension, and evaluate response to therapy. If renal function remains adequate, a high-protein, low-sodium, low-carbohydrate diet with increased fluid intake is recommended.

If the patient's blood pressure fails to respond to bed rest and sedation and persistently rises above 160/100 mm Hg, or if CNS irritability increases, magnesium sulfate may produce general sedation, promote diuresis, reduce blood pressure, and prevent convulsions. If these measures fail to improve the patient's condition, or if fetal life is endangered (as determined by stress or nonstress tests), cesarean section or oxytocin induction may be required to terminate the pregnancy.

Emergency treatment of eclamptic convulsions consists of immediate administration of diazepam I.V., followed by magnesium sulfate (I.V. drip), oxygen administration, and electronic fetal monitoring. After the patient's condition stabilizes, a cesarean section may be performed.

Adequate nutrition, good prenatal care, and control of preexisting hypertension during pregnancy decrease the incidence and severity of preeclampsia. Early recognition and prompt treatment of preeclampsia can prevent progression to eclampsia.

Special considerations

- Monitor regularly for changes in blood pressure, pulse rate, respiration, fetal heart tones, vision, level of consciousness, and deep tendon reflexes and for headache unrelieved by medication. Report changes immediately. Assess these signs before administering medications. Absence of patellar reflexes may indicate magnesium sulfate toxicity.
- Assess fluid balance by measuring intake and output and by checking daily weight.
- Observe for signs of fetal distress by closely monitoring the results of stress and nonstress tests.
- Instruct the patient to lie in a left lateral position to increase venous return, cardiac output, and renal blood flow.
- Keep emergency resuscitative equipment and drugs (including diazepam and magnesium sulfate) available in case of convulsions and cardiac or respiratory arrest. Also keep calcium gluconate at the bedside, since it counteracts the toxic effects of magnesium sulfate.
- To protect the patient from injury, maintain seizure precautions. Don't leave an unstable patient unattended.
- Assist with emergency medical treatment for the convulsive patient. Provide a quiet, darkened room until the patient's condition stabilizes, and enforce absolute bed rest. Carefully monitor administration of magnesium sulfate; give oxygen, as ordered. Don't administer anything by mouth. Insert an indwelling (Foley) catheter for accurate measurement of intake and output.
- Provide emotional support for the patient and family. If the patient's condition necessitates premature delivery, point out that infants of mothers with toxemia are usually small for gestational age but sometimes fare better than other premature babies of the same weight, possibly because they have developed adaptive responses to stress in utero.

Hydatidiform Mole

Hydatidiform mole is an uncommon chorionic tumor of the placenta. Its early signs—amenorrhea and uterine enlargement—mimic normal pregnancy; however, it eventually causes vaginal bleeding. Hydatidiform mole occurs in 1 in 1,500 to 2,000 pregnancies, most commonly in women over age 45. Incidence is highest in Oriental women.

With prompt diagnosis and appropriate treatment, prognosis is excellent; however, approximately 10% of patients with hydatidiform moles develop chorionic malignancy. Recurrence is possible in about 2% of cases.

Causes

The cause of hydatidiform mole is unknown, but death of the embryo and loss of fetal circulation seem to precede formation of the mole. Despite embryo death, maternal circulation continues to nourish the trophoblast, but loss of fetal circulation causes abnormal accumulation of fluid within the villi. This converts some or all of the chorionic villi into a mass of clear vesicles, resembling a bunch of grapes.

Signs and symptoms

The early stages of a pregnancy in which a hydatidiform mole develops typically seem normal, except that the uterus grows more rapidly than usual. The first obvious signs of trouble—absence of fetal heart tones, vaginal bleeding (ranging from spotting to hemorrhage), and lower abdominal cramps—mimic those of spontaneous abortion. The blood may contain hydatid vesicles; hyperemesis is likely, and signs and symptoms of preeclampsia are possible. Other possible complications of hydatidiform mole include anemia, infection, spontaneous abortion, uterine rupture, and choriocarcinoma.

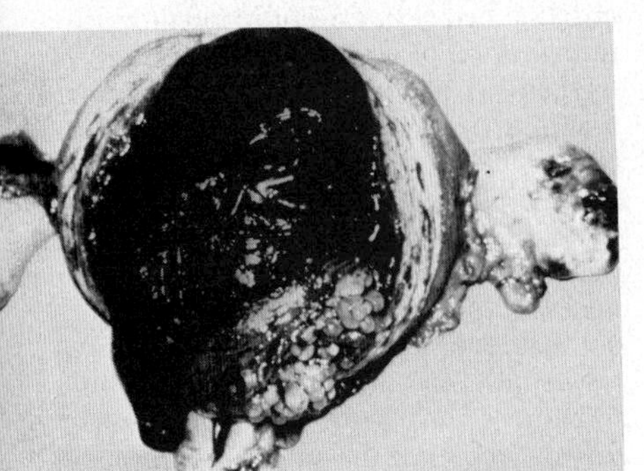

Uterine contents show grape-clustered chorionic villi and hyperplastic placental tissue characteristic of hydatidiform mole.

Diagnosis

Persistent bleeding and an abnormally enlarged uterus suggest hydatidiform mole. Diagnosis is based on the passage of hydatid vesicles that allow histologic confirmation. Without identification of hydatid vesicles, it's difficult to differentiate hydatidiform mole from other complications of pregnancy, particularly threatened abortion. Confirmation of hydatidiform mole requires dilation and curettage (D & C).

The following also support a diagnosis of hydatidiform mole:

- *Ultrasound* assesses uterine contents; use of a Doppler ultrasonic flowmeter demonstrates the absence of fetal heart tones.
- *Pregnancy test* shows elevated human chorionic gonadotropin (HCG) serum levels 100 or more days after the last menstrual period.
- Evidence of preeclampsia develops earlier in pregnancy than usual.
- *Hemoglobin* is decreased as a result of blood loss.
- *Chest X-ray* is negative for evidence of choriocarcinoma metastasis.
- *Arteriography* shows typical early venous shadows.

Treatment

Hydatidiform mole necessitates uterine evacuation via D & C, or, if this is ineffective, abdominal hysterectomy or suction curettage. Before evacuation, oxytocin I.V. promotes uterine contractions.

Postoperative treatment varies, depending on the amount of blood lost and complications. If no complications develop, hospitalization is usually brief, and normal activities can be resumed quickly, as tolerated.

Because of the possibility of choriocarcinoma development following hydatidiform mole, scrupulous follow-up care is essential. Such care includes monitoring HCG levels until they return to normal and taking chest X-rays to check for lung metastasis. Most doctors advise postponing another pregnancy until at least 1 year after HCG levels return to normal.

Special considerations

- Preoperatively, observe for signs of complications, such as hemorrhage and uterine infection, and vaginal passage of hydatid vesicles. Save any expelled tissue for laboratory analysis.
- Postoperatively, monitor vital signs, especially blood pressure, and check blood loss.
- Provide patient and family teaching, and give emotional support. Encourage the patient to express her feelings, and help her through the grieving for her lost infant.
- Instruct the patient to promptly report any new symptoms (for example, hemoptysis, cough, suspected pregnancy, nausea, vomiting, and vaginal bleeding).
- Stress the need for regular follow-up by HCG and chest X-ray monitoring, for early detection of possible malignant changes.
- Explain to the patient that she must use contraceptives to prevent pregnancy for at least 1 year after HCG levels return to normal and regular ovulation and menstrual cycles are reestablished.

TYPES OF HYSTERECTOMY

There are three types of hysterectomy: subtotal hysterectomy, total hysterectomy, and total hysterectomy with a salpingo-oophorectomy. The excised portion (which is shaded) varies in each one. In each of these procedures, however, the external genitalia and the vagina are left intact, and the woman is able to resume sexual relations.

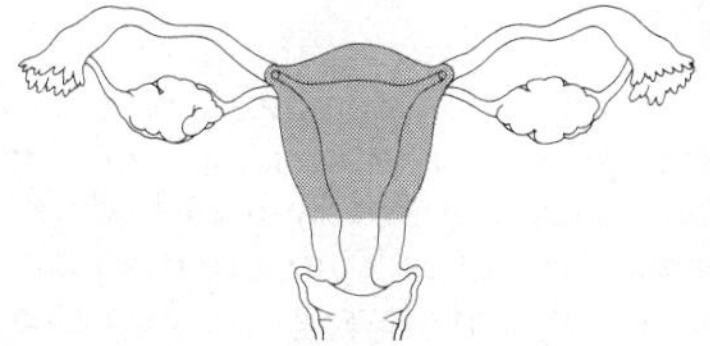

In a *subtotal hysterectomy,* all but the distal portion of the uterus is removed.

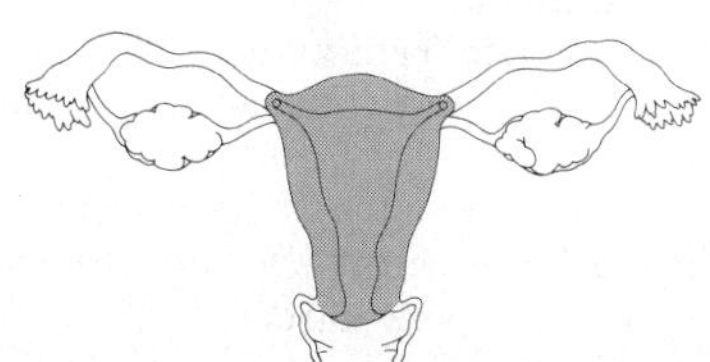

In a *total hysterectomy,* the entire uterus and the cervix are removed. This woman will no longer menstruate.

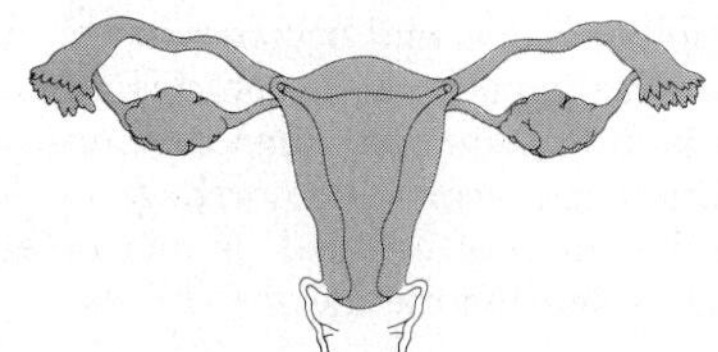

In a *total hysterectomy with a salpingo-oophorectomy,* the uterus, the cervix, the fallopian tubes, and the ovaries are removed. This woman will no longer menstruate.

Placenta Previa

In placenta previa, the placenta is implanted in the lower uterine segment, where it encroaches on the internal cervical os. This disorder, one of the most common causes of bleeding during the second half of pregnancy, occurs in approximately 1 in 200 pregnancies, more commonly in multigravidas than in primigravidas. Generally, termination of pregnancy is necessary when placenta previa is diagnosed in the presence of heavy maternal bleeding. Maternal prognosis is good if hemorrhage can be controlled; fetal prognosis depends on gestational age and amount of blood lost.

Causes

In placenta previa, the placenta may cover all (total, complete, or central), part (partial or incomplete), or a fraction (marginal or low-lying) of the internal cervical os. The degree of placenta previa depends largely on the extent of cervical dilation at the time of examination, because the dilating cervix gradually uncovers the placenta. Although the specific cause of placenta previa is unknown, factors that may affect the site of the placenta's attachment to the uterine wall include:

- early or late fertilization.
- receptivity and adequacy of the uterine lining.
- multiple pregnancy (the placenta requires a larger surface for attachment).
- previous uterine surgery.
- multiparity.
- advanced maternal age.

In placenta previa, the lower segment of the uterus fails to provide as much nourishment as the fundus. The placenta tends to spread out, seeking the blood supply it needs, and becomes larger and thinner than normal. Eccentric insertion of the umbilical cord often develops, for unknown reasons. Hemorrhage occurs as the internal cervical os effaces and dilates, tearing the uterine vessels.

Signs and symptoms

Placenta previa usually produces painless third trimester bleeding (often the first complaint). Various malpresentations occur because of the placenta's location, and interfere with proper descent of the fetal head. (The fetus remains active, however, with good heart tones.) Complications of placenta previa include shock, or maternal and fetal death.

Diagnosis

Special diagnostic measures that confirm placenta previa include:

- *ultrasound scanning* for placental position.
- *pelvic examination* (under a double setup because of the likelihood of hemorrhage), performed only immediately before delivery, to confirm diagnosis. In most cases, only the cervix is visualized.

Supportive findings include:

- minimal descent of the fetal presenting part.
- decreased hemoglobin (due to blood loss).
- radiologic testing (soft-tissue X-rays, femoral arteriography, retrograde catheterization, or radioisotope scanning or localization) to locate the placenta. However, these tests have limited value, are very risky, and are usually performed only when ultrasound is unavailable.

Treatment

Treatment of placenta previa is designed to assess, control, and restore blood loss; to deliver a viable infant; and to prevent coagulation disorders. Immediate therapy includes starting an I.V. using a large-bore catheter; drawing blood for hemoglobin and hematocrit, as well as type and cross match; initiating external electronic fetal monitoring; monitoring maternal blood pressure, pulse rate, and respirations; and assessing the amount of vaginal bleeding.

If the fetus is premature, following determination of the degree of placenta previa and necessary fluid and blood replacement, treatment consists of careful observation to allow the fetus more time to mature. If clinical evaluation confirms complete placenta previa, the patient is usually hospitalized due to the increased risk of hemorrhage. As soon as the fetus is sufficiently mature, or in case of intervening severe hemorrhage, immediate delivery by cesarean section may be necessary. Vaginal delivery is considered only when the bleeding is minimal and the placenta previa is marginal, or when the labor is rapid. Because of the possibility of fetal blood loss through the placenta, a pediatric team should be on hand during such delivery to immediately assess and treat neonatal shock, blood loss, and hypoxia.

Complications of placenta previa necessitate appropriate and immediate intervention.

Special considerations

- If the patient shows active bleeding because of placenta previa, a primary nurse should be assigned for continuous monitoring of maternal blood pressure, pulse rate, respirations, central venous pressure, intake and output, amount of vaginal bleeding, and fetal heart tones. Electronic monitoring of fetal heart tones is recommended.
- Prepare the patient and her family for a possible cesarean section and the birth of a premature infant. Thoroughly explain postpartum care, so the patient and her family know what measures to expect.
- Provide emotional support during labor. Because of the infant's prematurity, the patient may not be given analgesics, so labor pain may be intense. Reassure her of her progress throughout labor, and keep her informed of the fetus' condition. Although neonatal death is a possibility, continued monitoring and prompt management reduce this prospect.

THREE TYPES OF PLACENTA PREVIA

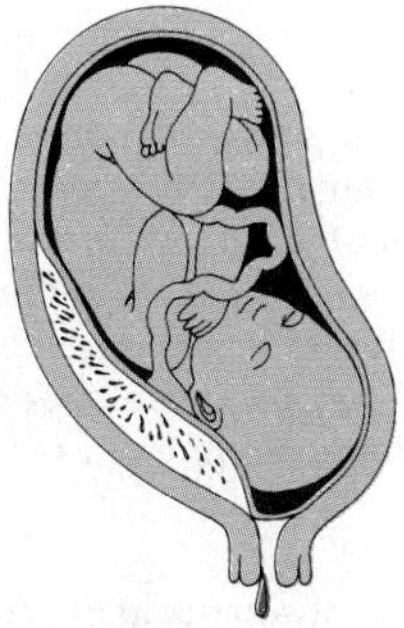

Low marginal implantation—A small placental edge can be felt through the internal os.

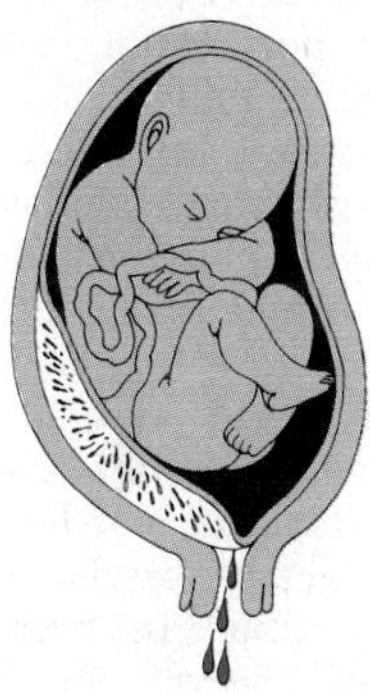

Partial placenta previa—Placenta partially caps the internal os.

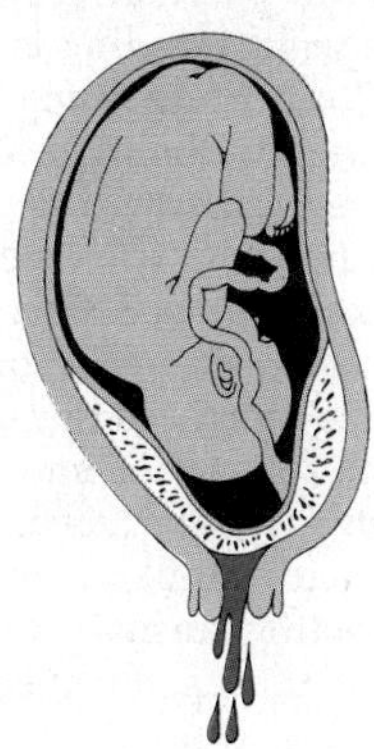

Total placenta previa—The internal os is covered entirely.

Abruptio Placentae

(Placental abruption)

In abruptio placentae, the placenta separates from the uterine wall prematurely, usually after the 20th week of gestation, producing hemorrhage. Abruptio placentae occurs most often in multigravidas—usually in women over age 35—and is a common cause of bleeding during the second half of pregnancy. Firm diagnosis, in the presence of heavy maternal bleeding, generally necessitates termination of pregnancy. Fetal prognosis depends on gestational age and amount of blood lost; maternal prognosis is good if hemorrhage can be controlled.

Causes

The cause of abruptio placentae is unknown. Predisposing factors include trauma—such as a direct blow to the uterus—placental site bleeding from a needle puncture during amniocentesis, chronic hypertension (which raises pressure on the maternal side of the placenta), acute toxemia, and pressure on the vena cava from an enlarged uterus.

In abruptio placentae, blood vessels at the placental bed rupture spontaneously, due to a lack of resiliency or changes in uterine vasculature. Hypertension complicates the situation, as does an enlarged uterus, which can't contract to seal off the torn vessels. Consequently, bleeding continues unchecked, possibly shearing off the placenta partially or completely. Bleeding is external or marginal (in 80% of patients) if a peripheral portion of the placenta separates from the uterine wall. Bleeding is internal or concealed (in the remaining 20%) if the central portion of the placenta becomes detached, in which case the still-intact peripheral portions trap the blood. As blood enters the muscle fibers, complete relaxation of the uterus becomes impossible, causing increased uterine tone and irritability. If bleeding into the muscle fibers is profuse, the uterus turns blue or purple, and the bleeding prevents it from contracting normally after delivery (Couvelaire uterus, or uteroplacental apoplexy).

Signs and symptoms

Abruptio placentae produces a wide range of clinical effects, depending on the extent of placental separation and the amount of blood lost from maternal circulation. Mild abruptio placentae (marginal separation) develops gradually and produces mild to moderate bleeding, vague lower abdominal discomfort, mild to moderate abdominal tenderness, and uterine irritability. Fetal heart tones remain strong and regular.

Moderate abruptio placentae (about 50% placental separation) may develop gradually or abruptly, and produces continuous abdominal pain, moderate dark red vaginal bleeding, a very tender uterus that remains firm between contractions, barely audible or irregular and bradycardic fetal heart tones, and possibly, signs of shock. Labor usually starts within 2 hours and often proceeds rapidly.

Severe abruptio placentae (nearly 70% placental separation) usually develops abruptly, and causes agonizing, unremitting uterine pain (often described as tearing or knifelike); a boardlike, tender uterus; moderate vaginal bleeding; rapidly progressive shock; and absence of fetal heart tones.

In addition to hemorrhage and shock, complications of abruptio placentae may include renal failure, disseminated intravascular coagulation (DIC), and maternal and fetal death.

Diagnosis

Diagnostic measures for abruptio placentae include observation of clinical features, pelvic examination (under double setup), and ultrasonography to rule out placenta previa. Decreased hemoglobin and platelet counts support the diagnosis. Periodic assays for fibrin split products aid in monitoring the progression of abruptio placentae and detect the development of DIC.

Treatment

Treatment of abruptio placentae is designed to assess, control, and restore the amount of blood lost; to deliver a viable infant; and to prevent coagulation disorders. Immediate measures for the patient with abruptio placentae include starting I.V. infusion (via large-bore catheter) of appropriate fluids (lactated Ringer's solution) to combat hypovolemia; drawing blood for hemoglobin and hematocrit determination and for type and cross match; initiating external electronic fetal monitoring; monitoring maternal blood pressure, pulse rate, and respirations; and assessing the amount of vaginal bleeding.

After determination of the severity of abruption and appropriate fluid and blood replacement, prompt delivery of the fetus by cesarean section is necessary if the fetus is alive but in distress. If the fetus is not in distress, monitoring continues; delivery is usually performed at the earliest sign of fetal distress. Because of the possibility of fetal blood loss through the placenta, a pediatric team should be on hand at delivery to immediately assess and treat the newborn for shock, blood loss, and hypoxia. If placental separation is severe and there are no signs of fetal life, vaginal delivery may be performed unless uncontrolled hemorrhage or other complications contraindicate it.

Complications of abruptio placentae require appropriate treatment. For example, DIC requires immediate intervention with heparin, platelets, and whole blood to prevent exsanguination.

Special considerations

- Check maternal blood pressure, pulse rate, respirations, central venous pressure, intake and output, and amount of vaginal bleeding every 10 to 15 minutes. Monitor fetal heart tones electronically.

DEGREES OF PLACENTAL SEPARATION IN ABRUPTIO PLACENTAE

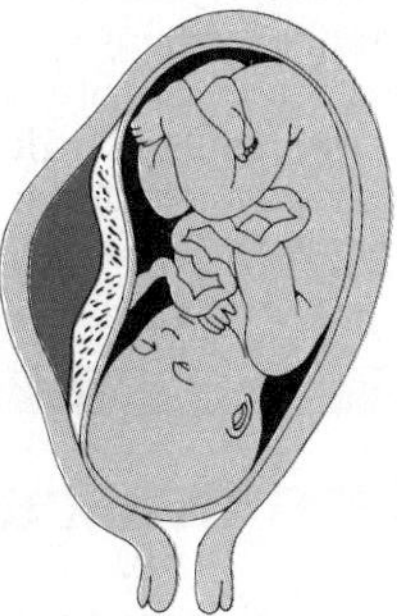

Mild separation with internal bleeding between placenta and uterine wall

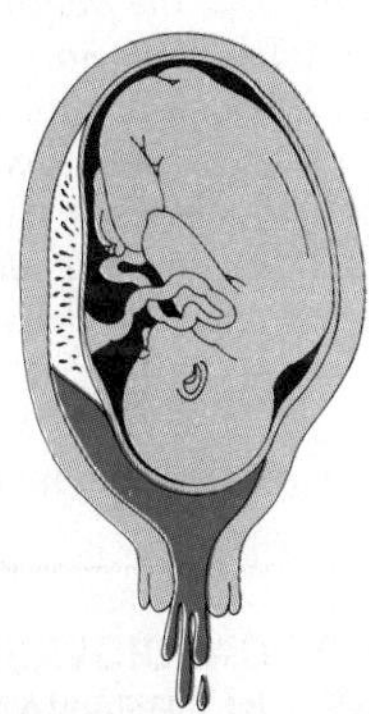

Moderate separation with external hemorrhage through the vagina

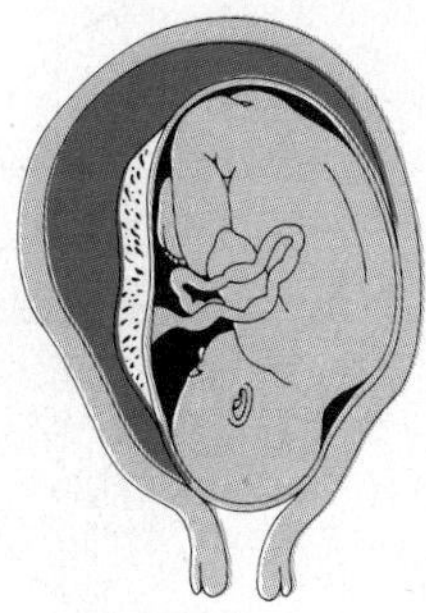

Severe separation with external hemorrhage

• Prepare the patient and family for cesarean section. Thoroughly explain postpartum care, so the patient and family know what to expect.
• If vaginal delivery is elected, provide emotional support during labor. Because of the infant's prematurity, the mother may not receive analgesics during labor and may experience intense pain. Reassure the patient of her progress through labor, and keep her informed of the fetus' condition.
• Tactfully suggest the possibility of neonatal death. Tell the mother the infant's survival depends primarily on gestational age, blood loss, and associated hypertensive disorders. Assure her that frequent monitoring and prompt management greatly reduce risk of fatality.

Cardiovascular Disease in Pregnancy

Cardiovascular disease ranks fourth (after infection, toxemia, and hemorrhage) among the leading causes of maternal death. The physiologic stress of pregnancy and delivery is often more than a compromised heart can tolerate and often leads to maternal and fetal mortality. Approximately 1% to 2% of pregnant females have cardiac disease, but the incidence is rising because medical treatment today allows more females with rheumatic heart disease and congenital defects to reach childbearing age. Prognosis for the pregnant patient with cardiovascular disease is good, with careful management. Decompensation is the leading cause of maternal death. Infant mortality increases with decompensation, since uterine congestion, insufficient oxygenation, and the elevated carbon dioxide content of the blood not only compromise the fetus, but also frequently cause premature labor and delivery.

Causes

Rheumatic heart disease is present in more than 80% of patients who develop cardiovascular complications. In the rest, these complications stem from congenital defects (10% to 15%) and coronary artery disease (2%).

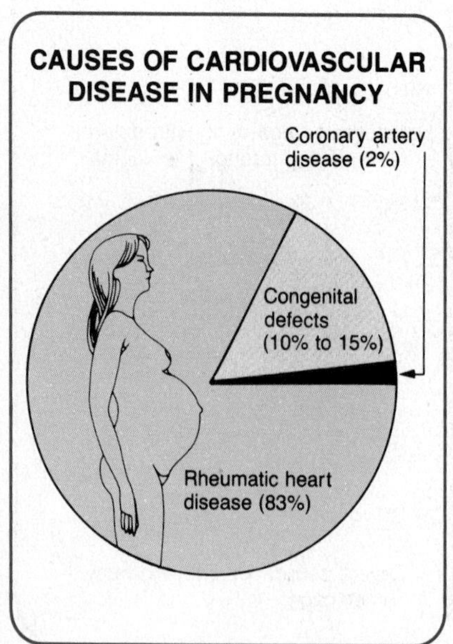

The diseased heart is sometimes unable to meet the normal demands of pregnancy: 25% increase in cardiac output, 40% to 50% increase in plasma volume, increased oxygen requirements, retention of salt and water, weight gain, and alterations in hemodynamics during delivery. This physiologic stress often leads to the heart's failure to maintain adequate circulation (decompensation). The degree of decompensation depends on the patient's age, the duration of cardiac disease, and the functional capacity of the heart at the outset of pregnancy.

Signs and symptoms

Typical clinical features of cardiovascular disease during pregnancy include distended neck veins, diastolic murmurs, moist basilar pulmonary rales, cardiac enlargement (discernible on percussion or as a cardiac shadow on chest X-ray), and cardiac dysrhythmias (other than sinus or paroxysmal atrial tachycardia). Other characteristic abnormalities may include cyanosis, pericardial friction rub, pulse delay, and pulsus alternans.

Decompensation may develop suddenly or gradually, with persistent rales at the lung bases. As it progresses, edema, increasing dyspnea on exertion, palpitations, a smothering sensation, and hemoptysis may occur.

Diagnosis

A diastolic murmur, cardiac enlargement, a systolic murmur of grade 3/6 intensity, and severe arrhythmia suggest cardiovascular disease. Determination of the extent and cause of the disease may necessitate electrocardiography, echocardiography (for valvular disorders, such as rheumatic heart disease), or phonocardiography. X-rays show cardiac enlargement and pulmonary congestion. Cardiac catheterization should be postponed until after delivery, unless surgery is necessary.

Treatment

The goal of antepartum management is to prevent complications and minimize the strain on the mother's heart, primarily through rest. This may require periodic hospitalization for patients with moderate cardiac dysfunction or with symptoms of decompensation, toxemia, or infection. Older women or those with previous decompensation may require hospitalization and bed rest throughout the pregnancy.

Drug therapy is often necessary and should always include the safest possible drug in the lowest possible dosage to minimize harmful effects to the fetus. Diuretics and drugs that increase blood pressure, blood volume, or cardiac output should be used with extreme caution. If an anticoagulant is needed, heparin is the drug of choice. Digitalis and common antiarrhythmics, such as quinidine and procainamide, are often required. The prophylactic use of antibiotics is reserved for patients who are susceptible to endocarditis.

A therapeutic abortion may be considered for patients with severe cardiac dysfunction, especially if decompensation occurs during the first trimester. Patients hospitalized with heart failure usually follow a regimen of digitalis, oxygen, rest, sedation, diuretics, and restricted intake of sodium and fluids. Patients in whom symptoms of heart failure do not improve after treatment with bed rest and digitalis may require cardiac surgery, such as valvotomy and commissurotomy. During labor, the patient may require oxygen and an analgesic, such as meperidine or morphine, for relief of pain and apprehension without undue depression of the fetus or herself. Depending on which procedure promises to be less stressful for the patient's heart, delivery may be vaginal or by cesarean section.

Bed rest and medications already instituted should continue for at least 1 week after delivery because of a high incidence of decompensation, cardiovascular collapse, and maternal death during the early puerperal period. These complications may result from the sudden release of intra-abdominal pressure at delivery and the mobilization of extracellular fluid for excretion, which increase the strain on the heart, especially if excessive interstitial fluid has accumulated. Breast-feeding is undesirable for patients with severely compromised cardiac dysfunction, because it increases fluid and metabolic demands on the heart.

Special considerations

- During pregnancy, stress the importance of rest and weight control to decrease the strain on the heart. Suggest a diet of limited fluid and sodium intake to prevent vascular congestion. Encourage the patient to take supplementary folic acid and iron to prevent anemia.
- During labor, watch for signs of decompensation, such as dyspnea and palpitations. Monitor pulse rate, respirations,

and blood pressure. Auscultate for rales every 30 minutes during the first phase of labor and every 10 minutes during the active and transition phases. Check carefully for edema and cyanosis, and assess intake and output. Administer oxygen for respiratory difficulty.

- Use electronic fetal monitoring to watch for the earliest signs of fetal distress.
- Keep the patient in a semirecumbent position. Limit her efforts to bear down during labor, which significantly raise blood pressure and stress the heart.
- After delivery, provide reassurance, and encourage the patient to adhere to her program of treatment. Emphasize the need to rest during her hospital stay.

Adolescent Pregnancy

In the United States, an estimated 1 million adolescents become pregnant each year. Since up to 70% of them don't receive adequate prenatal care, they are apt to develop special problems, and are known to have a significantly higher incidence of anemia, pregnancy-induced hypertension, and perinatal mortality. For example, pregnant adolescents are more likely to have babies who are premature or of low birth weight, with a higher neonatal mortality, and who are predisposed to injury at birth, childhood illness, and retardation or other neurologic defects. As a rule, the younger the mother, the greater the health risk for both mother and infant. Adolescents account for one third of all abortions performed in the United States.

Causes

Adolescent pregnancy is prevalent in all socioeconomic levels, and its contributing factors vary. Such factors may include ignorance about sexuality and contraception, increasing sexual activity at a young age, rebellion against parental influence, and a desire to escape an unhappy family situation and to fulfill emotional needs unmet by the family.

Signs and symptoms

Clinical manifestations of adolescent pregnancy are the same as those of adult

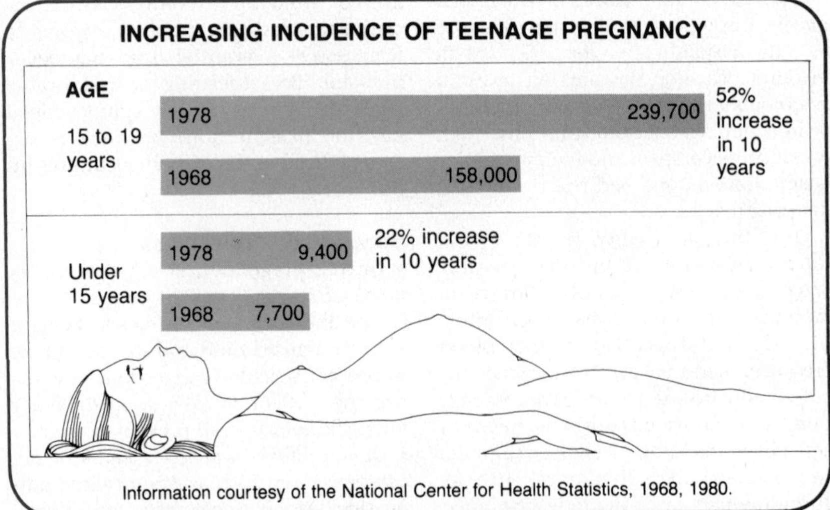

Information courtesy of the National Center for Health Statistics, 1968, 1980.

HOW MATERNAL DRUG USE AFFECTS INFANTS

An infant born to a drug-dependent mother risks developing certain medical problems during the first 8 months of life. These problems range from mild to severe withdrawal symptoms to a host of complications that affect virtually every body system. The onset and severity of adverse reactions varies with the type and amount of drugs the mother has been taking and for how long. However, *any* drug the mother takes, including over-the-counter products, alcohol, and illicit drugs, may cross the placenta and enter the fetal circulation, where its concentration is 50% to 100% higher than the maternal drug concentration. This chart lists some common adverse drug reactions and the body systems they affect.

BODY SYSTEM	ADVERSE DRUG REACTIONS
Gastrointestinal	Diarrhea, vomiting, colic, feeding problems, susceptibility to inguinal hernia
Respiratory	Bronchiolitis, croup, pneumonia, asthma
Neurologic	Nystagmus, squinting, abnormal head size, susceptibility to viral meningitis
Dermatologic	Moniliasis, susceptibility to bacterial skin infection, allergic dermatitis, seborrhea, ecchymoses, petechiae
Other	Failure to thrive, sudden infant death syndrome, otitis media

pregnancy (amenorrhea, nausea, vomiting, breast tenderness, fatigue). However, the pregnant adolescent is much more likely to develop complications such as poor weight gain during pregnancy, premature labor, pregnancy-induced hypertension, abruptio placentae, and preeclampsia. In addition, the infant is more likely to be of low birth weight. Some of these complications are related to the pregnant adolescent's physical immaturity, rapid growth, interest in fad diets, and generally poor nutrition; other complications may stem from the adolescent's need to deny her condition or to her ignorance of early signs of pregnancy, which often delays initiation of prenatal care.

Diagnosis

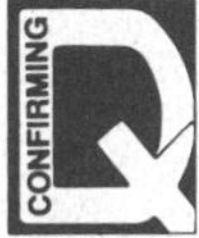

A pregnancy test showing human chorionic gonadotropin in the blood or urine and a pelvic examination confirm pregnancy. Auscultation of fetal heart sounds with a Doppler ultrasonic flowmeter or fetoscope and ultrasonography assess fetal gestational age.

Treatment and special considerations

The pregnant adolescent requires the standard prenatal care that is appropriate for an adult. However, she needs psychological support and close observation for signs of complications.

- Since you may be the first health care professional the pregnant adolescent encounters, you *must* help motivate her to follow sound medical advice without being judgmental, condescending, or threatening. Emphasize the importance of adhering to the prescribed diet, getting plenty of rest, and taking prescribed vitamin and iron supplements. Your understanding and support can ensure proper health care during the pregnancy for both mother and infant. Encourage her to ask questions and to express her feelings about the pregnancy. Answer her questions fully.
- Try to help the pregnant adolescent identify her own strengths and support systems for coping with pregnancy,

birth, and parenting.

- Prepare the patient and her partner for the physical and psychological process of labor and birth. Encourage attendance at prenatal classes: the use of educational films, hospital tours, and role-playing techniques will facilitate her cooperation with care providers.
- Following birth, encourage the patient to set realistic goals for the future. If she opts for adoption, make sure she clearly understands her legal rights and responsibilities. Allow the patient to care for the infant, as she desires.
- If the patient decides to raise the infant, help her make the transition from pregnancy to parenthood during the postpartum period. Facilitate bonding. Help her establish a realistic plan regarding childcare, parenting, returning to school or work, and her relationship with the infant's father.
- In the event of stillbirth or the newborn infant's death, help the patient through the grieving process.
- Before the patient is discharged, provide information on contraception.

Diabetic Complications During Pregnancy

Pregnancy places special demands on carbohydrate metabolism and causes the insulin requirement to increase, even in a healthy female. Consequently, pregnancy may lead to a prediabetic state, to the conversion of an asymptomatic subclinical diabetic state to a clinical one (gestational diabetes occurs in about 1% to 2% of all pregnancies), or to complications in a previously stable diabetic state.

Prevalence of diabetes mellitus increases with age. Maternal and fetal prognoses can be equivalent to those in nondiabetic females if maternal blood glucose is well controlled and ketosis and other complications are prevented. Infant morbidity and mortality depend on recognizing and successfully controlling hypoglycemia, which may develop within hours after delivery.

Causes

In diabetes mellitus, glucose is inadequately utilized either because insulin is not synthesized (as in a Type I, insulin-dependent diabetic) or because tissues are resistant to the hormonal action of endogenous insulin (as in a Type II, non-insulin-dependent diabetic). During pregnancy, the fetus relies on maternal glucose as a primary fuel source. Pregnancy triggers protective mechanisms that have anti-insulin effects: increased hormone production (placental lactogen, estrogen, and progesterone), which antagonizes the effects of insulin; degradation of insulin by the placenta; and prolonged elevation of stress hormones (cortisol, epinephrine, and glucagon), which raise blood glucose levels.

In a normal pregnancy, an increase in anti-insulin factors is counterbalanced by an increase in insulin production to maintain normal blood glucose levels. However, females who are prediabetic or diabetic are unable to produce sufficient insulin to overcome the insulin antagonist mechanisms of pregnancy, or their tissues are insulin-resistant. As insulin requirements rise toward term, the patient who is prediabetic may develop gestational diabetes, necessitating dietary management and, possibly, exogenous insulin to achieve glycemic control, whereas the patient who is insulin-dependent may need increased insulin dosage.

Signs and symptoms

Indications for diagnostic screening for maternal diabetes mellitus during pregnancy include obesity, excessive weight gain, excessive hunger or thirst, polyuria, recurrent monilial infections, glycosuria, previous delivery of a large infant, polyhydramnios, maternal hypertension, and a family history of diabetes.

Uncontrolled diabetes in a pregnant female can cause stillbirth, fetal anomalies, premature delivery, and birth of an infant who is large or small for gestational age. Such infants are predisposed to severe episodes of hypoglycemia shortly after birth. These infants may also develop hypocalcemia, hyperbilirubinemia, and respiratory distress syndrome.

Diagnosis

The prevalence of gestational diabetes makes careful screening for hyperglycemia appropriate in all pregnancies in each trimester. Abnormal fasting or postprandial blood glucose levels, and clinical signs and history suggest diabetes in patients not previously diabetic.

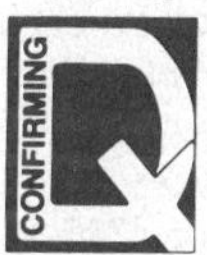

A 3-hour glucose tolerance test confirms diabetes mellitus when two or more values are above normal.

Procedures to assess fetal status include stress and nonstress tests, ultrasonography to determine fetal age and growth, measurement of urinary or serum estriols, and determination of the lecithin-sphingomyelin ratio from amniotic fluid to predict pulmonary maturity.

Treatment

Treatment of both the newly diagnosed and the established diabetic is designed to maintain blood glucose levels within acceptable limits through dietary management and insulin administration. Most females with overt diabetes mellitus require hospitalization at the beginning of pregnancy to assess physical status, to check for associated cardiac and renal disease, and to regulate diabetes.

For pregnant patients with diabetes, therapy includes:

- bimonthly visits to the obstetrician and the internist during the first 6 months of pregnancy. Weekly visits may be necessary during the third trimester.
- maintenance of blood glucose levels (60 to 120 mg/dl).
- frequent monitoring for glycosuria and ketonuria (ketosis presents a grave threat to the fetal central nervous system).
- weight control (gain not to exceed 3 to 3½ lb [1.36 to 1.59 kg] per month during the last 6 months of pregnancy).
- high-protein diet of 2 g/day/kg of body weight, or a minimum of 80 g/day during the second half of pregnancy; daily calorie intake of 30 to 40 calories/kg of body weight; daily carbohydrate intake of 200 g; and enough fat to provide 36% of total calories. However, vigorous calorie restriction can cause starvation ketosis.
- exogenous insulin if diet doesn't control blood glucose levels. Be alert for changes in insulin requirements from one trimester to the next and immediately postpartum. Oral hypoglycemic agents are contraindicated during pregnancy, because they may cause fetal hypoglycemia and congenital anomalies.

Generally, the optimal time for delivery is between 37 and 39 weeks' gestation. The insulin-dependent diabetic requires hospitalization prior to delivery, because bed rest promotes uteroplacental circulation and myometrial tone. In addition, hospitalization permits frequent monitoring of blood glucose levels and prompt intervention if complications develop.

Depending on fetal status and obstetrical history, the obstetrician may induce labor or perform a cesarean delivery. During labor and delivery, the patient with diabetes should receive continuous I.V. infusion of dextrose in water. Maternal and fetal status must be monitored closely throughout labor. The patient may benefit from half her prepregnancy dosage of insulin before a cesarean delivery. Her insulin requirement will fall markedly after delivery.

Special considerations

- Teach the newly diagnosed patient about diabetes, including dietary management, insulin administration, home monitoring of blood glucose or urine test-

ing for glucose and ketones, and skin and foot care. Instruct her to report ketonuria immediately.
• Evaluate the diabetic patient's knowledge about this disease, and provide supplementary patient teaching, as she requires. Inform the patient that frequent monitoring and adjustment of insulin dosage are necessary throughout the course of her pregnancy.
• Give reassurance that strict compliance to prescribed therapy should ensure a favorable outcome.
• Refer the patient to an appropriate social service agency if financial assistance is necessary because of prolonged hospitalization.
• Encourage medical counseling regarding the prognosis of future pregnancies.

ABNORMALITIES OF PARTURITION

Premature Labor

(Preterm labor)

Premature labor is onset of rhythmic uterine contractions that produce cervical change after fetal viability but before fetal maturity. It usually occurs between the 26th and 37th weeks of gestation. Approximately 5% to 10% of pregnancies end prematurely; about 75% of neonatal deaths and a great many birth defects stem from this disorder. Fetal prognosis depends on birth weight and length of gestation: infants weighing less than 1 lb 10 oz (750 g) and of less than 26 weeks' gestation have a survival rate of about 10%; infants weighing 1 lb 10 oz to 2 lb 3 oz (750 to 1,000 g) and of 27 to 28 weeks' gestation have a survival rate of more than 50%; those weighing 2 lb 3 oz to 2 lb 11 oz (1,000 to 1,250 g) and of more than 28 weeks' gestation have a 70% to 90% survival rate.

Causes

The possible causes of premature labor are many; they may include premature rupture of the membranes (occurs in 30% to 50% of premature labors), preeclampsia, chronic hypertensive vascular disease, hydramnios, multiple pregnancy, placenta previa, abruptio placentae, incompetent cervix, abdominal surgery, trauma, structural anomalies of the uterus, infections (such as rubella or toxoplasmosis), congenital adrenal hyperplasia, and fetal death.

Other important provocative factors:
• *Fetal stimulation:* Genetically imprinted information tells the fetus that nutrition is inadequate and that a change in environment is required for well-being; this provokes onset of labor.
• *Progesterone deficiency:* Decreased placental production of progesterone—thought to be the hormone that maintains pregnancy—triggers labor.
• *Oxytocin sensitivity:* Labor begins because the myometrium becomes hypersensitive to oxytocin, the hormone that normally induces uterine contractions.
• *Myometrial oxygen deficiency:* The fetus becomes increasingly proficient in obtaining oxygen, depriving the myometrium of the oxygen and energy it needs to function normally, thus making the myometrium irritable.
• *Maternal genetics:* A genetic defect in the mother shortens gestation and precipitates premature labor.

Signs and symptoms

Like labor at term, premature labor produces rhythmic uterine contractions, cervical dilation and effacement, possible rupture of the membranes, expulsion of the cervical mucous plug, and a bloody discharge.

Diagnosis

Premature labor is confirmed by the combined results of prenatal history, physical examination, presenting signs and symptoms, and ultrasonography (if available) showing the position of the fetus in relation to the mother's pelvis. Vaginal examination confirms progressive cervical effacement and dilation.

Treatment

Treatment is designed to suppress premature labor when tests show immature fetal pulmonary development, cervical dilation of less than 1½" (4 cm), and the absence of factors that contraindicate continuation of pregnancy. Such treatment consists of bed rest and, when necessary, drug therapy.

The following pharmacologic agents can suppress premature labor:

- *Beta-adrenergic stimulants* (isoxsuprine or ritodrine): Stimulation of the $beta_2$ receptors inhibits contractility of uterine smooth muscle. Side effects include maternal tachycardia and hypotension, and fetal tachycardia.
- *Magnesium sulfate:* Direct action on the myometrium relaxes the muscle. It also produces maternal side effects, such as drowsiness, slurred speech, flushing, decreased reflexes, decreased gastrointestinal motility, and decreased respirations. Fetal and neonatal side effects may include central nervous system (CNS) depression, decreased respirations, and decreased sucking reflex.

Maternal factors that jeopardize the fetus, making premature delivery the lesser risk, include intrauterine infection, abruptio placentae, placental insufficiency, and severe preeclampsia. Among the fetal problems that become more perilous as pregnancy nears term are severe isoimmunization and congenital anomalies.

Ideally, treatment for active premature labor should take place in a regional perinatal intensive care center, where the staff is specially trained to handle this situation. In such settings, the infant can remain close to his parents. (Community hospitals commonly lack the facilities for special neonatal care and transfer the infant alone to a perinatal center.)

Treatment and delivery necessitate intensive team effort, focusing on:

- continuous assessment of the infant's health through fetal monitoring.
- avoidance of sedatives and narcotics that might harm the infant. Morphine or meperidine may be required to minimize pain; these drugs have little effect on uterine contractions but depress CNS function and may cause fetal respiratory depression. These agents should be administered in the smallest dose possible and only when extremely necessary.
- avoidance of amniotomy, if possible, to prevent cord prolapse or damage to the infant's tender skull.
- maintenance of adequate hydration through I.V. fluids.

Prevention of premature labor requires good prenatal care, adequate nutrition, and proper rest. Insertion of a purse-string suture (cerclage) to reinforce an incompetent cervix at 14 to 18 weeks' gestation may prevent premature labor in patients with histories of this disorder.

Special considerations

A patient in premature labor requires close observation for signs of fetal or maternal distress, and comprehensive supportive care.

- During attempts to suppress premature labor, maintain bed rest and administer medications, as ordered. Give sedatives and analgesics sparingly, mindful of their potentially harmful effect on the fetus. Minimize the need for these drugs by providing comfort measures, such as frequent repositioning, and good perineal and back care.
- When administering beta-adrenergic stimulants, sedatives, and narcotics, monitor blood pressure, pulse rate, respirations, fetal heart rate, and uterine contraction pattern. Minimize side effects by keeping the patient in a lateral recumbent position as much as possible. Provide adequate hydration.
- When administering magnesium sulfate, monitor neurologic reflexes. Watch

the newborn for signs of magnesium toxicity, including neuromuscular and respiratory depression.

• Offer emotional support to the patient and family. Encourage the parents to express their fears concerning the infant's survival and health.

• During active premature labor, remember that the premature infant has a lower tolerance for the stress of labor and is much more likely to become hypoxic than the term infant. If necessary, administer oxygen to the patient through a nasal cannula. Encourage the patient to lie on her left side or sit up during labor; this position prevents caval compression, which can cause supine hypotension and subsequent fetal hypoxia. Observe fetal response to labor through continuous fetal monitoring. Prevent maternal hyperventilation; a rebreathing bag may be necessary. Continually reassure the patient throughout labor to help reduce her anxiety.

• Help the patient get through labor with as little analgesic and anesthetic as possible. To minimize fetal CNS depression, avoid administering analgesics when delivery seems imminent. Monitor fetal and maternal response to local and regional anesthetics.

• Explain all procedures. Throughout labor, keep the patient informed of her progress and the condition of the fetus. If the father is present during labor, allow the parents some time together to share their feelings.

• During delivery, instruct the patient to push only during contractions and only as long as she is told. Pushing between contractions is not only ineffective but can damage the premature infant's soft skull. A prepared resuscitation team, consisting of a doctor, nurse, respiratory therapist, and an anesthesiologist or anesthetist, should be in attendance to take care of the newborn immediately. Have resuscitative equipment available in case of neonatal respiratory distress.

• Inform the parents of their child's condition. Describe his appearance, and explain the purpose of any supportive equipment. Help them gain confidence in their ability to care for their child. Provide privacy, and encourage them to hold and feed the infant, when possible.

• As necessary, before the parents leave the hospital with the infant, refer them to a community health nurse who can help them adjust to caring for a premature infant.

Premature Rupture of the Membranes

Premature rupture of the membranes (PROM) is a spontaneous break or tear in the amniochorial sac before onset of regular contractions, resulting in progressive cervical dilation. PROM occurs in nearly 10% of all pregnancies over 20 weeks' gestation, and labor usually starts within 24 hours; more than 80% of these infants are mature. The latent period (between membrane rupture and onset of labor) is generally brief when the membranes rupture near term; when the infant is premature, this period is prolonged, which increases the risk of mortality from maternal infection (amnionitis, endometritis), fetal infection (pneumonia, septicemia), and prematurity.

Causes

Although the cause of PROM is unknown, malpresentation and contracted pelvis commonly accompany the rupture. Predisposing factors may include:

• poor nutrition and hygiene and lack of proper prenatal care

• incompetent cervix (perhaps as a result of abortions)

• increased intrauterine tension due to hydramnios or multiple pregnancies

• defects in the amniochorial mem-

branes' tensile strength.
- uterine infection.

Signs and symptoms

Typically, PROM causes blood-tinged amniotic fluid containing vernix particles to gush or leak from the vagina. Maternal fever, fetal tachycardia, and foul-smelling vaginal discharge indicate infection.

Diagnosis

Characteristic passage of amniotic fluid confirms PROM. Physical examination shows amniotic fluid in the vagina. Examination of this fluid helps determine appropriate management. For example, aerobic and anaerobic cultures and a Gram stain from the cervix reveal pathogenic organisms and indicate uterine or systemic infection.

Alkaline pH of fluid collected from the posterior fornix turns nitrazine paper deep blue. (The presence of blood can give a false-positive result.) If a smear of fluid is placed on a slide and allowed to dry, it takes on a fernlike pattern due to a high sodium and protein content of amniotic fluid. Staining the fluid with Nile blue sulfate reveals two categories of cell bodies. Blue-stained bodies represent shed fetal epithelial cells, while orange-stained bodies originate in sebaceous glands. Incidence of prematurity is low when more than 20% of cells stain orange.

Physical examination also determines the presence of multiple pregnancies. Fetal presentation and size should be assessed by abdominal palpation (Leopold's maneuvers).

Other data determine the fetus' gestational age:
- *historical:* date of last menstrual period, quickening
- *physical:* initial detection of unamplified fetal heart sound, measurement of fundal height above the symphysis, ultrasound measurements of fetal biparietal diameter
- *chemical:* tests on amniotic fluid, such as the lecithin-sphingomyelin (L/S) ratio (an L/S ratio greater than 2.0 indicates pulmonary maturity); foam stability (shake test) also indicates fetal pulmonary maturity.

Treatment

Treatment for PROM depends on fetal age and the risk of infection. In a term pregnancy, if spontaneous labor and vaginal delivery are not achieved within a relatively short time (usually within 24 hours after the membranes rupture), induction of labor with oxytocin is usually required; if induction fails, cesarean delivery is usually necessary. Cesarean hysterectomy is recommended with gross uterine infection.

Management of a preterm pregnancy of less than 34 weeks is controversial. However, with advances in technology, a conservative approach to PROM has now been proven effective. With a preterm pregnancy of 28 to 34 weeks, treatment includes hospitalization and observation for signs of infection (maternal leukocytosis or fever, and fetal tachycardia) while awaiting fetal maturation. If clinical status suggests infection, baseline cultures and sensitivity tests are appropriate. If these tests confirm infection, labor must be induced, followed by I.V. administration of antibiotics. A culture should also be made of gastric aspirate or a swabbing from the infant's ear, as antibiotic therapy may be indicated for the newborn as well. At such delivery, have resuscitative equipment available to treat neonatal distress.

Special considerations

- Teach the patient in the early stages of pregnancy how to recognize PROM. Make sure she understands that amniotic fluid doesn't always gush; it sometimes leaks slowly.
- Stress that she *must* report PROM immediately, since prompt treatment may prevent dangerous infection.
- Warn the patient not to engage in sexual intercourse or to douche after the membranes rupture.
- Before physical examination in suspected PROM, explain all diagnostic tests

and clarify any misunderstandings the patient may have. During the examination, stay with the patient and provide reassurance. Such examination requires sterile gloves and sterile lubricating jelly. *Don't* use iodophor antiseptic solution, since it discolors nitrazine paper and makes pH determination impossible.

• After the examination, provide proper perineal care. Send fluid samples to the laboratory promptly, since bacteriologic studies need immediate evaluation to be valid. If labor starts, observe the mother's contractions, and monitor vital signs every 2 hours. Watch for signs of maternal infection (fever, abdominal tenderness, and changes in amniotic fluid, such as foul odor or purulence) and fetal tachycardia. (Fetal tachycardia may precede maternal fever.) Report such signs immediately.

Cesarean Birth

(Cesarean section)

Cesarean birth is delivery of an infant by surgical incision through the abdomen and uterus. It can be performed as elective surgery or as an emergency procedure when conditions prohibit vaginal delivery. The rising incidence of cesarean birth coincides with recent medical and technologic advances in fetal and placental surveillance and care. In the United States, 9% to 16% of all pregnancies terminate in cesarean births, rising to 17% to 25% in perinatal centers that handle high-risk deliveries.

Causes

The most common reasons for cesarean birth are malpresentation (such as shoulder or face presentation), fetal distress, cephalopelvic disproportion ([CPD] the pelvis is too small to accommodate the fetal head), certain cases of toxemia, previous cesarean birth, and inadequate progress in labor (failure of induction).

Conditions causing fetal distress that indicate a need for cesarean birth include prolapsed cord with a live fetus, fetal hypoxia, abnormal fetal heart rate patterns, unfavorable intrauterine environment (from infection), and moderate to severe Rh isoimmunization. Less common maternal conditions that may necessitate cesarean birth include complete placenta previa, abruptio placentae, placenta accreta, malignant tumors, and chronic diseases in which delivery is indicated before term.

Cesarean birth may also be necessary if induction is contraindicated or difficult or if advanced labor increases the risk of morbidity and mortality.

In the case of a previous cesarean delivery, some doctors allow a subsequent vaginal delivery if the cesarean wasn't classic or due to CPD or if the original reason for the cesarean no longer exists. However, vaginal delivery risks uterine rupture if the uterus is scarred.

Diagnosis

Special tests and monitoring procedures provide early indications of the need for cesarean birth:

• *X-ray pelvimetry* reveals CPD and malpresentation.

• *Ultrasonography* shows pelvic masses that interfere with vaginal delivery and fetal position.

• *Amniocentesis* determines fetal maturity, Rh isoimmunization, fetal distress, and fetal genetic abnormalities.

• Auscultation of *fetal heart rate* (fetoscope, Doppler unit, or electronic fetal monitor) determines acute fetal distress.

Treatment

The most common type of cesarean birth is the *lower segment cesarean,* in which a transverse incision across the lower abdomen opens the visceral peritoneum over the uterus. The lower anterior uterine wall is then incised (transversely or longitudinally) behind the bladder. Since the peritoneum completely covers this part of the uterus, uterine seepage is reduced and, consequently, so is the risk of postpartum infection.

The *classic cesarean*—in which a longitudinal incision is made into the body of the uterus, extending into the fundus and opening the top of the uterus—is rarely performed, because it exaggerates the risk of infection and of uterine rupture in subsequent pregnancies. *Cesarean hysterectomy* removes the entire uterus and is reserved for cases such as malignant tumors, severe infection, and placenta accreta.

Patients may have general or regional anesthetic for surgery, depending on the extent of maternal or fetal distress. Possible maternal complications of cesarean delivery include respiratory tract infection, wound dehiscence, thromboembolism, paralytic ileus, hemorrhage, and genitourinary tract infection.

UTERINE INCISIONS FOR CESAREAN SECTION

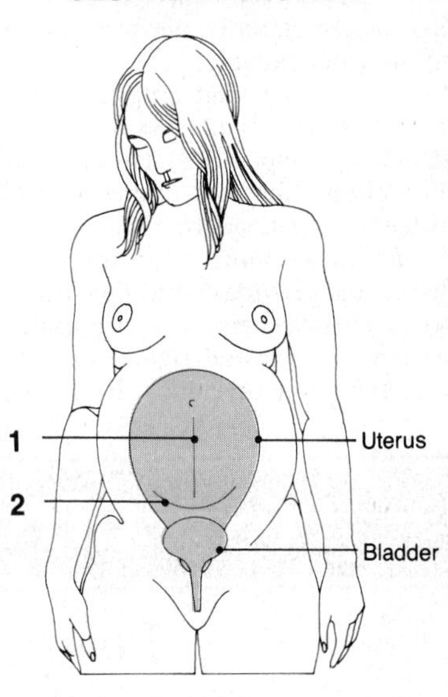

1. In *classic cesarean,* a vertical incision extends from the uterine fundus through the body, stopping above the level of the bladder.

2. In *lower segment cesarean,* the preferred method, a transverse incision is made across the lower abdomen and along the lower anterior uterine wall behind the bladder. This avoids incision of the peritoneum, reducing the risk of peritonitis.

Special considerations

Before cesarean delivery:

- Explain cesarean birth to the patient and her partner, and answer any questions they may have. Provide reassurance and emotional support. Cesarean birth often is performed after hours of labor have exhausted the patient.
- As ordered, administer preoperative medications.
- Prepare the patient by shaving her from below the breasts to the pubic region and the upper quarter of the anterior thighs. Make sure her bladder is empty, using an indwelling (Foley) catheter, as ordered. Insert an I.V. line for fluid replacement therapy, as ordered. Assess maternal temperature, pulse rate, respirations, and blood pressure and fetal heart rate.
- In the operating room, place the patient in a slight lateral position. Use of a 15° wedge reduces caval compression (supine hypotension) and subsequent fetal hypoxia.

After cesarean delivery:

- Check vital signs every 15 minutes until they stabilize. Maintain a patent airway. If general anesthetic was used, remain with the patient until she's responsive. If regional anesthetic was used, monitor the return of sensation to the legs.
- Encourage parent-infant bonding as soon as practical.
- Gently assess the fundus. Check the incision and lochia for signs of infection, such as a foul odor. Check frequently for bleeding, and report it immediately. Keep the incision clean and dry.

• Observe the infant for signs of respiratory distress (tachypnea, retractions, and cyanosis) until there is evidence of physiologic stability. Keep resuscitative equipment available.
• Assess intake and output (some patients have Foley catheters in place up to 48 hours postoperative). Observe the patient closely for indications of bladder fullness or urinary tract infection.
• Administer pain medication, as ordered, and provide comfort measures for breast engorgement, as appropriate. Offer reassurance and reduce anxiety by answering any questions. If the mother wishes to breast-feed, offer encouragement and help. Recognize afterpains in multiparas.
• Promote early ambulation to prevent cardiovascular and pulmonary complications.
• Provide psychological support. If the patient seems anxious about having had a cesarean delivery, encourage her to share her feelings with you. If appropriate, suggest that she participate in a cesarean birth sharing group. Encourage support from her family members as well.

POSTPARTUM DISORDERS

Puerperal Infection

A common cause of childbirth-related death, puerperal infection is an inflammation of the birth canal during the postpartum period or after abortion. It can occur as localized lesions of the perineum, vulva, and vagina, or it may spread, causing endometritis, parametritis, pelvic and femoral thrombophlebitis, and peritonitis. In the United States, puerperal infection develops in about 6% of maternity patients. Prognosis is good with treatment.

Causes

Microorganisms that commonly cause puerperal infection include streptococci, coagulase-negative staphylococci, *Clostridium perfringens, Bacteroides fragilis,* and *Escherichia coli.* Most of these organisms are considered normal vaginal flora but are known to cause puerperal infection in the presence of certain predisposing factors, which include:
• prolonged and premature rupture of the membranes.
• prolonged (more than 24 hours) or traumatic labor.
• frequent or unsanitary vaginal examinations or unsanitary delivery.
• invasive techniques, such as application of a fetal scalp electrode.
• intercourse after rupture of the membranes.
• retained products of conception.
• hemorrhage.
• maternal conditions, such as anemia or debilitation from malnutrition.

Signs and symptoms

A characteristic sign of puerperal infection is fever (at least 100.4° F. [38° C.]) that occurs after the first 24 hours postpartum on any 2 consecutive days up to the 11th day. This fever can spike as high as 105° F. (40.6° C.) and is commonly associated with chills, headache, malaise, restlessness, and anxiety.

Accompanying signs and symptoms depend on the extent and site of infection and may include:
• *local lesions of the perineum, vulva, and vagina:* pain, inflammation, edema of the affected area, dysuria, profuse purulent discharge.
• *endometritis:* heavy, sometimes foul-smelling lochia; tender, enlarged uterus; backache; severe uterine contractions

persisting after childbirth.

• *parametritis (pelvic cellulitis):* vaginal tenderness and abdominal pain and tenderness (pain may become more intense as infection spreads).

The inflammation may remain localized, may lead to abscess formation, or may spread through the blood or lymphatic system. Widespread inflammation may cause:

• *pelvic thrombophlebitis:* severe, repeated chills and dramatic swings in body temperature; lower abdominal or flank pain; and, possibly, a palpable tender mass over the affected area, which usually develops near the second postpartum week.

• *femoral thrombophlebitis:* pain, stiffness, or swelling in a leg or the groin; inflammation or shiny, white appearance of the affected leg; malaise; fever; and chills, usually beginning 10 to 20 days postpartum. These signs may precipitate pulmonary embolism.

• *peritonitis:* body temperature usually elevated, accompanied by tachycardia (greater than 140 beats per minute), weak pulse, hiccups, nausea, vomiting, and diarrhea; abdominal pain is constant and, possibly, excruciating.

Diagnosis

Development of the typical clinical features, especially fever within 48 hours after delivery, suggests diagnosis of puerperal infection.

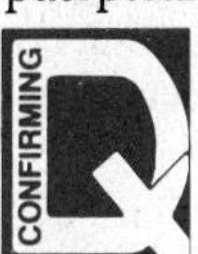

A culture of lochia, blood, incisional exudate (from cesarean incision or episiotomy), uterine tissue, or material collected from the vaginal cuff, revealing the causative organism, confirms the diagnosis. Within 36 to 48 hours, WBC count usually demonstrates leukocytosis (15,000 to 30,000/mm^3) and an increased sedimentation rate.

Typical clinical features usually suffice for diagnosis of endometritis and peritonitis. In parametritis, pelvic examination shows induration without purulent discharge; culdoscopy shows pelvic adnexal induration and thickening. Red, swollen abscesses on the broad

PUERPERAL INFECTION AND DR. IGNAZ SEMMELWEIS

Puerperal infection was well known throughout recorded history. Hippocrates, for example, wrote that puerperal infection resulted from the suppression of vaginal discharge. Its true cause remained unknown until Louis Pasteur's discoveries in microbiology, and puerperal infection persisted as a common cause of maternal death well into the 19th century.

In 1847, Dr. Ignaz Semmelweis, while working at a maternity hospital in Vienna, observed the dramatically low mortality from puerperal infection in a ward managed by midwives, compared to the high mortality in a ward managed by doctors. In the Vienna of his time, Dr. Semmelweis' colleagues went directly from dissecting cadavers to examining patients who were recovering from childbirth. He concluded that the doctors were spreading this fatal infection via their unwashed hands. He got dramatic proof of his theory when he saw a co-worker die of septicemia after accidentally cutting himself with a scalpel used during autopsy of a woman who had died of puerperal infection. As a result, Semmelweis required his staff to wash their hands with an antiseptic solution before examining maternity patients. During the first year of the hand-washing mandate, mortality from puerperal infection at Semmelweis' hospital dropped sharply from almost 12% to 3.8%.

Despite such dramatic results, Semmelweis' colleagues did not accept his theory for another 20 years—not until Pasteur's microbiologic theories and Lister's application of aseptic technique made Semmelweis' theory indisputable.

Almost coincidentally with Semmelweis' discovery, similar progress began in the United States. In an article published in 1843 in the *New England Journal of Medicine,* Oliver Wendell Holmes stressed the importance of adequate precautions by doctors and nurses to prevent puerperal infection.

ligaments are even more serious indications, since rupture leads to peritonitis.

Diagnosis of pelvic or femoral thrombophlebitis is suggested by characteristic clinical signs, venography, Doppler ultrasonography, Rielander's sign (palpable veins inside the thigh and calf), Payr's sign (pain in the calf when pressure is applied on the inside of the foot), and Homans' sign (pain on dorsiflexion of the foot with the knee extended).

Treatment

Treatment of puerperal infection usually begins with I.V. infusion of a broad-spectrum antibiotic to control the infection and prevent its spread while awaiting culture results. After identification of the infecting organism, a more specific antibiotic should be administered. (An oral antibiotic may be prescribed after hospital discharge.)

Ancillary measures include analgesics for pain; anticoagulants, such as heparin I.V., for thrombophlebitis and endometritis (after clotting time and partial thromboplastin time determine dosage); antiseptics for local lesions; and antiemetics for nausea and vomiting from peritonitis. Isolation or transfer from the maternity unit also may be indicated.

Supportive care includes bed rest, adequate fluid intake, I.V. fluids when necessary, and measures to reduce fever. Sitz baths and heat lamps may relieve discomfort from local lesions.

Surgery may be necessary to remove any remaining products of conception or to drain local lesions, such as an abscess in parametritis.

Management of femoral thrombophlebitis requires warm soaks, elevation of the affected leg to promote venous return, and observation for signs of pulmonary embolism. Rarely, recurrent pulmonary emboli from pelvic thrombophlebitis require laparotomy for plication of inferior vena cava and ovarian vein ligation.

Special considerations

- Monitor vital signs every 4 hours (more frequently if peritonitis has developed) and intake and output. Enforce strict bed rest.
- Frequently inspect the perineum. Assess the fundus, and palpate for tenderness (subinvolution may indicate endometritis). Note the amount, color, and odor of vaginal drainage, and document your observations.
- Administer antibiotics and analgesics, as ordered. Assess and document the type, degree, and location of pain, as well as the patient's response to analgesics. Give the patient an antiemetic to relieve nausea and vomiting, as necessary.
- Provide sitz baths and a heat lamp for local lesions. Change bed linen and perineal pads and under pads frequently. Keep the patient warm.
- Elevate the thrombophlebitic leg about 30°. *Don't* rub or manipulate it or compress it with bed linen. Provide warm soaks for the leg. Watch for signs of pulmonary embolism, such as cyanosis, dyspnea, and chest pain.
- Offer reassurance and emotional support. Thoroughly explain all procedures to the patient and family.
- If the mother is separated from her infant, provide her with frequent reassurance about his progress. Encourage the father to reassure the mother about the infant's condition as well.

To prevent puerperal infection:

- Maintain aseptic technique when performing a vaginal examination. Limit the number of vaginal examinations performed during labor. Take care to wash your hands thoroughly after each patient contact.
- Instruct all pregnant patients to call their doctors immediately when their membranes rupture. Warn them to avoid intercourse after rupture or leak of the amniotic sac.
- Keep the episiotomy site clean, and teach the patient how to maintain good perineal hygiene.
- Screen personnel and visitors to keep persons with active infections away from maternity patients.

Mastitis and Breast Engorgement

Mastitis (parenchymatous inflammation of the mammary glands) and breast engorgement (congestion) are disorders that may affect lactating females. Mastitis occurs postpartum in about 1%, mainly in primiparas who are breast-feeding. It occurs occasionally in nonlactating females and rarely in males. All breast-feeding mothers develop some degree of engorgement, but it's especially likely to be severe in primiparas. Prognosis for both disorders is good.

Causes

Mastitis develops when a pathogen that typically originates in the nursing infant's nose or pharynx invades breast tissue through a fissured or cracked nipple and disrupts normal lactation. The most common pathogen of this type is *Staphylococcus aureus;* less frequently,

PHYSIOLOGY OF LACTATION

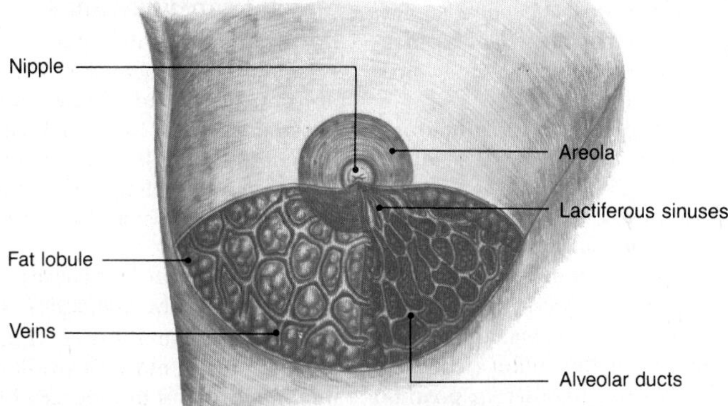

During pregnancy, progesterone and estrogen normally interact to suppress milk secretion while developing the breasts for lactation. Estrogen causes the breasts to grow by increasing their fat content; progesterone causes lobule growth and develops the alveolar cells' secretory capacity.

After childbirth, the mother's anterior pituitary gland secretes prolactin (suppressed during pregnancy), which helps the alveolar epithelium produce and release colostrum. Usually, within 3 days of prolactin release, the breasts secrete large amounts of milk rather than colostrum. The infant's sucking stimulates nerve endings at the nipple, initiating the let-down reflex that allows the expression of milk from the mother's breasts. Sucking also stimulates the release of another pituitary hormone, oxytocin, into the mother's bloodstream. This hormone causes alveolar contraction, which forces milk into the ducts and the lactiferous sinuses beneath the alveolar surface, making milk available to the infant. (It also promotes normal involution of the uterus.)

The infant's suckling provides the stimulus for both milk production and milk expression. Consequently, the more the infant breast-feeds, the more milk the breast produces. Conversely, the less sucking stimulation the breast receives, the less milk it produces.

it's *Staphylococcus epidermidis* or *beta-hemolytic streptococcus.* Rarely, mastitis may result from disseminated tuberculosis or the mumps virus. Predisposing factors include a fissure or abrasion on the nipple; blocked milk ducts; and an incomplete let-down reflex, usually due to emotional trauma. Blocked milk ducts can result from a tight bra or prolonged intervals between breast-feedings.

Causes of breast engorgement include venous and lymphatic stasis, and alveolar milk accumulation.

Signs and symptoms

Mastitis may develop anytime during lactation but usually begins 3 to 4 weeks postpartum, with fever (101° F. [38.3° C.], or higher in acute mastitis), malaise, and flulike symptoms. The breasts (or, occasionally, one breast) become tender, hard, swollen, and warm. Unless mastitis is treated adequately, it may progress to breast abscess.

Breast engorgement generally starts with onset of lactation (day 2 to day 5 postpartum). The breasts undergo changes similar to those in mastitis, and body temperature may be elevated. Engorgement may be mild, causing only slight discomfort, or severe, causing considerable pain. A severely engorged breast can interfere with the infant's capacity to feed due to his inability to position his mouth properly on the swollen, rigid breast.

Diagnosis

In a lactating female with breast discomfort or other signs of inflammation, cultures of expressed milk confirm generalized mastitis; cultures of breast skin surface confirm localized mastitis. Such cultures also determine appropriate antibiotic treatment. Obvious swelling of lactating breasts confirms engorgement.

Treatment

Antibiotic therapy, the primary treatment for mastitis, generally consists of penicillin G to combat staphylococcus; erythromycin or kanamycin is used for penicillin-resistant strains. Although symptoms usually subside 2 to 3 days after treatment begins, antibiotic therapy should continue for 10 days. Other appropriate measures include analgesics for pain and, rarely, when antibiotics fail to control the infection and mastitis progresses to breast abscess, incision and drainage of the abscess.

The goal of treatment of breast engorgement is to relieve discomfort and control swelling, and may include analgesics to alleviate pain, and ice packs and an uplift support to minimize edema. Rarely, oxytocin nasal spray may be necessary to release milk from the alveoli into the ducts. To facilitate breast-feeding, the mother may manually express excess milk before a feeding so the infant can grasp the nipple properly.

Special considerations

If the patient has mastitis:

- Isolate the patient and her infant to prevent the spread of infection to other nursing mothers. Explain mastitis to the patient and why isolation is necessary.
- Obtain a complete patient history, including a drug history, especially allergy to penicillin.
- Assess and record the cause and amount of discomfort. Give analgesics, as needed.
- Reassure the mother that breast-feeding during mastitis won't harm her infant, since he's the source of the infection. Tell her to offer the infant the affected breast first to promote complete emptying of the breast and prevent clogged ducts. However, if an open abscess develops, she must stop breast-feeding with this breast and use a breast pump until the abscess heals. She should continue to breast-feed on the unaffected side. Suggest applying a warm, wet towel to the affected breast or taking a warm shower to relax and improve her ability to breast-feed.
- To prevent mastitis and relieve its symptoms, teach the patient good health care, breast care, and breast-feeding habits. Advise her to always wash her hands before touching her breasts.
- Instruct the patient to combat fever by getting plenty of rest, drinking sufficient

PATIENT TEACHING AID

Tips for Effective Breast-Feeding

Dear Patient:
During pregnancy and lactation, good health care, breast care, and breast-feeding habits are essential.

- Maintain good nutrition and fluid intake, and get plenty of rest and sleep. Limit stress factors, which can inhibit your ability to breast-feed your infant.
- Don't use soap or other irritating substances on your breasts during your pregnancy. These agents remove protective oils. Toughen nipples during pregnancy by rolling them between your fingertips twice daily. Wear a comfortable support bra (not lowcut or tight) with protective pads. Keep your breasts dry and, when possible, open to the air.
- If you plan to breast-feed, begin as soon as your child is born. Breast-feed at regular intervals, including at least once during the night. Alternate breasts at each feeding. Relax in a comfortable position so the infant can suck effectively. If your breasts feel engorged, express excess milk manually. You may find that applying warm wet towels or taking a relaxing shower may help you to express milk more easily, or you may find it helpful to use a hand or electric breast pump. Avoid sleeping on your stomach, since this may cause mechanical milk stasis.
- If your nipples become dry and cracked, apply pure lanolin or a water-based cream if you're allergic to lanolin. Vitamins A and D ointment is sometimes recommended; if you use this, be sure to apply it only around the nipples and not to the duct openings.
- Wash your nipples thoroughly before breast-feeding.

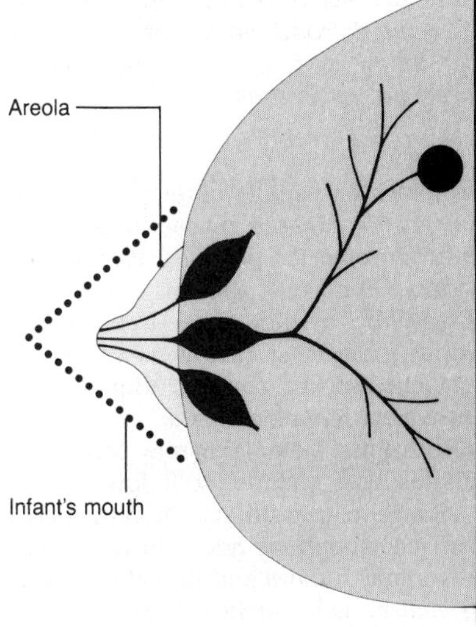

For effective breast-feeding, place the infant's mouth around but not directly on the areola.

fluids, and following prescribed antibiotic therapy.

If the patient has breast engorgement:

- Assess and record the level of discomfort. Give analgesics, and apply ice packs and a compression binder, as needed.
- Teach the patient how to express excess breast milk manually. She should do this just before nursing to enable the infant to get the swollen areola into his mouth. Caution against excessive expression of milk between feedings, as this stimulates milk production and prolongs engorgement.
- Explain that because breast engorgement is due to the physiologic processes of lactation, breast-feeding is the best remedy for engorgement. Suggest breast-feeding every 2 to 3 hours and at least once during the night.
- Ensure that the mother wears a well-fitted nursing bra, usually a size larger than she normally wears.

Galactorrhea

(Hyperprolactinemia)

Galactorrhea, inappropriate breast milk secretion, generally occurs 3 to 6 months after the discontinuation of breast-feeding (usually after a first delivery). It may also follow an abortion or may develop in a female who hasn't been pregnant; it rarely occurs in males.

Causes

Galactorrhea usually develops in a person with increased prolactin secretion from the anterior pituitary gland, with possible abnormal patterns of secretion of growth, thyroid, and adrenocorticotropic hormones. However, increased prolactin serum concentration doesn't always cause galactorrhea.

Additional factors that may precipitate this disorder include the following:

- *endogenous:* pituitary (high incidence with chromophobe adenoma), ovarian, or adrenal tumors and hypothyroidism. In males, galactorrhea usually results from pituitary, testicular, or pineal gland tumors.
- *idiopathic:* possibly from stress or anxiety, which causes neurogenic depression of the prolactin-inhibiting factor
- *exogenous:* breast stimulation, genital stimulation, or drugs (such as oral contraceptives, meprobamate, and phenothiazines).

Signs and symptoms

In the female with galactorrhea, milk continues to flow after the 21-day period that is normal after weaning. Galactorrhea may also be spontaneous and unrelated to normal lactation, or due to manual expression. Such abnormal flow is usually bilateral and may be accompanied by amenorrhea.

Diagnosis

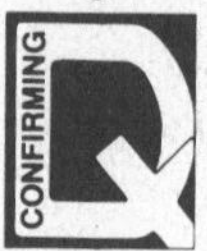

Characteristic clinical features and patient history (including drug and sex histories) confirm galactorrhea. Laboratory tests to help determine the cause include measurement of serum levels of prolactin, cortisol, thyroid-stimulating hormone, triiodothyronine, and thyroxine. CAT scan and, possibly, mammography may be indicated.

Treatment

Treatment varies according to the underlying cause and ranges from simple avoidance of precipitating exogenous factors, such as drugs, to treatment of tumors with surgery, radiation, or chemotherapy.

Therapy for idiopathic galactorrhea depends on whether or not the patient plans to have more children. If she does, treatment usually consists of bromocriptine; if she doesn't, oral estrogens (such as ethinyl estradiol) and progestins (such as progesterone) effectively treat this disorder. Idiopathic galactorrhea may recur after discontinuation of drug therapy.

Special considerations

- Watch for central nervous system abnormalities, such as headache, failing vision, and dizziness.
- Maintain adequate fluid intake, especially if the patient has a fever. However, advise the patient to avoid tea, coffee, and certain tranquilizers that may aggravate engorgement.
- Instruct the patient to keep her breasts and nipples clean.
- Tell the patient who is taking bromocriptine to report nausea, vomiting, dyspepsia, loss of appetite, dizziness, fatigue, numbness, and hypotension. To prevent gastrointestinal upset, advise her to eat small meals frequently and to take

this drug with dry toast or crackers. After treatment with this drug, milk secretion usually stops in 1 to 2 months, and menstruation recurs after 6 to 24 weeks.

HEMOLYTIC DISEASES OF THE NEWBORN

Hyperbilirubinemia

(Neonatal jaundice)

Hyperbilirubinemia, the result of hemolytic processes in the newborn, is marked by elevated serum bilirubin levels and mild jaundice. It can be physiologic (with jaundice the only symptom) or pathologic (resulting from an underlying disease). Physiologic jaundice is very common, and tends to be more common and more severe in certain ethnic groups (Chinese, Japanese, Koreans, American Indians), whose mean peak of unconjugated bilirubin is approximately twice that of the rest of the population. Physiologic jaundice is self-limiting; prognosis for pathologic jaundice varies, depending on the cause. Untreated, severe hyperbilirubinemia may result in kernicterus, a neurologic syndrome resulting from deposition of unconjugated bilirubin in the brain cells and characterized by severe neural symptoms. Survivors may develop cerebral palsy, epilepsy, or mental retardation or have only minor sequelae, such as perceptual-motor handicaps and learning disorders.

Causes

As erythrocytes break down at the end of their neonatal life cycle, hemoglobin separates into globin (protein) and heme (iron) fragments. Heme fragments form unconjugated (indirect) bilirubin, which binds with albumin for transport to liver cells to conjugate with glucuronide, forming direct bilirubin. Because unconjugated bilirubin is fat-soluble and cannot be excreted in the urine or bile, it may escape to extravascular tissue, especially fatty tissue and the brain, resulting in hyperbilirubinemia.

This pathophysiologic process may develop when:

- factors that disrupt conjugation and usurp albumin-binding sites include drugs such as aspirin, tranquilizers, and sulfonamides and conditions such as hypothermia, anoxia, hypoglycemia, and hypoalbuminemia.
- decreased hepatic function results in reduced bilirubin conjugation.
- increased erythrocyte production or breakdown results from hemolytic disorders, or Rh or ABO incompatibility.
- biliary obstruction or hepatitis results in blockage of normal bile flow.
- maternal enzymes present in breast milk inhibits the infant's glucuronyltransferase conjugating activity.

Signs and symptoms

The predominant sign of hyperbilirubinemia is jaundice, which does not become clinically apparent until serum bilirubin levels reach about 7 mg/100 ml. Physiologic jaundice develops 24 hours after delivery in 50% of term infants (usually day 2 to day 3) and 48 hours after delivery in 80% of premature infants (usually day 3 to day 5). It generally disappears by day 7 in term infants and by day 9 or day 10 in premature infants. Throughout physiologic jaundice, serum unconjugated bilirubin does not exceed 12 mg/100 ml. Pathologic jaundice may appear anytime after the first day of life and persists beyond 7 days with serum bilirubin levels greater than 12 mg/100 ml in a term infant, 15 mg/100 ml in a premature infant, or increasing more than 5 mg/100 ml in 24 hours.

UNDERLYING CAUSES OF HYPERBILIRUBINEMIA

When jaundice occurs during the first day of life:
- Blood type incompatibility (Rh, ABO, other minor blood groups)
- Intrauterine infection (rubella, cytomegalic inclusion body disease, toxoplasmosis, syphilis, and occasionally, bacteria such as *Escherichia coli*, staphylococcus, *Pseudomonas, Klebsiella, Proteus,* and streptococcus)

When jaundice occurs during the second or third day of life:
- Infection (usually from gram-negative bacteria)
- Polycythemia
- Enclosed hemorrhage (skin bruises, subdural hematoma)
- Respiratory distress syndrome (hyaline membrane disease)
- Heinz body anemia from drugs and toxins (vitamin K_3, sodium nitrate)
- Transient neonatal hyperbilirubinemia
- Abnormal RBC morphology
- Red cell enzyme deficiencies (glucose 6-phosphate dehydrogenase, hexokinase)
- Physiologic jaundice
- Blood group incompatibilities

When jaundice occurs during the fourth and fifth days of life:
- Breast-feeding, respiratory distress syndrome, maternal diabetes
- Crigler-Najjar syndrome (congenital nonhemolytic icterus)
- Gilbert syndrome

When jaundice occurs after one week of life:
- Herpes simplex
- Pyloric stenosis
- Hypothyroidism
- Neonatal giant cell hepatitis
- Infection (usually acquired in neonatal period)
- Bile duct atresia
- Galactosemia
- Choledochal cyst

Diagnosis

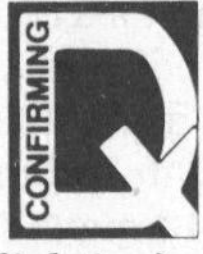

Jaundice and elevated levels of serum bilirubin confirm hyperbilirubinemia. Inspection of the infant in a well-lit room (without yellow or gold lighting) reveals a yellowish skin coloration, particularly in the sclerae. Jaundice can be verified by pressing the skin on the cheek or abdomen lightly with one finger, then releasing pressure and observing skin color immediately. Signs of jaundice necessitate measuring and charting serum bilirubin levels every 4 hours. Testing may include direct and indirect bilirubin levels, particularly for pathologic jaundice. Bilirubin levels that are excessively elevated or vary daily suggest a pathologic process.

Identifying the underlying cause of hyperbilirubinemia requires a detailed patient history (including prenatal history), family history (paternal Rh factor, inherited red cell defects), present infant status (immaturity, infection), and blood testing of the infant and mother (blood group incompatibilities, hemoglobin level, direct Coombs' test, hematocrit).

Treatment

Depending on the underlying cause, treatment may include phototherapy, exchange transfusions, albumin infusion, and possibly, drug therapy. Phototherapy is the treatment of choice for physiologic jaundice, and pathologic jaundice due to erythroblastosis fetalis (after the initial exchange transfusion). Phototherapy uses fluorescent light to decompose bilirubin in the skin by oxidation, and is usually discontinued after bilirubin levels fall below 10 mg/100 ml and continue to decrease for 24 hours. However, phototherapy is rarely the only treatment for jaundice due to a pathologic cause.

An exchange transfusion replaces the infant's blood with fresh blood (less than 48 hours old), removing some of the unconjugated bilirubin in serum. Possible indications for exchange transfusions include hydrops fetalis, polycythemia, erythroblastosis fetalis, marked reticulocytosis, drug toxicity, and jaundice that develops within the first 6 hours after birth.

Other therapy for excessive bilirubin levels may include albumin administration (1 g/kg of 25% salt-poor albumin), which provides additional albumin for binding unconjugated bilirubin. This may be done 1 to 2 hours before exchange or as a substitute for a portion of the plasma in the transfused blood.

Drug therapy, which is rare, usually consists of phenobarbital administered to the mother before delivery and to the newborn several days after delivery. This drug stimulates the hepatic glucuronide-conjugating system.

Special considerations

- Assess and record the infant's jaundice, and note the time it began. Report the jaundice and serum bilirubin levels immediately.

For the infant receiving phototherapy:

- Keep a record of how long each bilirubin light bulb is in use, since these bulbs require frequent changing for optimum effectiveness.
- Undress the infant, so his entire body surface is exposed to the light rays. Keep him 18″ to 30″ (45 to 75 cm) from the light source. Protect his eyes with shields that filter the light.
- Monitor and maintain the infant's body temperature; high and low temperatures predispose him to kernicterus. Remove the infant from the light source every 3 to 4 hours, and take off the eye shields. Allow his parents to visit and feed him.
- The infant usually shows a decrease in serum bilirubin level 1 to 12 hours after the start of phototherapy. When the infant's bilirubin level is less than 10 mg/100 ml and has been decreasing for 24 hours, discontinue phototherapy, as ordered. Resume therapy, as ordered, if serum bilirubin increases several milligrams per 100 ml, as it often does, due to a rebound effect.

For the infant receiving exchange transfusions:

- Prepare infant warmer and tray before the transfusion. Try to keep the infant quiet. Give him nothing by mouth for 3 to 4 hours before the procedure.
- Check the blood to be used for the exchange—type, Rh, age. Keep emergency equipment (resuscitative and intubation equipment, and oxygen) available. During the procedure, monitor respiratory and heart rates every 15 minutes; check the infant's temperature every 30 minutes. Continue to monitor vital signs every 15 to 30 minutes for 2 hours.
- Measure intake and output. Observe for cord bleeding and complications, such as hemorrhage, hypocalcemia, sepsis, and shock. Report serum bilirubin and hemoglobin levels. Bilirubin levels may rise, due to a rebound effect, within 30 minutes after transfusion, necessitating repeat transfusions.

To prevent hyperbilirubinemia:

- Maintain oral intake. Don't skip any feedings, since fasting stimulates the conversion of heme to bilirubin.
- Administer Rh_o (D) immune globulin (human), as ordered, to an Rh-negative mother after amniocentesis, or—to prevent hemolytic disease in subsequent infants—to an Rh-negative mother after the birth of an Rh-positive infant or after spontaneous or elective abortion.

Reassure parents that most infants experience some degree of jaundice. Explain hyperbilirubinemia, its causes, diagnostic tests, and treatment. Also, explain that the infant's stool contains some bile and may be greenish.

Erythroblastosis Fetalis

Erythroblastosis fetalis, a hemolytic disease of the fetus and newborn, stems from an incompatibility of fetal and maternal blood, resulting in maternal antibody activity against fetal red cells. Intrauterine transfusions can save 40% of fetuses with erythroblastosis. However, in severe, untreated erythroblastosis fetalis, prognosis is poor, especially if kernicterus develops. About 70% of these infants die, usually within the first week of life; survivors inevitably develop pronounced neu-

rologic damage (sensory impairment, mental deficiencies, cerebral palsy). Severely affected fetuses who develop hydrops fetalis—the most severe form of this disorder, associated with profound anemia and edema—are commonly stillborn; even if they are delivered live, they rarely survive longer than a few hours.

Causes and incidence

Although over 60 red cell antigens can stimulate antibody formation, erythroblastosis fetalis usually results from Rh isoimmunization—a condition that develops in approximately 7% of all pregnancies in the United States. Before the development of Rh_o (D) immune human globulin, this condition was an important cause of kernicterus and neonatal death.

During her first pregnancy, an Rh-negative female becomes sensitized (during delivery or abortion) by exposure to Rh-positive fetal blood antigens inherited from the father. A female may also become sensitized from receiving blood transfusions with alien Rh antigens, causing agglutins to develop; from inadequate doses of Rh_o (D); or from failure to receive Rh_o (D) after significant fetal-maternal leakage from abruptio placentae. Subsequent pregnancy with an Rh-positive fetus provokes increasing amounts of maternal agglutinating antibodies to cross the placental barrier, attach to Rh-positive cells in the fetus, and cause hemolysis and anemia. To

ABO INCOMPATIBILITY

ABO incompatibility—a form of fetomaternal incompatibility—occurs between mother and fetus in about 25% of all pregnancies, with highest incidence among Blacks. In about 1% of this number, it leads to hemolytic disease of the newborn. Although ABO incompatibility is more common than Rh isoimmunization, it is fortunately less severe. Low antigenicity of fetal or newborn ABO factors may account for the milder clinical effects.

Each blood group has specific antigens on RBCs and specific antibodies in serum. Maternal antibodies form against fetal cells when blood groups differ. Infants with group A blood, born of group O mothers, account for approximately 50% of all ABO incompatibilities. Unlike Rh isoimmunization, which always follows sensitization during a previous pregnancy, ABO incompatibility is likely to develop in a firstborn infant.

Blood Group	Antigens on RBCs	Antibodies in Serum	Most Common Incompatible Groups
A	A	Anti-B	Mother A, infant B or AB
B	B	Anti-A	Mother B, infant A or AB
AB	A and B	No antibodies	Mother AB, infant (no incompatibility)
O	No antigens	Anti-A and B	Mother O, infant A or B

Clinical effects of ABO incompatibility include jaundice, which usually appears in the newborn in 24 to 48 hours, mild anemia, and mild hepatosplenomegaly.

Diagnosis is based on clinical symptoms in the newborn, the presence of ABO incompatibility, a weak to moderately positive Coombs' test, and elevated serum bilirubin levels. Cord hemoglobin, and indirect bilirubin levels indicate the need for exchange transfusion. An exchange transfusion is done with blood of the same group and Rh type as that of the mother. Fortunately, because infants with ABO incompatibility respond so well to phototherapy, exchange transfusion is seldom necessary.

compensate for this, the fetus steps up the production of RBCs, and erythroblasts (immature RBCs) appear in the fetal circulation. Extensive hemolysis results in the release of large amounts of unconjugated bilirubin, which the liver is unable to conjugate and excrete, causing hyperbilirubinemia and hemolytic anemia.

Signs and symptoms

Jaundice usually isn't present at birth but may appear as soon as 30 minutes later or within 24 hours. The mildly affected infant shows mild to moderate hepatosplenomegaly and pallor. In severely affected infants who survive birth, erythroblastosis fetalis usually produces pallor, edema, petechiae, hepatosplenomegaly, grunting respirations, pulmonary rales, poor muscle tone, neurologic unresponsiveness, possible heart murmurs, a bile-stained umbilical cord, and yellow or meconium-stained amniotic fluid. Approximately 10% of untreated infants develop kernicterus from hemolytic disease and show symptoms such as anemia, lethargy, poor sucking ability, retracted head, stiff extremities, squinting, a high-pitched cry, and convulsions.

Hydrops fetalis causes extreme hemolysis, fetal hypoxia, heart failure (with possible pericardial effusion and circulatory collapse), edema (ranging from mild peripheral edema to anasarca), peritoneal and pleural effusions (with dyspnea and pulmonary rales), and green- or brown-tinged amniotic fluid (usually indicating a stillbirth).

Other distinctive characteristics of the infant with hydrops fetalis include enlarged placenta, marked pallor, hepatosplenomegaly, cardiomegaly, and ascites. Petechiae and widespread ecchymoses are present in severe cases, indicating concurrent disseminated intravascular coagulation. This disorder retards intrauterine growth, so the infant's lungs, kidneys, brain, and thymus are small, and despite edema, his body size is smaller than that of infants of comparable gestational age.

PREVENTION OF RH ISOIMMUNIZATION

Administration of Rh_o (D) immune human globulin to an unsensitized Rh-negative mother as soon as possible after the birth of an Rh-positive infant, or after a spontaneous or elective abortion prevents complications in subsequent pregnancies.

The following patients should be screened for Rh isoimmunization or irregular antibodies:

- all Rh-negative mothers during their first prenatal visit, and at 24, 28, 32, and 36 weeks' gestation.
- all Rh-positive mothers with histories of transfusion; a jaundiced baby; stillbirth; cesarean birth; induced abortion; placenta previa; or abruptio placentae.

Diagnosis

Diagnostic evaluation takes into account both prenatal and neonatal findings:

- maternal history (for erythroblastotic stillbirths, abortions, previously affected children, previous anti-Rh titers)
- blood typing and screening (titers should be taken frequently to determine changes in the degree of maternal immunization)
- paternal blood test (for Rh, blood group, and Rh zygosity)
- history of blood transfusion.

In addition, amniotic fluid analysis may show an increase in bilirubin (indicating possible hemolysis) and elevations in anti-Rh titers. Radiologic studies may show edema and, in hydrops fetalis, the halo sign (edematous, elevated, subcutaneous fat layers) and the Buddha position (fetus' legs are crossed).

Neonatal findings indicating erythroblastosis fetalis include:

- direct Coombs' test of umbilical cord blood to measure RBC (Rh-positive) antibodies in the newborn (positive only when the mother is Rh-negative and the fetus is Rh-positive).
- decreased cord hemoglobin count (less than 10 g), signaling severe disease.
- many nucleated peripheral RBCs.

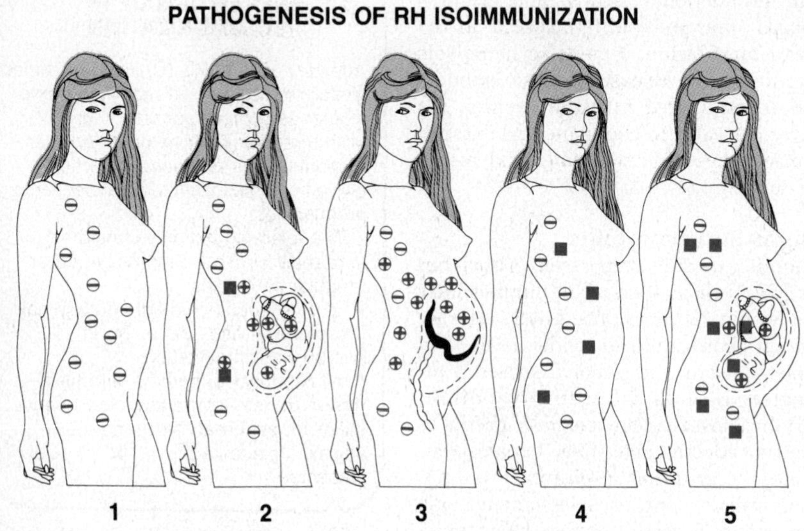

Fig. 1) Rh-negative woman prepregnancy. Fig. 2) Pregnancy with Rh-positive fetus. Fig. 3) Placental separation. Fig. 4) Postdelivery, mother becomes sensitized to Rh-positive blood and develops anti–Rh-positive antibodies (darkened squares). Fig. 5) During the next pregnancy with Rh-positive fetus, maternal anti–Rh-positive antibodies enter fetal circulation and attach to Rh-positive RBCs, subjecting them to hemolysis.

Treatment

Treatment depends on the degree of maternal sensitization and the effects of hemolytic disease on the fetus or newborn.

• *Intrauterine-intraperitoneal transfusion* is performed when amniotic fluid analysis suggests the fetus is severely affected and delivery is inappropriate due to fetal immaturity. A transabdominal puncture under fluoroscopy into the fetal peritoneal cavity allows infusion of group O, Rh-negative blood. This may be repeated every 2 weeks until the fetus is mature enough for delivery.

• *Planned delivery* is usually done 2 to 4 weeks before term date, depending on maternal history, serologic tests, and amniocentesis; labor may be induced from the 34th to 38th week of gestation. During labor, the fetus should be monitored electronically; capillary blood scalp sampling determines acid-base balance. Any indication of fetal distress necessitates immediate cesarean delivery.

• *Phenobarbital* administered during the last 5 to 6 weeks of pregnancy may lower serum bilirubin levels in the newborn.

• An *exchange transfusion* removes antibody-coated RBCs and prevents hyperbilirubinemia through removal of the infant's blood and replacement with fresh group O, Rh-negative blood.

• *Albumin infusion* aids in the binding of bilirubin, reducing the chances of hyperbilirubinemia.

• *Phototherapy* by exposure to ultraviolet light reduces bilirubin levels.

Neonatal therapy for hydrops fetalis consists of maintaining ventilation by intubation, oxygenation, and mechanical assistance, when necessary; and removal of excess fluid to relieve severe ascites and respiratory distress. Other appropriate measures include an exchange transfusion and maintenance of the infant's body temperature.

Gamma globulin that contains anti–

Rh-positive antibody (Rh_o [D]) can provide passive immunization, which prevents maternal Rh isoimmunization in Rh-negative females. However, it's ineffective if sensitization has already resulted from a previous pregnancy, abortion, or transfusion.

Special considerations

Structure the care plan around close maternal and fetal observation, explanations of diagnostic tests and therapeutic measures, and emotional support.

- Reassure the parents that they're not at fault in having a child with erythroblastosis fetalis. Encourage them to express their fears concerning possible complications of treatment.
- Before intrauterine transfusion, explain the procedure and its purpose. Before the transfusion, obtain a baseline fetal heart rate through electronic monitoring. Afterward, carefully observe the mother for uterine contractions and fluid leakage from the puncture site. Monitor fetal heart rate for tachycardia or bradycardia.
- During exchange transfusion, maintain the infant's body temperature by placing him under a heat lamp or overhead radiant warmer. Keep resuscitative and monitoring equipment handy, and warm blood before transfusion.
- Watch for complications of transfusion, such as lethargy, muscular twitching, convulsions, dark urine, edema, and change in vital signs. Watch for postexchange serum bilirubin levels that are usually 50% of preexchange levels (although these levels may rise to 70% to 80% of preexchange levels due to rebound effect). Within 30 minutes of transfusion, bilirubin may rebound, requiring repeat exchange transfusions.
- Measure intake and output. Observe for cord bleeding and complications, such as hemorrhage, hypocalcemia, sepsis, and shock. Report serum bilirubin and hemoglobin levels.
- To promote normal parental bonding, encourage parents to visit and to help care for the infant as often as possible.
- To prevent hemolytic disease in the newborn, evaluate all pregnant females for possible Rh incompatibility. Administer Rh_o (D) I.M., as ordered, to all Rh-negative, antibody-negative females following transfusion reaction or ectopic pregnancy, or during the second and third trimesters to patients with abruptio placentae, placenta previa, or amniocentesis.

Selected References

Andreyko, J.L., et al. "Results of Conservative Management of Premature Rupture of Membranes," *American Journal of Obstetrics and Gynecology* 148(5):600-04, March 1, 1984.

Bobak, Irene M., and Jensen, Margaret D. *Essentials of Maternity Nursing*. St. Louis: C.V. Mosby Co., 1984.

Brooten, Dorothy A., et al. "A Comparison of Four Treatments to Prevent and Control Breast Pain and Engorgement in Nonnursing Mothers," *Nursing Research* 32(4):225-29, July/August 1983.

Cashore, William J., and Oh, William. "Neonatal Jaundice. Exchange Transfusion, Phototherapy, or Observation?" *Consultant* 23(12):51-57, December 1983.

Holbrook, R.H., Jr., and Creasy, R.K. "Prevention of Preterm Delivery. The Important Role of Early Recognition," *Postgraduate Medicine* 75(8)177-85, June 1984.

Leach, Lynette, and Sproule, Valerie. "Meeting the Challenge of Cesarean Births," *Journal of Obstetric-Gynecologic-Neonatal Nursing* 13(3):191-95, May/June 1984.

McGregor, J., et al. "An Epidemic of 'Childbed Fever'," *American Journal of Obstetrics and Gynecology* 150(4):385-88, October 15, 1984.

Shortridge, L.A. "Using Ritodrine Hydrochloride to Inhibit Preterm Labor," *Journal of Maternal-Child Nursing* 8(1):58-61, January/February 1983.

16 Sexual Disorders

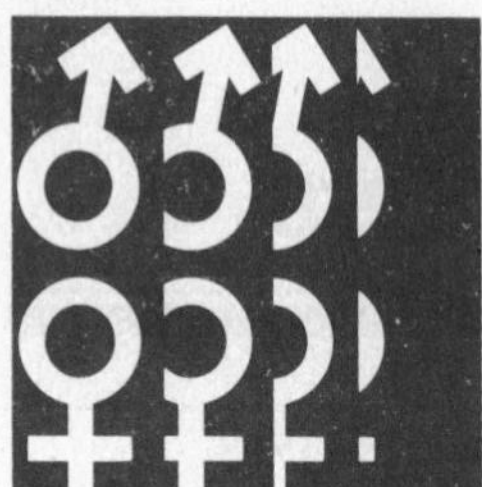

Sexual Disorders

Introduction

Sexuality is an integral human function that is inevitably colored and influenced by a host of interrelated factors. Its expression reflects the interaction of all the biological, psychological, and sociologic factors that affect a person's self-image and behavior.

Depending on these complex factors, human sexuality can be healthy and enriching, or it can be the source of mental and physical distress. J.W. Maddock, in *Postgraduate Medicine,* defines a sexually healthy person as one who meets the following criteria:

- His behavior agrees with his gender identity (persistent feeling of oneself as male or female).
- He can participate in a potentially loving or committed relationship.
- He finds erotic stimulation pleasurable.
- He can make decisions about his sexual behavior that are compatible with his values and beliefs.

Hazards to sexual health

An important group of sexually related disorders results from infection that is transmitted through sexual contact. These disorders include gonorrhea, syphilis, genital herpes, genital warts, trichomoniasis, chancroid, lymphogranuloma venereum, and nonspecific genitourinary infections caused by chlamydial, corynebacterial, or mycoplasmal organisms. Venereal diseases are among the most prevalent infections worldwide; gonorrhea and genital herpes are now reaching almost epidemic proportions in the United States.

Other sexually related disorders affect an individual's sexual ability or response and can have physical or psychological causes. In the female, such disorders are usually orgasmic dysfunction; in the male, erectile dysfunction.

Disorders of sexual behavior are more properly classified as psychiatric problems. These disorders, known as paraphilias, include voyeurism, exhibitionism, transvestitism, fetishism, masochism, sadism, necrophilia, pedophilia, and incest.

Physical assessment first

Physical assessment, primarily a diagnostic tool, can also serve as an excellent opportunity for patient teaching.

- During examination of the female, evaluate breast development (symmetry, contour, size), pubic hair distribution, and the development of external genitalia. Use a speculum to examine internal genitalia, including the cervix and vagina. Palpate the uterus and ovaries.
- During examination of the male, check pubic and axillary hair distribution. With a gloved hand, palpate the penis, scrotum, prostate gland, and rectum. Inspect the penis (shaft, glans, urethral

meatus) for lesions, swelling, inflammation, scars, or discharge. In the uncircumcised male, retract the foreskin to visualize the glans. Examine the scrotum for size, shape, and abnormalities, such as nodules or inflammation. Check for the presence of both testes (the left testis is often lower than the right).

PRODUCTION OF SPERMATOZOA

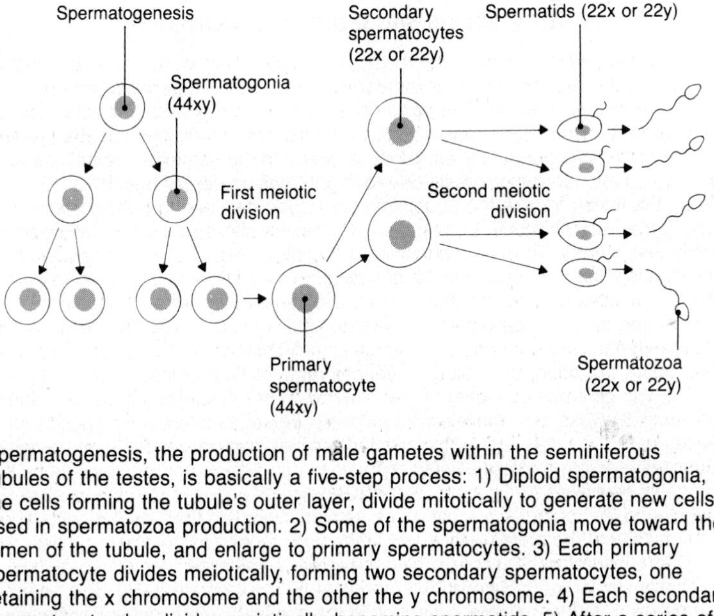

Spermatogenesis, the production of male gametes within the seminiferous tubules of the testes, is basically a five-step process: 1) Diploid spermatogonia, the cells forming the tubule's outer layer, divide mitotically to generate new cells used in spermatozoa production. 2) Some of the spermatogonia move toward the lumen of the tubule, and enlarge to primary spermatocytes. 3) Each primary spermatocyte divides meiotically, forming two secondary spermatocytes, one retaining the x chromosome and the other the y chromosome. 4) Each secondary spermatocyte also divides meiotically, becoming spermatids. 5) After a series of structural changes, the spermatids develop into mature spermatozoa.

MALE GENITALIA

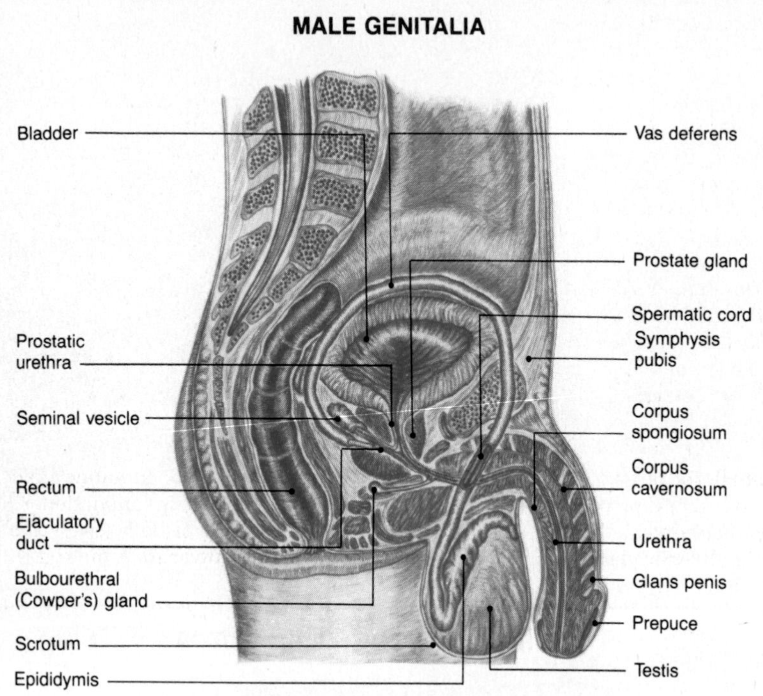

REVIEW OF MALE SEXUAL ANATOMY

The *scrotum,* which contains the testes, epididymis, and lower spermatic cords, maintains the proper testicular temperature for spermatogenesis through relaxation and contraction. The *penis* consists of three cylinders of erectile tissue: two corpora cavernosa, and the corpus spongiosum, which contains the urethra.

The *testes* (gonads, testicles) produce sperm in the seminiferous tubules, with complete spermatogenesis developing in most males by age 15 or 16. In the fetus, the testes form in the abdominal cavity and descend into the scrotum during the seventh month of gestation. The testes also secrete hormones, especially testosterone, in the interstitial cells (Leydig's cells). Testosterone affects the development and maintenance of secondary sex characteristics and sex drive. It also regulates metabolism, stimulates protein anabolism (encouraging skeletal growth and muscular development), inhibits pituitary secretion of the gonadotropins (follicle-stimulating hormone and interstitial cell-stimulating hormone), promotes potassium excretion, and mildly influences renal sodium reabsorption.

The *vas deferens* connects the *epididymis,* in which sperm mature and ripen for up to 6 weeks, and the *ejaculatory ducts.* (Vasectomy achieves sterilization by severing the vas deferens.) The *seminal vesicles,* two convoluted membranous pouches, secrete a viscous liquid of fructose-rich semen and prostaglandins that probably facilitates fertilization. The *prostate gland* secretes the thin alkaline substance that comprises most of the seminal fluid; this fluid also protects sperm from acidity in the male urethra and in the vagina, increasing sperm motility.

The *bulbourethral* (Cowper's) *glands* secrete an alkaline preejaculatory fluid, probably similar in function to that produced by the prostate gland. The *spermatic cords* are cylindrical fibrous coverings in the inguinal canal, containing the vas deferens, blood vessels, and nerves.

Sexual assessment: The history

Careful assessment helps identify the cause of a sexual problem as psychological or physical. A sexual history provides the basis for diagnosis and treatment, and may even prove informative and therapeutic to the patient.

- Ensure privacy, as for physical assessment. Allow sufficient time so the patient doesn't feel rushed.
- Approach a sexual history objectively. Remember, sexual health is relative; avoid making assumptions or judgments about the patient's sexual activities. Don't overreact to what the patient says.
- After listening to the patient, determine his level of sexual understanding, and phrase your questions in language he understands. Avoid technical terms, but don't talk down to him.
- Begin with the least threatening questions. Often, a menstrual or urologic history helps lead into a sexual history.
- Watch for clues to life-style and important life events that could predispose the patient to sexual problems.
- During the sexual history, be sensitive to nonverbal behavior that may provide clues to the patient's degree of trust, candor, understanding, and anxiety.
- Inquire about possible homosexual activity, a factor that can influence treatment of a condition such as gonorrhea.
- Ask the female patient if she has adequate lubrication during intercourse and if she has ever experienced orgasm or pain with sexual contact. Ask the male patient if he's ever had difficulties with erection or ejaculation.
- Ask about any current or past contraceptive practices.
- Try to utilize the history therapeutically by encouraging the patient to express his anxiety. Occasionally, these fears may be alleviated simply by providing factual information. Answer any questions the patient may have.

Therapy varies

Sex therapy can be a vital therapeutic tool for treating sexual dysfunctions. Before psychotherapy begins, history, physical examination, and appropriate treatment must rule out organic causes of sexual dysfunction. The major forms of sex therapy include psychoanalysis, behavioral therapy, group therapy, classic (Masters and Johnson) therapy, and Kaplan's sex therapy. The sex therapy appropriate to the patient depends on his problems, needs, and finances.

SEXUALLY TRANSMITTED DISEASES

Gonorrhea

A common venereal disease, gonorrhea is an infection of the genitourinary tract (especially the urethra and cervix) and, occasionally, the rectum, pharynx, and eyes. Untreated gonorrhea can spread through the blood to the joints, tendons, meninges, and endocardium; in females, it can also lead to chronic pelvic inflammatory disease (PID) and sterility. After adequate treatment, prognosis in both males and females is excellent, although reinfection is common. Incidence of gonorrhea is especially prevalent among unmarried persons and young people, particularly between ages 19 and 25.

Causes

Transmission of *Neisseria gonorrhoeae,* the organism that causes gonorrhea, almost exclusively follows sexual contact with an infected person. Children born of infected mothers can contract gonococcal ophthalmia neonatorum during passage through the birth canal. Children and adults with gonorrhea can contract gonococcal conjunctivitis by touching their eyes with contaminated hands.

Signs and symptoms

Although some infected males may be asymptomatic, after a 3- to 6-day incubation period, most develop symptoms of urethritis, including dysuria and purulent urethral discharge, with redness and swelling at the site of infection. Most infected females remain asymptomatic but may develop inflammation and a greenish-yellow discharge from the cervix—the most common gonorrheal symptoms in females. Other clinical features vary according to the site involved:

- *urethra:* dysuria, urinary frequency and incontinence, purulent discharge, itching, red and edematous meatus
- *vulva:* occasional itching, burning, and pain due to exudate from an adjacent infected area. Vulval symptoms tend to be more severe before puberty or after menopause.
- *vagina* (most common site in children over age 1): engorgement, redness, swelling, and profuse purulent discharge
- *pelvis:* severe pelvic and lower abdominal pain, muscular rigidity, tenderness, and abdominal distention. As the infection spreads, nausea, vomiting, fever, and tachycardia may develop in patients with salpingitis or PID.
- *liver:* right upper quadrant pain in patients with perihepatitis.

Other possible symptoms include pharyngitis, tonsillitis, and rectal burning, itching, and bloody mucopurulent discharge.

Gonococcal septicemia is more common in females than in males. Its characteristic signs include tender papillary skin lesions on the hands and feet; these lesions may be pustular, hemorrhagic, or necrotic. Gonococcal septicemia may also produce migratory polyarthralgia, and polyarthritis and tenosynovitis of the wrists, fingers, knees, or ankles. Untreated septic arthritis leads to progressive joint destruction.

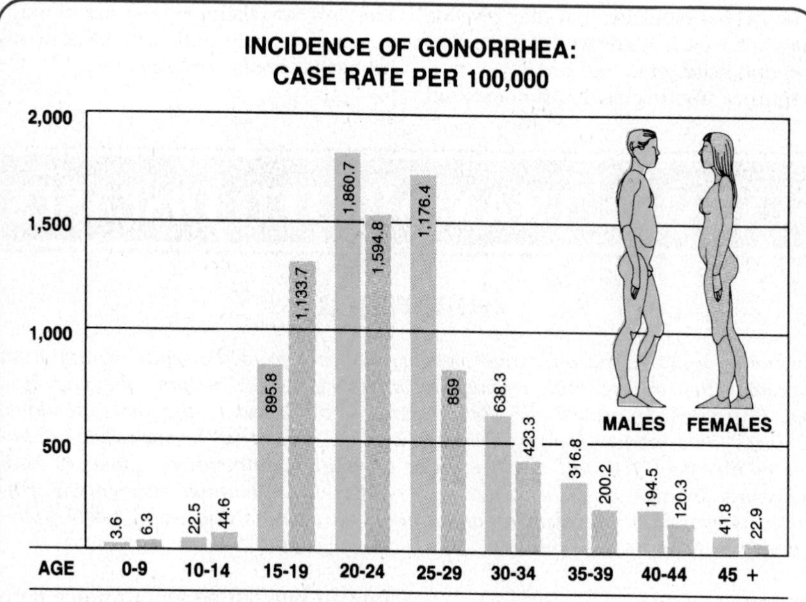

Source: *Sexually Transmitted Disease Statistics,* U.S. Dept. of Health and Human Services, Atlanta: Centers for Disease Control, 1984.

Signs of gonococcal ophthalmia neonatorum include lid edema, bilateral conjunctival infection, and abundant purulent discharge 2 to 3 days after birth. Adult conjunctivitis, most common in men, causes unilateral conjunctival redness and swelling. Untreated gonococcal conjunctivitis can progress to corneal ulceration and blindness.

Diagnosis

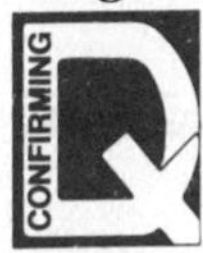

A culture from the site of infection (urethra, cervix, rectum, or pharynx), grown on a Thayer-Martin or Transgrow medium, usually establishes diagnosis by isolating the organism. A Gram stain showing gram-negative diplococci supports the diagnosis and may be sufficient to confirm gonorrhea in males.

Confirmation of gonococcal arthritis requires identification of gram-negative diplococci on smears made from joint fluid and skin lesions. Complement fixation and immunofluorescent assays of serum reveal antibody titers four times the normal rate. Culture of conjunctival scrapings confirms gonococcal conjunctivitis.

Treatment

Treatment of choice for uncomplicated gonorrhea (including gonorrhea during pregnancy) is 1 gram of probenecid P.O. to block penicillin excretion from the body, followed in 30 minutes by I.M. administration of 4.8 million units of aqueous procaine penicillin injected at two separate sites in a large muscle mass. If the patient is allergic to penicillin, tetracycline P.O. (contraindicated in pregnant women) or spectinomycin I.M. may be substituted.

Gonorrhea complicated by severe PID or septicemia requires I.V. antibiotic therapy with doxycycline and cefoxitin, for 4 to 6 days, followed by doxycycline P.O. for an additional 4 to 6 days. Outpatient therapy may consist of cefoxitin I.M., amoxicillin P.O., or ampicillin P.O., each with probenecid, followed by doxycycline P.O. for 10 to 14 days. Treatment of gonococcal conjunctivitis requires I.V. administration of penicillin G, accompanied by irrigation of the eye with penicillin G and saline solution.

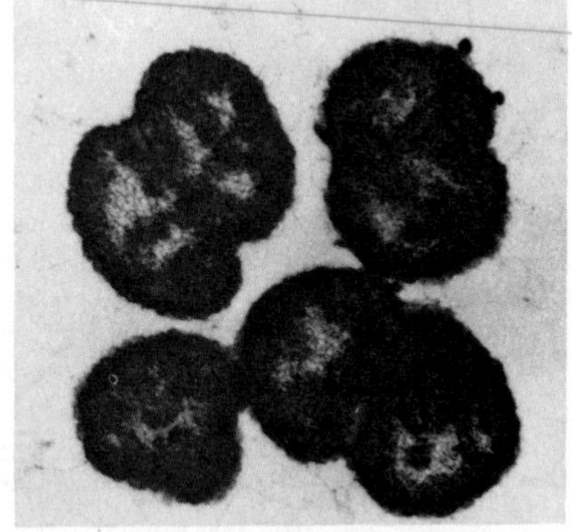

In gonorrhea, microscopic examination reveals gram-negative diplococcus—*Neisseria gonorrhoeae,* the causative organism.

To confirm cure of gonococcal infection, follow-up cultures are necessary 4 to 7 days after treatment and again in 6 months, or, in pregnant females, before delivery.

Routine instillation of 1% silver nitrate or erythromycin drops into the eyes of newborns has greatly reduced the incidence of gonococcal ophthalmia neonatorum.

Special considerations

- Before treatment, establish whether the patient has any drug sensitivities, especially to penicillin, and watch closely for drug reactions during therapy. Be prepared to treat anaphylaxis after parenteral administration of penicillin.
- Warn the patient that until cultures prove negative, he is still infectious and can transmit gonococcal infection. Double bag all soiled dressings and contaminated instruments; wear gloves when handling contaminated material and giving patient care. If the patient is being treated as an outpatient, advise the family to take precautions against infection. Isolate the patient with eye infection.
- In the patient with gonococcal ar-

thritis, apply moist heat to ease pain in affected joints.

- Urge the patient to inform sexual contacts of his infection so they can seek treatment also. Report all cases to the local public health authorities for follow-up on sexual contacts. Examine and test all persons exposed to gonorrhea, and children of infected mothers.
- Routinely instill two drops of 1% silver nitrate or erythromycin in the eyes of all newborns immediately after birth. Check newborns of infected mothers for signs of infection. Take specimens for culture from the infant's eyes, pharynx, and rectum.
- To prevent gonorrhea, tell patients to avoid anyone *suspected* of being infected, to use condoms during intercourse, and to avoid sharing washcloths or douche equipment.

Chlamydial Infections

Chlamydial infections—including urethritis in men, cervicitis in women, and lymphogranuloma venereum (LGV) in both—comprise a group of infections that are linked to one organism: Chlamydia trachomatis. *Such infections are the most common sexually transmitted diseases in the United States, afflicting an estimated 3 million Americans each year. Trachoma inclusion conjunctivitis, a chlamydial infection that occurs rarely in the United States, is a leading cause of blindness in Third World countries.*

Untreated, chlamydial infections can lead to such complications as acute epididymitis, salpingitis, pelvic inflammatory disease, and, eventually, sterility. In pregnant women, chlamydial infections are also associated with spontaneous abortion, premature delivery, and neonatal death, although a direct link with C. trachomatis *hasn't been established.*

Causes

Transmission of *C. trachomatis* primarily follows mucosal contact with an infected person. Because symptoms of many chlamydial infections don't appear until late in the course of the disease, sexual transmission of the organism often occurs unknowingly.

Children born of infected mothers may contract associated trachoma inclusion conjunctivitis, otitis media, and pneumonia during passage through the birth canal.

Signs and symptoms

Both men and women with chlamydial infections may be asymptomatic or may show signs of infection on physical examination. Individual signs and symptoms vary with the specific type of chlamydial infection and are determined by the organism's route of transmission to susceptible tissue.

The primary lesion of *LGV*—a painless vesicle or nonindurated ulcer, 2 to 3 mm in diameter—often goes unnoticed. After 1 to 4 weeks, regional lymphadenopathy develops, followed by inguinal lymph node swelling about 2 weeks later. Systemic symptoms, such as myalgia, headache, fever, chills, backache, and weight loss, may also occur.

In men with LGV, enlarged inguinal lymph nodes may become fluctuant, tender masses. Regional nodes draining the initial lesion may enlarge and appear as a series of bilateral buboes. Untreated buboes rupture and form sinus tracts that discharge a thick, yellow, granular secretion. Eventually, a scar forms or an indurated inguinal mass develops.

Women with LGV may develop iliac and sacral lymphatic obstruction, causing perineal edema. Occasionally, women develop genitoanorectal syndrome—characterized by mucopurulent rectal discharge and bloody diarrhea—which may be complicated by secondary bacterial infection. The rectal mucosa becomes edematous, ulcerated, and friable. Extensive cutaneous keloidal scarring often causes rectovaginal fistulas, rectal strictures, and perirectal abscesses.

In *proctitis*, patients may experience diarrhea, tenesmus, pruritus, bloody or mucopurulent discharge, and diffuse or discrete ulceration in the rectosigmoid colon.

In *cervicitis*, women may develop cervical erosion, mucopurulent discharge, pelvic pain, and dyspareunia. *Endometritis* or *salpingitis* may produce signs of pelvic inflammatory disease, such as pain and tenderness of the abdomen, cervix, uterus, and lymph nodes; chills; fever; vaginal discharge; and dysuria. Women with *urethral syndrome* may experience dysuria, pyuria, and urinary frequency.

In *epididymitis*, men may experience painful scrotal swelling and urethral discharge. Men with *prostatitis* may have lower back pain, urinary frequency, dysuria, nocturia, urethral discharge, and painful ejaculation. Men with *urethritis* may experience dysuria, erythema, tenderness of the urethral meatus, urinary frequency, pruritus, and urethral discharge, which may be copious and purulent or scant and clear or mucoid.

Diagnosis

Laboratory tests provide definitive diagnosis of individual chlamydial infections.

A swab culture from the site of infection (urethra, cervix, rectum) usually establishes diagnosis of urethritis, cervicitis, salpingitis, endometritis, and proctitis. Culture of aspirated blood, pus, or cerebrospinal fluid establishes diagnosis of epididymitis, prostatitis, and LGV. If the infection site is accessible, the doctor may first attempt direct visualization of cell scrapings or exudate with Giemsa stain or fluorescein-conjugated monoclonal antibodies, although tissue cell cultures are generally more sensitive and specific.

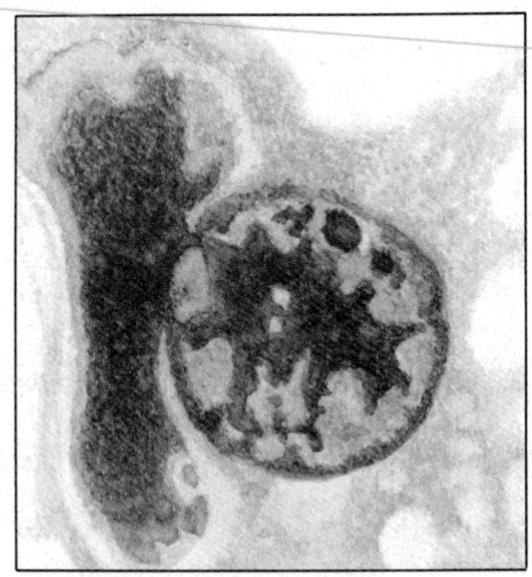

In chlamydial infections, microscopic examination reveals *Chlamydia trachomatis,* a unicellular parasite with a rigid cell wall.

Serologic tests to determine previous exposure to *C. trachomatis* include complement fixation and microimmunofluorescence (Micro IF) tests. Although the enzyme-linked immunosorbent assay is as effective as the Micro IF test at detecting *C. trachomatis* antibody, its value is uncertain.

Treatment

Recommended treatment is tetracycline, given P.O. for 7 to 21 days, or erythromycin or sulfamethoxazole, given P.O. for at least 7 days. Patients with LGV require extended treatment. In pregnant women with chlamydial infections, erythromycin (stearate base) is the treatment of choice, because of the adverse effects of tetracycline and sulfonamides on fetal growth and development.

Special considerations

- To prevent contracting a chlamydial infection, double-bag all soiled dressings and contaminated instruments, and wear gloves when handling contaminated material and giving patient care.
- Make sure the patient understands dosage requirements of prescribed med-

ications. Stress the importance of completing the course of drug therapy even after symptoms subside.

- To prevent reinfection during treatment, urge abstinence from intercourse or encourage use of condoms.
- Urge the patient to inform sexual contacts of his infection so they can seek treatment also. Report all cases to the local public health authorities for follow-up on sexual contacts.
- Check newborns of infected mothers for signs of infection. Take specimens for culture from the infant's eyes, nasopharynx, and rectum. (Positive rectal cultures will peak by 5 to 6 weeks postpartum.)

Genital Herpes

(Venereal herpes)

Genital herpes is an acute, inflammatory disease of the genitalia, resulting from infection with herpes simplex II virus. This infection is one of the most common recurring disorders of the genitalia. Prognosis varies according to the patient's age, the strength of his immune defenses, and the infection site. Primary genital herpes is usually self-limiting but may cause painful local or systemic disease. In newborns, in patients with weak immune defenses, and in those with disseminated disease, genital herpes is often severe, with complications and a high mortality.

Causes

Genital herpes is usually transmitted through sexual contact, but contamination from infected toilet seats, towels, and bathtubs also occurs. Pregnant females may transmit the infection to newborns during vaginal delivery. Such transmitted infection may be localized (for instance, in the eyes) or disseminated and may be associated with CNS involvement.

Signs and symptoms

After a 3- to 7-day incubation period, fluid-filled vesicles appear, usually on the cervix (the primary infection site) and, possibly, on the labia, perianal skin, vulva, or vagina of the female; on the glans penis, foreskin, or penile shaft of the male. Extragenital lesions may appear on the mouth or anus. In both males and females, the vesicles, usually painless at first, may rupture and develop into extensive, shallow, painful ulcers, creating redness, marked edema, and tender inguinal lymph nodes.

Other features of initial mucocutaneous infection include fever, malaise, dysuria, and, in the female, leukorrhea. Rare complications—which generally arise from extragenital lesions—include herpetic keratitis, which may lead to blindness, and potentially fatal herpetic encephalitis.

Diagnosis

Diagnosis is based on physical examination and patient history. Helpful (but nondiagnostic) measures include laboratory data showing increased antibody titers, smears of genital lesions showing atypical cells, and cytologic preparations (Tzank).

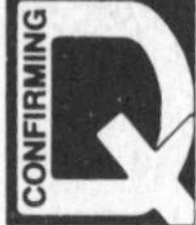

Diagnosis can be confirmed by demonstration of herpes simplex II virus in vesicular fluid, using tissue culture techniques.

Treatment

Acyclovir (Zovirax) has proven to be an effective treatment for genital herpes. Each of the three available dosage forms has a specific indication. A 5% acyclovir ointment is prescribed for first-time infections. I.V. administration may be required for patients who are hospitalized with severe genital herpes or who are immunocompromised and have potentially life-threatening herpes infections. Oral acyclovir may be prescribed for patients suffering from first-time infections or from recurrent outbreaks.

Special considerations

- Encourage the patient to get adequate rest and nutrition and to keep the lesions dry, except for applying prescribed medications using aseptic technique.
- Encourage the patient to avoid sexual intercourse during the active stage of this disease (while lesions are present). Urge the patient to seek medical examination for herpes for sexual partners.
- Advise the female patient to have a Pap smear taken every 6 months.
- Explain to the infected pregnant patient the risk to her newborn from vaginal delivery. Urge her to consider cesarean delivery.
- Refer patients to Herpes Resource Center, an American Social Health Association group, for support.

Genital Warts

(Venereal warts, condylomata acuminata)

Genital warts consist of papillomas, with fibrous tissue overgrowth from the dermis and thickened epithelial coverings. They are uncommon before puberty or after menopause.

Causes

Genital warts are usually transmitted through sexual contact and may result from the same papillomavirus that causes the common wart (verruca vulgaris). Genital warts grow rapidly in the presence of heavy perspiration, poor hygiene, or pregnancy; they often accompany other genital infections.

Signs and symptoms

After a 1- to 6-month incubation period (usually 2 months), genital warts develop on moist surfaces: in males, on the subpreputial sac, within the urethral meatus, and, less commonly, on the penile shaft; in females, on the vulva and on vaginal and cervical walls; in both sexes, papillomas spread to the perineum and the perianal area. These painless warts start as tiny red or pink swellings that grow (sometimes to 4" [10 cm]) and become pedunculated. Typically, multiple swellings give such warts a cauliflower appearance. If infected, these lesions become malodorous.

Diagnosis

Dark-field examination of scrapings from wart cells shows marked vascularization of epidermal cells, which helps to differentiate genital warts from condylomata lata.

Treatment

The initial goal of treatment is to eradicate associated genital infections. The warts may resolve spontaneously, but if treatment is necessary, topical drug therapy (20% podophyllum in tincture of benzoin or trichloroacetic acid) removes small warts. (Podophyllum is contraindicated in pregnancy.) Warts larger than 1" (2.5 cm) are generally removed by surgery, cryosurgery, electrocautery, or 5-fluorouracil cream debridement. Rarely, the patient's warts are excised and used to prepare a vaccine, which is then injected into the patient's body to try to create antibodies. Carbon dioxide laser treatment has also been proven effective.

Special considerations

- Tell the patient to wash off podophyllum with soap and water 4 to 6 hours after applying it. Recommend use of a condom during intercourse until healing is complete. Advise the patient to protect the surrounding tissue with petrolatum before using trichloroacetic acid.

• Emphasize other preventive measures, such as avoiding sex with an infected partner and regularly washing genitalia with soap and water. To prevent vaginal infection, advise the female patient to avoid feminine hygiene sprays, frequent douching, tight pants, nylon underpants, or panty hose.

• Encourage examination of the patient's sexual partners. Also advise female patients to have a Pap smear taken every 6 months.

Syphilis

A chronic, infectious, venereal disease, syphilis begins in the mucous membranes and quickly becomes systemic, spreading to nearby lymph nodes and the bloodstream. This disease, when untreated, is characterized by progressive stages: primary, secondary, latent, and late (formerly called tertiary). About 25,000 cases of syphilis, in primary and secondary stages, are reported annually in the United States, making it the third most prevalent reportable infectious disease. Incidence is highest among urban populations, especially in persons between ages 15 and 39. Untreated syphilis leads to crippling or death, but prognosis is excellent with early treatment.

Causes

Infection from the spirochete *Treponema pallidum* causes syphilis. Transmission occurs primarily through sexual contact during the primary, secondary, and early latent stages of infection. Prenatal transmission from an infected mother to her fetus is also possible.

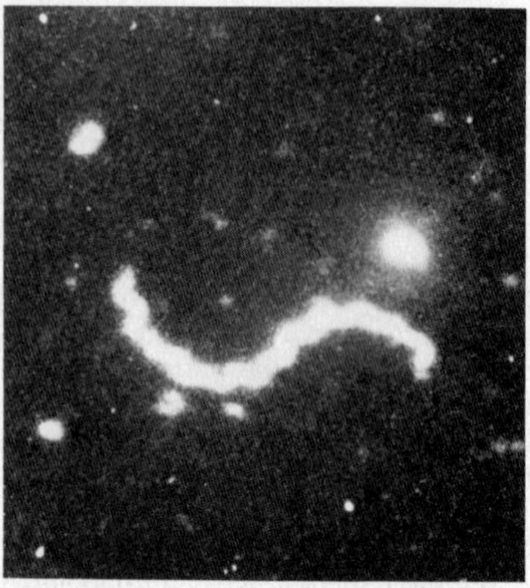

In syphilis, a dark-field examination that shows spiral-shaped bacterial organisms—*Treponema pallidum*—confirms diagnosis.

Signs and symptoms

Primary syphilis develops after an incubation period that generally lasts about 3 weeks. Initially, one or more chancres (small, fluid-filled lesions) erupt on the genitalia; others may erupt on the anus, fingers, lips, tongue, nipples, tonsils, or eyelids. These chancres, which are usually painless, start as papules and then erode; they have indurated, raised edges and clear bases. Chancres typically disappear after 3 to 6 weeks, even when untreated. They are usually associated with regional lymphadenopathy (unilateral or bilateral). In females, chancres are often overlooked because they often develop on internal structures—the cervix or the vaginal wall.

The development of symmetric mucocutaneous lesions and general lymphadenopathy signals the onset of *secondary syphilis,* which may develop within a few days or up to 8 weeks after onset of initial chancres. The rash of secondary syphilis can be macular, papular, pustular, or nodular. Lesions are of uniform size, well defined, and generalized. Macules often erupt between rolls of fat on the trunk and, proximally, on the arms, palms, soles, face, and scalp. In warm, moist areas (perineum, scrotum, vulva, between rolls of fat), the lesions enlarge and erode, producing highly contagious, pink, or grayish-white lesions (condylomata lata).

Mild constitutional symptoms of syphilis appear in the second stage, and may include headache, malaise, anorexia, weight loss, nausea, vomiting, sore throat, and possibly, slight fever. Alopecia may occur, with or without treatment, and is usually temporary. Nails become brittle and pitted.

Latent syphilis is characterized by an absence of clinical symptoms but a reactive serologic test for syphilis. Since infectious mucocutaneous lesions may reappear when infection is of less than 4 years' duration, early latent syphilis is considered contagious. Approximately two thirds of patients remain asymptomatic in the late latent stage, until death. The rest develop characteristic late-stage symptoms.

Late syphilis is the final, destructive but noninfectious stage of the disease. It has three subtypes, any or all of which may affect the patient: late benign syphilis, cardiovascular syphilis, and neurosyphilis. The lesions of late benign syphilis develop between 1 and 10 years after infection. They may appear on the skin, bones, mucous membranes, upper respiratory tract, liver, or stomach. The typical lesion is a gumma—a chronic, superficial nodule or deep, granulomatous lesion that is solitary, asymmetric, painless, and indurated. Gummas can be found on any bone—particularly the long bones of the legs—and in any organ. If late syphilis involves the liver, it can cause epigastric pain, tenderness, enlarged spleen, and anemia; if it involves the upper respiratory tract, it may cause perforation of the nasal septum or the palate. In severe cases, late benign syphilis results in destruction of bones or organs, which eventually causes death.

Cardiovascular syphilis develops about 10 years after the initial infection in approximately 10% of patients with late, untreated syphilis. It causes fibrosis of elastic tissue of the aorta and leads to aortitis, most often in the ascending and transverse sections of the aortic arch. Cardiovascular syphilis may be asymptomatic or may cause aortic regurgitation or aneurysm.

Symptoms of neurosyphilis develop in about 8% of patients with late, untreated syphilis and appear from 5 to 35 years after infection. These clinical effects consist of meningitis and widespread CNS damage that may include general paresis, personality changes, and arm and leg weakness.

Diagnosis

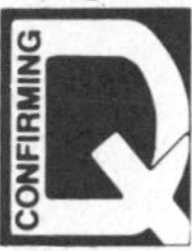

Identifying *T. pallidum* from a lesion on dark-field examination provides immediate diagnosis of syphilis. This method is most effective when moist lesions are present, as in primary, secondary, and prenatal syphilis. The Fluorescent Treponemal Antibody-Absorption (FTA-ABS) test identifies antigens of *T. pallidum* in tissue, ocular fluid, CSF, tracheobronchial secretions, and exudates from lesions. This is the most sensitive test available for detecting syphilis in all stages. Once reactive, it remains so permanently. Other appropriate procedures include the following:

• *Venereal Disease Research Laboratory* (VDRL) *slide test* and *Rapid Plasma Reagin* (RPR) *test* detect nonspecific antibodies. Both tests, if positive, become reactive within 1 to 2 weeks after the primary lesion appears, or 4 to 5 weeks after the infection begins.

• *CSF examination* identifies neurosyphilis when total protein level is above 40 mg/100 ml, VDRL slide test is reactive, and cell count exceeds five mononuclear cells/mm^3.

Treatment

Treatment of choice is administration of penicillin I.M. For early syphilis, treatment may consist of a single injection of penicillin G benzathine I.M. (2.4 million

PRENATAL SYPHILIS

A woman can transmit syphilis transplacentally to her unborn child throughout pregnancy. This type of syphilis is often called congenital, but prenatal is a more accurate term. Approximately 50% of infected fetuses die before or shortly after birth. Prognosis is better for infants who develop overt infection after age 2.

The infant with prenatal syphilis may appear healthy at birth, but usually develops characteristic lesions—vesicular, bullous eruptions, often on the palms and soles—3 weeks later. Shortly afterward, a maculopapular rash similar to that in secondary syphilis may erupt on the face, mouth, genitalia, palms, or soles. Condylomata lata often occur around the anus. Lesions may erupt on the mucous membranes of the mouth, pharynx, and nose. When the infant's larynx is affected, his cry becomes weak and forced. If the nasal mucous membranes are involved, he may also develop nasal discharge, which can be slight and mucopurulent or copious with blood-tinged pus. Visceral and bone lesions, liver or spleen enlargement with ascites, and nephrotic syndrome may also develop.

Late prenatal syphilis becomes apparent after age 2; it may be identifiable only through blood studies or may cause unmistakable syphilitic changes: screwdriver-shaped central incisors, deformed molars or cusps, thick clavicles, saber shins, bowed tibias, nasal septum perforation, eighth nerve deafness, and neurosyphilis.

In the infant with prenatal syphilis, VDRL titer, if reactive at birth, stays the same or rises, indicating active disease. The infant's titer drops in 3 months if the mother has received effective prenatal treatment. Absolute diagnosis necessitates dark-field examination of umbilical vein blood or lesion drainage.

An infant with abnormal CSF may be treated with aqueous crystalline penicillin G, I.M. or I.V., (50,000 units/kg of body weight/day divided in two doses for at least 10 days), or aqueous penicillin G procaine I.M. (50,000 units/kg of body weight/day for at least 10 days). An infant with normal CSF may be treated with a single injection of penicillin G benzathine (50,000 units/kg of body weight). When caring for a child with prenatal syphilis, record the extent of the rash, and watch for signs of systemic involvement, especially laryngeal swelling, jaundice, and decreasing urinary output.

units). Syphilis of more than 1 year's duration should be treated with penicillin G benzathine I.M. (2.4 million units/week for 3 weeks).

Patients who are allergic to penicillin may be treated successfully with tetracycline or erythromycin (in either case, 500 mg P.O. four times a day for 15 days for early syphilis; 30 days, for late infections). Tetracycline is contraindicated in pregnant females.

Special considerations

- Make sure the patient clearly understands the dosage schedule for medication.
- Stress the importance of completing the course of therapy even after symptoms subside.
- Check for history of drug sensitivity before administering the first dose. Promote rest and adequate nutrition.
- In secondary syphilis, keep lesions clean and dry. If they're draining, dispose of contaminated materials properly.
- In late syphilis, provide symptomatic care during prolonged treatment.
- In cardiovascular syphilis, check for signs of decreased cardiac output (decreased urinary output, hypoxia, decreased sensorium) and pulmonary congestion.
- In neurosyphilis, regularly check level of consciousness, mood, and coherence. Watch for signs of ataxia.
- Urge patients to seek VDRL testing after 3, 6, 12, and 24 months to detect possible relapse. Patients treated for la-

tent or late syphilis should receive blood tests at 6-month intervals for 2 years.

- Be sure to report all cases of syphilis to local public health authorities. Urge the patient to inform sexual partners of his infection so they can receive treatment also.

Trichomoniasis

A protozoal infection of the lower genitourinary tract, trichomoniasis affects about 15% of sexually active females and 10% of sexually active males. Incidence is worldwide. In females, the condition may be acute or chronic. Recurrence of trichomoniasis is minimized when sexual partners are treated concurrently.

Causes

Trichomonas vaginalis—a tetraflagellated, motile protozoan—causes trichomoniasis in females by infecting the vagina, the urethra, and, possibly, the endocervix, Bartholin's glands, Skene's glands, or the bladder; in males, it infects the lower urethra and, possibly, the prostate gland, seminal vesicles, or the epididymis.

T. vaginalis grows best when the vaginal mucosa is more alkaline than normal (pH about 5.5 to 5.8). Therefore, factors that raise the vaginal pH—use of oral contraceptives, pregnancy, bacterial overgrowth, exudative cervical or vaginal lesions, or frequent douching, which disturbs lactobacilli that normally live in the vagina and maintain acidity—may predispose to trichomoniasis.

Trichomoniasis is usually transmitted by intercourse; less often, by contaminated douche equipment or moist washcloths. Occasionally, the newborn of an infected mother develops the condition through vaginal delivery.

Signs and symptoms

Approximately 70% of females—including those with chronic infections—and most males with trichomoniasis are asymptomatic. In females, acute infection may produce variable signs, such as a gray or greenish-yellow and possibly profuse and frothy, malodorous vaginal discharge. Its other effects include severe itching, redness, swelling, tenderness, dyspareunia, dysuria, urinary frequency, and, occasionally, postcoital spotting, menorrhagia, or dysmenorrhea.

Such symptoms may persist for a week to several months and may be more pronounced just after menstruation or during pregnancy. If trichomoniasis is untreated, symptoms may subside, although *T. vaginalis* infection persists, possibly associated with an abnormal cytologic smear of the cervix.

In males, trichomoniasis may produce mild to severe transient urethritis, possibly with dysuria and frequency.

Diagnosis

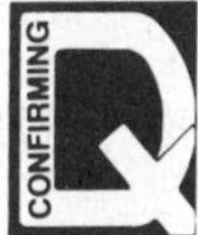

Direct microscopic examination of vaginal or seminal discharge is decisive when it reveals *T. vaginalis*, a motile, pear-shaped organism. Examination of clear urine specimens may also reveal *T. vaginalis*.

Physical examination of symptomatic females shows vaginal erythema; edema; frank excoriation; a frothy, malodorous, greenish-yellow vaginal discharge; and, rarely, a thin, gray pseudomembrane over the vagina. Cervical examination demonstrates punctate cervical hemorrhages, giving the cervix a strawberry appearance that is almost pathognomonic for this disorder.

Treatment

Metronidazole P.O., given to both sexual partners, effectively cures trichomoniasis. Metronidazole may be given in small doses for 7 days, or in a single, large dose. For females, a mild douche with a vinegar and water solution may help acidify vaginal pH.

Acidifying or antiseptic douches are useful to relieve symptoms in pregnant females with trichomoniasis. Such douches may minimize the extent of infection if used promptly. Metronidazole P.O. hasn't proven safe during pregnancy, especially in the first trimester. Pregnant patients may insert clotrimazole vaginal tablets at bedtime for 7 days.

After treatment, both sexual partners require a follow-up examination to check for residual signs of infection.

Special considerations

- Instruct the patient not to douche before being examined for trichomoniasis.
- To help prevent reinfection during treatment, urge abstinence from intercourse, or encourage the use of condoms. Tell the patient to use an acidic douche each day of treatment and to avoid using tampons.
- Warn the patient to abstain from alcoholic beverages while taking metronidazole, since alcohol consumption may provoke a disulfiram-type reaction (confusion, headache, cramps, vomiting, convulsions). Also, tell the patient this drug may turn urine dark brown.
- Caution the patient to avoid over-the-counter douches and vaginal sprays, since chronic use can alter vaginal pH.
- Tell the patient she can reduce the risk of genitourinary bacterial growth by wearing loose-fitting, cotton underwear that allows ventilation; bacteria flourish in a warm, dark, moist environment.
- To prevent newborns from contracting trichomoniasis, make sure pregnant females with this infection receive adequate treatment before delivery.

Chancroid

(Soft chancre)

Chancroid is a venereal disease characterized by painful genital ulcers and inguinal adenitis. This infection occurs worldwide but is particularly common in tropical countries; it affects males more often than females. Chancroidal lesions may heal spontaneously and usually respond well to treatment in the absence of secondary infections.

Causes

Chancroid results from *Hemophilus ducreyi,* a short, nonmotile, gram-negative streptobacillus. Poor personal hygiene may predispose males—especially those who are uncircumcised—to this disease. Chancroid is transmitted through sexual contact.

Signs and symptoms

After a 3- to 5-day incubation period, a small papule appears at the site of entry, usually the groin or inner thigh; in the male, it may appear on the penis; in the female, on the vulva, vagina, or cervix. Occasionally, this papule may erupt on the tongue, lip, breast, or navel. Such a papule (more than one may appear) rapidly ulcerates, becoming painful, soft, and malodorous; bleeds easily; and produces pus. It is gray and shallow, with irregular edges, and measures up to 1″ (2.5 cm) in diameter. Within 2 to 3 weeks, inguinal adenitis develops, creating suppurated, inflamed nodes that may rupture into large ulcers or buboes. Headache and malaise occur in 50% of patients. During the healing stage, phimosis may develop.

Diagnosis

Gram stain smears of ulcer exudate or bubo aspirate are 50% reliable; blood agar cultures are 75% reliable. Biopsy confirms diagnosis but is reserved for resistant cases or when malignancy is suspected. Dark-field examination and serologic testing rule out other venereal diseases (genital herpes, syphilis, lymphogranuloma venereum), which cause similar ulcers.

Treatment
Co-trimoxazole usually cures chancroid within 2 weeks. An alternative to sulfonamides, erythromycin may prevent detection of coexisting syphilis. Aspiration of fluid-filled nodes helps prevent infection from spreading.

Special considerations
- Make sure the patient is not allergic to sulfonamides or any other prescribed drug before giving the initial dose.
- Instruct the patient not to apply creams, lotions, or oils on or near genitalia or on other lesion sites.
- Tell the patient to abstain from sexual contact until healing is complete (usually about 2 weeks after treatment begins) and to wash the genitalia daily with soap and water. Instruct uncircumcised males to retract the foreskin to thoroughly cleanse the glans penis.
- To prevent chancroid, advise patients to avoid sexual contact with infected persons, to use condoms during sexual activity, and to wash the genitalia with soap and water after sexual activity.

CHANCROIDAL LESION

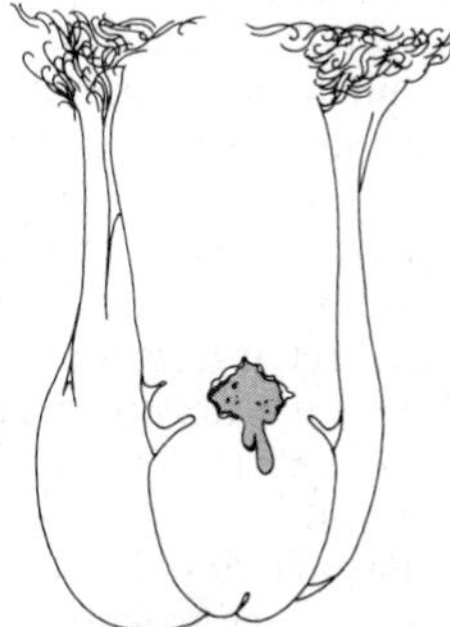

Chancroid produces a soft, painful chancre, similar to that of syphilis. Without treatment, it may progress to inguinal adenitis and formation of buboes.

Nonspecific Genitourinary Infections

Nonspecific genitourinary infections, including nongonococcal urethritis (NGU) in males and mild vaginitis or cervicitis in females, comprise a group of infections with similar manifestations that are not linked to a single organism. Such infections have become more prevalent since the mid-1960s and may be more widespread than gonorrhea. Prognosis is good if sexual partners are treated simultaneously.

Causes
In males, NGU often results from infection with *Chlamydia trachomatis* and *Ureaplasma urealyticum*. Such infection may also result from bacteria, such as staphylococci, diphtheroids, coliform organisms, and *Corynebacterium vaginale (Hemophilus vaginalis)*. Less frequently, infection may be related to preexisting strictures, neoplasms, and chemical or traumatic inflammation. Such infection spreads primarily through sexual intercourse.

Although less is known about nonspecific genitourinary infections in females, chlamydial or corynebacterial organisms may also cause these infections. A thin vaginal epithelium may predispose prepubertal and postmenopausal females to nonspecific vaginitis.

Signs and symptoms
NGU occurs 1 week to 1 month after coitus, with scant or moderate muco-

purulent urethral discharge, variable dysuria, and occasional hematuria. If untreated, NGU may lead to acute epididymitis. Subclinical urethritis may be found on physical examination, especially if the sex partner has a positive diagnosis.

Females with nonspecific genitourinary infections may experience persistent vaginal discharge, acute or recurrent cystitis for which no underlying cause can be found, or cervicitis with inflammatory erosion.

Both males and females with nonspecific genitourinary infections may be asymptomatic but show signs of urethral, vaginal, or cervical infection on physical examination.

Diagnosis

In males, microscopic examination of smears of prostatic or urethral secretions shows excess polymorphonuclear leukocytes but few, if any, specific organisms.

In females, cervical or urethral smears also reveal excess leukocytes and no specific organisms.

Treatment

Therapy for both sexes consists of oral tetracycline or erythromycin or of streptomycin followed by a sulfonamide. (Tetracycline is contraindicated in pregnant females.) For females, treatment may also include application of a sulfa vaginal cream. Cervicitis occasionally necessitates cryosurgery.

Special considerations

- Tell female patients to clean the pubic area before applying vaginal medication and to avoid using tampons during treatment.
- Make sure the patient clearly understands and strictly follows the dosage schedule for all prescribed medications.

To prevent nonspecific genitourinary infections:

- Tell patients to abstain from sexual contact with infected partners, to use condoms during sexual activity and follow appropriate hygienic measures afterward, and to void before and after intercourse.
- Encourage patients to maintain adequate fluid intake.
- Advise female patients to avoid routine use of douches and feminine hygiene sprays, tight-fitting pants or panty hose, insertion of foreign objects into the vagina, and deodorant tampons.
- Suggest female patients wear cotton underpants and remove them before going to bed.

FEMALE SEXUAL DYSFUNCTION

Arousal and Orgasmic Dysfunctions

Arousal dysfunction, one of the most severe forms of female sexual dysfunction, is an inability to experience sexual pleasure. Orgasmic dysfunction, the most common female sexual dysfunction, is an inability to achieve orgasm. Unlike the female with arousal dysfunction, the female with orgasmic dysfunction may have a desire for sexual activity and become aroused, but feels inhibited as she approaches orgasm. Both arousal and orgasmic dysfunctions are considered primary if they exist in a female who has never experienced sexual arousal or orgasm; they are secondary when some physical, mental, or situational condition has inhibited or obliterated a previously normal sexual function. Prognosis is good for temporary or mild dysfunctions resulting from misinformation or situational stress but is guarded for dysfunctions that result from intense anxiety, chronically discordant relationships, or psychologic disturbances.

Causes

Any of the following factors, alone or in combination, may cause arousal or orgasmic dysfunction:

• *drug use:* CNS depressants and oral contraceptives

• *disease:* general systemic illness, diseases of the endocrine or nervous system, or diseases that impair muscle tone or contractility

• *gynecologic factors:* chronic vaginal or pelvic infection, congenital anomalies, and genital malignancies

• *stress and fatigue*

• *inadequate or ineffective stimulation*

• *psychologic factors:* performance anxiety, guilt, depression, or unconscious conflicts about sexuality

• *discordant relationships:* poor communication, hostility or ambivalence toward the partner, fear of abandonment or of asserting independence, or boredom with sex.

All these factors may contribute to involuntary inhibition of the orgasmic reflex. Another crucial factor is the fear of losing control of feelings or behavior. Whether or not these factors produce sexual dysfunction and the type of dysfunction depend on how well the female copes with the resulting pressures. Physical factors alone rarely cause arousal or orgasmic dysfunction.

Signs and symptoms

The female with arousal dysfunction has limited or absent sexual desire and experiences little or no pleasure from sexual stimulation. Physical signs of this dysfunction include lack of vaginal lubrication or absence of signs of genital vasocongestion.

The female with orgasmic dysfunction reports an inability to achieve orgasm, either totally or under certain circumstances. Many females experience orgasm through masturbation or other means but not through intercourse alone. Others achieve orgasm with some partners but not with others.

Diagnosis

Thorough physical examination, laboratory tests, and medical history rule out physical causes of arousal or orgasmic dysfunction. In the absence of such causes, a complete psychosexual history is the most important tool for assessment. Such a history should include:

• detailed information concerning level of sex education and previous sexual response patterns.

• the patient's feelings during childhood and adolescence about sex in general and, specifically, about masturbation, incest, rape, sexual fantasies, and homosexual or heterosexual practices.

• contraceptive practices and reproductive goals.

• the nature of the patient's present relationship, including her partner's attitude toward sex.

• assessment of the patient's self-esteem and body image.

• any history of psychotherapy.

Treatment

Arousal dysfunction is difficult to treat, especially if the female has never experienced sexual pleasure. Therapy is designed to help the patient relax, to become aware of her feelings about sex, and to eliminate guilt and the fear of rejection. Specific measures usually include sensate focus exercises similar to those developed by Masters and Johnson, which emphasize touching and awareness of sensual feelings over body—not just genital sensations—and minimize the importance of intercourse and orgasm. Psychoanalytic treatment consists of free association, dream analysis, and discussion of life patterns to achieve greater sexual awareness. One behavioral approach attempts to correct maladaptive patterns through systematic desensitization to situations that provoke anxiety, partially by encouraging the patient to fantasize about these situations.

The goal in treating orgasmic dysfunction is to decrease or eliminate involuntary inhibition of the orgasmic reflex. Treatment may include experiential therapy, psychoanalysis, or behavior modification.

Treatment of primary orgasmic dysfunction may involve teaching the patient self-stimulation. Also, the therapist may teach distraction techniques, such as focusing attention on fantasies, breathing patterns, or muscular contractions to relieve anxiety. Thus, the patient learns new behavior through exercises she does in the privacy of her own home between sessions. Gradually, the therapist involves the patient's sexual partner in the treatment sessions, although some therapists treat the couple as a unit from the outset.

Treatment of secondary orgasmic dysfunction is designed to decrease anxiety and promote the factors necessary for the patient to experience orgasm. Sensate focus exercises are often used. The therapist should communicate an accepting and permissive attitude and help the patient understand that satisfactory sexual experiences don't always require coital orgasm.

Special considerations

• Be alert for clues to arousal or orgasmic dysfunction when obtaining a health history.

• Maintain an open, nonjudgmental attitude. Listen to the patient's problems sympathetically.

• Provide accurate information regarding sexual anatomy and physiology and sexual response patterns.

• Refer the patient to doctors, nurses, psychologists, social workers, and counselors trained in sex therapy. As a helpful guideline, inform the patient that the therapist's certification by the American Association of Sex Educators, Counselors, and Therapists, or by the American Society for Sex Therapy and Research usually assures quality treatment. If the therapist is not certified by one of these organizations, advise the patient to inquire about the therapist's training in sex counseling and therapy.

Dyspareunia

Dyspareunia is pain associated with intercourse. It may be mild, or severe enough to affect a female's enjoyment of intercourse. Dyspareunia is commonly associated with physical problems or, less commonly, with psychologically based sexual dysfunctions. Prognosis is good if the underlying disorder can be treated successfully.

Causes

Physical causes of dyspareunia include an intact hymen; deformities or lesions of the introitus or vagina; retroversion of the uterus; genital, rectal, or pelvic scar tissue; acute or chronic infections of the genitourinary tract; and disorders of the surrounding viscera (including residual effects of pelvic inflammatory disease or disease of the adnexal and broad ligaments). Among the many other possible physical causes are:

• endometriosis

• benign and malignant growths and tumors

• insufficient lubrication

• radiation to the area

• allergic reactions to diaphragms, condoms, or other contraceptives.

Psychological causes include fear of pain or of injury during intercourse, recollection of a previous painful experience, guilt feelings about sex, fear of pregnancy or of injury to the fetus during pregnancy, anxiety caused by a new sexual partner or technique, and mental or physical fatigue.

Signs and symptoms

Dyspareunia produces discomfort, ranging from mild aches to severe pain before, during, or after intercourse. It also may be associated with vaginal itching or burning.

Diagnosis

Physical examination and laboratory tests, which vary with the suspected cause, help determine the underlying disorder. Diagnosis also depends on a detailed sexual history and the answers to such questions as: When does the pain occur? Does it occur with certain positions or techniques, or at certain times during the sexual response cycle? Where does the pain occur? What is its quality, frequency, and duration? What factors relieve or aggravate it?

Treatment

Treatment of physical causes may include creams and water-soluble jellies for inadequate lubrication, appropriate medications for infections, excision of hymenal scars, and gentle stretching of painful scars at the vaginal opening with a medium-sized Graves speculum. The patient may be advised to change her coital position to reduce pain on deep penetration.

Methods for treating psychologically based dyspareunia vary with the particular patient. Psychotherapy may uncover hidden conflicts that are creating fears concerning intercourse. Sensate focus exercises de-emphasize intercourse itself and teach appropriate foreplay techniques. Education concerning appropriate methods of contraception can reduce fear of pregnancy; education concerning sexual activity during pregnancy can relieve fear of harming the fetus.

Special considerations

• Provide instruction concerning anatomy and physiology of the reproductive system, contraception, and the human sexual response cycle.
• When appropriate, provide advice and information on drugs that may affect the patient sexually, and on lubricating jellies and creams.
• Listen to the patient's complaints of sex-related pain, and maintain a sympathetic, nonjudgmental attitude toward her, which will encourage her to express her feelings without embarrassment.

Vaginismus

Vaginismus is involuntary spastic constriction of the lower vaginal muscles, usually from fear of vaginal penetration. This disorder may coexist with dyspareunia and, if severe, may prevent intercourse (a common cause of unconsummated marriages). Vaginismus affects females of all ages and backgrounds. Prognosis is excellent for a motivated patient who doesn't have untreatable organic abnormalities.

Causes

Vaginismus may be physical or psychologic in origin. It may occur spontaneously as a protective reflex to pain or result from organic causes, such as hymenal abnormalities, genital herpes, obstetric trauma, and atrophic vaginitis.

Psychologic causes may include:
• childhood and adolescent exposure to rigid, punitive, and guilt-ridden attitudes toward sex.
• fears resulting from painful or traumatic sexual experiences, such as incest or rape.
• early traumatic experience with pelvic examinations.
• phobias of pregnancy, venereal disease, or cancer.

Signs and symptoms

The female with vaginismus typically experiences muscle spasm with constriction and pain on insertion of any object into the vagina, such as a vaginal tampon, diaphragm, or speculum. She may profess total lack of sexual interest or a normal level of sexual desire (often characterized by sexual activity without intercourse).

Diagnosis

Diagnosis depends on sexual history and pelvic examination to rule out physical disorders. Sexual history must include early childhood experiences and family attitudes toward sex, previous and current sexual responses, contraceptive practices and reproductive goals, feelings about her sexual partner, and specifics about pain on insertion of any object into the vagina.

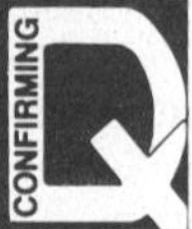

A carefully performed pelvic examination confirms diagnosis by showing involuntary constriction of the musculature surrounding the outer portion of the vagina.

Treatment

Treatment is designed to eliminate maladaptive muscular constriction and underlying psychologic problems. In Masters and Johnson therapy, the patient uses a graduated series of plastic dilators, which she inserts into her vagina while tensing and relaxing her pelvic muscles. The patient controls the time the dilator is left in place (if possible, she retains it for several hours) and the movement of the dilator. Together with her sexual partner, she begins sensate focus and counseling therapy to increase sexual responsiveness, improve communications skills, and resolve any underlying conflicts.

Kaplan therapy also uses progressive insertion of dilators or fingers (in vivo/desensitization therapy), with behavior therapy (imagining vaginal penetration until it can be tolerated) and, if necessary, psychoanalysis and hypnosis. Both Masters and Johnson, and Kaplan therapies report 100% cure; however, Kaplan states the patient and her partner may show other sexual dysfunctions that necessitate additional therapy.

Special considerations

- Since a pelvic examination may be painful for the patient with vaginismus, proceed gradually, at the patient's own pace. Support the patient throughout the pelvic examination, explaining each step before it is done. Encourage her to verbalize her feelings, and take plenty of time to answer her questions.
- Teach the patient about anatomy and physiology of the reproductive system, contraception, and human sexual response. This can be done quite naturally during the pelvic examination.
- Ask if the patient is taking any medications (antihypertensives, tranquilizers, steroids) that may affect her sexual response. If she has insufficient lubrication for intercourse, tell her about lubricating jellies and creams.

MALE SEXUAL DYSFUNCTION

Erectile Dysfunction

(Impotence)

Erectile dysfunction refers to a male's inability to attain or maintain penile erection sufficient to complete intercourse. The patient with primary impotence has never achieved a sufficient erection; secondary impotence, which is more common and less serious than the primary form, implies that, despite present inability, the patient has succeeded in completing intercourse in the past. Transient periods of impotence are not considered dysfunction and probably occur in half of adult males. Erectile dysfunction affects all age-groups but increases in frequency with age. Prognosis depends on the severity and duration of impotence and the underlying cause.

Causes

Psychogenic factors are responsible for approximately 50% to 60% of erectile dysfunction; organic factors, for the rest. In some patients, psychogenic and organic factors coexist, making isolation of the primary cause difficult.

Psychogenic causes may be intrapersonal, reflecting personal sexual anxieties, or interpersonal, reflecting a disturbed sexual relationship. Intrapersonal factors generally involve guilt, fear, depression, or feelings of inadequacy resulting from previous traumatic sexual experience, rejection by parents or peers, exaggerated religious orthodoxy, abnormal mother-son intimacy, or homosexual experiences. Interpersonal factors may stem from differences in sexual preferences between partners, lack of communication, insufficient knowledge of sexual function, or nonsexual personal conflicts. Situational impotence, a temporary condition, may develop in response to stress.

Organic causes may include chronic diseases, such as cardiopulmonary disease, diabetes, multiple sclerosis, or renal failure; spinal cord trauma; complications of surgery; drug- or alcohol-induced dysfunction; and, rarely, genital anomalies or CNS defects.

Signs and symptoms

Secondary erectile dysfunction is classified as follows:

- *Partial:* The patient is unable to achieve a full erection.
- *Intermittent:* The patient is sometimes potent with the same partner.
- *Selective:* The patient is potent only with certain females.

Some patients lose erectile function suddenly; others lose it gradually. If the cause is not organic, erection may still be achieved through masturbation.

Patients with psychogenic impotence may appear anxious, with sweating and palpitations, or they may become totally disinterested in sexual activity. Patients with psychogenic or drug-induced impotence may suffer extreme depression, which may cause the impotence or result from it.

Diagnosis

Personal sexual history provides the most useful clues in differentiating between organic and psychogenic factors and between primary and secondary impotence: Does the patient have intermittent, selective, nocturnal, or early-morning erections? Can he achieve erections through other sexual activity, such as masturbation or fantasizing? When did his dysfunction begin, and what was his life situation at that time? Did erectile problems occur suddenly or gradually? Is he taking large quantities of prescription or nonprescription drugs?

Diagnosis must rule out chronic disease, such as diabetes and other vascular, neurologic, or urogenital problems.

Treatment

Sex therapy, largely directed at reducing performance anxiety, may effectively cure psychogenic impotence. Such therapy should include both partners.

The course and content of sex therapy for impotence depend on the specific cause of the dysfunction and the nature of the male-female relationship. Usually, therapy includes the concept of sensate focus, which restricts the couple's sexual activity and encourages them to become more attuned to the physical sensations of touching. Sex therapy also includes improving verbal communication skills, eliminating unreasonable guilt, and reevaluating attitudes toward sex and sexual roles.

Treatment of organic impotence focuses on reversing the cause, if possible. If not, psychological counseling may help the couple deal realistically with their situation and explore alternatives for sexual expression. Certain patients suffering from organic impotence may benefit from surgically inserted inflatable or noninflatable penile implants.

Special considerations

- When you identify a patient with impotence or with a condition that may cause impotence, help him feel comfortable about discussing his sexuality. Assess his sexual health during your initial nursing history. When appropriate, refer him for further evaluation or treatment.
- After penile implant surgery, instruct the patient to avoid intercourse until the incision heals, usually in 6 weeks.

To help prevent impotence:

- Promote establishment of responsible health and sex education programs at primary, secondary, and college levels.
- Provide information about resuming sexual activity as part of discharge instructions for any patient with a condition that requires modification of daily activities. Such patients include those with cardiac disease, diabetes, hypertension, and COPD, and all postoperative patients.

Hypogonadism

Hypogonadism is a condition resulting from decreased androgen production in males, which may impair spermatogenesis (causing infertility) and inhibit the development of normal secondary sex characteristics. The clinical effects of androgen deficiency depend on age at onset.

Causes

Primary hypogonadism results directly from interstitial (Leydig's cell) cellular or seminiferous tubular damage due to faulty development or mechanical damage. This causes increased secretion of gonadotropins by the pituitary in an attempt to increase the testicular functional state and is therefore termed hypergonadotropic hypogonadism. It includes the following: Klinefelter's syndrome, Reifenstein's syndrome, male Turner's syndrome, Sertoli-cell–only syndrome, anorchism, orchitis, and sequelae of irradiation. Secondary hypogonadism results from faulty interaction within the hypothalamic-pituitary axis resulting in failure to secrete normal levels of gonadotropins, and is therefore termed hypogonadotropic hypogonadism. It includes the following: hypopituitarism, isolated follicle-stimulating hormone deficiency, isolated luteinizing hormone deficiency, Kallmann's syndrome, and Prader-Willi syndrome. Depending on the patient's age at onset, hypogonadism may cause eunuchism (complete gonadal failure) or eunuchoidism (partial failure).

Signs and symptoms

Although symptoms vary, depending on the specific cause of hypogonadism, some characteristic findings may include delayed closure of epiphyses and immature bone age; delayed puberty; infantile penis and small, soft testes; below-average muscle development and strength; fine, sparse facial hair; scant or absent axillary, pubic, and body hair; and a high-pitched, effeminate voice. In an adult, hypogonadism diminishes sex drive and potency and causes regression of secondary sex characteristics.

Diagnosis

Accurate diagnosis necessitates a detailed patient history, physical examination, and hormonal studies. Serum and urinary gonadotropin levels increase in primary, or hypergonadotropic, hypogonadism but decrease in secondary, or hypogonadotropic, hypogonadism. Other relevant hormonal studies include assessment of neuroendocrine functions, such as thyrotropin, adrenocorticotropin, growth hormone, and vasopressin levels. Chromosomal analysis may determine the specific causative syndrome. Testicular biopsy and semen analysis determine sperm production, identify impaired spermatogenesis, and assess low levels of testosterone.

Treatment
Treatment depends on the underlying cause and may consist of hormonal replacement, especially with testosterone, methyltestosterone, or human chorionic gonadotropin (HCG) for primary hypogonadism, and with HCG for secondary hypogonadism. Fertility cannot be restored after permanent testicular damage. However, eunuchism that results from hypothalamic-pituitary lesions can be corrected when administration of gonadotropins stimulates normal testicular function.

Special considerations
Because patients with hypogonadism tend to have multiple associated physical problems, the care plan should be tailored to meet their specific needs.

- When caring for an adolescent boy with hypogonadism, make every possible effort to promote his self-confidence. If he feels sensitive about his underdeveloped body, provide access to a private bathroom. Explain hypogonadism to his parents. Encourage them to express their concerns about their son's delayed development. Reassure them and the patient that effective treatment is available.
- Make sure the parents and the patient understand hormonal replacement therapy fully, including expected side effects such as acne and water retention.

Undescended Testes

(Cryptorchidism)

In this congenital disorder, one or both testes fail to descend into the scrotum, remaining in the abdomen, inguinal canal, or at the external ring. Although this condition may be bilateral, it more commonly affects the right testis. True undescended testes remain along the path of normal descent, while ectopic testes deviate from that path. If bilateral cryptorchidism persists untreated into adolescence, it may result in sterility, make the testes more vulnerable to trauma, and significantly increase the risk of testicular malignancy.

Causes
The mechanism whereby the testes descend into the scrotum is still unexplained. Some evidence is available to implicate hormonal factors—most likely androgenic hormones from the placenta, maternal or fetal adrenals, or the fetal immature testis, and, possibly, maternal progesterone or gonadotropic hormones from the maternal pituitary.

A popular but still unsubstantiated theory links undescended testes to the development of the gubernaculum, a fibromuscular band which connects the testes to the scrotal floor. In the normal male fetus, testosterone stimulates the formation of the gubernaculum. This band probably helps pull the testes into the scrotum by shortening as the fetus grows. Thus, cryptorchidism may result from inadequate testosterone levels or a defect in the testes or the gubernaculum.

Since the testes normally descend into the scrotum during the eighth month of gestation, cryptorchidism most commonly affects premature newborns. (It occurs in 30% of premature male newborns but in only 3% of those born at term.) In about 80% of affected infants, the testes descend spontaneously during the first year; in the rest, the testes may or may not descend later.

Signs and symptoms
In the young boy with unilateral cryptorchidism, the testis on the affected side

isn't palpable in the scrotum, and his scrotum may appear underdeveloped. On the unaffected side, the scrotum occasionally appears enlarged, as a result of compensatory hypertrophy. After puberty, uncorrected bilateral cryptorchidism prevents spermatogenesis and results in infertility, although testosterone levels remain normal.

Diagnosis

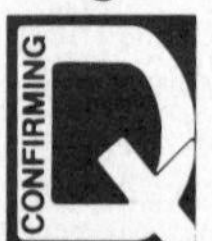

Physical examination confirms cryptorchidism after laboratory tests determine sex:

• *Buccal smear* determines genetic sex by showing a male sex chromatin pattern.
• *Serum gonadotropin* confirms the presence of testes by assessing the level of circulating hormone.

Treatment

If the testes don't descend spontaneously by age 1, surgical correction is generally indicated. Orchiopexy secures the testes in the scrotum and is commonly performed before the boy reaches age 4 (optimum age is 1 to 2 years). Orchiopexy prevents sterility, and excessive trauma from abnormal positioning. It also prevents harmful psychological effects. Rarely, human chorionic gonadotropin (HCG) I.M. may stimulate descent. However, hormonal therapy with HCG is ineffective if the testes are located in the abdomen.

Special considerations

• Encourage parents of the child with undescended testes to express their concern about his condition. Provide information about causes, available treatments, and ultimate effect on reproduction. Emphasize that, especially in premature infants, the testes may descend spontaneously.
• If orchiopexy is necessary, explain the surgery to the child, using terms he understands. Tell him that a rubber band may be taped to his thigh for about 1 week after surgery to keep the testis in place. Explain that his scrotum may swell but should not be painful.

After orchiopexy:

• Monitor vital signs and intake and output. Check dressings. Encourage coughing and deep breathing. Watch for urinary retention.
• Keep the operative site clean. Tell the child to wipe from front to back after defecating. If a rubber band has been applied to keep the testis in place, maintain tension, but check that it isn't too tight.
• Encourage parents to participate in postoperative care, such as bathing or feeding the child. Also urge the child to do as much for himself as possible.

Premature Ejaculation

Premature ejaculation refers to a male's inability to control the ejaculatory reflex during intravaginal containment, resulting in persistently early ejaculation. This common sexual disorder affects all age-groups.

Causes

Premature ejaculation may result from anxiety and is often linked to immature sexual experiences. Other psychological factors may include ambivalence toward or unconscious hatred of females, a negative sexual relationship in which the male unconsciously denies his partner sexual fulfillment, and guilty feelings about sex.

However, psychological factors aren't always the cause of premature ejaculation, since this disorder can occur in emotionally healthy males with stable, positive relationships. Rarely, premature ejaculation may be linked to an underlying degenerative neurologic disorder, such as multiple sclerosis, or an inflammatory process, such as posterior urethritis or prostatitis.

Signs and symptoms

Premature ejaculation may have a devastating psychological impact on some males, and they may exhibit signs of severe inadequacy or self-doubt, in addition to general anxiety and guilt. The patient may be unable to prolong foreplay, or he may have prolonged foreplay capacity but ejaculates as soon as intromission occurs. In other males, however, premature ejaculation may have little or no psychological impact. In such cases, the complaint lies solely with the sexual partner, who may believe that the male is indifferent to her sexual needs.

Diagnosis

Physical examination and laboratory test results are usually normal, since most males with this complaint are quite healthy. However, detailed sexual history can aid immeasurably in diagnosis. A history of adequate ejaculatory control in the absence of precipitating psychic trauma should arouse suspicion of an organic cause.

Treatment

Masters and Johnson have developed a highly successful, intensive program synthesizing insight therapy, behavioral techniques, and experiential sessions involving both sexual partners. The program is designed to help the patient focus on sensations of impending orgasm. The therapy sessions, which continue for 2 weeks or longer, typically include:

- *mutual physical examination,* which increases the couple's awareness of anatomy and physiology, while reducing shameful feelings about sexual parts of the body.
- *sensate focus,* which allows each partner, in turn, to caress the other's body, without intercourse, and to focus on the pleasurable sensations of touch.
- *Semans squeeze technique,* which helps the patient gain control of ejaculatory tension by having the woman squeeze his penis, with her thumb on the frenulum and her forefinger and middle finger on the dorsal surface, near the coronal ridge. At the male's direction, she applies and releases pressure every few minutes, during a touching exercise to delay ejaculation by keeping the male at an earlier phase of the sexual response cycle.

The *stop-and-start technique* helps delay ejaculation. With the female in the superior position, this method involves pelvic thrusting until orgasmic sensations start, then stopping and restarting to aid in control of ejaculation. Eventually, the couple is allowed to achieve orgasm.

Special considerations

- Encourage a positive self-image by explaining that premature ejaculation is a common disorder that does not reflect on the patient's masculinity.
- Assure the patient that the condition is reversible.
- Refer the patient to appropriate resources for therapy.

Testicular Torsion

Testicular torsion is an abnormal twisting of the spermatic cord, due to rotation of a testis or the mesorchium (a fold in the area between the testis and epididymis), which causes strangulation and, if untreated, eventual infarction of the testis. This condition is almost always (90%) unilateral. Testicular torsion is most common between ages 12 and 18, but it may occur at any age. Prognosis is good with early detection and prompt treatment.

Causes

Normally, the tunica vaginalis envelops the testis and attaches to the epididymis and spermatic cord. In *intravaginal torsion* (the most common type of testicular torsion in adolescents), testicular twisting may result from an abnormality of the tunica, in which the testis is abnormally positioned, or from a narrowing of the mesentery support. In *extravaginal torsion* (most common in neonates), loose attachment of the tunica vaginalis to the scrotal lining causes spermatic cord rotation above the testis. A sudden forceful contraction of the cremaster muscle may precipitate this condition.

TESTICULAR TORSION

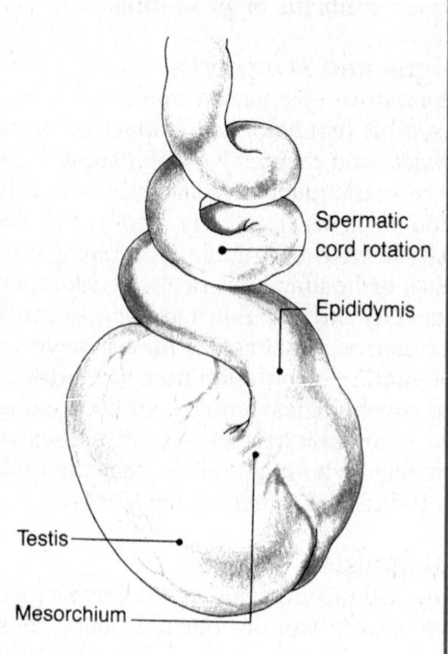

In extravaginal torsion, rotation of the spermatic cord above the testis causes strangulation and, eventually, infarction of the testis.

Signs and symptoms

Torsion produces excruciating pain in the affected testis or iliac fossa.

Diagnosis

Physical examination reveals tense, tender swelling in the scrotum or inguinal canal and hyperemia of the overlying skin. Doppler ultrasonography helps distinguish testicular torsion from strangulated hernia, undescended testes, or epididymitis.

Treatment

Treatment consists of immediate surgical repair by orchiopexy (fixation of a viable testis to the scrotum) or orchiectomy (excision of a nonviable testis).

Special considerations

- Promote the patient's comfort before and after surgery.
- After surgery, administer pain medication, as ordered. Monitor voiding, and apply an ice bag with a cover, to reduce edema. Protect the wound from contamination. Otherwise, allow the patient to perform as many normal daily activities as possible.

Male Infertility

Male infertility may be suspected whenever a couple fails to achieve pregnancy after about 1 year of regular unprotected intercourse. Approximately 40% to 50% of infertility problems in the United States are totally or partially attributed to the male. (See also FEMALE INFERTILITY, *pages 902 to 904.)*

Causes

Some of the factors that cause male infertility include:

- *varicocele*, a mass of dilated and tortuous varicose veins in the spermatic cord.

• *semen disorders,* such as volume or motility disturbances or inadequate sperm density.
• *proliferation of abnormal or immature sperm,* with variations in the size and shape of the head.
• *systemic disease,* such as diabetes mellitus, neoplasms, hepatic and renal diseases, and viral disturbances, especially mumps orchitis.
• *genital infection,* such as gonorrhea, tuberculosis, and herpes.
• *disorders of the testes,* such as cryptorchidism, Sertoli-cell–only syndrome, varicocele, and ductal obstruction (caused by absence or ligation of vas deferens or infection).
• *genetic defects,* such as Klinefelter's (chromosomal pattern XXY, eunuchoidal habitus, gynecomastia, small testes) or Reifenstein's syndrome (chromosomal pattern 46XY, reduced testosterone, azoospermia, eunuchoidism, gynecomastia, hypospadias).
• *immunologic disorders,* such as autoimmune infertility or allergic orchitis.
• *endocrine imbalance* (rare) that disrupts pituitary gonadotropins, inhibiting spermatogenesis, testosterone production, or both; such imbalances occur in Kallmann's syndrome, panhypopituitarism, hypothyroidism, and congenital adrenal hyperplasia.
• *chemicals* and *drugs* that can inhibit gonadotropins or interfere with spermatogenesis, such as arsenic, methotrexate, medroxyprogesterone acetate, nitrofurantoin, monoamine oxidase inhibitors, and some antihypertensives.
• *sexual problems,* such as erectile dysfunction, ejaculatory incompetence, or low libido.

Other factors may include age, occupation, and trauma to testes.

Signs and symptoms

The obvious indication of male infertility is, of course, failure to impregnate a fertile woman. Clinical features may include atrophied testes; empty scrotum; scrotal edema; varicocele or anteversion of the epididymis; inflamed seminal vesicles; beading or abnormal nodes on the spermatic cord and vas; penile nodes, warts, plaques, or hypospadias; and prostatic enlargement, nodules, swelling, or tenderness. In addition, male infertility is often apt to induce troublesome negative emotions in a couple—anger, hurt, disgust, guilt, and loss of self-esteem.

Diagnosis

Detailed patient history may reveal abnormal sexual development, delayed puberty, infertility in previous relationships, and a medical history of prolonged fever, mumps, impaired nutritional status, previous surgery, or trauma to genitalia. After a thorough patient history and physical examination, the most conclusive test for male infertility is semen analysis. Other laboratory tests include gonadotropin assay to determine integrity of pituitary gonadal axis, serum testosterone levels to determine end organ response to LH, urine 17-ketosteroid levels to measure testicular function, and testicular biopsy to help clarify unexplained oligospermia and azoospermia. Vasography and seminal vesiculography may be necessary.

Treatment

When anatomic dysfunctions or infections cause infertility, treatment consists of correcting the underlying problem. A varicocele requires surgical repair or removal. For patients with sexual dysfunctions, treatment includes education, counseling or therapy (on sexual techniques, coital frequency, and reproductive physiology), and proper nutrition with vitamin supplements. Decreased FSH levels may respond to vitamin B therapy; decreased LH levels, to chorionic gonadotropin therapy. Normal or elevated LH requires low dosages of testosterone. Decreased testosterone levels, decreased semen motility, and volume disturbances may respond to chorionic gonadotropin.

Patients with oligospermia who have a normal history and physical examination, normal hormonal assays, and no signs of systemic disease require emotional support and counseling, adequate nutrition, multivitamins, and selective therapeutic agents, such as clomiphene, chorionic gonadotropin, and low dosages of testosterone. Obvious alternatives to such treatment are adoption and artificial insemination.

Special considerations

- Educate the couple, as necessary, regarding reproductive and sexual functions and about factors that may interfere with fertility, such as the use of lubricants and douches.
- Urge men with oligospermia to avoid habits that may interfere with normal spermatogenesis by elevating scrotal temperature, such as wearing tight underwear and athletic supporters, taking hot tub baths, or habitually riding a bicycle. Explain that cool scrotal temperatures are essential for adequate spermatogenesis.
- When possible, advise infertile couples to join group programs to share their feelings and concerns with other couples who have the same problem.
- Help prevent male infertility by encouraging patients to have regular physical examinations, to protect gonads during athletic activity, and to receive early treatment for venereal diseases and surgical correction for anatomic defects.

Precocious Puberty in Males

In precocious puberty, boys begin to mature sexually before age 10. It can occur as true precocious puberty, *the most common form, with early maturation of the hypothalamic-pituitary-gonadal axis, development of secondary sexual characteristics, gonadal development, and spermatogenesis or as* pseudoprecocious puberty, *with development of secondary sexual characteristics without gonadal development. Boys with true precocious puberty reportedly have fathered children at as young an age as 7 years.*

In most boys with precocious puberty, sexual characteristics develop in essentially normal sequence; these children function normally when they reach adulthood.

Causes

True precocious puberty may be idiopathic (constitutional) or cerebral (neurogenic). In some patients, idiopathic precocity may be genetically transmitted as a dominant trait. Cerebral precocity results from pituitary or hypothalamic intracranial lesions that cause excessive secretion of gonadotropin.

Pseudoprecocious puberty may result from testicular tumors (hyperplasia, adenoma, or carcinoma) or from congenital adrenogenital syndrome. Testicular tumors create excessive testosterone levels; adrenogenital syndrome creates high levels of adrenocortical steroids.

Signs and symptoms

All boys with precocious puberty experience early bone development, causing initial growth spurt, early muscle development, and premature closure of the epiphyses, which results in stunted adult stature. Other features are adult hair pattern, penile growth, and bilateral enlarged testes. Symptoms of precocity due to cerebral lesions include nausea, vomiting, headache, visual disturbances, and internal hydrocephalus.

In pseudoprecocity caused by testicular tumors, adult hair patterns and acne develop. A discrepancy in testis size also occurs; the enlarged testis may be hard or may contain a palpable, isolated nodule. Adrenogenital syndrome produces adult skin tone, excessive hair (including beard), and deepened voice. A boy with this syndrome appears stocky and muscular; his penis, scrotal sac, and prostate are enlarged (but not the testes).

Diagnosis

Assessing the cause of precocious puberty requires a complete physical examination. Detailed patient history can help evaluate recent growth pattern, behavioral changes, family history of precocious puberty, or any hormonal ingestion.

In true precocity, laboratory results include the following:

• *Serum levels of luteinizing, follicle-stimulating, and adrenocorticotropic hormones* are elevated.
• *Plasma tests for testosterone* demonstrate elevated levels (equal to those of an adult male).
• *Evaluation of ejaculate* reveal presence of live spermatozoa.
• *Brain scan, skull X-rays, and EEG* can detect possible CNS tumors.
• *Skull and hand X-rays* reveal advanced bone age.

A child with an initial diagnosis of idiopathic precocious puberty should be reassessed regularly for possible tumors.

In pseudoprecocity, chromosomal karyotoype analysis demonstrates abnormal pattern of autosomes and sex chromosomes. Elevated 24-hour urinary 17-ketosteroids and other steroid excretion levels also indicate pseudoprecocity.

Treatment

Boys with idiopathic prococious puberty generally require no medical treatment and, except for stunted growth, suffer no physical complications in adulthood. Supportive psychological counseling is the most important therapy.

When precocious puberty is caused by tumors, the outlook is less encouraging. Brain tumors necessitate neurosurgery but commonly resist treatment and may prove fatal. Testicular tumors may be treated by removing the affected testis (orchiectomy). Malignant tumors additionally require chemotherapy and lymphatic radiation therapy, and have a poor prognosis.

Adrenogenital syndrome that causes precocious puberty may respond to lifelong therapy with maintenance doses of glucocorticoids (cortisol), to inhibit corticotropin production.

Special considerations

• Emphasize to parents that social and emotional development should remain consistent with the child's chronologic age, not with his physical development. Advise parents not to place unrealistic demands on the child or to expect him to act older than his age.
• Reassure the child that although his body is changing more rapidly than those of other boys, eventually they will experience the same changes. Help him feel less self-conscious about his differences. Suggest clothing that deemphasizes sexual development.
• Provide sex education for the child with true precocity.
• Explain the medication's side effects (cushingoid symptoms) to the child and parents.

Selected References

Corey, Lawrence. "The Diagnosis and Treatment of Genital Herpes," *Journal of the American Medical Association* 248(9):1041-49, September 3, 1982.

Kaplan, Helen S., et al. *The Evaluation of Sexual Disorders: Psychological and Medical Aspects*. New York: Brunner, Mazel, Inc., 1983.

Meyer, Jon K., and Schmidt, Chester M., Jr., eds. *Clinical Management of Sexual Disorders*, 2nd ed. Baltimore: Williams & Wilkins Co., 1983.

Thompson, Summer E., and Washington, A. Eugene. "Epidemiology of Sexually Transmitted Chlamydia Trachomatis Infections," *Epidemiologic Reviews* 5:96-123, 1983.

Uyeda, Charles T., et al. "Rapid Diagnosis of Chlamydial Infections with the Micro-Trak Direct Test," *Journal of Clinical Microbiology* 20(5):948-50, November 1984.

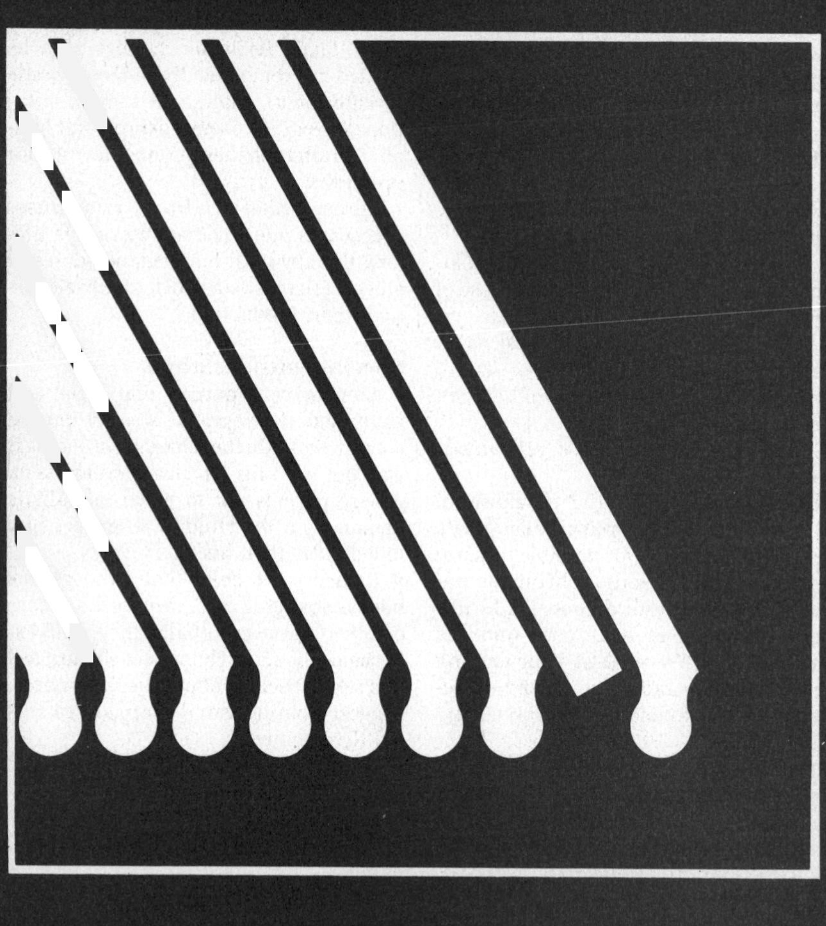

17 Hematologic Disorders

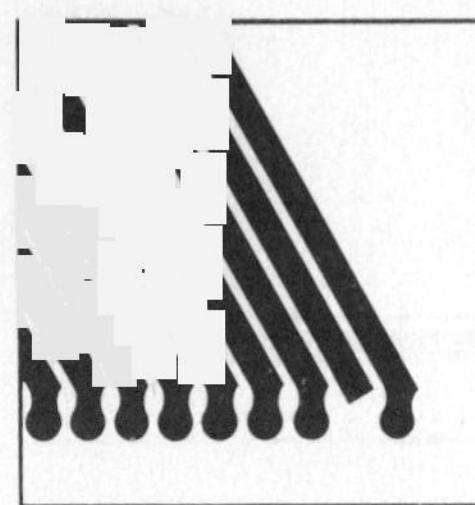

Hematologic Disorders

Introduction

Blood, one of the body's major fluid tissues, continuously circulates through the heart and blood vessels, carrying vital elements to every part of the body.

Blood basics

Blood performs several physiologically vital functions through its special components: the liquid portion (plasma), and the formed constituents (erythrocytes, leukocytes, thrombocytes) that are suspended in it. Erythrocytes (red blood cells [RBC]) carry oxygen to the tissues and remove carbon dioxide from them. Leukocytes (white blood cells [WBC]) participate in inflammatory and immune responses. Plasma (a clear, straw-colored fluid) carries antibodies and nutrients to tissues and carries waste away; coagulation factors in plasma, with thrombocytes (platelets), control clotting.

Typically, the average person has 5 to 6 liters of circulating blood that constitute 5% to 7% of body weight (as much as 10% in premature newborns). Blood is three to five times more viscous than water, with an alkaline pH of 7.35 to 7.45, and is either bright red (arterial blood) or dark red (venous blood), depending on the degree of oxygen saturation and the hemoglobin level.

Formation and characteristics

The process of blood formation by hematopoiesis occurs primarily in the bone marrow, where primitive blood cells (stem cells) produce the precursors of erythrocytes (normoblasts), leukocytes, and thrombocytes. During embryonic development, blood cells are derived from mesenchyma and form in the yolk sac. As the fetus matures, blood cells are produced in the liver, the spleen, and the thymus; by the fifth month of gestation, blood cells also begin to form in bone marrow. After birth, blood cells are usually produced only in the marrow.

Blood's function

The most important function of blood is to *transport oxygen* (bound to RBCs inside hemoglobin) from the lungs to the body tissues, and to *return carbon dioxide* from these tissues to the lungs. Blood also performs the following vital inflammatory and immunologic functions:

- production and delivery of antibodies (by way of WBCs) formed by plasma cells and lymphocytes
- transportation of granulocytes and monocytes to defend the body against pathogens by phagocytosis
- provision of complement, a group of immunologically important protein substances in plasma.

Blood's other functions include control of hemostasis by platelets, plasma, and coagulation factors that repair tissue injuries and prevent or halt bleeding;

acid-base and fluid balance; regulation of body temperature by carrying off excess heat generated by the internal organs for dissipation through the skin; and transportation of nutrients and regulatory hormones to body tissues, and of metabolic wastes to the organs of excretion (kidneys, lungs, and skin).

Blood dysfunction

Because of the rapid reproduction of bone marrow cells, and the short life span and minimal storage in the bone marrow of circulating cells, bone marrow cells and their precursors are particularly vulnerable to physiologic changes that can affect cell production. Resulting blood disorders may be primary or secondary, quantitative or qualitative, or both; they may involve some or all blood components. Quantitative blood disorders result from increased or decreased cell production or cell destruction; qualitative blood disorders stem from intrinsic cell abnormalities or plasma component dysfunction. Specific causes of blood disorders include trauma, chronic disease, surgery, malnutrition, drugs, exposure to toxins and radiation, and genetic and congenital defects that disrupt production and function. For example, depressed bone marrow production or mechanical destruction of mature blood cells can reduce the number of RBCs, platelets, and granulocytes, resulting in pancytopenia (anemia, thrombocytopenia, granulocytopenia). Increased production of multiple bone

COAGULATION FACTORS

FACTOR	SYNONYM	LOCATION
Factor I	Fibrinogen	Plasma
Factor II	Prothrombin	Plasma
Factor III	Tissue thromboplastin	Tissue cells
Factor IV	Calcium ion	Plasma
Factor V	Labile factor	Plasma
Factor VII	Stable factor	Plasma
Factor VIII	Antihemophilic globulin (AHG) or antihemophilic factor (AHF)	Plasma
Factor IX	Plasma thromboplastin component (PTC)	Plasma
Factor X	Stuart-Prower factor	Plasma
Factor XI	Plasma thromboplastin antecedent (PTA)	Plasma
Factor XII	Hageman factor	Plasma
Factor XIII	Fibrin stabilizing factor	Plasma

Adapted with permission from Ewald E. Selkurt, ed., BASIC PHYSIOLOGY FOR THE HEALTH SCIENCES (Boston: Little Brown & Co., 1975).

marrow components can follow myeloproliferative disorders.

Erythropoiesis

The tissues' demand for oxygen and the blood cells' ability to deliver it regulate RBC production. Consequently, hypoxia (or tissue anoxia) stimulates RBC production by triggering the formation and release of erythropoietin, a hormone (probably produced by the kidneys) that activates bone marrow to produce RBCs. Erythropoiesis may also be stimulated by androgens.

The actual formation of an erythrocyte begins with an uncommitted stem cell that may eventually develop into an RBC or a WBC. Such formation requires certain vitamins—B_{12} and folic acid—and minerals, such as copper, cobalt, and especially iron, which is vital to hemoglobin's oxygen-carrying capacity. Iron is obtained from various foods and is absorbed in the duodenum and upper jejunum, leaving any excess for temporary storage in reticuloendothelial cells, especially those in the liver. Iron excess is stored as ferritin and hemosiderin until it's released for use in the bone marrow to form new RBCs.

RBC disorders

RBC disorders include quantitative and qualitative abnormalities. Deficiency of RBCs (anemia) can follow any condition that destroys or inhibits the formation of these cells. Common factors leading to this deficiency include:

- drugs, toxins, ionizing radiation
- congenital or acquired defects that cause bone marrow aplasia and suppress general hematopoiesis (aplastic anemia) or erythropoiesis
- metabolic abnormalities (sideroblastic anemia)
- deficiencies of vitamins (vitamin B_{12} deficiency or pernicious anemia), iron, or minerals (iron, folic acid, copper, and cobalt deficiency anemias) that cause inadequate RBC production
- excessive chronic or acute blood loss (posthemorrhagic anemia)
- chronic illnesses, such as renal disease, malignancy, and chronic infections
- intrinsically or extrinsically defective red cells (sickle cell anemia, hemolytic transfusion reaction).

Comparatively few conditions lead to excessive numbers of red cells:

- abnormal proliferation of all bone marrow elements (polycythemia vera)
- a single-element abnormality (for instance, an increase in RBCs that results from erythropoietin excess, which in turn results from hypoxemia or pulmonary disease)
- decreased plasma cell volume, which causes an apparent corresponding increase—relative, not absolute—in RBC concentration.

Function of white cells

WBCs, or leukocytes, protect the body against harmful bacteria and infection, and are classified as granular leukocytes (basophils, neutrophils, and eosinophils) or nongranular leukocytes (lymphocytes, monocytes, and plasma cells). Usually, WBCs are produced in bone marrow; however, lymphocytes and plasma cells are produced in lymphoid tissue as well. Although WBCs have a poorly defined tissue life span, they generally have a circulating half-life of less than 6 hours. However, some monocytes may survive for weeks or months.

Normally, WBCs number between 5,000 and 10,000/mm^3 and comprise the following elements:

- *Neutrophils,* the predominant form of granulocyte, make up about 60% of WBCs; they help devour invading organisms by phagocytosis.
- *Eosinophils,* minor granulocytes, may defend against parasites and participate in allergic reactions.
- *Basophils,* minor granulocytes, may release heparin and histamine into the blood.
- *Monocytes,* along with neutrophils, help devour invading organisms by phagocytosis. They also help process antigens for lymphocytes and form macrophages in the tissues.
- *Lymphocytes* occur in two forms: B cells and T cells. B cells aid antibody

TWO TYPES OF LEUKOCYTES

I. GRANULAR

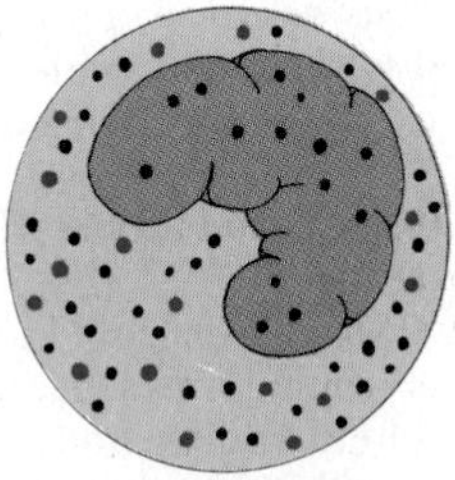

Basophil

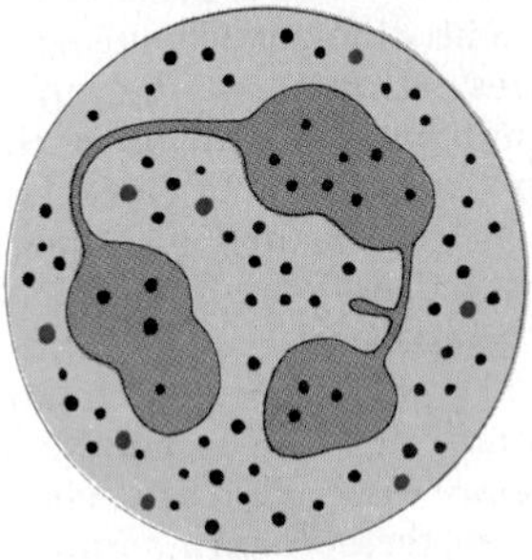

Neutrophil

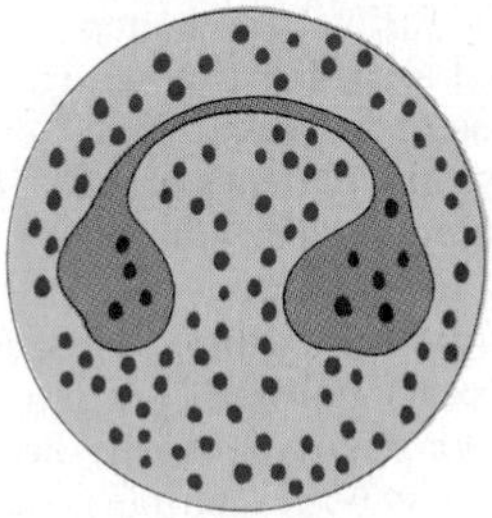

Eosinophil

II. NONGRANULAR

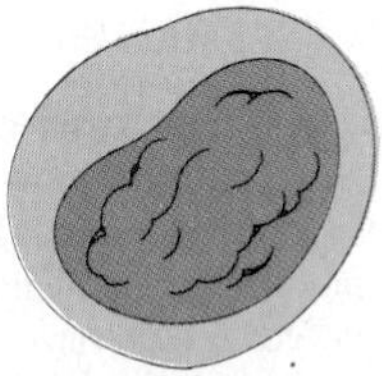

Lymphocyte

Leukocytes vary in size, shape, and number. Granulocytes are the most numerous and include basophils, containing cytoplasmic granules that stain readily with alkaline dyes; eosinophils, which stain with acidic dyes; and neutrophils, which are finely granular and recognizable by their multinucleated appearance. Lymphocytes and monocytes have few, if any, granulated particles in the cytoplasm.

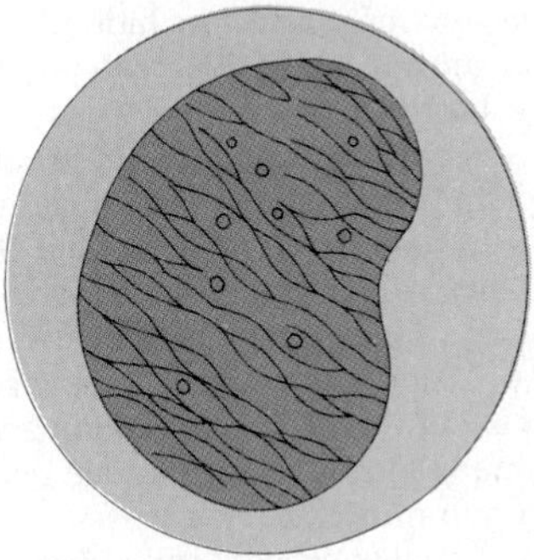

Monocyte

synthesis and T cells regulate cell-mediated immunity.

- *Plasma cells* develop from lymphocytes and produce antibodies.

A temporary increase in production and release of mature WBCs (leukemic reaction) is a normal response to infection. However, an abnormal increase of immature WBC precursors and their accumulation in bone marrow or lymphoid tissue is characteristic of leukemia. These nonfunctioning WBCs (blasts) provide no protection against infection, crowd out other vital components—RBCs, platelets, mature WBCs—and spill into the bloodstream, sometimes infiltrating organs and impairing organ functions.

WBC deficiencies may reflect inadequate cell production, drug reactions, ionizing radiation, infiltrated bone marrow (leukemia), congenital defects, aplastic anemia, folic acid deficiency, or hypersplenism. The major WBC deficiencies are granulocytopenia, lymphocytopenia, and, less frequently, monocytopenia, eosinophilia, and basophilia.

Platelets, plasma, and clotting

Platelets are small (2 to 4 microns in diameter), colorless, disk-shaped cytoplasmic fragments split from cells in bone marrow called megakaryocytes. These fragments, which have a life span of approximately 10 days, perform three vital functions:

- initiate contraction of damaged blood vessels to minimize blood loss
- form hemostatic plugs in injured blood vessels
- with plasma, provide materials that accelerate blood coagulation—notably platelet factor 3.

Plasma consists mainly of proteins (chiefly albumin, globulin, and fibrinogen) held in aqueous suspension. Other components of plasma include glucose, lipids, amino acids, electrolytes, pigments, hormones, respiratory gases (oxygen and carbon dioxide), and products of metabolism, such as urea, uric acid, creatinine, and lactic acid. Its fluid characteristics—including osmotic pressure, viscosity, and suspension qualities—depend on its protein content. Plasma components regulate acid-base balance and immune responses and mediate coagulation and nutrition.

In a complex process called hemostasis, platelets, plasma, and coagulation factors interact to control bleeding.

Hemostasis and the clotting mechanism

Hemostasis is the complex process by which the body controls bleeding. When a blood vessel ruptures, local vasoconstriction and platelet clumping (aggregation) at the site of the injury initially help prevent hemorrhage. This activation of the coagulation system, called extrinsic cascade, requires release of tissue thromboplastin from the damaged cells. However, formation of a more stable, secure clot requires initiation of the complex clotting mechanism known as the intrinsic cascade system. When this system becomes activated, prothrombin is converted to thrombin, which is necessary for creation of a fibrin clot.

Replacement therapy with blood components

Because of today's improved methods of collection, component separation, and storage, blood transfusions are being used more effectively than ever. Separating blood into components permits a single unit of blood to benefit several patients with different hematologic abnormalities. Component therapy allows patients who need blood transfusions for specific replacement of a deficient component to receive this replacement without risking transfusion reactions from other components.

Blood typing, cross matching, and histocompatibility locus antigen (HLA) typing are essential to safe, effective replacement therapy and minimize the risk of transfusion reactions. Blood typing determines the antigens present in the patient's RBCs by reaction with standardized sera. (Critical antigen groups are those of ABO and Rh factor.) Cross matching the patient's blood with transfusion blood before administration provides some assurance that the patient doesn't have antibodies against donor red cells. Occasionally, HLA typing may be helpful for the patient who needs long-term therapy with multiple transfusions. Usually, only family members can provide an appropriate match.

Bone marrow transplantation

One of the newest advances in treating acute leukemia and aplastic anemia, bone marrow transplantation is also used sometimes to treat severe combined immunodeficiency disease (SCID), Nezelof's syndrome, and Wiskott-Aldrich syndrome. In bone marrow transplantation, marrow from a twin or another HLA-identical donor (nearly always a

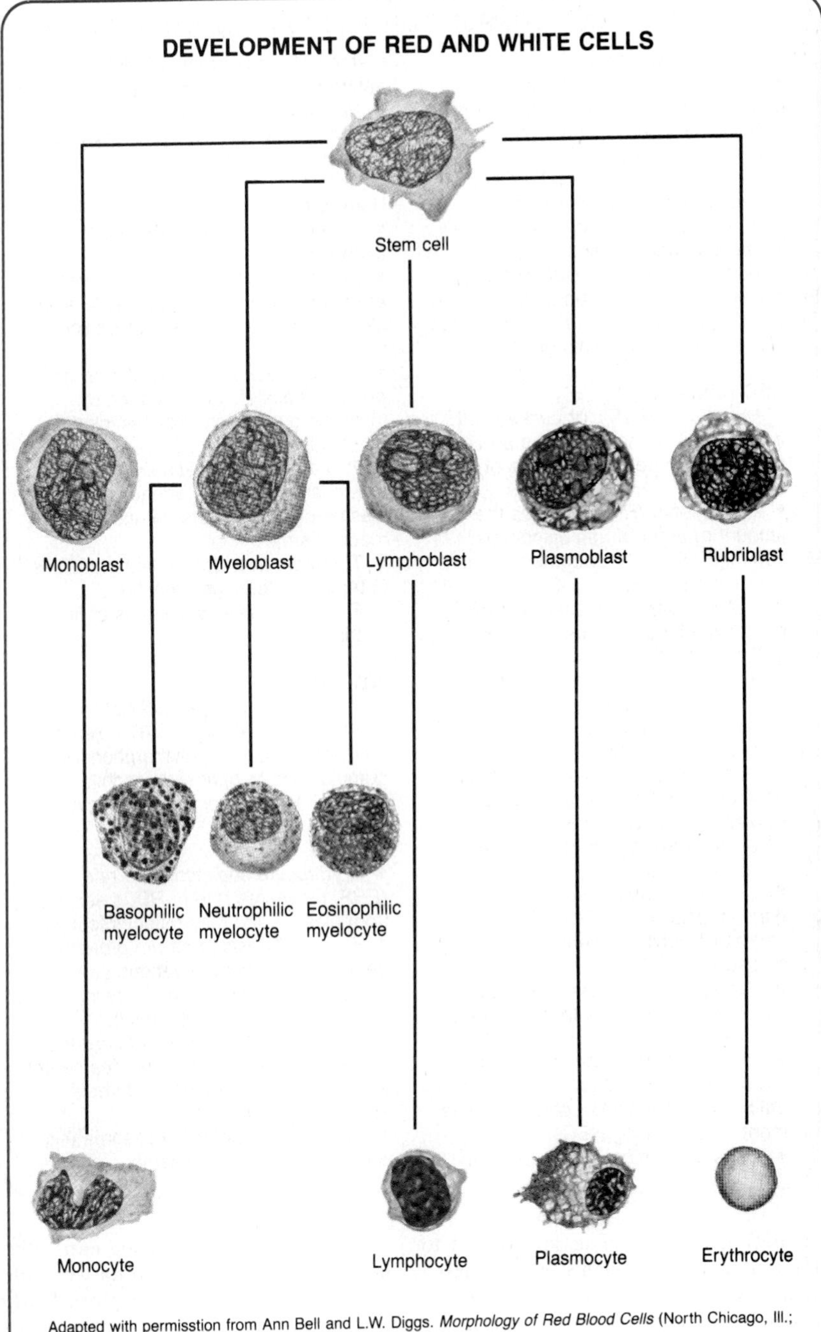

Adapted with permisstion from Ann Bell and L.W. Diggs. *Morphology of Red Blood Cells* (North Chicago, Ill.; Abbott Laboratories, 1978).

TESTS FOR BLOOD COMPOSITION, PRODUCTION, AND FUNCTION

Overall Composition

- *Peripheral blood smear* shows maturity and morphologic characteristics of blood elements and determines qualitative abnormalities.
- *Complete blood count (CBC)* determines the actual number of blood elements in relation to volume and quantifies abnormalities.
- *Bone marrow aspiration or biopsy* allows evaluation of hematopoiesis by showing blood elements and precursors, and abnormal or malignant cells.

RBC function

- *Hematocrit (HCT),* or packed cell volume (PCV), measures the percentage of RBCs per fluid volume of whole blood.
- *Hemoglobin (Hb)* measures the amount (grams) of hemoglobin per 100 ml of blood, to determine oxygen-carrying capacity.
- *Reticulocyte count* assesses RBC production by determining concentration of this erythrocyte precursor.
- *Schilling test* determines absorption of vitamin B_{12} (necessary for erythropoiesis) by measuring excretion of radioactive B_{12} in the urine.
- *Mean corpuscular volume (MCV)* describes the RBC in terms of size.
- *Mean corpuscular hemoglobin (MCH)* determines average amount of hemoglobin per RBC.
- *Mean corpuscular hemoglobin concentration (MCHC)* establishes average hemoglobin concentration in 100 ml packed RBCs.
- *Sugar-water test* assesses the susceptibility of RBCs to hemolyze with complement.
- *Direct Coombs' test* demonstrates the presence of IgG antibodies (such as antibodies to Rh factor) and/or complement on circulating RBCs.
- *Indirect Coombs' test,* a two-step test, detects the presence of IgG antibodies on RBCs in the serum.
- *Sideroblast test* detects stainable iron (available for hemoglobin synthesis) in normoblastic RBCs.

Hemostasis

- *Platelet count* determines number of platelets.
- *Bleeding time (Ivy bleeding time)* assesses capacity for platelets to stop bleeding in capillaries and small vessels.
- *Prothrombin time (Quick's test, pro time, PT)* assists in evaluation of thrombin generation (extrinsic clotting mechanism).
- *Partial thromboplastin time (PTT)* aids evaluation of the adequacy of plasma-clotting factors (intrinsic clotting mechanism).
- *Thrombin time* detects abnormalities in thrombin fibrinogen reaction.
- *Fibrinogen* assesses status of fibrin clotting.

WBC function

- *WBC count, differential* establishes quantity and maturity of WBC elements (neutrophils [called polymorphonuclear granulocytes or bands], basophils, eosinophils, lymphocytes, monocytes).

Plasma

- *Erythrocyte sedimentation rate (ESR)* measures rate of RBCs settling from plasma and may reflect infection.
- *Electrophoresis of serum proteins* determines amount of various serum proteins (classified by mobility in response to an electrical field).
- *Immunoelectrophoresis of serum proteins* separates and classifies serum antibodies (immunoglobins) through specific antisera.
- *Fibrinogen (Factor I)* measures this coagulation factor in plasma.

sibling) is transfused in an attempt to repopulate the recipient's bone marrow with normal cells. This procedure necessitates reverse isolation (preferably with laminar airflow) to prevent infection until the graft takes.

A hematologic disorder can affect nearly every aspect of the patient's life, perhaps resulting in life-threatening emergencies that require prompt medical treatment. With astute, sensitive care founded on a firm understanding of hematologic basics, you can help the patient survive such illnesses. In situations with poor prognoses, you can help the patient make the necessary adjustments to maintain an optimal quality of life.

ANEMIAS

Pernicious Anemia

(Addison's anemia)

Pernicious anemia is a megaloblastic anemia characterized by decreased gastric production of hydrochloric acid and deficiency of intrinsic factor (IF), a substance normally secreted by the parietal cells of the gastric mucosa that is essential for vitamin B_{12} absorption. The resulting deficiency of vitamin B_{12} causes serious neurologic, gastric, and intestinal abnormalities. Untreated pernicious anemia may lead to permanent neurologic disability and death.

Pernicious anemia primarily affects persons of northern European ancestry; in the United States, it's most common in New England and the Great Lakes region, due to ethnic concentrations. It's rare in children, blacks, and Asians. Onset is typically between ages 50 and 60; incidence rises with increasing age.

Causes

Familial incidence of pernicious anemia suggests a genetic predisposition. This disorder is significantly more common in patients with immunologically related diseases, such as thyroiditis, myxedema, and Graves' disease. These facts seem to support a widely held theory that an inherited autoimmune response causes gastric mucosal atrophy and, consequently, decreases hydrochloric acid and IF production. IF deficiency impairs vitamin B_{12} absorption. The resultant vitamin B_{12} deficiency inhibits the growth of all cells, particularly RBCs, leading to insufficient and deformed RBCs with poor oxygen-carrying capacity. It also impairs myelin formation, causing neurologic damage.

Signs and symptoms

Characteristically, pernicious anemia has an insidious onset but eventually causes an unmistakable triad of symptoms: weakness, sore tongue, and numbness and tingling in the extremities. The lips, gums, and tongue appear markedly bloodless. Hemolysis-induced hyperbilirubinemia may cause faintly jaundiced sclera and pale to bright yellow skin. In addition, the patient may become highly susceptible to infection, especially of the genitourinary tract.

Other systemic symptoms of pernicious anemia include the following:

- *GI:* Gastric mucosal atrophy and decreased hydrochloric acid production disturb digestion and lead to nausea, vomiting, anorexia, weight loss, flatulence, diarrhea, and constipation. Gingival bleeding and tongue inflammation may hinder eating and intensify anorexia.
- *CNS:* Demyelination caused by vitamin B_{12} deficiency initially affects the peripheral nerves but gradually extends to the spinal cord. Consequently, the neurologic effects of pernicious anemia may include neuritis; weakness in extremities; peripheral numbness and paresthesias; disturbed position sense; lack of coordination; ataxia; impaired fine finger movement; positive Babinski's and Romberg's signs; light-headedness; altered vision (diplopia, blurred vision), taste, and hearing (tinnitus); optic muscle atrophy; loss of bowel and bladder control; and, in males, impotence. Its ef-

fects on the nervous system may also produce irritability, poor memory, headache, depression, and delirium. Although some of these symptoms are temporary, irreversible CNS changes may have occurred before treatment.

• *Cardiovascular:* Increasingly fragile cell membranes induce widespread destruction of RBCs, resulting in low hemoglobin levels. The impaired oxygen-carrying capacity of the blood secondary to lowered hemoglobin leads to weakness, fatigue, and light-headedness. Compensatory increased cardiac output results in palpitations, wide pulse pressure, dyspnea, orthopnea, tachycardia, premature beats, and, eventually, congestive heart failure.

Diagnosis

A positive family history, typical ethnic heritage, and results of blood studies, bone marrow aspiration, gastric analysis, and the Schilling test establish the diagnosis. Laboratory screening must rule out other anemias with similar symptoms, such as folic acid deficiency anemia, since treatment differs. Diagnosis must also rule out vitamin B_{12} deficiency resulting from malabsorption due to gastrointestinal disorders, gastric surgery, radiation, or drug therapy.

Blood study results that suggest pernicious anemia include:

• decreased hemoglobin (4 to 5 g/100 ml) and decreased RBCs.

• increased mean corpuscular volume (MCV > 120); because larger-than-normal RBCs *each* contain increased amounts of hemoglobin, mean corpuscular hemoglobin concentration is also increased.

• possible low WBC and platelet counts, and large, malformed platelets.

• serum vitamin B_{12} assay levels less than 0.1 mcg/ml.

• elevated serum LDH.

Bone marrow aspiration reveals erythroid hyperplasia (crowded red bone marrow), with increased numbers of megaloblasts but few normally developing RBCs. Gastric analysis shows absence of free hydrochloric acid after histamine or pentagastrin injection.

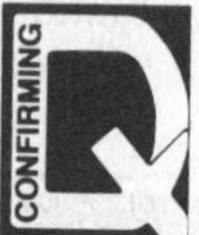

The Schilling test is the definitive test for pernicious anemia. In this test, the patient receives a small (0.5 to 2 mcg) oral dose of radioactive vitamin B_{12} after fasting for 12 hours. A larger (1 mg) dose of nonradioactive vitamin B_{12} is given I.M. 2 hours later, as a parenteral flush, and the radioactivity of a 24-hour urine specimen is measured. About 7% of the radioactive B_{12} dose is excreted in the first 24 hours; persons with pernicious anemia excrete less than 3%. (Generally, vitamin B_{12} is absorbed, and excess amounts are excreted in the urine; in pernicious anemia, the vitamin remains unabsorbed and is passed in the stool.) When the Schilling test is repeated with IF added, the test shows normal excretion of vitamin B_{12}.

Treatment

Early parenteral vitamin B_{12} replacement can reverse pernicious anemia, minimize complications, and may prevent permanent neurologic damage. These injections rarely cause side effects or induce an allergic response. An initial high dose of parenteral vitamin B_{12} causes rapid RBC regeneration. Within 2 weeks, hemoglobin should rise to normal, and the patient's condition should markedly improve. Since rapid cell regeneration increases the patient's iron requirements, concomitant iron replacement is necessary at this time to prevent iron deficiency anemia. After the patient's condition improves, vitamin B_{12} doses can be decreased to maintenance levels and given monthly. Because such injections must be continued for life, patients should learn self-administration.

If anemia causes extreme fatigue, the patient may require bed rest until hemoglobin rises. If hemoglobin is dangerously low, he may need blood transfusions, digitalis, a diuretic, and a low-sodium diet for congestive heart failure. Most important is the replacement of vitamin B_{12} to control the condition that led to this failure. Antibiotics help combat accompanying infections.

Special considerations

Supportive measures minimize the risk of complications and speed recovery. Patient and family teaching can promote compliance with lifelong vitamin B_{12} replacement.

- If the patient has severe anemia, plan activities, rest periods, and necessary diagnostic tests to conserve his energy. Monitor pulse rate often; tachycardia means his activities are too strenuous.
- To ensure accurate Schilling test results, make sure that all urine over a 24-hour period is collected and that the specimens are uncontaminated.
- Warn the patient to guard against infections, and tell him to report signs of infection promptly, especially pulmonary and urinary tract infections, since the patient's weakened condition may increase susceptibility.
- Provide a well-balanced diet, including foods high in vitamin B_{12} (meat, liver, fish, eggs, and milk). Offer between-meal snacks, and encourage the family to bring favorite foods from home.
- Since a sore mouth and tongue make eating painful, ask the dietitian to avoid giving the patient irritating foods. If these symptoms make talking difficult, supply a pad and pencil or some other aid to facilitate nonverbal communication; explain this problem to the family. Provide diluted mouthwash or, with severe conditions, swab the patient's mouth with tap water or warm saline solution.
- Warn the patient with a sensory deficit not to use a heating pad, since it may cause burns.
- If the patient is incontinent, establish a regular bowel and bladder routine. After the patient is discharged, a visiting nurse should follow up on this schedule and make adjustments, as needed.
- If neurologic damage causes behavioral problems, assess mental and neurologic status often; if necessary, give tranquilizers, as ordered, and apply a jacket restraint at night.
- Stress that vitamin B_{12} replacement isn't a permanent cure and that these injections *must* be continued for life, even after symptoms subside.
- To prevent pernicious anemia, emphasize the importance of vitamin B_{12} supplements for patients who've had extensive gastric resections or who follow strict vegetarian diets.

Folic Acid Deficiency Anemia

Folic acid deficiency anemia is a common, slowly progressive, megaloblastic anemia. It occurs most often in infants, adolescents, pregnant and lactating females, alcoholics, the elderly, and in persons with malignant or intestinal diseases.

Causes

Folic acid deficiency anemia may result from:

- *alcohol abuse* (alcohol may suppress metabolic effects of folate).
- *poor diet* (common in alcoholics, elderly persons living alone, and infants, especially those with infections or diarrhea).
- *impaired absorption* (due to intestinal dysfunction from disorders such as celiac disease, tropical sprue, regional jejunitis, or bowel resection).
- *bacteria* competing for available folic acid.
- *excessive cooking*, which can destroy a high percentage of folic acids in foods.
- *limited storage capacity* in infants.
- *prolonged drug therapy* (anticonvulsants, estrogens).
- *increased folic acid requirement* during pregnancy; during rapid growth in infancy (common because of recent increase in survival of premature infants);

FOODS HIGH IN FOLIC ACID CONTENT

Folic acid (pteroylglutamic acid, folacin) is found in most body tissues, where it acts as a coenzyme in metabolic processes involving one carbon transfer. It is essential for formation and maturation of RBCs and for synthesis of DNA. Although its body stores are comparatively small (about 70 mg), this vitamin is plentiful in most well-balanced diets.

However, because it's water-soluble and heat-labile, it's easily destroyed by cooking. Also, approximately 20% of folic acid intake is excreted unabsorbed. Insufficient daily folic acid intake (< 50 mcg/day) usually induces folic acid deficiency within 4 months. Below is a list of foods high in folic acid content.

FOOD	mcg/100 g
Asparagus spears	109
Beef liver	294
Broccoli spears	54
Collards (cooked)	102
Mushrooms	24
Oatmeal	33
Peanut butter	57
Red beans	180
Wheat germ	305

during childhood and adolescence (because of general use of folate-poor cow's milk); and in patients with neoplastic diseases and some skin diseases (chronic exfoliative dermatitis).

Signs and symptoms

Folic acid deficiency anemia gradually produces clinical features characteristic of other megaloblastic anemias, without the neurologic manifestations: progressive fatigue, shortness of breath, palpitations, weakness, glossitis, nausea, anorexia, headache, fainting, irritability, forgetfulness, pallor, and slight jaundice. Folic acid deficiency anemia does not cause neurologic impairment unless it's associated with vitamin B_{12} deficiency, as in pernicious anemia.

Diagnosis

The Schilling test and a therapeutic trial of vitamin B_{12} injections distinguish between folic acid deficiency anemia and pernicious anemia. Significant blood findings include macrocytosis, decreased reticulocyte count, abnormal platelets, and serum folate less than 4 mg/ml.

Treatment

Treatment consists primarily of folic acid supplements and elimination of contributing causes. Folic acid supplements may be given orally (usually 1 to 5 mg/day), or parenterally (to patients who are severely ill, have malabsorption, or are unable to take oral medication). Many patients respond favorably to a well-balanced diet.

Special considerations

- Teach the patient to meet daily folic acid requirements by including a food from each food group in every meal. If the patient has a severe deficiency, explain that diet only reinforces folic acid supplementation and isn't therapeutic by itself. Urge compliance with the prescribed course of therapy. Advise the patient not to stop taking the supplements when he begins to feel better.
- If the patient has glossitis, emphasize the importance of good oral hygiene. Suggest regular use of mild or diluted mouthwash and a soft toothbrush.
- Watch fluid and electrolyte balance, particularly in the patient who has severe diarrhea and is receiving parenteral fluid replacement therapy.
- Remember that anemia causes severe fatigue. Schedule regular rest periods until the patient is able to resume normal activity.
- To prevent folic acid deficiency anemia, emphasize the importance of a well-balanced diet high in folic acid. Identify alcoholics with poor dietary habits, and try to arrange for appropriate counseling. Tell mothers who are not breastfeeding to use commercially prepared formulas.

Aplastic or Hypoplastic Anemias

Aplastic or hypoplastic anemias result from injury to or destruction of stem cells in bone marrow or the bone marrow matrix, causing pancytopenia (anemia, granulocytopenia, thrombocytopenia) and bone marrow hypoplasia. Although often used interchangeably with other terms for bone marrow failure, aplastic anemias properly refer to pancytopenia resulting from the decreased functional capacity of a hypoplastic, fatty bone marrow. These disorders generally produce fatal bleeding or infection, particularly when they're idiopathic or stem from chloramphenicol or from infectious hepatitis. Mortality for aplastic anemias with severe pancytopenia is 80% to 90%.

Causes and incidence

Aplastic anemias usually develop when damaged or destroyed stem cells inhibit RBC production. Less commonly, they develop when damaged bone marrow microvasculature creates an unfavorable environment for cell growth and maturation. Approximately half of such anemias result from drugs, toxic agents (such as benzene and chloramphenicol), or radiation. The rest may result from immunologic factors (suspected but unconfirmed), severe disease (especially hepatitis), or preleukemic and neoplastic infiltration of bone marrow.

Idiopathic anemias may be congenital. Two such forms of aplastic anemia have been identified: congenital hypoplastic anemia (anemia of Blackfan and Diamond) develops between ages 2 months and 3 months; Fanconi's syndrome, between birth and age 10. In Fanconi's syndrome, chromosomal abnormalities are usually associated with multiple congenital anomalies—such as dwarfism, and hypoplasia of the kidneys and spleen. In the absence of a consistent familial or genetic history of aplastic anemia, researchers suspect that these congenital abnormalities result from an induced change in the development of the fetus.

Signs and symptoms

Clinical features of aplastic anemias vary with the severity of pancytopenia but often develop insidiously. Anemic symptoms include progressive weakness and fatigue, shortness of breath, headache, pallor, and, ultimately, tachycardia and congestive heart failure. Thrombocytopenia leads to ecchymosis, petechiae, and hemorrhage, especially from the mucous membranes (nose, gums, rectum, vagina) or into the retina or central nervous system. Neutropenia may lead to infection (fever, oral and rectal ulcers, sore throat) but without characteristic inflammation.

Diagnosis

Confirmation of aplastic anemia requires a series of laboratory tests:

• *RBCs* are usually normochromic and normocytic (although macrocytosis [larger than normal erythrocytes] and anisocytosis [excessive variation in erythrocyte size] may exist), with a total count of 1,000,000 or less. *Absolute reticulocyte count* is very low.

• *Serum iron* is elevated (unless bleeding occurs), but total iron-binding capacity is normal or slightly reduced. Hemosiderin is present, and tissue iron storage is visible microscopically.

• *Platelet, neutrophil, and WBC counts* fall.

• *Coagulation tests* (bleeding time), reflecting decreased platelet count, are abnormal.

• *Bone marrow biopsies* taken from several sites may yield a "dry tap" or show severely hypocellular or aplastic marrow, with a varying amount of fat, fibrous tissue, or gelatinous replacement; absence of tagged iron (since the iron is deposited in the liver rather than in bone

BONE MARROW TRANSPLANTATION

In bone marrow transplantation, usually 500 to 700 ml of marrow are aspirated from the pelvic bones of an HLA-compatible donor (allogeneic) or of the recipient himself during periods of complete remission (autologous). The aspirated marrow is filtered and then infused into the recipient in an attempt to repopulate his marrow with normal cells. This procedure has effected long-term, healthy survivals in about half the patients with severe aplastic anemia who have received such treatment. Transplantation may also be effective in treating patients with acute leukemia, certain immunodeficiency diseases, solid tumor malignancies, and genetic disorders, such as sickle cell anemia.

Because bone marrow transplantation carries serious risks, it requires reverse isolation, a primary nurse, and strict aseptic technique.

Before transplantation:

- After bone marrow aspiration is completed under local anesthetic, apply pressure dressings to the *donor's* aspiration sites. Observe the sites for bleeding. Relieve pain with analgesics and ice packs, as needed.
- Admit the patient (recipient) to a reverse isolation unit with laminar air flow, if possible. Obtain swabs for culture from each orifice. Give the patient an antiseptic bath and shampoo. Provide a sterile gown.
- Assess the patient's understanding of bone marrow transplantation. If necessary, correct any misconceptions, and provide additional information. Prepare the patient for an extended hospital stay, but encourage him by explaining the procedure's high success rate. Explain that radiation treatments and cyclophosphamide therapy are necessary to lower his body's resistance to the transplant.
- To suppress the patient's immune system, high-dose cyclophosphamide I.V. may be given for 2 days, with I.V. fluids, furosemide, and urine alkalinization to force diuresis and prevent hemorrhagic cystitis. During cyclophosphamide therapy, maintain the patient's urine pH between 7 and 9. Control nausea and vomiting with an antiemetic, such as prochlorperazine, as needed. Give allopurinol, as ordered, to prevent hyperuricemia resulting from tumor breakdown products. Since alopecia is a common side effect of high-dose cyclophosphamide therapy, encourage the patient to choose a wig or scarf before treatment begins.
- Total body irradiation (in one dose of 1000 rads or eight doses of 165 rads) follows chemotherapy, inducing total marrow aplasia. Warn the patient that cataracts, gastrointestinal disturbances, and sterility are possible side effects.

During marrow infusion:

- Monitor vital signs every 15 minutes for adverse reactions.
- Watch for complications of marrow infusion, such as pulmonary embolus and volume overload.
- Reassure the patient throughout the procedure.

After infusion is complete:

- Continue to monitor vital signs every 15 minutes for 2 to 4 hours after infusion, then every 4 hours. Watch for fever and chills, which may be the only signs of infection. Give prophylactic antibiotics, as ordered. To reduce the possibility of bleeding, don't administer medications rectally or intramuscularly.
- Administer methotrexate or cyclosporine, as ordered, to prevent graft-versus-host (GVH) reaction, a potentially fatal complication of transplantation. Watch for signs of GVH reaction, such as maculopapular rash, pancytopenia, jaundice, joint pain, and anasarca. Remember that unchecked GVH reaction may cause massive, fatal hemorrhage.
- Administer vitamins, steroids, and iron and folic acid supplements, as ordered. Blood products, such as platelets and packed RBCs, may also be indicated, depending on the results of daily blood studies.
- Give good mouth care every 2 hours. Use hydrogen peroxide and nystatin mouthwash, for example, to prevent candidiasis and other mouth infections. Also provide meticulous skin care, paying special attention to pressure points and open sites, such as aspiration and I.V. sites.

marrow) and megakaryocytes; and depression of erythroid elements.

Differential diagnosis must rule out paroxysmal nocturnal hemoglobinuria and other diseases in which pancytopenia is common.

Treatment

Effective treatment must eliminate any identifiable cause and provide vigorous supportive measures, such as packed red cell, platelet, and experimental HLA-matched leukocyte transfusions. Even after elimination of the cause, recovery can take months. Bone marrow transplantation is the treatment of choice for anemia due to severe aplasia and for patients who need constant RBC transfusions.

Reverse isolation is necessary to prevent infection in patients with low leukocyte counts. The infection itself may require specific antibiotics; however, these are not given prophylactically, because they tend to encourage resistant strains of organisms. Patients with low hemoglobin counts may need respiratory support with oxygen, in addition to blood transfusions.

Other appropriate forms of treatment include corticosteroids to stimulate erythroid production (successful in children, unsuccessful in adults), marrow-stimulating agents, such as androgens (which are controversial), and immunosuppressive agents (if the patient doesn't repspond to other therapy).

Special considerations

- If platelet count is low (less than 20,000/mm^3), prevent hemorrhage by avoiding I.M. injections, suggesting the use of an electric razor and a soft toothbrush, humidifying oxygen to prevent drying of mucous membranes (dry mucosa may bleed), and promoting regular bowel movements through the use of a stool softener and a proper diet to prevent constipation (which can cause rectal mucosal bleeding). Also, apply pressure to venipuncture sites until bleeding stops. Detect bleeding early by checking for blood in urine and stool and assessing skin for petechiae.
- Help prevent infection by washing your hands thoroughly before entering the patient's room, by making sure the patient is receiving a nutritious diet (high in vitamins and proteins) to improve his resistance, and by encouraging meticulous mouth and perianal care.
- Watch for life-threatening hemorrhage, infection, side effects of drug therapy, or blood transfusion reaction. Make sure routine throat, urine, and blood cultures are done regularly and correctly to check for infection. Teach the patient to recognize signs of infection, and tell him to report them immediately.
- If the patient has a low hemoglobin count, which causes fatigue, schedule frequent rest periods. Administer oxygen therapy, as needed. If blood transfusions are necessary, assess for a transfusion reaction by checking the patient's temperature and watching for the development of other signs, such as rash, hives, itching, back pain, restlessness, and shaking chills.
- Reassure and support the patient and family by explaining the disease and its treatment, particularly if the patient has recurring acute episodes. Explain the purpose of all prescribed drugs and discuss possible side effects, including which ones he should report promptly. Encourage the patient who doesn't require hospitalization to continue his normal life-style, with appropriate restrictions (such as regular rest periods), until remission occurs.
- To prevent aplastic anemia, monitor blood studies carefully in the patient receiving anemia-inducing drugs.
- Support efforts to educate the public about the hazards of toxic agents. Tell parents to keep toxic agents out of the reach of children. Encourage persons who work with radiation to wear protective clothing and a radiation-detecting badge and to observe plant safety precautions. Those who work with benzene (solvent) should know that 10 parts per million is the highest safe level and that a delayed reaction to benzene may develop.

Sideroblastic Anemias

Sideroblastic anemias comprise a group of heterogenous disorders with a common defect—failure to use iron in hemoglobin synthesis, despite the availability of adequate iron stores. These anemias may be hereditary or acquired; the acquired form, in turn, can be primary or secondary. Hereditary sideroblastic anemia often responds to treatment with pyridoxine. Correction of the secondary acquired form depends on the causative disorder; the primary acquired (idiopathic) form, however, resists treatment and usually proves fatal within 10 years after onset of complications or a concomitant disease.

Causes and incidence

Hereditary sideroblastic anemia appears to be transmitted by X-linked inheritance, occurring mostly in young males; females are carriers and usually show no signs of this disorder.

The acquired form may be secondary to ingestion of or exposure to toxins, such as alcohol and lead, or to drugs, such as isoniazid and chloramphenicol. It can also occur as a complication of other diseases, such as rheumatoid arthritis, lupus erythematosus, multiple myeloma, tuberculosis, and severe infections.

The primary acquired form, in which the cause is unknown, is most common in the elderly but occasionally develops in the young. It's often associated with thrombocytopenia or leukopenia.

In sideroblastic anemia, normoblasts (precursors of erythrocytes) fail to use iron to synthesize hemoglobin. As a result, iron deposits in the mitochondria of normoblasts, which are then termed ringed sideroblasts.

RINGED SIDEROBLAST

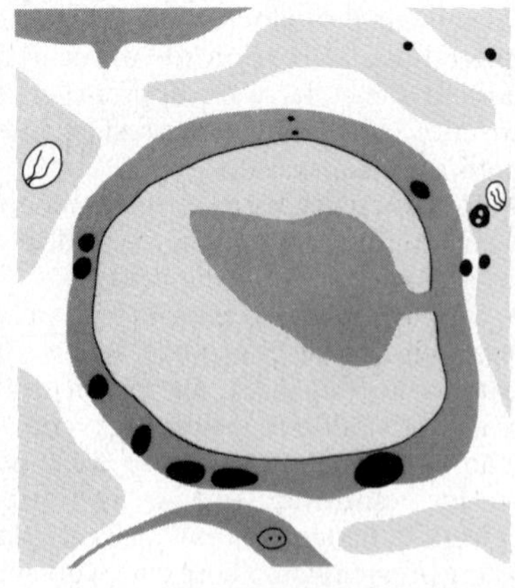

Electron microscopy shows large iron deposits in the mitochondria that surround the nucleus, forming the characteristic ringed sideroblast.

Signs and symptoms

Sideroblastic anemias usually produce nonspecific clinical effects, which may exist for several years before being identified. Such effects include anorexia, fatigue, weakness, dizziness, pale skin and mucous membranes, and, occasionally, enlarged lymph nodes. Heart and liver failure may develop due to excessive iron accumulation in these organs, causing dyspnea, exertional angina, slight jaundice, and hepatosplenomegaly. Hereditary sideroblastic anemia is associated with increased gastrointestinal absorption of iron, causing signs of hemosiderosis. Additional symptoms in secondary sideroblastic anemia depend upon the underlying cause.

Diagnosis

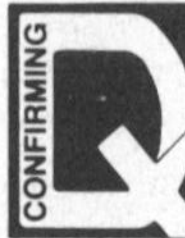

Ringed sideroblasts on microscopic examination of bone marrow aspirate, stained with Prussian blue or alizarin red dye, confirm this diagnosis. Microscopic examination of blood shows erythrocytes to be hypochromic or normochromic and slightly macrocytic. Red cell precursors may be megaloblastic, with anisocytosis (abnormal variation in RBC size) and poikilocytosis (abnormal variation in RBC shape). Unlike iron deficiency anemia, sideroblastic anemia lowers hemoglobin and raises serum iron and transferrin levels. In turn, faulty hemoglobin production raises urobilinogen and bilirubin levels. Platelets and leukocytes remain normal, but, occasionally, thrombocytopenia or leukopenia occurs.

Treatment

Treatment of sideroblastic anemias depends on the underlying cause. The hereditary form usually responds to several weeks of treatment with high doses of pyridoxine (vitamin B_6). The acquired secondary form generally subsides after the causative drug or toxin is removed or the underlying condition is adequately treated. Folic acid supplements may also be beneficial when concomitant megaloblastic nuclear changes in RBC precursors are present. Elderly patients with sideroblastic anemia—most commonly the primary acquired form—are less likely to improve quickly and are more likely to develop serious complications. Deferoxamine may be used to treat chronic iron overload in selected patients.

Carefully cross-matched transfusions (providing needed hemoglobin) or high doses of androgens are effective palliative measures for some patients with the primary acquired form of sideroblastic anemia. However, this form is essentially refractory to treatment and usually leads to death from acute leukemia or from respiratory or cardiac complications.

Some patients with sideroblastic anemia may benefit from phlebotomy to prevent hemochromatosis. Phlebotomy steps up the rate of erythropoiesis and uses up excess iron stores; thus, it reduces serum and total-body iron levels.

Special considerations

- Administer medications, as ordered. Teach the patient the importance of continuing prescribed therapy, even after he begins to feel better.
- Provide frequent rest periods if the patient becomes easily fatigued.
- If phlebotomy is scheduled, explain the procedure thoroughly to help reduce anxiety. If this procedure must be repeated frequently, provide a high-protein diet to help replace the protein lost during phlebotomy. Encourage the patient to follow a similar diet at home.
- Always inquire about the possibility of exposure to lead in the home (especially for children) or on the job.
- Identify patients who abuse alcohol; refer them for appropriate therapy.

Thalassemia

Thalassemia, a hereditary group of hemolytic anemias, is characterized by defective synthesis in the polypeptide chains necessary for hemoglobin production. Consequently, RBC synthesis is also impaired. Thalassemia is most common in persons of Mediterranean ancestry (especially Italian and Greek), but also occurs in blacks and persons from southern China, southeast Asia, and India.

β-Thalassemia is the most common form of this disorder, resulting from defective beta polypeptide chain synthesis. It occurs in three clinical forms: thalassemia major, intermedia, and minor. The severity of the resulting anemia depends on whether the patient is homozygous or heterozygous for the thalassemic trait. Prognosis for β-thalassemia varies. Patients with thalassemia major seldom survive to adulthood; children with thalassemia intermedia develop normally into adulthood, although puberty is usually delayed; persons with thalassemia minor can expect a normal life span.

Causes

Thalassemia major and *thalassemia intermedia* result from homozygous inheritance of the partially dominant autosomal gene responsible for this trait. *Thalassemia minor* results from heterozygous inheritance of the same gene. In all these disorders, total or partial deficiency of beta polypeptide chain production impairs hemoglobin synthesis and results in continual production of fetal hemoglobin, lasting even past the neonatal period.

Signs and symptoms

In thalassemia major (also known as Cooley's anemia, Mediterranean disease, and erythroblastic anemia), the infant is well at birth but develops severe anemia, bone abnormalities, failure to thrive, and life-threatening complications. Often, the first signs are pallor and yellow skin and scleras in infants aged 3 to 6 months. Later clinical features, in addition to severe anemia, include splenomegaly or hepatomegaly, with abdominal enlargement; frequent infections; bleeding tendencies (especially toward epistaxis); and anorexia.

Children with thalassemia major commonly have small bodies and large heads and may also be mentally retarded. Infants may have mongoloid features, because bone marrow hyperactivity has thickened the bone at the base of the nose. As these children grow older, they become susceptible to pathologic fractures, as a result of expansion of the marrow cavities with thinning of the long bones. They are also subject to cardiac arrhythmias, heart failure, and other complications that result from iron deposits in the heart and in other tissues from repeated blood transfusions.

THALASSEMIA MAJOR

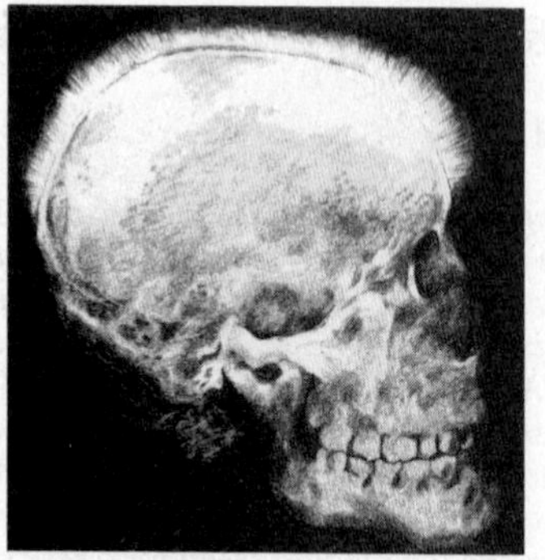

This X-ray shows a characteristic skull abnormality in thalassemia major: diploetic fibers extending from internal lamina.

Thalassemia intermedia comprises moderate thalassemic disorders in homozygotes. Patients with this condition show some degree of anemia, jaundice, and splenomegaly and, possibly, signs of hemosiderosis due to increased intestinal absorption of iron.

Thalassemia minor may cause mild anemia but usually produces no symptoms and is often overlooked.

Diagnosis

In thalassemia major, laboratory results show lowered RBCs and hemoglobin and elevated reticulocytes, bilirubin, and urinary and fecal urobilinogen. A low serum folate level indicates increased folate utilization by the hypertrophied bone marrow. A peripheral blood smear reveals target cells (extremely thin and fragile RBCs), pale nucleated RBCs, and marked anisocytosis. X-rays of the skull and long bones show a thinning and widening of the marrow space because of overactive bone marrow. The bones of the skull and vertebrae may appear granular; long bones may show areas of osteoporosis. The phalanges may also be deformed (rectangular or biconvex). Hemoglobin electrophoresis demonstrates a significant rise in Hb F and a slight increase in Hb A_2. Diagnosis must rule out iron deficiency anemia, which also produces hypochromia and microcytic RBCs.

In thalassemia intermedia, laboratory results show hypochromia and microcytic RBCs, but the anemia is less severe than that in thalassemia major. In thalassemia minor, laboratory results show hypochromia (slightly lowered hemoglobin) and microcytic (notably small) RBCs. Hemoglobin electrophoresis shows a significant increase in Hb A_2 and a moderate rise in Hb F.

Treatment

Treatment of thalassemia major is essentially supportive. For example, infections require prompt treatment with appropriate antibiotics. Folic acid supplements help maintain folic acid levels in the face of increased requirements. Transfusions of packed RBCs raise hemoglobin levels but must be used judiciously to minimize iron overload. Splenectomy and bone marrow transplantation have been tried, but their effectiveness has not been confirmed.

Thalassemia intermedia and thalassemia minor generally don't require treatment.

Iron supplements are contraindicated in all forms of thalassemia.

Special considerations

- During and after RBC transfusions for thalassemia major, watch for adverse reactions—shaking chills, fever, rash, itching, and hives.
- Stress the importance of good nutrition, meticulous wound care, periodic dental checkups, and other measures to prevent infection.
- Discuss with the parents of a young patient various options for healthy physical and creative outlets. Such a child must avoid strenuous athletic activity because of increased oxygen demand and the tendency toward pathologic fractures, but he may participate in less stressful activities.
- Teach parents to watch for signs of hepatitis and iron overload—always possible with frequent transfusions.
- Since parents may have questions about the vulnerability of future offspring, refer them for genetic counseling. Also, refer adult patients with thalassemia minor and thalassemia intermedia for genetic counseling; they need to recognize the risk of transmitting thalassemia major to their children if they marry another person with thalassemia. If such persons choose to marry and have children, all their children should be evaluated for thalassemia by age 1. Be sure to tell persons with thalassemia minor that their condition is benign.

Iron Deficiency Anemia

Iron deficiency anemia is caused by an inadequate supply of iron for optimal formation of RBCs, resulting in smaller (microcytic) cells with less color on staining. Body stores of iron, including plasma iron, decrease, as does transferrin, which binds with and transports iron. Insufficient body stores of iron lead to a depleted RBC mass and, in turn, to a decreased hemoglobin concentration (hypochromia) and decreased oxygen-carrying capacity of the blood. A common disease worldwide, iron deficiency anemia affects 10% to 30% of the adult population of the United States.

Causes and incidence

Iron deficiency anemia results from:

- inadequate dietary intake of iron (less than 1 to 2 mg/day), as in prolonged unsupplemented breast- or bottle-feeding of infants, or during periods of stress, such as rapid growth in children and adolescents.
- iron malabsorption, as in chronic diarrhea, partial or total gastrectomy, and malabsorption syndromes, such as celiac disease.
- blood loss secondary to drug-induced gastrointestinal bleeding (from anticoagulants, aspirin, steroids) or due to heavy menses, hemorrhage from trauma,

gastrointestinal ulcers, malignancy, or varices.
• pregnancy, in which the mother's iron supply is diverted to the fetus for erythropoiesis.
• intravascular hemolysis-induced hemoglobinuria or paroxysmal nocturnal hemoglobinuria.
• mechanical erythrocyte trauma caused by a prosthetic heart valve.

Iron deficiency anemia occurs most commonly in premenopausal women, infants (particularly premature or low–birth-weight infants), children, and adolescents (especially girls).

Signs and symptoms

Because of the gradual progression of iron deficiency anemia, many patients are initially asymptomatic, except for symptoms of any underlying condition. They tend not to seek medical treatment until anemia is severe. At advanced stages, decreased hemoglobin and the consequent decrease in the blood's oxygen-carrying capacity cause the patient to develop dyspnea on exertion, fatigue, listlessness, pallor, inability to concentrate, irritability, headache, and a susceptibility to infection. Decreased oxygen perfusion causes the heart to compensate with increased cardiac output and tachycardia.

In patients with chronic iron deficiency anemia, nails become spoon-shaped and brittle, the corners of the mouth crack, the tongue turns smooth, and the patient complains of dysphagia. Associated neuromuscular effects include vasomotor disturbances, numbness and tingling of the extremities, and neuralgic pain.

ABSORPTION AND STORAGE OF IRON

Iron, which is essential to erythropoiesis, is abundant throughout the body. Two thirds of total body iron is found in hemoglobin; the other third, mostly in the reticuloendothelial system (liver, spleen, bone marrow), with small amounts in muscle, blood serum, and body cells.

Adequate dietary ingestion of iron and recirculation of iron released from disintegrating red cells maintain iron supplies. The duodenum and upper part of the small intestine absorb dietary iron. Such absorption depends on gastric acid content, the amount of reducing substances (ascorbic acid, for example) present in the alimentary canal, and dietary iron intake. If iron intake is deficient, the body gradually depletes its iron stores, causing decreased hemoglobin and, eventually, symptoms of iron deficiency anemia.

Diagnosis

Blood studies (serum iron, total iron-binding capacity, ferritin levels) and stores in bone marrow may confirm iron deficiency anemia. However, the results of these tests can be misleading because of complicating factors, such as infection, pneumonia, blood transfusion, or iron supplements. Characteristic blood study results include:
• low hemoglobin levels (males, < 12g/100 ml; females, < 10g/100 ml)
• low hematocrit levels (males, < 47 ml/100 ml; females, < 42 ml/100 ml)
• low serum iron levels, with high binding capacity
• low serum ferritin levels
• low RBC count, with microcytic and hypochromic cells (in early stages, RBC count may be normal, except in infants and children)
• decreased mean corpuscular hemoglobin in severe anemia.

Bone marrow studies reveal depleted or absent iron stores (done by staining) and normoblastic hyperplasia.

Diagnosis must rule out other forms of anemia, such as those that result from thalassemia minor, malignancy, and chronic inflammatory, hepatic, and renal disease.

Prevention

Public health professionals can play a vital role in the prevention of iron deficiency anemia by:
• teaching the basics of a nutritionally balanced diet—red meats, green vegetables, eggs, whole wheat, iron-fortified

bread, and milk. (However, no food in itself contains enough iron to *treat* iron deficiency anemia; an average-sized person with anemia would have to eat at least 10 lb of steak daily to receive therapeutic amounts of iron.)

- emphasizing the need for high-risk individuals—such as premature infants, children under age 2, and pregnant women—to receive prophylactic oral iron, as ordered by a doctor. (Children under age 2 should also receive supplemental cereals and formulas high in iron.)
- assessing a family's dietary habits for iron intake and noting the influence of childhood eating patterns, cultural food preferences, and family income on adequate nutrition.
- encouraging families with deficient iron intake to eat meat, fish, or poultry; whole or enriched grain; and foods high in ascorbic acid.
- carefully assessing a patient's drug history, since certain drugs, such as pancreatic enzymes and vitamin E, may interfere with iron metabolism and absorption and since aspirin, steroids, and other drugs may cause gastrointestinal bleeding. (Teach patients who must take gastric irritants to take these medications with meals or milk.)

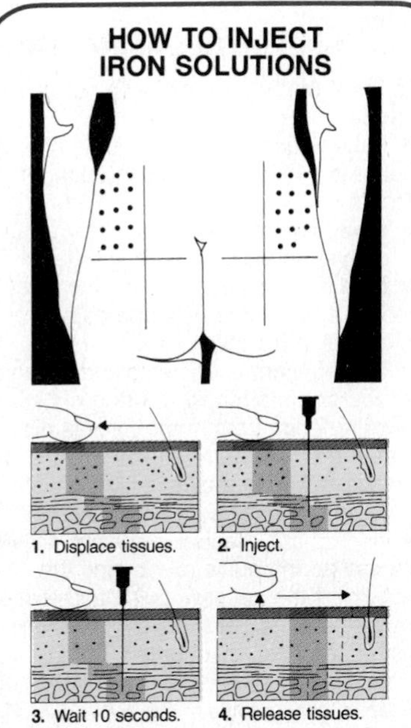
HOW TO INJECT IRON SOLUTIONS
1. Displace tissues.
2. Inject.
3. Wait 10 seconds.
4. Release tissues.

For deep I.M. injections of iron solutions, use the Z-track technique to avoid subcutaneous irritation and discoloration from leaking medication. Choose a 19- to 20-gauge, 5- to 7.5-cm (2- to 3-in) needle. After drawing up the solution, change to a fresh needle to avoid tracking the solution through to subcutaneous tissue. Allow 0.5 cc of air into the syringe.

Displace the skin, fat, and muscle at the injection site (in upper outer quadrant of buttocks only) firmly to one side. Cleanse the area, and insert the needle. Aspirate to check for entry into a blood vessel. Inject the solution slowly, followed by the 0.5 cc of air in the syringe. Wait 10 seconds, pull the needle straight out, and release tissues.

Apply direct pressure to the site, but don't massage it. Caution the patient against vigorous exercise for 15 to 30 minutes.

Treatment

The first priority of treatment is to determine the underlying cause of anemia. Once this is determined, iron replacement therapy can begin. Treatment of choice is an oral preparation of iron or a combination of iron and ascorbic acid (which enhances iron absorption). However, in some cases, iron may have to be administered parenterally—for instance, if the patient is noncompliant to the oral preparation, if he needs more iron than he can take orally, if malabsorption prevents adequate iron absorption, or if a maximum rate of hemoglobin regeneration is desired.

Because total dose I.V. infusion of supplemental iron is painless and requires fewer injections, it's usually preferred to I.M. administration. Pregnant patients and geriatric patients with severe anemia, for example, should receive a total dose infusion of iron dextran in normal saline solution over 8 hours. To minimize the risk of an allergic reaction to iron, an I.V. test dose of 0.5 ml should be given first.

Special considerations

- Monitor the patient's compliance with the prescribed iron supplement therapy.

SUPPORTIVE MANAGEMENT OF PATIENTS WITH ANEMIA

To meet the anemic patient's nutritional needs:

- If the patient is fatigued, urge him to eat small, frequent meals throughout the day.
- If he has oral lesions, suggest soft, cool, bland foods.
- If he has dyspepsia, eliminate spicy foods, and include milk and dairy products in his diet.
- If the patient is anorexic and irritable, encourage his family to bring his favorite foods from home (unless his diet is restricted) and to keep him company during meals, if possible.

To set limitations on activities:

- Assess the effect of a specific activity by monitoring pulse rate during the activity. If the patient's pulse accelerates rapidly and he develops hypotension with hypernoia, diaphoresis, light-headedness, palpitations, shortness of breath, or weakness, the activity is too strenuous.
- Tell the patient to pace his activities, and to allow for frequent rest periods.

To decrease susceptibility to infection:

- Use strict aseptic technique.
- Isolate the patient from infectious persons.
- Instruct the patient to avoid crowds and other sources of infection. Encourage him to practice good hand-washing technique. Stress the importance of receiving necessary immunizations and prompt medical treatment for any sign of infection.

To prepare the patient for diagnostic testing:

- Explain erythropoiesis, the function of blood, and the purpose of diagnostic and therapeutic procedures.
- Tell the patient how he can participate in diagnostic testing. Give him an honest description of the pain or discomfort he will probably experience.
- If possible, schedule all tests to avoid disrupting the patient's meals, sleep, and visiting hours.

To prevent complications:

- Observe for signs of bleeding that may exacerbate anemia. Check stool for occult bleeding. Assess for ecchymoses, gingival bleeding, and hematuria. Monitor vital signs frequently.
- If the patient is confined to strict bed rest, assist with range-of-motion exercises and frequent turning, coughing, and deep breathing.
- If blood transfusions are needed for severe anemia (hemoglobin less than 5 g/100 ml), give washed RBCs, as ordered, in partial exchange if evidence of pump failure is present. Carefully monitor for signs of circulatory overload or transfusion reaction. Watch for a change in pulse rate, blood pressure, or respirations, or onset of fever, chills, pruritus, or edema. If any of these signs develop, stop the transfusion and notify the doctor.
- Warn the patient to move about or change positions slowly to minimize dizziness induced by cerebral hypoxia.

Advise the patient not to stop therapy even if he feels better, since replacement of iron stores takes time.

- Advise the patient that milk or an antacid interferes with absorption but that vitamin C can increase absorption. Instruct the patient to drink liquid supplemental iron through a straw to prevent staining his teeth.
- Tell the patient to report any side effects of iron therapy, such as nausea, vomiting, diarrhea, or constipation, which may require a dosage adjustment.
- If the patient receives iron intravenously, monitor the infusion rate carefully, and observe for an allergic reaction. Stop the infusion and begin supportive treatment immediately if the patient shows signs of an adverse reaction. Also, watch for dizziness and headache and for thrombophlebitis around the I.V. site.
- Use the Z-track injection method when administering iron I.M. to prevent skin discoloration, scarring, and irritating iron deposits in the skin.
- Since an iron deficiency may recur, advise regular checkups.

POLYCYTHEMIAS

Polycythemia Vera

(Primary polycythemia, erythremia, polycythemia rubra vera, splenomegalic polycythemia, Vaquez-Osler disease)

Polycythemia vera is a chronic, myeloproliferative disorder characterized by increased RBC mass, leukocytosis, thrombocytosis, and increased hemoglobin concentration, with normal or decreased plasma volume. It usually occurs between

CLINICAL FEATURES OF POLYCYTHEMIA VERA

SYMPTOMS	CAUSES
Eye, ear, nose, and throat	
• Visual disturbances (blurring, diplopia, scotoma, engorged veins of fundus and retina) and congestion of conjunctiva, retina, retinal veins, oral mucous membrane	• Hypervolemia and hyperviscosity
• Epistaxis or gingival bleeding	• Engorgement of capillary beds
Central nervous system	
• Headache or fullness in the head, lethargy, weakness, fatigue, syncope, tinnitus, paresthesia of digits, and impaired mentation	• Hypervolemia and hyperviscosity
Cardiovascular	
• Hypertension	• Hypervolemia and hyperviscosity
• Intermittent claudication, thrombosis and emboli, angina, thrombophlebitis	• Hypervolemia, thrombocytosis, and vascular disease
• Hemorrhage	• Engorgement of capillary beds
Skin	
• Pruritus (especially after hot bath)	• Basophilia (secondary histamine release)
• Urticaria	• Altered histamine metabolism
• Ruddy cyanosis	• Hypervolemia and hyperviscosity due to congested vessels, increased oxyhemoglobin, and reduced hemoglobin
• Night sweats	• Hypermetabolism
• Ecchymosis	• Hemorrhage
Gastrointestinal and hepatic	
• Epigastric distress	• Hypervolemia and hyperviscosity
• Early satiety and fullness	• Hepatosplenomegaly
• Peptic ulcer pain	• Gastric thrombosis and hemorrhage
• Hepatosplenomegaly	• Congestion, extramedullary hemopoiesis, and myeloid metaplasia
• Weight loss	• Hypermetabolism
Respiratory	
• Dyspnea	• Hypervolemia and hyperviscosity
Musculoskeletal	
• Joint symptoms	• Increased urate production secondary to nucleoprotein turnover

ages 40 and 60, most commonly among males of Jewish ancestry; it rarely affects children or blacks and doesn't appear to be familial. Prognosis depends on age at diagnosis, treatment used, and complications. Mortality is high if polycythemia is untreated or is associated with leukemia or myeloid metaplasia.

Causes

In polycythemia vera, uncontrolled and rapid cellular reproduction and maturation cause proliferation or hyperplasia of all bone marrow cells (panmyelosis). The cause of such uncontrolled cellular activity is unknown, but it is probably due to a multipotential stem cell defect.

Signs and symptoms

Increased RBC mass results in hyperviscosity and inhibits blood flow to microcirculation. Subsequently, increased viscosity, diminished velocity, and thrombocytosis promote intravascular thrombosis. In its early stages, polycythemia vera usually produces no symptoms. (Increased hematocrit may be an incidental finding.) However, as altered circulation secondary to increased RBC mass produces hypervolemia and hyperviscosity, the patient may complain of a vague feeling of fullness in the head, headache, dizziness, and other symptoms, depending on the body system affected.

Paradoxically, hemorrhage is a complication of polycythemia vera. It may be due to defective platelet function or to hyperviscosity and the local effects from excess RBCs exerting pressure on distended venous and capillary walls.

Diagnosis

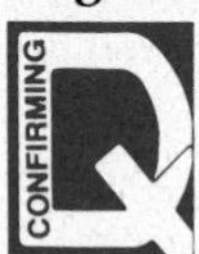

Laboratory studies confirm polycythemia vera by showing increased RBC mass and normal arterial oxygen saturation in association with splenomegaly or two of the following:

- thrombocytosis
- leukocytosis
- elevated leukocyte alkaline phosphatase level
- elevated serum vitamin B_{12} or unbound B_{12}-binding capacity.

Another common finding is increased uric acid production, leading to hyperuricemia and hyperuricuria. Other laboratory results include increased blood histamine, decreased serum iron concentration, and decreased or absent urinary erythropoietin. Bone marrow biopsy reveals panmyelosis.

Treatment

Phlebotomy, the primary treatment, can reduce red cell mass promptly. The frequency of phlebotomy and the amount of blood removed each time depends on the patient's condition. Typically, 350 to 500 ml of blood can be removed every other day until the patient's hematocrit is reduced to the low normal range. After repeated phlebotomies, the patient develops iron deficiency, which stabilizes red cell production and reduces the need for phlebotomy.

Phlebotomy doesn't reduce white cell or platelet count and won't control the hyperuricemia associated with marrow cell proliferation. For severe symptoms related to these manifestations, myelosuppressive therapy may be used. Radioactive phosphorus (^{32}P) or chemotherapeutic agents, such as melphalan, busulfan, or chlorambucil, can satisfactorily control the disease in most cases. However, these agents may cause leukemia, and should be reserved for older patients and those with serious problems not controlled by phlebotomy. Patients of any age who've had previous thrombotic problems should be considered for myelosuppressive therapy.

Special considerations

If the patient requires phlebotomy, explain the procedure, and reassure the patient that it will relieve distressing symptoms. Check blood pressure, pulse rate, and respirations. During phlebotomy, make sure the patient is lying down comfortably, to prevent vertigo and syncope. Stay alert for tachycardia, clamminess, or complaints of vertigo. If these effects occur, the procedure should be stopped.

- Immediately after phlebotomy, check blood pressure and pulse rate. Have the patient sit up for about 5 minutes before allowing him to walk; this prevents vasovagal attack or orthostatic hypotension. Also, administer 24 oz (720 ml) of juice or water.
- Tell the patient to watch for and report any symptoms of iron deficiency (pallor, weight loss, asthenia, glossitis).
- Keep the patient active and ambulatory to prevent thrombosis. If bed rest is absolutely necessary, prescribe a daily program of both active and passive range-of-motion exercises.
- Watch for complications: hypervolemia, thrombocytosis, and signs of an impending cerebrovascular accident (decreased sensation, numbness, transitory paralysis, fleeting blindness, headache, and epistaxis).
- Regularly examine the patient closely for bleeding. Tell him which are the most common bleeding sites (such as the nose, gingiva, and skin), so he can check for bleeding. Advise him to report any abnormal bleeding promptly.
- To compensate for increased uric acid production, give the patient additional fluids, administer allopurinol, as ordered, and alkalinize the urine to prevent uric acid calculi.
- If the patient has symptomatic splenomegaly, suggest or provide small, frequent meals, followed by a rest period, to prevent nausea and vomiting.
- Report acute abdominal pain immediately; it may signal splenic infarction, renal calculi, or abdominal organ thrombosis.

During myelosuppressive chemotherapy:

- Monitor CBC and platelet count before and during therapy. If leukopenia develops in an outpatient, warn him that his resistance to infection is low; advise him to avoid crowds, and make sure he knows the symptoms of infection. If leukopenia develops in a hospitalized patient who needs reverse isolation, follow your hospital's guidelines.
- Tell the patient about possible side effects (nausea, vomiting, and susceptibility to infection) that may follow administration of an alkylating agent. Alopecia may follow the use of busulfan, cyclophosphamide, and uracil mustard; sterile hemorrhagic cystitis may follow the use of cyclophosphamide (forcing fluids can prevent this side effect). Watch for and report all side effects. If nausea and vomiting occur, begin antiemetic therapy and adjust the patient's diet.

During treatment with ^{32}P:

- Explain the procedure to relieve anxiety. Tell the patient he may require repeated phlebotomies until ^{32}P takes effect. Make sure you have a blood sample for CBC and platelet count before beginning treatment. (Note: The health-care professional who administers ^{32}P should take radiation precautions to prevent contamination.)
- Have the patient lie down during I.V. administration (to facilitate the procedure and prevent extravasation) and for 15 to 20 minutes afterward.

Spurious Polycythemia

(Relative polycythemia, stress erythrocytosis, stress polycythemia, benign polycythemia, Gaisböck's syndrome, pseudopolycythemia)

Spurious polycythemia is characterized by increased hematocrit and normal or decreased RBC total mass; it results from decreasing plasma volume and subsequent hemoconcentration. This disease usually affects middle-aged persons and occurs more often in men than in women.

Causes

There are three possible causes of spurious polycythemia:

- *Dehydration:* Conditions that promote severe fluid loss decrease plasma levels and lead to hemoconcentration. Such conditions include persistent vomiting or diarrhea, burns, adrenocortical insufficiency, aggressive diuretic therapy, decreased fluid intake, diabetic acidosis, and renal disease.
- *Hemoconcentration due to stress:* Nervous stress leads to hemoconcentration by some unknown mechanism (possibly by temporarily decreasing circulating plasma volume or vascular redistribution of erythrocytes). This form of erythrocytosis (chronically elevated hematocrit) is particularly common in the middle-aged man who is a chronic smoker and a type A personality (tense, hard-driving, anxious).
- *High normal red cell mass and low normal plasma volume:* In many patients, an increased hematocrit merely reflects a normally high red cell mass and low plasma volume. This is particularly common in patients who are nonsmokers, are not obese, and have no history of hypertension.

Other factors that may be associated with spurious polycythemia include hypertension, thromboembolitic disease, elevated serum cholesterol and uric acid levels, and familial tendency.

Signs and symptoms

The patient with spurious polycythemia usually has no specific symptoms but may have vague complaints, such as headaches, dizziness, and fatigue. Less commonly, he may develop diaphoresis, dyspnea, and claudication.

Typically, the patient has a ruddy appearance, a short neck, slight hypertension, and a tendency to hypoventilate when recumbent. He shows no associated hepatosplenomegaly but may have cardiac or pulmonary disease.

Diagnosis

Hemoglobin and hematocrit levels, and RBC count are elevated; RBC mass, arterial oxygen saturation, and bone marrow are normal. Plasma volume may be decreased or normal. Hypercholesterolemia, hyperlipemia, or hyperuricemia may be present.

Spurious polycythemia is distinguishable from true polycythemia vera by its characteristic normal RBC mass, elevated hematocrit, and the absence of leukocytosis.

Treatment

The principal goals of treatment are to correct dehydration and to prevent life-threatening thromboembolism. Rehydration with appropriate fluids and electrolytes is the primary therapy for spurious polycythemia secondary to dehydration. Therapy must also include appropriate measures to prevent continuing fluid loss.

Special considerations

- During rehydration, carefully monitor intake and output to maintain fluid and electrolyte balance.
- To prevent thromboemboli in predisposed patients, suggest regular exercise and a low-cholesterol diet. Antilipemics may also be necessary. Reduced calorie intake may be required for the obese patient.
- Whenever appropriate, suggest counseling about the patient's work habits and lack of relaxation. If the patient is a smoker, make sure he understands how important it is that he stop smoking. Then, refer him to an antismoking program, if necessary.
- Emphasize the need for follow-up examinations every 3 to 4 months after leaving the hospital.
- Thoroughly explain spurious polycythemia, all diagnostic measures, and therapy. The hard-driving person predisposed to spurious polycythemia is likely to be more inquisitive and anxious than the average patient. Answer his questions honestly, but take care to reassure him that he can effectively control symptoms by complying with the prescribed treatment.

Secondary Polycythemia

(Reactive polycythemia)

Secondary polycythemia is a disorder characterized by excessive production of circulating RBCs due to hypoxia, tumor, or disease. It occurs in approximately 2 out of every 100,000 persons living at or near sea level; incidence rises among persons living at high altitudes.

Causes

Secondary polycythemia may result from increased production of erythropoietin. This hormone, which is possibly produced and secreted in the kidneys, stimulates bone marrow production of RBCs. This increased production may be an appropriate (compensatory) physiologic response to hypoxemia, which may result from:

- chronic obstructive pulmonary disease (COPD)
- hemoglobin abnormalities (such as carboxyhemoglobinemia, which is seen in heavy smokers)
- congestive heart failure (causing a decreased ventilation-perfusion ratio)
- right-to-left shunting of blood in the heart (as in transposition of the great vessels)
- central or peripheral alveolar hypoventilation (as in barbiturate intoxication or pickwickian syndrome)
- low oxygen content of air at high altitudes.

Increased production of erythropoietin may also be an inappropriate (pathologic) response to renal disease (such as renal vascular impairment, renal cysts, or hydronephrosis), to CNS disease (such as encephalitis and parkinsonism), to neoplasms (such as renal tumors, uterine myomas, or cerebellar hemangiomas), or to endocrine disorders (such as Cushing's syndrome, Bartter's syndrome, or pheochromocytomas). Rarely, secondary polycythemia results from a recessive genetic trait.

Signs and symptoms

In the hypoxic patient, suggestive physical findings include ruddy cyanotic skin, emphysema, hypoxemia without hepatosplenomegaly or hypertension. Clubbing of the fingers may occur if the underlying disease is cardiovascular. When secondary polycythemia isn't caused by hypoxemia, it's usually an incidental finding during treatment for an underlying disease.

Diagnosis

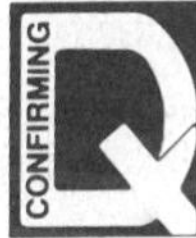

Laboratory values for secondary polycythemia include increased RBC mass, urinary erythropoietin, and blood histamine, with decreased or normal arterial oxygen saturation. Bone marrow biopsies reveal hyperplasia confined to the erythroid series. Unlike polycythemia vera, secondary polycythemia isn't associated with leukocytosis or thrombocytosis.

Treatment

The goal of treatment is correction of the underlying disease or environmental condition. In severe secondary polycythemia where altitude is a contributing factor, relocation may be advisable. If secondary polycythemia has produced hazardous hyperviscosity or if the patient doesn't respond to treatment for the primary disease, reduction of blood volume by phlebotomy may be effective. Emergency phlebotomy is indicated for prevention of impending vascular occlusion or before emergency surgery. In the latter case, it's usually advisable to remove excess RBCs and reinfuse the patient's plasma.

Because a patient with polycythemia has an increased risk of hemorrhage during and after surgery, elective surgery should be avoided until polycythemia is controlled. Generally, secondary polycythemia disappears when the primary disease is corrected.

Special considerations

- Keep the patient as active as possible to decrease the risk of thrombosis due to increased blood viscosity.
- Reduce calorie and sodium intake to counteract the tendency to hypertension.
- Before and after phlebotomy, check blood pressure with the patient lying down. After the procedure, give him approximately 24 oz (720 ml) of water or juice to drink. To prevent syncope, have him sit up for about 5 minutes before walking.
- Emphasize the importance of regular blood studies (every 2 to 3 months), even after the disease is controlled.
- Teach the patient and family about the underlying disorder. Help them understand its relationship to polycythemia and the measures needed to control both.

HEMORRHAGIC DISORDERS

Allergic Purpuras

(Henoch-Schönlein purpura, anaphylactoid purpura)

Allergic purpura, a nonthrombocytopenic purpura, is an acute or chronic vascular inflammation affecting the skin, joints, and gastrointestinal and genitourinary tracts, in association with allergy symptoms. When allergic purpura primarily affects the gastrointestinal tract, with accompanying joint pain, it is called Henoch-Schönlein syndrome or anaphylactoid purpura. However, the term allergic purpura applies to purpura associated with many other conditions, such as erythema nodosum. An acute attack of allergic purpura can last for several weeks and is potentially fatal (usually from renal failure); however, most patients do recover.

Fully developed allergic purpura is persistent and debilitating, possibly leading to chronic glomerulonephritis (especially following a streptococcal infection). Allergic purpura affects males more often than females and is most prevalent in children aged 3 to 7 years. Prognosis is more favorable for children than adults.

Causes

The most common identifiable cause of allergic purpura is probably an autoimmune reaction directed against vascular walls, triggered by a bacterial infection (particularly streptococcal infection). Typically, upper respiratory infection occurs 1 to 3 weeks before the onset of symptoms. Other possible causes include allergic reactions to some drugs and vaccines; allergic reactions to insect bites; and allergic reactions to some foods (such as wheat, eggs, milk, chocolate).

Signs and symptoms

Characteristic skin lesions of allergic purpura are purple, macular, ecchymotic, and of varying size and are caused by vascular leakage into the skin and mucous membranes. The lesions usually appear in symmetric patterns on the arms and legs and are accompanied by pruritus, paresthesia, and, occasionally, angioneurotic edema. In children, skin lesions are generally urticarial and expand and become hemorrhagic. Scattered petechiae may appear on the legs, buttocks, and perineum.

Henoch-Schönlein syndrome commonly produces transient or severe colic, tenesmus and constipation, vomiting, and edema or hemorrhage of the mucous membranes of the bowel, resulting in GI bleeding, occult blood in the stool, and, possibly, intussusception. Such GI abnormalities may *precede* overt, cutaneous signs of purpura. Musculoskeletal symptoms, such as rheumatoid pains and periarticular effusions, mostly affect the legs and feet.

In 25% to 50% of patients, allergic purpura is associated with genitourinary symptoms: nephritis; renal hemorrhages that may cause microscopic hematuria and disturb renal function; bleeding from the mucosal surfaces of the ureters, bladder, or urethra; and, occasionally, glomerulonephritis. Also possible are moderate and irregular fever, headache, anorexia, and localized edema of the hands, feet, or scalp.

PURPURIC LESIONS

Lesions of allergic purpura, such as those pictured on the foot and leg above, characteristically vary in size.

Diagnosis

No laboratory test clearly identifies allergic purpura (although WBC count and ESR are elevated). Diagnosis therefore necessitates careful clinical observation, often during the second or third attack. Except for a positive tourniquet test, coagulation and platelet function tests are usually normal. Small bowel X-rays may reveal areas of transient edema; tests for blood in the urine and stool are often positive. Increased BUN and creatinine may indicate renal involvement. Diagnosis must rule out other forms of nonthrombocytopenic purpura.

Treatment

Treatment is generally symptomatic; for example, severe allergic purpura may require steroids to relieve edema and analgesics to relieve joint and abdominal pain. Some patients with chronic renal disease may benefit from immunosuppression with azathioprine, along with identification of the provocative allergen. *Accurate allergy history is essential.*

Special considerations

- Encourage maintenance of an elimination diet to help identify specific allergenic foods, so these foods can be eliminated from the patient's diet.
- Monitor skin lesions and level of pain. Provide analgesics, as needed.
- Watch carefully for complications: GI and genitourinary tract bleeding, edema, nausea, vomiting, headache, hypertension (with nephritis), abdominal rigidity and tenderness, and absence of stool (with intussusception).
- To prevent muscle atrophy in the bedridden patient, provide passive or active range-of-motion exercises.
- Provide emotional support and reassurance, especially if the patient is temporarily disfigured by florid skin lesions.
- After the acute stage, stress the need for the patient to *immediately* report *any* recurrence of symptoms (recurrence is most common about 6 weeks after initial onset) and to return for follow-up urinalysis as scheduled.

Hereditary Hemorrhagic Telangiectasia

(Rendu-Osler-Weber disease)

Hereditary hemorrhagic telangiectasia is an inherited vascular disorder in which venules and capillaries dilate to form fragile masses of thin convoluted vessels (telangiectases), resulting in an abnormal tendency to hemorrhage. This disorder affects both sexes but may cause less severe bleeding in females.

Causes

Hereditary hemorrhagic telangiectasia is transmitted by autosomal dominant inheritance. It rarely skips generations. In its homozygous state, it may be lethal.

Signs and symptoms

Signs of hereditary hemorrhagic telangiectasia are present in childhood but increase in severity with age. Localized aggregations of dilated capillaries appear on the skin of the face, ears, scalp, hands, arms, and feet; under the nails; and on the mucous membranes of the nose, mouth, and stomach. These dilated capillaries cause frequent epistaxis, hemoptysis, and gastrointestinal bleeding, possibly leading to iron deficiency anemia. (In children, epistaxis is usually the first symptom.)

Characteristic telangiectases are violet, bleed spontaneously, may be flat or raised, blanch on pressure, and are nonpulsatile. They may be associated with vascular malformations such as arteriovenous fistulas. Visceral telangiectases are common in the liver, bladder, respiratory tract, and stomach. The type and distribution of these lesions are generally similar among family members.

Generalized capillary fragility, evidenced by spontaneous bleeding and spider hemangiomas of varying sizes, may exist without overt telangiectasia. Occasionally, vascular malformation may cause pulmonary arteriovenous fistulas; then, shunting of blood through the fistulas may lead to hypoxemia, recurring cerebral embolism, brain abscess, and clubbing of digits.

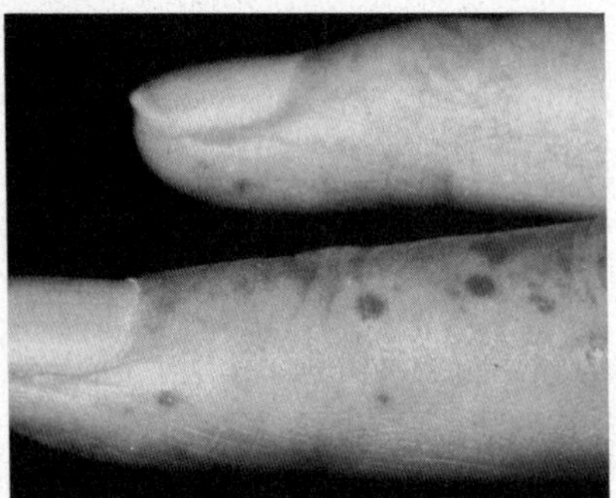

In hereditary hemorrhagic telangiectasia, localized aggregations of dilated capillaries may be flat or raised.

Diagnosis

Diagnosis rests on an established familial pattern of bleeding disorders and clinical evidence of telangiectasia and hemorrhage. Bone marrow aspiration showing depleted iron stores confirms secondary iron deficiency anemia. Hypochromic, microcytic anemia is common; abnormal platelet function may also be found. Coagulation tests are essentially irrelevant, though, because hemorrhage in telangiectasia results from vascular wall weakness.

Treatment

Supportive therapy includes blood transfusions and the administration of supplemental iron. Ancillary treatment includes applying pressure and topical hemostatic agents to bleeding sites; excising bleeding sites (when accessible); and protecting the patient from trauma and unnecessary bleeding.

Parenteral administration of supplemental iron enhances absorption to maintain adequate iron stores and prevents gastric irritation. Administering antipyretics or antihistamines before blood transfusion and using saline-washed cells, frozen blood, or other types of leukocyte-poor blood instead of whole blood transfusion, may prevent febrile transfusion reactions.

Special considerations

- If the patient is receiving a blood transfusion, stay with him during the first 15 minutes to observe for possible adverse reactions. Afterward, check again, every 15 minutes, for signs of febrile transfusion reaction (flushing, shaking chills, fever, headache, rash,

tachycardia, hypertension), since such a patient is quite susceptible to a reaction.
- Observe the patient for indications of gastrointestinal bleeding, such as hematemesis and melena. Instruct the patient to watch for and report such signs as well.
- If the patient requires an iron supplement, stress the importance of following dosage instructions and of taking oral iron with meals to minimize gastric irritation. Warn that iron turns stools dark green or black.
- Teach the patient and family how to manage minor bleeding episodes, especially recurrent epistaxis, and to recognize major ones that necessitate emergency intervention.

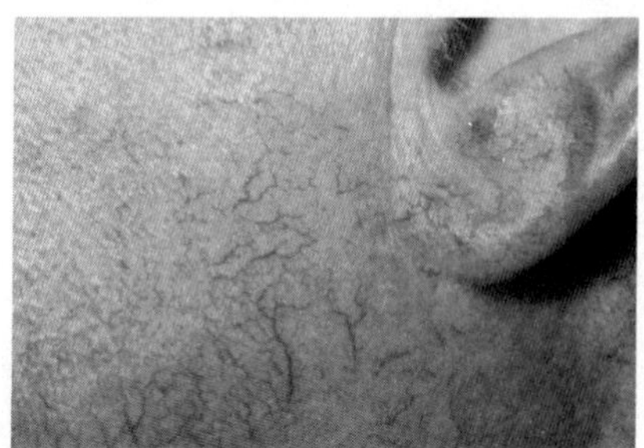

On the face shown above, spider hemangiomas reflect capillary fragility in hereditary hemorrhagic telangiectasia.

- Refer the patient for genetic counseling, as appropriate.

Thrombocytopenia

The most common cause of hemorrhagic disorders, thrombocytopenia is characterized by a deficient number of circulating platelets. Since platelets play a vital role in coagulation, this disease poses a serious threat to hemostasis. Prognosis is excellent in drug-induced thrombocytopenia if the offending drug is withdrawn; in such cases, recovery may be immediate. Otherwise, prognosis depends on response to treatment of the underlying cause.

Causes

Thrombocytopenia may be congenital or acquired; the acquired form is more common. In either case, it usually results from decreased or defective production of platelets in the marrow (such as occurs in leukemia, aplastic anemia, or toxicity with certain drugs) or from increased destruction outside the marrow caused by an underlying disorder (such as cirrhosis of the liver, disseminated intravascular coagulation, or severe infection). Less commonly, it results from sequestration (hypersplenism, hypothermia) or platelet loss. Acquired thrombocytopenia may result from certain drugs, such as quinine, quinidine, sulfisoxazole, chlorothiazide, hydrochlorothiazide, phenylbutazone, oxyphenbutazone, rifampin, heparin, cyclophosphamide, and vinblastine sulfate.

An idiopathic form of thrombocytopenia commonly occurs in children.

Signs and symptoms

Thrombocytopenia typically produces a sudden onset of petechiae or ecchymoses in the skin or bleeding into any mucous membrane (gastrointestinal, urinary, vaginal, or respiratory). As a result of such bleeding, the patient suffers malaise, fatigue, general weakness, and lethargy. In adults, large blood-filled bullae that are characteristic of thrombocytopenia appear in the mouth. In severe thrombocytopenia, hemorrhage may lead to tachycardia, shortness of breath, loss of consciousness, and death.

Diagnosis

Diagnosis necessitates a patient history (especially a drug history), physical examination, and laboratory tests. Coagulation tests show diminished platelet count (in adults, less than 200,000/ mm³), prolonged bleeding time, and normal prothrombin and partial thromboplastin times. If increased destruction of platelets is causing thrombocytopenia, bone marrow studies reveal a greater number of megakaryocytes (platelet precursors) and shortened platelet survival (several hours or days rather than the usual 7 to 10 days).

CAUSES OF DECREASED CIRCULATING PLATELETS

Diminished or defective production

Congenital
- Wiskott-Aldrich syndrome
- Maternal ingestion of thiazides
- Neonatal rubella
- Thrombopoietin deficiency

Acquired
- Aplastic anemia
- Marrow infiltration (acute and chronic leukemias, tumor)
- Nutritional deficiency (B_{12}, folic acid)
- Myelosuppressive agents
- Drugs that directly influence platelet production (thiazides, alcohol, hormones)
- Radiation
- Viral infections (measles, dengue)

Increased peripheral destruction

Congenital
- Nonimmune (prematurity, erythroblastosis fetalis, infection)
- Immune (drug sensitivity, maternal ITP)

Acquired
- Nonimmune (infection, DIC, thrombotic thrombocytopenic purpura)
- Immune (drug-induced, especially with quinine and quinidine; post-transfusion purpura; acute and chronic ITP; sepsis; alcohol)

Sequestration
- Hypersplenism
- Hypothermia

Loss
- Hemorrhage
- Extracorporeal perfusion

Adapted with permission from William J. Williams et al., HEMATOLOGY (New York: McGraw-Hill Book Co., 1977).

Treatment

Treatment varies with the underlying cause and may include corticosteroids to enhance vascular integrity. Removal of the offending agents in drug-induced thrombocytopenia or proper treatment of the underlying cause, when possible, is essential. Platelet transfusions are helpful only in treating complications of severe hemorrhage.

Special considerations

When caring for the patient with thrombocytopenia, take every possible precaution against bleeding.

- Protect the patient from trauma. Keep the side rails up, and pad them, if possible. Promote the use of an electric razor and a soft toothbrush. Avoid all invasive procedures, such as venipuncture or urinary catheterization, if possible. When venipuncture is unavoidable, be sure to exert pressure on the puncture site for at least 20 minutes or until the bleeding stops.
- Monitor platelet count daily.
- Test stool for guaiac; dipstick urine and emesis for blood.
- Watch for bleeding (petechiae, ecchymoses, surgical or gastrointestinal bleeding, menorrhagia).
- Warn the patient to avoid taking aspirin in any form, as well as other drugs that impair coagulation. Teach him how to recognize aspirin compounds that are listed on labels of over-the-counter remedies.
- Advise the patient to avoid straining at stool or coughing, as both can lead to increased intracranial pressure, possibly causing cerebral hemorrhage in the patient with thrombocytopenia. Provide a stool softener, if necessary.
- During periods of active bleeding, maintain the patient on strict bed rest, if necessary.
- When administering platelet concentrate, remember that platelets are extremely fragile, so infuse them quickly, using the administration set recommended by your blood bank.
- During platelet transfusion, monitor for febrile reaction (flushing, chills, fe-

ver, headache, tachycardia, hypertension). HLA-typed platelets may be ordered to prevent febrile reaction. If the patient has a history of minor reactions, he may benefit from acetaminophen and diphenhydramine before the transfusion.

• If thrombocytopenia is drug-induced, stress the importance of avoiding the offending drug.

• If the patient must receive long-term steroid therapy, teach him to watch for and report cushingoid symptoms (acne, moon face, hirsutism, buffalo hump, hypertension, girdle obesity, thinning arms and legs, glycosuria, and edema). Emphasize that steroid doses must be discontinued gradually. While the patient's receiving steroid therapy, monitor his fluid and electrolyte balance, and watch for infection, pathologic fractures, and mood changes.

FACTS ABOUT PLATELET CONCENTRATE

Contents:
• Platelets, WBCs, some plasma
• Random platelets (ABO matched)
• HLA platelets (HLA antigens typed for multiple transfusions)

Amount:
• 30 to 50 ml per donor
• 4 to 8 donor units given each time (each unit should raise the platelet count by 5,000/mm³)

Shelf life:
• 6 to 72 hours (best used within 24 hours)

Hepatitis risk:
• Same as with whole blood

Idiopathic Thrombocytopenic Purpura

Thrombocytopenia that results from immunologic platelet destruction is known as idiopathic thrombocytopenic purpura (ITP). This form of thrombocytopenia may be acute (postviral thrombocytopenia) or chronic (Werlhof's disease, purpura hemorrhagica, essential thrombocytopenia, autoimmune thrombocytopenia). Acute ITP usually affects children between ages 2 and 6; chronic ITP mainly affects adults under age 50, especially women between ages 20 and 40. Prognosis for acute ITP is excellent, with nearly four out of five patients recovering completely without specific treatment. Prognosis for chronic ITP is good; transient remissions lasting weeks or even years are common, especially among women.

Causes

ITP may be an autoimmune disorder, since antibodies that reduce the life span of platelets have been found in nearly all patients. The spleen probably helps to remove platelets modified by the antibody. Acute ITP usually follows a viral infection, such as rubella or chicken pox. ITP may also be drug-induced or associated with lupus erythematosus or pregnancy.

Signs and symptoms

ITP produces clinical features that are common to all forms of thrombocytopenia: petechiae, ecchymoses, and mucosal bleeding from the mouth, nose, or gastrointestinal tract. Generally, hemorrhage is the only abnormal physical finding. Purpuric lesions may occur in vital organs, such as the brain, and may prove fatal. In acute ITP, which commonly occurs in children, onset is usually sudden and without warning, causing easy bruising, epistaxis, and bleeding gums. Onset of chronic ITP is insidious.

Diagnosis

Platelet count less than 20,000/mm³ and prolonged bleeding time suggest ITP. Platelet size and morphologic appearance may be abnormal; anemia may be present if bleeding has occurred. As in thrombocytopenia, bone marrow studies show an abundance of megakaryocytes (platelet precursors) and a shortened circulating platelet survival time (several hours or days rather than the usual 7 to 10 days). Occasionally, platelet antibodies may be found in vitro, but this diagnosis is usually inferred from platelet survival data and the absence of an underlying disease.

Treatment

Corticosteroids, the initial treatment of choice, promote capillary integrity but are only temporarily effective in chronic ITP. Alternative treatments include immunosuppression (with vincristine sulfate, for example), plasmapheresis, and splenectomy in adults (85% successful). Before splenectomy, the patient may require blood, blood components, and vitamin K to correct anemia and coagulation defects. After splenectomy, he may need blood and component replacement, and platelet concentrate. Normally, however, platelets multiply spontaneously after splenectomy.

Special considerations

Patient care for ITP is essentially the same as for thrombocytopenia, with emphasis on teaching the patient to observe for petechiae, ecchymoses, and other signs of recurrence, especially following acute ITP.

Closely monitor patients receiving immunosuppressives (often given before splenectomy) for signs of bone marrow depression, infection, mucositis, gastrointestinal tract ulceration, and severe diarrhea or vomiting.

Platelet Function Disorders

Platelet function disorders are similar to thrombocytopenia but result from platelet dysfunction rather than platelet deficiency. They characteristically cause defects in platelet adhesion or procoagulation activity (ability to bind coagulation factors to their surface to form a stable fibrin clot). Such disorders may also create defects in platelet aggregation and thromboxane A_2 and may produce abnormalities by preventing the release of adenosine diphosphate (defective platelet release reaction). Prognosis varies widely.

Causes

Abnormal platelet function disorders may be inherited (autosomal recessive) or acquired. Inherited disorders cause bone marrow production of platelets that are ineffective in the clotting mechanism. Acquired disorders result from the effects of drugs, such as aspirin or carbenicillin; from systemic diseases, such as uremia; or from other hematologic disorders.

Signs and symptoms

Generally, the sudden appearance of petechiae or purpura or excessive bruising and bleeding of the nose and gums are the first overt signs of platelet function disorders. More serious signs are external hemorrhage, internal hemorrhage into the muscles and visceral organs, or excessive bleeding during surgery.

Diagnosis

Prolonged bleeding time in a patient with both a normal platelet count and normal clotting factors suggests this diagnosis. Determination of the defective mechanism requires a blood film and a platelet function test to measure platelet release reaction and aggregation. Depending on the type of platelet dysfunction, some or all of the test results may be abnormal.

Other typical laboratory findings are poor clot retraction and decreased pro-

PATIENT TEACHING AID

Precautions for Patients with Blood Clotting Problems

Because your doctor has prescribed anticoagulant medication, you must be careful to prevent bleeding. Here are some helpful tips:

DO'S

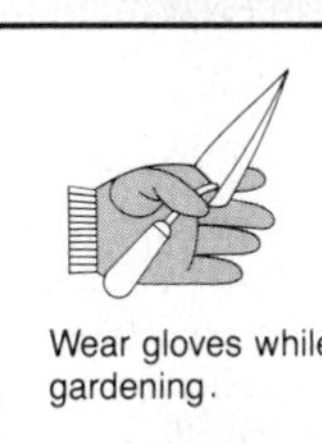

Wear gloves while gardening.

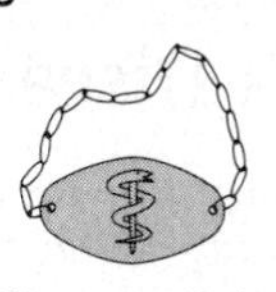

Wear a medical identification bracelet.

Use an electric shaver.

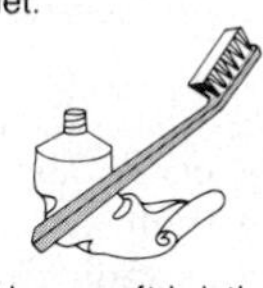

Use a soft-bristled toothbrush.

DON'TS

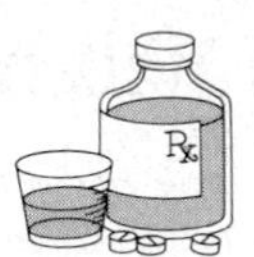

Don't self-medicate.

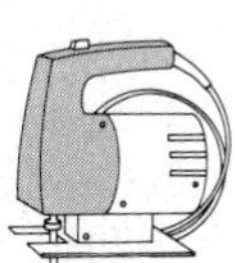

Don't use power tools.

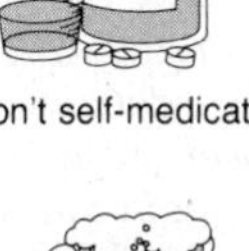

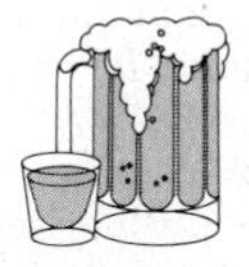

Don't use alcohol excessively.

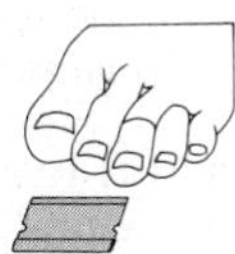

Don't trim calluses and corns.

This patient teaching aid may be reproduced by office copier for distribution to patients.

thrombin conversion. Baseline testing includes CBC and differential and appropriate tests to determine hemorrhage sites. In platelet function disorders, plasma clotting factors, platelet counts, and prothrombin, activated partial thromboplastin, and thrombin times are usually normal.

Treatment

Platelet replacement is the only satisfactory treatment for inherited platelet dysfunction. However, acquired platelet function disorders respond to adequate treatment of the underlying disease or discontinuation of damaging drug therapy. Plasmapheresis effectively controls bleeding caused by a plasma element that's inhibiting platelet function. During this procedure, one or more units of whole blood are removed from the patient; the plasma is removed from the whole blood, and the remaining packed RBCs are reinfused.

Special considerations

- Obtain an accurate patient history, including onset of bleeding, use of drugs (especially aspirin), and family history of bleeding disorders.
- Watch closely for bleeding from skin, nose, gums, GI tract, or an injury site.
- Help the patient avoid unnecessary trauma. Advise him to tell his dentist about this condition before undergoing oral surgery. (Also stress the need for good oral hygiene to help prevent such surgery.)
- Alert other care team members to the patient's hemorrhagic potential, especially before he undergoes diagnostic tests that may cause trauma and bleeding.
- Observe the patient undergoing plasmapheresis for hypovolemia, hypotension, tachycardia, vasoconstriction, and other signs of volume depletion.
- If platelet dysfunction is inherited, help the patient and family understand and accept the nature of this disorder. Teach them how to manage potential bleeding episodes. Warn them that petechiae, ecchymoses, and bleeding from the nose, gums, and GI tract signal ab-

normal bleeding and should be reported immediately.
- Tell the patient with a known coagulopathy or hepatic disease to avoid aspirin, aspirin compounds, and other agents that impair coagulation.
- Advise the patient to wear a medical identification bracelet or to carry a card identifying him as a potential bleeder.

Von Willebrand's Disease

Von Willebrand's disease is a hereditary bleeding disorder characterized by prolonged bleeding time, moderate deficiency of clotting Factor VIII$_{AHF}$ (antihemophilic factor), and impaired platelet function. This disease commonly causes bleeding from the skin or mucosal surfaces and, in females, excessive uterine bleeding. Bleeding may range from mild and asymptomatic to severe, potentially fatal hemorrhage. Prognosis, however, is usually good.

Causes and incidence

Unlike hemophilia, von Willebrand's disease is inherited as an autosomal dominant trait and occurs equally in males and females. One theory of pathophysiology holds that mild to moderate deficiency of Factor VIII and defective platelet adhesion prolong coagulation time. More specifically, this results from a deficiency of the von Willebrand factor (VWF), which appears to occupy the Factor VIII molecule and may be necessary for the production of Factor VIII and proper platelet function. Defective platelet function is characterized by:
- decreased agglutination and adhesion at the bleeding site.
- reduced platelet retention when filtered through a column of packed glass beads.
- diminished ristocetin-induced platelet aggregation.

Signs and symptoms

Von Willebrand's disease produces easy bruising, epistaxis, and bleeding from the gums. Severe forms of this disease may cause hemorrhage after laceration or surgery, menorrhagia, and gastrointestinal bleeding. Excessive postpartum bleeding is uncommon, because Factor VIII levels and bleeding time abnormalities become less pronounced during pregnancy. Massive soft-tissue hemorrhage and bleeding into joints rarely occur. Severity of bleeding may lessen with age, and bleeding episodes occur sporadically—a patient may bleed excessively after one dental extraction but not after another.

Diagnosis

Diagnosis is difficult, because symptoms are mild, laboratory values are borderline, and Factor VIII levels fluctuate. However, a positive family history and characteristic bleeding patterns and laboratory values help establish diagnosis. Typical laboratory data include:
- prolonged bleeding time (more than 6 minutes)
- slightly prolonged partial thromboplastin time (more than 45 seconds)
- absent or reduced levels of Factor VIII-related antigens (VIII$_{AGN}$), and low Factor VIII activity level
- defective in vitro platelet aggregation (using the ristocetin coagulation factor assay test)
- normal platelet count and normal clot retraction.

Treatment

The aims of treatment are to shorten bleeding time by local measures and to replace Factor VIII (and, consequently, VWF) by infusion of cryoprecipitate or blood fractions that are rich in Factor VIII.

During bleeding episodes and before

even minor surgery, I.V. infusion of cryoprecipitate or fresh-frozen plasma (in quantities sufficient to raise Factor VIII levels to 50% of normal) generally shortens bleeding time.

Special considerations

The care plan should include local measures to control bleeding and patient teaching to prevent bleeding, unnecessary trauma, and complications.

- After surgery, monitor bleeding time for 24 to 48 hours, and watch for signs of new bleeding.
- During a bleeding episode, elevate and apply cold compresses and gentle pressure to the bleeding site.
- Refer parents of affected children for genetic counseling.
- Advise the patient to consult the doctor after even minor trauma and before all surgery, to determine if replacement of blood components is necessary.
- Tell the patient to watch for signs of hepatitis within 6 weeks to 6 months after transfusion.
- Warn against using aspirin and other drugs that impair platelet function.
- If the patient has a severe form of this disease, instruct him to avoid contact sports.

Disseminated Intravascular Coagulation

(Consumption coagulopathy, defibrination syndrome)

Disseminated intravascular coagulation (DIC) occurs as a complication of diseases and conditions that accelerate clotting, causing small blood vessel occlusion, organ necrosis, depletion of circulating clotting factors and platelets, and activation of the fibrinolytic system. This, in turn, can provoke severe hemorrhage. Clotting in the microcirculation usually affects the kidneys and extremities but may occur in the brain, lungs, pituitary and adrenal glands, and gastrointestinal mucosa. Other conditions, such as vitamin K deficiency, hepatic disease, and anticoagulant therapy, may cause a similar hemorrhage. DIC is generally an acute condition but may be chronic in cancer patients. Prognosis depends on early detection and treatment, the severity of the hemorrhage, and treatment of the underlying disease or condition.

Causes

DIC may result from:

- *Infection:* gram-negative or gram-positive septicemia; viral, fungal, or rickettsial infection; protozoal infection (falciparum malaria).
- *Obstetric complications:* abruptio placentae, amniotic fluid embolism, retained dead fetus.
- *Neoplastic disease:* acute leukemia, metastatic carcinoma.
- *Disorders that produce necrosis:* extensive burns and trauma, brain tissue destruction, transplant rejection, hepatic necrosis.
- *Others:* heatstroke, shock, poisonous snakebite, cirrhosis, fat embolism, incompatible blood transfusion, cardiac arrest, surgery necessitating cardiopulmonary bypass, giant hemangioma, severe venous thrombosis, purpura fulminans.

It's not clear why such disorders lead to DIC; nor is it certain that they lead to it through a common mechanism. In many patients, the triggering mechanisms may be the entrance of foreign protein into the circulation, and vascular endothelial injury. Regardless of how DIC begins, the typical accelerated clotting results in generalized activation of prothrombin and a consequent excess of thrombin. Excess thrombin converts fibrinogen to fibrin, producing fibrin clots in the microcirculation. This process consumes exorbitant amounts of coagulation factors (especially fibrinogen, prothrombin, platelets, and Factor V and

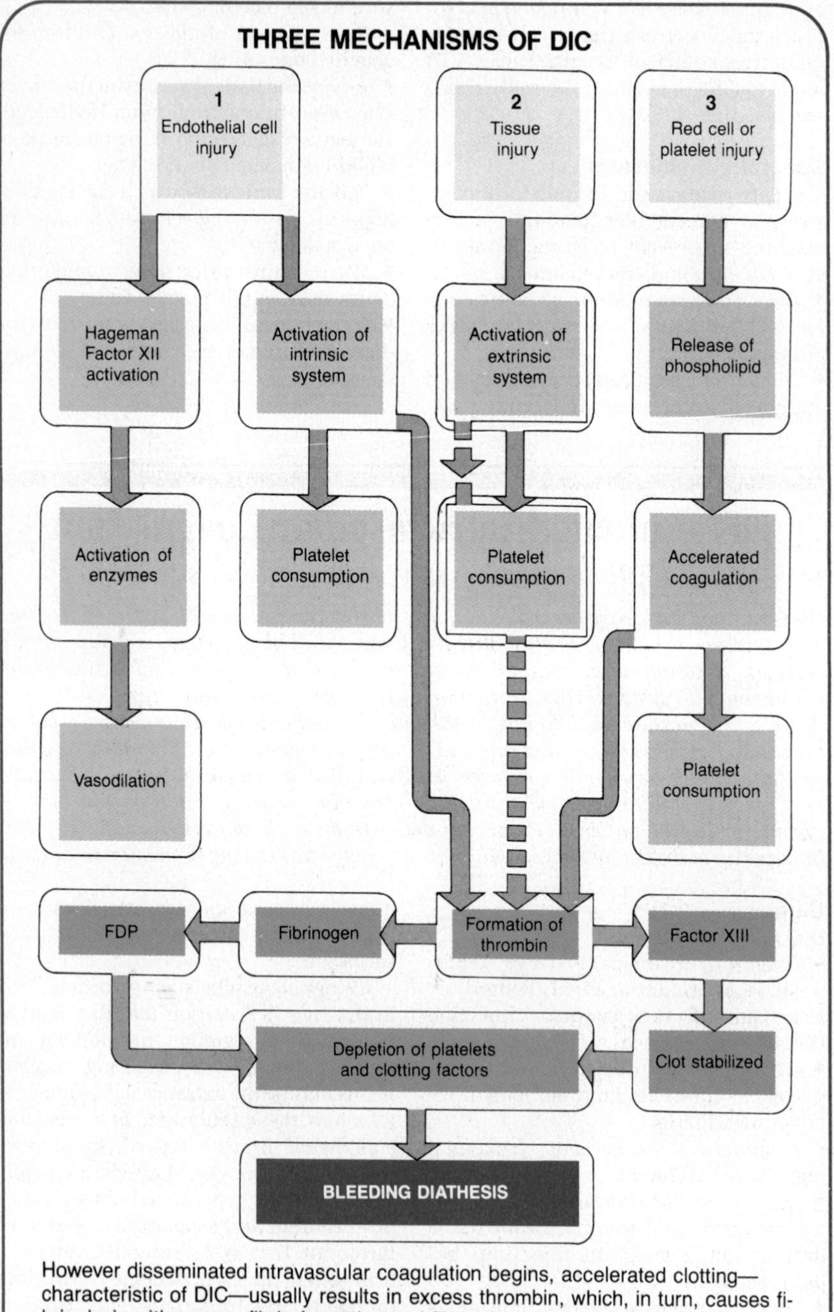

However disseminated intravascular coagulation begins, accelerated clotting—characteristic of DIC—usually results in excess thrombin, which, in turn, causes fibrinolysis with excess fibrin formation and fibrin degradation products (FDP), activation of fibrin-stabilizing factor (Factor XIII), consumption of platelet and clotting factors, and eventually, hemorrhage.

Factor VIII), causing hypofibrinogenemia, hypoprothrombinemia, thrombocytopenia, and deficiencies in Factor V and Factor VIII. Circulating thrombin activates the fibrinolytic system, which lyses fibrin clots into fibrin degradation products. The hemorrhage that occurs may be due largely to the anticoagulant activity of fibrin degradation products, as well as depletion of plasma coagulation factors.

Signs and symptoms

The most significant clinical feature of DIC is abnormal bleeding, *without* an accompanying history of a serious hemorrhagic disorder. Principal signs of such bleeding include cutaneous oozing, petechiae, ecchymoses, and hematomas caused by bleeding into the skin. Bleeding from sites of surgical or invasive procedures (such as incisions or I.V. sites) and from the gastrointestinal tract are equally significant signs, as are acrocyanosis and signs of acute tubular necrosis. Related symptoms and other possible effects include nausea, vomiting, dyspnea, oliguria, convulsions, coma, shock, failure of major organ systems, and severe muscle, back, and abdominal pain.

Diagnosis

Abnormal bleeding in the absence of a known hematologic disorder suggests DIC. Initial laboratory findings supporting a tentative diagnosis of DIC include:

- *prolonged prothrombin time:* > 15 seconds
- *prolonged partial thromboplastin time:* > 60 to 80 seconds
- *decreased fibrinogen levels:* < 150 mg%
- *decreased platelets:* < 100,000/mm^3
- *increased fibrin degradation products:* often > 100 mcg/ml.

Other supportive data include positive fibrin monomers, diminished levels of factors V and VIII, fragmentation of RBCs, and decreased hemoglobin (< 10 g/100 ml). Assessment of renal status demonstrates reduction in urinary output (< 30 ml/hour), and elevated BUN (> 25 mg/100 ml) and serum creatinine (> 1.3 mg/100 ml).

Final confirmation of the diagnosis may be difficult, because many of these test results also occur in other disorders (primary fibrinolysis, for example). Additional diagnostic measures determine the underlying disorder.

Treatment

Successful management of DIC necessitates prompt recognition and adequate treatment of the underlying disorder. Treatment may be supportive (when the underlying disorder is self-limiting, for example) or highly specific. If the patient isn't actively bleeding, supportive care alone may reverse DIC. However, active bleeding may require heparin I.V. and administration of blood, fresh-frozen plasma, platelets, or packed RBCs to support hemostasis.

Special considerations

Patient care must focus on early recognition of principal signs of abnormal bleeding, prompt treatment of the underlying disorders, and prevention of further bleeding.

- To prevent clots from dislodging and causing fresh bleeding, don't scrub bleeding areas. Use pressure, cold compresses, and topical hemostatic agents to control bleeding.
- Protect the patient from injury. Enforce complete bed rest during bleeding episodes. If the patient is very agitated, pad the side rails.
- Check all I.V. and venipuncture sites frequently for bleeding. Apply pressure to injection sites for at least 10 minutes. Alert other personnel to the patient's tendency to hemorrhage.
- Monitor intake and output hourly in acute DIC, especially when administering blood products. Watch for transfusion reactions and signs of fluid overload. To measure the amount of blood lost, weigh dressings and linen and record drainage. Weigh the patient daily, particularly if there is renal involvement.
- Watch for bleeding from the gastrointestinal and genitourinary tracts. If you

suspect intraabdominal bleeding, measure the patient's abdominal girth at least every 4 hours, and monitor closely for signs of shock.

• Monitor the results of serial blood studies (particularly hematocrit, hemoglobin, and coagulation times).

• Explain all diagnostic tests and procedures. Allow time for questions.

• Inform the family of the patient's progress. Prepare them for his appearance (I.V.s, nasogastric tubes, bruises, dried blood). Provide emotional support for the patient and family. As needed, enlist the aid of a social worker, chaplain, and other members of the health care team in providing such support.

MISCELLANEOUS DISORDERS

Granulocytopenia and Lymphocytopenia

(Agranulocytosis and lymphopenia)

Granulocytopenia is characterized by a marked reduction in the number of circulating granulocytes. Although this implies all the granulocytes (neutrophils, basophils, eosinophils) are reduced, granulocytopenia usually refers to decreased neutrophils. This disorder, which can occur at any age, is associated with infections and ulcerative lesions of the throat, gastrointestinal tract, other mucous membranes, and skin. Its severest form is known as agranulocytosis.

Lymphocytopenia, a rare disorder, is a deficiency of circulating lymphocytes (leukocytes produced mainly in lymph nodes).

In both granulocytopenia and lymphocytopenia, the total leukocyte count (WBC) may reach dangerously low levels, leaving the body unprotected against infection. Prognosis in both disorders depends on the underlying cause and whether it can be treated. Untreated, severe granulocytopenia can be fatal in 3 to 6 days.

Causes

Granulocytopenia may result from diminished production of granulocytes in bone marrow, increased peripheral destruction of granulocytes, or greater utilization of granulocytes. Diminished production of granulocytes in bone marrow generally stems from radiation or drug therapy; it's a common side effect of antimetabolites and alkylating agents and may occur in the patient who is hypersensitive to phenothiazines, sulfonamides (and some sulfonamide derivatives, such as chlorothiazide), antibiotics, and antiarrhythmic drugs. Drug-induced granulocytopenia usually develops slowly and typically correlates with the dosage and duration of therapy. Production of granulocytes also decreases in conditions such as aplastic anemia and bone marrow malignancies and in some hereditary disorders (infantile genetic agranulocytosis).

The growing loss of peripheral granulocytes is due to increased splenic sequestration, diseases that destroy peripheral blood cells (viral and bacterial infections), and drugs that act as haptens (carrying antigens that attack blood cells and causing acute idiosyncratic or non-dose-related drug reactions). Infections such as infectious mononucleosis may result in granulocytopenia because of increased utilization of granulocytes.

Similarly, lymphocytopenia may result from decreased production, increased destruction, or loss of lymphocytes. Decreased production of lymphocytes may be secondary to a genetic or a thymic abnormality or to immunodeficiency disorders, such as thymic dysplasia or ataxia-telangiectasia. Increased destruction of lymphocytes may be secondary to radiation or chemotherapy (alkylating agents). Loss of lymphocytes may follow postsurgical thoracic duct drainage, intestinal lymphangiectasia, or impaired intestinal lymphatic drainage (as in Whipple's disease).

Lymphocyte depletion can also result from elevated plasma corticoid levels (due to stress, ACTH or steroid treatment, or congestive heart failure). Other associated disorders: Hodgkin's disease, leukemia, aplastic anemia, sarcoidosis, myasthenia gravis, lupus erythematosus, protein-calorie malnutrition, renal failure, terminal cancer, tuberculosis and, in infants, severe combined immunodeficiency disease (SCID).

Signs and symptoms

Patients with granulocytopenia typically experience slowly progressive fatigue and weakness, followed by the sudden onset of signs of overwhelming infection (fever, chills, tachycardia, anxiety, headache, and extreme prostration); ulcers in the mouth or colon; pharyngeal ulceration, possibly with associated necrosis; pneumonia; and septicemia, possibly leading to mild shock. If granulocytopenia is caused by an idiosyncratic drug reaction, signs of infection develop abruptly, without slowly progressive fatigue and weakness.

Patients with lymphocytopenia may exhibit enlarged lymph nodes, spleen, and tonsils and signs of an associated disease.

Diagnosis

Diagnosis of granulocytopenia necessitates a thorough patient history to check for precipitating factors. Physical examination for clinical effects of underlying disorders is also essential.

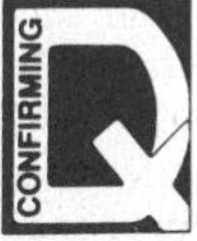

Marked reduction in neutrophils (less than 500/mm³ leads to severe bacterial infections) and a WBC lower than 2,000/mm³, with few observable granulocytes on CBC, confirm granulocytopenia.

Examination of bone marrow generally shows a scarcity of granulocytic precursor cells beyond the most immature forms, but this finding may vary, depending on the cause.

A lymphocyte count less than 1,500/mm³ in adults or less than 3,000/mm³ in children indicates lymphocytopenia. Identifying the cause by evaluation of the patient's clinical status, bone marrow and lymph node biopsies, or other appropriate diagnostic tests helps establish the diagnosis.

Treatment

Effective management of granulocytopenia must include identification and elimination of the cause, if possible. Treatment must also control infection until the bone marrow can generate more

TRANSFUSION OF WBC CONCENTRATE

Content: WBCs, a few RBCs, some plasma
Indication: to increase the patient's white cell mass
Amount: 250 to 500 ml/unit
Administration: through a blood filter
Risks: hepatitis, febrile reaction from leukoagglutinins, and respiratory reactions.

Administer antipyretics and antihistamines to help prevent adverse reactions. Stay with the patient during the transfusion. Observe for flushing, shaking chills, fever, headache, rash, tachycardia, and hypertension. Be sure the transfusion runs slowly—at least 2 hours. Don't stop the procedure because of hives or signs of a febrile reaction unless they are severe.

Symptoms of a respiratory reaction resemble those of pulmonary embolism: chest pain, dyspnea, and cyanosis. Such a reaction is generally due to the migration of white cells to the site of a pulmonary infection. If a respiratory reaction occurs, discontinue the transfusion and administer oxygen; the reaction usually subsides within an hour.

leukocytes. This often means drug or radiation therapy must be discontinued and antibiotic treatment begun immediately, even while awaiting results of culture and sensitivity tests. Treatment may also include antifungal preparations and transfusion of WBC concentrate. Spontaneous restoration of leukocyte production in bone marrow generally occurs within 1 to 3 weeks.

Treatment of lymphocytopenia includes eliminating the cause (such as alkylating drugs or thoracic drainage) and managing any underlying disorders (such as Hodgkin's disease). For infants with SCID, therapy may include bone marrow transplantation.

Special considerations

- Monitor vital signs frequently. Obtain cultures from blood, throat, urine, and sputum, as ordered. Give antibiotics, as scheduled.
- Explain the necessity of protective isolation (preferably with laminar air flow) to the patient and family. Teach proper hand-washing technique and how to correctly use gowns and masks. Prevent patient contact with staff members or visitors with respiratory tract infections.
- Maintain adequate nutrition and hydration, since malnutrition aggravates immunosuppression. Make sure the patient with mouth ulcerations receives a high-calorie liquid diet (for example, high-protein milk shakes). Offer a straw to make drinking less painful.
- Provide warm saline water gargles and rinses, analgesics, and anesthetic lozenges, since good oral hygiene promotes patient comfort and facilitates the healing process.
- Ensure adequate rest, which is essential to the mobilization of the body's defenses against infection. Provide good skin and perineal care.
- Monitor CBC and differential, blood culture results, serum electrolytes, intake and output, and daily weight.
- To help detect granulocytopenia and lymphocytopenia in the early, most treatable stages, monitor the WBC of any patient receiving radiation or chemotherapy. After the patient has developed bone marrow depression, he must zealously avoid exposure to infection.
- Advise the patient with known or suspected sensitivity to a drug that may lead to granulocytopenia or lymphocytopenia to alert medical personnel to this sensitivity in the future.

Hypersplenism

Hypersplenism is a syndrome marked by exaggerated splenic activity and possible splenomegaly. This disorder results in peripheral blood cell deficiency as the spleen traps and destroys peripheral blood cells.

Causes

Hypersplenism may be idiopathic (primary) or secondary to an extrasplenic disorder, such as chronic malaria, polycythemia vera, or rheumatoid arthritis. In hypersplenism, the spleen's normal filtering and phagocytic functions accelerate indiscriminately, automatically removing antibody-coated, aging, and abnormal cells, even though some cells may be functionally normal. The spleen may also temporarily sequester normal platelets and RBCs, withholding them from circulation. In this manner, the enlarged spleen may trap as much as 90% of the body's platelets and up to 45% of its RBC mass.

Signs and symptoms

Most patients with hypersplenism develop anemia, leukopenia, or thrombocytopenia, often with splenomegaly. They may contract bacterial infections frequently, bruise easily, hemorrhage spontaneously from the mucous membranes and gastrointestinal or genitourinary tract, and suffer ulcerations of the mouth, legs, and feet. They commonly develop fever, weakness, and palpitations. Patients with secondary hypersplenism may have other clinical abnormalities, depending on the underlying disease.

Diagnosis

Diagnosis requires evidence of abnormal splenic destruction or sequestration of RBCs or platelets, and splenomegaly.

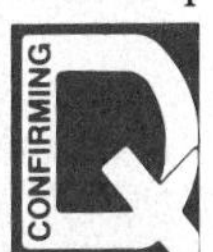

The most definitive test measures the accumulation of erythrocytes in the spleen and liver after I.V. infusion of chromium-labeled RBCs or platelets. A high spleen/liver ratio of radioactivity indicates splenic destruction or sequestration. Complete blood count shows decreased hemoglobin (as low as 4 g/100 ml), WBC (less than 4,000/mm^3), platelet count (less than 125,000), and reticulocyte count. Splenic biopsy, scan, and angiography may be useful; biopsy is hazardous, however, and should be avoided, if possible.

Treatment

Splenectomy is the treatment of choice if severe cytopenia (thrombocytopenia and granulocytopenia) occurs, but may be complicated by postoperative thromboembolic disease and infection. This procedure rarely cures the patient, especially if he has an underlying disease, but it does correct the effects of cytopenia. Occasionally, splenectomy may result in accelerated blood cell destruction in the bone marrow and liver. Secondary hypersplenism necessitates treatment of the underlying disease.

CAUSES OF SPLENOMEGALY

Infectious: acute (abscesses, subacute bacterial endocarditis), chronic (tuberculosis, malaria, Felty's syndrome)
Congestive: cirrhosis, thrombosis
Hyperplastic: hemolytic anemia, polycythemia vera
Infiltrative: Gaucher's, Niemann-Pick disease
Cystic/neoplastic: cysts, leukemia, lymphoma, myelofibrosis

Special considerations

- If splenectomy is scheduled, administer preoperative transfusions of blood or blood products (fresh-frozen plasma, platelets), as ordered, to replace deficient blood elements. Symptoms or complications of any underlying disorder should be treated also.
- Postoperatively, monitor vital signs. Check for any excessive drainage or apparent bleeding. Watch for infection, thromboembolism, and abdominal distention. Keep the nasogastric tube patent; listen for bowel sounds. Instruct the patient to perform deep breathing exercises, and encourage early ambulation to prevent respiratory complications and venous stasis.

Selected References

Erslev, Allan J., and Gabuzda, Thomas G. *Pathophysiology of Blood,* 2nd ed. Philadelphia: W.B. Saunders Co., 1979.

Hirsh, Jack, and Brain, Elizabeth A. *Hemostasis and Thrombosis: A Conceptual Approach,* 2nd ed. New York: Churchill Livingstone, 1983.

Hutchinson, Margaret McGahan. "Aplastic Anemia: Care of the Bone-Marrow-Failure Patient," *Nursing Clinics of North America* 18(3):543-51, September 1983.

Rifkind, R.A., et al. *Fundamentals of Hematology.* Chicago: Year Book Medical Pubs., 1984.

Thomson, Jean, ed. *Blood Coagulation and Haemostasis: A Practical Guide,* 2nd ed. New York: Churchill Livingstone, 1980.

Wintrobe, Maxwell M., et al. *Clinical Hematology,* 8th ed. Philadelphia: Lea & Febiger, 1981.

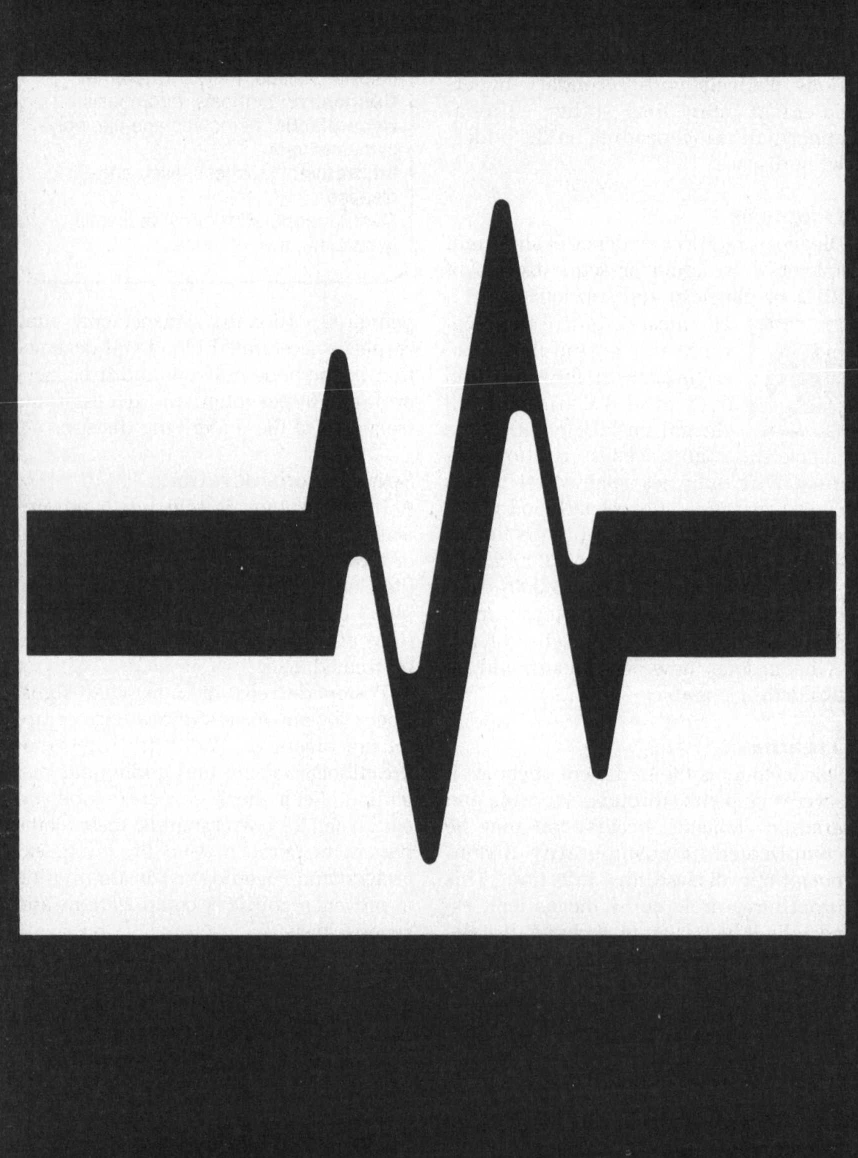

18 Cardiovascular Disorders

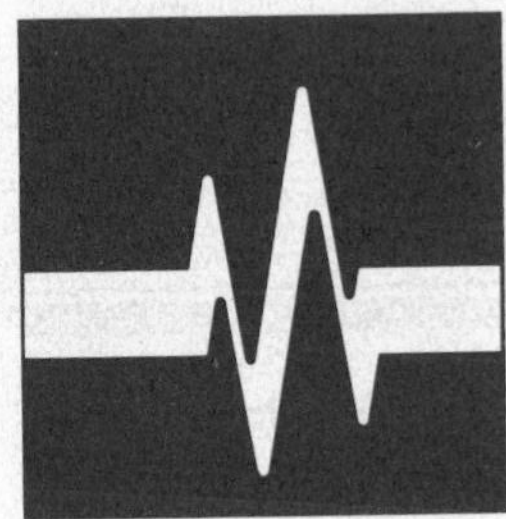

Cardiovascular Disorders

Introduction

The cardiovascular system begins its activity when the fetus is barely a month old and is the last to cease activity at the end of life. This system is so vital that its activity defines the presence of life.

Life-giving transport system

The heart, arteries, veins, and lymphatics form the cardiovascular network that serves as the body's transport system, bringing life-supporting oxygen and nutrients to cells, removing metabolic waste products, and carrying hormones from one part of the body to another. Often called the circulatory system, it may be divided into two branches: *pulmonary circulation,* in which blood picks up new oxygen and liberates the waste product carbon dioxide; and *systemic circulation* (includes coronary circulation), in which blood carries oxygen and nutrients to all active cells, while transporting waste products to the kidneys, liver, and skin for excretion. Circulation requires normal function of the heart, which propels blood through the system by continuous rhythmic contractions. Located behind the sternum, the heart is a muscular organ the size of a man's fist. It has three layers: the *endocardium*—the smooth inner layer; the *myocardium*—the thick, muscular middle layer that contracts in rhythmic beats; and the *epicardium*—the thin, serous membrane, or outer surface of the heart. Covering the entire heart is a saclike membrane called the *pericardium.* It has two layers: a *visceral* layer that is in contact with the heart and a *parietal,* or outer, layer. To prevent irritation when the heart moves against this layer during contraction, fluid lubricates the parietal pericardium.

The heart has four chambers: two thin-walled chambers called *atria* and two thick-walled chambers called *ventricles.* The atria serve as reservoirs during ventricular contraction (systole) and as booster pumps during ventricular relaxation (diastole). The left ventricle propels blood through the systemic circulation. The right ventricle, which forces blood through the pulmonary circulation, is much thinner than the left because it meets only one sixth the resistance.

Heart valves

Two kinds of valves work inside the heart: *atrioventricular* and *semilunar.* The atrioventricular valve between the right atrium and ventricle has three leaflets, or cusps, and three papillary muscles; hence, it's called the tricuspid valve. The atrioventricular valve between the left atrium and ventricle consists of two cusps shaped like a bishop's miter and two papillary muscles and is called the mitral valve. The tricuspid and mitral valves prevent blood backflow from the ventricles to the atria during ventricular contraction. The leaflets of both valves are attached to the papillary muscles of the ventricle by thin, fibrous bands called chordae tendineae; the leaflets separate and descend funnel-like into the ventricles during diastole, and are pushed upward and together during systole, to occlude the mitral and tricuspid orifices. The valves' action isn't entirely passive, since papillary muscles contract during systole and prevent the leaflets from prolapsing into the atria during ventricular contraction.

The two semilunar valves, which resemble half moons, prevent blood backflow from the aorta and pulmonary arteries into the ventricles when those chambers relax and fill with blood from the atria. These semilunar valves are referred to as aortic and pulmonic for their respective arteries.

The cardiac cycle

Diastole is the phase of ventricular relaxation and filling. As diastole begins, ventricular pressure falls below arterial pressure, and the aortic and pulmonic valves close. As ventricular pressure continues to fall below atrial pressure, the mitral and tricuspid valves open, and blood flows rapidly into the ventricle. Atrial contraction then increases the volume of ventricular filling by pumping up to 20% more blood into the ventricle. When systole begins, the ventricular muscle contracts, raising ventricular pressure above atrial pressure and closing the mitral and tricuspid valves. When ventricular pressure finally becomes greater than that in the aorta and pulmonary artery, the aortic and pulmonic valves open, and the ventricles eject blood. Ventricular pressure continues to rise as blood is expelled from the heart. As systole ends, the ventricles relax and stop ejecting blood, and ventricular pressure falls, closing both valves.

S_1 (the first heart sound) is heard as the ventricles contract and the atrioventricular valves close. S_1 is loudest at the apex of the heart, over the mitral area. S_2 (the second heart sound), which is normally rapid and sharp, occurs when the aortic and pulmonic valves close. S_2 is loudest at the base of the heart (second intercostal space on both sides of the sternum). Normally, the right heart valves close a fraction of a second later than the left valves because of lower pressures in the right ventricle and pulmonary artery. Identifying these components during auscultation is usually difficult, except when inspiration coincides with the end of systole or when a right bundle branch block exists. Either will cause a slightly prolonged right ventricle ejection time, when the delayed closing of the pulmonic valve is heard as a split S_2.

PULSE POINTS

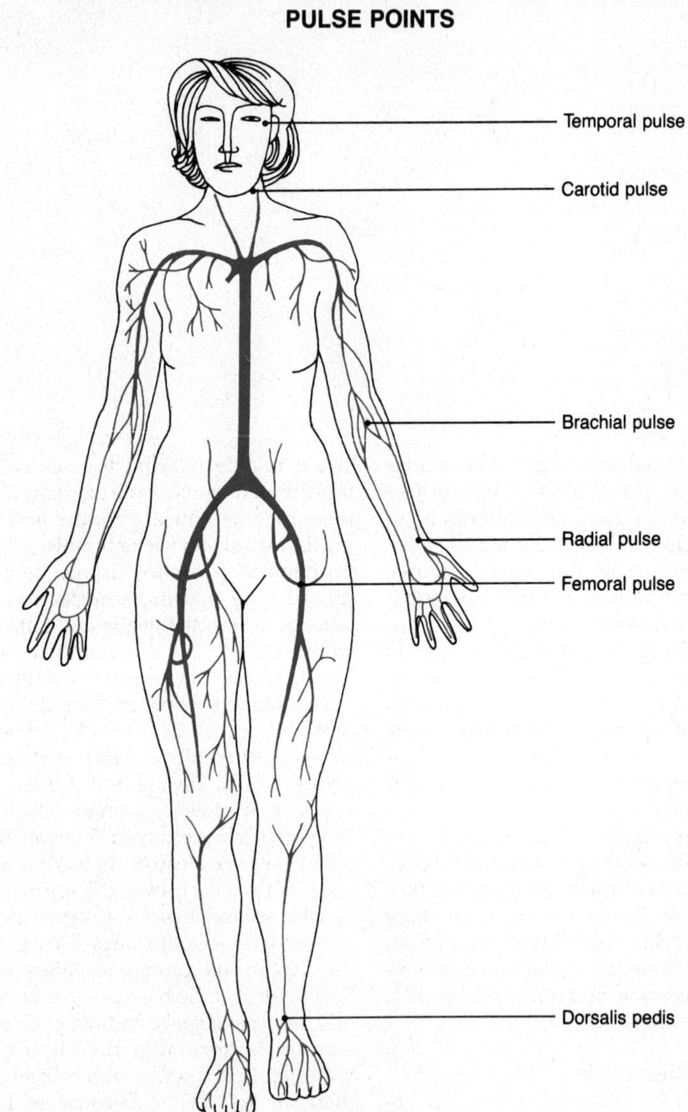

Peripheral pulse rhythm should correspond exactly to the auscultatory heart rhythm. The character of the pulse may offer useful information. For example, pulsus alternans, a strong beat followed by a weak one, can mean myocardial weakness. A water-hammer (or Corrigan's) pulse, a forceful bounding pulse best felt in the carotid arteries or in the forearm, accompanies increased pulse pressure—often with capillary pulsations of the fingernails (Quincke's sign). This pulse usually indicates patent ductus or aortic regurgitation.

Pulsus biferiens, a double peripheral pulse for every apical beat, can signal aortic stenosis, hyperthyroidism, or some other disease. Pulsus bigeminus is a coupled rhythm; you feel its beat in pairs. Pulsus paradoxus is exaggerated waxing and waning of the arterial pressure ($\geq$ 15 mmHg decrease in systolic blood pressure during inspiration).

Ventricular distention during diastole, which can occur in heart failure, creates low-frequency vibrations that may be heard as a third heart sound (S_3), or ventricular gallop. An atrial gallop (S_4) may appear at the end of diastole, just before S_1, if atrial filling is forced into a ventricle that has become less compliant or overdistended, or has a decreased ability to contract. A pressure rise and ventricular vibrations cause this sound.

Cardiac conduction

The heart's conduction system is composed of specialized cells capable of generating and conducting rhythmic electrical impulses to stimulate heart contraction. This system includes the sinoatrial (SA) node, the atrioventricular (AV) junction, the bundle of His and its bundle branches, and the ventricular conduction tissue and Purkinje's fibers.

Normally, the SA node controls the heart rate and rhythm at 60 to 100 beats/minute. Because the SA node usually depolarizes the fastest, it's the heart's pacemaker. If it defaults, another part of the system takes over. The AV junction may emerge at 40 to 60 beats/minute; the bundle of His and bundle branches at 30 to 40 beats/minute; and ventricular conduction tissue at 20 to 30 beats/minute.

Cardiac output

Cardiac output—the amount of blood pumped by the left ventricle into the aorta each minute—is calculated by multiplying the stroke volume (the amount of blood the left ventricle ejects during systole) by the heart rate (strokes per minute). When cellular demands increase, stroke volume or heart rate must increase.

Many factors affect the heart rate, such as exercise, pregnancy, and stress. When the sympathetic nervous system releases norepinephrine, the heart rate increases; when the parasympathetic system releases acetylcholine, it slows.

Stroke volume depends on the ventricle's blood volume and pressure at the end of diastole (preload), resistance to ejection (afterload), and the myocardium's contractile strength. Changes in preload, afterload, or contractile strength can alter the stroke volume.

PULSE AMPLITUDE SCALE

To record your patient's pulse amplitude, use this standard scale:

0: pulse not palpable.

+1: pulse is thready, weak, difficult to find, may fade in and out, and disappears easily with pressure.

+2: pulse is constant but not strong; light pressure must be applied or pulse will disappear.

+3: pulse considered normal. Is easily palpable, does not disappear with pressure.

+4: pulse is strong, bounding, and does not disappear with pressure.

Circulation and pulses

Blood circulates through three types of vessels: *arteries, veins,* and *capillaries.* The sturdy, pliable walls of the arteries adjust to the volume of blood leaving the heart. The major artery arching out of the left ventricle is the aorta. Its segments and subbranches ultimately divide into minute, thin-walled (one-cell thick) capillaries. Capillaries pass the blood to the veins, which return it to the heart. In the veins, valves prevent blood backflow.

Pulses are felt best wherever an artery runs near the skin and over a hard structure. Easily found pulses are:

- *radial artery:* anterolateral aspect of the wrist
- *temporal artery:* in front of the ear, above and lateral to the eye
- *common carotid artery:* neck (side)
- *femoral artery:* groin.

The lymphatic system also plays a role in the cardiovascular network. Originating in tissue spaces, the lymphatic system drains fluid and other plasma components that build up in extravascular spaces and reroutes them back to the circulatory system as lymph, a plasmalike fluid. Lymphatics also extract bacteria and foreign bodies.

Cardiovascular assessment

Physical assessment provides vital infor-

PATTERNS OF CARDIAC PAIN

PERICARDITIS	ANGINA	MYOCARDIAL INFARCTION
ONSET AND DURATION: • Sudden onset; continuous pain lasting for days; residual soreness	*ONSET AND DURATION:* • Gradual or sudden onset; pain usually lasts less than 15 minutes and not more than 30 minutes (average: 3 minutes)	*ONSET AND DURATION:* • Sudden onset; pain ½ to 2 hours; residual soreness 1 to 3 days
LOCATION AND RADIATION: • Substernal pain to left of midline; radiation to back or subclavicular area	*LOCATION AND RADIATION:* • Substernal or anterior chest pain, not sharply localized; radiation to back, neck, arms, jaws, even upper abdomen or fingers	*LOCATION AND RADIATION:* • Substernal, midline, or anterior chest pain; radiation to jaws, neck, back, shoulders, or one or both arms
QUALITY AND INTENSITY: • Mild ache to severe pain, deep or superficial; "stabbing," "knife-like"	*QUALITY AND INTENSITY:* • Mild-to-moderate pressure; deep sensation; varied pattern of attacks; "tightness," "squeezing," "crushing"	*QUALITY AND INTENSITY:* • Persistent, severe pressure; deep sensation; "crushing," "squeezing," "heavy," "oppressive"
SIGNS AND SYMPTOMS: • Precordial friction rub; increased pain with movement, inspiration, laughing, coughing; decreased pain with sitting or leaning forward (sitting up pulls the heart away from the diaphragm)	*SIGNS AND SYMPTOMS:* • Dyspnea, diaphoresis, nausea, desire to void, belching, apprehension	*SIGNS AND SYMPTOMS:* • Nausea, vomiting, apprehension, dyspnea, diaphoresis, increased or decreased blood pressure; gallop heart sound, "sensation of impending doom"
PRECIPITATING FACTORS: • Myocardial infarction or upper respiratory tract infection; no relation to effort	*PRECIPITATING FACTORS:* • Exertion, stress, eating, cold or hot and humid weather	*PRECIPITATING FACTORS:* • Occurrence at rest or during physical exertion or emotional stress

mation about cardiovascular status.

• First, observe for signs of underlying cardiovascular disorders, such as central cyanosis (disturbance in gas exchange), edema (congestive heart failure or valvular disease), and clubbing (congenital cardiovascular disease).

• Next, palpate the peripheral pulses bilaterally, and evaluate their rate, equality, and quality on a scale from 0 (absent) to 4+ (bounding).

• Inspect the carotid arteries for equal appearance. Palpate them individually for thrills (fine vibrations due to irregular blood flow), and listen for bruits.

• Check for pulsations in the jugular veins (more easily seen than felt). Watch for jugular venous distention—a possible sign of right heart failure, valvular stenosis, cardiac tamponade, or pulmonary embolism. Take blood pressure readings in both arms while the patient is lying, sitting, and standing.

• Systematically auscultate the anterior chest wall for each of the four heart sounds in the aortic area (second intercostal space at the right sternal border), pulmonic area (second intercostal space at the left sternal border), right ventricular area (lower half of the left sternal border), and mitral area (fifth intercostal space at the midclavicular line). For low-pitched sounds, use the bell of the stethoscope; for high-pitched sounds, the diaphragm. Carefully inspect each area for pulsations, and palpate for thrills. Check the location of apical pulsation for deviations in normal size (⅜" to ¾" [1 to 2 cm]) and position (in the mitral area)—possible signs of left ventricular hypertrophy, left-sided valvular disease, or right ventricular disease.

• Listen for the vibrating sound of turbulent blood flow through a stenotic or incompetent valve. Time the murmur to determine where it occurs in the cardiac cycle—between S_1 and S_2 (systolic), between S_2 and the following S_1 (diastolic), or throughout systole (holosystolic). Finally, listen for the scratching or squeaking of a pericardial friction rub.

Special cardiovascular tests

After a thorough history, physical examination, and clinical observation, special tests provide valuable diagnostic information.

Electrocardiography (EKG) is a primary tool for evaluating cardiac status. Through electrodes placed on the patient's limbs and over the precordium, an EKG measures electrical activity by recording currents transmitted by the heart. It can detect ischemia, conduction delay, chamber enlargement, and arrhythmias. In ambulatory electrocardiography, or Holter monitoring, a tape recording tracks as many as 100,000 cardiac cycles over a 12- or 24-hour period. This test is sometimes used to determine cardiac status after myocardial infarction, to assess the effectiveness of antiarrhythmic drugs, or to evaluate symptoms suggesting arrhythmia.

Chest X-rays may reveal cardiac enlargement and aortic dilation. Chest X-rays also assess pulmonary circulation. When pulmonary venous and arterial pressures rise, characteristic changes appear, such as dilation of the pulmonary venous shadows. When pulmonary venous pressure exceeds oncotic pressure of the blood, capillary fluid leaks into lung tissues, causing pulmonary edema. This fluid may settle in the alveoli, producing a butterfly pattern, or the lungs may appear cloudy or hazy; in the interlobular septa, sharp linear densities (Kerley's lines) may appear.

Exercise testing using a bicycle ergometer, treadmill, or short flight of stairs is a simple diagnostic procedure to determine cardiac response to physical stress. This type of test measures blood pressure and EKG changes during increasingly rigorous exercises. Myocardial ischemia, abnormal blood pressure response, or arrhythmias indicate failure of the circulatory system to adapt to exercise.

Cardiac catheterization evaluates chest pain, the need for coronary artery surgery or angioplasty, congenital heart defects, and valvular heart disease, and determines the extent of heart failure. Right heart catheterization involves threading a catheter through a vein into the right heart, pulmonary artery, and its branches in the lungs to measure right atrial, right ventricular, pulmonary artery, and pulmonary capillary wedge pressures. A pulmonary arterial thermodilution catheter can measure cardiac output. Left heart catheterization entails inserting a catheter into an artery and threading it retrogradely through the aorta into the left ventricle. *Ventriculography* during left heart catheterization involves injecting radiopaque dye into the left ventricle to measure ejection fraction (portion of ventricular volume ejected per beat) and to disclose abnormal heart wall motion or mitral valve incompetence.

In *coronary arteriography*, radiopaque material injected into coronary arteries allows cineangiographic visualization of coronary arterial narrowing or occlusion.

Digital subtraction angiography evaluates the coronary arteries using X-ray images that are digitally subtracted by computer. Time-based color enhancement shows blood flow in nearby areas.

Echocardiography uses echoes from pulsed high-frequency sound waves (ultrasound) to evaluate structures of the heart. A small transducer placed on the chest wall in various positions and angles acts as both transmitter and receiver. It provides information about valve leaflets, sizes and dimensions of heart chambers, and thicknesses and motions of the septum and the ventricular walls. It can also show intracardiac masses (atrial tumors and thrombi, for example), detect pericardial effusion, diagnose idiopathic hypertrophic subaortic stenosis, and estimate cardiac output and ejection fraction. Echocardiography can also evaluate possible aortic dissection when it involves the ascending aorta. Both M-mode and two-dimen-

EKG LEAD PLACEMENT

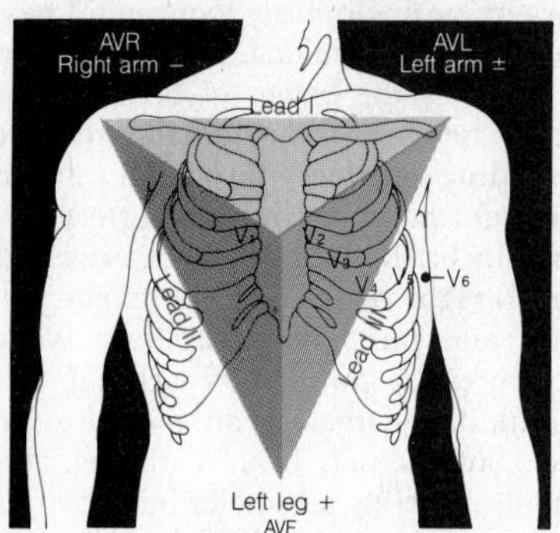

The twelve-lead EKG provides a three-dimensional view of cardiac activity through three sets of leads:

- Standard limb leads (I, II, III) record electrical activity from the heart to the extremities.
- Augmented leads (AVR, AVL, AVF) measure activity from the right and left shoulders and left leg.
- Precordial or chest leads (V_1 to V_6) show ventricular electrical activity.

sional echocardiography exist, but the latter has greater diagnostic abilities.

In *gated blood pool scan,* a radioactive isotope remains in the intravascular compartment, allowing measurement of stroke volume, ventricular ejection fraction, and wall motion. *Myocardial imaging* uses radioactive agents (most often thallium-201) to detect abnormalities in coronary artery perfusion. These agents concentrate in normally perfused myocardium but not in ischemic areas. Nonperfused areas, or "cold spots," may be permanent (scar tissue after myocardial infarction) or temporary (induced by transient ischemia). Thallium scanning with exercise tests identifies exercise-induced ischemia and evaluates abnormal findings on a stress EKG.

Acute infarct imaging documents muscle viability (not perfusion) through the use of technetium-labeled pyrophosphate. Unlike thallium, technetium accumulates only in irreversibly damaged myocardial tissue. Areas of necrosis appear as "hot spots" and can be detected only during acute infarction. This test determines the size and location of infarction but can produce false results.

Cardiac enzymes are cellular proteins released into the blood as a result of cell membrane injury. Their presence in the blood confirms acute myocardial infarction or severe cardiac trauma. All cardiac enzymes—creatine phosphokinase (CPK), lactic dehydrogenase (LDH), and serum glutamic-oxaloacetic transaminase (SGOT), for example—are also found in other cells. Fractionation of enzymes can determine the source of damaged cells. For example, three fractions of CPK are isolated, one of which (an isoenzyme called CPK-MB) is found only in cardiac cells. CPK-MB in the blood indicates injury to myocardial cells.

Peripheral arteriography consists of a fluoroscopic X-ray after arterial injection of contrast media. Similarly, *phlebography* defines the venous system after injection of contrast media into a vein. *Impedance plethysmography* evaluates the venous system to detect pressure changes transmitted to lower leg veins.

Ultrasound and *Doppler techniques* evaluate the peripheral vascular system and assess carotid disease.

Endomyocardial biopsy can detect cardiomyopathy, infiltrative myocardial diseases, and rejection of transplants. Under fluoroscopic control, a right ventricular biopsy is done via the right internal jugular vein. Less commonly, a left ventricular biopsy is done by retrograde arterial catheterization.

Electrophysiologic studies help diagnose conduction system disease and serious arrhythmias. Electronic induction and termination of arrhythmias aids drug selection. *Endocardial mapping* detects an arrhythmia's focus using a finger electrode. *Epicardial mapping* uses a computer and a fabric sock with electrodes that's slipped over the heart.

Managing cardiovascular disease

Patients with cardiovascular disease pose a tremendous challenge. Their sheer numbers alone compel a thorough understanding of cardiovascular anatomy, physiology, and pathophysiology. Anticipate a high anxiety level in cardiac patients, and provide support and reassurance, especially during stressful procedures such as cardiac catheterization.

Cardiac rehabilitation programs are widely prescribed, but are still controversial. Experts disagree about long-term benefits, yet most recommend that the rehabilitation program begin in the hospital and continue afterward on an outpatient basis. Helping the patient resume a satisfying life-style requires careful planning and comprehensive teaching. Inform the patient and his family about local hospitals and community organizations with cardiac rehabilitation programs that emphasize recognition, prevention, and treatment.

CONGENITAL ACYANOTIC DEFECTS

Ventricular Septal Defect

In ventricular septal defect (VSD), the most common congenital heart disorder, an opening in the septum between the ventricles allows blood to shunt between the left and right ventricles. VSD accounts for up to 30% of all congenital heart defects. Prognosis is good for defects that close spontaneously or are correctable surgically, but poor for untreated defects, which are sometimes fatal by age 1, usually from secondary complications.

Causes

In infants with VSD, the ventricular septum fails to close completely by the 8th week of gestation, as it would normally. VSD occurs in some infants with fetal alcohol syndrome, but a causal relationship has not been established. Although most children with congenital heart defects are otherwise normal, in some, VSD coexists with additional birth defects, especially Down's syndrome and other autosomal trisomies, renal anomalies, and such cardiac defects as patent ductus arteriosus and coarctation of the aorta. VSDs are located in the membranous or muscular portion of the ventricular septum and vary in size. Some defects close spontaneously; in other defects, the entire septum is absent, creating a single ventricle.

VSD isn't readily apparent at birth because right and left ventricular pressures are approximately equal, so blood doesn't shunt through the defect. As the pulmonary vasculature gradually relaxes, between 4 and 8 weeks after birth, right ventricular pressure decreases, allowing blood to shunt from the left to the right ventricle.

Signs and symptoms

Clinical features of VSD vary with the size of the defect, the effect of the shunting on the pulmonary vasculature, and the infant's age. In a small VSD, shunting is minimal, and pulmonary artery pressure and heart size remain normal. Such defects may eventually close spontaneously without ever causing symptoms.

Initially, large VSD shunts cause left atrial and left ventricular hypertrophy. Later, an uncorrected VSD will cause right ventricular hypertrophy due to increasing pulmonary vascular resistance. Eventually, biventricular congestive heart failure and cyanosis (from reversal of shunt direction) occur. Resulting cardiac hypertrophy may make the anterior chest wall prominent. A large VSD increases the risk of pneumonia.

Infants with large VSDs are thin, small, and gain weight slowly. They may develop congestive heart failure, with dusky skin; liver, heart, and spleen enlargement because of systemic venous congestion; diaphoresis; feeding difficulties; rapid, grunting respirations; and increased heart rate. They may also develop severe pulmonary hypertension. Fixed pulmonary hypertension may occur much later in life with right-to-left shunt (Eisenmenger complex), causing cyanosis and clubbing of the nail beds. The typical murmur associated with a VSD is blowing or rumbling and varies in frequency. In the newborn, a moderately loud early systolic murmur may be heard along the lower left sternal border. About the second or third day after birth, the murmur may become louder and longer. In infants, the murmur may be loudest near the base of the heart and may suggest pulmonary stenosis. A small VSD may produce a functional murmur or a characteristic loud, harsh systolic murmur. Moderate-sized and large VSDs produce audible murmurs (at least a grade 3 pansystolic), loudest at the fourth intercostal space, usually with a thrill. In addition, the pulmonic component of S_2 sounds loud and is widely split. Palpation reveals displacement of the point of maximal impulse to the left. When fixed pulmonary hypertension is present, a diastolic murmur may be audible on auscultation, the systolic murmur becomes quieter, and S_2 is greatly accentuated.

Diagnosis

Diagnostic findings include:

• *Chest X-ray* is normal in small defects; in large VSDs, it shows cardiomegaly, left atrial and left ventricular enlargement, and prominent pulmonary vascular markings.

• *EKG* is normal in children with small VSDs; in large VSDs, it shows left and right ventricular hypertrophy, suggesting pulmonary hypertension.

• *Echocardiography* may detect a large VSD and its location in the septum, estimate the size of a left-to-right shunt, suggest pulmonary hypertension, and identify associated lesions and complications.

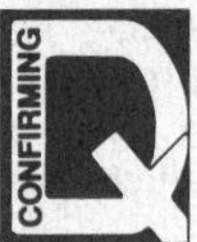

• *Cardiac catheterization* determines the size and exact location of the VSD, calculates the degree of shunting by comparing the blood oxygen saturation in each ventricle, determines the extent of pulmonary hypertension, and detects associated defects.

Treatment

Large defects usually require early surgical correction before irreversible pulmonary vascular disease develops. For small defects, surgery consists of simple suture closure. Moderate to large defects require insertion of a patch graft, using cardiopulmonary bypass.

If the child has other defects and will benefit from delaying surgery, pulmonary artery banding normalizes pressures and flow distal to the band and prevents pulmonary vascular disease, allowing postponement of surgery. (Pulmonary artery banding is done only when the child has other complications.) A rare complication of VSD repair is complete heart block from interference with the bundle of His during surgery. (Heart block may require temporary or permanent pacemaker implantation.)

Before surgery, treatment consists of:

• digoxin, sodium restriction, and diuretics to prevent congestive heart failure

• careful monitoring by physical examination, X-ray, and EKG to detect increased pulmonary hypertension, which, if it develops, indicates a need for early surgery

• measures to prevent infection (prophylactic antibiotics, for example, to prevent infective endocarditis).

Generally, postoperative treatment includes a brief period of mechanical ventilation. The patient will need analgesics and may also require diuretics to increase urine output, continuous infusions of nitroprusside or adrenergic agents to regulate blood pressure and cardiac output, and in rare cases, a temporary pacemaker.

Special considerations

Although the parents of an infant with VSD often suspect something is wrong with their child before diagnosis, they need psychological support to help them accept the reality of a serious cardiac disorder. Because surgery may take place months after diagnosis, parent teaching is vital to prevent complications until the child is scheduled for surgery or the defect closes. Thorough explanations of all tests are also essential.

- Instruct parents to watch for signs of congestive heart failure, such as poor feeding, sweating, and heavy breathing.
- If the child is receiving digoxin or other medications, tell the parents how to give it and how to recognize side effects. Caution them to keep medications out of the reach of all children.
- Teach parents to recognize and report early signs of infection and to avoid exposing the child to persons with obvious infections.
- Encourage parents to let the child engage in normal activities.
- Stress the importance of prophylactic antibiotics before and after surgery.

After surgery to correct VSD:

- Monitor vital signs and intake and output. Maintain the infant's body temperature with an overbed warmer. Give catecholamines, nitroprusside, and diuretics, as ordered; analgesics, as needed.
- Monitor central venous pressure, intraarterial blood pressure, and left atrial or pulmonary artery pressure readings. Assess heart rate and rhythm for signs of conduction block.
- Check oxygenation, particularly in a child who requires mechanical ventilation. Suction as needed to maintain a patent airway and to prevent atelectasis and pneumonia.
- Monitor pacemaker effectiveness, if needed. Watch for signs of failure, such as bradycardia and hypotension.
- Reassure parents, and allow them to participate in their child's care.

Atrial Septal Defect

In an atrial septal defect (ASD), an opening between the left and right atria allows shunting of blood between the chambers. Ostium secundum *defect (most common) occurs in the region of the fossa ovalis and, occasionally, extends inferiorly, close to the vena cava;* sinus venosus *defect occurs in the superior-posterior portion of the atrial septum, sometimes extending into the vena cava, and is almost always associated with abnormal drainage of pulmonary veins into the right atrium;* ostium primum, *a defect of the primitive septum, occurs in the inferior portion of the septum primum and is usually associated with atrioventricular valve abnormalities (cleft mitral valve) and conduction defects. ASD accounts for about 10% of congenital heart defects and appears almost twice as often in females as in males, with a strong familial tendency. Although ASD is usually a benign defect during infancy and childhood, delayed development of symptoms and complications makes it one of the most common congenital heart defects diagnosed in adults. Prognosis is excellent in asymptomatic persons, but poor in those with cyanosis caused by large, untreated defects.*

Causes

The cause of ASD is unknown. In this condition, blood shunts from left to right because left atrial pressure normally is slightly higher than right atrial pressure; this pressure difference forces large amounts of blood through a defect. The left-to-right shunt results in right heart volume overload, affecting the right atrium, right ventricle, and pulmonary arteries. Eventually, the right atrium enlarges, and the right ventricle dilates to accommodate the increased blood volume. If pulmonary artery hypertension develops because of the shunt (rare in children), increased pulmonary vascular resistance and right ventricular hypertrophy will follow. In some adult patients, irreversible (fixed) pulmonary artery hypertension causes reversal of the shunt direction, which results in unoxygenated blood entering the systemic circulation, causing cyanosis.

Signs and symptoms

ASD often goes undetected in preschoolers; such children may complain about feeling tired only after extreme exertion and may have frequent respiratory tract infections but otherwise appear normal and healthy. However, they may show growth retardation if they have large shunts. Children with ASD rarely develop congestive heart failure, pulmonary hypertension, infective endocarditis, or other complications. However, as adults, they usually manifest pronounced symptoms, such as fatigability and dyspnea on exertion, frequently to the point of severe limitation of activity (especially after age 40).

In children, auscultation reveals an early to midsystolic murmur, superficial in quality, heard at the second or third left intercostal space. In patients with large shunts—as a result of increased tricuspid valve flow—a low-pitched diastolic murmur is heard at the lower left sternal border, which becomes more pronounced on inspiration. Although the murmur's intensity is a rough indicator of the size of the left-to-right shunt, its low pitch sometimes makes it difficult to hear. Other signs include a fixed, widely split S_2, caused by delayed closure of the pulmonic valve, and a systolic click or late systolic murmur at the apex, resulting from mitral valve prolapse, which occasionally affects older children with ASD.

In older patients with large uncorrected defects and fixed pulmonary artery hypertension, auscultation reveals an accentuated S_2. A pulmonary ejection click and an audible S_4 may also be present. Clubbing and cyanosis become evident; syncope and hemoptysis may occur with severe pulmonary vascular disease.

Diagnosis

A history of increasing fatigue and characteristic physical features suggest ASD. The following findings confirm it:

- *Chest X-ray* shows an enlarged right atrium and right ventricle, a prominent pulmonary artery, and increased pulmonary vascular markings.
- *EKG* may be normal but often shows right axis deviation; prolonged P-R interval; varying degrees of right bundle branch block; right ventricular hypertrophy; atrial fibrillation (particularly in severe cases after age 30); and, in ostium primum, left axis deviation.
- *Echocardiography* measures the extent of right ventricular enlargement and may locate the defect. (Other causes of right ventricular enlargement must be ruled out.)

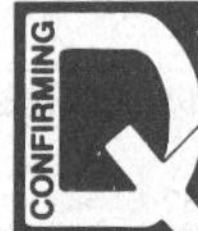

- *Cardiac catheterization* confirms ASD by demonstrating that right atrial blood is more oxygenated than superior vena cava blood—indicating a left-to-right shunt—and determines the degree of shunting and pulmonary vascular disease. Dye injection shows the ASD's size and location, the location of pulmonary venous drainage, and the A-V valves' competence.

Treatment and special considerations

Since ASD seldom produces complications in infants and toddlers, surgery can be delayed until they reach preschool or early school age. A large defect may need immediate surgical closure with sutures or a patch graft. Although experimental, treatment for a small ASD may involve insertion of an umbrellalike patch using a cardiac catheter instead of open heart surgery.

- Before cardiac catheterization, explain pre- and post-test procedures to the child and parents. If possible, use drawings or other visual aids to explain it to the child.

- As needed, teach the patient about antibiotic prophylaxis to prevent infective endocarditis.
- If surgery is scheduled, teach the child and parents about the ICU and introduce them to the staff. Show parents where they can wait during the operation. Explain postoperative procedures, tubes, dressings, and monitoring equipment.
- After surgery, closely monitor vital signs, central venous and intraarterial pressures, and intake and output. Watch for atrial arrhythmias, which may remain uncorrected.

Coarctation of the Aorta

Coarctation is a narrowing of the aorta, usually just below the left subclavian artery, near the site where the ligamentum arteriosum (the remnant of the ductus arteriosus, a fetal blood vessel) joins the pulmonary artery to the aorta. Coarctation may occur with aortic valve stenosis (usually of a bicuspid aortic valve) and with severe cases of hypoplasia of the aortic arch, patent ductus arteriosus, and ventricular septal defect. Generally, prognosis for coarctation of the aorta depends on the severity of associated cardiac anomalies; prognosis for isolated coarctation is good if corrective surgery is performed before this condition induces severe systemic hypertension or degenerative changes in the aorta.

Causes and incidence

Coarctation of the aorta may develop as a result of spasm and constriction of the smooth muscle in the ductus arteriosus as it closes. Possibly, this contractile tissue extends into the aortic wall, causing narrowing. The obstructive process causes hypertension in the aortic branches above the constriction (arteries that supply the arms, neck, and head) and diminished pressure in the vessels below the constriction.

Restricted blood flow through the narrowed aorta increases the pressure load on the left ventricle and causes dilation of the proximal aorta and ventricular hypertrophy. Untreated, this condition may lead to left heart failure and, rarely, to cerebral hemorrhage and aortic rupture. If ventricular septal defect accompanies coarctation, blood shunts left to right, straining the right heart. This leads to pulmonary hypertension and, eventually, right heart hypertrophy and failure.

Coarctation of the aorta accounts for about 7% of all congenital heart defects in children and is twice as common in males as in females. When it occurs in females, it's often associated with Turner's syndrome, a chromosomal disorder that causes ovarian dysgenesis.

Signs and symptoms

Clinical features vary with age. During the first year of life, when aortic coarctation may cause congestive heart failure, the infant displays tachypnea, dyspnea, pulmonary edema, pallor, tachycardia, failure to thrive, cardiomegaly, and hepatomegaly. Generally, heart sounds are normal unless a coexisting cardiac defect is present. Femoral pulses are absent or diminished.

If coarctation is asymptomatic in infancy, it usually remains so throughout adolescence, as collateral circulation develops to bypass the narrowed segment. During adolescence, this defect may produce dyspnea, claudication, headaches, epistaxis, and hypertension in the upper extremities despite collateral circulation. Frequently, it causes resting systolic hypertension and wide pulse pressure; high diastolic pressure readings are the same in both the arms and legs. Coarctation may also produce a visible aortic pulsation in the supra-

COARCTATION OF THE AORTA

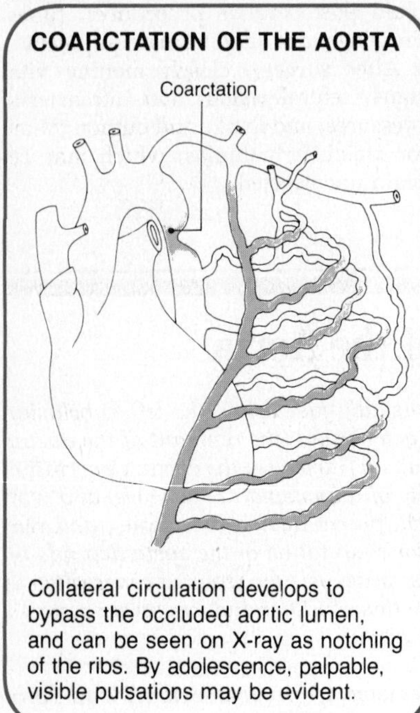

Collateral circulation develops to bypass the occluded aortic lumen, and can be seen on X-ray as notching of the ribs. By adolescence, palpable, visible pulsations may be evident.

sternal notch, a continuous systolic murmur, an accentuated S_2, and an S_4.

Diagnosis

The cardinal signs of coarctation of the aorta are resting systolic hypertension, absent or diminished femoral pulses, and wide pulse pressure. The following tests support this diagnosis:

- *Chest X-ray* may demonstrate left ventricular hypertrophy, congestive heart failure, a wide ascending and descending aorta, and notching of the undersurfaces of the ribs, due to extensive collateral circulation.
- *EKG* may eventually reveal left ventricular hypertrophy.
- *Echocardiography* may show increased left ventricular muscle thickness, coexisting aortic valve abnormalities, and the coarctation site.
- *Cardiac catheterization* and *aortography* are indicated. Cardiac catheterization evaluates collateral circulation and measures pressure in the right and left ventricles and in the ascending and descending aortas (on both sides of the obstruction); aortography locates the site and extent of coarctation.

Treatment

For an infant with congestive heart failure caused by coarctation of the aorta, treatment consists of medical management with digoxin and diuretics. If medical management fails, surgery may be needed. In general, the child's condition determines the timing of the surgery. Signs of congestive heart failure or hypertension may call for early surgery. If these signs don't appear, surgery usually occurs during the preschool years.

Before the operation, the child may require endocarditis prophylaxis or, if the child is older and has previously undetected coarctation, he may need antihypertensive therapy. During surgery, the doctor uses a flap of the left subclavian artery to reconstruct an unobstructed aorta.

Special considerations

- When coarctation in an infant requires rapid digitalization, monitor vital signs closely and watch for digitalis toxicity (poor feeding, vomiting).
- Balance intake and output carefully, especially if the infant is receiving diuretics with fluid restriction.
- Since the infant may not be able to maintain proper body temperature, regulate environmental temperature with an overbed warmer, if needed.
- Monitor blood glucose levels to detect possible hypoglycemia, which may occur as glycogen stores become depleted.
- Offer the parents emotional support and an explanation of the disorder. Also explain diagnostic procedures, surgery, and drug therapy. Tell parents what to expect postoperatively.
- For an older child, assess the blood pressure in his extremities regularly, explain any exercise restrictions, stress the need to take medications properly and to watch for side effects, and teach him about tests and other procedures.

After corrective surgery:

- Monitor blood pressure closely, using an intraarterial line. Take blood pressure in all extremities. Monitor intake and output.
- If the patient develops hypertension and requires nitroprusside or trimethaphan, administer it, as ordered, by continuous I.V. infusion, using an infusion pump. Watch for severe hypotension, and regulate the dosage carefully.
- Provide pain relief, and encourage a gradual increase in activity.
- Promote adequate respiratory functioning through turning, coughing, and deep breathing.
- Watch for abdominal pain or rigidity and signs of GI or urinary bleeding.
- If an older child needs to continue antihypertensives after surgery, teach him and his parents about them.
- Stress the importance of continued endocarditis prophylaxis.

Patent Ductus Arteriosus

The ductus arteriosus is a fetal blood vessel that connects the pulmonary artery to the descending aorta. In patent ductus arteriosus (PDA), the lumen of the ductus remains open after birth. This creates a left-to-right shunt of blood from the aorta to the pulmonary artery and results in recirculation of arterial blood through the lungs. Initially, PDA may produce no clinical effects, but in time it can precipitate pulmonary vascular disease, causing symptoms to appear by age 40. Prognosis is good if the shunt is small or surgical repair is effective. Otherwise, PDA may advance to intractable congestive heart failure, which may be fatal.

Causes and incidence

PDA affects twice as many females as males and is the most common congenital heart defect found in adults. Normally, the ductus closes within days to weeks after birth. Failure to close is most prevalent in premature infants, probably as a result of abnormalities in oxygenation or the relaxant action of prostaglandin E, which prevents ductal spasm and contracture necessary for closure. PDA often accompanies rubella syndrome and may be associated with other congenital defects, such as coarctation of the aorta, ventricular septal defect, and pulmonary and aortic stenoses.

In PDA, relative resistances in pulmonary and systemic vasculature and the size of the ductus determine the amount of left-to-right shunting. The left atrium and left ventricle must accommodate the increased pulmonary venous return, in turn increasing left heart filling pressure and workload and possibly causing congestive heart failure. In the final stages of untreated PDA, the left-to-right shunt leads to chronic pulmonary artery hypertension that becomes fixed and unreactive. This causes the shunt to reverse; unoxygenated blood thus enters systemic circulation, causing cyanosis.

Signs and symptoms

In infants, especially those who are premature, a large PDA usually produces respiratory distress, with signs of congestive heart failure due to the tremendous volume of blood shunted to the lungs through a patent ductus and the increased left heart workload. Other characteristic features may include heightened susceptibility to respiratory tract infections, slow motor development, and failure to thrive. Most children with PDA have no symptoms except cardiac ones. Others may exhibit signs of heart disease, such as physical underdevelopment, fatigability, and frequent respiratory infections. Adults with undetected PDA may develop pulmonary vascular disease and, by age 40, may display fatigability and dyspnea on exertion. About 10% of them also develop infective endocarditis.

Auscultation reveals the classic machinery murmur (Gibson murmur): a continuous murmur (during systole and diastole) best heard at the base of the heart, at the second left intercostal space under the left clavicle in 85% of children with PDA. This murmur may obscure S_2. However, with a right-to-left shunt, such a murmur may be absent. Palpation may reveal a thrill at the left sternal border and a prominent left ventricular impulse. Peripheral arterial pulses are bounding (Corrigan's pulse); pulse pressure is widened because of an elevation in systolic blood pressure and, primarily, a drop in diastolic pressure.

Diagnosis

- *Chest X-ray* shows increased pulmonary vascular markings, prominent pulmonary arteries, and enlargement of the left ventricle and aorta.
- *EKG* may be normal or may indicate left ventricular hypertrophy and, in pulmonary vascular disease, biventricular hypertrophy.
- *Echocardiography* detects and helps estimate the size of a PDA. It also reveals an enlarged left atrium and left ventricle, or right ventricular hypertrophy from pulmonary vascular disease.

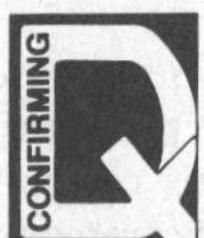

- *Cardiac catheterization* shows pulmonary arterial oxygen content higher than right ventricular content because of the influx of aortic blood. Increased pulmonary artery pressure indicates a large shunt or, if it exceeds systemic arterial pressure, severe pulmonary vascular disease. Catheterization allows calculation of blood volume crossing the ductus and can rule out associated cardiac defects. Dye injection definitively demonstrates PDA.

Treatment

Asymptomatic infants with PDA require no immediate treatment. Those with congestive heart failure require fluid restriction, diuretics, and digitalis to minimize or control symptoms. If these measures can't control congestive heart failure, surgery is necessary to ligate the ductus. If symptoms are mild, surgical correction is usually delayed until age 1. Before surgery, children with PDA require antibiotics to protect against infective endocarditis.

Other forms of therapy include cardiac catheterization to deposit a plug in the ductus to stop shunting, or administration of indomethacin I.V. (a prostaglandin inhibitor that is an alternative to surgery in premature infants) to induce ductus spasm and closure.

Special considerations

PDA necessitates careful monitoring, patient and family teaching, and emotional support.

- Watch carefully for signs of PDA in all premature infants.
- Be alert for respiratory distress symptoms resulting from congestive heart failure, which may develop rapidly in a premature infant. Frequently assess vital signs, EKG, electrolytes, and intake and output. Record response to diuretics and other therapy. Watch for signs of digitalis toxicity (poor feeding, vomiting).
- If the infant receives indomethacin for ductus closure, watch for possible side effects, such as diarrhea, jaundice, bleeding, and renal dysfunction.
- Before surgery, carefully explain all treatments and tests to parents. Include the child in your explanations. Arrange for the child and parents to meet the ICU staff. Tell them about expected I.V. lines, monitoring equipment, and postoperative procedures.
- Immediately after surgery, the child may have a central venous pressure catheter and an arterial line in place. Carefully assess vital signs, intake and output, and arterial and venous pressures. Provide pain relief, as needed.
- Before discharge, review instructions to the parents about activity restrictions based on the child's tolerance and energy levels. Advise parents not to become overprotective as their child's tolerance for physical activity increases.
- Stress the need for regular medical

follow-up examinations. Advise parents to inform any doctor who treats their child about his history of surgery for PDA—even if the child is being treated for an unrelated medical problem.

CONGENITAL CYANOTIC DEFECTS

Tetralogy of Fallot

Tetralogy of Fallot is a complex of four cardiac defects: ventricular septal defect (VSD), right ventricular outflow tract obstruction (pulmonary stenosis), right ventricular hypertrophy, and dextroposition of the aorta, with overriding of the VSD. Blood shunts right to left through the VSD, permitting unoxygenated blood to mix with oxygenated blood, resulting in cyanosis. Tetralogy of Fallot sometimes coexists with other congenital heart defects, such as patent ductus arteriosus or atrial septal defect. It accounts for about 10% of all congenital heart diseases and occurs equally in boys and girls. Before surgical advances made correction possible, approximately one third of these children died in infancy.

Causes

The cause of tetralogy of Fallot is unknown, but it results from embryologic hypoplasia of the outflow tract of the right ventricle and has been associated with fetal alcohol syndrome and the ingestion of thalidomide during pregnancy.

Signs and symptoms

The degree of pulmonary stenosis, interacting with the VSD's size and location, determines the clinical and hemodynamic effects of this complex defect. The VSD usually lies in the outflow tract of the right ventricle and is generally large enough to permit equalization of right and left ventricular pressures. However, the ratio of systemic vascular resistance to pulmonary stenosis affects the direction and magnitude of shunt flow across the VSD. Severe obstruction of right ventricular outflow produces a right-to-left shunt, causing decreased systemic arterial oxygen saturation, cyanosis, reduced pulmonary blood flow, and hypoplasia of the entire pulmonary vasculature. Increased right ventricular pressure causes right ventricular hypertrophy. Milder forms of pulmonary stenosis result in a left-to-right shunt or no shunt at all.

Generally, the hallmark of the disorder is cyanosis, which usually becomes evident within several months after birth but may be present at birth if the infant has severe pulmonary stenosis. Between ages 2 months and 2 years, children with tetralogy of Fallot may experience cyanotic, or "blue," spells. Such spells result from increased right-to-left shunting, possibly caused by spasm of the right ventricular outflow tract, increased systemic venous return, or decreased systemic arterial resistance.

Exercise, crying, straining, infection, or fever can precipitate blue spells. Blue spells are characterized by dyspnea; deep, sighing respirations; bradycardia; fainting; seizures; and loss of consciousness. Older children may also develop other signs of poor oxygenation, such as clubbing, diminished exercise tolerance, increasing dyspnea on exertion, growth retardation, and eating difficulties. These children habitually squat when they feel short of breath; this is thought to decrease venous return of unoxygenated blood from the legs and increase systemic arterial resistance.

Children with tetralogy of Fallot also risk developing cerebral abscesses, pulmonary thrombosis, venous thrombosis or cerebral embolism, and infective endocarditis.

In females with tetralogy of Fallot who live to childbearing age, incidence of spontaneous abortion, premature births, and low birth weight rises.

Diagnosis

In a patient with tetralogy of Fallot, auscultation detects a loud systolic heart murmur (best heard along the left sternal border), which may diminish or obscure the pulmonic component of S_2. In a patient with a large patent ductus, the continuous murmur of the ductus obscures the systolic murmur. Palpation may reveal a cardiac thrill at the left sternal border and an obvious right ventricular impulse. The inferior sternum appears prominent.

The results of special tests also support the diagnosis:

- *Chest X-ray* may demonstrate decreased pulmonary vascular marking, depending on the severity of the pulmonary obstruction, and a boot-shaped cardiac silhouette.
- *EKG* shows right ventricular hypertrophy, right axis deviation, and possibly right atrial hypertrophy.
- *Echocardiography* identifies septal overriding of the aorta, the VSD, and pulmonary stenosis, and detects the hypertrophied walls of the right ventricle.
- Laboratory findings reveal diminished arterial oxygen saturation and polycythemia (hematocrit may be more than 60%) if the cyanosis is severe and long-standing, predisposing the patient to thrombosis.

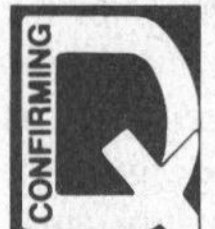

- *Cardiac catheterization* confirms diagnosis by visualizing pulmonary stenosis, the VSD, and the overriding aorta and ruling out other cyanotic heart defects. This test also measures the degree of oxygen saturation in aortic blood.

Treatment

Effective management of tetralogy of Fallot necessitates prevention and treatment of complications, measures to relieve cyanosis, and palliative or corrective surgery. During cyanotic spells, the knee-chest position and administration of oxygen and morphine improve oxygenation. Propranolol (a beta-adrenergic blocking agent) may prevent blue spells.

Palliative surgery is performed on infants with potentially fatal hypoxic spells. The goal of surgery is to enhance blood flow to the lungs to reduce hypoxia; this is often accomplished by joining the subclavian artery to the pulmonary artery (Blalock-Taussig procedure). Supportive measures include prophylactic antibiotics to prevent infective endocarditis or cerebral abscess administered before, during, and after bowel, bladder, or any other surgery or dental treatments. Management may also include phlebotomy in children with polycythemia.

Complete corrective surgery to relieve pulmonary stenosis and close the VSD, directing left ventricular outflow to the aorta, requires cardiopulmonary bypass with hypothermia to decrease oxygen utilization during surgery, especially in young children. An infant may have this corrective surgery without prior palliative surgery. It's usually done when progressive hypoxia and polycythemia impair the quality of his life, rather than at a specific age. However, most children require surgery before they reach school age.

Special considerations

- Explain tetralogy of Fallot to the parents. Inform them that their children will set their own exercise limits and will know when to rest. Make sure they understand that their child can engage in physical activity, and advise them not to be overprotective.
- Teach parents to recognize serious hypoxic spells, which can cause such things as dramatically increased cyanosis; deep, sighing respirations; and loss of consciousness. Tell them to place their child in the knee-chest position and to report such spells immediately. Emergency treatment may be necessary.
- To prevent infective endocarditis and

other infections, warn parents to keep their child away from persons with infections. Urge them to encourage good dental hygiene, and tell them to watch for ear, nose, and throat infections and dental caries, all of which necessitate immediate treatment. When dental care, infections, or surgery requires prophylactic antibiotics, tell parents to make sure the child completes the prescribed regimen.

• If the child requires medical attention for an unrelated problem, advise the parents to inform the doctor immediately of the child's history of tetralogy of Fallot since any treatment must take this serious heart defect into consideration.

• During hospitalization, alert the staff to the child's condition. Because of the right-to-left shunt through the VSD, treat I.V. lines like arterial lines. Remember, a clot dislodged from a catheter tip in a vein can cross the VSD and cause cerebral embolism. The same thing can happen if air enters the venous lines.

After palliative surgery:

• Monitor oxygenation and arterial blood gas (ABG) values closely in the ICU.

• If the child has undergone the Blalock-Taussig procedure, don't use the arm on the operative side for measuring blood pressure, inserting I.V. lines, or drawing blood samples, since blood perfusion on this side diminishes greatly until collateral circulation develops. Note this on the child's chart and at his bedside.

After corrective surgery:

• Watch for right bundle branch block or more serious disturbances of atrioventricular conduction and for ventricular ectopic beats.

• Be alert for other postoperative complications, such as bleeding, right heart failure, and respiratory failure. After surgery, transient congestive heart failure is common and may require treatment with digoxin and diuretics.

• Monitor left atrial pressure directly. A pulmonary artery catheter may also be used to check central venous and pulmonary artery pressures.

• Frequently check color and vital signs. Obtain ABG measurements regularly to assess oxygenation. As needed, suction to prevent atelectasis and pneumonia. Monitor mechanical ventilation.

• Monitor and record intake and output accurately.

• If atrioventricular block develops with a low heart rate, a temporary external pacemaker may be necessary.

• If blood pressure or cardiac output is inadequate, catecholamines may be ordered by continuous I.V. infusion. To decrease left ventricular workload, administer nitroprusside, if ordered. Provide analgesics, as needed.

• Keep the parents informed about their child's progress. After discharge, the child may require digoxin, diuretics, and other drugs. Stress the importance of complying with the prescribed regimen, and make sure the parents know how and when to administer these medications. Teach parents to watch for signs of digitalis toxicity (anorexia, nausea, vomiting). Prophylactic antibiotics to prevent infective endocarditis will still be required. Advise the parents to avoid becoming overprotective as the child's tolerance for physical activity rises.

Transposition of the Great Arteries

In this congenital heart defect, the great arteries are reversed: the aorta arises from the right ventricle and the pulmonary artery from the left ventricle, producing two noncommunicating circulatory systems (pulmonary and systemic). Transposition accounts for up to 5% of all congenital heart defects and often coexists with other congenital heart defects, such as ventricular septal defect (VSD), VSD with pulmonary stenosis (PS), atrial septal defect (ASD), and patent ductus arteriosus (PDA). It affects males two to three times more often than females.

Causes

Transposition of the great vessels results from faulty embryonic development, but the cause of such development is unknown. In transposition, oxygenated blood returning to the left side of the heart is carried back to the lungs by a transposed pulmonary artery; unoxygenated blood returning to the right side of the heart is carried to the systemic circulation by a transposed aorta.

Communication between the pulmonary and systemic circulations is necessary for survival. In infants with isolated transposition, blood mixes only at the patent foramen ovale and at the patent ductus arteriosus, resulting in slight mixing of unoxygenated systemic blood and oxygenated pulmonary blood. In infants with concurrent cardiac defects, greater mixing of blood occurs.

Signs and symptoms

Within the first few hours after birth, neonates with transposition of the great vessels and no other heart defects generally show cyanosis and tachypnea, which worsen with crying. After several days or weeks, such infants usually develop signs of congestive heart failure (gallop rhythm, tachycardia, dyspnea, hepatomegaly, and cardiomegaly). S_2 is louder than normal because the anteriorly transposed aorta is directly behind the sternum; often, however, no murmur can be heard during the first few days of life. Associated defects (ASD, VSD, or PDA) cause their typical murmurs and may minimize cyanosis but may also cause other complications (especially severe congestive heart failure). VSD with PS produces a characteristic murmur and severe cyanosis.

As infants with this defect grow older, cyanosis is their most prominent abnormality. However, they also develop diminished exercise tolerance, fatigability, coughing, clubbing, and more pronounced murmurs if ASD, VSD, PDA, or PS is present.

Diagnosis

- *Chest X-rays* are normal in the first days of life. Within days to weeks, right atrial and right ventricular enlargement characteristically cause the heart to appear oblong. X-rays also show increased pulmonary vascular markings, except when pulmonary stenosis coexists.
- *EKG* typically reveals right axis deviation and right ventricular hypertrophy but may be normal in a neonate.
- *Echocardiography* demonstrates the reversed position of the aorta and pulmonary artery, and records echoes from both semilunar valves simultaneously, due to aortic valve displacement. It also detects other cardiac defects.

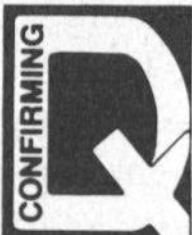

- *Cardiac catheterization* reveals decreased oxygen saturation in left ventricular blood and aortic blood; increased right atrial, right ventricular, and pulmonary artery oxygen saturation; and right ventricular systolic pressure equal to systemic pressure. Dye injection reveals the transposed vessels and the presence of any other cardiac defects.
- *Arterial blood gas measurements* indicate hypoxia and secondary metabolic acidosis.

Treatment

An infant with transposition may have atrial balloon septostomy (Rashkind procedure) during cardiac catheterization. This procedure enlarges the patent foramen ovale, which improves oxygenation by allowing greater mixing of the pulmonary and systemic circulations. Atrial balloon septostomy requires passage of a balloon-tipped catheter through the foramen ovale, and subsequent inflation and withdrawal across the atrial septum. This procedure alleviates hypoxia to a certain degree. Afterward, digoxin and diuretics can lessen congestive heart failure until the infant is ready to withstand corrective surgery (usually between birth and age 1). One of three

SURGICAL REPAIR OF TRANSPOSITION OF THE GREAT ARTERIES *(Mustard Procedure)*

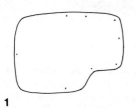

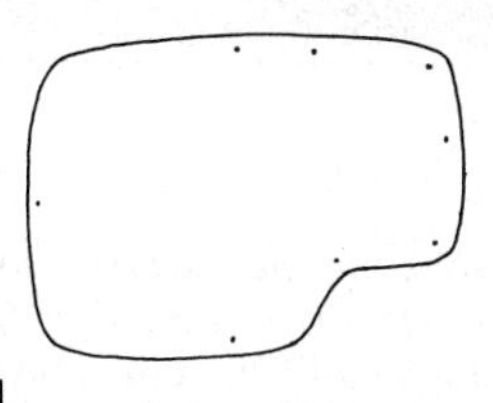

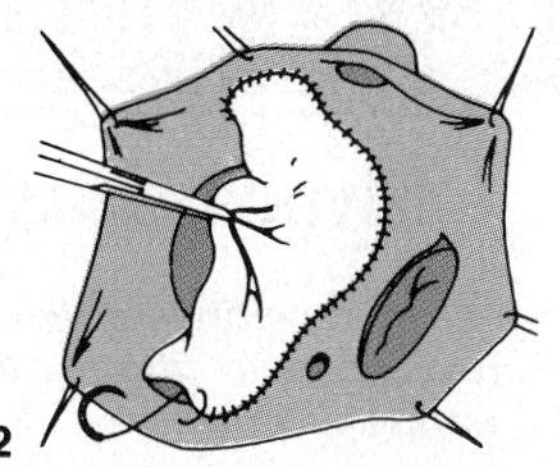

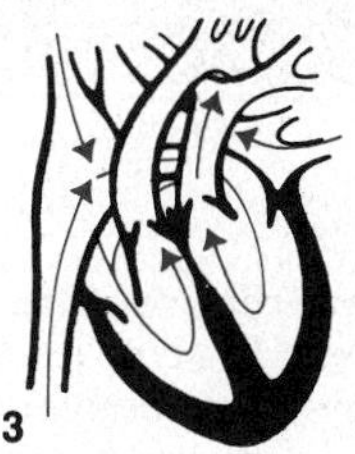

A Dacron patch (fig. 1) is sutured in the excised atrial septum (fig. 2) to divert pulmonary venous return to the tricuspid valve, and systemic venous return to the mitral valve (fig. 3).

surgical procedures can correct transposition, depending on the defect's physiology. The Mustard procedure replaces the atrial septum with a Dacron or pericardial partition that allows systemic venous blood to be channeled to the pulmonary artery—which carries the blood to the lungs for oxygenation—and oxygenated blood returning to the heart to be channeled from the pulmonary veins into the aorta. The Senning procedure accomplishes the same result, using the atrial septum to create partitions to redirect blood flow. In the arterial switch, or Jantene procedure, transposed arteries are surgically anastomosed to the correct ventricle. For this procedure to be successful, the left ventricle must be used to pump at systemic pressure, as it does in neonates or in children with a left ventricular outflow obstruction or a large VSD. Surgery also corrects other heart defects.

Special considerations

- Explain cardiac catheterization and all necessary procedures to the parents. Offer emotional support.
- Monitor vital signs, arterial blood gases, urinary output, and central venous pressure, watching for signs of congestive heart failure. Give digoxin and I.V. fluids, being careful to avoid fluid overload.
- Teach parents to recognize signs of congestive heart failure and digoxin toxicity (poor feeding, vomiting). Stress the importance of regular checkups to monitor cardiovascular status.
- Teach parents to protect their infant from infection and to give antibiotics.
- Tell the parents to let their child develop normally. They need not restrict activities; he'll set his own limits.
- If the patient is scheduled for surgery, explain the procedure to the parents and child, if old enough. Teach them about the ICU, and introduce them to the staff. Also explain postoperative care.
- Preoperatively, monitor arterial blood gases, acid-base balance, intake and output, and vital signs.

After corrective surgery:

- Monitor cardiac output by checking blood pressure, skin color, heart rate, urinary output, central venous and left atrial pressures, and level of consciousness. Report abnormalities or changes.
- Carefully measure arterial blood gases.
- To detect supraventricular conduction blocks and arrhythmias, monitor the patient closely. Watch for signs of atrioventricular blocks, atrial arrhythmias, and faulty sinoatrial function.
- After Mustard or Senning procedures, watch for signs of baffle obstruction, such as marked facial edema.
- Encourage parents to help their child assume new activity levels and independence. Teach them about postoperative antibiotic prophylaxis for endocarditis.

ACQUIRED INFLAMMATORY HEART DISEASE

Myocarditis

Myocarditis is focal or diffuse inflammation of the cardiac muscle (myocardium). It may be acute or chronic and can occur at any age. Frequently, myocarditis fails to produce specific cardiovascular symptoms or EKG abnormalities, and recovery is usually spontaneous, without residual defects. Occasionally, myocarditis is complicated by congestive heart failure and, rarely, leads to cardiomyopathy.

Causes

Myocarditis results from:

- *viral infections* (most common cause in the United States): Coxsackievirus A and B strains and, possibly, poliomyelitis, influenza, rubeola, rubella, and adeno- and echoviruses
- *bacterial infections:* diphtheria, tuberculosis, typhoid fever, tetanus, and staphylococcal, pneumococcal, and gonococcal infections
- *hypersensitive immune reactions:* acute rheumatic fever and postcardiotomy syndrome
- *radiation therapy:* large doses of radiation to the chest in treating lung or breast cancer
- *chemical poisons:* such as chronic alcoholism
- *parasitic infections:* especially South American trypanosomiasis (Chagas' disease) in infants and immunosuppressed adults; also, toxoplasmosis
- *helminthic infections:* such as trichinosis.

Signs and symptoms

Myocarditis usually causes nonspecific symptoms—such as fatigue, dyspnea, palpitations, and fever—that reflect the accompanying systemic infection. Occasionally, it may produce mild, continuous pressure or soreness in the chest (unlike the recurring, stress-related pain of angina pectoris). Although myocarditis is generally uncomplicated and self-limiting, it may induce myofibril degeneration that results in right and left heart failure, with cardiomegaly, neck vein distention, dyspnea, resting or exertional tachycardia disproportionate to the degree of fever, and supraventricular and ventricular arrhythmias. Sometimes myocarditis recurs or produces chronic valvulitis (when it results from rheumatic fever), cardiomyopathy, arrhythmias, and thromboembolism.

Diagnosis

Patient history commonly reveals recent febrile upper respiratory tract infection, viral pharyngitis, or tonsillitis. Physical examination shows supraventricular and ventricular arrhythmias, S_3 and S_4 gallops, a faint S_1, possibly a murmur of mitral regurgitation (from papillary muscle dysfunction), and, if pericarditis is present, a pericardial friction rub.

Laboratory tests can't unequivocally confirm myocarditis, but the following findings support this diagnosis:

- cardiac enzymes; elevated creatine phosphokinase (CPK), CPK isoenzyme (CPK_2), SGOT, and lactic dehydrogenase
- increased WBC and ESR
- elevated antibody titers (such as antistreptolysin O [ASO] titer in rheumatic fever).

EKG changes are the most reliable diagnostic aid, and typically show diffuse ST segment and T wave abnormalities as in pericarditis, conduction defects (prolonged P-R interval), and other supraventricular ectopic arrhythmias.

Stool and throat cultures may identify bacteria.

Endomyocardial biopsy provides a definitive diagnosis.

Treatment

Treatment includes antibiotics for bacterial infection, modified bed rest to decrease heart workload, and careful management of complications. Congestive heart failure requires restriction of activity to minimize myocardial oxygen consumption, supplemental oxygen therapy, sodium restriction, diuretics to decrease fluid retention, and digitalis to increase myocardial contractility. However, digitalis necessitates cautious administration, since some patients with myocarditis may show a paradoxical sensitivity to even small doses. Arrhythmias necessitate prompt but cautious administration of antiarrhythmics, such as quinidine or procainamide, since these drugs depress myocardial contractility. Thromboembolism requires anticoagulation therapy. Treatment with corticosteroids or other immunosuppressants is controversial and therefore limited to combatting life-threatening complications, such as intractable heart failure.

Special considerations

- Assess cardiovascular status frequently, watching for signs of congestive heart failure, such as dyspnea, hypotension, and tachycardia. Check for changes in cardiac rhythm or conduction.
- Observe for signs of digitalis toxicity (anorexia, nausea, vomiting, blurred vision, cardiac arrhythmias) and for complicating factors that may potentiate toxicity, such as electrolyte imbalance or hypoxia.
- Stress the importance of bed rest. Assist with bathing, as necessary; provide a bedside commode, since this stresses the heart less than using a bedpan. Give reassurance that activity limitations are temporary. Offer diversional activities that are physically undemanding.
- During recovery, recommend that the patient resume normal activities slowly and avoid competitive sports.

Endocarditis

(Infective endocarditis, bacterial endocarditis)

Endocarditis is an infection of the endocardium, heart valves, or cardiac prosthesis, resulting from bacterial (or, in intravenous drug abusers, fungal) invasion. This invasion produces vegetative growths on the heart valves, endocardial lining of a heart chamber, or the endothelium of a blood vessel that may embolize to the spleen, kidneys, central nervous system, and lungs. Untreated endocarditis is usually fatal, but with proper treatment, 70% of patients recover. Prognosis is worst when endocarditis causes severe valvular damage, leading to insufficiency and congestive heart failure, or when it involves a prosthetic valve.

Causes

Acute infective endocarditis usually results from bacteremia that follows septic thrombophlebitis, open heart surgery involving prosthetic valves, or skin, bone, and pulmonary infections. The most common causative organisms are group A nonhemolytic streptococcus (rheumatic endocarditis), pneumococcus, staphylococcus, and rarely, gonococcus. This form of endocarditis also occurs in intravenous drug abusers, possibly from *Staphylococcus aureus*, pseudomonas, *Candida*, or usually harmless skin saprophytes.

Subacute infective endocarditis typically occurs in persons with acquired valvular or congenital cardiac lesions. It can also follow dental, genitourinary, gynecologic, and gastrointestinal procedures. The most common infecting organisms are *Streptococcus viridans*, which normally inhabits the upper respiratory tract, and *Streptococcus faecalis* (enterococcus), generally found in gastrointestinal and perineal flora.

Preexisting rheumatic endocardial lesions are a common predisposing factor in bacterial endocarditis. Rheumatic endocarditis commonly affects the mitral valve; less frequently, the aortic or tricuspid valve; and rarely, the pulmonic valve.

In infective endocarditis, fibrin and platelets aggregate on the valve tissue and engulf circulating bacteria or fungi that flourish and produce friable verrucous vegetations. Such vegetations may cover the valve surfaces, causing ulceration and necrosis; they may also extend to the chordae tendineae, leading to their rupture and subsequent valvular insufficiency. Sometimes vegetations form on the endocardium, usually in areas altered by rheumatic, congenital, or syphilitic heart disease, although they may also form on normal surfaces.

Signs and symptoms

Early clinical features of endocarditis are nonspecific, and include weakness, fatigue, weight loss, anorexia, arthralgia, night sweats, and in 90% of patients, an intermittent fever that may recur for weeks. Endocarditis often causes a loud, regurgitant murmur typical of the underlying rheumatic or congenital heart disease. A suddenly changing murmur or the discovery of a new murmur in the presence of fever is a classic physical sign of endocarditis.

In about 30% of patients with subacute endocarditis, embolization from vegetating lesions or diseased valve tissue may produce typical features of splenic, renal, cerebral, or pulmonary infarction, or peripheral vascular occlusion:

- *splenic infarction:* pain in the upper left quadrant, radiating to the left shoulder; abdominal rigidity
- *renal infarction:* hematuria, pyuria, flank pain, decreased urinary output
- *cerebral infarction:* hemiparesis, aphasia, or other neurologic deficits
- *pulmonary infarction* (most common in right-sided endocarditis, which often occurs among intravenous drug abusers and after cardiac surgery): cough, pleuritic pain, pleural friction rub, dyspnea, and hemoptysis
- *peripheral vascular occlusion:* numbness and tingling in an arm, leg, finger, or toe, or signs of impending peripheral gangrene.

Other symptoms include petechiae of the skin (especially common on the upper anterior trunk) and the buccal, pharyngeal, or conjunctival mucosa, and splinter hemorrhages under the nails. Rarely, endocarditis produces Osler's nodes (tender, raised, subcutaneous lesions on the fingers or toes), Roth's spots (hemorrhagic areas with white centers on the retina), and Janeway lesions (purplish macules on the palms or soles).

PROSTHETIC VALVE ENDOCARDITIS

Increasing use of prosthetic heart valve implants has given rise to prosthetic valve endocarditis, an infection of the artificial valve along the suture line. This disorder can be either acute or subacute. Signs and symptoms usually are similar to those of other forms of endocarditis, although sometimes the only symptoms are fever and murmur from valve dysfunction. Treatment consists of antibiotic therapy and often, surgery to replace the infected prosthetic valve.

Diagnosis

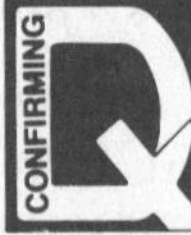

Three or more blood cultures during a 24- to 48-hour period identify the causative organism in up to 90% of patients. The remaining 10% may have negative blood cultures, possibly suggesting fungal infection. Other abnormal but nonspecific laboratory results include:

- elevated WBC
- abnormal histocytes (macrophages)
- elevated ESR
- normocytic, normochromic anemia

(in subacute bacterial endocarditis)
- rheumatoid factor, in about half of all patients with endocarditis.

Echocardiography may identify valvular damage; EKG may show atrial fibrillation and other arrhythmias that accompany valvular disease.

Treatment

The goal of treatment is to eradicate the infecting organism. Therapy should start promptly and continue over several weeks. Antibiotic selection is based on sensitivity studies of the infecting organism—or the probable organism, if blood cultures are negative. I.V. antibiotic therapy usually lasts about 4 weeks.

Supportive treatment includes bed rest, aspirin for fever and aches, and sufficient fluid intake. Severe valvular damage, especially aortic regurgitation or infection of cardiac prosthesis, may require corrective surgery if refractory heart failure develops.

DEGENERATIVE CHANGES OF ENDOCARDITIS

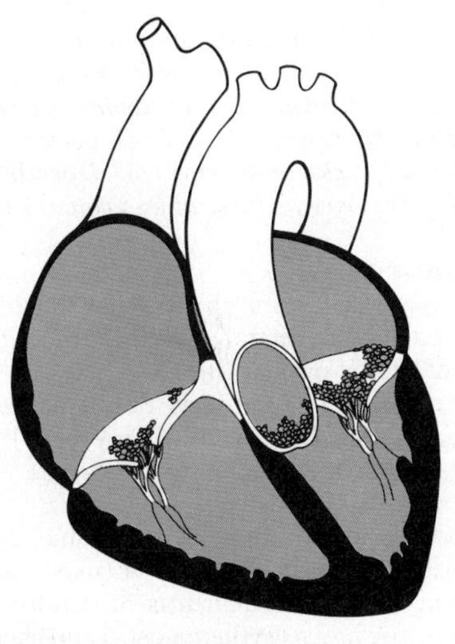

Typical vegetations on the endocardium produced by fibrin and platelet deposits on infection sites

Special considerations

- Before giving antibiotics, obtain a patient history of allergies. Administer antibiotics on time to maintain consistent antibiotic blood levels. Check dilutions for compatibility with other medications the patient is receiving, and use a solution that is compatible with drug stability. (For example, add methicillin to a buffered solution.)
- Observe for signs of infiltration or inflammation at the venipuncture site, possible complications of long-term I.V. administration. To reduce the risk of these complications, rotate venous access sites.
- Watch for signs of embolization (hematuria, pleuritic chest pain, upper left quadrant pain, or paresis), a common occurrence during the first 3 months of treatment. Tell the patient to watch for and report these signs, which may indicate impending peripheral vascular occlusion or splenic, renal, cerebral, or pulmonary infarction.
- Monitor the patient's renal status (including BUN, creatinine, and urinary output) to check for signs of renal emboli or drug toxicity.
- Observe for signs of congestive heart failure, such as dyspnea, tachypnea, tachycardia, rales, neck vein distention, edema, and weight gain.
- Provide reassurance by teaching the patient and family about this disease and the need for prolonged treatment. Tell them to watch closely for fever, anorexia, and other signs of relapse about 2 weeks after treatment stops. Suggest quiet diversionary activities to prevent excessive physical exertion.
- Make sure susceptible patients understand the need for prophylactic antibiotics before, during, and after dental work, childbirth, and genitourinary, gastrointestinal, or gynecologic procedures.
- Teach patients how to recognize symptoms of endocarditis, and tell them to notify the doctor immediately if such symptoms occur.

Pericarditis

Pericarditis is an inflammation of the pericardium, the fibroserous sac that envelops, supports, and protects the heart. It occurs in both acute and chronic forms. Acute pericarditis can be fibrinous or effusive, with purulent serous or hemorrhagic exudate; chronic constrictive pericarditis is characterized by dense fibrous pericardial thickening. Prognosis depends on the underlying cause but is generally good in acute pericarditis, unless constriction occurs.

Causes

Common causes of this disease include:
- bacterial, fungal, or viral infection (infectious pericarditis)
- neoplasms (primary, or metastases from lungs, breasts, or other organs)
- high-dose radiation to the chest
- uremia
- hypersensitivity or autoimmune disease, such as rheumatic fever (most common cause of pericarditis in children), systemic lupus erythematosus, and rheumatoid arthritis
- postcardiac injury, such as myocardial infarction (which later causes an autoimmune reaction [Dressler's syndrome] in the pericardium), trauma, or surgery that leaves the pericardium intact but causes blood to leak into the pericardial cavity
- drugs, such as hydralazine or procainamide
- idiopathic factors (most common in acute pericarditis).

Less common causes include aortic aneurysm with pericardial leakage, and myxedema with cholesterol deposits in the pericardium.

Signs and symptoms

Acute pericarditis typically produces a sharp and often sudden pain that usually starts over the sternum and radiates to the neck, shoulders, back, and arms. However, unlike the pain of myocardial infarction, pericardial pain is often pleuritic, increasing with deep inspiration and decreasing when the patient sits up and leans forward, pulling the heart away from the diaphragmatic pleurae of the lungs.

Pericardial effusion, the major complication of acute pericarditis, may produce effects of heart failure—such as dyspnea, orthopnea, and tachycardia—ill-defined substernal chest pain, and a feeling of fullness in the chest. If the fluid

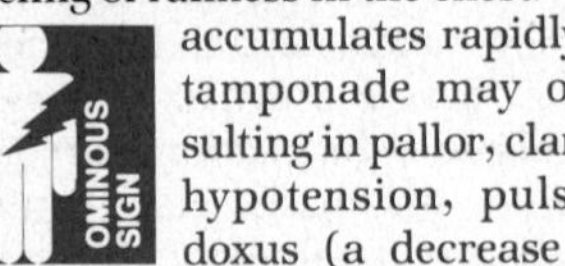

accumulates rapidly, cardiac tamponade may occur, resulting in pallor, clammy skin, hypotension, pulsus paradoxus (a decrease in blood pressure $\geqslant$ 15 mmHg during slow inspiration), neck vein distention, and eventually, cardiovascular collapse and death.

Chronic constrictive pericarditis causes a gradual increase in systemic venous pressure and produces symptoms similar to those of chronic right heart failure (fluid retention, ascites, hepatomegaly).

Diagnosis

Since pericarditis often coexists with other conditions, diagnosis of acute pericarditis depends on typical clinical features and elimination of other possible causes. A classic symptom, the pericardial friction rub, is a grating sound heard as the heart moves. It can usually be auscultated best during forced expiration, while the patient leans forward or is on his hands and knees in bed. It may have up to three components, corresponding to the timing of atrial systole, ventricular systole, and the rapid-filling phase of ventricular diastole. Occasionally, this friction rub is heard only briefly or not at all. Nevertheless, its presence, together with other characteristic features, is diagnostic of acute pericarditis. In addition if acute pericarditis has caused very large pericardial effusions, physical examination reveals increased cardiac dullness and diminished or absent apical impulse and distant heart sounds.

In patients with chronic pericarditis, acute inflammation or effusions do not occur—only restricted cardiac filling.

Laboratory results reflect inflammation and may identify its cause:
- normal or elevated WBC, especially in infectious pericarditis
- elevated ESR
- slightly elevated cardiac enzymes with associated myocarditis
- culture of pericardial fluid obtained by open surgical drainage or cardiocentesis (sometimes identifies a causative organism in bacterial or fungal pericarditis)
- EKG shows the following changes in acute pericarditis: elevation of ST segments in the standard limb leads and most precordial leads without significant changes in QRS morphology that occur with myocardial infarction; atrial ectopic rhythms, such as atrial fibrillation; and, in pericardial effusion, diminished QRS voltage.

Other pertinent laboratory data include BUN to check for uremia, antistreptolysin O titers to detect rheumatic fever, and a purified protein derivative skin test to check for tuberculosis. In pericardial effusion, echocardiography is diagnostic when it shows an echo-free space between the ventricular wall and the pericardium.

Treatment

The goal of treatment is to relieve symptoms and manage underlying systemic disease. In acute idiopathic pericarditis, postmyocardial infarction pericarditis, and post-thoracotomy pericarditis, treatment consists of bed rest as long as fever and pain persist and nonsteroidal drugs, such as aspirin and indomethacin, to relieve pain and reduce inflammation. If these drugs fail to relieve symptoms, corticosteroids may be used. Although corticosteroids produce rapid and effective relief, they must be used cautiously because episodes may recur when therapy is discontinued.

Infectious pericarditis that results from disease of the left pleural space, mediastinal abscesses, or septicemia requires antibiotics, surgical drainage, or both. If cardiac tamponade develops, the doctor may perform emergency pericardiocentesis. Signs of cardiac tamponade include pulsus paradoxus, neck vein distention, dyspnea, and shock.

Recurrent pericarditis may necessitate partial pericardectomy, which creates a "window" that allows fluid to drain into the pleural space. In constrictive pericarditis, total pericardectomy to permit adequate filling and contraction of the heart may be necessary. Treatment must also include management of rheumatic fever, uremia, tuberculosis, and other underlying disorders.

Special considerations

A patient with pericarditis needs complete bed rest. In addition, health care includes:
- assessing pain in relation to respiration and body position to distinguish pericardial pain from myocardial ischemic pain.
- placing the patient in an upright position to relieve dyspnea and chest pain; providing analgesics and oxygen; and reassuring the patient with acute pericarditis that his condition is temporary and treatable.
- monitoring for signs of cardiac compression or cardiac tamponade, possible complications of pericardial effusion. Signs include decreased blood pressure, increased central venous pressure, and pulsus paradoxus. Since cardiac tamponade requires immediate treatment, keep a pericardiocentesis set handy whenever pericardial effusion is suspected.
- explaining tests and treatments to the patient. If surgery is necessary, he should learn deep breathing and coughing exercises beforehand. Postoperative care is similar to that given following cardiothoracic surgery.

Rheumatic Fever and Rheumatic Heart Disease

Acute rheumatic fever is a systemic inflammatory disease of childhood, often recurrent, that follows a Group A beta-hemolytic streptococcal infection. Rheumatic heart disease refers to the cardiac manifestations of rheumatic fever, and includes pancarditis (myocarditis, pericarditis, and endocarditis) during the early acute phase and chronic valvular disease later. Long-term antibiotic therapy can minimize recurrence of rheumatic fever, reducing the risk of permanent cardiac damage and eventual valvular deformity. However, severe pancarditis occasionally produces fatal congestive heart failure during the acute phase. Of the patients who survive this complication, about 20% die within 10 years.

Causes and incidence

Rheumatic fever appears to be a hypersensitivity reaction to a Group A beta-hemolytic streptococcal infection, in which antibodies manufactured to combat streptococci react and produce characteristic lesions at specific tissue sites, especially in the heart and joints. Since very few persons (0.3%) with streptococcal infections ever contract rheumatic fever, altered host resistance must be involved in its development or recurrence. Although rheumatic fever tends to be familial, this may merely reflect contributing environmental factors. For example, in lower socioeconomic groups, incidence is highest in children between ages 5 and 15, probably as a result of malnutrition and crowded living conditions. This disease strikes most often during cool, damp weather in the winter and early spring. In the United States, it's most common in the northern states.

Signs and symptoms

In 95% of patients, rheumatic fever characteristically follows a streptococcal infection that appeared a few days to 6 weeks earlier. A temperature of at least 100.4° F. (38° C.) occurs, and most patients complain of migratory joint pain or *polyarthritis.* Swelling, redness, and signs of effusion usually accompany such pain, which most commonly affects the knees, ankles, elbows, or hips. In 5% of patients (generally those with carditis), rheumatic fever causes skin lesions such as *erythema marginatum,* a nonpruritic, macular, transient rash that gives rise to red lesions with blanched centers. Rheumatic fever may also produce firm, movable, nontender, *subcutaneous nodules* about 3 mm to 2 cm in diameter, usually near tendons or bony prominences of joints (especially the elbows, knuckles, wrists, and knees) and less often on the scalp and backs of the hands. These nodules persist for a few days to several weeks and, like erythema marginatum, often accompany carditis.

Later, rheumatic fever may cause transient *chorea,* which develops up to 6 months after the original streptococcal infection. Mild chorea may produce hyperirritability, a deterioration in handwriting, or inability to concentrate. Severe chorea causes purposeless, nonrepetitive, involuntary muscle spasms; poor muscle coordination; and weakness. Chorea always resolves without residual neurologic damage.

The most destructive effect of rheumatic fever is *carditis,* which develops in up to 50% of patients and may affect the endocardium, myocardium, pericardium, or the heart valves. Pericarditis causes a pericardial friction rub and, occasionally, pain and effusion. Myocarditis produces characteristic lesions called Aschoff's bodies (in the acute stages), and cellular swelling and fragmentation of interstitial collagen, leading to formation of a progressively fibrotic nodule and interstitial scars. Endocarditis causes valve leaflet swelling, erosion along the lines of leaflet closure, and blood, platelet, and fibrin deposits, which form beadlike vegetations. Endocarditis affects the mitral valve most often in females; the aortic, most often in males. In both females and males, endocarditis affects the tricuspid valves occasionally and the pulmonic only rarely.

Severe rheumatic carditis may cause congestive heart failure with dyspnea, upper right quadrant pain, tachycardia, tachypnea, a hacking nonproductive cough, edema, and significant mitral and aortic murmurs. The most common of such murmurs include:

- a systolic murmur of mitral regurgitation (high-pitched, blowing, holosystolic, loudest at apex, possibly radiating to the anterior axillary line)
- a midsystolic murmur due to stiffening and swelling of the mitral leaflet
- occasionally, a diastolic murmur of aortic regurgitation (low-pitched, rumbling, almost inaudible). Valvular disease may eventually result in chronic valvular stenosis and insufficiency, including mitral stenosis and regurgitation, and aortic regurgitation. In children, mitral insufficiency remains the major sequela of rheumatic heart disease.

Diagnosis

Diagnosis depends on recognition of one or more of the classic symptoms (carditis, polyarthritis, chorea, erythema marginatum, or subcutaneous nodules) and a detailed patient history. Laboratory data support the diagnosis:

- *WBC* and *ESR* may be elevated (especially during the acute phase); blood studies show slight anemia due to suppressed erythropoiesis during inflammation.
- *C-reactive protein* is positive (especially during acute phase).
- *Cardiac enzymes* may be increased in severe carditis.
- *Antistreptolysin O titer* is elevated in 95% of patients within 2 months of onset.
- *EKG* changes are not diagnostic; however, 20% of patients show a prolonged P-R interval.
- *Chest X-rays* show normal heart size (except with myocarditis, congestive heart failure, or pericardial effusion).
- *Echocardiography* helps evaluate valvular damage, chamber size, and ventricular function.
- *Cardiac catheterization* evaluates valvular damage and left ventricular function in severe cardiac dysfunction.

Treatment

Effective management eradicates the streptococcal infection, relieves symptoms, and prevents recurrence, reducing the chance of permanent cardiac damage. During the acute phase, treatment includes penicillin or (for patients with penicillin hypersensitivity) erythromycin. Salicylates, such as aspirin, relieve fever and minimize joint swelling and pain; if carditis is present or salicylates fail to relieve pain and inflammation, corticosteroids may be used. Supportive treatment requires strict bed rest for about 5 weeks during the acute phase with active carditis, followed by a progressive increase in physical activity, depending on clinical and laboratory findings and the response to treatment.

After the acute phase subsides, a monthly I.M. injection of penicillin G benzathine or daily doses of oral sulfadiazine or penicillin G may be used to prevent recurrence. Such preventive treatment usually continues for at least 5 years or until age 25. Congestive heart failure necessitates continued bed rest and diuretics. Severe mitral or aortic valvular dysfunction causing persistent congestive heart failure requires corrective valvular surgery, including commissurotomy (separation of the adherent, thickened leaflets of the mitral valve), valvuloplasty (repair of valve), or valve replacement (with prosthetic valve). Corrective valvular surgery is rarely necessary before late adolescence.

Special considerations

Because rheumatic fever and rheumatic heart disease require prolonged treatment, your care plan should include comprehensive patient teaching to promote compliance with the prescribed therapy.

• Before giving penicillin, ask the patient or (if the patient's a child) his parents if he's ever had a hypersensitive reaction to it. Even if the patient has never had a reaction to penicillin, warn that such a reaction is possible. Tell them to stop the drug and call the doctor immediately if the patient develops a rash, fever, chills, or other signs of allergy *at any time* during penicillin therapy.

• Instruct the patient and his family to watch for and report early signs of congestive heart failure such as dyspnea and a hacking, nonproductive cough.

• Stress the need for bed rest during the acute phase and suggest appropriate, physically undemanding diversions. After the acute phase, encourage the family and friends to spend as much time as possible with the patient to minimize boredom. Advise parents to secure tutorial services to help the child keep up with schoolwork during the long convalescence.

• Help parents overcome any guilt feelings they may have about their child's illness. Tell them that failure to seek treatment for streptococcal infection is common, since this illness often seems no worse than a cold. Encourage the parents and the child to vent their frustrations during the long, tedious recovery. If the child has severe carditis, help them prepare for permanent changes in the child's life-style.

• Teach the patient and family about this disease and its treatment. Warn parents to watch for and immediately report signs of recurrent streptococcal infection—sudden sore throat, diffuse throat redness and oropharyngeal exudate, swollen and tender cervical lymph glands, pain on swallowing, temperature of 101° to 104° F. (38.3° to 40° C.), headache, and nausea. Urge them to keep the child away from persons with respiratory tract infections.

• Promote good dental hygiene to prevent gingival infection. Make sure the patient and his family understand the need to comply with prolonged antibiotic therapy and follow-up care, and the need for additional antibiotics during dental surgery. Arrange for a visiting nurse to oversee home care, if necessary.

VALVULAR HEART DISEASE

Valvular Heart Disease

In valvular heart disease, two types of mechanical disruption can occur: stenosis, or narrowing, of the valve opening; or incomplete closure of the valve. They can result from such disorders as rheumatic endocarditis (most common), congenital defects, and inflammation and can lead to heart failure.

Valvular heart disease occurs in varying forms:

• *Mitral insufficiency:* In this form, blood from the left ventricle flows back into the left atrium during systole, causing the atrium to enlarge to accommodate the backflow. As a result, the left ventricle also dilates to accommodate the increased volume of blood from the atrium and to compensate for diminishing cardiac output. Ventricular hypertrophy and increased end-diastolic pressure result in increased pulmonary artery pressure, eventually leading to left and right ventricular failure.

• *Mitral stenosis:* Narrowing of the valve by valvular abnormalities, fibrosis, or calcification obstructs blood flow from the left atrium to the left ventricle. Consequently, left atrial volume and pres-

FORMS OF VALVULAR HEART DISEASE

CAUSES AND INCIDENCE	CLINICAL FEATURES	DIAGNOSTIC MEASURES
Mitral stenosis		
• Results from rheumatic fever (most common cause) • Most common in females • May be associated with other congenital anomalies	• Dyspnea on exertion, paroxysmal nocturnal dyspnea, orthopnea, weakness, fatigue, palpitations • Peripheral edema, jugular venous distention, ascites, hepatomegaly (right ventricular failure in severe pulmonary hypertension) • Rales, cardiac arrhythmias (atrial fibrillation), signs of systemic emboli • Auscultation reveals a loud S_1 or opening snap, and a diastolic murmur at the apex.	• Cardiac catheterization: diastolic pressure gradient across valve; elevated left atrial and pulmonary capillary wedge pressures (PCWP $>$ 15) with severe pulmonary hypertension and pulmonary arterial pressures; elevated right heart pressure; decreased cardiac output; and abnormal contraction of the left ventricle. May not be indicated in patients with isolated mitral stenosis with mild symptoms. • X-ray: left atrial and ventricular enlargement, enlarged pulmonary arteries, and mitral valve calcification • Echocardiography: thickened mitral valve leaflets, left atrial enlargement • Electrocardiography: left atrial hypertrophy, atrial fibrillation, right ventricular hypertrophy, and right axis deviation
Mitral insufficiency		
• Results from rheumatic fever, idiopathic hypertrophic subaortic stenosis (IHSS), mitral valve prolapse, myocardial infarction, severe left ventricular failure, ruptured chordae tendineae • Associated with other congenital anomalies, such as transposition of the great arteries • Rare in children without other congenital anomalies	• Orthopnea, dyspnea, fatigue, angina, palpitations • Peripheral edema, jugular vein distention, hepatomegaly (right ventricular failure) • Tachycardia, rales, pulmonary edema • Auscultation reveals a holosystolic murmur at apex, possible split S_2, and an S_3.	• Cardiac catheterization: mitral regurgitation, with increased left ventricular end-diastolic volume and pressure; increased atrial and pulmonary capillary wedge pressures; and decreased cardiac output • X-ray: left atrial and ventricular enlargement, pulmonary venous congestion • Echocardiography: abnormal valve leaflet motion, left atrial enlargement • Electrocardiography: may show left atrial and ventricular hypertrophy, sinus tachycardia, atrial fibrillation.

FORMS OF VALVULAR HEART DISEASE (continued)

CAUSES AND INCIDENCE	CLINICAL FEATURES	DIAGNOSTIC MEASURES
Tricuspid insufficiency		
• Results from right ventricular failure, rheumatic fever, and rarely, trauma and endocarditis • Associated with congenital disorders	• Dyspnea and fatigue • May lead to peripheral edema, jugular venous distention, hepatomegaly, and ascites (right ventricular failure) • Auscultation reveals possible S_3 and systolic murmur at lower left sternal border that increases with inspiration	• Right heart catheterization: high atrial pressure, tricuspid regurgitation, and decreased or normal cardiac output • X-ray: right atrial dilation, right ventricular enlargement • Echocardiography: shows systolic prolapse of tricuspid valve, right atrial enlargement • Electrocardiography: right atrial or right ventricular hypertrophy, atrial fibrillation
Tricuspid stenosis		
• Results from rheumatic fever • May be congenital • Associated with mitral or aortic valve disease • Most common in women	• May be symptomatic with dyspnea, fatigue, syncope • Possibly peripheral edema, jugular venous distention, hepatomegaly, and ascites (right ventricular failure) • Auscultation reveals diastolic murmur at lower left sternal border that increases with inspiration	• Cardiac catheterization: increased pressure gradient across valve, increased right atrial pressure, decreased cardiac output • X-ray: right atrial enlargement • Echocardiography: leaflet abnormality, right atrial enlargement • Electrocardiography: right atrial hypertrophy, right or left ventricular hypertrophy, atrial fibrillation
Pulmonic stenosis		
• Results from congenital stenosis of valve cusp or rheumatic heart disease (infrequent) • Associated with other congenital heart defects, such as tetralogy of Fallot	• Asymptomatic or symptomatic with dyspnea on exertion, fatigue, chest pain, syncope • May lead to peripheral edema, jugular venous distention, hepatomegaly (right ventricular failure) • Auscultation reveals a systolic murmur at the left sternal border, a split S_2 with a delayed or absent pulmonic component	• Cardiac catheterization: increased right ventricular pressure, decreased pulmonary artery pressure, and abnormal valve orifice • Electrocardiography: may show right ventricular hypertrophy, right axis deviation, right atrial hypertrophy, and atrial fibrillation

FORMS OF VALVULAR HEART DISEASE (continued)

CAUSES AND INCIDENCE	CLINICAL FEATURES	DIAGNOSTIC MEASURES
Pulmonic insufficiency		
• May be congenital or may result from pulmonary hypertension • May rarely result from prolonged use of pressure monitoring catheter in the pulmonary artery	• Dyspnea, weakness, fatigue, chest pain • Peripheral edema, jugular venous distention, hepatomegaly (right ventricular failure) • Auscultation reveals diastolic murmur in pulmonic area.	• Cardiac catheterization: pulmonary regurgitation, increased right ventricular pressure, associated cardiac defects • X-ray: right ventricular and pulmonary arterial enlargement • Electrocardiography: right ventricular or right atrial enlargement
Aortic insufficiency		
• Results from rheumatic fever, syphilis, hypertension, endocarditis, or may be idiopathic • Associated with Marfan's syndrome • Most common in males • Associated with ventricular septal defect, even after surgical closure	• Dyspnea, cough, fatigue, palpitations, angina, syncope • Pulmonary vein congestion, congestive heart failure, pulmonary edema (left ventricular failure), "pulsating" nail beds (Quincke's sign) • Rapidly rising and collapsing pulses (pulsus bifieriens), cardiac arrhythmias, wide pulse pressure in severe regurgitation • Auscultation reveals an S_3 and a diastolic blowing murmur at left sternal border. • Palpation and visualization of apical impulse in chronic disease	• Cardiac catheterization: reduction in arterial diastolic pressures, aortic regurgitation, other valvular abnormalities, and increased left ventricular end-diastolic pressure • X-ray: left ventricular enlargement, pulmonary venous congestion • Echocardiography: left ventricular enlargement, alterations in mitral valve movement (indirect indication of aortic valve disease), and mitral thickening • Electrocardiography: sinus tachycardia, left ventricular hypertrophy, left atrial hypertrophy in severe disease
Aortic stenosis		
• Results from congenital aortic bicuspid valve (associated with coarctation of the aorta), congenital stenosis of valve cusps, rheumatic fever, or atheroslerosis in the aged • Most common in males	• Dyspnea on exertion, paroxysmal nocturnal dyspnea, fatigue, syncope, angina, palpitations • Pulmonary venous congestion, congestive heart failure, pulmonary edema (left ventricular failure) • Diminished carotid pulses, decreased cardiac output, cardiac arrhythmias; may have pulsus alternans • Auscultation reveals systolic murmur heard at base or in carotids and, possibly, an S_4.	• Cardiac catheterization: pressure gradient across valve (indicating obstruction), increased left ventricular end-diastolic pressures • X-ray: valvular calcification, left ventricular enlargement, pulmonary venous congestion • Echocardiography: thickened aortic valve and left ventricular wall, possibly coexistent with mitral valve stenosis • Electrocardiography: left ventricular hypertrophy

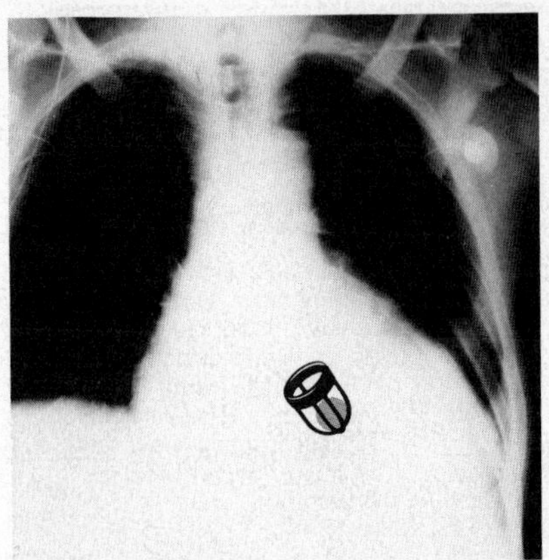

Severe valvular heart disease may require surgical insertion of a prosthetic mitral valve, such as the Starr Edwards valve illustrated in the X-ray above.

sure rise and the chamber dilates. Greater resistance to blood flow causes pulmonary hypertension, right ventricular hypertrophy, and, eventually, right ventricular failure. Also, inadequate filling of the left ventricle produces low cardiac output.

- *Aortic insufficiency:* Blood flows back into the left ventricle during diastole, causing a fluid overload in the ventricle, which, in turn, dilates and, ultimately, hypertrophies. The excess volume causes a fluid overload in the left atrium and, finally, in the pulmonary system. Left ventricular failure and pulmonary edema eventually result.
- *Aortic stenosis:* Increased left ventricular pressure attempts to overcome the resistance of the narrowed valvular opening. The added workload causes a greater demand for oxygen, while diminished cardiac output causes poor coronary artery perfusion, ischemia of the left ventricle, and eventually, left ventricular failure.
- *Pulmonic insufficiency:* Blood ejected into the pulmonary artery during systole flows back into the right ventricle during diastole, causing a fluid overload in the ventricle, ventricular hypertrophy, and, finally, right ventricular failure.
- *Pulmonic stenosis:* Obstructed right ventricular outflow causes right ventricular hypertrophy in an attempt to overcome resistance to the narrow valvular opening. Right ventricular failure ultimately results.
- *Tricuspid insufficiency:* Blood flows back into the right atrium during systole, decreasing blood flow to the lungs and left side of the heart. Cardiac output also lessens. Fluid overload in the right side of the heart can eventually lead to right ventricular failure.
- *Tricuspid stenosis:* Obstructed blood flow from the right atrium to the right ventricle causes the right atrium to dilate and hypertrophy. Eventually, this leads to right ventricular failure and increases pressure in the vena cava.

Treatment and special considerations

Treatment of valvular heart disease depends on the nature and severity of associated symptoms. For example, heart failure requires digoxin, diuretics, a sodium-restricted diet, and in acute cases, oxygen. Other appropriate measures include anticoagulant therapy to prevent thrombus formation around diseased or replaced valves, and prophylactic antibiotics before and after surgery or dental care.

If the patient has severe signs and symptoms that can't be managed medically, open heart surgery using cardiopulmonary bypass for valve replacement is indicated.

- Watch closely for signs of heart failure or pulmonary edema and side effects of drug therapy.
- Teach the patient about diet restrictions, medications, symptoms that should be reported, and the importance of consistent follow-up care.
- If the patient has surgery, watch for hypotension, arrhythmias, and thrombus formation. Monitor vital signs, arterial blood gases, intake, output, daily weights, blood chemistries, chest X-rays, and pulmonary artery catheter readings.

DEGENERATIVE CARDIOVASCULAR DISORDERS

Hypertension

Hypertension, an intermittent or sustained elevation in diastolic or systolic blood pressure, occurs as two major types: essential (idiopathic) hypertension, the most common, and secondary hypertension, which results from renal disease or another identifiable cause. Malignant hypertension is a severe, fulminant form of hypertension common to both types. Hypertension is a major cause of cerebrovascular accident, cardiac disease, and renal failure. Prognosis is good if this disorder is detected early and treatment begins before complications develop. Severely elevated blood pressure (hypertensive crisis) may be fatal.

Causes and incidence

Hypertension affects 15% to 20% of adults in the United States. If untreated, this disorder carries a high mortality. Risk factors for essential hypertension include family history, race (most common in blacks), stress, obesity, a high dietary intake of saturated fats or sodium, use of tobacco or oral contraceptives, sedentary life-style, and aging.

Secondary hypertension may result from renal vascular disease; pheochromocytoma; primary hyperaldosteronism; Cushing's syndrome; dysfunctions of the thyroid, pituitary, or parathyroid glands; coarctation of the aorta; pregnancy; and neurologic disorders.

Cardiac output and peripheral vascular resistance determine blood pressure. Increased blood volume, increased cardiac rate, increased stroke volume, or arteriolar vasoconstriction that increases peripheral resistance causes blood pressure to rise, but the relationship of these mechanisms to sustained hypertension is unclear. Increased blood pressure may also result from the breakdown or inappropriate response of mechanisms that intrinsically regulate it, as described below:

- Renin-angiotensin system is a neural mechanism that utilizes renin, a renal enzyme, to form angiotensin, a substance that directly produces vasoconstriction or indirectly stimulates the adrenal cortex to produce aldosterone, which, in turn, increases sodium reabsorption. Hypertonic-stimulated release of antidiuretic hormone (ADH) from the pituitary gland follows, in turn increasing water reabsorption, plasma volume, cardiac output, and blood pressure.
- Changes in renal arterial pressure stimulate autoregulation of the blood pressure by the kidneys. A decrease in pressure, for example, causes a decline in glomerular filtration rate and an increased tubular reabsorption of water, which increases blood volume, cardiac output, and finally blood pressure.
- When the blood pressure drops, baroreceptors (pressure receptors) in the aortic arch and carotid sinuses decrease their inhibition of the medulla's vasomotor center, which increases sympathetic stimulation of the heart by norepinephrine. This, in turn, increases cardiac output by strengthening the contractile force, increasing the heart rate, and augmenting peripheral resistance by vasoconstriction. Stress can also stimulate the sympathetic nervous system to increase cardiac output and peripheral vascular resistance.

Signs and symptoms

Hypertension usually does not produce clinical effects until vascular changes in the heart, brain, or kidneys occur. Severely elevated blood pressure damages

HYPERTENSIVE CRISIS

Hypertensive crisis is an acute, life-threatening rise in blood pressure (diastolic usually over 120 mm Hg). It may develop in hypertensive patients after abrupt discontinuation of antihypertensive medication; increased salt consumption; increased production of renin, epinephrine, and norepinephrine; and added stress. This emergency requires immediate and vigorous treatment to lower blood pressure and thereby prevent cerebrovascular accident, left heart failure, and pulmonary edema.

Hypertensive crisis produces severe and widespread symptoms, including headache, drowsiness, mental clouding, vomiting, focal neurologic signs (such as paresthesias), and, if pulmonary edema is present, shortness of breath and hemoptysis. Treatment to rapidly lower blood pressure and thereby prevent hypertensive encephalopathy may include vasodilators, such as I.V. nitroprusside, hydralazine, or diazoxide; a potent diuretic, such as furosemide; and a sympathetic blocker, such as methyldopa, trimethaphan, or phentolamine.

In the early stages of antihypertensive I.V. therapy, monitor blood pressure and heart rate frequently (as often as every 1 to 3 minutes with some drugs) for a precipitous drop, indicating hypersensitivity to the prescribed medications. Maintain blood pressure level, as ordered.

Keep the patient calm; administer a sedative, as ordered. Record intake and output accurately, and, if necessary, explain the reasons for fluid restriction. Watch closely for hypotension, and, until blood pressure is stable at a desirable level, check for signs of heart failure, such as tachycardia, tachypnea, dyspnea, pulmonary rales, S_3 or S_4 gallops, neck vein distention, cyanosis, edema, and oliguria.

the intima of small vessels, resulting in fibrin accumulation in the vessels, development of local edema, and possibly, intravascular clotting. Symptoms produced by this process depend on the location of the damaged vessels:

- brain: cerebrovascular accident
- retina: blindness
- heart: myocardial infarction
- kidneys: proteinuria, edema, and eventually, renal failure.

Hypertension increases the heart's workload, causing left ventricular hypertrophy and, later, left ventricular failure, congestive heart failure, pulmonary edema, and right heart failure.

Diagnosis

Serial blood pressure measurements on a sphygmomanometer of more than 140/90 in persons under age 50 or 150/95 in persons over age 50 confirm hypertension. During physical examination, auscultation may reveal bruits over the abdominal aorta and the carotid, renal, and femoral arteries; ophthalmoscopy reveals arteriovenous nicking and, in hypertensive encephalopathy, papilledema. Patient history and the following additional tests may show predisposing factors and help identify an underlying cause, such as renal disease:

- *Urinalysis:* Protein, RBCs, and WBCs may indicate glomerulonephritis.
- *Intravenous pyelography:* Renal atrophy indicates chronic renal disease; one kidney more than ⅝" (1.5 cm) shorter than the other suggests unilateral renal disease.
- *Serum potassium:* Levels less than 3.5 mEq/liter may indicate adrenal dysfunction (primary hyperaldosteronism).
- *BUN and creatinine:* BUN normal or elevated to more than 20 mg/100 ml and creatinine normal or elevated to more than 1.5 mg/100 ml suggest renal disease.

Other tests help detect cardiovascular damage and other complications:

- *EKG* may show left ventricular hypertrophy or ischemia.
- *Chest X-ray* may show cardiomegaly.

Treatment

Although essential hypertension has no cure, drugs and modifications in diet and life-style can control it. Drug therapy usually begins with a diuretic alone and beta-adrenergic blockers, other sympathetic blockers, or vasodilators added, as needed. Therapy may also include angiotensin converting enzyme and calcium channel blockers. Life-style and dietary changes may include weight loss, relaxation techniques, regular exercise, and restriction of sodium and saturated fat intake.

Treatment of secondary hypertension includes correcting the underlying cause and controlling hypertensive effects.

Special considerations

- To encourage compliance with antihypertensive therapy, suggest that the patient establish a daily routine for taking medication. Warn that uncontrolled hypertension may cause stroke and heart attack. Tell him to report drug side effects. Also, advise him to avoid high sodium antacids and over-the-counter cold and sinus medications, which contain harmful vasoconstrictors.
- Encourage a change in dietary habits. Help the obese patient plan a reducing diet; tell him to avoid high sodium foods (pickles, potato chips, canned soups, cold cuts) and table salt.
- Help the patient examine and modify his life-style (for example, by reducing stress and exercising regularly).

If a patient is hospitalized with hypertension:

- Find out if he was taking prescribed medication. If he wasn't, ask why. If the patient can't afford the medication, refer him to an appropriate social service agency. Tell the patient and family to keep a record of drugs used in the past, noting especially which ones were or were not effective. Suggest recording this information on a card so the patient can show it to his doctor.

When routine blood pressure screening reveals elevated pressure:

- make sure the cuff size is appropriate for the patient's upper arm circumference.
- take the pressure in both arms in lying, sitting, and standing positions.
- ask the patient if he smoked, drank a beverage containing caffeine, or was emotionally upset before the test.
- advise the patient to return for blood pressure testing at frequent and regular intervals.

To help identify hypertension and prevent untreated hypertension:

- participate in public education programs dealing with hypertension and ways to reduce risk factors. Encourage public participation in blood pressure screening programs. Routinely screen all patients, especially those at risk (blacks and persons with family histories of hypertension, stroke, or heart attack).

Coronary Artery Disease

The dominant effect of coronary artery disease is the loss of oxygen and nutrients to myocardial tissue because of diminished coronary blood flow. This disease is near epidemic in the Western world. Coronary artery disease occurs more often in men than in women, in whites, and in the middle-aged and the elderly. In the past, this disorder rarely affected women who were premenopausal, but that is no longer the case, perhaps because many women now take oral contraceptives, smoke cigarettes, and are employed in stressful jobs that used to be held exclusively by men.

Causes

Atherosclerosis is the usual cause of coronary artery disease. In this form of arteriosclerosis, fatty, fibrous plaques narrow the lumen of the coronary arteries, reduce the volume of blood that can

RELIEVING OCCLUSIONS WITH ANGIOPLASTY

For a patient with an occluded coronary artery, percutaneous transluminal coronary angioplasty (PTCA) can open it without opening the chest—an important advantage over bypass surgery. First, coronary angiography must confirm the presence and location of the arterial occlusion. Then, the doctor threads a guide catheter through the patient's femoral artery into the coronary artery under fluoroscopic guidance, as shown below.

When angiography shows the guide catheter positioned at the occlusion site, the doctor carefully inserts a smaller double-lumen balloon catheter through the guide catheter and directs the balloon through the occlusion (lower left). A marked pressure gradient will be obvious.

The doctor alternately inflates and deflates the balloon until an angiogram verifies successful arterial dilation (lower right) and the pressure gradient has decreased.

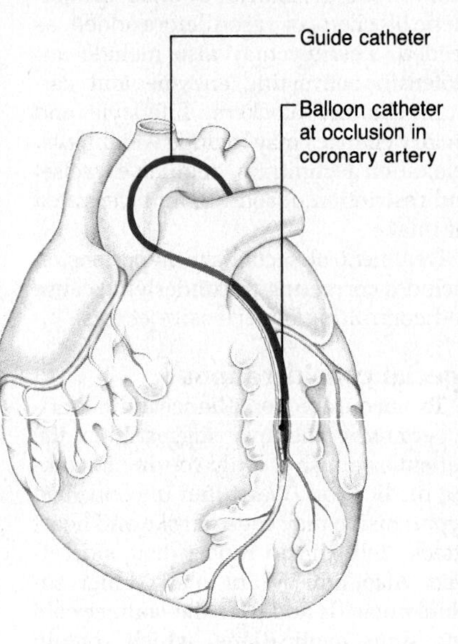

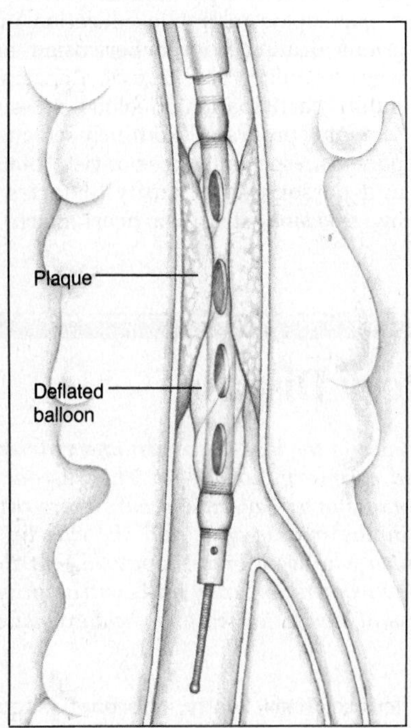

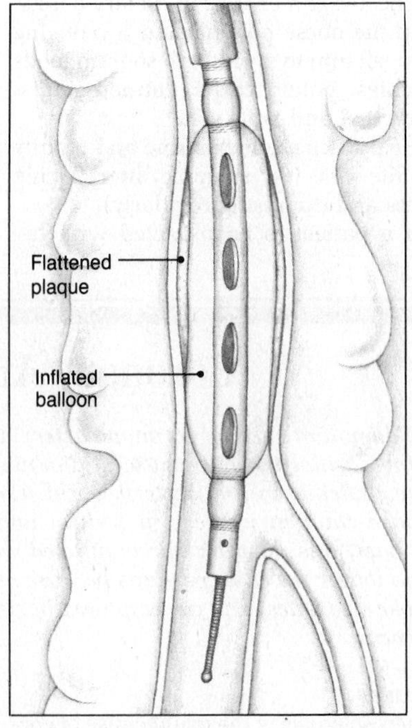

flow through them, and lead to myocardial ischemia. Plaque formation also predisposes to thrombosis, which can provoke myocardial infarction.

Atherosclerosis usually develops in high-flow, high-pressure arteries, such as those in the heart, brain, kidneys, and in the aorta, especially at bifurcation points. It has been linked to many risk factors: family history, hypertension, obesity, smoking, diabetes mellitus, stress, sedentary life-style, and high serum cholesterol and/or triglyceride levels.

Uncommon causes of reduced coronary artery blood flow include dissecting aneurysms, infectious vasculitis, syphilis, and congenital defects in the coronary vascular system. Coronary artery spasms may also impede blood flow.

Signs and symptoms

The classic symptom of coronary artery disease is angina, the direct result of inadequate flow of oxygen to the myocardium. It's usually described as a burning, squeezing, or crushing tightness in the substernal or precordial chest that radiates to the left arm, neck, jaw, or shoulder blade. Typically, the patient clenches his fist over his chest or rubs his left arm when describing the pain, which is often accompanied by nausea, vomiting, fainting, sweating, and cool extremities. Anginal episodes most often follow physical exertion but may also follow emotional excitement, exposure to cold, or a large meal.

Angina has three major forms: *stable* (pain is predictable in frequency and duration and can be relieved with nitrates and rest), *unstable* (pain increases in frequency and duration and is more easily induced), or *decubitus* (anginal pain recurs even at rest). Severe and prolonged anginal pain generally suggests myocardial infarction, with potentially fatal arrhythmias and mechanical failure.

Diagnosis

Patient history—including the frequency and duration of angina and the presence of associated risk factors—is crucial in evaluating coronary artery disease. Additional diagnostic measures include the following:

- *EKG during angina* shows ischemia and, possibly, arrhythmias, such as premature ventricular contraction. EKG is apt to be normal when the patient is painfree. Arrhythmias may occur without infarction, secondary to ischemia.
- *Treadmill or bicycle exercise test* may provoke chest pain and EKG signs of myocardial ischemia in response to physical exertion.
- *Coronary angiography* reveals coronary artery stenosis or obstruction, collateral circulation, and the arteries' condition beyond the narrowing.
- *Myocardial perfusion imaging* with thallium-201 during treadmill exercise detects ischemic areas of the myocardium, visualized as "cold spots."

Treatment

The goal of treatment in patients with angina is to either reduce myocardial oxygen demand or increase oxygen supply. Therapy consists primarily of nitrates, such as nitroglycerin (given sublingually, P.O., transdermally, or topically in ointment form), isosorbide dinitrate (sublingually or P.O.), beta-adrenergic blockers (P.O.), or calcium channel blockers (P.O.). Obstructive lesions may necessitate coronary artery bypass surgery using vein grafts. Angioplasty may be performed during cardiac catheterization to compress fatty deposits and relieve occlusion in patients with no calcification and partial occlusion. (See *Relieving Occlusions with Angioplasty.*) This procedure carries a certain risk, but its morbidity is lower than that for surgery. Laser angioplasty, a newer procedure, corrects occlusion by melting fatty deposits.

Because coronary artery disease is so widespread, prevention is of incalculable importance. Dietary restrictions aimed at reducing intake of calories (in obesity) and of salt, fats, and cholesterol serve to minimize the risk, especially when supplemented with regular exercise. Ab-

CORONARY ARTERY SPASM

In coronary artery spasm, a spontaneous, sustained contraction of one or more coronary arteries causes ischemia and dysfunction of the heart muscle. This disorder also causes Prinzmetal's angina and even myocardial infarction in patients with unoccluded coronary arteries.

The direct cause of coronary artery spasm is unknown, but possible contributing factors include:
- intimal hemorrhage into the medial layer of the blood vessel
- hyperventilation
- elevated catecholamine levels
- fatty buildup in lumen.

The major symptom of coronary artery spasm is angina. But unlike classic angina, this pain commonly occurs spontaneously and may not be related to physical exertion or emotional stress; it's also more severe, usually lasts longer, and may be cyclic, frequently recurring every day at the same time. Such ischemic episodes may cause arrhythmia, altered heart rate, lower blood pressure, and, occasionally, fainting due to diminished cardiac output. Spasm in the left coronary artery may result in mitral valve prolapse, producing a loud systolic murmur and, possibly, pulmonary edema, with dyspnea, crackles, and hemoptysis.

After diagnosis by coronary angiography and EKGs, the patient may receive calcium channel blockers (verapamil, nifedipine, or diltiazem) to reduce coronary artery spasm and to decrease vascular resistance; and nitrates, (nitroglycerin or isosorbide dinitrate) to relieve chest pain.

When caring for a patient with coronary artery spasm, explain all necessary procedures and teach him how to take his medications safely. For calcium antagonist therapy, monitor blood pressure, pulse rate, and EKG patterns to detect arrhythmias. For nifedipine and verapamil therapy, monitor digoxin levels and check for signs of digitalis toxicity. Because nifedipine may cause peripheral and periorbital edema, watch for fluid retention.

Because coronary artery spasm is sometimes associated with atherosclerotic disease, advise the patient to stop smoking, avoid overeating, use alcohol sparingly, and maintain a balance between exercise and rest.

stention from smoking and reduction of stress are also beneficial. Other preventive actions include control of hypertension (with sympathetic blocking agents, such as methyldopa and propranolol, or diuretics, such as hydrochlorothiazide); control of elevated serum cholesterol or triglyceride levels (with antilipemics, such as clofibrate); and measures to minimize platelet aggregation and the danger of blood clots (with aspirin or sulfinpyrazone).

Special considerations

- During anginal episodes, monitor blood pressure and heart rate. Take an EKG during anginal episodes and before administering nitroglycerin or other nitrates. Record duration of pain, amount of medication required to relieve it, and accompanying symptoms.
- Keep nitroglycerin available for immediate use. Instruct the patient to call immediately whenever he feels chest, arm, or neck pain.
- Before cardiac catheterization, explain the procedure to the patient. Make sure he knows why it is necessary, understands the risks, and realizes that it may indicate a need for surgery.
- After catheterization, review the expected course of treatment with the patient and family. Monitor the catheter site for bleeding. Also, check for distal pulses. To counter the diuretic effect of the dye, make sure the patient drinks plenty of fluids. Assess potassium levels.
- If the patient is scheduled for surgery, explain the procedure to the patient and family. Give them a tour of the ICU, and introduce them to the staff.
- After surgery, provide meticulous I.V.,

pulmonary artery catheter, and endotracheal tube care. Monitor blood pressure, intake and output, breath sounds, chest tube drainage, and EKG, watching for signs of ischemia and arrhythmias. Also, observe for and treat chest pain. Give vigorous chest physiotherapy and guide the patient in pulmonary toilet.

• Before discharge, stress the need to follow the prescribed drug regimen (antihypertensives, nitrates, antilipemics, for example), exercise program, and diet. Encourage regular, moderate exercise. Refer the patient to a self-help program to stop smoking.

Myocardial Infarction

(Heart attack)

In myocardial infarction (MI), reduced blood flow through one of the coronary arteries results in myocardial ischemia and necrosis. In cardiovascular disease, the leading cause of death in the United States and Western Europe, death usually results from the cardiac damage or complications of MI. Mortality is high when treatment is delayed, and almost half of sudden deaths due to an MI occur before hospitalization, within 1 hour of the onset of symptoms. Prognosis improves if vigorous treatment begins immediately.

Causes and incidence

Predisposing factors to coronary artery disease and, in turn, MI include:

• positive family history
• hypertension
• smoking
• elevated serum triglyceride and cholesterol levels
• diabetes mellitus
• obesity or excessive intake of saturated fats, carbohydrates, or salt
• sedentary life-style
• aging
• stress or a Type A personality (aggressive, ambitious, competitive attitude, addiction to work, chronic impatience).

Males are more susceptible to MI than females, although incidence is rising among females, especially those who smoke and take oral contraceptives.

The site of the MI depends on the vessels involved. Occlusion of the circumflex branch of the left coronary artery causes a lateral wall infarction; occlusion of the anterior descending branch of the left coronary artery, an anterior wall infarction. True posterior or inferior wall infarctions generally result from occlusion of the right coronary artery or one of its branches. Right ventricular infarctions can also result from right coronary artery occlusion, can accompany inferior infarctions, and may cause right heart failure. In transmural MI, tissue damage extends through all myocardial layers; in subendocardial MI, only in the innermost layer.

Signs and symptoms

The cardinal symptom of MI is persistent, crushing substernal pain that may radiate to the left arm, jaw, neck, or shoulder blades. Such pain is often described as heavy, squeezing, or crushing, and may persist for 12 hours or more. However, in some MI patients—particularly the elderly or diabetics—pain may not occur at all; in others, it may be mild and confused with indigestion. In patients with coronary artery disease, angina of increasing frequency, severity, or duration (especially when not precipitated by exertion, a heavy meal, or cold and wind) may signal an impending infarction.

Other clinical effects include a feeling of impending doom, fatigue, nausea, vomiting, and shortness of breath. The patient may experience catecholamine

COMPLICATIONS OF MYOCARDIAL INFARCTION

COMPLICATION	DIAGNOSIS	TREATMENT
Arrhythmias	• EKG shows premature ventricular contractions, ventricular tachycardia, or ventricular fibrillation; in inferior wall MI, bradycardia and junctional rhythms or AV block; in anterior wall MI, tachycardia or heart block.	• Antiarrhythmics, atropine, cardioversion, and pacemaker
Congestive heart failure	• In left heart failure, chest X-rays show venous congestion and cardiomegaly. • Catheterization shows increased pulmonary artery, pulmonary capillary wedge, and central venous pressure.	• Diuretics, vasodilators, inotropics, and cardiac glycosides
Cardiogenic shock	• Catheterization shows decreased cardiac output, and increased pulmonary artery and pulmonary capillary wedge pressures. • Signs are hypotension, tachycardia, decreased level of consciousness, decreased urinary output, neck vein distention, and cool, pale skin.	• I.V. fluids, vasodilators, cardiotonics, cardiac glycosides, intraaortic ballon pump (IABP), and beta-adrenergic stimulants
Mitral regurgitation	• Auscultation reveals crackles and apical holosystolic murmur. • Catheterization shows increased pulmonary artery and pulmonary capillary wedge pressures. • Dyspnea is prominent. • Echocardiogram shows valve dysfunction.	• Nitroglycerin, nitroprusside, IABP, and surgical replacement of the mitral valve and concomitant myocardial revascularization
Ventricular septal rupture	• In left-to-right shunt, auscultation reveals a harsh holosystolic murmur and thrill. • Catheterization shows increased pulmonary artery and pulmonary capillary wedge pressures. • Confirmation by increased oxygen saturation of right ventricle and pulmonary artery	• Surgical correction (may be postponed several weeks), IABP, nitroglycerin, or nitroprusside
Pericarditis or Dressler's syndrome	• Auscultation reveals a friction rub. • Chest pain is relieved by sitting up.	• Anti-inflammatory agents, such as aspirin or corticosteroids
Ventricular aneurysm	• Chest X-ray may show cardiomegaly. • EKG may show arrhythmias and persistent ST segment elevation. • Left ventriculography shows altered or paradoxical left ventricular motion.	• Cardioversion, antiarrhythmics, vasodilators, anticoagulants, cardiac glycosides, and diuretics. If conservative treatment fails to control complications, surgical resection is necessary.
Thromboembolism	• Severe dyspnea and chest pain or neurologic changes • Nuclear scan shows ventilation/perfusion mismatch. • Angiography shows arterial blockage.	• Oxygen, heparin, and endarterectomy

responses, such as coolness in extremities, perspiration, anxiety, and restlessness. Fever is unusual at the onset of an MI, but a low-grade temperature elevation may develop during the next few days. Blood pressure varies; hypo- or hypertension may be present.

The most common postmyocardial infarction complications include recurrent or persistent chest pain, arrhythmias, left ventricular failure (resulting in congestive heart failure or acute pulmonary edema), and cardiogenic shock. Unusual but potentially lethal complications that may develop soon after infarction include thromboembolism; papillary muscle dysfunction or rupture, causing mitral regurgitation; rupture of ventricular septum, causing ventricular septal defect; rupture of the myocardium; and ventricular aneurysm. Within 2 weeks to several months after infarction, Dressler's syndrome may develop, characterized by pericarditis, pericardial friction rub, chest pain, fever, and possibly, pleurisy or pneumonitis, and leukocytosis.

Diagnosis

A history of coronary artery disease, persistent chest pain, changes in EKG, and elevated serum enzyme (CPK-MB) levels over a 72-hour period usually confirm MI. Auscultation may reveal diminished heart sounds, gallops, and in papillary dysfunction, the apical systolic murmur of mitral regurgitation over the mitral valve area.

When clinical features are equivocal, it's essential to assume MI until special tests rule it out. Diagnostic laboratory results include the following:

- *serial 12-lead EKG:* EKG abnormalities may be absent or inconclusive during the first few hours following an MI. When present, characteristic abnormalities show serial ST-T changes in subendocardial MI and Q waves representing transmural MI.
- *serial serum enzymes:* creatine phosphokinase (CPK) is elevated, especially the CPK-MB isoenzyme, the cardiac muscle fraction of CPK.
- *echocardiography:* this test shows ventricular wall dyskinesia with a transmural MI.

Scans using I.V. technetium 99 can identify acutely damaged muscle by picking up radioactive nucleotide which appears as a "hot spot" on the film. They are useful in localizing a recent MI.

Treatment

The goals of treatment are to relieve chest pain, to stabilize heart rhythm, and to reduce cardiac workload. Arrhythmias, the predominant problem during the first 48 hours after the infarction, may require antiarrhythmics, possibly a pacemaker, and in rare instances, cardioversion.

Therapy includes:

- lidocaine for ventricular arrhythmias or, if lidocaine is ineffective, other drugs, such as procainamide, quinidine, bretylium, or disopyramide.
- atropine I.V. or a temporary pacemaker to treat heart block or bradycardia.
- nitroglycerin (sublingual, topical, transdermal, or I.V.); calcium channel blockers, such as nifedipine, verapamil, and diltiazem (sublingual, P.O., or I.V.); or isosorbide dinitrate (sublingual, P.O., or I.V.) to relieve pain by redistributing blood to ischemic area of myocardium, increasing cardiac output, and reducing myocardial workload.
- morphine or meperidine I.V. for pain and sedation.
- bed rest with bedside commode to decrease cardiac workload.
- oxygen administration (by face mask or nasal cannula) at a modest flow rate for 24 to 48 hours; a lower concentration is necessary if the patient has chronic obstructive pulmonary disease.
- pulmonary artery catheterization to detect left ventricular failure and to monitor response to treatment.
- drugs that increase contractility or blood pressure, or an intraaortic balloon pump for cardiogenic shock.
- thrombolytic therapy up to 6 hours after infarction, using intracoronary or systemic streptokinase (I.V.).

TREATING ACUTE M.I. WITH STREPTOKINASE

In the early stages of acute myocardial infarction (MI), therapy with the thrombolytic drug streptokinase can dissolve the clot in an occluded artery, restoring perfusion and limiting the size of an infarction. Here's how it works:

The doctor threads an arterial catheter through the major blood vessels to the patient's heart, and dye is injected to locate the clot. Then streptokinase infusion begins with a bolus dose of 10,000 to 20,000 units. Infusion may continue for several hours at a dosage ranging from 2,000 to 6,000 units/minute. During this time, angiography assesses the treatment's effectiveness.

Streptokinase works by hastening fibrinolysis. It joins with plasminogen to form a complex that then reacts with additional plasminogen to form plasmin, a proteolytic enzyme that dissolves the clot and relieves the occlusion. (See below.)

Because streptokinase alters the natural clotting mechanisms, it can produce hemorrhage, especially at the site of recent surgery, needle puncture, or trauma. Special considerations after streptokinase therapy include:

- avoiding I.M. or I.V. injections for 24 hours.
- maintaining alignment and immobility of the involved extremity: don't raise the head of the bed more than 15°.
- checking the infusion site for bleeding every 15 minutes for 1 hour, every 30 minutes for the next 2 hours, then once every hour until the catheter is removed.
- documenting pulse, color, temperature, and sensitivity of both extremities when checking the site for bleeding.
- applying direct pressure to the infusion site for at least 30 minutes after catheter removal. Assess the involved extremity distal to the pressure point, and keep the patient on bed rest for at least 6 hours with his leg straight and the head of the bed no higher than 15°.
- watching for signs and symptoms of GI bleeding.

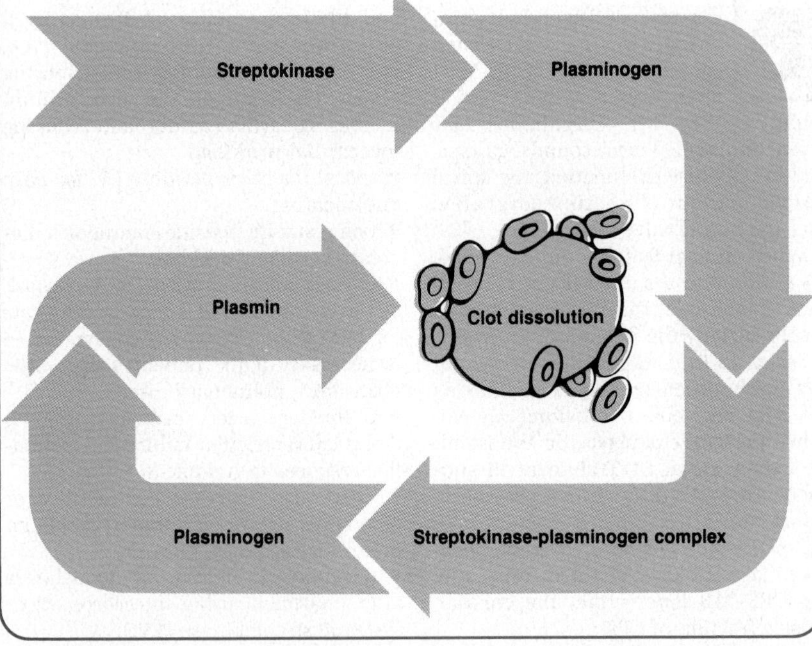

• beta-adrenergic blockers, such as propranolol and timolol, after acute MI to help prevent reinfarction.
• a relatively new inotropic drug, dobutamine, which is used to treat reduced myocardial contractility.

Special considerations

Care for patients who've suffered MI is directed toward detecting complications, preventing further myocardial damage, and promoting comfort, rest, and emotional well-being. Most patients with MI receive treatment in the critical care unit (CCU), under constant observation for complications.

• On admission to the CCU, monitor and record EKG, blood pressure, temperature, and heart and breath sounds.
• Assess pain, and administer analgesics, as ordered. Always record the severity and duration of pain. Avoid giving I.M. injections, since absorption from the muscle is unpredictable.
• Check the patient's blood pressure after giving nitroglycerin, especially the first dose.
• Frequently monitor EKG to detect rate changes or arrhythmias. Place rhythm strips in the patient's chart periodically for evaluation.
• During episodes of chest pain, obtain EKG, blood pressure, and pulmonary artery catheter measurements to determine changes.
• Watch for signs and symptoms of fluid retention (crackles, cough, tachypnea, edema), which may indicate impending heart failure. Carefully monitor daily weight, intake and output, respirations, serum enzymes, and blood pressure. Auscultate for adventitious breath sounds periodically (patients on bed rest frequently have atelectatic crackles, which may disappear after coughing) and for S_3 or S_4 gallops.
• Organize patient care and activities to maximize his periods of uninterrupted rest.
• Ask the dietary department to provide a clear liquid diet until nausea subsides. A low-cholesterol, low-sodium diet, without caffeine-containing beverages, may be ordered.
• Provide a stool softener to prevent straining at stool, which causes vagal stimulation and may slow heart rate. Allow the patient to use a bedside commode, and provide as much privacy as possible.
• Assist with range-of-motion exercises. If the patient is completely immobilized by a severe MI, turn him often. Antiembolism stockings help prevent venostasis and thrombophlebitis.
• Provide emotional support, and help reduce stress and anxiety; administer tranquilizers, as needed. Explain procedures and answer questions. An explanation of the CCU environment and routine can lessen the patient's anxiety. Involve his family as much as possible in his care.

Carefully prepare the MI patient for discharge:

• To promote compliance with prescribed medication regimen and other treatment measures, thoroughly explain dosages and therapy. Warn about drug side effects, and advise the patient to watch for and report signs of toxicity (anorexia, nausea, vomiting, and yellow vision, for example, if the patient is receiving digitalis).
• Review dietary restrictions with the patient. If he must follow a low-sodium or low-fat and low-cholesterol diet, provide a list of undesirable foods. Ask the dietitian to speak to the patient and his family.
• Counsel the patient to resume sexual activity progressively.
• Advise the patient about appropriate responses to new or recurrent symptoms.
• Advise the patient to report typical or atypical chest pain. Postinfarction syndrome may develop, producing chest pain that must be differentiated from recurrent MI, pulmonary infarct, or congestive heart failure.
• If the patient has a Holter monitor in place, explain its purpose and use.
• Stress the need to stop smoking. If necessary, refer the patient to a self-help group.

Congestive Heart Failure

Congestive heart failure (CHF) is a syndrome characterized by myocardial dysfunction that leads to impaired pump performance (diminished cardiac output) or to frank heart failure and abnormal circulatory congestion. Congestion of systemic venous circulation may result in peripheral edema or hepatomegaly; congestion of pulmonary circulation may cause pulmonary edema, an acute life-threatening emergency. Pump failure usually occurs in a damaged left ventricle (left heart failure) but may happen in the right ventricle (right heart failure) primarily, or secondary to left heart failure. Sometimes, left and right heart failures develop simultaneously. Although CHF may be acute (as a direct result of myocardial infarction), it's generally a chronic disorder associated with retention of salt and water by the kidneys. Advances in diagnostic and therapeutic techniques have greatly improved the outlook for patients with CHF, but prognosis still depends on the underlying cause and its response to treatment.

Causes

CHF may result from a primary abnormality of the heart muscle—such as an infarction—inadequate myocardial perfusion due to coronary artery disease, or cardiomyopathy. Other causes include:

- mechanical disturbances in ventricular filling during diastole when there's too little blood for the ventricle to pump, as in mitral stenosis secondary to rheumatic heart disease or constrictive pericarditis and atrial fibrillation.
- systolic hemodynamic disturbances, such as excessive cardiac workload due to volume overloading or pressure overload, that limit the heart's pumping ability. These disturbances can result from mitral or aortic regurgitation, which causes volume overloading, and aortic stenosis or systemic hypertension, which results in increased resistance to ventricular emptying.

Reduced cardiac output triggers three compensatory mechanisms: *ventricular dilation, hypertrophy,* and *increased sympathetic activity.* These mechanisms improve cardiac output at the expense of increased ventricular work. In *cardiac dilation,* an increase in end-diastolic ventricular volume (preload) causes increased stroke work and stroke volume during contraction, stretching cardiac muscle fibers beyond optimum limits and producing pulmonary congestion and pulmonary hypertension, which, in turn, lead to right ventricular failure.

In *ventricular hypertrophy,* an increase in muscle mass or diameter of the left ventricle allows the heart to pump against increased resistance (impedance) to the outflow of blood. An increase in ventricular diastolic pressure necessary to fill the enlarged ventricle may compromise diastolic coronary blood flow, limiting the oxygen supply to the ventricle, causing ischemia and impaired muscle contractility.

Increased sympathetic activity occurs as a response to decreased cardiac output and blood pressure by enhancing peripheral vascular resistance, contractility, heart rate, and venous return. Signs of increased sympathetic activity, such as cool extremities and clamminess, may indicate impending heart failure. Increased sympathetic activity also restricts blood flow to the kidneys, which respond by reducing the glomerular filtration rate and increasing tubular reabsorption of salt and water, in turn expanding the circulating blood volume. This renal mechanism, if unchecked, can aggravate congestion and produce overt edema.

Chronic CHF may worsen as a result of respiratory tract infections, pulmonary embolism, added emotional stress, increased salt or water intake, or failure to comply with prescribed therapy.

Signs and symptoms

Left heart failure produces fatigue and dyspnea (exertional, paroxysmal, nocturnal); right heart failure causes engorgement of veins (when the patient is upright, neck veins may appear distended, feel rigid, and show exaggerated pulsations) and hepatomegaly. Many patients complain of a slight but persistent cold and dry cough combined with wheezing, which may be confused with an allergic reaction.

Later symptoms include tachypnea; palpitations; dependent edema; unexplained, steady weight gain; nausea; chest tightness; slowed mental response; anorexia; hypotension; diaphoresis; narrow pulse pressure; pallor; and oliguria. Auscultation reveals a gallop rhythm (S_3) and crackles on inspiration; the liver may be palpable and slightly tender.

In later stages of congestive heart failure, dullness develops over the lung bases, as well as hemoptysis and cyanosis, marked hepatomegaly, pitting ankle edema, and in bedridden patients, edema over the sacrum.

Complications include pulmonary edema; venostasis, with predisposition to thromboembolism (especially with prolonged bed rest); cerebral insufficiency; and renal insufficiency, with severe electrolyte imbalance.

Diagnosis

- *EKG* reflects heart strain or enlargement, or ischemia. It may also reveal atrial enlargement, tachycardia, and extrasystoles, suggesting CHF.
- *Chest X-ray* shows increased pulmonary vascular markings, interstitial edema, or pleural effusion and cardiomegaly.
- *Pulmonary artery monitoring* demonstrates elevated pulmonary artery and capillary wedge pressures, which reflect left ventricular end-diastolic pressure in left heart failure, and elevated right atrial pressure or central venous pressure in right heart failure.

MANAGING PULMONARY EDEMA

INITIAL STAGE

SYMPTOMS
- Persistent cough
- Slight dyspnea/orthopnea
- Exercise intolerance
- Restlessness and anxiety
- Crackles at lung bases
- Diastolic gallop

SPECIAL CONSIDERATIONS
- Check color and amount of expectoration.
- Position patient for comfort and elevate head of bed.
- Auscultate chest for rales and S_3.
- Medicate, as ordered.
- Monitor apical and radial pulses.
- Assist patient to conserve strength.
- Provide emotional support (through all stages) for patient and family.

ACUTE STAGE

SYMPTOMS
- Acute shortness of breath
- Respirations—rapid, noisy (audible wheeze, crackles)
- Cough—more intense and productive of frothy, blood-tinged sputum
- Cyanosis—cold, clammy skin
- Tachycardia—arrhythmias
- Hypotension

SPECIAL CONSIDERATIONS
- Administer supplemental oxygen, as necessary (preferably by high concentration mask or intermittent positive-pressure breathing [IPPB]).
- Insert I.V., if not already done.
- Aspirate nasopharynx, as needed.
- Apply rotating tourniquets.
- Give nitrates, morphine, and potent diuretics (e.g., furosemide), as ordered.
- Insert indwelling (Foley) catheter.
- Calculate intake and output accurately.
- Draw blood to measure arterial blood gases.
- Attach cardiac monitor leads, and observe EKG.
- Reassure the patient.
- Keep resuscitation equipment available at all times.

ADVANCED STAGE

SYMPTOMS
- Decreased level of consciousness
- Ventricular arrhythmias; shock
- Diminished breath sounds

SPECIAL CONSIDERATIONS
- Be prepared for cardioversion.
- Assist with intubation and mechanical ventilation, and resuscitate, if necessary.

Treatment

The aim of therapy is to improve pump function by reversing the compensatory mechanisms producing the clinical effects. CHF can be controlled quickly by treatment consisting of:

- diuresis to reduce total blood volume and circulatory congestion
- prolonged bed rest
- digitalis to strengthen myocardial contractility
- vasodilators to increase cardiac output by reducing the impedance to ventricular outflow (afterload)
- antiembolism stockings to prevent venostasis and possible thromboembolism formation.

Pulmonary edema requires morphine, as a venodilator, to diminish blood return to the heart; supplemental oxygen; high Fowler's position; and possibly, rotating tourniquets for immediate decongestion by abruptly limiting venous return.

After recovery, the patient usually must continue taking digitalis and diuretics and must remain under medical supervision. If the patient with valve dysfunction has recurrent acute CHF, surgical replacement may be necessary.

Special considerations

During the acute phase of CHF:

- Place the patient in a Fowler's position and give him supplemental oxygen to help him breathe more easily.
- Weigh the patient daily (this is the best index of fluid retention), and check for peripheral edema. Also, carefully monitor I.V. intake and urinary output (especially in the patient receiving diuretics), vital signs (for increased respiratory rate, heart rate, and narrowing pulse pressure), and mental status. Auscultate the heart for abnormal sounds (S_3 gallop) and the lungs for crackles or rhonchi. Report changes immediately.
- Frequently monitor BUN, creatinine, and serum potassium, sodium, chloride, and magnesium levels.
- When using rotating tourniquets, check the patient's radial and pedal pulses often to ensure that the tourniquets aren't applied too tight. At the completion of tourniquet therapy, remove *one* tourniquet at a time to prevent a sudden upsurge in circulating volume.
- To prevent deep vein thrombosis due to vascular congestion, assist the patient with range-of-motion exercises. Enforce bed rest, and apply antiembolism stockings. Watch for calf pain and tenderness.

To prepare the patient for discharge:

- Advise the patient to avoid foods high in sodium, such as canned or commercially prepared foods and dairy products, to curb fluid overload.
- Instruct the patient that the potassium he loses through diuretic therapy must be replaced by taking a prescribed potassium supplement and eating high-potassium foods, such as bananas, apricots, and orange juice.
- Stress the need for regular checkups.
- Stress the importance of taking digitalis exactly as prescribed. Tell the patient to watch for and immediately report signs of toxicity, such as anorexia, vomiting, and yellow vision.
- Tell the patient to notify the doctor if pulse is unusually irregular or less than 60 beats per minute; or if he experiences dizziness, blurred vision, shortness of breath, a persistent dry cough, palpitations, increased fatigue, paroxysmal nocturnal dyspnea, swollen ankles, or decreased urinary output; or if he gains 3 to 5 lb (1.35 to 2.25 kg) in a week.

Dilated Cardiomyopathy

Dilated cardiomyopathy results from extensively damaged myocardial muscle fibers. This disorder interferes with myocardial metabolism and grossly dilates the ventricles without proportional compensatory hypertrophy, causing the heart to take on a globular shape and to contract poorly during systole. Dilated cardiomyopathy leads to intractable congestive heart failure, arrhythmias, and emboli. Since this disease is usually not diagnosed until it's in the advanced stages, prognosis is generally poor.

Causes

The cause of most cardiomyopathies is unknown. Occasionally, dilated cardiomyopathies are not primary myocardial diseases but rather result from myocardial destruction by toxic, infectious, or metabolic agents, such as certain viruses, endocrine and electrolyte disorders, and nutritional deficiencies. Other causes include muscle disorders (myasthenia gravis, progressive muscular dystrophy, myotonic dystrophy), infiltrative disorders (hemochromatosis, amyloidosis), and sarcoidosis.

Cardiomyopathy is a possible complication of alcoholism. In such cases, cardiomyopathy may improve somewhat with abstinence from alcohol but recurs when the patient resumes drinking. How viruses may induce cardiomyopathy is still unclear, but investigation is focused on a possible link between viral myocarditis and subsequent dilated cardiomyopathy, especially after infection with coxsackievirus B, poliovirus, and influenza virus.

Metabolic cardiomyopathies are related to endocrine and electrolyte disorders and nutritional deficiencies. Thus, dilated cardiomyopathy may develop in patients with hyperthyroidism, pheochromocytoma, beriberi (thiamine deficiency), and kwashiorkor (protein deficiency). Cardiomyopathy may also result from rheumatic fever, especially among children with myocarditis.

Ante- or postpartal cardiomyopathy may develop during the last trimester or within months after delivery. Its cause is unknown, but it occurs most frequently in multiparous women over age 30, particularly those with malnutrition or preeclampsia. In these patients, cardiomegaly and congestive heart failure may reverse with treatment, allowing a subsequent normal pregnancy. If cardiomegaly persists despite treatment, prognosis is extremely poor.

Signs and symptoms

In dilated cardiomyopathy, the heart ejects blood less efficiently than normal. Consequently, a large volume of blood remains in the left ventricle after systole, causing signs of congestive heart failure—both left-sided (shortness of breath, orthopnea, dyspnea on exertion, paroxysmal nocturnal dyspnea, fatigue, and an irritating dry cough at night) and right-sided (edema, liver engorgement, and jugular venous distention). Dilated cardiomyopathy also produces peripheral cyanosis, and sinus tachycardia or atrial fibrillation in some patients, secondary to low cardiac output. Auscultation reveals diffuse apical impulses, pansystolic murmur (mitral and tricuspid regurgitation secondary to cardiomegaly and weak papillary muscles), and S_3 and S_4 gallop rhythms.

Diagnosis

No single test confirms dilated cardiomyopathy. Diagnosis requires elimination of other possible causes of congestive heart failure and arrhythmias.

- *EKG* and *angiography* rule out ischemic heart disease; the EKG may also show biventricular hypertrophy, sinus tachycardia, atrial enlargement, and in 20% of patients, atrial fibrillation.
- *Chest X-ray* demonstrates cardiomegaly—usually affecting all heart chambers—pulmonary congestion, or pleural effusion.

Treatment

In dilated cardiomyopathy, the goal of treatment is to correct the underlying causes and to improve the heart's pumping ability with digitalis, diuretics, oxygen, and a restricted-sodium diet. Therapy may also include prolonged bed rest, selective use of steroids, and, possibly, pericardiotomy, which is still investigational. Vasodilators reduce preload and afterload, thereby decreasing conges-

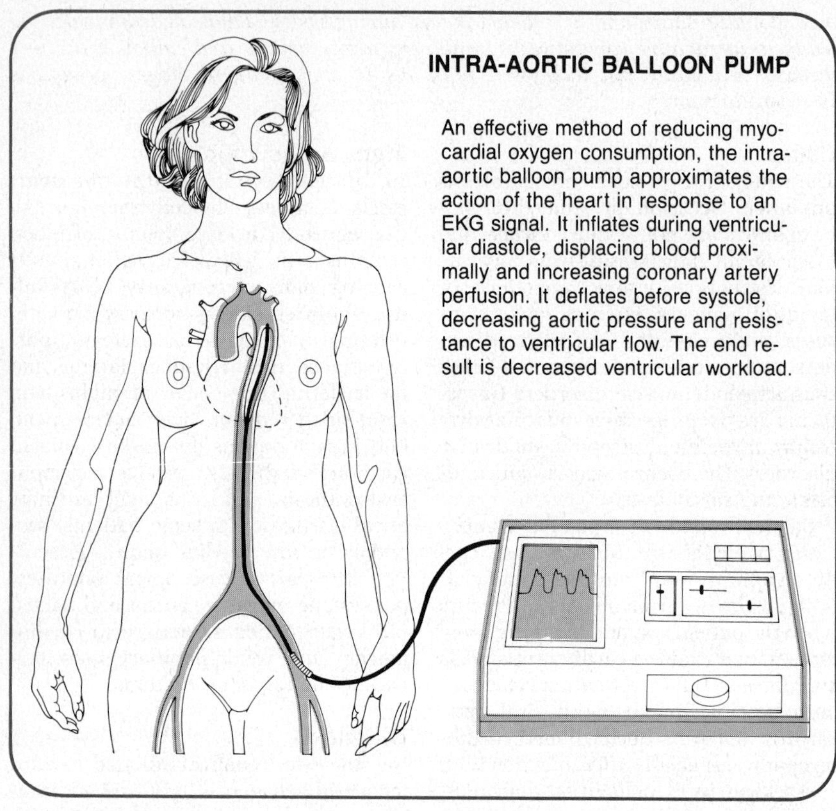

INTRA-AORTIC BALLOON PUMP

An effective method of reducing myocardial oxygen consumption, the intra-aortic balloon pump approximates the action of the heart in response to an EKG signal. It inflates during ventricular diastole, displacing blood proximally and increasing coronary artery perfusion. It deflates before systole, decreasing aortic pressure and resistance to ventricular flow. The end result is decreased ventricular workload.

tion and increasing cardiac output. Acute heart failure necessitates vasodilation with nitroprusside I.V. or nitroglycerin I.V. Long-term treatment may include prazosin, hydralazine, isosorbide dinitrate, and, if the patient is on prolonged bed rest, anticoagulants.

When these treatments fail, therapy may require a heart transplant for carefully selected patients.

Special considerations

In the patient with acute failure:

- Monitor for signs of progressive failure (decreased arterial pulses, increased neck vein distention) and compromised renal perfusion (oliguria, increased BUN and creatinine, and electrolyte imbalances). Weigh the patient daily.
- If the patient is receiving vasodilators, check blood pressure and heart rate frequently. If he becomes hypotensive, stop the infusion and place him supine, with legs elevated to increase venous return and to ensure cerebral blood flow.
- If the patient is receiving diuretics, monitor for signs of resolving congestion (decreased crackles and dyspnea) or too vigorous diuresis. Check serum potassium for hypokalemia, especially if therapy includes digitalis.
- Therapeutic restrictions and uncertain prognosis usually cause profound anxiety and depression, so offer support and let the patient express his feelings. Be flexible with visiting hours. If hospitalization is prolonged, try to obtain permission for the patient to spend occasional weekends away from the hospital.
- Before discharge, teach the patient about his illness and its treatment. Also, emphasize the need to restrict sodium intake, to watch for weight gain, and to

take digitalis as prescribed and watch for its toxic effects (anorexia, nausea, vomiting, yellow vision).

• Encourage family members to learn cardiopulmonary resuscitation since sudden cardiac arrest is possible.

Idiopathic Hypertrophic Subaortic Stenosis

This primary disease of cardiac muscle is characterized by disproportionate, asymmetric thickening of the interventricular septum, particularly in the anterior-superior part. In idiopathic hypertrophic subaortic stenosis (IHSS), cardiac output may be low, normal, or high, depending on whether stenosis is obstructive or nonobstructive. If cardiac output is normal or high, IHSS may go undetected for years; but low cardiac output may lead to potentially fatal congestive heart failure. The course of IHSS varies; some patients demonstrate progressive deterioration, while others remain stable for several years.

Causes

Despite being designated as idiopathic, in almost all cases, IHSS is inherited as a non–sex-linked autosomal dominant trait. Most patients with IHSS have obstructive disease, resulting from the combined effects of ventricular septal hypertrophy and the movement of the anterior mitral valve leaflet into the outflow tract during systole. Eventually, left ventricular dysfunction, due to rigidity and decreased compliance, causes pump failure.

Signs and symptoms

Generally, clinical features of IHSS don't appear until the disease is well advanced, when atrial dilation and, possibly, atrial fibrillation abruptly reduce blood flow to the left ventricle. Reduced inflow and subsequent low output may produce angina pectoris, arrhythmias, dyspnea, syncope, congestive heart failure, and sudden death. Auscultation reveals a medium-pitched systolic ejection murmur along the left sternal border and at the apex; palpation reveals a peripheral pulse with a characteristic double impulse (pulsus biferiens) and, with atrial fibrillation, an irregular pulse.

Diagnosis

Diagnosis of IHSS depends on typical clinical findings and the test results:

• *Echocardiography* (most useful) shows increased thickness of the interventricular septum and abnormal motion of the anterior mitral leaflet during systole, occluding left ventricular outflow in obstructive IHSS.

• *Cardiac catheterization* reveals elevated left ventricular end-diastolic pressure and, possibly, mitral insufficiency.

• *EKG* usually demonstrates left ventricular hypertrophy, ST segment and T wave abnormalities, deep waves (due to hypertrophy, not infarction), left anterior hemiblock, ventricular arrythmias, and, possibly, atrial fibrillation.

• *Phonocardiography* confirms an early systolic murmur.

Treatment

The goals of treatment of IHSS are to relax the ventricle and to relieve outflow tract obstruction. Propranolol, a beta-adrenergic blocking agent, slows heart rate and increases ventricular filling by relaxing the obstructing muscle, thereby reducing angina, syncope, dyspnea, and arrhythmias. However, propranolol may aggravate symptoms of cardiac decompensation. Atrial fibrillation necessitates cardioversion to treat the arrhythmia and, because of the high risk of systemic embolism, anticoagulant therapy until fibrillation subsides. Since vasodilators, such as nitroglycerin, reduce venous return by permitting pooling of blood in the periphery, decreasing ventricular volume and chamber size, and may cause further obstruction, they're contraindicated in patients with IHSS. Also contraindicated are sympathetic stimulators, such as isoproterenol, which enhance cardiac contractility and myocardial demands for oxygen, intensifying the obstruction.

If drug therapy fails, surgery is indicated. Ventricular myotomy (resection of the hypertrophied septum) alone or combined with mitral valve replacement may ease outflow tract obstruction and relieve symptoms. However, ventricular myotomy may cause complications, such as complete heart block and ventricular septal defect, and is experimental.

Special considerations

- Because syncope or sudden death may follow well-tolerated exercise, warn such patients against strenuous physical activity, such as running.
- Administer medication, as ordered. Caution: Avoid nitroglycerin, digitalis, or diuretics; they can worsen obstruction. Warn the patient not to stop taking propranolol abruptly, since doing so may cause rebound effects, resulting in myocardial infarction or sudden death. To determine the patient's tolerance for increased dosage of propranolol, take his pulse to check for bradycardia, and have him stand and walk around slowly, to check for orthostatic hypotension.
- Before dental work or surgery, administer prophylaxis for subacute bacterial endocarditis.
- Provide psychologic support. If the patient is hospitalized for a long time, be flexible with visiting hours, and encourage occasional weekends away from the hospital, if possible. Refer the patient for psychosocial counseling to help him and his family accept his restricted lifestyle and poor prognosis.
- If the patient is a child, have his parents arrange for him to continue his studies in the hospital.
- Since sudden cardiac arrest is possible, urge the patient's family to learn cardiopulmonary resuscitation.

Restrictive Cardiomyopathy

Restrictive cardiomyopathy, a disorder of the myocardial musculature, is characterized by restricted ventricular filling (the result of left ventricular hypertrophy) and endocardial fibrosis and thickening. If severe, it is irreversible.

Causes

An extremely rare disorder, primary restrictive cardiomyopathy is of unknown etiology. However, restrictive cardiomyopathy syndrome, a manifestation of amyloidosis, results from infiltration of amyloid into the intracellular spaces in the myocardium, endocardium, and subendocardium.

In both forms of restrictive cardiomyopathy, the myocardium becomes rigid, with poor distention during diastole, inhibiting complete ventricular filling, and fails to contract completely during systole, resulting in low cardiac output.

Signs and symptoms

Because it lowers cardiac output and leads to congestive heart failure, restrictive cardiomyopathy produces fatigue, dyspnea, orthopnea, chest pain, generalized edema, liver engorgement, peripheral cyanosis, pallor, and S_3 and/or S_4 gallop rhythms.

Diagnosis

- In advanced stages of this disease, *chest X-ray* shows massive cardiomegaly, affecting all four chambers of the heart.
- *Echocardiography* rules out constric-

tive pericarditis as the cause of restricted filling by detecting increased left ventricular muscle mass and differences in end-diastolic pressures between the ventricles.
• *EKG* may show low-voltage complexes, hypertrophy, or atrioventricular conduction defects.
• *Arterial pulsation* reveals blunt carotid upstroke with small volume.
• *Cardiac catheterization* demonstrates increased left ventricular end-diastolic pressure and rules out constrictive pericarditis as the cause of restricted filling.

Treatment

Although no therapy currently exists for restricted ventricular filling, digitalis, diuretics, and a restricted sodium diet are beneficial by easing the symptoms of congestive heart failure.

Oral vasodilators—such as isosorbide dinitrate, prazosin, and hydralazine—may control intractable congestive heart failure. Anticoagulant therapy may be necessary to prevent thrombophlebitis in the patient on prolonged bed rest.

Special considerations

• In the acute phase, monitor heart rate and rhythm, blood pressure, urinary output, and pulmonary artery pressure readings to help guide treatment.
• Give psychological support. Provide appropriate diversionary activities for the patient restricted to prolonged bed rest. Since a poor prognosis may cause profound anxiety and depression, be especially supportive and understanding, and encourage the patient to express his fears. Refer him for psychosocial counseling, as necessary, for assistance in coping with his restricted life-style. Be flexible with visiting hours whenever possible.
• Before discharge, teach the patient to watch for and report signs of digoxin toxicity (anorexia, nausea, vomiting, yellow vision); to record and report weight gain; and if sodium restriction is ordered, to avoid canned foods, pickles, smoked meats, and excessive use of table salt.

CARDIAC COMPLICATIONS

Hypovolemic Shock

(Hypovolemic shock syndrome)

In hypovolemic shock, reduced intravascular blood volume causes circulatory dysfunction and inadequate tissue perfusion. Without sufficient blood or fluid replacement, hypovolemic shock syndrome may lead to irreversible cerebral and renal damage, cardiac arrest, and, ultimately, death. Hypovolemic shock syndrome necessitates early recognition of signs and symptoms and prompt, aggressive treatment to improve prognosis.

Causes

Hypovolemic shock usually results from acute blood loss—about one fifth of total volume. Such massive blood loss may result from gastrointestinal bleeding, internal hemorrhage (hemothorax, hemoperitoneum), or external hemorrhage (accidental or surgical trauma) or from any condition that reduces circulating intravascular plasma volume or other body fluids, such as in severe burns. Other underlying causes of hypovolemic shock include intestinal obstruction, peritonitis, acute pancreatitis, ascites and dehydration from excessive perspiration, severe diarrhea or protracted vomiting, diabetes insipidus, diuresis, or inadequate fluid intake.

DO'S AND DON'TS FOR USING MAST EFFECTIVELY

MAST (Medical Anti-shock Trousers) counteracts bleeding and hypovolemia by slowing or stopping arterial bleeding; by forcing any available blood from the lower body to the heart, brain, and other vital organs; and by preventing return of the available circulating blood volume to the lower extremities.

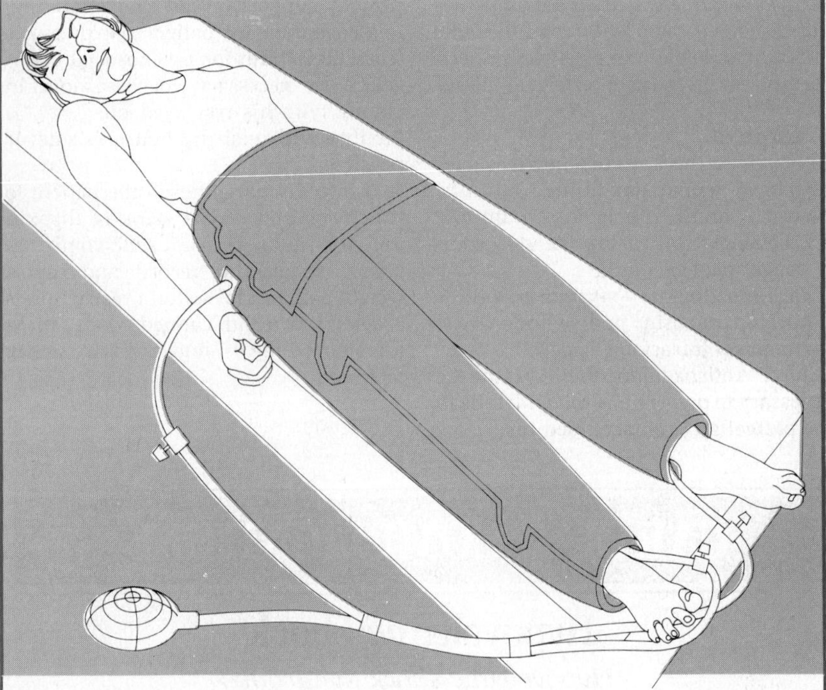

DO'S

- While patient is wearing MAST, monitor blood pressure, apical and radial pulse rates, and respirations; check extremities for pedal pulses, color, warmth, and numbness; and make sure MAST is not too constricting.
- Take MAST off only when a doctor is present, fluids are available for transfusion, and anesthesia and surgical teams are available.
- To clean, wash with warm soap and water, air dry and store.

DON'TS

- Don't apply MAST if positions or wounds show or suggest major intrathoracic or intracranial vascular injury; or if patient has open extremity bleeding, pulmonary edema, or trauma above the level of MAST application.
- When cleaning, don't autoclave or clean with solvents.

Signs and symptoms

Hypovolemic shock produces a syndrome of hypotension, with narrowing pulse pressure; decreased sensorium; tachycardia; rapid, shallow respirations; reduced urinary output (less than 25 ml/hour); and cold, pale, clammy skin. Metabolic acidosis with an accumulation of lactic acid develops as a result of tissue anoxia, as cellular metabolism shifts from aerobic to anaerobic pathways. Disseminated intravascular coagulation (DIC) is a possible complication of hypovolemic shock.

Diagnosis

No single symptom or diagnostic test establishes the diagnosis or severity of shock. Laboratory findings include:

- elevated potassium, serum lactate, and BUN levels.
- increased urine specific gravity (more than 1.020) and urine osmolality.
- decreased blood pH and PO_2, and increased PCO_2.

In addition, gastroscopy, aspiration of gastric contents through a nasogastric tube, and X-rays identify internal bleeding sites; coagulation studies may detect coagulopathy from DIC.

Treatment

Emergency treatment measures consist of prompt, adequate blood and fluid replacement to restore intravascular volume and raise blood pressure. Saline solution, then possibly plasma proteins (albumin), other plasma expanders, or lactated Ringer's solution, may produce volume expansion until whole blood can be matched. Application of Medical Anti-shock Trousers (MAST) may be helpful. Treatment may also include oxygen administration, identification of bleeding site, control of bleeding by direct measures (such as pressure and elevation of an extremity), and possibly, surgery.

Special considerations

Management of hypovolemic shock necessitates prompt, aggressive supportive measures, and careful assessment and monitoring of vital signs. Follow these priorities:

- Check for a patent airway and adequate circulation. If blood pressure and heart rate are absent, start cardiopulmonary resuscitation.
- Place the patient flat in bed, with his legs elevated about 30° to increase blood flow by promoting venous return to the heart.

PATHOPHYSIOLOGY OF HYPOVOLEMIC SHOCK

Normally, the body compensates for a loss of blood or fluid by constricting arteriolar beds, increasing heart rate and contractile force, and redistributing fluids. These compensation mechanisms are effective enough to maintain stable vital signs, even after a 10% blood loss. But by the time blood or fluid loss reaches 15% to 25%, these mechanisms fail to maintain cardiac output, and blood pressure drops.

Baroreceptors (pressure-sensitive stretch receptors) in the aorta and carotid bodies trigger sympathetic nerve fibers. As a result, the adrenals release norepinephrine and epinephrine, causing vasoconstriction, which sharply reduces the blood flow to peripheral muscle and some of the vital organs (kidneys, liver, and lungs). Some cells, therefore, no longer receive oxygen, and cellular metabolism shifts from aerobic to anaerobic pathways, producing an accumulation of lactic acid, which is not metabolized to yield needed energy. Impaired renal or hepatic function causes this acid to accumulate and results in metabolic acidosis.

To compensate for metabolic acidosis, the patient hyperventilates to exhale more CO_2 and, in doing so, induces respiratory alkalosis. Since he may be unable to maintain the physical exertion required for hyperventilation, he may eventually need respiratory support, either oxygen by mask or mechanical ventilation.

Eventually, the compensatory mechanisms that serve to maintain acid-base balance fail, and cellular function is severely impaired, leading to cell death and subsequent organ failure.

INVASIVE MONITORING IN HYPOVOLEMIC SHOCK

KIND OF MONITORING	TEST RESULTS	SIGNIFICANCE
Intraarterial pressure monitoring (for systemic arterial pressure)	• Hypotension (< 90 mmHg auscultatory systolic blood pressure) • Central blood pressure may be 10 to 20 mmHg higher than brachial reading.	• Impaired ventricular ejection or alterations in vascular compliance or resistance
Central venous pressure ([CVP]—a fair guide for I.V. fluid monitoring because of trend [increase or decrease] to fluid loading)	• Decreased central venous pressure (< 8 cm H_2O) • Reading may not reflect an accurate right ventricular filling pressure and does not reflect left heart function.	• Inadequate intravascular volume to produce a right ventricular filling pressure necessary for ventricular ejection
Pulmonary artery pressure The flow-directed, balloon-tipped, pulmonary artery thermodilution catheter is a quadruple-lumen catheter used to measure cardiac output, as well as right atrial, pulmonary artery, or pulmonary capillary wedge pressure (a reliable indicator of left heart function and fluid overload).	• Decreased right atrial, pulmonary artery, and pulmonary capillary wedge pressures (PCWP < 12 mmHg) • Reading reflects an accurate mean left atrial pressure. • Decreased cardiac output (with thermodilution catheter)	• Inadequate intravascular volume to produce a left ventricular filling pressure necessary for ventricular ejection

• Record blood pressure, pulse rate, peripheral pulses, and respirations, and other vital signs every 15 minutes, and EKG continuously. Systolic blood pressure less than 80 mmHg usually results in inadequate coronary artery blood flow, cardiac ischemia, arrhythmias, and further complications of low cardiac output. When blood pressure drops below 80 mmHg, increase the oxygen flow rate, and notify the doctor immediately. A progressive drop in blood pressure, accompanied by a thready pulse, generally signals inadequate cardiac output from reduced intravascular volume. Notify the doctor, and increase the infusion rate.

• Start I.V.s with normal saline or lactated Ringer's solution, using a large-bore catheter (14G), which allows easier administration of later blood transfusions. (*Caution:* Don't start I.V.s in the legs of a patient in shock who has suffered abdominal trauma, since infused fluid may escape through the ruptured vessel into the abdomen.)

• A Foley catheter may be inserted to measure hourly urinary output. If output is less than 30 ml/hour in adults, increase the fluid infusion rate, but watch for signs of fluid overload, such as an increase in pulmonary capillary wedge pressure (PCWP). Notify the doctor if urinary output does not improve. An osmotic diuretic, such as mannitol, may be ordered to increase renal blood flow and urinary output. Determine how much fluid to give by checking blood pressure, urinary output, central venous pressure (CVP), or PCWP. (To increase accuracy, CVP should be measured at the level of the right atrium, using the same reference point on the chest each time.)

• Draw an arterial blood sample to measure blood gas levels. Administer oxygen by face mask or airway to ensure adequate oxygenation of tissues. Adjust the oxygen flow rate to a higher or lower level, as blood gas measurements indicate.

- Draw venous blood for CBC, electrolytes, type and cross match, and coagulation studies.
- During therapy, assess skin color and temperature, and note any changes. Cold, clammy skin may be a sign of continuing peripheral vascular constriction, indicating progressive shock.
- Watch for signs of impending coagulopathy (petechiae, bruising, bleeding or oozing from gums or venipuncture sites).
- Explain all procedures and their purpose. Throughout these emergency measures, provide emotional support to the patient and family.

Cardiogenic Shock

Sometimes called pump failure, cardiogenic shock is a condition of diminished cardiac output that severely impairs tissue perfusion. It reflects severe left ventricular failure, and occurs as a serious complication in nearly 15% of all patients hospitalized with acute myocardial infarction. Cardiogenic shock typically affects patients whose area of infarction exceeds 40% of muscle mass; in such patients, the fatality rate may exceed 85%. Most patients with cardiogenic shock die within 24 hours of onset. Prognosis for those who survive is extremely poor.

Causes

Cardiogenic shock can result from any condition that causes significant left ventricular dysfunction with reduced cardiac output, such as myocardial infarction (most common), myocardial ischemia, papillary muscle dysfunction, or end-stage cardiomyopathy. Regardless of the underlying cause, left ventricular dysfunction sets into motion a series of compensatory mechanisms that attempt to increase cardiac output and, in turn, maintain vital organ function.

As cardiac output falls in left ventricular dysfunction, aortic and carotid baroreceptors initiate sympathetic nervous responses, which increase heart rate, left ventricular filling pressure, and peripheral resistance to flow, to enhance venous return to the heart. These compensatory responses initially stabilize the patient but later cause deterioration with rising oxygen demands of the already compromised myocardium. These events comprise a vicious circle of low cardiac output, sympathetic compensation, myocardial ischemia, and even lower cardiac output.

Signs and symptoms

Cardiogenic shock produces signs of poor tissue perfusion: cold, pale, clammy skin; a drop in systolic blood pressure to 30 mmHg below baseline, or a sustained reading below 80 mmHg not attributable to medication; tachycardia; rapid, shallow respirations; oliguria (less than 20 ml urine/hour); restlessness, and mental confusion and obtundation; narrowing pulse pressure; and cyanosis. Although many of these clinical features also occur in congestive heart failure and other shock syndromes, they are usually more profound in cardiogenic shock.

Diagnosis

Auscultation detects gallop rhythm, faint heart sounds, and possibly, if the shock results from rupture of the ventricular septum or papillary muscles, a holosystolic murmur. Other abnormal clinical findings include:

- *pulmonary artery pressure monitoring:* increased pulmonary artery pressure (PAP), and increased pulmonary capillary wedge pressure (PCWP), reflecting a rise in left ventricular end-diastolic pressure (preload) and increased resistance to left ventricular emptying (afterload) due to ineffective pumping and increased peripheral vascular resistance. Thermodilution technique measures decreased cardiac index (less than 2.2 liters/minute).

- *invasive arterial pressure monitoring:* hypotension due to impaired ventricular ejection
- *arterial blood gases:* may show metabolic acidosis and hypoxia
- *EKG:* possible evidence of acute myocardial infarction, ischemia, or ventricular aneurysm
- *enzyme levels:* elevated creatine phosphokinase (CPK), lactic dehydrogenase (LDH), SGOT, and SGPT, which point to myocardial infarction or ischemia and suggest congestive heart failure or shock. CPK and LDH isoenzymes determinations may confirm acute myocardial infarction.

Additional tests determine other conditions that can lead to pump dysfunction and failure, such as cardiac dysrhythmias, cardiac tamponade, papillary muscle infarct or rupture, ventricular septal rupture, pulmonary emboli, venous pooling (associated with venodilators and continuous intermittent positive-pressure breathing), and hypovolemia.

Treatment

The aim of treatment is to enhance cardiovascular status by increasing cardiac output, improving myocardial perfusion, and decreasing cardiac workload with combinations of various cardiovascular drugs and mechanical-assist techniques. Drug therapy may include dopamine I.V., a vasopressor that increases cardiac output, blood pressure, and renal blood flow; norepinephrine, when a more potent vasoconstrictor is necessary; and nitroprusside I.V., a vasodilator that may be used with a vasopressor to further improve cardiac output by decreasing peripheral vascular resistance (afterload) and reducing left ventricular end-diastolic pressure (preload). However, the patient's blood pressure must be adequate to support nitroprusside therapy and must be monitored closely.

The intraaortic balloon pump (IABP) is a mechanical-assist device that attempts to improve coronary artery perfusion and decrease cardiac workload. The inflatable balloon pump is surgically inserted through the femoral artery into the descending thoracic aorta. The balloon inflates during diastole to increase coronary artery perfusion pressure and deflates before systole (before the aortic valve opens) to reduce resistance to ejection (afterload) and therefore lessen cardiac workload. Improved ventricular ejection, which significantly improves cardiac output, and a subsequent vasodilation in the peripheral vasculature lead to lower preload volume.

When drug therapy and IABP insertion fail, treatment may require an experimental device—the ventricular assist pump or the artificial heart.

Special considerations

- At the first sign of cardiogenic shock, check the patient's blood pressure and heart rate. If the patient is hypotensive or is having difficulty breathing, make sure he has a patent I.V. line and a patent airway, and provide oxygen to promote tissue oxygenation. Notify the doctor immediately.
- Monitor arterial blood gases to measure oxygenation and detect acidosis from poor tissue perfusion. Increase oxygen flow as indicated by blood gas measurements. Check CBC and electrolytes.
- After diagnosis, monitor cardiac rhythm continuously. Assess skin color, temperature, and other vital signs often. Watch for a drop in systolic blood pressure to less than 80 mm Hg (usually compromising cardiac output further). Report hypotension immediately.
- A Foley catheter may be inserted to measure urinary output. Notify the doctor if output drops below 30 ml/hour.
- Using a pulmonary artery catheter, closely monitor PAP, PCWP, and if equipment is available, cardiac output. A high PCWP indicates congestive heart

NEW WAYS TO TREAT CARDIOGENIC SHOCK

Two experimental devices—the ventricular assist pump and the artificial heart—may help patients with cardiogenic shock who don't respond to drug therapy or IABP insertion.

Some centers use Pierce ventricular assist pumps (top) to maintain circulation in those who can't be weaned from cardiopulmonary bypass after open heart surgery. These sac-type pumps are fitted with tilting disk valves and powered pneumatically by periodic compression of the flexible sac. Each atrial appendage has a cannula that drains blood from the atria to the pumps. One pump propels the blood into the pulmonary artery; the other propels it into the aorta.

If a donor heart isn't available for transplantation in a patient with irreparable heart damage, he may receive an artificial heart, such as the Jarvik heart, shown at bottom. This device has two mechanical ventricles that are attached to the patient's aorta, pulmonary artery, and atria. Compressed air powers the heart, stimulating the internal diaphragms and valves to pump blood. After implantation, the artificial heart must work for the rest of the patient's life without malfunctioning or causing blood clots.

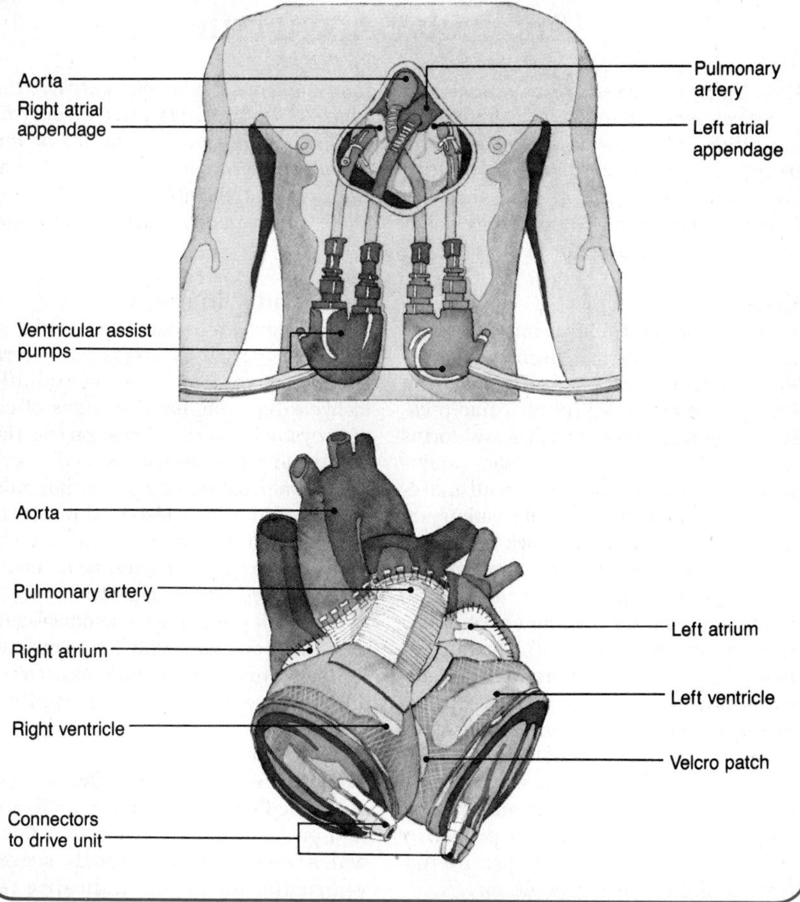

failure and should be reported immediately.

- When a patient is on the IABP, reposition him often and perform passive range-of-motion exercises to prevent skin breakdown. However, don't flex the patient's "ballooned" leg at the hip, since this may displace or fracture the catheter. Assess pedal pulses, and skin temperature and color to make sure circulation to the leg is adequate. Check the dressing on the insertion site frequently for bleeding, and change it according to hospital protocol. Also, check the site for hematoma or signs of infection, and culture any drainage.
- After the patient has become hemodynamically stable, the frequency of balloon inflation is gradually reduced to wean him from the IABP. During weaning, carefully watch for monitor changes, chest pain, and other signs of recurring cardiac ischemia and shock.
- Provide psychologic support. Since the patient and family may be anxious about the ICU, IABP, and other tubes and devices, offer reassurance. To ease emotional stress, plan your care to allow frequent rest periods, and provide for as much privacy as possible.

Ventricular Aneurysm

Ventricular aneurysm is an outpouching, almost always of the left ventricle, that produces ventricular wall dysfunction in about 20% of patients after myocardial infarction (MI). Ventricular aneurysm may develop within weeks after MI or may be delayed for years. Untreated ventricular aneurysm can lead to arrhythmias, systemic embolization, or congestive heart failure, and is potentially fatal. Resection improves prognosis in congestive heart failure or refractory patients who have developed ventricular arrhythmias.

Causes

When MI destroys a large muscular section of the left ventricle, necrosis reduces the ventricular wall to a thin sheath of fibrous tissue. Under intracardiac pressure, this thin layer stretches and forms a separate noncontractile sac (aneurysm). Abnormal muscular wall movement accompanies ventricular aneurysm and includes akinesia (lack of movement), dyskinesia (paradoxical movement), asynergia (decreased and inadequate movement), and asynchrony (uncoordinated movement). During systolic ejection, the abnormal muscular wall movements associated with the aneurysm cause the remaining normally functioning myocardial fibers to increase the force of contraction in order to maintain stroke volume and cardiac output. At the same time, a portion of the stroke volume is lost to passive distention of the noncontractile sac.

Signs and symptoms

Ventricular aneurysm may cause arrhythmias—such as premature ventricular contractions or ventricular tachycardia—palpitations, signs of cardiac dysfunction (weakness on exertion, fatigue, angina), and occasionally, a visible or palpable systolic precordial bulge. This condition may also lead to left ventricular dysfunction, with chronic congestive heart failure (dyspnea, fatigue, edema, rales, gallop rhythm, neck vein distention); pulmonary edema; systemic embolization; and with left ventricular failure, pulsus alternans. Ventricular aneurysms enlarge but rarely rupture.

Diagnosis

Persistent ventricular arrhythmias, onset of heart failure, or systemic embolization in a patient with left ventricular failure and a history of MI strongly suggests ventricular aneurysm. Indicative tests include the following:

• *Left ventriculography* reveals left ventricular enlargement, with an area of akinesia or dyskinesia (during cineangiography) and diminished cardiac function.
• *EKG* may show persistent ST-T wave elevations 2 weeks after infarction.
• *Chest X-ray* may demonstrate an abnormal bulge distorting the heart's contour if the aneurysm is large; the X-ray may be normal if the aneurysm is small.
• *Noninvasive nuclear cardiology scan* may indicate the site of infarction and suggest the area of aneurysm.
• *Echocardiography* shows abnormal motion in the left ventricular wall.

Treatment

Depending on the size of the aneurysm and the complications, treatment may necessitate only routine medical examination to follow the patient's condition or aggressive measures for intractable ventricular arrhythmias, congestive heart failure, and emboli.

Emergency treatment of ventricular arrhythmia includes antiarrhythmics I.V. or cardioversion. Preventive treatment continues with oral antiarrhythmics, such as procainamide, quinidine, or disopyramide.

Emergency treatment for congestive heart failure with pulmonary edema includes oxygen, digitalis I.V., furosemide I.V., morphine sulfate I.V., and, when necessary, nitroprusside I.V. and intubation. Maintenance therapy may include nitrates, prazosin, and hydralazine P.O. Systemic embolization requires anticoagulation therapy or embolectomy. Refractory ventricular tachycardia, heart failure, recurrent arterial embolization, and persistent angina with coronary artery occlusion may necessitate surgery, of which the most effective procedure is aneurysmectomy with myocardial revascularization.

Special considerations

• If ventricular tachycardia occurs, monitor blood pressure and heart rate. If cardiac arrest develops, initiate cardiopulmonary resuscitation (CPR) and call for assistance, resuscitative equipment, and medication.
• In a patient with congestive heart failure, closely monitor vital signs, heart sounds, intake and output, fluid and electrolyte balances, and BUN and creatinine levels. Because of the threat of systemic embolization, frequently check peripheral pulses and the color and temperature of extremities. Be alert for sudden changes in sensorium that indicate cerebral embolization and for any signs that suggest renal failure or progressive myocardial infarction.
• If arrhythmias necessitate cardioversion, use a sufficient amount of conducting jelly to prevent chest burns. If the patient is conscious, give diazepam I.V., as ordered, before cardioversion. Explain that cardioversion is a lifesaving method using brief electroshock to the heart. If the patient is receiving antiarrhythmics, check appropriate laboratory tests. For instance, if the patient takes procainamide, check antinuclear antibodies because this drug may induce symptoms that mimic lupus erythematosus.

If the patient is scheduled to undergo resection:

• Before surgery, explain expected postoperative care in the intensive care unit (including use of such things as endotracheal tube, ventilator, hemodynamic monitoring, chest tubes, and drainage bottle).
• After surgery, monitor vital signs, intake and output, heart sounds, and pulmonary artery catheter. Watch for signs of infection, such as fever and drainage.

To prepare the patient for discharge:

• Teach him how to check for pulse irregularity and rate changes. Encourage him to follow his prescribed medication regimen—even during the night—and to watch for side effects.
• Since arrhythmias can cause sudden death, refer the family to a community-based CPR training program.
• Provide psychologic support for the patient and family.

Cardiac Tamponade

In cardiac tamponade, a rapid, unchecked rise in intrapericardial pressure impairs diastolic filling of the heart. The rise in pressure usually results from blood or fluid accumulation in the pericardial sac. If fluid accumulates rapidly, this condition is commonly fatal and necessitates emergency lifesaving measures. Slow accumulation and rise in pressure, as in pericardial effusion associated with malignancies, may not produce immediate symptoms, since the fibrous wall of the pericardial sac can gradually stretch to accommodate as much as 1 to 2 liters of fluid.

Causes

Increased intrapericardial pressure and cardiac tamponade may be idiopathic (Dressler's syndrome) or may result from:

- effusion (in malignancy, bacterial infections, tuberculosis, and, rarely, acute rheumatic fever).
- hemorrhage from trauma (such as gunshot or stab wounds of the chest, and perforation by catheter during cardiac or central venous catheterization, or postcardiac surgery).
- hemorrhage from nontraumatic causes (such as rupture of the heart or great vessels, or anticoagulant therapy in a patient with pericarditis)
- acute myocardial infarction
- uremia.

Signs and symptoms

Cardiac tamponade classically produces increased venous pressure with neck vein distention, reduced arterial blood pressure, muffled heart sounds on auscultation, and pulsus paradoxus (an abnormal inspiratory drop in systemic blood pressure greater than 15 mm Hg). These classic symptoms represent failure of physiologic compensatory mechanisms to override the effects of rapidly rising pericardial pressure, which limits diastolic filling of the ventricles and reduces stroke volume to a critically low level. Generally, ventricular end-systolic volume is not changed significantly, since the contractile force of the ventricles remains intact even in severe tamponade. The increasing pericardial pressure is transmitted equally across the heart cavities, producing a matching rise in intracardiac pressure, especially atrial and end-diastolic ventricular pressures. Cardiac tamponade may also cause dyspnea, tachycardia, narrow pulse pressure, restlessness, and hepatomegaly, but the lung fields will be clear.

Diagnosis

Diagnosis usually relies on classic clinical features. Test results may include:

- *Chest X-ray* shows slightly widened mediastinum and cardiomegaly.
- *EKG* is rarely diagnostic of tamponade but is useful to rule out other cardiac disorders. It may reveal changes produced by acute pericarditis.
- *Pulmonary artery catheterization* detects increased right atrial pressure, right ventricular diastolic pressure, and central venous pressure.
- *Echocardiography* records pericardial effusion with signs of right ventricular and atrial compression.

Treatment

The goal of treatment is to relieve intrapericardial pressure and cardiac compression by removing accumulated blood or fluid. Pericardiocentesis (needle aspiration of the pericardial cavity) or surgical creation of an opening dramatically improves systemic arterial pressure and cardiac output with aspiration of as little as 25 ml of fluid. Such treatment necessitates continuous hemodynamic and EKG monitoring in the intensive care unit. Trial volume loading with temporary I.V. normal saline solution with albumin, and perhaps an inotropic drug, such as isoproterenol or dopamine, is necessary in the hypotensive patient to maintain cardiac output. Although these drugs normally improve myocardial function, they may further compromise an ischemic myocardium after myocardial infarction.

Depending on the cause of tamponade, additional treatment may include:
• *in traumatic injury:* blood transfusion or a thoracotomy to drain reaccumulating fluid or to repair bleeding sites
• *in heparin-induced tamponade:* the heparin antagonist protamine sulfate
• *in warfarin-induced tamponade:* vitamin K.

Special considerations

If the patient needs pericardiocentesis:
• Explain the procedure to the patient. Keep a pericardial aspiration needle attached to a 50 ml syringe by a three-way stopcock, an EKG machine, and an emergency cart with a defibrillator at the bedside. Make sure the equipment is turned on and ready for immediate use. Position the patient at a 45° to 60° angle. Connect the precordial EKG lead to the hub of the aspiration needle with an alligator clamp and connecting wire, and assist with fluid aspiration. When the needle touches the myocardium, you'll see an ST segment elevation or premature ventricular contractions.
• Monitor blood pressure and central venous pressure (CVP) during and after pericardiocentesis. Infuse I.V. solutions, as ordered, to maintain blood pressure. Watch for a decrease in CVP and a concomitant rise in blood pressure, which indicate relief of cardiac compression.
• Watch for complications of pericardiocentesis, such as ventricular fibrillation, vagovagal arrest, or coronary artery or cardiac chamber puncture. Closely monitor EKG changes, blood pressure, pulse rate, level of consciousness, and urinary output.

If the patient needs thoracotomy:
• Explain the procedure to the patient. Tell him what to expect postoperatively (chest tubes, drainage bottles, and administration of oxygen). Teach him how to turn, deep breathe, and cough.
• Give antibiotics, protamine sulfate, or vitamin K, as ordered.
• Postoperatively, monitor critical parameters, such as vital signs and arterial blood gases, and assess heart and breath sounds. Give pain medication, as ordered. Maintain the chest drainage system, and be alert for complications, such as hemorrhage and arrhythmias.

Cardiac Arrhythmias

(Cardiac dysrhythmias)

In cardiac arrhythmias, abnormal electrical conduction or automaticity changes heart rate and rhythm. Arrhythmias vary in severity, from those that are mild, asymptomatic, and require no treatment (such as sinus arrhythmia, in which heart rate increases and decreases with respiration) to catastrophic ventricular fibrillation, which necessitates immediate resuscitation. Arrhythmias are generally classified according to their origin (ventricular or supraventricular). Their effect on cardiac output and blood pressure, partially influenced by the site of origin, determines their clinical significance.

Causes

Arrhythmias may be congenital or may result from myocardial anoxia, infarction, hypertrophy of muscle fiber from hypertension or valvular heart disease, toxic doses of cardioactive drugs (such as digoxin and other cardiotonic glycosides), or degeneration of conductive tissue necessary to maintain normal heart rhythm (sick sinus syndrome).

CARDIAC ARRHYTHMIAS

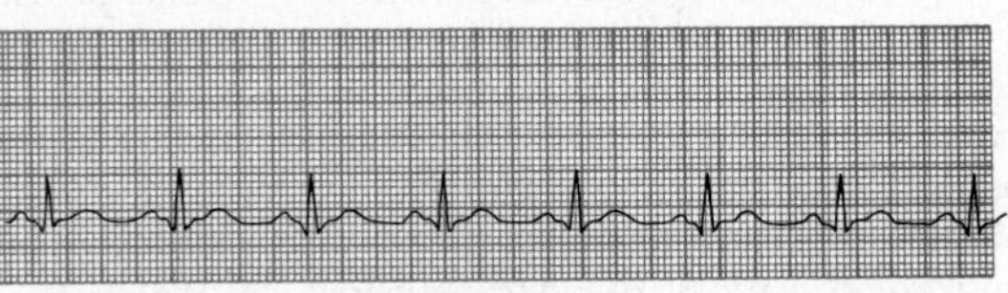

Normal sinus rhythm (NSR) **in adults**

- Ventricular and atrial rates of 60 to 100 beats per minute (BPM)
- QRS complexes and P waves regular and uniform
- P-R interval 0.12 to 0.2 seconds
- QRS duration < 0.12 seconds
- Identical atrial and ventricular rates, with constant P-R interval

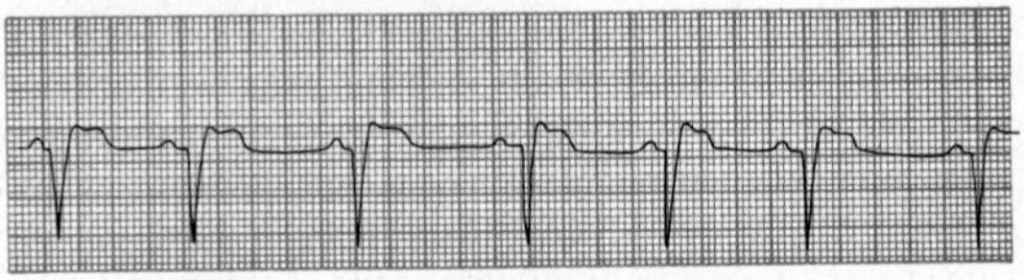

Sinus arrhythmia

CAUSES	DESCRIPTION	TREATMENT
• Usually a normal variation of NSR; associated with sinus bradycardia	• Slight irregularity of heartbeat, usually corresponding to respiratory cycle • Rate increases with inspiration and decreases with expiration.	• None

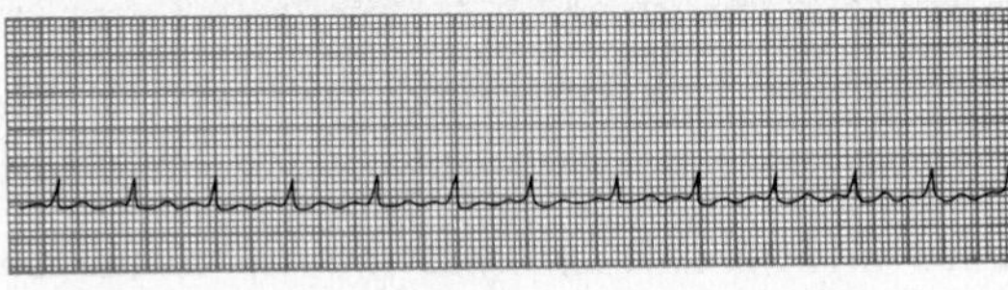

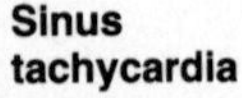

Sinus tachycardia

CAUSES	DESCRIPTION	TREATMENT
• Normal physiologic response to fever, exercise, anxiety, pain, dehydration; may also accompany shock, left ventricular failure, cardiac tamponade, anemia, hyperthyroidism, hypovolemia, pulmonary embolus • May result from treatment with vagolytic and sympathetic stimulating drugs	• Rate > 100 BPM; rarely, > 160 BPM • Every QRS wave follows a P wave.	• Correct underlying cause

CARDIAC ARRHYTHMIAS (continued)

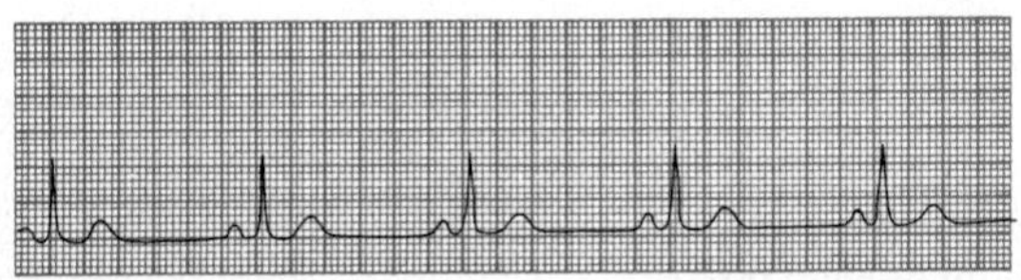

Sinus bradycardia

CAUSES	DESCRIPTION	TREATMENT
• Increased intracranial pressure; increased vagal tone due to bowel straining, vomiting, intubation, mechanical ventilation; sick sinus syndrome or hypothyroidism • Treatment with beta-blockers and sympatholytic drugs • May be normal in athletes	• Rate < 60 BPM • A QRS complex follows each P wave.	• For low cardiac output, dizziness, weakness, altered level of consciousness, or low blood pressure, 0.5 mg atropine every 5 minutes to total of 2.0 mg • Temporary pacemaker or isoproterenol, if atropine fails

Sinoatrial arrest or block (sinus arrest)

CAUSES	DESCRIPTION	TREATMENT
• Vagal stimulation, digitalis or quinidine toxicity • Often a sign of sick sinus syndrome	• NSR interrupted by unexpectedly prolonged P-P interval, often terminated by a junctional escape beat, or return to NSR • QRS complexes uniform but irregular	• A pacemaker for repeated episodes

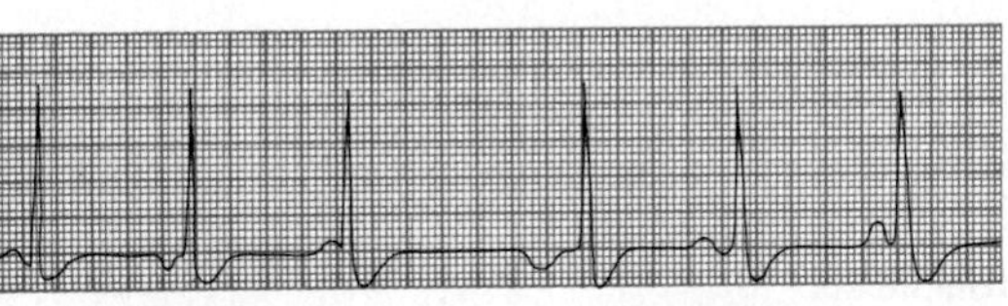

Wandering atrial pacemaker

CAUSES	DESCRIPTION	TREATMENT
• Seen in rheumatic pericarditis as a result of inflammation involving the SA node, digitalis toxicity, and sick sinus syndrome	• Rate varies • QRS complexes uniform in shape but irregular in rhythm • P waves irregular with changing configuration, indicating they're not all from sinus node or single atrial focus • P-R interval varies from short to normal.	• Patient should use digitalis cautiously. • No other treatment

CARDIAC ARRHYTHMIAS (continued)

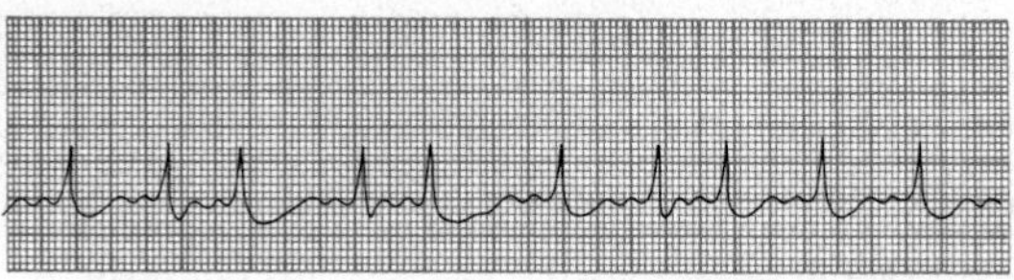

Premature atrial contraction (PAC)

CAUSES

- Congestive heart failure, ischemic heart disease, acute respiratory failure, or COPD
- May result from treatment with digitalis, aminophylline, or adrenergic drugs; or from anxiety or caffeine ingestion
- Occasional PAC may be normal.

DESCRIPTION

- Premature, abnormal-looking P waves
- QRS complexes follow, except in very early or blocked PACs.
- P wave often buried in the preceding T wave or can often be identified in the preceding T wave

TREATMENT

- If more than six times per minute or frequency is increasing, give digitalis, quinidine, or propranolol; after revascularization surgery, propranolol.
- Eliminate known causes, such as caffeine or drugs.

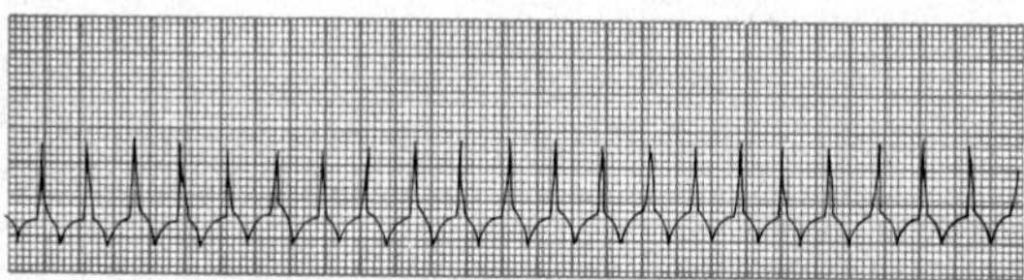

Paroxysmal atrial tachycardia (PAT) or paroxysmal supraventricular tachycardia (PSVT)

CAUSES

- Intrinsic abnormality of AV conduction system
- Congenital accessory atrial conduction pathway
- Physical or psychological stress, hypoxia, hypokalemia, caffeine, marijuana, stimulants, digitalis toxicity

DESCRIPTION

- Heart rate > 140 BPM; rarely exceeds 250 BPM
- P waves regular but aberrant; difficult to differentiate from preceding T wave
- Onset and termination of arrhythmia occur suddenly.
- May cause palpitations and light-headedness

TREATMENT

- Vagal maneuvers, sympathetic blockers (propranolol, quinidine), or calcium blockers (verapamil) to alter AV node conduction
- Elective cardioversion, if patient is symptomatic and unresponsive to drugs

Atrial flutter

CAUSES

- Heart failure, valvular heart disease, pulmonary embolism, digitalis toxicity, postoperative revascularization

DESCRIPTION

- Ventricular rate depends on degree of AV block (usually 60 to 100 BPM)
- Atrial rate 240 to 400 BPM and regular
- QRS complexes uniform in shape, but often irregular in rate
- P waves may have sawtooth configuration

TREATMENT

- Digitalis (unless arrhythmia is due to digitalis toxicity), propranolol, or quinidine
- May require synchronized cardioversion, atrial pacemaker, or vagal stimulation

CARDIAC ARRHYTHMIAS (continued)

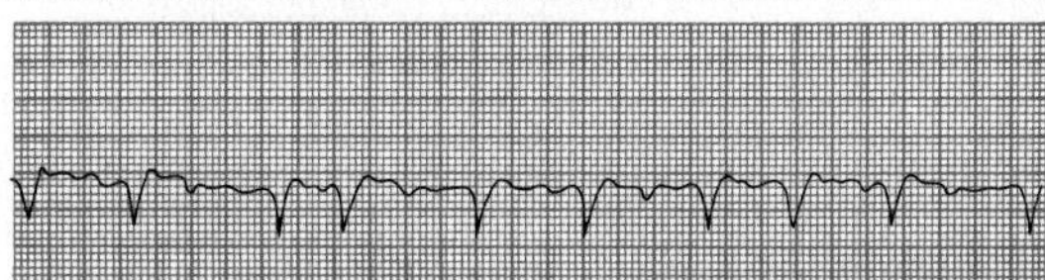

Atrial fibrillation

CAUSES

- Congestive heart failure, COPD, hyperthyroidism, sepsis, pulmonary embolus, mitral stenosis, digitalis toxicity (rarely), atrial irritation, post-coronary bypass or valve replacement surgery

DESCRIPTION

- Atrial rate > 400 BPM
- Ventricular rate varies
- QRS complexes uniform in shape, but at irregular intervals
- P-R interval indiscernible
- No P waves, or P waves appear as erratic, irregular baseline F waves
- Irregular QRS rate

TREATMENT

- Digitalis and quinidine to slow ventricular rate, and quinidine to convert rhythm to NSR; diuretics, such as furosemide, for congestive heart failure
- May require elective cardioversion for rapid rate

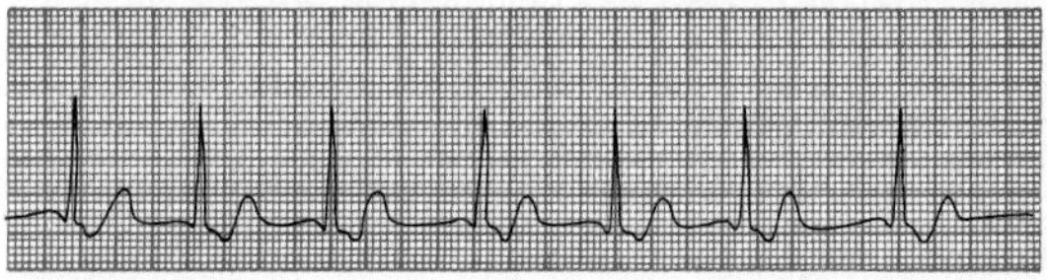

Nodal rhythm (AV junctional rhythm)

CAUSES

- Digitalis toxicity, inferior wall myocardial infarction or ischemia, hypoxia, vagal stimulation
- Acute rheumatic fever
- Valve surgery

DESCRIPTION

- Ventricular rate usually 40 to 60 BPM (60 to 100 BPM is accelerated junctional rhythm)
- P waves may precede, be hidden within (absent), or follow QRS; if visible, they're altered
- QRS duration is normal, except in aberrant conduction.
- Patient may be asymptomatic unless ventricular rate is very slow

TREATMENT

- Symptomatic
- Atropine, with slow rate
- If patient is taking digitalis, it is discontinued

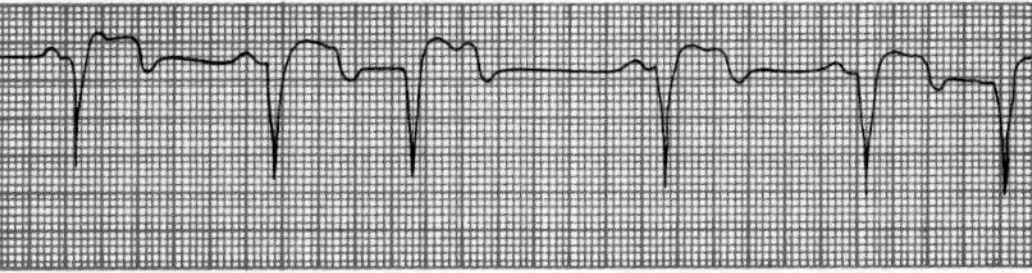

Premature nodal contractions (PNC) or junctional premature beats

CAUSES

- Myocardial infarction or ischemia, digitalis toxicity, caffeine ingestion, or amphetamines

DESCRIPTION

- QRS complexes of uniform shape but premature
- P waves irregular, with premature beat; may precede, be hidden within, or follow QRS

TREATMENT

- Correct underlying cause.
- Quinidine or disopyramide, as ordered
- If patient is taking digitalis, it may be discontinued.

CARDIAC ARRHYTHMIAS (continued)

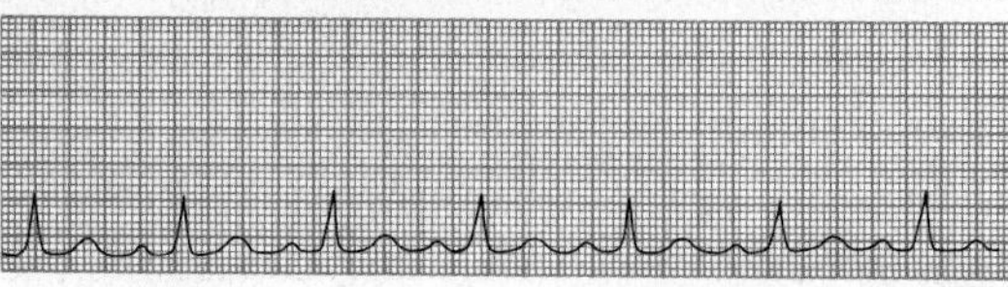

First-degree AV block

CAUSES

- Inferior myocardial ischemia or infarction, hypothyroidism, digitalis toxicity, potassium imbalance

DESCRIPTION

- P-R interval prolonged > 0.20 seconds
- QRS complex normal

TREATMENT

- Patient should use digitalis cautiously.
- Correct underlying cause. Otherwise, be alert for increasing block.

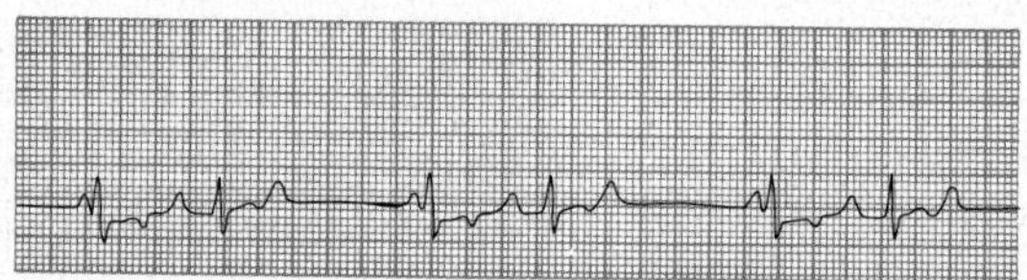

Second-degree AV block
Mobitz Type I (Wenckebach)

CAUSES

- *Mobitz Type I:* Inferior wall myocardial infarction, digitalis toxicity, vagal stimulation

DESCRIPTION

- *Mobitz Type I:* P-R interval becomes progressively longer with each cycle until QRS disappears (dropped beat). After a dropped beat, P-R interval is shorter. Ventricular rate is irregular; atrial rhythm, regular.

TREATMENT

- *Mobitz Type I:* Atropine, if patient is symptomatic
- Discontinue digitalis.

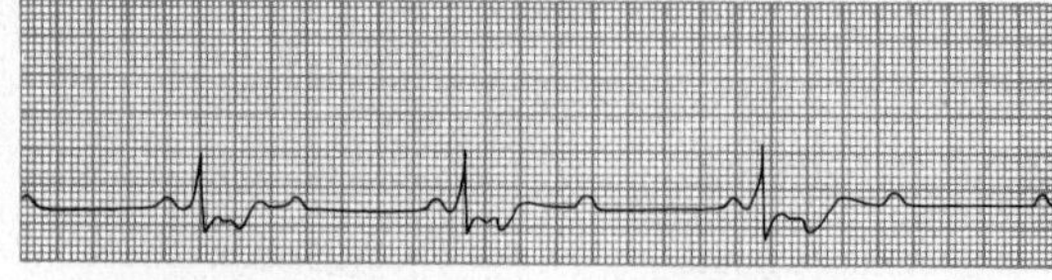

Second-degree AV block
Mobitz Type II

CAUSES

- *Mobitz Type II:* Degenerative disease of conduction system, ischemia of AV node in anterior myocardial infarction, digitalis toxicity, anteroseptal infarction

DESCRIPTION

- *Mobitz Type II:* P-R interval is constant, with QRS complexes dropped
- Ventricular rhythm may be irregular, with varying degree of block.
- Atrial rate regular

TREATMENT

- *Mobitz Type II:* Temporary pacemaker, sometimes followed by permanent pacemaker
- Atropine, for slow rate
- If patient is taking digitalis, it is discontinued.

CARDIAC ARRHYTHMIAS (continued)

Third-degree AV block
(complete heart block)

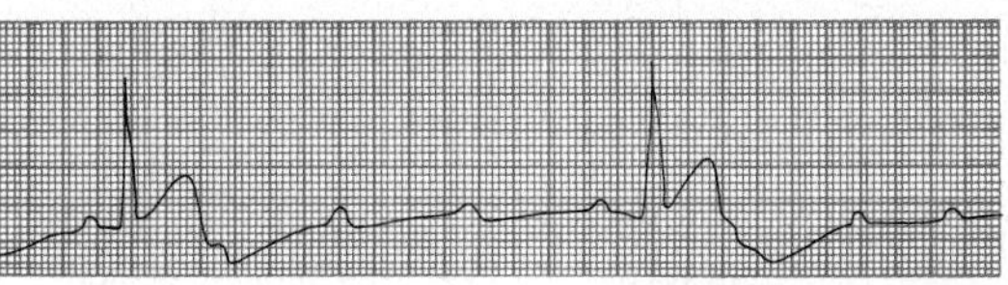

CAUSES
- Ischemic heart disease or infarction; postsurgical complications of mitral valve replacement; digitalis toxicity; hypoxia sometimes causing syncope due to decreased cerebral blood flow, as in Stokes-Adams syndrome

DESCRIPTION
- Atrial rate regular; ventricular rate, slow and regular
- No relationship between P waves and QRS complexes
- No constant P-R interval
- QRS interval normal (nodal pacemaker); wide and bizarre (ventricular pacemaker)

TREATMENT
- Usually requires temporary pacemaker, followed by permanent pacemaker
- Epinephrine or isoproterenol

Nodal tachycardia
(junctional tachycardia)

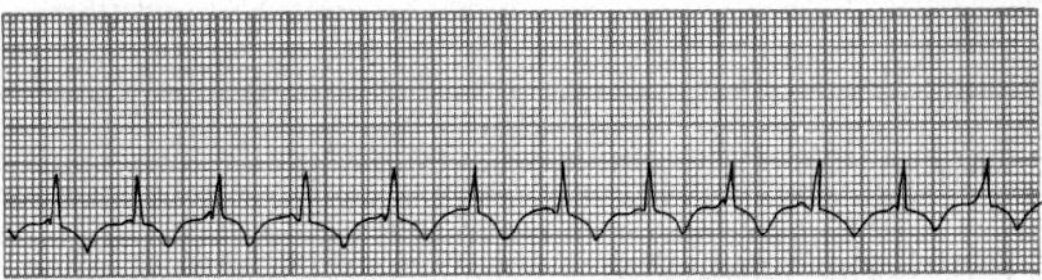

CAUSES
- Digitalis toxicity, myocarditis, cardiomyopathy, myocardial ischemia or infarct

DESCRIPTION
- Onset of rhythm often sudden, occurring in bursts
- Ventricular rate > 100 BPM
- Other characteristics same as junctional rhythm

TREATMENT
- Vagal stimulation
- Propranolol, quinidine, digitalis (if cause is not digitalis toxicity)
- Elective cardioversion

Premature ventricular contraction (PVC)

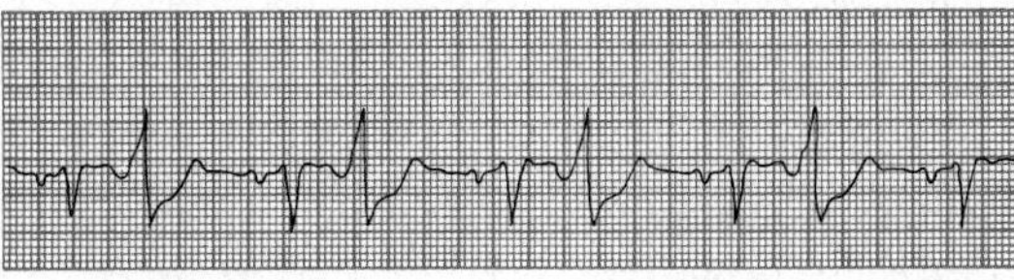

CAUSES
- Heart failure; old or acute myocardial infarction or contusion with trauma; myocardial irritation by ventricular catheter, such as a pacemaker; hypoxia, as in anemia and acute respiratory failure; drug toxicity (digitalis, aminophylline, tricyclic antidepressants, beta-adrenergics [isoproterenol or dopamine]); electrolyte imbalances (especially hypokalemia); psychological stress

DESCRIPTION
- Beat occurs prematurely, usually followed by a complete compensatory pause after PVC; irregular pulse.
- QRS complex wide and distorted
- Can occur singly, in pairs, or in threes; can alternate with normal beats; focus can be from one or more sites
- PVCs are most ominous when clustered, multifocal, with R wave on T pattern.

TREATMENT
- Lidocaine I.V. bolus and drip infusion; procainamide I.V. If induced by digitalis toxicity, stop this drug; if induced by hypokalemia, give potassium chloride I.V. Many other drugs may be used.

CARDIAC ARRHYTHMIAS (continued)

Ventricular tachycardia (VT)

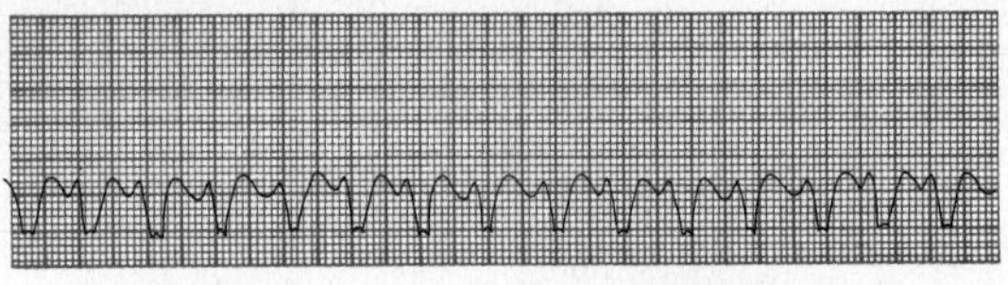

CAUSES
- Myocardial ischemia, infarction, or aneurysm; ventricular catheters; digitalis or quinidine toxicity; hypokalemia; hypercalcemia; anxiety

DESCRIPTION
- Ventricular rate 140 to 220 BPM; may be regular
- QRS complexes are wide, bizarre, and independent of P waves
- Usually no visible P waves
- Can produce chest pain, anxiety, palpitations, dyspnea, shock, coma, and death

TREATMENT
- CPR (if pulses are absent) followed by lidocaine I.V. (bolus and drip infusion) and countershock. Use synchronized cardioversion if pulse is present.
- Bretylium tosylate and procainamide

Ventricular fibrillation

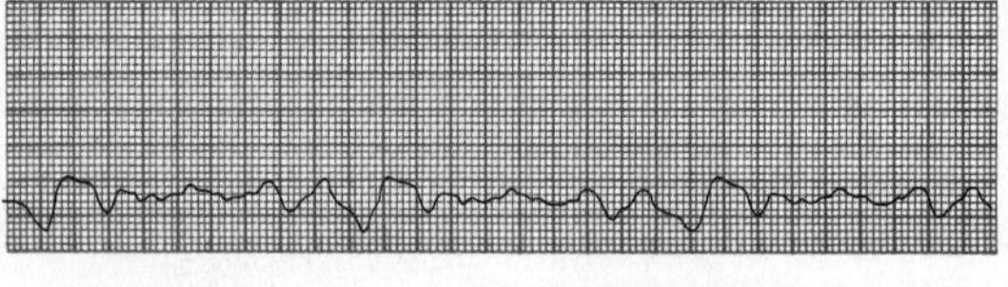

CAUSES
- Myocardial ischemia or infarction, untreated ventricular tachycardia, electrolyte imbalances (hypokalemia and alkalosis, hyperkalemia and hypercalcemia), digitalis or quinidine toxicity, electric shock, hypothermia

DESCRIPTION
- Ventricular rhythm rapid and chaotic
- QRS complexes wide and irregular; no visible P waves
- Loss of consciousness, with no peripheral pulses, blood pressure, or respirations; possible seizures; and sudden death

TREATMENT
- CPR
- Asynchronized countershock (200 to 300 watts/second) twice; if rhythm doesn't return, reshock (300 to 400 watts/second).
- Drugs, such as lidocaine or bretylium tosylate I.V. or procainamide

Ventricular standstill (asystole)

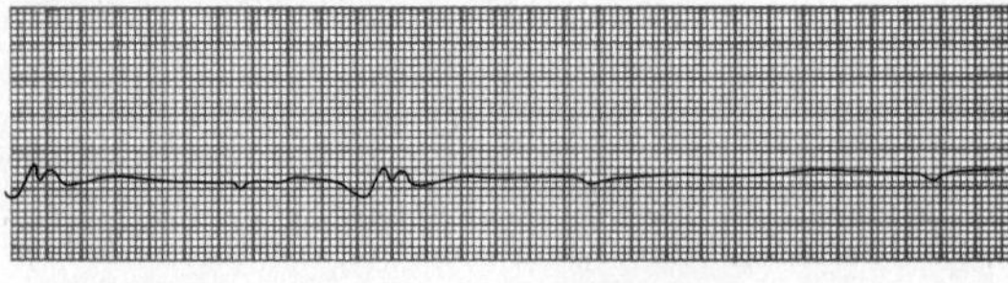

CAUSES
- Acute respiratory failure, myocardial ischemia or infarction, ruptured ventricular aneurysm, aortic valve disease, or hyperkalemia

DESCRIPTION
- Primary ventricular standstill—regular P waves, no QRS complexes
- Secondary ventricular standstill—QRS complexes wide and slurred, occurring at irregular intervals; agonal heart rhythm
- Loss of consciousness, with no peripheral pulses, blood pressure, or respirations

TREATMENT
- CPR
- Endotracheal intubation, pacemaker should be available
- Epinephrine, calcium gluconate, sodium bicarbonate, Isuprel, and atropine
- Cardiac monitoring

HOLTER MONITORING

Tape-recorded ambulatory electrocardiography (Holter monitoring) permits monitoring of all cardiac cycles over a prescribed period (usually 24 hours). This type of monitoring has proven useful for patients recuperating from myocardial infarctions, receiving antiarrhythmic drugs, or using pacemakers. It can record rate, rhythm, and conduction abnormalities as well as cardiac responses to typical environmental stimuli and is especially useful in diagnosing arrhythmias. Holter monitoring has many advantages:

- With minimal equipment, the patient can be hooked up to one or more EKG leads. (Equipment includes the monitor, its carrying case, a belt, skin electrodes, alcohol swabs, a blank cassette tape, a patient diary, and a test analysis report.)
- Leads are recorded on a tape in a portable cassette recorder that the patient can wear easily. After the recorder is connected to a cardiac monitor for test readings, the electrodes are attached to the patient, and he goes through a typical day with the Holter monitor in place. He is encouraged to engage in activities that usually precipitate symptoms and is instructed to keep a diary of the exact times of symptoms and activities and of any medication he takes, so the impact of these factors can be correlated with EKG patterns.
- With a high-speed computer scanner, the doctor can review 24 hours of tape in minutes to detect important rhythm changes. He can also correlate the patient's symptoms, such as light-headedness, with the documented arrhythmias.
- The Holter monitor can capture a sporadic arrhythmia that an office or stress-test EKG might miss.

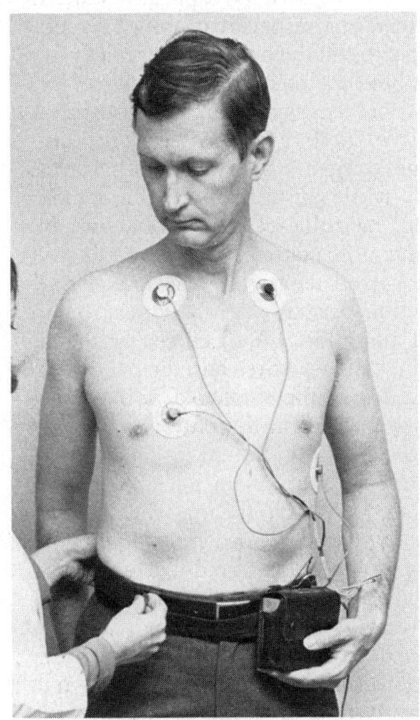

The Holter monitor should be strapped around the patient's waist to create a secure but comfortable fit. If the belt is too loose, the monitor's weight will pull on the electrodes.

Special considerations

- Assess an unmonitored patient for rhythm disturbances. If the patient's pulse is abnormally rapid, slow, or irregular, watch for signs of hypoperfusion, such as hypotension and diminished urinary output.
- Document any arrhythmias in a monitored patient, and assess for possible causes and effects.
- When life-threatening arrhythmias develop, rapidly assess the level of consciousness, respirations, and pulse, and initiate cardiopulmonary resuscitation, if indicated.
- Evaluate for altered cardiac output resulting from arrhythmias. Consider potentially progressive or ominous arrhythmias in determining your course of action. Administer medications, as ordered, and prepare to assist with medical procedures, if indicated (for ex-

ample, cardioversion).

- Monitor for predisposing factors—such as fluid and electrolyte imbalance—and signs of drug toxicity, especially with digoxin. If you suspect drug toxicity, report such signs to the doctor immediately and withhold the next dose.
- To prevent arrhythmias in a postoperative cardiac patient, provide adequate oxygen and reduce heart work load, while carefully maintaining metabolic, neurologic, respiratory, and hemodynamic status.
- To avoid temporary pacemaker malfunction, install a fresh battery before each insertion. Carefully secure the external catheter wires and the pacemaker box. Assess the threshold daily. Watch closely for premature contractions, a sign of myocardial irritation.
- To avert permanent pacemaker malfunction, restrict the patient's activity after insertion, as ordered. Monitor the pulse rate regularly, and watch for signs of decreased cardiac output.
- Warn the patient about environmental hazards, as indicated by the pacemaker manufacturer. Although hazards may not present a problem, in doubtful situations, 24-hour Holter monitoring may be helpful. Tell the patient to report lightheadedness or syncope, and stress the importance of regular checkups.

NORMAL CARDIAC CONDUCTION

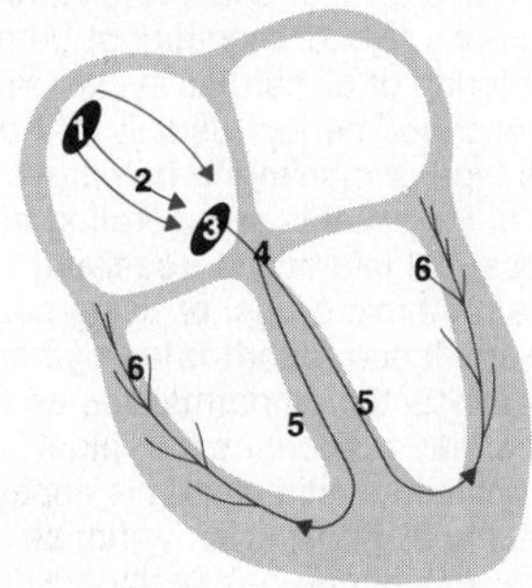

Each electrical impulse travels from the SA node (1) through the internodal tracts (2), producing atrial contraction. The impulse slows momentarily as it passes through the AV junction (3) to the bundle of His (4). Then, it descends the left and right bundle branches (5) and reaches Purkinje's fibers (6), stimulating ventricular contraction.

VASCULAR DISORDERS

Thoracic Aortic Aneurysm

Thoracic aortic aneurysm is an abnormal widening of the ascending, transverse, or descending part of the aorta. The aneurysm may be dissecting, *a hemorrhagic separation in the aortic wall, usually within the medial layer;* saccular, *an outpouching of the arterial wall, with a narrow neck; or* fusiform, *a spindle-shaped enlargement encompassing the entire aortic circumference. Some aneurysms progress to serious and, eventually, lethal complications, such as rupture of untreated thoracic dissecting aneurysm into the pericardium, with resulting tamponade.*

Causes and incidence

Commonly, a thoracic aortic aneurysm results from atherosclerosis, which weakens the aortic wall and gradually distends the lumen in this area. An intimal tear in the ascending aorta initiates dissecting aneurysm in about 60% of patients. Other causes include:

- infection (mycotic aneurysms) of the aortic arch and descending segments.
- congenital disorders, such as coarctation of the aorta.

- trauma, usually of the descending thoracic aorta, from an accident that shears the aorta transversely (acceleration-deceleration injuries).
- syphilis, usually of the ascending aorta (now uncommon because of antibiotics).
- hypertension (in dissecting aneurysm).

Thoracic aortic aneurysms are most common in men between ages 50 and 70; dissecting aneurysms, in blacks.

Signs and symptoms

The most common symptom of thoracic aortic aneurysm is pain. In dissecting aneurysm, such pain may be sudden in onset, with a tearing or ripping sensation in the thorax or the anterior chest. It may extend to the neck, shoulders, lower back, or abdomen, but rarely radiates to the jaw and arms.

Accompanying signs include syncope, pallor, sweating, shortness of breath, increased pulse rate, cyanosis, leg weakness or transient paralysis, diastolic murmur, and abrupt loss of radial and femoral pulses or wide variations in pulses or blood pressure between arms and legs. The patient appears to be in shock, but systolic blood pressure is often normal or significantly elevated.

Effects of thoracic aortic aneurysms (saccular or fusiform) vary according to the size and location of the aneurysm, and the compression, distortion, or erosion of surrounding structures, such as the lungs, trachea, larynx and recurrent laryngeal nerve, esophagus, and spinal nerves. An aneurysm in the ascending aorta may extend into the aortic root, causing aortic valve insufficiency and a diastolic murmur. This may signal a catastrophic event.

Other effects may include a substernal ache in the shoulders, lower back, or abdomen; marked respiratory distress (dyspnea, brassy cough, wheezing); hoarseness or loss of voice; dysphagia (rare); and, possibly, paresthesias or neuralgia. Aneurysms may rupture.

Diagnosis

Diagnosis relies on patient history, clinical features, and appropriate tests. In an asymptomatic patient, diagnosis often occurs accidentally, through posteroanterior and oblique chest X-rays showing widening of the aorta. Other tests help confirm aneurysm:

- *Aortography,* the most definitive test, shows the lumen of the aneurysm, its size and location, and the false lumen in dissecting aneurysm.
- *EKG* helps distinguish thoracic aneurysm from myocardial infarction.
- *Echocardiography* may help identify dissecting aneurysm of the aortic root.
- *Hemoglobin* may be normal or decreased, due to blood loss from a leaking aneurysm.
- *Computed tomography scanning* can confirm and locate the aneurysm and may be used to monitor its progression.
- *Magnetic resonance imaging* may aid diagnosis.

Treatment

Dissecting aortic aneurysm is an extreme emergency that requires prompt surgery and stabilizing measures: antihypertensives, such as nitroprusside; negative inotropic agents that decrease contractility force, such as propranolol; oxygen for respiratory distress; narcotics for pain; I.V. fluids; and, if necessary, whole blood transfusions.

Surgery is comparable to open heart surgery and consists of resecting the aneurysm, restoring normal blood flow through a Dacron or Teflon graft replacement, and, with aortic valve insufficiency, replacing the aortic valve.

Postoperative measures include careful monitoring and continuous assessment in the ICU, antibiotics, endotracheal and chest tubes, EKG monitoring, and pulmonary artery catheterization.

Special considerations

- Monitor blood pressure, pulmonary capillary wedge pressure, and central venous pressure. Assess pain, breathing, and carotid, radial, and femoral pulses.
- Make sure laboratory tests include CBC, differential, electrolytes, type and cross match for whole blood, arterial blood gas studies, and urinalysis.

TYPES OF AORTIC ANEURYSMS

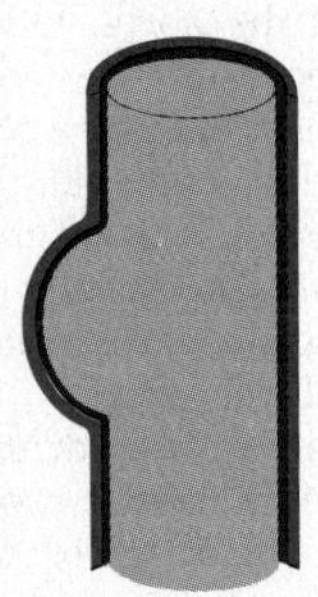

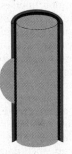

• *Saccular*—unilateral pouchlike bulge with a narrow neck

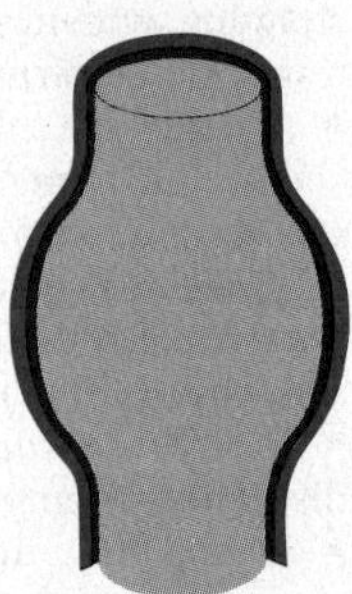

• *Fusiform*—a spindle-shaped bulge encompassing the entire diameter of the vessel

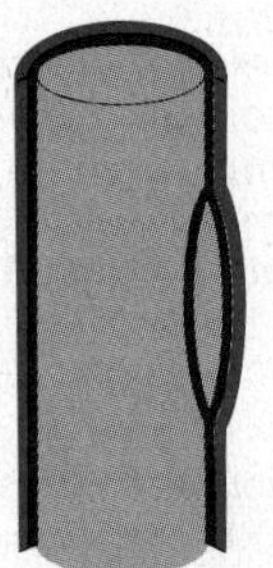

• *Dissecting*—a hemorrhagic separation of the medial layer of the vessel wall, which creates a false lumen

• *False aneurysm*—pulsating hematoma resulting from trauma and often mistaken for an abdominal aneurysm

• Insert a Foley catheter. Administer 5% dextrose in water or lactated Ringer's solution, and antibiotics, as ordered. Carefully monitor nitroprusside I.V.; use a separate I.V. line for infusion. Adjust the dose by slowly increasing the infusion rate. Meanwhile, check blood pressure every 5 minutes until it stabilizes. With suspected bleeding from aneurysm, give whole blood transfusion, as ordered.
• Explain diagnostic tests. If surgery is scheduled, explain the procedure and expected postoperative care (I.V.s, endotracheal and drainage tubes, cardiac monitoring, ventilation).

After repair of thoracic aneurysm:
• Carefully assess level of consciousness. Monitor vital signs, pulmonary artery and capillary wedge and central venous pressures, pulse rate, urinary output, and pain.
• Check respiratory function. Carefully observe and record type and amount of chest tube drainage, and frequently assess heart and lung sounds.
• Monitor I.V. therapy.
• Give medications, as ordered.
• Watch for signs of infection, especially fever, and excessive drainage on dressing.
• Assist with range-of-motion exercises of legs to prevent thromboembolic phenomenon due to venostasis during prolonged bed rest.
• After stabilization of vital signs and respiration, encourage and assist the patient in turning, coughing, and deep breathing. If necessary, provide intermittent positive pressure breathing to promote lung expansion. Help the patient walk as soon as he's able.
• Before discharge, ensure compliance with antihypertensive therapy by explaining the need for such drugs and the expected side effects. Teach the patient how to monitor his blood pressure. Refer him to community agencies for continued support and assistance, as needed.
• Throughout hospitalization, offer the patient and family psychologic support. Answer all questions honestly, and provide reassurance.

Abdominal Aneurysm

Abdominal aneurysm, an abnormal dilation in the arterial wall, generally occurs in the aorta between the renal arteries and iliac branches. Such aneurysms are four times more common in men than in women and are most prevalent in Caucasians aged 50 to 80. Over 50% of all persons with untreated abdominal aneurysms die, primarily from aneurysmal rupture, within 2 years of diagnosis; over 85%, within 5 years.

Causes

About 95% of abdominal aortic aneurysms result from arteriosclerosis; the rest, from cystic medial necrosis, trauma, syphilis, and other infections. These aneurysms develop slowly. First, a focal weakness in the muscular layer of the aorta (tunica media), due to degenerative changes, allows the inner layer (tunica intima) and outer layer (tunica adventitia) to stretch outward. Blood pressure within the aorta progressively weakens the vessel walls and enlarges the aneurysm.

Signs and symptoms

Although abdominal aneurysms usually don't manifest symptoms, most are evident (unless the patient is obese) as a pulsating mass in the periumbilical area, accompanied by a systolic bruit over the aorta. Some tenderness may be present on deep palpation. A large aneurysm may produce symptoms that mimic renal calculi, lumbar disk disease, and duodenal compression. Abdominal aneurysms rarely cause diminished peripheral pulses or claudication, unless embolization occurs.

Lumbar pain that radiates to the flank and groin from pressure on lumbar nerves may signify enlargement and imminent rupture. If the aneurysm ruptures into the peritoneal cavity, it causes severe, persistent abdominal and back pain, mimicking renal or ureteral colic. Signs of hemorrhage—such as weakness, sweating, tachycardia, and hypotension—may be subtle, since rupture into the retroperitoneal space produces a tamponade effect that prevents continued hemorrhage. Patients with such rupture may remain stable for hours before shock and death occur, although 20% die immediately.

Diagnosis

Since an abdominal aneurysm rarely produces symptoms, it's often detected accidentally as the result of an X-ray or a routine physical examination. Several

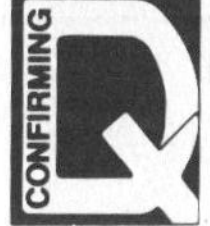

tests can confirm suspected abdominal aneurysm:

- *Serial ultrasound* (sonography) is accurate and allows determination of aneurysm size, shape, and location.
- *Anteroposterior and lateral X-rays* of the abdomen can detect aortic calcification, which outlines the mass, at least 75% of the time.
- *Aortography* shows the condition of vessels proximal and distal to the aneurysm and the extent of the aneurysm but may underestimate aneurysm diameter, because it visualizes only the flow channel and not the surrounding clot.

Treatment

Usually, abdominal aneurysm requires resection of the aneurysm and replacement of the damaged aortic section with a Dacron graft. If the aneurysm is small and asymptomatic, surgery may be delayed; however, small aneurysms may also rupture. Regular physical examination and ultrasound checks are necessary to detect enlargement, which may forewarn rupture. Large aneurysms or those that produce symptoms involve a significant risk of rupture and necessitate immediate repair. In patients with poor distal runoff, external grafting may be done.

COMMON FUSIFORM ABDOMINAL ANEURYSMS

During surgery, a prosthetic graft replaces or encloses weakened area.

BEFORE SURGERY	AFTER SURGERY
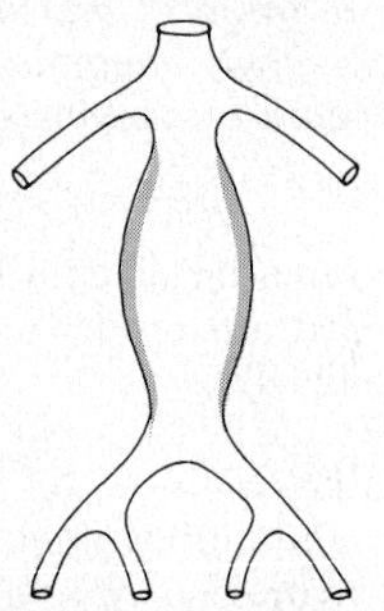	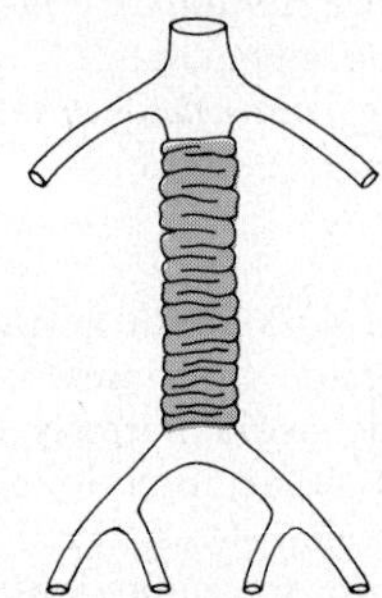
Aneurysm below renal arteries and above bifurcation	The prosthesis extends distal to the renal arteries to above the aortic bifurcation.
BEFORE SURGERY	AFTER SURGERY
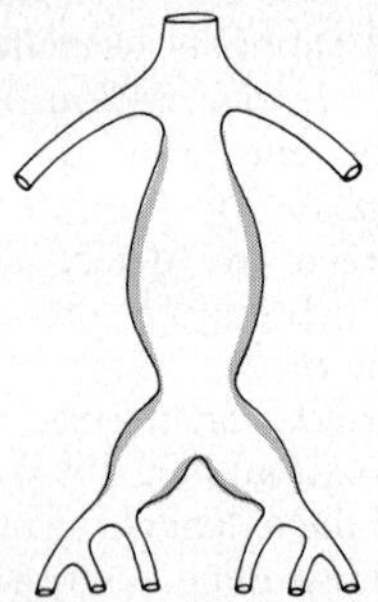	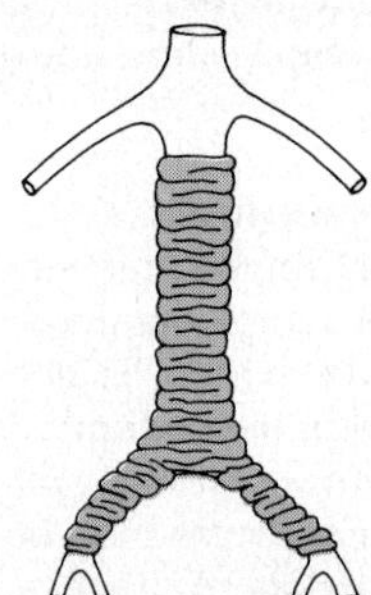
Aneurysm below renal arteries involving the iliac branches	The prosthesis extends to the common femoral arteries.
BEFORE SURGERY	AFTER SURGERY
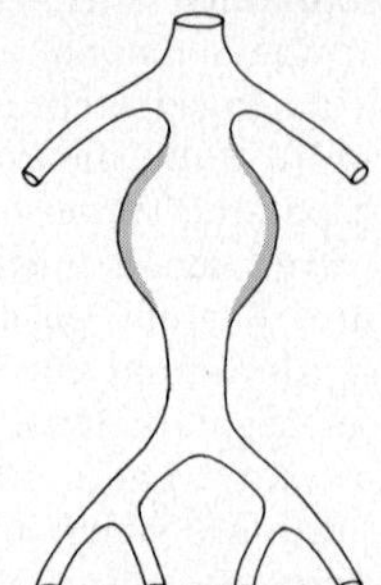	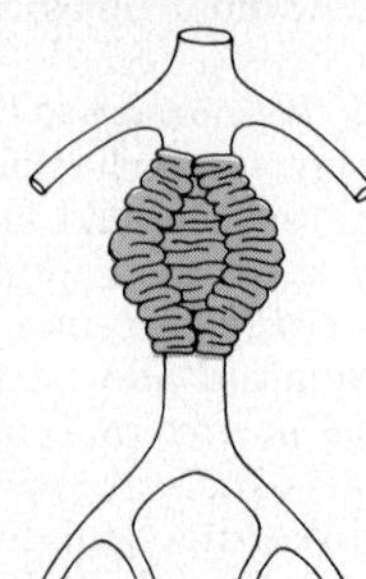
Small aneurysm in a patient with poor distal runoff (poor risk)	The external prosthesis encircles the aneurysm and is held in place with sutures.

Special considerations

Abdominal aneurysm requires meticulous preoperative and postoperative care, psychological support, and comprehensive patient teaching. Following diagnosis, if rupture is not imminent, elective surgery allows time for additional preoperative tests to evaluate the patient's clinical status.

- Monitor vital signs, and type and cross match blood.
- As ordered, obtain kidney function tests (BUN, creatinine, electrolytes), blood samples (CBC with differential), EKG and cardiac evaluation, baseline pulmonary function tests, and blood gases.
- Be alert for signs of rupture which may be immediately fatal. Watch closely for any signs of acute blood loss (decreasing blood pressure; increasing pulse and respiratory rate; cool, clammy skin; restlessness; and decreased sensorium).
- If rupture does occur, the first priority is to get the patient to surgery *immediately*. Medical antishock trousers may be used while transporting to surgery. Surgery allows direct compression of the aorta to control hemorrhage. Large amounts of blood may be needed during the resuscitative period to replace blood loss. In such a patient, renal failure due to ischemia is a major postoperative complication, possibly requiring hemodialysis.
- Before elective surgery, weigh the patient, insert a Foley catheter, an I.V., and assist with insertion of arterial line and pulmonary artery catheter to monitor fluid and hemodynamic balance. Give prophylactic antibiotics, as ordered.
- Explain the surgical procedure, and the expected postoperative care in the ICU for patients undergoing complex abdominal surgery (I.V.s, endotracheal and nasogastric intubation, mechanical ventilation).
- After surgery, in the ICU, closely monitor vital signs, intake and hourly output, neurologic status (level of consciousness, pupil size, sensation in arms and legs), and blood gases. Assess the depth, rate, and character of respirations and lung sounds at least every hour.
- Watch for signs of bleeding (increased pulse rate and respirations, hypotension), which may occur retroperitoneally from the graft site. Check abdominal dressings for excessive bleeding or drainage. Be alert for temperature elevations and other signs of infection. After nasogastric intubation for intestinal decompression, irrigate the tube frequently to ensure patency. Record the amount and type of drainage.
- Suction the endotracheal tube often. If the patient can breathe unassisted and has good lung sounds and adequate blood gases, tidal volume, and vital capacity 24 hours after surgery, he will be extubated and will require oxygen by mask. Weigh the patient daily to evaluate fluid balance.
- Help the patient walk as soon as he's able (generally the second day after surgery).
- Provide psychological support for the patient and family. Help ease their fears about the ICU, the threat of impending rupture, and surgery by providing appropriate explanations and answering all questions.

Femoral and Popliteal Aneurysms

(Peripheral arterial aneurysms)

Femoral and popliteal aneurysms are the end result of progressive atherosclerotic changes occurring in the walls (medial layer) of these major peripheral arteries. These aneurysmal formations may be fusiform *(spindle-shaped) or* saccular *(pouch-like), with fusiform occurring three times more frequently. They may be singular or multiple segmental lesions, often affecting both legs, and may accompany other*

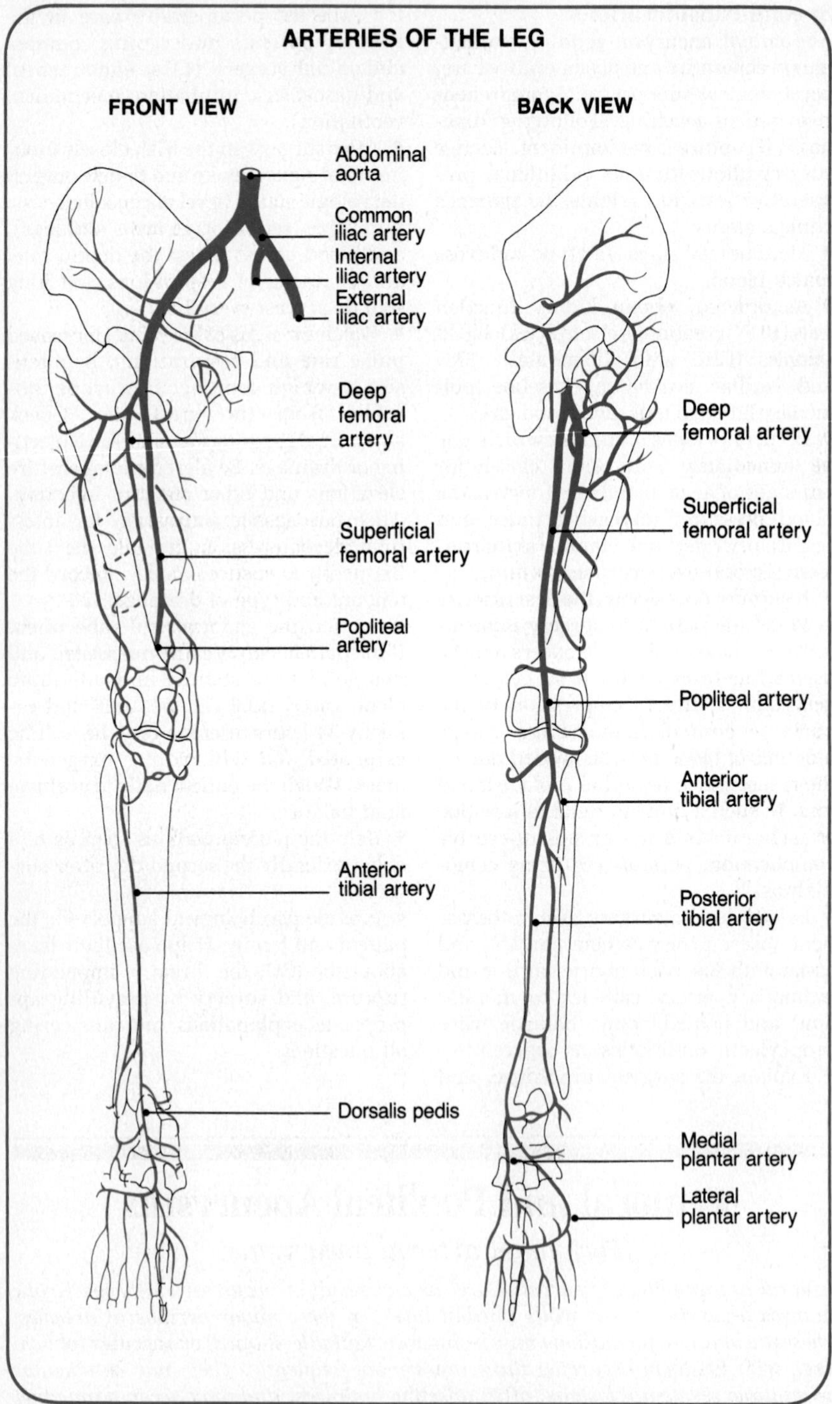
ARTERIES OF THE LEG
FRONT VIEW
BACK VIEW
Abdominal aorta
Common iliac artery
Internal iliac artery
External iliac artery
Deep femoral artery
Superficial femoral artery
Popliteal artery
Anterior tibial artery
Dorsalis pedis
Deep femoral artery
Superficial femoral artery
Popliteal artery
Anterior tibial artery
Posterior tibial artery
Medial plantar artery
Lateral plantar artery

arterial aneurysms located in the abdominal aorta or iliac arteries. This condition occurs most frequently in men over age 50. The clinical course is usually progressive, eventually ending in thrombosis, embolization, and gangrene. Elective surgery before complications arise greatly improves prognosis.

Causes

Femoral and popliteal aneurysms are usually secondary to atherosclerosis. Rarely, they result from congenital weakness in the arterial wall. They may also result from trauma (blunt or penetrating), bacterial infection, or peripheral vascular reconstructive surgery (which causes "suture line" aneurysms, whereby a blood clot forms a second lumen, also called false aneurysms).

Signs and symptoms

Popliteal aneurysms may cause pain in the popliteal space when they're large enough to compress the medial popliteal nerve, and edema and venous distention if the vein is compressed. Femoral and popliteal aneurysms can produce symptoms of severe ischemia in the leg or foot, due to acute thrombosis within the aneurysmal sac, embolization of mural thrombus fragments, and, rarely, rupture. Symptoms of acute aneurysmal thrombosis include severe pain, loss of pulse and color, coldness in the affected leg or foot, and gangrene. Distal petechial hemorrhages may develop from aneurysmal emboli.

Diagnosis

Diagnosis is usually confirmed by bilateral palpation that reveals a pulsating mass above or below the inguinal ligament in femoral aneurysm. When thrombosis has occurred, palpation detects a firm, nonpulsating mass. Arteriography or ultrasound may be indicated in doubtful situations. Arteriography may also detect associated aneurysms, especially those in the abdominal aorta and the iliac arteries. Ultrasound may be helpful in determining the size of the popliteal or femoral artery.

Treatment

Femoral and popliteal aneurysms require surgical bypass and reconstruction of the artery, usually with an autogenous saphenous vein graft replacement. Arterial occlusion that causes severe ischemia and gangrene may require leg amputation.

Special considerations

Before corrective surgery:

- Assess and record circulatory status, noting location and quality of peripheral pulses in the affected arm or leg.
- Administer prophylactic antibiotics or anticoagulants, as ordered.
- Discuss expected postoperative procedures, and review the explanation of the surgery.

After arterial surgery:

- Monitor carefully for early signs of thrombosis or graft occlusion (loss of pulse, decreased skin temperature and sensation, severe pain) and infection (fever).
- Palpate distal pulses at least every hour for the first 24 hours, then as frequently as ordered. Correlate these findings with preoperative circulatory assessment. Mark the sites on the patient's skin where pulses are palpable, to facilitate repeated checks.
- Help the patient walk soon after surgery, to prevent venostasis and possible thrombus formation.

To prepare the patient for discharge:

- Tell the patient to immediately report any recurrence of symptoms, since the saphenous vein graft replacement can fail or another aneurysm may develop.
- Explain to the patient with popliteal artery resection that swelling may persist for some time. If antiembolism stockings are ordered, make sure they fit properly, and teach the patient how to apply them. Warn against wearing constrictive apparel.
- If the patient is receiving anticoagulants, suggest measures to prevent bleeding, such as using an electric razor. Tell the patient to report any signs of bleeding

immediately (bleeding gums, tarry stools, easy bruising). Explain the importance of follow-up blood studies to monitor anticoagulant therapy. Warn him to avoid trauma, tobacco, and aspirin.

Thrombophlebitis

An acute condition characterized by inflammation and thrombus formation, thrombophlebitis may occur in deep (intermuscular or intramuscular) or superficial (subcutaneous) veins. Deep-vein thrombophlebitis affects small veins, such as the soleal venous sinuses, or large veins, such as the vena cava, and the femoral, iliac, and subclavian veins. This disorder is frequently progressive, leading to pulmonary embolism, a potentially lethal complication. Superficial thrombophlebitis is usually self-limiting and rarely leads to pulmonary embolism. Thrombophlebitis often begins with localized inflammation alone (phlebitis), but such inflammation rapidly provokes thrombus formation. Rarely, venous thrombosis develops without associated inflammation of the vein (phlebothrombosis).

Causes

A thrombus occurs when an alteration in the epithelial lining causes platelet aggregation and consequent fibrin entrapment of RBCs, WBCs, and additional platelets. Thrombus formation is more rapid in areas where blood flow is slower, due to greater contact between platelet and thrombin accumulation. The rapidly expanding thrombus initiates a chemical inflammatory process in the vessel epithelium, which leads to fibrosis. The enlarging clot may occlude the vessel lumen partially or totally, or it may detach and embolize, to lodge elsewhere in the systemic circulation.

Deep-vein thrombophlebitis may be idiopathic, but it usually results from endothelial damage, accelerated blood clotting, and reduced blood flow. Predisposing factors are prolonged bed rest, trauma, surgery, childbirth, and use of oral contraceptives, such as estrogens.

Causes of superficial thrombophlebitis include trauma, infection, I.V. drug abuse, and chemical irritation due to the extensive use of the I.V. route for medications and diagnostic tests.

Signs and symptoms

In both types of thrombophlebitis, clinical features vary with the site and length of the affected vein. Although deep-vein thrombophlebitis may occur asymptomatically, it may also produce severe pain, fever, chills, malaise, and possibly, swelling and cyanosis of the affected arm or leg. Superficial thrombophlebitis produces visible and palpable signs, such as heat, pain, swelling, rubor, tenderness, and induration along the length of the affected vein. Extensive vein involvement may cause lymphadenitis.

Diagnosis

Some patients may display signs of inflammation and, possibly, a positive Homans' sign (pain on dorsiflexion of the foot) during physical examination; others are asymptomatic. Consequently, essential laboratory tests include:

- *Doppler ultrasonography:* to identify reduced blood flow to a specific area and any obstruction to venous flow, particularly in iliofemoral deep-vein thrombophlebitis.
- *plethysmography:* to show decreased circulation distal to affected area; more sensitive than ultrasound in detecting deep-vein thrombophlebitis.
- *phlebography* (usually confirms diagnosis): to show filling defects and diverted blood flow.

Diagnosis must rule out arterial occlusive disease, lymphangitis, cellulitis, and myositis.

Diagnosis of superficial thrombophlebitis is based on physical examination (redness and warmth over affected area, palpable vein, and pain during palpation or compression).

Treatment

The goals of treatment are to control thrombus development, prevent complications, relieve pain, and prevent recurrence of the disorder. Symptomatic measures include bed rest, with elevation of the affected arm or leg; warm, moist soaks to the affected area; and analgesics, as ordered. After the acute episode of deep-vein thrombophlebitis subsides, the patient may begin to ambulate while wearing antiembolism stockings that were applied before he got out of bed.

Treatment may also include anticoagulants (initially, heparin; later, warfarin) to prolong clotting time. Full anticoagulant dose must be discontinued during any operative period, due to the risk of hemorrhage. After some types of surgery, especially major abdominal or pelvic operations, prophylactic doses of anticoagulants may reduce the risk of deep-vein thrombophlebitis and pulmonary embolism. For lysis of acute, extensive deep-vein thrombosis, treatment should include streptokinase. Rarely, deep-vein thrombophlebitis may cause complete venous occlusion, which necessitates venous interruption through simple ligation to vein plication, or clipping.

Therapy for severe superficial thrombophlebitis may include an anti-inflammatory drug, such as indomethacin, along with antiembolism stockings, warm soaks, and elevation of the patient's leg.

Special considerations

Patient teaching, identification of high-risk patients, and measures to prevent venostasis can prevent deep-vein thrombophlebitis; close monitoring of anticoagulant therapy can prevent serious complications, such internal hemorrhage.

CHRONIC VENOUS INSUFFICIENCY

Chronic venous insufficiency results from the valvular destruction of deep-vein thrombophlebitis, usually in the iliac and femoral veins, and occasionally, the saphenous veins. It's often accompanied by incompetence of the communicating veins at the ankle, causing increased venous pressure and fluid migration into the interstitial tissue. Clinical effects include chronic swelling of the affected leg from edema, leading to tissue fibrosis, and induration; skin discoloration from extravasation of blood in subcutaneous tissue; and stasis ulcers around the ankle.

Treatment of small ulcers includes bed rest, elevation of the legs, warm soaks, and antimicrobial therapy for infection. Treatment to counteract increased venous pressure, the result of reflux from the deep venous system to surface veins, may include compression dressings, such as a sponge rubber pressure dressing or a zinc gelatin boot (Unna's boot). This therapy begins after massive swelling subsides with leg elevation and bed rest.

Large stasis ulcers unresponsive to conservative treatment may require excision and skin grafting. Patient care includes daily inspection to assess healing. Other care measures are the same as for varicose veins.

- Enforce bed rest, as ordered, and elevate the patient's affected arm or leg. If you plan to use pillows for elevating the leg, place them so they support the entire length of the affected extremity to prevent possible compression of the popliteal space.
- Apply warm soaks to increase circulation to the affected area and to relieve pain and inflammation. Give analgesics to relieve pain, as ordered.
- Measure and record the circumference of the affected arm or leg daily, and compare this measurement to the other arm or leg. To ensure accuracy and consistency of serial measurements, mark the skin over the area and measure at the same spot daily.

VARICOSE VEINS

Varicose veins are dilated, tortuous veins, usually affecting the subcutaneous leg veins—the saphenous veins and their branches. They can result from congenital weakness of the valves or venous wall; from diseases of the venous system, such as deep-vein thrombophlebitis; from conditions that produce prolonged venostasis, such as pregnancy; or from occupations that necessitate standing for an extended period.

Varicose veins may be asymptomatic or produce mild to severe leg symptoms, including a feeling of heaviness; cramps at night; diffuse, dull aching after prolonged standing or walking; aching during menses; fatigability; palpable nodules; and with deep-vein incompetency, orthostatic edema and stasis pigmentation of the calves and ankles.

In mild to moderate varicose veins, antiembolism stockings or elastic bandages counteract pedal and ankle swelling by supporting the veins and improving circulation. An exercise program, such as walking, promotes muscular contraction and forces blood through the veins, thereby minimizing venous pooling. Severe varicose veins may necessitate stripping and ligation, or as an alternative to surgery, injection of a sclerosing agent into small affected vein segments.

To promote comfort and minimize worsening of varicosities:

- Discourage the patient from wearing constrictive clothing.
- Advise the patient to elevate his legs above heart level whenever possible and to avoid prolonged standing or sitting.

After stripping and ligation or after injection of a sclerosing agent:

- To relieve pain, administer analgesics, as ordered.
- Frequently check circulation in toes (color and temperature), and observe elastic bandages for bleeding. When ordered, rewrap bandages at least once a shift, wrapping from toe to thigh, with the leg elevated.
- Watch for signs of complications, such as sensory loss in the leg (which could indicate saphenous nerve damage), calf pain (thrombophlebitis), and fever (infection).

- Administer heparin I.V., as ordered, with an infusion monitor or pump to control the flow rate, if necessary.
- Measure partial thromboplastin time regularly for the patient on heparin therapy; prothrombin time for the patient on warfarin (therapeutic anticoagulation values for both are one and a half to two times control values). Watch for signs and symptoms of bleeding, such as dark, tarry stools; coffee-ground vomitus; and ecchymoses. Encourage the patient to use an electric razor and to avoid medications that contain aspirin.
- Be alert for signs of pulmonary emboli (rales, dyspnea, hemoptysis, sudden changes in mental status, restlessness, and hypotension).

To prepare the patient with thrombophlebitis for discharge:

- Emphasize the importance of follow-up blood studies to monitor anticoagulant therapy.
- If the patient is being discharged on heparin therapy, teach him or his family how to give subcutaneous injections. If he requires further assistance, arrange for a visiting nurse.
- Tell the patient to avoid prolonged sitting or standing to help prevent recurrence.
- Teach the patient how to properly apply and use antiembolism stockings. Tell him to report any complications, such as cold, blue toes.
- To prevent thrombophlebitis in high-risk patients, perform range-of-motion exercises while the patient is on bed rest, use intermittent pneumatic calf massage during lengthy surgical or diagnostic procedures, apply antiembolism stockings postoperatively, and encourage early ambulation.

Raynaud's Disease

Raynaud's disease is one of several primary arteriospastic disorders characterized by episodic vasospasm in the small peripheral arteries and arterioles, precipitated by exposure to cold or stress. This condition occurs bilaterally and usually affects the hands or, less often, the feet. Raynaud's disease is most prevalent in females, particularly between puberty and age 40. It is a benign condition, requiring no specific treatment and with no serious sequelae.

Raynaud's phenomenon, however, a condition often associated with several connective tissue disorders—such as scleroderma, systemic lupus erythematosus, or polymyositis—has a progressive course, leading to ischemia, gangrene, and amputation. Distinction between the two disorders is difficult, because some patients who experience mild symptoms of Raynaud's disease for several years may later develop overt connective tissue disease—especially scleroderma.

Causes

Although the cause is unknown, several theories account for the reduced digital blood flow: intrinsic vascular wall hyperactivity to cold, increased vasomotor tone due to sympathetic stimulation, and antigen-antibody immune response (the most probable theory, since abnormal immunologic test results accompany Raynaud's phenomenon).

Signs and symptoms

After exposure to cold or stress, the skin on the fingers typically blanches, then becomes cyanotic before changing to red and before changing from cold to normal temperature. Numbness and tingling may also occur. These symptoms are relieved by warmth. In long-standing disease, trophic changes, such as sclerodactyly, ulcerations, or chronic paronychia, may result. Although it's extremely uncommon, minimal cutaneous gangrene necessitates amputation of one or more phalanges.

Diagnosis

Clinical criteria that establish Raynaud's disease include skin color changes induced by cold or stress; bilateral involvement; absence of gangrene or, if present, minimal cutaneous gangrene; normal arterial pulses; and patient history of clinical symptoms of longer than 2 years' duration. Diagnosis must also rule out secondary disease processes, such as chronic arterial occlusive or connective tissue disease.

Treatment

Initially, treatment consists of avoidance of cold, mechanical, or chemical injury; cessation of smoking; and reassurance that symptoms are benign. Since drug side effects, especially from vasodilators, may be more bothersome than the disease itself, drug therapy is reserved for unusually severe symptoms. Such therapy may include phenoxybenzamine or reserpine. Sympathectomy may be helpful when conservative modalities fail to prevent ischemic ulcers and becomes necessary in less than 25% of patients.

Special considerations

- Warn against exposure to the cold. Tell the patient to wear mittens or gloves in cold weather or when handling cold items or defrosting the freezer.
- Advise the patient to avoid stressful situations and to stop smoking.
- Instruct the patient to inspect the skin frequently and to seek immediate care for signs of skin breakdown or infection.
- Teach the patient about drugs, their use, and their side effects.
- Provide psychological support and reassurance to allay the patient's fear of amputation and disfigurement.

Buerger's Disease

(Thromboangiitis obliterans)

Buerger's disease—an inflammatory, nonatheromatous occlusive condition—causes segmental lesions and subsequent thrombus formation in the small and medium arteries (and sometimes the veins), resulting in decreased blood flow to the feet and legs. This disorder may produce ulceration and, eventually, gangrene.

Causes

Although the cause of Buerger's disease is unknown, a definite link exists to smoking, suggesting a hypersensitivity reaction to nicotine. Incidence is highest among men of Jewish ancestry, aged 20 to 40, who smoke heavily.

Signs and symptoms

Buerger's disease typically produces intermittent claudication of the instep, which is aggravated by exercise and relieved by rest. During exposure to low temperature, the feet initially become cold, cyanotic, and numb; later, they redden, become hot, and tingle. Occasionally, Buerger's disease also affects the hands, possibly resulting in painful fingertip ulcerations. Associated signs and symptoms may include impaired peripheral pulses, migratory superficial thrombophlebitis, and, in later stages, ulceration, muscle atrophy, and gangrene.

Diagnosis

Patient history and physical examination strongly suggest Buerger's disease. Supportive diagnostic tests include:

- Doppler ultrasonography to show diminished circulation in the peripheral vessels
- plethysmography to help detect decreased circulation in the peripheral vessels
- arteriography to locate lesions and rule out atherosclerosis.

Treatment and special considerations

The primary goals of treatment are to relieve symptoms and prevent complications. Such therapy may include an exercise program that uses gravity to fill and drain the blood vessels or, in severe disease, a lumbar sympathectomy to increase blood supply to the skin. Amputation may be necessary for nonhealing ulcers, intractable pain, or gangrene.

- Strongly urge the patient to discontinue smoking permanently, to enhance the effectiveness of treatment. If necessary, refer him to a self-help group to stop smoking.
- Warn the patient to avoid precipitating factors, such as emotional stress, exposure to extreme temperatures, and trauma.
- Teach proper foot care, especially the importance of wearing well-fitting shoes and cotton or wool socks. Show the patient how to inspect his feet daily for cuts, abrasions, and signs of skin breakdown, such as redness and soreness. Remind him to seek medical attention immediately after any trauma.
- If the patient has ulcers and gangrene, enforce bed rest and use a padded footboard or bed cradle to prevent pressure from bed linens. Protect the feet with soft padding. Wash them gently with a mild soap and tepid water, rinse thoroughly, and pat dry with a soft towel.
- Provide emotional support. If necessary, refer the patient for psychological counseling to help him cope with restrictions imposed by this chronic disease. If he has undergone amputation, assess rehabilitative needs, especially regarding changes in body image. Refer him to physical therapists, occupational therapists, and social service agencies, as needed.

Arterial Occlusive Disease

Arterial occlusive disease is the obstruction or narrowing of the lumen of the aorta and its major branches, causing an interruption of blood flow, usually to the legs and feet. This disorder may affect the carotid, vertebral, innominate, subclavian, mesenteric, and celiac arteries. Occlusions may be acute or chronic, and often cause severe ischemia, skin ulceration, and gangrene.

Arterial occlusive disease is more common in males than in females. Prognosis depends on the location of the occlusion, the development of collateral circulation to counteract reduced blood flow, and, in acute disease, the time elapsed between occlusion and its removal.

Causes

Arterial occlusive disease is a frequent complication of atherosclerosis. The occlusive mechanism may be endogenous, due to emboli formation or thrombosis, or exogenous, due to trauma or fracture. Predisposing factors include smoking; aging; conditions such as hypertension, hyperlipemia, and diabetes; and family history of vascular disorders, myocardial infarction, or cerebrovascular accident.

Diagnosis

Diagnosis of arterial occlusive disease is usually indicated by patient history and physical examination.

Pertinent supportive diagnostic tests include the following:

- *Arteriography* demonstrates the type (thrombus or embolus), location, and degree of obstruction, and the collateral circulation. Arteriography is particularly useful in chronic disease or for evaluating candidates for reconstructive surgery.
- *Doppler ultrasonography* and *plethysmography* are noninvasive tests that, in acute disease, show decreased blood flow distal to the occlusion.
- *Ophthalmodynamometry* helps determine degree of obstruction in the internal carotid artery by comparing ophthalmic artery pressure to brachial artery pressure on the affected side. More than a 20% difference between pressures suggests insufficiency.
- *Electroencephalogram* and *computed tomography scan* may be necessary to rule out brain lesions.

Treatment

Generally, treatment of arterial occlusive disease depends on the cause, location, and size of the obstruction. For patients with mild chronic disease, treatment usually consists of supportive measures, elimination of smoking, hypertension control, and walking exercise. For patients with carotid artery occlusion, antiplatelet therapy may begin with dipyridamole and aspirin. For those with intermittent claudication caused by chronic arterial occlusive disease, pentoxifylline (Trental) may improve blood flow through the capillaries. This drug is particularly useful for patients who aren't good candidates for surgery.

Acute arterial occlusive disease usually necessitates surgery to restore circulation to the affected area. Appropriate surgical procedures may include the following:

- *Embolectomy:* In this procedure, a balloon-tipped Fogarty catheter is used to remove thrombotic material from the artery. Embolectomy is used mainly for mesenteric, femoral, or popliteal artery occlusion.
- *Thromboendarterectomy:* This procedure involves the opening of the artery and removal of the obstructing thrombus (atherosclerotic plaque) and the medial layer of the arterial wall. Thromboendarterectomy is usually performed after angiography, and is often used in con-

junction with autogenous vein or Dacron bypass surgery (femoral-popliteal or aortofemoral).

• *Patch grafting:* This procedure involves removal of the thrombosed arterial segment and replacement with an autogenous vein or Dacron graft.

• *Bypass graft:* In this procedure, blood flow is diverted through an anastomosed autogenous or woven Dacron graft to by-

ARTERIAL OCCLUSIVE DISEASE

SITE OF OCCLUSION	SIGNS AND SYMPTOMS
Carotid arterial system • Internal carotids • External carotids	Neurologic dysfunction: transient ischemic attacks (TIAs) due to reduced cerbral circulation produce unilateral sensory or motor dysfunction (transient monocular blindness, hemiparesis), possible aphasia or dysarthria, confusion, decreased mentation, and headache. These recurrent clinical features usually last 5 to 10 minutes but may persist up to 24 hours, and may herald a stroke. Absent or decreased pulsation with an auscultatory bruit over the affected vessels.
Vertebrobasilar system • Vertebral arteries • Basilar arteries	Neurologic dysfunction: TIAs of brain stem and cerebellum produce binocular visual disturbances, vertigo, dysarthria, and "drop attacks" (falling down without loss of consciousness). Less common than carotid TIA.
Innominate • Brachiocephalic artery	Neurologic dysfunction: signs and symptoms of vertebrobasilar occlusion. Indications of ischemia (claudication) of right arm; possible bruit over right side of neck.
Subclavian artery	Subclavian steal syndrome (characterized by the backflow of blood from the brain through the vertebral artery on the same side as the occlusion, into the subclavian artery distal to the occlusion); clinical effects of vertebrobasilar occlusion and exercise-induced arm claudication. Possible gangrene, usually limited to the digits.
Mesenteric artery • Superior (most commonly affected) • Celiac axis • Inferior	Bowel ischemia, infarct necrosis, and gangrene; sudden, acute abdominal pain; nausea and vomiting; diarrhea; leukocytosis; and shock due to massive intraluminal fluid and plasma loss.
Aortic bifurcation (saddle block occlusion, a medical emergency associated with cardiac embolization)	Sensory and motor deficits (muscle weakness, numbness, paresthesias, paralysis), and signs of ischemia (sudden pain; cold, pale legs with decreased or absent peripheral pulses) in both legs.
Iliac artery (Leriche's syndrome)	Intermittent claudication of lower back, buttocks, and thighs, relieved by rest; absent or reduced femoral or distal pulses; possible bruit over femoral arteries; impotence in males.
Femoral and popliteal artery (associated with aneurysm formation)	Intermittent claudication of the calves on exertion; ischemic pain in feet; pretrophic pain (heralds necrosis and ulceration); leg pallor and coolness; blanching of feet on elevation; gangrene; no palpable pulses in ankles and feet.

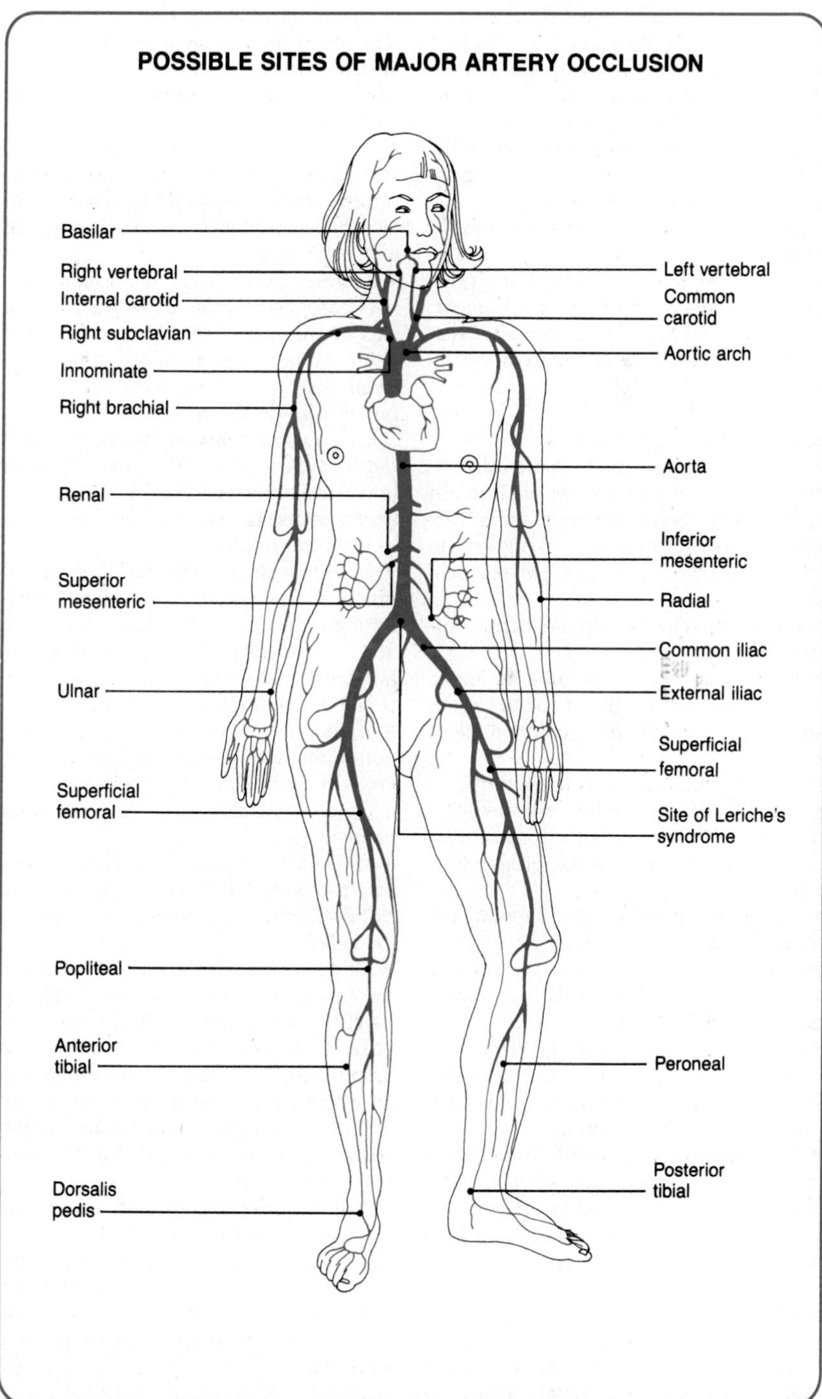
POSSIBLE SITES OF MAJOR ARTERY OCCLUSION
Basilar
Right vertebral
Internal carotid
Right subclavian
Innominate
Right brachial
Renal
Superior mesenteric
Ulnar
Superficial femoral
Popliteal
Anterior tibial
Dorsalis pedis
Left vertebral
Common carotid
Aortic arch
Aorta
Inferior mesenteric
Radial
Common iliac
External iliac
Superficial femoral
Site of Leriche's syndrome
Peroneal
Posterior tibial

pass the thrombosed arterial segment.
• *Lumbar sympathectomy:* Depending on the condition of the sympathetic nervous system, this procedure may be an adjunct to reconstructive surgery.

Amputation becomes necessary with failure of arterial reconstructive surgery or with the development of gangrene, uncontrollable infection, or intractable pain.

Other appropriate therapy includes heparin to prevent emboli (for embolic occlusion) and bowel resection after restoration of blood flow (for mesenteric artery occlusion).

Special considerations

• Provide comprehensive patient teaching, such as proper foot care. Explain all diagnostic tests and procedures. Advise the patient to stop smoking and to follow the prescribed medical regimen closely.

Preoperatively, during an acute episode:

• Assess the patient's circulatory status by checking for the most distal pulses and by inspecting his skin color and temperature.
• Provide pain relief, as needed.
• Administer heparin by continuous I.V. drip, as ordered. Use an infusion monitor or pump to ensure the proper flow rate.
• Wrap the patient's affected foot in soft cotton batting, and reposition it frequently to prevent pressure on any one area. Strictly avoid elevating or applying heat to the affected leg.
• Watch for signs of fluid and electrolyte imbalance, and monitor intake and output for signs of renal failure (urine output less than 30 ml/hour).
• If the patient has carotid, innominate, vertebral, or subclavian artery occlusion, monitor him for signs of cerebrovascular accident, such as numbness in an arm or leg and intermittent blindness.

Postoperatively:

• Monitor the patient's vital signs. Continuously assess his circulatory function by inspecting skin color and temperature and by checking for distal pulses. In charting, compare earlier assessments and observations. Watch closely for signs of hemorrhage (tachycardia, hypotension), and check dressings for excessive bleeding.
• In carotid, innominate, vertebral, or subclavian artery occlusion, assess neurologic status frequently for changes in level of consciousness or muscle strength and pupil size.
• In mesenteric artery occlusion, connect nasogastric tube to low intermittent suction. Monitor intake and output (low urine output may indicate damage to renal arteries during surgery). Check bowel sounds for return of peristalsis. Increasing abdominal distention and tenderness may indicate extension of bowel ischemia with resulting gangrene, necessitating further excision, or it may indicate peritonitis.
• In saddle block occlusion, check distal pulses for adequate circulation. Watch for signs of renal failure and mesenteric artery occlusion (severe abdominal pain), and for cardiac arrhythmias, which may precipitate embolus formation.
• In iliac artery occlusion, monitor urine output for signs of renal failure from decreased perfusion to the kidneys, as a result of surgery. Provide meticulous catheter care.
• In both femoral and popliteal artery occlusions, assist with early ambulation, but don't allow the patient to sit for an extended period.
• When caring for a patient who has undergone amputation, check the stump carefully for drainage. If drainage occurs, note and record its color and amount, and the time. Elevate the stump, as ordered, and administer adequate analgesic medication. Since phantom limb pain is common, explain this phenomenon to the patient.
• When preparing the patient for discharge, instruct him to watch for signs of recurrence (pain, pallor, numbness, paralysis, absence of pulse) that can result from graft occlusion or occlusion at another site. Warn him against wearing constrictive clothing.

Selected References

Adams, F.H., and Emmanouilides, G.C., eds. *Moss' Heart Disease in Infants, Children, and Adolescents,* 3rd ed. Baltimore: Williams & Wilkins Co., 1983.

Berne, R.M., and Levy, M.N. *Cardiovascular Physiology,* 4th ed. St. Louis: C.V. Mosby Co., 1981.

Braunwald, Eugene, M.D. *Heart Disease: A Textbook of Cardiovascular Medicine,* vol. 2. Philadelphia: W.B. Saunders Co., 1984.

Dec, William G., Jr., et al. "Active Myocarditis in the Spectrum of Acute Dilated Cardiomyopathies," *New England Journal of Medicine* 312(14):885, April 4, 1985.

Elenbaas, Robert M., ed. "Pharmacologic Management of Shock," *Critical Care Quarterly* 2:4, March 1980.

Guzzetta, C., and Dossey, B. *Cardiovascular Nursing: Bodymind Tapestry.* Philadelphia: J.B. Lippincott Co., 1983.

Hills, David, M.D., et al. *Manual of Clinical Problems in Cardiology with Annotated Key References.* Boston: Little, Brown & Co., 1981.

Hurst, J. Willis, et al. *The Heart.* New York: McGraw-Hill Book Co., 1982.

Loeb, J.M. "Cardiac Electrophysiology: Basic Concepts and Arrhythmogenesis," *Critical Care Quarterly* 7(2):9-19, September 1984.

Petersdorf, Robert G., et al. *Harrison's Principles of Internal Medicine,* 10th ed. New York: McGraw-Hill Book Co., 1983.

Sadler, Diane. *Nursing for Cardiovascular Health.* East Norwalk, Conn.: Appleton-Century-Crofts, 1984.

Schroeder, J.S., ed. *Invasive Cardiology.* Philadelphia: F.A. Davis Co., 1985.

Smith, J.B. *Pediatric Critical Care.* New York: John Wiley & Sons, 1983.

Stone, K., et al. "Understanding Calcium Channel Blockers," *Heart & Lung* 13(5):563-73, 1984.

Underhill, Sandra, et al. *Cardiac Nursing.* Philadelphia: J.B. Lippincott Co., 1983.

Williams, W.G., et al. "Early Experience with Arterial Repair of Transposition," *Annals of Thoracic Surgery* 32:8-15, 1981.

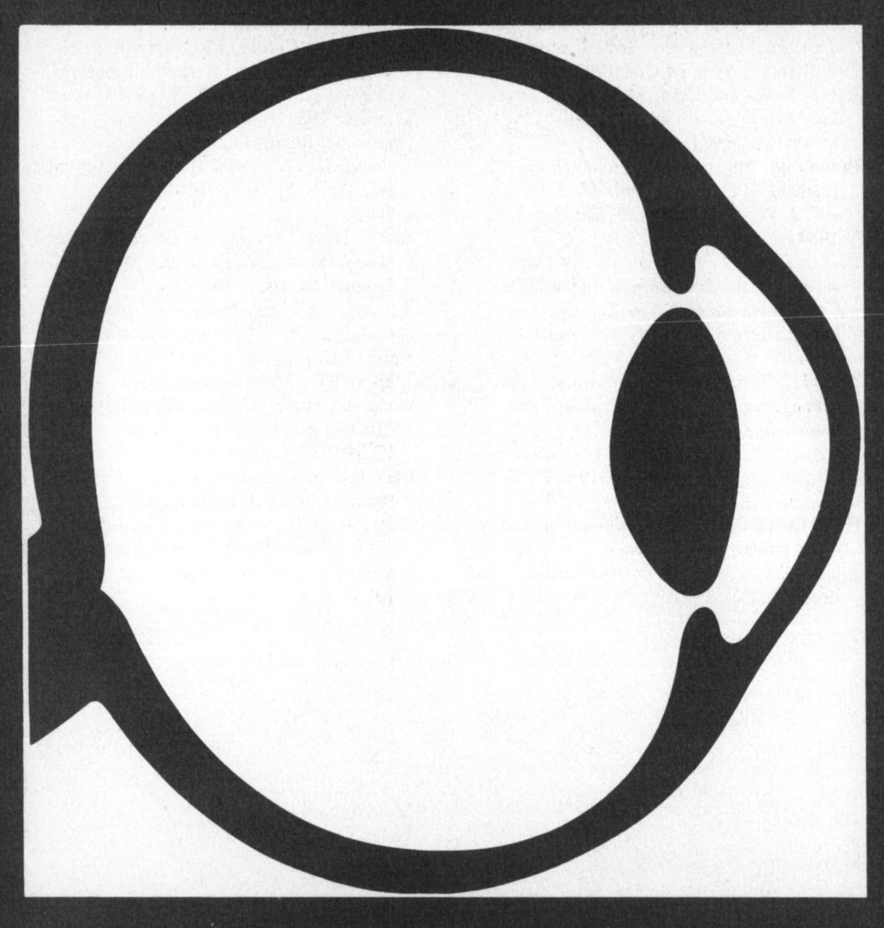

19 Eye Disorders

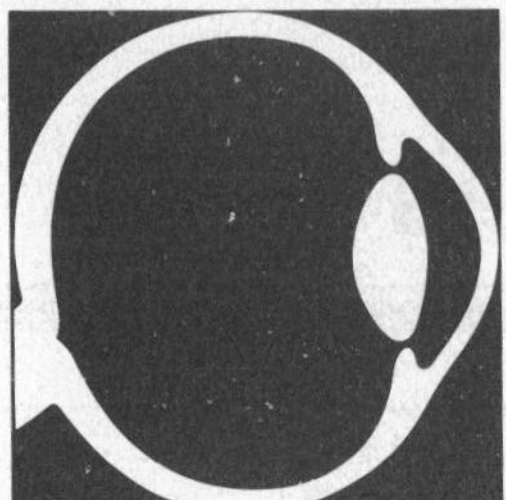

Eye Disorders

Introduction

Vision, the most complex sense, has recently been the focus of some of the greatest medical and surgical innovations. Disorders that affect the eye generally lead to vision loss or impairment; therefore, routine ophthalmic examinations and early treatment are essential.

Review of anatomy

The visual system consists mainly of the bony orbit, which houses the eye; the contents of the orbit, including the eyeball, optic nerves, extraocular muscles, cranial nerves, blood vessels, orbital fat, and lacrimal system; and the eyelids, which protect and cover the eye.

The *orbit* (or socket) encloses the eye in a protective recess in the skull. Its seven bones—frontal, sphenoid, zygomatic, maxilla, palatine, ethmoid, and lacrimal—form a cone, the apex of which points toward the brain; the cone's base forms the orbital rim. The periorbita covers the bones of the orbit.

Extraocular muscles hold the eyes in place and control their movement:

- *superior rectus:* primary function, rotates the eye upward; secondary function, adducts and rotates the eye inward
- *inferior rectus:* primary function, rotates the eye downward; secondary function, adducts and rotates the eye outward
- *lateral rectus:* primary function, turns the eye outward (laterally)
- *medial rectus:* primary function, turns the eye inward (medially)
- *superior oblique:* primary function, turns the eye downward; secondary function, abducts and rotates the eye inward
- *inferior oblique:* primary function, turns the eye upward; secondary function, abducts and turns the eye outward.

The actions of these muscles are mutually antagonistic: as one contracts, its opposing muscle relaxes.

Ocular layers

The eye has three structural layers: the sclera and cornea, the uveal tract, and the retina.

The *sclera* is the dense, white, fibrous outer protective coat of the eye. It meets the cornea at the limbus (corneoscleral junction) anteriorly, and the dural sheath of the optic nerve posteriorly. The lamina cribrosa is a sievelike structure composed of a few strands of scleral tissue that support the optic disk. The sclera is covered by the episclera, a thin layer of fine elastic tissue.

The *cornea* is the transparent, avascular, curved layer of the eye that is continuous with the sclera. The cornea consists of five layers: the epithelium, which contains sensory nerves; Bowman's membrane, the basement membrane for the epithelial cells; the stroma, or supporting tissue (90% of the corneal structure); Descemet's membrane, containing many elastic fibers; and the endothelium, a single layer of cells that acts as a pump to maintain proper hydration of the cornea. Aqueous humor bathes the surface of the cornea, maintaining intraocular pressure by volume and rate of outflow. The cornea's sole function is to refract light rays.

The middle layer of the eye, the *uveal tract,* is pigmented and vascular. It consists of the iris and the ciliary body in the anterior portion, and the choroid in the posterior portion. In the center of the iris is the pupil. The sphincter and dilator muscles control the amount of light that enters the eye through the pupil, while the pupil itself allows aqueous humor to flow from the posterior chamber

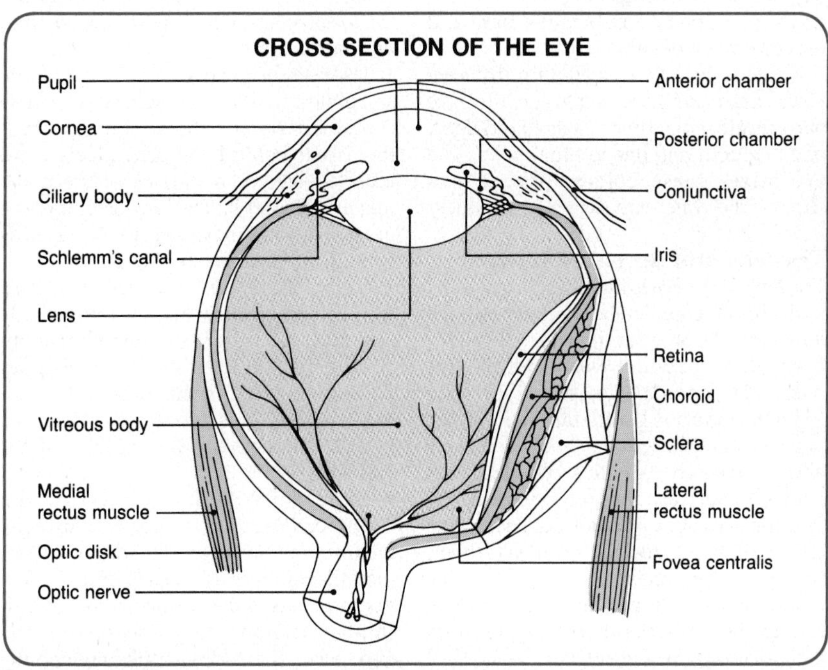

into the anterior chamber.

The anterior iris joins the posterior corneal surface at an angle, where many small collecting channels form the trabecular meshwork. Aqueous humor drains through these channels into an encircling venous system called the canal of Schlemm.

The *ciliary body,* which extends from the root of the iris to the ora serrata, produces aqueous humor and controls lens accommodation through its action on the zonules of Zinn. The *choroid,* the largest part of the uveal tract, is made up of blood vessels and is bound by Bruch's membrane.

The *retina,* the most essential structure, receives the light rays from all other parts of the eye. The retina extends from the ora serrata to the optic nerve; the retinal pigment epithelium (RPE) adheres lightly to the choroid. Located next to the RPE are rods and cones. Although both rods and cones are light receptors, they respond to light differently. Rods, scattered throughout the retina, respond to low levels of light and detect moving objects; cones, located in the fovea centralis, function best in brighter light and perceive finer details.

Three types of cones contain different visual pigments and react to specific light wavelengths: one type reacts to red light, one to green, and one to blue-violet. The eye mixes these colors into various shades; the cones can detect 150 shades.

The lens and accommodation

The *lens* of the eye is biconvex, avascular, and almost completely transparent; the lens capsule is a semipermeable membrane that can admit water and electrolytes. The lens changes shape for near (accommodation) and far vision. For near vision, the ciliary body contracts and relaxes the zonules, the lens becomes spherical, the pupil constricts, and the eyes converge; for far vision, the ciliary body relaxes, the zonules tighten, the lens becomes flatter, the eyes straighten, and the pupils dilate. The lens refines the refraction necessary to focus a clear image on the retina.

The *vitreous body,* which is 99% water and a small amount of insoluble protein, composes two thirds of the volume of the eye. This gelatinous body gives the eye its shape and contributes to the refraction of light rays. The vitreous is firmly attached to part of the ciliary body and to a small section of the retina; it contacts but doesn't adhere to the lens, zonules, retina, and optic nerve head.

Lacrimal network and eyelids

The lacrimal apparatus consists of the lacrimal gland, upper and lower canaliculi, lacrimal sac, and nasolacrimal duct. The gland, located in a shallow fossa beneath the superior temporal orbital rim, secretes tears, which keep the cornea and conjunctiva moist. These tears flow through 8 to 12 excretory ducts, and contain lysozyme, an enzyme that protects the conjunctiva from bacterial invasion. With every blink, the eyelids direct the flow to the inner canthus, where the tears pool and then drain through a tiny opening called the punctum. The tears then pass through the canaliculi and lacrimal sac and down the nasolacrimal duct, which opens into the nasal cavity.

The eyelids (palpebrae) consist of tarsal plates that are composed of dense connective tissue. The orbital septum—the fascia behind the orbicularis oculi muscle—acts as a barrier between the lids and the orbit. The levator palpebrae muscle elevates the upper lid. The eyelids contain three types of glands:

- *meibomian glands:* sebaceous glands in the tarsal plates that secrete an oily substance to lubricate the tear film; about 25 of these glands are found in the upper lid and about 20 in the lower lid
- *glands of Zeis:* modified sebaceous glands connected to the follicles of the eyelashes
- *Moll's glands:* ordinary sweat glands.

The *conjunctiva* is the thin mucous membrane that lines the eyelids (palpebral conjunctiva), folds over at the fornix, and covers the surface of the eyeball (bulbar conjunctiva). The ophthalmic and lacrimal arteries supply blood to the lids. The space between the open lids is the palpebral fissure; the juncture of the upper and lower lids is the canthus. The junction near the nose is called the nasal, medial, or inner canthus; the junction on the temporal side, the lateral or external canthus.

Depth perception

In normal binocular vision, a perceived image is projected onto the two foveae. Impulses then travel along the optic pathways to the occipital cortex, which perceives a single image. However, the cortex receives two images—each from a slightly different angle—giving the images perspective and providing depth perception.

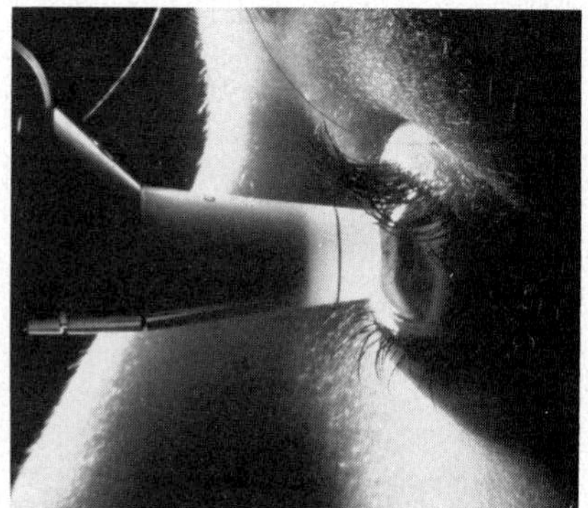

Applanation tonometry determines intraocular pressure by measuring the force required to flatten a small area of the central cornea.

Vision testing

Several tests assess visual acuity and identify visual defects:

- *Ishihara's test* determines color blindness by using a series of plates composed of a colored background, with a letter, number, or pattern of a contrasting color located in the center of each plate. The patient with deficient color perception can't perceive the differences in color or, consequently, the designs formed by the color contrasts.
- The *Snellen chart* or other eye charts evaluate visual acuity. Such charts use progressively smaller letters or symbols to determine central vision on a numerical scale. A person with normal acuity should be able to read the letters or recognize the symbols on the 20-foot line of the eye chart at a distance of 20 feet.
- *Ophthalmoscopy,* direct ophthalmoscopy or binocular indirect ophthalmoscopy, allows examination of the interior of the eye after the pupil has been dilated with a mydriatic.
- *Refraction tests* may be performed with or without cycloplegics. In cycloplegic refraction, eyedrops weaken the accommodative power of the ciliary muscle, which facilitates the use of an ophthalmoscope. A retinoscope directs a beam of light into the pupil; the light's shadow is neutralized by placing the appropriate lens in front of the eye.
- *Maddox rod test* assesses muscle dysfunction; it's especially useful to disclose and measure heterophoria (the tendency of the eyes to deviate).
- *Duction test* checks eye movement in all directions of gaze. While one eye is covered, the other eye follows a moving light. This test detects any weakness of rotation due to muscle paralysis or structural dysfunction.
- The *test for convergence* locates the breaking point of fusion. For this test, the examiner holds a small object in front of the patient's nose and slowly brings it closer to the patient. Normally, the patient can maintain convergence until the object reaches the bridge of the nose. The point at which the eyes "break" is termed the near point of convergence and is given a number.
- The *cover-uncover test* assesses muscle deviation. The patient stares at a small, fixed object—first, from a distance of 20′ (6 m); then, from 12″ (30 cm). The examiner covers the patient's eyes one at a time, noting any movement of the uncovered eye, the direction of any deviation, and the rate at which the eyes recover normal binocular vision when latent heterophoria is present. A corollary test, the *alternate cover test*, also tests for deviation.
- *Slit-lamp examination* allows a well-illuminated microscopic examination of

the eyelids and the anterior segment of the eyeball.

• *Visual field* tests the function of the retina, the optic nerve, and the optic pathways when both central and peripheral visual fields are examined.

• *Schiøtz tonometry* and *applanation tonometry* measure intraocular pressure. After instilling a local anesthetic in the patient's eye, the examiner places the Schiøtz tonometer lightly on the corneal surface and measures the indentation of the cornea produced by a given weight. Applanation tonometry gauges the force required to flatten, rather than indent, a small area of central cornea.

• *Gonioscopy* allows for direct visualization of the anterior chamber angle through use of a goniolens; the slit lamp is the light source and microscope.

• *Ophthalmodynamometry* measures the relative central retinal artery pressures and indirectly assesses carotid artery flow on each side.

• *Fluorescein angiography* evaluates the anatomic and physiologic states of the blood vessels in the choroid and the retina after I.V. injection of fluorescein dye; images of the dye-enhanced vasculature are recorded by rapid-sequence photographs of the fundus.

EYELIDS AND LACRIMAL DUCTS

Blepharitis

A common inflammation, especially in children, blepharitis produces a red-rimmed appearance of the margins of the eyelids. It's frequently chronic and often bilateral and can affect both upper and lower lids. It usually occurs as seborrheic (nonulcerative) blepharitis, characterized by greasy scales, or as staphylococcal (ulcerative) blepharitis, characterized by dry scales, with tiny ulcerated areas along the lid margins. Both types may coexist. Blepharitis tends to recur and become chronic. It can be controlled if treatment begins before onset of ocular involvement.

Causes and incidence

Seborrheic blepharitis generally results from seborrhea of the scalp, eyebrows, and ears; ulcerative blepharitis, from *Staphylococcus aureus* infection. (Persons with this infection may also be apt to develop chalazions and styes.) Blepharitis may also result from pediculosis (from *Phthirus pubis* or *Pediculus humanus capitis*) of the brows and lashes, which irritates the lid margins.

Signs and symptoms

Clinical features of blepharitis include itching, burning, foreign-body sensation, and sticky, crusted eyelids on waking. This constant irritation results in unconscious rubbing of the eyes (causing reddened rims) or continual blinking. Other signs include greasy scales in seborrheic blepharitis; flaky scales on lashes, loss of lashes, ulcerated areas on lid margins in ulcerative blepharitis; and nits on lashes in pediculosis.

Diagnosis

Diagnosis depends on patient history and characteristic symptoms. In ulcerative blepharitis, culture of ulcerated lid margin shows *S. aureus*. In pediculosis, examination of the lashes reveals nits.

Treatment

Early treatment is essential to prevent recurrence or complications. Treatment depends on the type of blepharitis:

• *seborrheic blepharitis:* daily shampooing (using a mild shampoo on a damp applicator stick or a washcloth) to remove scales from the lid margins; also,

frequent shampooing of the scalp and eyebrows
• *ulcerative blepharitis:* sulfonamide eye ointment or an appropriate antibiotic
• *blepharitis resulting from pediculosis:* removal of nits (with forceps), or application of ophthalmic physostigmine ointment as an insecticide (this may cause pupil constriction and, possibly, headache, conjunctival irritation, and blurred vision from the film of ointment on the cornea).

Special considerations

• Instruct the patient to remove scales from the lid margins daily, with an applicator stick or clean washcloth.
• Teach the patient the following method for applying warm compresses: First, run warm water into a clean bowl. Then, immerse a clean cloth in the water and wring it out. Then place the warm cloth against the closed eyelid (be careful not to burn the skin). Hold the compress in place until it cools. Continue this procedure for 15 minutes.
• If blepharitis results from pediculosis, check the patient's family and other contacts, and notify local health authorities.

Exophthalmos

(Proptosis)

Exophthalmos is the unilateral or bilateral bulging or protrusion of the eyeballs or their apparent forward displacement (with lid retraction). Prognosis depends on the underlying cause.

Causes

Exophthalmos commonly results from ophthalmic—not systemic—Graves' disease in which forward displacement of the eyeballs and lid retraction occur. Unilateral exophthalmos may also result from trauma (such as fracture of the ethmoid bone, which allows air from the sinus to enter the orbital tissue, displacing soft tissue and the eyeball). Exophthalmos may also stem from hemorrhage, varicosities, thrombosis, aneurysms, and edema, which similarly displace the eyeball(s).

Other systemic and ocular causes include the following:
• *infection:* orbital cellulitis, panophthalmitis, and infection of the lacrimal gland or orbital tissues
• *tumors and neoplastic diseases:* especially in children—rhabdomyosarcomas, leukemia, gliomas of the optic nerve, dermoid cysts, teratomas, metastatic neuroblastomas, and African lymphoma; in adults—lacrimal gland tumors, mucoceles, meningiomas, and metastatic carcinomas
• *parasitic cysts:* in surrounding tissue
• *paralysis of extraocular muscles:* relaxation of eyeball retractors, congenital macrophthalmia, and high myopia.

Signs and symptoms

The obvious effect is a bulging eyeball, commonly with diplopia, if extraocular muscle edema causes misalignment. A rim of the sclera may be visible around the limbus, and the patient may blink infrequently. Other symptoms depend on the cause: pain may accompany traumatic exophthalmos; a tumor may produce conjunctival hyperemia or chemosis; retraction of the upper lid predisposes to exposure keratitis. If exophthalmos is associated with cavernous sinus thrombosis, the patient may exhibit paresis of the muscles supplied by cranial nerves III, IV, and VI; limited ocular movement; and a septic-type (high) fever.

Diagnosis

Exophthalmos is obvious on physical examination; exophthalmometer readings

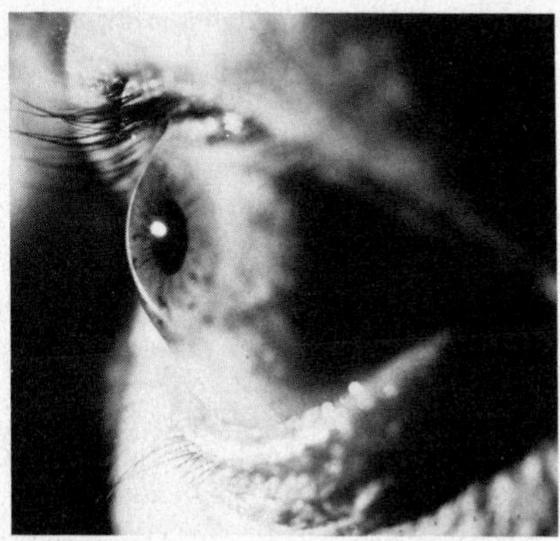

This photo of exophthalmos shows characteristic forward protrusion of the eye from the orbit.

confirm diagnosis by showing the degree of anterior projection and asymmetry between the eyes (normal bar readings range from 12 to 20 mm). Other diagnostic measures identify the cause:

- *X-rays* show orbital fracture or bony erosion by an orbital tumor.
- *CAT scan* detects pathology (lesions in the optic nerve, orbit, or ocular muscle) in the area within the orbit that is, relatively, radiologically blind.
- *Culture* of discharge from cellulitis or panophthalmitis determines the infecting organism; sensitivity testing indicates appropriate antibiotic therapy.
- *Biopsy* of orbital tissue may be necessary if initial treatment fails.

Treatment

The goal of treatment is to correct the underlying cause. For example, eye trauma may require cold compresses for the first 24 hours, followed by warm compresses, and prophylactic antibiotic therapy. After edema subsides, surgery may be necessary. Eye infection requires treatment with broad-spectrum antibiotics during the 24 hours preceding positive identification of the organism, followed by specific antibiotics. A patient with exophthalmos resulting from an orbital tumor may initially benefit from antibiotic or corticosteroid therapy. Eventually, however, surgical exploration of the orbit and, depending on the tumor, excision of the tumor, enucleation, or exenteration may be necessary. When primary orbital tumors, such as rhabdomyosarcoma, can't be fully excised as encapsulated lesions, radiation and chemotherapy may be used.

Treatment of Graves' disease may include antithyroid drug therapy or partial or total thyroidectomy to control hyperthyroidism; initial high doses of systemic corticosteroids, such as prednisone, for optic neuropathy; and, if lid retraction is severe, application of protective lubricants.

Surgery may include lateral tarsorrhaphy (suturing the lateral sections of the eyelids together) to correct lid retraction, or Krönlein's operation (removal of the superior and lateral orbital walls) to decompress the orbit. Such decompression is necessary if vision is threatened.

Special considerations

- Administer medication (steroids, antibiotics), as ordered, and carefully record the patient's response to therapy.
- Apply cold and warm compresses, as ordered, for fractures or other trauma.
- Provide postoperative care.
- Explain tests and procedures thoroughly to the patient and family.
- Give emotional support, especially to those with sudden exophthalmos.

Ptosis

Ptosis (drooping of the upper eyelid) may be congenital or acquired, unilateral or bilateral, constant or intermittent. Severe ptosis usually responds well to treatment; slight ptosis may require no treatment at all.

Causes and incidence

Congenital ptosis is transmitted as an autosomal dominant trait or results from a congenital anomaly in which the levator muscles of the eyelids fail to develop. This condition is usually bilateral.

Acquired ptosis may result from any of the following:

- *age* (senile ptosis), which causes loss of tone in the levator muscles, usually producing bilateral ptosis.
- *mechanical factors* that make the eyelid heavy, such as swelling caused by a foreign body on the palpebral surface of the eyelid or by edema, inflammation produced by a tumor or pseudotumor, or an extra fatty fold.
- *myogenic factors,* such as muscular dystrophy or myasthenia gravis (in which the defect seems to be in humoral transmission at the myoneural junction).
- *neurogenic (paralytic) factors* from interference in innervation of the eyelid by the oculomotor nerve (cranial nerve III), most commonly due to trauma, diabetes, or carotid aneurysm.
- *nutritional factors,* especially Wernicke's syndrome, due to severe chronic alcoholism, hyperemesis gravidarum, and other malnutrition-producing states.

Signs and symptoms

An infant with congenital ptosis has a smooth, flat upper eyelid, without the tarsal fold normally caused by the pull of the levator muscle; associated weakness of the superior rectus muscle is not uncommon.

The child with unilateral ptosis that covers the pupil can develop an amblyopic eye from disuse or lack of eye stimulation. In bilateral ptosis, the child may elevate his brow in an attempt to compensate, wrinkling his forehead in an effort to raise the upper lid. Also, the child may tilt his head backward to see.

In myasthenia gravis, ptosis results from fatigue and characteristically appears in the evening, but is relieved by rest. In addition to ptosis, oculomotor nerve damage produces a fixed, dilated pupil; divergent strabismus; and slight depression of the eyeball.

Diagnosis

A physical examination that consists of measuring palpebral fissure widths, range of lid movement, and relation of lid margin to upper border of the cornea will show the severity of ptosis. Diagnosis also includes tests to determine the underlying cause:

- *glucose tolerance test:* diabetes
- *edrophonium test:* myasthenia gravis (in acquired ptosis with no history of trauma)
- *ophthalmologic examination:* foreign bodies
- *patient history:* Wernicke's syndrome
- *cerebral arteriography:* aneurysm.

Treatment

Slight ptosis that doesn't produce deformity or loss of vision requires no treatment. Severe ptosis that interferes with vision or is cosmetically undesirable usually necessitates resection of the weak levator muscles. Surgery to correct congenital ptosis is usually performed at age 3 or 4, but it may be done earlier if ptosis is unilateral, since the totally occluded pupil may cause an amblyopic eye. If surgery is undesirable, special glasses with an attached suspended crutch on the frames may elevate the eyelid.

Effective treatment of ptosis also requires treatment of the underlying cause. For example, in patients with myasthenia gravis, neostigmine may be prescribed to increase the effect of acetylcholine and aid transmission of nerve impulses to muscles.

Special considerations

- Report any bleeding immediately. After surgery to correct ptosis, watch for blood on the pressure patch. (Some surgical procedures may not require a patch.) Apply ointment to the sutures, as prescribed.
- Emphasize to the patient and family the need to prevent accidental trauma to the surgical site until healing is complete (6 weeks). Suture line damage can precipitate recurrence of ptosis.

Orbital Cellulitis

Orbital cellulitis is an acute infection of the orbital tissues and eyelids that doesn't involve the eyeball. With treatment, prognosis is good; if cellulitis is not treated, infection may spread to the cavernous sinus or the meninges.

Causes and incidence

Orbital cellulitis is usually secondary to streptococcal, staphylococcal, or pneumococcal infection of nearby structures. These organisms then invade the orbit, frequently by direct extension through the sinuses (especially the ethmoidal sinus), the bloodstream, or the lymphatic ducts. Primary orbital cellulitis results from orbital trauma that permits entry of bacteria, such as an insect bite. It's most common in young children.

Signs and symptoms

Orbital cellulitis generally produces unilateral eyelid edema, hyperemia of the orbital tissues, reddened eyelids, and matted lashes. Although the eyeball is initially unaffected, proptosis develops later (because of edematous tissues within the bony confines of the orbit). Other indications include extreme orbital pain, impaired eye movement, chemosis, and purulent discharge from indurated areas. The severity of associated systemic symptoms (chills, fever, and malaise that may progress to marked debility) varies according to the cause.

Complications include posterior extension, causing cavernous sinus thrombosis, meningitis, or brain abscess, and, rarely, atrophy and subsequent loss of vision secondary to optic neuritis.

Diagnosis

Typical clinical features establish diagnosis. Wound culture and sensitivity testing determine the causative organism and specific antibiotic therapy. Other tests include *WBC count* (elevated from orbital tissue infection) and *ophthalmologic examination* (to rule out cavernous sinus thrombosis).

Treatment

Prompt treatment is necessary to prevent complications. Primary treatment consists of antibiotic therapy, depending on the results of culture and sensitivity tests. Systemic antibiotics (I.V., P.O.) and eye drops or ointment will be ordered. Supportive therapy consists of fluids; warm, moist compresses; and bed rest. If antibiotics fail, incision and drainage may be necessary.

Special considerations

- Monitor vital signs, and maintain fluid and electrolyte balance.
- Apply compresses every 3 to 4 hours to localize inflammation and relieve discomfort. Teach the patient to apply these compresses. Give pain medication, as ordered, after assessing pain level.
- Before discharge, stress the importance of completing prescribed antibiotic therapy. To prevent orbital cellulitis, tell the patient to maintain good general hygiene and to carefully cleanse abrasions and cuts that occur near the orbit. Urge early treatment of orbital cellulitis to prevent infection from spreading.

Dacryocystitis

Dacryocystitis is a common infection of the lacrimal sac. In adults, it results from an obstruction (dacryostenosis) of the nasolacrimal duct (most often in women over age 40) or from trauma; in infants, it results from congenital atresia of the nasolacrimal duct. Dacryocystitis can be acute or chronic and is usually unilateral.

Causes

The most common infecting organism in acute dacryocystitis is *Staphylococcus aureus* or, occasionally, beta-hemolytic streptococcus. In chronic dacryocystitis, *Streptococcus pneumoniae* and, sometimes, a fungus—such as *Candida albicans*—are the causative organisms.

In infants, atresia of the nasolacrimal ducts results from failure of canalization; or, in the first few weeks of life, from blockage when the membrane that separates the lower part of the nasolacrimal duct and the inferior nasal meatus fails to open spontaneously before tear secretion. It may also result from obstruction of the duct by gross abnormalities of the nasal bones.

Signs and symptoms

The hallmark of both acute and chronic forms of dacryocystitis is constant tearing. Other symptoms of acute dacryocystitis include inflammation and tenderness over the nasolacrimal sac; pressure over this area may produce purulent discharge from the punctum. In the chronic form, a mucoid discharge may be expressed from the tear sac.

Diagnosis

Clinical features and a physical examination suggest dacryocystitis. Culture of the discharged material demonstrates *Staphylococcus aureus* and, occasionally, beta-hemolytic streptococcus in acute dacryocystitis; *Streptococcus pneumoniae* or *C. albicans* in the chronic form. WBC may be elevated in the acute form; in the chronic form, it's generally normal. An X-ray after injection of a radiopaque medium (dacryocystography) locates the atresia.

Treatment

Treatment of acute dacryocystitis consists of application of warm compresses, and topical and systemic antibiotic therapy. Chronic dacryocystitis may eventually require dacryocystorhinostomy.

Therapy for nasolacrimal duct obstruction in an infant consists of careful massage of the area over the lacrimal sac 4 times a day for 2 to 3 months. If this fails to open the duct, dilation of the punctum and probing of the duct are necessary. Postoperative management requires a pressure patch over the area of the eye.

Special considerations

- Check patient history for possible allergy to antibiotics before giving them. Stress the need for precise compliance with prescribed antibiotic therapy.
- Tell the adult patient what to expect after surgery: he must lie on the operative side, with his arm behind him and his head tilted forward on a pillow, to facilitate drainage of blood. This position keeps the sinuses on the opposite side free of secretions and aids breathing.
- Monitor blood loss by counting dressings used to collect the blood.
- Apply ice compresses postoperatively. After the patch is removed (24 to 48 hours after surgery), place a small adhesive bandage over the suture line to protect it from damage.

Chalazion

A chalazion is a granulomatous inflammation of a meibomian gland in the upper or lower eyelid. This common eye disorder is characterized by localized swelling and usually develops slowly over several weeks. A chalazion may become large enough to press on the eyeball, producing astigmatism; a large chalazion seldom subsides spontaneously. It's generally benign and chronic, and can occur at any age; in some patients, it's apt to recur.

Causes
Obstruction of the meibomian (sebaceous) gland duct causes a chalazion.

Signs and symptoms
A chalazion occurs as a painless, hard lump that usually *points toward* the conjunctival side of the eyelid. Eversion of the lid reveals a red or red-yellow elevated area on the conjunctival surface.

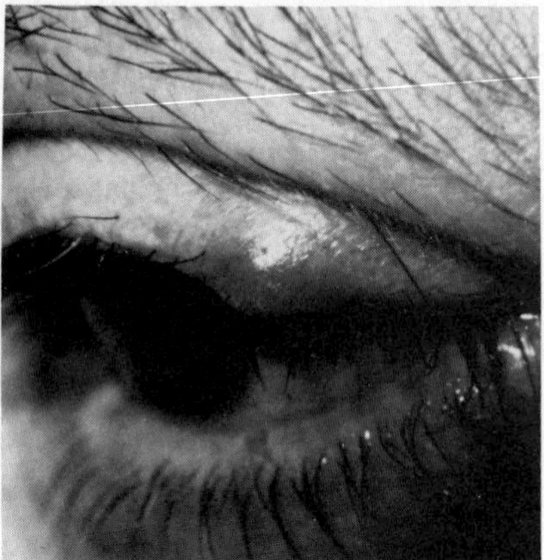

Chalazion, a nontender granulomatous inflammation of a meibomian gland on the upper eyelid.

Diagnosis
Diagnosis requires visual examination and palpation of the eyelid, revealing a small bump or nodule. Persistently recurrent chalazions, especially in an adult, necessitate biopsy to rule out meibomian cancer.

Treatment and special considerations
Initial treatment consists of application of warm compresses to open the lumen of the gland and, occasionally, instillation of sulfonamide eye drops. If such therapy fails, or if the chalazion presses on the eyeball or causes a severe cosmetic problem, incision and curettage under local anesthetic may be necessary. After such surgery, a pressure eye patch applied for 8 to 24 hours controls bleeding and swelling. After removal of the patch, treatment again consists of warm compresses applied for 10 to 15 minutes, 2 to 4 times daily, and antimicrobial eye drops or ointment to prevent secondary infection.

- Teach proper lid hygiene to the patient disposed to chalazions (water and mild baby shampoo applied with a cotton applicator).
- Instruct the patient how to properly apply *warm* compresses: Take special care to avoid burning the skin; always use a clean cloth; discard used compresses. Tell the patient to start applying warm compresses at the first sign of lid irritation, to increase the blood supply and keep the lumen open.

Stye
(Hordeolum)

A localized, purulent staphylococcal infection, a stye can occur externally (in the lumen of the smaller glands of Zeis or in Moll's glands) or internally (in the larger meibomian gland). A stye can occur at any age. Generally, this infection responds well to treatment but tends to recur. If untreated, a stye can eventually lead to cellulitis of the eyelid.

Signs and symptoms
Typically, a stye produces redness, swelling, and pain. An abscess frequently forms at the lid margin, with an

eyelash pointing outward from its center.

Diagnosis

Visual examination generally confirms this infection. Culture of purulent material from the abscess usually reveals a staphylococcal organism.

Treatment

Treatment consists of warm compresses applied for 10 to 15 minutes, 4 times a day for 3 to 4 days, to facilitate drainage of the abscess, to relieve pain and inflammation, and to promote suppuration. Drug therapy includes a topical sulfonamide or antibiotic eye drops or ointment and, occasionally, a systemic antibiotic. If conservative treatment fails, incision and drainage may be necessary.

Special considerations

- Instruct the patient to use a clean cloth for each application of warm compresses and to dispose of it or launder it separately to prevent spreading this infection to family members. For the same reason, the patient should avoid sharing towels and washcloths.
- Warn against squeezing the stye; this spreads the infection and may cause cellulitis.
- Teach the patient or family members the proper technique for instilling eye drops or ointments into the cul-de-sac of the lower eyelid.

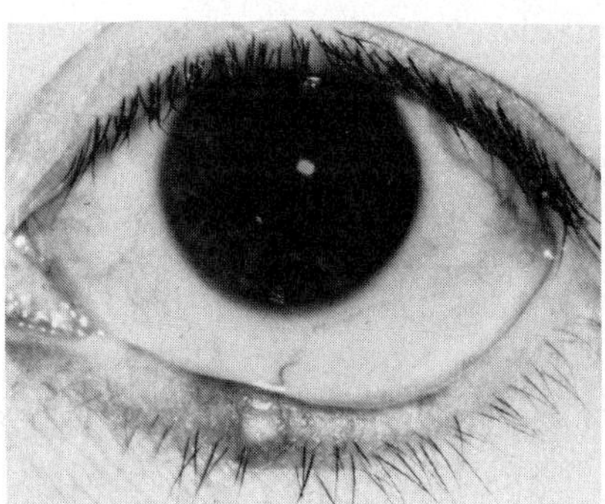

A stye is a localized red, swollen, and tender abscess of the lid glands.

CONJUNCTIVA

Inclusion Conjunctivitis

(Inclusion blennorrhea)

A fairly common disease, inclusion conjunctivitis is an acute ocular inflammation resulting from infection by Chlamydia trachomatis. *Although inclusion conjunctivitis occasionally becomes chronic, prognosis is generally good.*

Causes

C. trachomatis (an organism of the psittacosis-lymphogranuloma, venereum-trachoma group that may be a large, atypical virus) usually infects the urethra in males and the cervix in females and is transmitted during sexual activity. Since contaminated cervical secretions infect the eyes of the neonate during birth, inclusion conjunctivitis is an important cause of ophthalmia neonatorum. Rarely, inclusion conjunctivitis results from autoinfection, when an infected person transfers the virus from his genitourinary tract to his own eyes.

Signs and symptoms

Inclusion conjunctivitis develops 5 to 10 days after contamination (it takes longer to develop than gonococcal ophthalmia). In a newborn, the lower eyelids redden, and a thick, purulent discharge develops. In children and adults, follicles appear inside the lower eyelids; such follicles don't form in infants because the lymphoid tissue is not yet well developed. Children and adults also develop preauricular lymphadenopathy and, as a complication, otitis media. Inclusion conjunctivitis may persist for weeks or months, possibly with superficial corneal involvement. In newborns, pseudomembranes may form, which can lead to conjunctival scarring.

Diagnosis

Clinical features and a history of sexual contact with an infected individual suggest inclusion conjunctivitis.

Examination of Giemsa-stained conjunctival scraping reveals cytoplasmic inclusion bodies in conjunctival epithelial cells, many polymorphonuclear leukocytes, and a negative culture for bacteria.

Treatment

Treatment consists of eye drops of 1% tetracycline in oil, erythromycin ophthalmic ointment, or sulfonamide eye drops 5 or 6 times daily for 2 weeks for infants, and oral tetracycline or erythromycin for 3 weeks for adults. In severe disease, adults may require concomitant systemic sulfonamide therapy.

Special considerations

- Keep patient's eyes as clean as possible, using strict aseptic technique. Clean the eyes from the inner to the outer canthus. Apply warm soaks, as needed. Record amount and color of drainage.
- Remind the patient not to rub his eyes, which can irritate them.
- If the patient's eyes are sensitive to light, keep the room dark or suggest that he wear dark glasses. Provide appropriate diversionary activities.

To prevent further spread of inclusion conjunctivitis:

- Wash hands thoroughly before and after administering eye medications.
- Suggest genital examination of the mother of an infected newborn or of any adult with inclusion conjunctivitis.
- Obtain a history of recent sexual contacts, so they can be examined for inclusion conjunctivitis.

Conjunctivitis

Conjunctivitis is characterized by hyperemia of the conjunctiva due to infection, allergy, or chemical reactions. This disorder usually occurs as benign, self-limiting pinkeye; it may also be chronic, possibly indicating degenerative changes or damage from repeated acute attacks. In the Western hemisphere, conjunctivitis is probably the most common eye disorder.

Causes

The most common causative organisms are the following:

- *bacterial: Staphylococcus aureus, Streptococcus pneumoniae, Neisseria gonorrhoeae, Neisseria meningitidis*
- *chlamydial: Chlamydia trachomatis* (inclusion conjunctivitis)
- *viral:* adenovirus types 3, 7, and 8; herpes simplex virus, type 1.

Other causes include allergic reactions to pollen, grass, topical medications, air pollutants, smoke, or unknown seasonal allergens (vernal conjunctivitis); occupational irritants (acids and alkalies); rickettsial diseases (Rocky Mountain spotted fever); parasitic diseases caused by *Phthirus pubis, Schistosoma haematobium;* and, rarely, fungal infections.

Vernal conjunctivitis (also called seasonal or warm-weather conjunctivitis) results from allergy to an unidentified allergen. This form of conjunctivitis is bilateral; it usually begins before puberty and persists for about 10 years. It is sometimes associated with other signs of allergy commonly related to grass or pollen sensitivity.

An idiopathic form of conjunctivitis may be associated with certain systemic diseases, such as erythema multiforme, chronic follicular conjunctivitis (orphan's conjunctivitis), and thyroid disease. Conjunctivitis may be secondary to pneumococcal dacryocystitis or canaliculitis due to candidal infection.

Signs and symptoms

Conjunctivitis commonly produces hyperemia of the conjunctiva, sometimes accompanied by discharge, tearing, pain, and, with corneal involvement, photophobia. It generally doesn't affect vision. Conjunctivitis usually begins in one eye and rapidly spreads to the other by contamination of towels, washcloths, or the patient's own hand.

Acute bacterial conjunctivitis (pinkeye) usually lasts only 2 weeks. The patient typically complains of itching, burning, and the sensation of a foreign body in his eye. The eyelids show a crust of sticky, mucopurulent discharge. If the disorder is due to *N. gonorrhoeae,* however, the patient exhibits a profuse, purulent discharge.

Viral conjunctivitis produces copious tearing with minimal exudate, and enlargement of the preauricular lymph node. Some viruses follow a chronic course and produce severe disabling disease, while others last 2 to 3 weeks.

Diagnosis

Physical examination reveals injection of the bulbar conjunctival vessels. In children, possible systemic symptoms include sore throat or fever.

Monocytes are predominant in stained smears of conjunctival scrapings if conjunctivitis is caused by a virus. Polymorphonuclear cells (neutrophils) predominate if conjunctivitis is due to bacteria; eosinophils, if it's allergy-related. Culture and sensitivity tests identify the causative bacterial organism and indicate appropriate antibiotic therapy.

Treatment

Treatment of conjunctivitis varies with the cause. Bacterial conjunctivitis requires topical application of the appropriate antibiotic or sulfonamide. Although viral conjunctivitis resists treatment, a sulfonamide or broad-spectrum antibiotic eye drops may prevent secondary infection. Herpes simplex infection generally responds to treatment with idoxuridine or vidarabine ointment, but the infection may persist for 2 to 3 weeks. Treatment of vernal (allergic) conjunctivitis includes administration of vasoconstrictor eye drops, such as epinephrine; cold compresses to relieve itching; and, occasionally, oral antihistamines.

Instillation of 1% silver nitrate into the eyes of newborns prevents gonococcal conjunctivitis.

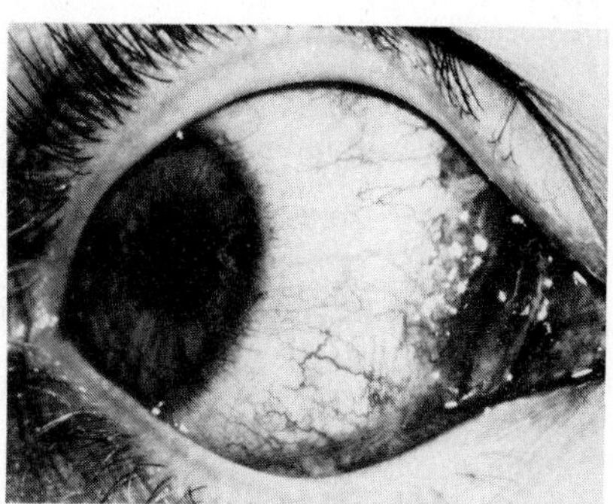

Allergy, infection, or physical or chemical trauma can cause an inflammation of the conjunctiva, which produces redness, pain, swelling, lacrimation, and possible discharge.

Special considerations

- Teach proper hand-washing technique, since some forms of conjunctivitis are highly contagious. Stress the risk of spreading infection to family members by sharing washcloths, towels, and pillows. Warn against rubbing the infected eye, which can spread the infection to the other eye and to other persons.
- Apply warm compresses and therapeutic ointment or drops, as ordered. Do not irrigate eye, as this will spread infection. Have the patient wash his hands before he uses the medication, and use clean washcloths or towels frequently so

he doesn't infect his other eye.
- Teach the patient to instill eye drops and ointments correctly—without touching the bottle tip to his eye or lashes.
- Stress the importance of safety glasses for the patient who works near chemical irritants.
- Notify public health authorities if cultures show *N. gonorrhoeae.*

Trachoma

The most common cause of blindness in underdeveloped areas of the world, trachoma is a chronic form of keratoconjunctivitis. This infection is usually confined to the eye but can also localize in the urethra. Although trachoma itself is self-limiting, it causes permanent damage to the cornea and conjunctiva; severe trachoma may lead to blindness, especially if a secondary bacterial infection develops. Early diagnosis and treatment (before trachoma results in scar formation) ensure recovery but without immunity to reinfection. Trachoma is prevalent in Africa, Latin America, and Asia, particularly in children; in the United States, it is prevalent among the American Indians of the Southwest.

Causes

Trachoma results from infection by *Chlamydia trachomatis,* an organism once thought to be a virus, but now thought to be more closely related to bacteria. These chlamydial organisms, described as nonmotile, obligate intracellular parasites, are transmitted from eye to eye by flies and gnats in endemic areas.

Trachoma is spread by close contact between family members or among schoolchildren. Other prediposing factors include poverty and poor hygiene due to lack of water.

Signs and symptoms

Trachoma begins with a mild infection resembling bacterial conjunctivitis (visible conjunctival follicles, red and edematous eyelids, pain, photophobia, tearing, and exudation).

After about 1 month, if the infection is untreated, conjunctival follicles enlarge into inflamed papillae that later become yellow or gray. At this stage, small blood vessels invade the cornea under the upper lid.

Eventually, severe scarring and contraction of the eyelids cause entropion; the eyelids turn inward and the lashes rub against the cornea, producing corneal scarring and visual distortion. Severe conjunctival scarring may obstruct the lacrimal ducts and cause dry eyes.

Diagnosis

Follicular conjunctivitis with corneal infiltration, and upper lid or conjunctival scarring suggest trachoma, especially in endemic areas, when these symptoms persist longer than 3 weeks.

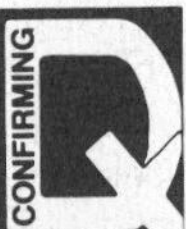

Microscopic examination of a Giemsa-stained conjunctival scraping confirms diagnosis by showing cytoplasmic inclusion bodies, some polymorphonuclear reaction, plasma cells, Leber's cells (large macrophages containing phagocytosed debris), and follicle cells.

Treatment and special considerations

Primary treatment of trachoma consists of 3 to 4 weeks of topical or systemic antibiotic therapy with tetracycline, erythromycin, or sulfonamides. (Tetracycline is contraindicated in pregnant females because it may adversely affect the fetus, and in children under age 7, in whom it may discolor teeth permanently.) Severe entropion requires surgical correction.

Patient teaching is essential:

- Emphasize the importance of hand washing and making the best use of available water supplies to maintain good personal hygiene. To prevent trachoma, warn patients not to allow flies or gnats to settle around the eyes.
- Because no definitive preventive measure exists (vaccines offer temporary and partial protection, at best), stress the need for strict compliance with the prescribed drug therapy.
- If ordered, teach the patient or family members how to instill eye drops correctly.

CORNEA

Keratitis

Keratitis, inflammation of the cornea, may be acute or chronic, superficial or deep. Superficial keratitis is fairly common and may develop at any age. Prognosis is good, with treatment. Untreated, recurrent keratitis may lead to blindness.

Causes

Keratitis usually results from infection by herpes simplex virus, type 1 (known as dendritic keratitis). It may also result from exposure, due to the patient's inability to close his eyelids, or from congenital syphilis (interstitial keratitis). Less commonly, it stems from bacterial and fungal infections.

Signs and symptoms

Usually unilateral, keratitis produces opacities of the cornea, mild irritation, tearing, and photophobia. If the infection is in the center of the cornea, it may produce blurred vision. When keratitis results from exposure, it usually affects the lower portion of the cornea.

Diagnosis

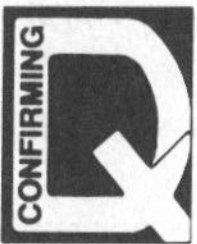

Slit-lamp examination confirms keratitis. If keratitis is due to herpes simplex virus, staining the eye with a fluorescein strip produces one or more small branchlike (dendritic) lesions; touching the cornea with cotton reveals reduced corneal sensation. Vision testing may show slightly decreased acuity. Patient history may reveal a recent infection of the upper respiratory tract accompanied by cold sores.

Treatment

Treatment of acute keratitis due to herpes simplex virus consists of idoxuridine eye drops and ointment or vidarabine ointment; treatment of recurrent herpetic keratitis, trifluridine. A broad-spectrum antibiotic may prevent secondary bacterial infection. Chronic dendritic keratitis may respond more quickly to vidarabine. Long-term topical therapy may be necessary. (Corticosteroid therapy is contraindicated in dendritic keratitis or any other viral or fungal disease of the cornea.) Treatment for fungal keratitis consists of natamycin.

Keratitis due to exposure requires application of moisturizing ointment to the exposed cornea and of a plastic bubble eye shield or eye patch. Treatment for severe corneal scarring may include keratoplasty (cornea transplantation).

Special considerations

- Look for keratitis in patients predisposed to cold sores. Explain that stress, trauma, fever, colds, and overexposure to the sun may trigger flare-ups.
- Protect the exposed corneas of unconscious patients by cleaning the eyes daily, applying moisturizing ointment, or covering the eyes with an eye shield.

Corneal Abrasion

A corneal abrasion is a scratch on the surface epithelium of the cornea, often caused by a foreign body. An abrasion, or foreign body in the eye is the most common eye injury. With treatment, prognosis is usually good.

Causes

A corneal abrasion usually results from a foreign body, such as a cinder or a piece of dust, dirt, or grit, that becomes embedded under the eyelid. Even if the foreign body is washed out by tears, it may still injure the cornea. Small pieces of metal that get in the eyes of workers who don't wear protective glasses quickly form a rust ring on the cornea and cause corneal abrasion. Such abrasions also commonly occur in the eyes of persons who fall asleep wearing hard contact lenses.

A corneal scratch produced by a fingernail, a piece of paper, or other organic substance may cause a persistent lesion. The epithelium doesn't always heal properly, and a recurrent corneal erosion may develop, with delayed effects more severe than the original injury.

Signs and symptoms

Typically, corneal abrasions produce redness, increased tearing, a sensation of "something in the eye," and because the cornea is richly endowed with nerve endings from the trigeminal nerve (cranial nerve V), pain disproportionate to the size of the injury. A corneal abrasion may affect visual acuity, depending on the size and location of the injury.

Diagnosis

History of eye trauma or prolonged wearing of contact lenses, and typical symptoms suggest corneal abrasion.

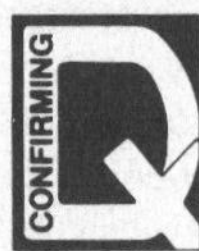

Staining the cornea with fluorescein stain confirms the diagnosis: The injured area appears green when examined with a flashlight. Slit-lamp examination discloses the depth of the abrasion.

Examining the eye with a flashlight may reveal a foreign body on the cornea; the eyelid must be everted to check for a foreign body embedded under the lid.

Before beginning treatment, a test to determine visual acuity provides a medical baseline and a legal safeguard.

Treatment and special considerations

Removal of a deeply embedded foreign body is done with a foreign body spud, using a topical anesthetic. A rust ring on the cornea can be removed with an ophthalmic burr, after applying a topical anesthetic. When only partial removal is possible, re-epithelialization lifts the ring again to the surface and allows complete removal the following day.

Treatment also includes instillation of broad-spectrum antibiotic eyedrops in the affected eye every 3 to 4 hours. Initial application of a pressure patch prevents further corneal irritation when the patient blinks.

- Assist with examination of the eye. Check visual acuity before beginning treatment.
- If a foreign body is visible, irrigate the eye with normal saline solution.
- Tell the patient with an eyepatch to leave the patch in place for 24 to 48 hours. Warn that wearing a patch alters depth perception, so advise caution in everyday activities, such as climbing stairs or stepping off a curb.
- Reassure the patient that the corneal epithelium usually heals in 24 to 48 hours.
- Stress the importance of instilling antibiotic eyedrops, as ordered, since an untreated corneal infection can lead to ulceration and permanent loss of vision. Teach the patient the proper way to instill eye medications.

• Emphasize the importance of safety glasses to protect workers' eyes from flying fragments. Also review instructions for wearing and caring for contact lenses, to prevent further trauma.

Corneal Ulcers

A major cause of blindness worldwide, ulcers produce corneal scarring or perforation. They occur in the central or marginal areas of the cornea, vary in shape and size, and may be singular or multiple. Marginal ulcers are the most common form. Prompt treatment (within hours of onset) can prevent visual impairment.

Causes

Corneal ulcers generally result from bacterial, viral, or fungal infections. Common bacterial sources include *Staphylococcus aureus, Pseudomonas aeruginosa, Streptococcus viridans, Streptococcus (Diplococcus) pneumoniae,* and *Moraxella liquefaciens;* viral sources, herpes simplex type 1, variola, vaccinia, and varicella-zoster viruses; common fungal sources, *Candida, Fusarium,* and *Cephalosporium.*

Other causes include trauma, exposure, reactions to bacterial infections, toxins, and allergens. Tuberculoprotein causes a classic phlyctenular keratoconjunctivitis; vitamin A deficiency results in xerophthalmia; and fifth cranial nerve lesions, neurotropic ulcers.

Signs and symptoms

Typically, corneal ulceration begins with pain (aggravated by blinking), followed by increased tearing. Eventually, central corneal ulceration produces pronounced visual blurring. The eye may appear injected, from congestion in the conjunctival blood vessels. Purulent discharge is possible with a bacterial ulcer.

Diagnosis

Patient history—possibly indicating trauma—and examination, using a flashlight, that reveals irregular corneal surface suggest corneal ulcer. Exudate may be present on the cornea, and a hypopyon (accumulation of white cells or pus in the anterior chamber) may produce cloudiness or color change.

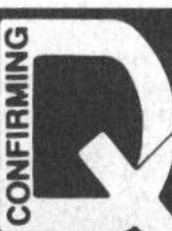

Fluorescein dye, instilled in the conjunctival sac, stains the outline of the ulcer and confirms the diagnosis.

Culture and sensitivity testing of corneal scraping may identify the causative bacteria or fungus, and indicate appropriate antibiotic or antifungal therapy.

Treatment and special considerations

Generally, treatment consists of systemic and topical broad-spectrum antibiotics until culture results identify the causative organism. The goals of treatment are to eliminate the underlying cause of the ulcer and to relieve pain:

• *infection by P. aeruginosa:* polymyxin B and gentamicin, administered topically and by subconjunctival injection, or carbenicillin and tobramycin I.V. Since this type of corneal ulcer spreads so rapidly, it can cause corneal perforation and loss of the eye within 48 hours. Immediate treatment and isolation of hospitalized patients are required. *Note:* Treatment of a corneal ulcer due to bacterial infection should *never* include an eye patch, since patching creates the dark, warm, moist environment ideal for bacterial growth.

• *herpes simplex type 1 virus:* hourly topical application of idoxuridine or vidarabine. Corneal ulcers resulting from a viral infection often recur; in which case, trifluridine becomes the treatment of choice.

• *varicella-zoster virus:* topical sulfonamide ointment applied three to four times daily to prevent secondary infection. These lesions are unilateral, following the pathway of the fifth cranial nerve, and are quite painful. Give analgesics, as ordered. Associated anterior uveitis requires cycloplegic eye drops. Watch for signs of secondary glaucoma (increased intraocular pressure, transient vision loss, and halos around lights).

- *fungi:* topical instillation of natamycin for *Fusarium, Cephalosporium,* and *Candida.*
- *hypersensitivity reactions:* topical corticosteroids, such as dexamethasone and hydrocortisone.
- *hypovitaminosis A:* correction of dietary deficiency or gastrointestinal malabsorption of vitamin A.
- *neurotropic ulcers or exposure keratitis:* frequent instillation of artificial tears or lubricating ointments and use of a plastic bubble eye shield.

Prompt treatment is essential for all forms of corneal ulcer, to prevent complications and permanent visual impairment.

UVEAL TRACT, RETINA, AND LENS

Uveitis

Uveitis is inflammation of one uveal tract. It occurs as anterior uveitis, which affects the iris (iritis), or both the iris and the ciliary body (iridocyclitis); as posterior uveitis, which affects the choroid (choroiditis), or both the choroid and the retina (chorioretinitis); or as panuveitis, which affects the entire uveal tract. Although clinical distinction is not always possible, anterior uveitis occurs in two forms—granulomatous and nongranulomatous. Granulomatous uveitis was once thought to be caused by tuberculosis bacilli; nongranulomatous uveitis, by streptococcus. Although this is not true, the terms are still used. Untreated anterior uveitis progresses to posterior uveitis, causing scarring, cataracts, and glaucoma. With immediate treatment, anterior uveitis usually subsides after a few days to several weeks; however, recurrence is likely. Posterior uveitis generally produces some residual visual loss and marked blurring of vision.

Causes

Typically, uveitis is idiopathic. But it can result from allergy, bacteria, viruses, fungi, chemicals, trauma, or surgery; or from systemic diseases, such as rheumatoid arthritis, ankylosing spondylitis, and toxoplasmosis.

Signs and symptoms

Anterior uveitis produces moderate to severe eye pain; severe ciliary injection; photophobia; tearing; a small, nonreactive pupil; and blurred vision (due to the increased number of cells in the aqueous humor). It sometimes produces deposits on the back of the cornea that may be seen in the anterior chamber. Onset may be acute or insidious.

Posterior uveitis begins insidiously, with complaints of slightly decreased or blurred vision or floating spots. The iris may adhere to the lens, causing posterior synechia and pupillary distortion; pain and photophobia may occur. Posterior uveitis may be acute or chronic; it may appear with secondary cataracts, glaucoma, or retinal detachment.

Diagnosis

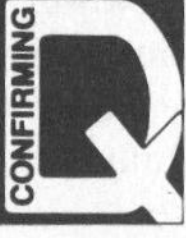

In anterior and posterior uveitis, a slit-lamp examination shows a "flare and cell" pattern, which looks like light passing through smoke.

GRANULOMATOUS AND NONGRANULOMATOUS UVEITIS

FACTOR	GRANULOMATOUS	NONGRANULOMATOUS
Location	• Any part of uveal tract, but usually the posterior part	• Anterior portion: iris, ciliary body
Onset	• Insidious	• Acute
Pain	• None or slight	• Marked
Photophobia	• Slight	• Marked
Course	• Chronic	• Acute
Prognosis	• Fair to poor	• Good
Recurrence	• Occasional	• Common

Adapted with permission from Lillian S. Brunner and Doris S. Suddarth, TEXTBOOK OF MEDICAL-SURGICAL NURSING (Philadelphia: J.B. Lippincott Co., 1980).

It also shows an increased number of cells over the inflamed area. With a special lens, slit-lamp examination can also identify active inflammatory fundus lesions involving the retina and/or choroid. These lesions may also be identified by ophthalmoscopic examination.

In posterior uveitis, serologic tests can tell if toxoplasmosis is the cause.

Treatment

Uveitis requires vigorous and prompt management, which includes treatment of any known underlying cause; and application of a topical cycloplegic, such as 1% atropine sulfate, and of topical and subconjunctival corticosteroids. For severe uveitis, therapy includes oral systemic corticosteroids. However, long-term steroid therapy can cause a rise in intraocular pressure (IOP) and/or cataracts. So, carefully monitor IOP during acute inflammation. If IOP rises, therapy should include an antiglaucoma medication, such as the beta-blocker timolol, or a carbonic anhydrase inhibitor, such as acetazolamide (Diamox).

Special considerations

- Encourage rest during the acute phase.
- Teach the patient the proper method of instilling eye drops.
- Suggest the use of dark glasses to ease the discomfort of photophobia.
- Instruct the patient to watch for and report side effects of systemic corticosteroid therapy (edema, muscle weakness).
- Stress the importance of follow-up care because of the strong likelihood of recurrence. Tell the patient to seek treatment immediately, at first signs of iritis.

Retinal Detachment

Retinal detachment occurs when the layers of the retina become separated, creating a subretinal space. This space then fills with fluid, called subretinal fluid (SRF). Retinal detachment usually involves only one eye, but may involve the other eye later. Surgical reattachment is often successful. However, prognosis for good vision depends upon the area of the eye that's been affected.

Causes

Any retinal tear or hole allows the liquid vitreous to seep between the retinal layers, separating the retina from its choroidal blood supply. In adults, retinal detachment usually results from degenerative changes of aging, which cause a spontaneous retinal hole. Predisposing factors include myopia, cataract surgery, and trauma. Perhaps the influence of trauma explains why retinal detachment is twice as common in males. Retinal detachment may also result from seepage of fluid into the subretinal space (due to inflammation, tumors, or systemic diseases, such as accelerated hypertension or circulatory disorders) or from traction that's placed on the retina by vitreous bands or membranes (due to proliferative diabetic retinopathy, posterior uveitis, or a traumatic intraocular foreign body).

Retinal detachment is rare in children, but can occur as a result of retinopathy of prematurity, tumors (retinoblastomas), or trauma. It can also be inherited, usually in association with myopia.

Signs and symptoms

Initially, the patient may complain of floating spots and recurrent flashes of light. But as detachment progresses, he experiences gradual, painless vision loss. The patient may describe vision loss as a veil, curtain, or cobweb that eliminates a portion of the visual field.

Diagnosis

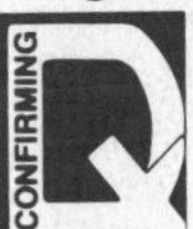

Diagnosis depends on ophthalmoscopy after full pupil dilation. Examination shows the usually transparent retina as gray and opaque. In severe detachment, examination reveals folds in the retina and a ballooning out of the area. Indirect ophthalmoscopy is also used to search the retina for tears and holes.

Treatment

Treatment depends on the location and severity of the detachment. It may include

SURGICAL CORRECTION OF RETINAL DETACHMENT

In scleral buckling, cryotherapy (cold therapy), photocoagulation (laser therapy), or diathermy (heat therapy) creates a sterile inflammatory reaction that seals the retinal hole and causes retinal readherence. The surgeon then places a silicone plate or sponge—called an explant—over the site of reattachment, and holds it in place with a circling band. The pressure exerted on the explant indents (buckles) the eyeball and gently pushes the choroid and retina closer together.

restricting eye movements (through bed rest, sedation, and, if the patient's macula is threatened, a pressure patch) and positioning the head so the tear or hole is below the rest of the eye. A hole in the peripheral retina can be treated with cryotherapy; a hole in the posterior portion, with laser therapy. Retinal detachment rarely heals spontaneously; surgery, consisting of scleral buckling, is necessary to reattach the retina.

Special considerations

- Provide emotional support, since the patient may be understandably distraught because of his loss of vision.
- To prepare the patient for surgery, wash his face with no-tears shampoo, and cut off his eyelashes to lower the risk of infection. Give antibiotics and cycloplegic/mydriatic eye drops, as ordered.
- Postoperatively, position the patient on his back or on his unoperated side. Elevating the head of the bed may make him feel more comfortable. Allow him to use the bathroom after complete recovery from anesthesia. But discourage him from straining at stool or bending down unnecessarily; these actions can raise IOP. Tell him to avoid activities that may cause him to bump his eye.
- After removing the pressure patch, gently cleanse the eye with cycloplegic eye drops and steroid/antibiotic eye drops, as ordered. Use cold compresses to decrease swelling and pain.
- Administer medications for pain, p.r.n. Notify the patient's doctor if pain persists. Teach the patient and his family how to properly instill eye drops, and stress the importance of compliance and follow-up care. Suggest dark glasses to compensate for light sensitivity.

Vascular Retinopathies

Vascular retinopathies are noninflammatory retinal disorders that result from interference with the blood supply to the eyes. The four distinct types of vascular retinopathy are central retinal artery occlusion, central retinal vein occlusion, diabetic retinopathy, and hypertensive retinopathy.

Causes and incidence

The retinal arteries feed the capillaries and thus maintain blood circulation in the retina. When one of these vessels becomes obstructed, diminished blood flow causes visual deficits.

Central retinal artery occlusion may be idiopathic or may result from embolism, atherosclerosis, infection (syphilis, rheumatic fever), or conditions that retard blood flow, such as temporal arteritis, massive hemorrhage, carotid occlusion, and heart failure. Central retinal artery occlusion is rare, usually occurs unilaterally, and most commonly affects the elderly.

Causes of *central retinal vein occlusion* include external compression of the retinal vein, trauma, diabetes, phlebitis, thrombosis, granulomatous diseases, generalized infection, inflammation of the orbit or the sinuses, gastrointestinal bleeding, glaucoma, and atherosclerosis. This form of vascular retinopathy is most prevalent in the elderly.

Diabetic retinopathy has two forms—nonproliferative (early-appearing background) and proliferative (late-appearing)—and results from juvenile or adult diabetes. Microcirculatory changes occur more rapidly when diabetes is poorly controlled. About 75% of patients with juvenile diabetes develop retinopathy within 20 years of onset of diabetes. In patients with adult diabetes, incidence increases with the duration of diabetes. For example, 80% of patients who have had diabetes for 20 to 25 years develop retinopathy. This condition is a leading cause of acquired adult blindness.

DIAGNOSTIC TESTS FOR VASCULAR RETINOPATHIES

CENTRAL RETINAL ARTERY OCCLUSION	CENTRAL RETINAL VEIN OCCLUSION	DIABETIC RETINOPATHY	HYPERTENSIVE RETINOPATHY
• **Ophthalmoscopy (direct or indirect):** shows emptying of retinal arterioles during transient attack. • **Slit-lamp examination:** within 2 hours of onset, shows clumps or segmentation in artery; later, milky white retina around disk due to swelling and necrosis of ganglion cells caused by reduced blood supply; also shows cherry-red spot in macula that subsides after several weeks. • **Ophthalmodynamometry:** approximately measures the relative pressures in the central retinal arteries and indirectly assesses internal carotid artery obstruction. • **Ultrasonography:** reveals condition of blood vessels in the neck. • **Digital subtraction angiography (DSA):** evaluates carotid occlusion with no need for arteriography. • **Physical examination:** reveals underlying cause.	• **Opthalmoscopy (direct or indirect):** shows retinal hemorrhage, retinal vein engorgement, white patches among hemorrhages, edema around the disk. • **Ultrasonography:** confirms or rules out occlusion of blood vessels. • **Physical examination:** reveals underlying cause.	• **Slit-lamp examination:** shows thickening of retinal capillary walls. • **Indirect ophthalmoscopy:** shows retinal changes such as microaneurysms (earliest change), retinal hemorrhages and edema, venous dilation and twisting, exudates, vitreous hemorrhage, proliferation of fibrin into vitreous due to retinal holes, growth of new blood vessels, and microinfarcts of nerve fiber layer. • **Fluorescein angiography:** shows leakage of fluorescein from dilated vessels and differentiates between microaneurysms and true hemorrhages. • **History:** of diabetes.	• **Ophthalmoscopy (direct or indirect):** in early stages, shows hard, shiny deposits, tiny hemorrhages, and elevated arterial blood pressure; in late stages, cotton wool patches, exudates, retinal edema, papilledema due to ischemia and capillary insufficiency, hemorrhages, and microaneurysms. • **History:** of hypertension.

Hypertensive retinopathy results from prolonged hypertensive disease, producing retinal vasospasm, and consequent damage and narrowing of the arteriolar lumen.

Signs and symptoms

Central retinal artery occlusion produces sudden, painless, unilateral loss of vision (partial or complete). It may follow amaurosis fugax or transient episodes of unilateral loss of vision lasting from a few seconds to minutes, probably due to vasospasm. This condition typically causes permanent blindness. However, some patients experience spontaneous resolution within hours and regain partial vision.

Central retinal vein occlusion causes reduced visual acuity, allowing perception of only hand movement and light. This condition is painless, except when it results in secondary neovascular glaucoma (uncontrolled proliferation of weak blood vessels). Prognosis is poor—5% to 20% of patients with this type of vascular retinopathy develop secondary glaucoma within 3 to 4 months after occlusion.

Nonproliferative diabetic retinopathy produces changes in the lining of the retinal blood vessels that cause the vessels to leak plasma or fatty substances, which decrease or block blood flow (nonperfusion) within the retina. This disorder may also produce microaneurysms and

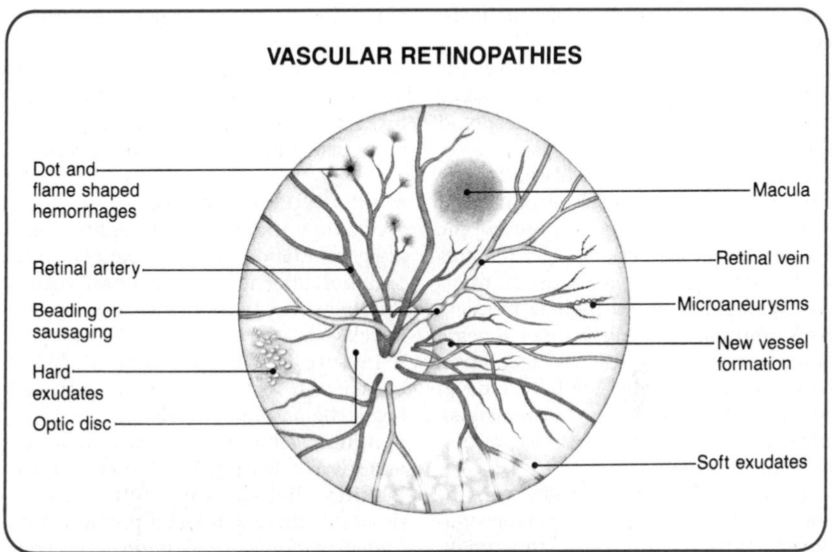

small hemorrhages. Although nonproliferative retinopathy causes no symptoms in some patients, in others leakage of fluid into the macular region causes significant loss of central visual acuity (necessary for reading and driving) and diminished night vision.

Proliferative diabetic retinopathy produces fragile new blood vessels on the disk (neovascularization of the disk) and elsewhere in the fundus (neovascularization elsewhere). These vessels can grow into the vitreous and then rupture, causing vitreous hemorrhage with corresponding sudden vision loss. Scar tissue that may form along the new blood vessels can pull on the retina, causing macular distortion and even retinal detachment.

Symptoms of hypertensive retinopathy depend on location of retinopathy. For example, mild visual disturbances, such as blurred vision, result from retinopathy located near the macula. Without treatment, prognosis is poor (50% of patients become blind within 5 years). With treatment, prognosis varies with the severity of the disorder. Severe, prolonged disease eventually produces blindness; mild, prolonged disease, visual defects.

Diagnosis

Appropriate diagnostic tests depend on the type of vascular retinopathy. (See *Diagnostic Tests for Vascular Retinopathies* on page 1142.) Diagnostic evaluation should always include determination of visual acuity and ophthalmoscopic examination.

Treatment

No particular treatment has been shown to control central retinal artery occlusion. However, an attempt is made to release the occlusion into the peripheral circulation. To reduce intraocular pressure, therapy includes acetazolamide 500 mg. I.V. or I.M.; eyeball massage, using a Goldman-type goniolens; and, possibly, anterior chamber paracentesis. Therapy also includes inhalation of carbogen (95% oxygen and 5% carbon dioxide) to improve retinal oxygenation. Because inhalation therapy may be given hourly for up to 48 hours, the patient should be hospitalized so his vital signs can be monitored closely.

Therapy for central retinal vein occlusion may include aspirin, which acts as a mild anticoagulant. Therapy sometimes includes stronger anticoagulants, such as heparin and warfarin; however, many disagree about the use of these drugs.

Laser photocoagulation can reduce the risk of neovascular glaucoma for some patients whose eyes have widespread capillary nonperfusion.

Treatment of nonproliferative diabetic retinopathy consists of controlling the patient's blood sugar level to prevent the disease from progressing. For patients with early symptoms of microaneurysms, therapy should include frequent eye examinations (3 to 4 times a year) to monitor their condition. For children with diabetes, therapy should include an eye examination by an ophthalmologist, either 3 to 5 years after the onset of diabetes or at puberty.

The best treatment for proliferative diabetic retinopathy is laser photocoagulation, which cauterizes the weak, leaking blood vessels. Laser treatment may be focal (aimed directly at new blood vessels) or panretinal (placing as many as 2,000 burns throughout the peripheral retina). Despite such treatment, neovascularization doesn't always regress, and vitreous hemorrhage, with or without retinal detachment, may follow. If the leaked blood isn't absorbed in 3 to 6 months, vitrectomy may be performed to restore partial vision.

In addition to many of these therapies, treatment for hypertensive retinopathy includes control of blood pressure with appropriate drugs, diet, and exercise.

Special considerations

- Arrange for *immediate* ophthalmologic evaluation when a patient complains of sudden, unilateral loss of vision. Blindness may be permanent if treatment is delayed.
- Be sure to monitor a patient's blood pressure if he complains of occipital headache and blurred vision.
- Administer acetazolamide I.M. or I.V., as ordered. During inhalation therapy, monitor vital signs carefully. Discontinue this therapy if blood pressure fluctuates markedly or if patient becomes dysrhythmic or disoriented.
- Encourage a diabetic patient to comply with prescribed diet, exercise, and medication regimen to prevent diabetic retinopathy.
- For a patient with hypertensive retinopathy, stress the importance of complying with antihypertensive therapy.

Cataract

A common cause of vision loss, a cataract is a gradually developing opacity of the lens or lens capsule of the eye. Cataracts commonly occur bilaterally, with each progressing independently. Exceptions are traumatic cataracts, which are usually unilateral, and congenital cataracts, which may remain stationary. Cataracts are most prevalent in persons over age 70, as part of aging. Prognosis is generally good; surgery improves vision in 95% of affected persons.

Causes

Cataracts have various causes:

- *Senile cataracts* develop in the elderly, probably because of changes in the chemical state of lens proteins.
- *Congenital cataracts* occur in newborns as genetic defects or due to maternal rubella during the first trimester.
- *Traumatic cataracts* develop after a foreign body injures the lens with sufficient force to allow aqueous or vitreous humor to enter the lens capsule.
- *Complicated cataracts* occur secondary to uveitis, glaucoma, retinitis pigmentosa, detached retina, or, in the course of a systemic disease, such as diabetes, hypoparathyroidism or atopic dermatitis. They can also result from ionizing radiation or infrared rays.
- *Toxic cataracts* result from drug or

chemical toxicity with ergot, dinitrophenol, naphthalene, and phenothiazines or from galactose in patients with galactosemia.

Signs and symptoms

Typically, a patient with a cataract experiences painless, gradual blurring and loss of vision. As the cataract progresses, the normally black pupil turns milky white. Some patients see halos around lights and blinding glare from headlights when they drive at night; others complain of poor reading vision, and of an unpleasant glare and poor vision in bright sunlight. Patients with central opacities can see better in dim light than in bright light because the cataract is nuclear, and, as the pupils dilate, patients can see around the lens opacity.

Diagnosis

On examination, shining a penlight on the pupil reveals the white area behind the pupil (unnoticeable until the cataract is advanced) and suggests a cataract.

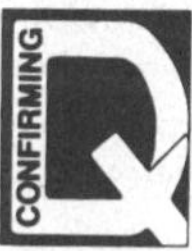

Ophthalmoscopy or slit-lamp examination confirms the diagnosis by revealing a dark area in the normally homogeneous red reflex.

Treatment

Treatment consists of surgical extraction of the opaque lens and postoperative correction of visual deficits. The current trend is to perform the surgery as a 1-day procedure.

Surgical procedures include the following:

- *Extracapsular cataract extraction*, the most common procedure, removes the anterior lens capsule and cortex, leaving the posterior capsule intact. With this procedure, a posterior chamber intraocular lens (IOL) is implanted where the patient's own lens used to be. (A posterior chamber IOL is the most common type now used in the United States.) This procedure is used for patients of all ages.
- *Intracapsular cataract extraction* removes the entire lens within the intact capsule by cryoextraction (the moist lens sticks to an extremely cold metal probe for easy and safe removal with gentle traction). Once the lens is removed, an IOL is implanted in either the pupil or the anterior chamber. If an IOL implant isn't used, the visual deficit is corrected with contact lenses or aphakic glasses.
- *Phacoemulsification* fragments the lens with ultrasonic vibrations and aspirates the pieces; occasionally, this is performed on patients under age 30.
- *Discission and aspiration* can still be used for children with soft cataracts, but this procedure has largely been replaced by the use of multifunction suction cutting instruments.

Possible complications of surgery include loss of vitreous (during surgery), wound dehiscence from loosening of sutures and flat anterior chamber or iris prolapse into the wound, hyphema, pupillary block glaucoma, retinal detachment, and infection.

A patient with an IOL implant may experience improved vision once the eye patch is removed; however, the IOL corrects distance vision only. The patient will also need either corrective reading glasses or a corrective contact lens, which will be fitted 4 to 8 weeks after surgery.

Where no IOL has been implanted, the patient may be given temporary aphakic cataract glasses; in about 4 to 8 weeks, he'll be refracted for his own glasses.

Some patients who have an extracapsular cataract extraction develop a secondary membrane in the posterior lens capsule (which has been left intact), and that causes decreased visual acuity. But this membrane can be removed by the Nd:YAG laser, which cuts an area out of the center of the membrane, thereby restoring vision. However, laser therapy alone cannot be used to remove a cataract.

Special considerations

After surgery to extract a cataract:

- Because the patient will be discharged after he recovers from anesthesia, remind him to return for a checkup the next day and warn him to avoid activities that increase intraocular pressure, such as straining.

- Urge the patient to protect the eye from accidental injury by wearing an eye shield (a plastic or metal shield with perforations) or glasses during the day, and an eye shield at night.
- Administer antibiotic ointment or drops to prevent infection and steroids to reduce inflammation, or combination steroid/antibiotic eye drops.
- Watch for the development of complications, such as iris prolapse, a sharp pain in the eye, or hyphema, and report them immediately.
- Before discharge, teach correct instillation of eye drops, and instruct the patient to notify the doctor immediately if he experiences sharp eye pain. Caution him about activity restrictions, and advise him that it takes several weeks before he will receive his corrective reading glasses or lenses.

Retinitis Pigmentosa

Retinitis pigmentosa is a genetically induced, progressive destruction of the retinal rods, resulting in atrophy of the pigment epithelium and eventual blindness. Incidence ranges from 1 in 2,000 to 1 in 7,000 live births. Retinitis pigmentosa often accompanies other hereditary disorders in several distinct syndromes; the most common is Laurence-Moon-Biedl syndrome, typified by visual destruction from retinitis pigmentosa, obesity, mental retardation, polydactyly, and hypogenitalism.

Causes

About 80% of children with retinitis pigmentosa inherit it as an autosomal recessive trait. Onset occurs before age 20, initially affecting night and peripheral vision, and progresses inevitably—sometimes rapidly—to blindness before age 50. Retinitis pigmentosa can also be transmitted as an X-linked trait, producing the least common but most severe form of the disease, usually causing blindness before age 40.

Typically, in all forms of retinitis pigmentosa, the retinal rods slowly deteriorate; subsequently, the rest of the retina and pigment epithelium atrophy. Clumps of pigment resembling bone corpuscles aggregate in the equatorial region of the retina and later involve the macular and peripheral areas. In advanced stages, the retinal arterioles narrow, and the disk looks pale and waxy.

Signs and symptoms

Generally, night blindness occurs while the patient is in his teens. As the disease progresses, his visual field gradually constricts, causing tunnel or "gun-barrel" vision and, possibly, other ocular disorders, such as cataracts, choroidal sclerosis, macular degeneration, glaucoma, keratoconus, or scotomata (blind spots). Eventually, blindness follows invasion of the macula.

Diagnosis

A detailed family history may imply predisposition to retinitis pigmentosa. In a patient whose history suggests this condition, the following tests help confirm diagnosis.

- *Electroretinography* shows a retinal response time slower than normal or absent.
- *Visual field testing* (using a tangent screen) detects ring scotomata.
- *Fluorescein angiography* visualizes white dots (areas of dyspigmentation) in the epithelium.
- *Ophthalmoscopy* may initially show normal fundi but later reveals characteristic black pigmentary disturbance.

Treatment

Although extensive research continues, no cure exists for retinitis pigmentosa.

Special considerations

• Teach the patient and family what they need to know about retinitis pigmentosa. Explain that it's hereditary, and suggest genetic counseling for adults who risk transmitting it to their children.
• Tell the patient to wear dark glasses in bright sunlight. Warn him that he might not be able to drive a car at night. (Special new glasses can help patients with retinitis pigmentosa see at night but are experimental and expensive.)
• Refer the patient to a social service agency or to the National Retinitis Pigmentosa Foundation for information and for counseling to prepare him for eventual blindness. If the patient is willing, arrange for him to learn braille.
• Since the prospect of blindness is frightening, your emotional support and guidance are indispensable.

MISCELLANEOUS

Optic Atrophy

Optic atrophy, or degeneration of the optic nerve, can develop spontaneously (primary) or follow inflammation or edema of the nerve head (secondary). Some forms of this condition may subside without treatment, but degeneration of the optic nerve is irreversible.

Causes

Optic atrophy usually results from CNS disorders, such as:
• pressure on the optic nerve from aneurysms or intraorbital or intracranial tumors (descending optic atrophy)
• optic neuritis, in multiple sclerosis, retrobulbar neuritis, and tabes.

Other causes include retinitis pigmentosa; chronic papilledema and papillitis; congenital syphilis; glaucoma; central retinal artery or vein occlusion that interrupts the blood supply to the optic nerve, causing degeneration of ganglion cells (ascending optic atrophy); trauma; and ingestion of toxins, such as methanol and quinine.

Symptoms and diagnosis

Optic atrophy produces painless loss of either visual field or visual acuity, or both. Loss of vision may be abrupt or gradual, depending on the cause.

Slit-lamp examination and ophthalmoscopy confirm the diagnosis, although use of an opthalmoscope gives a better view. Slit-lamp examination reveals a pupil that reacts sluggishly to direct light stimulation. Ophthalmoscopy shows pallor of the nerve head from loss of microvascular circulation in the disk and deposit of fibrous or glial tissue. Visual field testing reveals a scotoma and, possibly, major visual field impairment.

Treatment and special considerations

Optic atrophy is irreversible, so treatment generally consists of correcting the underlying cause to prevent further vision loss. Steroids may be given to decrease inflammation and swelling, if a space-occupying lesion is the cause. In multiple sclerosis, resulting optic neuritis often subsides spontaneously.
• Provide symptomatic care during diagnostic procedures and treatment. Assist the patient who is visually compromised to perform daily activities.
• Explain all procedures, to minimize anxiety. Offer emotional support to help the patient deal with loss of vision.

Extraocular Motor Nerve Palsies

Extraocular motor nerve palsies are dysfunctions of the third, fourth, and sixth cranial nerves. The oculomotor (third cranial) nerve innervates the inferior, medial, and superior rectus muscles; the inferior oblique extraocular muscles; the pupilloconstrictor muscles; and the levator palpebrae muscles. The trochlear (fourth cranial) nerve innervates the superior oblique muscles; the abducens (sixth cranial) nerve innervates the lateral rectus muscles. The superior oblique muscles control downward rotation, intorsion, and abduction of the eye. Complete dysfunction of the third cranial nerve is called total oculomotor ophthalmoplegia and may be associated with other CNS abnormalities.

Causes

The most common causes of extraocular motor nerve palsies are diabetic neuropathy and pressure from an aneurysm or brain tumor. Other causes of these disorders vary, depending on the cranial nerve involved:

- *Third nerve (oculomotor) palsy* (acute ophthalmoplegia) also results from brain stem ischemia or other cerebrovascular disorders, poisoning (lead, carbon monoxide, botulism), alcohol abuse, infections (measles, encephalitis), trauma to the extraocular muscles, myasthenia gravis, or tumors in the cavernous sinus area.
- *Fourth nerve (trochlear) palsy* also results from closed-head trauma (blow-out fracture) or sinus surgery.
- *Sixth nerve (abducens) palsy* also results from increased intracranial pressure, brain abscess, meningitis, arterial brain occlusion, infections of the petrous bone (rare), lateral sinus thrombosis, myasthenia gravis, and thyrotropic exophthalmos.

Signs and symptoms

The most characteristic clinical effect of extraocular motor nerve palsies is diplopia of recent onset, which varies in different visual fields, depending on the muscles affected.

Typically, the patient with third nerve palsy exhibits ptosis, exotropia (eye looks outward), pupil dilation, and unresponsiveness to light; the eye is unable to move and cannot accommodate.

The patient with fourth nerve palsy displays diplopia and an inability to rotate the eye downward or upward. Such a patient develops ocular torticollis (wryneck) from repeatedly tilting his head to the affected side to compensate for vertical diplopia.

Sixth nerve palsy causes one eye to turn; the eye cannot abduct beyond the midline. To compensate for diplopia, the patient turns his head to the unaffected side and develops torticollis.

Diagnosis

Diagnosis necessitates a complete neuro-ophthalmologic examination and a thorough patient history. Differential diagnosis of third, fourth, or sixth nerve palsy depends on the specific motor defect exhibited by the patient.

For all extraocular motor nerve palsies, skull X-rays and CAT scans rule out tumors. The patient is also evaluated for an aneurysm or diabetes. If sixth nerve palsy results from infection, culture and sensitivity tests identify the causative organism and determine specific antibiotic therapy.

Treatment and special considerations

Identification of the underlying cause is essential, since treatment of extraocular motor nerve palsies varies accordingly. Neurosurgery is necessary if the cause is a brain tumor or an aneurysm. For infection, massive doses of antibiotics I.V. may be appropriate. After treatment of the primary condition, the patient may need to perform exercises that stretch the neck muscles to correct acquired torticollis. Other treatment and care are symptomatic.

Nystagmus

Nystagmus is recurring, involuntary eyeball movement. Such movement may be horizontal, vertical, rotating, or mixed; it produces blurred vision and difficulty in focusing. Nystagmus is classified according to eye movement characteristics and may be jerking or pendular. Prognosis varies with the underlying cause.

Causes

Although nystagmus may be congenital, it is usually an acquired disorder. *Jerking nystagmus,* the most common type, results from excessive stimulation of the vestibular apparatus in the inner ear or from lesions of the brain stem or cerebellum. This disorder occurs in acute labyrinthitis, Ménière's disease, multiple sclerosis, vascular lesions (especially in patients with hypertension), and any inflammation of the brain (such as encephalitis and meningitis). Jerking nystagmus may also result from drug and alcohol toxicity, and congenital neurologic disorders.

Pendular nystagmus results from improper transmission of visual impulses to the brain in the presence of corneal opacification, high astigmatism, congenital cataract or congenital anomalies of the optic disk, or bilateral macular lesions. Additional causes of pendular nystagmus include optic atrophy and albinism.

Signs and symptoms

In jerking nystagmus, the eyeballs oscillate faster in one direction than in the other; in pendular nystagmus, horizontal movements are approximately equal in both directions. If nystagmus results from a localized lesion, it may be unilateral; if from systemic disease, it's usually bilateral.

Diagnosis

The opticokinetic drum test is useful in diagnosing the underlying cause of nystagmus. In this test, the patient looks at a rapidly rotating, vertically striped drum—first at the stripes themselves, then quickly in the direction from which the stripes are coming, producing a normal jerking movement of the eyeballs. The absence of such a response suggests a CNS disturbance (such as a brain stem lesion).

Injecting warm or cold water into the external ear canal (caloric stimulation) also can precipitate nystagmus in an unaffected person. In patients with labyrinthine disorders, the response is abnormal (hypoactive or hyperactive) or absent.

Positional testing involves quickly changing the patient's position from supine to upright and turning his head from side to side, precipitating nystagmus. The direction of the nystagmus response aids diagnosis.

Treatment and special considerations

The goal of treatment of nystagmus is to correct the underlying cause, if possible. Unfortunately, the underlying cause often has no known cure (for example, brain stem lesions or multiple sclerosis). Eyeglasses can correct visual disturbances, such as high astigmatism. The patient can help himself see by positioning his head in a certain way; if he can't focus with both eyes, he can turn his head and use only one eye.

When caring for a patient with nystagmus, be sure to:

- explain testing procedures thoroughly

to lessen anxiety and help ensure his cooperation.
• provide emotional support for the patient with nystagmus of rapid onset, since the disorder may be caused by a brain stem lesion or some other severe neurologic disturbance.

Strabismus

(Squint, heterotropia, cross-eye, walleye)

Strabismus is a condition of eye malalignment due to the absence of normal, parallel, or coordinated eye movement. In children, it may be concomitant, in which the degree of deviation doesn't vary with the direction of gaze; inconcomitant, in which the degree of deviation varies with the direction of gaze; congenital (present at birth or during the first 6 months); or acquired (present during the first 2½ years.) Strabismus can also be latent (phoria), apparent when the child is tired or sick, or manifest (tropia). Tropias are categorized into four types: esotropia (eyes deviate inward), exotropia (eyes deviate outward), hypertropia (eyes deviate upward), and hypotropia (eyes deviate downward). Prognosis for correction varies with the timing of treatment and the onset of the disease. Muscle imbalances may be corrected by glasses, patching, or surgery, depending on the cause. However, residual defects in vision and extraocular muscle alignment may persist even after treatment. Strabismus affects about 2% of the population. Incidence of strabismus is higher in patients with CNS disorders, such as cerebral palsy, mental retardation, and Down's syndrome.

Causes

Strabismus is frequently inherited, but its cause is unknown. Controversy exists over whether or not amblyopia (lazy eye) causes or results from strabismus. In adults, strabismus may result from trauma. Strabismic amblyopia is characterized by a loss of central vision in one eye that typically results in esotropia (due to fixation in the dominant eye and suppression of images in the deviating eye). Strabismic amblyopia may result from hyperopia (farsightedness) or anisometropia (unequal refractive power). Esotropia may result from muscle imbalance and may be congenital or acquired. In accommodative esotropia, the child's attempt to compensate for the farsightedness affects the convergent reflex, and the eyes cross. Malalignment of the eyes leads to suppression of vision in one of the eyes, causing amblyopia if it develops early in life, before bifoveal fixation is established.

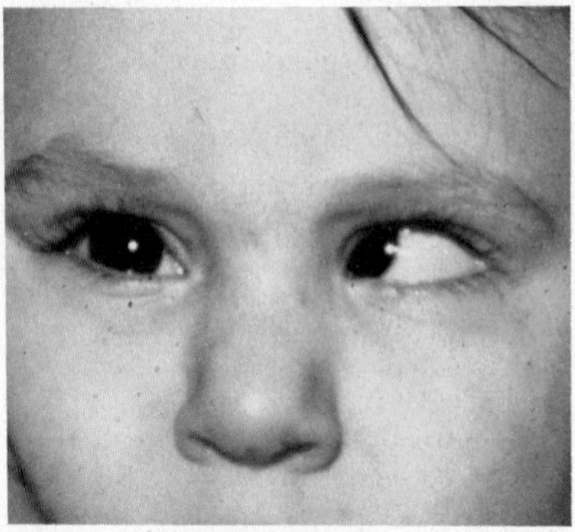

Note the medial deviation of the patient's left eye in this photo of esotropia.

Signs and symptoms

Malalignment of the eyes can be detected by external eye examination when deviation is obvious or by ophthalmoscopic observation of the corneal light reflex in the center of the pupils.

In addition, strabismus causes diplopia and other visual disturbances, which is often the reason that the patient seeks medical help.

Diagnosis

Parents of children with strabismus will typically seek medical advice. Older persons with strabismus commonly seek treatment to correct double vision or to improve appearance. A careful, detailed history is essential not only for the diagnosis, but also for the prognosis and treatment of strabismus. Ophthalmologic tests help diagnose strabismus:

- *Visual acuity test* evaluates the degree of visual defect.
- *Hirschberg's method* detects malalignment. The patient fixes his gaze on a light at a distance of about 13 inches, as the examiner observes the light decentered in the deviating eye.
- *Retinoscopy* determines refractive error; usually done with pupils dilated.
- *Maddox rods test* assesses specific muscle involvement.
- *Convergence test* shows distance at which convergence is sustained.
- *Duction test* reveals limitation of eye movement.
- *Cover-uncover test* demonstrates eye deviation and the rate of recovery to original alignment.
- *Alternate-cover test* shows intermittent or latent deviation.
- *Neurologic examination* determines whether condition is muscular or neurologic in origin, and should be performed if the onset of strabismus is sudden or if the CNS is involved.

Treatment

Initial treatment depends on the type of strabismus. For strabismic amblyopia, therapy includes patching the normal eye and prescribing corrective glasses to keep the eye straight and to counteract farsightedness (especially in accommodative esotropia). Surgery is often necessary for cosmetic and psychological reasons to correct strabismus due to basic esotropia, or residual accommodative esotropia after correction with glasses. Timing of surgery varies with individual circumstances. For example, a 6-month-old infant with equal visual acuity and a large esotropia will have the deviation corrected surgically. But a child with unequal visual acuity and an acquired deviation will have the affected eye patched until visual acuity is equal, *then* undergo surgery.

Surgical correction includes recession (moving the muscle posteriorly from its original insertion) or resection (shortening the muscle). Possible complications include overcorrection or undercorrection, slipped muscle, and perforation of the globe. Postoperative therapy may include patching the affected eye and applying combination antibiotic/steroid eye drops. Eye exercises and corrective glasses may still be necessary; surgery may have to be repeated.

Special considerations

- Postoperatively, discourage a child from rubbing his eyes.
- Gently wipe the child's tears, which will be serosanguineous. Parents may become upset by this aspect of surgery; reassure them that this is normal.
- Administer antiemetics, if necessary.
- Apply antibiotic ointment to the affected eye. Teach the patient or his parents how to instill the ointment.
- Because this surgery is usually a one-day procedure, most children are discharged after they recover from anesthesia; encourage compliance with recommended follow-up care.

Glaucoma

Glaucoma is a group of disorders characterized by an abnormally high intraocular pressure, which can damage the optic nerve. If untreated, it can lead to a gradual vision loss and, ultimately, blindness. Glaucoma occurs in several forms: chronic open-angle (primary), acute closed-angle, congenital (inherited as an autosomal recessive trait), and secondary to other causes.

Glaucoma affects 2% of the U.S. population over age 40 and accounts for 12% of all cases of new blindness in the U.S. Its incidence is highest among blacks. Prognosis is good with early treatment.

NORMAL FLOW OF AQUEOUS HUMOR

Aqueous humor, a transparent fluid produced by the ciliary epithelium of the ciliary body, flows from the posterior chamber to the anterior chamber through the pupil. Here it flows peripherally, and filters through the trabecular meshwork to the canal of Schlemm, through which the fluid ultimately enters venous circulation.

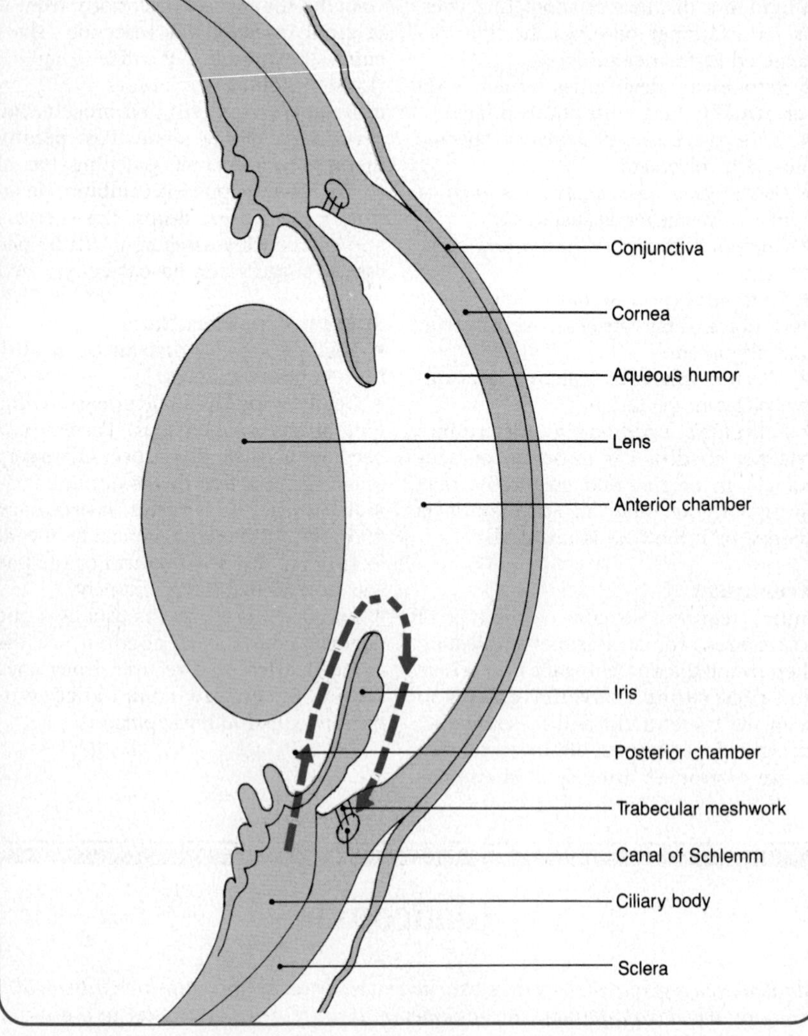

Causes and incidence

Chronic open-angle glaucoma results from overproduction of aqueous humor or obstruction to its outflow through the trabecular meshwork or the canal of Schlemm. This form of glaucoma is frequently familial in origin, and affects 90% of all patients with glaucoma.

Acute closed-angle (narrow-angle) glaucoma results from obstruction to the outflow of aqueous humor due to anatomically narrow angles between the anterior iris and the posterior corneal surface, shallow anterior chambers, a thickened iris that causes angle closure on pupil dilation, or a bulging iris that presses on the trabeculae, closing the angle (peripheral anterior synechiae).

Secondary glaucoma can result from uveitis, trauma, or drugs (such as steroids.) Neovascularization in the angle can result from vein occlusion or diabetes.

Signs and symptoms

Chronic open-angle glaucoma is usually bilateral, with insidious onset and a slowly progressive course. Symptoms appear late in the disease and include mild aching in the eyes, loss of peripheral vision, seeing halos around lights, and reduced visual acuity (especially at night) that is uncorrectable with glasses.

Acute closed-angle glaucoma typically has a rapid onset, constituting an ophthalmic emergency. Symptoms may include unilateral inflammation and pain, pressure over the eye, moderate pupil dilation that is nonreactive to light, a cloudy cornea, blurring and decreased visual acuity, photophobia, and seeing halos around lights. Increased intraocular pressure may induce nausea and vomiting, which may cause glaucoma to be misinterpreted as gastrointestinal distress. Unless treated promptly, this acute form of glaucoma produces blindness in 3 to 5 days.

Diagnosis

Loss of peripheral vision and disk changes confirm that glaucoma is present. Relevant diagnostic tests include:

- *tonometry* (using an applanation, Schiøtz, or pneumatic tonometer). This test measures the intraocular pressure (IOP) and provides a baseline for reference. Normal IOP ranges from 8 to 21 mm Hg. However, patients who fall in this normal range can develop signs and symptoms of glaucoma, and patients who have abnormally high pressure may have no clinical effects. Fingertip tension is another way to measure IOP. On gentle palpation of closed eyelids, one eye feels harder than the other in acute closed-angle glaucoma.
- *slit-lamp examination.* The slit lamp provides a look at the anterior structures of the eye, including the cornea, iris, and lens.
- *gonioscopy.* By determining the angle of the anterior chamber of the eye, gonioscopy enables differentiation between chronic open-angle glaucoma and acute closed-angle glaucoma. The angle is normal in chronic open-angle glaucoma. However, in older patients partial closure of the angle may also occur, so that two forms of glaucoma may coexist.

BLINDNESS

Blindness affects 28 million people worldwide. In the United States, blindness is legally defined as optimal visual acuity of 20/200 or less in the better eye after best correction, or a visual field not exceeding 20° in the better eye.

According to the World Health Organization, the most common causes of preventable blindness worldwide are trachoma, onchocerciasis (roundworm infection transmitted by a blackfly and other species of *Simulium*), and xerophthalmia (dryness of conjunctiva and cornea from vitamin A deficiency).

In the United States, the most common causes of acquired blindness are glaucoma, senile macular degeneration, and diabetic retinopathy. However, incidence of blindness from glaucoma is decreasing due to early detection and treatment. Rarer causes of acquired blindness include herpes simplex keratitis, cataracts, and retinal detachment.

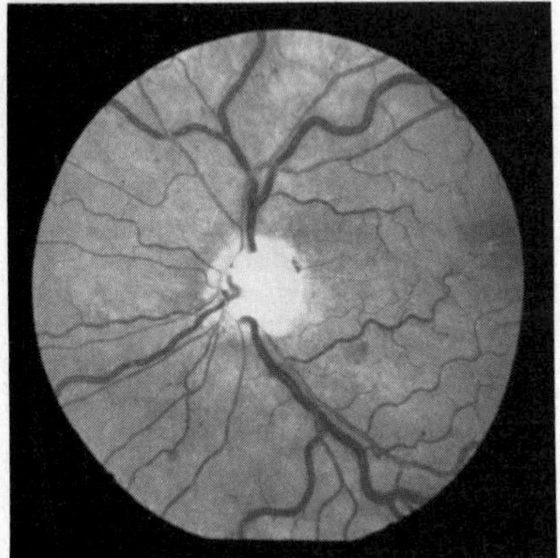

Ophthalmoscopy and slit-lamp examination show cupping of the optic disk characteristic of chronic glaucoma.

- *ophthalmoscopy*. This test provides a look at the fundus, where cupping and atrophy of the optic disk are visible in chronic open-angle glaucoma. These changes appear later in chronic closed-angle glaucoma, if the disease is not brought under control. A pale disk appears in acute closed-angle glaucoma.
- *perimetry or visual field tests*. The extent of chronic open-angle deterioration is evaluated by determining peripheral vision loss.
- *fundus photography*. Photographic recordings can monitor the disk for any changes.

Treatment

For chronic open-angle glaucoma, treatment initially decreases aqueous humor production through beta-blockers, such as timolol (contraindicated for asthmatics or patients with bradycardia) or betaxolol (Betoptic), a beta-1 blocker; epinephrine to lower intraocular pressure; or diuretics, such as acetazolamide. Drug treatment also includes miotic eyedrops, such as pilocarpine, to facilitate the outflow of aqueous humor. Patients who are unresponsive to drug therapy may be candidates for argon laser trabeculoplasty (ALT) or a surgical filtering procedure called trabeculectomy, which creates an opening for aqueous outflow. In ALT, an argon laser beam is focused on the trabecular meshwork of an open angle. This produces a thermal burn that changes the surface of the meshwork and increases the outflow of aqueous humor. In trabeculectomy, a flap of sclera is dissected free to expose the trabecular meshwork. Then, this discrete tissue block is removed and a peripheral iridectomy is performed. This produces an opening for aqueous outflow under the conjunctiva, creating a filtering bleb.

Acute closed-angle glaucoma is an ocular emergency requiring immediate treatment to lower the high IOP. If pressure doesn't decrease with drug therapy, laser iridotomy or surgical peripheral iridectomy must be performed promptly to save the patient's vision. Iridectomy relieves pressure by excising part of the iris to reestablish aqueous humor outflow. A prophylactic iridectomy is performed a few days later on the other eye to prevent an acute episode of glaucoma in the normal eye. Preoperative drug therapy lowers IOP with acetazolamide, pilocarpine (constricts the pupil, forcing the iris away from the trabeculae, allowing fluid to escape), and I.V. mannitol (20%) or oral glycerin (50%) to force fluid from the eye by making the blood hypertonic. Severe pain may necessitate narcotic analgesics.

Special considerations

- Stress the importance of meticulous compliance with prescribed drug therapy to prevent disk changes, loss of vision, and an increase in IOP.
- For the patient with acute closed-angle glaucoma, give medications, as ordered, and prepare him physically and psychologically for laser iridotomy or surgery.
- Postoperative care after peripheral iridectomy includes cycloplegic eye drops to relax the ciliary muscle and to decrease inflammation, thus preventing adhesions. *Note:* Cycloplegics must be used only in the affected eye. The use of these drops in the normal eye may precipitate an attack of acute closed-angle glaucoma in this eye, threatening the pa-

tient's residual vision.

• Encourage ambulation immediately after surgery.

• Following surgical filtering, postoperative care includes dilation and topical steroids to rest the pupil.

• Stress the importance of glaucoma screening for early detection and prevention. All persons over age 35, especially those with family histories of glaucoma, should have an annual tonometric examination.

Selected References

Boyd-Monk, Heather, "Examining the External Eye," Part 1, *Nursing80* 10(5):58-62, May 1980.

Ciolino, N., and Horowitz, J. "What Diabetics Need to Know About Their Risk of Blindness," *Sight Saving: Journal for Blindness Prevention Professionals and Volunteers* 52(1):2-5, 1983.

Conn, Howard F., and Conn, Rex B., Jr. *Current Diagnosis*. Philadelphia: W.B. Saunders Co., 1980.

Duane, Thomas, ed. *Clinical Ophthalmology*. New York: Harper & Row Publishers, 1985.

Harley, Robinson D., ed. *Pediatric Ophthalmology*, Philadelphia: W.B. Saunders Co., 1983.

Jay, Walter M., and Calvert, Jon C. "The Child with Strabismus," *AFP Practical Therapeutics* 23(4):156-62, April 1981.

Luckman, J., and Sorensen, K.C. *Medical/Surgical Nursing*, 2nd ed. Philadelphia: W.B. Saunders Co., 1980.

MacFaden, J.S. "Caring for the Patient with a Primary Retinal Detachment," *American Journal of Nursing* 80(5):920-21, May 1980.

Perrin, Elizabeth D. "Laser Therapy for Diabetic Retinopathy," *American Journal of Nursing* 80(4):664-65, April 1980.

Saunders, William H., et al. *Nursing Care in Eye, Ear, Nose and Throat Disorders*, 4th ed. St. Louis: C.V. Mosby Co., 1979.

Shields, Jerry A., and Augsburger, James J. "Current Approaches to the Diagnosis and Management of Retinoblastoma," *Survey of Ophthalmology* 25(6):347-72, May/June 1981.

Vaughan, Daniel, and Asbury, Taylor. *General Ophthalmology*, 10th ed. Los Altos, Calif.: Lange Medical Pubs., 1983.

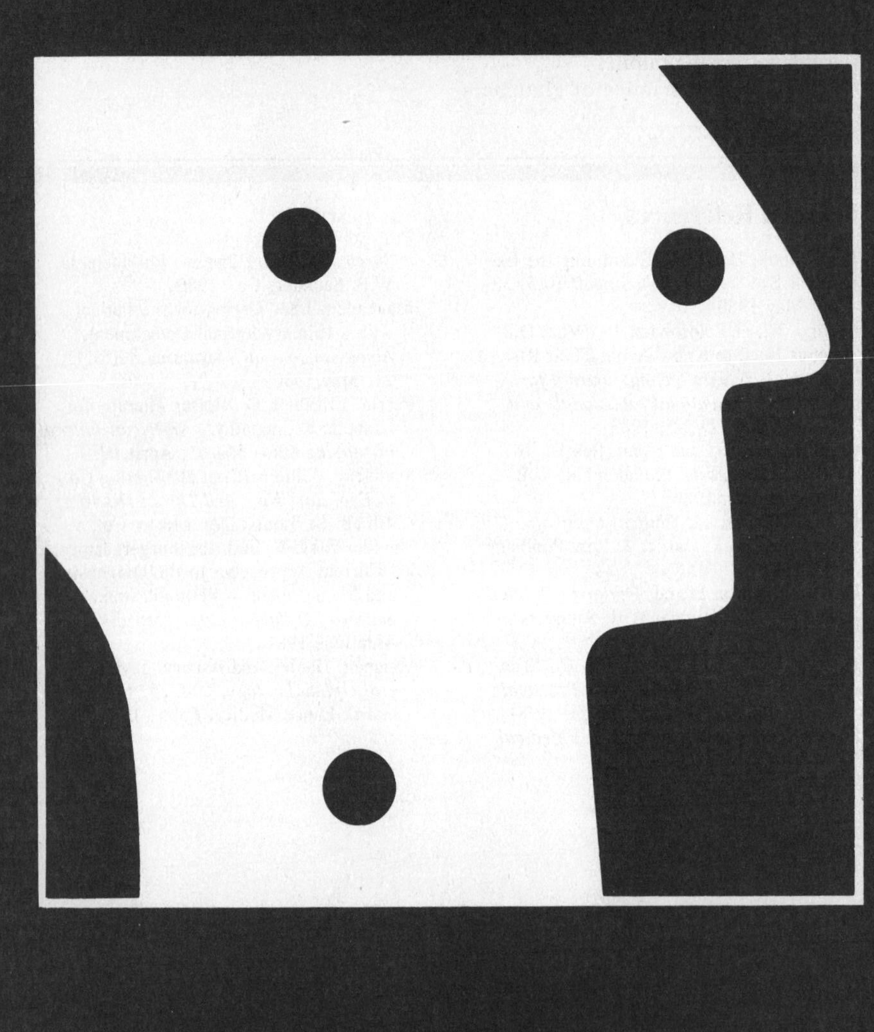

20 Ear, Nose, and Throat Disorders

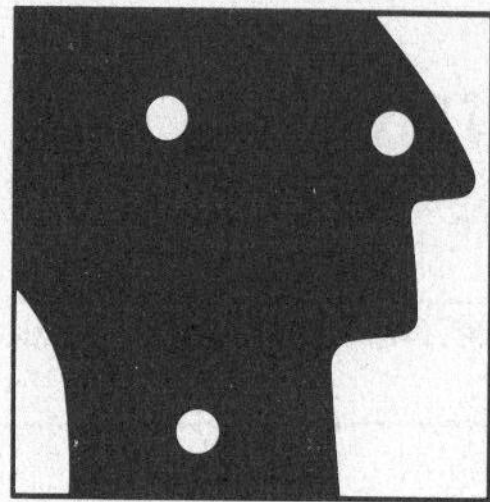

Ear, Nose, and Throat Disorders

Introduction

Most ear, nose, and throat disorders rarely prove fatal (except for those resulting from neoplasms, epiglottitis, and neck trauma) but may cause serious social, cosmetic, and communication problems. Untreated hearing loss or deafness can drastically impair ability to interact with society. Ear disorders also have the ability to impair equilibrium. Nasal disorders can cause changes in facial features and interfere with breathing and tasting. Diseases arising in the throat may threaten airway patency and interfere with speech. In addition, these disorders can cause considerable discomfort and pain for the patient and require thorough assessment and prompt treatment.

The ear

Hearing begins when sound waves reach the tympanic membrane, which then vibrates the ossicles in the middle ear cavity. The stapes transmits these vibrations to the perilymphatic fluid in the inner ear by vibrating against the oval window. The vibrations then pass across the cochlea's fluid receptor cells, in the basilar membrane, stimulating movement of the hair cells of the organ of Corti and initiating auditory nerve impulses to the brain.

The inner ear structures also maintain the body's equilibrium and balance through the fluid in the semicircular canals. This fluid is set in motion by body movement and stimulates nerve cells that line the canals. These cells, in turn, transmit impulses to the brain by way of the vestibular branch of the acoustic nerve.

Although the ear can respond to sounds that vibrate at frequencies from 20 to 20,000 hertz (Hz), the range of normal speech is from 250 to 4,000 Hz, with 70% falling between 500 and 2,000 Hz. The ratio between sound intensities, the decibel (db), is the lowest volume at which any given sound can be heard. A faint whisper registers 10 to 15 db; average conversation, 50 to 60 db; a shout, 85 to 90 db. Hearing damage may follow exposure to sounds louder than 90 db.

Assessment

After obtaining a thorough patient history of ear disease, inspect the auricle and surrounding tissue for deformities, lumps, and skin lesions. Ask the patient if he has ear pain. If you see inflammation, check for tenderness by moving the auricle and pressing on the tragus and the mastoid process. Check the ear canal for excessive cerumen, discharge, or foreign bodies.

Ask the patient if he's had episodes of vertigo or blurred vision. To test for vertigo, have the patient stand on one foot and close his eyes, or have him walk a straight line with his eyes closed. Ask him if he always falls to the same side and if the room seems to be spinning.

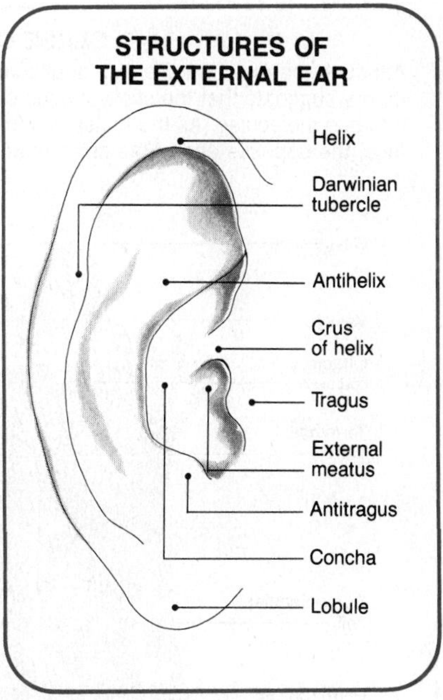

Audiometric testing

Audiometric testing evaluates hearing and determines the type and extent of hearing loss. The simplest but least reliable method for judging hearing acuity consists of covering one of the patient's ears, standing 18″ to 24″ (45 to 60 cm) from the uncovered ear, and whispering a short phrase or series of numbers. (Block the patient's vision to prevent lip reading.) Then ask the patient to repeat the phrase or series of numbers. To test hearing at both high and low frequencies, repeat the test in a normal speaking voice. (As an alternative, you can hold a ticking watch to the patient's ear.)

If you identify a hearing loss, further testing is necessary to determine if the loss is conductive or sensorineural. A conductive loss can result from faulty bone conduction (inability of the eighth cranial nerve to respond to sound waves traveling through the skull) or faulty air conduction (impaired transmission of sound through ear structures to the auditory nerve and, ultimately, the brain).

The following tests assess bone and air conduction:

- *Rinne test:* The base of a lightly vibrating tuning fork is placed on the mastoid process (bone conduction [BC]). Then the fork is moved to the front of the meatus, where the patient should continue to hear the vibrations (air conduction [AC]). The patient must determine which sounds louder. In a positive Rinne test, AC is greater than BC, usually indicating sensorineural loss. In a negative Rinne test, BC is greater than AC, and may suggest a conductive loss.
- *Weber test* (used for testing unilateral

hearing loss): The handle of a lightly vibrating tuning fork is placed on the midline of the forehead. Normally, the patient should hear sounds equally in both ears. With conductive hearing loss, sound lateralizes (localizes) to the ear with the poorest hearing. With sensorineural loss, sound lateralizes to the better functioning ear.

After identification of the hearing loss as conductive, sensorineural, or mixed, further audiometric testing determines the extent of hearing loss. These audiometric tests include pure tone audiometry, speech audiometry, impedance audiometry, and tympanometry.

• *Pure tone audiometry* uses an audiometer to produce a series of pure tones of calibrated loudness (db) at different frequencies (125 to 8,000 Hz). These test tones are conveyed to the patient's ears through headphones or a bone conduction (sound) vibrator. Speech threshold represents the loudness at which a person with normal hearing can perceive the tone. Both AC and BC are measured for each ear, and the results are plotted on a graph. If hearing is normal, the line is plotted at 0 db. In adults, normal hearing may range from 0 to 25 db.

• *Speech audiometry* uses the same technique as pure tone audiometry, but with speech, instead of pure tones, transmitted through the headset. (A person

SENSE OF SMELL

Although the exact mechanism of olfactory perception is unknown, the most likely theory suggests that the sticky mucus covering the olfactory cells traps airborne odorous molecules. As the molecules fit into appropriate receptors on the cell surface, the opposite end of the cell transmits an electrical impulse to the brain.

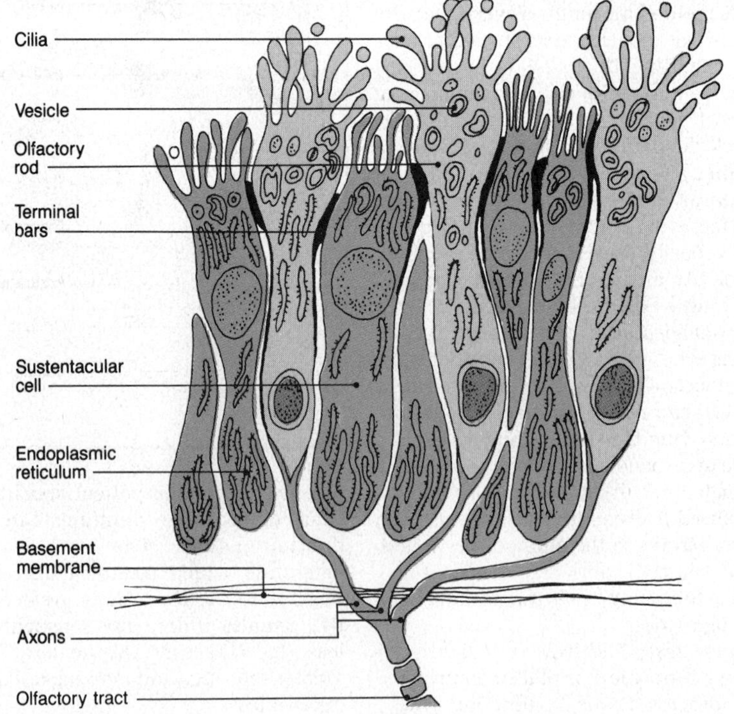

with normal hearing can hear and repeat 88% to 100% of transmitted words.)

- *Impedance audiometry* detects middle ear pathology, precisely determining the degree of tympanic membrane and middle ear mobility. One end of the impedance audiometer, a probe with three small tubes, is inserted into the external canal; the other end is attached to an oscillator. One tube delivers a low tone of variable intensity, the second contains a microphone, and the third, an air pump. A mobile tympanic membrane reflects minimal sound waves and produces a low-voltage curve on the graph. A tympanic membrane with decreased mobility reflects maximal sound waves and produces a high-voltage curve.
- *Tympanometry*, using the impedance audiometer, measures tympanic membrane compliance to air pressure variations in the external canal and determines the degree of negative pressure in the middle ear.

The nose

As air travels between the septum and the turbinates, it touches sensory hairs (cilia) in the mucosal surface, which then add, retain, or remove moisture and particles in the air to ensure delivery of humid, bacteria-free air to the pharynx and lungs. In addition, when air touches the mucosal cilia, the resultant stimulation of the first cranial nerve sends nerve impulses to the olfactory area of the frontal cortex, providing the sense of smell.

Assessment

Check the external nose for redness, edema, lumps, tumors, or poor alignment. Marked septal cartilage depression may indicate saddle deformity due to septal destruction from trauma or congenital syphilis; extreme lateral deviation, from injury. Red nostrils may indicate frequent nose blowing caused by allergies or infectious rhinitis. Dilated, engorged blood vessels may suggest alcoholism or constant exposure to the elements. A bulbous, discolored nose may be a sign of rosacea.

With a nasal speculum and adequate lighting, check nasal mucosa for pallor and edema or redness and inflammation, dried mucous plugs, furuncles, and polyps. Also, look for abnormal appearance of capillaries and a deviated or perforated septum. Check for nasal discharge (assess color, consistency, and odor) and blood. Profuse, thin, watery discharge may indicate allergy or cold; excessive, thin, purulent discharge may indicate cold or chronic sinus infection.

Check for sinus inflammation by applying pressure to the nostrils, orbital rims, and cheeks. Pain after pressure applied above the upper orbital rims indicates frontal sinus irritation; pain after pressure applied to the cheeks, maxillary sinus irritation.

The throat

Parts of the throat include the pharynx, epiglottis, and larynx. The pharynx is the passageway for food to the esophagus and air to the larynx. The epiglottis diverts material away from the glottis during swallowing. The larynx produces sounds by vibrating expired air through the vocal cords. Changes in vocal cord length and air pressure affect pitch and voice intensity. The larynx also stimulates the vital cough reflex when a foreign body touches its sensitive mucosa.

Assessment

Using a bright light and a tongue blade, inspect the patient's mouth and throat. Look for inflammation or white patches, and any irregularities on the tongue or throat. Assess vital signs and respiratory status. Make sure the patient's airway isn't compromised. Watch for and immediately report signs of respiratory distress (dyspnea, tachycardia, tachypnea, inspiratory stridor, restlessness) and changes in voice or in skin color, such as circumoral or nail-bed cyanosis. The main diagnostic test used in throat assessment is a culture to identify the infection-causing organism.

EXTERNAL EAR

Otitis Externa

(External otitis, swimmer's ear)

Otitis externa, inflammation of the skin of the external ear canal and auricle, may be acute or chronic. It is most common in the summer. With treatment, acute otitis externa usually subsides within 7 days—although it may become chronic—and tends to recur.

Causes and incidence

Otitis externa usually results from bacteria, such as *Pseudomonas*, *Proteus vulgaris*, streptococci, and *Staphylococcus aureus* and, sometimes, fungi, such as *Aspergillus niger* and *Candida albicans* (fungal otitis externa is most common in the Tropics). Occasionally, chronic otitis externa results from dermatologic conditions, such as seborrhea or psoriasis. Predisposing factors include:

- swimming in contaminated water; cerumen creates a culture medium for the waterborne organism.
- cleaning the ear canal with a cotton swab, bobby pin, finger, or other foreign objects; this irritates the ear canal and possibly introduces the infecting microorganism.
- exposure to dust, hair care products, or other irritants, which causes the patient to scratch his ear, excoriating the auricle and canal.
- regular use of earphones, earplugs, or earmuffs, which trap moisture in the ear canal, creating a culture medium for infection.
- chronic drainage from a perforated tympanic membrane.

Signs and symptoms

Acute otitis externa characteristically produces moderate to severe pain that is exacerbated by manipulation of the auricle or tragus, clenching the teeth, opening the mouth, or chewing. Its other clinical effects may include fever, foul-smelling aural discharge, regional cellulitis, and partial hearing loss.

Fungal otitis externa may be asymptomatic, although *A. niger* produces a black or gray, blotting paper–like growth in the ear canal. In chronic otitis externa, pruritus replaces pain, which may lead to scaling and skin thickening. Aural discharge may also occur.

Diagnosis

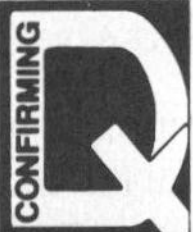

Physical examination confirms otitis externa. In acute otitis externa, otoscopy reveals a swollen external ear canal (sometimes to the point of complete closure), periauricular lymphadenopathy (tender nodes in front of the tragus, behind the ear, or in the upper neck), and, occasionally, regional cellulitis.

In fungal otitis externa, removal of growth shows thick, red epithelium. Microscopic examination or culture and sensitivity tests can identify the causative organism and determine antibiotic treatment. Pain on palpation of the tragus or auricle distinguishes acute otitis externa from otitis media.

In chronic otitis externa, physical examination shows thick red epithelium in the ear canal. Severe chronic otitis externa may reflect underlying diabetes mellitus, hypothyroidism, or nephritis.

Treatment

To relieve the pain of acute otitis externa, treatment includes heat therapy to the periauricular region (heat lamp; hot, damp compresses; heating pad), aspirin

DIFFERENTIAL DIAGNOSIS OF ACUTE OTITIS EXTERNA AND ACUTE OTITIS MEDIA

ACUTE OTITIS EXTERNA (PREVALENT IN SUMMER)

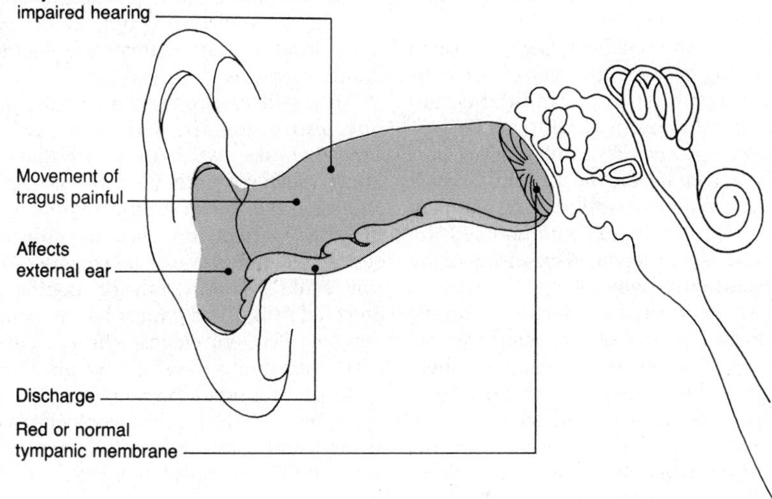

ACUTE OTITIS MEDIA (PREVALENT IN WINTER)

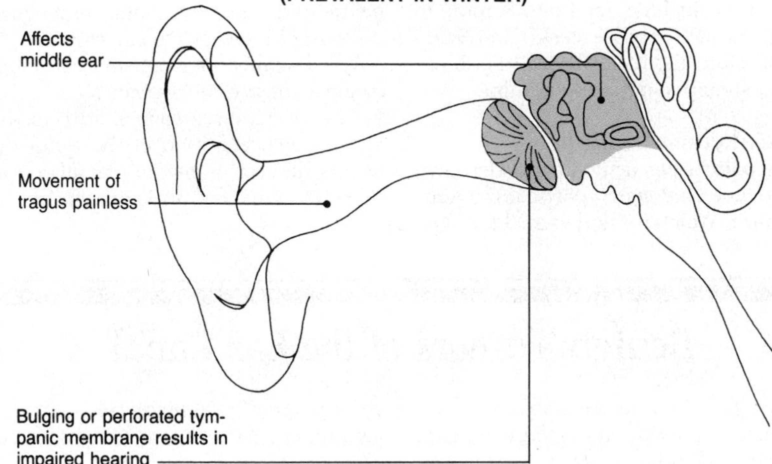

or acetaminophen, and codeine. Instillation of antibiotic eardrops (with or without hydrocortisone) follows cleansing of the ear and removal of debris. If fever persists or regional cellulitis develops, a systemic antibiotic is necessary.

As with other forms of this disorder, fungal otitis externa necessitates careful cleansing of the ear. Application of a keratolytic or 2% salicylic acid in cream containing nystatin may help treat otitis externa resulting from candidal organisms. Instillation of slightly acidic eardrops creates an unfavorable environment in the ear canal for most fungi, as well as *Pseudomonas*. No specific treatment exists for otitis externa caused by *A. niger*, except repeated cleansing of the ear canal with baby oil.

In chronic otitis externa, primary treatment consists of cleansing the ear and removing debris. Supplemental therapy includes instillation of antibiotic eardrops or application of antibiotic ointment or cream (neomycin, bacitracin, or polymyxin, possibly combined with hydrocortisone). Another ointment contains phenol, salicylic acid, precipitated sulfur, and petrolatum and produces exfoliative and antipruritic effects.

For mild chronic otitis externa, treatment may include instilling antibiotic eardrops once or twice weekly and wearing specially fitted earplugs while showering, shampooing, or swimming.

Special considerations

If the patient has acute otitis externa:

- Monitor vital signs, particularly temperature. Watch for and record the type and amount of aural drainage.
- Remove debris and gently cleanse the ear canal with mild Burow's solution (aluminum acetate). Place a wisp of cotton soaked with solution into the ear, and apply a saturated compress directly to the auricle. Afterward, dry the ear gently but thoroughly. (In severe otitis externa, such cleansing may be delayed until after initial treatment with antibiotic eardrops.)
- To instill eardrops in an adult, pull the pinna upward and backward to straighten the canal. To ensure that the drops reach the epithelium, insert a wisp of cotton moistened with eardrops.
- If the patient has chronic otitis externa, cleanse the ear thoroughly. Use wet soaks intermittently on oozing or infected skin. If the patient has a chronic fungal infection, cleanse the ear canal well, then apply an exfoliative ointment.

To prevent otitis externa:

- Suggest using lamb's wool earplugs coated with petrolatum, to keep water out of the ears when showering or shampooing.
- Tell the patient to wear earplugs or to keep his head above water when swimming; to instill two or three drops of 3% boric acid solution in 70% alcohol before and after swimming, to toughen the skin of the external ear canal.
- Warn against cleaning the ears with cotton swabs or other objects.
- Urge prompt treatment of otitis media to prevent perforation of the tympanic membrane, (otitis media may also lead to the more benign otitis externa).

Benign Tumors of the Ear Canal

Benign tumors may develop anywhere in the ear canal. Common types include keloids, osteomas, and sebaceous cysts; their causes vary. These tumors rarely become malignant, and, with proper treatment, prognosis is excellent.

Signs and symptoms

A benign ear tumor is usually asymptomatic, unless it becomes infected, in which case pain, fever, or inflammation may result. (Pain is often a sign of malignancy.) If the tumor grows large enough

CAUSES AND CHARACTERISTICS OF BENIGN EAR TUMORS

TUMOR	CAUSES AND INCIDENCE	CHARACTERISTICS
Keloid	• Surgery or trauma, such as ear-piercing • Most common in Blacks	• Hypertrophy and fibrosis of scar tissue • Commonly recurs
Osteoma	• Idiopathic growth • Predisposing factor, swimming in cold water • Three times more common in males than in females • Seldom occurs before adolescence	• Bony outgrowth from wall of external auditory meatus • Usually bilateral and multiple (exostoses)
Sebaceous cyst	• Obstruction of a sebaceous gland	• Painless mass filled with oily, fatty, glandular secretions • May occur on external ear (especially postauricular area) and outer one third of external auditory canal

to obstruct the ear canal by itself or through accumulated cerumen and debris, it may cause hearing loss and the sensation of pressure.

Diagnosis

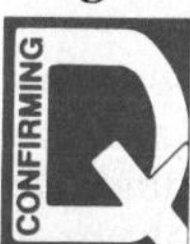

Clinical features and patient history suggest a benign tumor of the ear canal; otoscopy confirms it. To rule out malignancy, the doctor may perform a biopsy.

Treatment

Generally, a benign tumor requires surgical excision if it obstructs the ear canal, is cosmetically undesirable, or becomes malignant.

Treatment of keloids may include surgery followed by repeated injections of long-acting steroids into the suture line. Excision must be complete, but even this may not prevent recurrence.

Surgical excision of an osteoma consists of elevating the skin from the surface of the bony growth and shaving the osteoma with a mechanical burr or drill.

Prior to surgery, a sebaceous cyst requires preliminary treatment with antibiotics, to reduce inflammation. To prevent recurrence, excision must be complete, including the sac or capsule of the cyst.

Special considerations

Since treatment of benign ear tumors generally doesn't require hospitalization, focus your care on giving emotional support and providing appropriate patient teaching so that the patient follows his therapeutic plan properly when he's at home.

- Thoroughly explain diagnostic procedures and treatment to the patient and his family. Reassure them and answer any questions they may have.
- After surgery, instruct the patient in good aural hygiene. Until his ear is completely healed, advise him not to insert anything in his ear or allow water to get in it. Suggest that he cover his ears with a cap when showering.
- Teach the patient how to recognize signs of infection, such as pain, fever, localized redness, and swelling. If he detects any of these signs, instruct him to report them immediately.

MIDDLE EAR

Otitis Media

Otitis media, inflammation of the middle ear, may be suppurative or secretory, acute or chronic. Acute otitis media is common in children; its incidence rises during the winter months, paralleling the seasonal rise in nonbacterial respiratory tract infections. With prompt treatment, prognosis for acute otitis media is excellent; however, prolonged accumulation of fluid within the middle ear cavity causes chronic otitis media, with possible perforation of the tympanic membrane. Chronic suppurative otitis media may lead to scarring, adhesions, and severe structural or functional ear damage; chronic secretory otitis media, with its persistent inflammation and pressure, may cause conductive hearing loss.

Causes

Otitis media results from disruption of eustachian tube patency. In the suppurative form, respiratory tract infection, allergic reaction, or positional changes (such as holding an infant supine during feeding) allow nasopharyngeal flora to reflux through the eustachian tube and colonize the middle ear. Suppurative otitis media usually results from bacterial infection with pneumococcus, *Hemophilus influenzae* (the most common cause in children under age 6), beta-hemolytic streptococci, staphylococci (most common cause in children age 6 and older), and gram-negative bacteria. Predisposing factors include the normally wider, shorter, more horizontal eustachian tubes and increased lymphoid tissue in children, and anatomic anomalies, such as cleft palate. Chronic suppurative otitis media results from inadequate treatment of acute otitis episodes or from infection by resistant strains of bacteria.

Secretory otitis media results from obstruction of the eustachian tube. This causes a buildup of negative pressure in the middle ear that promotes transudation of sterile serous fluid from blood vessels in the membrane of the middle ear. Such effusion may be secondary to eustachian tube dysfunction from viral infection or allergy. It may also follow barotrauma (pressure injury caused by inability to equalize pressures between the environment and the middle ear), such as that during rapid aircraft descent in a person with an upper respiratory tract infection or during rapid underwater ascent in scuba diving (barotitis media). Chronic secretory otitis media follows persistent eustachian tube dysfunction from mechanical obstruction (adenoidal tissue overgrowth, tumors), edema (allergic rhinitis, chronic sinus infection), or inadequate treatment of acute suppurative otitis media.

Signs and symptoms

Clinical features of acute suppurative otitis media include severe, deep, throbbing pain (from pressure behind the tympanic membrane); signs of upper respiratory tract infection (sneezing, coughing); mild to very high fever; hearing loss (usually mild and conductive); dizziness; nausea; and vomiting. Other possible effects include bulging of the tympanic membrane, with concomitant erythema, and purulent drainage in the ear canal from tympanic membrane rupture. However, many patients are asymptomatic.

Acute secretory otitis media produces severe conductive hearing loss—which varies from 15 to 35 db, depending on the thickness and amount of fluid in the middle ear cavity—and, possibly, a sensation of fullness in the ear and popping, crackling, or clicking sounds on swallowing or with jaw movement. Accumulation of fluid may also cause the patient to hear an echo when he speaks and to experience a vague feeling of top heaviness. However, acute secretory otitis media is frequently asymptomatic.

Chronic otitis media usually begins in childhood and persists into adulthood. Its cumulative effects include thickening and scarring of the tympanic membrane; decreased or absent tympanic membrane mobility; cholesteatoma (a cystlike mass in the middle ear); and, with chronic suppurative otitis media, painless purulent discharge. Associated conductive hearing loss varies with the size and type of tympanic membrane perforation and ossicular destruction. Complications may include abscesses (brain, subperiosteal, and epidural), sigmoid sinus or jugular vein thrombosis, septicemia, meningitis, suppurative labyrinthitis, facial paralysis, and otitis externa.

Diagnosis

In acute suppurative otitis media, otoscopy reveals obscured or distorted bony landmarks of the tympanic membrane. Pneumatoscopy can show decreased tympanic membrane mobility, but this procedure is painful with an obviously bulging, erythematous tympanic membrane. The pain pattern is diagnostically significant: in acute suppurative otitis media, for example, pulling the auricle *doesn't* exacerbate the pain.

In acute secretory otitis media, otoscopy demonstrates tympanic membrane retraction, which causes the bony landmarks to appear more prominent. This examination also detects clear or amber fluid behind the tympanic membrane, possibly with a meniscus and bubbles. If hemorrhage into the middle ear has occurred, as in barotrauma, the tympanic membrane appears blue-black.

In chronic otitis media, patient history discloses recurrent or unresolved otitis media. Otoscopy shows thickening and sometimes scarring, and decreased mobility of the tympanic membrane; pneumatoscopy, decreased or absent tympanic membrane movement. History of recent air travel or scuba diving suggests barotitis media.

Treatment

In acute suppurative otitis media, antibiotic therapy includes ampicillin or amoxicillin for infants, children, and adults. For those who are allergic to penicillin derivatives, therapy may include cefaclor or co-trimoxazole. Aspirin or acetaminophen are given to control pain and fever. Severe, painful bulging of the tympanic membrane usually necessitates myringotomy. Broad-spectrum antibiotics can help prevent acute suppurative otitis media in high-risk patients, such as children with recurring episodes of otitis. However, in patients with recurring otitis, antibiotics must be used sparingly and with discretion, to prevent development of resistant strains of bacteria.

In acute secretory otitis media, inflation of the eustachian tube by performing Valsalva's maneuver several times a day may be the only treatment required. Otherwise, nasopharyngeal decongestant therapy may be helpful. It should continue for at least 2 weeks and, sometimes, indefinitely, with periodic evaluation. If decongestant therapy fails, myringotomy and aspiration of middle ear fluid are necessary, followed by insertion of a polyethylene tube into the tympanic membrane, for immediate and prolonged equalization of pressure. The tube falls out spontaneously after 9 to 12 months. Concomitant treatment of the underlying cause (such as elimination of allergens, or adenoidectomy for hypertrophied adenoids) may also be helpful in correcting this disorder.

Treatment of chronic otitis media includes antibiotics for exacerbations of acute otitis media, elimination of eustachian tube obstruction, treatment of otitis externa (when present), myringoplasty (tympanic membrane graft) and tympanoplasty to reconstruct middle ear structures when thickening and scarring are present, and, possibly, mastoidectomy. When present, cholesteatoma requires excision.

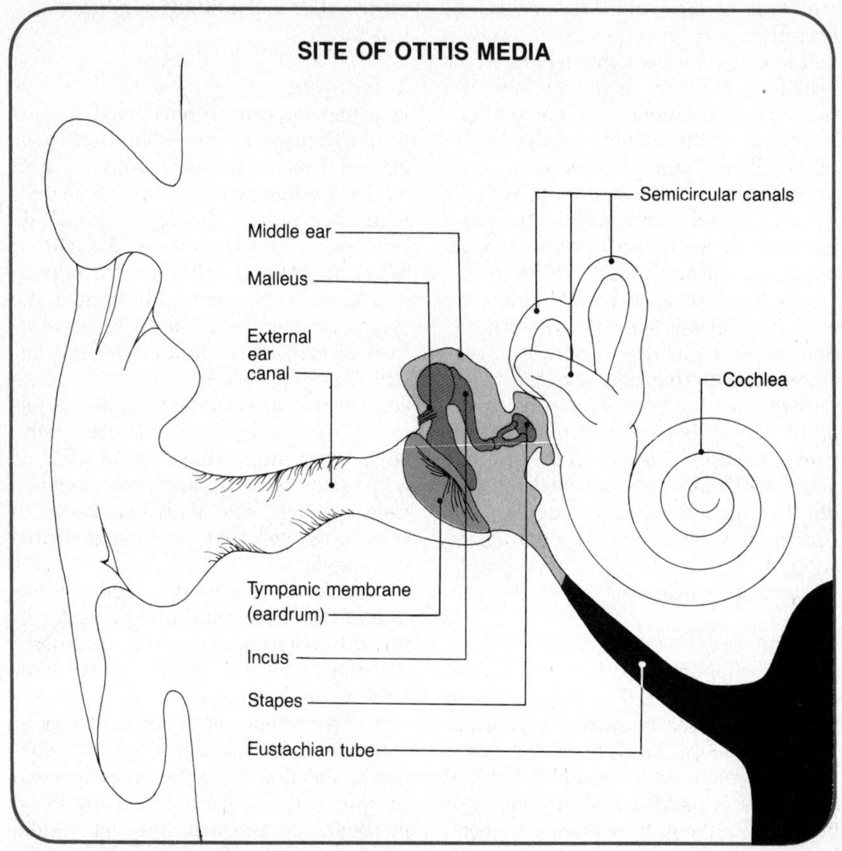

Special considerations

- Explain all diagnostic tests and procedures. After myringotomy, maintain drainage flow. Don't place cotton or plugs deep in the ear canal; however, sterile cotton may be placed loosely in the external ear to absorb drainage. To prevent infection, change the cotton whenever it gets damp, and wash hands before and after giving ear care. Watch for and report headache, fever, severe pain, or disorientation.
- After tympanoplasty, reinforce dressings, and observe for excessive bleeding from the ear canal. Administer analgesics, as needed. Warn the patient against blowing his nose or getting the ear wet when bathing.
- Encourage the patient to complete the prescribed course of antibiotic treatment. If nasopharyngeal decongestants are ordered, teach correct instillation.
- Suggest application of heat to the ear to relieve pain.
- Advise the patient with acute secretory otitis media to watch for and immediately report pain and fever—signs of secondary infection.

To prevent otitis media:

- Teach recognition of upper respiratory tract infections and encourage early treatment.
- Instruct parents not to feed their infant in a supine position or put him to bed with a bottle. This prevents reflux of nasopharyngeal flora.
- To promote eustachian tube patency, instruct the patient to perform Valsalva's maneuver several times daily.

Mastoiditis

Mastoiditis is a bacterial infection and inflammation of the air cells of the mastoid antrum. Although prognosis is good with early treatment, possible complications include meningitis, facial paralysis, brain abscess, and suppurative labyrinthitis.

Causes and incidence

Bacteria that cause mastoiditis include pneumococcus (usually in children under age 6), *Hemophilus influenzae,* beta-hemolytic streptococci, staphylococci, and gram-negative organisms. Mastoiditis is usually a complication of chronic otitis media and, less frequently, of acute otitis media. An accumulation of pus under pressure in the middle ear cavity results in necrosis of adjacent tissue and extension of the infection into the mastoid cells. Chronic systemic diseases or immunosuppression may also lead to mastoiditis.

Signs and symptoms

Primary clinical features include a dull ache and tenderness in the area of the mastoid process, low-grade fever, and a thick, purulent discharge that gradually becomes more profuse, possibly leading to otitis externa. Postauricular erythema and edema may push the auricle out from the head; pressure within the edematous mastoid antrum may produce swelling and obstruction of the external ear canal, causing conductive hearing loss.

Diagnosis

X-rays of the mastoid area reveal hazy mastoid air cells; the bony walls between the cells appear decalcified. Examination shows a dull, thickened, and edematous tympanic membrane, if the membrane isn't concealed by obstruction. During examination, the external ear canal is cleaned; persistent oozing into the canal indicates perforation of the tympanic membrane.

Treatment

Treatment of mastoiditis consists of intense parenteral antibiotic therapy. If bone damage is minimal, myringotomy drains purulent fluid and provides a specimen of discharge for culture and sensitivity testing. Recurrent or persistent infection, or signs of intracranial complications necessitate simple mastoidectomy. This procedure involves removal of the diseased bone and cleansing of the affected area, after which a drain is inserted.

A chronically inflamed mastoid requires radical mastoidectomy (excision of the posterior wall of the ear canal, remnants of the tympanic membrane, and the malleus and incus [although these bones are usually destroyed by infection before surgery]). The stapes and facial nerve remain intact. Radical mastoidectomy, which is seldom necessary because of antibiotic therapy, does not drastically affect the patient's hearing because significant hearing loss precedes surgery. With either surgical procedure, the patient continues oral antibiotic therapy for several weeks after surgery and hospital discharge.

Special considerations

- After simple mastoidectomy, give pain medication, as needed. Check wound drainage, and reinforce dressings (the surgeon usually changes the dressing daily and removes the drain in 72 hours). Check the patient's hearing, and watch for signs of complications, especially infection (either localized or extending to the brain); facial nerve paralysis, with unilateral facial drooping; bleeding; and vertigo, especially when the patient stands.
- After radical mastoidectomy, the wound is packed with petrolatum gauze or gauze treated with an antibiotic oint-

ment. Give pain medication before the packing is removed, on the fourth or fifth postoperative day.

• Because of stimulation to the inner ear during surgery, the patient may feel dizzy and nauseated for several days afterward. Keep the side rails up, and assist the patient with ambulation. Also, give antiemetics, as ordered and as needed.

• Before discharge, teach the patient and family how to change the dressing, and tell them to avoid getting it wet. Urge compliance with prescribed antibiotic treatment, and promote regular follow-up care.

Otosclerosis

The most common cause of conductive deafness, otosclerosis is the slow formation of spongy bone in the otic capsule, particularly at the oval window. It occurs in at least 10% of Caucasians, and is twice as prevalent in females as in males, usually between ages 15 and 30. With surgery, prognosis is good.

Causes

Otosclerosis appears to result from a genetic factor transmitted as an autosomal dominant trait; many patients with this disorder report family histories of hearing loss (excluding presbycusis). Pregnancy may trigger onset of this condition.

Signs and symptoms

Spongy bone in the otic capsule immobilizes the footplate of the normally mobile stapes, disrupting the conduction of vibrations from the tympanic membrane to the cochlea. This causes slowly progressive unilateral hearing loss, which may advance to bilateral deafness. Other symptoms include tinnitus (low and medium pitch) and paracusis of Willis (hearing conversation better in a noisy environment than in a quiet one).

Diagnosis

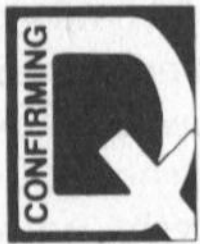

Early diagnosis is based on a Rinne test that shows bone conduction lasting longer than air conduction (normally, the reverse is true). As otosclerosis progresses, bone conduction also deteriorates. Audiometric testing reveals hearing loss ranging from 60 db, in early stages, to total loss, as the disease advances. Weber's test detects sound lateralizing to the more affected ear. Physical examination reveals a normal tympanic membrane.

Treatment

Generally, treatment consists of stapedectomy (removal of the stapes) and insertion of a prosthesis, to restore partial or total hearing. This procedure is performed on only one ear at a time, beginning with the ear that has suffered greater damage. Postoperatively, treatment includes hospitalization for 2 to 3 days and antibiotics to prevent infection. If stapedectomy is not possible, a hearing aid (air conduction aid with molded ear insert receiver) enables the patient to hear conversation in normal surroundings, although this therapy isn't as effective as stapedectomy.

Special considerations

• During the first 24 hours following surgery, keep the patient lying flat, with his head turned so that the affected ear faces upward (to maintain the position of the graft). Enforce bed rest for 48 hours. Since the patient may be dizzy, keep the side rails up, and gradually assist him with ambulation. Assess for pain and vertigo, which may be relieved with repositioning or prescribed medication.

• Before discharge, instruct the patient to avoid loud noises and sudden pressure changes (such as those that occur while diving or flying) until healing is complete (usually 6 months). Advise the patient not to blow his nose for at least 1 week to prevent contaminated air and bacteria from entering the eustachian tube.

• Stress the importance of protecting the ears against cold; avoiding any activities that provoke dizziness, such as straining, bending, or heavy lifting; and if possible, avoiding contact with anyone who has an upper respiratory tract infection. Teach the patient and family how to change the external ear dressing (eye or gauze pad) and care for the incision. Emphasize the need to complete the prescribed antibiotic regimen and to return for scheduled follow-up care.

Infectious Myringitis

Acute infectious myringitis is characterized by inflammation, hemorrhage, and effusion of fluid into the tissue at the end of the external ear canal and the tympanic membrane. This self-limiting disorder (resolving spontaneously within 3 days to 2 weeks) often follows acute otitis media or upper respiratory tract infection and frequently occurs epidemically in children.

Chronic granular myringitis, a rare inflammation of the squamous layer of the tympanic membrane, causes gradual hearing loss. Without specific treatment, this condition can lead to stenosis of the ear canal, as granulation extends from the tympanic membrane to the external ear.

Causes

Acute infectious myringitis usually follows viral infection, but may also result from infection with bacteria, (pneumococcus, *Hemophilus influenzae*, beta-hemolytic streptococci, staphylococci) or any other organism that may cause acute otitis media. Myringitis is a rare sequela of atypical pneumonia caused by *Mycoplasma pneumoniae*. The cause of chronic granular myringitis is unknown.

Signs and symptoms

Acute infectious myringitis begins with severe ear pain, commonly accompanied by tenderness over the mastoid process. Small, reddened, inflamed blebs form in the canal, on the tympanic membrane, and with bacterial invasion, in the middle ear. Fever and hearing loss are rare unless fluid accumulates in the middle ear or a large bleb totally obstructs the external auditory meatus. Spontaneous rupture of these blebs may cause bloody discharge. Chronic granular myringitis produces pruritus, purulent discharge, and gradual hearing loss.

Diagnosis

Diagnosis of acute infectious myringitis is based on physical examination showing characteristic blebs, and typical patient history. Culture and sensitivity testing of exudate identify any secondary infection present. In chronic granular myringitis, physical examination may reveal granulation extending from the tympanic membrane to the external ear.

Treatment and special considerations

Hospitalization is usually not required for acute infectious myringitis. Treatment consists of measures to relieve pain: analgesics, such as aspirin or acetaminophen, and application of heat to the external ear are usually sufficient, but severe pain may necessitate use of codeine. Systemic or topical antibiotics prevent or treat secondary infection. Incision of blebs and evacuation of serum and blood may relieve pressure and help drain exudate but do not speed recovery.

Treatment of chronic granular myringitis consists of systemic antibiotics or local anti-inflammatory antibiotic combination eardrops, and surgical excision and cautery. If stenosis is present, surgical reconstruction is necessary.

- Stress the importance of completing prescribed antibiotic therapy.
- Teach the patient how to instill topical antibiotics (eardrops). When necessary, explain incision of blebs.
- To help prevent acute infectious myringitis, advise early treatment of acute otitis media.

INNER EAR

Ménière's Disease

(Endolymphatic hydrops)

Ménière's disease, a labyrinthine dysfunction, produces severe vertigo, sensorineural hearing loss, and tinnitus. It usually affects adults, men slightly more often than women, between ages 30 and 60. After multiple attacks over several years, this disorder leads to residual tinnitus and hearing loss.

Causes

Although its etiology is unknown, this disease may result from overproduction or decreased absorption of endolymph, which causes endolymphatic hydrops or endolymphatic hypertension, with consequent degeneration of the vestibular and cochlear hair cells. This condition may stem from autonomic nervous system dysfunction that produces a temporary constriction of blood vessels supplying the inner ear. In some women, premenstrual edema may precipitate attacks of Ménière's disease.

Signs and symptoms

Ménière's disease produces three characteristic effects: severe vertigo, tinnitus, and sensorineural hearing loss. Fullness or blocked feeling in the ear is also quite common. Violent paroxysmal attacks last from 10 minutes to several hours. During an acute attack, other symptoms include severe nausea, vomiting, sweating, giddiness, and nystagmus. Also, vertigo may cause loss of balance and falling to the affected side. To lessen these symptoms, the patient may assume a characteristic posture—lying on the unaffected ear and looking in the direction of the affected ear. Initially, the patient may be asymptomatic between attacks, except for residual tinnitus that worsens during an attack. Such attacks may occur several times a year, or remissions may last as long as several years. Eventually, these attacks become less frequent, as hearing loss progresses (usually unilateral), and they may cease when hearing loss is total.

Diagnosis

Presence of all three typical symptoms suggests Ménière's disease. Audiometric studies indicate a sensorineural hearing loss and loss of discrimination and recruitment. Electronystagmography, and X-rays of the internal meatus may be necessary for differential diagnosis.

Treatment

Treatment with atropine may stop an attack in 20 to 30 minutes. Epinephrine or diphenhydramine may be necessary in a severe attack; dimenhydrinate, meclizine, diphenhydramine, or diazepam may be effective in a milder attack.

Long-term management includes use of a diuretic or vasodilator, and restricted sodium intake. Prophylactic antihistamines or mild sedatives (phenobarbital, diazepam) may also be helpful. If Ménière's disease persists after more than 2 years of treatment or produces incapacitating vertigo, surgical destruction of the affected labyrinth may be necessary. This procedure permanently relieves symptoms but at the expense of irreversible hearing loss.

Special considerations

If the patient's in the hospital during an attack of Ménière's disease:

- Advise him against reading and exposure to glaring lights, to reduce dizziness.
- Keep the side rails of the patient's bed up to prevent falls. Tell him not to get out of bed or walk without assistance.
- Instruct the patient to avoid sudden position changes and any tasks that vertigo makes hazardous, because an attack can begin quite rapidly.

Before surgery:

- If the patient is vomiting, record fluid intake and output and characteristics of emesis. Administer antiemetics, as ordered, and give small amounts of fluid frequently.
- Explain diagnostic tests and offer reassurance and emotional support.

After surgery:

- Record intake and output carefully.
- Tell the patient to expect dizziness and nausea for 1 to 2 days after surgery.
- Give prophylactic antibiotics and antiemetics, as ordered.

Labyrinthitis

Labyrinthitis, an inflammation of the labyrinth of the inner ear, frequently incapacitates the patient by producing severe vertigo that lasts for 3 to 5 days; symptoms gradually subside over a 3- to 6-week period. This disorder is rare, although viral labyrinthitis is often associated with upper respiratory tract infections.

Causes

Labyrinthitis results from the same organisms that cause acute febrile diseases, such as pneumonia, influenza, and, especially, chronic otitis media. In chronic otitis media, cholesteatoma formation erodes the bone of the labyrinth, allowing bacteria to enter from the middle ear. Toxic drug ingestion is another possible cause of labyrinthitis.

Signs and symptoms

Since the inner ear controls both hearing and balance, this infection typically produces severe vertigo (with any movement of the head) and sensorineural hearing loss. Vertigo begins gradually but peaks within 48 hours, causing loss of balance and falling in the direction of the affected ear. Other associated signs and symptoms include spontaneous nystagmus, with jerking movements of the eyes toward the unaffected ear; nausea, vomiting, and giddiness; with cholesteatoma, signs of middle ear disease; and with severe bacterial infection, purulent drainage. To minimize symptoms such as giddiness and nystagmus, the patient may assume a characteristic posture—lying on the side of the unaffected ear and looking in the direction of the affected ear.

Diagnosis

Typical clinical picture and history of upper respiratory tract infection suggest labyrinthitis. Typical diagnostic measures include culture and sensitivity testing to identify the infecting organism, if purulent drainage is present, and audiometric testing.

When an infectious etiology can't be found, additional testing must be done to rule out a brain lesion or Ménière's disease.

Treatment

Symptomatic treatment includes bed rest,

with the head immobilized between pillows; meclizine P.O. to control vertigo; and massive doses of antibiotics to combat diffuse purulent labyrinthitis. Oral fluids can prevent dehydration from vomiting; for severe nausea and vomiting, I.V. fluids may be necessary.

When conservative management fails, treatment necessitates surgical excision of the cholesteatoma and drainage of the infected areas of the middle and inner ear. Prevention is possible by early and vigorous treatment of predisposing conditions, such as otitis media and any local or systemic infection.

Special considerations

- Keep the side rails up to prevent falls.
- If vomiting is severe, administer antiemetics, as ordered. Record intake and output, and give I.V. fluids, as ordered.
- Reassure the patient that recovery is certain but may take as long as 6 weeks. Tell the patient that during this time he should limit activities that vertigo may make hazardous, such as climbing a ladder or driving a car.

Hearing Loss

Hearing loss results from a mechanical or nervous impediment to the transmission of sound waves. The major forms of hearing loss are classified as conductive loss (interrupted passage of sound from the external ear to the junction of the stapes and oval window); sensorineural loss (impaired cochlea or acoustic [eighth cranial] nerve dysfunction, causing failure of transmission of sound impulses within the inner ear or brain); or mixed (combined dysfunction of conduction and sensorineural transmission). Hearing loss may be partial or total and is calculated from the American Medical Association formula: hearing is 1.5% impaired for every decibel that the pure tone average exceeds 25 db.

Causes and incidence

Congenital hearing loss may be transmitted as a dominant, autosomal dominant, autosomal recessive, or sex-linked recessive trait. Hearing loss in neonates may also result from trauma, toxicity, or infection during pregnancy or delivery. Predisposing factors include a family history of hearing loss or known hereditary disorders (otosclerosis, for example), maternal exposure to rubella or syphilis during pregnancy, use of ototoxic drugs during pregnancy, prolonged fetal anoxia during delivery, and congenital abnormalities of the ears, nose, or throat. Premature or low–birth-weight infants are most likely to have structural or functional hearing impairments; those with serum bilirubin levels greater than 20 mg/100 ml also risk hearing impairment from the toxic effect of high serum bilirubin levels on the brain. In addition, trauma during delivery may cause intracranial hemorrhage and damage the cochlea or acoustic nerve.

Sudden deafness refers to sudden hearing loss in a person with no prior hearing impairment. This condition is considered a medical emergency, because prompt treatment may restore full hearing. Its causes and predisposing factors may include:

- acute infections, especially mumps (most common cause of unilateral sensorineural hearing loss in children), and other bacterial and viral infections, such as rubella, rubeola, influenza, herpes zoster, and infectious mononucleosis; and mycoplasma infections.
- metabolic disorders (diabetes mellitus, hypothyroidism, hyperlipoproteinemia).
- vascular disorders, such as hypertension, arteriosclerosis.
- head trauma or brain tumors.
- ototoxic drugs (tobramycin, strepto-

mycin, quinine, gentamicin, furosemide, ethacrynic acid).
• neurologic disorders (multiple sclerosis, neurosyphilis).
• blood dyscrasias (leukemia and hypercoagulation).

Noise-induced hearing loss, which may be transient or permanent, may follow prolonged exposure to loud noise (85 to 90 db) or brief exposure to extremely loud noise (greater than 90 db). Such hearing loss is common in workers subjected to constant industrial noise and in military personnel, hunters, and rock musicians.

Presbycusis, an otologic effect of aging, results from a loss of hair cells in the organ of Corti. This disorder causes sensorineural hearing loss, usually of high-frequency tones.

Signs and symptoms

Although congenital hearing loss may produce no obvious signs of hearing impairment at birth, deficient response to auditory stimuli generally becomes apparent within 2 to 3 days. As the child grows older, hearing loss impairs speech development.

Sudden deafness may be conductive, sensorineural, or mixed, depending on etiology. Associated clinical features depend on the underlying cause.

Noise-induced hearing loss causes sensorineural damage, the extent of which depends on the duration and intensity of the noise. Initially, the patient loses perception of certain frequencies (around 4,000 Hz) but, with continued exposure, eventually loses perception of all frequencies.

Presbycusis usually produces tinnitus and the inability to understand the spoken word.

Diagnosis

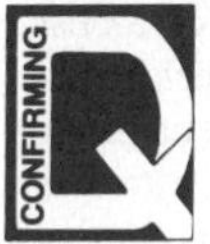

Patient, family, and occupational histories and a complete audiologic examination usually provide ample evidence of hearing loss and suggest possible causes or predisposing factors. The Weber, the Rinne, and specialized audiologic tests differentiate between conductive and sensorineural hearing loss.

Treatment

After identifying the underlying cause, therapy for congenital hearing loss refractory to surgery consists of developing the patient's ability to communicate through sign language, speech reading, or other effective means. Measures to prevent congenital hearing loss include aggressively immunizing children against rubella, to reduce the risk of maternal exposure during pregnancy; educating pregnant women about the dangers of exposure to drugs, chemicals, or infection; and careful monitoring during labor and delivery to prevent fetal anoxia.

Treatment of sudden deafness requires prompt identification of the underlying cause. Prevention necessitates educating patients and health-care professionals about the many causes of sudden deafness and the ways to recognize and treat them.

In persons with noise-induced hearing loss, overnight rest usually restores normal hearing in those who have been exposed to noise levels greater than 90 db for several hours; but not in those who have been exposed to such noise repeatedly. As hearing deteriorates, treatment must include speech and hearing rehabilitation, since hearing aids are rarely helpful. Prevention of noise-induced hearing loss requires public recognition of the dangers of noise exposure and insistence on the use, as mandated by law, of protective devices, such as earplugs, during occupational exposure to noise.

Presbycusis usually requires the use of a hearing aid.

Special considerations

• When speaking to a patient with hearing loss who can read lips, stand directly in front of him, with the light on your face, and speak slowly and distinctly. Approach the patient within his visual range, and elicit his attention by raising your arm or waving; touching him may be unnecessarily startling.

• Make other staff members and hospital personnel aware of the patient's handicap and his established method of communication. Carefully explain all diagnostic tests and hospital procedures in a way the patient understands.

• Make sure the patient with a hearing loss is in an area where he can observe unit activities and persons approaching, since such a patient depends totally on visual clues.

• When addressing an older patient, speak slowly and distinctly in a low tone; avoid shouting.

• Provide emotional support and encouragement to the patient learning to use a hearing aid. Teach him how the aid works and how to maintain it.

• Refer children with suspected hearing loss to an audiologist or otolaryngologist for further evaluation.

• To help prevent hearing loss, watch for signs of hearing impairment in patients receiving ototoxic drugs. Emphasize the danger of excessive exposure to noise; stress the danger of exposure to drugs, chemicals, and infection (especially rubella) to pregnant women; and encourage the use of protective devices in a noisy environment.

Motion Sickness

Motion sickness is characterized by loss of equilibrium, associated with nausea and vomiting that result from irregular or rhythmic movements or from the sensation of motion. Removal of the stimulus restores normal equilibrium.

Causes and incidence

Motion sickness may result from excessive stimulation of the labyrinthine receptors of the inner ear by certain motions, such as those experienced in a car, boat, plane, or swing. The disorder may also be caused by confusion in the cerebellum from conflicting sensory input; visual stimulus (a moving horizon) conflicts with labyrinthine perception. Predisposing factors include tension or fear, offensive odors, or sights and sounds associated with a previous attack. Motion sickness from cars, elevators, trains, and swings is most common in children; from boats and airplanes, in adults. Persons who suffer from one kind of motion sickness are not necessarily susceptible to other types.

Signs and symptoms

Typically, motion sickness induces nausea, vomiting, headache, dizziness, fatigue, diaphoresis, and, occasionally, difficulty in breathing, leading to a sensation of suffocation. These symptoms usually subside when the precipitating stimulus is removed, but they may persist for several hours or days.

Treatment and special considerations

The best way to treat the disorder is to stop the motion that's causing it. If this isn't possible, the patient will benefit from lying down, closing his eyes, and trying to sleep. Antiemetics, such as dimenhydrinate, cyclizine, meclizine, and scopolamine (transdermal patch), may prevent or relieve motion sickness.

• Tell the patient to avoid exposure to precipitating motion whenever possible. The traveler can minimize motion sickness by sitting where motion is least apparent (near the wing section in an aircraft, in the center of a boat, or in the front seat of an automobile). Instruct him to keep his head still and his eyes closed or focused on a distant and stationary object. An elevated car seat may help prevent motion sickness in a child, by allowing him to see out the front window.

• Instruct the patient to avoid eating or drinking for at least 4 hours before traveling and to take an antiemetic 30 to 60 minutes before traveling or to apply a transdermal scopolamine patch at least 4 hours before traveling. Tell the patient with prostate enlargement or glaucoma to consult a doctor or pharmacist before taking antiemetics.

NOSE

Epistaxis

(Nosebleed)

Epistaxis may be either a primary disorder or secondary to another condition. Such bleeding in children generally originates in the anterior nasal septum and tends to be mild. In adults, such bleeding is most likely to originate in the posterior septum and can be severe. Epistaxis is twice as common in children as in adults.

Causes

Epistaxis usually follows trauma from external or internal causes: a blow to the nose, nose picking, or insertion of a foreign body. Less commonly, it follows polyps; acute or chronic infections, such as sinusitis or rhinitis, which cause congestion and eventual bleeding of the capillary blood vessels; or inhalation of chemicals that irritate the nasal mucosa.

Predisposing factors include anticoagulant therapy; hypertension; chronic use of aspirin; high altitudes and dry climates; sclerotic vessel disease; Hodgkin's disease; scurvy; vitamin K deficiency; rheumatic fever; and blood dyscrasias, such as hemophilia, purpura, leukemia, and some anemias.

Signs and symptoms

Blood oozing from the nostrils usually originates in the anterior nose and is bright red. Blood from the back of the throat originates in the posterior area and may be dark or bright red (often mistaken for hemoptysis due to expectoration). Epistaxis is generally unilateral, except when due to dyscrasia or severe trauma. In severe epistaxis, blood may seep behind the nasal septum; it may also appear in the middle ear and in the corners of the eyes.

Associated clinical effects depend on the severity of bleeding. Moderate blood loss may produce light-headedness, dizziness, and slight respiratory difficulty; severe hemorrhage causes a drop in blood pressure, rapid and bounding pulse, dyspnea, pallor, and other indications of progressive shock. Bleeding is considered severe if it persists longer than 10 minutes after pressure is applied and may cause blood loss as great as 1 liter/hour in adults.

Diagnosis

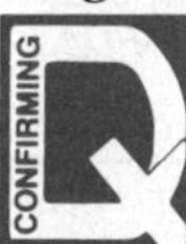

Although simple observation confirms epistaxis, inspection with a bright light and nasal speculum is necessary to locate the site of bleeding.

Relevant laboratory values include:

- gradual reduction in hemoglobin and hematocrit (often inaccurate immediately following epistaxis, due to hemoconcentration).
- decreased platelet count in a patient with blood dyscrasia.
- prothrombin time and partial thromboplastin time showing a coagulation time twice the control, due to a bleeding disorder or anticoagulant therapy.

Diagnosis must rule out underlying systemic causes of epistaxis, especially disseminated intravascular coagulation and rheumatic fever. Bruises or concomitant bleeding elsewhere probably indicates a hematologic disorder.

INSERTION OF AN ANTERIOR-POSTERIOR NASAL PACK

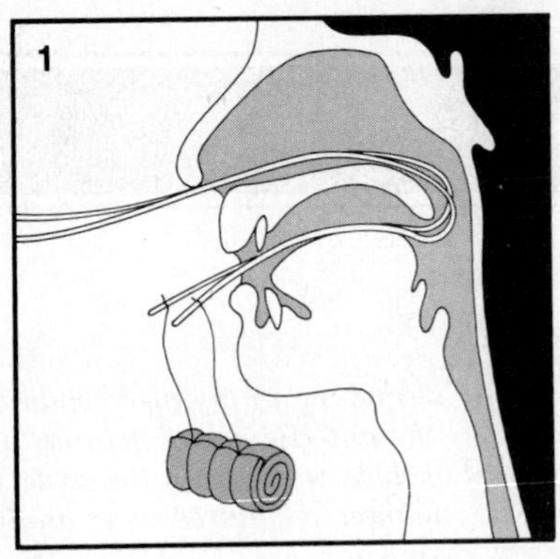

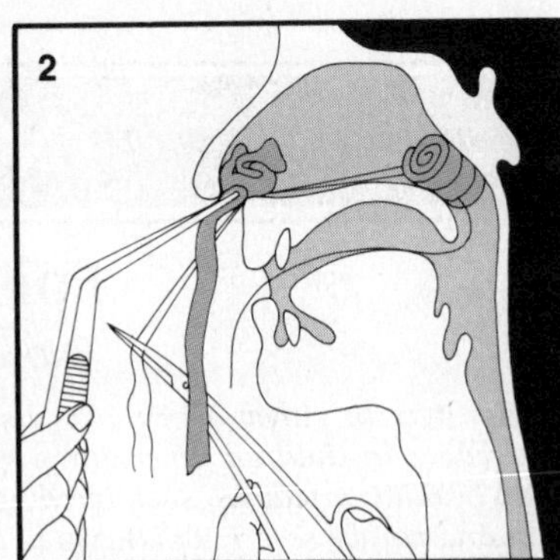

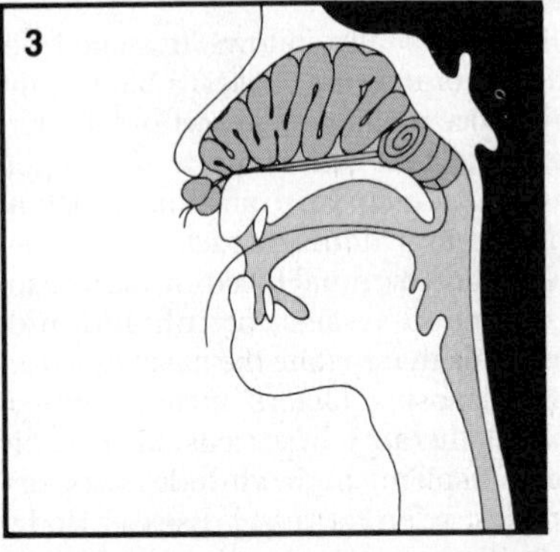

The first step in the insertion of an anterior-posterior nasal pack is the insertion of catheters in the nostrils. After drawing the catheters through the mouth, a suture from the pack is tied to each (fig. 1), which positions the pack in place as the catheters are drawn back through the nostrils. While the sutures are held tightly, packing is inserted into the anterior nose (fig. 2). The sutures are then secured around a dental roll; the middle suture extends from the mouth (fig. 3) and is tied to the cheek.

Treatment

For anterior bleeding, treatment consists of application of a cotton ball saturated with epinephrine to the bleeding site, external pressure, followed by cauterization with electrocautery or silver nitrate stick. If these measures don't control the bleeding, petrolatum gauze nasal packing may be needed.

For posterior bleeding, therapy includes gauze packing inserted through the nose, or postnasal packing inserted through the mouth, depending on the bleeding site. (Gauze packing generally remains in place for 24 to 48 hours; postnasal packing, 3 to 5 days.) An alternate method, the nasal balloon catheter, also controls bleeding effectively. Antibiotics may be appropriate if packing must remain in place for longer than 24 hours. If local measures fail to control bleeding, additional treatment may include supplemental vitamin K and, for severe bleeding, blood transfusions and surgical ligation of a bleeding artery.

Special considerations

To control epistaxis:

- Elevate the patient's head 45°.
- Compress the soft portion of the nostrils against the septum continuously for 5 to 10 minutes. Apply an ice collar or cold, wet compresses to the nose. If bleeding continues after 10 minutes of pressure, notify the doctor.
- Administer oxygen, as needed.

• Monitor vital signs and skin color; record blood loss.
• Instruct patient to breathe through the mouth. Tell him not to swallow blood, to talk, or to blow his nose.
• Keep vasoconstrictors, such as phenylephrine, handy.
• Reassure the patient and family that epistaxis usually *looks* worse than it is.

To prevent recurrence of epistaxis:
• Instruct the patient not to pick his nose or insert foreign objects in it. Emphasize the need for follow-up examinations and periodic blood studies after an episode of epistaxis. Advise prompt treatment of nasal infection or irritation, to prevent recurring nose trauma.
• Suggest humidifiers for persons who live in dry climates or at high elevations or whose homes are heated with circulating hot air.

Septal Perforation and Deviation

Perforated septum, a hole in the nasal septum between the two air passages, usually occurs in the anterior cartilaginous septum but may occur in the bony septum. Deviated septum, a shift from the midline, is common in most adults. This condition may be severe enough to obstruct the passage of air through the nostrils. With surgical correction, prognosis for either perforated or deviated septum is good.

Causes and incidence

Generally, perforated septum is caused by traumatic irritation, most commonly from excessive nose picking; less frequently, from repeated cauterization for epistaxis or from penetrating septal injury. It may also result from perichondritis, an infection that gradually erodes the perichondrial layer and cartilage, finally forming an ulcer that perforates the septum. Other causes of septal perforation include syphilis, tuberculosis, untreated septal hematoma, inhalation of irritating chemicals, snorting cocaine, chronic nasal infections, nasal carcinoma, granuloma, and chronic sinusitis.

Deviated septum commonly develops during normal growth, as the septum shifts from one side to the other. Consequently, few adults have perfectly straight septa. Nasal trauma resulting from a fall, a blow to the nose, or surgery further exaggerates the deviation. Congenital deviated septum is rare.

Signs and symptoms

A small septal perforation is usually asymptomatic but may produce a whistle on inspiration. A large perforation causes rhinitis, epistaxis, nasal crusting, and watery discharge.

The patient with a deviated septum may develop a crooked nose, as the midline deflects to one side. The predominant symptom of severe deflection, however, is nasal obstruction. Other manifestations include a sensation of

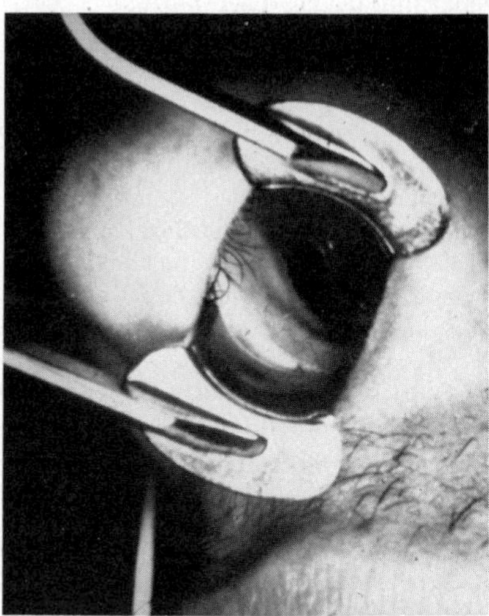
In the photograph above, the nasal septum shows obvious perforation of the cartilage between the two air passages.

fullness in the face, shortness of breath, nasal discharge, recurring epistaxis, infection, sinusitis, and headache.

Diagnosis

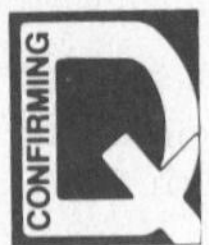

Although clinical features suggest septal perforation or deviation, confirmation requires inspection of the nasal mucosa with bright light and a nasal speculum.

Treatment

Symptomatic treatment of perforated septum includes decongestants to reduce nasal congestion by local vasoconstriction, local application of lanolin or petrolatum to prevent ulceration and crusting, and antibiotics to combat infection. Surgery may be necessary to graft part of the perichondrial layer over the perforation. Also, a plastic or Silastic "button" prosthesis may be used to close the perforation.

Symptomatic treatment of deviated septum usually includes analgesics to relieve headache; decongestants to minimize secretions; and as necessary, vasoconstrictors, nasal packing, or cautery to control hemorrhage. Manipulation of the nasal septum at birth can correct congenital deviated septum.

Corrective surgical procedures include:

- *reconstruction of the nasal septum by submucous resection* to reposition the nasal septal cartilage and relieve nasal obstruction.
- *rhinoplasty* to correct nasal structure deformity by intranasal incisions.
- *septoplasty* to relieve nasal obstruction and enhance cosmetic appearance.

Special considerations

- In the patient with perforated septum, use a cotton applicator to apply petrolatum to the nasal mucosa to minimize crusting and ulceration.
- Warn the patient with perforation or severe deviation against blowing his nose. To relieve nasal congestion, instill saline nosedrops and suggest use of a humidifier. Give decongestants, as ordered.
- To treat epistaxis, elevate the head of the bed, provide an emesis basin, and instruct the patient to expectorate any blood. Compress the outer portion of the nose against the septum for 10 to 15 minutes, and apply ice packs. If bleeding persists, notify the doctor.
- If corrective surgery is scheduled, prepare the patient to expect postoperative facial edema, periorbital bruising, and nasal packing, which remains in place for 12 to 24 hours. The patient must breathe through his mouth. After surgery for deviated septum, the patient may also have a splint on his nose.
- To reduce or prevent edema and promote drainage, place the patient in semi-Fowler's position, and use a cool-mist vaporizer to liquefy secretions and facilitate normal breathing. To lessen facial edema and pain, place crushed ice in a rubber glove or a small ice bag, and apply the glove or ice bag intermittently over the eyes and nose for 24 hours.
- Because the patient is breathing through his mouth, provide frequent and meticulous mouth care.
- Change the mustache dressing or drip pad, as needed. Record the color, consistency, and amount of drainage. While nasal packing is in place, expect slight, bright red drainage, with clots. After packing is removed, watch for purulent discharge, an indication of infection.
- Watch for and report excessive swallowing, hematoma, or a falling or flapping septum (depressed, or soft and unstable septum). Intranasal examination is necessary to detect hematoma formation. Any of these complications requires surgical correction.
- Administer sedatives and analgesics, as ordered. Because of its anticoagulant properties, aspirin is contraindicated after surgery for septal deviation or perforation.
- Noseblowing may cause bruising and swelling even after nasal packing is removed. After surgery, the patient must limit physical activity for 2 or 3 days, and if he's a smoker, he must stop smoking for at least 2 days.

Sinusitis

Sinusitis, inflammation of the paranasal sinuses, may be acute, subacute, chronic, allergic, or hyperplastic. Acute sinusitis usually results from the common cold and lingers in subacute form in only about 10% of patients. Chronic sinusitis follows persistent bacterial infection; allergic sinusitis accompanies allergic rhinitis; hyperplastic sinusitis is a combination of purulent acute sinusitis and allergic sinusitis or rhinitis. Prognosis is good for all types.

Causes and incidence

Sinusitis usually results from bacterial infection (*Hemophilus influenzae,* anaerobes) or, less frequently, from viral infection. Bacterial invasion generally occurs when a cold spreads to the sinuses. Excessive nose blowing during an acute infection forces infected material into the sinuses.

Predisposing factors include any condition that interferes with drainage and ventilation of the sinuses, such as chronic nasal edema, deviated septum, viscous mucus, or nasal polyps. Bacterial invasion may also result from swimming in contaminated water.

Signs and symptoms

The primary indication of *acute sinusitis* is nasal congestion, followed by a gradual buildup of pressure in the affected sinus. For 24 to 48 hours after onset, nasal discharge may be present and later become purulent. Associated symptoms include malaise, sore throat, headache, and low-grade fever (temperature of 99° to 99.5° F. [37.2° to 37.5° C.]).

Characteristic pain depends on the affected sinus: maxillary sinusitis causes pain over the cheeks and upper teeth; ethmoid sinusitis, pain over the eyes; frontal sinusitis, pain over the eyebrows; and sphenoid sinusitis (rare), pain behind the eyes.

Purulent nasal drainage that continues longer than 3 weeks after an acute infection subsides suggests *subacute sinusitis.* Other clinical features of the subacute form include a stuffy nose, vague facial discomfort, fatigue, and a nonproductive cough.

The effects of *chronic sinusitis* are similar to those of acute sinusitis, but the chronic form causes continuous mucopurulent discharge.

The effects of *allergic sinusitis* are the same as those of allergic rhinitis. In both conditions, the prominent symptoms are sneezing, frontal headache, watery nasal discharge, and a stuffy, burning, itchy nose.

In *hyperplastic sinusitis,* bacterial growth on diseased tissue causes pronounced tissue edema; thickening of the mucosal lining and the development of mucosal polyps produce chronic stuffiness of the nose, and headaches.

Diagnosis

The following measures are useful in diagnosing sinusitis:

- *Nasal examination* reveals inflammation and pus.
- *Sinus X-rays* reveal cloudiness in the affected sinus, air-fluid levels, or thickened mucosal lining.
- *Antral puncture* promotes drainage and removal of purulent material. It may also provide a specimen for culture and sensitivity identification of the infecting organism, but this is rarely done.
- *Transillumination* allows inspection of the sinus cavities by passing a light through them; purulent drainage prevents passage of light.

Treatment

Antibiotics are the primary treatment for the patient with acute sinusitis. Analgesics may be prescribed to relieve pain. Other appropriate measures include vasoconstrictors, such as epinephrine or phenylephrine, to decrease nasal secretions. Steam inhalation also promotes vasoconstriction, in addition to encouraging drainage.

Antibiotics are necessary to combat persistent infection. Amoxicillin or ampicillin are usually the antibiotics of choice. Local applications of heat may help to relieve pain and congestion.

In subacute sinusitis, antibiotic therapy is also the primary treatment. As in acute sinusitis, vasoconstrictors may lessen nasal secretions.

Treatment of allergic sinusitis must include treatment of allergic rhinitis—administration of antihistamines, identification of allergens by skin testing, and desensitization by immunotherapy. Severe allergic symptoms may require treatment with corticosteroids and epinephrine.

In both chronic sinusitis and hyperplastic sinusitis, antihistamines, antibiotics, and a steroid nasal spray may relieve pain and congestion. If irrigation fails to relieve symptoms, one or more sinuses may require surgery.

SURGERY FOR CHRONIC AND HYPERPLASTIC SINUSITIS

For maxillary sinusitis:
- *Nasal window procedure* creates an opening in the sinus, allowing secretions and pus to drain through the nose.
- *Caldwell-Luc procedure* removes diseased mucosa in the maxillary sinus through an incision under the upper lip.

For chronic ethmoid sinusitis:
- *Ethmoidectomy* removes all infected tissue through an external or intranasal incision into the ethmoidal sinus.

For sphenoid sinusitis:
- *External ethmoidectomy* removes infected ethmoidal sinus tissue through a crescent-shaped incision, beginning under the inner eyebrow and extending along the side of the nose.

For chronic frontal sinusitis:
- *Fronto-ethmoidectomy* removes infected frontal sinus tissue through an extended external ethmoidectomy.
- *Osteoplastic flap* drains the sinuses through an incision across the skull, behind the hairline.

Special considerations

- Enforce bed rest, and encourage the patient to drink plenty of fluids, to promote drainage. Don't elevate the head of the bed more than 30°.
- To relieve pain and promote drainage, apply warm compresses continuously, or 4 times daily for 2-hour intervals. In addition, give analgesics and antihistamines, as needed.
- Watch for and report complications, such as vomiting, chills, fever, edema of the forehead or eyelids, blurred or double vision, and personality changes.
- If surgery is necessary, tell the patient what to expect postoperatively: a nasal packing will be in place for 12 to 24 hours following surgery; he'll have to breathe through his mouth and won't be able to blow his nose. After surgery, monitor for excessive drainage or bleeding, and watch for complications.
- To prevent edema and promote drainage, place the patient in semi-Fowler's position. To relieve edema and pain, and minimize bleeding, apply ice compresses or a rubber glove filled with ice chips over the nose, and iced saline gauze over the eyes. Continue these measures for 24 hours.
- Frequently change the mustache dressing or drip pad, and record the consistency, amount, and color of drainage (expect scant, bright red, and clotty drainage).
- Because the patient will be breathing through his mouth, provide meticulous mouth care.
- Tell the patient that even after the packing is removed, nose blowing may cause bleeding and swelling. If the patient is a smoker, instruct him not to smoke for at least 2 to 3 days following surgery.
- Tell the patient to finish the prescribed antibiotics, even if his symptoms disappear.

Nasal Polyps

Benign and edematous growths, nasal polyps are usually multiple, mobile, and bilateral. Nasal polyps may become large and numerous enough to cause nasal distention and enlargement of the bony framework, possibly occluding the airway. They are more common in adults than in children and tend to recur.

Causes

Nasal polyps are usually produced by the continuous pressure resulting from a chronic allergy that causes prolonged mucous membrane edema in the nose and sinuses. Other predisposing factors include chronic sinusitis, chronic rhinitis, and recurrent nasal infections.

Signs and symptoms

Nasal obstruction is the primary indication of nasal polyps. Such obstruction causes anosmia, a sensation of fullness in the face, nasal discharge, and shortness of breath. Associated clinical features are usually symptomatic of allergic rhinitis.

Diagnosis

Diagnosis of nasal polyps is aided by the following tests:

- *X-rays of sinuses and nasal passages* reveal soft tissue shadows over the affected areas.
- *Examination with a nasal speculum* shows a dry, red surface, with clear or gray growths. Large growths may resemble tumors.

Nasal polyps occurring in children require further testing to rule out cystic fibrosis.

Treatment

Generally, treatment consists of corticosteroids (either by direct injection into the polyps or by local spray) to temporarily reduce the polyp. Treatment of the underlying cause may include antihistamines to control allergy, and antibiotic therapy if infection is present. Local application of an astringent shrinks hypertrophied tissue. However, medical management alone is rarely effective.

Consequently, the treatment of choice is polypectomy (intranasal removal of the nasal polyp with a wire snare), usually performed under a local anesthetic. Continued recurrence may require surgical opening of the ethmoidal and the maxillary sinuses, and evacuation of diseased tissue.

Special considerations

- Administer antihistamines, as ordered, for the patient with allergies. Prepare the patient for scheduled surgery by telling him what to expect postoperatively, such as nasal packing for 1 to 2 days after surgery.

After surgery:

- Monitor for excessive bleeding or other drainage, and promote patient comfort.
- Elevate the head of the bed to facilitate breathing, reduce swelling, and promote adequate drainage. Change the mustache dressing or drip pad, as needed, and record the consistency, amount, and color of nasal drainage.
- Intermittently apply ice compresses over the nostrils to lessen swelling, prevent bleeding, and relieve pain.
- If nasal bleeding occurs—most likely after packing is removed—elevate the head of the bed, monitor vital signs, and advise the patient not to swallow blood. Compress the outside of the nose against the septum for 10 to 15 minutes. If bleeding persists, notify the doctor immediately. Nasal packing may be necessary.

To prevent nasal polyps, instruct patients with allergies to avoid exposure to allergens and to take antihistamines at the first sign of an allergic reaction. Also, advise them to avoid overuse of nose drops and sprays.

Nasal Papillomas

A papilloma is a benign epithelial tissue overgrowth within the intranasal mucosa. Inverted papillomas grow into the underlying tissue, usually at the junction of the antrum and the ethmoidal sinus; they generally occur singly but sometimes are associated with a squamous cell malignancy. Exophytic papillomas, which also tend to occur singly, arise from epithelial tissue, commonly on the surface of the nasal septum. Both types of papillomas are most prevalent in males. Recurrence is likely, even after surgical excision.

Causes

A papilloma may arise as a benign precursor of a neoplasm or as a response to tissue injury or viral infection, but its cause is unknown.

Signs and symptoms

Both inverted and exophytic papillomas typically produce symptoms related to unilateral nasal obstruction—stuffiness, postnasal drip, headache, shortness of breath, dyspnea, and, rarely, severe respiratory distress, nasal drainage, and infection. Epistaxis is most likely to occur with exophytic papillomas.

Diagnosis

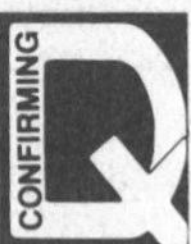

On examination of the nasal mucosa, inverted papillomas usually appear large, bulky, highly vascular, and edematous; color varies from dark red to gray; consistency, from firm to friable. Exophytic papillomas are commonly raised, firm, and rubbery; pink to gray; and securely attached by a broad or pedunculated base to the mucous membrane. Histologic examination of excised tissue confirms the diagnosis.

Treatment

The most effective treatment is wide surgical excision or diathermy, with careful inspection of adjacent tissues and sinuses to rule out extension. Aspirin or acetaminophen, and decongestants may relieve symptoms.

Special considerations

- If bleeding occurs, raise the head of the bed, and instruct the patient to expectorate blood into an emesis basin. Compress the sides of the nose against the septum for 10 to 15 minutes, and, if necessary, apply ice compresses to the nose. If bleeding doesn't stop, notify the doctor.
- Check for airway obstruction. Place your hand under the patient's nostrils to assess air exchange, and watch for signs of mild shortness of breath.
- If surgery is scheduled, tell the patient what to expect postoperatively: that his nostrils will probably be packed and that he'll have to breathe through his mouth. Instruct him not to blow his nose. (Packing is usually removed 12 to 24 hours after surgery.)

Postoperatively:

- Monitor vital signs and respiratory status. As needed, administer analgesics and facilitate breathing with a cool-mist vaporizer. Provide good mouth care.
- Frequently change the mustache dressing or drip pad, to ensure proper absorption of drainage. Record type and amount of drainage. While the nasal packing is in place, expect scant, usually bright red, clotted drainage. Remember that the amount of drainage often increases for a few hours after the packing is removed.
- Because papillomas tend to recur, tell the patient to seek medical attention at the first sign of nasal discomfort, discharge, or congestion that doesn't subside with conservative treatment.
- Encourage regular follow-up visits to detect early signs of recurrence.

Adenoid Hyperplasia

(Adenoid hypertrophy)

A fairly common childhood condition, adenoid hyperplasia is enlargement of the lymphoid tissue of the nasopharynx. Normally, adenoidal tissue is small at birth (3/4" to 1 1/4" [2 to 3 cm]), grows until the child reaches adolescence, and then begins to slowly atrophy. In adenoid hyperplasia, however, this tissue continues to grow.

Causes

Although the precise cause of adenoid hyperplasia is unknown, contributing factors may include heredity, repeated infection, chronic nasal congestion, persistent allergy, insufficient aeration, and inefficient nasal breathing. Inflammation resulting from repeated infection increases the patient's risk of respiratory obstruction.

Signs and symptoms

Typically, adenoid hyperplasia produces symptoms of respiratory obstruction, especially mouth breathing, snoring at night, and frequent, prolonged nasal congestion. Persistent mouth breathing during the formative years produces distinctive changes in facial features—a slightly elongated face, open mouth, highly arched palate, shortened upper lip, and a vacant expression.

Occasionally, the child is incapable of mouth breathing, snores loudly at night, and may eventually show effects of nocturnal respiratory insufficiency, such as intercostal retractions and nasal flaring; this may lead to pulmonary hypertension and cor pulmonale. Adenoid hyperplasia can also obstruct the eustachian tube and predispose to otitis media, which in turn can lead to fluctuating conductive hearing loss. Stasis of nasal secretions from adenoidal inflammation can lead to sinusitis.

Diagnosis

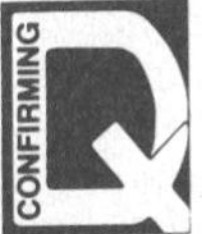

Nasopharyngoscopy or rhinoscopy confirms adenoid hyperplasia by visualizing abnormal tissue mass. Lateral pharyngeal X-rays show obliteration of the nasopharyngeal air column.

Treatment

Adenoidectomy is the treatment of choice of adenoid hyperplasia and is commonly recommended for the patient with prolonged mouth breathing, nasal speech, adenoid facies, recurrent otitis media, constant nasopharyngitis, and nocturnal respiratory distress. This procedure usually eliminates recurrent nasal infections and ear complications and reverses any secondary hearing loss.

Special considerations

Focus your care plan on sympathetic preoperative care and diligent postoperative monitoring.

Before surgery:

- Describe the hospital routine and arrange for the patient and parents to tour relevant areas of the hospital.
- Explain adenoidectomy to the child, using illustrations, if necessary, and detail the recovery process. Reassure him that he'll probably need to be hospitalized only two nights. If hospital protocol allows, encourage one parent to stay with the child and participate in his care.

After surgery:

- Maintain a patent airway. Position the child on his side, with head down, to prevent aspiration of draining secretions. Frequently check the throat for bleeding. Be alert for vomiting of old, partially digested blood ("coffee ground"). Closely monitor vital signs, and report excessive bleeding, rise in pulse rate, drop in blood pressure, tachypnea, and restlessness.
- If no bleeding occurs, offer cracked ice or water when the patient is fully awake.
- Tell the parents that their child may temporarily have a nasal voice.

Velopharyngeal Insufficiency

Velopharyngeal insufficiency results from failure of the velopharyngeal sphincter to close properly during speech, giving the voice a hypernasal quality and permitting nasal emission (air escape during pronunciation of consonants). Velopharyngeal insufficiency commonly occurs in persons who undergo cleft palate surgery and those with submucous cleft palates. Middle ear disease and hearing loss frequently accompany this disorder.

Causes

Velopharyngeal insufficiency can result from an inherited palate abnormality (short palate, pharyngomegaly, submucous cleft palate), or it can be an acquired disorder from tonsillectomy, adenoidectomy, or palatal paresis.

Signs and symptoms

Generally, this condition causes unintelligible speech, marked by hypernasality, nasal emission, poor consonant definition, and a weak voice. The patient experiences dysphagia, and, if velopharyngeal insufficiency is severe, he may regurgitate through the nose.

Diagnosis

Fiberoptic nasopharyngoscopy, which permits monitoring of velopharyngeal patency during speech, suggests this diagnosis. Ultrasound scanning, which shows air-tissue overlap, reflects the degree of velopharyngeal sphincter incompetence (an opening greater than 20 mm^2 results in unintelligible speech).

Treatment

Treatment consists of corrective surgery, usually at age 6 or 7. The preferred surgical method is the *pharyngeal flap procedure,* which diverts a tissue flap from the pharynx to the soft palate. Other appropriate surgical procedures include:

- *palatal push-back,* which separates the hard and soft palates to allow insertion of an obturator, thus lengthening the soft palate.
- *pharyngoplasty,* which rotates pharyngeal flaps to lengthen the soft palate and narrow the pharynx.
- *augmentation pharyngoplasty,* which narrows the velopharyngeal opening by enlarging the pharyngeal wall with a retropharyngeal implant.
- *velopharyngeal sphincter reconstruction,* which uses free muscle implantation to reconstruct the sphincter.

Surgery eliminates hypernasality and nasal emission, but speech maladjustments persist and usually necessitate speech therapy, depending on the patient's age. Immediate postoperative therapy includes antibiotics and a clear, liquid diet for the first 3 days, followed by a soft diet for 2 weeks.

Special considerations

- After surgery for velopharyngeal insufficiency, maintain a patent airway (nasopharynx edema may obstruct the airway). Position the patient on his side, and suction the dependent side of his mouth, avoiding the pharynx.
- Control postoperative agitation, which may provoke pharyngeal bleeding, with sedation, as ordered.
- Administer high-humidity oxygen, as ordered.
- Monitor vital signs frequently, and report any changes immediately. Observe for bleeding from the mouth or nose. Check intake and output, and watch for signs of dehydration.
- Advise the patient that speech therapy, if ordered, requires time and effort on his part, but with persistence and practice, his speech will improve. Before discharge, emphasize the importance of completing the prescribed antibiotic therapy.

THROAT

Pharyngitis

The most common throat disorder, pharyngitis is an acute or chronic inflammation of the pharynx. It is widespread among adults who live or work in dusty or very dry environments, use their voices excessively, habitually use tobacco or alcohol, or suffer from chronic sinusitis, persistent coughs, or allergies.

Causes

Pharyngitis is caused by a virus (90% of patients) or bacteria (most often streptococcus, especially in children). Acute pharyngitis may precede the common cold or other communicable diseases; chronic pharyngitis is often an extension of nasopharyngeal obstruction or inflammation.

Signs and symptoms

Pharyngitis typically produces a sore throat and slight difficulty in swallowing. Oddly, swallowing saliva is usually more painful than swallowing food. Pharyngitis may also cause the sensation of a lump in the throat, as well as a constant, aggravating urge to swallow. Associated features may include mild fever, headache, and muscle and joint pain (especially in bacterial pharyngitis). Uncomplicated pharyngitis usually subsides in 3 to 10 days.

Diagnosis

Physical examination of the pharynx reveals generalized redness and inflammation of the posterior wall, and red, edematous mucous membranes studded with white or yellow follicles. Exudate is usually confined to the lymphoid areas of the throat, sparing the tonsillar pillars. Throat culture may identify bacterial organisms, if they are the cause of the inflammation.

Treatment

Treatment of acute viral pharyngitis is usually symptomatic, and consists mainly of rest, warm saline gargles, throat lozenges containing a mild anesthetic, plenty of fluids, and analgesics, as needed. If the patient can't swallow fluids, hospitalization may be required, for I.V. hydration.

Bacterial pharyngitis necessitates rigorous treatment with penicillin—or another broad-spectrum antibiotic, if the patient is allergic to penicillin—since streptococcus is the chief infecting organism. Antibiotic therapy should continue for 48 hours after visible signs of infection have disappeared, or for at least 7 to 10 days.

Chronic pharyngitis requires the same supportive measures as acute pharyngitis but with greater emphasis on eliminating the underlying cause, such as an allergen. Preventive measures include adequate humidification and avoiding excessive exposure to air conditioning. In addition, the patient should be urged to stop smoking.

Special considerations

- Administer analgesics and warm saline gargles, as ordered and as appropriate. Encourage the patient to drink plenty of fluids (up to 2,500 ml/day). Monitor intake and output scrupulously, and watch for signs of dehydration (cracked lips, dry mucous membranes, low urinary output). Provide meticulous mouth care to prevent dry lips and oral pyoderma, and maintain a restful environment.
- Obtain throat cultures, and administer antibiotics, as ordered. If the patient has acute bacterial pharyngitis, emphasize the importance of completing the full course of antibiotic therapy. Teach the patient with chronic pharyngitis how

to minimize sources of throat irritation in the environment, such as using a bedside humidifier. Refer the patient to a self-help group to stop smoking, if appropriate.

Tonsillitis

Tonsillitis, or inflammation of the tonsils, can be acute or chronic. The uncomplicated acute form usually lasts 4 to 6 days and commonly affects children between ages 5 and 10. The presence of proven chronic tonsillitis justifies tonsillectomy, the only effective treatment. Tonsils tend to hypertrophy during childhood and atrophy after puberty.

Causes

Tonsillitis generally results from infection with beta-hemolytic streptococci but can result from other bacteria or viruses.

Signs and symptoms

Acute tonsillitis commonly begins with a mild to severe sore throat. A very young child, unable to complain about a sore throat, may stop eating. Tonsillitis may also produce dysphagia, fever, swelling and tenderness of the lymph glands in the submandibular area, muscle and joint pain, chills, malaise, headache, and pain (frequently referred to the ears). Excess secretions may elicit the complaint of a constant urge to swallow; the back of the throat may feel constricted. Such discomfort usually subsides after 72 hours.

Chronic tonsillitis produces a recurrent sore throat and purulent drainage in the tonsillar crypts. Frequent attacks of acute tonsillitis may also occur. Complications include obstruction from tonsillar hypertrophy and peritonsillar abscess.

Diagnosis

Diagnostic confirmation requires a thorough throat examination that reveals:

- generalized inflammation of the pharyngeal wall.
- swollen tonsils that project from between the pillars of the fauces and exude white or yellow follicles.
- purulent drainage when pressure is applied to the tonsillar pillars.
- possible edematous and inflamed uvula.

Culture may determine the infecting organism and indicate appropriate antibiotic therapy. Leukocytosis is also usually present. Differential diagnosis rules out infectious mononucleosis and diphtheria.

Treatment

Treatment of acute tonsillitis requires rest, adequate fluid intake, administration of aspirin or acetaminophen, and for bacterial infection, antibiotics. When the causative organism is Group A beta-hemolytic streptococcus, penicillin is the drug of choice (erythromycin or another broad-spectrum antibiotic may be given if the patient is allergic to penicillin). To prevent complications, antibiotic therapy should continue for 10 days. Chronic tonsillitis or the development of complications (obstructions from tonsillar hypertrophy, peritonsillar abscess) may require a tonsillectomy, but only after the patient has been free of tonsillar or respiratory tract infections for 3 to 4 weeks.

Special considerations

- Despite dysphagia, urge the patient to drink plenty of fluids, especially if he has a fever. Offer a child ice cream and flavored drinks and ices. Suggest gargling to soothe the throat, unless it exacerbates pain. Make sure the patient and parents understand the importance of completing the prescribed course of antibiotic therapy.

• Before tonsillectomy, explain to the adult patient that a local anesthetic prevents pain but allows a sensation of pressure during surgery. Warn the patient to expect considerable throat discomfort and some bleeding postoperatively.

• For the pediatric patient, keep your explanation simple and nonthreatening. Show the child the operating and recovery rooms, and briefly explain the hospital routine. Most hospitals allow one parent to stay with the child.

• Postoperatively, maintain a patent airway. To prevent aspiration, place the patient on his side. Monitor vital signs frequently, and check for bleeding. Immediately report excessive bleeding, increased pulse rate, or dropping blood pressure. After the patient is fully alert and the gag reflex has returned, allow him to drink water. Later, urge him to drink plenty of nonirritating fluids, to ambulate, and to take frequent deep breaths to prevent pulmonary complications. Give pain medication, as needed.

• Before discharge, provide the patient or parents with written instructions on home care. Tell them to expect a white scab to form in the throat between 5 and 10 days postoperatively, and to report bleeding, ear discomfort, or a fever that lasts longer than 3 days.

Throat Abscesses

Throat abscesses may be peritonsillar (quinsy) or retropharyngeal. Peritonsillar abscess forms in the connective tissue space between the tonsil capsule and constrictor muscle of the pharynx. Retropharyngeal abscess, or abscess of the potential space, forms between the posterior pharyngeal wall and prevertebral fascia. With treatment, the prognosis for both types of abscesses is good.

Causes and incidence

Peritonsillar abscess is a complication of acute tonsillitis, usually after streptococcal or staphylococcal infection. It occurs more often in adolescents and young adults than in children.

Acute retropharyngeal abscess results from infection in the retropharyngeal lymph glands, which may follow an upper respiratory tract bacterial infection. Because these lymph glands, present at birth, begin to atrophy after age 2, acute retropharyngeal abscess most commonly affects infants and children under age 2.

Chronic retropharyngeal abscess results from tuberculosis of the cervical spine (Pott's disease) and may occur at any age.

Signs and symptoms

Key symptoms of peritonsillar abscess include severe throat pain, occasional ear pain on the same side as the abscess, and tenderness of the submandibular gland. Dysphagia causes drooling. Trismus may occur as a result of edema and infection spreading from the peritonsillar space to the pterygoid muscles. Other effects include fever, chills, malaise, rancid breath, nausea, muffled speech, dehydration, cervical adenopathy, and localized or systemic sepsis.

Clinical features of retropharyngeal abscess include pain, dysphagia, fever, and, when the abscess is located in the upper pharynx, nasal obstruction; with a low-positioned abscess, dyspnea, progressive inspiratory stridor (from laryngeal obstruction), neck hyperextension, and, in children, drooling and muffled crying. A very large abscess may press on the larynx, causing edema, or may erode into major vessels, causing sudden death from asphyxia or aspiration.

Diagnosis

Diagnosis of peritonsillar abscess begins with a patient history of staphylococcal

PATIENT TEACHING AID

Gargling with Warm Salt Water

Dear Patient:
Following an incision to drain a throat abscess, you may be instructed to gargle with warm salt water. Proper gargling helps relieve throat irritation, remove secretions, and promote healing. Here's how to do it:

- Run tap water until it's 100° to 120° F. (37.8° to 48.9° C.). You should try to gargle with water that's as warm as you can stand it.
- Mix 1 cup of warm tap water with 1 to 2 teaspoonfuls of salt. Stir until it's dissolved.
- Take a mouthful of this solution and tip your head back, allowing the fluid to flow gently against the walls of your throat.
- Agitate the solution at the back of your throat by forcing air through it. Do this for as long as you can.
- Spit out this mouthful of salt water and repeat this process three more times. (You don't have to gargle the whole cup.)

or streptococcal infection. Examination of the throat shows swelling of the soft palate on the abscessed side, with displacement of the uvula to the opposite side; red, edematous mucous membranes; and tonsil displacement toward the midline. Culture may reveal streptococcal or staphylococcal infection.

Diagnosis of retropharyngeal abscess is based on patient history of nasopharyngitis or pharyngitis and on physical examination revealing a soft, red bulging of the posterior pharyngeal wall. X-rays show the larynx pushed forward and a widened space between the posterior pharyngeal wall and vertebrae. Culture and sensitivity tests isolate the causative organism and determine the appropriate antibiotic.

Treatment

For early-stage peritonsillar abscess, large doses of penicillin or another broad-spectrum antibiotic are necessary. For late-stage abscess, with cellulitis of the tonsillar space, primary treatment is usually incision and drainage under a local anesthetic, followed by antibiotic therapy for 7 to 10 days. Tonsillectomy, scheduled no sooner than 1 month after healing, prevents recurrence but is recommended only after several episodes.

In acute retropharyngeal abscess, the primary treatment is incision and drainage through the pharyngeal wall. In chronic retropharyngeal abscess, drainage is performed through an external incision behind the sternomastoid muscle. During incision and drainage, strong, continuous mouth suction is necessary to prevent aspiration of pus. Postoperative drug therapy includes antibiotics (usually penicillin) and analgesics.

Special considerations

- Be alert for signs of respiratory obstruction (inspiratory stridor, dyspnea, increasing restlessness, or cyanosis). Keep emergency airway equipment nearby.
- Explain drainage procedure to the patient or his parents. Since the procedure is generally done under a local anesthetic, the patient may be apprehensive.
- Assist with incision and drainage. To allow easy expectoration and suction of pus and blood, place the patient in a semirecumbent or sitting position.

After incision and drainage:

- Give antibiotics, analgesics, and antipyretics, as ordered. Stress the importance of completing the full course of prescribed antibiotic therapy.
- Monitor vital signs, and report any significant changes or bleeding. Assess

pain and treat accordingly.

- If the patient is unable to swallow, ensure adequate hydration with I.V. therapy. Monitor fluid intake and output, and watch for dehydration.
- Provide meticulous mouth care. Apply petrolatum to the patient's lips. Promote healing with warm saline gargles or throat irrigations for 24 to 36 hours after incision and drainage. Encourage adequate rest.

Vocal Cord Paralysis

Vocal cord paralysis results from disease of or injury to the superior or, most often, the recurrent laryngeal nerve.

Causes

Vocal cord paralysis commonly results from the accidental severing of the recurrent laryngeal nerve or of one of its extralaryngeal branches, during thyroidectomy. Other causes include pressure from an aortic aneurysm or from an enlarged atrium (in patients with mitral stenosis), bronchial or esophageal carcinoma, hypertrophy of the thyroid gland, trauma (such as neck injuries), and neuritis due to infections or metallic poisoning.

Vocal cord paralysis can also result from hysteria and, rarely, lesions of the central nervous system.

Signs and symptoms

Signs and symptoms of vocal cord paralysis depend on whether the paralysis is unilateral or bilateral, and on the position of the cord or cords when paralyzed. Unilateral paralysis, the most common form, may cause vocal weakness and hoarseness. Bilateral paralysis typically produces vocal weakness and incapacitating airway obstruction if the cords become paralyzed in the adducted position.

Diagnosis

Patient history and characteristic features suggest vocal cord paralysis.

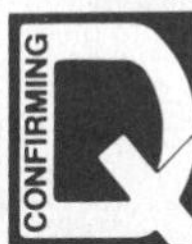

Visualization by indirect laryngoscopy shows one or both cords fixed in an adducted or partially abducted position, and confirms the diagnosis.

Treatment

Treatment of unilateral vocal cord paralysis consists of injection of Teflon into the paralyzed cord, under direct laryngoscopy. This procedure enlarges the cord and brings it closer to the other cord, which usually strengthens the voice and protects the airway from aspiration. Bilateral cord paralysis in an adducted position generally necessitates tracheotomy to restore a patent airway.

Alternative treatments for adult patients include arytenoidectomy to open the glottis, and lateral fixation of the arytenoid cartilage through an external neck incision. Excision or fixation of the arytenoid cartilage improves airway patency but produces residual voice impairment.

Treatment of hysterical aphonia may include psychotherapy and, for some patients, hypnosis.

Special considerations

If the patient chooses direct laryngoscopy and Teflon injection, explain these procedures thoroughly. Tell him these measures will improve his voice but won't restore it to normal.

Many patients with bilateral cord paralysis prefer to keep a tracheostomy instead of having an arytenoidectomy; their voices are generally better with a tracheostomy alone than after corrective surgery.

If the patient is scheduled to undergo a tracheotomy:

- Explain the procedure thoroughly, and

offer reassurance. Since the procedure is performed under a local anesthetic, the patient may be apprehensive.

- Teach the patient how to suction, clean, and change the tracheostomy tube.
- Reassure the patient that he can still speak by covering the lumen of the tracheostomy tube with his finger or a tracheostomy plug.

If the patient elects to have an arytenoidectomy, explain the procedure thoroughly. Advise the patient that the tracheostomy will remain in place until the edema has subsided and the airway is patent.

Vocal Cord Nodules and Polyps

Vocal cord nodules result from hypertrophy of fibrous tissue and form at the point where the cords come together forcibly. Vocal cord polyps are chronic, subepithelial, edematous masses. Both nodules and polyps have good prognoses, unless continued voice abuse causes recurrence, with subsequent scarring and permanent hoarseness.

Causes and incidence

Vocal cord nodules and polyps usually result from voice abuse, especially in the presence of infection. Consequently, they're most common in teachers, singers, and sports fans, and in energetic children (ages 8 to 12) who continually shout while playing. Polyps are common in adults who smoke, live in dry climates, or have allergies.

Signs and symptoms

Nodules and polyps inhibit the approximation of vocal cords and produce painless hoarseness. The voice may also develop a breathy or husky quality.

VOCAL CORD NODULES

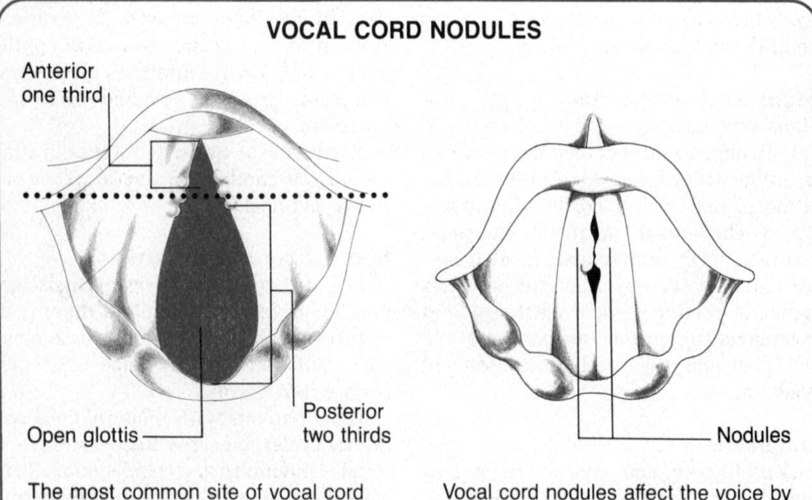

The most common site of vocal cord nodules is the point of maximal vibration and impact (junction of the anterior one third and the posterior two thirds of the vocal cord).

Vocal cord nodules affect the voice by inhibiting proper closure of the vocal cords during phonation.

Diagnosis

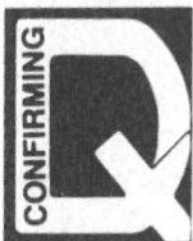

Persistent hoarseness suggests vocal cord nodules and polyps; visualization by indirect laryngoscopy confirms it. In the patient with vocal cord nodules, laryngoscopy initially shows small red nodes; later, white solid nodes on one or both cords. In the patient with polyps, laryngoscopy reveals unilateral or, occasionally, bilateral, sessile or pedunculated polyps of varying size, anywhere on the vocal cords.

Treatment

Conservative management of small vocal cord nodules and polyps includes humidification, speech therapy (voice rest, training to reduce the intensity and duration of voice production), and treatment of any underlying allergies.

When conservative treatment fails to relieve hoarseness, nodules or polyps require removal under direct laryngoscopy. Microlaryngoscopy may be done for small lesions, to avoid injuring the vocal cord surface. If nodules or polyps are bilateral, excision may be performed in two stages: one cord is allowed to heal before excision of polyps on the other cord. Two-stage excision prevents laryngeal web, which occurs when epithelial tissue is removed from adjacent cord surfaces, and these surfaces grow together. For children, treatment consists of speech therapy. If possible, surgery should be delayed until the child is old enough to benefit from voice training, or until he can understand the need to abstain from voice abuse.

Special considerations

- Postoperatively, stress the importance of resting the voice for 10 days to 2 weeks while the vocal cords heal. Provide an alternative means of communication—Magic Slate, pad and pencil, or alphabet board. Place a sign over the bed to remind visitors that the patient shouldn't talk. Mark the intercom so other hospital personnel are aware the patient can't answer. Minimize the need to speak by trying to anticipate the patient's needs.
- If the patient is a smoker, encourage him to stop smoking entirely or, at the very least, to refrain from smoking during recovery from surgery.
- Utilize a vaporizer to increase humidity and decrease throat irritation.
- Make sure the patient receives speech therapy after healing, if necessary, since continued voice abuse causes recurrence of growths.

Laryngitis

A common disorder, laryngitis is acute or chronic inflammation of the vocal cords. Acute laryngitis may occur as an isolated infection or as part of a generalized bacterial or viral upper respiratory tract infection. Repeated attacks of acute laryngitis cause inflammatory changes associated with chronic laryngitis.

Causes and incidence

Acute laryngitis usually results from infection or excessive use of the voice, an occupational hazard in certain vocations (teaching, public speaking, singing, for example). It may also result from leisuretime activities (such as cheering at a sports event), inhalation of smoke or fumes, or aspiration of caustic chemicals. Causes of chronic laryngitis include chronic upper respiratory tract disorders (sinusitis, bronchitis, nasal polyps, allergy), mouth breathing, smoking, constant exposure to dust or other irritants, and alcohol abuse.

Signs and symptoms

Acute laryngitis typically begins with hoarseness, ranging from mild to complete loss of voice. Associated clinical features include pain (especially when swallowing or speaking), dry cough, fever, laryngeal edema, and malaise. In chronic laryngitis, persistent hoarseness is usually the only symptom.

Diagnosis

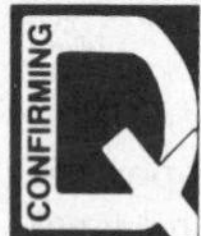

Indirect laryngoscopy confirms diagnosis by revealing red, inflamed, and occasionally, hemorrhagic vocal cords, with rounded rather than sharp edges, and exudate. Bilateral swelling may be present, which restricts movement but doesn't cause paralysis.

Treatment

Primary treatment consists of resting the voice. For viral infection, symptomatic care includes analgesics and throat lozenges for pain relief. Bacterial infection requires antibiotic therapy. Severe, acute laryngitis may necessitate hospitalization. Occasionally, when laryngeal edema results in airway obstruction, tracheotomy may be necessary. In chronic laryngitis, effective treatment must eliminate the underlying cause.

Special considerations

- Explain to the patient why he should not talk, and place a sign over the bed to remind others of this restriction. Provide a Magic Slate or a pad and pencil for communication. Mark the intercom panel so other hospital personnel are aware the patient can't answer. Minimize the need to talk by trying to anticipate the patient's needs.
- Suggest the patient maintain adequate humidification by using a vaporizer or humidifier during the winter; by avoiding air conditioning during the summer (because it dehumidifies); by using medicated throat lozenges; and by not smoking. Urge completion of prescribed antibiotics.
- Obtain a detailed patient history, to help determine the cause of chronic laryngitis. Encourage modification of predisposing habits.

Juvenile Angiofibroma

An uncommon disorder, juvenile angiofibroma is a highly vascular, nasopharyngeal tumor made up of masses of fibrous tissue that contain many thin-walled blood vessels. These tumors are found primarily in adolescent males and are extremely rare in females. Incidence is higher in Egypt, India, Southeast Asia, and Kenya than in the United States and Europe. Prognosis is good with treatment.

Causes

Although its cause is unknown, juvenile angiofibroma has been identified as a type of hemangioma. This tumor grows on one side of the posterior nares and may completely fill the nasopharynx, nose, paranasal sinuses, and possibly the orbit. More often sessile than polypoid, juvenile angiofibroma is nonencapsulated and invades surrounding tissue.

Signs and symptoms

Juvenile angiofibroma produces unilateral or bilateral nasal obstruction and severe recurrent epistaxis, usually between ages 7 and 21. Recurrent epistaxic episodes eventually cause secondary anemia. Associated effects include purulent rhinorrhea, facial deformity, and nasal speech. Serous otitis media and hearing loss may result from eustachian tube obstruction.

Diagnosis

A nasopharyngeal mirror or nasal speculum permits visualization of the tumor, which appears as a blue mass in the nose or nasopharynx. X-rays show a bowing of the posterior wall of the maxillary sinus. Angiography determines the size and location of the tumor and also shows the source of vascularization. Biopsy of the tumor is contraindicated because of the danger of hemorrhage.

Treatment

Several surgical methods are used, ranging from avulsion to cryosurgical techniques. Surgical excision is preferred after embolization with Teflon or absorbable gelatin sponge, to decrease vascularization. Whichever surgical method is used, this tumor must be removed in its entirety and not in pieces. Preoperative hormonal therapy may decrease the tumor's size and vascularity. Blood transfusions may be necessary during avulsion. Radiation therapy produces only a temporary regression in an angiofibroma but is the treatment of choice if the tumor has expanded into the cranium or orbit. Because the tumor is multilobular and locally invasive, symptomatic recurrences are common (about 30% of patients) during the first year after treatment, but are uncommon after 2 years.

Special considerations

- Explain all diagnostic and surgical procedures. Provide emotional support; severe epistaxis frightens many persons to the point of panic. Check hemoglobin and hematocrit for anemia.
- After surgery, report excessive bleeding immediately. Make sure an adequate supply of typed and cross-matched blood is available for transfusion.
- Monitor for any change in vital signs. Provide good oral hygiene, and use a bedside vaporizer bedside to raise humidity.
- During blood transfusion, watch for transfusion reactions, such as fever, chills, or a rash. If any of these reactions occur, discontinue the blood transfusion and notify the doctor immediately.
- Teach the family how to apply pressure over the affected area, and instruct them to seek immediate medical attention if bleeding occurs after discharge. Stress the importance of providing adequate humidification at home to keep nasal mucosa moist.

Selected References

Bluestone, Charles D., and Stool, Sylvan S., eds. *Pediatric Otolaryngology,* vols. 1 and 2. Philadelphia: W.B. Saunders Co., 1983.

DeWeese, David D., and Saunders, William H. *Textbook of Otolaryngology,* 6th ed. St. Louis: C.V. Mosby Co., 1982.

English, Gerald, ed. "Otolaryngology," *Loose Leaf Reference Services,* vols. 1-5. Philadelphia: J.B. Lippincott Co., 1985.

Hall, Ian S., and Colman, Bernard S. *Diseases of the Nose, Throat, and Ear,* 12th ed. New York: Churchill Livingstone, 1981.

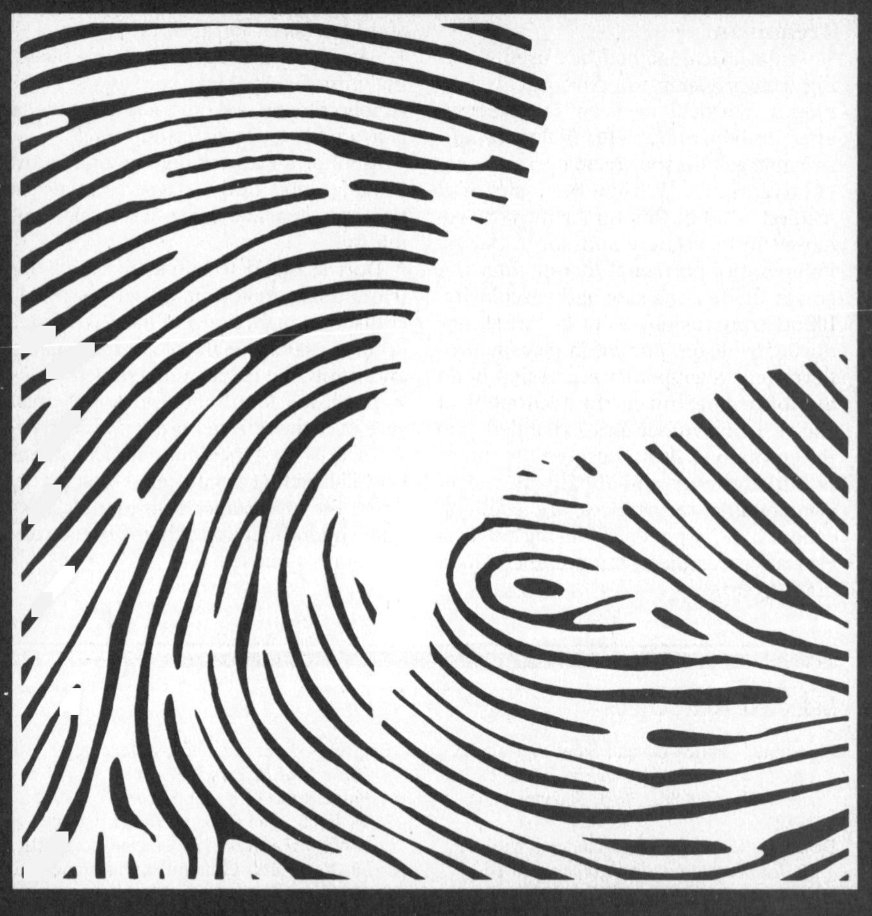

21 Skin Disorders

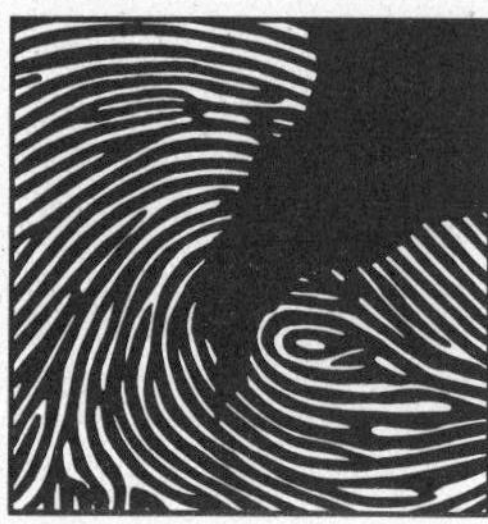

Skin Disorders

Introduction

Skin is man's front-line protective barrier between internal structures and the external environment. It's tough, resilient, and virtually impermeable to aqueous solutions, bacteria, or toxic compounds. It also performs many vital functions. Skin protects against trauma, regulates body temperature, serves as an organ of excretion and sensation, and synthesizes vitamin D in the presence of ultraviolet light. Skin varies in thickness and other qualities from one part of the body to another, which often accounts for the distribution of skin diseases.

Skin has three primary layers: *epidermis, dermis,* and *subcutaneous tissue.* The epidermis—the outermost layer—as its primary function, produces keratin. This layer is generally thin but is thicker in areas subject to constant pressure or friction, such as the soles and palms. Epidermis contains two sublayers: the *stratum corneum,* an outer, horny layer of keratin that protects the body against harmful environmental substances and restricts water loss; and the *cellular stratum,* where keratin cells are synthesized. The *basement membrane* lies beneath the cellular stratum and joins the epidermis to the dermis.

The cellular stratum, the deepest layer of the epidermis, consists of the *basal layer,* where mitosis takes place; the *stratum spinosum,* where cells begin to flatten, and fibrils—precursors of keratin—start to appear; and the *stratum granulosum,* made up of cells containing deeply staining granules of keratohyalin, which are generally thought to become the keratin that forms the stratum corneum. A skin cell moves from the basal layer of the cellular stratum to the stratum corneum in about 14 days. After another 14 days, normal wear and tear on the skin cause it to slough off. The epidermis also contains melanocytes, which produce the melanin that gives the skin its color, and a yellow pigment called carotene.

The *dermis,* the second primary layer of the skin, consists of three fibrous proteins, fibroblasts, and an intervening ground substance. The proteins are collagen, which strengthens the skin to prevent it from tearing; elastin to give it resilience; and reticulin, which helps make up the basement membrane. The ground substance contains primarily jellylike mucopolysaccharides; this substance makes the skin soft and compressible. Two distinct layers comprise the dermis: the papillary dermis (top layer) and the reticular dermis (bottom layer).

Subcutaneous tissue, the third primary layer of the skin, consists mainly of fat (containing mostly triglycerides), which provides heat, insulation, shock absorption, and a reserve of calories. Both sensory and motor nerves (autonomic fibers) are found in the dermis and the subcutaneous tissue.

Appendages: Nails, glands, and hair

Nails are epidermal cells converted to hard keratin. The bed on which the nail rests is highly vascular, making the nail appear pink; the whitish, crescent-shaped area extending beyond the proximal nail fold, called the lunula—most visible in the thumbnail—marks the end of the matrix, the site of mitosis and of nail growth.

Sebaceous glands, found everywhere on the body except the palms and soles, serve as appendages of the dermis. These glands generally excrete sebum into hair follicles, but in some cases, they empty directly onto the skin surface. Sebum is an oily substance that helps keep the skin and hair from drying out and prevents water and heat loss. Sebaceous glands abound on the scalp, forehead, cheeks, chin, back, and genitalia, and may be stimulated by sex hormones—primarily testosterone.

Appendages found in the dermis and the subcutaneous tissue include *eccrine* and *apocrine glands,* and *hair.* Eccrine sweat glands open directly onto the skin and regulate body temperature. Innervated by sympathetic nerves, these sweat glands are distributed throughout the body, except for the lips, ears, and parts of the genitalia. They secrete a solution made up mostly of water and sodium chloride; the prime stimulus for eccrine gland secretion is heat. Other stimuli include muscular exertion and emotional stress.

Apocrine sweat glands appear chiefly in the axillae and genitalia; they are responsible for producing body odor and are stimulated by emotional stress. The sweat produced is sterile but undergoes bacterial decomposition on the skin surface. These glands become functional after puberty. (Ceruminous glands, located in the external ear canal, appear to be modified sweat glands and secrete a waxy substance known as cerumen.)

Hair grows on most of the body, except for the palms, the soles, and parts of the genitalia. An individual hair consists of a shaft (a column of keratinized cells), a root (embedded in the dermis), the hair follicle (the root and its covering), and the hair papilla (a loop of capillaries at the base of the follicle). Mitosis at the base of the follicle causes the hair to grow, while the papilla provides nourishment for mitosis. Small bundles of involuntary muscles known as arrectores pilorum cling to hair follicles. When these muscles contract, usually during moments of fear or shock, the hairs stand on end, and the person is said to have goose bumps or gooseflesh. Melanin in the outer layer of the hair shaft gives the

PRIMARY SKIN LESIONS

MACULE
(flat, circumscribed area with change in normal skin)

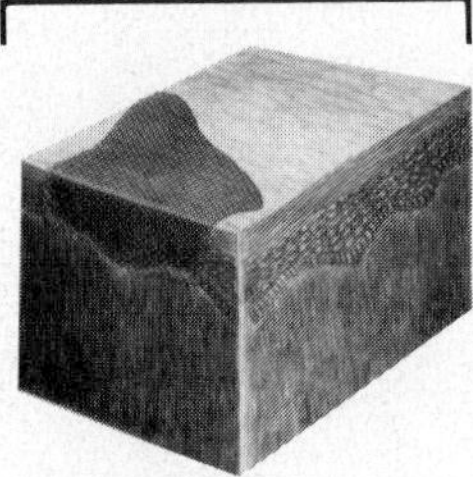

Patch (usually > 1 cm)—flat area of skin with change in color

VESICLE
(serous fluid-filled lesion)

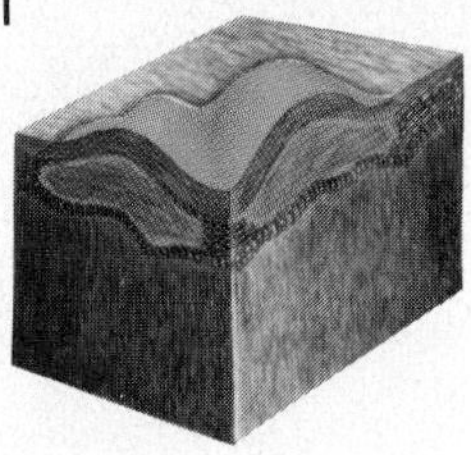

Bulla (> 1 cm)—larger circumscribed area containing free serous fluid

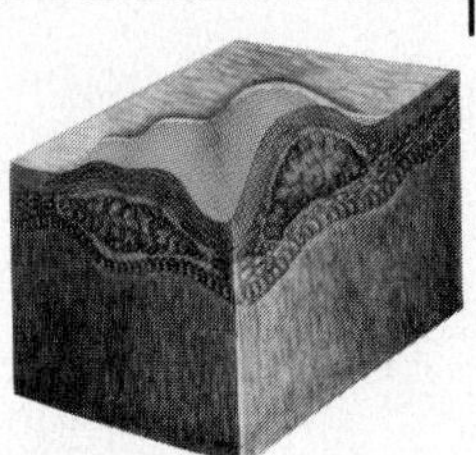

Pustule (size varies)—lesion containing purulent fluid

PAPULE
(solid, elevated mass)

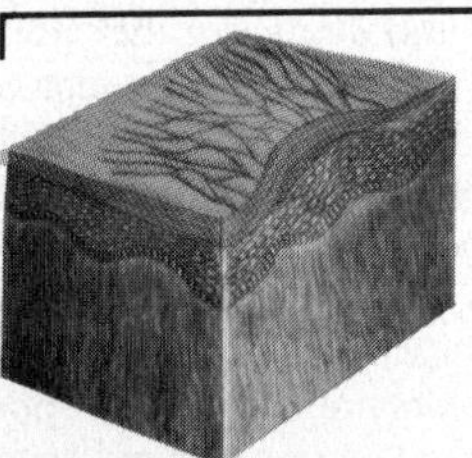

Plaque—formed by confluence of papules

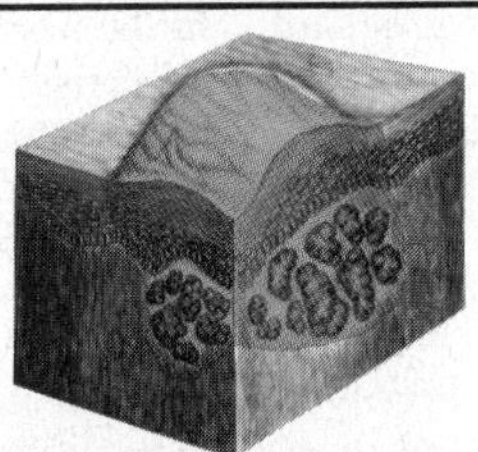

Nodule or tumor (usually > 1 cm)—palpable, solid, and round

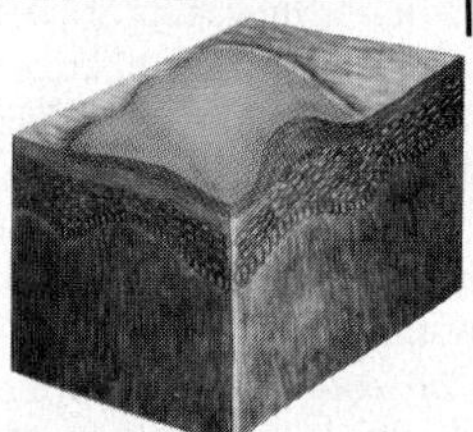

Wheal—circumscribed area of edema, usually transient

hair its distinctive color, which is directly related to the number of melanocytes (melanin-producing cells) in the hair bulb.

Vascular influence

Skin contains a vast arteriovenous network, extending from subcutaneous tissue to the dermis. These blood vessels provide oxygen and nutrients to sensory nerves (which control touch, temperature, and pain), motor nerves (which control the activities of sweat glands, the arterioles, and smooth muscles of the skin), and skin appendages. Blood flow also influences skin coloring, since the amount of oxygen carried to capillaries in the dermis can produce transient changes in color. For example, decreased oxygen supply can turn the skin pale or bluish; increased oxygen can turn it pink or ruddy.

Assessing skin disorders

Assessment begins with a thorough patient history to determine whether a skin disorder is an acute flare-up, recurrent problem, or chronic condition. Ask the patient how long he's had the disorder; how a typical flare-up or attack begins; whether or not it itches; and what medications—systemic or topical—have been used to treat it. Also, find out if any family members, friends, or contacts have the same disorder, and if the patient lives or works in an environment that could cause the condition.

When examining a patient with a skin disorder, be sure to look everywhere—mucous membranes, hair, scalp, axillae, groin, palms, soles, nails. Note moisture, temperature, texture, thickness, mobility, edema, turgor, and any irregularities in skin color. Look for skin lesions; if you find a lesion, record its color, size, and location. Try to determine which is the primary lesion—the one that appeared first—which always starts in normal skin. The patient might be able to point it out.

If more than one lesion is in evidence, note the pattern of distribution. Lesions can be localized (isolated), regional, general, or universal (total), involving the entire skin, hair, and nails. Also, observe whether the lesions are unilateral or bilateral, symmetric or asymmetric, and note the arrangement of the lesions (clustered or linear configuration, for example).

Diagnostic aids

After simple observation, and examination of the affected area of the skin with a dermatoscope, for morphologic detail, the following clinical diagnostic techniques may help to identify skin disorders:

- *Diascopy*, in which a lesion is covered with a microscopic slide or piece of clear plastic, helps determine whether dilated capillaries or extravasated blood is causing the redness of a lesion.
- *Sidelighting* shows minor elevations or depressions in lesions; it also helps determine the configuration and degree of

SECONDARY CHANGES IN PRIMARY SKIN LESIONS

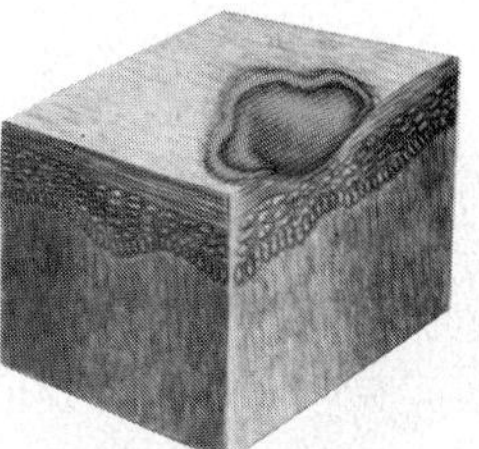

Erosion—circumscribed, partial loss of epidermis

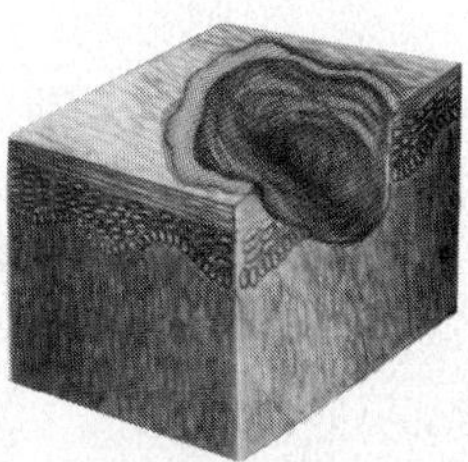

Ulcer—irregularly sized and shaped excavations penetrating into dermis

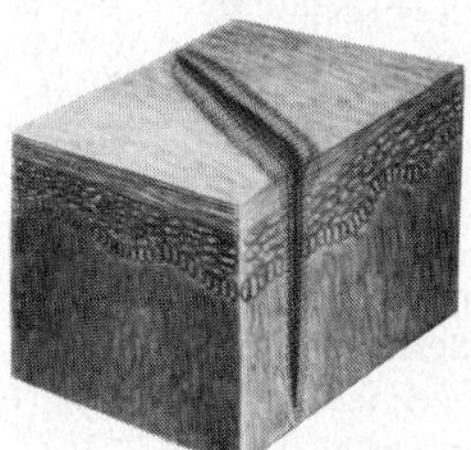

Fissure—linear ulcer

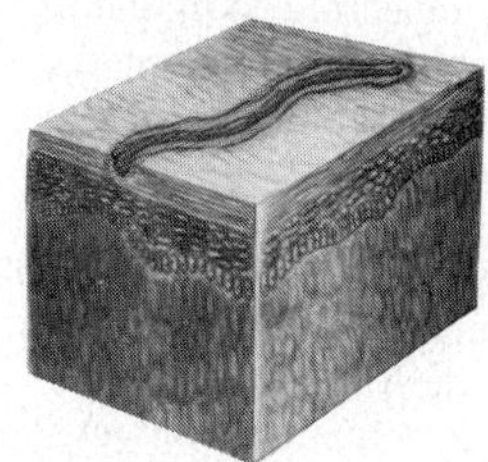

Excoriation—abrasion or scratch mark (linear break produced manually)

SECONDARY CHANGES IN PRIMARY SKIN LESIONS

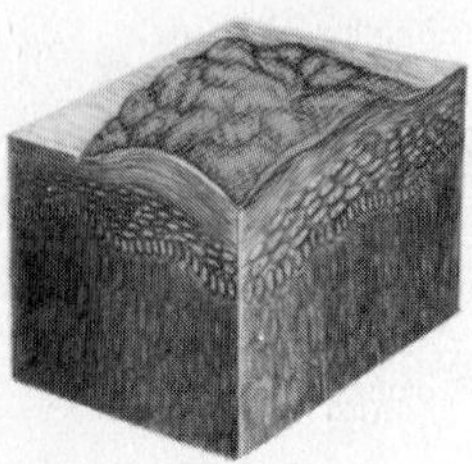

Crust—variously colored masses of exudate from skin

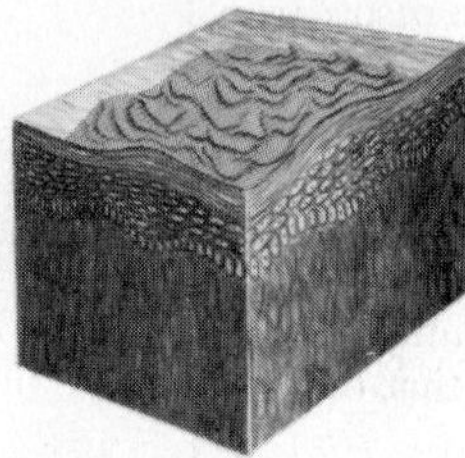

Scale—loose fragments of keratin in stratum corneum

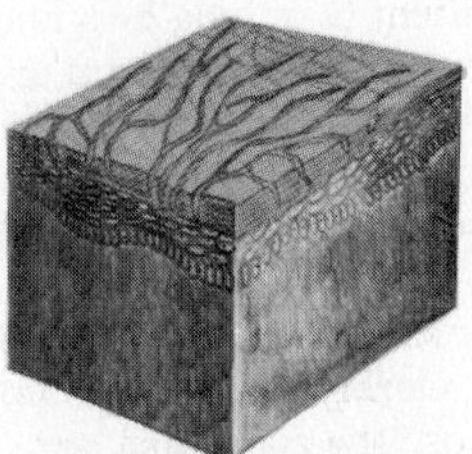

Lichenification—thick and roughened skin, exaggerated skin lines

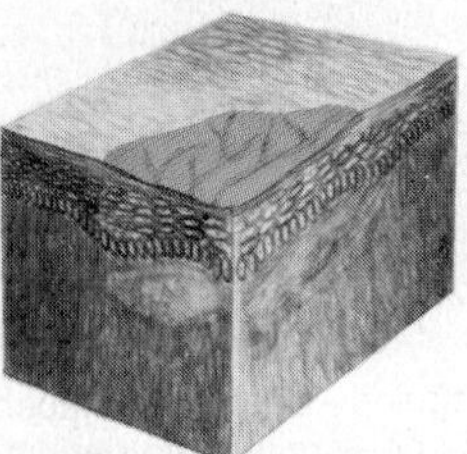

Atrophy—thin skin without normal markings

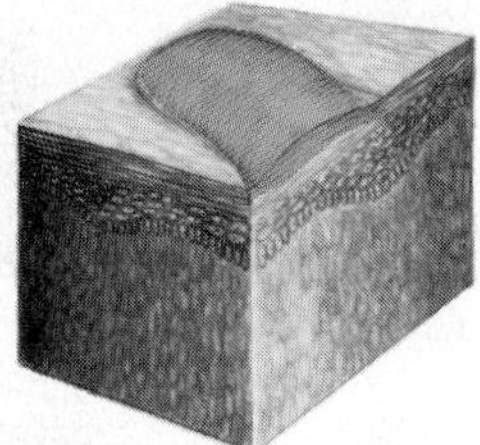

Scar—permanent fibrous tissue at site of healed injury

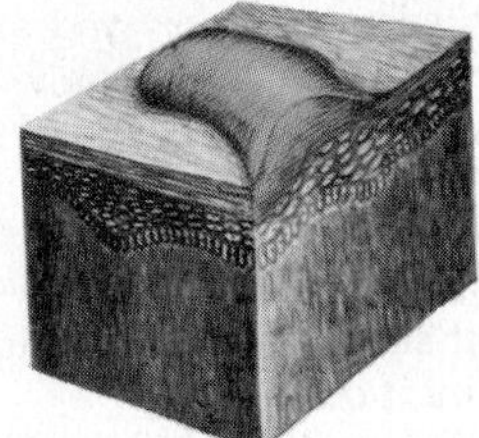

Keloid—hypertrophied scar

eruption.

• *Subdued lighting* highlights the difference between normal skin and circumscribed lesions that are hypo- or hyperpigmented.
• *Microscopic immunofluorescence* identifies immunoglobulins and elastic tissue in detecting skin manifestations of immunologically mediated disease.
• *Potassium hydroxide preparations* permit examination for mycelia in fungal infections.
• *Gram's stains and exudate cultures* help identify the organism responsible for an underlying infection.
• *Patch tests* identify contact sensitivity (usually with dermatitis).
• *Biopsy* determines histology of cells, and may be diagnostic, confirmatory, or inconclusive, depending on the disease.

Special considerations

When assessing a skin disorder, keep in mind its distressing social and psychologic implications. Unlike internal disorders, such as cardiac disease or diabetes mellitus, a skin condition is usually obvious and disfiguring. Understandably, the psychologic implications are most acute when skin disorders affect the face—especially during adolescence, an emotionally turbulent time of life. But such disorders can also create tremendous psychologic problems for adults. A skin disease often interferes with a person's ability to work because the condition affects the hands or because it distresses the patient to such an extent that he can't function.

For these reasons, be empathetic and accepting. Above all, don't be afraid to touch such a patient; most skin disorders are not contagious. Touching the patient naturally and without hesitation helps show your acceptance of the dermatologic condition. Such acceptance is no less important than your patient teaching about the disease, and your guidance and help with carrying out prescribed treatment.

BACTERIAL INFECTION

Impetigo

(Impetigo contagiosa)

A contagious, superficial skin infection, impetigo occurs in nonbullous and bullous forms. This vesiculopustular eruptive disorder spreads most easily among infants, young children, and the elderly. Predisposing factors such as poor hygiene, anemia, malnutrition, and a warm climate favor outbreaks of this infection, most of which occur during the late summer and early fall. Impetigo can complicate chickenpox, eczema, or other skin conditions marked by open lesions.

Causes

Beta-hemolytic streptococcus usually produces nonbullous impetigo; coagulase-positive *Staphylococcus aureus* generally causes bullous impetigo.

Signs and symptoms

Streptococcal impetigo typically begins with a small red macule that turns into a vesicle, becoming pustular in a matter of hours. When the vesicle breaks, a characteristic thick yellow crust forms from the exudate. Autoinoculation may cause satellite lesions to appear. Other clinical features include pruritus, burning, and regional lymphadenopathy.

A rare but serious complication of streptococcal impetigo is glomerulonephritis. Infants and very young children may develop aural impetigo or otitis externa, but the lesions usually clear without treatment in 2 to 3 weeks, unless an underlying disorder, such as eczema, is present.

In *staphylococcal impetigo,* a thin-walled vesicle opens, and a thin, clear crust forms from the exudate. As in the streptococcal form, the lesion consists of a central clearing, circumscribed by an outer rim—much like a ringworm lesion—and commonly appears on the face or other exposed areas. Both forms usually produce painless itching, and may appear simultaneously and be clinically indistinguishable.

Diagnosis

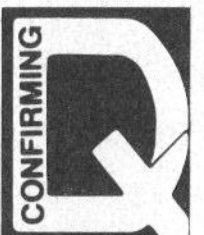

Characteristic lesions suggest impetigo; microscopic visualization of the causative organism in a Gram's stain of vesicle fluid usually confirms *S. aureus* infection and justifies anti-

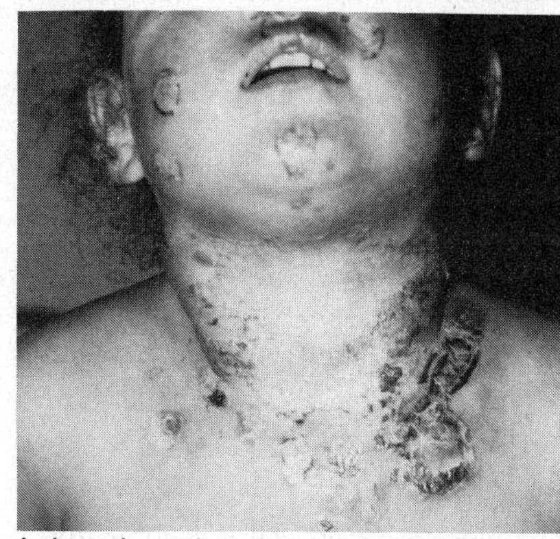

In impetigo, when the vesicles break, crust forms from the exudate. This infection is especially contagious among young children.

ECTHYMA

Ecthyma is a superficial skin infection that usually causes scarring. It generally results from infection by beta-hemolytic streptococcus. Ecthyma differs from impetigo in that its characteristic ulcer results from deeper penetration of the skin by the infecting organism (involving the lower epidermis and dermis), and the overlying crust tends to be piled high (1 to 3 cm). These lesions often occur on the posterior aspects of the thighs and buttocks. Autoinoculation can transmit ecthyma to other parts of the body, especially to sites that have been scratched open. (Ecthyma often results from the scratching of chigger bites.) Therapy is basically the same as for impetigo, beginning with removal of the crust, but response may be slower. Widespread ulcers may require parenteral antibiotics.

biotic therapy. Culture and sensitivity testing of fluid or denuded skin may indicate the most appropriate antibiotic, but therapy should not be delayed for laboratory results, which can take 3 days. WBC may be elevated in the presence of infection.

Treatment

Generally, treatment consists of systemic antibiotics (usually penicillin, or erythromycin for patients who are allergic to penicillin), which also help prevent glomerulonephritis. Therapy also includes removal of the exudate by washing the lesions two to three times a day with soap and water, or for stubborn crusts, warm soaks or compresses of normal saline or a diluted soap solution before application of topical antibiotics (usually polymyxin B and bacitracin). Topical antibiotics are less effective than systemic antibiotics.

Special considerations

- Urge the patient not to scratch, since this exacerbates impetigo. Advise parents to cut the child's fingernails. Give medications, as ordered; remember to check for penicillin allergy. Stress the need to continue prescribed medications even after lesions have healed.
- Teach the patient or family how to care for impetiginous lesions. To prevent further spread of this highly contagious infection, encourage frequent bathing using a bactericidal soap. Tell the patient not to share towels, washcloths, or bed linens with family members. Emphasize the importance of following proper handwashing technique.
- Check family members for impetigo. If this infection is present in a schoolchild, notify his school.

Folliculitis, Furunculosis, and Carbunculosis

Folliculitis is a bacterial infection of the hair follicle that causes the formation of a pustule. The infection can be superficial (follicular impetigo or Bockhart's impetigo) or deep (sycosis barbae). Folliculitis may also lead to the development of furuncles (furunculosis), commonly known as boils, or carbuncles (carbunculosis). Prognosis depends on the severity of the infection and on the patient's physical condition and ability to resist infection.

Causes

The most common cause of folliculitis, furunculosis, or carbunculosis is coagulase-positive *Staphylococcus aureus*. For furunculosis, predisposing factors include an infected wound elsewhere on the body, poor personal hygiene, debilitation, diabetes, exposure to chemicals (cutting oils), and management of skin lesions with tar or with occlusive therapy, using steroids. Furunculosis generally follows folliculitis exacerbated by irritation, pressure, friction, or perspiration. Carbunculosis follows persistent *S. aureus* infection and furunculosis.

Signs and symptoms

Pustules of folliculitis usually appear on the scalp, arms, and legs in children; on the face of bearded men (sycosis barbae); and on the eyelids (styes). Deep folliculitis may be painful.

Folliculitis may progress to the hard, painful nodules of furunculosis, which commonly develop on the neck, face, axillae, and buttocks. For several days these nodules enlarge, and then rupture, discharging pus and necrotic material. After the nodules rupture, pain subsides, but erythema and edema may persist for days or weeks.

Carbunculosis is marked by extremely painful, deep abscesses that drain through multiple openings onto the skin surface, usually around several hair follicles. Fever and malaise may accompany these lesions.

Diagnosis

The obvious skin lesion confirms follicu-

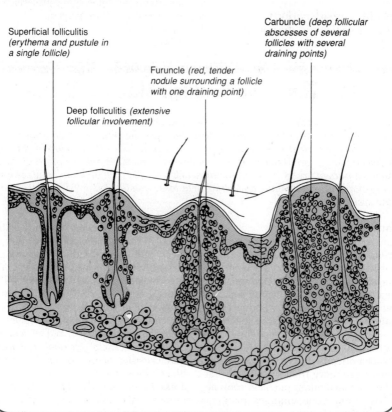

FORMS OF BACTERIAL SKIN INFECTION

Degree of hair follicle involvement in bacterial skin infection ranges from superficial erythema and pustule of a single follicle to deep abscesses (carbuncles) involving several follicles.

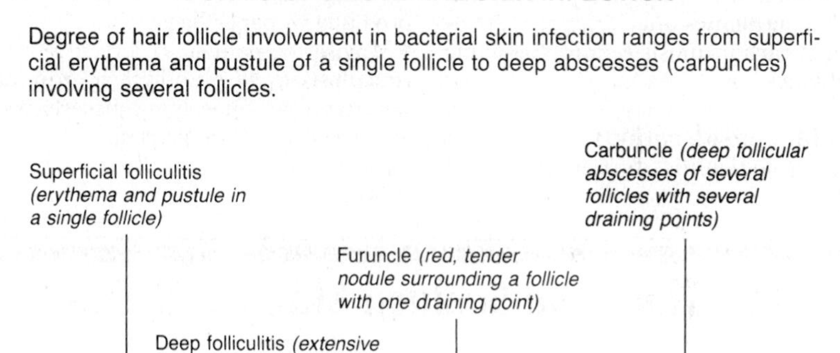

litis, furunculosis, or carbunculosis. Wound culture shows *S. aureus.* In carbunculosis, patient history reveals preexistent furunculosis. CBC may show elevated WBC (leukocytosis).

Treatment

Treatment of folliculitis consists of cleansing the infected area thoroughly with soap and water; applying hot, wet compresses to promote vasodilation and drainage of infected material from the lesions; topical antibiotics, such as bacitracin and polymyxin B; and in recurrent infection, systemic antibiotics.

Furunculosis may also require incision and drainage of ripe lesions after application of hot, wet compresses, and topical antibiotics after drainage. Treatment of carbunculosis requires systemic antibiotics.

Special considerations

Care for folliculitis, furunculosis, and carbunculosis is basically supportive, and emphasizes patient teaching of scrupulous personal and family hygiene, dietary modifications (reduced intake of sugars and fats), and precautions to prevent spreading infection.

- Caution the patient never to squeeze a boil, since this may cause it to rupture into the surrounding area.
- To avoid spreading bacteria to family members, urge the patient not to share his towel and washcloth. Tell him that these items should be boiled in hot water before being reused. The patient should change his clothes and bedsheets daily, and these also should be washed in hot water. Encourage the patient to change dressings frequently and to discard them promptly in paper bags.
- Advise the patient with recurrent furunculosis to have a physical examination, since an underlying disease, such as diabetes, may be present.

Staphylococcal Scalded Skin Syndrome

A severe skin disorder, staphylococcal scalded skin syndrome (SSSS) is marked by epidermal erythema, peeling, and necrosis that give the skin a scalded appearance. SSSS is most prevalent in infants aged 1 to 3 months but may develop in children; it's uncommon in adults. This disease follows a consistent pattern of progression, and most patients recover fully. Mortality is 2% to 3%, with death usually resulting from complications of fluid and electrolyte loss, sepsis, and involvement of other body systems.

Causes

The causative organism in SSSS is Group 2 *Staphylococcus aureus,* primarily phage type 71. Predisposing factors may include impaired immunity and renal insufficiency—present to some extent in the normal neonate, due to immature development of these systems.

Signs and symptoms

SSSS can often be traced to a prodromal upper respiratory tract infection, possibly with concomitant purulent conjunctivitis. Cutaneous changes progress through three stages:

- *Erythema:* Erythema becomes visible, usually around the mouth and other orifices, and may spread in widening circles over the entire body surface. The skin becomes tender; Nikolsky's sign (sloughing of the skin when friction is applied) may appear.
- *Exfoliation* (24 to 48 hours later): In the more common, localized form of this disease, superficial erosions and minimal crusting occur, generally around body orifices, and may spread to exposed areas of the skin. In the more severe forms of this disease, large, flaccid bullae erupt and may spread to cover ex-

IDENTIFYING STAPHYLOCOCCAL SCALDED SKIN SYNDROME

Staphylococcal scalded skin syndrome is a severe skin disorder that commonly affects infants and children. The illustration below shows the typical scalded skin appearance, with areas of denuded skin found in an infant.

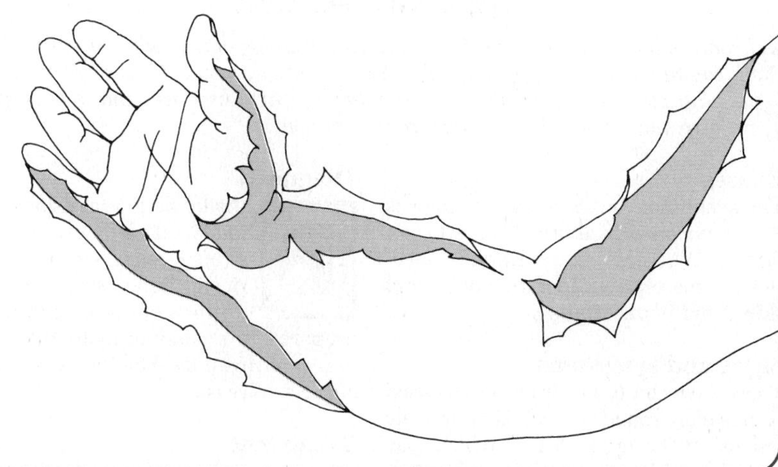

tensive areas of the body. These bullae eventually rupture, revealing sections of denuded skin.

• *Desquamation:* In this final stage, affected areas dry up, and powdery scales form. Normal skin replaces these scales in 5 to 7 days.

Diagnosis

Diagnosis requires careful observation of the three-stage progression of this disease. Results of exfoliative cytology and biopsy aid in differential diagnosis, ruling out erythema multiforme and drug-induced toxic epidermal necrolysis, both of which are similar to SSSS. Isolation of Group 2 *S. aureus* on cultures of skin lesions confirms the diagnosis. However, skin lesions sometimes appear sterile.

Treatment and special considerations

Treatment includes systemic antibiotics—usually penicillinase-resistant penicillin—to prevent secondary infections, and replacement measures to maintain fluid and electrolyte balance.

• Provide special care for the neonate, if required, including placement in a warming infant incubator to maintain body temperature and provide isolation.

• Carefully monitor intake and output to assess fluid and electrolyte balance. In severe cases, I.V. fluid replacement may be necessary.

• Check vital signs. Be especially alert for a sudden rise in temperature, indicating sepsis, which requires prompt, aggressive treatment.

• Maintain skin integrity. Use strict aseptic technique to preclude secondary infection, especially during the exfoliative stage, because of open lesions. To prevent friction and sloughing of the skin, leave affected areas uncovered or loosely covered. Place cotton between severely affected fingers and toes to prevent webbing.

• Administer warm baths and soaks during the recovery period. Gently debride exfoliated areas.

• Reassure parents that complications are rare and residual scars are unlikely.

FUNGAL INFECTION

Tinea Versicolor

(Pityriasis versicolor)

A chronic, superficial, fungal infection, tinea versicolor may produce a multicolored rash, commonly on the upper trunk. This condition, primarily a cosmetic defect, usually affects young persons, especially during warm weather, and is most prevalent in tropical countries. Recurrence is common.

Causes

The agent that causes tinea versicolor is *Pityrosporon orbiculare (Microsporum furfur).* Whether this condition is infectious or merely a proliferation of normal skin fungi is uncertain.

Signs and symptoms

Tinea versicolor typically produces raised or macular, round or oval, slightly scaly lesions on the upper trunk, which may extend to the lower abdomen, neck, arms, and rarely, the face. These lesions are usually tawny but may range from hypopigmented (white) patches in dark-skinned patients to hyperpigmented (brown) patches in fair-skinned patients. Some areas don't tan when exposed to sunlight, causing the cosmetic defect for which most persons seek medical help. Inflammation, burning, and itching are possible but usually absent.

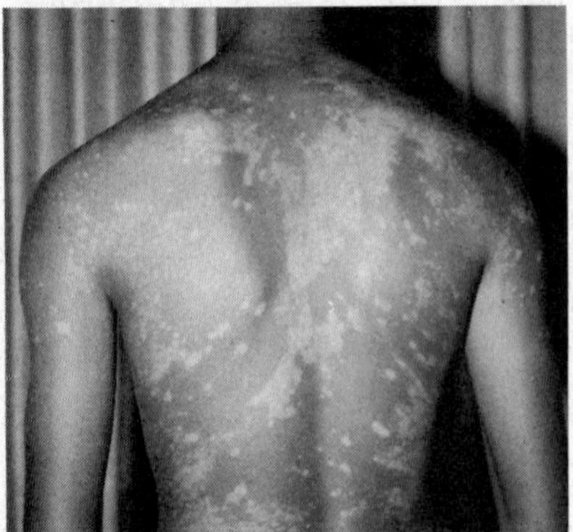

In dark-skinned patients, tinea versicolor causes hypopigmented areas (white patches) that fail to tan.

Diagnosis

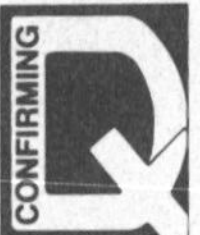

Visualization of lesions during Wood's light examination strongly suggests tinea versicolor; microscopic examination of skin scrapings prepared in potassium hydroxide solution confirms it by showing hyphae and clusters of yeast.

Treatment

The most economical and effective treatment is selenium sulfide lotion 2.5% applied once a day for 7 days. It's left on the skin for 10 minutes, then rinsed off thoroughly. In persistent cases, therapy may require a single 12-hour application of this lotion followed by weekly cleansing with an antifungal soap (3% sulfur and 20% salicylic acid). Either treatment may cause temporary redness and irritation.

More expensive treatments include topical antifungals, such as tolnaftate, applied twice daily for a month; and oral antifungals, such as griseofulvin and ketoconazole.

Special considerations

- Instruct the patient to apply selenium sulfide lotion, as ordered.
- Assure the patient that once his fungal infection is cured, discolored areas will gradually blend in after exposure to the sun or ultraviolet light.
- Since recurrence of tinea versicolor is common, advise the patient to watch for new areas of discoloration.

Dermatophytosis

(Ringworm)

Dermatophytosis may affect the scalp (tinea capitis), body (tinea corporis), nails (tinea unguium), feet (tinea pedis), groin (tinea cruris), and bearded skin (tinea barbae). Tinea infections are quite prevalent in the United States and are usually more common in males than in females. With effective treatment, the cure rate is very high, although about 20% of infected persons develop chronic conditions.

Causes

Tinea infections (except for tinea versicolor) result from dermatophytes (fungi) of the genera *Trichophyton, Microsporum,* and *Epidermophyton.*

Transmission can occur directly (through contact with infected lesions) or indirectly (through contact with contaminated articles, such as shoes, towels, or shower stalls).

Signs and symptoms

Lesions vary in appearance and duration. *Tinea capitis,* which mainly affects children, is characterized by small, spreading papules on the scalp, causing patchy hair loss with scaling. These papules may progress to inflamed, pus-filled lesions (kerions).

Tinea corporis produces flat lesions on the skin at any site except the scalp, bearded skin, or feet. These lesions may be dry and scaly or moist and crusty; as they enlarge, their centers heal, causing the classic ring-shaped appearance. In *tinea unguium* (onychomycosis), infection typically starts at the tip of one or more toenails (fingernail infection is less common) and produces gradual thickening, discoloration, and crumbling of the nail, with accumulation of subungual debris. Eventually, the nail may be destroyed completely.

Tinea pedis causes scaling and blisters between the toes. Severe infection may result in inflammation, with severe itching and pain on walking. A dry, squamous inflammation may affect the entire sole. *Tinea cruris* (jock itch) produces red, raised, sharply defined, itchy lesions in the groin that may extend to the buttocks, inner thighs, and the external genitalia. Warm weather and tight clothing encourage fungus growth. *Tinea barbae* is an uncommon infection that affects the bearded facial area of men.

Diagnosis

Microscopic examination of lesion scrapings prepared in potassium hydroxide solution usually confirms tinea infection. Other diagnostic procedures include Wood's light examination for some types of tinea capitis, and culture of the infecting organism; however, culturing may delay treatment.

Treatment

Tinea infections usually respond to treatment with griseofulvin P.O., which is especially effective in tinea infections of the skin, hair, and nails; tinea pedis requires concomitant use of a topical agent. (Griseofulvin is contraindicated in the patient with porphyria; it may also necessitate an increase in dosage during anticoagulant [warfarin] therapy.) Topical application of antifungals, such as clotrimazole, miconazole, haloprogin, or tolnaftate for localized infections, is also effective. Supportive measures include open wet dressings, removal of scabs and scales, and application of keratolytics, such as salicylic acid, to soften and remove hyperkeratotic lesions of the heels or soles.

Special considerations

Management of tinea infections requires application of topical agents, observation for sensitivity reactions, observation for secondary bacterial infections, and patient teaching.

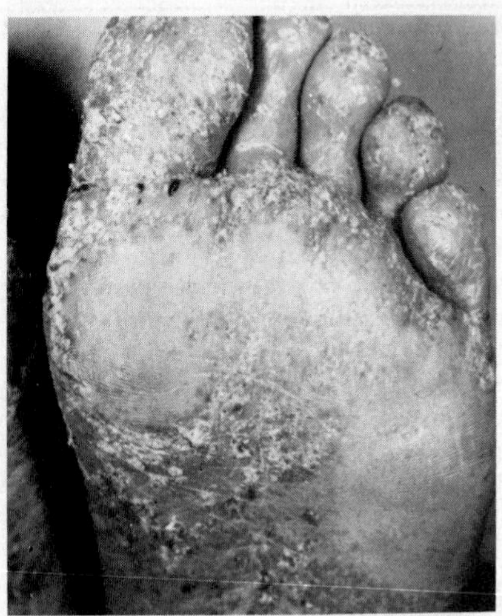

Dermatophytosis of the feet (tinea pedis) is popularly called athlete's foot. This infection causes macerated, scaling lesions, which may spread from the interdigital spaces to the sole. Diagnosis must rule out other possible causes of signs and symptoms; for example, eczema, psoriasis, contact dermatitis, and maceration by tight, ill-fitting shoes.

Specific care varies by site of infection:

- For tinea capitis: Keep topical medications away from the patient's eyes. Discontinue medications if condition worsens, and notify doctor. Use good hand-washing technique, and teach the patient to do the same. To prevent spread of infection to others, advise him to wash his towels, bedclothes, and combs frequently in hot water, and to avoid sharing them. Suggest that family members be checked for tinea capitis.
- For tinea corporis: Use abdominal pads between skin folds for the patient with excessive abdominal girth; change pads frequently. Check the patient daily for excoriated, newly denuded areas of skin. Apply open wet dressings two or three times daily to decrease inflammation and help remove scales.
- For tinea unguium: Keep nails short and straight. Gently remove debris under the nails with an emery board. Prepare the patient for prolonged therapy and possible side effects of griseofulvin, such as headache, nausea, vomiting, and photosensitivity.
- For tinea pedis: Encourage the patient to expose his feet to air whenever possible, and to wear sandals or leather shoes and clean cotton socks. Instruct the patient to wash his feet twice daily and, after drying them thoroughly, to evenly apply an antifungal powder to absorb perspiration and prevent excoriation. In severe infection, it may be necessary for the patient to disinfect his socks in boiling water.
- For tinea cruris: Instruct the patient to dry the affected area thoroughly after bathing and to evenly apply antifungal powder. Advise him to wear loose-fitting clothing, which should be changed frequently and laundered in hot water. Suggest sitz baths to relieve itching.
- For tinea barbae: Suggest that the patient let his beard grow (whiskers may be trimmed with scissors, not a razor). If the patient insists that he must shave, advise him to use an electric razor instead of a blade.

PARASITIC INFESTATIONS

Scabies

An age-old skin infection, scabies results from infestation with Sarcoptes scabiei *var.* hominis *(itch mite), which provokes a sensitivity reaction. It occurs worldwide, is predisposed by overcrowding and poor hygiene, and can be endemic.*

Causes

Mites can live their entire life cycles in the skin of humans, causing chronic infection. The female mite burrows into the skin to lay her eggs, from which larvae emerge to copulate and then reburrow under the skin.

Transmission of scabies occurs through skin contact or venereally. The adult mite can survive without a human host for only 2 or 3 days.

Signs and symptoms

Typically, scabies causes itching, which intensifies at night. Characteristic lesions are usually excoriated and may appear as erythematous nodules. These threadlike lesions are approximately 3/8" long and generally occur between fingers, on flexor surfaces of the wrists, on elbows, in axillary folds, at the waistline, on nipples in females, and on genitalia in males. In infants, the burrows (lesions) may appear on the head and neck.

Intense scratching can lead to severe excoriation and secondary bacterial infection. Itching may become generalized secondary to sensitization.

Diagnosis

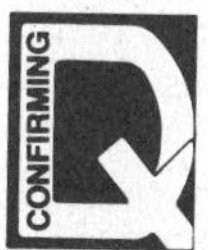

Visual examination of the contents of the scabietic burrow may reveal the itch mite. If not, a drop of mineral oil placed over the burrow, followed by superficial scraping and examination of expressed material under a low-power microscope, may reveal ova, or mite feces. However, excoriation or inflammation of the burrow often makes such identification difficult. If scabies is strongly suspected but diagnostic tests offer no positive identification of the mite, skin clearing with a therapeutic trial of a pediculicide confirms the diagnosis.

Treatment

Generally, treatment of scabies consists of bathing with soap and water, followed by application of a pediculicide. Lindane cream should be applied in a thin layer over the entire skin surface and left on for 8 to 12 hours. Because this cream is not ovicidal, this application must be repeated in 1 week. Another pediculicide, crotamiton cream, may be applied twice in 48 hours.

Approximately 10% of a pediculicide is absorbed systemically; therefore, a 6% to 10% solution of sulfur, which is less toxic, applied for 3 consecutive days is an alternative therapy for infants and pregnant females. Widespread bacterial infections require systemic antibiotics.

Persistent pruritus is usually due to mite sensitization or contact dermatitis, which may develop from repeated use of pediculicides rather than from continued infection. An antipruritic emollient or topical steroid can reduce itching; intralesional steroids may resolve erythematous nodules.

Special considerations

- Instruct the patient to apply lindane cream from the neck down, covering his entire body. (He may need assistance to reach all body areas.) Afterward, he must wait about 15 minutes before dressing and must avoid bathing for 24 hours. Contaminated clothing and linens must be washed or dry-cleaned.
- Tell the patient not to apply lindane cream if his skin is raw or inflamed. Advise him that if skin irritation or hypersensitivity reaction develops, he should notify the doctor immediately,

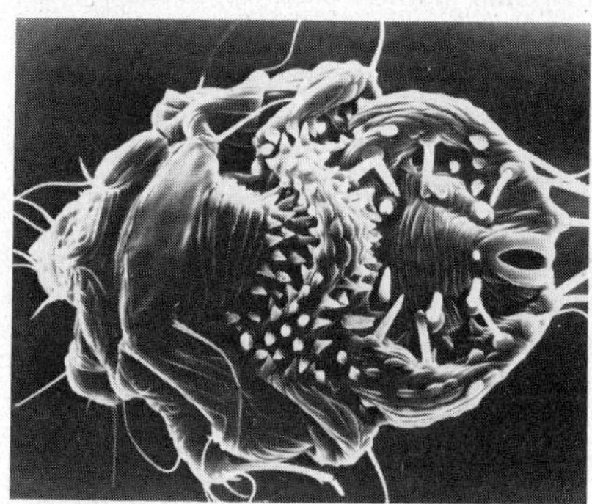

Sarcoptes scabiei—the itch mite—has a hard shell and measures a microscopic 0.1 mm.

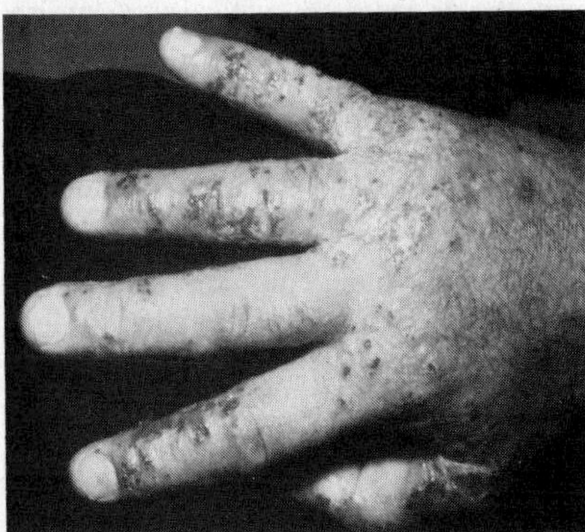
This photo of scabies lesions shows erythematous nodules with excoriation. These lesions are usually highly pruritic.

discontinue using the drug, and wash it off his skin thoroughly.
- Suggest that family members and other close personal contacts of the patient be checked for possible symptoms.
- If a hospitalized patient has scabies, prevent transmission to other patients: Practice good hand-washing technique or wear gloves when touching the patient; observe wound and skin precautions for 24 hours after treatment with a pediculicide; gas autoclave blood pressure cuffs before using them on other patients; isolate linens until the patient is noninfectious; and thoroughly disinfect the patient's room after discharge.

Cutaneous Larva Migrans

(Creeping eruption)

Cutaneous larva migrans is a skin reaction to infestation by nematodes (hookworms or roundworms) that usually infect dogs and cats. This parasitic infection most often affects persons who come in contact with infected soil or sand, such as children and farmers. Eruptions associated with cutaneous larva migrans clear completely with treatment.

Causes
Under favorable conditions—warmth, moisture, sandy soil—hookworm or roundworm ova present in feces of affected animals (such as dogs and cats) hatch into larvae, which can then burrow into human skin on contact. After penetrating its host, the larva becomes trapped under the skin, unable to reach the intestines to complete its normal life cycle.

Then the parasite begins to move around, producing the peculiar, tunnel-like lesions that are alternately meandering and linear, reflecting the nematode's persistent and unsuccessful attempts to escape its host.

Signs and symptoms
A transient rash or, possibly, a small vesicle appears at the point of penetration, usually on an exposed area that has come in contact with the ground, such as the feet, legs, or buttocks. The incubation period may be weeks or months, or the parasite may be active almost as soon as it enters the skin.

As the parasite migrates, it etches a noticeable thin, raised, red line on the skin, which may become vesicular and encrusted. Pruritus quickly develops, often with crusting and secondary infection following excoriation. The larva's apparently random path can cover from 1 mm to 1 cm a day. Penetration of more than one larva may involve a much larger area of the skin, marking it with many tracks.

Diagnosis
Characteristic migratory lesions strongly suggest cutaneous larva migrans. (See photograph of skin lesions on page 1213.) A thorough patient history usually reveals contact with warm, moist soil within the past several months.

Treatment
Cutaneous larva migrans infections may require administration of 50 mg/kg thiabendazole P.O. for 2 or 3 days. Tell the patient that side effects of systemic thiabendazole include nausea, vomiting, abdominal pain, and dizziness.

Special considerations
Prevention requires patient teaching about the existence of these parasites, sanitation of beaches and sandboxes, and proper pet care.

Give reassurance that larva migrans lesions usually clear 1 to 2 weeks after treatment, especially if the patient is sensitive about his appearance. Stress the importance of adhering to the treatment regimen exactly as ordered.

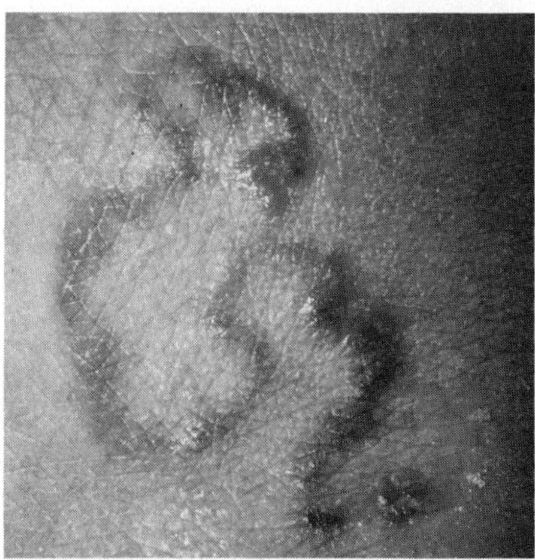
In cutaneous larva migrans, as the parasite migrates, it etches a noticeable red line on the skin. These lesions are thin, raised, and alternately meandering and linear.

Pediculosis

Pediculosis is caused by parasitic forms of lice: Pediculus humanus *var.* capitis *causes pediculosis capitis (head lice);* Pediculus humanus *var.* corporis *causes pediculosis corporis (body lice); and* Phthirus pubis *causes pediculosis pubis (crab lice). These lice feed on human blood and lay their eggs (nits) in body hairs or clothing fibers. After the nits hatch, the lice must feed within 24 hours or die; they mature in about 2 to 3 weeks. When a louse bites, it injects a toxin into the skin that produces mild irritation and a purpuric spot. Repeated bites cause sensitization to the toxin, leading to more serious inflammation. Treatment can effectively eliminate lice.*

Causes and incidence
P. humanus var. *capitis* (most common species) feeds on the scalp and, rarely, in the eyebrows, eyelashes, and beard. This form of pediculosis is caused by overcrowded conditions and poor personal hygiene, and commonly affects children, especially girls. It spreads through shared clothing, hats, combs, and hairbrushes.

P. humanus var. *corporis* lives in the seams of clothing, next to the skin, leaving only to feed on blood. Common causes include prolonged wearing of the same clothing (which might occur in cold climates), overcrowding, and poor personal hygiene. It spreads through shared clothing and bedsheets.

P. pubis is primarily found in pubic

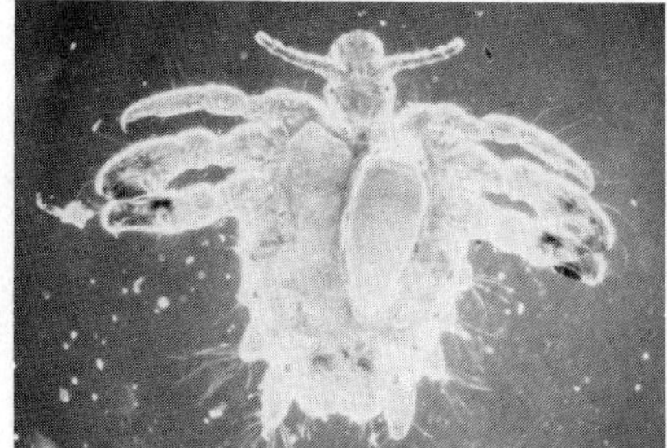
Phthirus pubis (pubic or "crab" louse) is slightly translucent; its first set of legs is shorter than its second and third.

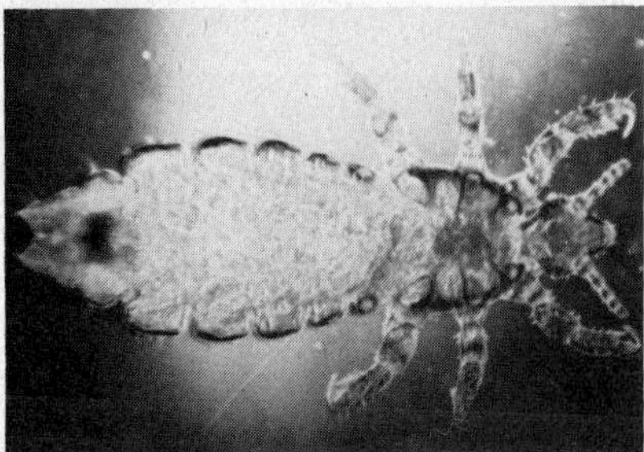

Pediculus humanus var. *corporis* (body louse) has a long abdomen, and all its legs are approximately the same length.

hairs, but this species may extend to the eyebrows, eyelashes, and axillary or body hair. Pediculosis pubis is transmitted through sexual intercourse or by contact with clothes, bedsheets, or towels harboring lice.

Signs and symptoms

Clinical features of pediculosis capitis include itching; excoriation (with severe itching); matted, foul-smelling, lusterless hair (in severe cases); occipital and cervical lymphadenopathy; and a rash on the trunk, probably due to sensitization. Adult lice migrate from the scalp and deposit oval, gray-white nits on hair shafts.

Pediculosis corporis initially produces small red papules (usually on the shoulders, trunk, or buttocks), which change to urticaria from scratching. Later, rashes or wheals (probably a sensitivity reaction) may develop. Untreated pediculosis corporis may lead to dry, discolored, thickly encrusted, scaly skin, with bacterial infection and scarring. In severe cases, headache, fever, and malaise may accompany cutaneous symptoms.

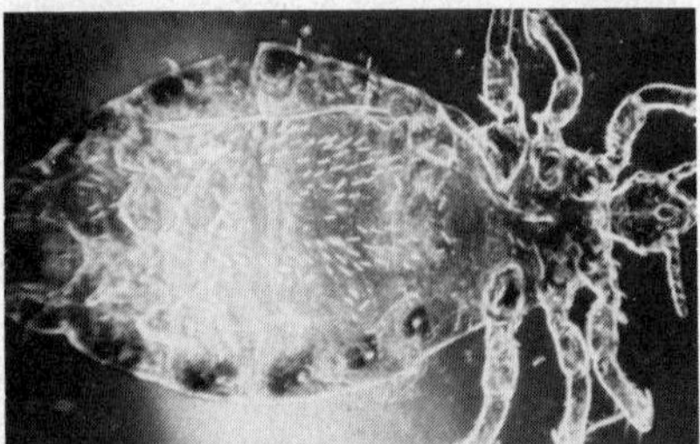

Pediculus humanus var. *capitis* (head louse) is similar in appearance to *P. humanus* var. *corporis*.

Pediculosis pubis causes skin irritation from scratching, which is usually more obvious than the bites. Small gray-blue spots (maculae caeruleae) may appear on the thighs or upper body.

Diagnosis

Pediculosis is visible on physical examination:

- *in pediculosis capitis:* oval, grayish nits that can't be shaken loose like dandruff (the closer the nits are to the end of the hair shaft, the longer the infection has been present, since the ova are laid close to the scalp)
- *in pediculosis corporis:* characteristic skin lesions; nits found on clothing
- *in pediculosis pubis:* nits attached to pubic hairs, which feel coarse and grainy to the touch.

Treatment

For pediculosis capitis, treatment consists of lindane cream rubbed into the scalp at night, then rinsed out in the morning with lindane shampoo (this treatment should be repeated the following night). A fine-tooth comb dipped in vinegar removes nits from hair; washing hair with ordinary shampoo removes crustations.

Pediculosis corporis requires bathing with soap and water to remove lice from the body; in severe infestation, treatment with lindane may be necessary. Lice may be removed from clothes by washing, ironing, or dry-cleaning. Storing clothes for more than 30 days or placing them in dry heat of 140° F. (60° C.) kills lice. If clothes can't be washed or changed, application of 10% DDT or 10% lindane powder is effective.

Treatment of pediculosis pubis includes application of lindane cream or lotion (which is then left on for 24 hours), or shampooing with lindane shampoo. Treatment should be repeated in 1 week. Clothes and bedsheets must be laundered to prevent reinfestation.

Special considerations

- Instruct patients how to use the creams, ointments, powders, and shampoos that can eliminate lice. To prevent self-infestation, avoid prolonged contact with the patient's hair, clothing, and bedsheets.
- Ask the patient with pediculosis pubis for a history of recent sexual contacts, so that they can be examined and treated.
- To prevent the spread of pediculosis to other hospitalized persons, examine all high-risk patients on admission, especially the elderly who depend on others for care, those admitted from nursing homes, or persons living in crowded conditions.

FOLLICULAR & GLANDULAR DISORDERS

Acne Vulgaris

An inflammatory disease of the sebaceous follicles, acne vulgaris primarily affects adolescents, although lesions can appear as early as age 8. Although acne strikes boys more often and more severely, it usually occurs in girls at an earlier age and tends to affect them for a longer period, sometimes into adulthood. Prognosis is good with treatment.

Causes

The cause of acne is unknown, but theories regarding dietary influences (including the nearly universally held "chocolate causes acne" theory) appear to be groundless. Research now centers on hormonal dysfunction and oversecretion of sebum as possible primary causes.

Predisposing factors include the use of oral contraceptives (many females experience an acne flare-up during their first few menstrual cycles on oral contraceptives or after they stop using them); certain medications, including corticosteroids, adrenocorticotropic hormone, androgens, iodides, bromides, trimethadione, phenytoin, isoniazid, lithium, and halothane; cobalt irradiation; or hyperalimentation therapy. Other predisposing factors are exposure to heavy oils, greases, or tars; trauma or rubbing from tight clothing; cosmetics; emotional stress; or unfavorable climate.

More is known about the pathogenesis of acne. Androgens stimulate sebaceous gland growth and production of sebum, which is secreted into dilated hair follicles that contain bacteria. The bacteria, usually *Propionibacterium acnes* and *Staphylococcus epidermidis*—which are normal skin flora—secrete lipase. This enzyme interacts with sebum to produce free fatty acids, which provoke inflammation. Also the hair follicles produce more keratin, which joins with the sebum to form a plug in the dilated follicle.

Signs and symptoms

The acne plug may appear as a closed comedo, or whitehead (if it doesn't protrude from the follicle and is covered by the epidermis), or as an open comedo, or blackhead (if it does protrude and isn't covered by the epidermis). The black coloration is caused by the melanin or pigment of the follicle. Rupture or leakage of an enlarged plug into the dermis produces inflammation and characteristic acne pustules, papules, or, in severe forms, acne cysts or abscesses. Chronic, recurring lesions produce acne scars.

Diagnosis

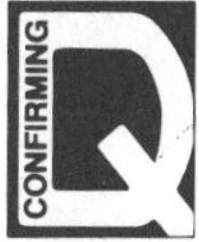

The appearance of characteristic acne lesions, especially in an adolescent patient, confirms the presence of acne vulgaris.

Treatment

Common therapy for severe acne includes benzoyl peroxide, a powerful antibacterial, alone or in combination with tretinoin, a keratolytic (retinoic acid or topical vitamin A); both agents may irritate the skin. Topical antibiotics, such as tetracycline, erythromycin, and clindamycin, may prove helpful in reducing the effects of acne.

Systemic therapy consists primarily of antibiotics, usually tetracycline, to decrease bacterial growth until the patient is in remission; then a lower dosage is used for long-term maintenance. Tetracycline is contraindicated during pregnancy because it discolors the teeth of the fetus. Erythromycin is an alternate for these patients. Exacerbation of pustules or abscesses during either type of antibiotic therapy requires a culture to identify a possible secondary bacterial infection.

Oral isotretinoin (Accutane), a newer treatment, combats acne by inhibiting sebaceous gland function and keratinization. But because of its severe side effects, the 16- to 20-week course of isotretinoin is limited to those with severe papulopustular or cystic acne who don't respond to conventional therapy. Women of childbearing age should not take isotretinoin unless they use contraceptives, because birth defects can occur.

Females with particularly stubborn acne may benefit from the administration of estrogens to inhibit androgen activity. However, this method of treatment is usually a last resort, since improvement rarely occurs before 2 to 4 months and exacerbations may follow its discontinuation.

Other treatments for acne vulgaris include intralesional corticosteroid injections, exposure to ultraviolet light (but never when a photosensitizing agent, such as tretinoin, is being used), cryotherapy, or surgery.

Special considerations

For those with acne, the main focus of your care is on patient teaching about the disorder as well as its treatment and prevention.

- Check the patient's drug history, since certain medications, such as oral contraceptives, may cause an acne flare-up.
- Try to identify predisposing factors which may be eliminated or modified, such as emotional stress.
- Explain the causes of acne to the patient and family. Make sure they understand the prescribed treatment is more likely to improve acne than a strict diet and fanatic scrubbing with soap and water. In fact, overzealous washing can worsen the lesions. Provide written instructions regarding treatment.
- Instruct the patient receiving tretinoin to apply it at least 30 minutes after washing the face and at least 1 hour before bedtime. Warn against using this medication around the eyes or lips. After treatments, the skin should look pink and dry. If it appears red or starts to peel, the preparation may have to be weakened or applied less often. Advise the patient to avoid exposure to sunlight or to use a sunscreening agent. If the prescribed regimen includes tretinoin and benzoyl peroxide, avoid skin irritation by using one preparation in the morning and the other at night.
- Instruct the patient to take tetracycline on an empty stomach and not to take it along with antacids or milk since it interacts with their metallic ions and is poorly absorbed.
- If the patient is taking isotretinoin, tell him to avoid vitamin A supplements, which can worsen any side effects. Also teach him how to deal with the dry skin and mucous membranes that usually occur during treatment.
- Inform the patient that acne takes a long time to clear—even years for complete resolution. Encourage him to continue local skin care even after acne clears. Explain the side effects of all medications.
- Pay special attention to the patient's perception of his physical appearance, and offer emotional support.

Hirsutism

A distressing disorder usually found in women and children, hirsutism is the excessive growth of body hair, typically in an adult male distribution pattern. This condition commonly occurs spontaneously but may also develop as a secondary disorder of various underlying diseases. It must always be distinguished from hypertrichosis. Prognosis varies with the cause and the effectiveness of treatment.

Causes

Idiopathic hirsutism probably stems from a hereditary trait, since the patient usually has a family history of the disorder. Causes of secondary hirsutism include endocrine abnormalities related to pituitary dysfunction (acromegaly, precocious puberty), adrenal dysfunction (Cushing's disease, congenital adrenal hyperplasia, or Cushing's syndrome), and ovarian lesions (such as polycystic ovary syndrome); and iatrogenic factors (such as use of minoxidil, androgen steroids, or testosterone).

Signs and symptoms

Hirsutism typically produces enlarged hair follicles as well as enlargement and hyperpigmentation of the hairs themselves. Excessive facial hair growth is the complaint for which most patients seek medical help. The pattern of hirsutism varies widely, depending on the patient's race and age. An elderly woman, for example, commonly shows increased hair growth on the chin and upper lip. In secondary hirsutism, signs of masculinization may appear—deepening of the voice, increased muscle mass, increased size of genitalia, menstrual irregularity, and decreased breast size.

Diagnosis

Family history of hirsutism, absence of menstrual abnormalities or signs of masculinization, and a normal pelvic examination strongly suggest idiopathic hirsutism. Tests for secondary hirsutism depend on associated symptoms that suggest an underlying disorder.

Treatment

At the patient's request, treatment of idiopathic hirsutism consists of eliminating excess hair by scissors, shaving, depilatory creams, or removal of the entire hair shaft with tweezers or wax. Bleaching with hydrogen peroxide may also be satisfactory. Electrolysis, a slow and expensive process, can destroy hair bulbs permanently, but it works best when only a few hairs need to be removed. (A history of keloid formation contraindicates this procedure.) Hirsutism due to elevated androgen levels may require low dose dexamethasone, oral

HYPERTRICHOSIS

Hypertrichosis is a localized or generalized condition in males and females that is marked by excessive hair growth. Localized hypertrichosis usually results from local trauma, chemical irritation, or hormonal stimulation; pigmented nevi (Becker's nevus, for example) may also contain hairs. Generalized hypertrichosis results from neurologic or psychiatric disorders, such as encephalitis, multiple sclerosis, concussion, anorexia nervosa, or schizophrenia; contributing factors include juvenile hypothyroidism, porphyria cutanea tarda, and the use of drugs such as phenytoin.

Hypertrichosis lanuginosa is a generalized proliferation of fine, lanugo-type hair (sometimes called down, or woolly hair). Such hair may be present at birth but generally disappears shortly thereafter. This condition may become chronic, with persistent lanugo-type hair growing over the entire body, or may develop suddenly later in life; it is very rare and usually results from malignancy.

contraceptives, or antiandrogens. They vary in effectiveness.

Treatment of secondary hirsutism varies depending on the nature of the underlying disorder.

Special considerations

Care for patients with idiopathic hirsutism focuses on emotional support and patient teaching; care for patients with secondary hirsutism depends on the treatment of the underlying disease.

- Provide emotional support by being sensitive to the patient's feelings about her appearance.
- Watch for signs of contact dermatitis in patients being treated with depilatory creams, especially the elderly. Also, watch for infection of hair follicles after hair removal with tweezers or wax.
- Suggest consulting a cosmetologist about makeup or bleaching agents.

Alopecia

Alopecia, or hair loss, usually occurs on the scalp; hair loss elsewhere on the body is less common and less conspicuous. In the nonscarring form of this disorder (noncicatricial alopecia), the hair follicle can generally regrow hair. But scarring alopecia usually destroys the hair follicle, making hair loss irreversible.

Causes and incidence

The most common form of nonscarring alopecia is male-pattern alopecia, which appears to be related to androgen levels and to aging. Genetic predisposition commonly influences time of onset, degree of baldness, speed with which it spreads, and pattern of hair loss. Male-pattern alopecia may also occur in women, but it's rarely severe.

Other forms of nonscarring alopecia include:

- *physiologic alopecia* (usually temporary): sudden hair loss in infants, loss of straight hairline in adolescents, and diffuse hair loss after childbirth
- *alopecia areata* (idiopathic form): generally reversible and self-limiting; occurs most frequently in young and middle-aged adults of both sexes
- *trichotillomania:* compulsive pulling out of one's own hair; most common in children.

Predisposing factors of nonscarring alopecia also include radiation, many types of drug therapies and drug reactions, bacterial and fungal infections, psoriasis, seborrhea, and endocrine disorders, such as thyroid, parathyroid, and pituitary dysfunctions.

Scarring alopecia causes irreversible hair loss. It may result from physical or chemical trauma or chronic tension on a hair shaft, such as braiding or rolling the hair. Diseases that produce alopecia include destructive skin tumors, granulomas, lupus erythematosus, scleroderma, follicular lichen planus, and severe bacterial or viral infections, such as folliculitis or herpes simplex.

Signs and symptoms

In male-pattern alopecia, hair loss is gradual and usually affects the thinner, shorter, and less pigmented hairs of the frontal and parietal portions of the scalp. In women, hair loss is generally more diffuse; completely bald areas are uncommon but may occur.

Alopecia areata affects small patches of the scalp but may also occur as alopecia totalis, which involves the entire scalp, or as alopecia universalis, which involves the entire body. Although mild erythema may occur initially, affected areas of scalp or skin appear normal. "Exclamation point" hairs (loose hairs with dark, rough, brushlike tips on narrow, less pigmented shafts) occur at the periphery of new patches. Regrowth initially appears as fine, white, downy hair, which is replaced by normal hair.

In trichotillomania, patchy, incomplete areas of hair loss with many broken hairs appear on the scalp but may occur on other areas, such as the eyebrows.

Diagnosis

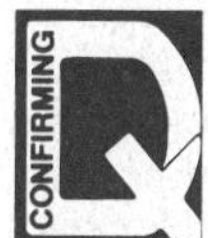

Physical examination is usually sufficient to confirm alopecia. In trichotillomania, an occlusive dressing can establish diagnosis by allowing new hair to grow, revealing that the hair is being pulled out. Diagnosis must also identify any underlying disorder.

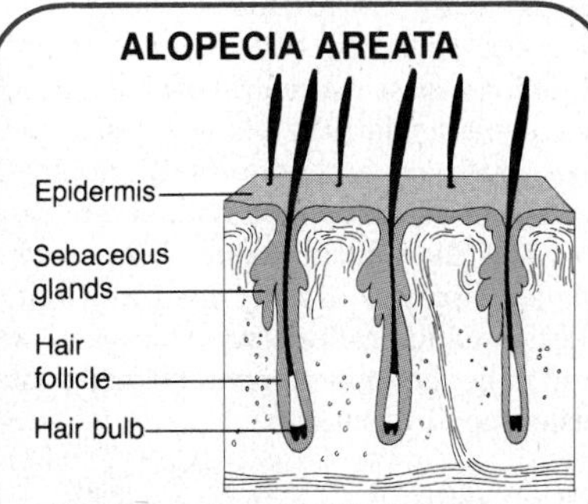

"Exclamation point" hairs often border new patches of alopecia areata. Not seen in any other type of alopecia, these hairs indicate the patch is expanding.

Treatment

Topical application of minoxidil, a peripheral vasodilator more typically used as an oral antihypertensive, has limited success in treating male-pattern alopecia. An alternate treatment is surgical redistribution of hair follicles by autografting.

In alopecia areata, minoxidil is more effective, although treatment is often unnecessary, as spontaneous regrowth is common. Intralesional corticosteroid injections are beneficial for small patches and may produce regrowth in 4 to 6 weeks. In trichotillomania, an occlusive dressing encourages normal hair growth, simply by identifying the cause of hair loss. Treatment of other types of alopecia varies according to the underlying cause.

Special considerations

- Reassure a woman with male-pattern alopecia that it doesn't lead to total baldness. Suggest wearing a wig.
- If the patient has alopecia areata, explain the disorder and give reassurance that complete regrowth is possible.

Rosacea

A chronic skin eruption, rosacea produces flushing and dilation of the small blood vessels in the face, especially the nose and cheeks. Papules and pustules may also occur but without the characteristic comedones of acne vulgaris. Rosacea is most common in white women between ages 30 and 50. When it occurs in men, however, it's usually more severe and often associated with rhinophyma, which is characterized by dilated follicles and thickened, bulbous skin on the nose. Ocular involvement may result in blepharitis, conjunctivitis, uveitis, or keratitis. Rosacea usually spreads slowly and rarely subsides spontaneously.

Causes

Although the cause of rosacea is unknown, stress, infection, vitamin deficiency, and endocrine abnormalities can aggravate this condition. Anything that produces flushing—for example, hot beverages, such as tea or coffee; tobacco; alcohol; spicy foods; physical activity; sunlight; and extreme heat or cold—can also aggravate rosacea.

Signs and symptoms
Rosacea generally begins with periodic flushing across the central oval of the face, accompanied later by telangiectasias, papules, pustules, and nodules. Rhinophyma is commonly associated with severe rosacea but may occur alone. Rhinophyma usually appears first on the lower half of the nose, and produces red, thickened skin and follicular enlargement. Related ocular lesions are uncommon.

Diagnosis

Typical vascular and acneiform lesions—without the comedones characteristically associated with acne vulgaris—and rhinophyma in severe cases confirm rosacea.

Treatment and special considerations
Treatment of the acneiform component of rosacea consists of tetracycline P.O. in gradually decreasing doses as symptoms subside. Topical application of hydrocortisone ointment reduces erythema and inflammation. Other treatment may include electrolysis to destroy large, dilated blood vessels, and removal of excess tissue in patients with rhinophyma.
• Instruct the patient to avoid hot beverages, alcohol, and other possible causes of flushing.
• Assess the effect of rosacea on body image. Since it's always apparent on the face, your support and reassurance are essential.

DISORDERS OF PIGMENTATION

Vitiligo

Marked by stark-white skin patches that may cause a serious cosmetic problem, vitiligo results from the destruction and loss of pigment cells. This condition affects about 1% of the U.S. population, usually persons between ages 10 and 30, with peak incidence around age 20. It shows no racial preference, but the distinctive patches are most prominent in Blacks. Vitiligo doesn't favor one sex; however, women tend to seek treatment more often than men. Repigmentation therapy, which is widely used in treating vitiligo, may necessitate several summers of exposure to sunlight; the effects of this treatment may not be permanent.

Causes
Although the cause of vitiligo is unknown, inheritance seems a definite etiologic factor, since about 30% of patients with vitiligo have family members with the same condition. Other theories implicate enzymatic self-destructing mechanisms, autoimmune mechanisms, and abnormal neurogenic stimuli.

Some link exists between vitiligo and several other disorders that it often accompanies—thyroid dysfunction, pernicious anemia, Addison's disease, aseptic meningitis, diabetes mellitus, photophobia, hearing defects, alopecia areata, and halo nevi.

The most frequently reported precipitating factor is a stressful physical or psychologic event—severe sunburn, surgery, pregnancy, loss of job, bereavement, or some other source of distress. Chemical agents, such as phenols and catechols, may also cause this condition.

Signs and symptoms
Vitiligo produces depigmented or stark-white patches on the skin; on fair-skinned Caucasians, these are almost imperceptible. Lesions are usually bilaterally symmetric with sharp borders, which, occasionally, are raised and hyperpigmented. These unique patches generally

appear over bony prominences, around orifices (eyes, mouth), within body folds, and at sites of trauma. The hair within these lesions may also turn white. Since hair follicles and certain parts of the eyes also contain pigment cells, vitiligo may be associated with premature gray hair and ocular pigmentary changes.

Diagnosis

Diagnosis requires accurate history of onset and of associated illnesses, family history, and observation of characteristic lesions. Other skin disorders, such as tinea versicolor, must be ruled out.

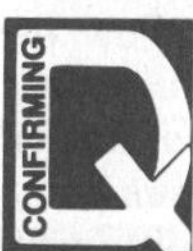

In fair-skinned patients, Wood's light examination in a darkened room detects vitiliginous patches; depigmented skin reflects the light, while pigmented skin absorbs it. If autoimmune or endocrine disturbances are suspected, laboratory studies (thyroid indexes, for example) are appropriate.

Treatment

Repigmentation therapy combines systemic and topical psoralen compounds (methoxsalen and trioxsalen) with exposure to sunlight or artificial ultraviolet light, wavelength A (UVA). New pigment rises from hair follicles and appears on the skin as small freckles, which gradually enlarge and coalesce. Body parts containing few hair follicles (such as the fingertips) may resist this therapy.

Since psoralens and UVA affect the entire skin surface, systemic therapy enhances the contrast between normal and vitiliginous skin. Therefore, white, vitiliginous areas are accented by normal skin, which tans darker than usual (use of sunscreen on normal skin may minimize the contrast, while also preventing sunburn).

Depigmentation therapy is suggested for patients with vitiligo affecting over 50% of the body surface. A cream containing 20% monobenzone permanently destroys pigment cells in unaffected areas of the skin and produces a uniform skin tone. This medication is applied initially to a small area of normal skin once daily to test for unfavorable reactions (contact dermatitis, for example). In the absence of adverse effects, the patient begins applying the cream twice daily to those areas he wishes to depigment first. *Note:* Depigmentation is permanent and results in extreme sensitivity to sunlight.

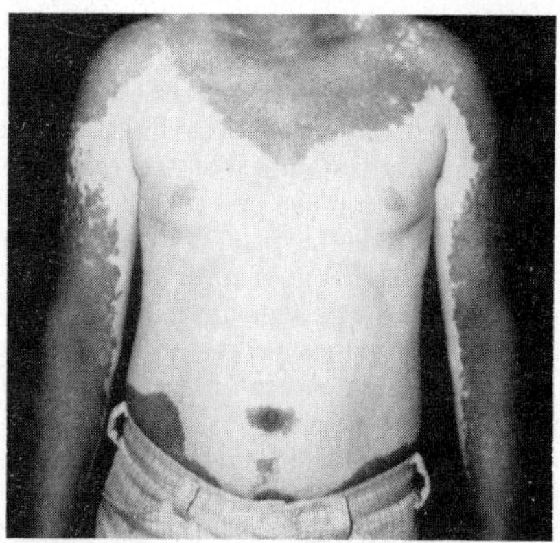

This photo shows characteristic depigmented skin patches in vitiligo. These patches are usually bilaterally symmetric, with distinct borders.

Commercial cosmetics may also help deemphasize vitiliginous skin. Some patients prefer dyes because these remain on the skin for several days, although the results are not always satisfactory. Although often impractical, complete avoidance of exposure to sunlight through the use of screening agents and protective clothing may minimize vitiliginous lesions in whites.

Special considerations

- Instruct the patient to use psoralen medications three or four times weekly. (*Note:* Systemic psoralens should be taken 2 hours before exposure to sun; topical solutions should be applied 30 to 60 minutes before exposure.) Warn him to use a sunscreen (SPF 8 to 10) to protect both affected and normal skin during exposure and to wear sunglasses after taking the medication. If periorbital areas require exposure, tell the patient to keep his eyes closed during treatment.
- Suggest that the patient receiving depigmentation therapy wear protective

clothing and use a sunscreen (SPF 15). Explain the therapy thoroughly, and allow the patient plenty of time to decide whether to undergo this treatment. Make sure he understands that the results of depigmentation are permanent and that he must thereafter protect his skin from the adverse effects of sunlight.

- Caution the patient about buying commercial cosmetics or dyes without trying them first, since some may not be suitable.
- For the child with vitiligo: Modify repigmentation therapy to avoid unnecessary restrictions. Tell parents to give the initial dose of psoralen medication at 1 p.m. and then let the child go out to play as usual. After this, medication should be given 30 minutes earlier each day of treatment, provided the child's skin doesn't turn more than slightly pink from exposure. If marked erythema develops, parents should discontinue treatment and notify the doctor. Eventually, the child should be able to take the medication at 9:30 a.m. and play outdoors the rest of the day without side effects. Tell the parents the child should wear clothing that permits maximum exposure of vitiliginous areas to the sun.
- Remind patients undergoing repigmentation therapy that exposure to sunlight also darkens normal skin. After being exposed to UVA for the prescribed amount of time, the patient should apply a sunscreen if he plans to be exposed to sunlight also. If sunburn occurs, advise the patient to discontinue therapy temporarily and to apply open wet dressings (using thin sheeting) to affected areas for 15 to 20 minutes, four or five times daily or as necessary for comfort. After application of wet dressings, allow the skin to air-dry. Suggest application of a soothing lubricating cream or lotion while the skin is still slightly moist.
- Reinforce patient teaching with written instructions.
- Be sensitive to the patient's emotional needs, but avoid promoting unrealistic hope for a total cure.

Melasma

(Chloasma, mask of pregnancy)

A patchy, hypermelanotic skin disorder, melasma poses a serious cosmetic problem. Although it tends to occur equally in all races, the light-brown color characteristic of melasma is most evident in dark-skinned whites. Melasma affects females more often than males; it may be chronic but is never life-threatening.

Causes

The cause of melasma is unknown. Histologically, hyperpigmentation results from increased melanin production, although the number of melanocytes remains normal. Melasma may be related to the increased hormonal levels associated with pregnancy, ovarian carcinoma, and the use of oral contraceptives. Progestational agents, phenytoin, and mephenytoin may also contribute to this disorder. Exposure to sunlight stimulates melasma, but it may develop without any apparent predisposing factor.

Signs and symptoms

Typically, melasma produces large, brown, irregular patches, symmetrically distributed on the forehead, cheeks, and sides of the nose. Less commonly, these patches may occur on the neck, upper lip, and temples.

Diagnosis

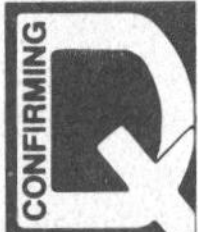

Observation of characteristic dark patches on the face usually confirms melasma. Patient history may reveal predisposing factors.

Treatment and special considerations

Treatment consists primarily of application of bleaching agents containing 2% to 4% hydroquinone, to inhibit melanin synthesis. This medication is applied twice daily for up to 8 weeks. Adjunctive measures include topical steroids, avoidance of sunlight, use of sunblockers, and discontinuation of oral contraceptives.

- Instruct the patient to avoid sunlight by using sunscreens and wearing protective clothing. Advise him that bleaching agents may achieve the desired effect but may require periodic treatments to maintain it. Cosmetics may help mask deep pigmentation.
- Reassure the patient that melasma is treatable. Serial photographs help show the patient that patches are improving.

Photosensitivity Reactions

A photosensitivity reaction is a skin eruption that can be a toxic or allergic response to light alone or light and chemicals. A phototoxic *reaction is a dose-related primary response. A* photoallergic *reaction is an uncommon, acquired immune response that isn't dose related—even slight exposure can cause a severe reaction.*

Causes

Certain chemicals can cause a photosensitivity reaction, including dyes, coal tar, furocoumarin compounds found in plants, and drugs such as phenothiazines, sulfonamide, sulfonylureas, tetracycline, griseofulvin, and thiazides. Berlock dermatitis, a specific photosensitivity reaction, results from use of oil of bergamot—a common component of perfumes, colognes, and pomades.

Signs and symptoms

Immediately after exposure, a phototoxic reaction causes a burning sensation followed by erythema, edema, desquamation, and hyperpigmentation. Berlock dermatitis produces an acute reaction with erythematous vesicles that later becomes hyperpigmented.

Photoallergic reactions may take one of two forms. Developing 2 hours to 5 days after light exposure, polymorphous light eruption (PMLE) produces erythema, papules, vesicles, urticaria, and eczematous lesions on exposed areas; pruritus may persist for 1 to 2 weeks. Solar urticaria begins minutes after exposure and lasts about an hour; erythema and wheals follow itching and burning sensations.

Diagnosis

Characteristic skin eruptions and patient history of recent exposure to light or certain chemicals suggest a photosensitivity reaction. A photopatch test for ultraviolet A and B (UVA and UVB) may aid diagnosis and identify the causative light wavelength. Other studies must rule out connective tissue disease, such as lupus erythematosus and porphyrias.

Treatment and special considerations

For many patients, treatment involves a sunscreen, protective clothing, and minimal exposure to sunlight. For others, progressive exposure to sunlight can thicken the skin and produce a tan that interferes with photoallergens and prevents further eruptions.

Antimalarial drugs, beta-carotene, and PUVA (psoralen and UVA) may be used to treat PMLE. Treatment for solar urticaria may also require PUVA. Although hyperpigmentation usually fades in several months, hydroquinone preparations can hasten the process. To prevent reactions, advise the patient to avoid prolonged exposure to light.

INFLAMMATORY REACTION

Dermatitis

Dermatitis, inflammation of the skin, occurs in several forms: atopic (discussed here), contact, chronic, seborrheic, nummular, exfoliative, and stasis dermatitises (discussed below). Atopic dermatitis (atopic or infantile eczema, neurodermatitis constitutionalis, Besnier's prurigo) is a chronic inflammatory response often associated with other atopic diseases, such as bronchial asthma, allergic rhinitis, and chronic urticaria. It usually develops in infants and toddlers between ages 1 month and 1 year, commonly in those with strong family histories of atopic disease. These children often acquire other atopic disorders as they grow older. Typically, this form of dermatitis subsides spontaneously by age 3 and stays in remission until prepuberty (ages 10 to 12), when it often flares up again.

Causes and incidence

Atopic dermatitis is the cutaneous manifestation of a delayed, cell-mediated allergic response (not a T cell disease, but related to IgE), resulting from the same allergens (pollen, wool, silk, fur, ointment, detergent, or perfume) that provoke other atopic diseases. Such allergens also include certain foods, particularly wheat, milk, and eggs. Atopic dermatitis tends to flare up in response to extremes in temperature and humidity. Other causes of flare-ups are sweating and psychologic stress.

In approximately 70% of patients with atopic dermatitis, positive skin tests and

DERMATITIS AND ECZEMA

TYPE	CAUSES	SIGNS AND SYMPTOMS
Seborrheic dermatitis 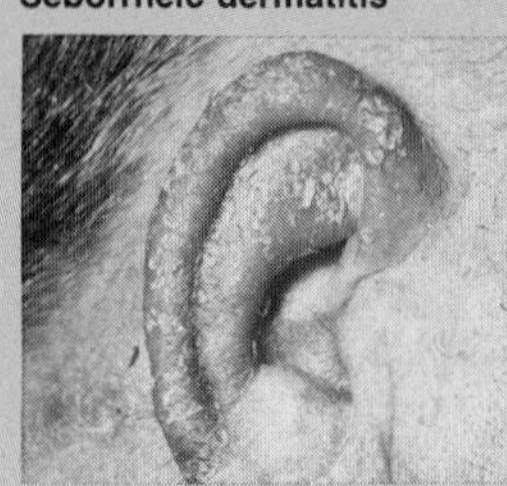	• Unknown; stress, and neurologic conditions may be predisposing factors	• Eruptions in areas with many sebaceous glands (usually scalp, face, and trunk) and in skin folds • Itching, redness, and inflammation of affected areas; lesions may appear greasy; fissures may occur • Indistinct, occasionally yellowish, scaly patches from excess stratum corneum (dandruff may be a mild seborrheic dermatitis)
Nummular dermatitis 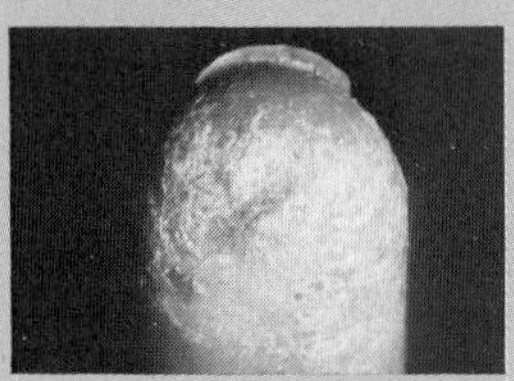	• Possibly precipitated by stress; or dryness, irritants, or scratching	• Round, nummular (coin-shaped) lesions, usually on arms and legs, with distinct borders of crusts and scales • Possible oozing and severe itching • Summertime remissions common, with wintertime recurrence

carefully controlled food elimination diets identify at least one allergen but rarely determine the primary cause.

An important secondary cause of atopic dermatitis is irritation, which seems to change the epidermal structure, allowing IgE activity to increase. Consequently, chronic skin irritation usually continues even after exposure to the allergen has ended or after the irritation has been systemically controlled.

Signs and symptoms

Atopic skin lesions generally begin as erythematous areas on excessively dry skin. In children, such lesions typically appear on the forehead, cheeks, and extensor surfaces of the arms and legs; in adults, at flexion points (antecubital fossa, popliteal area, and neck). During flare-ups, pruritus and scratching cause edema, vesiculation (sometimes vesicles are pus-filled), and scaling. Eventually, chronic atopic lesions lead to multiple areas of dry, scaly skin, with white dermatographia, blanching, and lichenification.

Common secondary conditions associated with atopic dermatitis include viral, fungal, or bacterial infections, and ocular disorders. Because of intense pruritus, the upper eyelid is commonly hyperpigmented and swollen, producing a double fold under the lower lid (Morgan's, Dennie's, or Mongolian fold). Atopic cataracts usually develop between ages 20 and 40. Kaposi's varicelliform eruption, a potentially fatal generalized viral infection, may develop if the patient with atopic dermatitis comes in contact with a person who has herpes simplex.

Diagnosis

Positive family history of allergy and chronic inflammation suggest atopic dermatitis. Typical distribution of skin lesions rules out other inflammatory skin lesions, such as diaper rash (lesions confined to the diapered area), seborrheic dermatitis (no pigmentation changes, or lichenification occurs in chronic lesions), and chronic contact dermatitis (lesions affect hands and forearms, sparing antecubital and popliteal areas). Serum IgE levels are elevated.

DIAGNOSIS	TREATMENT AND INTERVENTION
• Patient history and physical findings, especially distribution of lesions in sebaceous gland areas, confirm seborrheic dermatitis. • Diagnosis must rule out psoriasis.	• Removal of scales with frequent washing and shampooing with selenium sulfide suspension (most effective), zinc pyrithione, or tar and salicylic acid shampoo • Application of fluorinated steroids to nonhairy areas
• Physical findings and patient history confirm nummular dermatitis; a middle-aged or older patient may have a history of atopic dermatitis. • Diagnosis must rule out fungal infections, atopic or contact dermatitis, and psoriasis.	• Elimination of known irritants • Measures to relieve dry skin: increased humidification; limited frequency of baths and use of bland soap and bath oils; and application of emollients • Application of wet dressings in acute phase • Topical steroids (occlusive dressing or intralesional injections) for persistent lesions • Tar preparations and antihistamines to control itching • Antibiotics for secondary infection • Other intervention similar to atopic dermatitis

DERMATITIS AND ECZEMA (continued)

TYPE	CAUSES	SIGNS AND SYMPTOMS
Contact dermatitis 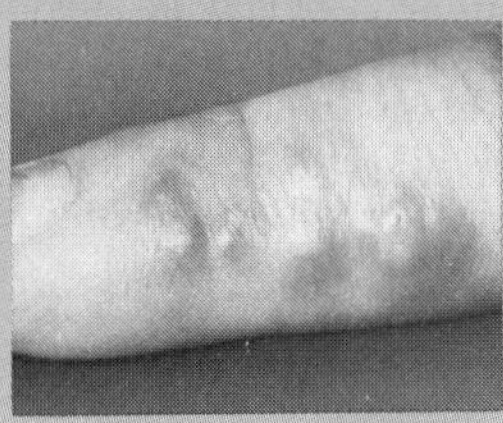	• Mild irritants: chronic exposure to detergents or solvents • Strong irritants: damage on contact with acids or alkalis • Allergens: sensitization after repeated exposure	• Mild irritants and allergens: erythema, and small vesicles that ooze, scale, and itch • Strong irritants: blisters and ulcerations • Classic allergic response: clearly defined lesions, with straight lines following points of contact • Severe allergic reaction: marked edema of affected areas
Chronic dermatitis 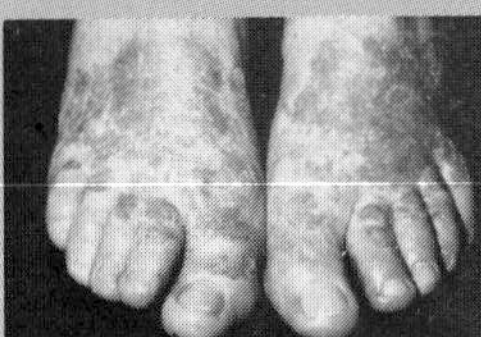	• Usually unknown but may result from progressive contact dermatitis • Secondary factors: trauma, infections, redistribution of normal flora, photosensitivity, and food sensitivity, which may perpetuate this condition	• Thick, lichenified, single or multiple lesions on any part of the body (often on the hands) • Inflammation and scaling • Recurrence follows long remissions.
Localized neurodermatitis (lichen simplex chronicus, essential pruritus) 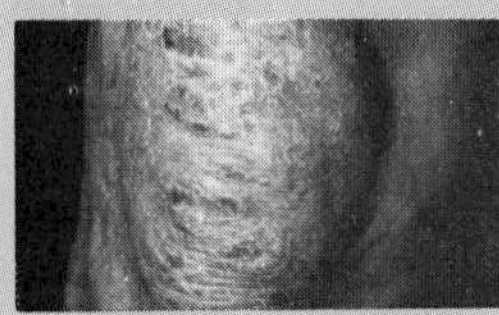	• Chronic scratching or rubbing of a primary lesion or insect bite, or other skin irritation	• Intense, sometimes continual scratching • Thick, sharp-bordered, possibly dry, scaly lesions, with raised papules • Usually affects easily reached areas, such as ankles, lower legs, anogenital area, back of neck, and ears
Exfoliative dermatitis 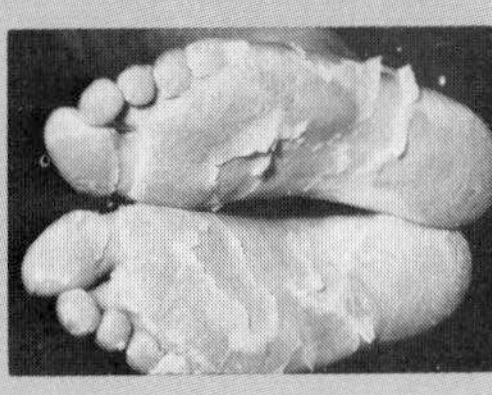	• Usually, preexisting skin lesions progress to exfoliative stage, such as in contact dermatitis, drug reaction, lymphoma, or leukemia.	• Generalized dermatitis, with acute loss of stratum corneum, and erythema and scaling • Sensation of tight skin • Hair loss • Possible fever, sensitivity to cold, shivering, gynecomastia, and lymphadenopathy
Stasis dermatitis 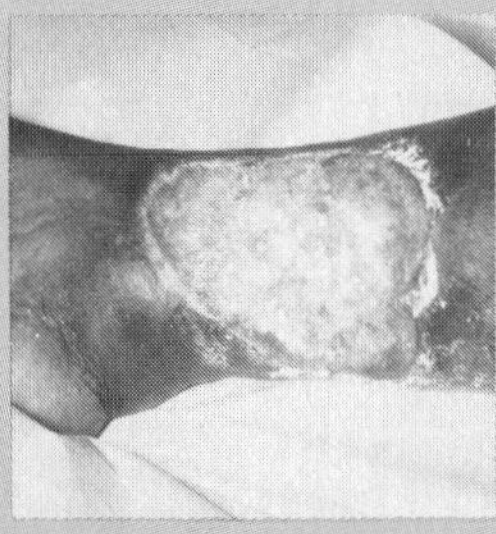	• Secondary to peripheral vascular diseases affecting legs, such as recurrent thrombophlebitis and resultant chronic venous insufficiency	• Varicosities and edema common, but obvious vascular insufficiency not always present • Usually affects the lower leg, just above internal malleolus, or sites of trauma or irritation • Early signs: dusky red deposits of hemosiderin in skin, with itching and dimpling of subcutaneous tissue. Later signs: edema, redness, and scaling of large area of legs • Fissures, crusts, and ulcers may develop

DIAGNOSIS	TREATMENT AND INTERVENTION
• Patient history • Patch testing to identify allergens • Shape and distribution of lesions suggest contact dermatitis.	• Elimination of known allergens and decreased exposure to irritants; wearing protective clothing, such as gloves; and washing immediately after contact with irritants or allergens • Topical anti-inflammatory agents (including steroids), systemic steroids for edema and bullae, antihistamines, and local applications of Burow's solution (for blisters) • Sensitization to topical medications may occur. • Other intervention similar to atopic dermatitis
• No characteristic pattern or course; diagnosis relies on detailed patient history and physical findings.	• Same as for contact dermatitis • Antibiotics for secondary infection • Avoidance of excessive washing and drying of hands, and of accumulation of soaps and detergents under rings • Use of emollients with topical steroids
• Physical findings confirm diagnosis.	• Lesions disappear about 2 weeks after scratching stops. • Fixed dressing or Unna's boot, to cover affected area • Steroids under occlusion or by intralesional injection • Antihistamines and open wet dressings • Emollients • Inform patient about underlying cause.
• Diagnosis requires identification of the underlying cause.	• Hospitalization, with protective isolation and hygienic measures to prevent secondary bacterial infection • Open wet dressings, with colloidal baths • Bland lotions over topical steroids • Maintenance of constant environmental temperature to prevent chilling or overheating • Careful monitoring of renal and cardiac status • Systemic antibiotics and steroids • Other intervention similar to atopic dermatitis
• Diagnosis requires positive history of venous insufficiency and physical findings, such as varicosities.	• Measures to prevent venous stasis: avoidance of prolonged sitting or standing, use of support stockings, and weight reduction in obesity • Corrective surgery for underlying cause • After ulcer develops, encourage rest periods, with legs elevated; open wet dressings; Unna's boot (zinc gelatin dressing provides continuous pressure to affected areas); antibiotics for secondary infection after wound culture.

Treatment and special considerations

Effective treatment of atopic lesions consists of eliminating allergens and avoiding irritants, extreme temperature changes, and other precipitating factors; local and systemic measures relieve itching and inflammation. Topical application of a corticosteroid cream, especially after bathing, often alleviates inflammation. Between steroid doses, application of petrolatum can help retain moisture. Systemic corticosteroid therapy should be used only during extreme exacerbations. Weak tar preparations and ultraviolet B light therapy are used to increase the thickness of the stratum corneum. Antibiotics are appropriate if a bacterial agent has been cultured.

- Warn that drowsiness is possible with the use of antihistamines to relieve daytime itching. If nocturnal itching interferes with sleep, suggest methods for inducing natural sleep, such as drinking a glass of warm milk, to prevent overuse of sedatives.
- Complement medical treatment by helping the patient set up an individual schedule and plan for daily skin care. Instruct the patient to limit bathing, according to the severity of the lesions. Tell him to bathe with a special nonfatty soap and tepid water but to avoid using any soap when lesions are acutely inflamed. Advise the patient to shampoo frequently and apply corticosteroid cream afterward, to keep his fingernails short to limit excoriation and secondary infections caused by scratching, and to lubricate his skin after a tub bath.
- To help clear lichenified skin, apply occlusive dressings (such as plastic film) intermittently, and secure them with nonallergenic tape.
- Inform the patient that irritants, such as detergents and wool, and emotional stress exacerbate atopic dermatitis.
- Be careful not to show any anxiety or revulsion when touching the lesions during treatment. Help the patient accept his altered body image, and encourage him to verbalize his feelings. Remember, coping with disfigurement is extremely difficult, especially for children and adolescents. Arrange for counseling, if necessary, to help the patient deal with the disease more effectively.

MISCELLANEOUS DISORDERS

Toxic Epidermal Necrolysis

(Scalded skin syndrome)

Toxic epidermal necrolysis (TEN) is a rare, severe skin disorder that causes epidermal erythema, superficial necrosis, and skin erosions. The skin appears to be scalded; hence the term scalded skin syndrome. Mortality is high (30%), especially among the debilitated and the elderly. Reepithelialization is slow, and residual scarring is common. TEN primarily affects adults.

Causes

The immediate cause of this disease is still obscure, but it may be a reaction to a toxin, an allergen, or both. TEN usually results from a drug reaction—most commonly to butazones, sulfonamides, penicillins, barbiturates, and hydantoins—but may be linked to other drugs as well. TEN may reflect an immune response or may be related to overwhelming physiologic stress, (coexisting sepsis, neoplastic diseases, and drug treatment). Airborne toxins, such as carbon monoxide, have also been linked to TEN.

Signs and symptoms

Early symptoms of TEN include inflammation of the mucous membranes, a burning sensation in the conjunctivae, malaise, fever, and generalized skin tenderness. After such prodromal symptoms, TEN erupts in three phases:

- diffuse, erythematous rash
- vesiculation and blistering
- large-scale epidermal necrolysis and desquamation.

Large, flaccid bullae that rupture easily expose extensive areas of denuded skin, permitting loss of tissue fluids and electrolytes, and widespread systemic involvement. Systemic complications may include bronchopneumonia, pulmonary edema, gastrointestinal and esophageal hemorrhage, shock, renal failure, sepsis, and disseminated intravascular coagulation; these conditions markedly increase the mortality.

Diagnosis

Diagnosis is based on clinical status at the peak stage of disease. Nikolsky's sign (skin sloughs off with slight friction) is present in erythematous areas. Culture and Gram's stain of lesions determine whether infection is present. Supportive findings include leukocytosis, elevated transaminase (SGOT and SGPT) levels, albuminuria, and fluid and electrolyte imbalances.

Exfoliative cytology and biopsy aid in ruling out erythema multiforme and exfoliative dermatitis.

Treatment and special considerations

Treatment consists of high-dose systemic corticosteroids and maintenance of fluid and electrolyte balance with I.V. fluid replacement. Frequent determinations of hemoglobin and hematocrit, electrolytes, serum proteins, and blood gases are necessary.

- Monitor vital signs, central venous pressure, and urinary output. Watch for signs of renal failure (decreased urinary output) and bleeding. Report temperature elevations immediately, and obtain blood cultures and sensitivity tests promptly, as ordered, to detect and treat septic infection.
- Prevent secondary infection. Protective isolation and prophylactic antibiotic therapy may be necessary.
- Maintain skin integrity as much as possible. Patient should not wear clothing and should be covered loosely to prevent friction and sloughing of skin. A turning frame is helpful.
- Administer analgesics, as needed. Applying cool, sterile compresses may relieve some discomfort.
- Provide frequent eye care to remove exudate. Ocular lesions are common.
- Provide emotional support for the patient and family.

Warts

(Verrucae)

Warts are common, benign, viral infections of the skin and adjacent mucous membranes. Although their incidence is highest in children and young adults, warts may occur at any age. Prognosis varies: some warts disappear readily with treatment; others necessitate more vigorous and prolonged treatment.

Causes

Warts are caused by infection with the human papillomavirus, a group of ether-resistant, DNA-containing papovaviruses. Mode of transmission is probably through direct contact, but autoinoculation is possible.

Signs and symptoms

Clinical manifestations depend on the

REMOVING WARTS BY ELECTROSURGERY

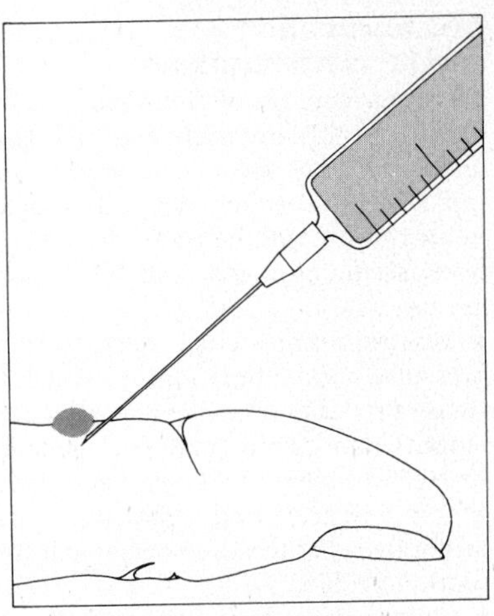

1. Injection of 1% to 2% lidocaine under and around the wart, avoiding wart itself

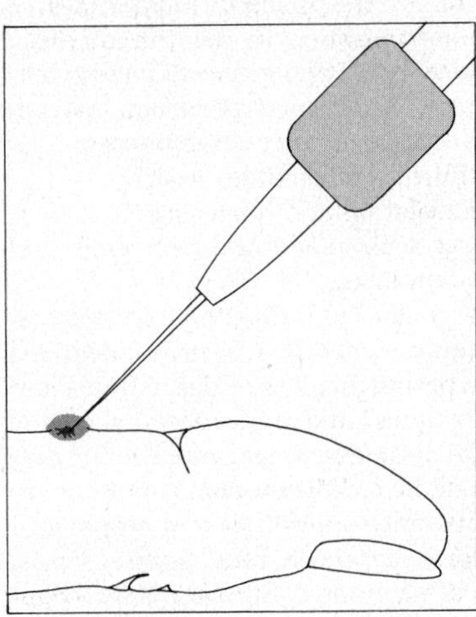

2. Desiccation of the wart

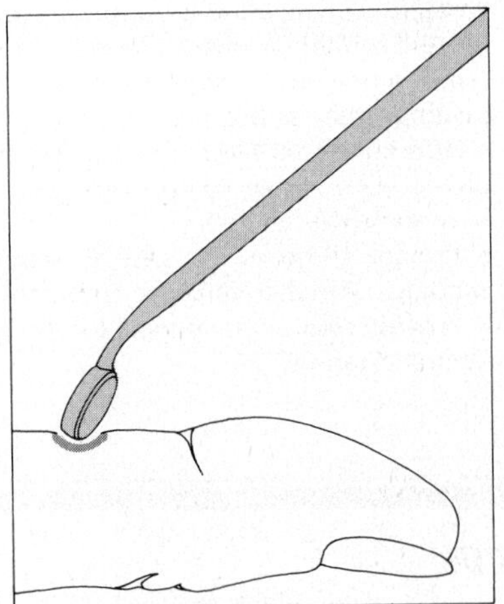

3. Removal of the wart tissue with a curette and small, curved scissors

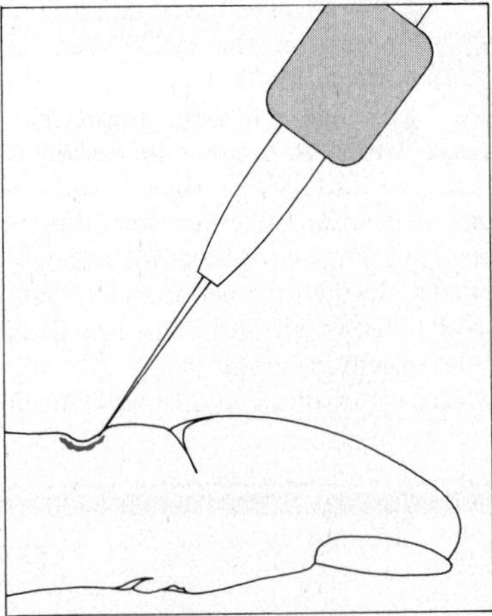

4. Light desiccation of the area to control bleeding and prevent recurrence

type of wart and its location:

- *common* (verruca vulgaris): rough, elevated, rounded surface; appears most frequently on extremities, particularly hands and fingers; most prevalent in children and young adults
- *filiform:* single, thin, threadlike projection; commonly occurs around the face and neck
- *periungual:* rough, irregularly shaped, elevated surface; occurs around edges of finger- and toenails. When severe, the wart may extend under the nail and lift it off the nailbed, causing pain.

• *flat:* multiple groupings of up to several hundred slightly raised lesions with smooth, flat, or slightly rounded tops; common on the face, neck, chest, knees, dorsa of hands, wrists, and flexor surfaces of the forearms; usually occur in children but can affect adults. Distribution is often linear, because these warts can spread from scratching or shaving.
• *plantar:* slightly elevated or flat; occurs singly or in large clusters (mosaic warts), primarily at pressure points of the feet
• *digitate:* fingerlike, horny projection arising from a pea-shaped base; occurs on scalp or near hairline
• *condyloma acuminatum* (moist wart): usually small, pink to red, moist, and soft; may occur singly or in large cauliflowerlike clusters on the penis, scrotum, vulva, and anus. Although this type of wart may be transmitted through sexual contact, it's not always venereal in origin.

Diagnosis

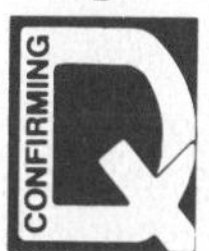

Visual examination usually confirms diagnosis. Plantar warts can be differentiated from corns and calluses by certain distinguishing features. Plantar warts obliterate natural lines of the skin, may contain red or black capillary dots that are easily discernible if the surface of the wart is shaved down with a scalpel, and are painful on application of pressure. Both plantar warts and corns have a soft, pulpy core surrounded by a thick callous ring; plantar warts and calluses are flush with the skin surface.

Recurrent anal warts require sigmoidoscopy to rule out internal involvement, which may necessitate surgery.

Treatment and special considerations

Treatment of warts varies according to location, size, number, pain level (present and projected), history of therapy, the patient's age, and compliance with treatment. Most persons eventually develop an immune response that causes warts to disappear spontaneously and require no treatment.

Treatment may include:
• *Electrodesiccation and curettage:* High-frequency electric current destroys the wart, and is followed by surgical removal of dead tissue at the base and application of an antibiotic ointment (such as polysporin), covered with a bandage, for 48 hours. This method is effective for common, filiform, and, occasionally, plantar warts.
• *Cryotherapy:* Liquid nitrogen or solid carbon dioxide kills the wart; the resulting dried blister is removed several days later. If initial treatment isn't successful, it can be repeated at 2- to 4-week intervals. This method is useful for either periungual warts or for common warts on the face, extremities, penis, vagina, or anus.
• *Acid therapy* (primary or adjunctive): The patient applies plaster patches impregnated with acid (such as 40% salicylic acid plasters), or acid drops (such as 5% to 16.7% salicylic and lactic acid in flexible collodion) every 12 to 24 hours for 2 to 4 weeks. This method is not recommended for areas where perspiration is heavy or that are likely to get wet, or for exposed body parts where patches are cosmetically undesirable.
• *25% podophyllum in compound with tincture of benzoin (for venereal warts):* For protection, cover adjacent unaffected skin with dimethicone or petrolatum before each treatment. The solution is then applied on moist warts. The patient must lie still while it dries, leave it on for 4 hours, and then wash it off with soap and water. Treatment may be repeated every 3 to 4 days and, in some cases, must be left on a maximum of 24 hours, depending on the patient's tolerance. Apply triamcinolone cream 0.1% to relieve post-treatment inflammation.

The use of antiviral drugs is under investigation; suggestion and hypnosis are occasionally successful, especially with children. Conscientious adherence to prescribed therapy is essential. The patient's sexual partner may also require treatment.

Psoriasis

Psoriasis is a chronic, recurrent disease marked by epidermal proliferation. Its lesions, which appear as erythematous papules and plaques covered with silvery scales, vary widely in severity and distribution. It affects about 2% of the population in the United States, and incidence is higher among Caucasians than other races. Although this disorder is most common in adults, it may strike at any age, including infancy. Psoriasis is characterized by recurring remissions and exacerbations. Flare-ups are often related to specific systemic and environmental factors but may be unpredictable; they can usually be controlled with therapy.

Causes

The tendency to develop psoriasis is genetically determined. Researchers have discovered significantly higher than normal incidence of certain histocompatibility antigens (HLA) in patients with psoriasis, suggesting a possible autoimmune deficiency. Onset of disease is also influenced by environmental factors. Trauma can trigger the isomorphic effect, or Koebner's phenomenon, in which lesions develop at sites of injury. Infections, especially those resulting from beta-hemolytic streptococcus, may cause a flare of guttate (drop-shaped) lesions. Other contributing factors include pregnancy, endocrine changes, climatic conditions (cold weather tends to exacerbate psoriasis), and emotional stress.

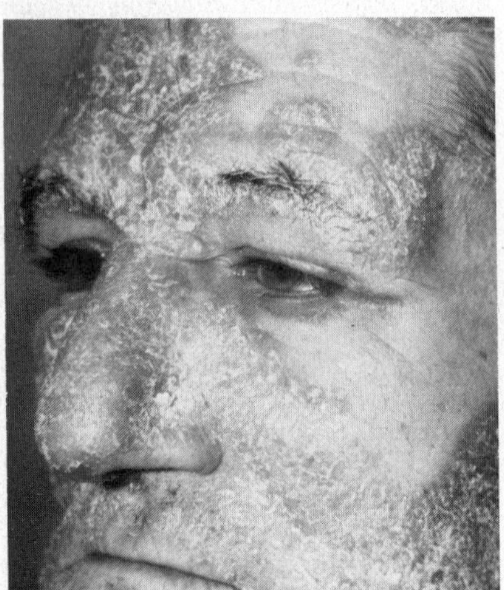

In this patient with psoriasis, plaques consisting of silver scales cover a large area of the face.

Generally, a skin cell takes 14 days to move from the basal layer to the stratum corneum, where after 14 days of normal wear and tear, it's sloughed off. The life cycle of a normal skin cell is 28 days, compared to only 4 days for a psoriatic skin cell. This markedly shortened cycle doesn't allow time for the cell to mature. Consequently, the stratum corneum becomes thick and flaky, producing the cardinal manifestations of psoriasis.

Signs and symptoms

The most common complaint of the patient with psoriasis is itching and, occasionally, pain from dry, cracked, encrusted lesions. Psoriatic lesions are erythematous and usually form well-defined plaques, sometimes covering large areas of the body. Such lesions most commonly appear on the scalp, chest, elbows, knees, back, and buttocks. The plaques consist of characteristic silver scales that either flake off easily or can thicken, covering the lesion. Removal of psoriatic scales frequently produces fine bleeding points (Auspitz sign). Occasionally, small guttate lesions appear, either alone or with plaques; these lesions are typically thin and erythematous, with few scales.

Widespread shedding of scales is common in exfoliative or erythrodermic psoriasis and may also develop in chronic psoriasis.

Rarely, psoriasis becomes pustular, taking one of two forms. In localized pustular psoriasis (Barber), pustules appear on the palms and soles, and remain sterile until opened. In generalized pustular psoriasis (Von Zumbusch), which often occurs with fever, leukocytosis, and malaise, groups of pustules coalesce to form lakes of pus on the skin. These pustules also remain sterile until opened and commonly involve the tongue and oral mucosa.

In approximately 30% of patients, psoriasis spreads to the fingernails (more often than the toenails), producing small indentations or pits, and yellow or brown discoloration. In severe cases, the accumulation of thick crumbly debris under the nail causes the nail to separate from the nailbed.

Many patients with psoriasis develop arthritic symptoms, usually in one or more joints of the fingers or toes, or sometimes in the sacroiliac joints, which may progress to spondylitis. Such patients may complain of morning stiffness. Joint symptoms show no consistent linkage to the course of the cutaneous manifestations of psoriasis; they demonstrate remissions and exacerbations similar to those of rheumatoid arthritis.

Diagnosis

Diagnosis depends on patient history, appearance of the lesions, and, if needed, the results of skin biopsy. Typically, serum uric acid level is elevated, due to accelerated nucleic acid degradation, but indications of gout are absent. HLA antigens 13 and 17 may be present.

Treatment

Treatment depends on the type of psoriasis, the extent of the disease and the patient's response to it, and what effect the disease has on the patient's life-style. No permanent cure exists, and all methods of treatment are merely palliative.

Removal of psoriatic scales necessitates application of occlusive ointment bases, such as petrolatum, salicylic acid preparations, or preparations containing urea. These medications soften the scales, which can then be removed by scrubbing carefully with a soft brush in an oatmeal or salt bath.

Methods to retard rapid cell production include exposure to ultraviolet light (wavelength B [UVB] or natural sunlight) to the point of minimal erythema. Tar preparations or crude coal tar itself may be applied to affected areas about 15 minutes before exposure or may be left on overnight and wiped off the next morning. A thin layer of petrolatum may be applied before UVB exposure. In fact, it's the most common treatment for generalized psoriasis. Exposure time can increase gradually. Outpatient or day treatment with UVB avoids long hospitalizations and prolongs remission.

Steroid creams are useful to control psoriasis. A potent fluorinated steroid works well, except on the face and intertriginous areas. These creams require application three or four times a day, preferably after washing or bathing to facilitate absorption, and possibly with occlusive dressings—plastic wrap, plastic gloves or booties, or a vinyl exercise suit—especially overnight. Small, stubborn plaques that resist local treatment may require intralesional steroid injections. Anthralin, combined with a paste mixture, may be used for well-defined plaques but must not be applied to unaffected areas, because it may cause an allergic reaction; it also stains the skin. It's often used concurrently with steroids; anthralin is applied at night and steroids during the day.

In a patient with severe chronic psoriasis, the Goeckerman regimen—which combines tar baths and UVB treatments—may help achieve remission and clear the skin in 3 to 5 weeks. The Ingram technique is a variation of this treatment, using anthralin instead of tar. A program called PUVA combines administration of methoxsalen with exposure to ultraviolet light, wavelength A (UVA). As a last resort, a cytotoxin, usually methotrexate, may help severe, refractory psoriasis.

Low-dosage antihistamines, oatmeal baths, emollients (perhaps with phenol and menthol), and open wet dressings may help relieve pruritus. Aspirin and local heat help alleviate the pain of psoriatic arthritis; severe cases may require nonsteroidal anti-inflammatory drugs, such as indomethacin.

Therapy for psoriasis of the scalp often consists of a tar shampoo, followed by application of a steroid lotion while the hair is still wet. No effective treatment exists for psoriasis of the nails. The nails usually improve as skin lesions improve.

Special considerations

Design your patient's care plan to include patient teaching, careful monitoring for side effects of therapy, and sympathetic support.

- Make sure the patient understands his prescribed therapy; provide written instructions to avoid confusion. Teach correct application of prescribed creams and lotions. A steroid cream, for example, should be applied in a thin film and rubbed into the skin until the cream disappears. Steroid creams are usually covered with an occlusive dressing and left on overnight. Anthralin and tar should be applied with a downward motion to avoid rubbing it into the follicles. Gloves should be worn, since anthralin stains the skin. After application, the patient may dust himself with powder to prevent anthralin from rubbing off on his clothes. Warn the patient never to put an occlusive dressing over anthralin. Suggest use of mineral oil, then soap and water, to remove anthralin. Caution the patient to avoid scrubbing his skin vigorously, to prevent Koebner's phenomenon. If a medication has been applied to the scales to soften them, suggest the patient use a soft brush to remove them.
- Watch for side effects, especially allergic reactions to anthralin, atrophy and acne from steroids, and burning, itching, nausea, and squamous cell epitheliomas from PUVA. Evaluate the patient on methotrexate weekly for RBC, WBC, and platelet counts, since cytotoxins may cause hepatic or bone marrow toxicity. Liver biopsy may be done to assess the effects of methotrexate.
- Caution the patient receiving PUVA therapy to stay out of the sun on the day of treatment, and to protect his eyes with sunglasses that screen UVA for 24 hours after treatment. Tell him to wear goggles during exposure to this light.
- Be aware that psoriasis can cause psychologic problems. Assure the patient that psoriasis is not contagious, and although exacerbations and remissions occur, they're controllable with treatment. However, be sure he understands there is no cure. Also, since stressful situations tend to exacerbate psoriasis, help the patient learn to cope with these situations. Explain the relationship between psoriasis and arthritis, but point out that psoriasis causes no other systemic disturbances. Refer all patients to the National Psoriasis Foundation, which provides information and directs patients to local chapters.

Lichen Planus

A benign but pruritic skin eruption, lichen planus usually produces scaling, purple papules, marked by white lines or spots. Such eruptions occur most often in middle-aged persons and are uncommon in the young or elderly. Lichen planus, a relatively rare disorder, is found in all geographic areas, with equal distribution among races. In most patients, it resolves spontaneously in 6 to 18 months; in a few, chronic lichen planus may persist for several years.

Causes

The cause of lichen planus is unknown, but possible causes may include a virus, an immunologic defect, or psychogenic factors, such as fatigue or severe emotional stress. Eruptions similar to lichen planus have been induced by certain chemicals and drugs.

Signs and symptoms

Lichen planus may develop suddenly or insidiously. Initial lesions commonly appear on the arms or legs, and evolve into the generalized eruption of flat, glistening, purple papules, marked with white lines or spots (Wickham's striae). These lesions may be linear, due to scratching, or coalesce into plaques. Lesions often affect the mucous membranes (especially the buccal mucosa), male genitalia, and less often, the nails. Mild-to-severe pruritus is common.

Diagnosis

Although characteristic skin lesions frequently establish the diagnosis of lichen planus, confirmation may necessitate skin biopsy.

Treatment

Treatment is essentially symptomatic. The goal of therapy is to relieve itching with topical fluorinated steroids, with occlusive dressings; intralesional injections of steroids; oatmeal baths; and antihistamines. Vitamin A in the form of retinoic acid may shrink lesions but is not generally recommended. Systemic corticosteroids, given in early acute stages, may shorten the duration of the disease. If a drug is suspected as the cause, it should be discontinued. Treatment of lichen planus associated with emotional stress may require counseling to identify stressors and teach more effective coping mechanisms.

Special considerations

- Administer medications, as ordered, and inform the patient of possible side effects, especially drowsiness produced by antihistamines.
- Provide emotional support, and reassure the patient that lichen planus, although annoying, is usually a benign, self-limiting condition.

Corns and Calluses

Usually located on areas of repeated trauma (most often the feet), corns and calluses are acquired skin conditions marked by hyperkeratosis of the stratum corneum. Prognosis is good with proper foot care.

Causes and incidence

A corn is a hyperkeratotic area that usually results from external pressure, such as that from ill-fitting shoes, or less commonly, from internal pressure, such as that caused by a protruding underlying bone (due to arthritis, for example). A callus is an area of thickened skin, generally found on the foot or hand, produced by external pressure or friction. Persons whose activities produce repeated trauma (for example, manual laborers or guitarists) commonly develop calluses.

The severity of a corn or callus depends on the degree and duration of trauma.

Signs and symptoms

Both corns and calluses cause pain through pressure on underlying tissue by localized thickened skin. Corns contain a central keratinous core, are smaller and more clearly defined than calluses, and are usually more painful. The pain they cause may be dull and constant or sharp when pressure is applied. "Soft" corns are caused by the pressure of a bony prominence. They appear as whitish thickenings and are commonly found between the toes, most often in the fourth interdigital web. "Hard" corns are sharply delineated and conical, and appear most frequently over the dorsolateral aspect of the fifth toe.

AIDS FOR RELIEVING PAINFUL PRESSURE

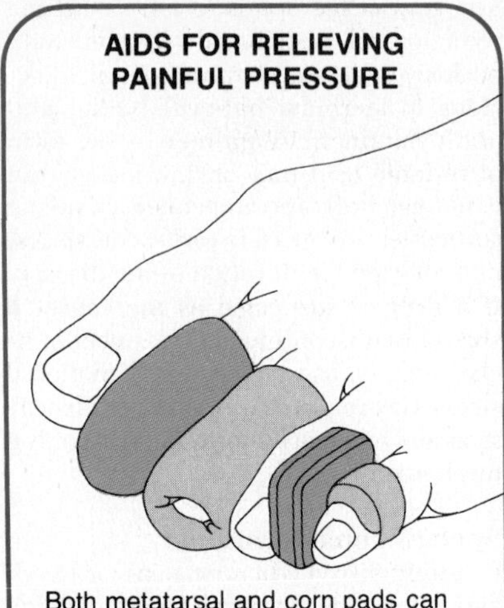

Both metatarsal and corn pads can help relieve painful pressure. Commercial products available include, from left to right, foam toe cap, foam toe sleeve, soft corn shield, and hard corn (fifth toe) shield.

Calluses have indefinite borders and may be quite large. They usually produce dull pain on pressure, rather than constant pain. Although calluses commonly appear over plantar warts, they're distinguished from these warts by normal skin markings.

Diagnosis

Diagnosis depends on careful physical examination of the affected area and on patient history revealing chronic trauma.

Treatment

Surgical debridement may be performed to remove the nucleus of a corn, usually under a local anesthetic. In intermittent debridement, keratolytics—usually 40% salicylic acid plasters—are applied to affected areas. Injections of corticosteroids beneath the corn may be necessary to relieve pain. However, the simplest and best treatment is essentially preventive—avoidance of trauma. Corns and calluses disappear after the source of trauma has been removed. Metatarsal pads may redistribute the weight-bearing areas of the foot; corn pads may prevent painful pressure.

Patients with persistent corns or calluses require referral to a podiatrist or dermatologist; those with corns or calluses caused by a bony malformation, as in arthritis, require orthopedic consultation.

Special considerations

- Teach the patient how to apply salicylic acid plasters. Make sure the plaster is large enough to cover the affected area. Place the sticky side down on the foot, then cover the plaster with adhesive tape. Plasters are usually taken off after an overnight application but may be left in place for as long as 7 days. After removing the plaster, the patient should soak the area in water and abrade the soft, macerated skin with a towel or pumice stone. He should then reapply the plaster, and repeat the entire procedure until he has removed all the hyperkeratotic skin. Warn the patient against removing corns or calluses with a sharp instrument, such as a razor blade.
- Advise the patient to wear properly fitted shoes. Suggest the use of metatarsal or corn pads to relieve pressure. Refer to a podiatrist, dermatologist, or orthopedist, if necessary.
- Assure the patient that good foot care can correct this condition.

Pityriasis Rosea

An acute, self-limiting, inflammatory skin disease, pityriasis rosea produces a "herald" patch—which usually goes undetected—followed by a generalized eruption of papulosquamous lesions. Although this noncontagious disorder may develop at any age, it's most apt to occur in adolescents and young adults. Incidence rises in the spring and fall.

Causes

The cause of pityriasis rosea is unknown, but the brief course of the disease and the virtual absence of recurrence suggest a viral agent or an autoimmune disorder.

Signs and symptoms

Pityriasis typically begins with an erythematous "herald" patch, which may appear anywhere on the body. Although this slightly raised, oval lesion is about 2 to 6 cm in diameter, approximately 25% of patients don't notice it. A few days to several weeks later, yellow-tan or erythematous patches with scaly edges (about 0.5 to 1 cm in diameter) erupt on the trunk and extremities—and sometimes on the face, hands, and feet in adolescents. Eruption continues for 7 to 10 days, and the patches persist for 2 to 6 weeks. Occasionally, these patches are macular, vesicular, or urticarial. A characteristic of this disease is the arrangement of lesions along body cleavage lines, producing a pattern similar to that of a pine tree. Accompanying pruritus is usually mild but may be severe.

Diagnosis

Characteristic skin lesions support the diagnosis. Differential diagnosis must also rule out secondary syphilis (through serologic testing), dermatophytosis, and drug reaction.

Treatment and special considerations

Treatment focuses on relief of pruritus, with emollients, oatmeal baths, antihistamines, and occasionally, exposure to ultraviolet light or sunlight. Topical steroids in a hydrophilic cream base may be beneficial. Rarely, if inflammation is severe, systemic corticosteroids may be required.

- Reassure the patient that pityriasis rosea is noncontagious, that spontaneous remission usually occurs in 2 to 6 weeks, and that lesions generally don't recur.
- Urge the patient not to scratch. Advise him that hot baths may intensify itching. Encourage the use of antipruritics.

Hyperhidrosis

Hyperhidrosis is the excessive secretion of sweat from the eccrine glands. It usually occurs in the axillae (typically after puberty) and on the palms and soles (often starting during infancy or childhood).

Causes

Genetic factors may contribute to the development of hyperhidrosis, and in susceptible individuals, emotional stress appears to be the most prominent cause. Increased CNS impulses may provoke excessive release of acetylcholine, producing a heightened sweat response. Exercise and a hot climate can cause profuse sweating in these patients. Certain drugs, such as antipyretics, emetics, meperidine, and anticholinesterase, have been known to increase sweating.

In addition, hyperhidrosis often occurs as a clinical manifestation of an underlying disorder. Infections and chronic diseases, such as tuberculosis, malaria, or lymphoma, may cause excessive nighttime sweating. A person with diabetes often demonstrates hyperhidrosis during a hypoglycemic crisis. Other predisposing conditions include pheochromocytomas; cardiovascular disorders, such as shock or heart failure; CNS disturbances (most often lesions of the hypothalamus); withdrawal from drugs or alcohol; menopause; and Graves' disease.

Signs and symptoms

Axillary hyperhidrosis frequently produces such extreme sweating that patients often ruin their clothes in 1 day and develop contact dermatitis from clothing dyes; similarly, hyperhidrosis of the soles can easily damage a pair of shoes. Profuse sweating from both the soles and palms hinders the patient's ability to work and interact socially. Patients with this condition often report increased emotional strain.

Diagnosis

Clinical observations and patient history confirm hyperhidrosis.

Treatment

Treatment of choice is application of 20% aluminum chloride in absolute ethanol. (Most antiperspirants contain a 5% solution.) Formaldehyde may also be used but may lead to allergic contact sensitization. Glutaraldehyde produces less contact sensitivity than formaldehyde but stains the skin; it's used more often on the feet than on the hands, as a soak or applied directly several times a week and then weekly, as needed. Therapy sometimes includes anticholinergics, except in patients with glaucoma or prostatic hypertrophy. Severe hyperhidrosis unresponsive to conservative therapy may require local axillary removal of sweat glands or, as a last resort, a cervicothoracic or lumbar sympathectomy.

Special considerations

Provide support and reassurance since hyperhidrosis may be socially embarrassing. Tell the patient to apply aluminum chloride in absolute ethanol nightly to dry axillae, soles, or palms. The area should be covered with plastic wrap for 6 to 8 hours, preferably overnight, then washed with soap and water. Repeat this procedure for several nights, until profuse daytime sweating subsides. Frequency of treatments can then be reduced. Advise the patient with hyperhidrosis of the soles to wear leather sandals and white or colorfast cotton socks.

Decubitus Ulcers

(Pressure sores, bedsores)

Decubitus ulcers are localized areas of cellular necrosis that occur most often in the skin and subcutaneous tissue over bony prominences. These ulcers may be superficial, caused by local skin irritation with subsequent surface maceration, or deep, originating in underlying tissue. Deep lesions often go undetected until they penetrate the skin; but, by then, they've usually caused subcutaneous damage.

Causes

Pressure, particularly over bony prominences, interrupts normal circulatory function and causes most decubitus ulcers. The intensity and duration of such pressure governs the severity of the ulcer; pressure exerted over an area for a moderate period (1 to 2 hours) produces tissue ischemia and increased capillary pressure, leading to edema and multiple small-vessel thromboses. An inflammatory reaction gives way to ulceration and necrosis of ischemic cells. In turn, necrotic tissue predisposes to bacterial invasion and subsequent infection.

The patient's position determines the pressure exerted on the tissues. For example, if the head of the bed is elevated, or the patient assumes a slumped position, gravity pulls his weight downward and forward. This shearing force causes deep ulcers due to ischemic changes in the muscles and subcutaneous tissues, and occurs most often over the sacrum

SPECIAL AIDS FOR PREVENTING AND TREATING DECUBITUS ULCERS

Pressure relief aids:

- *Gel flotation pads* disperse pressure over a greater skin surface area; convenient and adaptable for home and wheelchair use.
- *Water mattress* distributes body weight equally but is heavy and awkward; "mini" water beds (partially filled rubber gloves or plastic bags) help in small areas, such as heels.
- *Alternating pressure mattress* contains tubelike sections, running lengthwise, that deflate and reinflate, changing areas of pressure. Use mattress with a single untucked sheet, since layers of linen decrease its effectiveness.
- *Egg crate mattress* minimizes area of skin pressure with its alternating areas of depression and elevation: soft, elevated foam areas cushion skin; depressed areas relieve pressure. This mattress should be used with a single, loosely tucked sheet and is adaptable for home and wheelchair use. If the patient is incontinent, cover mattress with the provided plastic sleeve.
- *Spanco mattress* has polyester fibers with silicon tubes to decrease pressure without limiting the patient's position. It has no weight limitation.
- *Sheepskin* is soft, dry, absorbent, and easy to clean. It should be in direct contact with the patient's skin. It's available in sizes to fit elbows and heels and is adaptable to home use.
- *Clinitron bed* supports the patient at a subcapillary pressure point and provides a warm, relaxing therapeutic airflow. The bed is filled with beads that move when the air flows. It eliminates friction and maceration.
- *Turning bed* (such as Stryker or Foster frame, CircOlectric bed, and Roto-Rest) is ineffective without adjuvant therapy. It also limits free movement and is expensive.

Topical agents:

- Gentle soap
- Dakins solution
- Zinc oxide cream
- Absorbable gelatin sponge
- Granulated sugar (mechanical irritant to enhance granulation)
- Dextranomer (inert, absorbing beads)
- Karaya gum patches
- Topical antibiotics (*only* when infection is confirmed by culture and sensitivity tests)
- Silver sulfadiazine cream (antimicrobial agent)
- Povidone-iodine packs (remain in place until dry)
- Water vapor–permeable dressings.

Avoid these skin-damaging agents:

- Harsh alkali soaps
- Alcohol-based products (can cause vasoconstriction)
- Tincture of benzoin (may cause painful erosions)
- Hexachlorophene (may irritate the central nervous system)
- Petrolatum gauze.

and ischial tuberosities.

Predisposing conditions for decubitus ulcers include altered mobility, inadequate nutrition (leading to weight loss and subsequent reduction of subcutaneous tissue and muscle bulk), and a breakdown in skin or subcutaneous tissue (as a result of edema, incontinence, fever, pathologic conditions, or obesity).

Signs and symptoms

Decubitus ulcers commonly develop over bony prominences. Early features of superficial lesions are shiny, erythematous changes over the compressed area, caused by localized vasodilation when pressure is relieved. Superficial erythema progresses to small blisters or erosions and, ultimately, to necrosis and ulceration.

An inflamed area on the skin's surface may be the first sign of underlying damage when pressure is exerted between deep tissue and bone. Bacteria in a com-

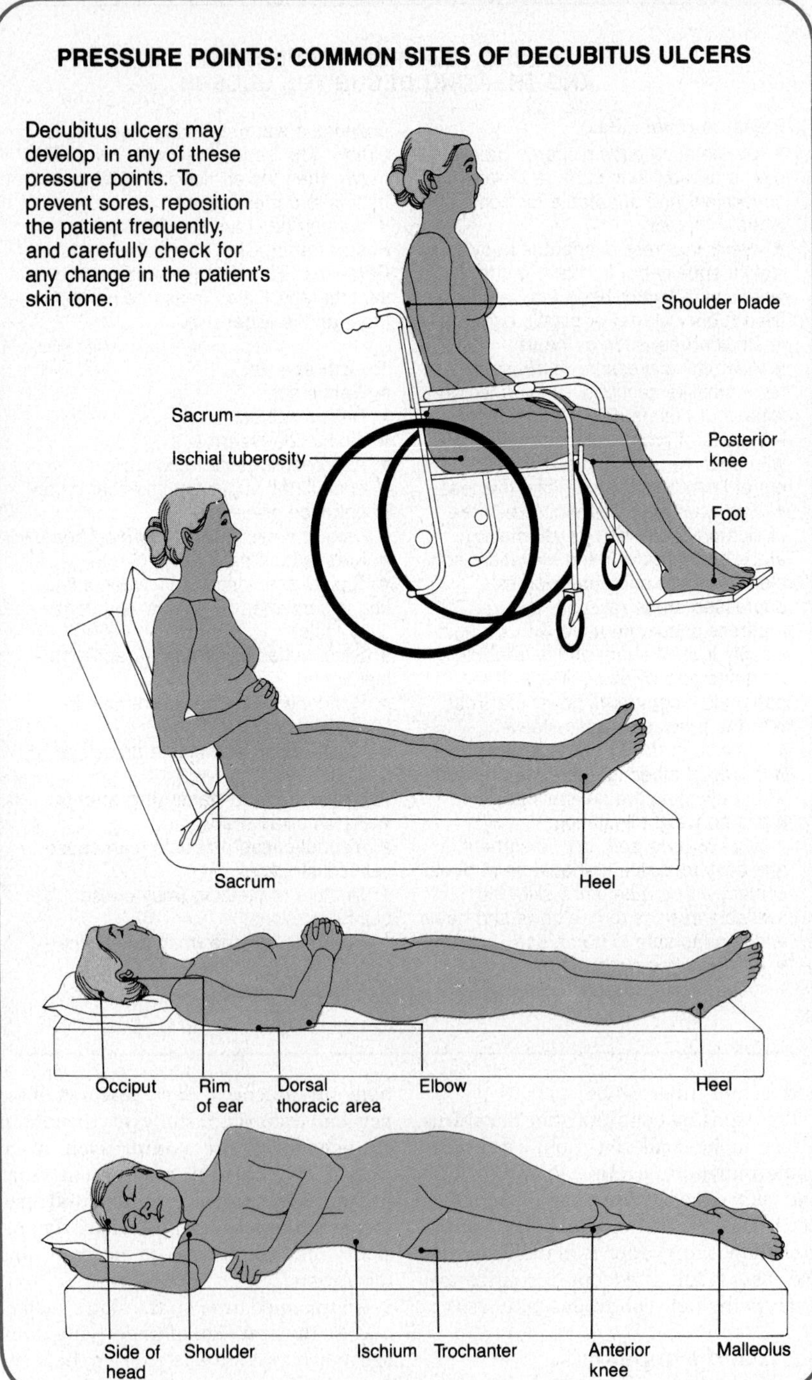
PRESSURE POINTS: COMMON SITES OF DECUBITUS ULCERS
Decubitus ulcers may develop in any of these pressure points. To prevent sores, reposition the patient frequently, and carefully check for any change in the patient's skin tone.
Shoulder blade
Sacrum
Ischial tuberosity
Posterior knee
Foot
Sacrum
Heel
Occiput
Rim of ear
Dorsal thoracic area
Elbow
Heel
Side of head
Shoulder
Ischium
Trochanter
Anterior knee
Malleolus

pressed site cause inflammation and, eventually, infection, which leads to further necrosis. A foul-smelling, purulent discharge may seep from a lesion that penetrates the skin from beneath. Infected, necrotic tissue prevents healthy granulation of scar tissue; a black eschar may develop around and over the lesion.

Diagnosis

Decubitus ulcers are obvious on physical examination. Wound culture and sensitivity testing of the exudate in the ulcer identify infecting organisms and antibiotics that may be needed. If severe hypoproteinemia is suspected, total serum protein values and serum albumin studies may be appropriate.

Treatment and special considerations

Successful treatment must relieve pressure on the affected area, keep the area clean and dry, and promote healing.

- During each shift, check the skin of bedridden patients for possible changes in color, turgor, temperature, and sensation. Examine an existing ulcer for any change in size or degree of damage. When using pressure relief aids or topical agents, explain their function to the patient.
- Prevent pressure sores by repositioning the bedridden patient at least every 2 hours around the clock. Minimize the effects of a shearing force by using a footboard and by not raising the head of the bed to an angle that exceeds 60°. Keep the patient's knees slightly flexed for short periods. Perform passive range-of-motion exercises, or encourage the patient to do active exercises, if possible.
- To prevent pressure sores in immobilized patients, use pressure relief aids on their beds.
- Give meticulous skin care. Keep the skin clean and dry without the use of harsh soaps. Gently massaging the skin around the affected area—not on it—promotes healing. Rub moisturizing lotions into the skin thoroughly to prevent maceration of the skin surface. Change bed linens frequently for patients who are diaphoretic or incontinent.
- Clean open lesions with a 3% solution of hydrogen peroxide or normal saline solution. Dressings, if needed, should be porous and lightly taped to healthy skin. Debridement of necrotic tissue may be necessary to allow healing. One method is to apply open wet dressings and allow them to dry on the ulcer. Removal of the dressings mechanically debrides exudate and necrotic tissue. Other methods include surgical debridement with a fine scalpel blade and chemical debridement using proteolytic enzyme agents.
- Encourage adequate intake of food and fluids to maintain body weight and promote healing. Consult with the dietary department to provide a diet that promotes granulation of new tissue. Encourage the debilitated patient to eat frequent, small meals that include protein- and calorie-rich supplements. Assist weakened patients with their meals.

Selected References

Arndt, Kenneth A. *Manual of Dermatologic Therapeutics*, 3rd ed. Boston: Little, Brown & Co., 1983.

Braverman, Irwin M. *Skin Signs of Systemic Disease*. Philadelphia: W.B. Saunders Co., 1981.

Fitzpatrick, Thomas B., et al. *Dermatology in General Medicine: Update One*. New York: McGraw-Hill Book Co., 1982.

Moschella, Samuel L., et al. *Dermatology*, 2nd ed., vols. 1 and 2. Philadelphia: W.B. Saunders Co., 1985.

Sauer, G.C. *Manual of Skin Diseases*, 4th ed. Philadelphia: J.B. Lippincott Co., 1980.

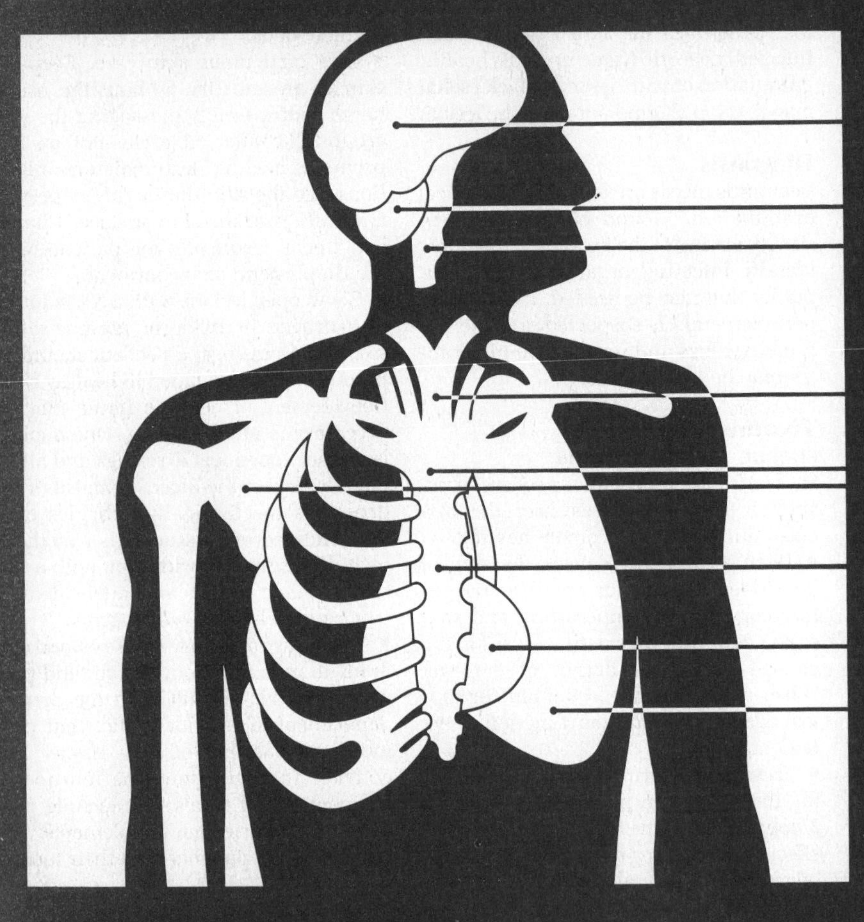

Appendices and Index

RARE DISEASES

DISEASE	DEFINITION AND CHARACTERISTICS
African trypanosomiasis: sleeping sickness	Febrile illness that may be Gambian—typically found in west and central Africa—or Rhodesian—a more virulent type found in east Africa
Akureyri disease: benign myalgic encephalomyelitis	Acute encephalitic/myelitic process marked by symptoms of damage to the white matter of the brain or spinal cord
Albarrán's disease: colibacilluria	Presence of *Escherichia coli* in the urine may be associated with cystitis, pyelonephritis, and asymptomatic bacteremia; symptoms may include frequency, with burning and bladder pain.
Albers-Schönberg disease: osteopetrosis	Rare bone disorder marked by disorganization of bone structure that causes dense sclerotic bones vulnerable to recurrent fractures. Malignant variant begins in utero and progresses rapidly to cause marked anemia, hydrocephalus, cranial nerve involvement, hepatosplenomegaly, and fatal infection. Benign variant causes milder anemia and fewer neurologic abnormalities.
American trypanosomiasis: Chagas' disease	Febrile illness prevalent in Mexico, Central America, and South America. Often benign in adults, although cardiomyopathy may develop. Can be severe in children
Anthrax: woolsorters' disease	Acute bacterial infection affecting people who have contact with contaminated animals or their hides, bones, fur, hair, or wool
Arc-welders' disease: siderosis	Benign pneumoconiosis that can occur in iron ore miners, welders, metal grinders, and polishers from the inhalation and retention of iron
Armstrong's disease: lymphocytic choriomeningitis (LCM)	Central nervous system and influenzalike illness that may be associated with rash, arthritis, or orchitis. A zoonotic virus that causes meningitis and encephalitis. (Incidence rises in winter, when mice move indoors.) Probable port of entry is through the respiratory tract. Viremia occurs and LCM virus crosses the blood-brain barrier.
Balanitis	Inflammation of the glans penis, which slowly develops an erosive and possibly gangrenous lesion that may extend to the penile shaft
Balanoposthitis: fourth venereal disease	Ulcerative inflammation of the glans penis and prepuce; granuloma inguinale
Baló's disease: leukoencephalitis periaxialis concentrica	Atypical form of Schilder's disease (see also Schilder's disease) causing concentric demyelination; most common in immunodeficient persons
Barometer-maker's disease: chronic mercurial poisoning	Soreness of gums, loosening of teeth, salivation, fetid breath, griping diarrhea, weakness, and death
Basal cell carcinoma of the eye	Common extraorbital cancer affecting the eyelid, conjunctivae, and cornea
Basel disease: keratosis follicularis, Darier's disease	Any skin condition marked by formation of horny growths

CAUSE	TREATMENT
Trypanosoma transmitted by tsetse fly bite	Suramin for patients with central nervous system (CNS) involvement; melarsoprol for those without
Damage chiefly to white matter of brain or spinal cord secondary to perivascular cellular infiltration and perivenous myelination that may follow measles and smallpox, or vaccination against smallpox and rabies	Discontinuation of smallpox vaccine, use of measles vaccine to eliminate postinfectious encephalomyelitis, use of killed duck embryo vaccine for postrabies vaccination to decrease encephalomyelitis
Usually transmitted by fecal contamination, but airborne and fomes contamination are possible. Can be prevented by limited use of indwelling (Foley) catheters associated with rigorous aseptic technique; isolation of infectious patients; appropriate use of antibiotics, steroids, and cytotoxics in infection-prone patients; and increased fluid intake to flush urinary tract.	Antibiotic treatment selected according to results of in vitro sensitivity tests. *E. coli* is sensitive to gentamicin (90%), ampicillin (85% to 90%), tetracycline (75%), streptomycin (50%), and high concentrations of penicillin (50%).
Malignant variant transmitted as autosomal recessive trait; benign variant transmitted as autosomal dominant trait. Increased bone mass secondary to defect in remodeling bone, resulting in thickened cortices (increased density). Bone is mechanically abnormal and fractures easily.	Transfusion of nucleated marrow cells from a healthy, clinically normal donor (almost always a sibling); associated splenectomy may decrease erythrocyte destruction and increase erythrocytic life span and effectiveness.
Trypanosoma cruzi transmitted by the reduviid beetle	Nifurtimox
Bacillus anthracis	High-dose penicillin; isolation
Inhalation and retention of iron after exposure to iron oxide fumes and dust	Limiting or preventing exposure to iron dust or fumes prevents progression of this disease.
Viral infection that follows exposure to food or dust contaminated by rodents. Can be prevented by careful hand washing (although mode of transmission may be airborne)	Supportive and symptomatic management
Sexual or other mode of transmission of *Borrelia vincentii*, streptococci, staphylococci, *Neisseria gonorrhoeae*, or *Candida albicans*	Penicillin or tetracycline; circumcision may be necessary.
Sexual or other mode of transmission of *Borrelia vincentii*, streptococci, straphylococci, *Neisseria gonorrhoeae*, or *Candida albicans*	Penicillin or tetracycline; circumcision may be necessary.
Viral infection from the papovaviruses	Supportive and symptomatic management; invariably fatal
Mercury poisoning resulting from chronic exposure to mercury or its vapors	Evacuate stomach, lavage with milk or sodium bicarbonate, but treat with BAL (dimercaprol) as soon as possible to prevent fatal progression.
Unknown, but predisposing factors include sunlight, radiation, chemicals, and other carcinogens	Surgery; radiation therapy may be necessary.
Unknown	No specific therapy, but keratolytic lotions and moistening skin to prevent cracking, drying, and skin breakdown may be useful.

(continued)

RARE DISEASES *(continued)*

DISEASE	DEFINITION AND CHARACTERISTICS
Bateman's disease: molluscum contagiosum	Mildly contagious skin disease marked by formation of small, waxy globular epithelial tumors containing semifluid caseous matter or of solid masses on the face, eyelids, breasts, and inner surfaces of thighs and genitalia
Bauxite workers' disease: bauxite pneumoconiosis, Shaver's disease	Occupational disorder causing rapid and progressive pneumoconiosis and leading to empyema; may be accompanied by pneumothorax
Behr's disease: degeneration of the macula retinae	Familial spastic paraplegia with or without optic atrophy; hyperactive tendon reflexes and sensory disturbances in adolescents and adults
Black disease	Rare infectious necrotic hepatitis
Blinding filarial disease: onchocerciasis, "river blindness"	Invasion of eye tissues by the filarial worm, which is enclosed in fibrous cysts or nodules
Bouillaud's disease: endocarditis	Rheumatic endocarditis
Breisky's disease: kraurosis vulvae	Vulval atrophy and dryness of skin and mucous membranes
Brill-Zinsser disease	Relapse of typhus, which can occur years after the primary attack
Brown-Symmers disease	Acute serous encephalitis in children
Bruck's disease	Condition marked by deformity of the bones, multiple fractures, ankylosis of joints, and atrophy of muscles
Budd-Chiari syndrome	Hepatic vein obstruction that impairs blood flow out of the liver, producing massive ascites and hepatomegaly
Bulimia	Obsessive eating associated with ritualistic vomiting and purging to maintain a desired weight level. Leads to electrolyte imbalance and may impair hepatic and renal function
Burkitt's tumor: Burkitt's lymphoma	Undifferentiated malignant lymphoma that usually begins as a large mass in the jaw (African Burkitt's) or as an abdominal mass (American Burkitt's)
Castellani's disease: bronchospirochetosis	Hemorrhagic bronchitis, bronchopulmonary inflammation of the bronchial mucous membrane; usually follows the common cold
Cat-scratch fever: cat-scratch disease, nonbacterial regional lymphadenitis, benign lymphoreticulosis	Subacute self-limiting disease characterized by a primary local lesion and regional lymphadenopathy
Central core disease of muscle	Rare muscle disease in which severe hypotonia causes weakness and arrests motor development in infancy. A central core in each muscle fiber is diagnostic.
Charrin's disease	Pyogenic infections causing formation of blue pus; may cause urinary tract infections or otitis externa

CAUSE	TREATMENT
A large virus of the pox group	Incision and drainage of tumor contents, followed by cleansing with iodine base solution
Inhalation of dust particles of alumina and silica (bauxite)	Elimination of exposure to bauxite
Hereditary form of cerebellar ataxia	No confirmed treatment; vitamin B therapy sometimes indicated
Clostridium novyi	Immediate surgical debridement and antibiotic therapy (usually 20 mU/day of penicillin by continuous I.V. infusion)
Onchocerca volvulus transmitted by the blackfly *(Simulium* and *Eusimulium)*	Diethylcarbamazine destroys microfilaria but has little effect on the adult worm. Antihistamines treat possible allergic reactions. This condition leads to blindness despite treatment.
Delayed sequel to pharyngeal infection of group B streptococci	No specific cure; supportive therapy to reduce mortality/morbidity
Probable hypoestrogenism	Surgery
Rickettsia prowazekii	Tetracycline; doxycycline; chloramphenicol; analgesics; antipyretics
Viral pathogens (rabies, measles, mumps, rubella, influenza)	Supportive care; control of intracranial pressure; correction of metabolic problems, disseminated intravascular coagulation, bleeding, renal failure, pulmonary emboli, and pneumonia; invariably fatal
Unknown	Symptomatic and supportive management
Any condition that obstructs blood flow from hepatic veins	Symptomatic management with diuretics and fluid restriction; surgery to shunt hepatic blood flow
Abnormal mental state marked by overwhelming obsession with food; compulsion to eat may be related to low blood glucose levels.	Treatment difficult but successful at special clinics. Hypnotherapy used occasionally.
Unknown, but Epstein-Barr virus suspected	Chemotherapy; radiation therapy; surgical resection in extensive local disease
Spirochete infection	Bed rest and fluid intake; antipyretics, analgesics, and antibiotics; nebulization; humidified therapy
Unknown agent transmitted by cats to humans	Symptomatic management
Transmitted as autosomal dominant trait	Symptomatic and supportive management
Pseudomonas aeruginosa	Increased fluid intake to flush urinary tract; appropriate antibiotics; vitamin C to increase glomerular filtration rate

(continued)

DISEASE	DEFINITION AND CHARACTERISTICS
Chester's disease: xanthomatosis	Excessive accumulation of lipids in the long bones, marked by the formation of foam cells in skin lesions
Chiari-Frommel disease: Frommel's disease	Postpartum condition marked by uterine atrophy, persistent lactation, galactorrhea, prolonged amenorrhea, and low levels of urinary estrogen and gonadotropin
Choriocarcinoma	Rapidly metastasizing malignant tumor of placental tissue that typically causes profuse vaginal and intraabdominal bleeding
Chromomycosis: chromoblastomycosis	Slow-spreading fungal infection of the skin and subcutaneous tissues. It produces cauliflowerlike lesions on the legs or arms and may spread to the brain, causing an abscess.
Cockayne's syndrome	Hereditary syndrome consisting of dwarfism, with retinal atrophy and deafness, associated with progeria, prognathism, mental retardation, and photosensitivity
Concato's disease	Progressive malignant polyserositis, with large effusions into the pericardium, pleura, and peritoneum
Conradi's disease: dysplasia epiphysealis punctata	Abnormal development of the secondary bone-forming center; marked by depressions or pinpoint structures
Contact ulcers	Erosions on the laryngeal mucosa over the vocal cords, producing hoarseness and mild dysphagia. Ulcers cause gradual tissue necrosis.
Copper deficiency anemia: hypocupremia	Nutritional deficiency that impairs hemoglobin synthesis and causes shortness of breath, pallor, fatigue, edema, poor wound healing, and anorexia. If prolonged, it can cause poor mental development in infants and mental deterioration in adults.
Crocq's disease: acrocyanosis	Symmetrical cyanosis of the hands and feet; distinguished from Raynaud's disease by persistent discoloration
Csillag's disease: lichen sclerosis et atrophicus	Acute inflammatory dermatitis, such as heat rash, prickly heat, miliaria rubra; chronic atrophic and lichenoid dermatitis
Czerny's disease	Joint pain, with swelling
Darier's disease: keratosis follicularis	Skin condition marked by excessive formation of horny growths, usually on the trunk, face, ears, nasolabial furrows, and scalp
Dengue: breakbone or dandy fever	Acute febrile disease endemic during the warmer months in the tropics and subtropics. Rarely fatal, unless it progresses to hemorrhagic shock syndrome
Deutschländer's disease	Tumor of the metatarsal bones
Diamond-skin disease: swine erysipelas	Acute febrile vascular disease, causing localized swelling and inflammation of the skin and subcutaneous tissue
Dubois' disease: congenital syphilis	Multiple thymic abscesses in congenital syphilis
Duhring's disease: dermatitis herpetiformis	Chronic inflammatory disease marked by erythematous, papular, vesicular, bullous, or pustular lesions, with tendency to grouping and associated with itching and burning
Dukes' disease: fourth disease	Marked by myalgia, headache, fever, pharyngitis, conjunctivitis, generalized adenopathy and desquamation following confluent raised erythema

CAUSE	TREATMENT
Disturbances of lipid metabolism	Unknown
Possibly pituitary dysfunction or tumor	Treatment of underlying illness
Possible causes include hydatidiform mole, abortion, fetal-maternal histoincompatibility, inherited factors, or infections.	Chemotherapy; radiation therapy; hysterectomy
Phialophora verrucosa, Fonsecaea pedrosoi, and *Cladosporium carrioni*	Lesion removal with liquid nitrogen, electrocoagulation, or surgery; intralesional injections of amphotericin B
Transmitted as autosomal recessive trait	Effective treatment unknown; symptomatic management; establishment of protective environment
Mycobacterium tuberculosis	Thoracentesis and parenteral or oral antitubercular antibiotics, such as para-aminosalicylate and ethionamide
Hereditary	Supportive management, ensuring adequate calcium intake
Vocal strain, laryngeal trauma, or emotional stress	Supportive management with absolute voice rest, adequate humidification, and aerosol therapy
Diseases associated with low protein levels; substantial protein loss; decreased gastrointestinal absorption of copper; total parenteral nutrition without copper supplement; or Wilson's disease	Copper sulfate; supportive management of associated symptoms
Vasospastic disturbance of smaller arterioles of the skin from unknown cause	Reassurance and protection from exposure to cold; vasodilators may be prescribed for cosmetic reasons.
Keratin obstruction of sweat ducts	Symptomatic management, including cool environment, application of calamine lotion, and desquamation by ultraviolet rays
Serous effusion in a joint space or cavity	Treatment of inflammation; aspiration of joint space
Unknown	Systemic antibiotics can induce temporary amelioration.
Group B arboviruses transmitted by the female *Aedes* mosquito	Nonaspirin analgesics; I.V. fluid replacement
Unknown	Surgery
Streptococcus pyogenes; capillary congestion follows dilatation of superficial capillaries resulting from stress, inflammation, or external heat stimulation.	Penicillin or erythromycin; application of cool magnesium sulfate compresses; aspirin for pain; and fluid replacement, as needed
Treponema pallidum, a spirochete transmitted by venereal contact	Penicillin, or in allergic patients, oxytetracycline, chlortetracycline, or erythromycin
Cause unknown; most prevalent in males	Removal of sources of reflex irritation; application of antiseptic to excoriated areas
Most likely a viral exanthema of Coxsackie-Echo group	Symptomatic and supportive management

(continued)

DISEASE	DEFINITION AND CHARACTERISTICS
Dupré's disease: meningism	Noninflammatory irritation of the brain and spinal cord, with symptoms simulating meningitis
Durand's disease	Marked by headache, with upper respiratory tract, meningeal, and gastrointestinal tract symptoms
Duroziez's disease: congenital mitral stenosis	Narrowing orifice of the mitral valve that obstructs blood flow from atrium to ventricle
Eales's disease	Condition marked by recurrent hemorrhages into the retina and vitreous, mainly affecting males in the second and third decades of life
Economo's disease: lethargic encephalitis, Vienna encephalitis, sleeping sickness	Epidemic encephalitis marked by increasing languor, apathy, and drowsiness, progressing to lethargy; usually occurs in winter
Elevator disease	Respiratory distress affecting persons who work in grain elevators; a form of occupational pneumoconiosis
Engel-Recklinghausen disease: hyperparathyroidism, osteitis fibrosa cystica generalisata	Fibrous degeneration of bone, with the formation of cysts and fibrous nodules on bone affected
Engman's disease	Infectious eczematoid dermatitis
Eosinophilic endomyocardial disease: Löffler's endocarditis, Löffler's syndrome	Benign self-limiting pneumonitis marked by transient eosinophilic infiltration of the lungs and associated with marked eosinophilia in the blood and sputum, involving endocardium and myocardium
Epstein's disease: pseudodiphtheria, mononucleosis	Classic heterophil-positive infectious mononucleosis, occasionally complicated by neurologic diseases, i.e., encephalitis or transverse myelitis
Erysipeloid	Acute, self-limiting skin infection most common in butchers, fishermen, and others who handle infected material
Erythrasma	Superficial, bacterial skin infection that usually affects the skin folds, especially in the groin, axillae, and toe webs
Eulenburg's disease: myotonia congenita, Thomsen's disease	Slowly progressive disease of the skeletal muscles; similar to muscular dystrophy
Extrapulmonary tuberculosis	Infectious disease that can affect any organ, but most commonly strikes the lymphatic system, meninges, genitourinary tract, pericardium, gastrointestinal tract, peritoneum, bones and joints, larynx, and the pleura
Fabry's disease	Extremely painful systemic disorder related to a deficiency in the enzyme alpha-galactosidase and characterized by glycolipid accumulations in body tissues
Fifth disease: erythema infectiosum	Contagious form of macula, showing rose-colored eruptions diffused over the skin.
File-cutters' disease	Lead poisoning from inhalation of particles of lead that arise during file cutting
Fish-skin disease	Condition of dry and scaly skin resembling fish skin; several forms, including vulgaris and lamellar

CAUSE	TREATMENT
Unknown	Symptomatic and supportive management
Viral infection	Symptomatic and supportive management
Congenital	Surgical management, if possible; otherwise, supportive management
Possible causes include sickle-cell anemia, tuberculosis, or obscure vasculitis	Treatment of underlying causes
Arthropod-borne virus or sequela of influenza, rubella, varicella, or vaccinia	Symptomatic management, including appropriate antibiotics for secondary infection
Inhalation of dust particles, causing irritation and inflammation of respiratory tract	Elimination of exposure to dust
Marked osteoclastic activity secondary to parathyroid hyperfunction, with calcium/phosphorus metabolic disturbances	Control of parathyroid hyperactivity
Endogenous and exogenous agents	Topical application of corticosteroids, bath oils, lubricants, and topical antibiotics for secondary infections
Tubercle bacillus, privet pollen, *Ascaris, Trichinella*	Antibiotics for secondary endocarditis or myocarditis
Epstein-Barr virus	Symptomatic management, including appropriate antibiotics; generally benign course
Erysipelothrix insidiosa transmitted by contact with infected meat, fish, poultry or animal hides, bones, or manure	Penicillin G or erythromycin
Corynebacterium minutissimum	Keratolytics; topical antibiotics
Transmitted as autosomal dominant trait	Treatment comparable to that for muscular dystrophy
Mycobacterium tuberculosis; extension of pulmonary tuberculosis to adjacent tissues	Isoniazid; ethambutol; rifampin
Transmitted as an X-linked recessive trait	Symptomatic management with low-dosage phenytoin or carbamazepine; possibly renal transplantation
Capillary congestion from dilatation of superficial capillaries caused by nerves, heat, sunburn, and general inflammation	Symptomatic treatment
Inhalation of lead particles	Avoidance of exposure to lead
Congenital	Effective treatment unknown

DISEASE	DEFINITION AND CHARACTERISTICS
Fish-slime disease	Rapidly progressive septicemia following a puncture wound by the spine of a fish
Flax-dresser's disease	Pulmonary disorder of flax-dressers
Flecked retina disease	Group of retinal disorders, including fundus flavimaculatus, fundus albipunctatus, drusen, and congenital macular degeneration; all may be primary abnormalities of retinal pigment epithelium.
Fleischner's disease	Inflammation of bone and cartilage affecting the middle phalanges of the hand
Frankl-Hochwart's disease: polyneuritis cerebralis menieriformis	Recurrent, progressive symptoms, including progressive deafness, ringing in the ears, dizziness, and a sensation of fullness/pressure in the ears; vertigo
Friedländer's disease: endarteritis obliterans	Chronic, progressive thickening of the intima, leading to stenosis or obstruction of the lumen
Friedreich's disease: paramyoclonus multiplex, Friedreich's ataxia	Tremors resembling those in multiple sclerosis, with evidence of cerebellar involvement of its pathways
Fürstner's disease: pseudospastic paralysis	Excessive tone and spasticity of muscles; exaggeration of tendon reflexes but loss of superficial reflexes; positive Babinski's reflex
Gensoul's disease: Ludwig's angina	Infection of the sublingual and submandibular spaces, characterized by brawny induration of the submaxillary region, edema of the sublingual floor of the mouth, and elevation of the tongue
Geotrichosis	Fungal infection affecting the mouth, throat, lungs, or intestines
Gerlier's disease: endemic paralytic vertigo, paralyzing vertigo	Nervous system disorder in farm workers and stable workers, marked by pain, vertigo, paresis, and muscle contractions
Gliomas of the optic nerve	Slow-growing tumor that causes progressive vision loss
Glossopharyngeal neuralgia	Disease of the ninth cranial (glossopharyngeal) nerve that produces paroxysms of pain in the ear, posterior pharynx, or base of the tongue or the jaws
Glucose-6-phosphate dehydrogenase (G6PD) deficiency	Deficiency of red blood cell enzyme, which causes anemia. Common in people of African or Mediterranean descent
Graefe's disease: ophthalmoplegia progressiva	Gradual paralysis of the eye, affecting first one eye muscle, then the other
Grinder's disease: pneumoconiosis	Permanent deposition of particles in the lungs
Habermann's disease	Sudden onset of a polymorphous skin eruption of macules, papules, and occasionally vesicles, with hemorrhage
Haff disease	Condition affecting fishermen of the Haff lagoon, which joins the Baltic Sea; characterized by severe pain in the extremities, with accompanying weakness and weariness with myoglobinuria
Hagner's disease	Obscure bone disease resembling acromegaly, associated with increased soft-tissue growth after puberty; increased metabolic rate, with increased sweating and sebaceous activity
Heavy-chain disease	Neoplasms of the lymphoplasmacytes, in which abnormal proliferation occurs among cells that produce immunoglobulins, causing incomplete heavy chains and no light chains in their molecular structure

CAUSE	TREATMENT
Septic substances introduced into blood through puncture wound	Supportive and symptomatic management of septicemia and secondary infections
Inhalation of flax particles	Avoidance of exposure to flax
Congenital	Supportive and symptomatic management
Unknown	Anti-inflammatory agents (including steroids in severe cases) and analgesics
Inflammation of the nerves (of the membranous labyrinth)	Bed rest and antihistamines
Trauma, pyogenic bacterial infection, infective thrombi, or syphilis	Endarterectomy
CNS damage secondary to trauma, or infection	Treatment of underlying disease
Lesions of upper motor neurons or cerebrum	Treatment of underlying disease
Usually abscesses of the second and third mandibular molars	Large doses of penicillin; significant airway obstruction may require tracheotomy.
Geotrichum candidum	Gentian violet for oral, throat, or intestinal infections; oral potassium iodide for pulmonary infections
Disease of the internal ear from pressure of cerumen on the drum membrane	Symptomatic management; scopolamine for combatting nausea
Unknown	Surgical excision; radiation therapy
Unknown	Surgery; carbamazepine; phenytoin
Transmitted as an X-linked trait	Transfusions
Usually secondary to brain lesions	Treatment of underlying disease, corrective lenses
Inhalation of dust particles	Irreversible pulmonary disease; eliminating exposure to dust particles can prevent further irritation of tissues.
Virus resembling smallpox	Supportive management; isolation may be necessary.
Arsenic poisoning from waste water of cellulose factories; by direct contact with or ingestion of fish that have been exposed to toxins	Supportive and symptomatic management
Growth hormone–secreting tumors that develop after puberty	Management of cardiovascular complications; surgery for large tumors and irradiation (proton beam or heavy particle treatment and supravoltage)
Possible causes include microorganisms and immune deficiency syndrome due to malnutrition or genetic predisposition.	Supportive and palliative management with chemotherapy, radiation therapy, antibiotics, and steroids

(continued)

DISEASE	DEFINITION AND CHARACTERISTICS
Heerfordt's disease: uveoparotid fever	Variant of sarcoidosis
Hemangioma of the eye	In children, tumors are not encapsulated, grow quickly in the first year, and then regress by about age 7. In adults, tumors are encapsulated.
Hemochromatosis: bronze diabetes, Recklinghausen-Applebaum disease	Disorder characterized by iron overload in parenchymal cells, leading to cirrhosis; diabetes; cardiomegaly with congestive heart failure and dysrhythmias; and increased skin pigmentation
Hemoglobin C–thalassemia disease	Simultaneous heterozygosity from hemoglobin C and thalassemia; characterized by mild hemolytic anemia and persistent splenomegaly
Henderson-Jones disease: osteochondromatosis	Presence of numerous benign cartilaginous tumors in the joint cavity or in the bursa of a tendon sheath
Hereditary spherocytosis	Anemia resulting in increased red blood cell membrane permeability and intracellular hypertonicity, characterized by slight jaundice, splenomegaly, and cholelithiasis
Heubner's disease	Syphilitic inflammation of tunica intima of cerebral arteries
Hodgson's disease	Aneurysmal dilatation of the proximal aorta, resulting in cardiac hypertrophy
Hoffa's disease	Proliferation of fatty tissue (solitary lipoma) in the knee joint
Huchard's disease	Chronic arterial hypertension
Hünermann's disease: dysplasia epiphysealis punctata	Failure of ossification of center in bone formation
Hutchinson-Gilford disease: progeria	Premature old age marked by small stature, wrinkled skin, and gray hair, with attitude and appearance of old age in very young children
Hutinel's disease	Tuberculous pericarditis, with cirrhosis of the liver in children
Hydatid disease	Hepatic infection marked by development of expanding cysts (hydatid cysts); cysticercosis by *Taenia solium*
Hydatid disease, alveolar	Invasion and destruction of tissue as endogenous budding of cysts form an aggregate over the affected organ—usually the liver—and may metastasize
Hydatid disease, unilocular	Infection causing marked formation of single or multiple unilocular cysts
Iceland disease: epidemic neuromyasthenia, benign myalgic encephalomyelitis	Marked by headaches, muscle pain, low-grade fever, lymphadenopathy, fatigue, and paresthesia; outbreaks occur in summer, usually in young women
Intestinal lymphangiectasia	Dilation and possible rupture of intestinal lymphatic vessels, resulting in hypoproteinemia and steatorrhea due to loss of fat and albumin into the intestinal lumen
Isambert's disease	Acute miliary tuberculosis of the larynx and pharynx

CAUSE	TREATMENT
Impaired regulation of thymus-derived lymphocytes (T cells) and bone marrow-derived lymphocytes (B cells)	Adrenal corticosteroids to suppress inflammation and control symptoms
Unknown	Surgical excision for adults. (Children need no treatment.)
Erythropoietic disorders, hepatic disorders that increase iron absorption, autosomal recessive inheritance	Phlebotomy to remove excess iron
Hereditary and congenital	Supportive management, including transfusions for severe anemia, and folate therapy
Irritation and trauma	Resection of tumor, with curettage and bone grafts
Transmitted as autosomal dominant trait	Splenectomy
Treponema pallidum	Supportive management, including antibiotic therapy
Degenerative process involving the elastic and muscular components of the medial layer; hypertension, aortic dissection, trauma	Surgery
Tissue trauma	Aspiration or surgery
Arteriosclerosis	Supportive management, including reduction of arterial pressure
Unknown	Supportive and symptomatic management
Acquired immunodeficiency; sarcoma meningiomas	No known treatment
Mycobacterium tuberculosis	Tuberculostatic agents
Ingestion of fish or meat contaminated by larvae of tapeworms of the genus *Echinococcus* or fecal-oral route of *Taenia solium*	Antilarval treatment with thiabendazole steroids
Infection by *Echinococcus multilocularis* (larvae)	Symptomatic management and surgery; usually fatal
Infestation by *Echinococcus granulosus* (larvae); hydatid tapeworm in dogs and cats	Symptomatic management; surgery
Infection probable but possibly psychosocial phenomenon	Symptomatic management
Congenital or may be acquired when obstruction, valvular heart disease, or constrictive pericarditis increases pressure on the lymphatics	No-fat diet; replacement of dietary sources of long-chain triglycerides with medium-chain triglycerides
Mycobacterium tuberculosis	Tuberculostatic agents

(continued)

RARE DISEASES *(continued)*

DISEASE	DEFINITION AND CHARACTERISTICS
Jaffe-Lichtenstein disease: cystic osteofibromatosis	Form of polyostotic fibrous dysplasia marked by an enlarged medullary cavity with a thin cortex, which is filled with fibrous tissue (fibroma)
Jakob-Creutzfeldt disease spastic pseudoparalysis, Creutzfeldt-Jakob syndrome:	Rapidly progressive dementia developing between ages 40 and 65; accompanied by neurologic symptoms, such as myoclonic jerking, ataxia, aphasia, visual disturbances, and paralysis. EEG is abnormal early, with a distinct pattern useful for diagnosis.
Jaksch's disease: anemia pseudoleukemica infantum	Syndrome of anisocytosis, peripheral red blood cell immaturity, leukocytosis, and hepatosplenomegaly that usually occurs in children under age 3
Jansen's disease: metaphyseal dysostosis	Skeletal abnormality with nearly normal epiphyses in which the metaphyseal tissues are replaced by masses of cartilage
Jensen's disease: retinochoroiditis juxtapapillaris	Inflammation of the retina and choroid marked by small inflammatory areas on the fundus close to the papilla
Juvenile angiofibroma	Highly vascular, nasopharyngeal tumor that causes nasal obstruction and severe recurrent epistaxis
Keratoconus	Degenerative eye disorder typified by thinning and anterior protrusion of the cornea
Kienböck's disease: (1) lunatomalacia, (2) traumatic syringomyelia	(1) Slowly progressive osteochondrosis of the semilunar (carpal lunate) bone from avascular necrosis; (2) cavity formation in the spinal cord
Kirkland's disease	Acute throat infection, with regional lymphadenitis
Knight's disease	Perianal infection following skin abrasion (so called because of prevalence in equestrians)
Köhler's bone disease: tarsal scaphoiditis, epiphysitis juvenilis	Osteochondrosis of the tarsal navicular bone in children; onset about age 5
Krabbe's disease: globoid cell leukodystrophy	Rapidly progressive cerebral demyelination, with large globoid bodies in the white matter, associated with irritability, rigidity, tonic seizures, convulsions, blindness, deafness, and progressive mental deterioration
Kugelberg-Welander disease: juvenile progressive muscular atrophy	Slowly progressive muscular atrophy resulting from lesions of the anterior horns of the spinal cord; usual onset in preschool or adolescent years
Kümmell's disease: posttraumatic spondylitis	Intercostal neuralgia, with spinal pain and motor disturbances in the legs
Kuru	Chronic, progressive, and fatal neurologic disease found only in New Guinea
Kyrle's disease	Form of follicular disease marked by keratotic pegs in the hair follicles and eccrine ducts, penetrating the epidermis and extending into the corium, causing foreign-body reaction and pain
Larsen's disease: Larsen-Johansson disease	Accessory center of ossification within the patella, associated with flat facies and short metacarpals
Leiner's disease: erythroderma desquamativum	Generalized exfoliative dermatitis and erythroderma, chiefly affecting newborn breast-fed infants; probably identical to severe seborrheic dermatitis

CAUSE	TREATMENT
May be a lipoid granuloma	Symptomatic and supportive management; surgerv
Probably related to a latent virus; may be dependent on genetically determined susceptibility to a common agent, common environment, or familial dietary habits	Effective treatment unknown; symptomatic and supportive management that establishes a protective environment; invariably fatal
Malnutrition, chronic infection, malabsorption, hemoglobinopathies	Treatment of underlying causes
Unknown	Surgery
Unknown; probably an autoimmune process	Steroids may induce improvements.
Unknown	Surgery
Transmitted as an autosomal recessive trait	Hard contact lenses or glasses with high astigmatic correction; corneal transplant may be necessary.
(1) Degenerative process, precipitated by trauma; (2) trauma	(1) Immobilization of wrist for several months; if ineffective, surgery; (2) possibly surgery
Unknown	Appropriate antibiotics and symptomatic management
Trauma	Symptomatic management
Unknown but trauma suspected	Protection of foot from excessive use or trauma. If pain is severe, plaster cast may be required for 6 to 8 weeks. Complete spontaneous recovery may occur.
Familial	Symptomatic management; death by age 2
Transmitted as autosomal recessive or dominant trait	Supportive management; normal life span probable
Compression fracture of the vertebrae	Management of fracture; extension of spine
Slow virus thought to be associated with cannibalism	No effective treatment; invariably fatal
Unknown	Symptomatic management
Unknown	Supportive management; surgery
Allergic, hereditary, and psychogenic causes suspected	Symptomatic management

(continued)

RARE DISEASES *(continued)*

DISEASE	DEFINITION AND CHARACTERISTICS
Leishmaniasis	Group of infectious disorders: Old World and New World cutaneous leishmaniasis are self-limiting; kala-azar and New World mucocutaneous leishmaniasis are sometimes fatal.
Lenegre's disease	Acquired complete heart block
Leptospirosis	Infectious disease that causes such things as meningitis, hepatitis, nephritis, or febrile disease. May be mild (anicteric) or severe (icteric or Weil's disease)
Lesch-Nyhan syndrome	Disorder of purine metabolism marked by mental and physical retardation, spastic cerebral palsy, and compulsive self-mutilation of fingers and lips by biting; hyperuricemia and excessive uricaciduria
Letterer-Siwe disease: nonlipid reticuloendotheliosis	Hemorrhagic tendency, with eczematoid skin eruptions, lymph node enlargement, hepatosplenomegaly, and progressive anemia
Lewandowsky-Lutz disease	Widespread red or red-violet lesions resembling verruca plana, having a tendency to become malignant
Lichtheim's disease	Subacute degeneration of the spinal cord, associated with pernicious anemia
Little's disease	Form of cerebral spastic paralysis and stiffness of the limbs, associated with muscle weakness, convulsions, bilateral athetosis, and mental deficiencies
Lung fluke disease: *Paragonimus westermani, Paragonimus heterotrema*	Parasitic hemoptysis, or oriental hemoptysis from pulmonary cysts
MacLean-Maxwell disease	Chronic condition of the calcaneus, marked by enlargement of the posterior third and by sensitivity to pressure
Macroglobulinemia: Waldenström's macroglobulinemia	Neoplastic disease of plasma and lymphoid cells that produces IgM antibodies. May be asymptomatic or have diverse signs and symptoms
Magitot's disease	Osteoperiostitis of the alveoli of the teeth
Malibu disease: surfers' nodules	Hyperplastic, fibrosing granulomas occurring over bony prominences of the feet and legs of surfers
Malignant melanoma of the eye	Malignant tumor stemming from the melanocytes in the uvea, retina, or iris
Maple syrup urine disease	Enzyme defect in the metabolism of the branched chain amino acids, resulting in mental and physical retardation, feeding difficulties, and a characteristic odor of urine
Marburg disease: Marburg virus disease	Severe viral disease, characterized by skin lesions, conjunctivitis, enteritis, hepatitis, encephalitis, and renal failure
Marie-Strümpell disease: Bekhterev's disease, rheumatoid spondylitis	Progressive immobility of sacroiliac joints, paravertebral soft tissues, and spinal articulations; most prevalent in males, ages 10 to 30
Marie-Tooth disease	Progressive neuropathic (peroneal) muscular atrophy
Marion's disease	Obstruction of the posterior urethra resulting from muscular hypertrophy of the bladder neck or absence of the flexiform dilator fibers
Martin's disease	Periosteoarthritis of the foot
Maxcy's disease	Rickettsial infection endemic in southeastern United States

CAUSE	TREATMENT
Leishmania transmitted by sand fly bites	Antimony sodium gluconate, cycloguanil pamoate, or amphotericin B
Primary degeneration of the conduction system	Artificial pacemaker; supportive management
Leptospira transmitted by contact with water, soil, food, or vegetation contaminated with urine from an infected lower mammal	Penicillin, tetracycline, or erythromycin
Defective enzyme transmitted by female carriers as sex-linked recessive trait	Symptomatic and supportive management, including protective restraints; usually fatal in childhood
Probably transmitted as autosomal recessive trait	Symptomatic and supportive treatment of anemia
Virus identical to or closely related to the virus of common warts	No effective treatment
Vitamin B_{12} deficiency	Correction of vitamin B_{12} deficiency
Congenital; birth trauma, fetal anoxia, or maternal illness during pregnancy	Preventive measures and symptomatic management
Infestation by trematodes or flukes	Parasitotropic agents; symptomatic and supportive management of hemoptysis
Trauma	Supportive shoes; avoidance of prolonged standing; surgery
Unknown, but genetic predisposition suspected	Alkylating agents, such as chlorambucil, cyclophosphamide, or melphalan. Asymptomatic patients need no specific therapy.
Usually secondary to gingivitis	Steroid therapy for extreme inflammation; antibiotics for secondary infection
Repeated trauma from surfboard	Supportive shoes; avoidance of prolonged standing
Unknown	Surgical excision; eye enucleation
Transmitted as autosomal recessive trait	Supportive management
Exposure to African green monkeys	Symptomatic and supportive management; usually fatal
Unknown; hereditary predisposition possible	Management to suppress pain and inflammation; supportive maintenance of a functional posture
Unknown	Surgery
Congenital	Surgery
Trauma, excessive walking	Supportive shoes; avoidance of prolonged standing
Rickettsieae	Treatment of underlying disease

(continued)

RARE DISEASES *(continued)*

DISEASE	DEFINITION AND CHARACTERISTICS
Medullary cystic disease: familial juvenile nephronophthisis	Congenital renal disorder marked by cyst formation, primarily in the medulla and the corticomedullary junction
Megaloblastic anemia	Complication of pregnancy, resulting from folic acid deficiency that alters the nucleic acid production needed for erythrocyte maturation in bone marrow
Meyer-Betz disease: idiopathic, spontaneous, or familial myoglobinuria	Myoglobinuria, which may be precipitated by strenuous exertion or possibly by infection, and marked by tenderness, swelling, and muscle weakness
Microdrepanocytic disease	Sickle-cell thalassemia; anemia involving simultaneous heterozygosity for hemoglobin and thalassemia
Milroy's disease	Chronic lymphatic obstruction, causing lymphedema of the legs; sometimes associated with edema of the arms, trunk, and face
Minamata disease	Severe neurologic disorder characterized by peripheral and circumoral paresthesia, ataxia, mental disabilities, and loss of peripheral vision
Minor's disease	Hematomyelia, involving the central parts of the spinal cord; marked by sudden onset of flaccid paralysis, with sensory disturbances
Morton's toe: metatarsalgia	Metatarsal pain
Mozer's disease: myelosclerosis	Sclerosis of the spinal cord; obliteration of the normal marrow cavity by the formation of small spicules of bone
Mule spinner's disease	Warts or ulcers, especially on the scrotum, that tend to become malignant; common among operators of spinning mules in cotton mills
Mushroom picker's disease	Allergic respiratory disease of persons working with moldy compost prepared for growing mushrooms
Mycetoma: maduromycosis, Madura foot	Chronic infection of the skin, subcutaneous tissues, and bone, usually affecting the foot
Niemann-Pick disease	Metabolic disorder resulting in abnormal accumulation of sphingomyelin in reticuloendothelial cells. Most common in those of Eastern European Jewish ancestry, it occurs in five different phenotypes, each with slightly different symptoms.
Norrie's disease: atrophia bulborum hereditaria	Bilateral blindness resulting from retinal malformation, with mental retardation and deafness
Olivopontocerebellar atrophy	Progressively deteriorating neurologic disease marked by ataxia, dysarthria, and an action tremor that develops late in middle life; often mistaken for mental illness; usually normal deep tendon reflexes; associated with occasional rigidity and other extrapyramidal signs
Opitz's disease	Thrombophlebitic splenomegaly
Otto's disease: arthrokatadysis	Osteoarthritic protrusion of the acetabulum
Owren's disease: parahemophilia	Rare hemorrhagic tendency resulting from deficiency of coagulation Factor V
Paas's disease	Familial disorder marked by skeletal deformities, such as coxa valga, shortening of phalanges, scoliosis, and spondylitis
Paracoccidioidomycosis: South American blastomycosis	Fungal infection of the skin, lungs, mucous membranes, lymphatics, and viscera, seen primarily in the tropical forests of Colombia, Venezuela, and Brazil

CAUSE	TREATMENT
Transmitted as autosomal recessive or dominant trait	Symptomatic management; transplantation or dialysis
Pregnancy, which increases demand for folic acid. Predisposing factors may include poor diet and overcooking of food.	Folic acid with iron supplement; diet high in vitamins and protein
Unknown; familial tendencies possible	Bed rest; anti-inflammatory agents; steroids in extreme cases; analgesics for pain
Hereditary transmission	Management of anemia
Congenital and hereditary	Surgery
Alkyl mercury poisoning	Avoidance of causative agents; supportive and symptomatic management; usually fatal
Unknown	Treatment of underlying disease; supportive management
Abnormality of the foot, or osteochondrosis	Supportive shoes; analgesics
Unknown	Surgery
Unknown	Surgery
Airborne irritant, usually mold	Supportive and symptomatic management
Allescheria boydii or an *Actinomycetales* bacteria	Sulfonamides; or penicillin or tetracycline
Transmitted as autosomal recessive disorder	Supportive and symptomatic management; possibly splenectomy
Transmitted as X-linked trait	Unknown
Transmitted as autosomal or recessive trait	No effective treatment; death usually follows pneumonia secondary to loss of cough reflex.
Thrombosis of the splenic vein	Symptomatic and supportive management, including anticoagulation
Degenerative changes, probably hereditary	Surgery, if night traction and rest ineffective
Transmitted as autosomal recessive trait	Supportive management
Hereditary	Unknown
Paracoccidioides brasiliensis	Long-term sulfonamide therapy; amphotericin B

(continued)

RARE DISEASES *(continued)*

DISEASE	DEFINITION AND CHARACTERISTICS
Paroxysmal nocturnal hemoglobinuria	Acquired abnormality in red blood cell membrane that increases susceptibility to lytic action of normal plasma components
Patella's disease	Pyloric stenosis, following fibrous stenosis in patients with tuberculosis
Pearl-worker's disease	Recurrent inflammation of bone, with hypertrophy
Pelizaeus-Merzbacher disease: sudanophilic leukodystrophy	Hyperplastic centrolobar sclerosis marked by nystagmus, ataxia, tremors, choreoathetotic movements, parkinsonian facies, and mental deterioration; begins early in life, predominantly in males
Pellegrini's disease: Pellegrini-Stieda disease, Köhler-Pellegrini-Stieda disease	Semilunar bony formation in the upper portion of the medial lateral ligament of the knee
Pemphigus	Chronic blistering disease that causes superficial and deep lesions. Pemphigus vulgaris, the most common form of this disease, can be fatal.
Perrin-Ferraton disease	Snapping hip
Plaster-of-Paris disease	Limb atrophy after prolonged enclosure in a plaster splint
Pneumatic hammer disease	Vasospastic disease of the hands
Poncet's disease	Rheumatic symptoms associated with tuberculosis
Pulseless disease	Progressive obliteration of the brachiocephalic trunk and the left subclavian and left common carotid arteries above their origin on the aortic arch (loss of pulse in both arms)
Purtscher's disease	Retinal angiopathy, with edema, hemorrhage, and exudation
Q fever	Acute systemic disease that strikes people who are exposed to cattle, sheep, or goats
Rat-bite fever	Gram-negative bacterial infection that occurs 1 to 3 weeks after bite from an infected rat or mouse
Recklinghausen's disease of bone: osteitis fibrosa cystica	Presence of fibrous nodules on affected bones
Refsum's disease	Defect in metabolism of phytanic acid, marked by chronic polyneuritis, retinitis pigmentosa, and cerebellar signs (mild ataxia) with persistent elevation of protein in cerebrospinal fluid
Retinoblastoma	Tumor arising from retinal gum cells. Most common eye tumor in children
Rhabdomyosarcoma	Rapidly growing mass on inner part of upper eyelid, causing restricted eye movement without vision loss
Rhinosporidiosis	Fungal infection producing painless, vascularized, friable, and often large, tumorlike lesions. Most common in Ceylon and India
Rickettsialpox	Mild self-limiting disease characterized by lesions and fever
Ritter's disease	Dermatitis exfoliativa neonatorum
Robles' disease	Onchocerciasis of the fibroid nodules, lymph, subcutaneous connective tissue, and eyes
Roger's disease	Presence of small asymptomatic ventricular septal defects
Rummo's disease: Wenckebach's disease	Downward displacement of the heart (cardioptosis)

CAUSE	TREATMENT
Infection, immunization, iron administration, aplastic anemia, or leukemia	Transfusions
Secondary to tuberculosis	Surgery
Inhalation of pearl dust	Avoidance of exposure to pearl dust
Familial transmission as a sex-linked recessive trait	No effective treatment; invariably fatal in several years
Trauma	Surgical correction; supportive management
Unknown	Corticosteroids; immunosuppressives
Unknown	No effective treatment
Prolonged immobilization	Removal of cast; use or exercise of the affected limb
Prolonged trauma from use of pneumatic hammer	Avoidance of trauma
Mycobacterium tuberculosis	Tuberculostatic agents
Arteriosclerosis; loss of pulse in both arms	Surgery
Trauma—usually a crushing injury to the chest	Treatment of underlying injury and supportive management
Coxiella burnetii	Tetracycline or chloramphenicol
Streptobacillus moniliformis or *Spirillum minor*	Penicillin G procaine, tetracycline, or streptomycin
Marked osteoclastic activity secondary to parathyroid hyperfunction	Control of parathyroid hyperfunction
Hereditary transmission as autosomal recessive trait	Symptomatic and supportive management
Transmitted as autosomal dominant trait	Enucleation; radiation therapy
Unknown	Radiation therapy; surgical excision
Rhinosporidium seeberi	Electrocauterization or surgical excision
Rickettsia akari transmitted by bites of mites carried by infected mice	Tetracycline or chloramphenicol; antipyretics; analgesics; increased fluid intake
Unknown	Unknown
Onchocerca volvulus	Parasitotropic agents
Congenital	Surgery, if defects become symptomatic
Probably congenital	Unknown

(continued)

DISEASE	DEFINITION AND CHARACTERISTICS
Rust's disease	Tuberculous spondylitis of the cervical vertebrae
Sacroiliac disease	Chronic inflammation of the sacroiliac joint, associated with tuberculosis
Schanz's disease	Inflammation of the Achilles tendon
Schilder's disease: leukoencephalopathy	Diffuse degeneration of the brain in infancy or adolescence, characterized by loss of myelin and progressive loss of cerebral function, leading to spasticity, optic neuritis, blindness, and dementia
Scholz's disease: leukoencephalopathy	Demyelination of the white substance of the brain, producing sensory aphasia, cortical blindness, deafness, weakness, spasticity of the limbs, and eventually complete paralysis and dementia
Schridde's disease	Generalized edema; abnormal accumulation of serous fluid in the cellular tissue or in a body cavity
Sever's disease	Epiphysitis of the calcaneus
Shuttlemaker's disease	Faintness, shortness of breath, headaches, and nausea
Silo-filler's disease	Pulmonary inflammation, often associated with acute pulmonary edema
Smith-Strang disease	Defective methionine absorption, resulting in white hair, mental retardation, convulsions, attacks of hyperpnea, and characteristic odor of urine
Soft-tissue sarcoma	Soft-tissue malignancy of muscle, fat, connective tissue, blood vessels, and synovium, composed of tightly packed cells similar to embryonic connective tissue
Sponge-diver's disease	Burning, itching, erythema, necrosis, and ulceration of skin common in Mediterranean divers
Stargardt's disease	Degeneration of the macula lutea, marked by rapid loss of visual activity and abnormal appearance and pigmentation of the macular area
Strümpell-Leichtenstern disease: hemorrhagic encephalitis	Lateral sclerosis, in which spasticity is limited to the legs
Swediaur's disease: Schwediauer's disease	Inflammation of the calcaneal bursa
Tangier disease	Deficiency of high-density lipoprotein in the serum, with storage of cholesterol esters in the tonsils and other tissues
Tarabagan disease	Plague in humans
Thiemann's disease	Vascular necrosis of the phalangeal epiphysis, resulting in deformity of the interphalangeal joints
Thomson's disease: Rothmund-Thomson syndrome	Developmental hyperkeratotic lesions and xerodermatous changes
Tommaselli's disease	Pyrexia and hematuria
Toxocariasis: visceral larva migrans, VLM	Chronic, frequently mild syndrome common in children, involving roundworm migration from the intestine to various organs and tissues

CAUSE	TREATMENT
Mycobacterium tuberculosis	Tuberculostatic agents
Mycobacterium tuberculosis	Tuberculostatic agents
Trauma	Symptomatic management with anti-inflammatory agents, steroids, analgesics
Unknown; possibly familial	Symptomatic and supportive management; invariably fatal
Transmitted as X-linked recessive trait	Symptomatic and supportive management
Congenital	Management of fluid and electrolyte balance; symptomatic and supportive management
Inflammation secondary to trauma, irritation	Treatment of underlying cause
Inhalation of wood dust	Supportive respiratory management; avoidance of exposure to wood dust
Inhalation of oxides of nitrogen and other gases that collect in silos	Supportive respiratory management; avoidance of exposure to silo gases
Transmitted as autosomal recessive trait	Unknown
Unknown	Surgical resection; radiation therapy; chemotherapy
Irritation by toxins of sea anemones of the *Sagartia* and *Actinia* genera	Symptomatic management, with local application of calamine lotion and treatment with antihistamines for hives and itching
Hereditary transmission	Corrective lenses as symptomatic treatment; supportive management
Hereditary transmission	Supportive management
Irritation of bursa	Symptomatic management, with application of warm moist heat, anti-inflammatory agents, and analgesics
Excessive cholesterol intake	Reduction of serum cholesterol levels
Bite of an ectoparasite of the Mongolian marmot (tarabagan)	Parasitotropic agent
Familial tendency	Unknown
Hereditary transmission	Unknown
Quinine toxicity	Discontinue quinine; symptomatic and supportive management
Ingestion of *Toxocara* larvae	Thiabendazole; diethylcarbamazine citrate

(continued)

RARE DISEASES *(continued)*

DISEASE	DEFINITION AND CHARACTERISTICS
Trench fever: Wolhynia fever, shin bone fever, His-Werner disease, quintana fever	Self-limiting illness occuring sporadically in Eastern Europe, Asia, North Africa, and Mexico, and producing multiple symptoms
Trevor's disease	Dysplasia epiphysealis hemimelica
Trichuriasis: whipworm disease	Nematode infection of the cecum and the anterior parts of the large intestine, producing various gastrointestinal effects
Tropical sprue	Gastrointestinal disorder that causes atrophy of the small intestine and produces malabsorption, malnutrition, and folic acid deficiency. It occurs mainly in Puerto Rico, Cuba, Haiti, Hong Kong, and India.
Tularemia: deer fly fever, rabbit fever, Ohara's disease (in Japan)	Acute, gram-negative infection that has five forms—ulceroglandular, oculoglandular, typhoidal (enteric), oropharyngeal (pneumonic), and glandular—each with varying symptoms
Typhus, endemic: murine, rat, or flea typhus	Mild form of typhus, causing systemic illness
Typhus, epidemic: European, classic, or louse-borne typhus	Acute systemic illness that may lead to death
Typhus, scrub: Japanese river or flood fever, tsutsugamushi fever	Acute systemic disease occuring almost exclusively in the western Pacific, Japan, and Southeast Asia
Tyrosinemia	*Hereditary form:* results in liver failure and renal tubular failure, hypoglycemia, rickets, darkening of the skin, and mild mental retardation; occasionally causes liver cancer *Transient form:* usually in premature newborns, marked by elevation of blood tyrosine
Tyzzer's disease	Necrotic lesions of liver and intestine
Verneuil's disease	Syphilitic disease of the bursae
Vidal's disease	Lichen simplex chronicus; pruritic, discrete, confluent, lichenoid, papular eruptions
Volkmann's disease	Tibiotarsal dislocation, causing deformity of the foot
Von Hippel-Lindau disease	Phakomatosis characterized by angiomatosis of the retina, cerebellum, spinal cord, and less commonly cysts of the pancreas, kidneys, and other viscera; onset usually in third decade and marked by symptoms of retina or cerebral tumors
Wegner's disease	Osteochondritic separation of the epiphyses
Werdnig-Hoffmann paralysis: progressive muscular atrophy of infancy	Progressive degeneration of anterior horn cells and bulbar motor nuclei in a fetus or infant. Onset marked by hypotonia, with abducted and externally rotated hips and flexed knees; reflexes absent. Later marked by accessory use of respiratory muscles
Whipple's disease: intestinal lipodystrophy, lipophagia granulomatosis	Gastrointestinal disorder characterized by chronic diarrhea and progressive wasting
White-spot disease: lichen sclerosus et atrophicus	Characterized by irregular flat-topped papules with keratotic plugging. Often asymptomatic but may cause itching, soreness, and atrophy, especially in genital areas

CAUSE	TREATMENT
Rochalimaea quintana transmitted by body lice	Analgesics; antipyretics; delousing with lindane or other pediculicide
Unknown	Unknown
Ingestion of food contaminated with nematoid ova	Mebendazole
Unknown	Tetracycline or oxytetracycline; phthalysulfathiazole; diphenoxylate with atropine sulfate
Francisella tularensis transmitted by contact with secretions of an infected animal; bite of a tick, deer fly, or flea that feeds on these animals; or ingestion of contaminated water or meat	Streptomycin, kanamycin, or gentamicin
Rickettsia typhi transmitted by bites of infected fleas or lice, or by inhalation of contaminated flea feces	Tetracycline, doxycycline, or chloramphenicol; analgesics; antipyretics
Rickettsia prowazekii transmitted by *Pediculus humanus*	Tetracycline, doxycycline, or chloramphenicol; analgesics; antipyretics; delousing with lindane or other pediculicide
Rickettsia tsutsugamushi transmitted by mite larvae	Chloramphenicol or tetracycline
Autosomal recessive trait, resulting in excess of tyrosine in blood and urine	Tyrosine restriction; liver transplant may be successful; otherwise, fatal early in childhood
Bacillus piliformis transmitted through contact with rodents or dogs	Symptomatic management and appropriate antibiotics
Treponema pallidum	Early treatment of syphilis
Psychogenic origin suspected	Unknown
Congenital	Surgery
Transmitted as autosomal dominant trait	Early surgical intervention
Congenital syphilis	Effective treatment of syphilis during pregnancy
Transmitted as autosomal recessive trait	Symptomatic and supportive management; no effective treatment. Death usually occurs in a year, but if disease is limited to legs, progression is slower.
Unknown	Penicillin G procaine; streptomycin; tetracycline; corticosteroids
Unknown but often associated with white females; some familial incidence	Symptomatic management

(continued)

RARE DISEASES *(continued)*

DISEASE	DEFINITION AND CHARACTERISTICS
Wilms' tumor: congenital nephroblastoma, embryonal adenomyosarcoma	Malignant mixed tumors of the kidneys, primarily affecting children. Major signs are abdominal mass, enlarged abdomen, hypertension, and vomiting.
Witkop's disease: Witkop-Von Sallmann disease	Benign intraepithelial dyskeratosis affecting the oral mucosa and bulbar conjunctiva
Wolman's disease	Xanthomatosis in infants; associated with calcification of the adrenal glands, failure to thrive, vomiting, diarrhea, hepatomegaly, splenomegaly, and foam cells in skin lesions and bone marrow
Yaws: frambesia tropica	Chronic relapsing infection characterized by lesions and systemic signs and symptoms
Yellow fever	Arbovirus infection that causes sudden illness accompanied by fever, slow pulse rate, and headache. Endemic in tropical Africa and Central and South America
Zygomycosis: phycomycosis; mucormycosis	Fungal infection most often seen in immunocompromised patients. Several forms exist: rhinocerebral, gastrointestinal, pulmonary, and disseminated mucormycosis.

CAUSE	TREATMENT
Unknown	Surgery; radiation therapy; chemotherapy
Hereditary	No effective treatment; symptomatic management depending on severity
Transmitted as autosomal recessive trait	No known treatment; invariably fatal
Treponema pertenue	Penicillin in aluminum monostearate 2%, oxytetracycline, or chlortetracycline
Arbovirus transmitted by the *Aedes* mosquito	High-protein, high-carbohydrate liquid diet; analgesics; sedatives; antipyretics; bed rest
Zygomycetes	Amphotericin B; surgery

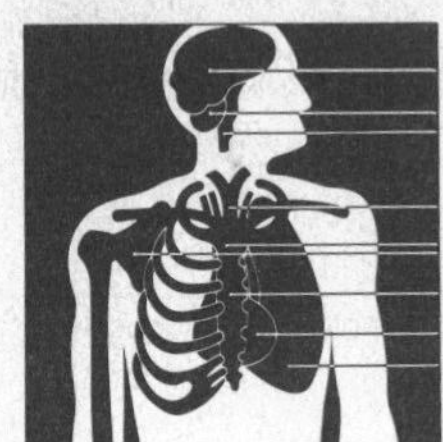

Acknowledgments

p. 9 Ashley Montagu, *The Elephant Man, A Study in Human Dignity.* New York: E.P. Dutton, 1979.

p. 10 © Carroll H. Weiss, RBP, 1980.

p. 23 (upper right) © Carroll H. Weiss, RBP, 1973.

p. 55 Paul A. Cohen.

p. 66 © Carroll H. Weiss, RBP, 1980.

p. 95 Photo courtesy: Roswell Park Memorial Institute, Department of Urologic Oncology, Buffalo.

p. 117 © Carroll H. Weiss, RBP, 1980.

p. 118 © Carroll H. Weiss, RBP, 1980.

p. 123 (upper right) © Carroll H. Weiss, RBP, 1980.

p. 123 (lower right) © Carroll H. Weiss, RBP, 1980.

p. 151 Photo courtesy: Ivan L. Roth, University of Georgia, Athens.

p. 155 Photo courtesy: Ivan L. Roth, University of Georgia, Atlanta.

p. 182 Photo courtesy: Centers for Disease Control, Atlanta.

p. 184 © Alfred T. Lamme, 1973.

p. 194 © Carroll H. Weiss, RBP, 1978.

p. 203 © Carroll H. Weiss, RBP, 1980.

p. 217 © Carroll H. Weiss, RBP, 1980.

p. 229 Photo courtesy: Centers for Disease Control, Atlanta.

p. 233 © Carroll H. Weiss, RBP, 1976.

p. 258 American College of Surgeons, Committee on Trauma, *Prophylaxis against Tetanus in Wound Management,* April 1984.

p. 280 © Camera MD Studios, Inc., 1980.

p. 290 Photo courtesy: *Consultant Magazine,* Greenwich, Conn.: Cliggott Publishing Co., 1972.

p. 297 © Carroll H. Weiss, RBP, 1980.

p. 302 Tom McHugh/Photo Researchers.

p. 303 Photo courtesy: *Consultant Magazine,* Greenwich, Conn.: Cliggott Publishing Co., 1971.

p. 305 © Carroll H. Weiss, RBP, 1980.

p. 339 © Carroll H. Weiss, RBP, 1980.

p. 527 © Carroll H. Weiss, RBP, 1980.

p. 531 © Carroll H. Weiss, RBP, 1980.

p. 547 Photo courtesy: Eleanor M. Brower, RN, and Clyde L. Nash, Jr., MD, St. Luke's Hospital Spine Center, Cleveland.

p. 573 © Robert Ford, RBP, 1976.

p. 582 Photo courtesy: Lucy Rorke, MD, Children's Hospital, Philadelphia.

p. 630 © Carroll H. Weiss, RBP, 1980.

p. 654 Photo courtesy: Marc S. Lapayowker, MD, Temple University Hospital, Philadelphia.

p. 670 Photo courtesy: Marc S. Lapayowker, MD, Temple University Hospital, Philadelphia.

p. 712 © Carroll H. Weiss, RBP, 1973.

p. 787 Photo courtesy: *Consultant Magazine,* Greenwich, Conn.: Cliggott Publishing Co., 1977.

p. 792 Photo courtesy: *Consultant Magazine,* Greenwich, Conn.: Cliggott Publishing Co., 1974.

p. 830 Photo courtesy: *Consultant Magazine,* Greenwich, Conn.: Cliggott Publishing Co., 1974.

p. 833 Photos courtesy: *Consultant Magazine,* Greenwich, Conn.: Cliggott Publishing Co., 1975.

p. 835 © Robert Ford, RBP, 1976.

p. 852 © Carroll H. Weiss, RBP, 1980.

p. 866 Photo courtesy: Majorie Beyers and Susan Dudas, *The Clinical Practice of Medical-Surgical Nursing.* Boston: Little, Brown & Co., 1977. Ron Hurst, Photographer.

p. 867 Photo courtesy: Marjorie Beyers and Susan Dudas, *The Clinical Practice of Medical-Surgical Nursing.* Boston: Little, Brown & Co., 1977. Ron Hurst, Photographer.

p. 918 Photo courtesy: Sharon R. Reeder, et al., *Maternity Nursing.* Philadelphia: J.B. Lippincott Co., 1976.

p. 959 Photo courtesy: Centers for Disease Control, Atlanta.

p. 961 Adapted from microscopic photos. Abbott Laboratories.

p. 964 Photo courtesy: Centers for Disease Control, Atlanta.

p. 1014 © Carroll H. Weiss, RBP, 1980.

p. 1015 © Carroll H. Weiss, RBP, 1980.

p. 1062 Photo courtesy: Peter G. Lavine, MD, Crozer-Chester Medical Center, Chester, Pa.

p. 1099 Paul A. Cohen.

p. 1123 © Muriel Laban Nussbaum, 1977.

p. 1126 © Carroll H. Weiss, RBP, 1980.

p. 1130 © Carroll H. Weiss, RBP, 1980.

p. 1131 Photo courtesy: Heather Boyd-Monk, RN, Wills Eye Hospital, Philadelphia.

p. 1133 Photo courtesy: Wills Eye Hospital, Philadelphia.

p. 1150 © Tom Merrill, 1977.

p. 1154 © Muriel Laban Nussbaum, 1977.

p. 1179 Photo courtesy: *Consultant Magazine,* Greenwich, Conn.: Cliggott Publishing Co., 1978.

p. 1203 © Carroll H. Weiss, RBP, 1980.

p. 1208 © Carroll H. Weiss, RBP, 1980.

p. 1210 Photo courtesy: Evelina A. Bernardino, MD, Dermatology Department, St. Mary Hospital, Langhorne, Pa.

p. 1211 © Christopher Papa, MD, 1978.

p. 1212 © Carroll H. Weiss, RBP, 1980.

p. 1213 (upper right) © Carroll H. Weiss, RBP, 1980.

p. 1213 (lower right) Photo courtesy: Reed and Carnrick, Kenilworth, N.J.

p. 1214 Photos courtesy: Reed and Carnrick, Kenilworth, N.J.

p. 1221 © Carroll H. Weiss, RBP, 1980.

p. 1224 © Carroll H. Weiss, RBP, 1977, 1980.

p. 1226 © Carroll H. Weiss, RBP, 1978, 1980.

p. 1232 © Carroll H. Weiss, RBP, 1980.

Index

Boldface page numbers indicate major entries; i refers to an illustration, t to a table.

Boldface page numbers indicate major entries; i refers to an illustration, t to a table.

Boldface page numbers indicate major entries; i refers to an illustration, t to a table.

B

C

Boldface page numbers indicate major entries; i refers to an illustration, t to a table.

Boldface page numbers indicate major entries; i refers to an illustration, t to a table.

Boldface page numbers indicate major entries; i refers to an illustration, t to a table.

D

Boldface page numbers indicate major entries; i refers to an illustration, t to a table.

Boldface page numbers indicate major entries; i refers to an illustration, t to a table.

Boldface page numbers indicate major entries; i refers to an illustration, t to a table.

F

G

H

I

Boldface page numbers indicate major entries; i refers to an illustration, t to a table.

J

K

L

Boldface page numbers indicate major entries; i refers to an illustration, t to a table.

M

Boldface page numbers indicate major entries; i refers to an illustration, t to a table.

O

P

Boldface page numbers indicate major entries; i refers to an illustration, t to a table.

Boldface page numbers indicate major entries; i refers to an illustration, t to a table.

Boldface page numbers indicate major entries; i refers to an illustration, t to a table.

S

Boldface page numbers indicate major entries; i refers to an illustration, t to a table.

T

Boldface page numbers indicate major entries; i refers to an illustration, t to a table.

U

W

X

Y

Z

SOURCES OF MORE INFORMATION AND HELP

ALCOHOLISM

Al-Anon Family Group Headquarters, 1372 Broadway, New York, N.Y. 10018; (212) 302-7240
Alateen World Service Headquarters, 1372 Broadway, New York, N.Y. 10018; (212) 302-7240
General Service Board of Alcoholics Anonymous (AA), 468 Park Ave., S., New York, N.Y., 10016, (212) 686-1100

ANOREXIA NERVOSA

Anorexia Nervosa and Associated Disorders (ANAD), Box 7, Highland Park, Ill. 60035; (312) 831-3438

ARTHRITIS

Arthritis Foundation (AF), 1314 Spring St., N.W., Atlanta, Ga. 30309; (404) 872-7100
American Rheumatism Association (ARA), c/o AF

AUTISM

National Society for Autistic Children and Adults, 1234 Massachusetts Ave., N.W., Suite 1017, Washington, D.C. 20005; (202) 783-0125

BIRTH DEFECTS

March of Dimes Birth Defects Foundation (MDBDF), 1275 Mamaroneck Ave., White Plains, N.Y. 10605; (914) 428-7100

BLINDNESS

American Foundation for the Blind (AFB), 15 W. 16th St., New York, N.Y. 10011; (212) 620-2000

CANCER

American Cancer Society (ACS), 90 Park Ave., New York, N.Y. 10016; (212) 599-8200
International Association of Laryngectomees (IAL), c/o American Cancer Society
Reach to Recovery Foundation, c/o American Cancer Society
United Ostomy Association (UOA), 2001 W. Beverly Blvd., Los Angeles, Calif. 90057; (213) 413-5510

CEREBRAL PALSY

United Cerebral Palsy Association, Inc., 66 E. 34th St., New York, N.Y. 10016; (212) 481-6300

CYSTIC FIBROSIS

Cystic Fibrosis Foundation (CFF), 6000 Executive Blvd., Suite 510, Rockville, Md. 20852; (800) 344-4823

DIABETES

American Association of Diabetes Educators (AADE), 500 N. Michigan Ave., Suite 1400, Chicago, Ill. 60611; (312) 661-1700
American Diabetes Association (ADA), National Service Center, 1600 Duke Street, Alexandria, Va. 22314; (800) 232-3472
Juvenile Diabetes Foundation International (JDFI), 60 Madison Ave., 4th Floor, New York, N.Y. 10010; (212) 889-7575

EPILEPSY

Epilepsy Foundation of America (EFA), 4351 Garden City Dr., Landover, Md. 20785; (301) 459-3700

HEMOPHILIA

National Hemophilia Foundation (NHF), 110 Green St., Room 406, New York, N.Y. 10012; (212) 219-8180

HUNTINGTON'S DISEASE

Huntington's Disease Foundation of America (HDFA), 140 W. 22nd St., 6th Floor, New York, N.Y. 10011; (212) 242-1968
National Huntington's Disease Association (NHDA), 1182 Broadway, Suite 402, New York, N.Y. 10001; (212) 684-2781

INFECTIOUS DISEASES

Centers for Disease Control, 1600 Clifton Rd., N.E., Atlanta, Ga. 30333; (404) 329-3311

Simon & Schuster Handbook for Writers will help you become a better writer by answering the questions that come up as you write. Use the following tools to quickly find the information you need:

- The **Brief Contents** here lists all the parts and chapters in the handbook.
- The **Detailed Contents** inside the back cover shows the chapter sections as well as chapters and parts.
- The **Index** lists all handbook topics covered in alphabetic order. Find your topic, note the page number, and then turn to that page to locate your information quickly.
- **Quick Boxes** throughout the book give you an easy way to skim and access the most common and important issues that will come up as you write.
- The **Terms Glossary** at the end of the book defines important terms related to writing and grammar. Every word printed in SMALL CAPITAL LETTERS is defined in the glossary.
- **Proofreading Marks** and **Response Symbols** that your instructor may use to mark your writing appear on the last page of the book. Refer to these lists to find the section of the handbook that will help you edit and proofread your work.
- The **eText version** of the handbook provides many links to additional resources. For example,

  Video tutorials show key concepts in writing, grammar, and research.

  Audio podcasts explain common grammar and punctuation issues.

  Exercises offer opportunities for online practice.

  Model documents provide examples of different kinds of writing.

Simon & Schuster
Handbook for Writers

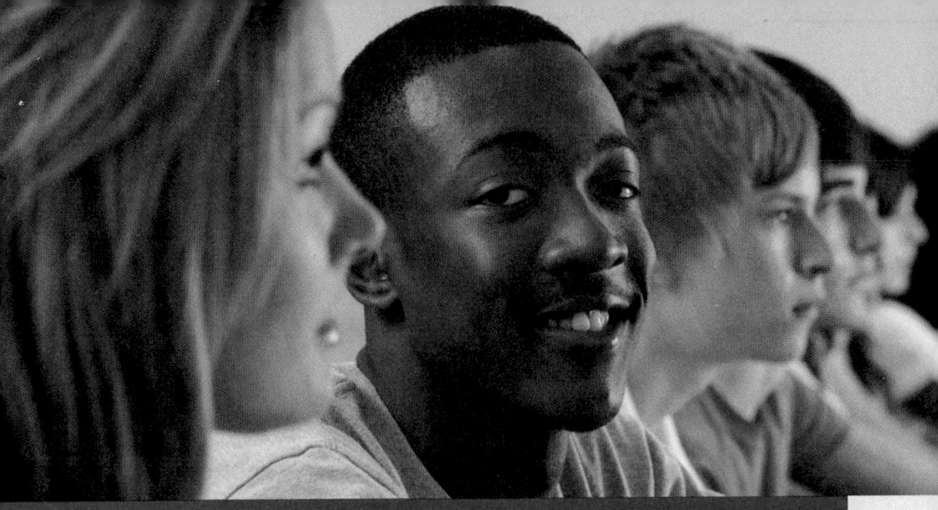

Why Do You Need This New Edition?

Here are seven features that you'll find only in the new edition of the *Simon & Schuster Handbook for Writers*:

1. Eight new chapters provide advice on writing commonly assigned papers—personal essays, informative writing, process analysis, cause and effect analysis, textual analysis, arguments, proposal and solution essays, and evaluations. Each chapter helps you identify your audience and purpose, gives you a Frame chart to organize your paper, provides Sentence and Paragraph Guides to help you develop common writing moves, and presents an annotated model paper (Part 2).
2. A new chapter on evaluating sources provides five key questions to ask about each of your research sources so that you use only credible, reliable sources in your papers. Each question includes a chart that contrasts characteristics of reliable versus questionable sources as well as examples (Ch. 23).
3. An expanded chapter on using sources in a research paper helps you decide what to do when your sources agree, partly agree, or disagree with one another. Sentence and Paragraph Guides demonstrate common moves you can make to transition among different sources while building your own argument (Ch. 18).
4. A new chapter "Ten Troublesome Mistakes Writers Make" highlights the most common grammar and punctuation errors and examples and exercises help you identify and correct these errors in your own writing (Ch. 2).
5. A new chapter, "Writing About Readings," covers summary, response, analysis/interpretation, and synthesis essays, emphasizing how often assignments, not just in formal research papers, require writing about texts (Ch. 20).
6. Completely updated MLA, APA, CM, and CSE documentation styles show you how to document and cite your sources. Examples for electronic sources like e-readers, wikis, and tweets help you accurately cite increasingly common types of new sources (Chs. 25–27).
7. Media-rich eText versions of the handbook provide videos, animations, model documents, and exercises to create a rich, interactive learning experience. You can access additional resources online to help you write effectively and correctly.

Simon & Schuster
Handbook for Writers

TENTH EDITION

LYNN QUITMAN TROYKA

DOUGLAS HESSE

PEARSON

Boston Columbus Indianapolis New York San Francisco Upper Saddle River
Amsterdam Cape Town Dubai London Madrid Milan Munich Paris Montreal Toronto
Delhi Mexico City Sao Paulo Sydney Hong Kong Seoul Singapore Taipei Tokyo

Senior Acquisitions Editor: Lauren A. Finn
Senior Development Editor: Marion B. Castellucci
Editorial Assistant: Shannon Kobran
Executive Marketing Manager: Thomas DeMarco
Senior Supplements Editor: Donna Campion
Executive Digital Producer: Stefanie A. Snajder
Digital Manager: Janell Lantana
Digital Editor: Sara Gordus
Production Manager: Savoula Amanatidis
Project Coordination, Text Design, and Electronic Page Makeup: Laserwords
Cover Designer/Manager: John Callahan
Cover Image: *Enclosed Field with Rising Sun, Saint-Remy 1889* Vincent van Gogh (1853–1890/Dutch) Oil on canvas Private Collection, © SuperStock/SuperStock
Photo Researcher: Integra–New York
Senior Manufacturing Buyer: Dennis J. Para
Printer and Binder: R. R. Donnelley and Sons Company–Crawfordsville
Cover Printer: Lehigh-Phoenix Color Corporation–Hagerstown

For permission to use copyrighted material, grateful acknowledgment is made to the copyright holders on pp. C-1–C-2, which are hereby made part of this copyright page.

Library of Congress Cataloging-in-Publication Data
Troyka, Lynn Quitman
Simon & Schuster handbook for writers / Lynn Quitman Troyka, Douglas Hesse. — 10th ed.
p.cm.
Includes index.
ISBN 978-0-205-90360-3 (student ed.) — ISBN 0-205-90360-6 (student ed.)
1. English language—Rhetoric—Handbooks, manuals, etc. 2. English language—Grammar—Handbooks, manuals, etc. 3. Report writing—Handbooks, manuals, etc. I. Hesse, Douglas Dean. II. Title. III. Title: Simon and Schuster handbook for writers. IV. Title: Handbook for writers.
PE1408.T696 2012
808'.042—dc23
2012030985

---

10 9 8 7 6 5 4 3 2 1—DOC—15 14 13 12

Student Edition
ISBN-10: 0-205-90360-6
ISBN-13: 978-0-205-90360-3

Instructor's Review Copy
ISBN-10: 0-321-84660-5
ISBN-13: 978-0-321-84660-0

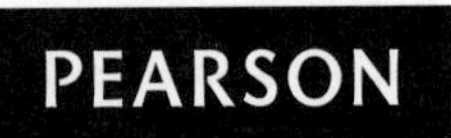

www.pearsonhighered.com

In memory of David Troyka,
my sweetheart and
husband of 47 years

LYNN QUITMAN TROYKA

To Don and Coral Hesse

DOUG HESSE

FINDING WHAT YOU NEED ON A PAGE

The runninghead shows the last section on the current page.

Chapter and section

What works in writing a first draft? **5G** 75

Section heading indicates new section of a chapter.

5G What works in writing a first draft?

Drafting means getting ideas onto paper or into the computer, in sentences and paragraphs. A draft is a version of the paper; experienced writers produce several drafts. The early ones focus on generating ideas, whereas later versions focus on developing and polishing ideas. But you can't polish something that doesn't exist, so your goal on the first draft is just producing words. Don't expect perfection; the pressure to "get it right the first time" can paralyze you.

Words in bold or SMALL CAPITAL LETTERS are discussed in various places in the book and are defined in the Terms Glossary.

Quick Box 4.6

Questions for analyzing genre

- What is the PURPOSE of the writing?
- Who is the apparent AUDIENCE?
- Are there clearly identified parts of individual works? Are there headings, for example?

Quick Boxes highlight key information.

NO **Approaching the island, a mountainous rock wall** was terrifying.

This sentence suggests that the mountainous wall was approaching the island.

YES Approaching the island, **we** saw a terrifying mountainous rock wall.

Examples show how to apply a rule.

ESOL Tip: If the cultural background of your readers differs from yours, you might find it difficult to estimate how much your readers know about your topic. To get a better idea of your readers' backgrounds, you might browse for information on the Internet or discuss your topic with people who might know more than you do about your readers' backgrounds.

ESOL icons call out information of particular use for multilingual students.

13. Article in a Newspaper with Print Version: Database

Hesse, Monica. "Falling in Love with St. Andrews, Scotland." *Washington Post* 24 Apr. 2011. *LexisNexis Academic*. Web. 3 Oct. 2011.

14. Article in a Newspaper with Print Version: Direct Online Access

Hesse, Monica. "Falling in Love with St. Andrews, Scotland." *Washington Post.* Washington Post, 22 Apr. 2011. Web. 3 Oct. 2011.

Citation examples are color-coded for clarity.

The runninghead shows the last section on the current page.

Chapter and section

11C What is a frame for an informative essay?

Section heading indicates new section of a chapter.

Informative essays can be organized in many ways. Here's a frame you can adapt to the specifics of your assignments.

Watch the Video

Listen to the Podcast

eText icons for video, audio, and exercise, and document resources provide links to additional instruction and practice online.

Frame for an Informative Essay

Introductory paragraph(s)

- **Capture your readers' interest** by using one of the strategies for writing effective introductory paragraphs (see 6C).
- **Present your thesis statement**, making sure it gives the central point of the essay (see 5F).

Body paragraph(s): background information

- **Provide background** for the information in your essay. This might follow the introductory paragraph or come later in the essay at a point when the background is more relevant.
- **Start with a topic sentence** that clearly relates to your thesis statement and leads logically to the information in the paragraph (see 6E).

Frames charts show you how to organize typical college papers.

Sentence and Paragraph Guides

- People experienced with __________ advise that the public needs to know __________ so that everyone can __________.
- __________ captured my interest because __________.
- People generally consider __________, __________, and __________ as the major components of information about __________.
- In addition to __________, __________ plays a major role in __________.

Sentence and paragraph guides help you think out moves writers make.

Alert: There are readers who aren't very well educated, and, sadly, there are readers who are prejudiced or narrow minded. Unless your instructor assigns otherwise, uninformed or biased readers usually aren't the audiences for college writing. ●

Alerts call attention to important rules and best practices.

INTRODUCTION TO STUDENTS

As writers, many of you have much in common with both of us. Sure, we've been at it longer, so we've had more practice, and most rules have become cemented in our heads. However, we share with you a common goal: to put ideas into words worthy of someone else's reading time. So that you can know us better as practicing writers, we'd each like to share a personal story with you.

From Doug: I first glimpsed the power of writing in high school, when I wrote sappy—but apparently successful—love poems. Still, when I went to college, I was surprised to discover all I didn't know about writing. Fortunately, I had good teachers and developed lots of patience. I needed it. I continue to learn from my colleagues, my students, and my coauthor, Lynn.

From Lynn: When I was an undergraduate, questions about writing nagged at me. One day, browsing in the library, I found a dust-covered book with the words *handbook* and *writing* in its title. Such books weren't common in those days, so I read it hungrily. Back then, I never imagined that someday I might write such a book myself. Now that we've completed the tenth edition of the *Simon & Schuster Handbook for Writers*, I'm amazed that I ever had the nerve to begin. This proves to me—and I hope to you—that anyone can write. Students don't always believe that. I hope you will.

We welcome you as our partners in the process of writing. We hope that the pages of this handbook will help you give voice to your thoughts, in school and in life. Please know that you're welcome always to write us at 2LTROYKA@gmail.com or dhesse@du.edu with comments about this handbook and about your experiences as a writer. We promise to answer.

Lynn Quitman Troyka

Doug Hesse

PREFACE

This tenth edition of the *Simon & Schuster Handbook for Writers* provides all the information students need about writing, from writing college papers to using and documenting sources, from writing online to writing using visuals, and from mastering grammar to using correct punctuation. We designed the *Simon & Schuster Handbook* for easy use and speedy entrée into all topics, welcoming students into a conversation about becoming better writers.

WHAT'S NEW IN THE TENTH EDITION?

- **Eight new chapters, "Frames for College Writing,"** advise students on commonly assigned papers. They offer guidance on the personal essay, informative writing, process analysis, cause and effect analysis, textual analysis, argument, proposal and solution, and evaluation. They include a discussion of audience and purpose, a frames chart illustrating a typical organization, sentence/paragraph guides that help develop common writing moves, and an annotated sample student paper (Part 2).
- **A new chapter on evaluating sources** emphasizes five critical thinking questions for students. For each question, a chart contrasts the characteristics of reliable versus questionable sources while illustrations of sample sources show those qualities in practice (Ch. 23).
- **New sections on synthesizing researched sources** in a paper helps students decide what to do when multiple sources agree, partly agree, or disagree. Sentence and paragraph guides demonstrate common moves writers make to transition among different sources while building their arguments (sections 18F–18L).
- **A new chapter "Ten Troublesome Mistakes Writers Make" with interactive online resources** highlights for students the most common grammar and punctuation mistakes, alerting them to key areas that they might otherwise overlook in what can seem a sea of grammar rules. This overview of common mistakes provides additional examples to help students identify and correct these errors in their own writing (Ch. 2). In the e-textbook, online videos provide interactive instruction, practice, and remediation of the ten troublesome mistakes.
- **A new chapter, "Writing About Readings,"** covers the summary essay, response essay, and synthesis essay, emphasizing the importance of writing about readings in many college assignments, not just in formal research papers (Ch. 20).

- **A new chapter "Ten Top Tips for College Writers"** suggests ten fundamental writing practices and encourages students to keep basic rhetorical principles at the forefront of their writing, to record source information immediately during research, and more (Ch. 1).
- **MLA, APA, CM, and CSE documentation examples** have been completely updated, and examples of electronic sources like e-readers and wikis help students accurately cite increasingly common types of new sources (Chs. 25–27). All citation examples are color coded for clarity.
- **More than 40 new exercises** support students with opportunities to apply what they've learned about grammar and punctuation as well as thinking and writing strategies.
- **New media enhancements in the e-textbook** link students to videos, animations, model documents, and exercises to create a rich, interactive learning experience. Resources that reinforce and extend the instructional content in the *Simon & Schuster Handbook* let students access additional help and assessment as needed and support students who have different learning styles. See E-textbook Resources on page xi for more information.

OTHER FEATURES OF THE HANDBOOK

- **Authoritative advice about grammar, punctuation, and mechanics** provides comprehensive and clear explanations with plentiful examples of correct usage.
- **Quick Boxes** highlight and summarize key content throughout the text, providing quick access to important strategies, suggestions, and examples to improve student writing.
- **Extensive samples of student writing** include 18 full academic essays and complete workplace documents to illustrate key elements of various types of writing and help students apply them in their own writing.
- **Annotated source illustrations** show students how to identify citation information in a range of typical sources—journal articles, web pages, and books—and how to arrange that information into correct MLA and APA citations.
- **Support for multilingual writers** includes seven stand alone chapters devoted to areas of special concern, as well as ESOL Tips integrated throughout the handbook and embedded within specific grammar, research, and writing topics.
- **Contemporary emphasis on visual and media literacy** includes coverage of reading visuals critically (Ch. 3), using photos and graphics to support a verbal text (Ch. 7), searching for images (Ch. 20), using multimedia in

presentations (Ch. 61), and writing in online environments such as blogs and wikis (Ch. 62).

- **Thoughtful, up-to-date documentation** coverage includes more MLA, APA, and CMS example citations than most other comparable titles.
- **The Terms Glossary** provides a convenient cross-referencing system: key terms are boldfaced and defined where they first appear in this book, and are thereafter presented in small capital letters—providing visual cues to readers when more complete definitions can be found in the Terms Glossary.

PRINT AND ELECTRONIC FORMATS

The tenth edition of the *Simon & Schuster Handbook* is available both in print and as an e-textbook in the following formats:

Pearson eText. An interactive online version of the *Simon & Schuster Handbook* is available in MyWritingLab. This eText brings together the many resources of MyWritingLab with the instruction and content of this successful handbook to create an enriched, interactive learning experience for students. See below for more on the eText resources.

CourseSmart e-textbook. Students can subscribe to the *Simon & Schuster Handbook* at CourseSmart.com. The format of the eText allows students to search the text, bookmark passages, save their own notes, and print reading assignments that incorporate lecture notes.

Android and iPad e-textbooks. Android and iPad versions of the text provide the complete handbook and the electronic resources described below.

E-textbook resources

Marginal icons in the handbook's eText, CourseSmart, iPad, Android, and print versions link to a wealth of electronic resources in MyWritingLab:

- Exercises from the handbook as well as additional exercises in MyWritingLab offer ample opportunities to help students sharpen their writing, grammar, and research skills.
- Video tutorials illustrate key concepts, offering tips and guidance on critical reading, evaluating sources, avoiding plagiarism, and many other topics.
- Audio podcasts discuss common questions about grammar, usage, punctuation, and mechanics.
- Sample documents illustrate the range of writing students do in composition classes, their other courses, the workplace, and the community.

MYWRITINGLAB

MyWritingLab empowers student writers to improve their writing, grammar, research, and documentation skills by uniquely integrating an e-text of the *Simon & Schuster Handbook for Writers* and book-specific resources with market-leading instruction, multimedia tutorials, exercises, and assessment.

Students can use MyWritingLab on their own, benefiting from self-paced diagnostics and a personal learning path that recommends the instruction and practice each student needs to improve his or her writing skills. Instructors can use MyWritingLab in ways that best complement their courses and teaching styles. They can recommend it to students for self-study, track student progress, or leverage the power of administrative features to be more effective and save time. The assignment builder and commenting tools, developed specifically for writing instruction, bring instructors closer to their student writers, make managing assignments more efficient, and put powerful assessment within reach. To learn more, visit MyWritingLab online or ask your Pearson representative.

SUPPLEMENTS

- **Instructor's Manual.** *Instructor's Resource Manual to accompany the Simon & Schuster Handbook for Writers, Tenth Edition* offers practical, hands-on advice for new and experienced composition instructors for organizing their syllabi, planning, and teaching.
- **The *Simon & Schuster Handbook* Exercise Answer Key.** Contains answers to the many exercises and activities in the *Simon & Schuster Handbook.*
- **Student Workbook.** *Workbook for Writers* has additional instruction and exercises for the writing, research, and grammar sections.

If you would like additional information about supplements for your composition course(s), please contact your Pearson sales representative.

ACKNOWLEDGMENTS

With this tenth edition of the *Simon & Schuster Handbook for Writers*, we heartily thank all those students who, to our great luck, have landed in our writing courses. We yearly learn from them how to stay up to date with students' needs and concerns as writers. We greatly admire how they strive to write skillfully, think critically, and communicate successfully. We especially thank the individual students who have given us permission to make them "published authors" by including their exemplary writing in this handbook.

We also are grateful to our many colleagues who have helped us with their criticisms, suggestions, and encouragement. In particular, we thank: Kaye Brown, Owensboro Community and Technical College; Anita P. Chirco, Keuka

College; Linda De Roche, Wesley College; Jason DePolo, North Carolina A&T State University; Christopher Ervin, Western Kentucky University; Joshua W. Everett, Central Texas College; Eric Fish, Northeast State Community College; Gary Heba, Bowling Green State University; Rebecca Heintz, Polk State College; Tina Hultgren, Kishwaukee College; Shanie Latham, Jefferson College; Nancy McGee, Macomb Community College; Joan Reeves, Northeast Alabama Community College; and Marcella Remund, University of South Dakota.

A project as complicated as the *Simon & Schuster Handbook* cannot be completed without the expertise and dedication of many professionals. We thank all the exceptional people at Pearson who facilitated this new edition. We're especially endebted to Marion Castellucci, Senior Development Editor, for her splendid vision and disciplined leadership; we thank also Paul Sarkis, Development Editor, Lauren Finn, Senior Acquisitions Editor, and Joe Opiela, Senior Vice President and Editorial Director for English. We appreciate the several contributions of Geoff Stacks. We wish to call special attention to the admirable work of Michael Montagna, a fellow faculty member, for reviewing, clarifying, and streamlining our grammar sections.

Doug values Lynn Troyka's vast knowledge, skill, dedication to teaching, and patience. He appreciates the support of all his colleagues in the writing program at the University of Denver, the knowledge and dedication embodied in the memberships of CCCC, TYCA, and WPA, and the hardworking team at Pearson. He further states, "My children, Monica, Andrew, and Paige, amaze me with their creativity, as does the very best writer I know: Becky Bradway, my wife."

Lynn wishes first to pay tribute to David Troyka, her beloved husband of 47 years, who inspired her to enjoy teaching and writing along with their amazing adventures in barely explored parts of the world. She thanks also her coauthor Doug Hesse for his gentle friendship and wisdom while writing the new 7th edition of *Quick Access Reference for Writers* and this newest edition of the *Simon & Schuster Handbook for Writers.* For their energetic, clever thoughts on logos, ethos, and pathos, she thanks Lynn Reid and Elisa Ham. For their unwavering support and love, Lynn also thanks Ida Morea, her steadfast friend and Administrative Assistant for 18 years; Kristen and Dan Black, her amazing daughter and son-in-law, and their superb children, Lindsey and Ryan; Bernice Joseph, her "adopted" sister and anchor of an amazing family: Mauricia Joseph, and Rachael and Eric Thomas, and their gifted children Nickyla, Nicholas, and Nehemiah; Michael Burns and his wife, Janelle James; and her grand pals Alice, Melanie, Avery, Jimmy, Gitam, Ian, Gavin, Hy Cohen, Doug Young, Andrene, Tzila, Susan, Rose, and Amanda.

Lynn Quitman Troyka
Doug Hesse

ABOUT THE AUTHORS

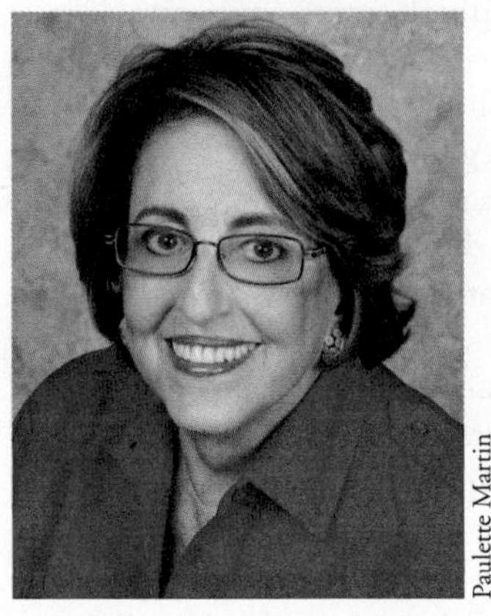
Paulette Martin

Lynn Quitman Troyka

Lynn Quitman Troyka, Adjunct Professor of English in the MA Program in Language and Literature at the City College (CCNY) of the City University of New York (CUNY), taught freshman English and basic writing for many years at Queensborough Community College. Dr. Troyka is a past chair of the Conference on College Composition and Communication (CCCC); the College Section of the National Council of Teachers of English (NCTE); and the Writing Division of the Modern Language Association (MLA). She has won many awards for teaching, scholarship, and service, and has conducted hundreds of faculty workshops about teaching writing and its relation to college-level reading.

"This information," says Dr. Troyka, "tells what I've done, not who I am. I am a teacher. Teaching is my life's work, and I love it."

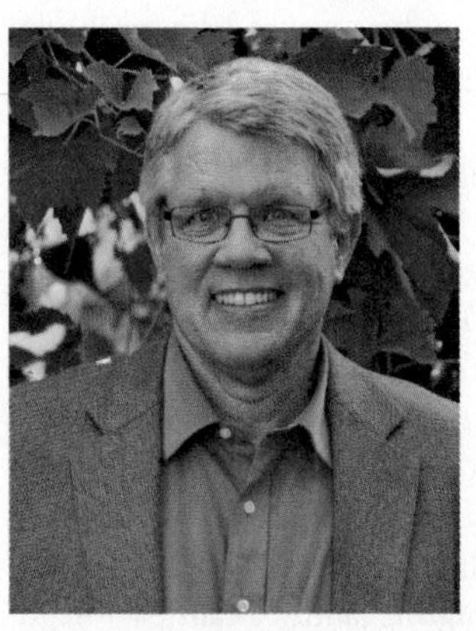

Doug Hesse

Douglas Hesse is Professor of English and Executive Director of Writing at the University of Denver, one of only thirty writing programs to receive the CCCC Certificate of Excellence. Dr. Hesse is a past chair of the CCCC, the nation's largest association of college writing instructors. A past president, as well, of the Council of Writing Program Administrators (WPA), Dr. Hesse edited *WPA: Writing Program Administration.* He has served on the NCTE executive committee, chaired the MLA Division on Teaching as a Profession, and served on the MLA Committee on Contingent Labor. Author of nearly sixty articles and book chapters, he has been named University Distinguished Scholar at the University of Denver.

"Of various awards I've received," says Dr. Hesse, "the one that matters most is Distinguished Humanities Teacher. That one came from my students and suggests that, in however small a way, I've mattered in their education and lives."

Simon & Schuster
Handbook for Writers

PART

1

Writing Situations and Processes

1 Ten Top Tips for College Writers

Quick Points You will learn to

➤ Focus on ten elements to improve your college writing.

Lynn, having taught writing and teachers of writing for over 30 years, has always surveyed her students at the close of each term by asking, "What tips for writers that you've learned this term have proved most helpful?" She has seen approximately 7,200 responses. After considering the most frequent advice Doug has given thousands of writers, he found his students had a lot in common with Lynn's. Our combined results are shown in Quick Box 1.1, starting with the top favorite tip.

Quick Box 1.1

Ten top tips for college writers

1. Be specific by thinking of RENNS: **R**easons, **E**xamples, **N**ames, **N**umbers, and the five **S**enses (see 6F).
2. Create a personal system to record writing ideas that pop into your head.
3. Use essay frames and sentence and paragraph guides as aids to writing (see Chapters 10–17).
4. Stay focused on the concepts of "purpose" and "audience" throughout your writing process (see 4B and 4C).
5. Weave *logos* (logic), *ethos* (credibility), and *pathos* (emotion) into your writing (see 3B).
6. Engage your readers by presenting and then complicating a topic.
7. Play the "believing game" and the "doubting game" (see page 8).
8. Record source information the very first time you find a source, even if you're not sure you will use it (see Chapters 21–22).
9. Welcome feedback about your writing (see Chapter 9).
10. Avoid slipping into "textspeak" in your writing.

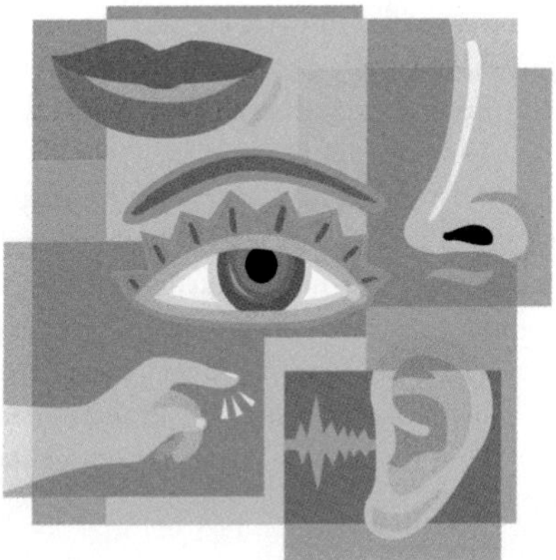

■ TIP 1. Be specific: use RENNS.

Successful college writing moves back and forth between main ideas, usually stated in TOPIC SENTENCES,* and specific details. The letters "RENNS" start words that lead to specific details: **R**easons, **E**xamples, **N**ames, **N**umbers, and the five **S**enses (sight, sound, smell, taste, and touch). You might include emotions along with the five senses when they fit your topic. Only some RENNS need to appear as specific details in a piece of writing. For more on RENNS with additional examples, see 6F.

Here's a paragraph that uses specific details to describe an environmental disaster.

> On April 20, 2010, an oil drilling rig in the Gulf of Mexico **Numbers**
> exploded, killing 11 workers and causing a huge oil spill that **Names**
> leaked 340,000 gallons a day of crude oil into the waters 40
> miles southeast of the Louisiana coast. Because the rig, called **Reasons**
> The Deepwater Horizon, sat half submerged so that it could
> extract more oil per day than a surface rig, the spilled oil
> went into deeper water than ever in the history of oil spills.
> The devastation of life below, on, and above the water was
> unusually widespread because the Gulf's strong currents
> spread the oil over large areas. Coral beds that live in darker **Examples**
> waters far below the surface died quickly as oil fell onto their
> fragile formations. Fish such as flounder and monkfish that
> normally live in deep water were quickly suffocated by the
> oil entering their gills. On the surface, microorganisms such
> as algae and krill, vital to oxygen in the water and food for

---

* Words printed in SMALL CAPITAL LETTERS are discussed elsewhere in the text and are defined in the Terms Glossary at the back of the book.

many types of whales, were wiped out. Sea life closer to shore, such as dolphins, turtles, and seals, died slowly, coated in the thick oil that seeped into their mouths and skin. Sea grasses and kelp, near-shore nesting sites for many species, wilted and died in the oil. And who can forget photographs of oil-coated pelicans, guillemots, and other sea birds held by human hands rushing against time to wash off the thick, sticky crude oil from feathers, bills, and feet? Or the videos of people weeping silently, angry at the sight of the dead birds and turtles that could not be saved? The oil poured out of the explosion site for over a month, creating the second worst environmental disaster in the United States.

Senses and emotions

TIP 2. Create a personal system to record writing ideas that pop into your head.

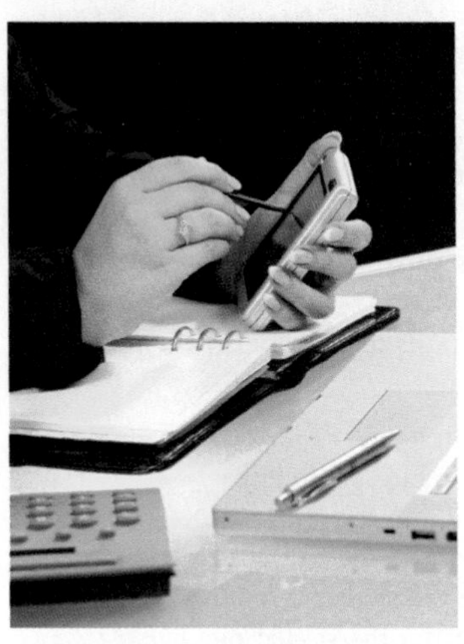

Writers often find that ideas pop into their heads while they're thinking of something else. You might be doing your laundry, driving your car or riding on a bus, or waking up in the middle of the night. Those ideas can slip through your fingers like snowflakes if you don't save them right away. We urge you to devise a recording system that suits your lifestyle. It might be a paper pad and a pencil, a cell phone, a small recording device, or a combination of these.

From time to time, check what you've saved because one idea might lead you to expanded or new thoughts. And while you're writing each of your assignments, consider whether some of what you've saved might fit in well with the current project. For more on brainstorming a topic and other techniques to help you plan your writing, see 5E.

TIP 3. If you're unsure how to approach a writing assignment, check Part 2, "Frames for College Writing."

The eight essay frames in Part 2 of this handbook introduce you to different types of college writing assignments and immerse you in a variety of practical techniques to help you think clearly and write effectively. Our purpose is to give you sufficient general guidance so that you can concentrate on your own concerns: building a good THESIS STATEMENT, writing paragraphs that relate to your thesis statement and topic sentences, and making sure that you're staying on topic. For lots of information about eight different essay types, see Chapters 10–17. Also, for frame information to help you write research papers, see Chapter 24.

■ TIP 4. Stay focused on the concepts of "purpose" and "audience" throughout your writing process.

All human communication starts with a PURPOSE: to explain something, to describe an experience, to mount an argument that you hope will persuade, or to inspire someone to take action or think in new ways. Your AUDIENCE is the person or people you're reaching out to with your words. To write successfully in college, begin thinking about your topic—whether assigned by an instructor or chosen on your own—by consciously deciding from the start

- What is your purpose?
- Who is your audience?

Develop this habit until it flows naturally each time you start a writing assignment. One excellent way to check yourself is to participate in class-sponsored peer review sessions, so that other students read your writing and tell you whether they can discern the purpose of your writing and your intended audience. For more about the concepts of purpose and audience, see sections 4B and 4C.

In the following excerpt, the author's *purpose* is to give helpful advice; her *audience* is people who want to write.

> If you dream of writing the screenplay for next summer's blockbuster movie, keep in mind one thing: writing is work. Oh, it can be enjoyable and immensely satisfying work, but you have to put in the time, often when you'd rather be doing something else. You'll need to put your butt in a chair, your hands on the keyboard, and crank out words—not just now and then, but pretty regularly, at least several minutes most days of the week, for weeks, months, even years. You see, it's that constant practice over time that gets you to the level of experts. Of course, you can learn some strategies and techniques that can help you be competent with specific kinds of writing. But for really good writing, the paragraphs of professional prose that win book contracts and screen credits, you'll need to work at it, just like all the rest of us.
>
> —Kiri Irvin, "You Just Can't Toss This Stuff Off"

TIP 5. Weave logical, ethical, and emotional appeals into your writing.

The advice that Greek philosopher Aristotle gave 2,300 years ago to people who wanted to persuade others is still excellent guidance for writers today. Aristotle taught that all effective communication needs three qualities:

- **Logical appeal (in Greek, *logos*).** Writers need to make statements that are logical so that the audience can accept and believe them.
- **Ethical appeal (*ethos*).** Writers need to choose words that communicate good character and integrity so their readers feel confident they're reading the ideas of someone who can be trusted and is not trying to manipulate them.
- **Emotional appeal (*pathos*).** Writers need to use words to establish an emotional connection with the audience.

Without these three qualities, readers will not easily accept the message being offered by the writer. Weaving all three qualities into your writing takes practice. You need to dig into yourself to make sure you're being honest, refraining from distorting information, showing personal humility, and exhibiting an understanding of the human condition. For more about the logical, ethical, and emotional appeals, see section 4B.

The following paragraph uses only a few words to communicate a logical position (*logos*), engages in a bit of self-mockery that conveys humility (*pathos*), and shows that the writer is honest and forthright in accepting her position in relation to others (*ethos*).

> Wearing a canvas jumpsuit zipped up to my neck, I must have looked as though I was stepping onto the set of *ET: The ExtraTerrestrial*, but my actual destination was Madison Avenue, home to some of the fanciest boutiques in New York City. The bright blue jumpsuit I wore was far from high fashion; it was sized for a full-grown man, and it ballooned about my slender frame. My blonde hair was pulled back in a pony tail, and the only label I displayed was the bold-lettered logo on my back: Ready, Willing, & Able. I was suited up to collect trash from the sidewalks of New York.
>
> —Zoe Shewer, "Ready, Willing, and Able"

Logical appeal. The author states the facts logically.

Ethical appeal. The author describes herself honestly; she isn't concerned about appearing unattractive.

Emotional appeal. The author has become a street cleaner, which many people consider undignified.

TIP 6. Engage your readers by presenting and then complicating a topic.

One way to capture and hold readers' attention is to present and then complicate a topic. A simple procession of details to support the **generalization** in a topic sentence can bore readers. When you introduce a complication into your ideas, you lure your readers to think more deeply about a topic, a habit of mind that greatly enhances the pleasure people get from reading. If you can't resolve the complication, you can close your discussion by acknowledging that the complication remains, and, by implication, you can invite your readers to think more about it on their own.

Here's a paragraph that contains a topic sentence as its generalization and specific details to support it. The complicating sentence is shown in boldface. By the end of the essay, the author doesn't smooth over the stark differences in worldviews that he presents, but he acknowledges them and suggests readers will see future evidence of their impact.

> The world can be divided in many ways—rich and poor, democratic and authoritarian—but one of the most striking is the divide between societies with an individualistic mentality and the ones with a collectivist mentality. **This divide goes deeper than economics into the way people perceive the world.** If you show an American an image of a fish tank, the American will usually describe the biggest fish in the tank and what it is doing. If you ask a Chinese person to describe a fish tank, the Chinese will usually describe the context in which the fish swim. These experiments have been done over and over again, and the results reveal the same underlying pattern. Americans usually see individuals; Chinese and other Asians see contexts.
>
> —David Brooks, "Harmony and the Dream"

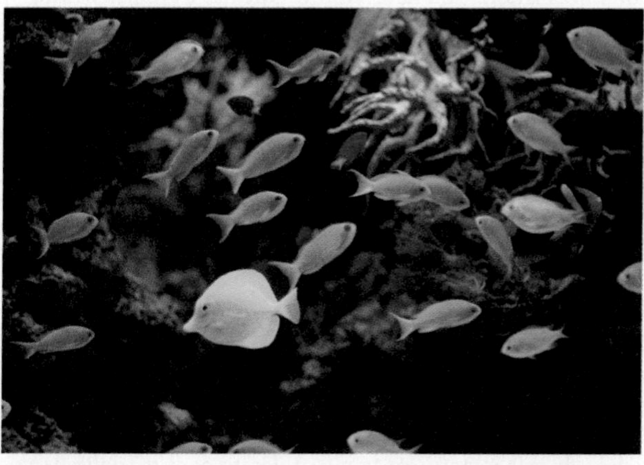

■ TIP 7. Play the "believing game" and the "doubting game."

The "believing game" comes in handy when you're brainstorming and drafting your writing. If you suddenly feel you have nothing to say, or you think your ideas aren't smart enough or your writing isn't good enough, turn on your ability to believe. Push yourself to become confident that you have something worth saying and the right to say it. Write boldly. Believing can propel you to get enough on paper to start your revising processes.

The "doubting game" is the flip side of the believing game. It's invaluable when you really don't want to bother doing any more with an essay—even though you know there's room for improvement. At these times, the doubting game can jump-start your revision process by turning up the volume of that quiet little voice, the one you'd like to ignore, that whispers maybe you had better look over your work one last time before you hand it in—perhaps you need more specific details or maybe you've cited one of your sources incorrectly. If you're like most professional writers, chances are you'll find holes that need filling or flaws you want to fix.

■ TIP 8. Record source information the very first time you find a source, even if you're not sure you will use it.

At the very moment you access a source, take an extra few minutes to record publication information so that you won't need to retrace your steps later on. Retracking down sources can take days, meaning wasted time and destructive stress. Use a master checklist of the publication details you'll need for the DOCUMENTATION STYLE you'll be using. Record that information every time. Never put it off. Even if a source seems irrelevant to the focus of your topic, force yourself to note its publication information. You never know! One day as you're writing you might suddenly realize you do indeed want to use that source.

Another important reason for recording publication information from the start is it helps you avoid unintentional PLAGIARISM. With the exact source information, you can always go back to it to make sure that you're not claiming an author's words as your own, or that your summary or paraphrase uses too many of the author's own words. For more about what publication information to record, see section 21M.

■ TIP 9. Welcome feedback about your writing.

Feedback about your writing from your instructor, your classmates, and other trusted readers can be invaluable when you want to improve your writing. Avoid reacting defensively or becoming resentful when you hear constructive criticism. If this is hard for you to tolerate or if it frightens you at first,

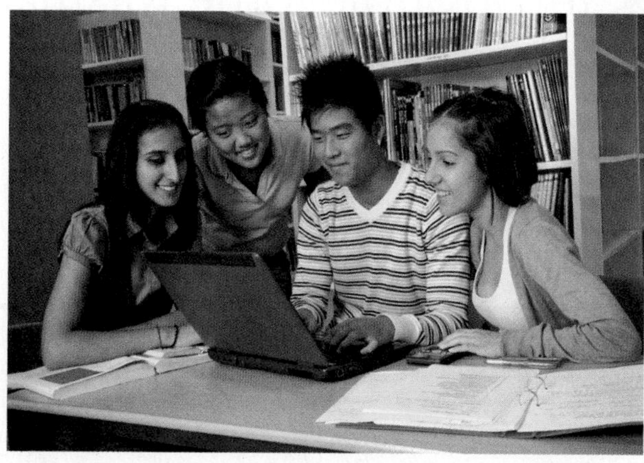

discipline yourself to listen to the comments and consider the points made. You might see possibilities you didn't notice on your own. Similarly, you can help others see their writing with new eyes.

Of course, always remember that you are the author, the one to make the final choice about whether to use each suggestion. (Please note that because some instructors require students refrain from asking for feedback about their writing before handing it in, be sure to check the teacher's policy in each of your writing classes.) For more about receiving feedback on your writing and giving feedback to others about their writing, see sections 9C–9D.

■ TIP 10. Avoid slipping into "textspeak" in your writing.

Textspeak is a coined term for shortening words, mostly by omitting vowels, in informally written text and chat messages. It's quicker to type "2morrow" or "cu soon." Of course, people who text know that texting forms aren't acceptable in ACADEMIC WRITING. Yet after a while for many people, textspeak starts to look normal, and it creeps without notice into their formal writing. Students particularly seem to allow textspeak to slip into their writing in blogged entries for class. Professors expect blogs for class to be written with serious, formal intent. Little will annoy your instructors and peer readers as much as assignments written in textspeak, so monitor your college writing carefully.

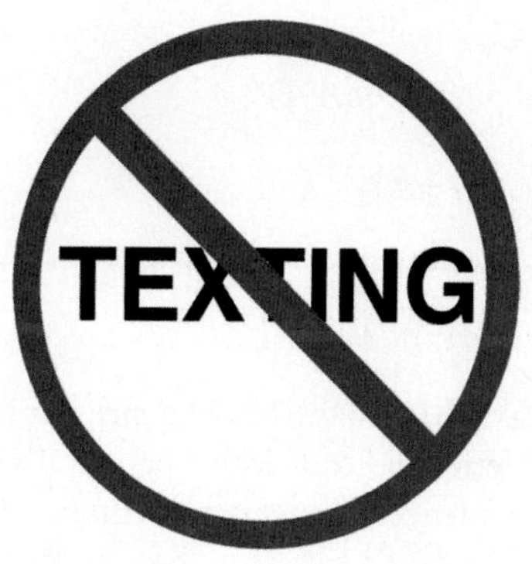

2 Ten Troublesome Mistakes Writers Make

Quick Points You will learn to

➤ Recognize and correct ten common errors in writing.

Ten troublesome mistakes tend to pop up frequently in college students' writing because students often forget what they learned years before. Most stand out more in written than in spoken English. We urge you to work through the quick review in this chapter to check whether any of these ten errors gives you trouble. If you see any, put aside some time right away to learn to recognize and eliminate them. You'll also find a full chapter on each error in this handbook (the chapter numbers are in parentheses in Quick Box 2.1).

Quick Box 2.1

Ten troublesome mistakes in writing

1. Sentence fragments instead of complete sentences (see Chapter 33)
2. Comma-spliced sentences and run-on sentences (see Chapter 34)
3. Subject–verb disagreement (see Chapter 31)
4. Pronoun–antecedent disagreement (see Chapter 31, sections 31O–31T)
5. Pronouns unclear in what they refer to (see Chapter 30, sections 30L–30N)
6. Illogical sentence shifts (see Chapter 36)
7. Modifiers placed incorrectly (see Chapter 35)
8. Homonyms misused (see Chapter 49, section 49F)
9. Commas misused (see Chapter 42)
10. Apostrophes misused (see Chapter 45)

1. Sentence fragments

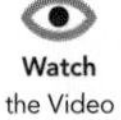

A **sentence fragment** is a written mistake that looks like a sentence but isn't one. Even though it starts with a capital letter and ends with a period, it's not a sentence. It's only a group of words. Sentence fragments are written errors created by three types of incomplete word groups. Chapter 33 lists the types and shows how to turn them into complete sentences.

NO **When** companies show employees respect**.**

The fragment starts with *when*, a SUBORDINATING CONJUNCTION, and is only a group of words.

YES **When** companies show employees respect**,** the best workers rarely quit.

The fragment is joined with a complete sentence.

NO A positive working atmosphere most employees productive and happy**.**

The fragment lacks a VERB and is only a group of words.

YES A positive working atmosphere **keeps** most employees productive and happy**.**

Keeps, a verb, completes the sentence.

2. Comma splices and run-on sentences

Watch the Video

Comma splices and run-on sentences are written mistakes that look almost alike. A **comma-spliced sentence** uses only a comma between two complete sentences. A **run-on sentence** uses no punctuation between two complete sentences. These errors disappear with any one of three fixes: placing a period or semicolon between the two sentences; writing a CONJUNCTION with needed punctuation between the two sentences; or turning one of the sentences into a DEPENDENT CLAUSE. Chapter 34 describes the types of comma splices and run-on sentences and explains how to revise them correctly.

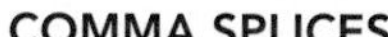

COMMA SPLICES

NO Bad bosses quickly stand out in workplaces**,** they scream impatiently at everyone.

YES Bad bosses quickly stand out in workplaces**.** They scream impatiently at everyone.

A period replaces the comma, which corrects the error. A semicolon also works.

YES Bad bosses quickly stand out in workplaces**, for** they scream impatiently at everyone.

Inserting the COORDINATING CONJUNCTION ***for*** corrects the error.

YES Bad bosses quickly stand out in workplaces **because** they scream impatiently at everyone.

The SUBORDINATING CONJUNCTION ***because*** turns the second sentence into a dependent clause, which corrects the error. The comma is dropped.

YES **Because** they scream impatiently at everyone**,** bad bosses quickly stand out in workplaces.

The SUBORDINATING CONJUNCTION ***because*** turns the second sentence into a dependent clause, which corrects the error. Now the dependent clause comes before the complete sentence, so the comma is retained.

RUN-ON SENTENCES

NO Bad bosses quickly stand out in workplaces they scream impatiently at everyone.

YES Bad bosses quickly stand out in workplaces**.** They scream impatiently at everyone.

A period or semicolon between the two sentences corrects the error.

YES Bad bosses quickly stand out in workplaces**, for** they scream impatiently at everyone.

A comma and the COORDINATING CONJUNCTION ***for*** correct the error.

YES Bad bosses quickly stand out in workplaces **because** they scream impatiently at everyone.

The SUBORDINATING CONJUNCTION ***because*** turns the second sentence into a dependent clause, which corrects the error.

YES **Because** they scream impatiently at everyone**,** bad bosses quickly stand out in workplaces.

The SUBORDINATING CONJUNCTION ***because*** turns the second sentence into a dependent clause, which corrects the error. Now the dependent clause comes before the complete sentence and is followed by a comma.

■ 3. Mistakes in subject–verb agreement

Watch the Video

A mistake in subject–verb agreement occurs when a VERB and its SUBJECT are mismatched, often within one sentence. This error, in written as well as spoken English, often occurs when singulars and plurals are mixed incorrectly. Chapter 31 explains all the ways subject–verb agreement errors occur and shows how to correct them.

NO **Effective leaders** in business **knows** how to motivate people to excel.

YES **Effective leaders** in business **know** how to motivate people to excel.

The plural subject ***Effective leaders*** matches the plural verb ***know***.

YES **An effective leader** in business **knows** how to motivate people to excel.

The singular subject ***Effective leader*** matches the singular verb ***knows***.

4. Mistakes in pronoun–antecedent agreement

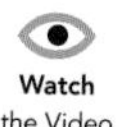

Pronoun–antecedent agreement errors occur when a PRONOUN and its ANTECEDENT are mismatched. A pronoun—such as *it, its, they*, and *their*—takes the place of a NOUN; an antecedent is the specific noun that a pronoun replaces in the same sentence or a nearby sentence. Errors in pronoun–antecedent agreement, in written as well as spoken English, often occur when singulars and plurals are mixed incorrectly. Chapter 31, sections 31O–31T, explains all the ways mistakes in pronoun–antecedent agreement occur and shows how to correct them.

NO My office partner admired my new computer **monitors** for **its** sleek design.

YES My office partner admired my new computer **monitors** for **their** sleek design.

The plural antecedent ***monitors*** matches the plural pronoun ***their***.

YES My office partner admired my new computer **monitor** for **its** sleek design.

The singular subject ***monitor*** matches the singular pronoun ***its***.

5. Unclear pronoun reference

Unclear pronoun reference, in written as well as spoken English, is a mistake that happens when the noun to which a pronoun—often *it, they, them*—refers is not obvious. Chapter 30, sections 30L–30N, describes the sentence structures that often have unclear pronoun reference problems and explains how to revise them correctly.

NO The construction supervisors paid little attention to the bricklayers when **they** were distracted.

They is an unclear pronoun reference. Who is distracted, the ***construction supervisors*** or the ***bricklayers?***

YES When the construction supervisors were distracted, ***they*** paid little attention to the bricklayers.

They clearly refers to the ***construction supervisors.***

NO Experienced bricklayers waste little motion to preserve their energy so that they can finish an entire section of wall without taking a break. **This** creates a sturdy wall.

This is an unclear pronoun reference. Is the wall sturdy because the bricklayers wasted little motion to preserve their energy or because the bricklayers finished an entire section without taking a break?

YES So that the wall they build is sturdy, experienced bricklayers waste little motion to preserve their energy so that they can finish an entire wall section without taking a break.

This is eliminated when the revised sentence makes clear how bricklayers can create a sturdy wall.

6. Illogical shifts within sentences

Watch the Video

Illogical shifts within sentences are mistakes, in written as well as spoken English, that occur midsentence when a category of word, such as the verb, changes form for no reason. In addition to verb tenses, other categories of words need to remain consistent within sentences as well as in groups of sentences. Chapter 36 shows how shifts create unclear writing and how they can be avoided.

NO Our union representative **explained** the new salary schedule and then **allows** time for questions.

YES Our union representative **explained** the new salary schedule and then **allowed** time for questions.

YES Our union representative **explains** the new salary schedule and then **allows** time for questions.

In the correct sentences, both verbs are in same tense, either PAST TENSE or PRESENT TENSE.

7. Mistakes with modifiers

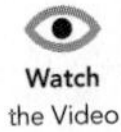
Watch the Video

Mistakes with MODIFIERS are more obvious in written than spoken English. Such errors happen when a modifier is placed in the wrong spot in a sentence, thereby muddling the meaning. Misplaced modifiers and dangling modifiers are two of the four types of incorrect placements for modifiers. Chapter 35 explains all four and how to correct them.

MISPLACED MODIFIER

NO The consultant who observed our meeting **only** took notes with a pen.

YES The consultant who observed our meeting took notes **only** with a pen.

Modifier ***only*** belongs with ***pen*** to clarify that nothing else was used to take notes.

NO The consultant took notes with a pen **sporting a large handlebar mustache**.

YES The consultant **sporting a large handlebar mustache** took notes with a pen.

The mustache belongs to the consultant, not the pen.

DANGLING MODIFIER

NO Studying our company's budget projection, the numbers predicted bankruptcy.

Numbers after the comma says that numbers can study.

YES Studying our company's budget projection, I saw that the numbers predicted bankruptcy.

I saw after the comma says that a person is studying.

8. Mistakes with homonyms

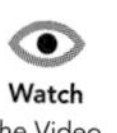

Mistakes with HOMONYMS are obvious in written English more than in spoken English. Homonyms are words that sound alike, but they have different meanings and spellings. We advise you to compile your own personal list of the homonyms that you habitually mix up. Then set aside time to master the correct usage of each word. Although an almost overwhelming number of homonym sets turn up in any Internet search, you need be concerned only with those that give you trouble. Chapter 49, section 49F, lists the homonym sets most frequently confused.

NO **Its** important **too** lock **you're** office door and **right** a note **four** the guards if you have **all ready** turned off the heat.

Simply to illustrate common homonym errors, we exaggerate how many show up in one sentence.

YES **It's** important **to** lock **your** office door and **write** a note **for** the guards if you have **already** turned off the heat.

9. Comma errors

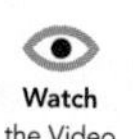

Comma errors are written, not spoken, mistakes. Commas clarify meaning for readers, especially when a sentence contains both major and minor information. Currently, commas turn up in published writing far less frequently than they did only 20 years ago. As a writer, beware of the suggestion to insert a comma whenever you pause because everyone speaks and thinks at different rates. This fact is particularly noticeable when people gather from different parts of the United States and Canada, or when a person's native language isn't English.

We suggest that you copy and carry with you the major rules for using commas, listed in Quick Box 42.1 on pages 620–621. The more you check this list of rules, the more quickly you'll know it by heart. Chapter 42 presents and explains all rules for comma use in written English.

To help you start, here's a list you'll probably master quite quickly—the five spots where a comma *never* belongs.

- Never after *such as*, but before it, it's fine: *Our office staff enjoyed perks**, such as** free coffee, tea, and hot chocolate.*
- Never before *than* in a comparison: *That company's truck was safer **than** ours.*
- Never between a subject and verb written close together: ***Our firm's maternity leave program** is **enlightened**.*
- Never immediately after a subordinating conjunction, and only after a clause that starts with one: ***Because** I developed a nasty cold**,** I left work early.*
- Never before an opening parenthesis, but after a closing parenthesis, it's fine: *When an office's intercom system works by public announcements **(people tend to ignore alerts by telephone),** everyone's concentration suffers.*

10. Apostrophe errors

Watch the Video

Apostrophe errors are written, not spoken, mistakes. Apostrophes serve only two purposes: they indicate possession (the president's car; the president's schedule), and they indicate missing letters in contractions (isn't). For complete information about apostrophes, see Chapter 45.

NO The main **office's** are closed for the evening.

YES The main **offices** are closed for the evening.

Apostrophes never create plural words.

NO The security guard **patrol's** the building every hour.

YES The security guard **patrols** the building every hour.

Apostrophes are never involved with verbs.

NO The security guards **do'nt** need dogs to help them.

YES The security guards **don't** need dogs to help them.

If you write a contraction, place an apostrophe only where a letter is omitted.

3 Thinking, Reading, and Analyzing Images Critically

Quick Points You will learn to

- Use critical thinking when examining ideas (see 3A).
- Recognize and use the logical, ethical, and emotional appeals (see 3B).
- Reason inductively and deductively (see 3H).
- Recognize logical fallacies (see 3I).

3A What is critical thinking?

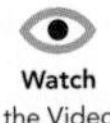
Watch the Video

Thinking isn't something people choose to do, any more than fish choose to live in water. But although thinking may come naturally, critical thinking demands more. **Critical thinking** means thoroughly examining ideas, readings, or images. It means identifying weaknesses, strengths, connections, and implications.

For example, consider the claim, "Because climate change is natural, we shouldn't worry about it." It's true that the earth's climate has varied over the millennia, but critical readers won't immediately accept the claim without further thought. They might ask, for example, whether the conditions that caused climate change in the past are the same ones causing it today. It could prove true that we shouldn't worry about climate change (though scientists almost universally agree we should), so a critical reader might ultimately accept the original claim—but not without careful analysis.

The word *critical* here has a neutral meaning. It doesn't mean taking a negative view or finding fault. Quick Box 3.1 lists questions that critical thinkers ask themselves.

Quick Box 3.1

Questions critical thinkers ask themselves

- Do I insist on examining an idea from all sides?
- Do I resist easy solutions that are being pushed at me?
- Do I face up to uncomfortable truths?
- Do I insist on factual accuracy?
- Do I remain open to ideas that don't fit with what I'm used to believing?
- Do I insist on clarity?
- Do I insist on hearing "the whole story," not just one point of view?
- Do I resist being hurried to make up my mind?

3B How can understanding rhetorical principles help critical thinking?

Rhetoric is the art and skill of speaking and writing effectively. If you understand three central principles of rhetoric—the **persuasive appeals**—you can greatly enhance your ability to think critically. Often the three are called by their Greek names: *logos*, meaning logic; *ethos*, meaning credibility; and *pathos*, meaning empathy or compassion. These appeals turn up in most material you read, see, hear, or run into every day. To recognize them in action, see Quick Box 3.2 (page 18).

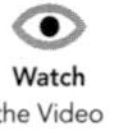
Watch the Video

Quick Box 3.2

Three central principles of rhetoric: the persuasive appeals

- **Logical appeals** (*logos*) evoke a rational response. People use them when they
  - Demonstrate sound reasoning.
  - Define terms.
  - Give accurate facts and statistics.
  - Use relevant quotations from experts and authorities.
  - Use deductive and inductive reasoning well (see 3I).
  - Use effective evidence (see 6F).
- **Ethical appeals** (*ethos*) evoke confidence in the writer's reliability and trustworthiness. People use them when they
  - Show respect by using appropriate language and tone.
  - Are fair-minded.
  - Are well informed and sincere.
  - Are open to a variety of perspectives.
  - Use reliable sources (see Chapter 23).
- **Emotional appeals** (*pathos*) stir emotions, passion, or compassion. People use them when they
  - Reflect values that call upon one's "better self."
  - Use concrete details and descriptive or figurative language to create mental pictures.
  - Add a sense of humanity and reality.
  - Appeal to hearts more than minds, but never manipulate with biased or slanted language.

Figure 3.1 is an example of these principles in action. It is an excerpt from the Web site of Doctors Without Borders, an organization dedicated to providing medical and humanitarian help. Perhaps most obvious are the emotional appeals, with the descriptions of malnourished children. For logical appeals the writer includes very specific information about medical processes (the "MUAC test") and treatments (the use of "ORS [oral rehydration salts] and zinc sulphate"). The medical terminology enhances the writer's ethical appeals, strengthening his

Figure 3.1 Three rhetorical appeals in action.

South Sudan: "These People Tell Us That They Are Desperate"

DECEMBER 9, 2011

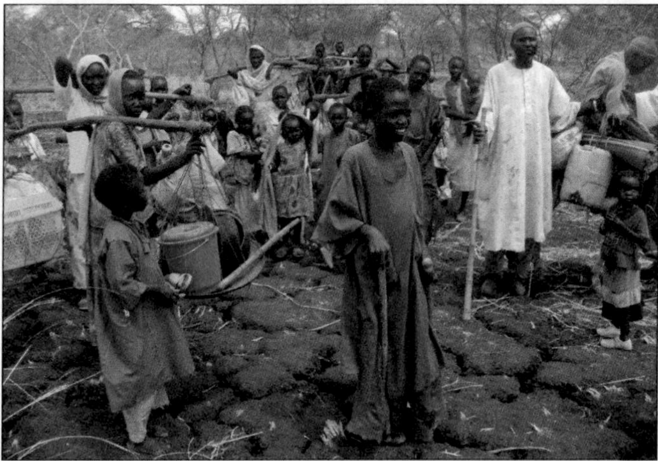

Some of the thousands of refugees in Doro.

South Sudan © Jean-Marc Jacobs

Robert Mungai Maina, from Kenya, has eight years of professional experience as a clinical officer. He has worked with Doctors Without Borders/Médecins Sans Frontières (MSF) in South Sudan for the past five months, and was assigned to the emergency team working in the Doro refugee camp last week. Here, he describes what he has seen.

"Many of the patients that we see in our clinic have respiratory diseases. This is because most of the refugees are sleeping outside without anything to cover themselves. . . .

We are also seeing malnourished children, some with moderate and some with severe malnutrition. They don't come with any particular complaint. You have to spot them. The child might come with diarrhea or a cough but the mother will not say to you, "this child is malnourished." So we do the MUAC test, the criterion that we use for detecting malnutrition in children. We measure their middle upper left arm using a measuring tape with a colored scale.

Yesterday I did a consultation with a mother who had one-year-old twins, both coughing and with fever. They both had severe malnutrition. She is still breastfeeding but doesn't have enough milk because she's not feeding herself well. She is just eating sorghum mixed with hot water to make a porridge, which is carbohydrates, nothing else. . . . We started both of the twins on specially formulated therapeutic food and one of them, who has frequent diarrhea, we started on ORS (oral rehydration salts) and zinc sulphate. . . .

I try my level best to do what I can do for them. Those who are sick, we take care of them and do the follow-up to make sure they get the right treatment. I tell them to come back any time they have a medical problem. That's what we are here to do."

credibility as someone who can characterize the problem accurately. The writer's credentials and his careful, quiet tone also build his ethical appeals.

3C How can I break down the critical thinking process?

Quick Box 3.3 describes the general steps of critical thinking. Expect sometimes to combine them, reverse their order, and return to parts of the process you thought you had completed.

Quick Box 3.3

Steps in the critical thinking process

1. **Summarize.** Comprehend the **literal meaning**: the "plain" meaning on the surface of the material. Be able to extract and restate the main message or central point or to accurately and objectively describe an image, event, or situation. Add nothing. Read "on the lines" (see 3D).
2. **Analyze.** Break ideas component parts. Figure out how each idea contributes to the overall meaning. Read "between the lines" for INFERENCES; look to see what's implied by the ideas, even if not stated (see 3E).
3. **Synthesize.** Connect what you've summarized and analyzed with your prior knowledge or experiences, with other ideas or perspectives, or with other readings (see 3F).
4. **Evaluate.** Read "beyond the lines." Judge the quality of the material or form your own informed opinion about it. Answer such questions as, "Is it reasonable? Fair? Accurate? Convincing? Ethical? Useful? Comprehensive? Important?" (see 3G).

3D How do I summarize or comprehend?

To summarize or comprehend, first, try to understand the basic, literal meaning of an idea, argument, or reading. The following activities can help.

3D.1 Read closely and actively

Reading is an active process, an interaction between the page or screen and your brain. The secret to reading closely and actively is to **annotate**. Annotating means writing notes to yourself in a book or article's margins, inserting comments electronically, or keeping a separate file or notebook about your reading. **Close reading** means annotating for content. You might, for

Figure 3.2 Example of close reading (blue) and active reading (black).

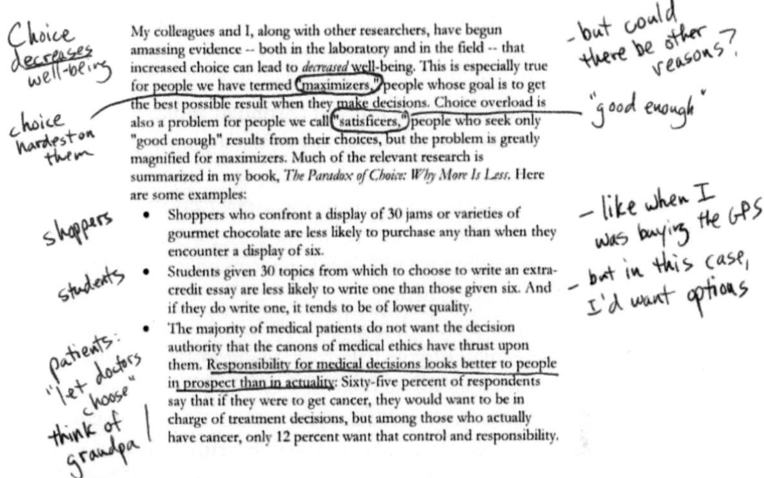
My colleagues and I, along with other researchers, have begun amassing evidence -- both in the laboratory and in the field -- that increased choice can lead to *decreased* well-being. This is especially true for people we have termed "maximizers," people whose goal is to get the best possible result when they make decisions. Choice overload is also a problem for people we call "satisficers," people who seek only "good enough" results from their choices, but the problem is greatly magnified for maximizers. Much of the relevant research is summarized in my book, *The Paradox of Choice: Why More Is Less.* Here are some examples:

- Shoppers who confront a display of 30 jams or varieties of gourmet chocolate are less likely to purchase any than when they encounter a display of six.
- Students given 30 topics from which to choose to write an extra-credit essay are less likely to write one than those given six. And if they do write one, it tends to be of lower quality.
- The majority of medical patients do not want the decision authority that the canons of medical ethics have thrust upon them. Responsibility for medical decisions looks better to people in prospect than in actuality: Sixty-five percent of respondents say that if they were to get cancer, they would want to be in charge of treatment decisions, but among those who actually have cancer, only 12 percent want that control and responsibility.

example, use the margin to number steps in a process or summarize major points. **Active reading** means annotating to make connections between the material and your own knowledge or experiences. This is your chance to converse on paper with the writer.

Figure 3.2 is an example of one kind of annotated reading, a section from "The Tyranny of Choice," an essay printed in Exercise 3-1. The student has written notes in the margin in two colors of ink. The blue ink shows close reading, and the black ink shows active reading.

Figure 3.3 (page 22) is another kind of annotation, using a double entry method. In the left column the student put close reading or content notes. The right column has active reading or synthesis notes.

● **EXERCISE 3-1** Annotate the following essay. Depending on your instructor's directions, either follow the annotation example in Figure 3.2, the double-entry example in Figure 3.3, or try both.

"THE TYRANNY OF CHOICE"
Barry Schwartz

Does increased affluence and increased choice mean we have more happy people? Not at all. Three recently published books—by the psychologist David Myers, the political scientist Robert E. Lane, and the journalist Gregg Easterbrook—point out how the growth of material affluence has not brought with it an increase in subjective well-being. Indeed, they argue that we are actually experiencing a *decrease* in well-being.

Why are people increasingly unhappy even as they experience greater material abundance and freedom of choice? Recent psychological research suggests that increased choice may itself be part of the problem.

It may seem implausible that there can be too much choice. As a matter of logic, it would appear that adding options will make no one worse off and is bound to make someone better off. If you're content choosing among three different kinds of breakfast cereal, or six television stations, you can simply ignore the dozens or hundreds that get added to your supermarket shelves or cable provider's menu. Meanwhile, one of those new cereals or TV stations may be just what some other person was hoping for. Given the indisputable fact that choice is good for human well-being, it seems only logical that if some choice is good, more choice is better.

Logically true, yes. Psychologically true, no. My colleagues and I, along with other researchers, have begun amassing evidence—both in the laboratory and in the field—that increased choice can lead to *decreased* well-being. This is especially true for people we have termed "maximizers," people whose goal is to get the best possible result when they make decisions. Choice overload is also a problem for people we call "satisficers," people who seek only "good enough" results from their choices, but the problem is greatly magnified for maximizers. Much of the relevant research

Figure 3.3 Double entry notebook example.

Content Notes	Synthesis Notes
--increased wealth and choice hasn't made people happier	
--14 million people fewer than in 1974 report being "very happy"	I wonder if people define happiness different today than they did 30-40 years ago
--depression and suicide has increased, especially among young people	Scary. There could be lots of causes, and I wonder if wealth and choice are the most important
--demand for counseling has increased at colleges	Could it be that more students seek counseling? Maybe need was there before but people didn't act.

is summarized in my book, *The Paradox of Choice: Why More Is Less.* Here are some examples:

- Shoppers who confront a display of 30 jams or varieties of gourmet chocolate are less likely to purchase *any* than when they encounter a display of six.
- Students given 30 topics from which to choose to write an extra-credit essay are less likely to write one than those given six. And if they do write one, it tends to be of lower quality.
- The majority of medical patients do not want the decision authority that the canons of medical ethics have thrust upon them. Responsibility for medical decisions looks better to people in prospect than in actuality: Sixty-five percent of respondents say that if they were to get cancer, they would want to be in charge of treatment decisions, but among those who actually have cancer, only 12 percent want that control and responsibility.
- Maximizing college seniors send out more résumés, investigate more different fields, go on more job interviews, and get better, higher paying jobs than satisficers. But they are less satisfied with the jobs, and are much more stressed, anxious, frustrated, and unhappy with the process.

These examples paint a common picture: Increasing options does not increase well-being, especially for maximizers, even when it enables choosers to do better by some objective standard. We have identified several processes that help explain why increased choice decreases satisfaction. Greater choice:

- Increases the burden of gathering information to make a wise decision.
- Increases the likelihood that people will regret the decisions they make.
- Increases the likelihood that people will *anticipate* regretting the decision they make, with the result that they can't make a decision at all.
- Increases the feeling of missed opportunities, as people encounter the attractive features of one option after another that they are rejecting. ●

3D.2 Read systematically

Reading systematically helps you pay attention. It's tempting to read quickly and carelessly, especially when you run up against long or complicated readings. Here's a three-part plan to help you read systematically.

1. **Preview:** Before you begin reading, start making **predictions** and jot down your questions.
   - For books, first look at the table of contents. What topics are included? What seems to be the main emphasis? If there's an introduction or preface, skim it.

- For chapters, or Web sites, first read all the headings, both large and small. Look for call-outs (quotations or excerpts in boxes or in the margins) and for figures, tables, and boxes.
- Check for introductory notes. Is there an abstract (a summary of the entire piece)? A note about the author? Other information?
- Jot a few questions that you expect—or hope—the reading will answer.

2. **Read:** Read the material closely and actively (see 3D.1). Identify the main points and start thinking about how the writer supports them. Annotate as you read.
3. **Review:** Go back to questions you jotted during previewing. Did the reading answer them? If not, either your predictions could have been wrong, or you didn't read carefully; reread to determine which.

Quick Box 3.4 lists more ways to help your reading comprehension.

Alert: The speed at which you read depends on your purpose. When you're hunting for a particular fact, you might skim the page until you find what you want. When you read about a subject you know well, you might read somewhat rapidly, slowing down only when you come to new material. When you're unfamiliar with the subject, you need to work slowly to give your mind time to absorb the new material. ●

Quick Box 3.4

More ways to help reading comprehension

- **Make associations.** Link new material to what you already know. You may even find it helpful to read an encyclopedia article or an easier book or article on the subject first to build your knowledge base.
- **Simplify tough sentences.** If the author's writing style is complex, break long sentences into several shorter ones or reword them into a simpler style.
- **Make it easy for you to focus.** Do whatever it takes to concentrate.
- **Allot the time you need.** We know it's tough to balance classes, work, and social or family activities, but allow sufficient time to read, reflect, reread, and study.
- **Master the vocabulary.** As you encounter new words, try to figure out their meanings from context clues. See if definitions (called a *glossary*) are at the end of the reading. Have a good dictionary at hand or access an online dictionary site like dictionary.com.

3E How do I analyze readings?

To analyze something is to break it into parts, just as a chemist does, for example, to figure out the compounds in a particular mixture. Quick Box 3.5 explains how.

Quick Box 3.5

Strategies for analysis

1. Identify the key assertions or claims (see 3E.1).
2. Separate facts from opinions (see 3E.2).
3. Identify rhetorical appeals (see 3B and 3E.3).
4. Identify the evidence (see 3E.4).
5. Identify cause and effect (see 3E.5).
6. Describe the tone, and look for bias (see 3E.6).
7. Identify inferences and assumptions (see 3E.7).
8. Identify implications (see 3E.8).

3E.1 Identify the key assertions or claims

Most writings are a combination of main ideas and the evidence, examples, or illustrations provided to support them. The most important idea is the writing's THESIS STATEMENT, which states the main idea for the whole piece. Identifying main ideas is crucial to evaluating how well the writer supports them.

3E.2 Separate facts from opinions

Distinguish **fact** from **opinion**.

- Facts are statements that can be checked objectively by observation, experiment, or research.

  EXAMPLE:

  Abraham Lincoln was the sixteenth president of the United States.

- Opinions are statements open to debate.

  EXAMPLE:

  Abraham Lincoln is the greatest U.S. president who ever lived.

Most statements are not so easy to discern as the ones given here about Abraham Lincoln. For example, is the statement, "All people desire a steady income," a fact or an opinion? If read without reflection, it can seem a fact. However, critical readers realize that although it's common for people to equate success with a constant stream of money, some individuals prefer a more freewheeling approach to life. They may work hard, save money, and then travel for months, not working at all. Thus the statement is an opinion because although it's accurate for most people, it isn't true for all.

Problems arise when a writer blurs the distinction between fact and opinion. Critical readers recognize the difference.

● **EXERCISE 3-2** Working individually or with a collaborative group, decide which of the following statements are facts and which are opinions. When the author and source are provided, explain how that information influenced your judgment.

1. The life of people on earth is better now than it has ever been—certainly much better than it was 500 years ago.

   —Peggy Noonan, "Why Are We So Unhappy When We Have It So Good?"

2. The fast food industry pays the minimum wage to a higher proportion of its workers than any other American industry.

   —Eric Schlosser, *Fast Food Nation*

3. Grief, when it comes, is nothing we expect it to be.

   —Joan Didion, *The Year of Living Dangerously*

4. History is the branch of knowledge that deals systematically with the past.

   —*Webster's New World College Dictionary*, Fourth Edition

5. In 1927, F. E. Tylcote, an English physician, reported in the medical journal *Lancet* that in almost every case of lung cancer he had seen or known about, the patient smoked.

   —William Ecenbarger, "The Strange History of Tobacco"

6. Trucks that must travel on frozen highways in Alaska for most of the year now sometimes get stuck in the mud as the permafrost thaws.

   —Al Gore, *An Inconvenient Truth*

7. You change laws by changing lawmakers.

—Sissy Farenthold, political activist, *Bakersfield Californian*

8. A critical task for all of the world's religions and spiritual traditions is to enrich the vision—and the reality—of the sense of community among us.

—Joel D. Beversluis, *A Sourcebook for Earth's Community of Religions* ●

3E.3 Identify rhetorical appeals

As we explained in 3B, writers use logical, ethical, and emotional appeals to persuade readers. Identifying how each of these appear in a reading is a key step to evaluating whether material is reasonable or fair.

3E.4 Identify the evidence

Evidence consists of facts, examples, the results of formal studies, and the opinions of experts. A helpful step in analysis is to identify the kind of evidence used for any claims or opinions—or where evidence is missing.

You might especially look for how the writer uses primary or secondary sources. **Primary sources** are firsthand evidence based on your own or someone else's original work or direct observation. Primary sources can take the form of experiments, surveys, interviews, memoirs, observations (such as in ETHNOGRAPHIES), original creative works (for example, poems, novels, paintings and other visual art, plays, films, or musical compositions). **Secondary sources** report, describe, comment on, or analyze the experiences or work of others. Quick Box 3.6 (page 28) illustrates the difference.

Secondary sources sometimes don't represent original material accurately, whether intentionally or by accident. For example, suppose a primary source concluded, "It would be a mistake to assume that people's poverty level reflects their intelligence," while a secondary source represents this as, "People's poverty level reflects their intelligence." Problem! This is a distortion. Examining the quality of sources is so important that we devote all of Chapter 23 to this topic.

● **EXERCISE 3-3** Individually or with a group, choose one of the following thesis statements and list the kinds of primary and secondary sources you might consult to support the thesis (you can guess intelligently, rather than checking to make sure that the sources exist). Then, decide which sources in your list would be primary and which secondary.

THESIS STATEMENT 1:

People who regularly perform volunteer work lead happier lives than those who don't.

THESIS STATEMENT 2:

Whether someone regularly performs volunteer work or not ultimately has no effect on their happiness. ●

Quick Box 3.6

Examples of differences between primary and secondary sources

Primary Source	Secondary Source
Professor Fassi interviews thirty single parents and reports his findings in a journal article.	*Time* magazine summarizes Professor Fassi's study in a longer article on single parents.
Medical researcher Molly Cameron publishes the results of her experiments with a new cancer drug in the *New England Journal of Medicine.*	*The Washington Post* runs an article that summarizes findings from Cameron's study.
The National Assessment of Educational Progress publishes test results on the reading abilities of ninth graders.	National Public Radio refers to the NAEP study in a story on reading in America.
A team of researchers at Bowling Green State University survey 2,259 Ohio citizens about their voting patterns and write an article explaining their findings.	Scholar Maya Dai conducts a study of politics in Colorado; in her review of literature section of her study, she summarizes the Bowling Green study, along with studies in four other states.
Rosa Rodriguez writes a memoir about life as a migrant worker.	Writer Phil Gronowski discusses Rodriguez's memoir in his daily blog.
Gerhard Richter exhibits his paintings at the Art Institute of Chicago.	The *Chicago Tribune* publishes a review of Richter's exhibition.

Once you've identified the evidence used to support claims, you can evaluate it by asking the questions in Quick Box 3.7.

Quick Box 3.7

Questions for analyzing evidence

- **Is the evidence sufficient?** A claim with no support should alert you to a possible problem. As a further rule, the more evidence, the better. Readers have more confidence in the results of a survey that draws on a hundred respondents rather than on ten.
- **Is the evidence representative?** Evidence is representative if it is typical. For example, a pollster surveying national political views would not get representative evidence by interviewing people only in Austin, Texas, because that group doesn't represent the regional, racial, political, and ethnic makeup of the entire U.S. electorate.
- **Is the evidence relevant?** Relevant evidence is directly related to the conclusion you're drawing. Suppose you read that one hundred high school students who watched television for more than two hours a day earned significantly lower scores on a college entrance exam than one hundred students who didn't. Can you conclude that all students who watch less television are more successful after college? Not necessarily.
- **Is the evidence accurate?** Accurate evidence is correct and complete. To be accurate, evidence must come from a reliable source. If someone includes a figure (for example, "The average new college graduate earns $78,000 per year"), ask yourself where that figure comes from. (NOTE: We just made up that $78,000 figure; we wish it were true! According to the *New York Times*, the median salary for new college grads in 2010 was $27,000.)
- **Is the evidence qualified?** Reasonable evidence doesn't make extreme claims. Claims that use words such as *all, always, never*, and *certainly* are disqualified if even one exception is found. Conclusions are more sensible and believable when they are qualified with words such as *some, many, may, possibly, often*, and *usually*.

3E.5 Identify cause and effect

Cause and effect describes the relationship between one event (cause) and another event that happens as a result (effect). The relationship also works in reverse: One event (effect) results from another event (cause).

Quick Box 3.8 (page 30) gives brief advice for assessing claims of cause and effect.

Quick Box 3.8

Assessing cause and effect

- **Is there a clear relationship between events?** Imagine this sequence: First the wind blows; then a door slams; then a pane of glass in the door breaks. You conclude that the wind caused the glass to break. But CHRONOLOGICAL ORDER merely implies a cause-and-effect relationship. Perhaps it was windy, but actually someone slammed the door or threw a baseball through the glass. The fact that B happened after A doesn't prove that A caused B.
- **Is there a pattern of repetition?** To establish that A causes B, every time A is present, B must occur. The need for repetition explains why the U.S. Food and Drug Administration (FDA) runs thousands of clinical trials before approving a new medicine.
- **Are there multiple causes and/or effects?** Avoid oversimplification. Multiple causes and/or effects are typical of real life. For example, it would be oversimplification to state that high unemployment is strictly due to poor schools.

● **EXERCISE 3-4** For each of the following sentences, explain how the effect might not be a result of the cause given.

EXAMPLE

The number of shoppers downtown increased because the city planted more trees there.

Explanation: Of course, planting trees might have made the downtown more attractive and drawn more shoppers. However, perhaps there are other reasons: new stores opening, more parking, a suburban mall closed down, and so on.

1. Attendance at baseball games declined because the team raised prices.
2. Test scores improved because the school instituted a dress code.
3. Amy Williams got elected to Congress because she was the smartest candidate. ●

3E.6 Describe tone, bias, and point of view

Tone emerges from a writer's use of words and ways of presenting ideas. Just as our voices emit certain tones when we're happy, bored, sad, or excited, so do our words. Tone can be serious, respectful, friendly, humorous, slanted, sarcastic, or angry. Consider the difference between, "Would you please refrain from doing that?" and "Knock it off right now!"

When their tone is extreme, writers may be seeking to manipulate readers rather than to have them think logically.

NO Urban renewal must be stopped. Greedy politicians are ruining this country, and money-hungry capitalists are robbing law-abiding citizens.

YES Urban renewal may revitalize our cities, but it can also cause serious problems. When developers wish to revitalize decaying neighborhoods, they must also remember that they're displacing people who don't want to leave familiar homes.

In addition, you'll want to detect **bias**, also known as prejudice. When writing is distorted by hatred or distrust of individuals, groups of people, or ideas, critical readers want to suspect the accuracy and fairness of the material.

Considering the writer's **point of view**, the situation from which he or she is writing, can open up new perspectives. For example, consider the statement, "Freedom isn't the ability to do what you want but rather the ability to do what you should." If you were told this statement was made by a third-world dictator, you would interpret it differently than if you were told it was made by a leader of the American Legion (which it actually was).

Although considering point of view can help you draw inferences, take care that you don't fall prey to the LOGICAL FALLACY of personal attack (see 3H). Just because a position was stated by someone you don't like doesn't mean that the position is wrong.

● **EXERCISE 3-5** Identify any bias and prejudice in the following paragraph. Then, rewrite the paragraph so that it presents the same basic point of view but with a more reasonable tone.

> Once again we see the consequences of babying college students. Now these spoiled kids want the library to be open later at night. They claim it's for homework, but anyone who's not a fool know they really just want to hang out and hit on each other while pretending to study. Hey, I have an idea. They should drag their lazy carcasses out of bed at a decent hour and get to the library first thing in the morning. Of course, that will never happen as long as they continue to party, watch television, and play games all night. ●

3E.7 Identify inferences and assumptions

When you read for **inferences**, you're trying to understand what's suggested or implied but not explicitly stated. Here's an example.

> The band finally appeared an hour after the concert was scheduled to start. The lead singer spent the first two songs staring at the stage and mumbling into his microphone, before finally looking at the audience and saying, "It's great to be here in Portland." The only problem was that they were playing in Denver. At that point the crowd was too stunned even to boo. I started texting some friends to see if they had better options for the evening.
>
> —Jenny Shi, student

Literally, this paragraph describes what happened at a concert. But there's clearly more going on. Among the inferential meanings are that (1) the band wasn't very enthusiastic about this concert; and (2) this wasn't a very pleasant experience for Jenny.

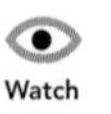
Watch the Video

An **assumption** is a statement or idea that writers expect readers to accept as true without proof. For example, in writing this handbook, we assume that students are open to advice about how to write successfully. (You are, aren't you?) Critical readers need to take time to uncover and examine **unstated assumptions.**

3E.8 Identify implications

An implication takes the form, "If this is true (or if this happens), then that might also be true (or that might be the consequence.)" One way to consider implications, especially for readings that contain a proposal, is to ask, "Who might benefit from an action, and who might lose?" For example, consider the following short argument.

> Because parking downtown is so limited, we should require anyone putting up a new building to construct a parking lot or contribute to parking garages.

It doesn't take much to infer who might benefit: people who are looking for places to park. Who might lose? More room for parking means less room for building, so the downtown could sprawl into neighborhoods. More parking can encourage more driving, which contributes to congestion and pollution.

● **EXERCISE 3-6** Consider the implications of the following short argument, focusing on who might gain and lose from the following proposal: "In an effort to cut tuition costs, Machiavelli College will increase its enrollment from 5,000 students to 10,000 over the next four years by reducing the admissions requirements and increasing the number of students who don't require financial aid and can pay full price." ●

● **EXERCISE 3-7** Read the following passage, then (1) list all literal information, and (2) list all assumptions and implications.

EXAMPLE

The study found many complaints against the lawyers were not investigated, seemingly out of a "desire to avoid difficult cases."

—Norman F. Dacey

Literal information: Few complaints against lawyers are investigated.

Assumptions or implications: The term *difficult cases* implies a cover-up: Lawyers, or others in power, hesitate to criticize lawyers for fear of being sued or for fear of a public outcry if the truth about abuses and errors were revealed.

[T]he sexual balance of power in the world is changing, slowly but surely. New evidence can be found in the 2007 World Development Indicators from the World Bank. It is something to celebrate.

The most obvious changes are in education. In 2004 girls outnumbered boys at secondary schools in almost half the countries of the world (84 of 171). The number of countries in which the gap between the sexes has more or less disappeared has risen by a fifth since 1991. At university level, girls do better still, outnumbering boys in 83 of 141 countries. They do so not only in the rich world, which is perhaps not surprising, but also in countries such as Mongolia and Guyana where university education for anyone is not common.

—*The Economist*, "A Man's World?" ●

3F How do I synthesize?

Watch the Video

To **synthesize** is to put things together. It happens when you connect the ideas you generate through analysis with things you know from readings or experience. We discuss synthesis at great length in Chapter 20.

3G How do I evaluate?

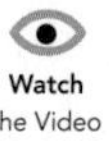

The final step in critical thinking is evaluation. **Evaluation** requires an overall assessment of the the writer's reasoning, evidence, and fairness. Quick Box 3.9 (page 34) lists questions to help you evaluate ideas generated by analysis.

3H How do I use inductive and deductive reasoning?

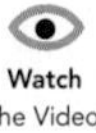

Two thought patterns, inductive reasoning and deductive reasoning, can help you think critically.

Quick Box 3.9

Questions to move from analysis and synthesis to evaluation

- How does the argument connect to other ideas, readings, or experiences? Do they support, complicate, or contradict each other (see 3F)?
- Does the argument use rhetorical appeals effectively and fairly? In particular, does it rely too much on emotional appeals (see 3E.3)?
- Is the evidence provided sufficent, representative, relevant, accurate, and qualified (see Quick Box 3.7)?
- Are any claims about cause and effect reasonable (see 3E.5)?
- Is the tone reasonable? Is the argument free from bias (see 3E.6)?
- Are the inferences and assumptions reasonable (see 3E.7)?
- Are the implications of the argument reasonable and desirable (see 3E.8)?
- Does the argument use inductive or deductive reasoning effectively (see 3H)?
- Is the argument free of logical fallacies (see 3I)?

3H.1 Inductive reasoning

Inductive reasoning moves from specific, explicit facts or instances to broad general principles. For example, suppose you go to the Registry of Motor Vehicles closest to your home to renew your driver's license, and you stand in line for two hours. A few months later, you return to the same location to get new license plates and again stand in a two-hour line. Your friends have had similar experiences. You conclude, therefore, that all offices of the Registry of Motor Vehicles are inefficient. Your conclusion is based on inductive reasoning, from your specific experiences to your general judgment.

As a critical thinker, you might ask whether the conclusion is an absolute truth. It is not. The conclusion is only a statement of probability. After all, perhaps another Registry of Motor Vehicles office is so well run that no one ever stands in line for more than ten minutes. Quick Box 3.10 lists the characteristics of inductive reasoning.

3H.2 Deductive reasoning

Deductive reasoning moves from general claims, called **premises**, to a specific conclusion. The three-part structure of two premises and a conclusion is known as a **syllogism**.

Quick Box 3.10

Features of inductive reasoning

- Inductive reasoning begins with specific evidence—facts, observations, or experiences—and moves to a general conclusion.
- Inductive reasoning is based on a sampling of facts, not on the whole universe of related facts.
- The conclusions in inductive reasoning are considered reliable or unreliable, but never true or false.
- The advantage of inductive reasoning is that you can speculate on the unknown based on what's known.

PREMISE 1 Students who don't study fail Professor Sanchez's exams.
PREMISE 2 My friend didn't study.
CONCLUSION My friend failed Professor Sanchez's exams.

Premises in syllogism can be facts or ASSUMPTIONS. Assumptions need close scrutiny. Because some assumptions are based on incorrect information, a critical thinker needs to evaluate each premise—that is, each assumption—carefully. When the conclusion logically follows from premises, a deductive argument is **valid** or acceptable. When the conclusion doesn't logically follow from the premises, a deductive argument is invalid.

VALID—DEDUCTIVE REASONING EXAMPLE 1

PREMISE 1 When it snows, the streets get wet. [fact]
PREMISE 2 It is snowing. [fact]
CONCLUSION Therefore, the streets are getting wet. [valid]

INVALID—DEDUCTIVE REASONING EXAMPLE 2

PREMISE 1 When it snows, the streets get wet. [fact]
PREMISE 2 The streets are getting wet. [fact]
CONCLUSION Therefore, it is snowing. [invalid]

Deductive argument 2 is invalid because even though the two premises are facts, the conclusion is wrong. After all, the streets can be wet for many reasons other than snow: from rain, from street-cleaning trucks that spray water, or from people washing their cars.

INVALID—DEDUCTIVE REASONING EXAMPLE 3

PREMISE 1	Learning a new language takes hard work.
PREMISE 2	Nicholas has learned to speak Spanish.
CONCLUSION	Nicholas worked hard to learn Spanish.

Deductive argument 3 is invalid because it rests on a wrong assumption: not everyone has to work hard to learn a new language; some people—for example, young children—learn new languages easily. Therefore, Nicholas might have learned Spanish effortlessly.

As a critical thinker, whenever you encounter an assumption, either stated or unstated, you need to check whether it's true. If it isn't, the reasoning is flawed. Quick Box 3.11 lists the characteristics of deductive reasoning.

Quick Box 3.11

Features of deductive reasoning

- Deductive reasoning moves from the general to the specific. Its three-part structure, called a syllogism, consists of two premises and a conclusion drawn from them.
- Deductive reasoning is valid if its conclusion follows logically from its premises.
- In deductive reasoning, if one or both premises state an assumption, the truth of the assumption needs to be proven before the truth of the reasoning can be established.
- The conclusion in deductive reasoning can be judged true or false.
  - If both premises are true, and the conclusion follows logically from them, the conclusion is true.
  - If either premise is false, the conclusion is false.
- Deductive reasoning can build stronger arguments than inductive reasoning as long as any assumptions in the premises can be proven to be true.

● **EXERCISE 3-8** Working individually or with a peer-response group, determine whether each conclusion listed is valid or invalid. Be ready to explain your answers. For help, consult section 3H.

1. Faddish clothes are expensive.
   This shirt is expensive.
   This shirt must be part of a fad.

2. When a storm is threatening, the Coast Guard issues small-craft warnings.

   A storm is threatening.

   The Coast Guard will issue small-craft warnings.

3. The Pulitzer Prize is awarded to outstanding literary works.

   The Great Gatsby never won a Pulitzer Prize.

   The Great Gatsby isn't an outstanding literary work.

4. All states send representatives to the U.S. Congress.

   Puerto Rico sends a representative to the U.S. Congress.

   Puerto Rico is a state.

5. Finding a good job requires patience.

   Sherrill is patient.

   Sherrill will find a good job. ●

3l What are logical fallacies?

Logical fallacies are statements with defective reasoning based on irrational ideas. For example, suppose you see a teenager driving dangerously over the speed limit on a crowded highway. You would be irrational if you decided that all teens drive dangerously. The label for this type of flawed statement is *hasty generalization*, which is one of the most common logical fallacies.

Critical thinking calls for making sure arguments aren't based on logical fallacies. To avoid falling prey to manipulation, study the following list of the most common logical fallacies.

- **Hasty generalization** occurs when someone draws a conclusion based on inadequate evidence. Stereotyping is a common example of hasty generalization. For example, it is faulty to come to the conclusion that *all college students leave bad tips at restaurants* based on a few experiences with some students who have.
- The **either-or fallacy**, also called the *false dilemma*, limits the choices to only two alternatives when more exist. For example, *Either stop criticizing the president or move to another country* falsely implies that completely supporting elected officials is a prerequisite for living in America, to the exclusion of other options.
- A **false analogy** claims that two items are alike when actually they are more different than similar. The statement *If we can put a man on the moon, we should be able to find a cure for cancer* is faulty because space science is very different from biological science.

- A **false cause** asserts that one event leads to another when in fact the two events may be only loosely or coincidentally related. A common type of false cause is called *post hoc, ergo propter hoc*, which is Latin for "after this, therefore because of this." For example, *Ever since we opened that new city park, the crime rate has increased* suggests that the new park caused a change in criminal activity. There are many more likely causes.
- **Slippery slope** arguments suggest that an event will cause a "domino effect," a series of uncontrollable consequences. Some argue that the anti–gun control and pro-choice movements use the slippery slope fallacy when they say that *any* limitation of individual rights will inevitably lead to the removal of other civil rights.
- A **personal attack**, also known as an *ad hominem attack*, criticizes a person's appearance, personal habits, or character instead of dealing with the merits of the individual's argument. The following example is faulty because the writer attacks the person rather than the person's argument: *If Senator Williams had children of her own, we could take seriously her argument against permanently jailing all child abusers.*
- The **bandwagon** effect, also known as an *ad populum appeal*, implies that something is right because everyone else is doing it. An example is a teenager asking, "Why can't I go to the concert next week? All my friends are going."
- **False authority** means citing the opinion of an "expert" who has no claim to expertise about the subject at hand. Using celebrities to advertise products unrelated to their careers is a common example of this tactic.
- An **irrelevant argument** is also called a *non sequitur*, which is Latin for "it does not follow." This flaw occurs when a conclusion does not follow from the premise: *Ms. Chu is a forceful speaker, so she will be an outstanding mayor.* Ms. Chu's speaking style does not entirely reflect her administrative abilities.
- A **red herring** is a fallacy of distraction. Sidetracking an issue by bringing up totally unrelated issues can distract people from the truth. The following question diverts attention from the issue of homelessness rather than arguing about it: *Why worry about the homeless situation when we should really be concerned with global warming?*
- **Begging the question** is also called *circular reasoning*. The supporting reasons only restate the claim. For example, in the statement *We shouldn't*

increase our workers' salaries because then our payroll would be larger, the idea of *increased salaries* and a *larger payroll* essentially state the same outcome; the reason simply restates the claim rather than supporting it.

- **Emotional appeals**, such as appeals to fear, tradition, or pity, substitute emotions for logical reasoning. These appeals attempt to manipulate readers by reaching their hearts rather than their heads. The following statement attempts to appeal to readers' pity rather than their logic: *This woman has lived in poverty all her life; she is ill and has four children at home to care for, so she should not be punished for her crimes.*
- **Slanted language** involves biasing the reader by using word choices that have strong positive or negative connotations. Calling a group of people involved in a political rally a *mob* elicits a negative response from readers, whereas referring to the group as *concerned citizens* receives a positive response.

● **EXERCISE 3-9** Following are comments posted to a newspaper Web site. Working alone or with a peer-response group, do a critical analysis of each, paying special attention to logical fallacies.

1. I oppose the plan to convert the abandoned railroad tracks into a bicycle trail. Everyone knows that the only reason the mayor wants to do this is so that she and her wealthy friends can have a new place to play. No one I know likes this plan, and if they did, it would probably be because they're part of the wine and cheese set, too. The next thing you know, the mayor will be proposing that we turn the schools into art museums or the park into a golf course. If you're working hard to support a family, you don't have time for this bike trail nonsense. And if you're not working hard, I don't have time for you.

   —Mike1218

2. I encourage everyone to support the bicycle trail project. Good recreation facilities are the key to the success of any community. Since the bike trail will add more recreation opportunities, it will guarantee the success of our town. Remember that several years ago our neighbors over in Springfield decided not to build a new park, and look what happened to their economy, especially that city's high unemployment rate. We can't afford to let the same thing happen to us. People who oppose this plan are narrow-minded, selfish, and almost unpatriotic. As that great patriot John Paul Jones said, "I have not yet begun to fight."

   —Bikerdude ●

3J How can I view images with a critical eye?

Watch the Video

You can view images critically in the same way that you can read texts critically by using summary, analysis, synthesis, and evaluation (Quick Box 3.3). For example, look at Figure 3.4 with a critical eye.

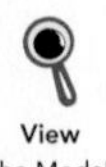

View the Model Document

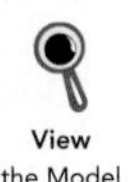

View the Model Document

- *Summarizing* the picture, as well as viewing it literally, you can see—at a minimum—a park with some men playing football, with some geese in the front.
- *Analyzing* the picture, as well as viewing it inferentially, you can "read between the lines" to see that it's fairly rich with layers of meaning. For example, you can tell from the leaves on the ground and the color in some trees, the bareness of others, that it's fall. You can tell the football game is probably happening in a park, not a football field because there are no goal posts or stands. The fact that at least three people are wearing football jerseys indicates that this game was planned, not something that just happened spontaneously. The fact that the geese are milling around on the field suggests either that the game hasn't yet started or that it's been a pretty quiet affair. In fact, the relationship between the geese and players is the most interesting part of the photograph. Notice how the clump of four geese on the right, with a fifth separated to the left mirrors the group of players on the right, with a separate player on

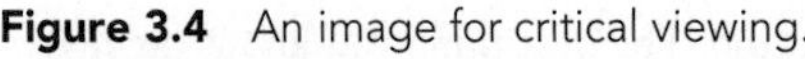

Figure 3.4 An image for critical viewing.

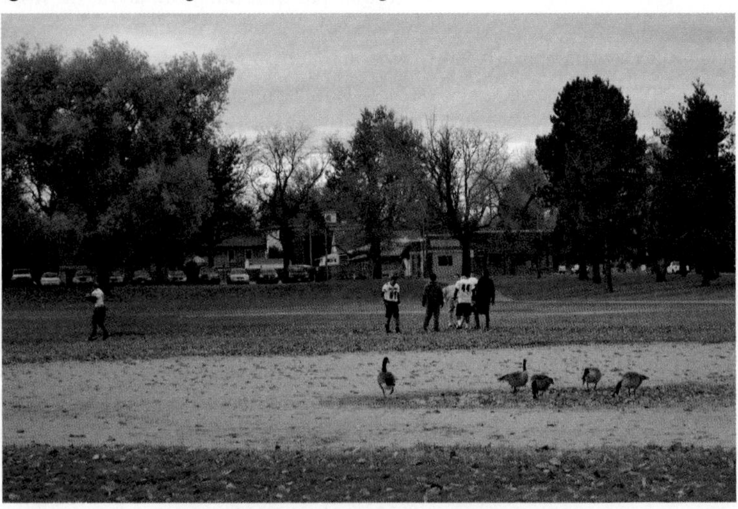

the left. Notice how a couple players have their heads down, as do three of the geese. Now ask yourself, "Why might the photographer have chosen to frame the picture this way, with the geese in front, players in back? What message (perhaps a humorous one) might the photographer have been trying to convey about football—or about geese?"

- *Synthesizing* the picture, you can connect what you've analyzed and inferred to your previous knowledge and experiences, readings, or even other images.
- *Evaluating* the picture is the last step in viewing it critically. You can speak of how the visual "struck" you at first glance; how it did or didn't gain depth of meaning as you analyzed it; and how it lent itself to synthesis within the realms of your personal experience and education.

See Quick Box 3.12.

Quick Box 3.12

Some helpful questions for analyzing visual images

- What does the image show?
- What are its parts? Do the parts belong together (like a lake, trees, and mountains), or do they contrast with one another (such as a woman in a fancy dress sitting on a tractor)? What might be the significance of the relationships among the parts?
- If there is a foreground and a background in the image, what is in each, and why?
- If the image is a scene, what seems to be going on? What might be its message? If the image seems to be part of a story, what might have happened before or after?
- How do the people, if any, seem to be related?
- If the image has a variety of shadings, colorings, and focuses, what's sharply in focus, blurry, bright, in shadows, colorful, or drab? How do such differences call attention to various parts of the image?
- Can you think of any connections between the image and things you've experienced or learned from school, work, reading, or other aspects of your life?
- What is your evaluation of the image?

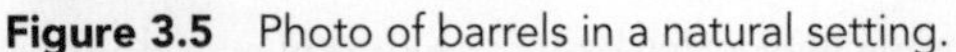

Figure 3.5 Photo of barrels in a natural setting.

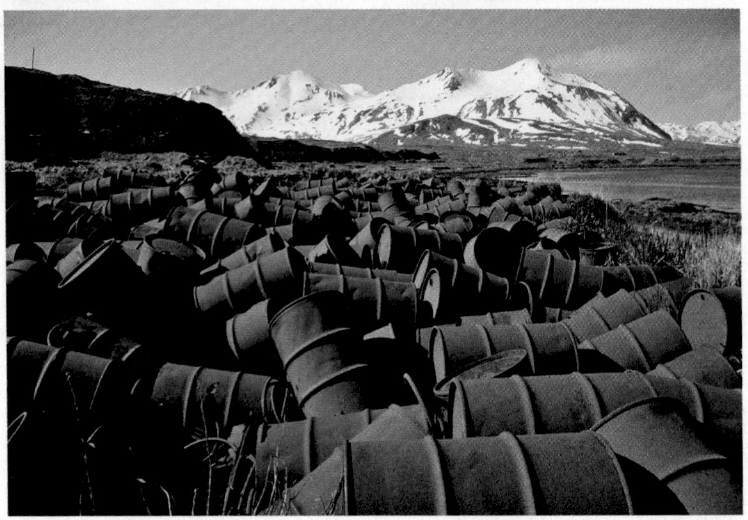

3K How can images persuade?

Because they convey lots of information in a small space, and because they can generate powerful emotional responses, images play a strong role in persuasion. (Just think about advertising!) Sometimes persuasion comes through a single well-chosen image: a picture of a bruised child's face demonstrates the cruelty of child abuse; a picture of a grateful civilian hugging a soldier seeks to show that a military action is just and good.

Figure 3.5 is a photograph of a pile of rusted barrels in a beautiful natural setting. The contrast between the barrels and the snow-covered mountains in the background, the lake, and the blue sky is stark and alarming. The barrels stand between viewers and the stunning scenery; they can't be ignored. The photographer has created this juxtaposition to persuade you—but to what purpose? Perhaps this photo makes an argument against pollution. Perhaps it's a statement against industrial development. Perhaps it emphasizes that people can act carelessly. Images can't state what they mean, although they can move viewers in certain fairly predictable directions.

● **EXERCISE 3-10** Working individually or with a peer-response group, use critical thinking and the questions in Quick Box 3.10 to consider one or both of the following photographs: Figure 3.6 and Figure 3.7. Write either informal notes or a miniessay, according to what your instructor requires.

Figure 3.6 Photo of houses against a city skyline.

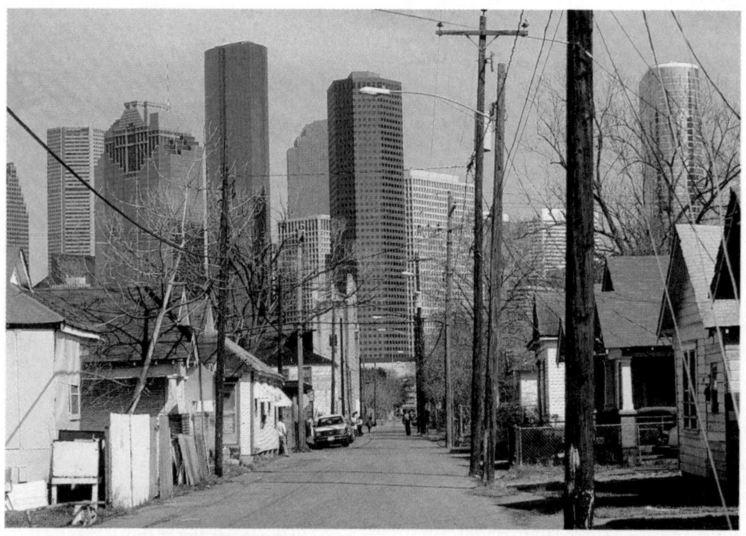

Figure 3.7 Photo of students at a university gate.

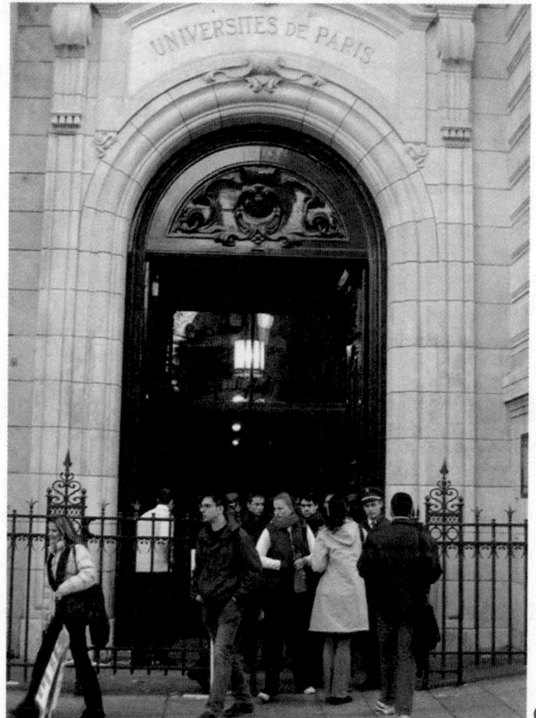

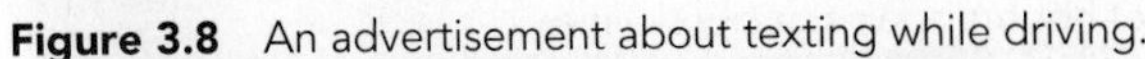

Figure 3.8 An advertisement about texting while driving.

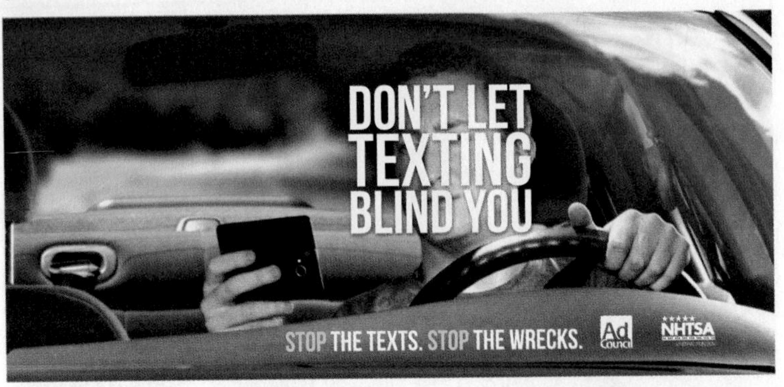
DON'T LET
TEXTING
BLIND YOU
STOP THE TEXTS. STOP THE WRECKS.
Ad Council
NHTSA

3L How can I analyze words combined with images?

Many texts—from Web pages to advertisements, posters, brochures, and so on—are **multimodal** in that they combine words and images. (See Chapters 7 and 63.) These texts can take advantage of logical and ethical appeals, in addition to the emotional appeals readily created by pictures alone. Critically analyzing multimodal texts means considering the images (see Quick Box 3.12) and the words separately, and then analyzing how the two elements combine to create a single effect. Figure 3.8 shows a simple example.

A critical thinker asks, "What is the relationship between the words and the image(s)?" and "Why did the writer choose this particular image for these particular words?"

- Sometimes words and images reinforce one another. A poster with several sentences about poverty, for example, may have a picture of an obviously malnourished person.
- Other times, words and images contrast with one another for effect. Think of a picture of a belching smokestack accompanied by a caption that says, "Everyone deserves fresh air."
- Occasionally, a text might contain images simply to add visual interest. A little decoration is sometimes fine, but always be wary of images that seem simply to be thrown in for the sake of including an image.

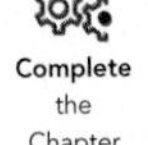
Complete the Chapter Exercises

● **EXERCISE 3-11** Working individually or with a peer-response group, use critical thinking to analyze one of the visual arguments that follow in Figures 3.9 and 3.10. Write either informal notes or a miniessay, according to what your instructor requires.

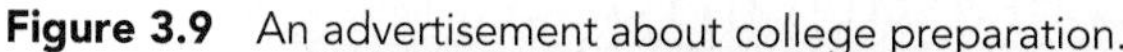

Figure 3.9 An advertisement about college preparation.

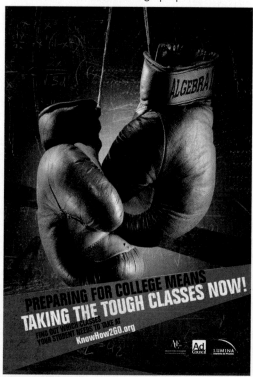

Figure 3.10 An advertisement about saving money.

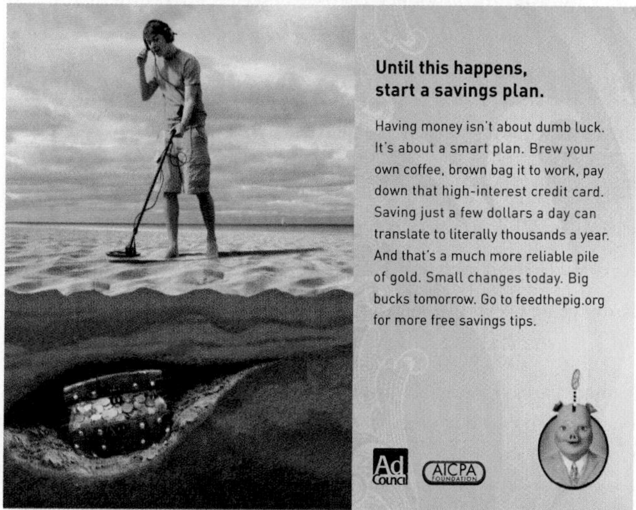

4 Understanding College and Other Writing Situations

Quick Points You will learn to

- Use "purpose" and "audience" in your writing (see 4B).
- Use "role" and "genre" in your writing (see 4C–4D).

4A What is a writing situation?

Consider two situations: (1) you're texting a message to a friend or (2) you're completing a research paper for a history class. In both cases, you're writing, but if you're going to be successful, the results need to be very different. A history paper in the short, casual style of a text message definitely won't impress a professor. Similarly, texting friends in long paragraphs followed by a works cited page would make them impatient (and likely wonder who's stolen your phone). For each task they encounter, effective writers analyze the **writing situation:** a combination of several elements, most importantly your purpose (see 4B) and audience (see 4C). Then they adjust their writing to fit that situation. Quick Box 4.1 lists elements of writing situations.

Understanding a writing situation guides your WRITING PROCESS and shapes your final draft. For example, consider the following task: "In a five-page paper for a political science course, describe government restrictions on

Quick Box 4.1

Elements of writing situations

- **Topic:** What will be the subject of your writing (see 5C)?
- **Purpose:** What should the writing accomplish (see 4B)?
- **Audience:** Who are your main readers (see 4C)?
- **Role:** How do you want your audience to perceive you (see 4D)?
- **Genre:** What form or type of writing do readers expect (see 4E)?
- **Context and Special Requirements:** When and how will your writing be read? Do you have requirements such as length, format, or due dates (see 4F)?

giving to political campaigns." Your INFORMATIVE purpose would require careful research and an objective, serious style, complete with a list of works cited or references, in a paper that explains without judging or arguing. In contrast, imagine the following assignment: "Write a 300-word newspaper editorial arguing that people should (or shouldn't) be allowed to give as much money as they want to a political candidate." As a short editorial, your writing would reflect your PERSUASIVE purpose for a public audience. It would state and explain a position quickly, probably have an energetic style, and include no list of references. The rest of this chapter discusses the other elements of writing situations.

● **EXERCISE 4-1** Either in a class discussion or in a short paper, explain how these different situations would result in different kinds of writing: a résumé and cover letter; a research paper for a sociology course; an e-mail to a friend about that sociology paper; a poster for an upcoming concert; a newspaper editorial; a newspaper news article; an essay exam; a movie review. ●

4B What does "purpose" mean for writing?

A writer's **purpose** is the reason he or she is writing. It's the general result that he or she wants the writing to achieve. Quick Box 4.2 lists five major purposes for writing.

Quick Box 4.2

Purposes for writing

- To express yourself (see 4B.1)
- To build connections (see 4B.2)
- To entertain readers (see 4B.3)
- To inform readers (see 4B.4)
- To persuade readers (see 4B.5)

The purpose of most college writing is to **inform** and to **persuade**.

4B.1 What is expressive writing?

Expressive writing is writing to convey your thoughts, experiences, feelings, or opinions. Some expressive writing is for your eyes only, as in diaries, personal journals, or exploratory drafts. Some expressive writing just blows off

Figure 4.1 A blog written for friends.

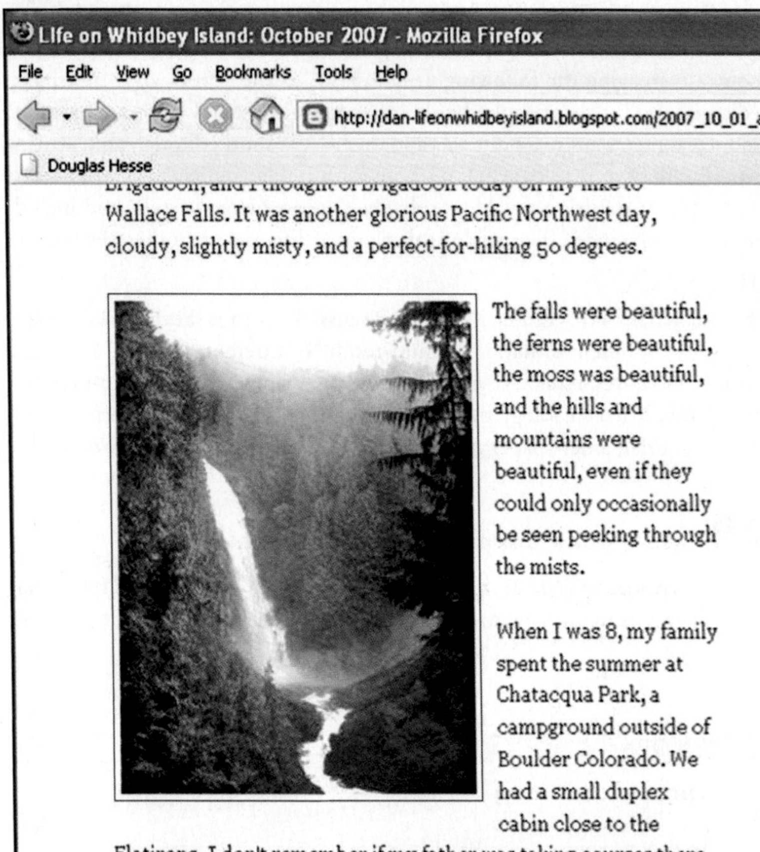

steam. For example, writing that "Congressman Jameson is a total idiot" might make an author feel good, but simply expressing that belief won't change many minds. At best, it lets people know where you stand. Finally, some expressive writing has the purpose of engaging or entertaining readers. We say more about this kind of writing in section 4B.3.

4B.2 What is writing to connect?

In our connected digital world, people do a lot of writing simply to connect to others. They tweet messages, put status updates on social networking sites, comment on others' postings, and share notes, photos, and videos.

Why? Mostly to maintain friendships or relationships. Digital communication has enlivened, this purpose, which is as old as writing personal letters or sticking a child's finger painting on a refrigerator door. Yes, channels like Facebook and Twitter, often do impart information and do try to persuade others. However, their main purpose is to establish and deepen human contact. For example, Figure 4.1 is part of a blog kept by Doug's friend, Dan.

4B.3 What is writing to entertain and engage?

Why do people write novels, movie scripts, comic strips, or jokes? For many reasons, perhaps, but the most important is to entertain. And why do people read sports pages, romances, or horror novels? Mainly for enjoyment. Much writing happens to entertain, and much reading occurs not because people *have* to do it but because they *want* to. Of course, there is "light" entertainment and "serious" entertainment; after all, for all the messages in *Romeo and Juliet*, Shakespeare wrote it for an audience who bought theatre tickets.

Personal essays are a form of expressive writing written for wider readership. Chapter 10 provides advice on writing them.

4B.4 What is writing to inform?

The essential goal of informative writing is to educate your readers about observations, ideas, facts, scientific data, and statistics. Like all good educators, therefore, you want to present your information clearly, accurately, completely, and fairly. Quick Box 4.3 (page 50) gives you a checklist to assess your informative writing. But first, here's a paragraph written to inform.

> "Diamonds in the rough" are usually round and greasy looking. But diamond miners are in no need of dark glasses to shield them from the dazzling brilliance of the mines for quite another reason: even in a diamond pipe, there is only one part diamond per 14 million parts of worthless rock. Approximately 46,000 pounds of earth must be mined and sifted to produce the half-carat gem you might be wearing. No wonder diamonds are expensive!
>
> —Richard B. Manchester, "Diamonds"

As informative writing, this paragraph works because it focuses clearly on its TOPIC (diamonds in the rough), presents facts that can be verified (who, what, when, where), and is written in a reasonable tone.

Informative writing comes in many types and varieties. Chapter 11, for example, provides general advice for writing informative essays. Chapter 12 discusses process essays, Chapter 13 cause and effect analysis, and Chapter 14 textual analysis.

Quick Box 4.3

Questions important to informative writing

- Is its information clear?
- Does it present facts, ideas, and observations that can be verified?
- Does its information seem complete and accurate?
- Does it explain ideas or concepts clearly and effectively?
- Is the writer's TONE reasonable and free of distortions (see 3E.6)?

4B.5 What is writing to persuade?

Persuasive writing, also called *argumentative* writing, seeks to persuade readers to support a particular opinion. When you write to persuade, you deal with debatable topics—those that people can consider from more than one point of view. Your goal is to change your readers' minds—or at least to bring their opinions closer to yours. You want your audience to think beyond their present position (for example, reasoning why national security should—or shouldn't—limit individual rights) or to take action (for example, register to vote). Examples of persuasive writing include newspaper editorials, letters to the editor, opinion essays in magazines, reviews, sermons, advertising, fund-raising letters, books that argue a point of view, business proposals, and so on.

Argument is a frequent purpose for college writing. We discuss common types of argument in three chapters: Chapter 15: Argument Essays (covering general principles, strategies, and examples), Chapter 16: Proposal and Solution Essays, and Chapter 17: Evaluation Essays.

In general, persuasive writing means you need to move beyond merely stating your opinion. You need to support your opinion by using specific, illustrative details to back up your claims and assertions, as you can see in the following short passage:

> Our nation's economic and democratic future depends on preparing more students to succeed in college, work and life. We must engage all students in meaningful and rigorous academic work in high school and prepare more of them to succeed in college.
>
> Connecting studies to real-world issues through learning communities is a proven way to get students engaged and motivated. But there is a difference between providing students with good learning environments that include fellow students with similar interests and narrowing students' options

by tracking especially less-advantaged students into career-oriented paths in high school.

The fact is that many of the well-paying jobs that today's ninth graders might have 10 years from now do not yet exist—and the technical demands of all jobs are changing so rapidly that narrowing one's academic focus too early won't prepare one well for college and will diminish rather than enhance one's employability over the long term.

The key to success in the global economy is having the broad capacities and knowledge developed by a solid liberal education. In an economy fueled by innovation, these capabilities have, in fact, become America's most valuable economic asset.

—Debra Humphreys, "Give Students Broad Education, Not Narrow Vocational Tracks"

As persuasive writing, this passage works because it provides factual information on school and work; it expresses a point of view that resides in sound reasoning; it offers a logical line of reasoning; and it tries to get the reader to agree with the point of view. Quick Box 4.4 lists questions to assess persuasive writing.

Quick Box 4.4

Persuasive writing

- Does it present a point of view about which opinions vary?
- Does it support its point of view with specifics?
- Does it provide sound reasoning and logic?
- Are the parts of its argument clear?
- Does it intend to evoke a reaction from the reader?

● **EXERCISE 4-2** For each paragraph, decide what the dominant purpose is for each of the following paragraphs. Use the information in section 4B to explain your answers.

A. Trees are living archives, carrying within their structure a record not only of their age but also of precipitation and temperature for each year in which a ring was formed. The record might also include the marks of forest fires, early frosts and, incorporated into the wood itself, chemical elements the tree removed from its environment. Thus, if we only knew how to unlock its secrets, a tree could tell us a great deal about what was happening in its neighborhood from the time of its beginning. Trees can tell us what was happening before written records became available. They also have a great deal to tell us about our future. The records of past climate that they contain can help us to understand the natural forces that produce our weather, and this, in turn, can help us plan.

—James S. Trefil, "Concentric Clues from Growth Rings Unlock the Past"

B. Actual physical location threatens to evaporate everywhere we look. Information, we are everywhere taught, has annihilated distances. Surgeons can cut you open from a thousand miles away. Facsimile Las Vegas casinos deliver Rome and New York on the same daily walk. You don't have to go to the office to go to the office. You can shop in your kitchen and go to school in your living room. And, sadly enough, when you actually do go out shopping, one mall seems much like another. For what actually matters, physicality doesn't matter anymore. Even with money; now, we are told, information about money is more important than the actual green.

—Richard Lanham, *The Economics of Attention*

C. I've had it with hipsters. I've had it with their skinny jeans and their plastic glasses. I've had it with their smug superiority over everyone else—at least as they see it. They pay stupid amounts of money drinking cheap beer just because it's trendy. They decide a restaurant is popular and cram it like sheep until the poor regulars no longer feel welcome. I wish they'd all decide to stick to one neighborhood, concentrating the idiocy there.

—Rod Bateman, student

D. Soybeans. The smell hangs thick over Decatur, like a lollipop left to melt on a heat register—sweet and sticky and almost nauseating. Locals are used to this: the scent of money, Archer Daniels Midland, jobs. Midwestern and rural as corn, soybeans are fillers in ice cream and gasoline.

—Becky Bradway, *Pink Houses and Family Taverns* ●

● **EXERCISE 4-3** Consulting section 4B, write on each of these topics twice, once to inform and once to persuade your reader: reality television, part-time jobs, a current movie. Your instructor can tell you if you should write paragraphs or short papers. Be prepared to discuss how your two treatments of each topic differ. ●

4C What does "audience" mean for writing?

Your **audience** consists of everyone who will read your writing, but it especially refers to **readers** to whom you're most directly aiming your words. For example, anyone can try to read an issue of *The New England Journal of Medicine*, but that publication is aimed at doctors and medical researchers. An article about how to treat a certain illness would be written very differently if, instead of doctors, the audience consisted of parents whose children had that illness. The article would be even more different if it were written for children themselves. Effective writers know they need to adjust their writing for different audiences. The questions in Quick Box 4.5 (page 54) will help you analyze your audience for a particular writing situation.

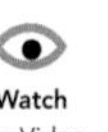
Watch the Video

There are four general kinds of audiences:

- General educated audiences (see 4C.1)
- Specialist audiences (see 4C.2)
- Your instructor (who represents your general or specialized readers) (see 4C.3)
- Your peers (classmates, coworkers, friends, or others like yourself) (see 9A)

4C.1 What is a general educated audience?

A general educated audience is composed of experienced readers who regularly read newspapers, magazines, and books, whether in print or on the screen. They read not just because they have to but because they want to be an informed citizen. These readers typically have a basic knowledge of many subjects and are likely to understand something about your topic. If your writing contains too many technical details or unusual references, your writing may confuse and alienate them. Consequently, for general educated readers you need to avoid using uncommon terms without plainly defining or explaining them.

General educated readers usually approach a piece of writing expecting to become interested in it, to learn something, or to see a subject from a perspective other than their own. As a writer, work to fulfill those expectations.

Alert: There are readers who aren't very well educated, and, sadly, there are readers who are prejudiced or narrow minded. Unless your instructor assigns otherwise, uninformed or biased readers usually aren't the audiences for college writing. ●

Quick Box 4.5

Ways to analyze your audience

IN WHAT SETTING ARE THEY READING?

- Academic setting? Specifically, what subject?
- Workplace setting? Specifically, what business area?
- Public setting? Specifically, what form of communication? (newspaper? blog? poster?)

WHO ARE THEY?

- Age, gender, economic situation
- Ethnic backgrounds, political philosophies, religious beliefs
- Roles (student, parent, voter, wage earner, property owner, veteran, and others)
- Interests, hobbies

WHAT DO THEY KNOW?

- General level of education
- Specific level of knowledge about topic: Do they know less than you about the subject? As much as you about the subject? More than you about the subject?
- Beliefs: Is the audience likely to agree with your point of view? Disagree with your point of view? Have no opinion about the topic?
- Interests: Is the audience eager to read about the topic? Open to the topic? Resistant to or not interested in the topic?

WHAT IS THEIR RELATIONSHIP TO YOU?

- Distance and formality: Do you know your audience personally or not?
- Authority: Does your reader have the authority to judge or evaluate you (a supervisor at work, a teacher)? Do you have the authority to evaluate your reader, or does this not apply?

4C.2 What is a specialist audience?

A specialist audience is composed of readers who have a thorough knowledge of specific subjects or who are particularly committed to certain interests or viewpoints. Many people are experts in their occupational fields, and some become experts in areas that simply interest them, such as astronomy or raising orchids.

Specialist readers may also share certain assumptions and beliefs. For example, suppose you're writing for an audience of immigrants to the United States who feel strongly about keeping their cultural traditions alive. You can surely assume your readers know those traditions well, so you won't need to describe and explain the basics. Similarly, if you intend to argue that immigrants should abandon their cultural traditions in favor of U.S. practices, you'll want to write respectfully about their beliefs. Examples of specialized audiences include

- Members of specific academic disciplines, such as chemistry, political science, art history;
- People in specific professions, such as finance, education, engineering;
- People with common interests or hobbies, such as fans of certain television shows, of cooking, of NASCAR;
- People with common political beliefs (conservatives, liberals, independents) or views (on health care, the environment, immigration);
- People with common experiences, such as veterans, single parents, athletes.

ESOL Tips: (1) If you do not share a cultural background with your readers, it may be difficult for you to estimate how much your readers know about your topic. Discussing your topic with friends or classmates might help you decide what background information you need to include in your paper.

(2) As someone from a non–U.S. culture, you might be surprised—even offended—by the directness with which people speak and write in the United States. If so, we hope you'll read our open letter—it introduces Part 8 of this handbook—to multilingual students about honoring their cultures. U.S. writers and readers expect language and style that are very direct, straightforward, and without embellishment (as compared with the styles of many other cultures). U.S. college instructors expect essays in academic writing to contain a thesis statement (usually at the end of the introductory paragraph). They further expect your writing to contain an organized presentation of information that moves tightly from one paragraph to the next, with generalizations that you always back up with strong supporting details, and with an ending paragraph that presents a logical conclusion to your discussion. Also, for writing in the United States, you need to use so-called edited American English. This means following the

rules used by educated speakers. In reality, the United States has a rich mixture of grammar systems, but academic writing nevertheless requires edited American English. ●

4C.3 What is my instructor's role as audience?

As your audience, your instructor functions in three ways. First, your instructor assumes the role of your target audience by reading and responding to your writing as though he or she is one of your intended general or specific readers. Second, your instructor acts as a coach who is dedicated to helping improve your writing. Third, your instructor evaluates your final drafts.

Although instructors know that few students are experienced writers or experts on the subjects they write about, they expect your writing to reflect that you've taken the time to learn something worthwhile about a topic and then to write about it clearly. Don't assume that your instructor can mentally fill in what you leave out of your writing. Indeed, you might think that it's wrong, even insulting to your instructor, if you explain things in depth. However, instructors—indeed, all readers—can't be mind readers, and they expect students' writing to fully explore their chosen topic.

4D What is role in writing?

It may surprise you to learn that you can take on different **roles** (personalities or identities) for different writing situations. For example, suppose you're trying to persuade readers to save energy.

- You might emphasize your role as a prospective parent who is personally worried about energy for your future children.
- You might present yourself as a conservationist concerned about the environment.
- You might present yourself as someone giving budget advice to consumers.

The point is that the role your readers see can affect how they react to your argument. For example, some readers unfortunately dismiss students as young or naive. So, you might want to emphasize your role as a voter or a taxpayer on some issue, not your role as a student. Both of us (Lynn and Doug) have found that sometimes it's useful if readers know that we're professors, but other times it's not. Some readers are intimidated by professors, whereas some other readers think professors are "impractical" or lack the ability to identify with them. We hope neither are true.

4E What is genre in writing?

To say that a writing fits in a particular **genre** means that it can be grouped with others in a category of writings that share features in common. You might be most familiar with the genres of and distinctions between poetry, fiction, and drama. However, there are many other genres of writing. Consider the following list:

A term or research paper

A resume

A lab report

A personal essay

A newspaper editorial

A job application letter

A movie review

A Web site

A reader encountering each genre would expects to see certain characteristics. For example, imagine that you turned in a lab report that began, "It was a warm, sunny April afternoon as I walked into the chemistry lab, shivering with gleeful anticipation at the prospect of titrating beakers full of colorful substances, arrayed on the lab bench like dancers in a Broadway musical." Your chemistry instructor would almost certainly give you a low grade for failing to write something that fit the objective and precise genre of a lab report.

The best way to understand the type of writing that you've been assigned is to look at some examples. The main reason we've put in so many examples of actual writing, especially in Chapters 10 to 17 but also throughout the book, is that students learn best from seeing what real writers actually do. Quick Box 4.6 (page 58) lists questions that help you analyze pieces that represent a genre.

Alert: Terms that describe different types of writing are often used interchangeably. Most instructors attach specific meanings to each one; we've listed several terms. If your instructor's use of terms isn't clear, ask for clarification. For example, the words *essay*, *theme*, and *composition* usually—but not always—refer to written works of about 500 to 1,500 words. *Essay* is probably the most common. Similarly, the word *paper* can mean anything from a few paragraphs to a complex research project; it often refers to longer works. Finally, the general term *piece of writing* can refer to all types of writing. ●

Quick Box 4.6

Questions for analyzing genre

- What is the PURPOSE of the writing?
- Who is the apparent AUDIENCE?
- Are there clearly identified parts of individual works? Are there headings, for example?
- What kind of evidence or sources seem to count in this genre? Readings? Author's experiences? Measurements or data? Observations?
- What is the TONE or style of works in the genre? Formal? Informal? Friendly? Stuffy? Cautious? Energetic?
- What seems to be the writer's role? For example, is he or she an impartial observer who keeps in the background or a center of attention whose experience and personality are on display?
- What DOCUMENTATION STYLE, if any, does it use?

For centuries, formal writing has consisted of essays and reports containing paragraphs of connected words. These texts will always remain essential, and you need to master them. However, computers have enabled different kinds of genres, and we list some of them in Quick Box 4.7. Don't worry if your knowledge about producing any of these types of writing is limited. Instructors who require such projects can tell you how to proceed.

4F What are context and special requirements in writing?

Context refers to the circumstances in which your readers will encounter your writing. For example, persuading people to buy fuel-efficient cars when gas costs $2 per gallon is very different than when it costs over $4. Arguing that we should have a military draft is different in a time of war than in a time of peace.

Special requirements are practical matters such as how much time you're given to complete an assignment, the required length of your writing, the format of your final draft, and so on. For example, your audience expects more from an assignment that you had a week to complete than from one written in class. In the second case, your readers realize you had to write in relative haste, though no one ever accepts sloppy or careless work. Make sure you know—and follow—all special requirements.

Complete the Chapter Exercises

Quick Box 4.7

Some digital genres

BLOGS Short for We**b logs**, the term refers to messages that writers post in sites that anyone can read on the Internet. Blogs can be personal, such as daily reflections written for an audience of friends and family, or they can be on cultural, political, social, scientific or other topics and intended general educated or specialized audiences.

WIKIS A Web site that allows multiple readers to change its content. We explain how to write in wikis in section 63C.

PRESENTATION SLIDES Visuals created with software such as PowerPoint to be projected or viewed on screens. They can incorporate both words and images. Chapter 62 provides advice on creating presentations.

PODCASTS Sound files that can be shared over the Internet. Many podcasts are miniature essays or commentaries that their writers have carefully polished and then read, as a script.

VIDEOS Digital cameras or smartphones allow people to convey ideas or information through short movies on sites like YouTube and elsewhere. Similar to podcasts, effective videos are often built around carefully written and narrated scripts and often contain titles or captions. We discuss composing in digital environments in Chapter 63.

PORTFOLIOS A collection of several of your own texts that you've chosen to represent the range of your skills and abilities. They can appear on paper or in digital form. See Chapter 8.

5 Essential Processes for Writing

Quick Points You will learn to

- Adapt the writing processes to your own needs (see 5A).
- Think like a writer, especially about your purpose and audience (see 5B).
- Use different strategies to develop ideas (see 5C–5D).
- Write an effective thesis statement (see 5E).
- Use outlines to help you write (see 5F).

5A What are writing processes?

Many people assume that a real writer can magically write a finished product, word by perfect word. Experienced writers know that writing is a process, a series of activities that starts the moment they begin thinking about a topic and ends when they complete a final draft. In addition, experienced writers are aware that good writing is actually rewriting—again and yet again. Their drafts contain additions, deletions, rewordings, and rearrangements. Figure 5.1 shows how we drafted and revised the first few sentences of this chapter.

Figure 5.1 Draft and revision of the first paragraph in Chapter 5.

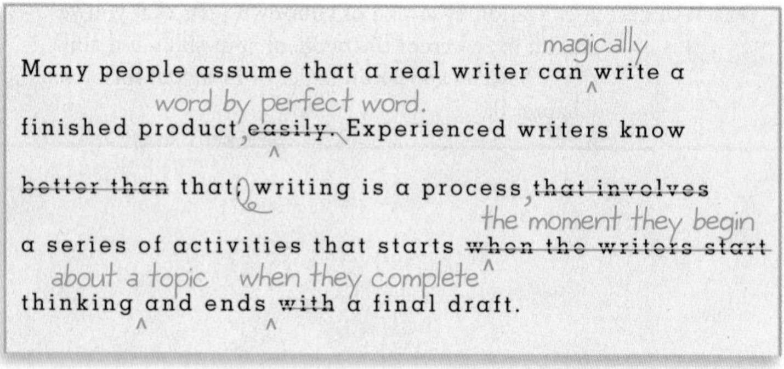

magically
Many people assume that a real writer can ^ write a
word by perfect word.
finished product, ~~easily.~~ Experienced writers know
~~better than~~ that writing is a process, ~~that involves~~
the moment they begin
a series of activities that starts ~~when the writers start~~
about a topic when they complete
thinking and ends ~~with~~ a final draft.

Quick Box 5.1

Steps in the writing process

- **Planning** means you think like a writer (see 5B); select a topic (see 5C); determine your purpose and audience (see 4B and 4C); develop ideas about your topic (see 5D); compose a tentative thesis statement (see 5E); and consider using an outline (see 5F).
- **Drafting** means you compose your ideas into sentences and paragraphs (see 5G).
- **Revising** means rewriting your drafts, often more than once (see 5I).
- **Editing** means you check for the correctness of your surface-level features, including grammar, spelling, punctuation, and mechanics (see 5J).
- **Proofreading** means you carefully scrutinize your final draft to fix errors (see 5K).

All writers adapt their **writing processes** to suit their personalities as well as specific WRITING SITUATIONS. For typical steps in the writing process, see Quick Box 5.1. Although these steps are listed separately, few writers in the real world work in lockstep order. They know that the steps overlap and double back on themselves, as the circles and arrows in Figure 5.2 show.

What is the major difference between weak writers and successful ones? The good ones refuse to give up. Good writing takes time. As you discover your personal preferences for your writing process, be patient with yourself. Remember that experienced writers sometimes struggle with ideas that are difficult to express, sentences that won't take shape, and words that aren't precise. When that becomes frustrating, they put their writing aside for a while and return later with the "new eyes" that only distance makes available.

Figure 5.2 Visualizing the writing process.

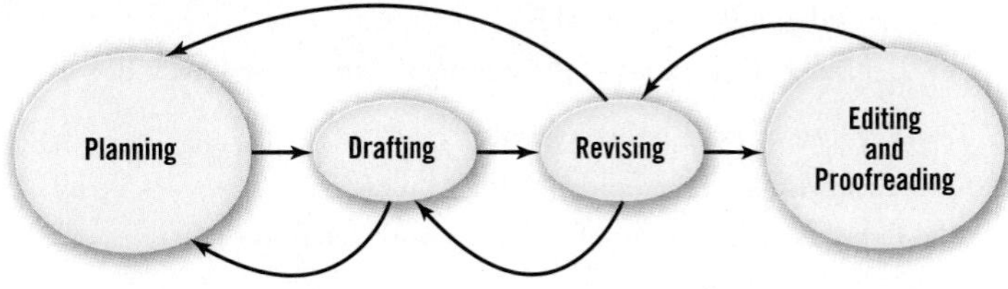

5B How do I think like a writer?

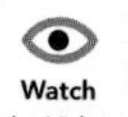

Quick Box 5.2 summarizes effective writers' habits of mind and practices.

Quick Box 5.2

How to think like a writer

***Think** by engaging in writers' habits of mind*

- Realize that writing takes time.
- Know that writing requires focused attention free of distractions.
- Recognize that all writing involves rewriting, often many times (see 5L).
- Believe that the physical act of writing helps ideas spring to mind (see 5D).
- Think critically (see Chapter 3).

***Think** by completely understanding the task at hand*

- Read writing assignments completely. Then reread them.
- Estimate how long you'll need for
  - Planning (see 5C–5H)
  - Drafting (see 5G)
  - Revising (see 5I)
  - Editing (see 5J)
  - Proofreading (see 5K)
- Calculate and set aside the total time you'll need to complete the assignment.

***Think** by analyzing the writing task*

- Think about your topic (see 5C).
- Consider multiple ways to develop your topic (see 5D).
- Think carefully about your thesis statement (see 5E).
- Consider outlining (see 5F).
- Consider all elements of the writing situation (see Quick Box 4.1).

***Think** of writing as an ongoing process*

- Use revising opportunities to their fullest.
- Expect to edit and proofread your work carefully.

5C How do I begin planning?

Begin every writing assignment by carefully analyzing the writing situation you're given. Some assignments are very specific. For example, here's an assignment that leaves no room for choice: "In a 500-word article for an audience of seventh graders, explain how oxygen is absorbed in the lungs." More often, however, writing-class assignments aren't nearly as specific as that one.

5C.1 Selecting your own topic or purpose

If you have to choose a **topic**, take time to think through your ideas. Avoid getting so deeply committed to one topic that you cannot change to a more suitable topic in the time allotted.

Beware of topics so broad that they lead to well-meaning but vague generalizations (for example, "Education is necessary for success"). Also, beware of topics so narrow that they lead nowhere after a few sentences.

GENERAL TOPIC	Marriage
TOO BROAD	What makes a successful marriage?
TOO NARROW	Couples can go to a municipal hall to get married.
APPROPRIATE	Compromise is vital for a happy marriage.

Suppose your assignment doesn't indicate a writing purpose—for example, "Write an essay on exercising." Here, you're expected to choose a purpose. Will you try to explain to a general educated audience why some people exercise regularly and others don't? Will you try to persuade a specialized audience of nonexercising college students to start? Will you summarize the current literature on exercise to inform an audience of school nurses? Considering different audiences and purposes can help you find a topic angle that engages you.

5C.2 Broadening a narrow topic

You know a topic is too narrow when you realize there's little to say after a few sentences. When faced with a too-narrow topic, think about underlying concepts. For example, suppose you want to write about the television show *American Idol*. If you chose "*American Idol* debuted in 2002," you'd be working with a single fact rather than a topic. To expand beyond such a narrow thought, you could think about a general area that your fact fits into—say, the impact of television shows on popular culture. Although that is too broad to be useful, you're headed in the right direction. You might arrive at a suitable topic like, "What impact has *American Idol* had on popular music since it began broadcasting in 2002?" Depending on your WRITING SITUATION (4A), you might need to narrow your idea further by focusing on one aspect, such as how the appearances and behaviors of performers affected what people expect on stage.

5C.3 Narrowing a broad topic

Narrowing a broad topic calls for you to break the topic down into subtopics. For example, if you're assigned "relationships" as the topic for a 1,000-word essay, you'd be too broad if you chose "What kinds of relationships are there?" You'd be too narrow if you came up with "Alexandra and Gavin have dated for two years." You'd probably be on target with a subtopic such as "In successful relationships, people learn to accept each other's faults." Here are two more examples.

SUBJECT	*music*
WRITING SITUATION	freshman composition class informative purpose instructor as audience 500 words; one week
POSSIBLE TOPICS	"How music affects moods" "The main characteristics of country music" "The types of songs in Disney animations"

SUBJECT	*cities*
WRITING SITUATION	sociology course persuasive purpose peers and then instructor as audience 950 to 1,000 words; ten days
POSSIBLE TOPICS	"The importance of public transportation" "Discomforts of city living" "How open spaces enhance the quality of city life"

5D How can I develop ideas about my topic?

When you're looking for ideas to develop your topics, try the strategies in Quick Box 5.3. Experiment to find out which strategies you find most helpful, adapting to your PURPOSE and AUDIENCE for each new writing assignment.

Quick Box 5.3

Strategies for developing ideas

- Freewriting and focused freewriting (see 5D.1)
- Brainstorming (see 5D.2)
- Asking and answering structured questions (see 5D.3)
- Clustering, also called "mapping" (see 5D.4)
- Writing in a journal or a blog (see 5D.5)
- Chatting with other people (see 5D.6)
- Read, browse, or search (see 5D.7)

5D.1 Freewriting

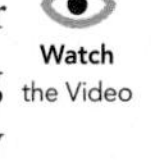

Freewriting is writing nonstop. You write down whatever comes into your mind without stopping to wonder whether the ideas are good or the spelling is correct. When you freewrite, don't interrupt the flow. Don't censor any thoughts. Don't delete.

The physical act of writing triggers ideas, memories, and insights. Freewriting works best if you set a goal—perhaps writing for fifteen minutes or filling one or two pages. Keep going until you reach that goal, even if you have to write one word repeatedly until a new word comes to mind. Sometimes your writing might seem mindless, but often interesting ideas will startle or delight you.

In **focused freewriting**, you write from a specific starting point—a sentence from your general freewriting, an idea, a quotation, or anything else you choose. Except for this initial focal point, focused freewriting is the same as regular freewriting. See where your thoughts take you. Just keep moving forward.

5D.2 Brainstorming

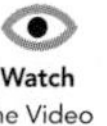

Brainstorming means listing everything that comes to mind about your topic. Don't censor your thoughts. Let your mind roam, and jot down all ideas that flow logically or that simply pop into your head. After you've brainstormed for a while, look over your lists for patterns. If you don't have enough to work with, choose one item in your list and brainstorm from there. Next, move the items, even if loosely related, into groups. Discard items that don't fit into any group.

Here's some brainstorming by student Carol Moreno, whose essay about the benefits for women of learning to lift weights appears in Chapter 11. Carol grouped the items marked here with an asterisk and used them in her second paragraph.

*women don't want masculine-looking muscles

how much weight is safe for a woman to lift?

how long does it take?

*women's muscles grow long, not bulky

how to bend down for lifting?

*firm muscles are attractive

free weights or machines?

*exercise type—anaerobic

*exercise type—aerobic exercise

injuries

*toning the body

● **EXERCISE 5-1** Here's a list brainstormed for a writing assignment. The topic was "Ways to promote a new movie." Working individually or in a peer-response group, look over the list and group the ideas. You'll find that some ideas don't fit into a group. Then, add any other ideas you have to the list.

previews in theaters
TV ads
provocative
movie reviews
how movie was made
sneak previews
word of mouth
suspense
book the movie was based on
locations
Internet trailers
adventure
newspaper ads
stars
director
topical subject
special effects
dialogue
excitement
photography
Facebook page ●

5D.3 Asking and answering structured questions

Asking and answering structured questions can stimulate you to think of ideas for developing your topic. One popular question set consists of those journalists use: *Who? What? Where? When? Why? How?*

Here's how Alex Garcia used the journalists' questions to start him writing about why organic foods are worth the cost, shown in Chapter 15:

Who are the people who care about the benefits of eating organic foods?

What are typical foods people prefer to be organically grown?

Where did the idea of organic foods originate?

When did organic foods become popular?

Why do organic foods cost more than nonorganic foods?

How are organic foods processed?

Another generative question set was developed years ago by rhetorician Richard Young and his colleagues.

- What are the major characteristics of the topic?
- What's the topic's history? How has the topic changed recently? How might the topic change in the future?
- To what categories does the topic belong? How does the topic fit into a larger context?
- How does the topic relate to other aspects of culture or ideas? How is the topic similar or different?

Some of these questions, in addition to the journalists' questions, helped Alex Garcia develop his essay about organic foods in Chapter 15:

What are the major characteristics of organic foods?

What's the history of growing organic food, and how has the process changed?

How might it change in the future?

What are larger contexts for organically grown food, such as being related to overall health issues?

How does interest in organically grown food connect to other aspects of our culture?

5D.4 Clustering

Clustering, also called *mapping*, is a visual form of brainstorming. Write your topic in the middle of a sheet and then circle it. Next, move out from the middle circle by drawing lines with circles at the end of each line. Put in each circle a subtopic or detail related to the main topic. If a subtopic or detail in a given circle has further subtopics, draw lines and circles fanning out from that circle. Continue using this method as far as it can take you.

Watch the Video

Though you might not include in your essay all the subtopics and details in your map, chances are that some the material might come in handy. For example, here's the map that Miguel Sanz drew to help him think of ideas for the second paragraph of his essay about auditioning to be in a musical.

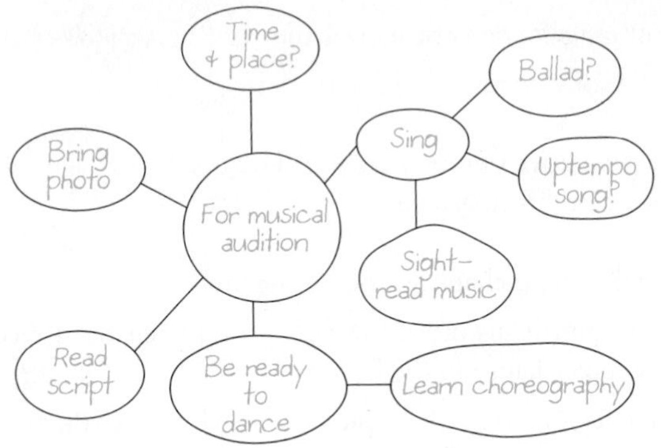

5D.5 Writing in a journal or blog

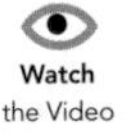

Writing in a journal or blog every day for 5 to 10 minutes is like having a conversation with yourself. The habit of regular writing makes getting started easier and gets you used to expressing yourself through words.

Draw on your thoughts, experiences, observations, dreams, reactions to your course work, or responses to something you've read recently. Use a paper notebook or a computer, depending on what's most handy and pleasurable for you. One good use for your journal or blog is to serve as a source of topics for essays as well as related supporting specifics.

5D.6 Chatting

Chatting with others means talking with them—but with a targeted purpose. Talk about your topic, and toss around ideas. Keep paper, or your journal or computer, at hand so that you'll be sure to jot down the ideas as they emerge. Little is as frustrating as remembering you'd had a good idea—but you've now forgotten it. Chatting today has come to mean more than only talking. You can chat online through texting, messaging, e-mail, and other electronic forums. Digital chats not only stimulate your thinking but also put ideas into words.

5D.7 Reading or browsing

Reading newspapers, magazines, or books, whether in print or online, provides a constant source of ideas. Experienced writers do this all the time. Check out online versions of newspapers or magazines every day, especially national papers like the *New York Times* or *Washington Post*. Follow blogs on topics you find interesting. Spend time in the PERIODICALS or new books section of a library or browse a bookstore; just looking at covers, images, or contents can generate fresh ideas.

● **EXERCISE 5-2** Try each structured technique for discovering and compiling ideas discussed in 5D. Use your own topics or select from the suggestions here.

1. Professions and job prospects
2. An important personal decision
3. Professional sports
4. Advertisements on television
5. What you want in a life partner ●

5E How can a thesis statement help me plan?

A **thesis statement** serves as the central, controlling point for most college writing assignments. A thesis statement gives readers a general preview of what they can expect to read about. The basic requirements of a thesis statement are listed in Quick Box 5.4 (page 70), but just as a complete essay doesn't appear in full bloom in a first draft, so too the first draft of a thesis statement is tentative. As you revise your essay, continually check your thesis statement to make sure that it goes well with the content of your essay. If you find a mismatch, revise one or the other—or perhaps both.

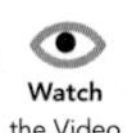

In writing "Women Can Pump Iron Too," shown in Chapter 11, student Carol Moreno describes how with the right training woman can become strong by lifting free weights. She uses the idiom "pumping iron," a commonly used term in gyms. Her thesis statement evolved from a thin assertion to a full one that makes her message clear.

NO I think women can pump iron like men.

This has too little information.

NO If trained, any woman can get strong.

The concept of lifting weights is gone; "any" is too broad.

Quick Box 5.4

Basic requirements for a thesis statement

1. It states the essay's subject—the topic of the writing.
2. It states the essay's **assertion** or **claim**, putting forward the central message or point.
3. It leads to the essay's TOPIC SENTENCES (see 6E) that start the essay's BODY PARAGRAPHS (see 6D).
4. It usually comes at the end of the INTRODUCTORY PARAGRAPH (see 6C).
5. It uses clear, straightforward language without IRONY or SARCASM.
6. It might lay out the major subdivisions of a topic, but a more graceful technique is to imply them rather than stating them outright.
7. It avoids common mistakes in writing a thesis statement:
   a. Don't use it to give a fact that leads nowhere.
   b. Don't say you're not an expert in your topic; your readers expect you to have learned enough about it to write your essay.
   c. Don't announce your essay's PURPOSE with words such as "The purpose of this essay is . . . "
   d. Don't refer back to your essay's title using words such as "This is an important issue . . ." or "My essay is called 'XYZ' because . . ."

NO In spite of thinking only men can "pump iron," women can also do it with the right training.

This repeats the essay's title rather than give its central message.

YES With the right training, women can "pump iron" to build strength.

Captures the central message of Moreno's essay, meets the thesis statement requirements, and avoids the pitfalls listed in in Quick Box 5.7.

Following are three other examples.

TOPIC ***Reality television***

NO There are many kinds of reality television shows.

YES A common feature of reality television shows is a villain, a contestant that viewers love to hate.

TOPIC ***Public transportation***

NO Public transportation has many advantages.

YES Investing in public transportation pays strong benefits in environmental quality, economic development, and social interactions.

TOPIC ***Deceptive advertising***

NO Deceptive advertising can cause many problems for consumers.

YES Deceptive advertising costs consumers not only their money but also their health.

● **EXERCISE 5-3** Each set of sentences offers several versions of a thesis statement. Within each set, the thesis statements progress from weak to strong. Work individually or with a group to explain why the first three choices in each set are weak and the last is best.

A. 1. Advertising is complex.
   2. Magazine advertisements appeal to readers.
   3. Magazine advertisements must be creative and appealing to all readers.
   4. To appeal to readers, magazine advertisements must skillfully use language, color, and design.

B. 1. Soccer is a widely played sport.
   2. Playing soccer is fun.
   3. Soccer requires various skills.
   4. Playing soccer for fun and exercise requires agility, stamina, and teamwork.

C. 1. We should pay attention to the environment.
   2. We should worry about air pollution.
   3. Automobile emissions cause air pollution.
   4. Congress should raise emissions standards for passenger cars and SUVs.

D. 1. Cell phones are popular.
   2. People use cell phones in many situations.
   3. The increased use of cell phones causes problems.
   4. Using cell phones while driving should be illegal. ●

5F How can outlining help me plan?

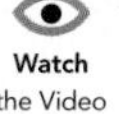

An **outline** is a structured, sequential list of the contents of a text. Some instructors require an outline with assignments, but others don't. Always ask. When given a choice, some students never outline, whereas others find that outlining helps them write. Figure out what works best for you by experimenting.

For example, you might like to use outlines for some, but not all, types of writing assignments (see Chapters 10–17). Also, you might find that outlining helps at different stages of your writing process: perhaps before DRAFTING to help you flesh out, pull together, and arrange material; or perhaps during REVISION to help you check your flow of thought or make sure you haven't gone off the topic.

An **informal outline** does not follow the numbering and lettering conventions of a formal outline. It often looks like a BRAINSTORMING list, with ideas jotted down in a somewhat random order. Here's an informal outline for the second paragraph of student Yanggu Cui's argument essay, "A Proposal to Improve Fan Behavior at Children's Games" (see Chapter 16).

Sample Informal Outline

little league games

parents on sidelines

softball, baseball, soccer

parents yell at officials

insult opposing team

A **formal outline** follows long-established conventions for using numbers and letters to show relationships among ideas. No one outline format is endorsed for MLA STYLE, but instructors generally prefer the format used in Quick Box 5.5. Outlines usually don't show the content of introductory

Quick Box 5.5

Outline formats

FORMAT OF TRADITIONAL FORMAL OUTLINE

Thesis statement: Present the entire thesis statement.

I. First main idea
    A. First subordinate idea
        1. First reason or example
        2. Second reason or example
            a. First supporting detail
            b. Second supporting detail
    B. Second subordinate idea
II. Second main idea

continued >>

Quick Box 5.5 (continued)

EXAMPLE: FORMAL SENTENCE OUTLINE

This outline goes with the second paragraph of student Yanggu Cui's argument essay, "A Proposal to Improve Fan Behavior at Children's Games" (see Chapter 16).

Thesis statement: The league organizers need to bring an end to this kind of abuse, and the best way to do so is by requiring parents to sign a code of good behavior.

I. For decades, parents have proudly watched their sons and daughters play little league softball, baseball, soccer, and other sports.

   A. In recent years, the parents who attend little league games have become more vocal on sidelines.

   B. Parents who used to shout encouragement and congratulations to their children and the teams are now rude.

      1. They scream protests about the coaches' decisions.

      2. They yell insults at the opposing team.

      3. They hurl threats at officials, many of whom are young.

EXAMPLE: FORMAL TOPIC OUTLINE

This outline goes with the second paragraph of Yanghgu Cui's argument essay, "A Proposal to Improve Fan Behavior at Children's Games" (see Chapter 16).

Thesis Statement: The league organizers need to bring an end to this kind of abuse, and the best way to do so is by requiring parents to sign a code of good behavior.

I. Parents at little league softball, baseball, soccer, and other sports.

   A. Parents vocal on sidelines.

   B. Parents not encouraging but rude.

      1. Protesting coaches' decisions.

      2. Insulting the opposing team.

      3. Threatening officials.

and concluding paragraphs, but some instructors want them included, so always ask.

To compose a formal outline, always use at least two subdivisions at each level—no I without a II, no A without a B, etc. If a level has only one subdivision, either integrate it into the higher level or expand it into two subdivisions.

In addition, all subdivisions need to be at the same level of generality: don't pair a main idea with a subordinate idea or a subordinate idea with a supporting detail. In format, use PARALLELISM so that each outline item starts with the same PART OF SPEECH.

A formal outline can be a **sentence outline**, of only complete sentences, or a **topic outline**, of only words and PHRASES. Be careful never to mix the two styles in one outline. Quick Box 5.5 shows both types.

● **EXERCISE 5-4** Here is one section of a sentence outline. Individually or with your peer-response group, revise it into a topic outline. Then, be ready to explain why you prefer using a topic outline or a sentence outline as a guide to writing.

Thesis statement: Taxpayers should demand more investment in public transportation.

I. The current level of public transportation is inadequate everywhere.
  A. Cities need the ability to move lots of residents.
    1. Increased population in large cities causes transportation pressures.
    2. Some cities have responded well.
    3. Most cities have responded poorly.
  B. People need to move easily and cheaply between cities and towns.
    1. Cars are the only way to reach many cities and towns.
    2. It is easier and less expensive to travel in Europe.

II. The lack of public transportation causes many problems.
  A. Driving individual cars increases pollution.
  B. Space for building new roads and highways is limited.
  C. Congestion on city streets limits productivity.
  D. Many people aren't able to drive themselves.
    1. Young or elderly people may not drive.
    2. Many people cannot afford cars.

III. Improving public transportation is possible.
  A. Cities can expand bus services and light rail services.
  B. The United States can develop a wider national rail service.
  C. Although improvements are costly, we can afford them.
    1. We can reallocate money from building new roads.
    2. Building and running transportation creates jobs and adds to our tax base.
    3. Individual savings will offset any tax increases. ●

5G What works in writing a first draft?

Drafting means getting ideas onto paper or into the computer, in sentences and paragraphs. A draft is a version of the paper; experienced writers produce several drafts. The early ones focus on generating ideas, whereas later versions focus on developing and polishing ideas. But you can't polish something that doesn't exist, so your goal on the first draft is just producing words. Don't expect perfection; the pressure to "get it right the first time" can paralyze you. On the other hand, remember that a first draft isn't a final draft, even if it looks like it's finished. Rather, it's the basis for REVISING, EDITING, and PROOFREADING, as shown in Figure 5.3.

Here are three alternatives for writing a first draft.

- Write a discovery draft. Put aside any planning notes and use FOCUSED FREEWRITING about your topic. When you finish the first draft, you can consult your notes.
- Write a structured draft. Consult your planning notes or an OUTLINE as you write, but don't allow yourself to stall at a part you don't like. Signal you want to return to it, and keep on going.
- Combine using a DISCOVERY DRAFT and a STRUCTURED DRAFT. Start with a discovery draft, and when stalled, switch to a structured draft. Or do the reverse.

The direction of drafting is forward. Keep pressing ahead. If a spelling, a word choice, or a sentence bothers you, use a signal that says you want to check it later—underline it, highlight it in a color, or switch it to capital letters. Type a note to yourself in brackets, [like this], but charge onward. Research proves that the physical act of writing without pausing makes ideas and connections among them "pop into people's heads unbidden."

Figure 5.3 Using a first draft for later revising, editing, and proofreading.

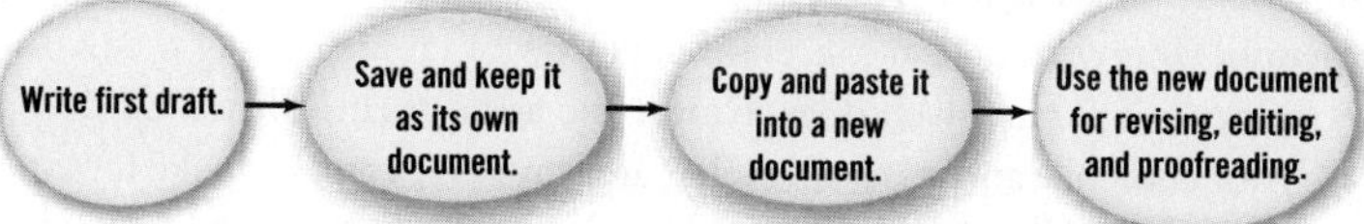
Write first draft.
Save and keep it as its own document.
Copy and paste it into a new document.
Use the new document for revising, editing, and proofreading.

Here are some drafting problems and possible solutions.

MY DRAFTING PROBLEM: I open a blank document, write a few words, don't like them, delete them, and start again, repeatedly.

SOLUTION: Open a new document, darken your computer screen, and type without stopping. When you think you have a complete first draft, save it. Then lighten your computer screen to see what you've written.

MY DRAFTING PROBLEM: I start out well, but soon I see that I'm going off the topic.

SOLUTION: Mark the spot with a highlighter or a large arrow showing a direction change (⤵). Consult your notes or outline and get right back onto the topic.

MY DRAFTING PROBLEM: I'm writing only general statements and no specifics, but I can't think of any supporting examples or details as I go along.

SOLUTION: Keep on writing. When you revise, you can concentrate on supplying the supporting details.

5H How do I get over writer's block?

Watch the Video

If you're afraid or otherwise feel unable to start writing, perhaps you're being stopped by **writer's block**. You want to get started but somehow can't. Often, writer's block occurs because the writer harbors a fear of being wrong. But the only thing "wrong" about a first draft is if the page or screen is empty, so don't worry! If you get blocked, try the suggestions in Quick Box 5.6.

5I How does revision work?

Watch the Video

REVISING is rewriting. The word *revision* breaks down into *re-vision*, literally, "again vision": to see again with fresh eyes. During DRAFTING you suspended judgment of your writing, but for revision, you switch to evaluating the writing you've done so far. How well does it meet the assignment? How well does it address your audience and purpose? What are ways that you can make it better? As you revise, keep all your drafts and notes. You might want to go back to an earlier revision and use part of it. Quick Box 5.7 (page 78) shows the major types of revision, and the levels you can apply them in your paper.

Quick Box 5.6

Ways to overcome writer's block

- **Start in the middle.** Rather than start at the beginning of your essay, start with the body paragraph you feel will be easiest or most interesting for you to write.
- **Visualize yourself writing, moving your fingers across the keyboard.** Top athletes always use visualizing, imagining themselves mechanically going though each motion involved in their sport. Visualize yourself writing easily.
- **Write an e-mail about your topic to a friend, even if you don't send it.** Write informally. Be playful with your language or ideas. Loosen up.
- **Write a draft to a different, "easier" audience.** If it feels scary to write to your instructor or an academic audience, imagine you're writing for someone much younger or someone who knows nothing about the topic. You can revise that writing later.
- **Call a friend or relative to chat about your topic.** Ask if they'll give you a few minutes to chat with you about your topic, inviting them to disagree or argue with you.
- **Play the role of someone else, and write to yourself about your topic.** Take on someone else's identity—an expert or teacher or friend—and pretend "they" are explaining the topic to you.
- **Imagine a scene or sound that relates to your topic.** Start to write by describing what you see or hear. Allow yourself to sink into the environment of that scene or sound.

In revising you work on the overarching elements of your essay. Save the last two steps—editing and proofreading—until after you've finished revising the draft. This tactic is important: "premature editing" distracts writers too soon from the content of their material.

5I.1 Using your thesis statement or title to guide revision

To use your THESIS STATEMENT as a guide your revision, ask at the end of every body paragraph, "Does the topic sentence and content of this paragraph relate to my thesis statement?" If they do not, revise the thesis statement, your paragraph, or both.

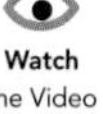
Watch the Video

Quick Box 5.7

Types and levels of revision

Type \ Level	Word	Sentence	Paragraph	Idea
Add Insert words, sentences, paragraphs ideas.				
Subtract Cut whatever goes off the topic or is repetitive.				
Replace Substitute more effective words or ideas for less effective ones				
Move Change the order of things, from sentences to paragraphs, to find the most effective arrangement.				

Your essay **title** is an important part of revising, so create a working title during your first draft. Use it consistently as a checkpoint as your essay evolves. A **direct title** tells exactly what the essay will be about: for example, "Why We're Going Less Often to the Movies." An **indirect title** hints at an essay's topic: "Can We Really Afford It?" Such an indirect title can capture a reader's interest as long as the connection is not too obscure. For example, this indirect title would not work: "Too Much and Getting Worse." Never tack on a title at the last minute.

Alert: A title stands alone. Don't open an essay with a reaction to the title or with an opening sentence that is a continuation of the title. For example, the following would be an inappropriate first sentence in student Cheryl Cusack's essay "Why We're Going Less Often to the Movies" in Chapter 13: "It's too expensive these days." Such an opening sentence is improper because it leans on the essay's title, and "It" is an unclear PRONOUN REFERENCE. ●

5I.2 Considering style and tone to guide revision

As you revise your writing, you want to consider *how* you say something as well as *what* you're saying. You create the STYLE of your writing by how you shape sentence structures and how you choose to address readers. TONE involves using the right words to deliver your meaning.

Chapters 37 to 40 cover style and tone in greater detail.

5I.3 Other revision aids

Probably the best source of ideas for revision is feedback that your instructor or a careful peer reviewer provides on a draft. Keep in mind that any comments your instructor makes are designed to help you get better. Take them seriously, and recognize this feedback as a gift. Revision checklists, like the one in Quick Box 5.8 (page 80), can also focus your attention as you revise your writing.

Here's a section of the earliest draft of the fifth paragraph in student Cheryl Cusack's essay "Why We're Going Less Often to the Movies" in Chapter 13.

> Ticket prices are very high, with the national average at $8.00. Throw in purchasing refreshments, and a night at the movies for a couple can reach $40.00. What about a family of four? Given the recent troubles in our economy, movies are out of reach for many.

If you compare this earliest draft with Cheryl's final draft, you see that in her revision (a) she's inserted a topic sentence to start the paragraph to tie into the essay's other topic sentences and its thesis statement; (b) she's more specific about the average price; (c) she's more specific by converting her question into a sentence so that she can use a number: "twice that"; (d) she's expanded her last sentence. In section 5L we provide a complete early draft of Cheryl's essay.

5J How does editing work?

Editing comes after you've revised the content and organization of your paper to your critical satisfaction. Some people use the terms *editing* and *revising* interchangeably, but these terms refer to very different steps. Revising refers to making changes that affect the content, meaning, and organization of a paper. In contrast, editing means finding and fixing errors you've made in grammar, spelling, punctuation, capitals, numbers, italics, and abbreviations. Some instructors call these *surface-level features*. When do you know you've finished revising and are ready to edit? Ask yourself, "Is there anything else I can do to improve the content, organization, and development of this draft?" If the answer is no, you're ready to edit.

Quick Box 5.8

Revision checklist

Your goal is to answer *yes* to each question on the following list. If you answer *no*, you need to revise your writing accordingly. The section numbers in parentheses tell you where to look in this handbook for help.

1. Is your essay topic suitable and sufficiently narrow (see 5C)?
2. Does your thesis statement effectively focus on your topic and purpose (see Quick Box 5.4)?
3. Does your essay show that you are aware of your audience (see Quick Box 4.5)?
4. Have you checked for places where your reader would be confused or need more information?
5. Have you checked for places where a skeptical reader would not be convinced?
6. Is your essay arranged effectively?
7. Have you checked for material that strays off the topic?
8. Does your introduction prepare your reader for the rest of the essay (see 6C)?
9. Do your body paragraphs express main ideas in topic sentences as needed (see 6E)? Are your main ideas clearly related to your thesis statement?
10. Do you provide specific, concrete support for each main idea (see 6F)?
11. Do you use transitions and other techniques to connect ideas within and between paragraphs (see 6G and 6I)?
12. Does your conclusion give your essay a sense of completion?

Slapdash editing distracts and annoys your reader; lowers that reader's opinion of you and what you say in your essay; and, in a college assignment, usually earns a lower grade. The best editors work slowly and methodically. Whenever you question your use of a rule or a writing technique, look it up in this handbook. Use the Index at the back of this handbook to find the page for the exact rule or technique you want to check.

Using an editing checklist—either one provided by your instructor or one based on Quick Box 5.9—can help you find errors by moving through editing systematically.

You may also want to ask friends, classmates, or colleagues with a good "editing eye" to read your papers and circle anything they think you need to check for correctness.

Quick Box 5.9

Editing

Your goal is to answer *yes* to each of the following questions. If you answer *no*, you need to edit. The numbers in parentheses tell you which chapters in this handbook to go to for more information.

1. Are your sentences concise (see Chapter 40)?
2. Are your sentences interesting? Do you use parallelism, variety, and emphasis correctly and to increase the impact of your writing (see Chapters 38–39)?
3. Have you used exact words (see 37F)?
4. Is your usage correct and your language appropriate (see Chapter 37)?
5. Have you avoided sexist or stereotypical language (see 37I)?
6. Is your grammar correct (see Chapters 28–36)?
7. Is your spelling correct (see Chapter 49)?
8. Have you used commas correctly (see Chapter 42)?
9. Have you used all other punctuation correctly (see Chapters 41 and 43–47)?
10. Have you used capital letters, italics, abbreviations, and numbers correctly (see Chapter 48)?
11. Have you used the appropriate citation and documentation formats (see Chapters 25–27)?

Alert: Be careful relying on the editing features in word processing programs or apps. Many of them are wrong or outdated. For example, some versions of Microsoft Word flag correct contractions when your choice is correct. When in doubt, consult this handbook.

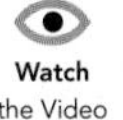

Spell-check programs can both help and hinder. They help when they spot a misspelled or mistyped word (for example, if you type "abot" for "about"). However, they don't spot a wrong word (for example, if you type "form" but mean "from"), so if you rely only on them, your paper can still have mistakes.

Thesaurus programs give you **synonyms** for words. You need to select the ones that fit well into your particular sentences. Many offered synonyms have slightly different meanings than what you intend, so never use one that's unfamiliar or that you know only vaguely. Always first look it up in your dictionary. Misused words make readers assume you don't know what you are saying or that you're trying to show off. ●

5K What strategies can I use to proofread?

Watch the Video

Proofreading is a careful, line-by-line reading of a final, clean version of your writing. Always proofread for errors and correct them before you hand in a paper. If you find errors during proofreading, always print a fresh, clean copy of your work.

Almost all writers proofread more effectively on a printed page rather than on a screen, so print your pages whenever possible for proofreading purposes. If you cannot help working onscreen, try highlighting a small section of your writing at a time so that you are visually separating it from the rest of the screen.

Here are effective proofreading strategies that are popular with many writers.

- Proofread with a ruler held just under the line you are reading so that you can focus on one line at a time.
- Start at the end of a paragraph or the end of your essay and read each sentence in reverse order or word by word, to avoid being distracted by the content.
- Read your final draft aloud so that you see and/or hear errors.
- Look especially carefully for omitted letters and words.
- Watch out for repeated words (*the* or *and* are common repeats).
- Keep lists of spelling, punctuation, or grammar errors that you often make. For example, you may know you have trouble keeping *to, too*, and *two* straight. Consult those lists before you revise, edit, and proofread so that you look specifically for those personal troublemakers.

5L A student's draft essay with revision notes

Cheryl Cusack received the following assignment: "Write an essay for a general educated audience in which you analyze the cause of a current situation or behavior in our society. Your essay should be 500–1000 words." After freewriting and brainstorming, Cheryl decided to write on the topic of movie attendance and why it is falling. We've included Cheryl's first draft here, and we've included her final draft in Chapter 13. When you look carefully at these drafts, you'll see that she did substantial revisions between them. We've included some of her revision notes.

Cheryl's First Draft

Cheryl Cusack

The Problem with Movies Today

Better title?

The other day I heard that total movie attendance keeps going down. This surprised me because there seem to be more movies showing now than ever. There's certainly more movie advertising, and the popularity of the Oscars and other awards suggests that people are interested in the movies. Movie stars show up all the time on the news and on entertainment programs. So, it's surprising that people aren't going to movies. The purpose of this paper will be to explain what people aren't going to the movies.

Need to check attendance figures

Improve thesis. This one will do for a start.

One reason is that ticket prices are very high, with the national average at $8.00. Throw in purchasing refreshments, and a night at the movies for a couple can reach $40.00. What about a family of four? Given the recent troubles in our economy, movies are out of reach for many.

Another reason is that the movies are bad. I recently saw *Tinker, Tailor, Soldier, Spy*, and I haven't been so bored in all my life. There was almost no action in the movie, just a lot of slow talking. Of course, at the other end of the spectrum, having a lot of action doesn't necessarily make a good movie, either. At Christmas I saw the sequel to *Sherlock Holmes*, and there was scarcely a minute when Robert Downey Jr. or Jude Law weren't punching someone in the face or escaping some calamity. The problem in Sherlock Holmes was that the plot didn't make much sense. It was just an excuse for fights and explosions. Even though there are lots of movies out there, not many of them are very good.

My taste might not be shared by others. Drop this?

But there were good movies, too.

continued >>

Needs more details.

A third reason is that going to the movies is no longer a special experience. People behave rudely in movie theaters. In addition to watching previews, which are actually OK, people now have to watch endless commercials. You can get that experience at home.

Can I expand?

A fourth reason is that there are new forms of entertainment. There are hundreds of channels on cable TV these days, with many of them running movies. Plus, you can rent movies, so if you just wait a couple of months, you can see a film in the privacy of your own home and for a fraction of the cost. Movies just can't compete with that.

Not a very interesting conclusion

As you can see, there are four reasons why people are going less often to movies: cost, quality, lack of a special experience, and competition for other forms of entertainment. Unless movie makers can address each of these four problems, it won't be long until movie theaters close down.

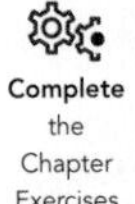

Complete the Chapter Exercises

—Put the best idea last. Maybe that's the experience?

Writing Paragraphs, Shaping Essays

Quick Points You will learn to

- Write effective paragraphs (see 6C–6K).
- Use topic sentences (see 6E).
- Use rhetorical patterns to help you write paragraphs (see 6H).

6A How do I shape essays?

A good essay has an effective beginning, middle, and end. The key word is *effective*. Beginnings interest your reader and create expectations for the rest of the essay, usually through a THESIS STATEMENT. Middles explain or provide arguments for the thesis, usually through a series of statements and supporting details or evidence. Endings provide closure. They make readers feel that the writing achieved its purpose and that the writer had a skilled sense of the audience to the very end.

6B How do paragraphs work?

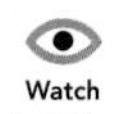

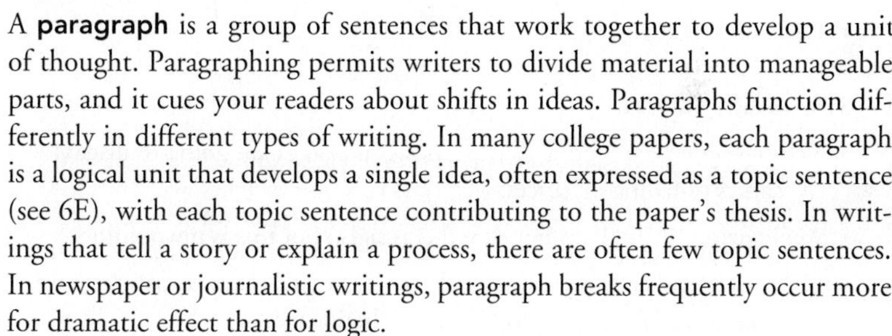

A **paragraph** is a group of sentences that work together to develop a unit of thought. Paragraphing permits writers to divide material into manageable parts, and it cues your readers about shifts in ideas. Paragraphs function differently in different types of writing. In many college papers, each paragraph is a logical unit that develops a single idea, often expressed as a topic sentence (see 6E), with each topic sentence contributing to the paper's thesis. In writings that tell a story or explain a process, there are often few topic sentences. In newspaper or journalistic writings, paragraph breaks frequently occur more for dramatic effect than for logic.

6C How can I write effective introductory paragraphs?

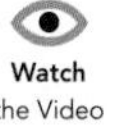

An **introductory paragraph** leads the reader to sense what's ahead. It also, if possible, attempts to arouse a reader's interest in the topic.

A THESIS STATEMENT is an important component in most introductions. Many instructors require students to place the thesis statement at the end of the opening paragraph. Doing so disciplines students to state early the central point of the essay. Professional writers don't necessarily include a thesis statement in their introductory paragraphs. Most have the skill to maintain a line of thought without overtly stating a main idea.

Be careful not to tack on a sloppy introduction at the last minute. That doesn't mean you have to write an introduction first; you might put down ideas and a thesis to start, then return during the revision process to write a full, polished introduction. Quick Box 6.1 (page 86) lists strategies to use and pitfalls to avoid for introductory paragraphs.

Quick Box 6.1

Introductory paragraphs

STRATEGIES TO USE

- Provide relevant background information.
- Relate a brief interesting story or anecdote.
- Give one or more pertinent—perhaps surprising—statistics.
- Ask one or more provocative questions.
- Use an appropriate quotation.
- Define a KEY TERM.
- Present one or more brief examples.
- Draw an ANALOGY.

STRATEGIES TO AVOID

- Writing statements about your purpose, such as "I am going to discuss the causes of falling oil prices."
- Apologizing, as in "I am not sure this is right, but this is my opinion."
- Using overworked expressions, such as "Haste makes waste, as I recently discovered" or "According to Webster's dictionary."

Here's an introductory paragraph that uses two brief examples to lead into the thesis statement at the end of the paragraph.

> 1 On seeing another child fall and hurt himself, Hope, just nine months old, stared, tears welling up in her eyes, and crawled to her mother to be comforted—as though she had been hurt, not her friend. When 15-month-old Michael saw his friend Paul crying, Michael fetched his own teddy bear and offered it to Paul; when that didn't stop Paul's tears, Michael brought Paul's security blanket from another room. Such small acts of sympathy and caring, observed in scientific studies, are leading researchers to trace the roots of empathy—the ability to share another's emotions—to infancy, contradicting a long-standing assumption that infants and toddlers were incapable of these feelings. **Thesis**
>
> —Daniel Goleman, "Researchers Trace Empathy's Roots to Infancy"

Paragraph 2 opens with an interesting fact and image (the brain as oatmeal).

2 Arguably the greatest mysteries in the universe lie in the three-pound mass of cells, approximately the consistency of oatmeal, that reside in the skull of each of us. It has even been suggested that the brain is so complex that our species is smart enough to fathom everything except what makes us so smart; that is, the brain is so cunningly designed for intelligence that it is too stupid to understand itself. We now know that is not true. The mind is at last yielding its secrets to persistent scientific investigation. We have learned more about how the mind works in the last twenty-five years than we did in the previous twenty-five hundred. **Thesis**

—Daniel T. Willingham, *Why Don't Students Like School?*

In paragraph 3, the writer asks a direct question and next puts the reader in a dramatic situation to arouse interest in the topic.

3 What should you do? You're out riding your bike, playing golf, or in the middle of a long run when you look up and suddenly see a jagged streak of light shoot across the sky, followed by a deafening clap of thunder. Unfortunately, most outdoor exercisers don't know whether to stay put or make a dash for shelter when a thunderstorm approaches, and sometimes the consequences are tragic.

—Gerald Secor Couzens, "If Lightning Strikes"

● **EXERCISE 6-1** Write an introduction for each of the three essays informally outlined here. Then, for more practice, write one alternative introduction for each. For help, see section 6C.

1. Play at school

   Thesis statement: School recesses today differ tremendously from recess a generation ago.

   Body paragraph 1: types of recess activities thirty years ago

   Body paragraph 2: types of games now, including ultimate frisbee

   Body paragraph 3: other activities, including climbing walls and free running

2. Cell phones

   Thesis statement: Cell phones have changed how some people behave in public.

   Body paragraph 1: driving

   Body paragraph 2: restaurants

   Body paragraph 3: movies and concerts

   Body paragraph 4: sidewalks, parks, and other casual spaces

3. Identity theft

   Thesis statement: Taking some simple precautions can reduce the danger of identity theft.

   Body paragraph 1: discarding junk mail

   Body paragraph 2: watching store purchases

   Body paragraph 3: Internet security ●

6D What are body paragraphs?

In most **academic writing**, each **body paragraph**, the several paragraphs between an introductory paragraph (see 6C) and a concluding paragraph (see 6K), consists of a main idea and support for that idea. What separates most good writing from bad is the writer's ability to move back and forth between main ideas and specific details. To be effective, a body paragraph needs development and coherence. Development consists of detailed and sufficient support for the paragraph's main idea (see 6F). Coherence means that all the ideas in the paragraph connect to each other and that the sentences progress smoothly (see 6G). Paragraph 4 is an example of an effective body paragraph.

> The Miss Plastic Surgery contest, trumpeted by Chinese promoters as
> "the world's first pageant for artificial beauties," shows the power of cosmetic
> surgery in a country that has swung from one extreme to another when it comes
> to the feminine ideal. In the 10th century, Emperor Li Yu ordered his consort
> 4 to bind her feet; women practiced the painful ritual for more than 900 years
> in the belief that small feet were more alluring. In contrast, at the height of the
> Cultural Revolution in the 1960s and 1970s, Maoist officials condemned any
> form of personal grooming or beautification as "unrevolutionary" and regularly
> beat women for owning hairbrushes, wearing blush, or painting their nails.
>
> —Abigail Haworth, "Nothing about These Women Is Real"

The main idea stated in the TOPIC SENTENCE (see 6E) is developed with detailed examples. The content of every sentence ties into the content of the other sentences, and the paragraph *coheres*—sticks together—because of the use of transitional phrases ("In the 10th century" and "In contrast," for example).

6E What are topic sentences?

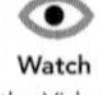
Watch the Video

A **topic sentence** contains the main idea of a paragraph and controls its content. Often, the topic sentence comes at the beginning of a paragraph, though not always. Professional writers, because they have the skill to carry the reader along without explicit signposts, sometimes decide not to use topic sentences. However, instructors often require students to use topic sentences to help them stay focused and coherent.

TOPIC SENTENCE STARTING A PARAGRAPH

When paragraphs begin with a topic sentence, readers know immediately what to expect, as in paragraph 5.

5 Music patronage was at a turning point when Mozart went to Vienna in the last part of the eighteenth century. **Topic sentence** Many patrons of music continued to be wealthy aristocrats. Haydn's entire career was funded by a rich prince. Mozart's father and, for a time, Mozart himself were in the employ of another prince. But when Mozart went to Vienna in 1781, he contrived to make a living from a variety of sources. In addition to performances at aristocratic houses and commissions for particular works, Mozart gave piano and composition lessons, put on operas, and gave many public concerts of his own music.

—Jeremy Yudkin, "Composers and Patrons in the Classic Era"

TOPIC SENTENCE ENDING A PARAGRAPH

When a topic sentence ends a body paragraph, the sentences need to lead up to it clearly.

6 The third most popular language in America—after English and Spanish—is American Sign Language (ASL). It is a visual-gestural language composed of a collection of coded gestures based on a system developed in France in the eighteenth century. It was brought to the United States by Thomas Hopkins Gallaudet, a young Congregational minister from Connecticut. After traveling to France and learning about this system of signing, Gallaudet returned to the United States, bringing a young French deaf-signing teacher, Laurent Clerc, with him. Together they developed sign language system that blended French signs with American signs. As a legacy, today deaf people in both France and the United States can recognize similarities in the signs they use. **Topic sentence**

—Roger E. Axtell, *Gestures: The Do's and Taboos of Body Language around the World*

TOPIC SENTENCE IMPLIED, NOT STATED

Some paragraphs work even without a topic sentence. Yet, most readers can catch the main idea anyway. The implied topic sentence of paragraph 7 might be stated something like, "Filmmakers tend to care more about characters and action than about facts."

7 It is easy to identify with the quest for a secret document, somewhat harder to do so with a heroine whose goal is identifying and understanding the element radium, which is why in dramatic biography writers and directors end up reverting to fiction. To be effective, the dramatic elements must, and finally will, take precedence over any "real" biographical facts. We viewers do not care—if we wanted to know about the element radium, we would read a book on the element radium. When we go to the movies to see *The Story of Marie Curie* we want to find out how her little dog Skipper died.

—David Mamet, *Three Uses of the Knife: On the Nature and Purpose of Drama*

● **EXERCISE 6-2** Working individually or with a group, identify the topic sentences in the following paragraphs. If the topic sentence is implied, write the point the paragraph conveys. For help, consult section 6E.

8 A. A good college program should stress the development of high-level reading, writing, and mathematical skills and should provide you with a broad historical, social, and cultural perspective, no matter what subject you choose as your major. The program should teach you not only the most current knowledge in your field but also—just as important—prepare you to keep learning throughout your life. After all, you'll probably change jobs, and possibly even careers, at least six times, and you'll have other responsibilities, too—perhaps as a spouse and as a parent and certainly as a member of a community whose bounds extend beyond the workplace.

—Frank T. Rhodes, "Let the Student Decide"

9 B. The once majestic oak tree crashes to the ground amid the destructive flames, as its panic-stricken inhabitants attempt to flee the fiery tomb. Undergrowth that formerly flourished smolders in ashes. A family of deer darts furiously from one wall of flame to the other, without an emergency exit. On the outskirts of the inferno, firefighters try desperately to stop the destruction. Somewhere at the source of this chaos lies a former campsite containing the cause of this destruction—an untended campfire. This scene is one of many that illustrate how human apathy and carelessness destroy nature.

—Anne Bryson, student

10 C. Rudeness isn't a distinctive quality of our own time. People today would be shocked by how rudely our ancestors behaved. In the colonial period, a French traveler marveled that "Virginians don't use napkins, but they wear silk cravats, and instead of carrying white handkerchiefs, they blow their noses either with their fingers or with a silk handkerchief that also serves as a cravat, a napkin, and so on." In the 19th century, up to about the 1830s, even very distinguished people routinely put their knives in their mouths. And when people went to the theater, they would not just applaud politely—they would chant, jeer, and shout. So, the notion that there's been a downhill slide in manners ever since time began is just not so.

—"Horizons," *U.S. News & World Report* ●

6F How can I develop my body paragraphs?

You develop a BODY PARAGRAPH by supplying detailed support for the main idea communicated by your TOPIC SENTENCE (6E), whether stated or implied. **Paragraph development** is not merely repeating the main idea using other words. When this happens, you're merely going around in circles.

To check whether you are providing sufficient detail in a body paragraph, use the **RENNS** Test. Each letter in the made-up word *RENNS* cues you to remember a different kind of supporting detail at your disposal, as listed in Quick Box 6.2 (page 92). Of course, not every paragraph needs all five kinds of RENNS details, nor do the supporting details need to occur in the order of the letters in *RENNS*. Paragraph 11 contains three of the five types of RENNS details. Identify the topic sentence and as many RENNS as you can before reading the analysis that follows the paragraph.

11 Between 1910 and 1920, "The Rubber Capital of the World" was the fastest-growing city in the nation, thanks to a booming automobile industry. Akron, Ohio, had a few crucial features that helped it thrive as a hub. It was not only located close to auto makers, it also had water power and cheap coal to draw on. During the peak years, more than 300 rubber companies called the city home, but most died off in the fierce pricing competition. Then, in the 1970s, French manufacturer Michelin introduced the longer-lasting radial tire. In Akron, profits slipped and plants closed. Goodyear Tire & Rubber Co. is now the only major tire company that still has headquarters in Akron.

—Wall Street Journal research "Akron, Ohio"

In paragraph 11, the first sentence serves as the topic sentence. Supporting details for that main idea include reasons, examples, numbers, and names.

Quick Box 6.2

The RENNS test: checking for supporting details

R = **Reasons** provide support.

- Jules Verne, a nineteenth-century writer of science fiction, amazes readers today **because he imagined inventions impossible to develop until recent years**.

E = **Examples** provide support.

- **For example**, he predicted submarines and moon rockets.

N = **Names** provide support.

- He forecast that the moon rockets would take off from an area in the **state of Florida**.

N = **Numbers** provide support.

- Specifically, he declared as the point of departure **27 degrees North Latitude and 5 degrees West Longitude**.

S = **Senses**—sight, sound, smell, taste, touch—provide support.

- Today, space vehicles are **heard blasting off** from Cape Kennedy, only eighty miles from the site Verne chose.

The writer provides reasons for growth (there was a booming auto industry; Akron was close to auto makers; there was water power and cheap coal) and examples (Michelin introducing the radial tire). The writer also provides numbers (300 rubber companies) and names (Rubber Capital of the World; Akron, Ohio; Goodyear Tire & Rubber Co.).

● **EXERCISE 6-3** Working individually or with a peer-response group, look again at the paragraphs in Exercise 6-2. Identify the RENNS in each paragraph. For help, consult 6F. ●

6G How can I create coherence in paragraphs?

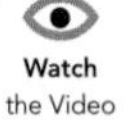

A paragraph is coherent when its sentences connect in content and relate to each other in form and language. To show you broken **coherence**, in paragraph 12 we've deliberately inserted two sentences (the fourth and the next to last) that go off the topic and ruin a perfectly good paragraph, shown as paragraph 13. (Neither a personal complaint about stress nor hormones produced by men and women during exercise belong in a paragraph defining different kinds of stress.)

NO Stress has long been the subject of psychological and physiological speculation. In fact, more often than not, the word itself is ill defined and overused, meaning different things to different people. Emotional stress, for
example, can come about as the result of a family argument or the death
of a loved one. Everyone says, "Don't get stressed," but I have no idea
12 how to do that. Environmental stress, such as exposure to excessive heat
or cold, is an entirely different phenomenon. Physiologic stress has been
described as the outpouring of the steroid hormones from the adrenal
glands. During exercise, such as weightlifting, males and females produce
different hormones. Whatever its guise, a lack of a firm definition of stress
has seriously impeded past research.

YES Stress has long been the subject of psychological and physiological speculation. In fact, more often than not, the word itself is ill defined and overused, meaning different things to different people. Emotional stress, for
13 example, can come about as the result of a family argument or the death
of a loved one. Environmental stress, such as exposure to excessive heat
or cold, is an entirely different phenomenon. Physiologic stress has been
described as the outpouring of the steroid hormones from the adrenal
glands. Whatever its guise, a lack of a firm definition of stress has seriously
impeded past research.

—Herbert Benson, MD, *The Relaxation Response*

Techniques for achieving coherence are listed in Quick Box 6.3.

Quick Box 6.3

Techniques for achieving coherence

- Using appropriate transitional expressions (see 6G.1)
- Using pronouns when possible (see 6G.2)
- Using **deliberate repetition** of a key word (see 6G.3)
- Using parallel structures (see 6G.4)
- Using coherence techniques to create connections among paragraphs (see 6G.5)

6G.1 Using transitional expressions for coherence

Transitional expressions are words and phrases that express connections among ideas, both within and between paragraphs. Common transitional expressions are listed in Quick Box 6.4 (page 94).

Quick Box 6.4

Transitional expressions and the relationships they signal

ADDITION	also, in addition, too, moreover, and, besides, furthermore, equally important, then, finally
EXAMPLE	for example, for instance, thus, as an illustration, namely, specifically
CONTRAST	but, yet, however, nevertheless, nonetheless, conversely, in contrast, still, at the same time, on the one hand, on the other hand
COMPARISON	similarly, likewise, in the same way
CONCESSION	of course, to be sure, certainly, granted
RESULT	therefore, thus, as a result, so, accordingly, consequently
SUMMARY	hence, in short, in brief, in summary, in conclusion, finally
TIME	first, second, third, next, then, finally, afterward, before, soon, later, meanwhile, subsequently, immediately, eventually, currently
PLACE	in the front, in the foreground, in the back, in the background, at the side, adjacent, nearby, in the distance, here, there

- Vary your choices of transitional words. For example, instead of always using *for example*, try *for instance*.
- When choosing a transitional word, make sure it correctly says what you mean. For instance, don't use *however* in the sense of *on the other hand* if you mean *therefore* in the sense of *as a result*

Alert: In ACADEMIC WRITING, set off a transitional expression with a comma, unless the expression is one short word (see 42C). ●

Paragraph 14 demonstrates how transitional expressions (shown in **bold**) enhance a paragraph's COHERENCE. The TOPIC SENTENCE is the final sentence.

Before the days of television, people were entertained by exciting radio shows such as *Superman, Batman*, and "War of the Worlds." **Of course**, the listener was required to pay careful attention to the story if all details were to be
14 comprehended. **Better yet**, while listening to the stories, listeners would form their own images of the actions taking place. When the broadcaster would give brief descriptions of the Martian space ships invading earth, **for example**, every

member of the audience would imagine a different space ship. **In contrast**, television's version of "War of the Worlds" will not stir the imagination at all, for everyone can clearly see the actions taking place. All viewers see the same space ship with the same features. Each aspect is clearly defined, and **therefore**, no one will imagine anything different from what is seen. **Thus**, television can't be considered an effective tool for stimulating the imagination.

—Tom Paradis, "A Child's Other World"

6G.2 Using pronouns for coherence

PRONOUNS—words that refer to nouns or other pronouns—allow readers to follow your train of thought from one sentence to the next without boring repetition. For example, this sentence uses no pronouns and therefore has boring repetition: *After Gary Hanson, now 56, got laid off from* ***Gary Hanson's*** *corporate position in 2003,* ***Gary Hanson, Gary Hanson's*** *wife, Susan, and* ***Gary Hanson's*** *son, John, now 54 and 27, respectively, wanted to do a spot of cleaning.* Paragraph 15 illustrates how pronouns (shown in **bold**) contribute to COHERENCE.

After Gary Hanson, now 56, got laid off from **his** corporate position in
2003, **he, his** wife, Susan, and **his** son, John, now 54 and 27, respectively,
15 wanted to do a spot of cleaning. Though **they** are hard at work, **they** are not
scrubbing floors or washing windows. **They** are running **their** very own house-
cleaning franchise, *The Maids Home Services,* which **they** opened in February.

—Sara Wilson, "Clean House: Getting Laid Off from His Corporate Job Gave This Franchisee a Fresh Start"

6G.3 Using deliberate repetition for coherence

Repetition of key words or phrases is a useful way to achieve COHERENCE in a paragraph. The word or phrase usually appears first in the paragraph's TOPIC SENTENCE and then again throughout the paragraph. Use this technique sparingly to avoid being monotonous. Paragraph 16 contains repeated words and phrases (shown in **bold**).

Anthropology, broadly defined, is the study of **humanity**, from its
evolutionary origins millions of years ago to its present great numbers
and worldwide diversity. Many other disciplines, of course, share with
anthropology a focus on one aspect or another of **humanity**. **Like** sociology,
16 economics, political science, psychology, and other behavioral and social
sciences, **anthropology** is concerned with the way people organize their lives
and relate to one another in interacting, interconnected groups—societies—
that share basic beliefs and practices. **Like** economists, **anthropologists are**
interested in society's material foundations—in how people produce and

distribute food and other valued goods. **Like** sociologists, **anthropologists are interested in** the way people structure their relations in society—in families, at work, in institutions. **Like** political scientists, **anthropologists are interested in** power and authority: who has them and how they are allocated. And, **like** psychologists, **anthropologists are interested in** individual development and the interaction between society and individual people.

—Nancy Bonvillain, "The Study of Humanity"

6G.4 Using parallel structures for coherence

Parallel structures are created when grammatically equivalent forms are used in series, usually of three or more items, but sometimes only two (see Chapter 39). The repeated parallel structures reinforce connections among ideas, and they add both tempo and sound to the sentence.

In paragraph 17, the author uses several parallel structures (shown in **bold**):

17 Our skin is what stands between us and the world. If you think about it, no other part of us makes contact with something not us, but the skin. It imprisons us, but it also **gives us** individual shape, **protects us** from invaders, **cools us down** or **heats us up** as need be, **produces** vitamin D, **holds** in our body fluids. Most amazing, perhaps, is that it can mend itself when necessary, and it is constantly renewing itself. Weighing from six to ten pounds, it's **the largest organ of the body**, and **the key organ of sexual attraction**. Skin can take a startling variety of shapes: claws, spines, hooves, feathers, scales, hair. It's waterproof, washable, and elastic.

—Diane Ackerman, *A Natural History of the Senses*

● **EXERCISE 6-4** Working individually or with a peer-response group, locate the coherence techniques in each paragraph. Look for transitional expressions, pronouns, deliberate repetition, and parallel structures. For help, consult 6G.

18 A. Kathy sat with her legs dangling over the edge of the side of the hood. The band of her earphones held back strands of straight copper hair that had come loose from two thick braids that hung down her back. She swayed with the music that only she could hear. Her shoulders raised, making circles in the warm air. Her arms reached out to her side; her open hands reached for the air; her closed hands brought the air back to her. Her arms reached over her head; her opened hands reached for a cloud; her closed hands brought the cloud back to her. Her head moved from side to side; her eyes opened and closed to the tempo of the tunes. Kathy was motion.

—Claire Burke, student

19 B. Newton's law may have wider application than just the physical world. In the social world, racism, once set into motion, will remain in motion unless acted upon by an outside force. The collective "we" must be the outside force. We must fight racism through education. We must make sure every school has the resources to do its job. We must present to our children a culturally diverse curriculum that reflects our pluralistic society. This can help students understand that prejudice is learned through contact with prejudiced people, rather than with the people toward whom the prejudice is directed.

—Randolph H. Manning, "Fighting Racism with Inclusion" ●

● **EXERCISE 6-5** Working individually or with a peer-response group, use RENNS (see 6F) and techniques for achieving coherence (see 6G) to develop three of the following topic sentences into paragraphs. When finished, list the RENNS and the coherence techniques you used in each paragraph.

1. Video games reflect current concerns in our culture.
2. The content of trash in the United States says a great deal about U.S. culture.
3. Reality shows on television tend to have several common elements.
4. In many respects, our culture is very wasteful.
5. College students face several true challenges. ●

6H How can rhetorical patterns help me write paragraphs?

Rhetorical patterns (sometimes called *rhetorical strategies*) are techniques for presenting ideas clearly and effectively in academic and other situations. Quick Box 6.5 (page 98) lists the common rhetorical strategies at your disposal.

NARRATIVE

Narrative writing tells a story. A *narration* relates what is happening or what has happened. Paragraph 20 is an example.

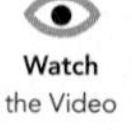
Watch the Video

20 Gordon Parks speculates that he might have spent his life as a waiter on the North Coast Limited train if he hadn't strolled into one particular movie house during a stopover in Chicago. It was shortly before World War II began, and on the screen was a hair-raising newsreel of Japanese planes attacking a gunboat. When it was over the camera operator came out on stage and the audience cheered. From that moment on Parks was determined to become a photographer. During his next stopover, in Seattle, he went into a pawnshop and purchased his first camera for $7.50. With that small sum, Parks later proclaimed, "I had bought what was to become my weapon against poverty and racism." Eleven years later, he became the first black photographer at *Life* magazine.

—Susan Howard, "Depth of Field"

Quick Box 6.5

Common rhetorical patterns of thought (strategies) for paragraphs

- Narrative
- Description
- Process
- Examples
- Definition
- Analysis
- Classification
- Comparison and contrast
- Analogy
- Cause-and-effect analysis

DESCRIPTION

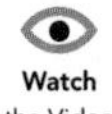
Watch the Video

Writing a **description** is a rhetorical strategy that appeals to a reader's senses—sight, sound, smell, taste, and touch. *Descriptive writing* paints a picture in words. Paragraph 21 is an example.

21 Walking to the ranch house from the shed, we saw the Northern Lights. They looked like talcum powder fallen from a woman's face. Rouge and blue eye shadow streaked the spires of a white light which exploded, then pulsated, shaking the colors down—like lives—until they faded from sight.

—Gretel Ehrlich, "Other Lives"

PROCESS

Writing about a **process** reports a sequence of actions or pattern by which something is done or made. A process usually proceeds in **chronological order**—first do this, then do that. A process's complexity dictates the level of detail in the writing. For example, paragraph 22 provides an overview of a complicated process.

22 Making chocolate isn't as simple as grinding a bag of beans. The machinery in a chocolate factory towers over you, rumbling and whirring. A huge cleaner first blows the beans away from their accompanying debris—sticks and stones, coins and even bullets can fall among cocoa beans being bagged. Then they go into another machine for roasting. Next comes separation in a winnower, shells

sliding out one side, beans falling from the other. Grinding follows, resulting in chocolate liquor. Fermentation, roasting, and "conching" all influence the flavor of chocolate. Chocolate is "conched"—rolled over and over against itself like pebbles in the sea—in enormous circular machines named conches for the shells they once resembled. Climbing a flight of steps to peer into this huge, slow-moving glacier, I was expecting something like molten mud but found myself forced to conclude it resembled nothing so much as chocolate.

—Ruth Mehrtens Galvin, "Sybaritic to Some, Sinful to Others"

EXAMPLES

A paragraph developed by **examples** presents particular instances of a larger category. Paragraph 23 is an example of this strategy. On the other hand, sometimes one extended example, often called an **illustration**, is useful. Paragraph 24 is an example of this technique.

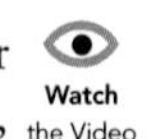

23 Certain numbers have magical properties. E, pi and the Fibonacci series come quickly to mind—if you are a mathematician, that is. For the rest of us, the magic numbers are the familiar ones that have something to do with the way we keep track of time (7, say, and 24) or something to do with the way we count (namely, on 10 fingers). The "time numbers" and the "10 numbers" hold remarkable sway over our lives. We think in these numbers (if you ask people to produce a random number between one and a hundred, their guesses will cluster around the handful that end in zero or five) and we talk in these numbers (we say we will be there in five or ten minutes, not six or 11).

—Daniel Gilbert, "Magic By Numbers"

24 He was one of the greatest scientists the world has ever known, yet if I had to convey the essence of Albert Einstein in a single word, I would choose *simplicity*. Perhaps an anecdote will help. Once, caught in a downpour, he took off his hat and held it under his coat. Asked why, he explained, with admirable logic, that the rain would damage the hat, but his hair would be none the worse for its wetting. This knack of going instinctively to the heart of the matter was the secret of his major scientific discoveries—this and his extraordinary feeling for beauty.

—Banesh Hoffman, "My Friend, Albert Einstein"

DEFINITION

When you define something, you give its meaning. **Definition** is often used together with other rhetorical strategies. If, for example, you were explaining how to build a picture frame (process), you'd probably want to define *mitre box*, a tool needed for the project. You can also develop an entire paragraph by using definition, called an extended definition. An extended definition

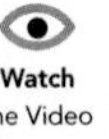

discusses the meaning of a word or concept in more detail than a dictionary definition. Sometimes a definition tells what something is not, as well as what it is.

25 When it comes to soft skills, most people think they are all about those warm-and-fuzzy people skills. Yes, it's true that people skills are a part of the equation, but that's just for starters. While hard skills refer to the technical ability and the factual knowledge needed to do the job, soft skills allow you to more effectively use your technical abilities and knowledge. Soft skills encompass personal, social, communication, and self-management behaviors. They cover a wide spectrum of abilities and traits: being self-aware, trustworthiness, conscientiousness, adaptability, critical thinking, attitude, initiative, empathy, confidence, integrity, self-control, organizational awareness, likeability, influence, risk taking, problem solving, leadership, time management, and then some. Quite a mouthful, eh? These so-called soft skills complement the hard ones and are essential for success in the rough-and-tumble workplace.

—Peggy Klaus, *The Hard Truth about Soft Skills*

ANALYSIS

Analysis, sometimes called *division*, divides things up into their parts. It usually starts, often in its topic sentence, by identifying one subject and continues by explaining the subject's distinct parts, as in paragraph 26.

26 Jazz is by its very nature inexact, and thus difficult to define with much precision: humble in its roots, yet an avenue to wealth and fame for its stars; improvised anew with each performance, but following a handful of tried-and-true formulas; done by everybody but mastered by an elite few; made by African Americans, but made the definition of its age by white bands—and predominantly white audiences. Jazz is primarily an instrumental idiom, but nearly all jazz is based on songs with words, and there are great jazz singers. "If you have to ask what jazz is," said Louis Armstrong, "you'll never know."

—D. Kern Holoman, "Jazz"

CLASSIFICATION

Watch the Video

Classification groups items according to an underlying, shared characteristic. Paragraph 27 groups—classifies—interior violations of building-safety codes.

27 A public health student, Marian Glaser, did a detailed analysis of 180 cases of building code violation. Each case represented a single building, almost all of which were multiple-unit dwellings. In these 180 buildings, there were an incredible total of 1,244 different recorded violations—about seven per building. What did the violations consist of? First of all, over one-third of the violations were exterior defects: broken doors and stairways, holes in the walls, sagging roofs, broken chimneys, damaged porches, and so on. Another one-third were

interior violations that could scarcely be attributed to the most ingeniously destructive rural southern migrant in America. There were, for example, a total of 160 instances of defective wiring or other electrical hazards, a very common cause of the excessive number of fires and needless tragic deaths in the slums. There were 125 instances of inadequate, defective, or inoperable plumbing or heating. There were 34 instances of serious infestation by rats and roaches.

—William Ryan, "Blaming the Victim"

COMPARISON AND CONTRAST

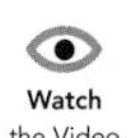

A paragraph developed by *comparison* deals with similarities; a paragraph developed by *contrast* deals with differences. **Comparison and contrast** writing is usually organized one of two ways: You can use *point-by-point organization*, which moves back and forth between the items being compared; or you can use *block organization*, which discusses one item completely before discussing the other. Quick Box 6.6 lays out the two patterns visually.

Quick Box 6.6

Comparison and contrast

POINT-BY-POINT STRUCTURE

Student body: college A, college B
Curriculum: college A, college B
Location: college A, college B

BLOCK STRUCTURE

College A: student body, curriculum, location
College B: student body, curriculum, location

Paragraph 28 is structured point by point.

28 The world can be divided in many ways—rich and poor, democratic and authoritarian—but one of the most striking is the divide between the societies with an **individualist mentality** and the ones with a **collective mentality**. This is a divide that goes deeper than economics into the way people perceive the world. If you show an **American** an image of a fish tank, the **American** will usually describe the biggest fish in the tank and what it is doing. If you ask a **Chinese** person to describe a fish tank, the **Chinese** will usually describe the context in which the fish swim. These sorts of experiments have been done over and over again, and the results reveal the same underlying pattern. **Americans** usually see individuals; **Chinese** and other Asians see contexts.

—David Brooks "Harmony and the Dream"

Paragraph 29 uses the block pattern for comparison and contrast. The writer first discusses games and then business (each key word is in **boldface**).

Games are of limited duration, take place on or in fixed and finite sites, and are governed by openly promulgated rules that are enforced on the spot by neutral professionals. Moreover, they're performed by relatively evenly matched teams that are counseled and led through every move by seasoned hands. Scores are kept, and at the end of the game, a winner is declared.
29 **Business** is usually a little different. In fact, if there is anyone out there who can say that the business is of limited duration, takes place on a fixed site, is governed by openly promulgated rules that are enforced on the spot by neutral professionals, competes only on relatively even terms, and performs in a way that can be measured in runs or points, then that person is either extraordinarily lucky or seriously deluded.

—Warren Bennis, "Time to Hang Up the Old Sports Clichés"

ANALOGY

An **analogy** is an extended comparison between objects or ideas that aren't normally associated. Analogy is particularly effective in explaining new concepts because readers can compare to what is familiar.

30 Casual dress, like casual speech, tends to be loose, relaxed, and colorful. It often contains what might be called "slang words": blue jeans, sneakers, baseball caps, aprons, flowered cotton housedresses, and the like. These garments could not be worn on a formal occasion without causing disapproval, but in ordinary circumstances, they pass without remark. "Vulgar words" in dress, on the other hand, give emphasis and get immediate attention in almost any circumstances, just as they do in speech. Only the skillful can employ them without some loss of face, and even then, they must be used in the right way. A torn, unbuttoned shirt or wildly uncombed hair can signify strong emotions: passion, grief, rage, despair. They're most effective if people already think of you as being neatly dressed, just as the curses of well-spoken persons count for more than those of the customarily foul-mouthed do.

—Alison Lurie, *The Language of Clothes*

CAUSE-AND-EFFECT ANALYSIS

Watch the Video

Causes lead to an event or an effect, and effects result from causes. Paragraph 31 discusses the causes of economic collapses.

Many collapses of the past appear to have been triggered, at least in part, by ecological problems: people inadvertently destroyed their environmental
31 resources. But societies are not doomed to collapse because of environmental damage. Some societies have coped with their problems, whereas others have not. But I know of no case in which a society's collapse can be attributed simply

to environmental damage; there are always complicating factors. Among them are climate change, the role of neighbors (who can be friendly or hostile), and most important, the ways people respond to their environmental problems.

—Jared Diamond, "Collapse: Ecological Lessons in Survival"

● **EXERCISE 6-6** Working individually or with a peer-response group, decide what rhetorical strategies are used in each of paragraphs 32–35. Choose from any one or a combination of narrative, description, process, example, definition, analysis, classification, comparison and contrast, analogy, and cause and effect. For help, consult 6H.

32 A. Another way to think about metamessages is that they frame a conversation, much as a picture frame provides a context for the images in the picture. Metamessages let you know how to interpret what someone is saying by identifying the activity that is going on. Is this an argument or a chat? Is it helping, advising, or scolding? At the same time, they let you know what position the speaker is assuming in the activity, and what position you are being assigned.

—Deborah Tannen, *You Just Don't Understand*

33 B. I retain only one confused impression from my earliest years: it's all red, and black, and warm. Our apartment was red: the upholstery was of red moquette, the Renaissance dining-room was red, the figured silk hangings over the stained-glass doors were red, and the velvet curtains in Papa's study were red too. The furniture in this awful sanctum was made of black pear wood; I used to creep into the kneehole under the desk and envelop myself in its dusty glooms; it was dark and warm, and the red of the carpet rejoiced my eyes. That is how I seem to have passed the early days of infancy. Safely ensconced, I watched, I touched, I took stock of the world.

—Simone de Beauvoir, *Memoirs of a Dutiful Daughter*

34 C. In the case of wool, very hot water can actually cause some structural changes within the fiber, but the resulting shrinkage is minor. The fundamental cause of shrinkage in wool is felting, in which the fibers scrunch together in a tighter bunch, and the yarn, fabric, and garment follow suit. Wool fibers are curly and rough-surfaced, and when squished together under the lubricating influence of water, the fibers wind around each other, like two springs interlocking. Because of their rough surfaces, they stick together and can't be pulled apart.

—James Gorman, "Gadgets"

D. Lacking access to a year-round supermarket, the many species—from ants to wolves—that in the course of evolution have learned the advantages of hoarding must devote a lot of energy and ingenuity to protecting their stashes from marauders. Creatures like beavers and honeybees, for example, hoard food to get them through cold winters. Others, like desert rodents that face food scarcities throughout the year, must take advantage of the
35 short-lived harvests that follow occasional rains. For animals like burying beetles that dine on mice hundreds of times their size, a habit of biting off more than they can chew at the moment forces them to store their leftovers. Still others, like the male MacGregor's bowerbird, stockpile goodies during mating season so they can concentrate on wooing females and defending their arena d'amour.

—Jane Brody, "A Hoarder's Life: Filling the Cache—and Finding It" ●

6I What is a transitional paragraph?

Transitional paragraphs form a bridge between one long discussion on a single topic that requires a number of paragraphs and another discussion, usually lengthy, of another topic. Paragraph 36 is an example of a transitional paragraph that allows the writer to move from a long discussion of anger to a long discussion of possible remedies.

So is there any hope for you and your anger? Is there any reason to believe
36 that you will be able to survive the afternoon commute without screaming or tailgating or displaying choice fingers?

—Andrew Santella, "All the Rage"

6J What are effective concluding paragraphs?

Watch the Video

A **concluding paragraph** ends the discussion smoothly by following logically from the essay's introductory paragraph (see 6C) and the essay's body paragraphs (see 6D). A conclusion that is hurriedly tacked on is a missed opportunity to provide a sense of completion and a finishing touch that adds to the whole essay. Quick Box 6.7 lists strategies for concluding your essay as well as strategies to avoid.

The same writers who wait to write their introductory paragraph until they've drafted their body paragraphs often also wait to write their concluding paragraph until they've drafted their introduction. They do this to coordinate the beginning and end so that they can make sure they don't repeat the same strategy in both places.

Paragraph 37 is a concluding paragraph that summarizes the main points of an essay.

Quick Box 6.7

Strategies for concluding paragraphs

STRATEGIES TO TRY

- Adapt a strategy from those used for introductory paragraphs (see 6C)—but be careful to choose a different strategy for your introduction and conclusion.
- Relate a brief concluding interesting story or anecdote.
- Give one or more pertinent—perhaps surprising—concluding statistics.
- Ask one or more provocative questions for further thought.
- Use an appropriate quotation to sum up the THESIS STATEMENT.
- Redefine a key term for emphasis.
- Use an ANALOGY that summarizes the thesis statement.
- Use a SUMMARY of the main points, but only if the piece of writing is longer than three to four pages.
- Use a statement that urges awareness by the readers.
- Use a statement that looks ahead to the future.
- Use a call to readers.

STRATEGIES TO AVOID

- Introducing new ideas or facts that belong in the body of the essay
- Rewording your introduction
- Announcing what you've discussed, as in "In this paper, I have explained why oil prices have dropped."
- Making absolute claims, as in "I have proved that oil prices don't affect gasoline prices."
- Apologizing, as in "Even though I'm not an expert, I feel my position is correct."

Now the equivalent to molecule fingerprints, DNA profiles have indeed
proven to be valuable investigative tools. As the FBI Laboratory continues to
37 develop innovative technologies and share its expertise with criminal justice
professionals worldwide, it takes great strides in bringing offenders to swift and
sure justice, while clearing innocent individuals and protecting crime victims.

—"DNA Profiling Advancement: The Use of DNA Profiles in Solving Crimes," *The FBI Law Enforcement Bulletin*

Paragraph 38 is a concluding paragraph from an essay on the potential collapse of public schools. It looks ahead to the future and calls for action that involves taking control of them.

> Our schools provide a key to the future of society. We must take control
> **38** of them, watch over them, and nurture them if they are to be set right again. To do less is to invite disaster upon ourselves, our children, and our nation.
>
> —John C. Sawhill, "The Collapse of Public Schools"

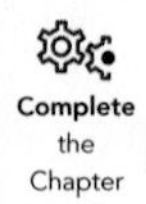
Complete the Chapter Exercises

● **EXERCISE 6-7** Working individually or in a group, return to Exercise 6-1, in which you wrote introductory paragraphs for three informally outlined essays. Now, write a concluding paragraph for each. ●

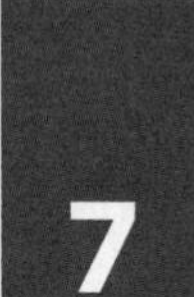

7 Designing Documents

Quick Points You will learn to

- Identify the elements of good document design (see 7A–7C).
- Use text and headings effectively (see 7D).
- Use photographs and other visuals for a purpose (see 7E–7F).
- Lay out the pages of a document (see 7G).

7A What is document design?

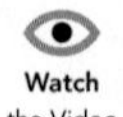
Watch the Video

Document design refers to the physical appearance of your writing. Design focuses on how a document looks rather than on what it says, although how we present information affects how others understand and respond to it. Quick Box 7.1 lists the elements of document design.

Alert: Most instructors are very particular about the design and format of papers for their courses. They want certain margins, spacing, fonts, headings, and so on. It's disrespectful not to follow their directions—and it can also harm your grade! ●

Quick Box 7.1

Elements of document design

Text—Fonts, type sizes, and highlighting (see 7C)

Headings—(see 7D)

Images—Photographs or illustrations (see 7E)

Visuals—Tables or charts as well as features like lines, arrows, or boxes (see 7F)

White Space—Empty areas for emphasis (see 7G)

Layout—The relationships among the previous elements (see 7G)

7B What are basic principles of design?

The basic principles of design are unity, variety, balance, and emphasis. Quick Box 7.2 describes how to check for these principles.

Quick Box 7.2

Checklist for document design

- **Unity:** Do all elements in my document work together visually with effective consistency?
- **Variety:** Have I introduced design elements, where appropriate, that break up monotony and add interest, such as headings or illustrations?
- **Balance:** Are the parts of my document in proportion to one another?
- **Emphasis:** Does my document design draw attention to key information?

The flyer that a student produced for the environmental group Sustain! in Figure 7.1 (page 108) reflects the four design principles.

7C How do I design with text?

Text consists of letters and words. You need to decide which font you'll use. Also called typefaces, fonts fall into two major categories. **Serif** fonts have little "feet" or finishing lines at the top and bottom of each letter; **sans serif** fonts (*sans* is French for "without") don't. Times New Roman is serif; Arial is sans serif.

Figure 7.1 Flyer that has unity, variety, balance, and emphasis.

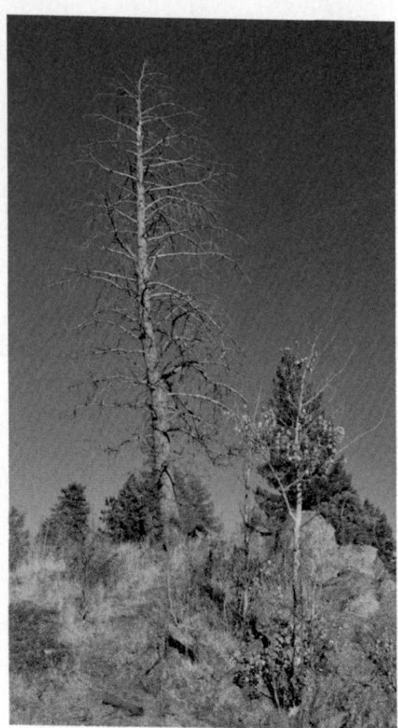

Sustain!

Please join a new environmental action group, Sustain!

Our Goals

- Raise environmental awareness on campus
- Implement sustainable practices
- Have fun together!

Meetings

The second Tuesday of each month at 7:00 pm in 727 Aspen Hall

Next Event

"The Grim Future of Landfills"
Dr. Kathleen Glenn
Trash Action Research
7:00 pm October 13
727 Aspen Hall

More information?

Megan Bateman, President
megman444@wombatmail.com

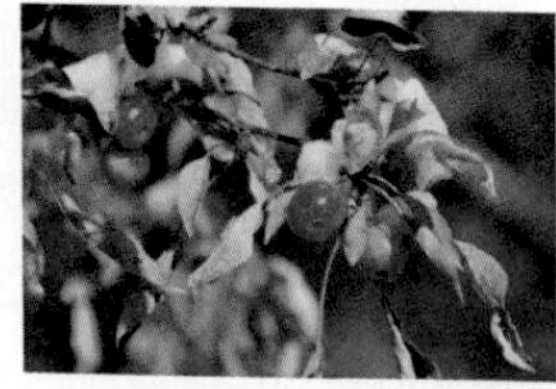

Fonts come in different sizes that are measured in "points." There are 72 points in an inch. For body text in longer documents, use 10- to 12-point serif typefaces. Avoid using playful fonts (**Comic Sans MS**) or simulated handwriting fonts (*Monotype Corsiva*) in academic and business writing. Twelve-point Times New Roman usually is best for academic writing.

8 point 12 point 16 point 24 point

7C.1 Highlighting text

Highlighting draws attention to key words or elements of a document. You can highlight in various ways, but the one guideline that applies in all cases is this: Use moderation.

BOLDFACE, ITALICS, AND UNDERLINING

Italics and underlining—they serve the same purpose—have special functions in writing (for example, to indicate titles of certain works), but they're also useful for emphasis and for headings. **Boldface** is reserved for heavy emphasis.

BULLETED AND NUMBERED LISTS

Bulleted and numbered lists are useful when you discuss a series of items or steps in a complicated process or when you want to summarize key points or guidelines. Bullets are small dots or marks in front of each entry.

COLOR

You can change the color of text for emphasis or you can highlight a text segment. Take time, however, to judge whether color helps accomplish your purpose. Use color sparingly for variety and emphasis. For college writing, use black text.

7C.2 Justifying text

When you make your text lines even in relation to the left or right margin, you **justify** them. There are four kinds of justification, or ways to line up text lines on margins: left, right, centered, and full, as shown here. Most academic and business documents are left-justified.

Left-justified text (text aligns on the left)

Right-justified text (text aligns on the right)

Center-justified text (text aligns in the center)

Full-justified text (both left and right justified to full length, or measure, of the line of type)

7C.3 Indentation

When you move text in from the left margin, you are indenting. Using the ruler line in your word processing program to control indentations makes it easier to make global changes in your indentation. The top arrow of the bar sets the paragraph indentation, and the bottom arrow sets the indentation for everything else in the paragraph.

7D How do I use headings?

Headings clarify how you've organized your material and tell your readers what to expect in each section. Longer documents, including handbooks (like this one), reports, brochures, and Web pages, use headings to break content into chunks that are easier to read and understand. In ACADEMIC WRITING, APA STYLE favors headings, and MLA STYLE tends to discourage them. Following are some guidelines for writing and formatting headings.

- **Create headings in a slightly larger type than the type size in the body of your text.** You can use the same or a contrasting typeface, as long as it coordinates visually and is easy to read.
- **Keep headings brief and informative.**
- **Change the format for headings of different levels.** Think of levels in headings the way you think of items in an OUTLINE. First-level headings show main divisions. Second-level headings divide material that appears under first-level headings, and so on.
- **Use parallel structure.** All headings at the same level should be grammatically similar. For example, you might make all first-level headings questions and all second-level headings noun phrases. Quick Box 7.3 presents common types of headings.

7E How can I incorporate photographs?

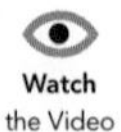
Watch the Video

Digital cameras and the Internet have made it cheap and easy to take photographs and circulate them. As a result, pictures can sometimes enhance a variety of documents.

7E.1 Finding photographs

Every Internet browser has a way to search for images, which you can then copy and paste into a document. However, there are three crucial considerations.

Quick Box 7.3

Common types of headings

- **Noun phrases can cover a variety of topics.**
  - Executive Branch of Government
- **Questions can evoke reader interest.**
  - When and How Does the President Use the Veto Power?
- **Gerunds and *-ing* phrases can explain instructions or solve problems.**
  - Submitting the Congressional Budget
- **Imperative sentences can give advice or directions.**
  - Identify a Problem

- **Copyright and permissions.** Just because you find something on the Web doesn't mean you can do whatever you want with it. Getting permission from its owner or maker is important. Generally, you're okay to use an image one time for a class project that will not appear anywhere else, especially online. But to be extra careful—and often to find better images—consider using online "stock photo" sites (such as istockphoto .com or gettyimages.com) that have hundreds of thousands of images available for small fees or even free.
- **Quality.** Many images you find through a browser search are low resolution or poor quality. They may look fine online, but if you print them in a document they're often fuzzy. That's another reason to use stock photos.
- **Documentation.** Regardless of how you've found an image, you must document it in your Works Cited or References page. (See Chapters 25 to 27.)

7E.2 Taking photographs

Sometimes it's easier and more effective just to take a picture yourself. Consider your camera as a drafting tool. Take multiple pictures of each subject, using different camera settings and zooms so that you can choose the best one. Your main subject should fill most of the image; a common mistake is having people get lost against a background that's too large.

7E.3 Adjusting photographs

It's fine to adjust an image by making it lighter or darker, fixing colors, and making other changes. A very useful adjustment is cropping, which means removing some parts of the image. Figure 7.2 presents two versions of the same image, creating two different meanings.

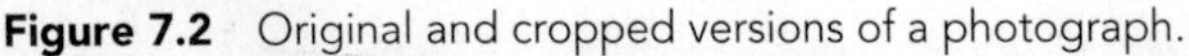

Figure 7.2 Original and cropped versions of a photograph.

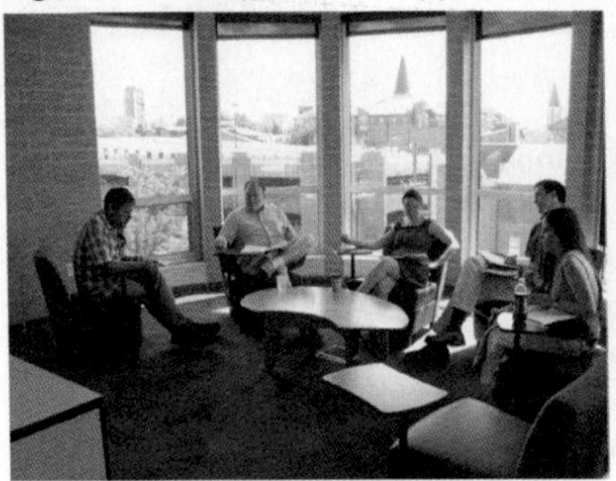

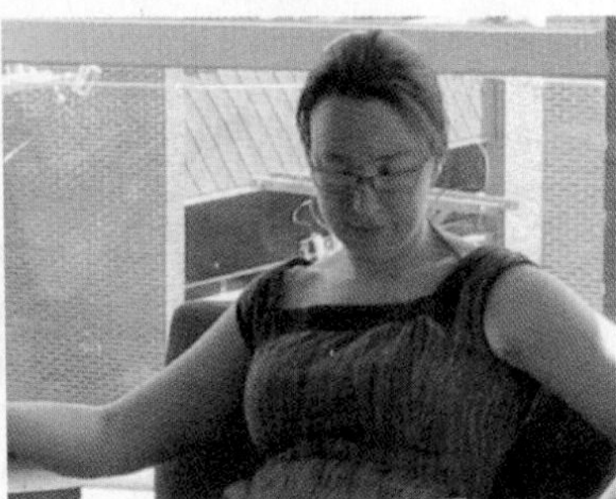

PLACING PHOTOGRAPHS

How you place photographs in relation to text is an important part of layout. Unless an image is the width of the page itself, it's generally more effective to wrap the text around it. (Look for "picture tools" or formatting commands in your word processing program.) Figure 7.3 shows a picture centered by itself, whereas Figure 7.4 shows a more effective version in which that same

Figure 7.3 Photograph simply inserted and centered

Without a doubt, the best pitcher in baseball in 2011 was Justin Verlander of the Detroit Tigers. Verlander won the American League Cy Young and the Most Valuable Player Awards, something that almost never had happened previously. He had 250 strikeouts, won 24 games, with only five losses, and had an earned run average of 2.40.

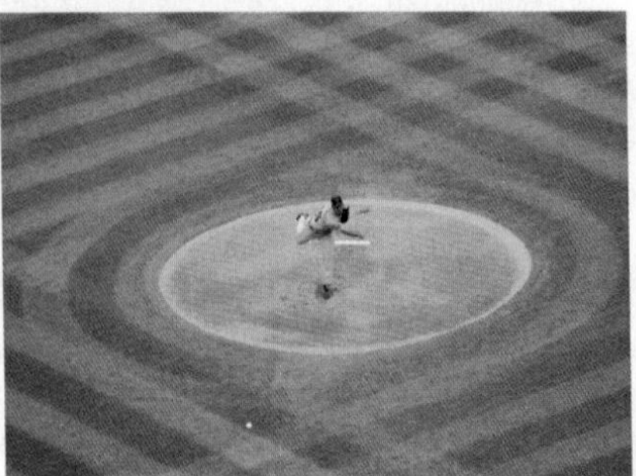

Figure 7.4 Photograph wrapped by text

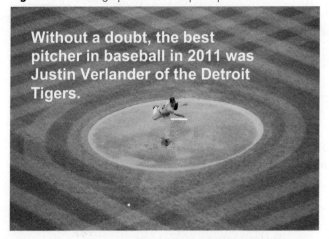

Without a doubt, the best pitcher in baseball in 2011 was Justin Verlander of the Detroit Tigers. Verlander won the American League Cy Young and the Most Valuable Player Awards, something that almost never had happened previously. He had 250 strikeouts, won 24 games, with only five losses, and had an earned run average of 2.40.

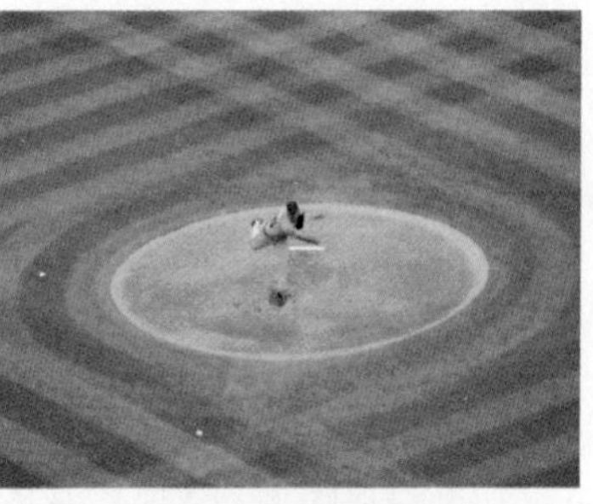

Figure 7.5 Photograph with text superimposed on it.

Without a doubt, the best pitcher in baseball in 2011 was Justin Verlander of the Detroit Tigers.

picture is wrapped by text. Of course, digital technologies offer a third possibility, useful in posters, brochures, etc.: placing words over the picture, as Figure 7.5 shows.

7F How can I incorporate other visuals?

Visuals, also called graphics, often can condense, compare, and display information more effectively than words.

7F.1 Charts, graphs, and tables

- **Bar graphs** compare values, such as the number of different majors at a college, as shown in the graph at right.

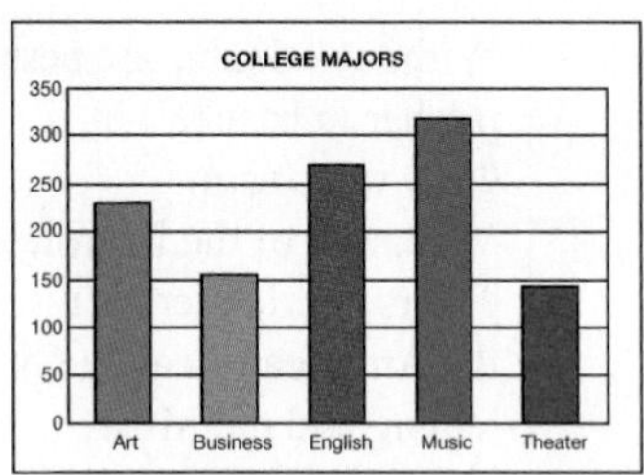

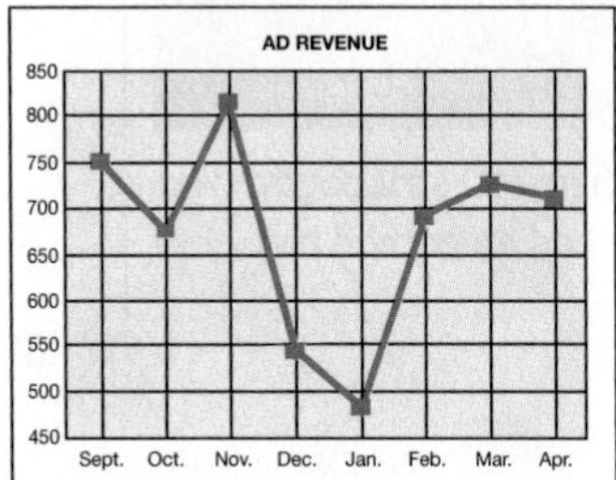

- **Line graphs** indicate changes over time. For example, advertising revenue is shown over an eight-month period in the graph at left.

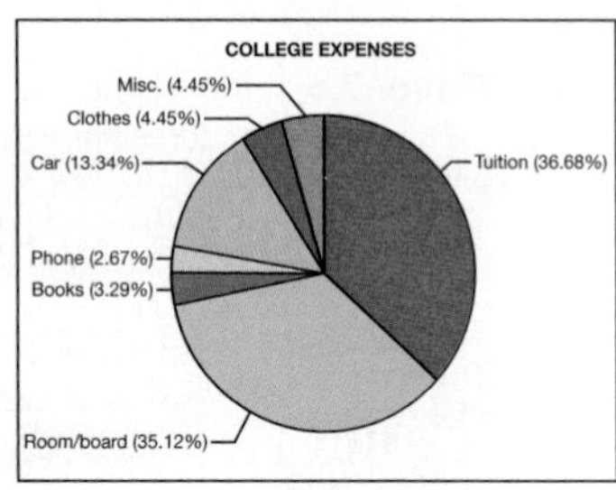

- **Pie charts** show the relationship of each part to a whole, such as a typical budget for a college student, as shown in the chart at right.

- **Tables** present data in list form, as shown here, allowing readers to grasp a lot of information at a glance.

TABLE 1 STUDENT RATINGS OF SUSTAINABILITY, BY TERM

Semester	Students rating sustainability as important	Percentage of All Students
Fall 2011	2,321	65.8%
Spring 2012	2,892	72.3%
Fall 2012	3,425	78.1%

Number figures and tables, if there are more than one, and number them sequentially. Quick Box 7.4 offers guidelines for using visuals in your documents.

Quick Box 7.4

Guidelines for using visuals

- **Design all visuals to be simple and uncluttered.**
- **Include a heading or caption for each visual.**
- **Never use unnecessary visuals.** Visuals should clearly enhance your purpose, not simply decorate your document.
- **Consider your audience and their sensibilities.** You don't want to offend or confuse your readers.
- **Credit your source if an image or visual isn't your own.** Always avoid PLAGIARISM by crediting your SOURCE. If you plan to use a visual for anything other than a class project, you need to obtain written permission from the copyright holder.

7G What is page layout?

Layout is the arrangement of text, visuals, color, and space on a page. You'll want to arrange these elements so that you follow the basic principles of design (see 7B). White space, the part of your document that has neither text nor visuals, allows readers to read your document more easily. Quick Box 7.5

Quick Box 7.5

Guidelines for positioning text and visuals

- Consider the size of visuals in placing them so they don't cluster at the top or the bottom of a page. In other words, avoid creating a page that's top heavy or bottom heavy.
- To create balance in a document, imagine it as divided into halves, quarters, or eighths. As you position text or images in the spaces, see which look full, which look empty, and whether the effect seems visually balanced.
- Avoid splitting a chart or table between one page and the next, if at all possible. If it runs slightly more than a page, look for ways to adjust spacing or reduce wording. If you have no choice but to continue a chart or table, then on the second page repeat the title and add the word *continued* at the top.
- Create various layouts, and look at their strengths and weaknesses. Ask others to tell you what they like best and least about each.

explains how to position text and visuals. (Also see Figures 7.3, 7.4, and 7.5 for some options.)

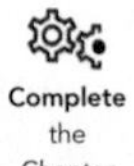
Complete the Chapter Exercises

● **EXERCISE 7-1** Figure 7.6 shows a very poorly designed poster advertising events for The Civic Society. Working alone or in a small group, explain all the design problems you see with this poster, and suggest improvements. You might even draw a rough sketch of how the improved poster might look.

Figure 7.6 A poorly designed poster for The Civic Society.

The American City
Explorations by The Civic Society

2013-2014 Events

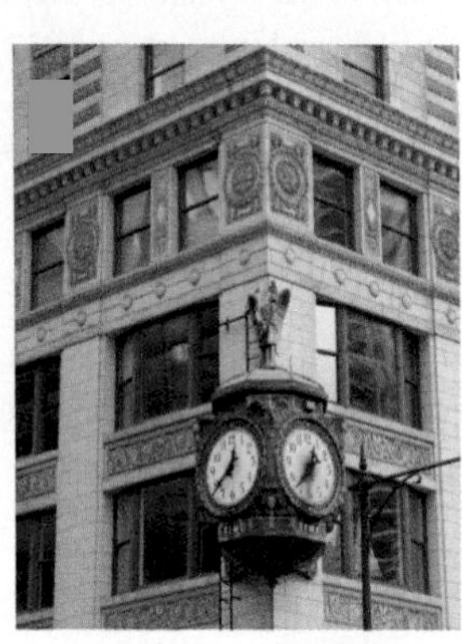

The Civic Society is dedicated to fostering conversations about important issues of the day. This year's series will investigate the **potentials** and the **challenges** facing America's cities.

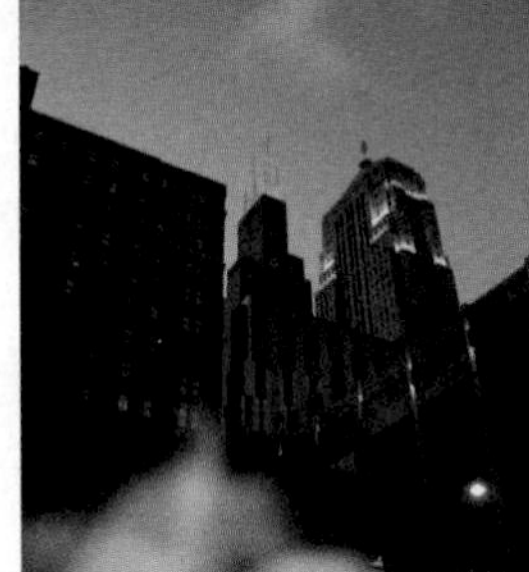

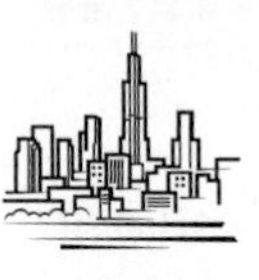

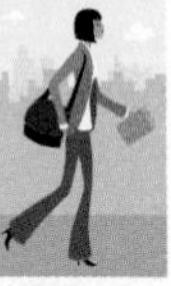

Public Lectures
September 15
"Architecture for a New Age."
Professor Amy Osburn, Chicago.
November 15
"Leisure and Work in Urban Neighborhoods." Bruce McCartney, Philadelphia.
January 15
"The Challenges of Transportation." Sasha Fedukovich, Seattle.
All lectures are at 7:00 pm in Wilmer Auditorium, 1338 State Street.

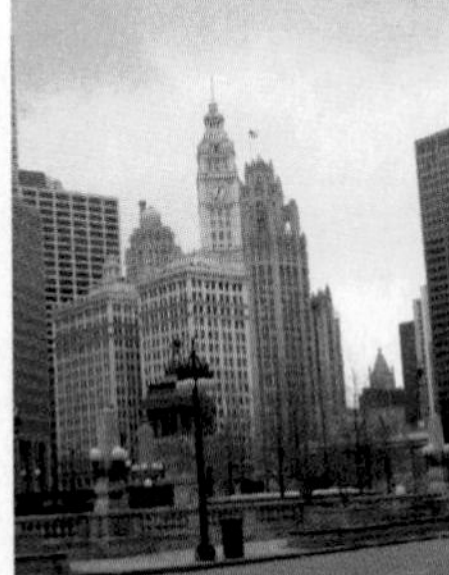

Contact us for more information at
civicsociety@civicgerb.org

8 Creating a Writing Portfolio

Quick Points You will learn to

- Plan a writing portfolio that shows your writing skill (see 8A–8B).
- Write a self-reflective essay or letter to introduce a portfolio (see 8C).
- Present a paper or digital portfolio (see 8D).

8A What is a writing portfolio?

A **writing portfolio** is a collection of your writing (see Quick Box 8.1). It is often a required final project in a writing course, so you need to keep track of all writing from the first day of class. Carefully date everything you write: all drafts of every paper, project, and exam. Preserve all your computer files, clearly labeled for future reference, and keep backups.

Quick Box 8.1

What's in a writing portfolio?

- Some or all of your writings completed for a course, according to your instructor's requirements (see 8B)
- An essay or letter of self-reflection to discuss what you've learned about yourself as a writer and your writing (see 8C)
- A list of all items in the portfolio
- An appealing format, whether paper-based (see 8D) or digital (see 8E)

8B What writing do I include in a portfolio?

Read your portfolio assignment carefully to understand the purpose your instructor has in mind. Three types of portfolio are most common.

- **Portfolios that demonstrate your general writing ability** Consider this kind of assignment: "Present three works that best display your strengths as a writer." You'll want, of course, to choose what you consider is your best writing; however, if the course called for you to demonstrate the range of your abilities, you might want to include an example of a risk you took to stretch as a writer.

- **Portfolios that demonstrate your range of responses** Consider another kind of situation: "Create a portfolio of three works that demonstrates how you're able to write for different AUDIENCES and PURPOSES." Here, you want to choose examples that respond to more than one WRITING SITUATION and one FRAME.
- **Portfolios that demonstrate your improvement as a writer** Consider a third kind of portfolio: "Select four examples of your writing from this semester that demonstrate how your writing has developed." In this case, your instructor wants to see your improvement. You might choose writings from the beginning, middle, and end of the course; or, you might choose both early and revised drafts from the same paper.

8C How do I write my self reflection?

Quick Box 8.2 explains how to structure a self-reflection.

Quick Box 8.2

Structure of a self-reflective essay or letter

1. Opening paragraph introduces yourself as a writer and makes a generalization about the writing in your portfolio.
2. A paragraph, either here or after the set of BODY PARAGRAPHS described in item 3, discusses how you have evolved, or have not evolved, as a writer during the course. Specific examples refer to discussions with peers, your instructor, or other teachers.
3. A set of body paragraphs, each referring to a separate piece of writing in your portfolio and explaining why you chose to include it. If you do this systematically, your reader knows precisely which piece of writing you're discussing in each paragraph.
4. Concluding paragraph wraps up your self-reflection. You might mention the goals you've set for yourself as a writer in your future.

EXCERPT FROM A STUDENT'S REFLECTIVE ESSAY

Following is the opening section of a student's reflective essay for his portfolio. Here is the assignment he received: "Create a portfolio in which you select three papers from the course that best demonstrate your abilities and your development as a writer in this course. Please write a reflective essay of two to three pages in which you explain and analyze the papers you've chosen and what they reveal about your writing."

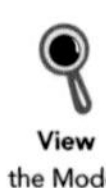

View the Model Document

During the 2013 fall semester, I completed five papers in English 101, revising each of them several times based on responses from my peers and feedback from my instructor. In the beginning, I was very frustrated. I was getting low grades, but I had been told in high school my writing was excellent. After a few weeks in this class, I came to realize my critical thinking about our topics was too superficial and my peers didn't always understand what I thought was clear in my writing. I'm leaving this course with a different kind of confidence as a writer, based on the strengths the three papers in this portfolio demonstrate.

Opening introduces writer and writings in portfolio

One quality apparent in these papers is my ability to adjust writings for different audiences, both academic and general. For example, "Analyzing the Merits of Organic Produce" addresses an academic readership, specifically members of the scientific community reading a review of the literature. This can be seen in my consistent use of APA citation style and a scholarly tone suitable for experts, as in my opening sentence, "Research on the health values of organic produce over nonorganic reveals that this issue remains unresolved" (Johnson, 2006; Akule, 2007). The paper begins bluntly and directly because I decided scholars would require little orientation and would value my getting right to the point. Stressing that "research . . . reveals" emphasizes my ethos as a careful scholar, a quality reinforced by my including two citations. Academic readers will value this ethos more than they would an opinionated or informal one. The objective and cautious tone of "remains unresolved" differs from a more casual phrase like "is messy." In contrast, my paper "Is That Organic Apple Really Worth It?" is aimed at a more general audience, such as readers of a weekly news magazine. That paper uses scenes and examples designed to engage readers with a friendly tone. On pages seven and eight, for example, I include an interview with organic grower Jane Treadway in which I describe the setting. . . .

Generalization

Specific example

Quotation

Explanation of specific example

Another specific example

8D How do I format a writing portfolio?

8D.1 Paper portfolios

Paper portfolios can come in several formats, from a set of papers stapled or clipped together to writings collected in a folder or a binder. Add page numbers and a list of contents so that readers can locate your writings. Follow any further specific directions from your instructor. For an example of a cover page that includes contents, see Figure 8.1.

Figure 8.1 Print portfolio cover page, with contents.

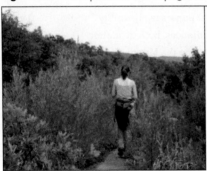

"Paths to Progress"

Portfolio by

Alba Carmen

WRIT 1133: Writing and Research

Casey Sampson, Instructor

May 30, 2012

Contents

Figure 8.2 Opening screen of a student's digital portfolio.

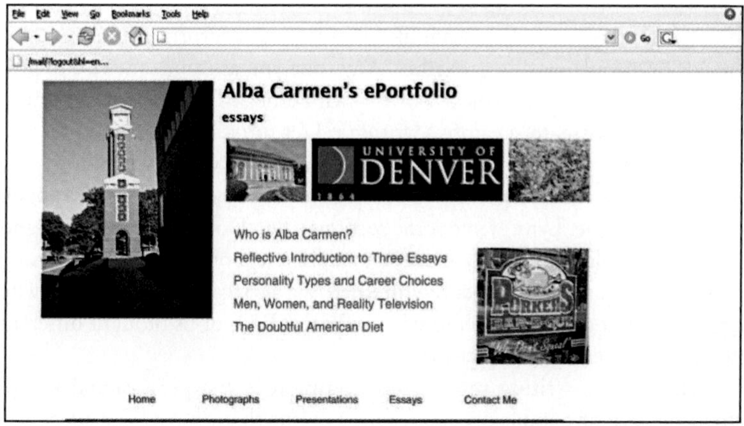

8D.2 Digital portfolios

A **digital portfolio** is a collection of several texts in electronic format. Unlike paper portfolios, digital versions contain links between—and within—individual texts; they can be modified and shared easily and cheaply; and they can be put online for public reading. Figure 8.2 shows the opening screen of one student's digital portfolio for a first semester writing course. Note that all the titles function as links to the papers themselves.

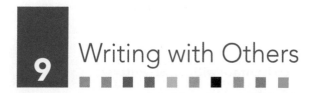

9 Writing with Others

Quick Points You will learn to

- Collaborate with other writers (see 9A–9B).
- Give useful feedback to others (see 9C).
- Benefit from others' help (see 9D).
- Participate effectively in online discussions (see 9E).

9A What is writing with others?

Although writing may often seem like a lonely act, a surprising amount of it depends on people working together. Any time you ask someone else to give you feedback for revision, you're working with others. The other person could be a friend, a classmate, a campus writing center tutor, or an instructor.

A more direct kind of writing with others happens when two or more people **collaborate** (work together) to complete a single project. This handbook is a prime example. Lynn wrote some sections, then Doug revised them—and vice versa. We planned the book over e-mail, in telephone calls, and in person. Drafts flew back and forth over the Internet. We also worked with editors who suggested—and sometimes required—revisions. Each of us brought different knowledge, experience, and talents.

Collaborative writing projects are common in the professional world. Often, the size or complexity of a project means that only a team of people can accomplish it in the given amount of time.

Collaborative writing assignments are also popular in college courses; small groups are commonly asked to brainstorm a topic together before individual writing tasks, to discuss various sides of a debatable topic, to share reactions to a reading, or so on. Collaborative experience you gain in college is a skill that employers value.

Alert: Some instructors and students use the terms *peer-response group* and *collaborative writing* to mean the same thing. In this handbook, we assign the terms to two different situations. We use *collaborative writing* (see 9B) for students writing a paper together in a group. We use *peer-response group* (see 9C) for students getting together in small groups to help one another write and revise. ●

9B How can I collaborate with other writers?

Three qualities are essential to collaborative writing.

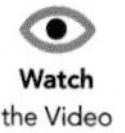
Watch the Video

1. **Careful planning.** Your group needs to decide when and how it will meet (in person, in a telephone call, in an online discussion); what steps it will follow and what the due dates will be; what technology you'll use; and who will be responsible for what. You'll also probably find it useful to assign people basic roles such as leader (or facilitator) and recorder (or secretary).
2. **Clear communication.** Open and honest communication is vital, and people need to build a productive and trusting atmosphere. Keep

notes for every meeting. If people disagree over the group's decisions, the group should resolve that disagreement before moving on. You'll also find it effective to ask for regular brief reports from each group member.

3. **A fair division of labor.** Almost nothing causes bad feelings more quickly than when some group members feel like they're doing more than their share. There are two basic ways to divide tasks:

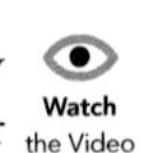

   A. Divide according to the different steps in the writing process. One or more people can be in charge of generating ideas or conducting research; one or more can be in charge of writing the first draft; one or more can be in charge of revising; and one or more may be in charge of editing, proofreading, and formatting the final draft. It's hard to separate these tasks cleanly, however, and we warn that writing the first draft usually requires more effort than any other element.
   B. Assign part of the project to each person. Many projects can be broken into sections, and using an outline (see 5G) can help you see what those sections are. Each person can then plan, write, revise, and edit a section, and the other members can serve as a built-in peer-response group to make suggestions for revision. This approach can have the advantage of distributing the work more cleanly at the outset, but it often takes a lot of work at the end to stitch the parts together.

See Quick Box 9.1 (pp. 124–125) for some guidelines for collaborative writing.

● **EXERCISE 9-1** Working in a small group, plan how your group might proceed on one or more of the following collaborative projects, satisfying each of the three essential criteria for group work. (*Note:* You don't actually have to complete the project; the purpose of this exercise is to develop your planning skills.)

- A report for a public audience in which you explain trends in social media
- A research project in which you analyze the religious views of students on your campus
- A persuasive paper in which you argue whether the United States should pass laws to make it harder for American companies to move jobs to other countries

Be prepared to explain your planning to your instructor or to class members in a way that shows your group has been thoughtful and thorough. ●

Quick Box 9.1

Guidelines for collaborative writing

STARTING

1. Learn each other's names and exchange contact information.
2. Participate actively. During discussions, help set a tone that encourages everyone to participate. Conversely, help the group set limits if someone dominates the discussions or makes all the decisions.
3. As a group, assign everyone work to be done between meetings. Distribute the responsibilities as fairly as possible. Also, decide whether to choose one discussion leader or to rotate leadership.
4. Make decisions regarding the technology you'll use. Make sure everyone can access all word processing documents. Decide if you'll share materials via e-mail attachments, flash drives, a shared document like GoogleDocs, or even through a WIKI (see 62C). Help any group members who are unfamiliar with these processes.
5. Set a timeline and deadlines. Agree on what to do if someone misses a deadline.

PLANNING

6. After discussing the project, brainstorm as a group or use structured techniques for discovering ideas. Agree on the ideas that seem best. Repeat the process, if needed.
7. As a group, divide the project into parts and distribute assignments fairly.
8. As a group, OUTLINE or otherwise sketch a preliminary overview of the project.
9. As you work on your part of the project, prepare progress reports for your group.

DRAFTING

10. Draft a THESIS STATEMENT. Each member of the group can draft a possible thesis statement, but the group needs early to agree on one version. Your group might revise the thesis statement after the whole paper has been drafted, but using a preliminary version starts everyone in the same direction.
11. Draft the paper using one of the strategies described above for dividing tasks. Share draft materials among all group members. For most group meetings, it will be important to have copies for everyone.

continued >>

Quick Box 9.1 (continued)

REVISING

12. Read over the drafts. Are all the important points included?
13. Use the revision checklist (see Quick Box 5.8), and work either as a group or by assigning portions to subgroups. If different people have drafted different sections, COHERENCE should receive special attention in revision, as should the introduction and the conclusion.
14. Agree on a final version. Either work as a group, or assign someone to prepare the final draft and make sure every group member has a copy.

EDITING AND PROOFREADING

15. Use the editing checklist (see Quick Box 5.9) to double-check for errors. No matter how well the group has performed, a sloppy final version reflects negatively on the entire group.
16. As a group, review printouts of the final draft. Use everyone's eyes for proofreading.
17. If your instructor asks, be prepared to describe your personal contribution to the project and to describe or evaluate the contributions of others.

9C How can I give useful feedback to others?

There are two main ways to give feedback to other writers. One is in a small group of three to five people (usually), who together discuss each group member's draft out loud. Another way is to work in pairs, providing oral or written comments for each other.

9C.1 Working in peer-response groups

A peer is an "equal": another writer like you. Participating in a **peer-response group** makes you part of a respected tradition of colleagues helping colleagues. Professional writers often seek comments from other writers to improve their rough drafts. As a member of a peer-response group, you're not expected to be a writing expert. Rather, you're expected to offer responses as a practiced reader and as a fellow student writer who understands what writers go through.

Alert: Some instructors use the term *workshopping* for peer response. The term comes from creative-writing programs, sometimes called "Writers' Workshops." ●

Peer-response groups are set up in different ways.

1. Students pass around and read one another's drafts silently, writing down reactions or questions in the margins or on a response form created by the instructor. Figure 9.1 shows an example of a response form.
2. Students read drafts aloud, and then others respond orally or in writing.

Figure 9.1 A peer-response group form.

Peer Response Questions and Directions

Reviewer's name: ______________________________

Writer's name: ______________________________

Directions to ***Writer****: Please choose three questions you'd like the reviewer to address. Circle them. After you receive feedback, write a half-page synthesis and plan for revision.*

Directions to ***Reviewer****: Please read the work and provide clear and detailed answers to each of the THREE questions to which the writer has asked you to respond. Continue on the back, if needed.*

1. How can this writer make the central argument of this essay stronger, clearer, or more easily accessible to readers?

2. Identify any paragraphs whose purpose is unclear or that seem to be working at cross purposes, and explain how the writer can revise them to make the purpose clear.

3. Does the sequence of the argument build successfully? If not, suggest a way to reorder it and identify transitions that may need clarifying.

4. Writers can offer their readers guidance in a number of ways, such as clearly defining their terms, explaining exactly how the evidence supports their claims, etc. **Identify places in this essay where these forms of guidance could be stronger, and explain specifically how the writer can strengthen them.**

5. Are there places in which you feel the textures or structures of language are serving the writer's purpose effectively? Are there places in which the language could be modified?

3. In yet another arrangement, students provide focused responses to only one or two features of each draft (perhaps each member's thesis statement, or topic sentences and supporting details, for example).

If your instructor gives you directions, follow them carefully. The guidelines in Quick Box 9.2 will also help you.

Quick Box 9.2

Guidelines for participating in peer-response groups

Always take an upbeat, constructive attitude, whether you're responding to someone else's writing or receiving responses from others.

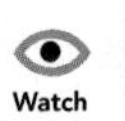

- Think of yourself as a coach, not a judge.
- Consider all writing by your peers as "works in progress."
- After hearing or reading a peer's writing, summarize it briefly to check that both of you are clear about what the peer actually wrote. (It's useful to know when you thought you were saying one thing but people thought you meant something else.)
- Start with what you think is well done. No one likes to hear only negative comments.
- Be honest in your suggestions for improvement.
- Base your responses on an understanding of the writing process, and remember that you're reading drafts, not finished products. All writing can be revised.
- Give concrete and specific responses. General comments such as "This is good" or "This is weak" don't offer much help. Describe specifically what is good or weak.
- Follow your instructor's system for recording your comments so that your peer can recall what you said. For example, one group member might take notes from the discussion; the group should take care that they're accurate.

9C.2 Giving peer response as an individual

Often an instructor will have two people exchange drafts and provide responses and suggestions to each other. All the general guidelines for peer response in groups apply to situations when you're the only person giving feedback, especially being helpful, specific, and polite.

You might find it useful to play a role if you feel awkward about giving reactions or suggestions to a classmate—especially if you think that some critical comments will help revision. For example, instead of responding as yourself, pretend that you're a skeptical member of the writer's target audience. Respond as that person would, even in his or her voice. However, you should still aim to be constructive. Of course, you could also take the opposite role, responding as someone who agrees with the writer; that role can be particularly helpful if you personally disagree with a draft's position. If you're playing a role as you respond, you should make that clear to the writer.

As with peer response, your instructor may have you use a response form or follow a set of questions. (See Figure 9.1.) Here are some specific questions you might find useful for giving peer feedback:

- What part of the paper was most interesting or effective?
- If you had to remove one paragraph, which would you sacrifice, and why?
- If you had to rearrange two parts of the paper, which would you change, and why?
- What is one additional fact, argument, or piece of information that might improve the paper?

Another good strategy is for the writer to generate a couple of questions that he or she would particularly like the reviewer to answer. Avoid questions that require only a *yes* or *no* response. For example:

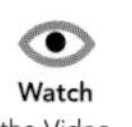

NOT HELPFUL Is paragraph two on page three effective?

HELPFUL How can I improve paragraph two on page three?

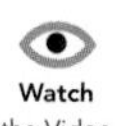

NOT HELPFUL Do you like my tone in the paper?

HELPFUL How would you describe my tone in this paper?

Instead of answering specific questions, the instructor might ask you simply to write to the author about the strengths and weaknesses of the draft. Such responses can take the form of a letter to the author, as in Figure 9.2. Our students usually find that if they're thoughtful while writing open responses to others, they get useful responses in return.

EXERCISE 9-2

1. Choose a paper that you're writing (or have written). Create a set of questions that you would ask a peer reviewer to answer about that paper.
2. Show your questions to someone else in your class. Ask them to comment on how well those questions might generate constructive comments; ask them to suggest additional questions.

Figure 9.2 An example of one student's peer response.

Directions. I'll pair you up with another student. Your task is to write a letter in which you play the role of someone who disagrees with the author of the paper; explain as carefully as you can why you disagree. State your own arguments and explain why they lead to a different conclusion. Now, I want you to be polite about this; don't indulge in the extreme language we looked at earlier in the course. However, to be helpful to the author you should be as persuasive as possible—even if you're playing a role that you actually disagree with. Send this letter by e-mail, with a copy to me (dhesse@du.edu).

Dear Leslie,

To begin with I thought your paper was very thorough and well thought out. It was lengthy and covered all the important things you needed to. But as I've been asked to take the role of someone who disagrees, then offer constructive criticism, there are some things that I think would help clarify and convince your readers who are on the fence about your position.

Your argument is that sex education in schools needs to be complete and that "abstinence only" education is inadequate. You use a lot of statistics and surveys. This is good, it added credibility and "scientific reasoning," but when I see these, I wonder where you found these studies and whether they are themselves factual? You reiterated multiple times that abstinence-only educators use statistics that are untrue or slanted to favor their position. How does the reader know that you haven't made your own facts up or slanted them in your favor? My suggestion would be to label your studies and discuss where they came from and why they're credible. If one of them is from a government agency, you can include the address so if the reader wanted to they could verify the facts. I'm not accusing you of doing this, but it would only make your paper more believable.

Because I am a strong believer in no sex before marriage, I worry about giving students too much information. I think that sex before marriage causes more problems than it solves. I do believe that giving out specific advice about contraception can encourage people to engage in sex before they are ready. Instead we should encourage students to wait. Can you prove to me that having information doesn't lead to early sexual activity?

You stated on page two that a study found that consensual sex between two teenagers had no mental health effects on them. I disagree with this finding. Regardless of age and relationship status of the two parties involved, someone often gets hurt by casual sex. If there was a relationship before, it has the potential to be destroyed due to the new baggage. If one of the parties involved uses it as a one night stand and the other person really liked the other, he or she suffers emotional distress that could be extreme. Actually, I'm not sure this point belongs in your paper; because it's contoversial, I wonder if your paper would be stronger without it.

Sincerely,
Stephen

9D How can I benefit from others' help?

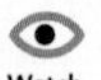
Watch the Video

We offer you three pieces of advice from our own experiences.

1. Keep in mind that most students don't like to criticize their peers. They worry about being impolite or inaccurate, or losing someone's friendship. Try, therefore, to cultivate an attitude that encourages your peers to respond as freely and as helpfully as possible. It's particularly important to show that you can listen without getting upset or defensive.
2. Realize that most people can be a little defensive about even the best-intentioned and most tactful criticism. Of course, if a comment is purposely mean, you and all the others in your peer-response group have every right to say so.
3. Listen and resist any urge to interrupt during a comment or to jump in to react. A common rule in many writing workshops is that the paper's author must remain silent until the group has finished its responses and discussion.
4. Ask for clarification if a comment isn't clear or is too general.

Finally, no matter what anyone says about your writing, you keep ownership of your writing always, and you don't have to make every suggested change. Use only the comments that you think can move you closer to reaching your intended AUDIENCE and PURPOSE. Of course, if a comment from your instructor points out a definite problem, and if you choose to ignore it, that could affect your grade.

ESOL Tip: International students might feel especially uncomfortable about responding to peers. Please know, however, that peer-response groups are fairly common in U.S. schools and at jobs because people usually think that "two heads are better than one." Sharing and questioning others' ideas—as well as how they are expressed in writing—is an honorable tradition in North American colleges, so please feel free to participate fully and politely. In fact, some instructors grade students on their participation in such activities. ●

9E How can I participate effectively in online discussions?

You might take a course that happens entirely online, where discussion takes place through e-mail, a class blog, or a course management system like Blackboard. However, even traditional courses often have an online component.

There are two kinds of online discussions. In synchronous discussions, all the participants are online at the same time. The discussions are scheduled in advance, and everyone meets online in "real time" for a specific amount of time. In asynchronous discussions, participants are online at different times. The discussion is usually open for hours or days, and there may be long periods of time between individual messages. Quick Box 9.3 contains some additional guidelines about online discussions.

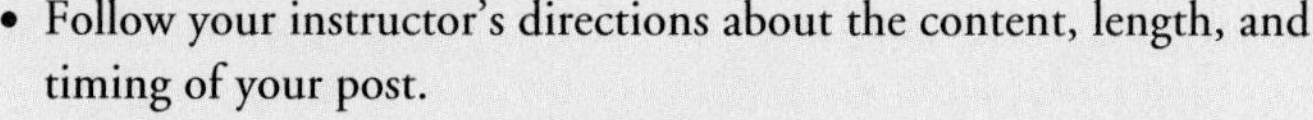

Quick Box 9.3

Guidelines for online discussions

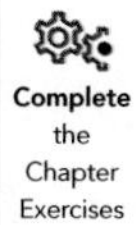

Complete the Chapter Exercises

- Follow your instructor's directions about the content, length, and timing of your post.
- Write in complete sentences and paragraphs, unless specifically instructed to do otherwise. Academic discussions are more formal than messages between friends.
- Provide a context for your remarks. You might begin by summarizing a point from a reading before giving your opinion. Your contribution should be able to stand on its own, or it should clearly connect to the rest of the conversation.
- Respond to other writers. Discussions work better when people are actually discussing. If someone makes a particularly good point, say so—and explain why. If you disagree with someone, politely explain why you disagree, and be sure to support your reasoning.
- Be polite and work for the good of the discussion. When people aren't meeting face-to-face, they can be rude—even when they don't mean to be. You need to work extra hard to make sure that your TONE is constructive and helpful.

PART

2

Frames for College Writing

Frames for College Writing

Essay **frames** are guides that suggest how to develop and structure an effective college essay. We offer frames for eight types of essays, the ones most frequently assigned in college writing courses. Each frame lays out how the elements of essays can combine to create the greatest possible unity, clarity, and impact. Each frame is followed by a complete student essay, with annotations to show how the essay works, along with the writer's thinking that includes integrating the three persuasive appeals of logical reasoning (*logos*), ethical credibility (*ethos*), and compassionate emotions (*pathos*).

Before each frame, we thoroughly explain how the writing process works for that type of essay. First, we discuss that type's PURPOSE* and probable AUDIENCE and then list specific strategies for planning and revising it. Following each frame is a collection of sentence and paragraph guides that offer hands-on experience with the language moves expected in ACADEMIC WRITING.

In using the frames and guides, you must adapt them to the specifics of each of your writing assignments. Although we place the eight essay types in separate chapters, we hope you use them flexibly and creatively.

10 Personal Essays

Quick Points You will learn to

- Describe key elements of a personal essay (see section 10A).
- Apply the writing process to a personal essay (see 10B).
- Adapt frames and guides for a personal essay to your own needs (see 10C).

10A What is a personal essay?

Personal essays narrate one or more true experiences to reveal something worth knowing about their writers' lives or ideas. Personal essays often use stories and explain what they mean. The trick in writing a personal essay for audiences

* Words printed in SMALL CAPITAL LETTERS are discussed elsewhere in the text and are defined in the Terms Glossary at the back of the book.

wider than your family and friends is to narrate your experiences so that readers care about not only what happened but also what you thought of it.

What makes a personal essay effective are specific details and an engaging STYLE and TONE (see 37A). Consider the following example.

NO I can remember my father driving our car into a filling station at the edge of Birmingham. Two miles after we passed a particular motel, he would turn onto Callahan drive, which was a gravel road.

YES After lunch, our father would fold up his map and tuck it in the felt visor until we pulled into the filling station on the outskirts of Birmingham. Are we there yet? We had arrived when we saw the Moon Winx Motel sign—a heart-stopping piece of American road art, a double-sided neon extravaganza; a big taxicab-yellow crescent with a man-in-the-moon on each side, a sly smile, a blue eye that winked, and that blatant misspelling that "x" that made us so happy.

—Emily Hiestand, *Angela the Upside-Down Girl*

10A.1 Purpose

Personal essays mainly have an expressive or literary purpose that's designed to engage and enlighten readers. The best personal essays have a message or point that they reveal artistically. (For more about purposes for writing, see 4B.)

10A.2 Audience

People tend to read personal essays for "serious pleasure." They want to be entertained by true stories, especially by the way the writer tells them, but they also want to encounter thoughts and ideas. Work for a mixture of scene, in which you explain the action or setting in detail, and SUMMARY, in which you cover events quickly so that you can get to the interesting stuff. (For more about audience, see 4C.)

10B How do I plan and revise personal essays?

Generating ideas

- Concentrate on getting the basic story down. Perhaps imagine you're writing to a friend who's interested in your story.
- Try creating detailed scenes. Work on describing the physical setting in detail and perhaps use some dialogue so that readers can get a sense of being there. In descriptive words, recreate the place, time, and people who were involved, to allow readers to form their opinion of the scene.

Revising

- Does your story and its details convey your impression of the experience? Be sure to "show, not tell."
- Do you need more specific details (see "RENNS" 6F)?
- Would your essay benefit if you included some dialogue?

10C What is a frame for a personal essay?

The basic shape of a personal essay is a story, but it will also probably have some commentary or reflection (when you "step back" and explain what it all means). Here is a possible frame for a personal essay to adapt to the specifics of your assignment.

Frame for a Personal Essay

Introductory paragraph(s): Dramatic scene from the story

- **Capture your readers' attention** with an event or significant detail.
- (1) **Describe a specific scene or action** at the start of your story; (2) begin with the end of the story, OR (3) begin at a dramatic point in the middle of the story. Each way creates a different kind of suspense.
- **Use your THESIS STATEMENT** to give readers a preview of the central point of your narrative.

Background

- **Explain the background** of the story, the general setting, the time and place it happened.
- **Include here, if you wish, some reflection** or the point of your experience.

Rest of the story

- **Tell what happened** in several paragraphs.
- **Keep your story going** if you started at its beginning. However, if you started at the middle or end, be sure to return to the beginning so that you tell the whole story. Use a mixture of SUMMARY (covering time in a few sentences) and scene (slowing down and including details and dialogue).

(*continued*)

Personal Essay Frame (cont.)

Reflection or analysis

- **Explain what readers can learn** from this event—about you, about other people or human nature, about situations, ideas, institutions, etc.

Optional: Include related experience or event

- **Include a second experience** or story that relates to your main one, or an event in the news, someone else's story, or an historical situation.
- **Include your reflection or analysis** of the related material.
- **Connect any related material** to your main story.

Conclusion

- **Include a final detail, a final observation**, a restatement of the main message of your story, or relate what happened after your story ended as long as it flows smoothly with the rest of your paragraph.

10D What sentence and paragraph guides can help generate ideas?

Adapt these sentence and paragraph guides to your PURPOSE and AUDIENCE.

Sentence and Paragraph Guides

- One day [incident, event, experience, etc.] in particular stands out because ___________.
- The experience of ___________ ultimately taught me [helped me realize, illustrated how] ___________.
- At first, this event might have seemed ___________, but on deeper reflection it was ___________.
- The most interesting [strangest, disturbing, humorous, perplexing, etc.] thing about the experience was ___________. That was because ___________. Furthermore, ___________.

10E A student's personal essay

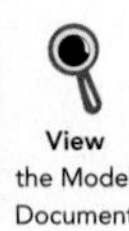

View the Model Document

Neuchterlein 1

Samantha Neuchterlein

WRIT 1622

Dr. Hesse

2 Feb. 2012

Saved by Technology—or Distracted by It?

Dramatic opening starts in the middle of the story, making readers wonder how the writer got there and what will happen. Embeds an emotional appeal (*pathos*).

In the late afternoon of a cold January day, Kurt and I were struggling through deep snow. We had slung our skis over our shoulders and had spent the past hour hiking up the face of a mountain, searching for familiar territory. It would be getting dark soon, and we were lost.

Ethical appeal (*ethos*) hints at the character and human side of the writer.

Paragraph of reflection and analysis with point at the end.

I have often exaggerated that my smartphone has "saved my life." Usually these perilous moments happen when, for example, a calendar notice pops up to remind me that I have a meeting with a teacher in fifteen minutes that I had totally forgotten. Recently though, my friend and his iPhone actually saved my life. Well, maybe that's a little extreme but the phone certainly helped. In the process, however, I had a disturbing realization about the way technology has infiltrated our lives.

Paragraph explains context, introducing the people and setting the background.

A few Saturdays ago, I joined two friends, Kurt and Carter, for a day of skiing. We left our dorms at the University of Denver before dawn to drive two hours west, to the Arapahoe Basin ski area. The sun came up as we neared the Continental Divide, bathing the high peaks in pink and gold light. It was a spectacular cloudless morning with temperatures in the teens, and the brilliant skies promised a great day on the slopes.

continued >>

Neuchterlein 2

By early afternoon we had completed several runs and had just taken the lift up to the top of the mountain. Standing at 12,000 feet, we stared at the backside, considering several options in the Montezuma Bowl. One was the tempting area out of bounds, the unpatrolled and unofficial slopes where signs warned us of dangers, including death. Most skiers have a love affair with untouched powder, fluffy snow with no tracks that surrounds you in a shimmering white cocoon as you swoosh through it. Any powder had long since been packed down on Arapahoe's ski runs, but out of bounds everything was still clean and pure. So, naturally (and foolishly) the three of us ducked under the ropes and hurtled down uncharted territory.

Writer summarizes most of the day so that she can focus on the most dramatic events. In this paragraph and the next, she slows down to provide details.

Logical explanation (*logos*) of the situation.

At first it was terrific. The fresh snow squeaked with each turn that sent up white sparkling waves, as we dodged boulders and looked for a path down. We called to each other in delight. But after about fifteen turns, things changed. Carter got split off from Kurt and me, and suddenly the untouched terrain became unskiable, over sixty degrees steep, with cliffs and drop-offs. Although we had started above tree line, our path was now blocked with lodgepole pines. Going further would have been even more suicidal, so we stopped.

Writer combines logical appeal (*logos*) with ethical and emotional appeals (*ethos* and *pathos*).

Details give a clear picture of the situation.

"What's our plan?" Kurt asked.

"Our best hope is hiking up."

So we took off our skis and began trudging back up toward the edge of the boundary. Ski boots, deep snow, and thin air are a bad combination, especially when you're trying to climb a thousand feet and it's getting late. After nearly an hour

continued >>

Neuchterlein 3

and a half, we were exhausted. It was around five o'clock, well after the lifts had closed, dusk was falling, and it was getting colder. Suddenly, Kurt's cell phone rang. He quickly ripped off his gloves thinking it was Carter. However, it was the ski patrol. Kurt told them that we had climbed back to the edge of bounds and would be back at the bottom momentarily. Two ski patrollers met us near the lift, which they started to get us out of the back bowl. One said, "We got your phone numbers from your friend. He's OK. He's skiing down with other patrollers."

Dialogue creates immediacy. Writer maintains emotional (*pathos*) and ethical (*ethos*) appeals.

Forty-five minutes later, when we finally all met at the car, Carter explained more or less how he and his iPhone had saved us from a cold night in the middle of the woods. When he had realized that he was lost and much too far away from the resort, he took out his iPhone to check if there was 3G. There was. The first thing he Googled was when the sun would set at his location. 5:30. He had about an hour and a half of sunlight left. He then Googled the phone number for Arapahoe Basin ski patrol, called them, and said he was in the middle of the woods, split from his friends. He gave them our phone numbers, emailed his coordinates, and sat down waiting. "So I was sitting in the snow in the middle of the woods, waiting for them, going through my iTunes library trying to decide which song I'd like to die listening to." The three of us got a laugh out of this, but later I got thinking.

Writer shows the logic of the situation (*logos*).

Dialogue shows Carter's character, rather than telling us about it.

Carter's comment is the epitome of how technology has infiltrated our daily life. At all times, even a situation where someone is contemplating his "pre-death ritual," technology affects our decisions. Rather than thinking of his family or his

continued >>

Neuchterlein 4

life's accomplishments, Carter was caught between Dr. Dre and Eminem's "Forgot About Dre" and the classic by Kanye West, "Higher." Our unique thoughts and experiences are overshadowed by a small rectangle of plastic and metal. Even in an extreme moment, we're not entirely in that moment. Although this technology certainly holds the power to take us out of danger, as that day on the mountain showed, it also can distract us from our very lives.

This paragraph begins the writer's reflection of thinking back on her friend's comment and what it might signify.

That night on the dark drive back to Denver, we listened to music. We told each other the story of that afternoon over and over, remembering details, sharing thoughts. We knew that our irresponsibility in going out of bounds had cost others trouble and effort, but we also knew we got a great story out of it. It was a story we would tell with some guilt, but we would happily tell it anyway. Beyond that, I knew that I had seen two sides of our reliance on technology, which can both save us and distract us from ourselves.

Concluding paragraph includes both the end of the story and more reflection. It ends with a powerful sentence, a logical statement (*logos*).

11 Informative Essays

Quick Points You will learn to

- Describe key elements of informative essays (see 11A).
- Apply the writing process to an informative essay (see 11B).
- Adapt frames and guides for an informative essay to your own needs (see 11C).

11A What are informative essays?

Watch the Video

When you write an informative essay, you play the role of an expert on the topic you're assigned or you choose.

11A.1 Purpose

Your PURPOSE in writing an informative essay is solely to give your readers information about your topic in a logical sequence, written clearly and engagingly. If the assignment asks only for information, don't add an argument.

Although assignments might not include the word *informative*, you can usually figure out the purpose from the wording. (For more about purposes for writing, see 4B.)

11A.2 Audience

To give information, you want to consider whether your readers might be specialists on your topic. If you can't know this, you're safest in assuming that your audience consists of nonspecialists, which means you need to present full information for people who have no background in your topic. Your readers hope to learn not only the basics of your topic but also sufficient, interesting specifics to hold their interest. (For more about audience, see 4C.)

11B How do I plan and revise informative essays?

Generating ideas

- Do some reading or talk to people knowledgeable about your topic.
- Find published sources (see Chapter 22) that have useful, interesting information about your topic, remembering to use only reliable, credible sources, quote them carefully, and avoid PLAGIARISM (see Chapters 18 and 19).

Revising

- Have you included the right amount of information if your audience members are specialists in your topic? Conversely, if your audience members aren't specialists on your topic, have you provided sufficient information?
- Have you answered "Why is this information important or significant?"
- Have you used specific details to make your information come alive (for example, see 6F)?

11C What is a frame for an informative essay?

Informative essays can be organized in many ways. Here's a frame you can adapt to the specifics of your assignments.

Frame for an Informative Essay

Introductory paragraph(s)

- **Capture your readers' interest** by using one of the strategies for writing effective introductory paragraphs (see 6C).
- **Present your THESIS STATEMENT,** making sure it gives the central point of the essay (see 5F).

Body paragraph(s): background information

- **Provide background** for the information in your essay. This might follow the introductory paragraph or come later in the essay at a point when the background is more relevant.
- **Start with a TOPIC SENTENCE** that clearly relates to your thesis statement and leads logically to the information in the paragraph (see 6E).

Body paragraph(s)

- **Present sections of information**, divided into logical groups, generally one to a paragraph.
- **Start each paragraph with a topic sentence** that clearly relates to the essay's thesis statement and leads logically to the information in the paragraph (see 6E).
- **Support each topic sentence with specific details**—use RENNS (see 6F).

Conclusion

- **Bring the essay to a logical conclusion**, using one of the strategies for writing effective concluding paragraphs (see 6G).

11D What are sentence and paragraph guides for an informative essay?

Adapt the sentence and paragraph guides on page 144 to your PURPOSE and AUDIENCE.

Sentence and Paragraph Guides

- People experienced with ___________ advise that the public needs to know ___________ so that everyone can ___________.
- ___________ captured my interest because ___________.
- People generally consider ___________, ___________, and ___________ as the major components of information about ___________.
- In addition to ___________, ___________ plays a major role in ___________.
- For many people, the most compelling information about ___________ is ___________. However, they often overlook ___________. That aspect is important because ___________.
- Other important information about ___________ is ___________.
- In conclusion, ___________.
- After considering all the information available about ___________, we can conclude that ___________.

11E A student's informative essay

Moreno 1

Carol Moreno

English 1122

Professor Fleming

12 Feb. 2012

Weight Lifting for Women

Introductory paragraph uses ethical and emotional appeals (*ethos* and *logos,* telling an anecdote to set the stage for the essay's information.

Last summer, after my grandmother fell and broke her hip, I wanted to help care for her. Because she was bedridden, she needed to be lifted at times. I was shocked to discover that I could not lift her fragile frame of 90 pounds without my brother's help. At least I could tend to her in other ways,

continued >>

Moreno 2

especially by reading aloud to her, which she loved. Still, my pride was hurt, so I signed up for a Physical Education class at the local community college in weight lifting for women. The course brochure captured my interest immediately because it said that women can indeed "pump iron" as long as they learn how to do so properly.

Thesis statement presents writer's point of view about the topic.

What excited me the most about the weight lifting course for women was that my career goal was to be a nurse. Once my two children were old enough to go to school all day, I intended to start my studies. Nursing care for the elderly had always appealed to me. My experience with my grandmother proved how important physical strength would be in nursing. Although in the United States the elderly usually are not revered as much as they are in Asian countries, I had great respect for my grandparents. They all lived nearby, and I would seek them out to tell me their life stories. For example, my grandmother who had broken her hip had lived in Nairobi, Kenya, for ten years as a U.S. Trade Representative to various African countries. She had to have been a strong, resourceful woman. Not being able to lift her when she was ill really upset me.

Topic sentence ties into the thesis statement and the information in this paragraph about the writer's career goal.

Background body paragraph tells how the writer's career goal fits with her experience with her grandmother.

Specific details name a location and job.

The first fact that I learned in my course for women lifting weights was we can rely on our biology to protect us from developing masculine-looking muscle mass. Women's bodies produce only small amounts of the hormones that enlarge muscles in men. If women want to be bodybuilders and compete for titles such as Ms. Olympia and Ms. International, they need to take supplements to alter their chemistry so

Topic sentence ties into thesis statement and leads into information about biology.

Specific details name two titles.

continued >>

Moreno 3

that their muscles become bulkier rather than longer. The students in my class did not want that look. We wanted smooth, firm muscles, not massive bulges. Aside from gaining nicer looking muscles, some students said from the start that they expected the course to help them lose weight. Our teacher had disappointing news for them. Muscles actually weigh more than fat. The good news was that when our flab turned into muscle, we would lose inches from our limbs and waist. Those students might not weigh less, but they would look slimmer.

Specific details give factual information.

Striving for strength can end in injury unless weight lifters learn the safe use of free weights and weight machines. Free weights are barbells, the metal bars that round metal weights can be attached to at each end. To be safe, no matter how little the weight, lifters must never raise a barbell by bending at the waist. Instead, they should squat, grasp the barbell, and then use their leg muscles to straighten into a standing position. To avoid a twist that can lead to serious injury, lifters must use this posture: head erect and facing forward, back and neck aligned. The big advantage of weight machines, which use weighted handles and bars hooked to wires and pulleys, is that lifters must use them sitting down. Therefore, machines like the Nautilus and Universal actually force lifters to keep their bodies properly aligned, which drastically reduces the chance of injury.

Writer uses logical appeal (*logos*).

Once a weight lifter understands how to lift safely, she needs a regimen personalized to her physical needs. Because benefits come from "resistance," which is the stress that lifting weight puts on a muscle, no one has to be strong to get

continued >>

Moreno 4

started. A well-planned, progressive weight-training program begins with whatever weight a person can lift comfortably and gradually adds to the base weight as she gets stronger. What builds muscle strength is the number of repetitions, or "reps," the lifter does, not necessarily the addition of weight. Our instructor helped the women, who ranged from 18 to 43, scrawny to pudgy, and couch potato to superstar, to develop a program that was right for our individual weight, age, and overall level of conditioning. Everyone's program differed in how much weight to start out with and how many reps to do for each exercise. Our instructor urged us to not try more weight or reps than our programs called for, even if our first workouts seemed too easy. This turned out to be good advice because those of us who did not listen woke up the next day feeling as though evil forces had twisted our bodies.

Writer uses specific details for an emotional appeal (*pathos*).

Writer uses humor for ethical appeal (*ethos*).

In addition to fitting a program to her physical capabilities, a female weight lifter needs to design an individual routine to fit her personal goals. Most students in my class wanted to improve their upper body strength, so we focused on exercises to strengthen our arms, shoulders, abdomens, and chests. Each student worked on specifically tailored exercises to isolate certain muscle groups. Because muscles toughen up and grow when they are rested after a workout, our instructor taught us to alternate muscle groups on different days. For example, a student might work on her arms and abdomen one day and then her shoulders and chest the next day. Because I had had such trouble lifting my grandmother, I added exercises to strengthen my legs

Topic sentence ties back to the essay's thesis statement and uses transition "in addition."

Specific details give factual information about biology.

Writer uses ethical appeal (*ethos*).

continued >>

Moreno 5

Closing sentence sums up the discussion and leads into the concluding paragraph.

Opening sentence starts drawing the essay to a logical end.

Specific detail ties into the introductory paragraph.

Specific details wrap up the student's experience.

Concluding sentences tie back to the essay's thesis statement and end with a humor.

and back. Another student had hurt her neck in a car crash, so she added exercises that focused exclusively on her neck and upper shoulders. Someone else who was planning to be a physical therapist added finger and hand-strengthening routines. By the middle of the term, we each had our specific, personal routine to use during class and continue once the term ended.

At the end of our 10 weeks of weight training, we had to evaluate our progress. Was I impressed! I felt ready to lift the world. If my grandmother were still bedridden, I could lift her with ease. When I started, I could not lift 10 pounds over my head twice. Midterm, I could lift that much only for four repetitions. By the end of the course, I could lift 10 pounds over my head for 15 repetitions, and I could lift 18 pounds for two repetitions. Also, I could swim laps for 20 sustained minutes instead of the five I had barely managed at first. In conclusion, I am so proud of my accomplishments that I still work out three or four times a week. I am proof that any woman can benefit from "pumping iron." After all, there isn't anything to lose—except some flab.

12 Process Essays

Quick Points You will learn to

- Describe key elements of a process essay (see 12A).
- Apply the writing process to a process essay (see 12B).
- Adapt frames and guides for a process essay to your own needs (see 12C).

12A What is a process essay?

Process essays explain how to do or understand things that involve an ordered sequence of steps. Indeed, some process writing takes the form of simple lists. However, your instructors expect an essay with complete sentences, not lists. For example, these topics require a human touch that only sentences can deliver: "how to buy a used car," "how to comfort a friend who has lost a loved one," or "how to decorate an apartment when you have little money."

12A.1 Purpose

The PURPOSE (see 4B) of most process essays is INFORMATIVE (see 4B.4); they tell readers how to do something. Clarity is vital. When a process can be done more than one way, a secondary purpose is to persuade the reader that your approach is superior to others. In such cases, you not only explain steps, but you also give reasons why your strategy is best.

12A.2 Audience

What does your AUDIENCE (see 4C) already know about the information in your essay? That's the most important question as you're writing process essays. If your readers don't know what an Allen wrench is, you'll have to explain that basic tool before telling readers how to use it. On the other hand, if you go into great detail telling a chemist what it means to "titrate 50 mL of aqueous solution," you'll both use unnecessary words and insult her.

12B How do I plan and revise process essays?

Generating Ideas

- Break the process you're explaining into the best possible order of steps. You can try different sequences on yourself until you find the one that makes most sense, or ask some friends to try to follow your directions and comment.
- Pay close attention to what your readers already know—or don't know. Check always for terms you need to define.
- Anticipate common mistakes or problems that people might encounter, and explain what to look for, or what to do, in those situations.

Revising

- Are the steps in the best order, or do they require more detailed explanations? Be sure to provide enough discussion so that your material makes sense.
- Do you have too much explanation or detail in some sections of your essay and not enough in others?
- Might pictures, drawings, or other graphics help your readers?
- Would using numbers or headings for the sections in your essay help your readers?
- Is your final THESIS STATEMENT a concise preview of the process you explain in your essay?

12C What is a frame for a process essay?

Process essays are usually organized in time order. Here's a process essay frame you can adapt to the specifics of your assignment.

Frame for a Process Essay

Introductory paragraph(s)

- **Lead into your topic** by engaging your readers' attention (see 6C).
- **Explain your topic**, and give an overview of the process, what the results will be, and any benefits of this process. (If appropriate, state the number of steps involved.)
- **Use your THESIS STATEMENT** to note the outcome of the process, which can be the payoff to the reader of the essay.

(continued)

Process Essay Frame (cont.)

Body paragraphs

- **Give each step its own paragraph**, unless the step is very short.
- **Use a TOPIC SENTENCE** as the first sentence of each paragraph to introduce the step.
- **Follow the topic sentence** with sentences that offer clarifications, anticipate difficulties, provide reasons for doing this step, and so on.

Conclusion

- **Explain the outcome** of the process, perhaps how the readers will know whether they're successful in following the process to its conclusion.
- **Mention other ways of executing** the process, if appropriate, and give reasons why the process you have described is the preferable one.

12D What are sentence and paragraph guides for process essays?

Sentences and paragraphs in process essays signal the order of events, explain steps, or offer solutions or outcomes. Adapt these sentence and paragraph guides to your PURPOSE and AUDIENCE.

Sentence and Paragraph Guides

- The first (second, third, etc.) step is ____________.
- Next, you __________.
- Finally, __________.
- The most important thing to keep in mind at this step is __________.
- An alternative at this point is to __________. The advantage of that alternative is _____. However, the disadvantage is ______.
- A problem that might arise is ________. One solution is ______. Another solution is ______. For example, you might ______.
- One indication that you have been successful is _____. Another is ______. However, the most important is _____.

12E A student's process essay

Sanz 1

Miguel Sanz

Professor Taczak

English A

11 Feb. 2012

Opens with an attention-getting sentence. Appeals to the readers emotions (*pathos*).

The last sentence is a thesis that forecasts the general shape of the essay.

Headings quickly show the parts of the process.

Paragraph begins with a step clearly labeled first. The following sentences elaborate what requirements might exist.

Writer shows he's a credible source about the process, which is an ethical appeal (*ethos*).

"Next" signals the second step. The writer provides specific illustrations for choosing the right kind of song.

Auditioning for a Musical

If you've always had a secret desire to perform on Broadway with Neil Patrick Harris or Sutton Foster, you'll need to get started somewhere. Musical productions at your college or, even better, your local community theater offer your best opportunity. Knowing how the audition process works will help you get ready and calm your nerves. The process has two phases: one before the audition, the other the day of the audition itself.

Before the Audition

First, you need to learn the specific requirements for your audition. Knowing the time and place is obvious, of course. But will you need to prepare a song or two? If so, should it be an up-tempo song, a ballad, or both? You might also have to sight-read from the score. You'll almost certainly need to read part of a scene from a script, and you'll likely have to learn a little choreography for a dance audition. Sometimes you'll need to bring a headshot (a shoulders-up photograph) of yourself. In any case, be clear about everything you'll need to do; you won't be as nervous.

Next, well in advance, choose a song for your audition. Find one that fits the musical; in most cases, it's best not to choose a song from the musical itself, unless you're specifically asked to do so. Generally, this means that if the show is a

continued >>

Sanz 2

"classic" one being revived, like *South Pacific*, *Guys and Dolls*, or *The Sound of Music*, you'll want a song from that era. If it's a more contemporary show, like *Rent* or *Avenue Q*, you'll want a more modern tune. The song should showcase the best qualities of your voice. Once you choose a song, be sure to rehearse with a pianist because you need to be comfortable singing with the accompanist at the audition.

About the same time, if you may need a headshot, which is a picture of your face only, arrange to have it taken. Dozens of people will probably audition, and the people casting the show find it helpful to associate a face with their notes on each person. They may want people of a certain age or look for each part, and pictures provide good records. You can pay a professional photographer quite a bit of money for a quality studio session, and if you're a professional actor, that's a good investment. However, for most college or community theaters, a friend who is good with a camera can take an effective portrait. Just choose a fairly plain background and make sure that your face is well lit on all sides.

The writer again states the step in a clear topic sentence, then provides details and explanations.

Writer shows sensitivity to the actor's finances, which again shows he's a credible person.

Next, familiarize yourself with the script, if you know the name of the show. If you don't know the show well, get a sense of the characters in it, their relation to other characters, and the plot. Why? You'll likely be asked to read a scene, so it will help you "get in character" if you aren't reading the scene cold in front of the director. You may even be able to figure out which scenes are the best candidates for auditions. See if you can find a score so you can get familiar with songs you might have to sight-read. Of course, if the show is an original one for which you can get no script, see if you can tactfully find out the type

Because readers might wonder why the step is important, the writer answers this question directly.

The writer uses a logical appeal (*logos*) concerning how to handle not having a script.

continued >>

Sanz 3

The heading and following paragraph signal shift to the second phase.

of musical and look over existing scripts of that type. Whatever you can do to prepare yourself will help you be comfortable at the audition.

On the Day of the Audition

Practical information, along with a little humor, reveals the writer's awareness of his possible emotional impact of his advice (*pathos*) and helps establish his credibility (*ethos*).

On the day of the audition itself, a few preparations will help. Most important, dress appropriately. You want to look your best, of course, but you also need to be ready to move. Overly tight or revealing clothing won't do you much good. The most important thing is wearing proper shoes. Neither stiletto heels nor tennis shoes are useful for the dance part of the audition. The bottoms of your shoes should allow you to slide without their being slippery. Sexism prevails on stage; men almost always need to be taller than women with whom they're partnered. Sorry.

By giving specific information, the writer uses a personal touch to anticipate the fears or anxieties the reader might have, which is an emotional appeal (*pathos*).

Show up on time or a little early. Bring a copy of your audition music. You'll need to sign in, which usually consists of filling out a data sheet about yourself. That includes name, address, and contact information, of course, but you'll also be asked your height and weight (for both costuming and casting purposes). Resist the urge to lie. The information sheet will also ask you about your previous acting or performing experiences. Don't panic if you don't have much to put down, especially if you're trying out for a community production. High school productions, dance or music lessons, choirs you've sung with: all of these are reasonable to list.

Giving a popular analogy can help people understand the situation better.

Now comes the audition itself. Usually, everyone who is auditioning will sit together in the theater. (You've seen this on *American Idol*, for example.) The casting team will be there, too. This always includes the director, the music director, and

continued >>

Sanz 4

the choreographer, but there might be others. Someone will call people up one at a time. Generally, you'll be asked to sing first, but this can vary. Quite often you'll only sing 16 bars of your song, so expect to be interrupted. Say thank you and return to your seat. Most theater people are quite friendly, even if they have to give disappointing news. Try not to be nervous; of course, that's much easier said than done! After everyone has sung, different combinations of actors will be called to the stage to read scenes. After everyone has read, the choreographer may teach the group a few simple steps, let them practice, and then have small groups perform the routine. Especially in community theaters, remember that very few people have dance training. In such situations, you aren't expected to be a professional.

Here is another place where the writer tries to be personal and reassuring.

The process is almost finished. After the audition, the casting team will announce the results, but almost never does that happen the same day. It can be the next day or even longer. Most productions include a round of call-backs, which are just what they sound like. The director asks a few people to return for a second round of auditioning so that he or she can gather more information and make tough decisions.

This sentence cues readers that they're nearing the end. The essay has used chronological order throughout.

If you get cast, congratulations! Your efforts have paid off, and you're on your way to Broadway—or at least to a lot of fun. But if you don't get chosen, it's not the end of the world. You've gained some valuable experience, and you've almost certainly met some interesting and friendly people who share some of your passions. Look for the next audition call!

Concluding paragraph explains the outcome of a successful process but also addresses a failure. Tone shows ethical and emotional appeals (*ethos* and *pathos*) in action.

13 Essays Analyzing Cause or Effect

Quick Points You will learn to

- ➤ Describe key elements of a cause or effect essay (see 13A).
- ➤ Apply the writing process to a cause or effect essay (see 13B).
- ➤ Adapt frames and guides for a cause or effect essay to your own needs (see 13C).

13A What is an essay analyzing cause or effect?

An essay that analyzes **cause** explains why a particular event or situation happened. Why did a certain candidate lose the election? Why has a certain musician become popular?

An essay that analyzes **effect** explains what happened or might happen as a result of a particular action or idea. If we increase or decrease taxes, what will happen to the economy? If I study nursing, what will my life be like?

13A.1 Purpose

Essays that focus on cause or effect can be either

- Mainly INFORMATIVE, providing information and ideas to help readers understand a situation or idea (see 4B.4). Mainly informative essays have an element of argument. Many events have several possible causes, and you need to show readers why the ones you've identified are the best. The same is true for effects. After all, predicting the future is usually open to debate.
- Mainly PERSUASIVE, convincing readers that your explanation of causes or effects is reasonable (see 4B.5).

In writing both kinds of essays, you need to identify good reasons and support them.

13A.2 Audience

Three important questions will help you write for your AUDIENCE (see 4C):

- **How much do your readers know about the topic?** Decide how much background information or explanation you need to provide.

- **What do your readers already believe about the topic?** If your audience already accepts some causes or effects as true, then you know you face certain challenges if you want to propose different ones.
- **How interested are your readers in the topic?** For some readers, questions on their minds like, "Who cares?" or "So what?" are significant, so you'll want to find ways to create interest in your topic.

13B How do I plan and revise essays that analyze cause or effect?

Generating Ideas

- **Brainstorm as many causes or effects as possible**. Some ideas might end up being silly, but get them down first before you pass judgment.
- **Look for possible causes by exploring various categories:** events; attitudes or beliefs; popular culture; social developments or behaviors; economic conditions; and so on.
- **Look for possible effects in related situations**. Did something like this happen in the past? How is the present situation like (and not like) the previous one? What might be the possible social, legal, economic, or personal effects?
- **Develop as many reasons, illustrations, or examples as you can for each cause or effect**. Decide if you need to do research to find facts, gather information, or seek expert perspectives.
- **Choose the one cause or effect** that looks most promising for your essay.
- See section 3E.5 for more advice on analyzing cause and effect.

Revising

- **Consider your audience.** Is the information or ideas that your readers will need to know clear? (In contrast, do your readers already know some of your content, so that you need to trim?)
- **Play the doubting game.** Imagine someone saying, "Sure, that's a possible cause, (or effect) but the real cause (or effect) is ________________." How would you answer?
- **Ask, "So what?"** Ask youself what's important or interesting about knowing that X caused Y, or that if Y happens, then Z is likely to follow? Make that clear in your essay.
- **Examine the order in which you presented your material.** What is your reason for putting them in the order you did? Is it the best order?
- Is your final THESIS STATEMENT a concise preview of your essay?

13C What are frames for essays that analyze cause or effect?

The frame we offer here suggests not only how you might use these structures to organize your essay but also how you can generate ideas.

Frame for a Cause or Effect Essay

Introductory paragraph(s)

- **Explain the event, situation, idea**, etc., that you're analyzing.
- **Explain why understanding** its cause(s)/effect(s) is important or interesting.
- **Give your main point or THESIS STATEMENT**, explaining why the cause or effect in your essay is significant.

Background or context
(Optional if your topic can be explained in introduction)

- **Use a TOPIC SENTENCE** to start each major body paragraph.
- **Provide further information** that readers need to understand the topic.
- **Include history, facts, or circumstances**, if appropriate.

Your main cause(s)/effect(s)

In each paragraph:

- **State the cause(s)/effect(s)** you identify as the strongest or most interesting
- **Use RENNS** to generate support for your reasons (see 6F).
- **Use a TOPIC SENTENCE** to start each major body paragraph.

Possible alternative causes/effects; place this before or after your main cause(s) or effect(s)

- **Discuss some possible explanations/outcomes** that you don't think are the best ones.
- **Comment on their strengths** but make sure to show their weaknesses.

Or

- **If there are multiple causes or effects**, discuss the less important ones, giving reasons why they're reasonable.
- **Use a TOPIC SENTENCE** to start each major body paragraph.
- **Generally devote one paragraph** to all your alternative or secondary causes or effects. However, if they are complicated, you might write a paragraph on each one.

(*continued*)

Frame for a Cause or Effect Essay (cont.)

Conclusion

- **Summarize the cause/effect** you've identified as strongest.

Or

- **If you explained multiple causes and effects**, explain how they relate to or combine with one another.
- **Explain insights or advantages** that readers get from understanding this cause or effect, or explain what might be the consequences of this knowledge.

13D What are sentence and paragraph guides for essays that analyze cause or effect?

Adapt these guides to your PURPOSE and AUDIENCE.

Sentence and Paragraph Guides

- Of three [or however many] possible causes [or effects], the most important one is ____.
- Although it might appear that the causes [or effects] of ____ were ____ or even ____, the most significant cause [effect] was actually ____.
- Recognizing that the most likely effect of ____ will be ____ should lead to us to ____.
- Two [or however many] primary reasons that ______ is the most likely cause [effect] of ____ are ____ and ____.
- One possible cause [effect] is ____. This cause is reasonable because ____. For example, it helps explain ____. However, the cause is weak/has limitations because ____. Still, it's worth considering because ____.
- The most important result of this action [or decision or belief] will be ____. One reason is ____. Noted scholar ____ points out that ____. A second reason is ____. After all, this situation is closely related to ____ , and in that case the result was _____. Some people will argue that ____ can't happen because of ____. However, their argument is weak because ____.
- Someone people contend that ____ is the main cause [will be the actual effect] of ____. They argue that ____. However, they fail to take into account ____. Furthermore, they ignore such evidence as ____. Therefore, although _____ has some attractive [promising, credible] aspects, we should reject it as a satisfactory [convincing, accurate] cause.

13E A student's essay analyzing cause

Cusack 1

Cheryl Cusack

Writing 100

Professor Leake

24 Feb. 2012

Why We're Going Less Often to the Movies

Introduction. Explains topic and creates interest.

Good use of RENNS (see 6F) for specific details.

Thesis statement

On December 31, 2010, when someone purchased the last ticket for the last showing of a movie (perhaps *Little Fockers*), that year's annual box office results were complete. They showed that 5.2% fewer Americans attended movies in 2010 than did in 2009 ("Yearly"). What accounts for that significant decline in attendance? After all, the number of movies released increased in 2010. The films were heavily advertised, and they featured the kinds of stars that moviegoers have long flocked to see. Among the possible causes of the attendance decline are the types of films released, the cost, and the existence of other forms of entertainment. However, the most significant cause is actually the poor quality of the movie theater experience itself.

Writer presents information logically (*logos*), which carries an ethical appeal (*ethos*).

Writer gives specific details using RENNS (see 6F), and in so doing appeals to logic (*logos*).

Movies have been a mainstay of American entertainment for over a century. According to figures gathered by Box Office Mojo, an industry group based in Burbank, California, we spend nearly $10 billion buying tickets each year, not to mention billions more on popcorn and snacks. Audiences have generally increased in the past thirty years, from about a billion tickets sold in 1980 to about 1.3 billion in 2010. However, even this number is down from the peak of 1.6 billion tickets sold in 2002.

One possible reason is that the quality and variety of movies themselves has declined. Quality is a subjective thing, of

continued >>

Cusack 2

course. Still, the movies released in 2010 seem to have a wide range of appeals. Consider that year's top ten films: *Toy Story 3, Alice in Wonderland; Iron Man 2; The Twilight Saga: Eclipse; Harry Potter and the Deathly Hallows Part 1; Inception; Despicable Me; Shrek Forever After; How to Train Your Dragon;* and *Tangled*. Together they show a range from action adventure to family features, including some popular series and franchises. Lack of quality and variety don't seem to have been a problem.

Paragraph introducing possible cause and explaining why it's not satisfactory.

Cost might be a better reason. Ticket prices have continued to increase, to a national average of $8.00 and, of course, much higher many places. Throw in modest refreshments and travel costs, and a night at the movies for a couple can easily be $40. A family of four can spend almost twice that. Given recent troubles in our economy, movies may have priced themselves out of reach for many. However, at other times of financial stress, including the Great Depression of the 1930s, people still went to movies. Cost can account for some, but not all of the decline.

Paragraph introducing second possible cause and explaining its strengths and weaknesses.

Once again, writer uses RENNS (see 6F) to give specific details that support her topic sentence and the essay's thesis statement.

More plausible is the rise of alternative forms of entertainment, especially at home. Video sales and rentals have gone from tapes and DVDs at stores like Blockbuster, to mail distribution through services like Netflix, to today's instant online access. Not only is the cost cheaper (for much less than the price of one night at the theater, people can have unlimited access to a month of movies), but also the number of titles available far exceeds what's playing at the local multiplex. Even with that, people would likely pay for a quality and kind of movie experience superior to the one they can get at home. That leads to the most important reason movie attendance is declining.

Paragraph introducing third possible cause and explaining its strengths and weaknesses.

continued >>

Cusack 3

Paragraph introducing the cause that the student thinks is most important and provides a reason and support.

The quality of the movie theater experience these days is terrible. Consider, first, the advertising. While previews have been around for a long time and have even been welcome entertainments in their own right, they are now joined by ads for everything from body sprays, to new cars, to joining the U.S. Army. Some commercials that you see on television you also see on the big screen. The combination of ads and previews now creates a gauntlet of twenty or more minutes before you even see the first frame of Brad Pitt or Gwyneth Paltrow. Unlike at home, you can't fast forward.

A particularly accurate statement that appeals to the emotions (*pathos*).

Paragraph provides a second reason and support.

Equally distracting is the behavior of others in the theater. Listening to cell phone conversations or watching the bright screens of people texting, networking, or whatever is standard. Some people talk to companions as if they were sitting in a basement or backyard, not in a place where others have paid eight bucks—and not to listen to them. Being annoyed is one thing, but paying to be annoyed is another thing altogether.

The writer is pleasantly blunt about her feelings.

Conclusion. Suggests who should care about this analysis and why.

Unless the movie industry can restore some of the atmosphere of being in the theater, the combination of cost, quality, and alternatives will continue to feed the decline of attendance. Perhaps this is no one's concern except the theater owners' themselves, along with the people who work for them. However, it would be sad to see a vital part of American public life disappear just because we aren't willing to keep some things special, some things part of what used to be the magic of the movies.

A clear statement of the writer's opinion using appeals of logic, ethics, and emotions (*logos*, *ethos*, and *pathos*).

continued >>

Cusack 4

Work Cited

"Yearly Box Office." *Box Office Mojo*. IMDB.com, 15 Feb. 2012. Web. 17 Feb. 2012.

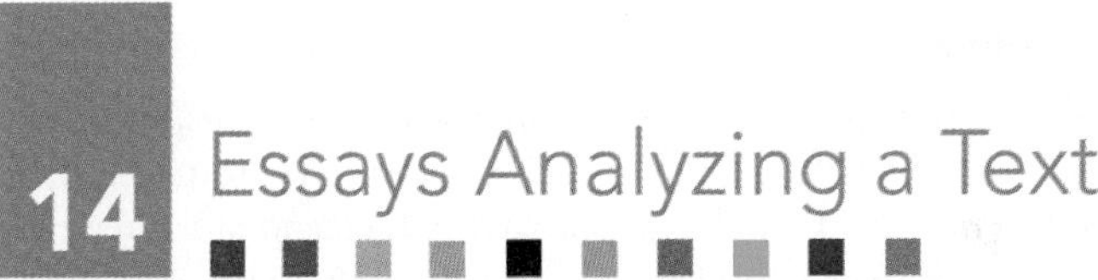

14 Essays Analyzing a Text

Quick Points You will learn to

- Describe key elements of textual analysis essays (see 14A).
- Apply the writing process to your textual analysis (see 14B).
- Adapt frames and guides for a textual analysis to your own needs (see 14C).

14A What is textual analysis?

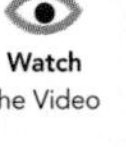

Watch the Video

A **textual analysis** essay is either (a) a content analysis that explains the meaning of a text, such as an article, a book, a Web site, a poem, a script, a song, or so on; or (b) a rhetorical analysis that explains how a text works to achieve a certain purpose or effect. Some textual analyses combine the two. Examples of textual analysis are papers that explain, for example, how women are portrayed in popular songs; what biases are evident in a politician's speech; or how characters, themes, imagery, or word choices develop meaning in a short story. To analyze a text, use this four-step process.

1. **Make sure you understand the text** by reading or viewing it carefully and critically (see Chapter 3) and perhaps doing research to understand its context.
2. **Identify the text's separate elements or features**, such as ideas, words, figures of speech, evidence, and references. Pay attention to patterns or connections between elements.

3. **Explain the meaning of the elements** you've identified. What INFERENCES can you make from them?
4. **Explain the meaning that you've identified** by providing evidence and using sound reasoning.

14A.1 Purpose

Textual analyses can have two purposes. Descriptive analyses explain some features or patterns, what they mean, and how they function. Evaluative analyses to describe features as well as judge them. (For more about purposes for writing, see 4B.)

14A.2 Audience

Many audiences of textual analysis are academic: your instructors, other students, people who read scholarly journals, and so on. At times, textual analysis can also have a broader public audience, such as for book and movie reviews.

Whether your audience is academic or popular, take care to explain the text that's your focus, using SUMMARY or DESCRIPTION. Remember always that your readers will probably not have the text you're discussing in front of them nor will they be as familiar with the text as you are. Still, one major pitfall in writing a textual analysis is offering almost exclusively only SUMMARY and sacrificing analysis and evaluation. (For more about audience, see 4C.)

14B How do I generate ideas for a rhetorical or content analysis?

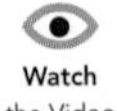
Watch the Video

Usually, your instructors will assign a text to analyze, but sometimes you need to choose the specific text from a broad category, such as an advertisement, a newspaper editorial, or a Web site. If so, choose a text with enough features and elements to support a suitable analysis.

14B.1 Generating ideas for a rhetorical analysis

A basic **rhetorical analysis** explains how the writer tries to influence his or her readers. It focuses on the three major rhetorical principles, also called the three persuasive appeals (see 3B): logic (*logos*), ethical credibility (*ethos*), and compassion and empathy (*pathos*).

14B.2 Generating ideas for a content analysis

A **content analysis** focuses on the "what" of a text—its ideas or meanings—rather than on the "how." It can answer questions such as how images or ideas in the text relate to each other, and if there are repetitions of images or phrases, why is this done? what evidence does the writer use or exclude?

14B.3 Revising

- Do you use QUOTATION, SUMMARY, PARAPHRASE, or DESCRIPTION to explain the elements of the text you've identified?
- Do you discuss why you've identified those elements or how they tie to your THESIS STATEMENT?
- Is your analysis structured effectively? (See 14C.)
- Have you used appropriate CITATIONS? Do you have an appropriate WORKS CITED or REFERENCES page (see Chapters 25–27)?

14C What is a frame for a textual analysis?

Essays of textual analysis can be organized in many ways. Here's a possible frame you can adapt to the specifics of your assignments.

Frame for a Textual Analysis

Introductory paragraph

- **Capture your readers' interest** by using one of the strategies for writing effective introductory paragraphs (see 6C).
- **Present your THESIS STATEMENT**, making sure it states the point of your analysis and offers your readers a concise preview of your essay (see 5F).

Paragraph(s) summarizing the text

- **Characterize the text you're analyzing**. Provide information that readers will need to understand the text you're analyzing.
- **Summarize the source** and, if appropriate, information about its context: where it was published, what its purpose and audience was, etc.

Body paragraphs analyzing the text

- **Start each paragraph with a TOPIC SENTENCE** that makes a point about the text you're discussing.
- **Support each topic sentence** with specific information from the text, using quotations, summaries, or paraphrases.
- **Include discussion or explanation** that makes clear why you included the example and how it supports your topic sentence.

(*continued*)

Textual Analysis Frame (cont.)

Evaluative paragraphs (if your assignment requires you to evaluate)

- **Start each paragraph with a topic sentence.** The topic sentence should judge the success or quality of an element you've analyzed.
- **Support topic sentences with reasons.** Include reasons and explanations that convince readers your judgment is acceptable.

Conclusion

- **Wrap up the essay.** Readers should finish the essay clearly understanding the points you've made. Most important, make clear why your analysis matters.

Works Cited or References

- **Include a Works Cited or References page.** Because you're analyzing a text, your readers will need clear information on how to find it. Follow the required style: MLA, APA, or Chicago.

14D What are some sentence and paragraph guides for textual analysis?

Adapt these guides to your PURPOSE and AUDIENCE.

Sentence and Paragraph Guides

- The writer attempts to ___________ primarily by using the strategy of ___________.
- The most significant feature (interesting aspect/important quality/etc.) of this text is ___________ because ___________.
- The writer uses emotional [or logical or ethical] appeals to create a sense of ___________ in readers. Consider for example the statement that "___________" or the statement that "___________." The language of these passages suggests ___________ because ___________. Consider, for example, how different the emotional appeals would be if the wording had been ___________.
- A noteworthy pattern in the text is ___________. For example, at one point the writer states ___________. At another she asserts ___________. At a third, she claims ___________. This pattern is significant because ___________.
- Reading this text through ___________'s theory that ___________ reveals a key meaning.

14E A student's textual analysis

Gotlin-Sheehan 1

Matt Gotlin-Sheehan

Professor Hesse

WRIT 1622

17 Nov. 2011

Rhetorical Strategies in Two Airport Security Web Sites

Is the current level of security screening at American airports a patriotic way to safeguard travelers, or is it a ruthless assault by power-crazed bureaucrats? Most people are somewhere between these two positions; they might be annoyed by things they have to do to board a plane, but they find the experience reasonable and serving a good purpose. Other people, though, hold an extreme view. For example, the group We Won't Fly protests, "We will not be treated like criminals," while the federal government's Transportation Security Administration (TSA), soothes, "Your safety is our priority." Analyzing the web sites of these two groups reveals not only contrasting messages but also quite different rhetorical strategies for delivering them.

Opening sentence captures attention by stating two options.

Thesis statement sets up promise to discuss both the content and the strategies of two different texts.

Airport security measures changed drastically following the September 11, 2001, attacks. Previously, private companies performed airport security and passenger screenings. However, in November 2001 the Transportation Security Administration (TSA) was created to standardize security practices and promote safer travel. In the decade that followed, a few incidents and threats persuaded the TSA to enhance their measures, culminating in full-body scanners and passenger pat downs. These practices have been the subject of intense scrutiny, criticism, and ridicule, especially over the Internet.

Paragraph of background information orients readers.

continued >>

Gotlin-Sheehan 2

Topic sentence tells readers this paragraph will give arguments against the current level of airport security.

Wewontfly.com voices anger over airport security. The ultimate point of the site is to convince visitors that the TSA security procedures are invasive. Adorned with aggressive imagery, such as mock scanner images underneath a foreboding red "no" symbol, the site has bold headlines: "Act Now. Travel With Dignity" and "Stop Flying Until the Scanners and Gropers are Gone." Characterizing the screening agents as "gropers" associates them with sex offenders and criminals, not faithful public servants, and it casts travelers as innocent victims. This strong language is reinforced by the "distressed" fonts used for the headlines on the page, as seen in Figure 1.

Writer appeals to logic (*logos*) with information and emotions (*pathos*) by quoting inflammatory language.

The main rhetorical strategy is to arouse readers' emotions. The page calls the TSA "ineffective and dangerous" as well as a "health risk." The site claims that security scanners may cause radiation poisoning, and that screeners don't change gloves between pat-downs, increasing the chance of spreading harmful contagion like lice. The emotional appeals are heightened by passenger stories reported on the site's blog. In one of them, a passenger named Elizabeth narrates in detail how she was "a victim of a government

Emotional appeals (*pathos*) are focus of this paragraph.

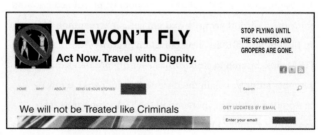

Figure 1 Heading from the home page for http://wewontfly .com.

Inserting a screen capture of the Web site provides a helpful visual. It also confirms the writers' credibility (*ethos*) by showing a concrete example.

continued >>

Gotlin-Sheehan 3

sanctioned sexual assault." Another anonymous poster explains that she had once been raped, so that being touched against her will, as during a search, was traumatic. Because physical modesty is a strong cultural value and people regard sexual assault as a particularly offensive crime, these stories might upset people. They imply that, if disturbing things can happen in such graphic detail to others, they can also happen to me, my friends, or family.

Two specific examples arouse readers' sense of compassion, an aspect of an emotional appeal (*pathos*).

In general, the site uses examples and stories rather than statistics or other kinds of evidence to support its claims. As a result, logical appeals are minimal. Consider the following argument:

> Al-Qaeda is an agile, networked organization. It's peer-to-peer. The TSA is a top-down, lumbering bureaucracy. Al-Qaeda operatives are passionate and motivated. TSA employees are order-takers. There is simply no contest between these two types of organizational structures. It's like David and Goliath, the Viet Cong vs the US Army, Luke vs the Death Star. The TSA is structurally incapable of defending against this threat, just as the US Army was structurally incapable of defeating the Viet Cong.

To make the point most clearly, the writer includes an extended block quotation.

Many readers will probably find the analogies between the TSA and Goliath, the American army in Vietnam, and the Death Star clever, perhaps even convincing. However, the site provides no evidence to support these claims. The TSA may or may not be a "lumbering bureaucracy," but there aren't enough facts or evidence in this paragraph to make an informed judgment about the truth of this claim.

Writer explains and analyzes. Thus, the writer uses a logical appeal (*logos*).

continued >>

Gotlin-Sheehan 4

Transitional sentence to the next text also serves as a topic sentence for the paragraph.

The TSA (www.tsa.gov) site also uses emotional and ethical appeals, but to a very different effect. Featuring smooth, clean lines, soothing shades of blue, and calming photos of empty airports, the site implies "It's all cool. Relax!" The site's banner features the slogan "Your Safety Is Our Priority," and information for travelers and the media, along with explanations of "Our Approach" suggest that the TSA has nothing to hide. The site is easy to navigate, looks clean, and presents visitors with extensive information, in a systematic manner. Figure 2 shows a page from the site.

Topic sentence announces the theme of the paragraph, which goes on to provide examples, using quotations and discussion.

The TSA tries to project a personality of friendship and common purpose. It identifies employees as "your neighbors, friends, and relatives" who work hard so that "you and your family can travel safely." Rather than being distant or harsh bureaucrats, TSA workers are presented as just like us, sharing our values and interested in our safety. The site portrays them as hard working. They "look for bombs," "inspect rail cars," and "patrol subways." A worker "saves a life" or "helps a stranded motorist," suggesting that the TSA goes beyond faithfully performing assigned duties to help people in need. These techniques are designed to provide comfort to, and instill confidence in, the TSA.

The writer saves the most important rhetorical strategy, logic (*logos*), for this paragraph, introducing it with a clear topic sentence.

However, the most striking rhetorical strategy on the TSA site is the extensive use of logical appeals. The information available ranges from poll results and surveys to news articles and television reports from credible sources like *USA Today*. An entire tab is devoted to "Research," which is divided into three main headings and fourteen subheadings, each of which lists numerous facts. "Screening Statistics," for example, notes that,

continued >>

Gotlin-Sheehan 5

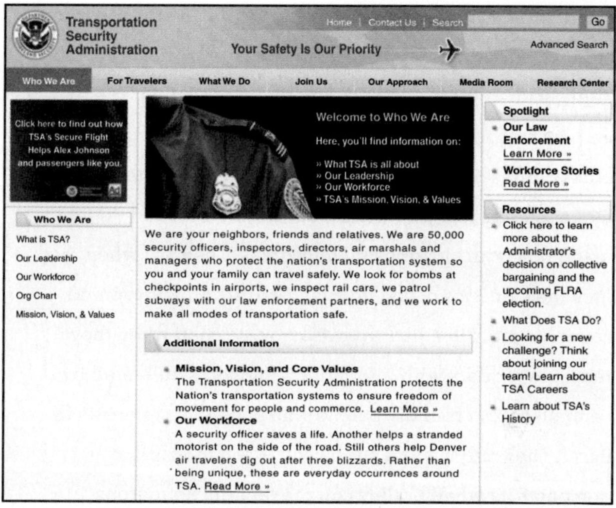

Figure 2 Page from TSA Web site: www.tsa.gov/who_we_are/index.shtm.

Inserting a screen capture of the Web site provides a helpful visual element. It also confirms the writers' credibility (*ethos*) by showing a concrete example.

"We screened 708,400,522. The average wait time was 3.79 minutes and the average peak wait time was 11.76 minutes." Clearly, then, the TSA site puts a strong emphasis on knowledge. Suggesting that airline passengers understand TSA security policies *before* they arrive at the airport seems designed to make people less upset by surprise procedures. "What to know before you go" explains various traveling scenarios, and a search bar tells passengers whether they can take particular items through a checkpoint. The strategy seems to be one of overwhelming travelers with mountains of information so that TSA looks like it's thorough, open, and cooperative, and that travelers have nothing to fear.

Writer uses RENNS (see 6F) to give readers specific details to bring the material alive.

The two Web sites will succeed with different types of visitors. Chances are that an anti-government activist will

continued >>

Gotlin-Sheehan 6

Once again, the writer goes beyond simply summarizing to include discussion of its meaning.

distrust the extensive information on the TSA site. Likewise, a staunch supporter of U.S. security measures after 9/11 would likely scoff at *We Won't Fly's* emotional outbursts. The two sites employ rhetorical strategies that reinforce their audience's biases. Sites like www.wewontfly.com succeed when they make readers feel threatened, uncomfortable, and angry by using powerful slogans and anecdotes. They fail when they lack the evidence of just how legitimate and widespread concerns are. Sites like www.tsa.gov succeed when they reassure readers with information and facts delivered by competent and friendly people who have their interests in mind. They may be less successful when they fail to demonstrate whether they can prevent the dangerous situations they're trying to prevent.

A balanced conclusion that uses a logical appeal (*logos*) and shows the that writer is fair minded, an emotional appeal (*ethos*).

Gotlin-Sheehan 7

Works Cited appears alone on the next page in the actual paper.

Works Cited

Transportation Security Administration. "Who We Are." *Transportation Security Administration*, 2011. Web. 15 Nov. 2011.

Wewontfly.com. 2011. Web. 15 Nov. 2011.

15 Argument Essays

Quick Points You will learn to

➤ Describe key elements of arguments (see 15A).
➤ Apply the writing process to an argument (see 15B).
➤ Adapt frames and guides for an argument to your own needs (see 15C).

15A What is an argument?

A written ARGUMENT consists of

- A THESIS STATEMENT (also called a *claim*) that clearly presents the topic to be debated in the essay and sets forth the writer's opinion regarding that topic

Watch the Video

- **Support** for the writer's position on the debatable topic, consisting of reasons, with EVIDENCE, EXAMPLES, and logical explanations to back them up

If you were to judge the nature of arguments only by the popular media, you might think arguments are simply name-calling or fighting. For college-level writing, however, arguments need to demonstrate CRITICAL THINKING and sound reasoning (see Chapter 3).

15A.1 Purpose

The goal of your argument essay is try to convince readers to believe or do something. In some instances, you can't reasonably expect to change a person's mind, especially on highly controversial issues like capital punishment or a woman's right to choose. In those cases, your purpose is to demonstrate that your position is thoughtful and reasoned.

Sometimes instructors assign students a position to argue. In such cases, even if you personally disagree with it, you need to reason logically and effectively.

If instructors tell you to select your own topic, choose one suitable for college writing. For example, "Should public libraries block certain Web sites?" is worthy of a college-level essay. In contrast, "Which color is best for baseball caps?" is not. (For more about purposes for writing, see 4B.)

Arguments fall into four general categories, as explained in Quick Box 15.1.

Quick Box 15.1

Purposes and types of arguments

- **Definition arguments** persuade readers to interpret a term or concept in a particular way. Is something a "work of art," or is it "obscene"? Is assisted suicide "murder" or "a medical procedure" or an "act of kindness"? What characteristics must a film have to be called a romantic comedy?
- **Evaluation arguments** persuade readers that something is good or bad, worthwhile or a waste of time, or better or worse than other things like it. We explain evaluation arguments further in Chapter 17.
- **Cause and effect arguments** take two different forms. One argues that a situation results from a particular cause. For example, you might argue that certain causes are responsible for homelessness. Another argues that an action will have a specific effect. For example, you might argue that building more nuclear power plants would reduce global warming.
- **Proposal or solution arguments** convince readers that a particular solution to a problem or a particular way of addressing a need is best. For more about proposal and solution arguments, see Chapter 16.

15A.2 Audience

More than any other kind of writing, arguments require being sensitive to readers' interests and needs. What are their values, viewpoints, and assumptions? As you present your argument, you want to demonstrate your command of CRITICAL THINKING, especially how you carefully avoid LOGICAL FALLACIES. The approach most commonly used for such arguments is known as **classical argument**. Section 15C offers you a frame for it.

Some readers hold extreme or one-sided opinions. Your arguments can rarely change the minds of such people. Still, you're expected to demonstrate that you can use sound reasoning and avoid logical fallacies. If you think that your audience is likely to read your point of view with hostility, you might consider using the approach to argument known as **Rogerian argument**. It's based on psychologist Carl Rogers's communication principles, which suggest that even hostile readers can respect your position, if you show that you understand their viewpoint and treat it with respect. Section 15C offers you a frame for a Rogerian argument. For more about audience, see 4C.

15B How do I plan and revise arguments?

Generating ideas

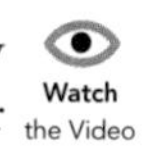

- Make sure your topic is open to debate. For example, "We will eventually run out of fossil fuels" is not a debatable topic. "We should require car makers to increase mileage by 50 percent" is.
- Check that your topic is open to debate by testing whether it answers a question that could receive more than one possible answer.

TOPIC	Students at Mitchler College must study a foreign language.
DEBATABLE QUESTION	Should Mitchler College require students to study a foreign language?
FIRST ANSWER	Mitchler College should not require students to study a foreign language.
SECOND ANSWER	Mitchler College should require students to study a foreign language.
THIRD ANSWER	Mitchler College should require all business majors to study a foreign language.
	All answers show that the topic is open to debate.

Alex Garcia, the biology major who wrote the argument essay that appears in section 15E, was interested in whether organic food was really better. Here's how Alex progressed from topic to claim to thesis statement.

DEBATABLE QUESTION	Are organic foods better than regular foods?
MY POSITION	I think people should buy organic foods when they can.
THESIS STATEMENT (FIRST DRAFT)	It is good for people to buy organic foods. This is a preliminary thesis statement. It clearly states the writer's position, but the word *good* is vague.
THESIS STATEMENT (SECOND DRAFT)	To achieve health benefits and improve the quality of the environment, organic foods should be purchased by consumers. This revised thesis statement is better because it states the writer's claim as well as a reason for the claim. However, it suffers from a lack of conciseness and from the unnecessary passive construction "should be purchased."
THESIS STATEMENT (FINAL DRAFT)	Research shows that the health and environmental benefits of organic foods outweigh their extra costs. This final version works well because it states the writer's claim clearly and concisely, with verbs all in the active voice. This thesis statement is suitable for the time and length given in the assignment. It also meets the requirements for a thesis statement given in Quick Box 5.4.

- Use the three persuasive appeals, explained in 3B: logical appeal (*logos*), ethical appeal (*ethos*), and emotional appeal (*pathos*).
- Use CRITICAL THINKING techniques. One strategy for generating and analyzing logical appeals was developed by philosopher Stephen Toulmin and is explained in Quick Box 15.2.
- Ask yourself *why* you take the position you do on your debatable topic. When you respond, "Because . . . ," you're ready to offer reasons. Arrange your possible reasons in logical order, which might suitably become TOPIC SENTENCES of your paragraphs.
- List the pros (in favor) and cons (against) your position.
- Consider evidence that could be useful: facts, statistics, expert testimony, personal experience, analogies, and so on.
- Decide whether support for your position involves research. (See Chapters 21–23.)

Revising

- Does your essay take a clear position on your debatable topic?
- Do your reasons and evidence support your argument?
- Is your evidence sufficient, representative, relevant, and accurate (see 23D)?
- Do you use logical, emotional, and ethical appeals (*logos, pathos*, and *ethos*) appropriately to convince your audience (see 3B)?
- Have you avoided logical fallacies (see 3I)?

Quick Box 15.2

Toulmin model for analyzing arguments

1. **Look for CLAIMS.** Identify all the main assertions in an argument.
2. **Identify and evaluate data (support).** The term *data* refers to evidence or support. Claims are unsupported if they have no data or if the data are weak.
3. **Identify warrants.** WARRANTS are the assumptions, often unstated, that connect data or reasons to claims. For example, in "We should not elect Daniels as mayor because she is divorced," the warrant (which is unstated) is, "Divorced people shouldn't be elected." Certainly that is open to debate. On the other hand, in "We should elect Daniels as mayor because she served in the Military," the warrant (which is stated) is "Military service is good preparation for public office."

- Have you anticipated objections or counterarguments that others might have?
- Is your tone reasonable, thoughtful, and fair?

15C What are frames for arguments?

Successful arguments can take many forms. We present here two possible frames—one for classical argument and one for Rogerian argument—to adapt to the specifics of your assignments.

Frame for a Classical Argument

Introductory paragraph(s)

- **Capture your readers' interest** by using one of the strategies for writing effective introductory paragraphs (see 6C).
- **Present your THESIS STATEMENT**, making sure it makes the central point that you will argue.

Body paragraph(s): background information

- **Provide background** for the information in your essay. This might follow the introductory paragraph or come later in the essay at a point when the background is more relevant.
- **Start with a TOPIC SENTENCE** that clearly relates to your thesis statement and leads logically to the information in the paragraph.

Body paragraphs: Reasons to support your claim

- **Present reasons for your argument**, one to a paragraph. If a reason is very complicated, use two paragraphs divided at a logical point.
- **Start each paragraph with a topic sentence** that states your reason.
- **Support each topic sentence** with evidence, examples, and reasoning (see RENNS, 6F).

Body Paragraphs: Rebuttal

- **Present objections and answer them**. State reasons that someone might give against your position. Answer these criticisms by explaining why your position is stronger.
- **Start each paragraph with a topic sentence** that helps your readers follow your line of reasoning.

Conclusion

- **Wrap up the essay**, often with a summary of the argument.
- **Present an elaboration of the argument's significance**, or a call to action for the readers or use one of the strategies for an effective concluding paragraph listed in Quick Box 6.8.

Frame for a Rogerian Argument

Introductory paragraph(s)

- **Capture your readers' interest** by using one of the strategies for writing effective introductory paragraphs (see 6C).
- **Present your thesis statement**, making sure it makes the central point that you will argue.

Body paragraph(s): Establish common ground with readers

- **Explain the issue**, acknowledging that some readers probably don't agree with you.
- **Explain the points of agreement** you and your readers probably share concerning underlying problems or issues.
- **Summarize opposing positions** and even acknowledge ways that some of them may be desirable. This may take one paragraph or several, depending on the complexity of the issue.
- **Start each paragraph with a TOPIC SENTENCE** that ties into your thesis statement and previews the content of the paragraph.

Body paragraphs: Reasons to support your claim

- **Present reasons for your claim**, one to a paragraph.
- **Start each paragraph with a topic sentence** that states your reason.
- **Support each topic sentence** with evidence, examples, and reasoning.

Conclusion

- **Use an engaging strategy** for a concluding paragraph (see 6J).
- **Summarize why your position is preferable** to your opponent's. Use a reasonable tone.

15D What are some sentence and paragraph guides for arguments?

Adapt these guides to your PURPOSE and AUDIENCE.

Sentence and Paragraph Guides

- The main reason [the most compelling argument] is ___________. Recent statistics show that ___________. These statistics are important because ___________.

Argument Guides (cont.)

- Many experts support this position. For example, ___________, who is ___________, has argued "___________." ___________ makes a similar point by explaining ___________. The significance of this quotation is ___________.
- I understand that my opponents believe ___________. I respect their reasoning that ___________ and also that ___________. In fact, one thing we have in common is ___________.
- Some people might oppose my position by arguing that ___________. They might explain that ___________, and they might point to support such as ___________. However, this argument fails to take into account ___________. Furthermore, other evidence suggests a different conclusion, namely ___________. Ultimately, this opposing argument is unconvincing because ___________.

15E A student's argument essay

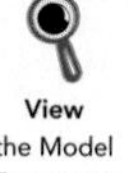

View the Model Document

Garcia 1

Alex Garcia

Professor Brosnahan

WRIT 1122

4 Oct. 2012

Why Organic Foods Are Worth the Cost

Judging from cable television, many Americans apparently like talking about or watching food being made almost as much as eating it. A mainstay of these cooking programs and competitions, from *Top Chef* to *Iron Chef*, is an emphasis on fine ingredients. Beyond the caviar, truffles, and lobster, however, one small quality gets big attention: organic. Increasingly, that word matters not only on the Food Network but also in supermarkets, where displays of similar fruits and vegetables differ by cost and a tiny sticker reading "organic."

Writer uses a popular reference to get readers' attention and introduces a key debatable question.

continued >>

Garcia 2

Are organics worth the extra money, especially when budgets are tight? Have American consumers simply fallen victim, yet again, to peer pressure and advertising? After all, even the United States Department of Agriculture (USDA) "makes no claims that organically produced food is safer or more nutritious than conventionally produced food." Despite all the confusion, current research shows that the health and environmental benefits of organic foods outweigh their extra costs.

Thesis statement

Organic foods are produced without using most chemical pesticides, without artificial fertilizers, without genetic engineering, and without radiation (USDA). In the case of organic meat, poultry, eggs, and dairy products, the animals are raised without antibiotics or growth hormones. As a result, people sometimes use the term "natural" instead of "organic," but "natural" is less precise. Before 2002, people could never be quite sure what they were getting when they bought supposedly organic food, unless they bought it directly from a farmer they knew personally. In 2002, the USDA established standards that food must meet in order to be labeled and sold as organic.

Writer provides background information, making sure that readers understand what "organic" means.

Organic foods do tend to cost more than nonorganic, even up to 50% more (Zelman), mainly because they are currently more difficult to mass-produce. Farmers who apply pesticides often get larger crops from the same amount of land because there is less insect damage. Artificial fertilizers tend to increase the yield, size, and uniformity of fruits and vegetables, and herbicides kill weeds that compete with desirable crops for

A second paragraph of background information. Because cost is a key issue, this entire paragraph explains why organic foods are expensive.

continued >>

Garcia 3

sun, nutrients, and moisture. Animals that routinely receive antibiotics and growth hormones tend to grow more quickly and produce more milk and eggs. In contrast, organic farmers have lower yields and, therefore, higher costs. These get passed along as higher prices to consumers.

Still, the extra cost is certainly worthwhile in terms of health benefits. Numerous studies have shown the dangers of pesticides for humans. An extensive review of research by the Ontario College of Family Physicians concludes that "Exposure to all the commonly used pesticides . . . has shown positive associations with adverse health effects" (Sanborn et al. 173). The risks include cancer, psychiatric effects, difficulties becoming pregnant, miscarriages, and dermatitis. Carefully washing fruits and vegetables can remove some of these dangerous chemicals, but according to the prestigious journal *Nature*, even this does not remove all of them (Giles 797). An extensive review of research by medical professor Denis Lairon found that "the vast majority (94–100%) of organic food does not contain any pesticide residues (38). Certainly, if there's a way to prevent these poisons from entering our bodies, we should take advantage of it. The few cents saved on cheaper food can quickly disappear in doctors' bills needed to treat conditions caused or worsened by chemicals.

Topic sentence introduces health benefits.

Writer uses an emotional appeal (*pathos*) and gives the first main reason in support of the thesis. Details explain the dangers of pesticides in foods, and three expert studies provide support.

Organic meat, poultry, and dairy products can address another health concern: the diminishing effectiveness of antibiotics. In the past decades, many kinds of bacteria have become resistant to drugs, making it extremely difficult to treat some kinds of tuberculosis, pneumonia, staphylococcus

A second reason in favor of organic foods. The writer uses careful reasoning to explain.

continued >>

Garcia 4

infections, and less serious diseases ("Dangerous" 1). True, this has happened mainly because doctors have over-prescribed antibiotics to patients who expect a pill for every illness. However, routinely giving antibiotics to all cows and chickens means that these drugs enter our food chain early, giving bacteria lots of chances to develop resistance. A person who switches to organic meats won't suddenly experience better results from antibiotics; the benefit is a more gradual one for society as a whole. However, if we want to be able to fight infections with effective drugs, we need to reserve antibiotics for true cases of need and discourage their routine use in animals raised for food. Buying organic is a way to persuade more farmers to adopt this practice.

Writer uses logical, ethical, and emotional appeals (*logos*, *ethos*, and *pathos*).

Another benefit of organic foods is also a societal one: Organic farming is better for the environment. In his review of several studies, Colin Macilwain concluded that organic farms nurture more and diverse plants and animals than regular farms (797). Organic farms also don't release pesticides and herbicides that can harm wildlife and run into our water supply, with implications for people's health, too. Macilwain notes that those farms also can generate less carbon dioxide, which will help with global warming; also, many scientists believe that organic farming is more sustainable because it results in better soil quality (798). Once again, these benefits are not ones that you will personally experience right away. However, a better natural environment means a better quality of living for everyone and for future generations.

Writer explains a third reason, again using an expert source in support.

By arousing the "better self" of readers, the writer uses an ethical appeal (*ethos*).

Some critics point out that organic products aren't more nutritious than regular ones. Four years ago, media star and

continued >>

Garcia 5

physician Sanjay Gupta, for example, found the medical evidence for nutritional advantages is "thin" (60), and the *Tufts University Health and Nutrition Letter* reported that the research on nutritional benefits is mixed, ("Is Organic" 8). However, other studies differ. For example, research shows that organically raised tomatoes have higher levels of flavonoids, nutrients that have many health benefits (Mitchell et al.). More recently, both Denis Lairon and Walter J. Crinnion found higher levels of several nutrients in organic found. Nutritional value, which includes qualities such as vitamins and other beneficial substances, is a different measure than food safety. Even if the nutritional evidence is uncertain, food safety from avoiding chemicals and environmental quality remain convincing reasons to purchase organic food.

One point has to be conceded. Claims that organic foods taste better are probably groundless. Researchers at Cornell University gave people identical chips, yogurt, and cookies but labeled some of them "organic" and others "regular." People rated the organic ones as better tasting even though there was no difference ("Even Organic"). Labels clearly shape our perceptions.

Despite considerable benefits for purchasing organic products, consumers have to make individual purchasing decisions. There are no simple ways to measure that spending fifty cents more on a cantaloupe will improve my quality of life by fifty cents. However, there is a position between all organics and none. The nonprofit Environmental Working Group identifies a dozen types of organic produce (including apples, strawberries, and spinach) as safer and worth the extra cost,

Writer acknowledges an objection and even cites expert opinions that contradict his argument. However, he counters those objections and concludes with a strong comment in support of organic foods.

Writer uses logical appeal (*logos*) to try to convince his readers.

Writer concedes a possible objection. This builds an ethical case (*ethos*) by showing writer is open-minded.

Concluding paragraph returns to issues of cost in the thesis statement, summarizes the reasons the paper has provided, and ends with a strong call for action.

continued >>

Garcia 6

but they conclude another dozen are not, including bananas, pineapples, and onions (Zelman). The bottom line is that countless people are rightly concerned these days about our personal health and the health of the world in which we live. It's nearly impossible to put a value on a sustainable, diverse natural environment and having the physical health to enjoy it. The long-term benefits of buying organic, for anyone who can reasonably afford to, far outweigh the short-term savings in the checkout line.

The writer ends by appealing to logic, ethics, and emotions (*logos, ethos,* and *pathos*).

Garcia 7

Works Cited

In an actual paper, the Works Cited appears alone on a new page.

"Dangerous Bacterial Infections Are on the Rise." *Consumer Reports on Health* (Nov. 2007): 1–4. Print.

Crinnion, Walter J. "Organic Foods Contain Higher Levels of Certain Nutrients, Lower Levels of Pesticides, and May Provide Health Benefits for the Consumer." *Alternative Medicine Review* 15.1 (Apr. 2010): 4–12. Web. 14 Sept. 2011.

"Even Organic Cookies and Chips Enjoy Health 'Halo'." *Tufts University Health and Nutrition Letter* 29.5 (July 2011): 3. Web. 12 Sept. 2011.

Giles, Jim. "Is Organic Food Better for Us?" *Nature* 428.6985 (2004): 796–97. Print.

continued >>

Garcia 8

Gupta, Sanjay, and Shahreen Abedin. "Rethinking Organics." *Time* (20 Aug. 2007): 60. Print.

"Is Organic Food Really More Nutritious?" *Tufts University Health and Nutrition Letter* (Sept. 2007): 8. Web. 25 Sept. 2011.

Lairon, Denis. "Nutritional Quality and Safety of Organic Food. A Review." *Agronomy for Sustainable Development* 30 (2010): 33–41. Web. 14 Sept. 2011.

Macilwain, Colin. "Is Organic Farming Better for the Environment?" *Nature* 428.6985 (2004): 797–98. Print.

Mitchell, Alyson E., et al. "Ten-Year Comparison of the Influence of Organic and Conventional Crop Management Practices on the Content of Flavonoids in Tomatoes." *Journal of Agricultural Food Chemistry* 55.15 (2007): 6154–59. Web. 30 Sept. 2011.

United States. Dept. of Agriculture. "Organic Food Labels and Standards: The Facts." National Organic Program. Jan. 2007. Web. 26 Sept. 2011.

Sanborn, Margaret, et al. *Pesticides Literature Review: Systematic Review of Pesticide Human Health Effects.* Toronto: Ontario College of Family Physicians, 2004. Web. 28 Sept. 2011.

Zelman, Kathleen M. "Organic Food—Is 'Natural' Worth the Extra Cost?" *WebMD*. 2007. Web. 17 Sept. 2011.

16 Proposal or Solution Essays

Quick Points You will learn to

- Describe key elements of a proposal or solution essay (see 16A).
- Apply the writing process to a proposal or solution essay (see 16B).
- Adapt frames and guides for a proposal or solution essay to your own needs (see 16C).

16A What are proposal or solution essays?

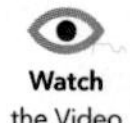

Proposal or solution essays are specific types of ARGUMENTS (see Chapter 15) that require you to do three things:

1. Convince readers that a particular problem or opportunity exists and requires action.
2. Propose a specific solution or course of action and offer reasons for proposing it.
3. Defend your solution or proposal as better than others.

16A.1 Purpose

Proposal or solution essays seek to persuade readers to act on a solution. In your essay, you need to address the problem you want to write about, your proposed solution(s), and the beliefs your readers hold about them. Here are two examples:

A. Problem: Students can't get the classes they need to graduate on time.

Solution 1: The college should offer more courses by either (a) hiring more faculty, or (b) having faculty teach more students.

Solution 2: The college should increase its number of popular or required courses by cutting unpopular or elective courses.

Solution 3: The college should change graduation requirements.

B. Problem: Unemployment is high.

Solution 1: The government should hire unemployed people to build roads, bridges, parks, and other public projects.

Solution 2: The government should reward businesses that hire people to work in this country or penalize businesses that send jobs overseas.

Solution 3: Workers should be less choosey about the jobs they will accept, or they should start their own businesses.

The preceding examples list several possible solutions, but no doubt you can think of others. Which solution would be best? Why? (For more about purposes for writing, see 4B.)

16A.2 Audience

Consult Quick Box 16.1 for four considerations of audience specifically for problem or solution essays. For more about audience, see 4C.

Quick Box 16.1

Four aspects of audience for problem or solution essays

1. **The audience doesn't know or agree that a problem exists.** Here explaining the problem is your most important task. You want to increase public awareness so that the desperate need for solutions becomes obvious, but your solution isn't your central concern.
2. **The audience generally agrees on a problem—but not on a solution.** Here you explain the problem briefly and spend your time and energy on writing about the value of your solution.
3. **The audience believes there's a problem, but it favors a different solution.** Here you emphasize why your solution is better (for instance, more practical, easier to achieve, less expensive) than theirs.
4. **The audience is in a direct position to act versus an indirect position.** Here you target your argument to the audience that has direct power to act or indirect power to influence.

16B How do I plan and revise proposal or solution arguments?

Consult section 15B for advice useful for generating arguments and their support, or use these questions for proposal or solution essays.

- **What caused the problem?** Complex problems usually have many possible causes so take time to brainstorm a list.
- **What are possible solutions?** Because each cause might have a different solution, don't rush into settling on one of them. Allow yourself time to be creative.
- **Why is your solution effective?** Who needs to be involved? What do they need to do? When? How? Why?
- **Why is your solution feasible?** A solution is feasible when it is practical and affordable. For example, we could solve poverty by giving every poor person $50,000 a year, but that's not feasible.
- **What are drawbacks of other solutions?** Apply questions of effectiveness and feasibility to all solutions to reveal weaknesses in alternative proposals. Also, you might consider unintended effects or results.
- **What will happen if people don't act?** This question can generate an effective conclusion and be a good source of emotional appeals (*pathos*).

Revising

- Have you established that there's a problem that needs a solution?
- Is your solution effective, feasible, and better than others?
- Have you used evidence that is sufficient, representative, relevant, and accurate (see Quick Box 3.7)?
- Have you used appropriate logical, emotional, and ethical appeals (*logos, pathos*, and *ethos;* see 3B)?
- Is your TONE reasonable, thoughtful, and fair?

16C What is a frame for a proposal or solution essay?

Here is a possible proposal/solution essay frame to adapt to the specifics of your assignments.

Frame for a Proposal or Solution Essay

Introductory paragraph(s)

- **Capture your readers' interest** in your topic by using one of the strategies for writing effective introductory paragraphs (see 6C).
- **Introduce** a problem or opportunity.
- **Present your** THESIS STATEMENT, making sure it proposes an action or solution (see 5F).

Body paragraph(s): Background information

- **Provide background information.** Note: If the background isn't complicated, your essay might move directly to persuading readers that a problem exists.
- **Start each paragraph with a** TOPIC SENTENCE that clearly relates to your thesis statement and leads logically to the information in the paragraph (see 6E).

Body paragraphs: Persuade readers that a problem exists

- **Explain the problem that exists**, grouping the parts of the problem effectively within separate paragraphs.
- **Start each paragraph with a** TOPIC SENTENCE that makes clear what you will explain in the paragraph.
- **Support each topic sentence** with evidence, examples, and reasoning.
- **If your emphasis is on the solution** because the problem is well known, keep this section short.

Solution paragraph(s)

- **Explain why your solution will be effective and feasible.**
- **Divide parts of your solution** into sensible paragraphs, starting each one with a topic sentence that leads into the point you are making.
- **If your emphasis is on the problem**, keep this section short.

Rebuttal paragraph(s): Place here or immediately before your solution

- **Present alternative solutions and refute them.** State other possible solutions and explain why they aren't as good as yours. Answer possible criticisms.
- **Again, if your emphasis is on the problem**, keep this section short.

Conclusion

- **Wrap up the essay** with one of the strategies for concluding paragraphs in 6J.
- **Summarize** your problem or solution.
- **Make a call to action** or portray the negative consequences of not acting or the clear benefits of adopting your solution.

16D What are some sentence and paragraph guides for proposal/solution essays?

Adapt these guides to your PURPOSE and AUDIENCE.

Sentence and Paragraph Guides

- The best way to solve the problem of ___________ is by ___________.
- To address the problem of ___________, ___________ (we, you, the city council, the board, parking services, etc.) should ___________.
- There are ___________ reasons the current situation is a problem. The first is ___________. The second is ___________. However, the most important is ___________.
- The most effective and practical solution to this problem is ___________. One result of implementing this solution would be ___________. That's because ___________. Another outcome would be ___________. A potential difficulty of this solution is ___________. However, we can overcome that difficulty by ___________.
- Some other possible solutions would be to ___________ or to ___________. The first is problematic because ___________. The second is impractical because _____. My solution is preferable to both alternatives because ___________.
- Failing to take this action will have several negative consequences. First, ___________. Furthermore, ___________.

16E A student's solution essay

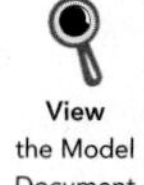

View the Model Document

Cui 1

Yanggu Cui

Professor Leade

Writing 102

10 Dec. 2012

A Proposal to Improve Fan Behavior at Children's Games

Quotations get readers' attention and lead to the introduction.

"Ref, you're an idiot!"

"You're blind as a bat and twice as stupid!"

continued >>

Cui 2

"Get a life, ref!"

"I'll see you after the game!"

Those were just a few yells I heard from the sidelines of a soccer game last Saturday. I wasn't watching a professional match or even a high school one. Instead, it was my eight year old cousin's game in the Arapahoe Recreation League. The referee wasn't a 30 year old professional but, rather, a skinny high school girl who seemed to be fifteen or sixteen. The people yelling weren't drunken guys in sweatshirts or even coaches with red faces and bulging neck veins; instead, they were moms and dads drinking lattes. The league organizers need to bring an end to this kind of abuse, and the best way to do so is by requiring all parents to sign a code of good behavior.

Details create emotional appeals (*pathos*) by giving a picture of the events.

Introductory paragraph sets up the problem. In the thesis sentence at the end of the paragraph, the writer presents a solution.

Parents for decades have proudly watched their sons and daughters play little league softball, baseball, soccer, and other sports. In recent years, these sports have gotten more competitive, with more games, longer seasons, more practices, and greater expectations for winning. One result is that parents have gotten more vocal on the sidelines, not only yelling encouragement for Julio and Jenny but also screaming protests at coaches, the opposing team, and officials. Almost every call against their team is greeted by a loud disbelief, at best, and insults or threats, at worst.

By invoking parents with children, the writer appeals to emotions (*pathos*) and provides context on the issue.

The current level of fan abuse is troubling for at least four reasons. First, it discourages officials, especially younger ones who are just learning the job themselves. No one fears making a wrong call more than someone who is just gaining experience as a referee. If parents make the job so unpleasant

Topic sentence announces four reasons for convincing readers that a problem exists and is a logical appeal (*logos*).

continued >>

Cui 3

that kids making minimum wage stop doing it, the games will come to a halt. Second, it makes what should be a fun recreational experience for all into an ordeal. Rather than paying attention to the game, players and spectators alike get distracted by the drama on the sidelines, even getting nervous that a physical confrontation or fight might occur. Third, it embarrasses the kids themselves. Parents might feel like their kids appreciate and value someone sticking up for them, but the truth of the matter is that most children would rather not have that particular kind of attention.

Each reason receives a brief explanation. Numbering them creates clarity.

The fourth, and most distressing, problem is that fan abuse warps the nature of the game itself. At a time when participating, having fun, and learning new skills should be primary, young players get the clear message that only winning matters, winning at all costs. Rather than assuming that officials and others are trying their best to be impartial and fair, kids are being taught that people are incompetent and malicious. Rather than assuming that sometimes in life we make mistakes that get penalized, but life goes on, kids learn that they are rarely, if ever at fault. Rather than accepting adversity, even if sometimes it's wrong, kids learn to dwell on every hardship. The result is that, instead of learning lessons valuable for a happy life, kids learn to be intolerant and bitter, and they learn it from their parents.

The writer keeps the most important reason for last and devotes an entire paragraph to explaining it in detail.

Writer uses ethical and emotional appeals (*ethos* and *pathos*) by showing the negative influence on children.

It would be nice to assume that merely talking to parents would control the situation, but the situation actually requires a more active solution. The Arapahoe Recreational League should adopt a code of conduct for all parents, in the form of an agreement they must sign. This code should indicate

Writer introduces the solution and provides an explanation using a logical appeal (*logos*).

continued >>

Cui 4

fan behaviors that are approved and encouraged; these would include yelling encouragement or congratulations for all players. The code would also specify behaviors that are banned; these would include taunting or criticizing players, coaches, and officials. Children whose parents refuse to sign would not be allowed to participate.

Granted, merely signing a code of conduct will not prevent all abuse. However, it gives a clear mechanism to end it once it happens. If there's a violation, officials can stop the game, and ask the coach of the team with offending parents to remind them of the code they signed. If extreme behavior continues, the official can stop the game for an extended period, and if it still persists, he or she can declare a forfeit and end the game. This series of events puts responsibility on the parents, who cannot claim they didn't understand the consequences, and it puts a clear end to the abuse.

Writer strengthens her ethical appeal (*ethos*) by recognizing some limitations. She goes on to explain how the solution would be effective.

Other solutions have been proposed in different leagues. The most extreme is to ban spectators from even attending games. While a ban would surely prevent fan abuse, it would unfairly penalize those many parents who are good sports and supportive spectators. Plus, who wants to deprive people from seeing an important part of their children, grandchildren, and friends' childhood? Another solution has been to require spectators to be absolutely silent during games. This solution, while also potentially successful, deprives players and parents alike of the joys of praise and encouragement.

Topic sentence acknowledges other possible solutions and explains their shortcomings.

I urge you, then, to adopt my solution. Having a code of conduct will reduce fan abuse, restore some of the fun to

continued >>

Cui 5

The essay concludes with a call to action that has a logical appeal (*logos*). It shows the benefits of the solution and portrays the consequences of not adopting it.

our games, and keep them in perspective as fun, not battles. Failing to take this action would worsen the attitude that winning is everything and leave children even less prepared for the inevitable disappointments and struggles of life. Ultimately, it might eventually result in empty fields with no one willing to endure threats and insults from spectators who lack the discipline and perspective to behave in ways that their own children deserve.

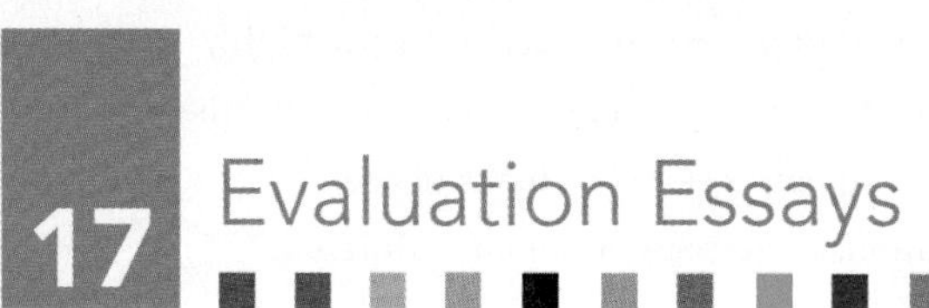

17 Evaluation Essays

Quick Points You will learn to

- ➤ Describe key elements of an evaluation (see 17A).
- ➤ Apply the writing process to an evaluation (see 17B).
- ➤ Adapt frames and guides for an evaluation to your own needs (see 17C).

17A What are evaluation essays?

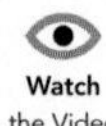
Watch the Video

EVALUATION essays judge the quality of a text, object, individual, or event by providing reasons and support. Here are typical categories of evaluations:

- **Reviews.** Movie, concert, book, theater, television, architecture, restaurant, product, or art reviews are all evaluations. They answer questions such as: Is that play worth seeing? Will certain readers like that book? Is the current season of this television series as good as last year's?

- **Recommendations or performance reviews.** Letters of recommendation and/or reviews of performances evaluate peoples' qualifications for a particular job or how well they've done it.
- **Critical analyses.** A critical analysis judges ideas, recommendations, or proposals. It assesses whether an argument is sound or whether an informative text is accurate or useful. It answers questions such as, "Do the facts support the writer's claims? Is the writer fair and reasonable? Is the recommended action practical and more effective than other actions?"

17A.1 Purpose

Evaluations have mainly an argumentative purpose although they also inform readers about what is being evaluated. (For more about purpose, see 4B.)

17A.2 Audience

Audiences for evaluations can be as small as a single person (such as an employee's annual job evaluation) or as large as the general public who reads a magazine or blog. (For more about audience, see 4C). If your audience is general, the questions below will help you.

- **What will readers already know about your subject?** Are they familiar with the text, object, individual, or event being evaluated? Do you need to explain your subject in detail, or is a brief explanation sufficient?
- **What might readers already believe about your subject?** Most people think fondly of *The Wizard of Oz,* so if you argue that Judy Garland played Dorothy poorly, be aware that readers might disagree with you.
- **What are the circumstances in which your readers will read your evaluation?** For an academic audience, including scholars like your instructor, you need to be scholarly and your TONE relatively formal. You might need research to support your position. On the other hand, for a popular blog, your tone can be more informal, but you still need sound reasons for your position.

17B How do I plan and revise evaluation essays?

Several questions can generate ideas for evaluations. Although we've arranged them here according to types, they can be mixed in the order you find most effective.

Generating ideas for reviews

- What seems to be the main purpose of the author, director, artist, etc.? How well was it achieved? Is that purpose worthwhile?
- Was the plot plausible? Interesting? Original?
- Were characters interesting and effective? In other words, if you infer that viewers are supposed to like, hate, or sympathize with them, can they?
- How well did the setting work, including what it looked like, its lighting, sounds, any music, etc.? (These questions apply to restaurants, galleries, or other settings, too.)
- What other works does this particular one resemble? Does it compare well? Why or why not?

Generating ideas for performance evaluations

- What specific qualities are needed to perform a particular job? Does the individual have those qualities? How can you tell?
- What are examples of the person's main strengths? Main weaknesses?
- How does this person compare with others in similar positions?
- What advice do you have for this person or anyone working with him or her?

Generating ideas for critical analyses

- Is the support the writer gives for his or her claims reasonable? Sufficient?
- Are there missing facts, viewpoints, or interpretations?
- Who would agree and who would disagree with the text? On what basis? How right would people be who disagree?
- If the text proposes an action, would it work? Is it practical? Is it the best one available?

Revising

- Does your THESIS STATEMENT present a clear judgment of the text, object, person, or event you're evaluating?
- Will your readers have a clear understanding of the text, object, person, or event you're summarizing? Have you given enough detail but not too much?
- Do you give and support reasons for your evaluation?

- Do you take into account your audience's knowledge, belief, and expectations?
- If your evaluation is mostly negative, have you tried to acknowledge possible strengths? If your evaluation is mostly positive, have you tried to acknowledge possible critiques?
- Do you need to include a WORKS CITED or REFERENCES page? If so, is it formatted correctly, with proper in-text citations (see Chapters 25–27)?

17C What is a frame for an evaluation essay?

Here is a possible frame for an evaluation essay to adapt to your assignments.

Frame for an Evaluation Essay

Introductory paragraph(s)

- **Capture your readers' interest** in your topic by using one of the strategies for writing effective introductory paragraphs (see 6C).
- **Present your THESIS STATEMENT**, making sure it states your overall evaluation (see 5F).

Background paragraph(s):

- **Clearly explain what you're evaluating**. Give a brief objective overview by providing a brief plot summary if you're evaluating a book, play, movie, etc.; providing a description of an event or object; introducing the person if you're writing a recommendation.

Body paragraphs: Stating evaluations

- **Start each paragraph with a TOPIC SENTENCE** that states a reason that ties in logically to your thesis statement.
- **Support each topic sentence** with examples, evidence, and reasoning (including SUMMARIES or QUOTATIONS, if appropriate).
- **Include as many paragraphs as there are reasons** for your evaluation. If a reason is especially complicated, or if you have extensive examples or explanations, you might divide it into two or more paragraphs.
- **Save your most important evaluation for last**. Building toward your most powerful judgment will leave readers with the best reason for believing you.

(*continued*)

Evaluation Frame (cont.)

Rebuttal or "conceding" paragraph(s): Place either after your evaluating paragraphs, as in this frame; or immediately after your background paragraph(s) above.

- **Present alternative evaluations and refute them**. If it seems practical, state some reasons why others might disagree with your evaluations, and explain why your evaluation is still strong.
- **[optional] Concede some points**. To concede a point means to admit that it's valid. If it seems practical and honest, and you think it will make your readers more receptive to your evaluation, concede a positive point or two (if your overall evaluation is negative) or concede a negative point or two (if you're positive). Still, explain why your overall evaluation is reasonable.

Conclusion

- **Wrap up the essay with an engaging strategy** for concluding paragraphs (see 6J).
- **Summarize your point of view.**
- **Give your readers a recommendation,** such as buy this, don't attend that, hire this person, don't accept this argument, etc.

17D What are some sentence and paragraph guides for evaluations?

Adapt these guides to your PURPOSE and AUDIENCE.

Sentence and Paragraph Guides

- Despite a few redeeming qualities, this ___________ (book, movie, CD, etc.) is ultimately ___________ (disappointing, frustrating, etc.).
- Four qualities are especially strong. First, ___________. Second, ___________. Third, ___________. Most important, however, is ___________.
- Admittedly, ___________ has a couple of strong features. For example, ___________. In addition, ___________. However, even taking these into consideration, the total effect is not enough to overcome an overall weakness. That is primarily because ___________.

Evaluation Guides (cont.)

- The author's strongest point is ___________. The idea is effective because ___________. For example, she ___________, as is clear from the statement that "___________."
- ___________'s most impressive quality is her [or his] ability to ___________. That quality came through most clearly when ___________. Although other employees might have ___________, ___________ instead chose to ___________.

17E A student's evaluation essay

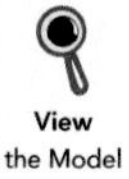

View the Model Document

Pietruszynski 1

Kelly Pietruszynski

Communications 100

Professor Moeller

12 Nov. 2012

The Worthy *Rise of the Planet of the Apes*

In the famous scene at the end of the 1968 movie *The Planet of the Apes*, Charlton Heston rides along a desolate beach until he comes across the top of the Statue of Liberty buried in the sand. At that moment, he and the movie's audience realize that the planet on which he's been stranded, where apes rule humans, is actually Earth in the future. That successful original movie led to sequels and even a remake in 2001, starring Mark Wahlberg. But not until the 2011 film *Rise of the Planet of the Apes* did we get any explanation of how the strange future came to be. The result is a satisfying film well worth seeing.

Opening paragraph stirs interest by giving some background, ending with a thesis sentence that states the evaluation the writer will support.

Rise of the Planet of the Apes is set in contemporary San Francisco. Will Rodman (played by James Franco) is a scientist

continued >>

Pietruszynski 2

who develops a drug meant to grow new brain cells and, as a result, cure diseases like Alzheimer's. Through a series of events, Rodman adopts and raises an ape exposed to that drug. Caesar (the ape) demonstrates human-like intelligence that eventually gets him in trouble, resulting in his being imprisoned with a number of apes, gorillas, and orangutans in a medical testing facility. After being exposed to another drug, the entire colony of apes develops intelligence and escapes, led by Caesar.

The writer summarizes the movie's plot so that readers have a clear context for the writer's arguments.

One impressive quality of this movie is the plot. Admittedly, any attempt to explain how apes become intelligent and humans stupid is finally going to stretch credibility. However, *Rise of the Planet of the Apes* is fairly plausible. Because finding a cure for Alzheimer's and related diseases is such a strong interest in our society, we can easily imagine extensive research and animal testing. To the plot's credit, the ape's intelligence breakthrough isn't sudden and miraculous. Even after Caesar is exposed to the drug, years pass while he lives with Will, allowing him to accumulate human experiences and intelligence. We see conflict development in Caesar between the world of nature and the world of human society, and his mistreatment at the hands of cruel humans, especially a keeper named Dodge explains why the apes eventually turn against humans.

Topic sentence gives one reason for the evaluation. The rest of this paragraph supports the topic sentence.

An appeal to logic as well as ethics (*logos* and *ethos*).

This plot benefits from exceptional camera work and special effects. There are powerfully breathtaking scenes. For example, when Will takes Caesar to play in a redwood forest, the size and scope of the trees as Caesar climbs through them is stunning. When the apes later escape, we see them swarm through the trees on San Francisco streets; or, rather, we see

Topic sentence gives a second reason for the evaluation. Note the transitional connection to the previous paragraph.

continued >>

Pietruszynski 3

the trees shuddering, as the apes are invisible among them, which is a more suggestive effect. The final battle takes place with dramatic fury on Golden Gate Bridge. But some of the best camera work depicts quiet scenes, not energetic ones. In one profound scene, Caesar is alone in the attic. Through a small window, he watches children play on the street far below, and the camera angle and distance creates a powerful sense of isolation and loneliness.

The writer uses an emotional appeal here (*pathos*)

The best special effect is Caesar himself. While the original movie had actors wearing masks and makeup that won an Academy Award in 1969, *Rise of the Planet of the Apes* uses motion capture computer graphics. Andy Serkis (who played Gollum in *Lord of the Rings*) wore multiple computer sensors while acting the role of Caesar. The results were translated by skilled technicians and powerful computers into extraordinarily realistic images. The apes look like real animals, not actors in costumes. Most impressive are the emotions conveyed. At various times, Caesar looks happy, sad, confused, scheming, and so on. The effects alone are worth seeing.

Topic sentence ties back to the previous paragraph and explains one effect in detail.

Writer uses an emotional appeal (*pathos*) to urge readers to see the movie.

The movie's most impressive quality, however, is the way it establishes relationships between its characters. Will lives with his father, played by John Lithgow, who has Alzheimer's, and you can see not only the loving relationship between the two of them, but also Lithgow and Caesar. Indeed, Caesar gets into trouble at one point because he comes to the ailing man's defense. The most important relationship, of course, is between Will and Caesar, which develops fairly convincingly as identical to one between father and son. The relationship is

Topic sentence states the third reason in support of the thesis. Note that the writer saved what she thought was the best reason for last.

continued >>

Writer uses an ethical and emotional appeal (*ethos* and *pathos*).

complete with struggles for autonomy that characterize human families, as children move through adolescence and parents try to find the right combination of discipline and independence. As a result, we identify with and care about Will and Caesar. Instead of just being an action flick, *Rise* has emotional depth.

Transitional sentence moves into some counterarguments.

Topic sentence for this paragraph comes in the middle to connect the opening three sentences to three sentences that acknowledge why some might disagree with the writer's evaluation.

There are silly relationships, too. It's hard to imagine what Will's love interest, an attractive veterinarian played by Frieda Pinto, sees in him. He's so obsessed with his work and his family situation, that I can't see her putting up with him through the several years in which the movie unfolds. This is just one of several negative elements of the film. Critics can accurately point out that the villains in the film are just too extreme, from the evil animal keepers, to an angry neighbor, to the ultimate bad guy, the director of Will's lab who pursues profits at any cost. Also, the final battle scenes clash a little with the rest of the movie. The director seems to trade subtle relationships and characterizations for chases and explosions.

Concluding paragraph uses a logical appeal (*logos*) by saying this isn't a perfect movie, summarizes the writer's positive review, and ends on a strong recommendation.

Rise of the Planet of the Apes, then, is hardly a perfect movie. However, it is an entertaining and thoughtful one. It provides a plausible origin story for the entire series of films, delivering a solid plot, great special effects, and engaging relationships. As with any science fiction, viewers have to go along with certain premises. Because this movie makes you willing to do so, it's well worth seeing.

PART

3

Source-Based Writing

18 Quoting, Paraphrasing, and Summarizing

Quick Points You will learn to

- Use quotations effectively (see 18B).
- Integrate sources using paraphrasing and summarizing (see 18C–18D).
- Synthesize two or more sources (see 18F–18L).

18A How can I integrate sources into my writing?

You integrate sources into your writing when you combine information or ideas from other writers with your own. To integrate sources well, you use three techniques: QUOTATION (see 18B), PARAPHRASE (see 18C), and SUMMARY (see 18D). The techniques are essential for SYNTHESIZING sources (see 18F to 18L). Mastering them allows you to write smooth, effective papers that avoid PLAGIARISM: stealing or representing someone else's words or ideas as your own (see Chapter 19).

18B How can I use quotations effectively?

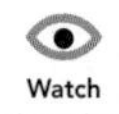

A **quotation** is the exact words of a source enclosed in quotation marks (see Chapter 46). Well-chosen quotations can lend a note of authority and enliven a document with someone else's voice.

Avoid adding too many quotations, however. If more than a quarter of your paper consists of quotations, you make readers suspect that you haven't bothered to develop your own thinking. Quick Box 18.1 provides guidelines for using quotations. All examples are in MLA documentation style.

18B.1 Making quotations fit smoothly with your sentences

When you use quotations, the greatest risk you take is that you'll end up with incoherent, choppy sentences. You can avoid this problem by making the words you quote fit smoothly with three aspects of your writing: grammar, style, and logic. Here are some examples of sentences that don't mesh well with quotations, followed by a revised version.

Quick Box 18.1

Guidelines for using quotations

- Use quotations from authorities on your subject to support or refute what you've written.
- Never use a quotation to present your THESIS STATEMENT or a TOPIC SENTENCE.
- Choose a quotation only for the following reasons.

  Its language is particularly appropriate or distinctive.

  Its idea is particularly hard to paraphrase accurately.

  Its authority comes from a source that is especially important for support.

  Its words are open to interpretation.
- Never allow quotations to make up a quarter or more of your paper. Instead, rely on PARAPHRASE (see 18C) and SUMMARY (see 18D).
- Quote accurately. Always check a quotation against the original source—and then recheck it.
- Integrate quotations smoothly into your writing (see 18B.1–18B.4).
- Document quotations carefully.
- Avoid plagiarism (see Chapter 19).

SOURCE

Turkle, Sherry. *Alone Together: Why We Expect More from Technology and Less from Each Other*. New York: Basic Books, 2011. Print.

ORIGINAL (TURKLE'S EXACT WORDS)

Digital connections and the sociable robot may offer the illusion of companionship without the demands of friendship. Our networked life allows us to hide from each other, even as we are tethered to each other. [from page 1]

GRAMMAR PROBLEM

Turkle explains how relying on network communication "illusion of companionship without the demands of friendship" (1).

STYLE PROBLEM

Turkle explains that digital connections and the lives of robots "offer the illusion of companionship without the demands of friendship" (1).

LOGIC PROBLEM

Turkle explains networked connections "without the demands of friendship" (1).

ACCEPTABLE SMOOTH USE OF QUOTATION

Turkle explains that networked connections "may offer the illusion of companionship without the demands of friendship" (1).

18B.2 Using brackets to add words

One way to fit a quotation smoothly into your writing is to add a word or very brief phrase to the quotation by placing it in brackets—[ ]—so that it fits seamlessly with the rest of your sentence.

ORIGINAL (TURKLE'S EXACT WORDS)

If we divest ourselves of such things, we risk being coarsened, reduced. [from page 292]

QUOTATION WITH EXPLANATORY BRACKETS

"If we divest ourselves of such things [as caring for the sick], we risk being coarsened, reduced" (Turkle 292).

18B.3 Using ellipses to delete words

Another way to fit a quotation smoothly into your sentence is to use ellipses. Delete the part of the quotation that is causing the problem, and mark the omission by using ELLIPSIS POINTS. When you use ellipses to delete troublesome words, make sure that the remaining words accurately reflect the source's meaning and that your sentence still flows smoothly.

ORIGINAL (TURKLE'S EXACT WORDS)

The idea of addiction, with its one solution that we know we won't take, makes us feel hopeless. [from page 294]

QUOTATION USING ELLIPSIS

Turkle notes that "the idea of addiction . . . makes us feel hopeless" (294).

18B.4 Integrating author names, source titles, and other information

A huge complaint instructors have about student papers is that quotations sometimes are simply stuck in, for no apparent reason. Without context-setting information, the reader can't tell exactly why the writer included a particular quotation. Also, always be sure your readers can tell who said each group of quoted words in your writing.

SOURCE

Wright, Karen. "Times of Our Lives." *Scientific American* Sept. 2002: 58-66. Print.

ORIGINAL (WRIGHT'S EXACT WORDS)

In human bodies, biological clocks keep track of seconds, minutes, days, months and years. [from page 66]

PROBLEM: DISCONNECTED QUOTATION

The human body has many subconscious processes. People don't have to make their hearts beat or remind themselves to breathe. "In human bodies, biological clocks keep track of seconds, minutes, days, months and years" (Wright 66).

ACCEPTABLY CONNECTED QUOTATION

The human body has many subconscious processes. People don't have to make their hearts beat or remind themselves to breathe. However, other processes are less obvious and perhaps more surprising. Karen Wright observes, for example, "In human bodies, biological clocks keep track of seconds, minutes, days, months and years" (66).

Quick Box 18.2 lists other strategies for working quotations smoothly into your paper by integrating the author's name, the source title, or other information into your writing.

Quick Box 18.2

Strategies for smoothly fitting quotations into your sentences

- Mention in your sentence (before or after the quotation) the name of the author you're quoting.
- Mention in your sentence the title of the work you're quoting from.
- If the author of a quotation is a noteworthy figure, mention the author's credentials.
- Add your own introductory analysis to the quotation.
- Combine any of the previous four strategies.

Applying strategies from Quick Box 18.2, here are some examples, using a quotation from Karen Wright.

AUTHOR'S NAME

Karen Wright explains that "in human bodies, biological clocks keep track of seconds, minutes, days, months and years" (66).

AUTHOR'S NAME AND SOURCE TITLE

Karen Wright explains in "Times of Our Lives" that "in human bodies, biological clocks keep track of seconds, minutes, days, months and years" (66).

AUTHOR'S NAME AND CREDENTIALS

Karen Wright, an award-winning science journalist, explains that "in human bodies, biological clocks keep track of seconds, minutes, days, months and years" (66).

AUTHOR'S NAME WITH STUDENT'S INTRODUCTORY ANALYSIS

Karen Wright reviews evidence of surprising subconscious processes, explaining that "in human bodies, biological clocks keep track of seconds, minutes, days, months and years" (66).

● **EXERCISE 18-1** Working individually or with a group, read the following original material, from page 295 of *Deep Water: The Gulf Oil Disaster and the Future of Offshore Drilling*, published in 2011 by the National Commission on the BP Deepwater Horizon Oil Spill and Offshore Drilling. Then, read items 1 through 4 and explain why each is an incorrect use of a quotation. Next, revise each numbered sentence so that it correctly uses a quotation. End each quotation with this MLA-STYLE parenthetical reference: (National 295).

> Yet growing demand for oil around the world, particularly in the huge and rapidly developing economies of Asia, ensures heightened competition for supplies, putting upward pressure on oil prices. That poses a long-term challenge for the United States, which is not and cannot be self-sufficient in oil supply.

UNACCEPTABLE USES OF QUOTATIONS

1. Demand for oil is increasing globally. "That poses a long-term challenge for the United States, which is not and cannot be self-sufficient in oil supply" (National 295).
2. One obvious cause is that "the huge economies of Asia are putting upward pressure on prices" (National 295).

3. A difficult situation, "that poses a long-term challenge for the United States" (National 295).
4. In the 1990s, "that poses a long-term challenge for the United States" (National 295). ●

● **EXERCISE 18-2** Integrate each of the following quotations into a sentence using one of the strategies in Quick Box 18.2. Use at least two different strategies as you complete the exercise; you may use only part of the quotation if doing so fits your strategy. The author of all the quotations is Thomas Larson. Larson is a journalist who has lectured across America about the classical music composer Samuel Barber. The citation for the source is

Larson, Thomas. *The Saddest Music Ever Written: The Story of Samuel Barber's* Adagio for Strings. New York, Pegasus, 2010. Print.

EXAMPLE

Original: "Sad music must be seductive enough to induce the state of sorrow" (226).

Integrated quotation 1: As Thomas Larson points out, "Sad music must be seductive enough to induce the state of sorrow" (226).

Integrated quotation 2: An expert on the composer Samuel Barber notes that "Sad music must be seductive enough to induce the state of sorrow" (Larson 226).

1. "'Gloomy Sunday,' written in 1933 and recorded by Billie Holiday in 1941, is quite sad" (218).
2. "The Internet Movie Database lists thirty films and TV shows in which the *Adagio* has appeared" (204).
3. "Higher art has a higher calling" (227).
4. "Like the book before and the TV and computer after it, the radio . . . changed the way our grandparents experienced the world" (22).
5. "The *Adagio* is a sound shrine to music's power to evoke emotion" (7). ●

18C How can I write good paraphrases?

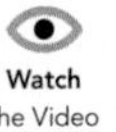
Watch the Video

A **paraphrase** precisely restates in your own words the written or spoken words of someone else. Paraphrase only passages that carry ideas you need to reproduce in detail to explain a point or support an argument. Avoid trying to paraphrase more than a paragraph or two; for longer passages, use summary (see 18D). Quick Box 18.3 (page 210) offers advice for paraphrasing.

Here is an example of an unacceptable paraphrase and an acceptable one. The first paraphrase is unacceptable because the highlighted words have been plagiarized. The second paraphrase is acceptable. It captures the meaning of the original in the student's own words.

Quick Box 18.3

Guidelines for writing paraphrases

- Never use a paraphrase to present your THESIS STATEMENT or a TOPIC SENTENCE.
- Say what the source says, but no more.
- Reproduce the source's sequence of ideas and emphases.
- Use your own words, phrasing, and sentence structure to restate the material. If some technical words in the original have only awkward synonyms, quote the original words—but do so sparingly.
- Read your sentences over to make sure they don't distort the source's meaning.
- Expect your material to be as long as the original or even slightly longer.
- Integrate your paraphrase into your writing so that it fits smoothly.
- Avoid PLAGIARISM (see Chapter 19).
- Document your paraphrase carefully.

SOURCE

Hulbert, Ann. "Post-Teenage Wasteland?" *New York Times Magazine* 9 Oct. 2005: 11–12. Print.

ORIGINAL (HULBERT'S EXACT WORDS)

[T]he available data suggest that the road to maturity hasn't become as drastically different as people think—or as drawn out, either. It's true that the median age of marriage rose to 25 for women and almost 27 for men in 2000, from 20 and 23, respectively, in 1960. Yet those midcentury figures were record lows (earnestly analyzed in their time). Moreover, Americans of all ages have ceased to view starting a family as the major benchmark of grown-up status. When asked to rank the importance of traditional milestones in defining the arrival of adulthood, poll respondents place completing school, finding full-time employment, achieving financial independence and being able to support a family far above actually wedding a spouse or having kids. The new perspective isn't merely an immature swerve into selfishness; postponing those last two steps is good for the future of the whole family. [from page 11]

UNACCEPTABLE PARAPHRASE (HIGHLIGHTED WORDS ARE PLAGIARIZED)

Data suggest that the road to maturity hasn't changed as much as people think. True, the median age of marriage was 25 for women and 27 for men in 2000, up from 20 and 23 in 1960. Yet those 1960 figures were record lows. Furthermore, Americans have stopped regarding beginning a family as the signpost of grown-up status. When they were asked to rank the importance of traditional benchmarks for deciding the arrival of adulthood, people rated graduating from school, finding a full-time job, gaining financial status, and being a breadwinner far above marrying or having kids. This new belief isn't merely immature selfishness; delaying those last two steps is good for the future of the whole family (Hulbert 11).

ACCEPTABLE PARAPHRASE

According to Ann Hulbert, statistics show that people are wrong when they believe our society is delaying maturity. She acknowledges that between 1960 and 2000, the median age at which women married rose from 20 to 25 (for men it went from 23 to 27), but points out that the early figures were extreme lows. Hulbert finds that Americans no longer equate adulthood with starting a family. Polls show that people rank several other "milestones" above marriage and children as signaling adulthood. These include finishing school, securing a full-time job, and earning enough to be independent and to support a family. Hulbert concludes that we should regard postponing marriage and children not as being selfish or immature but as investing in the family's future (11).

● **EXERCISE 18-3** Working individually or with your peer-response group, read the original material given here, a paragraph from page 34 of *What Technology Wants* by Kevin Kelly (New York: Viking, 2010. Print). Then, read the unacceptable paraphrase, and point out each example of plagiarism. Finally, write your own paraphrase, starting it with a phrase naming Kelly and ending it with this parenthetical reference: (34).

ORIGINAL (KELLY'S EXACT WORDS)

Most hunter-gatherers clustered into family clans that averaged about 25 related people. Clans would gather in larger tribes of several hundred at seasonal feasts or camping groups. One function of the tribes was to keep genes moving through intermarriage. Population was spread thinly. The average density of a tribe was less than .01 person per square kilometer in cooler climes.

The 200 to 300 folk in your greater tribe would be the total number of people you'd meet in your lifetime. (34)

UNACCEPTABLE PARAPHRASE

Kevin Kelly says that most hunter-gatherers lived in groups that averaged about 25 related people. Clans would gather tribes of several hundred at seasonal feasts or gatherings. The larger tribes allowed intermarriage, which meant more diversity in the gene pool. Population was spread thinly. Fewer than .01 person lived per square kilometer in cooler climates. The 200 to 300 people in your tribe would be the complete number of individuals you'd meet in your lifetime (34). ●

18D How can I summarize?

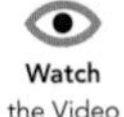
Watch the Video

A **summary** differs from a paraphrase (see 18C) in an important way: Whereas a paraphrase restates the original material in its entirety, a summary states only the main points of the original source in a much briefer fashion. A summary doesn't include supporting evidence or details. As a result, a summary is much shorter than a paraphrase. Summarizing is the technique you'll probably use most frequently to integrate sources. Quick Box 18.4 explains how to summarize effectively.

Here's an example of an unacceptable summary and an acceptable one.

SOURCE

Tanenbaum, Leora. *Catfight: Women and Competition*. New York: Seven Stories, 2002. Print.

ORIGINAL (TANENBAUM'S EXACT WORDS)

Until recently, most Americans disapproved of cosmetic surgery, but today the stigma is disappearing. Average Americans are lining up for procedures—two-thirds of patients report family incomes of less than $50,000 a year—and many of them return for more. Younger women undergo "maintenance" surgeries in a futile attempt to halt time. The latest fad is Botox, a purified and diluted form of botulinum toxin that is injected between the eyebrows to eliminate frown lines. Although the procedure costs between $300 and $1000 and must be repeated every few months, roughly 850,000 patients have had it performed on them. That number will undoubtedly shoot up now that the FDA has approved Botox for cosmetic use. Even teenagers are making appointments with plastic surgeons. More than 14,000 adolescents had plastic

Quick Box 18.4

Guidelines for summarizing

- Identify the main points, and take care not to alter the meaning of the original source.
- Don't be tempted to include your opinions; they don't belong in a summary.
- Never use a summary to present your THESIS STATEMENT or a TOPIC SENTENCE.
- Keep your summary as short as possible to accomplish your purpose.
- Integrate summarized material smoothly into your writing.
- Use your own words. If you need to use key terms or phrases from the source, include them in quotation marks, but otherwise put everything into your own words.
- Document the original source accurately.
- Avoid PLAGIARISM (see Chapter 19).

surgery in 1996, and many of them are choosing controversial procedures such as breast implants, liposuction, and tummy tucks, rather than the rhinoplasties of previous generations. [from pages 117–118]

UNACCEPTABLE SUMMARY (HIGHLIGHTED WORDS ARE PLAGIARIZED)

Average Americans are lining up for surgical procedures. The latest fad is Botox, a toxin injected to eliminate frown lines. This is an insanely foolish waste of money. Even teenagers are making appointments with plastic surgeons, many of them for controversial procedures such as breast implants, liposuction, and tummy tucks (Tanenbaum 117–18).

ACCEPTABLE SUMMARY

Tanenbaum explains that plastic surgery is becoming widely acceptable, even for Americans with modest incomes and for younger women. Most popular is injecting the toxin Botox to smooth wrinkles. She notes that thousands of adolescents are even requesting controversial surgeries (117–18).

The unacceptable summary has several major problems: It doesn't isolate the main point. It plagiarizes by taking much of its language directly from the source and it includes the writer's interpretation. The acceptable summary concisely isolates the main point, puts the source into the writer's own words, calls attention to the author by including her name in the summary, and remains objective throughout.

DEGREES OF SUMMARY

The degree to which your summary compresses the original source depends on your situation and assignment. For example, you can summarize an entire 500-page book in a single sentence, in a single page, or in five or six pages. Following are two different levels of summary based on the same source.

SOURCE

[Note: We included the text of this article in section 3D, on pages 21–23]

Schwartz, Barry. "The Tyranny of Choice." *Chronicle of Higher Education.* Chronicle of Higher Education, 23 Jan. 2004. Web. 3 Apr. 2011.

SUMMARY IN A SINGLE SENTENCE

Research finds that people with large numbers of choices are actually less happy than people with fewer choices (Schwartz).

SUMMARY IN 50 TO 100 WORDS

Research finds that people with large numbers of choices are actually less happy than people with fewer choices. Although the amount of wealth and number of choices have increased during the past thirty years, fewer Americans report themselves as being happy, and depression, suicide, and mental health problems have increased. While some choice is good, having too many choices hinders decision making, especially among "maximizers," who try to make the best possible choices. Research in shopping, education, and medical settings shows that even when people eventually decide, they experience regret, worrying that the options they didn't choose might have been better (Schwartz).

Notice that the longer summary begins with the same sentence as the short one; leading a summary with the reading's main idea is effective. One decision to make in summary writing is whether to refer to the author or to leave him or her out, as in the earlier examples. Check if your instructor has a preference. The previous example could be rewritten as follows:

SUMMARY THAT INCLUDES THE AUTHOR'S NAME

In "The Tyranny of Research," Barry Schwartz explains that people with large numbers of choices are actually less happy than people with fewer choices. Although the amount of wealth and number of choices have increased during the past thirty years, Schwartz notes that fewer Americans report themselves as being happy, and depression, suicide, and mental health problems have increased.

Instructors sometimes assign a paper that consists entirely of writing a summary. We discuss that kind of assignment in section 20B.

● **EXERCISE 18-4** Working individually or with your peer-response group, read the following original material from pages 23–24 of *Quiet: The Power of Introverts in a World that Can't Stop Talking* by Susan Cain (New York: Crown, 2012. Print). Then, read the unacceptable summary. Point out each example of plagiarism. Finally, write your own summary, starting it with a phrase mentioning Cain and ending it with this parenthetical reference: (4).

ORIGINAL (CAIN'S EXACT WORDS)

It makes sense that so many introverts hide from themselves. We live with a value system that I call the Extrovert Ideal—the omnipresent belief that the ideal self is gregarious, alpha, and comfortable in the spotlight. The archetypal extrovert prefers action to contemplation, risk-taking to heed-taking, certainty to doubt. He favors quick decisions, even at the risk of being wrong. She works well in teams and socializes in groups. We like to think that we value individuality, but all too often we admire one *type* of individual—the kind who's comfortable "putting himself out there." [from page 4]

UNACCEPTABLE, PLAGIARIZED SUMMARY

The Extrovert Ideal is the omnipresent belief that the ideal self is gregarious, favoring action, risks, and decisions. Extroverts work well in teams and socialize in groups. People too often admire one *type* of person despite thinking they value individuality. (4) ●

18E Which verbs can help me weave source material into my sentences?

Use the verbs in Quick Box 18.5 appropriately according to their meanings in your sentences.

Quick Box 18.5

Useful verbs for integrating quotations, paraphrases, and summaries

acknowledges	contrasts	illustrates	recommends
agrees	declares	implies	refutes
analyzes	demonstrates	indicates	rejects
argues	denies	insists	remarks
asserts	describes	introduces	reports
begins	develops	maintains	reveals
believes	discusses	means	says
claims	distinguishes	notes	shows
comments	between	notices	specifies
compares	among	observes	speculates
complains	emphasizes	offers	states
concedes	establishes	points out	suggests
concludes	explains	prepares	supports
confirms	expresses	promises	supposes
considers	finds	proves	wishes
contends	focuses on	questions	writes
contradicts	grants	recognizes	

18F What is synthesizing sources?

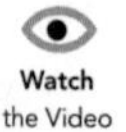
Watch the Video

When you SYNTHESIZE sources, you connect them to one another and to your own thinking, in an original paper. The resulting text needs to be more than just a succession of summaries. Your CRITICAL THINKING (see Chapter 3) skills help you synthesize, as do QUOTING, SUMMARIZING, and PARAPHRASING (see 18B–18D).

The following example shows how student Devon Petersen synthesized two sources. Read source 1 and source 2 to familiarize yourself with the information he read.

SOURCE 1

Shishmaref is melting into the ocean. Over the past 30 years, the Inupiaq Eskimo village, perched on a slender barrier island 625 miles north of Anchorage, has lost 100 ft. to 300 ft. of coastline—half of it since 1997. As Alaska's climate warms, the permafrost beneath the beaches is thawing and the sea ice is thinning, leaving its 600 residents increasingly vulnerable to violent storms. One house has collapsed, and 18 others had to be moved to higher ground, along with the town's bulk-fuel tanks.

—Margot Roosevelt, "Vanishing Alaska"

SOURCE 2

Since 2000 more than 6.5 million acres have perished in the U.S., turning forests into meadows in almost a dozen states. The culprit: the pine beetle, a fingernail-size bug that's become more voracious as the planet warms. Once a balanced part of forest life, the tree-eating insect now usually survives the winter, starts feeding earlier in the spring, and continues to plunder late into the fall.

—Jim Robbins, "Global Warming Kills Forests in Colorado"

Now read Devon's synthesis. Notice that he used summary (see 18B) and paraphrase (see 18C). Also look at how the first sentence in his synthesis weaves the sources together with a new concept.

EXAMPLE OF A SYNTHESIS OF TWO SOURCES

Global warming is affecting both the natural and artificial worlds. Rising temperatures have allowed pine beetles to survive winters and thrive, killing over 6.5 millions of forests (Robbins 8). Climate change has also altered life for residents of Arctic regions. For example, eighteen families in Shishmaref, Alaska, had to move their houses away from the coast because the permafrost under the beaches had thawed (Roosevelt 68).

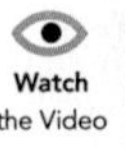

—Devon Petersen, student

In his synthesis, Devon also used in-text citations (in MLA STYLE). In the Works Cited list at the end of his paper, Devon listed full source information for both sources. To learn how to document your sources, see Chapters 25 through 27.

SOURCES LISTED ON DEVON'S WORKS CITED PAGE

Robbins, Jim. "Global Warming Kills Forests in Colorado." *Newsweek* 19 Apr. 2010: 8. Print.

Roosevelt, Margot. "Vanishing Alaska." *Time* 4 Oct. 2004: 68–70. Print.

● **EXERCISE 18-5** Write a one-paragraph synthesis of the passage by Barry Schwartz published in section 3D, pages 21–23, and the following opening to a short article by Ronni Sandroff, editor of *Consumer Reports on Health:*

Last time I dropped by my pharmacy in search of a decongestant, I was stopped cold by the wall-sized display of remedies. The brands I had used in the past had multiplied into extended families of products. Yes, I saw *Contac, Excedrin, Tylenol,* and *Vicks,* but each brand came in multiple versions. Products for severe colds, coughs and colds, and headache and flu abounded, and there were further choices: gels, tablets, capsules, extended release, extra strength. I was eager to just grab a product and go, but to find the right one I had to dig out my reading glasses and examine the fine print.

—Ronni Sandroff, "Too Many Choices" ●

18G What are possible relationships between sources?

Knowing five relationships between sources can help you go beyond simply listing or summarizing your sources. Those relationships are

- **Different Subtopic:** Sources are on same broad subject but about different subtopics.
- **Agreement:** Two sources make the same basic point, though perhaps in different words.
- **Part Agreement:** Two sources mostly agree but differ a little bit.
- **Disagreement:** Two sources disagree.
- **General and Specific:** One source offers specific information that either supports or contradicts a more general point in a second source.

In the next five sections of this chapter, we explain each relationship. We present quotations from two different readings on a common topic, and we follow them with CONTENT NOTES (21P) that a student took on each reading. Next, we suggest a sentence or paragraph guide that shows how you might synthesize the readings. Finally, we give an example of a paragraph that shows this synthesis.

18H What can I do when sources are about different subtopics?

You will likely find sources that present different subtopics of the same broad subject. For example, as you research career options, one source might discuss salaries, another might discuss workplace environments, and a third might discuss expectations for job openings. When student Matthew Yan was researching how the Internet has affected the way we get information (you'll see part of his paper in Chapter 24), among the sources he found were these.

Source A	Source B
"While new technology eases connections between people, it also, paradoxically, facilitates a closeted view of the world, keeping us coiled tightly with those who share our ideas. In a world that lacks real gatekeepers and authority figures . . . conspiracy theories, myths, and outright lies may get the better of many of us." (17–18) Manjoo, Farhad. *True Enough: Learning to Live in a Post-Fact Society*. Hoboken, NJ: Wiley. 2008. Print.	"CNN used to be a twenty-four-hour news outlet shown only on TV. The *New York Times* and the *Wall Street Journal* were simply newspapers. But on the Internet today, they are surprisingly similar. . . . Online, the lines between television and newspapers have blurred—and soon the same will be said about books, movies, TV shows, and more." (14) Bilton, Nick. *I Live in the Future & Here's How It Works*. New York: Crown Business, 2010. Print.
Content Note	**Content Note**
Manjoo 17–18 —although technology can connect us to others, it can also allow us to communicate only with people that agree with us; we might be susceptible to lies [paraphrase]	Bilton 14 —TV network and newspaper sites have become similar on the Internet. Examples: CNN and *NY Times*, *WSJ* [summary]

Following each source, you can see the content note that Matthew wrote. Notice how he included the kind of note he took in brackets (see 47C).

One possible sentence/paragraph guide for sources on different subtopics

There are (one, two, or however many) important considerations for (aspects of, reasons for, etc.) __________. One is ______ [from Source A] __________. A second is ______ [from Source B] ________.

EXAMPLE

There are two important developments in the way we receive news online. One is that, even though it is easier to connect to information, we tend to seek people with whom we already agree (Manjoo 17–18). A second, as Nick Bilton notes, is that distinctions between types of news sources on the Internet are disappearing (14).

18l What can I do when sources agree?

Sources agree when they present similar information or make the same point. Of course, if sources are truly repetitious, you might use only one. Sometimes, however, including multiple similar sources strengthens your point. Here is an example.

Source A	Source B
"Our study confirmed the well-known gender gap in gaming, verifying that this overall trend also occurs among college students. Seventy percent of male undergraduates had played a digital game the week of the survey, compared to only one quarter of the females. The majority of women fell in the category of non-gamers, those who had not played a game in over 6 months, or never." (Winn 10) Winn, Jillian, and Carrie Heeter. "Gaming, Gender, and Time: Who Makes Time to Play?" *Sex Roles* 61 (2009): 1–13. Web. 9 May 2011.	"Women proportionally were more likely than men to only play an hour or less per week. . . . Twenty-one percent of the women and 68% of the men played two or more hours per week." (Ogletree 539) Ogletree, Shirley Matile, and Ryan Drake. "College Students' Video Game Participation and Perceptions: Gender Differences and Implications." *Sex Roles* 56 (2007): 537–42. Web. 9 May 2011.
Content Notes	**Content Notes**
Winn 10 —70% of male students played video games; 25% of female [summary]	Ogletree —68% of men and 21% of women played 2 or more hour per week [summary]

One possible sentence/paragraph guide for synthesizing sources that agree

A and B reach the same conclusion (provide similar information, argue the same point, reach the same conclusion etc.) about ____________. A explains that ____________. B found that ____________.

EXAMPLE

Researchers Winn and Heeter and researchers Ogletree and Drake reached the same conclusion that men play video games more extensively than women. Winn and Heeter found that 70% of male students but only 25% of females regularly play games (10). In a study of how many hour per week students play, Ogletree and Drake learned that 68% of men and only 21% of women play two or more hours per week (539).

A REVISION (TO MAKE THIS MORE EFFECTIVE)

Two studies show that men play video games more extensively than women. Winn and Heeter found that 70% of male students but only 25% of females regularly play games (10). In a study of how many hour per week students play, Ogletree learned that 68% of men and only 21% of women play two or more hours per week (539).

18J What can I do when sources partly agree?

Often sources generally agree with each other but cite different evidence or emphasize slightly different conclusions. Here is an example.

Source A	Source B
"[M]ore males reportedly developed leadership skills as a result of playing video games as opposed to females. More males also reported that playing video games helped them develop skills that will help them in the workplace, such as the ability to work as a team member, to collaborate with others and the ability to provide directions to others." (Thirunarayanan, 324) Thirunarayanan, M. O., Manuel Vilchez, Liala Abreu, Cyntianna Ledesma, and Sandra Lopez. "A Survey of Video Game Players in a Public, Urban Research University." *Educational Media International* 47.4 (2009): 311–27. Web. 9 May 2011.	"Games make it easy to build stronger social bonds with our friends and family. Studies show that we like and trust someone better after we play a game with them—even if they beat us. And we're more likely to help someone in real life after we've helped them in an online game." (McGonigal) McGonigal, Jane. "Be a Gamer, Save the World." *Wall Street Journal.* Dow Jones, 22 Jan. 2011. Web. 9 May 2011.
Content Note	**Content Note**
Thirunarayanan, 324 —more men said they learn leadership and team member skills than women said they did [summary]	McGonigal —games build social connections like trust and willingness to help others [summary]

One possible sentence or paragraph guide to use when sources partly agree

Scholars generally agree (conclude, share the opinion, or demonstrate, etc.) that ____________. However, a difference between them is ________. A emphasizes (asserts, believes, etc.) _________. B, on the other hand, emphasizes ______.

EXAMPLE

Scholars generally agree that playing video games can have some positive social effects. However, they differ as to who benefits most. Jane McGonigal asserts that games build social connections such as trust and the willingness to help others, suggesting this is true for all players. Thirunarayanan et al., on the other hand, found that men believe they learn leadership and team member skills more than women say they do (324).

18K What can I do when sources disagree?

Because people can disagree on everything from whether certain laws should be passed to whether certain movies are any good, it's no surprise that sources can disagree, too. Here is an example.

Source A	Source B
"Imagine that everything stays 99 percent the same, that people continue to consume 99 percent of the television they used to, but 1 percent of that time gets carved out for producing and sharing. The connected population still watches well over a trillion hours of TV a year; 1 percent of that is more than one hundred Wikipedias' worth of participation per year." (Shirky 23)	"With hundreds of thousands of visitors a day, Wikipedia has become the third most visited site for information and current events; a more trusted source for news than the CNN or BBC Web sites, even though Wikipedia has no reporters, no editorial staff, and no experience in news-gathering. It's the blind leading the blind—infinite monkeys providing infinite information for infinite readers, perpetuating the cycle of misinformation and ignorance." (Keen 4)
Shirky, Clay. *Cognitive Surplus, Creativity and Generosity in a Connected Age*. New York: Penguin, 2010. Print.	Keen, Andrew. *The Cult of the Amateur*. New York: Doubleday, 2007. Print.

Content Note	Content Note
Shirky 23 —If people used even 1% of time they spend watching TV instead to produce content for the Web they'd create "one hundred Wikipedia's worth" each year [paraphrase and quotation]	Keen 4 —Wikipedia used more for information and current events than CNN or the BBC —no professionals writing for W. —writers are "infinite monkeys" who create "misinformation and ignorance" [summary and quotation]

One possible sentence/paragraph guide to use for sources that disagree

There are two different perspectives (positions, interpretations, or opinions, etc.) about __________. A says __________________. B, on the other hand, says _________________.

However, your writing will be stronger if you go a step further and use critical thinking to understand the nature of the disagreement. For example:

- Writers might disagree because they use different facts or information (or no information at all!).
- Writers might disagree when they use the same information but interpret it differently.
- Writers might operate with different assumptions or perspectives.

A stronger sentence/paragraph guide for sources that disagree

There are two different perspectives (positions, interpretations, or opinions, etc.) about __________. A says __________________. B, on the other hand, says _________________. They disagree mainly because they cite different facts (interpret information differently, operate with different assumptions). A points to ____________, while B ______________. On this point, B's [or A's] perspective is more convincing because __________.

EXAMPLE

There are two different opinions about Wikipedia. Clay Shirky is enthusiastic and notes that if people diverted just 1% of their TV watching time to writing for the Web, they could generate "one hundred Wikipedia's worth" of content each year (23). Andrew Keen, on the other hand, sees Wikipedia writers as "infinite monkeys" who only spread "misinformation and ignorance" (4). They disagree mainly because they have different assumptions about the quality of Wikipedia entries. Shirky believes it is generally fine, while Keen sees almost nothing of value.

REVISED VERSION, WITH MORE EFFECTIVE WORDING

Some writers find Wikipedia a reason for celebration, while others declare it a cause for despair. Clay Shirky hopes people will divert just 1% of their TV watching time to writing for the Web, which could generate "one hundred Wikipedia's worth" of content each year (23). That possibility would trouble Andrew Keen, who characterizes those writers as "infinite monkeys" who only spread "misinformation and ignorance" (4). Shirky and Keen assume quite different things about quality of knowledge on Wikipedia. Keen has considerably less faith in the ability of people to write accurate information.

18L What can I do when one source is more specific than the other one?

1. **When a specific source supports a more general idea in another source.** Sometimes a source provides examples, illustrations, or evidence that support a more general point in another. Here is an example:

Source A	Source B
"Old media is facing extinction." (Keen 9) Keen, Andrew. *The Cult of the Amateur*. New York: Doubleday, 2007. Print.	"In 2008, paid newspaper circulation in the United States fell to 49.1 million, the lowest number since the late 1960s and well below the peak of 60 million reached in the 1990s, when the internet was just starting to come into its own." (Bilton 6) Bilton, Nick. *I Live in the Future & Here's How It Works*. New York: Crown Business, 2010. Print.
Content Note	**Content Note**
Keen 9 "Old media is facing extinction" [quotation]	Bilton 6 —newspaper circulation was 60 million in the 1990s, 49.1 million in 2008 [summary]

Two useful sentence/paragraph guides when a specific source supports a general one

A observes (claims, argues, concludes, etc.) that ______________. B provides an example (a set of data, some information, etc.) to support this observation. B states that _________.

or

According to B, _______________. This illustrates A's concept (point, claim, conclusion) that ________.

EXAMPLE

According to Nick Bilton, newspaper circulation declined over ten million between the 1990s and 2008, from 60 million to 49.1 million subscribers (6). His figures illustrate Andrew Keen's observation that "Old media is facing extinction" (9).

2. **When a specific source contradicts a more general idea in another source.** As we've noted, sources can disagree with each other at the level of ideas or claims. Sometimes, however, specific information in one source can contradict a more general point made in another. This can happen when writers make a claim but offer no proof or when they offer partial or different evidence. Here's an example:

Source A	Source B
"But college students are, in fact, getting lazier. 'Aggregate time spent studying by full-time college students declined from about 24 hours per week in 1961 to about 14 hours per week in 2004,' Babcock writes, citing his own research." (de Vise)	"Nationally, approximately 80 percent of community college students work, and they work an average of 32 hours per week. Research indicates that working a few hours each week is actually beneficial to students' persistence and success, provided that they are in school full time and attending consistently. However, to succeed academically, experts suggest working no more than 15–20 hours per week." (Zomer 2)
de Vise, Daniel. "Grade Inflation is Making Students Lazier." *washingtonpost.com/college-inc.* Washington Post, 22 July 2010. Web. 9 May 2011.	Zomer, Saffron. *Working Too Hard to Make the Grade*. Sacramento, CA: California Public Interest Research Group, 2009. Web. 9 May 2011.

(*continued*)

Content Note	Content Note
de Vise —college students getting "lazier;" they studied 7 hours a week less in 2004 than in 1961 [summary]	Zomer 2 —80% of CC students work average of 32 hours/week —some work is good, but should be no more than 15–20 hours [summary]

One useful sentence/paragraph guide when specific information contradicts a general claim

Evidence suggests (proves, demonstrates, etc.) that A's claim that _______________ is wrong (incomplete, overstated, etc.) B shows that _______________.

EXAMPLE

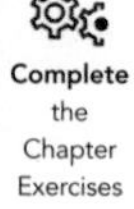
Complete the Chapter Exercises

Daniel de Vise's claim that college students are getting lazier fails to recognize complete information. De Vise points to students studying seven hours per week less in 2004 than in 1961. However, he fails to take into account how much students are now working. For example, 80% of community college students now work an average of 32 hours per week, even though experts recommend working no more than 20 hours per week (Zomer 2). Far from being lazy, college students are working hard, perhaps with less time for studying.

19 Avoiding Plagiarism

Quick Points You will learn to

- Identify plagiarism (see 19A).
- Use techniques to avoid the different types of plagiarism (see 19B).

19A What is plagiarism?

To use SOURCES well, you need to learn how to incorporate others' words and ideas into your own papers accurately, effectively, and honestly. This last skill is especially important, so that you avoid **plagiarism**, which is presenting another person's words, ideas, or visual images as if they were your own. Plagiarizing, like stealing, is a form of academic dishonesty or cheating. It's a serious offense that can be grounds for a failing grade or expulsion from a college. Beyond that, you're hurting yourself. If you're plagiarizing, you're not learning.

Watch the Video

Plagiarism isn't just something that college instructors get fussy about. In the workplace, it can get you fired. Plagiarism at work also has legal implications; using someone else's intellectual property without permission or credit is a form of theft that may land you in court. Furthermore, plagiarism in any setting—academic, business, or civic—hurts your credibility and reputation. Quick Box 19.1 lists the major types of plagiarism.

Quick Box 19.1

Types of plagiarism

You're plagiarizing if you . . .

- Buy a paper from an Internet site, another student or writer, or any other source.
- Turn in any paper that someone else has written, whether the person has given it to you, you've downloaded it from the Internet, or you've copied it from any other source.
- Change selected parts of an existing paper and claim the paper as your own.
- Neglect to put quotation marks around words that you quote directly from a source, even if you list the source in your Works Cited or References.
- Type or paste into your paper any key terms, phrases, sentences, or longer passages from another source without using documentation to tell precisely where the material came from.
- Use ideas or reasoning from a source without correctly citing and documenting that source, even if you put the ideas into your own words. (See 19E.)
- Combine ideas from many sources and pass them off as your own without correctly citing and documenting the sources.
- Use photographs, charts, figures, or other visual images from anyone (colleagues, organizations, Web sites, and so on) without crediting and documenting them.

Never assume that your instructor won't detect plagiarism. Instructors have a keen eye for writing styles that differ from the ones students generally produce and from your own style in particular. Instructors can check your work against online paper providers or materials, look up sources, or check with their colleagues.

ESOL Tip: Perhaps you come from a country or culture that considers it acceptable for students to copy the writing of experts and authorities. Some cultures, in fact, believe that using another's words, even without citing them, is a sign of respect or learning. However, this practice is unacceptable in American colleges.

19B How do I avoid plagiarism?

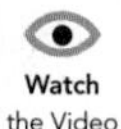

Watch the Video

The first step in avoiding plagiarism is to learn the techniques of quoting (see 18B), paraphrasing (see 18C), and summarizing (see 18D) source materials. The second step is to document sources correctly. A third step is to take advantage

Quick Box 19.2

Strategies for avoiding plagiarism

- Acknowledge and document when you're using the ideas, words, or images of others.
- Become thoroughly familiar with the documentation style your instructor requires you to use (see Chs. 25–27).
- Follow a consistent notetaking system. Use different colors, or some other coding system, to distinguish three different types of material.
  1. **Quotations** from a source; write clear, even oversized quotation marks so you can't miss them later (documentation required)
  2. **Material you have paraphrased, summarized**, or otherwise drawn from a source (documentation required)
  3. **Your own thoughts**, triggered by what you have read or experienced (no documentation required; see 20D)
- Immediately when you quote, paraphrase, or summarize in your draft, include the appropriate in-text citation, and add the source to your Works Cited or References. Don't wait to do this later.
- As part of editing and proofreading, look carefully at your paper for any places that might need documentation.
- Consult your instructor if you're unsure about any aspect of the documentation process.

of the learning opportunities your instructor may build into assignments. Many instructors require students to hand in a WORKING BIBLIOGRAPHY or ANNOTATED BIBLIOGRAPHY, a research log, working notes, a copy of the sources, or a draft (see 21G). Quick Box 19.2 suggests some practical steps you can take to avoid plagiarism.

19C How do I avoid plagiarism when using Internet sources?

You might be tempted to download a paper from the Internet. Don't. That kind of intellectual dishonesty can get you into real trouble. We've been dismayed to hear that some students believe if they buy a paper or hire someone else to write it, the paper is "theirs." No. It's not. This is clearly plagiarism.

Watch the Video

Even if you have absolutely no intention of plagiarizing, being careless can easily lead to trouble. Quick Box 19.3 suggests some ways you can avoid plagiarism when you're working on the Internet.

Quick Box 19.3

Guidelines for avoiding plagiarism when using Internet sources

- Never copy material from an online source and paste it directly into your paper without taking great care. You can too easily lose track of which language is your own and which comes from a source. If you have to copy and paste a direct quotation or visual, immediately place quotation marks around the material. Be sure to document the source at the same time, or you may forget to do it later or do it incorrectly.
- Keep downloaded or printed material separate from your own writing, even if you intend to quote, summarize, or paraphrase the material. Use another color or a much larger font as a visual reminder that this isn't your work.
- Summarize or paraphrase materials *before* you include them in your paper. Document the sources of summarized passages at the same time.
- Use an Internet service to check a passage you're not sure about. If you're concerned that you may have plagiarized by mistake, use Google to search one or two sentences that concern you. To make this work, always place quotation marks around the sentences you want to check when you type them into the search window.

19D What don't I have to document?

You don't have to document common knowledge or your own thinking. Common knowledge is information that most educated people know, although they might need to remind themselves of certain facts by looking them up in a reference book. For example, you would not need to document statements like these:

- George W. Bush was the U.S. president before Barack Obama.
- Mercury is the planet closest to the sun.
- Water boils at 212°F.
- All the oceans on our planet contain saltwater.

A very important component of a paper that doesn't need documentation is *your own thinking*. It consists of your ANALYSIS, SYNTHESIS, and evaluation of new material as you read or observe it.

19E How do I document ideas?

You need to document everything that you learn from a source, including ideas or reasoning. Expressing others' ideas in your own words doesn't release you from the obligation to tell exactly where you got them. Consider the following example.

SOURCE

Silberman, Steve. "The Placebo Problem." *The Best American Science Writing 2010*. Ed. Jerome Groopman and Jesse Cohen. New York: Ecco, 2010. 31–44. Print.

ORIGINAL (SILBERMAN'S EXACT WORDS)

The fact that an increasing number of medications are unable to beat sugar pills has thrown the industry into crisis. The stakes could hardly be higher. In today's economy, the fate of a long-established company can hang on the outcome of a handful of tests. (33)

PLAGIARISM EXAMPLE

The fact that more and more drugs are unable to beat sugar pills has caused problems. Much is at stake. Currently, the future of established companies can depend on the outcome of a handful of tests.

Even though the student changed some wording in the preceding example, the ideas aren't original to her. The highlighted phrases are especially problematic examples of plagiarism because they're Silberman's exact wording. To avoid plagiarism the student needs both to document the source and to use quotation marks to show Silberman's wording.

1. CORRECT EXAMPLE USING QUOTATION, PARAPHRASE, AND DOCUMENTATION

Steve Silberman claims that the increasing success of placebos "has thrown the [drug] industry into crisis." The market is so competitive that even "a handful of tests" can determine whether a company survives (33).

2. CORRECT EXAMPLES USING SUMMARY AND DOCUMENTATION

A. Steve Silberman argues that the success of placebos challenges drug company profits (33).

B. The success of placebos challenges drug company profits (Silberman 33).

In correct example 1, the writer has properly integrated Silberman's ideas through quotation and paraphrase, and she has included an in-text citation that points to her Works Cited page. In correct example 2A, the writer summarizes the idea, including the author's name in the sentence and a parenthetical citation. In correct example 2B, she also summarizes, but here she includes the author's name as part of the parenthetical citation.

● **EXERCISE 19-1** Following the quoted passage here are three passages. Each passage is plagiarized. For each one (1) explain why it is plagiarism, and (2) revise the passage so that it no longer is plagiarized.

ORIGINAL (SARAH NASSAUER'S EXACT WORDS)

How the check is brought to the table can make diners grumble. Some guests want the check without asking, some feel rushed if a check is placed on the table before they ask. When researchers asked customers which restaurant service mistake is worst in terms of overall satisfaction, they said not promptly settling the check when the guest is ready to leave, or problems with the check amount. (This complaint was second only to messing up the food order.) The research, which surveyed 491 people who had dined at a table-service restaurant within the past month, was published in the *Cornell Hospitality Quarterly* in 2010.

Nassauer, Sarah. "How Waiters Read Your Table." *Wall Street Journal.* Dow Jones, 22 Feb. 2012. Web. 9 April 2012.

PLAGIARIZED PASSAGES

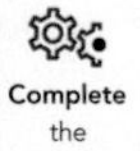
Complete the Chapter Exercises

1. If a waiter brings a check too soon, some guests are upset. However, other guests don't feel they should have to ask for the check.
2. When researchers asked customers which restaurant serve mistake is worst in terms of overall satisfaction, they said not promptly settling the check when the guest is ready to leave (Nassauer).
3. Restaurant customers reported being most bothered by waiters "not promptly settling the check" at the end of the meal. ●

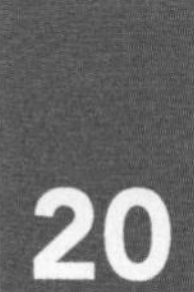

20 Writing About Readings

Quick Points You will learn to

➤ Write summary and response essays (see 20B–20C).
➤ Write analysis essays (see 20D).
➤ Write essays that apply readings (see 20E).

20A What are typical assignments for writing about readings?

Although much college writing requires using techniques for integrating sources (QUOTATION, PARAPHRASE, SUMMARY, and SYNTHESIS, which we explain in Chapter 18), some assignments focus entirely on writing about reading. Some common types of papers are summary essays (see 20B), response essays (see 20C), analysis essays (see 20D), and essays that apply readings (see 20E). Research paper assignments require finding and synthesizing multiple sources. Chapters 21 to 24 give extensive advice about RESEARCH writing.

20B How do I write a summary essay?

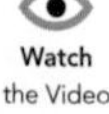
Watch the Video

Your instructors may assign papers that consist entirely of summary. Although some students may consider writing summaries as simple or obvious, we've found it takes practice and skill to do them well.

Here is specific advice for writing a summary paper.

1. **Generating ideas**
   - Identify TOPIC SENTENCES or main ideas, separating them from examples or illustrations. You want to focus on the main ideas.
   - Take notes in your own words, then put the source away. Write from your notes, going back to check the original only after you've written a first draft.
2. **Shaping and drafting**
   - Begin with a sentence that summarizes the entire reading, unless you're writing a particularly long summary.
   - Follow the order of the original.
   - Summarize proportionally. Longer and more important aspects of the original source need to get more space and attention in your summary.
   - Include a Works Cited (see Chapter 25) or References (see Chapter 26) page, depending on the required DOCUMENTATION STYLE.
3. **Revising your summary**
   - Have I maintained objectivity throughout?
   - Have I put ideas into my own words?
   - Is the summary proportional?
   - Is documentation accurate?
   - Can I make any statements more CONCISE (see Chapter 40)?

A STUDENT'S SUMMARY ESSAY

Brian Jirak received the assignment to write a 200-word summary of an article.

Jirak 1

Brian Jirak

Economics 101

Professor Connolly

15 Jan. 2012

continued >>

Jirak 2

Summary of "Living by Default"

In "Living by Default," James Surowiecki argues that there is a double standard regarding defaulting on loans. When corporations like American Airlines do so, analysts call them "very smart" (44). However, when homeowners don't pay mortgages, they are called deadbeats.

Surowiecki notes that millions of American homeowners owe far more than their homes are worth, so that paying the mortgage is "like setting a pile of money on fire every month" (44). Still, most people keep doing so. Why? Although one reason is worry about damaging their credit ratings, the more important reason is that people feel ashamed not to pay.

While Surowieki generally agrees that people should pay debts, he believes that if we consider it reasonable for corporations to walk away from loans, we should think the same for homeowners. Of course, banks and corporations could help by changing loans or modifying debts, but they choose not to. Surowieki calls them hypocritical for scolding homeowners when they have done worse. In the end, he suggests it might make sense for people just to stop paying on bad mortgages, because it may force banks to change their ways.

Jirak 3

Work Cited

Surowiecki, James. "Living by Default." *The New Yorker*. 19 and 26 Dec. 2011. 44. Print.

20C How do I write a response essay?

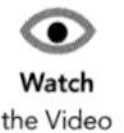

A **response** essay has two missions: to provide a SUMMARY of a source and to make statements—supported by reasons—about the source's ideas or quality. Responses may

1. Comment on a work's accuracy, logic, or conclusions. ("Is this history of hip-hop music accurate?" "Is this argument about requiring military service convincing?")
2. Present the writer's reaction to a source. ("I found the ideas in the reading shocking/intriguing/confusing/promising, etc.")
3. Focus on a work's form, or genre ("How well does this poem satisfy the requirements of a sonnet?").
4. Explain a reading's relation to other works ("Is this novel better than that novel?") or to the "real" world ("To what extent does this article accurately portray student life?").

Quick Box 20.1 explains elements of effective response essays.

Quick Box 20.1

Effective response essays

- Include a clear and concise summary of the source.
- State agreements, disagreements, or qualified agreements. (In a qualified agreement, you accept some points but not others.)
- Provide reasons and evidence for your statements.

Try the following processes for writing responses.

1. **Generating ideas**
   - Use ACTIVE READING and CRITICAL READING (see 3D) to identify the main points and generate reactions to the source.
   - Use techniques for ANALYZING (see 3E), drawing INFERENCES (see 3G), and assessing reasoning processes (see 3G–3I).
   - Discuss or debate the source with another person. Discussions and debates can get your mind moving. If in your writing you use that other person's ideas, be sure to give the person credit as a source.

2. **Shaping and drafting**
   - Write a SUMMARY of the material's main idea or central point.
   - Write a thesis statement that provides a smooth TRANSITION between the summary and your response. Your thesis clearly signals the beginning of your response.
   - Respond based on your prior knowledge, experience, reading, or research.

3. **Revising your response**

   Respond to the following questions as you consider revisions.
   - Have I combined summary and response? Have I explained my response in a way that readers will find thoughtful and convincing?
   - Have I fulfilled all DOCUMENTATION requirements? See Chapters 25–27 for coverage of four DOCUMENTATION STYLES (MLA, APA, CM, and CSE). Ask your instructor which style to use.

A STUDENT EXAMPLE

Here is student Kristin Boshoven's short response to Barry Schwartz's essay, "The Tyranny of Choice." We printed Schwartz's essay in section 3D, on pages 21–23, and we included Kristin's summary of that essay in 18D, on page 214. Note that Kristin incorporates the summary before using her own experience and her general knowledge to respond.

Boshoven 1

Kristin Boshoven

English 101

Professor Lequire

12 Apr. 2011

Too Much Choice: Disturbing but Not Destructive

Barry Schwartz argues that people with large numbers of choices are actually less happy than people with fewer

continued >>

Boshoven 2

choices. Although the amount of wealth and choice has increased during the past thirty years, studies show that fewer Americans report themselves as being happy. Depression, suicide, and mental health problems have increased. While some choice is good, too many choices hinder decision making, especially among people who Schwartz calls "maximizers," people who try to make the best possible choices. Research in shopping, education, and medical settings shows that even when people eventually decide, they experience regret, worrying that the options they didn't choose might have been better.

Although Schwartz cites convincing evidence for his claims, he ultimately goes too far in his conclusions. Excessive choice does seem to make life harder, not easier, but it alone can't be blamed for whatever unhappiness exists in our society.

My own experience supports Schwartz's finding that people who have thirty choices of jam as opposed to six often don't purchase any. A week ago I decided to buy a new smart phone. When we went to the store, we were confronted with twenty different models, and even though a helpful salesperson explained the various features, I couldn't make up my mind. I decided to do more research, which was a mistake. After reading reviews in everything from *Consumer Reports* to the *New York Times*, I am close to making a decision. However, I have a sinking feeling that as soon as I buy a phone, I'll learn that another choice would have been better, or mine will drop $50 in price. I could relate similar experiences trying to choose

continued >>

Boshoven 3

which movie to see, which dentist to visit, and so on. I suspect others could, too, which is why I find Schwartz's argument convincing at this level.

However, when he suggests that the increase of choice is a source of things like depression and suicide, he goes too far. Our society has undergone tremendous changes in the past forty or fifty years, and many of those changes are more likely to cause problems than the existence of too much choice. For example, workers in the 1950s through the 1970s could generally count on holding jobs with one company as long as they wanted, even through retirement. A 1950s autoworker, for example, might not have been thrilled with his job (and these were jobs held almost exclusively by men), but at least he could count on it, and it paid enough to buy a house and education for his family. The economic uncertainties of the past decade have meant that workers—and now women as well as men—do not have the same job stability they once did.

Although I agree that too many choices can lead to anxiety and even unhappiness, there are larger factors. If Americans report more depression and suicide than previously, a more likely candidate is economic and social uncertainty, not having too many kinds of cereal on the grocery store shelves.

continued >>

Boshoven 4

Work Cited

Schwartz, Barry. "The Tyranny of Choice." *Chronicle of Higher Education*. Chronicle of Higher Education, 23 Jan. 2004. Web. 3 Apr. 2011.

20D What are analysis or interpretation essays?

Analysis and interpretation are TEXTUAL ANALYSIS. An analysis identifies elements or parts of a source and explains how those elements work. An interpretation explains a reading's possible meaning by stating and defending an idea that perhaps isn't obvious. Textual analyses are so important in college writing that we devote an entire chapter to writing them (see Chapter 14). Literature instructors may assign you to write a literary interpretation. Chapter 58 can help you with that kind of writing. Meanwhile, Quick Box 20.2 reviews features of effective analyses or interpretation.

Quick Box 20.2

Effective analyses or interpretations

- Have a thesis that states the main idea of the analysis or interpretation.
- Refer to specific elements (sentences, examples, ideas, etc.) of the source, using quotation, paraphrase, or summary.
- Explain the meaning of the elements identified.

20D.1 Essays that report quantitative information

Some essays that analyze readings require writers to translate quantitative date into words and to explain what they mean. Quantitative information comes in the form of numbers. These essays require two activities: reporting and analyzing.

When reporting data, you need clearly and objectively to translate numbers into words. To illustrate this kind of writing, we've included part of a paper here, in which student Marcus Kapuranis reports information from the National Survey of Student Engagement.

SAMPLE STUDENT REPORT OF QUANTITATIVE DATA

Marcus Kapuranis

English 1122

Professor Bateman

24 May 2012

Diversity of Student Experiences Reported in the National Survey of Student Engagement

Part of the 2007 National Survey of Student Engagement (NSSE) asked college freshmen and seniors to report on their experiences with people different from themselves. These differences included racial and ethnic backgrounds as well as attitudes and beliefs, and the final report provides not only totals for each group of students but also a breakdown of responses according to types of college. Responses to three questions, shown in Figure 1, provide a clear picture of the national situation.

When asked how often they had serious conversations with students whose religious beliefs, personal opinions, or values differed from their own, 12% of first year students

Figure 1 Student experiences with difference.

First-Year Students Seniors (in percentages)		DRU-VH		DRU-H		DRU		Master's-L		Bac-DIV		Top 10%		NSSE 2007	
Had serious conversations with students who are very different from you in terms of their religious beliefs, political opinions, or personal values	Never	10	8	12	10	12	10	13	11	15	11	8	6	12	10
	Sometimes	33	33	33	35	34	35	34	35	37	38	29	30	34	35
	Often	31	31	30	30	29	28	29	29	28	28	30	33	29	30
	Very often	27	27	26	26	25	27	24	25	21	23	33	32	25	26
Had serious conversations with students of a different race or ethnicity than your own	Never	14	11	15	12	15	12	18	14	19	15	11	8	16	12
	Sometimes	34	34	34	35	35	33	34	34	37	38	31	32	34	35
	Often	28	29	27	28	27	28	26	27	24	26	28	28	27	28
	Very often	24	27	24	26	23	26	22	25	20	21	31	32	23	25
Institutional emphasis: Encouraging contact among students from different economic, social, and racial or ethnic backgrounds	Very little	12	21	14	20	14	18	14	18	15	19	11	17	13	19
	Some	33	36	34	36	32	34	32	35	33	36	29	35	33	35
	Quite a bit	33	27	32	28	32	29	33	29	32	37	33	28	32	28
	Very much	22	16	21	16	22	19	21	18	21	18	27	20	22	17

continued >>

Kapuranis 2

reported "never," 34% said "sometimes," 29% said "often," and 25% said "very often." In response to the same question, seniors reported similarly. 10% said "never," 35% said "sometimes," 30% said "often," and 26% said "very often."

The NSSE study also broke the responses down according to type of institution. There are three categories of "Doctoral Research University" (DRU): those that have "very high" (VH) research levels, those that have "high" (H), and others. There are three categories of "Master's Universities," Large, Medium, and Small (L, M, S), and two categories of "Baccalaureate Colleges," traditional liberal arts and sciences colleges (AS) and those that have a broader range of course and programs (DIV). (This particular study didn't survey two-year colleges, although the *Two-Year College Survey of Student Engagement* does.) The findings across the institutional types were fairly comparable, with the largest differences between traditional liberal arts colleges and medium-size master's universities. The liberal arts colleges had the fewest students (8%) reporting "never" talking to diverse students and most students (30%) reporting "very often" doing so. In contrast the medium-sized master's colleges had the most students (16%) reporting "never" talking to diverse students and the second fewest (22%) reporting "very often."

A second question asked students to report how frequently they had serious conversations with someone of a different race or ethnicity . . .

continued >>

Kapuranis 3

Work Cited

NSSE: National Survey of Student Engagement. *Experiences That Matter: Enhancing Student Learning and Success Annual Report 2007*. Center for Postsecondary Research, Indiana University, 2007. Web. 14 May 2012.

In his report, Marcus opens with a brief overview of the study. When he starts summarizing its findings, he moves from the big picture to the more detailed, and he takes care to explain information (such as the institutional types) that would be unclear to his audience. He selects the most important information, which takes some judgment. Most important for this type of writing, he remains objective.

Important Elements of Reporting Data

- Clear and accurate translations of numbers into language.
- Judicious selection and summary of data to report.
- Objective reporting, unless your task is to go a step further to analyze or interpret.

Advice on Process

1. **Generating**
   - Ask yourself what readers most need to see or recognize in the data.
   - If you're stuck, begin by trying to put everything into sentences. You probably won't want to keep all these sentences in your final draft because it would get boring; however, you should start writing rather than stare at a blank page.

2. **Shaping and drafting**
   - In the first paragraph, provide a summary or overview of the data you're reporting. Tell its source, how it was gathered, and its purpose. Your thesis will generally forecast the kind of information that follows.

- Group pieces of related information. Each grouping will potentially become a paragraph.
- Create or reproduce any charts or tables that would be too wordy to translate into language.

3. **Revising**
   - Do your words accurately report the main information?
   - Will your readers better understand the information through your language?
   - Have you made the writing as interesting as you can, given the limitations of maintaining objectivity?
   - Have you documented the source(s) accurately?

20D.2 Essays that analyze quantitative information

Most essays go beyond reporting information to analyzing and interpreting it: drawing conclusions about what the information means. Marcus Kapuranis's paper reports how frequently first-year students and seniors had serious conversations with people different from them. Here is what a paragraph analyzing that data might say:

> In terms of how often they had serious conversations with students whose religious beliefs, personal opinions, or values differ from their own, first-year students and seniors were disappointingly similar. For example, 34% of first years said "sometimes," almost identical to the 35% of seniors, and 25% of first years said "very often," almost identical to 26% of seniors. The reason this is disappointing is that four years in college seem to have had little effect on students in this dimension. If one of the purposes of college is to have students learn from new knowledge and experiences, one would expect an increase in the frequency of serious encounters with different types of people. Apparently, this isn't happening.

Notice that the analysis emphasizes why the results are disappointing and provides reasons for that interpretation.

Important Elements of Quantitative Information Analyses

- A clear report of the data
- Statements that make interpretations, inferences, or evaluations of the data
- Reasoning and support that convince readers that your statements are justified

Advice on Process

1. **Generating**
   - Follow strategies for generating reports of data.
   - Use techniques for analysis and making inferences (see 3E).
   - Brainstorm. For example, try to write five different statements about what the information means or what its implications might be. Many of them will be silly or invalid, but don't let that stop you. At least one or two will probably be worthwhile.
2. **Shaping and drafting**
   - Your basic organization will be a summary of the data (report) followed by analysis. However, you don't want to summarize everything up front—just the most important materials. During your analysis, you'll want to quote or cite some of the data, and it becomes boring to see the information twice.
3. **Revising**
   - Have you been fair and accurate in presenting the information?
   - Have you considered alternative interpretations?
   - Have you provided clear and convincing explanations for any analytic, interpretive, or evaluative comments?
   - Have you documented your paper appropriately?

● **EXERCISE 20-1** Following are two tables of data from the General Social Survey. Table A reports responses from the 1970s and Table B from the 2000s. Write a 100- to 300-word analysis of the findings.

Figure 20.2 Data tables from the general social survey.

"Men are better suited for politics than are women"

A. 1970's results, by two age groups, by percent

	18-40	41-89	TOTAL
AGREE	38.3	55.9	47.5
DISAGREE	61.7	44.1	52.5
Total Percent	100.0	100.0	100.0
(Total N)	(2,418)	(2,612)	(5,030)

B. 2000's results, by two age groups, by percent

	18-40	41-89	TOTAL
AGREE	20.7	25.5	23.4
DISAGREE	79.3	74.5	76.6
Total Percent	100.0	100.0	100.0
(Total N)	(1,480)	(1,915)	(3,395)

SDA: Survey Documentation and Analysis. "General Social Survey Quick Tables." <http://sda.berkeley.edu/archive.htm>

20E How do I write essays that apply readings?

Some assignments require you to apply ideas or concepts from one reading to another source. Four example assignments will make this clearer.

1. How does Smith's theory of social deviance explain the behaviors of the criminals who are portrayed in Jones's book?
2. Based on your own experiences, are Beaudoin's categories of high school cliques accurate and sufficient?
3. Which symptoms of depression, as explained by Kho, does the narrator of *The Bell Jar* seem to display? Which does she not?
4. Kevin Sarkis argues that baseball pitchers have progressed further than batters in the past fifty years. Analyze statistics in *The Baseball Abstract* to either confirm or disprove his claim.

Instructors assign essays of application for three reasons.

1. To test how well you grasp concepts; being able to apply an idea to a new situation demonstrates your deeper understanding of it.
2. To help you analyze information in a way you might not have considered. For example, suppose you're asked to apply an article that theorizes gender determines the roles assumed by children at play to your own observations. You would pay attention to that situation differently if asked to apply a different theory—for example, that physical size determines play roles.
3. To have you test a theory or explanation to see if it fits a situation.

The following advice will help you write essays that apply readings.

1. **Generating ideas**
    - Brainstorm a list of all the possible ways your target information or situation illustrates or "fits" the ideas from your reading.
    - Brainstorm a list of ways your information or situation disproves or complicates the ideas from your reading.
2. **Shaping and drafting**
    - Begin your essay by introducing your topic, the reading, and the source to which you're applying the reading.
    - Write a thesis that states how reading helps interpret your other target source or how your source illustrates, supports, or contradicts the reading.
    - Summarize the reading briefly.

- Summarize your target source.
- Include paragraphs to support your thesis, giving reasons for your assertion.

3. **Revising your essay**
   - Have you explained your sources accurately and efficiently?
   - Have you written a strong thesis and provided reasons and support?

AN EXAMPLE OF A STUDENT ESSAY APPLYING A READING

Carlotta Torres received the following assignment.

> Choose a recent movie, television show, or book that has a female action hero. Analyze that character using ideas from Gladys Knight's book *Female Action Heroes*. Your purpose, in a paper of 500 to 750 words, is to explain how well Knight's ideas describe the character in the source you're analyzing.

Carlotta chose to focus on the movie *X-Men: First Class*.

Torres 1

Carlotta Torres

English 101

Professor Parrish

22 October 2011

The Complicated Character of Raven in *X-Men: First Class*

For most of the twentieth century, heroes and superheroes in action movies were mostly men, from Superman and Batman to Spiderman and Wolverine, joined by only a few characters like Wonder Woman. However, from the last part of the century to the present, women superheroes have become more frequent. In *Female Action Heroes*, Gladys L. Knight explains the qualities of contemporary women characters, especially as they developed in the past three decades. The recent movie *X-Men: First Class* includes both a female villain, the character

continued >>

Torres 2

Emma Frost, and a female hero, Raven. Raven complicates the qualities that Knight has identified.

Knight describes the transition of women in films from being "weak, unintelligent, and needing to be rescued" at the turn of the twentieth century (xvi) to being tough, smart and independent by the end, including in action films, where they have emerged as heroes. The character Ellen Ripley in the *Alien* film series shows this change most clearly. In defeating alien monsters, Ripley represents "second wave feminism," Knight claims. Ripley is tough, unemotional, and stronger than her male companions in space (xx). Knight contends that female heroes in the 1990's to the present are different, with many of them characterized less by masculine toughness than by "youthfulness, girliness, and combativeness" (xxi). She points to Buffy the Vampire Slayer and Lara Croft as examples. Even as female heroes become more athletic and powerful, they continue having "all-impossible beautiful and svelte figure[s]," and they reflect "third-wave feminism, with its advocacy of looking good and being powerful" (xxi).

X-Men: First Class explains the origins in the early 1960's of the popular team of superheroes, the X-Men, whose mutations give them special powers. The group's leader, a telepath named Charles Xavier, identifies and recruits people with mutant powers, including characters named Banshee, whose impossibly loud voice can destroy buildings, and Beast, who has hands instead of feet and who possesses tremendous agility and strength. However, the first mutant that Xavier

continued >>

Torres 3

meets is a girl named Raven. Raven is a shape shifter; she can assume the exact appearance, manners, and voice of anyone else.

Although Raven matches some of Gladys Knight's description of modern heroes, she doesn't fit them all. Raven is certainly beautiful, even if in an odd way. Her natural form is as a dark blue woman whose skin has elaborate patterns of ridges and swirls. When she appears in this form, she is nude; although her skin color and texture camouflage specific bodily details, her figure is clearly curvy and sexy. Raven is smart and powerful, too. At a crucial point in the movie, for example, she imitates the lead villain, which confuses a situation long enough to let the X-Men escape. However, Raven lacks the confidence of modern female heroes as Knight depicts them. Although she is the main female hero of the movie, she is secondary to Xavier and the other male hero, Magneto. Most important, she alternates between being proud of her natural form and being ashamed of it; she even considers taking a drug that promises to make her "normal." In the end, she embraces who she is, but this decision brings a powerful change: she turns from good to evil, changing her name to Mystique in the process.

The character Raven may signal another stage of development in female action movie heroes. Instead of being purely beautiful, powerful, and in control, Raven has doubts. Her unconventional beauty causes problems, and in the end she decides to use her powers against society. In this way, Raven resembles problematic male film superheroes like

continued >>

Torres 4

Batman, who is a dark outsider whose powers don't necessarily bring him happiness. Perhaps Gladys Knight will have to write a new chapter for female action heroes like Raven.

Torres 5

Works Cited

Knight, Gladys L. *Female Action Heroes: A Guide to Women in Comics, Video Games, Film, and Television*. Santa Barbara, CA: Greenwood, 2010. Google eBook, 2010. Web. 14 Oct. 2011.

X-Men: First Class. Dir. Matthew Vaughn. Twentieth Century Fox, 2011. Film.

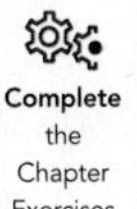

Complete the Chapter Exercises

PART

4

Research and Documentation

21 Starting and Planning Research Projects

Quick Points You will learn to

- Understand purposes of research (see 21A–21C).
- Plan the steps of a research project (see 21D).
- Choose a research topic and refine a research question (see 21E–21H).
- Identify two main types of research papers (see 21I–21J).
- Develop a search strategy (see 21K).
- Understand field research (see 21L).
- Create a bibliography, an annotated bibliography, and content notes (see 21M–21O).

21A What is research?

Research is a systematic process of gathering information to answer a question. You're doing research when you're trying to decide which college to attend or which smartphone to buy.

How much research you will do for a writing assignment can vary, depending on your AUDIENCE*, PURPOSE, and type of writing (see Ch. 5; Chs. 10–17). However, any writing might benefit from a little research. Consider these original and revised statements.

ORIGINAL Most people own a cell phone these days.

RESEARCHED According to the Pew Research Center, 84% of American adults owned a cell phone in 2011 (Purcell 2).

WORK CITED

Purcell, Kristen, Lee Rainie, Tom Rosenstiel, and Amy Mitchell. "How Mobile Devices are Changing Community Information Environments." *Pew Internet Project*. Pew Research Center, 14 Mar. 2011. Web. 20 Apr. 2011.

* Words printed in small capital letters are discussed elsewhere in the text and are defined in the Terms Glossary at the back of the book.

In the second version, the writer uses research to answer the question, "How many people own cell phones?" See Quick Box 21.1.

Quick Box 21.1

Reasons for doing research

- **To find a single fact.** Sometimes you simply need to answer a direct question of "How much?" or "When?" or "Where?" or "Who?"
  - How does the cost of college today compare to the cost twenty years ago?
- **To understand an issue or situation more broadly.** Sometimes you need to learn basic information as well as the range of viewpoints or opinions on a particular topic.
  - What are the effects of globalization?
- **To gather current information.** You may need to bring together the most current information. A **review of the literature** is a comprehensive synthesis of the latest knowledge on a particular topic.
  - What treatments are possible for diabetes?
- **To identify a specific opinion or point of view.** You might want to find out what the people who disagree with you believe—and why. You can then defend your position. Of course, you might also look for experts who support your view.
  - What are the arguments for colleges restricting student Internet downloads?
- **To create new knowledge.** Researchers make new knowledge as well as find existing knowledge. Chemists and biologists as well as psychologists, sociologists, journalists, and others do this kind of research. They conduct experiments, surveys, interviews, and observations. For instance, if you were writing a guide to coffee houses in a certain area for a sociology course, you'd need to visit all of them, take notes, and present your findings to readers.

● **EXERCISE 21-1** The following paragraph has a number of general statements. Generate a list of all the possible research questions you might pursue to strengthen the paragraph.

EXAMPLE

"If we fail to act on climate change, our coastal cities will be damaged by rising ocean levels."

POSSIBLE QUESTIONS How will climate change affect oceans? How much will oceans rise? Which cities will be affected? How?

In a troubling reversal of roles, boys are now considerably more at risk in school than are girls. Girls used to be denied many opportunities in schools and colleges, as boys enjoyed several unfair advantages. Now, however, girls are graduating from high schools at much higher rates. They are performing better on standardized tests and entering colleges and universities at much higher levels, to the extent that several colleges now have programs specifically targeted to attract and admit more male students. Women substantially outnumber men in admission to medical and law schools. A number of factors is responsible, but unless we take actions to ensure academic quality and success for both boys and girls, we will need to create affirmative action programs for men. ●

21B What is a source?

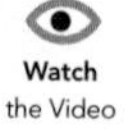
Watch the Video

A **source** is any form of information that provides ideas, examples, or evidence. One broad category is PUBLISHED SOURCES: books, articles, Web sites, and so on. You find published sources by searching library and other databases; we explain how in Chapter 22, and we explain how to judge the quality of published sources in Chapter 23. A second broad category of sources is FIELD RESEARCH, studies that you carry out directly yourself through experiments, observations, interviews, or surveys as we explain in section 21C.

Sources are either primary or secondary, as we explain in Quick Box 3.6, on page 28.

Suppose you are researching student attitudes toward American policy in the Middle East. Surveying several students would be primary research. Consulting scholars' books and articles about student attitudes toward the Middle East would be secondary research. Your decision to use primary or secondary sources depends on your research question or the requirements of your assignment. For her paper in Chapter 26, Leslie Palm conducted primary research by analyzing several video games and secondary research by reading scholarly articles.

21C What is a research paper?

A **research paper** (sometimes called a *term paper*) is a specific kind of researched writing common in many college courses. It most commonly requires the SYNTHESIS of published sources (see Chapter 22). See Quick Box 21.2.

Quick Box 21.2

Steps in most research projects

1. **Develop a research question.** What is the question that you need to answer by conducting research? Some questions might be very specific, such as when you're looking for a piece of data; for example, "How much methane is produced by dairy cattle in the United States?" Other questions are broad and complex; for example, or "How might the depiction of schools on television influence people's decisions to become teachers?" See section 21F for more about effective research questions.
2. **Decide what kinds of sources will best answer your question.** Will you need PUBLISHED SOURCES, or the results of field research (see 21L)?
3. **Develop a search strategy.** Develop a plan for finding the sources you need (see 21K).
4. **Gather and evaluate sources.** Try to accumulate more than enough materials so that you feel confident you can answer your research question (see Chapter 22). As you do so, it's crucial to use good and credible sources (see Chapter 23).
5. **Take notes on your source materials.** Take CONTENT NOTES about your sources, using summary, quotation, and paraphrase (see 21P).
6. **Draft, revise, edit, and proofread your paper.** Chapter 24 explains how to apply the general writing processes presented in Chapter 5 specifically to writing research papers.

21D How do I plan a research project?

If you feel overwhelmed by the prospect of writing an extended research project, you're not alone. Dividing your project into steps makes the process less intimidating. Giving yourself target deadlines along the way keeps you on track. Quick Box 21.3 (pages 256–257) shows how you can plan a research project.

Alert: While the steps in Quick Box 21.3 are generally true for writing research papers, the process doesn't always occur in a straight line. For example, during the drafting process, writers often discover the need to go back and find some additional sources, or even to revise their thesis statement. Being flexible will help your research process go better. ●

Quick Box 21.3

Sample schedule for a research project

Assignment received ________

Assignment due date ________

PLANNING	FINISH BY (DATE)
1. Choose a topic suitable for research (see 21E).	________
2. Draft my research question (see 21F).	________
3. Start my research log (see 21G).	________
4. Understand my writing situation (see 21H) and type of research paper (see 21I).	________
5. Determine what documentation style I need to use (see 21J).	________
RESEARCHING	
6. Plan my SEARCH STRATEGY, and modify as necessary (see 21K).	________
7. Decide if I need or am required to conduct field research; if so, plan those tasks (see 21M).	________
8. Locate and evaluate published sources (see Chs. 22 and 23).	________
9. Compile a working bibliography (see 21M) or annotated bibliography (see 21O).	________
10. Determine whether online software can be useful for me to track sources (see 21N).	________
11. Take content notes from sources I find useful (see 21P).	________
WRITING	
12. Draft my thesis statement (see 24B).	________
13. Review my content notes and determine relations between sources (see 21P).	________
14. Create an outline, as required or useful (see 24C) or use a research paper frame (see 24E).	________
15. Draft my paper (see 24D).	________
16. Use correct in-text citations (see 25B–C, 26B–C, 27A, 35A).	________

continued >>

Quick Box 21.3 (continued)

17. Compile my final bibliography (Works Cited or References), using the documentation style required (see 25A–B, 26A–B, 27). ________
18. Revise my paper (see 24G). ________
19. Edit and proofread paper for content, lack of plagiarism, in-text citations, bibliography, and format (see 24H). ________

21E How do I choose a research topic?

Sometimes college instructors assign specific topics; other times you get to choose. When you need to select your own research topic:

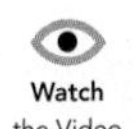

- Select a topic that interests you. It will be your companion for quite a while, perhaps most of a term.
- Choose a sufficiently narrow topic that will allow you to be successful within the time and length given by the assignment. Avoid topics that are too broad.

  NO Emotions
  YES How people respond to anger in others.

  NO Social networking
  YES The effect of Facebook on physical relationships

- Choose a topic that your readers will perceive as significant. Avoid trivial topics that prevent you from investigating ideas, analyzing them critically, or synthesizing complex concepts.

  NO Kinds of fast food
  YES The relation between fast food and obesity

The freedom to choose any topic you want can sometimes lead to research topic block. Don't panic. Instead, use some of the following strategies for generating ideas.

- **Talk with others.** Ask instructors or other experts in your area of interest what issues currently seem hot to them. Ask them to recommend readings or the names of authorities on those issues.
- **Browse the Internet.** Browse SUBJECT DIRECTORIES found in some Web search engines (see 23E).
- **Pay attention to news and current events.** Regularly browse newspapers or magazines (print or online), blogs, or social network channels.

- **Browse textbooks in your area of interest.** Read the table of contents and major headings. As you narrow your focus, note the names of important books and experts, often mentioned in reference lists at the end of chapters or at the back of the book.
- **Read encyclopedia articles** about your area of interest, its subcategories, and possible ideas for real investigation. Even Wikipedia can be useful as a starting place—but only as a starting place—be sure to read the Alert in section 22H. Never, however, stop with the encyclopedia—it is too basic for college-level research.
- **Browse the library or a good bookstore.** Look at books and popular magazines to find subjects that interest you. Also, skim academic journals in fields that interest you.

21F What is a research question?

A **research question** provides a clear focus for your research and a goal for your WRITING PROCESS. For example, you can more successfully research the question "How do people become homeless?" than you can research the broad topic of "homelessness." Some questions can lead to a final, definitive answer (for example, "How does penicillin destroy bacteria?"). Others can't (for example, "Is softball a better sport than volleyball?").

You may often find that you need to refine your question, as in the following example.

1. What is the current situation regarding homelessness?
2. What are the causes of homelessness in the United States?
3. Are the reasons for homelessness today the same reasons that existed twenty-five years ago?

Compared to the first broad question, the third is more focused. Because the third question is more complicated, it provides a better focus for your research writing.

The answer to your research question usually, but not always, appears in your THESIS STATEMENT (see Ch. 5). Sometimes, however, your thesis statement simply suggests or hints at your answer, especially when the answer is long or complicated.

21G What is a research log?

A **research log**, which is a diary of your research process, can be useful for keeping yourself organized and on track. Research logs can also show instructors and others how carefully and thoroughly you've worked. To set one up, follow these steps:

Figure 21.1 A selection from the research log of Andrei Gurov, who wrote the paper in 25G.

November 17: Finished reading Brown's book, The Déjà Vu Experience. Great source. I wonder if he's published anything more recently. Will meet with reference librarian this afternoon to identify sources.

November 18: Followed librarian's suggestion and searched the PsycINFO database for more recent articles. Found a chapter by Brown in a 2010 book that looks promising.

- Create a "Research Log" file or folder on your computer or use a separate notebook.
- Record each step in your search for information. Enter the date; your search strategies; the gist of the information you discovered; the details of exactly where you found it; and exactly where you filed your detailed notes. This step is crucial if you ever, which you often will, need to retrace your steps.
- Write down the next step you think you should take when you return to your research.
- Decide when you're ready to move away from gathering material to organizing it or to writing about it.
- Write down your thoughts and insights as you move through the research and writing processes.

Although much of what you write in your research log will never find its way into your paper, it will greatly increase your efficiency. Figure 21.1 shows a page from Andrei Gurov's research log for his paper in Chapter 25.

21H How does the writing situation shape my research paper?

Your TOPIC, PURPOSE, AUDIENCE, ROLE, and special considerations (see 4A) all influence your research paper. If you receive an assignment to argue for a position but instead you inform readers about possible positions, your paper will fall short. The same would happen if you were assigned to write a ten-page paper, in MLA style, for an audience of people knowledgeable on a certain topic and instead you wrote fifteen pages in APA style, for a very general audience. When you receive a research paper assignment, make sure to understand the required writing situation.

AUDIENCES for research papers can vary. Your instructor, of course, is always an audience. However, in most cases he or she will read as a representative of other, larger audiences, and you'll want to meet their expectations. For example, if you're writing about the topic of déjà vu for a specialized audience (see 4C) that knows psychology and expects your paper to have the characteristics of writing in that field, your research paper will differ slightly from one on the very same topic but for a general educated audience (see 4C).

21I What are two main types of research papers?

Most research papers are either informative or argumentative. Informative research papers explain a topic by SYNTHESIZING several sources (see 20E). Your goal is to gather and clarify information for your readers. Informative research papers answer questions like, "What is the current state of knowledge about X?" or "What are the current controversies or positions about Y?"

Argumentative research papers go a step further. In these papers, you choose a topic on which intelligent people have different positions, identify and analyze sources, and argue the position that appears best. You back up your reasons with support. Argumentative research papers answer questions like, "What is the best course of action regarding X?" or "Why should I believe Y?" Section 24E presents two FRAMES for research papers to guide you.

21J What documentation style should I use?

A **documentation style** is a system for providing information about each source you use. Documentation styles vary from one academic discipline to another. The types are

MLA (Modern Language Association) STYLE (see Ch. 25): Humanities

APA (American Psychological Association) STYLE (see Ch. 26): Social sciences

CM (*Chicago Manual*) STYLE (see Ch. 27): Various disciplines, generally in the humanities

CSE (Council of Science Editors) STYLE (see Ch. 27): Many natural sciences

If you don't know which style to use, ask your instructor. Use only one documentation style in each piece of writing.

At the start determine the required documentation style. This helps you write down the exact details you need to document your sources. You'll need to document all sources. If you're doing field research, your instructor may have special requirements for documentation, such as asking you to submit your research notes or results from observations, questionnaires, surveys, interviews, or anything else that has produced your primary data.

21K What is a search strategy?

A **search strategy** is an organized procedure for locating and gathering sources to answer your research question. Using a search strategy helps you work more systematically and quickly. If you are doing FIELD RESEARCH, see 21L. Here are three frequently used search strategies for PUBLISHED SOURCES. You can switch or combine these strategies or even create your own.

QUESTIONING METHOD	Useful when you have a topic. Brainstorm to break your overall research question into several smaller questions, then find sources to answer each of them. This method has the advantage of allowing you to see if your sources cover all the areas important to your research question. Generating a list of questions like this can give your search a direction and purpose.
EXPERT METHOD	Useful when your topic is specific and narrow. Start with articles or books by an expert in the field. You might want to interview an expert on the topic.
CHAINING METHOD	Useful when your topic is a general one. Start with reference books and bibliographies in current articles or WEB SITES; use them to link to additional sources. Keep following the links until you reach increasingly expert sources. Alternatively, talk with people who have some general knowledge of your topic and ask them to refer you to experts they might know.

Start and complete your search as soon as possible after you get your assignment. Early in your process you may discover sources that take time to obtain (for example, through an interlibrary loan).

One more piece of advice: Evaluate your topic before getting too far along in your search. Rather than spend endless hours simply gathering sources, take time to read and analyze some of your materials to make sure your topic will work. Your research log (see 21G) can be useful for this purpose.

21L What is field research?

Field research involves going into real-life situations to observe, survey, interview, or participate in some activity firsthand. As a field researcher, you might go to a factory, a lecture, a day-care center, or a mall—anywhere that people engage in everyday activities. You might also interview experts and other relevant individuals. Finally, you might observe and describe objects, such as paintings or buildings, or performances and events, such as concerts or television shows.

21L.1 Surveying

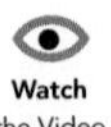
Watch the Video

Surveys use questions to gather information about peoples' experiences, situations, or opinions. Multiple-choice or true/false questions are easy for people to complete and for researchers to summarize and report. Open-ended questions, in which people are asked to write responses, require more effort. However, they sometimes provide more complete or accurate information. For advice, see Quick Box 21.4.

When you report findings from a survey, keep within your limitations. For example, if the only people who answer your survey are students at a particular campus, you can't claim they represent "all college students."

Quick Box 21.4

Guidelines for developing a survey

1. Define what you want to learn.
2. Identify the appropriate types and numbers of people to answer your survey so that you get the information you need.
3. Write questions to elicit the information.
4. Phrase questions so that they are easy to understand.

   NO Recognizing several complex variables, what age generally do you perceive as most advantageous for matrimony?

   YES What do you think is the ideal age for getting married?
5. Make sure that your wording does not imply what you want to hear.

   NO Do irresponsible and lazy deadbeats deserve support from hard-working and honest taxpayers?

   YES Should we provide benefits to unemployed people?
6. Decide whether to include open-ended questions that allow people to write their own answers.
7. Test a draft of the questionnaire on a small group of people. If any question is misinterpreted or difficult to understand, revise and retest it.

Alert: Online tools can help you distribute and analyze surveys easily. Two popular free services for small surveys are Zoomerang and SurveyMonkey. You go to the service's site, enter your survey questions, and then receive a URL to send participants. After you receive responses, you can go back to the site to download the results or do some analysis. ●

21L.2 Interviewing

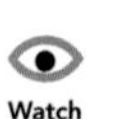

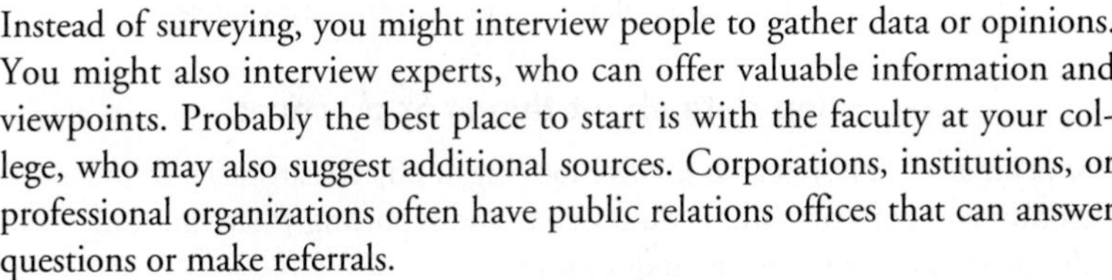

Instead of surveying, you might interview people to gather data or opinions. You might also interview experts, who can offer valuable information and viewpoints. Probably the best place to start is with the faculty at your college, who may also suggest additional sources. Corporations, institutions, or professional organizations often have public relations offices that can answer questions or make referrals.

Make every attempt to conduct interviews in person so that you can observe body language and facial expressions. However, if distance is a problem, you can conduct interviews over the phone or online. Quick Box 21.5 provides suggestions for conducting interviews.

Quick Box 21.5

Conducting research interviews

- Arrange the interview well in advance, do background research, prepare specific questions, and show up on time.
- Rehearse how to ask your questions without reading them (perhaps highlight the key words). Looking your interviewee in the eye as you ask questions establishes ease and trust. If you're interviewing on the telephone, be organized and precise.
- Take careful notes, listening especially for key names, books, Web sites, or other sources.
- Create a shortcut symbol or letter for key terms you expect to hear during the interview. This cuts down on the time needed to look away from your interviewee.
- Use standard paper so that you have room to write. (Many people are annoyed when others type while they're talking.)
- Bring extra pens or pencils.
- Never depend on recording an interview. People have become reluctant to permit such recording.

21L.3 Observing people and situations

Anthropologists, education or marketing researchers, sociologists, and other scholars conduct research by observing people and situations. For observations of behavior (for example, fans at a game or tourists at a museum), take notes during the activity. Try to remain objective so that you can see things clearly. One strategy is to take notes in a two-column format. On the left, record only objective observations; on the right, record comments or possible interpretations. Figure 21.2 is an example of a double-column note strategy.

21L.4 Gathering data about things or practices

Some kinds of field research involve looking at objects, artifacts, or practices, describing or counting what you observe, and reporting what you find. Consider these two sample research questions:

1. How are women portrayed on the covers of fashion magazines?
2. Are characters with foreign-sounding names or accents in current movies more likely to be heroes or villains?

Figure 21.2 A double-column set of notes.

Notes	Comment/Analyses
Small conference room; round table covered with papers	
JP suggests fundraising plan	JP seems nervous. Her normal behavior, or is it this situation?
AR and CT lean forward; SM leans back	
SM interrupts JP's plan, asks for more; CT silent	The fact that JP and AR are women might explain SM's response. Or is it that he's more senior?
JP continues proposal	
SM looks out window, taps pencil	Seems to have made up his mind. A power move?

You might be able to answer these questions by finding published sources, interviewing experts, or using existing means. However, it is more likely that you'd need to collect this information yourself, by directly and systematically looking at examples. For sample question one above, you'd need to examine dozens of magazine covers. For sample question two above, you'd need to view several movies. Quick Box 21.6 summarizes steps for this kind of research.

Quick Box 21.6

Research using direct observations

1. Identify your research question.
2. Identify the sample (the group of individual examples) that you're going to examine, count, describe, or analyze.
3. Develop a system for recording your observations.
4. Look for patterns, make conclusions, or draw inferences after recording all observations.
5. Explore questions such as "Why are things as I found them?" or "What might be the implications of my findings?"

● **EXERCISE 21-2** For each of the research questions, what kinds of research would be appropriate? If more than one type would work, explain all that apply.

1. What types of television programs most appeal to college students?
2. Do men and women behave differently in fast-food restaurants?
3. What factors led to the genocide in Rwanda in the 1990s?
4. What are the working conditions in a job that interests me?
5. How do clothing displays in upscale stores differ from clothing displays in discount stores? ●

21M What is a working bibliography?

A **working bibliography** is a preliminary list of the sources you gather in your research. It contains information about each source and where others might find it. Here's a list of basic elements to include (for more detailed information about documenting specific types of sources, see Chapters 25–27).

ELEMENTS OF A CITATION TO RECORD

Books	**Periodical Articles**	**Online Sources**
Author(s)	Author(s)	Author(s) (if available)
Title of book	Title of article; digital object identifier (doi), if any	Title of document
Publisher and place of publication	Name of periodical, volume number, issue number	Name of Web site or database; editor or sponsor of site
Year of publication	Date of issue	Date of electronic publication
Call number	Page numbers of article	Electronic address (URL)
Print or Web version?	Print or Web version?	Date you accessed the source

Begin your working bibliography as soon as you start identifying sources. If your search turns up very few sources, you may want to change your topic. If it reveals a vast number, you'll want to narrow your topic or choose a different one. Expect to add and drop sources throughout the research process. As a rough estimate, your working bibliography needs to be about twice as long as the list of sources you end up using.

You can record your working bibliography on note cards or on a computer. On the one hand, note cards are easy to sift through and rearrange. At the end of your WRITING PROCESS, you can easily alphabetize them to prepare your final bibliography. Write only one source on each card (see Figure 21.3).

On the other hand, putting your working bibliography on a computer saves having to type your list of sources later. Clearly separate one entry from another. You can organize the list alphabetically, by author, or by subtopics.

Whichever method you use, when you come across a potential source, immediately record the information exactly as you need it to fulfill the requirements of the DOCUMENTATION STYLE your assignment requires. Spending a few extra moments at this stage can save you hours of retracing your steps and frustration later on.

Figure 21.3 Bibliographic entry in MLA format.

Brown, Alan S. and Elizabeth J. Marsh. "Digging into Déjà Vu: Recent Research on Possible Mechanisms." The Psychology of Learning and Motivation: Advances in Research and Theory. Ed. Brian H. Ross. Burlington: Academic P, 2010, 33–62. Web. 20 Nov. 2011.

21N How might online software help me create bibliographies or organize sources?

Several software programs allow you to store bibliographic information about your sources. You can then access this information and organize it in many ways. For example, a program like NoodleBib or RefWorks lets you type in information (author, title, publisher, and so on) about each source you find. Then, with a click of a button, you can generate an MLA-style "Works Cited" page, an APA-style "References" page, or a bibliography in other formats. You can export the bibliography into the paper you're writing, without having to retype. Of course, you're still responsible for the accuracy of any bibliography you generate with this software.

Furthermore, these programs allow you to import citations directly from many databases. That means you never have to type them. Check to see if your library gives you access to bibliographic software, or use an application like NoodleBib (Figure 21.4.)

Other online tools can help you collect, store, access, and organize materials you find on the Web. For example, Diigo (http://www.diigo.com/) allows you to store URLs or even copies of Web pages so you always have access to them from any device that connects to the Internet (see Figure 21.5). You can tag each entry (add descriptive words so you can search for particular topics later), and you can highlight or add notes. You can share your bibliographies with others, which can be helpful for group projects. We have one caution. Because this software makes it so easy to gather materials, it can be tempting to avoid analysis. Analysis, however, is vital to making sources your own (see Chs. 4 and 14).

Figure 21.4 Page showing the start of a project in NoodleBib

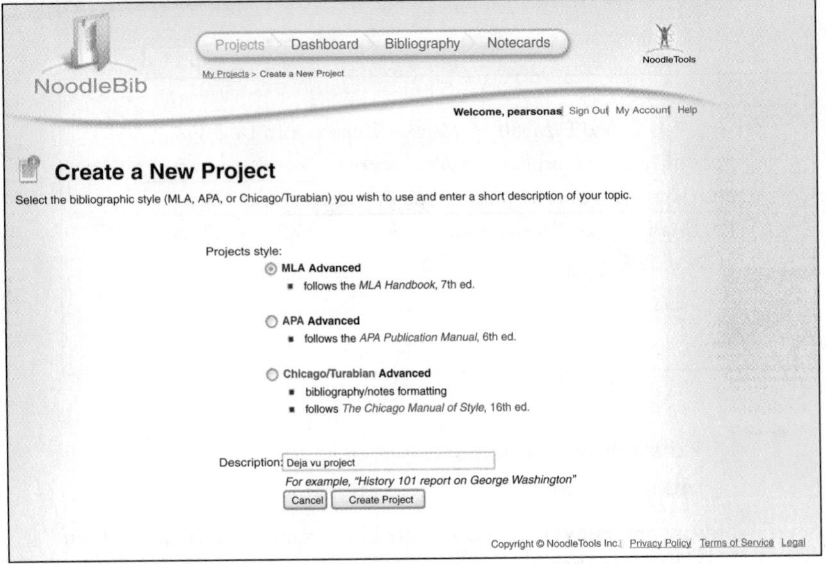

Figure 21.5 Example of a source management system.

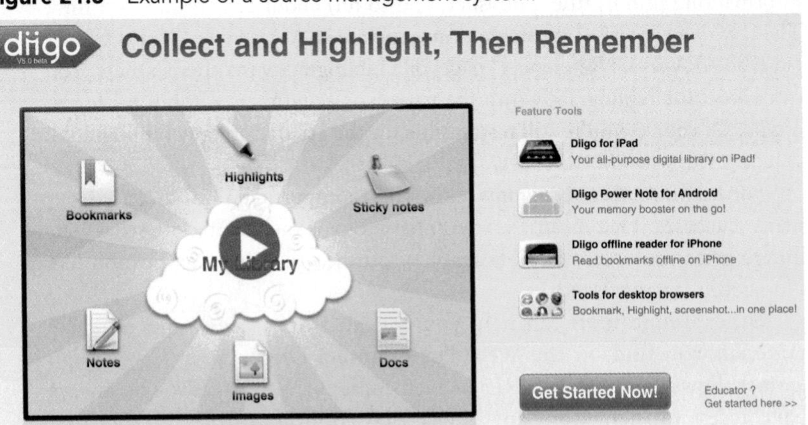

21O What is an annotated bibliography?

View the Model Document

An **annotated bibliography** includes not only publishing information about your sources but also a brief summary and perhaps a commentary. We suggest you include three types of information:

1. the thesis or a one-sentence summary;
2. the main claims or arguments in support of the thesis;

Figure 21.6 Section from an annotated bibliography in MLA style.

Brown, Alan S. and Elizabeth J. Marsh. "Digging into Déjà Vu: Recent Research on Possible Mechanisms." *The Psychology of Learning and Motivation: Advances in Research and Theory*. Ed. Brian H. Ross. Burlington: Academic P, 2010, 33-62. Web. 20 Nov. 2011.

This chapter summarizes laboratory research that tried to explain déjà vu. The authors discuss three theories. "Split perception" refers to people seeing part of a scene before seeing the whole. "Implicit memory" refers to people having had a previous experience that, however, is stored in their memories imprecisely, so they remember only the sensation and not the scene. "Gestalt familiarity" refers to having experienced something very familiar to the present setting.

Carey, Benedict. "Déjà Vu: If It All Seems Familiar, There May Be a Reason." *New York Times* 14 Sept. 2004: F1+. *LexisNexis*. Web. 11 Nov. 2011.

Scientific research shows that déjà vu is a common and real phenomenon, even if its causes are unclear. Perhaps the best explanation is that people have had a similar previous experience that they have since forgotten.

3. the kind of evidence used in the source. For example, does the source report facts or results from formal studies? Are these PRIMARY SOURCES or SECONDARY SOURCES?

Instructors sometimes require annotated bibliographies as a step in research projects, or they sometimes assign them as separate projects in their own right. Whether it's assigned or not, you may find making an annotated bibliography helps you better understand sources. Figure 21.6 shows part of an annotated bibliography using MLA-style documentation.

21P How do I take content notes?

When you write **content notes**, you record information from your sources. Writing content notes is a crucial bridge between finding and evaluating sources (see Chs. 22 and 23) and moving on to drafting your paper. Understanding

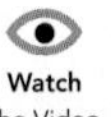

some basic strategies and procedures will make taking content notes more efficient and effective. On each index card or computer document

- Put a heading (title and author) that gives a precise link to one of your bibliography items.
- Keep careful track of what ideas came from each source if you use a computer document. Create a document called "Research Project Notes" and then create a heading for each source you use. Always include the author and page at the beginning or end of each note you type into a document.
- Include the page numbers from which you're taking notes unless an online source has no page numbers.
- Do one of three things for every note: (1) copy the exact words from a source, enclosing them in quotation marks; (2) write a paraphrase; or (3) write a summary. To avoid PLAGIARISM keep track of the kind of note you're taking. You might use the code *Q* for QUOTATION, *P* for PARAPHRASE, and *S* for SUMMARY.
- Record your own reactions and ideas separately. Use critical thinking skills (see Chapter 3). Record what might be useful from the source. Does it provide an example? An idea? A fact? Take care to differentiate your ideas from those in your sources. If you don't, you risk plagiarizing. You might write your own thoughts in a different color ink (note card) or font (computer).

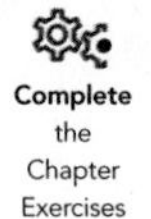

Figure 21.7 shows one of Andrei Gurov's note cards for his research paper in section 25G.

Figure 21.7 Bibliographic entry in MLA format.

Brown, Alan S. "The Déjà Vu Illusion." Current Directions in Psychological Science 13.6 (2004): 256–59. Print.

Summary: Recent advances in neurology and the study of cognitive illusions reveal that two seemingly separate perceptual events are indeed one.

Comment: This is the part that grabs my attention. How could this be?

22 Finding Published Sources

Quick Points You will learn to

- Identify the different types of published sources (see 22A).
- Locate sources using libraries, databases, and online tools (see 22B–22J).

22A What kinds of published sources are there?

Published sources refer to books, articles, documents, and other writings that appear online or in print. Because most college research writing relies on published sources, we've written this chapter to explain how to find them. The sheer number and types of published sources today can be confusing. However, you can clarify things by asking two questions: Is the source "scholarly" or "popular"? Quick Box 22.1 (page 272) helps you decide. Is the source "edited" or "unedited"? Quick Box 22.2 (page 273) explains the differences.

Popular sources can be high quality, especially if they're edited and from serious publishers or periodicals (such as *The New York Times* or *The Atlantic Monthly*). Unedited sources can be useful, too, but because no editor has selected or reviewed them, you should judge them carefully. Chapter 23 explains how to evaluate all your sources.

22B How can libraries help me?

In an age when the Web contains billions of pages of information, it might seem almost prehistoric to talk about libraries. After all, so much is now available online. Still, many sources, especially scholarly ones, are available only through the library. Notice that we've said "through" the library, not necessarily "in" it. That's because many library sources and services are available through the Internet to students or registered users. Watch the Video

In many respects, the function that a library performs is even more important than the physical building. Librarians and scholars have systematically gathered and organized sources so you can find the best ones efficiently and reliably. You can access and search electronic catalogs, **indexes,** and databases

Quick Box 22.1

Scholarly sources versus popular sources

Scholarly Sources	Popular Sources
Examples: Journal articles; books published by university presses; professional organization Web sites	**Examples:** Newspapers and magazines; general Web sites and blogs
Audience: Scholars, experts, researchers, students	**Audience:** General readers; people who may be interested but don't necessarily have specific knowledge or expertise
Purpose: To provide cutting-edge ideas and information supported by research	**Purpose:** To entertain; to translate expert information for general readers; to persuade
Authors: Researchers; professors; content experts; professionals	**Authors:** Journalists or freelance writers; hobbyists or enthusiasts; people from all walks of life
Characteristics: Citations and bibliographies show sources of ideas; sources explain research methods and limitations of conclusions	**Characteristics:** Rarely include citations or bibliographies; may refer to people or sources in the body of the work
Where published: Appear in scholarly books and periodicals or on Web sites maintained by professional organizations	**Where published:** Appear in popular books and periodicals; blogs; personal or informal Web sites
How you find them: Mainly through DATABASES	**How you find them:** Sometimes through databases; often through SEARCH ENGINES

from computers with the library itself or, in many cases, by connecting to the library via the Internet. If you have remote access, you'll probably have to log in with an ID and password. Our point is that you might be able use library-based sources without ever setting foot in the building.

Still, the building itself continues to be a vital place for all research. One key advantage of going to the library is your chance to consult with librarians face-to-face. Helping is their profession. Never hesitate to ask how to proceed or where to find a resource. Quick Box 22.3 lists ten useful questions.

Quick Box 22.2

Edited versus unedited sources

Edited	Unedited
Examples: Periodicals; books from a publisher; organizational or professional Web site	**Examples:** Personal blogs and Web sites; online comments or discussion postings; self-published books
Selection: An editor or other professional has evaluated and chosen the work to publish	**Selection:** The individual publishes the work him or herself (for example, in a blog)
Accuracy/Quality: Reviewed by an editor or expert readers	**Accuracy/Quality:** Not reviewed by others before publication.
Publisher: A periodical, book publisher, or professional organization	**Publisher:** The author him- or herself (as in blogs or discussion posts) or perhaps a special-interest group
How you find them: Mainly through databases or catalogs	**How you find them:** Mainly through search engines; unedited works almost never appear in databases

Quick Box 22.3

Top ten questions to ask a librarian

1. Do I need to log in to use the library's computer system? If so, how?
2. Can I access the library's computer system from home or off campus?
3. How do I search the library's catalog?
4. Can I find books directly on the shelves, or do I have to request them? How do I check out materials?
5. How can I use an electronic version of a book, if the library has one?
6. What databases would you recommend when I'm looking for scholarly sources on topic X?
7. What might be the best keywords or search strategy when I'm searching databases for sources on topic X?
8. How can I keep track of sources I find? E-mail them to myself? Print a list of citations? Use source management software?
9. How do I get copies of articles or other sources I've found?
10. Is there a way for me to access or order a copy if our library doesn't own a source I need?

22C What are search engines and databases?

Using search engines and using databases are two related, but different, ways to find published sources.

22C.1 Search engines

Watch the Video

Search engines are programs designed to hunt the Web for sources on specific topics by using KEYWORDS (see 22D) or subject directories (see 22E). Once you use a **browser** (a program like Internet Explorer, Firefox, or Safari) to get on the Web, you can use a search engine like Google (www.google.com) or Yahoo! (www.yahoo.com). Of course, if you know a specific Web address—called a **URL**, for Universal (or Uniform) Resource Locator—you can type it directly in a search box. Quick Box 22.4 offers tips for using search engines.

Because anyone can put anything on the Web, the Web is a rich source of information. However, it also makes finding what you need difficult, and it opens the possibility of encountering inaccurate or biased materials. In addition, many articles and documents, especially those published in scholarly journals or some edited periodicals, can't be found on the Web through search engines. To find them, you need to use databases, as explained next.

Quick Box 22.4

Tips on using Web search engines

- Use keyword combinations or BOOLEAN EXPRESSIONS (see Quick Box 22.5).
- Try using more than one search engine because different search engines will provide different results for the same search.
- Go to the toolbar at the top of the screen and click on "Bookmark" and then click on "Add" when you find a useful site. This will make it easy for you to return to a good source. Or use social networking software (see 21N) to gather your sources.
- Use the "History" function on your browser to revisit sites.
- Sources on the Web come in various formats. Most common are Web pages in html (Hypertext Markup Language) format. However, you may also encounter Word or Excel documents, PowerPoint slides, or PDF (portable document format) files.

22C.2 Databases

Databases are collections of sources that experts or librarians have gathered. You find databases mostly in libraries or through library **Web sites,** and you search them mainly by using keywords. We explain how in section 22D. Sources that you identify through databases are usually more reliable and appropriate than sources you find by simply browsing the Web. Therefore, we recommend that you search a database as part of any college research project.

Watch the Video

Alert: Google Scholar is a site within Google that does pretty much what it announces: lists scholarly sources, including books and articles, that are on the Web. It functions somewhat like a database. ●

Most college libraries subscribe to one or more database services, such as EBSCO, ProQuest, and FirstSearch. Your library's Web site will show the resources it has available. Because the college pays for these services, you don't have to, but you'll need an ID or password to use them. Commonly, your student number serves as your ID, but check with a librarian to see what's required at your college. Figure 22.1 shows a college library Web site.

Figure 22.1 College library Web site.

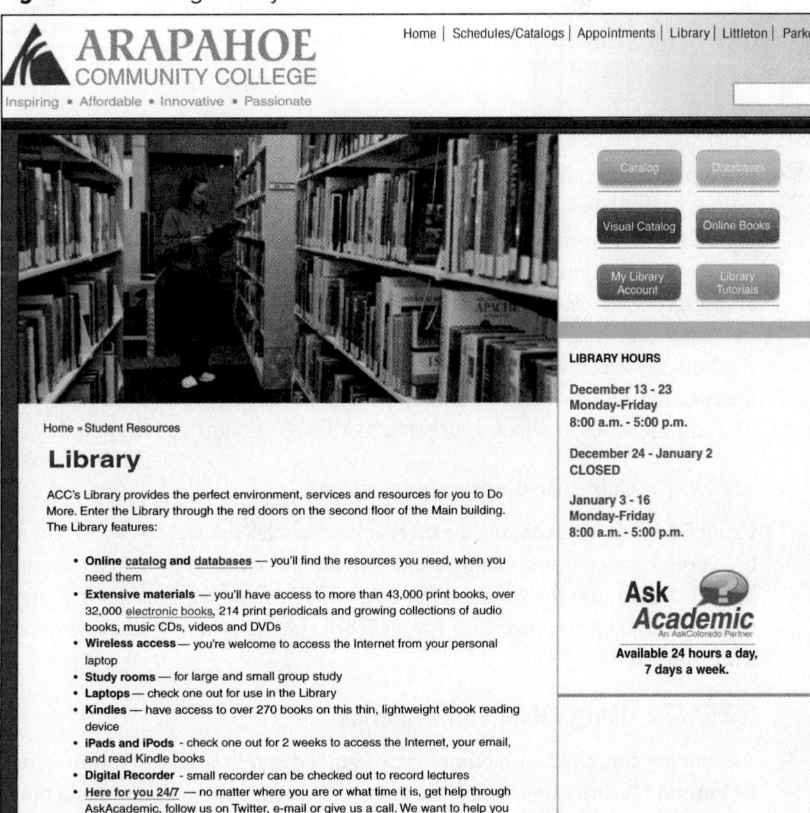

General databases include sources from a broad range of periodicals and books, both popular and scholarly. General databases are suitable for academic research projects. Just take care to focus on scholarly sources and well-regarded popular publications. Large libraries have many general databases. A common one is *Academic Search Premier*.

Specialized databases focus on specific subject areas or disciplines. They list books and articles published by and for expert readers. Some examples include *Art Abstracts, MLA International Bibliography, PsycINFO*, and *Business Abstracts*.

Each source in a DATABASE contains bibliographic information, including a title, author, date of publication, and publisher (in the case of books or reports) or periodical (in the case of articles). The entry might also provide a summary or a list of contents.

● **EXERCISE 22-1** Working either individually or as part of a group, access your library's Web site. List all the types of information available. In particular, list the indexes and databases you can search and the subject areas each one covers. Note whether any of the databases have full-text versions of articles. ●

22D How do I use search engines and databases?

Keywords (also called descriptors or identifiers) are your pathways to finding sources in databases, catalogs, and Web sites. Keywords are the main words in a source's title or words that an author or editor has identified as most important to its topic and content. Figure 22.2 shows three screens from a keyword search of *PsycINFO* on *déjà vu*. Andrei Gurov consulted this source while working on the paper that appears in section 25G.

You can search with a single keyword, but often that will generate far toow many or far too few hits. Combinations of keywords can solve both problems. You can use BOOLEAN EXPRESSIONS or ADVANCED SEARCHES.

22D.1 Using Boolean expressions

Using **Boolean expressions** means that you search a database or search engine by typing keyword combinations that narrow and refine your search. To combine keywords, use the words *AND, OR*, and *NOT* (or symbols that represent those words). Quick Box 22.5 (page 278) explains how to search with keywords more effectively.

22D.2 Using advanced searches

Advanced searches (sometimes called guided searches) allow you to search by entering information in a form. A typical search involves selecting a range of dates of publication (for example, after 2010 or between 1990 and 1995)

Figure 22.2 Keyword search of *déjà vu* in a database.

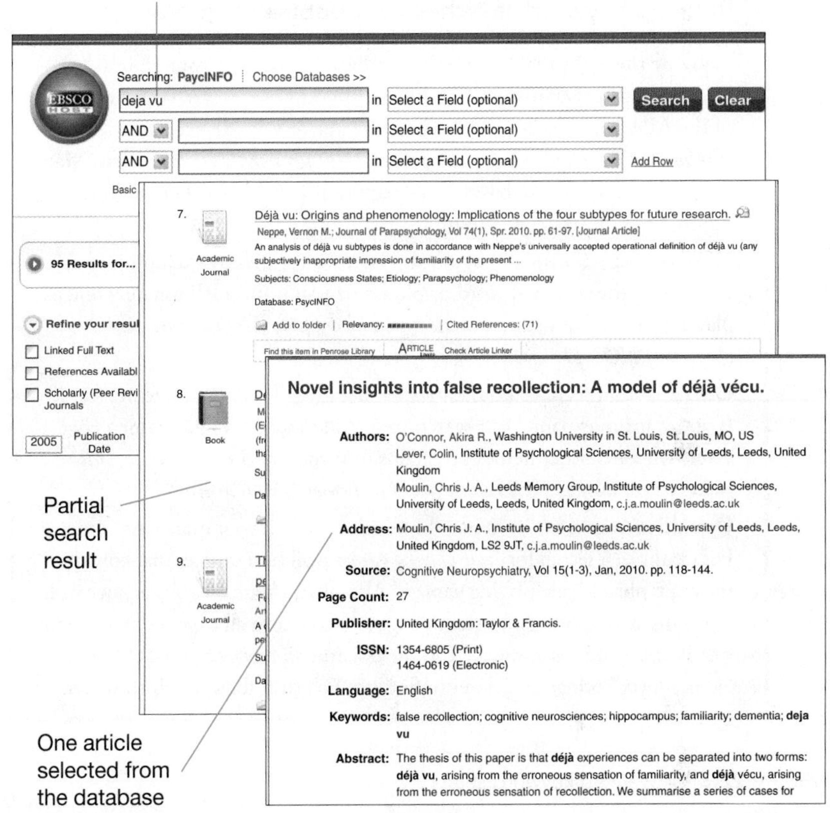

and specifying only a certain language (such as English) or format (such as books). Figure 22.3 (page 278) shows a search for sources that have *déjà vu* in their titles and use *false memory* as another keyword but are not about *crime.*

22E How do I use subject directories?

Subject directories provide an alternative to keyword searches. These directories are lists of topics (education, computing, entertainment, and so on) or resources and services (shopping, travel, and so on), with links to sources on them. Most search engines, and some library catalogs or databases, have one or more subject directories. In addition, there are independent subject directories. Some examples are *Educator's Reference Desk* (http://www.eduref.org), *Library of Congress* (http://www.loc.gov), and *Refdesk.com* (http://www.refdesk.com).

Quick Box 22.5

Refining keyword searches with Boolean expressions

AND or the + ("plus") symbol: Narrows the focus of your search because both keywords must be found. If you were researching the topic of the APA paper in 26I (how women characters are depicted in video games), try the expression *video games AND women AND characters*. Many search engines and databases don't require the word *AND* between terms. Figure 22.4 illustrates the results.

NOT or the – ("minus") symbol: Narrows a search by excluding texts containing the specified word or phrase. If you want to eliminate women playing games from your search, type *video games AND women AND characters NOT players*.

Or: Expands a search's boundaries by including more than one keyword. If you want to expand your search to include sources about women characters who are either heroes or villains in game, try the expression *video games AND women AND characters OR heroes OR villains*.

Quotation marks (" "): Direct the search to match your exact word order. For example, a search for *"role playing games"* will find sources that contain the exact phrase "role playing games." Also, if you search for *James Joyce* without using quotation marks, search engines will return all pages containing the words *James* and *Joyce* anywhere in the document; however, a search using "James Joyce" brings you closer to finding Web sites about the Irish writer.

Figure 22.3 Advanced keyword search.

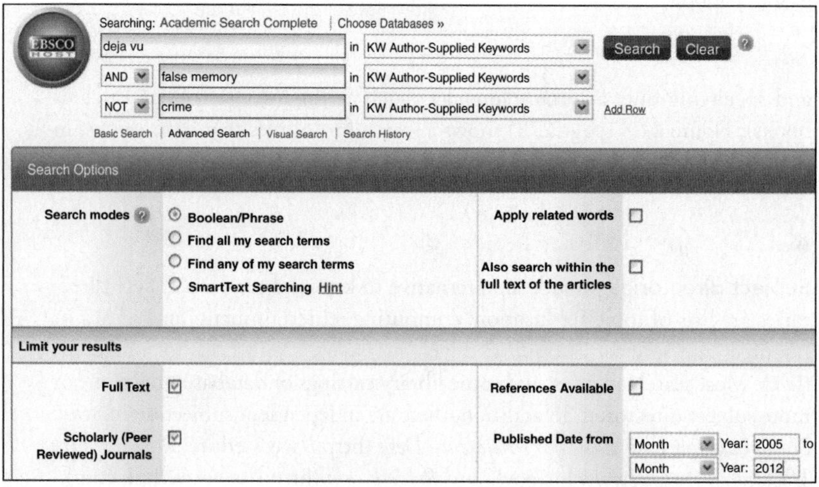

Figure 22.4 A Venn diagram showing overlaps among video games, women, and characters.

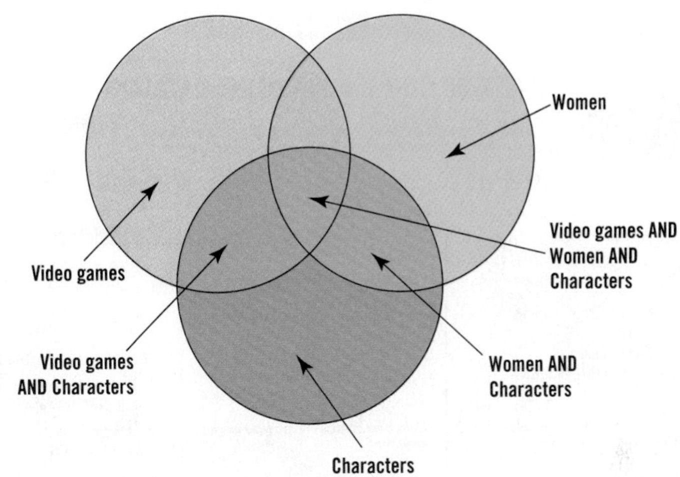

Clicking on a general category in a subject directory will take you to lists of increasingly specific categories. Eventually, you'll get a list of Web pages on the most specific subtopic you select.

22F How do I find books?

A library's **catalog**, which lists its holdings (its entire collection), exists as a computer database in almost every modern library. To find a book, you can search by author, by title, by subject, or by keyword. Figure 22.5 shows the home page for a typical **book catalog**, this one at the Library of Congress. Note that it allows you to search by title, author, subject, CALL NUMBER, or keyword; to search particular indexes; or to search using Boolean expressions.

Suppose a source recommends that you find a book by the author, Tim Wu, but you don't know its title. A screen on your library's computer will have a place for you to type *Wu, Tim* in a space for "author." (Usually, you enter last name, then first name, but first check which system your library uses.) If your library owns any books by Tim Wu, the computer will display their titles and other bibliographic information, such as the library call number. Then you can use the call number to request the book or to find it yourself. Figure 22.6 shows results from search for books by author Tim Wu.

Among the books you might find when searching for "Wu, Tim" is *The Master Switch: The Rise and Fall of Information Empires* (New York: Knopf, 2010. Print.). Suppose you know that book's title but not its author and want to see if your library owns a copy. Find the place to type in the title. In some

Figure 22.5 Library of Congress online catalog.

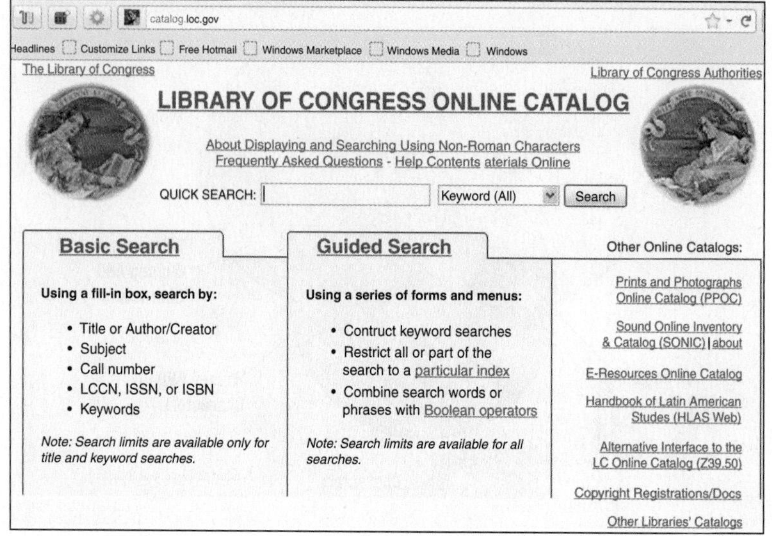

Figure 22.6 Results of an author search for Tim Wu.

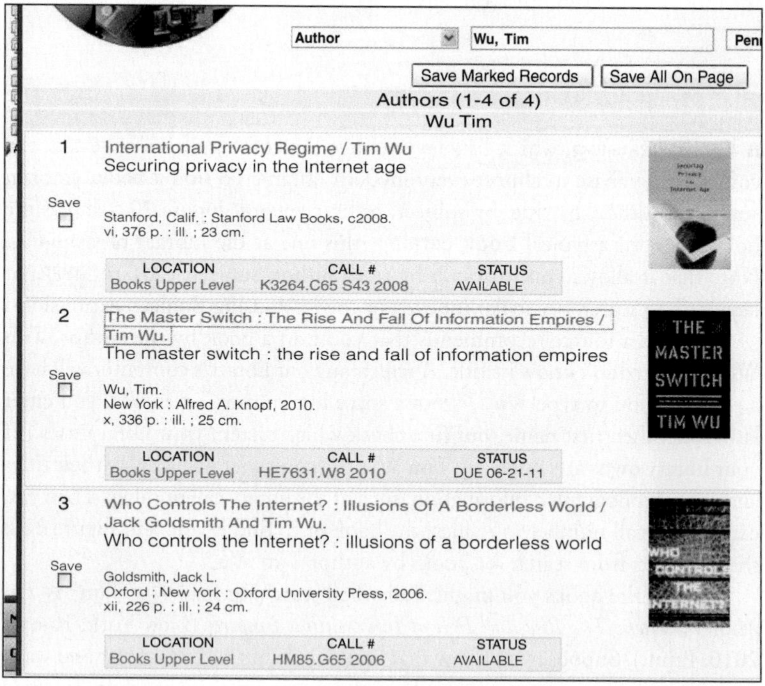

Author | Wu, Tim | Pen

Save Marked Records | Save All On Page

Authors (1-4 of 4)

Wu Tim

1 International Privacy Regime / Tim Wu
Securing privacy in the Internet age

Save

Stanford, Calif. : Stanford Law Books, c2008.
vi, 376 p. : ill. ; 23 cm.

LOCATION	CALL #	STATUS
Books Upper Level	K3264.C65 S43 2008	AVAILABLE

2 The Master Switch : The Rise And Fall Of Information Empires / Tim Wu.
The master switch : the rise and fall of information empires

Save

Wu, Tim.
New York : Alfred A. Knopf, 2010.
x, 336 p. : ill. ; 25 cm.

LOCATION	CALL #	STATUS
Books Upper Level	HE7631.W8 2010	DUE 06-21-11

3 Who Controls The Internet? : Illusions Of A Borderless World / Jack Goldsmith And Tim Wu.
Who controls the Internet? : illusions of a borderless world

Save

Goldsmith, Jack L.
Oxford ; New York : Oxford University Press, 2006.
xii, 226 p. : ill. ; 24 cm.

LOCATION	CALL #	STATUS
Books Upper Level	HM85.G65 2006	AVAILABLE

systems, you don't type articles (*a, an, the*), so then you would type in only *"Master Switch Rise Fall Information Empires."*

Suppose, however, you don't know an author's name or a book title. You have only a research topic. In this case, you need to search by subject, using the terms listed in the *Library of Congress Subject Headings (LCSH)*. The *LCSH* is a multivolume catalog available in the reference section of every library. A version of the information in the *LCSH* is online at http://authorities.loc.gov.

Finally, you may wish to search by keyword in your library's holdings. You could find Wu's book using the keywords *information, media, technology*, and so on. A sample book catalog keyword search is shown in Figure 22.7.

Scan the results to identify promising sources. When you select a record (usually by clicking on it or on a box next to it), you encounter detailed information about the source, as we illustrate in Figure 22.8 (page 282).

Some libraries allow you to print out this information, send it to your e-mail account, download it, or use online software (see 21N). Whether you choose one of these options or copy the information directly into your WORKING BIBLIOGRAPHY, it's crucial to record the **call number** exactly as it appears, with all numbers, letters, and decimal points. The call number tells where the book is located in the library's stacks (storage shelves). If you're researching in

Figure 22.7 A catalog search using keywords.

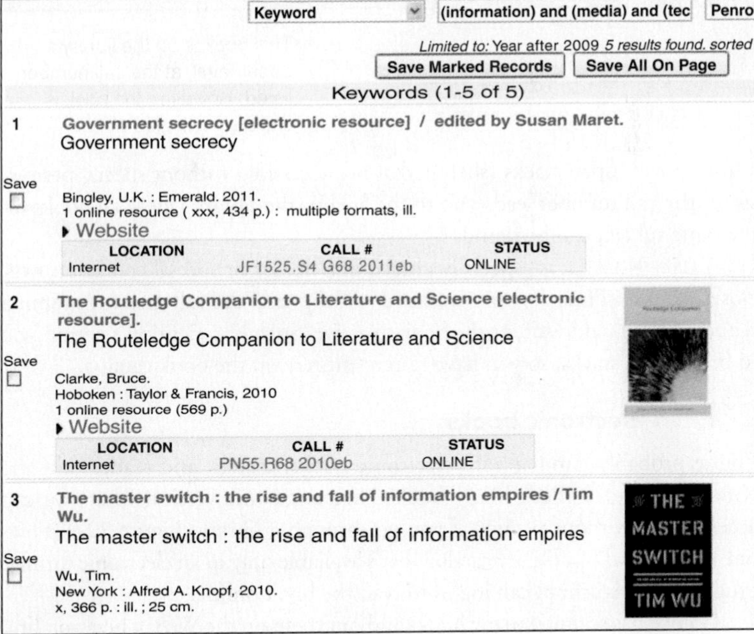

Figure 22.8 Detailed book record in a library catalog.

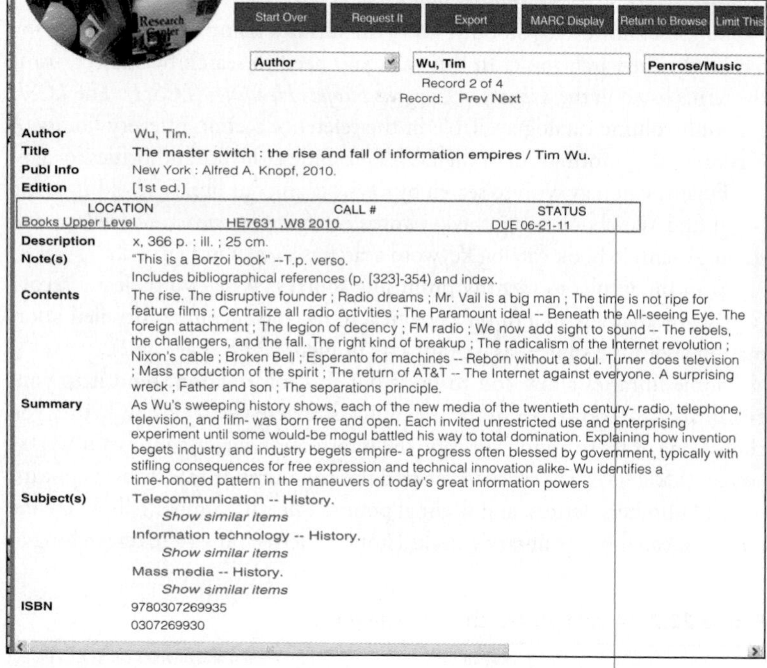

This book is on the library's upper level, at the call number listed. However, the book is currently checked out.

a library with open stacks (shelves that are accessible without special permission), the call number leads you to the area in the library where all books on the same subject can be found.

A CALL NUMBER is especially crucial in a library or special collection with closed stacks, a library where you hand in a slip in at the call desk (or submit a request online) and wait for the book to arrive. Such libraries don't permit you to browse the stacks, so you have to rely entirely on the book catalog.

22F.1 Electronic books

You're probably familiar with electronic books, tablets, and readers like the Kindle, Nook, or iPad. Many books have electronic versions that you can access—and without paying, if you go through a library. Figure 22.9 shows one book found in a library catalog that's available only in an electronic format. Students at this school can log in to read the book online.

Google has scanned many books and put them on the Web, where you find them by searching Google Books. Even if you find a book you want online,

Figure 22.9 Book available only online.

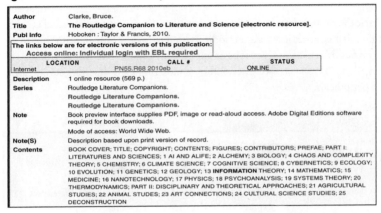

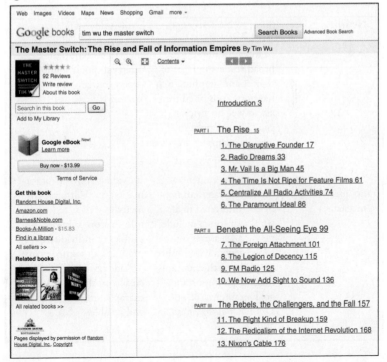

Author	Clarke, Bruce.
Title	**The Routledge Companion to Literature and Science [electronic resource].**
Publ Info	Hoboken : Taylor & Francis, 2010.

The links below are for electronic versions of this publication:
Access online: Individual login with EBL required

LOCATION	CALL #	STATUS
Internet	PN55.R68 2010eb	ONLINE

Description	1 online resource (569 p.)
Series	Routledge Literature Companions. **Routledge Literature Companions.** **Routledge Literature Companions.**
Note	Book preview interface supplies PDF, image or read-aloud access. Adobe Digital Editions software required for book downloads. Mode of access: World Wide Web.
Note(S)	Description based upon print version of record.
Contents	BOOK COVER; TITLE; COPYRIGHT; CONTENTS; FIGURES; CONTRIBUTORS; PREFAE; PART I: LITERATURES AND SCIENCES; 1 AI AND ALIFE; 2 ALCHEMY; 3 BIOLOGY; 4 CHAOS AND COMPLEXITY THEORY; 5 CHEMISTRY; 6 CLIMATE SCIENCE; 7 COGNITIVE SCIENCE; 8 CYBERNETICS; 9 ECOLOGY; 10 EVOLUTION; 11 GENETICS; 12 GEOLOGY; 13 **INFORMATION** THEORY; 14 MATHEMATICS; 15 MEDICINE; 16 NANOTECHNOLOGY; 17 PHYSICS; 18 PSYCHOANALYSIS; 19 SYSTEMS THEORY; 20 THERMODYNAMICS; PART II: DISCIPLINARY AND THEORETICAL APPROACHES; 21 AGRICULTURAL STUDIES; 22 ANIMAL STUDES; 23 ART CONNECTIONS; 24 CULTURAL SCIENCE STUDIES; 25 DECONSTRUCTION

unless it's very old, only a portion of it will be available. If you're lucky, it will be the part you want; otherwise, you'll need to find the entire book through other means. Figure 22.10 shows the Google Books contents for *The Master Switch.*

Figure 22.10 Google Books contents for *The Master Switch.*

Web Images Videos Maps News Shopping Gmail more ▾

Google books | tim wu the master switch | Search Books | Advanced Book Search

The Master Switch: The Rise and Fall of Information Empires By Tim Wu

★★★★★
92 Reviews
Write review
About this book

Search in this book | Go
Add to My Library

Google eBook New!
Learn more

Buy now - $13.99

Terms of Service

Get this book
Random House Digital, Inc.
Amazon.com
Barnes&Noble.com
Books-A-Million - $15.83
Find in a library
All sellers >>

Related books

All related books >>

Pages displayed by permission of Random House Digital, Inc.. Copyright

Contents ▾

Introduction 3

PART I The Rise 15

1. The Disruptive Founder 17
2. Radio Dreams 33
3. Mr. Vail Is a Big Man 45
4. The Time Is Not Ripe for Feature Films 61
5. Centralize All Radio Activities 74
6. The Paramount Ideal 86

PART II Beneath the All-Seeing Eye 99

7. The Foreign Attachment 101
8. The Legion of Decency 115
9. FM Radio 125
10. We Now Add Sight to Sound 136

PART III The Rebels, the Challengers, and the Fall 157

11. The Right Kind of Breakup 159
12. The Redicalism of the Internet Revolution 168
13. Nixon's Cable 176

22G How do I find periodicals?

Periodicals are edited magazines, journals, and newspapers published periodically, that is, at set intervals. Periodicals used to appear only in print, but many now publish electronic versions or appear only online. You find periodicals by searching DATABASES (see 22C, 22D). Quick Box 22.6 describes several types of periodicals.

Quick Box 22.6

Types of periodicals

Type	Characteristics	Useful for
Journal	Scholarly articles written by experts for other experts; usually focus on one academic discipline; published relatively infrequently; examples are *College Composition and Communication* and *American Journal of Public Health*.	The most reliable expert research on a particular subject; detailed articles and extensive bibliographies that can point to other sources or experts; may also have book reviews
News magazines	Short to modest-length articles on current events or topics of interest to a broad readership; lots of photos and graphics; may have opinions or editorials, as well as reviews; generally are published weekly; examples are *Time* and *Newsweek*	Easily understandable and timely introductions to current topics; often can point to more expert sources, topics, and keywords
Special-interest or "lifestyle" magazines	Written for audiences (including fans and hobbyists) interested in a particular topic; include news and features on that topic; generally published monthly, with entertainment as an important goal; examples include *Outside*, *Rolling Stone*, *Wired*	Providing "how-to" information on their topics of focus, as well as technical information or in-depth profiles of individuals, products, or events; many include reviews related to emphasis; the more serious examples are well written and reliable

continued >>

Quick Box 22.6 (continued)

Type	Characteristics	Useful for
"Intellectual" or literary magazines	Publish relatively longer articles that provide in-depth analysis of issues, events, or people; may include creative work as well as nonfiction; aimed at a general, well-educated audience; usually published monthly; examples include *The Atlantic, Harper's, The New Yorker*	Learning about a topic in depth but in a way more accessible than scholarly journals; becoming aware of major controversies and positions; learning who experts are and what books or other sources have been published; reading arguments on topics
Trade magazines	Focus on particular businesses, industries, and trade groups; discuss new products, legislation, or events that will influence individuals or businesses in that area; examples include *National Hog Farmer, Sound and Video Contractor*	Specialized information focusing on applying information or research in particular settings; seeing how specific audiences or interest groups may respond to a particular position
Newspapers	Publish articles about current news, sports, and cultural events; contain several sections, including opinions and editorials, lifestyle, sports; most appear daily; examples are *The Washington Post, The DeWitt, Iowa, Observer*	Very current information; national newspapers (such as *The New York Times*) cover world events and frequently have analysis and commentary; local newspapers cover small happenings you likely won't find elsewhere; opinion sections and reviews are sources of ideas and positions

22G.1 Locating articles themselves

Databases help you find information about sources, but the important question is how do you get your hands on the source itself? Often you can find an online full-text version of the article to read, download, or print. A full-text version may be either in HTML format or PDF; the listing will tell you which one. If you have a choice, we recommend using the PDF version, which is easier to cite because it has the layout of a print article, including page numbers.

Sometimes, however, you need to find a printed copy of the periodical. Often the listing in the database will say whether your library owns a copy and what its call number is. Otherwise, you'll need to check if the periodical is listed in the library's CATALOG; search for the periodical name you want (for example, *American Literature* or *The Economist*).

Use the periodical's call number to find it in the library. To find the specific article you want, look for the issue in which the article you need appears. For advice on locating sources that you library doesn't own, see the Alert on page 289.

● **EXERCISE 22-2** Use two databases that are available through your library to conduct two searches for one or more of the following terms. (Alternatively, your instructor may suggest a different term or have you pursue a topic of your own choosing.)

Suggested terms for searching (with type of specialized database to consult in parentheses): memory (psychology); globalization (business, economics, sociology); cloning (biology); climate change (geology, geography, political science); obesity (medicine, psychology).

If possible, choose one general and one specialized database. Compile a brief report that compares the sources you generate. You might address questions like these: How many sources did each search turn up? Is there any overlap? What kinds of periodicals are represented in each database? What access does your library provide to the several sources you find most interesting in each search? ●

Alert: If you're generating lots of hits, restrict your search to the past year or two. ●

22H How do I use reference works?

Reference works include encyclopedias, almanacs, yearbooks, fact books, atlases, dictionaries, biographical reference works, and bibliographies. Reference works are the starting point for many college researchers—but they're no more than a starting point. *General* reference works provide information on a vast number of subjects, but without much depth. *Specialized* reference works provide information on selected topics, often for more expert or professional audiences.

22H.1 General reference works

General reference works help researchers identify useful keywords for subject headings and online catalog searches. In addition, they are excellent sources for finding examples and verifying facts.

Most widely used reference works are available in electronic versions. Check your library's Web site to see what's available online through a subscription the library has purchased. For example, you may find a subscription to the *Gale Virtual Reference Library*, which allows libraries to make up to 1,000 reference books available to users online. Alternatively, search the Web (for example, *Encyclopaedia Britannica* is at http://www.britannica.com). Be aware that often you have to pay a fee for works you don't access through the library.

GENERAL ENCYCLOPEDIAS

Articles in general scholarly encyclopedias, such as the *Encyclopaedia Britannica*, can give you helpful background information, the names of major experts in the field, and, often, a brief BIBLIOGRAPHY on the subject.

Alert: A Note on *Wikipedia*. *Wikipedia* is an unedited source that almost anyone can modify. The accuracy and quality of information it contains, therefore, must always be investigated further. Still, *Wikipedia* is often a possible starting place for some quick information on a topic. For example, Doug, like many professionals and even professors, will occasionally check *Wikipedia* to learn names, concepts, or basic information on a particular topic. But *Wikipedia* is only a starting place, a way to get oriented. You need to find other sources that serve you better for college-level research. As important, your ETHOS is weak when you use *Wikipedia* extensively. Your readers will suspect you haven't taken the time or responsibility to find more scholarly sources. You surely want to avoid that suspicion. We strongly recommend, then, that you use *Wikipedia* only to get some first impressions of a research topic, then find and use other, better recognized sources. ●

ALMANACS, YEARBOOKS, AND FACT BOOKS

Often available both in print and online, almanacs, yearbooks, and fact books are huge compilations of facts and figures. Examples include the *World Almanac, Facts on File*, and the annual *Statistical Abstract of the United States* (accessed online through http://www.census.gov).

ATLASES AND GAZETTEERS

Atlases (such as the *Times Atlas of the World*) contain maps of our planet's continents, seas, and skies. Gazetteers (such as the *Columbia Gazetteer of the World*) provide comprehensive geographical information on topography, climates, populations, migrations, natural resources, and so on.

DICTIONARIES

Dictionaries define words and terms. In addition to general dictionaries, specialized dictionaries exist in many academic disciplines.

BIOGRAPHICAL REFERENCE WORKS

Biographical reference books give brief factual information about famous people—their accomplishments along with pertinent events and dates in their lives. Biographical references include the *Who's Who* series and the *Dictionary of American Biography*.

BIBLIOGRAPHIES

Bibliographies are guides to sources on particular topics. They list books, articles, documents, films, and other resources and provide publication information so that you can find those sources. Annotated or critical bibliographies describe and evaluate the works that they list.

22H.2 Specialized reference works

Specialized reference works provide authoritative and specific information on selected topics, often for more expert researchers. These works are usually appropriate for college-level research because the information is more advanced and detailed.

Here are a few examples of specialized references:

Dictionary of American Biography
Encyclopedia of Banking and Finance
Encyclopedia of Chemistry
Encyclopedia of Religion
Encyclopedia of the Biological Sciences
International Encyclopedia of Film
New Grove Dictionary of Music and Musicians
Oxford Companion to the Theatre

22I How can I find images?

If you need or want to include images in a research paper, you have three options. A keyword search through the "Images" menu on Google or Yahoo! will generate links to images as they appear in sites and documents across the Internet. However, there are ethical and, sometimes, even legal concerns in using what you find this way (see 7E.1).

A good alternative to general Internet searches is to use a "stock photo" Web site. These are services like iStockphoto.com or GettyImages.com that have gathered thousands, even millions, of photographs, which you can browse by category or keyword. For a small fee you can purchase the use of an image from these sites. (There are a few "free" sites, too.)

Finally, your library may provide access to image archives or databases. Ask a librarian.

22J How do I find government documents?

Government publications are available in astounding variety. You can find information on laws and legal decisions, regulations, population, weather patterns, agriculture, national parks, education, and health, to name just a few topics. Most government documents are available online.

- The Government Printing Office maintains its searchable *Catalog of U.S. Government Publications* at http://www.gpoaccess.gov/index.html.
- THOMAS, a service of the Library of Congress, offers information about legislation at http://thomas.loc.gov/.
- A directory of all federal government sites that provide statistical information is at http://www.fedstats.gov.
- The LexisNexis database service provides access to a huge number of other governmental reports and documents. For example, the Congressional Information Service indexes all papers produced by congressional panels and committees.

Alert: Almost no library will contain every source that you need. However, many libraries are connected electronically to other libraries' book catalogs, giving you access to additional holdings. Often you or a librarian can request materials from other libraries through interlibrary loan (generally free of charge). ●

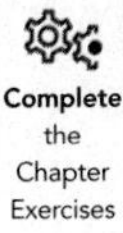
Complete the Chapter Exercises

23 Evaluating Sources

Quick Points You will learn to

- ➤ Evaluate sources (see Ch. 23).
- ➤ Find useful sources (see 23A–23F).

Not all sources are created equal. We don't just mean the differences explained in Chapter 22 between books, PERIODICALS, and Web sites, or between scholarly and popular sources. Sources also differ in quality. Some present information that has been carefully gathered and checked. Others report information, even rumor, that is second- or third-hand and, worse, perhaps not even based in fact.

Some sources make claims that are accompanied by strong evidence and reasoning. Others make claims based only on opinion, or they use information illogically. Some are written by experts wanting to advance knowledge. Others are produced by people wanting to promote special interests however they can, even if it means ignoring data, oversimplifying issues, or overpromising results. Some sources have been reviewed by experts and published only after passing standards. Others appear without anyone judging their quality.

You don't want to conduct research and organize it for writing, only to have weak sources hurt your ETHOS and weaken your paper. Therefore, you want to evaluate each source you find by asking the questions in Quick Box 23.1.

Quick Box 23.1

Five questions for evaluating sources

1. How did you find the source? (See 23A.)
2. Is the publisher authoritative? (See 23B.)
3. Is the author qualified to write about the topic? (See 23C.)
4. Does the source have sufficient and credible evidence? (See 23D.)
5. Does the source pass other critical thinking tests? (See 23E.)

23A How did you find the source?

Sources that you find through DATABASES, especially databases you access through a library Web site (see 22B), are more likely to be good than sources found through a general Google search. If a source is in a database, it has passed a level of review. It comes from a book or periodical that has been edited and checked for quality. Certainly you can find useful sources through a general search, but you'll have to work harder to sort strong ones from weak.

For example, suppose you want to research the safety of vaccines. (We illustrate the range of options in Figure 23.1 (pages 292–293), where a student has done four different searches.) A Google search will produce thousands of sources. Some of them will be reliable; many will not. If, instead, you search a library database like Academic Search Premier, you'll still find hundreds of sources, but these will mainly be of higher quality. The most authoritative sources will come from a college library's CATALOG or a scholarly database that specializes in a specific field, such as Medlines, which is created for physicians, researchers, and other medical professionals.

23B Is the publisher authoritative?

The publisher is the company or group ultimately responsible for a book, periodical, or Web site. Authoritative publishers produce journals, respected magazines and newspapers, and books from university and other major presses. Professional organizations sponsor authoritative Web sites.

Figure 23.1 Four searches with less to more reliable results.

A. Least Reliable:
A general Google search

A site that expresses the strong opinion that doctors cause autism. You'd have to check this one carefully.

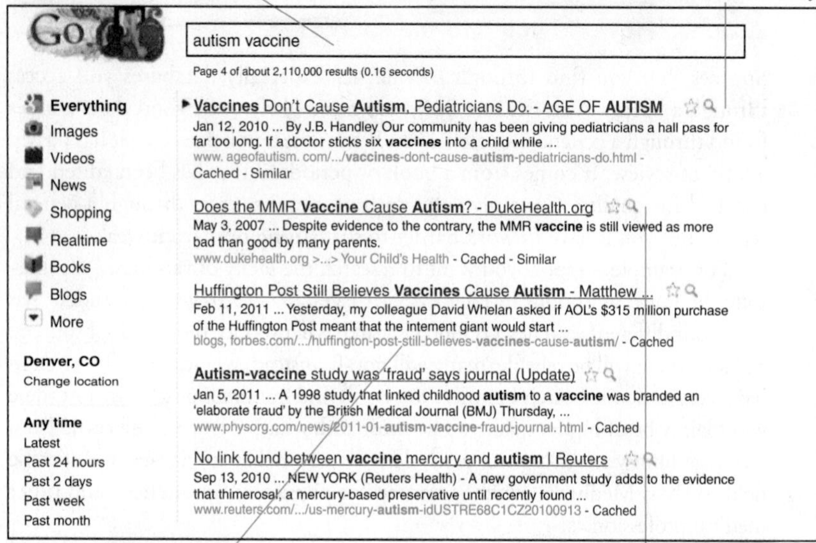

Blogs can have opinions unsupported by facts. Check carefully.

The name and the .org domain suggests that it might be associated with Duke University.

B. More Reliable:
A Google Scholar Search

Sources on this page come from journals in the field, which are edited and written by experts.

Google scholar | autism vaccines | Search | Advanced Scholar Search

Scholar | Articles and patents | anytime | include citations | Create email alert

Autism and thimerosal-containing **vaccines**: lack of consistent evidence for an association — U. of Denver fulltext
P Stehr-Green, P Tull, M Strllfeld... - American journal of ..., 2003 - cat.inist.fr
Background: In 1999, concerns were raised that **vaccines** containing the preservative Thimerosal might increase the risk of **autism** and/or other neurodevelopmental disorders. Methods: Between the mid-1980s through the late-1990s, we compared the prevalence/incidence of **autism** ...
Cited by 177 - Related articles - All 5 versions

... comparative evaluation of the effects of MMR immunization and mercury doses from thimerosal-containing childhood **vaccines** on the population prevalence of **autism** ...
DA Geier... - ... medical journal of experimental and clinical ... , 2004 - ncbi.nlm.nih.gov
BACKGROUND: The purpose of the study was to evaluate the effects of MMR immunization and mercury from thimerosal-containing childhood **vaccines** on the prevalence of **autism**.
MATERIAL/METHODS: Evaluations of the Biological Surveillance Summaries of the ...
Cited by 66 - Related articles - Check Library Holdings - BL Direct - All 10 versions

Thimerosal and the occurrence of **autism**: negative ecological evidence from Danish population-based data — [PDF] from pkids.org; U. of Denver fulltext
KM Madsen, MB Lauritsen, CB Pedersen... -Pediatrics, 2003 - Am Acad Psdiatrics
... Our ecological data do not support a correlation between thimerosal-containing **vaccines** and the incidence of **autism**. Key Words: **autism** • vaccine • thimerosal • mercury • population • epidemiology. ... Diseases Home page Does Thimerosal in **Vaccines** Cause **Autism**? ...
Cited by 146 - Related articles - BL Direct - All 32 versions

Vaccines and **autism** revisited--the Hannah Poling case — U. of Denver fulltext
PA Offit - New England Journal of Medicine, 2008 - content.nejm. org
Injury Compensation Program (VICP) and won. On March 6, 2008, the Polings took their case to the public. Standing before a bank of micro- phones from several major news organizations, Jon Poling said that "the results in this case may well signify a landmark ...
Cited by 28 - Related articles - Bl Direct - All 7 versions

Full text versions show that these are articles, not Web sites.

The sources are somewhat old, however, for medical research.

Database includes popular sources like newspaper articles, which will be easier to understand.

C. Also Reliable: A search using a common college library database

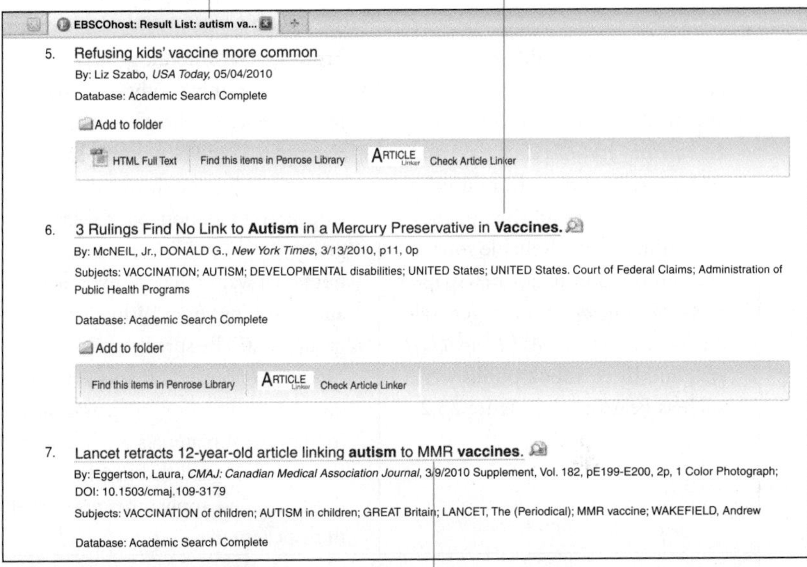
EBSCOhost: Result List: autism va...

5. Refusing kids' vaccine more common
By: Liz Szabo, *USA Today*, 05/04/2010
Database: Academic Search Complete
Add to folder
HTML Full Text | Find this items in Penrose Library | ARTICLE Linker Check Article Linker

6. 3 Rulings Find No Link to **Autism** in a Mercury Preservative in **Vaccines.**
By: McNEIL, Jr., DONALD G., *New York Times*, 3/13/2010, p11, 0p
Subjects: VACCINATION; AUTISM; DEVELOPMENTAL disabilities; UNITED States; UNITED States. Court of Federal Claims; Administration of Public Health Programs
Database: Academic Search Complete
Add to folder
Find this items in Penrose Library | ARTICLE Linker Check Article Linker

7. Lancet retracts 12-year-old article linking **autism** to MMR **vaccines.**
By: Eggertson, Laura, *CMAJ: Canadian Medical Association Journal*, 3/9/2010 Supplement, Vol. 182, pE199-E200, 2p, 1 Color Photograph; DOI: 10.1503/cmaj.109-3179
Subjects: VACCINATION of children; AUTISM in children; GREAT Britain; LANCET, The (Periodical); MMR vaccine; WAKEFIELD, Andrew
Database: Academic Search Complete

Database also includes scholarly sources like journal articles. These PRIMARY SOURCES will have most authoritative research but can sometimes be difficult.

D. Expert: A search using a database designed for experts in a field

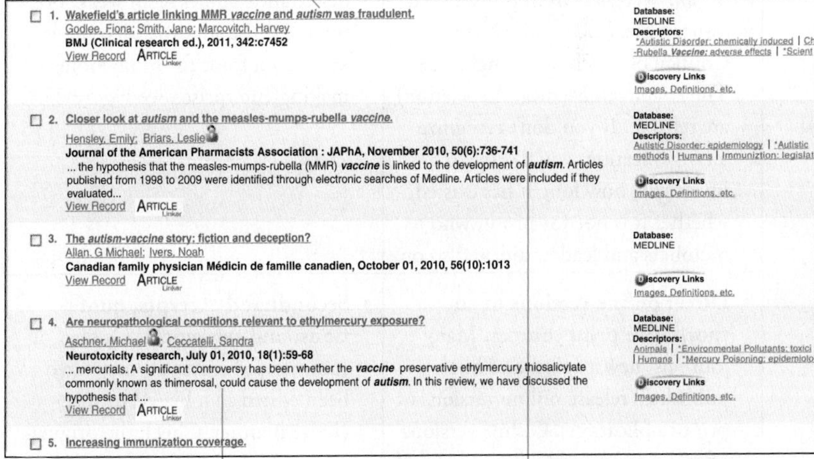
1. Wakefield's article linking MMR *vaccine* and *autism* was fraudulent.
Godlee, Fiona; Smith, Jane; Marcovitch, Harvey
BMJ (Clinical research ed.), 2011, 342:c7452
View Record ARTICLE Linker
Database: MEDLINE
Descriptors: *Autistic Disorder: chemically induced | Ch -Rubella *Vaccine:* adverse effects | *Scient
Discovery Links
Images, Definitions, etc.

2. Closer look at *autism* and the measles-mumps-rubella *vaccine*.
Hensley, Emily; Briars, Leslie
Journal of the American Pharmacists Association : JAPhA, November 2010, 50(6):736-741
... the hypothesis that the measles-mumps-rubella (MMR) ***vaccine*** is linked to the development of ***autism***. Articles published from 1998 to 2009 were identified through electronic searches of Medline. Articles were included if they evaluated...
View Record ARTICLE Linker
Database: MEDLINE
Descriptors: Autistic Disorder: epidemiology | *Autistic methods | Humans | Immuniztion: legislat
Discovery Links
Images, Definitions, etc.

3. The *autism-vaccine* story: fiction and deception?
Allan, G Michael; Ivers, Noah
Canadian family physician Médicin de famille canadien, October 01, 2010, 56(10):1013
View Record ARTICLE Linker
Database: MEDLINE
Discovery Links
Images, Definitions, etc.

4. Are neuropathological conditions relevant to ethylmercury exposure?
Aschner, Michael; Ceccatelli, Sandra
Neurotoxicity research, July 01, 2010, 18(1):59-68
... mercurials. A significant controversy has been whether the ***vaccine*** preservative ethylmercury thiosalicylate commonly known as thimerosal, could cause the development of ***autism***. In this review, we have discussed the hypothesis that ...
View Record ARTICLE Linker
Database: MEDLINE
Descriptors: Animals | *Environmental Pollutants: toxici | Humans | *Mercury Poisoning: epidemiolo
Discovery Links
Images, Definitions, etc.

5. Increasing immunization coverage.

Short descriptions provide some information about article contents.

All articles in this database come from scholarly journals, and many report research.

Is the publisher authorative?

Reliable sources are . . .	Questionable sources are . . .
• **From reputable publishers.** Generally, encyclopedias, textbooks, and academic journals (*Journal of Counseling and Development*) are authoritative. Books from university and other established presses are authoritative. Reliable sources are published in major newspapers (*The Washington Post*); in general-readership magazines (*Time, Harpers*); and by textbook publishers such as Pearson. See Figure 23.2.	• **From special-interest groups.** Some groups exist only to advance a narrow interest or political viewpoint. Examples would be a group existing only to legalize marijuana or one to stop all immigration. Special-interest groups might publish useful sources, but you'll want to check their facts and reasoning. Ask, "Why does the group exist?" Be sure to question its motives, especially if it asks you to take a specific action, such as donate money. See if materials published by the group are included in scholarly databases, and apply other tests listed in this chapter.
• **Web sites from educational, not-for-profit, or government organizations.** One sign is an Internet address ending in *.edu, .gov,* or a country abbreviation such as *.ca* or *.uk*. Web sites from professional associations (such as the National Council of Teachers of English or The American Medical Association) are reliable. If you don't recognize an organization, you'll want to investigate how long it has existed, whether it is not-for-profit, who its members and leaders are, and so on.	• **Web sites from commercial enterprises** that end in *.com*. These sites may or may not provide evidence or list sources for claims they make. If they fail to do so, or if the evidence and sources seem weak, don't use them. Be sure the Web site is not only a front for some money-making enterprise. See Figure 23.3.
• **Direct online versions of authoritative print sources.** Many journals, newspapers, and book publishers release online versions of print publications. Online versions of authoritative publications are reliable.	• **Secondhand excerpts, quotations, and references.** Quoted or summarized materials may have been edited in a biased or inaccurate manner. Check the original. Figure 23.4 illustrates a problem that can occur with secondhand materials.

Figure 23.2 A commercial (nonscholarly) book and a scholarly book.

Commercial Book

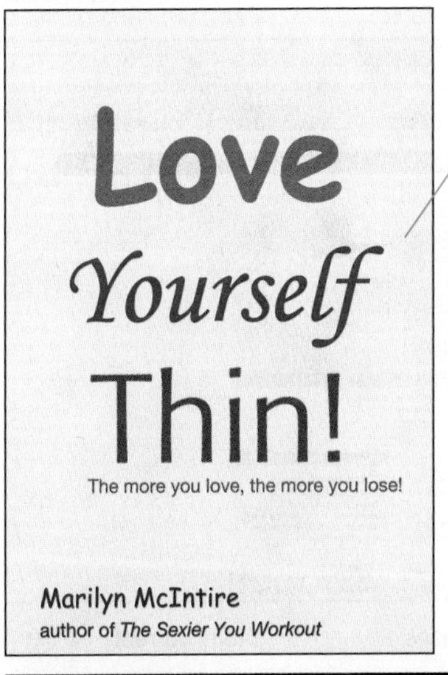

A self-help book that gives diet and relationship advice and promises results. The publisher also sponsors a commercial Web site focusing on spin-off products. This is not a scholarly source.

McIntire, Marilyn. *Love Yourself Thin!* Ankeny, IA: Maddie, 2012. Print.

Scholarly Book

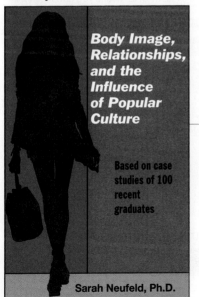

A scholarly book that reports findings from a research study of body image and relationships among young college graduates. The publisher is a university press.

Neufeld, Sarah. *Body Image, Relationships, and the Influence of Popular Culture.* Evergreen, CO: Evans UP, 2012. Print.

Figure 23.3 An authoritative Web site and a questionable Web site.

An authoritative Web site

A .gov URL signals government sponsorship.

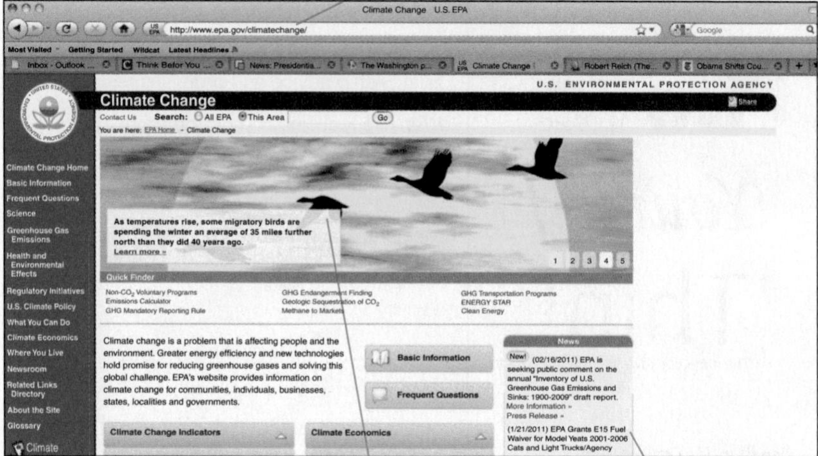

Site points to a wide range of information.

Site emphasizes facts.

Site is current.

A questionable Web site

A .com URL means you should check the nature and motives of the group.

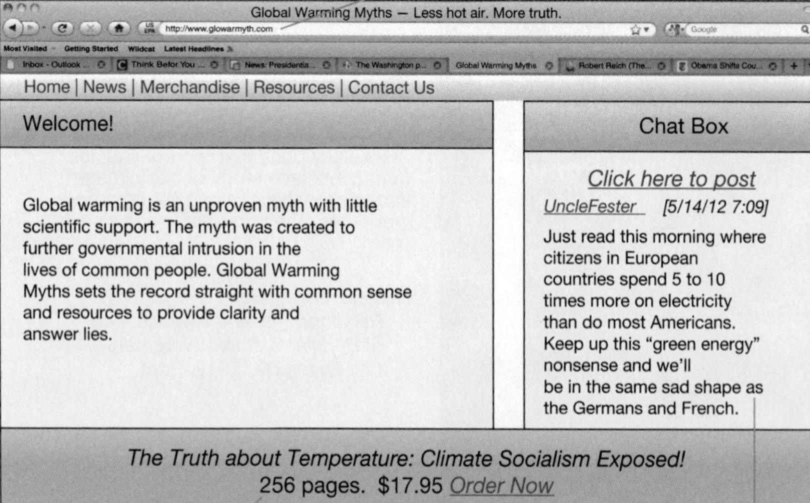

Advertising.

Chat box will contain information that hasn't been reviewed.

Note: Site might have worthy information, but it needs checking.

Figure 23.4 A section from an original article and a misused quotation from that article.

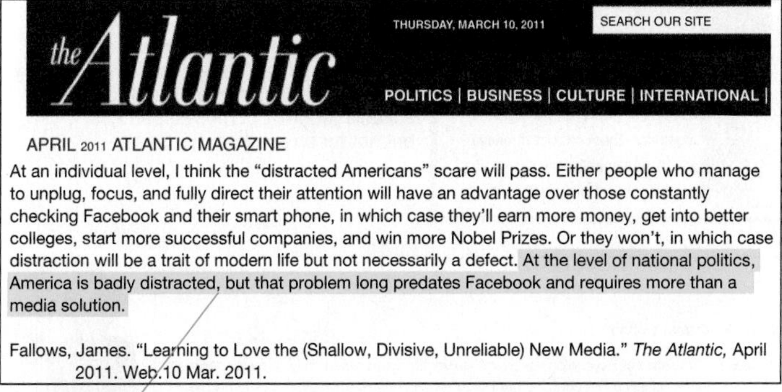

the Atlantic
THURSDAY, MARCH 10, 2011
SEARCH OUR SITE
POLITICS | BUSINESS | CULTURE | INTERNATIONAL |

APRIL 2011 ATLANTIC MAGAZINE

At an individual level, I think the "distracted Americans" scare will pass. Either people who manage to unplug, focus, and fully direct their attention will have an advantage over those constantly checking Facebook and their smart phone, in which case they'll earn more money, get into better colleges, start more successful companies, and win more Nobel Prizes. Or they won't, in which case distraction will be a trait of modern life but not necessarily a defect. At the level of national politics, America is badly distracted, but that problem long predates Facebook and requires more than a media solution.

Fallows, James. "Learning to Love the (Shallow, Divisive, Unreliable) New Media." *The Atlantic,* April 2011. Web. 10 Mar. 2011.

Comment on original: In the original full article from *The Atlantic*, a serious magazine for general readers, James Fallows agrees that Americans are distracted when it comes to politics, but he does not blame the Internet for that situation.

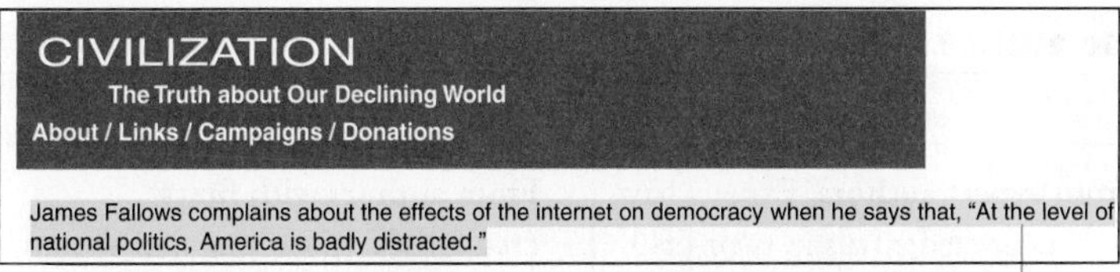

CIVILIZATION
The Truth about Our Declining World
About / Links / Campaigns / Donations

James Fallows complains about the effects of the internet on democracy when he says that, "At the level of national politics, America is badly distracted."

Comment on misused quotation: The Civilization Web site misrepresents Fallows. By using only part of his quotation, it makes him express exactly the opposite of what he actually wrote. It would be a serious mistake to quote this site.

23C Is the author qualified to write about the topic?

Anyone can express an opinion or argue a course of action, but writers worth quoting or summarizing have knowledge and expertise about their topics. Often, their credentials appear in an introduction, at the bottom of the first page, or at the end of an article. Look for an "About the Author" statement in a book; a short biography on a Web site; or a "Contributors" note (see Figure 23.5). Sometimes, however, you might need to do a little investigating to learn about the author.

ESOL Tip: The definition of "authority" can differ across cultures. However, in the United States, a source must meet specific criteria to be considered authoritative. It must appear in a scholarly book or journal; its author must have a degree, title, or license; or other authorities must seek his or her knowledge. A source is not reliable simply because the author or speaker is an influential or well-known member of the community, claims to have knowledge about a topic, or publishes material in print or online.

Figure 23.5 An author with scholarly credentials and an author without.

Start Loving Life!

Hi! I'm **Marilyn McIntire**, motivational speaker, fitness guru, relationship coach, and author. My life has been an astonishing adventure, and yours can be, too. Let's walk this journey together! Check me out whenever you need inspiration, advice, and a good laugh. —Rainbow joys, Marilyn

If you were writing an academic paper on dieting and evaluating the two books in Figure 23.2 (page 295), the credentials of Sarah Neufeld would be much more credible. (Marilyn McIntire's credentials would be suitable for other purposes, perhaps, but not for an academic paper.)

Sarah Neufeld

Psychology Department Chair

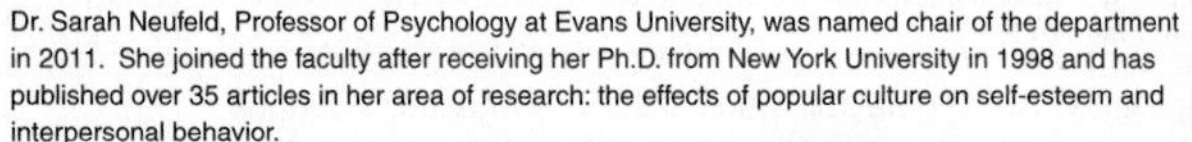

Dr. Sarah Neufeld, Professor of Psychology at Evans University, was named chair of the department in 2011. She joined the faculty after receiving her Ph.D. from New York University in 1998 and has published over 35 articles in her area of research: the effects of popular culture on self-esteem and interpersonal behavior.

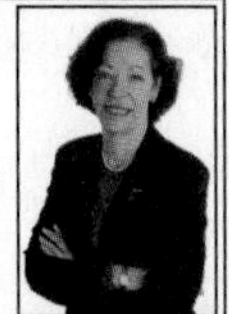

Is the author qualified to write about the topic?

Reliable sources are . . .	Questionable sources are . . .
• **From expert authors.** Experts have degrees or credentials in their field. Biographical material in the source may list these credentials. If in doubt, look up the author in a biographical dictionary, search online for a resume or bio, or search a database. Check if the author's name appears in other reliable sources; do others cite him or her? Check whether there is contact information for questions or comments.	• **From authors with fuzzy credentials.** A warning sign should flash when you can't identify who has produced a source. Discussion threads, anonymous blogs, and similar online postings are questionable when they don't give qualifying information. Check that listed credentials fit the topic. Just because someone has a graduate degree in history, for example, doesn't qualify him or her to give medical advice.

23D Does the source have sufficient and accurate evidence?

If an author expresses a point of view but offers little evidence to back up that position, reject the source. See Figure 23.6 for an example of how sources use evidence.

Figure 23.6 Source that cites evidence and source that does not.

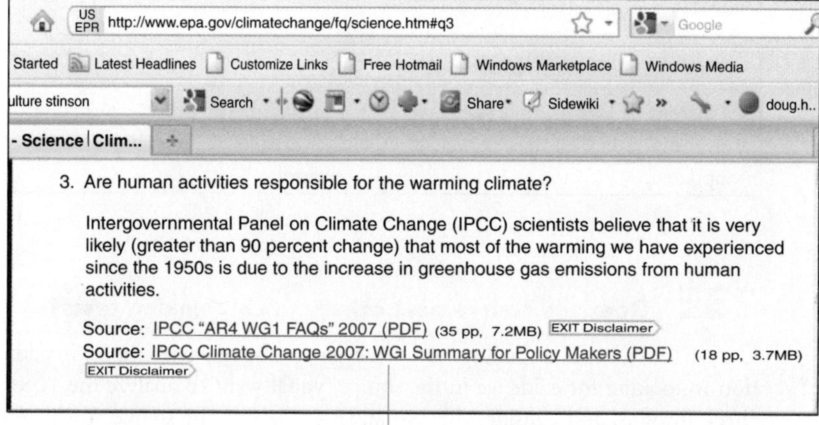

The Environmental Protection Agency provides specific facts, and the source of those facts.

> RedDawn [6/13/2012]
> So it's been hot and the global warming clones are screeming again. Big deal. many scientists show that theres no proof we're making the world warmer, just google it if you want to know the truth. If the temperatures increasing, its because of natural causes not pollution, smoke, etc. Politicians wont give money to real scientists to prove it. Common sense, people!

This posting, from a blog, makes claims but provides no evidence, simply telling readers to "just google it."

The source has some proofreading errors, substitutes name-calling for reasoning, and has other logical fallacies.

Does the source have sufficient and accurate evidence?

Reliable sources are . . .	Questionable sources are . . .
• **Well supported with evidence.** The writer cites clear and plentiful facts and reasons to support assertions.	• **Unsupported or biased.** They carry assertions that have little or no supporting evidence.
• **Factually accurate.** Listed are the sources for statistics, quotations, and other information. You (or anyone else) could look them up to check their accuracy.	• **Factually questionable.** Although they may include statistics or other information, they fail to identify who generated them or how. You have no way to check facts because the writer failed to provide this information.

(*continued*)

Reliable sources are . . .	Questionable sources are . . .
• **Current.** Information is recent or, in the case of Web sites, regularly updated.	• **Outdated.** You don't want to cite 20-year-old medical advice, for example.

23E Does the source pass other critical thinking tests?

Use CRITICAL THINKING skills when you evaluate a source (see Ch. 3). In addition to looking for evidence in the source, you'll want to analyze the TONE, check for BIAS, and consider the ASSUMPTIONS behind the source. You'll certainly want to check for LOGICAL FALLACIES (see Ch. 3). Figure 23.7 shows a Web site with a fairly balanced tone and one that is more biased.

Figure 23.7 A source with balanced tone and a source with biased tone.

Balanced tone

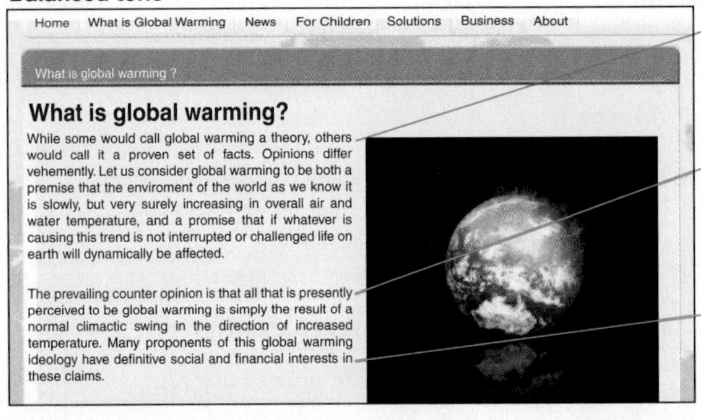

The writer acknowledges there is a difference of opinion.

The writer summarizes the point of view with which he or she disagrees.

There is a slight element of bias in saying that people have an ideology.

Biased tone

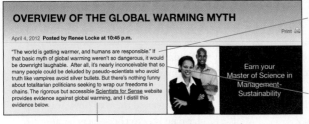

The writer relies on name-calling rather than acknowledging others.

The comparison to "vampires avoid silver bullets" gets readers' attention, but it's hardly respectful.

At least the writer promises to send readers to a "rigorous but accessible" informational site. You would have to evaluate that site to be sure.

Does the source pass other critical thinking tests?

Reliable sources are . . .	Questionable sources are . . .
• **Balanced in tone.** The author is respectful of others and creates a sense of fairness.	• **Biased in tone.** Some warning signs of biased tone are name-calling, sarcasm, stereotyping, or absolute assertions about matters that are open to interpretation.
• **Balanced in treatment.** Even if they advocate a particular position, credible sources acknowledge different viewpoints. For example, they summarize contradictory evidence.	• **One-sided.** Sources that omit any mention or fair summary of competing views or information may be unreliable, especially if they openly ridicule competing positions.
• **Logical.** The source draws fair conclusions from evidence. The reasoning is clear.	• **Full of logical fallacies.** See section 3I.
• **Well-edited**. The source has been proofread and is free of grammatical errors.	• **Marked by errors.** Beware if the source has typos or sloppy errors.

23F How do strategies for evaluating sources work together?

The most important quality of any reliable source is to be based on facts, evidence, and clear reasoning. If you're using sources that you find through library databases, from authoritative publishers or groups, and from expert writers, then the sources are likely to be reliable. You still need to think critically about them. On the other hand, if you're using sources that you find through general searches, from questionable publishers or organizations, or from writers with unclear expertise, then you have to work hard. You have to make sure that the facts, evidence, and reasoning are all solid.

24 Drafting and Revising a Research Paper

Quick Points You will learn to

➤ Write and revise a research paper (see following sections).

24A How does the writing process apply to research papers?

DRAFTING and REVISING a research paper is like drafting and revising any piece of writing (see Ch. 5). However, you need extra time to write a research paper because you need to demonstrate that:

- You've followed the steps of the research process (see Chs. 21–22).
- You've evaluated your SOURCES (see Ch. 23).
- You haven't PLAGIARIZED (see Ch. 19).
- You've correctly employed QUOTATIONS, PARAPHRASES, and SUMMARIES (see Ch. 18).
- You've moved beyond summary to SYNTHESIS so that your sources are interwoven with each other and with your own thinking, not merely listed one by one (see 18F–18L).
- You've used DOCUMENTATION accurately. (For MLA STYLE, see Chapter 25; for APA STYLE, see Chapter 26; for other documentation styles, see Chapter 27.)

24B How do I draft a thesis statement for a research paper?

A THESIS STATEMENT in a research paper sets out the central theme, which you need to sustain throughout the paper. As with any piece of writing, your research paper must fulfill the promise of its thesis statement. Remember that a good thesis statement makes an assertion that conveys your point of view about your topic and foreshadows the content of your paper.

One way to start your thesis statement is to try to convert your RESEARCH QUESTION into a preliminary thesis statement. Another way is to ask yourself whether the material you've gathered from sources can effectively support your thesis statement. If your answer is "no," you want to revise your thesis statement, conduct further research, or do both.

Here are examples of subjects narrowed to topics, focused into research questions, and then cast as thesis statements.

SUBJECT	***nonverbal communication***
TOPIC	Personal space
RESEARCH QUESTION	How do standards for personal space differ among cultures?
INFORMATIVE THESIS STATEMENT	Everyone has expectations concerning the use of personal space, but accepted distances for that space are determined by each person's culture.
PERSUASIVE THESIS STATEMENT	To prevent intercultural misunderstandings, people must be aware of cultural differences in standards for personal space.

SUBJECT	***computers***
TOPIC	artificial intelligence
RESEARCH QUESTION	How close are researchers to developing artificial intelligence in computers?
INFORMATIVE THESIS STATEMENT	Scientists disagree about whether computers need emotions to have artificial intelligence.
PERSUASIVE THESIS STATEMENT	Because emotions play a strong role in human intelligence, computers must have emotions before they can truly have artificial intelligence.

Andrei Gurov (whose research paper appears in section 25G) revised his preliminary thesis statement twice before he felt that it expressed the point he wanted to make. Andrei also took the key step of checking that he would be able to support it sufficiently.

FIRST PRELIMINARY THESIS STATEMENT

Déjà vu can be explained by a variety of scientific theories.

Andrei realized that this draft thesis would lead to a paper that would merely list, paragraph by paragraph, each theory, and that the paper would lack synthesis.

SECOND PRELIMINARY THESIS STATEMENT

Many people believe feelings of déjà vu have mysterious origins, but science has shown this is not true.

Andrei liked this statement better because it began to get at the complexity of the topic, but he wanted to work on it more because he felt the second part was too general.

FINAL THESIS STATEMENT

Although a few people today still prefer to believe that feelings of déjà vu have mysterious or supernatural origins, recent research in cognitive psychology and the neurosciences has shed much rational light on the phenomenon.

24C How do I outline a research paper?

Some, though not all, instructors require an OUTLINE of your research paper, either before you hand in the paper or along with the paper (see 5G). In such cases, your instructor is probably expecting you to be working from an outline as you write your drafts. Your research log can come in handy when you group ideas in an outline, especially for a first draft of your paper. To see a topic outline of Andrei Gurov's research paper, turn to section 25G.

24D How do I draft a research paper?

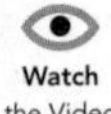
Watch the Video

You need to expect to write several drafts of your research paper. The first draft is a chance to discover new insights and fresh connections. Then use your first draft to revise into more developed and polished further drafts. Here are some ways to write your first draft.

- **Some researchers work from a source map.** They organize their notes into topics and determine the relationship between sources.
- **Some researchers work with their notes at hand.** They organize CONTENT NOTES into broad categories by creating a separate group for each topic. Each category then becomes a section of the first draft. This method often reveals any gaps in information that call for additional research. Also, you may discover that some of your research doesn't fit your topic or thesis statement. If so, put it aside; it might be useful in a later draft.
- **Some writers generate a list of questions that their paper needs to address.** Then they answer each question, one at a time, looking for the content notes that will help them. For example, writing on the topic of déjà vu, some possible questions might be, "What is déjà vu? What are possible explanations for it? Are there any benefits or dangers of déjà vu?" Generating and answering questions can be a very useful way of turning a mass of information into manageable groupings.
- **Some researchers stop at various points and use FREEWRITING to get their ideas into words.** Researchers who use this method say that it helps them to recognize when they need to adjust their research question or change their search. After a number of rounds of researching and freewriting, these researchers find that they can write their complete first draft relatively easily.

- **Some researchers review their sources and create an OUTLINE before drafting (see 5G).** Some find a FORMAL OUTLINE helpful, whereas others use a less formal approach.
- **Some researchers use a frame to guide their drafting (see 24E).**

24E What are frames for research papers?

Although all research papers seek to answer a question, some are mainly informative, others are mainly persuasive, and still others are a mix. We offer two possible frames for research papers in this section.

Frame for an Informative Research Paper

Introductory paragraph(s)

- **Establish why your topic is important or interesting**. Consider, "Why does this matter? To whom does this matter? What might happen if we resolve this issue one way versus another?"
- **Your THESIS STATEMENT needs to make clear** how you will answer your research question.

Body paragraph(s): background information

- **Provide the history or background of your topic**. Why is it a problem or concern at this time?

Body paragraphs: Explanations of topics

- **Discuss the main subtopics** of your general topic in a paragraph with a clear TOPIC SENTENCE.
- **If a subtopic is lengthy**, it may require more than one paragraph.

Body Paragraphs: Complications

- **Discuss what is controversial or in dispute.** What do people disagree about? Why? Do they dispute facts? Interpretations? Causes? Effects or implications? Solutions?

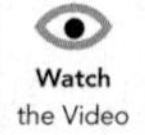
Watch the Video

Conclusion

- **Wrap up your topic.** What questions or issues remain? What are areas for further research or investigation? What might readers do with this information?

Works Cited or References

- **If you are using MLA STYLE,** include a list of Works Cited (see Ch. 25); if you are using APA style, include a References list (see Ch. 26).

For an example of an informative research paper, see the MLA STYLE research paper in section 25G.

Frame for an Argumentative Research Paper

Introductory paragraph(s)

- **Establish why your topic is important or interesting**. Consider, "Why does this matter? To whom does this matter? What might happen if we resolve this issue one way versus another?"
- **Your THESIS STATEMENT needs to make clear** how you will answer your research question.

Body paragraph(s): background information

- **Provide the history or background of your topic**. Why is it a problem or concern at this time?

Body paragraph(s): Agreement among sources

- **Discuss points of agreement**. What is uncontroversial or widely accepted?
- **Depending on the size or nature of the topic,** this may be one or several paragraphs.

Body paragraph(s): Complications

- **Discuss what is controversial or in dispute**. What do people disagree about? Why? Do they dispute facts? Interpretations? Causes? Effects or implications? Solutions?

Body paragraph(s): Arguments

- **Present your arguments**. What reasons do you have for your position or proposed action? State each reason as a TOPIC SENTENCE, and provide evidence and support in the paragraph.
- **If you have extensive support** for a particular reason, you might need more than one paragraph.

Conclusion

- **Wrap up your argument.** Why is your position or proposal best? What actions should follow?

Works Cited or References

- **If you are using MLA STYLE,** include a list of Works Cited (see Ch. 25); if you are using APA style, include a References list (see Ch. 26).

For an example of an argumentative research paper in MLA STYLE, see Chapter 15. For an example of an argumentative research paper in APA STYLE, see section 26I.

24F How do I revise a research paper?

To revise your research paper, before you write each new draft, read your previous draft with a sharp eye. Assess all of the features listed in Quick Box 24.1. For best results, take a break for a few days (or at least a few hours) before beginning this process. Consider asking a few people you respect to read and react to a draft (see 9D).

Quick Box 24.1

Revision checklist for a research paper

If the answer to a question in this checklist is no, you need to revise. The section numbers in parentheses tell you where to find helpful information.

WRITING

✓ Does your introductory paragraph lead effectively into the material (see 6C)?

✓ Have you met the basic requirements for a written thesis statement (see 5F)?

✓ Do your thesis statement and the content of your paper address your research question(s) (see 24B)?

✓ Have you developed effective body paragraphs (see 6F)?

✓ Do your ideas follow sensibly and logically within each paragraph and from one paragraph to the next (see 6G)?

✓ Does the concluding paragraph end your paper effectively (see 6J)?

✓ Does your paper satisfy a critical thinker (see Ch. 3)?

RESEARCH

✓ Have you fully answered your research question (see 21F)?

✓ Have you evaluated the quality of your sources? Do you have the kinds of sources that are appropriate for academic writing (see Ch. 23)?

✓ Have you used quotations, paraphrases, and summaries well (see Ch. 19)?

✓ Have you integrated your source material well without plagiarizing (see Chs. 18 and 20)?

One key to revising any research paper is to examine carefully the evidence you've included. **Evidence** consists of facts, statistics, expert studies and opinions, examples, and stories. Use RENNS (see 6F) to develop paragraphs more fully. Identify each of the points you have made in your paper, including your THESIS STATEMENT and all your subpoints. Then ask the following questions.

- **Is the evidence sufficient?** To be sufficient, evidence can't be thin or trivial. As a rule, the more evidence you present, the more convincing your thesis will be to readers.
- **Is the evidence representative?** Representative evidence is customary and normal, not based on exceptions.
- **Is the evidence relevant?** Relevant evidence relates directly to your thesis or topic sentence. It never introduces unrelated material.
- **Is the evidence accurate?** Accurate evidence is correct, complete, and up to date. It comes from a reliable source. Equally important, you present it honestly, without distorting or misrepresenting it.
- **Is the evidence reasonable?** Reasonable evidence is not phrased in extreme language and avoids sweeping generalizations. Reasonable evidence is free of LOGICAL FALLACIES (see 3I).

24G How do I edit and format a research paper?

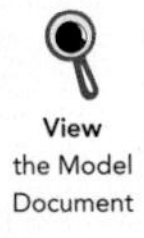

As with every paper, you'll want to make sure that there are no errors in grammar, punctuation, or mechanics. You'll want to check your style and tone. Research papers have additional requirements in documentation, citation, and format. Quick Box 24.2 lists questions to ask.

Quick Box 24.2

Editing and formatting checklist for a research paper

- ✓ Is the paper free of errors in grammar, punctuation, and mechanics?
- ✓ Are your style and tone effective?
- ✓ Have you used the correct format in your parenthetical references (see 25A or 26A)?
- ✓ Does each of your parenthetical references tie into an item in your Works Cited list (MLA STYLE) or References list (APA STYLE) at the end of your paper or follow CM or CSE styles (see Ch. 25, 26, or 27)?
- ✓ Does the paper exactly match the format you've been assigned to follow? Check margins, spacing, title, headings, page numbers, font, and so on (see 25F or 26F).

25 MLA Documentation with Case Study

Quick Points You will learn to

- Use MLA in-text parenthetical documentation (see 25B and 25C).
- Create an MLA Works Cited page (see 25D and 25E).
- Format your paper according to MLA guidelines (see 25F).

MLA In-Text Citation Directory

MLA Works Cited List Directory

25A What is MLA documentation style?

A DOCUMENTATION STYLE* is a standard format that writers use to tell readers what SOURCES they used and how readers can locate them. Different disciplines follow different documentation styles. The one most frequently used in the humanities is from the Modern Language Association (MLA).

MLA style requires writers to document their sources in two connected, equally important ways.

1. Within the body of the paper, you need to use parenthetical documentation, as described in sections 25B and 25C.
2. At the end of the paper, you need to provide a list of the sources you used in your paper. This list is called "Works Cited," as described in 25D and 25E.

The guidelines and examples in this chapter are based on the Seventh Edition of *The MLA Handbook for Writers of Research Papers* (2009), which is the most current edition. If you need more information regarding MLA STYLE updates, check http://www.mla.org. See Quick Box 25.1 on pages 317–320 for more guidance on following these requirements.

25B What is MLA in-text parenthetical documentation?

MLA-style **parenthetical documentation** (also called **in-text citations**) places source information in parentheses within the sentences of your research papers. This information—given each time you SUMMARIZE, PARAPHRASE, or

* Words printed in SMALL CAPITAL LETTERS are discussed elsewhere in the text and are defined in the Terms Glossary at the back of the book.

use a QUOTATION from source materials—signals materials used from sources and enables readers to find the originals. (See Chapter 18 for information on how to quote, paraphrase, and summarize.)

Author name cited in text; page number cited in parentheses If you include an author's name (or, if none, the title of the work) in the sentence to introduce your source material, you include in parentheses only the page number where you found the material:

> According to Brent Staples, IQ tests give scientists little insight into intelligence (293).

For readability and good writing technique, try to introduce the names of authors (or titles of sources) in your own sentences.

Author name and page number cited in parentheses If you don't include the author's name in your sentence, you need to insert it in the parentheses, before the page number. Use no punctuation between the author's name and the page number:

> IQ tests give scientists little insight into intelligence (Staples 293).

25B.1 Placement of parenthetical reference

When possible, position a parenthetical reference at the end of the quotation, summary, or paraphrase it refers to. The best position is at the end of a sentence, unless that would place it too far from the source's material. When you do place the parenthetical reference at the end of a sentence, insert it before the sentence-ending period.

When you cite a quotation enclosed in quotation marks, place the parenthetical information after the closing quotation mark but before sentence-ending punctuation.

> Coleman summarizes research that shows that "the number, rate, and direction of time-zone changes are the critical factors in determining the extent and degree of jet lag symptoms" (67).

25B.2 Block quotations: longer than four lines

The one exception to the rule of putting parenthetical information before sentence-ending punctuation concerns quotations that you set off in block style, meaning one inch from the left margin. (MLA requires that quotations longer than four typed lines be handled this way.) For block quotations, put the parenthetical reference after the period.

Bruce Sterling worries that people are pursuing less conventional medical treatments, and not always for good reasons:

> Medical tourism is already in full swing. Thailand is the golden shore for wealthy, sickly Asians and Australians. Fashionable Europeans head to South Africa for embarrassing plastic surgery. Crowds of scrip-waving Americans buy prescription drugs in Canada and Mexico. (92)

If you're quoting part of a paragraph or one complete paragraph, don't indent the first line of quoted words any extra space beyond the one inch of the entire block. But if you quote more than one paragraph, indent the first line of each paragraph—including the first if it's a complete paragraph from the source—an additional quarter inch.

25C What are examples of MLA parenthetical citations?

The directory at the beginning of this tab corresponds to the numbered examples in this section. Most of these examples show the author's name or the title included in the parenthetical citation, but remember that it's usually more effective to include that information in your sentence.

1. One Author

Give an author's name as it appears on the source: for a book, on the title page; for an article, directly below the title or at the end of the article.

> IQ tests give scientists little insight into intelligence (Staples 293).

2. Two or Three Authors

Give the names in the same order as in the source. Spell out *and.* For three authors, use commas to separate the authors' names.

> As children get older, they begin to express several different kinds of intelligence (Todd and Taylor 23).

> Another measure of emotional intelligence is the success of inter- and intrapersonal relationships (Voigt, Dees, and Prigoff 14).

3. More Than Three Authors

If your source has more than three authors, you can name them all or use the first author's name only, followed by *et al.*, either in a parenthetical reference or in your sentence. *Et al.* is an abbreviation of the Latin *et alii,* meaning "and others." Don't underline or italicize *et al.* Note that no period follows *et,* but one follows *al.*

> Emotional security varies, depending on the circumstances of the social interaction (Carter et al. 158).

4. More Than One Source by an Author

When you use two or more sources by the same author, include the title of the individual source in each citation. In parenthetical citations, you can use a shortened version of the title. (The Works Cited listing requires the whole title.) For example, in a paper using two of Howard Gardner's works, *Frames of Mind: The Theory of Multiple Intelligences* and "Reflections on Multiple Intelligences: Myths and Messages," use *Frames* and "Reflections," respectively. In shortening titles be sure they aren't ambiguous to readers, and always start with the word by which the work is alphabetized in your WORKS CITED list. Separate the author's name and the title with a comma, but don't use punctuation between the title and page number.

> Although it seems straightforward to think of multiple intelligences as multiple approaches to learning (Gardner, *Frames* 60–61), an intelligence is not a learning style (Gardner, "Reflections" 202–03).

When you incorporate the title into your own sentences, use the full title, though you can omit a subtitle. After the first mention, you can shorten the title.

5. Two or More Authors with the Same Last Name

Use each author's first initial and full last name in each parenthetical citation. If both authors have the same first initial, use the full first name in all instances.

> According to Anne Cates, psychologists can predict how empathetic an adult will be from his or her behavior at age two (41), but other researchers disagree (T. Cates 171).

6. Group or Corporate Author

When a corporation or other group is named as the author of a source you want to cite, use the corporate name the same way you would an author's name.

> A five-year study shows that these tests are usually unreliable (Boston Women's Health Collective 11).

7. Work Cited by Title

If no author is named, use only the title. If the title is long, shorten it. Here's an in-text citation for an article titled "Are You a Day or Night Person?"

> The "morning lark" and "night owl" descriptions typically are used to categorize the human extremes ("Are You" 11).

8. Multivolume Work

If you use more than one volume of a multivolume work, include the relevant volume number in each citation. Separate the volume number and page number with a colon followed by a space.

Although Amazon forest dwellers had been exposed to these viruses by 1900 (Rand 3: 202), Borneo forest dwellers escaped them until the 1960s (Rand 1: 543).

9. Novel, Play, Short Story, or Poem

Literary works frequently appear in different editions. When you cite material from literary works, provide the part, chapter, act, scene, canto, stanza, or line numbers. This usually helps readers locate what you're referring to more easily than do page numbers alone. Unless your instructor tells you not to, use arabic numerals for these references, even if the literary work uses roman numerals. For novels that use part and/or chapter numbers, include them after page numbers. Use a semicolon after the page number but a comma to separate a part from a chapter.

Flannery O'Connor describes one character in *The Violent Bear It Away* as "divided in two—a violent and a rational self" (139; pt. 2, ch. 6).

For plays that use them, give act, scene, and line numbers. Use periods between these numbers. For short stories, use page numbers.

Among the most quoted of Shakespeare's lines is Hamlet's soliloquy beginning "To be, or not to be: that is the question" (3.1.56).

The old man in John Collier's "The Chaser" says about his potions, "I don't deal in laxatives and teething mixtures . . ." (79).

For poems and songs, give canto, stanza, and/or line numbers. Use periods between these numbers.

In "To Autumn," Keats's most melancholy image occurs in the lines "Then in a wailful choir the small gnats mourn / Among the river swallows" (3.27–28).

10. Bible or Sacred Text

Give the title of the edition you're using, the book (in the case of the Bible), and the chapter and verse. Spell out the names of books in sentences, but use abbreviations in parenthetical references.

He would certainly benefit from the advice in Ephesians to "get rid of all bitterness, rage, and anger" (*New International Version Bible*, 4.31).

He would certainly benefit from the advice to "get rid of all bitterness, rage, and anger" (*New International Version Bible*, Eph. 4.31).

11. Work in an Anthology or Other Collection

You may want to cite a work you have read in a book that contains many works by various authors and that was compiled or edited by someone other than the person you're citing. Your in-text citation should include the author of the selection you're citing and the page number. For example, suppose you want to cite the poem "Several Things" by Martha Collins, in a literature text edited by Pamela Annas and Robert Rosen. Use Collins's name and the title of her work in the sentence and the line numbers (see item 9) in a parenthetical citation.

> In "Several Things," Martha Collins enumerates what could take place in the lines of her poem: "Plums could appear, on a pewter plate / A dead red hare, hung by one foot. / A vase of flowers. Three shallots" (2–4).

12. Indirect Source

When you want to quote words that you found quoted in someone else's work, put the name of the person whose words you're quoting into your own sentence. Give the work where you found the quotation either in your sentence or in a parenthetical citation beginning with *qtd. in*.

> Martin Scorsese acknowledges the link between himself and his films: "I realize that all my life, I've been an outsider. I splatter bits of myself all over the screen" (qtd. in Giannetti and Eyman 397).

13. Two or More Sources in One Reference

If more than one source has contributed to an idea, opinion, or fact in your paper, cite them all. An efficient way to credit all is to include them in a single parenthetical citation, with a semicolon separating each source.

> Once researchers agreed that multiple intelligences existed, their next step was to try to measure or define them (West 17; Arturi 477; Gibbs 68).

14. An Entire Work

References to an entire work usually fit best into your own sentences.

> In *Convergence Culture*, Henry Jenkins explores how new digital media create a culture of active participation rather than passive reception.

15. Electronic Source with Page Numbers

The principles that govern in-text citations of electronic sources are exactly the same as the ones that apply to books, articles, or other sources. When an electronically accessed source identifies its author, use the author's name for parenthetical references. If no author is named, use the title of the source. When an electronic source has page numbers, use them exactly as you would the page numbers of a print source.

> Learning happens best when teachers truly care about their students' complete well-being (Anderson 7).

16. Electronic Source without Page Numbers

Many online sources don't number pages. In such cases, simply refer to those works in their entirety. Try to include the name of the author in your sentence.

> In "What Is Artificial Intelligence?" John McCarthy notes that the science of artificial intelligence includes efforts beyond trying to simulate human intelligence.

25D What are MLA guidelines for a Works Cited list?

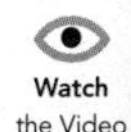

In MLA-style DOCUMENTATION, the **Works Cited** list gives complete bibliographic information for each SOURCE used in your paper. Include all—but only—the sources from which you quote, paraphrase, or summarize. Quick Box 25.1 gives general information about the Works Cited list. The rest of this chapter gives models of many specific kinds of Works Cited entries.

Quick Box 25.1

Guidelines for an MLA-style Works Cited list

See 25G for a sample student Works Cited list.

TITLE

Use "Works Cited" (without quotation marks), centered, as the title.

PLACEMENT OF LIST

Start a new page numbered sequentially with the rest of the paper, following the Notes pages, if any.

CONTENT AND FORMAT

Include all sources quoted from, paraphrased, or summarized in your paper. Start each entry on a new line and at the regular left margin. If the entry uses more than one line, indent the second and all following lines one-half inch from the left margin. Double-space all lines.

SPACING AFTER PUNCTUATION

Use one space after a period, unless your instructor asks you to use two. Always put only one space after a comma or a colon.

ARRANGEMENT OF ENTRIES

Alphabetize by author's last name. If no author is named, alphabetize by the title's first significant word (ignore *A*, *An*, and *The*).

continued >>

Quick Box 25.1 (continued)

AUTHORS' NAMES

Use first names and middle names or middle initials, if any, as given in the source. Don't reduce to initials any name that is given in full. For one author or the first-named author in multiauthor works, give the last name first. Use the word *and* with two or more authors. List multiple authors in the order given in the source. Use a comma between the first author's last and first names and after each complete author name except the last, which ends with a period: Fein, Ethel Andrea, Bert Griggs, and Delaware Rogash.

Include *Jr., Sr., II,* or *III* but no other titles or degrees before or after a name. For example, an entry for a work by Edward Meep III, MD, and Sir Richard Bolton would start like this: Meep, Edward, III, and Richard Bolton.

CAPITALIZATION OF TITLES

Capitalize all major words and the first and last words of all titles and subtitles. Don't capitalize ARTICLES (*a, an, the*), PREPOSITIONS, COORDINATING CONJUNCTIONS, or *to* in INFINITIVES in the middle of a title. These rules also apply to the titles of your own papers.

SPECIAL TREATMENT OF TITLES

Use quotation marks around titles of shorter works (poems, short stories, essays, articles). Use italics for the titles of longer works (books, periodicals, plays).

When a book title includes the title of another work that is usually in italics (such as a novel, play, or long poem), the preferred MLA style is not to italicize the incorporated title: *Decoding* Jane Eyre.

If the incorporated title is usually enclosed in quotation marks (such as a short story or short poem), keep the quotation marks and italicize the complete title of the book: *Theme and Form in "I Shall Laugh Purely": A Brief Study.*

Drop *A, An,* or *The* as the first word of a periodical title.

PLACE OF PUBLICATION

If several cities are listed for the place of publication, give only the first. MLA doesn't require US state names, so give only the city name. For an unfamiliar city outside the United States, include an abbreviated name of the country or Canadian province. If there is no place of publication, use "N.p."

PUBLISHER

Use shortened names for publishers as long as they're clear: *Random* for *Random House.* For companies named for more than one person, name only the first: *Prentice* for *Prentice Hall.* For university presses, use the capital letters

continued >>

Quick Box 25.1 (continued)

U and *P* (without periods) instead of the words *University* and *Press:* Oxford UP, U of Chicago P

PUBLICATION MONTH ABBREVIATIONS

Abbreviate all publication months except *May, June,* and *July*. Use the first three letters followed by a period (*Dec., Feb.*) except for September (*Sept.*).

PAGE RANGES

Give the page range—the starting page number and the ending page number, connected by a hyphen—of any paginated electronic source and any paginated print source that is part of a longer work (for example, a chapter in a book, an article in a journal). The range indicates that the cited work is on those pages and all pages in between. If that is not the case, use the style shown next for discontinuous pages (see below). In either case, use numerals only, without the word *page* or *pages* or the abbreviation *p.* or *pp.*

Use the full second number in a range through 99. Above that, use only the last two digits for the second number unless it would be unclear: 103–04 is clear, but 567–02 is not, so use the full numbers 567–602.

DISCONTINUOUS PAGES

A source has discontinuous pages when the source is interrupted by material that's not part of the sections of the source you're using (for example, an article beginning on page 32 but continued on page 54). Use the starting page number followed by a plus sign (+): 32+.

MEDIUM OF PUBLICATION

Include the medium (the type) of publication for each Works Cited entry. For example, every entry for a print source must include "Print" at the end, followed by a period. Every source from the World Wide Web must include *Web* at the end, followed by a period and the date of access. The medium of publication can be broadcast sources (*Television, Radio*), sound recordings (*CD, LP, Audiocassette*), as well as films, DVDs, live performances, musical scores and works of visual art, and so on. If required, certain supplementary bibliographic information like translation information, name of a book series, or the total number of volumes in a set should follow the medium of publication.

ISSUE AND VOLUME NUMBERS FOR SCHOLARLY JOURNALS

Include both an issue and volume number for each Works Cited entry for scholarly journals. This applies both to journals that are continuously paginated and those that are not.

continued >>

Quick Box 25.1 (continued)

URLs IN ELECTRONIC SOURCES

Entries for online citations should include the URL only when the reader probably could not locate the source without it. If the entry does require a URL, enclose it in angle brackets <like this>. Put the URL before the access date and end it with a period. If your computer automatically creates a hyperlink when you type a URL, format the URL to look the same as the rest of the entry. In applications like Microsoft Word, you can use the command "remove hyperlink," which you can find on the "Insert" menu or by right-clicking on the hyperlink. If a URL must be divided between two lines, only break the URL after a slash even if a line runs short. Do not use a hyphen.

25E What are MLA examples for sources in a Works Cited list?

The directory at the beginning of this chapter corresponds to the numbered examples in this section. Not every possible documentation model is here. You may find that you have to combine features of models to document a particular source. You will also find more information in the *MLA Handbook for Writers of Research Papers*. Figure 25.1 provides another tool to help you find the Works Cited model you need: a decision-making flowchart.

PERIODICALS

You can read periodical articles in four different formats. Some articles appear in all print and electronic versions; others are published in only one or two formats.

1. **Print.**
2. **Digital version in a database.** You most commonly access these sources through a DATABASE such as EBSCO or Academic Search Premier, which your library purchases.
3. **Digital version with direct online access.** Without going through a database, you access these sources directly on the Web, either by entering a specific URL or clicking on links provided by a search. (Of course, many other Web sources are not from periodicals; we explain them in examples 76–88.)
4. **Digital version on a digital reader.** Many devices allow you to access online content. These include e-readers like Kindle or Nook, computers or tablet computers (like iPads), or smart phones (like Android).

Figure 25.1 Decision-making flowchart for finding the right MLA citation format.

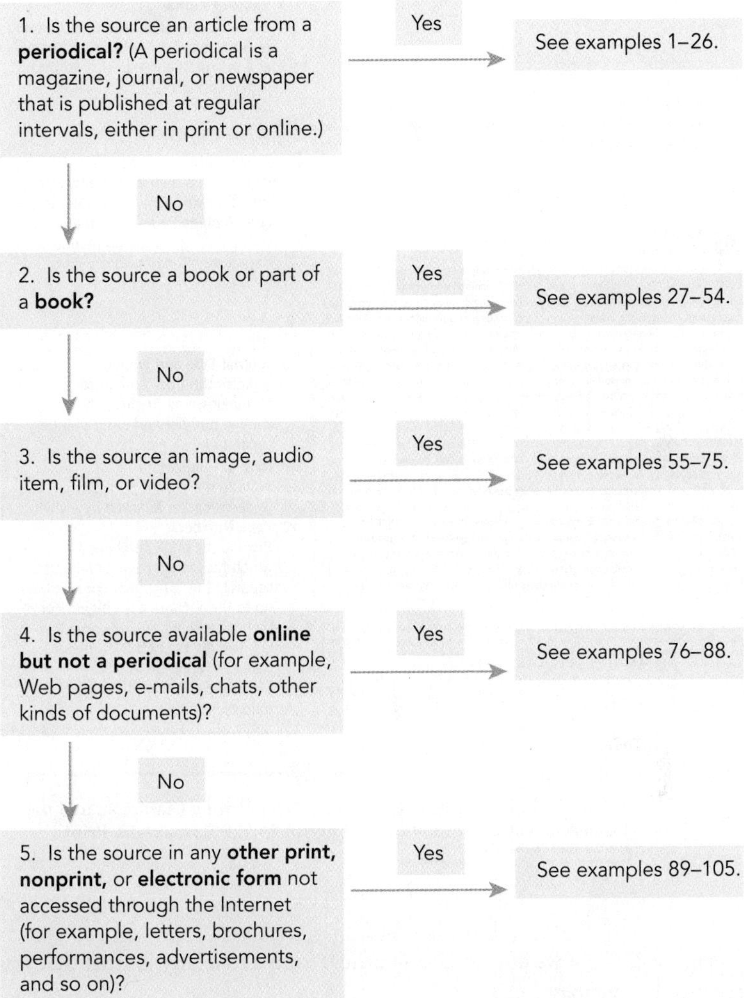

1. Is the source an article from a **periodical?** (A periodical is a magazine, journal, or newspaper that is published at regular intervals, either in print or online.)
Yes
See examples 1–26.
No
2. Is the source a book or part of a **book?**
Yes
See examples 27–54.
No
3. Is the source an image, audio item, film, or video?
Yes
See examples 55–75.
No
4. Is the source available **online but not a periodical** (for example, Web pages, e-mails, chats, other kinds of documents)?
Yes
See examples 76–88.
No
5. Is the source in any **other print, nonprint,** or **electronic form** not accessed through the Internet (for example, letters, brochures, performances, advertisements, and so on)?
Yes
See examples 89–105.

Citations for periodical articles contain three major parts: author, title of article, and publication information. The publication information differs according to not only the type of source (such as an editorial or a cartoon; see 16, below) but also how you access it (print, Web, and so on). If you access a source on the Web, you must include your date of access.

Figure 25.2 shows how to cite a print article from a scholarly journal.

Figure 25.2 Print article from a scholarly journal.

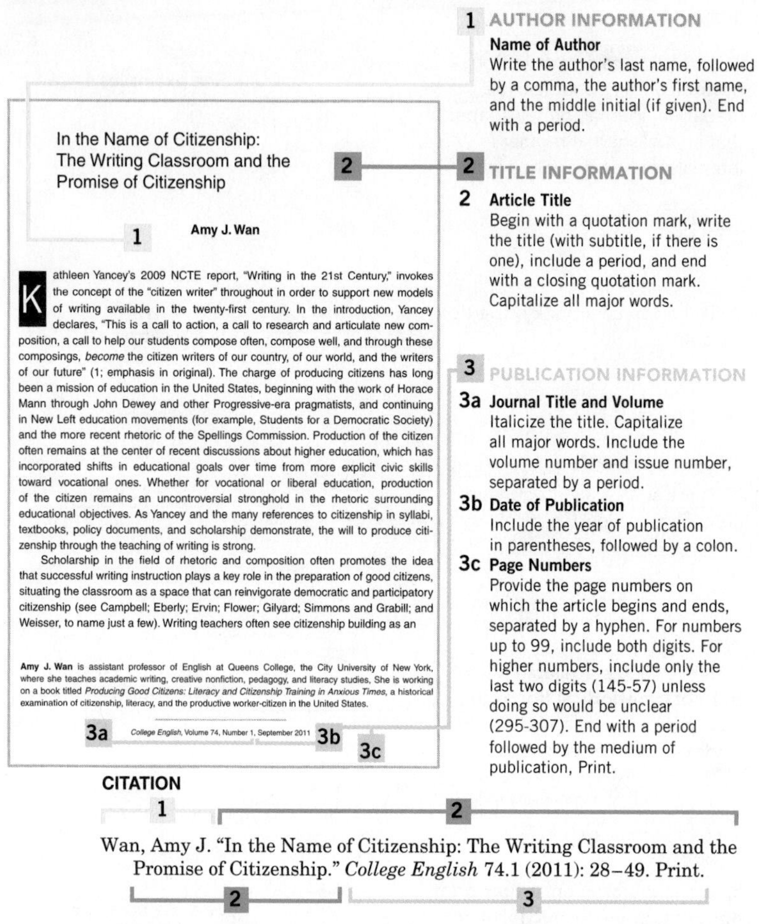

In the Name of Citizenship: The Writing Classroom and the Promise of Citizenship

Amy J. Wan

Kathleen Yancey's 2009 NCTE report, "Writing in the 21st Century," invokes the concept of the "citizen writer" throughout in order to support new models of writing available in the twenty-first century. In the introduction, Yancey declares, "This is a call to action, a call to research and articulate new composition, a call to help our students compose often, compose well, and through these composings, *become* the citizen writers of our country, of our world, and the writers of our future" (1; emphasis in original). The charge of producing citizens has long been a mission of education in the United States, beginning with the work of Horace Mann through John Dewey and other Progressive-era pragmatists, and continuing in New Left education movements (for example, Students for a Democratic Society) and the more recent rhetoric of the Spellings Commission. Production of the citizen often remains at the center of recent discussions about higher education, which has incorporated shifts in educational goals over time from more explicit civic skills toward vocational ones. Whether for vocational or liberal education, production of the citizen remains an uncontroversial stronghold in the rhetoric surrounding educational objectives. As Yancey and the many references to citizenship in syllabi, textbooks, policy documents, and scholarship demonstrate, the will to produce citizenship through the teaching of writing is strong.

Scholarship in the field of rhetoric and composition often promotes the idea that successful writing instruction plays a key role in the preparation of good citizens, situating the classroom as a space that can reinvigorate democratic and participatory citizenship (see Campbell; Eberly; Ervin; Flower; Gilyard; Simmons and Grabill; and Weisser, to name just a few). Writing teachers often see citizenship building as an

Amy J. Wan is assistant professor of English at Queens College, the City University of New York, where she teaches academic writing, creative nonfiction, pedagogy, and literacy studies, She is working on a book titled *Producing Good Citizens: Literacy and Citizenship Training in Anxious Times*, a historical examination of citizenship, literacy, and the productive worker-citizen in the United States.

College English, Volume 74, Number 1, September 2011

1
2
3a
3b
3c
1 AUTHOR INFORMATION
Name of Author
Write the author's last name, followed by a comma, the author's first name, and the middle initial (if given). End with a period.
2 TITLE INFORMATION
2 Article Title
Begin with a quotation mark, write the title (with subtitle, if there is one), include a period, and end with a closing quotation mark. Capitalize all major words.
3 PUBLICATION INFORMATION
3a Journal Title and Volume
Italicize the title. Capitalize all major words. Include the volume number and issue number, separated by a period.
3b Date of Publication
Include the year of publication in parentheses, followed by a colon.
3c Page Numbers
Provide the page numbers on which the article begins and ends, separated by a hyphen. For numbers up to 99, include both digits. For higher numbers, include only the last two digits (145-57) unless doing so would be unclear (295-307). End with a period followed by the medium of publication, Print.
CITATION
1
2
Wan, Amy J. "In the Name of Citizenship: The Writing Classroom and the Promise of Citizenship." *College English* 74.1 (2011): 28–49. Print.
2
3

Figure 25.3 shows how to cite an article from a scholarly journal that was accessed in a database.

Figure 25.4 (page 324) shows how to cite an article from a periodical that appears on the Web.

1. Article in a Scholarly Journal: Print

Williams, Bronwyn T. "Seeking New Worlds: The Study of Writing beyond Our Classrooms." *College Composition and Communication* 62.1 (2010): 127–46. Print.

Provide both volume and issue number, if available.

Figure 25.3 Article from a scholarly journal accessed in a database.

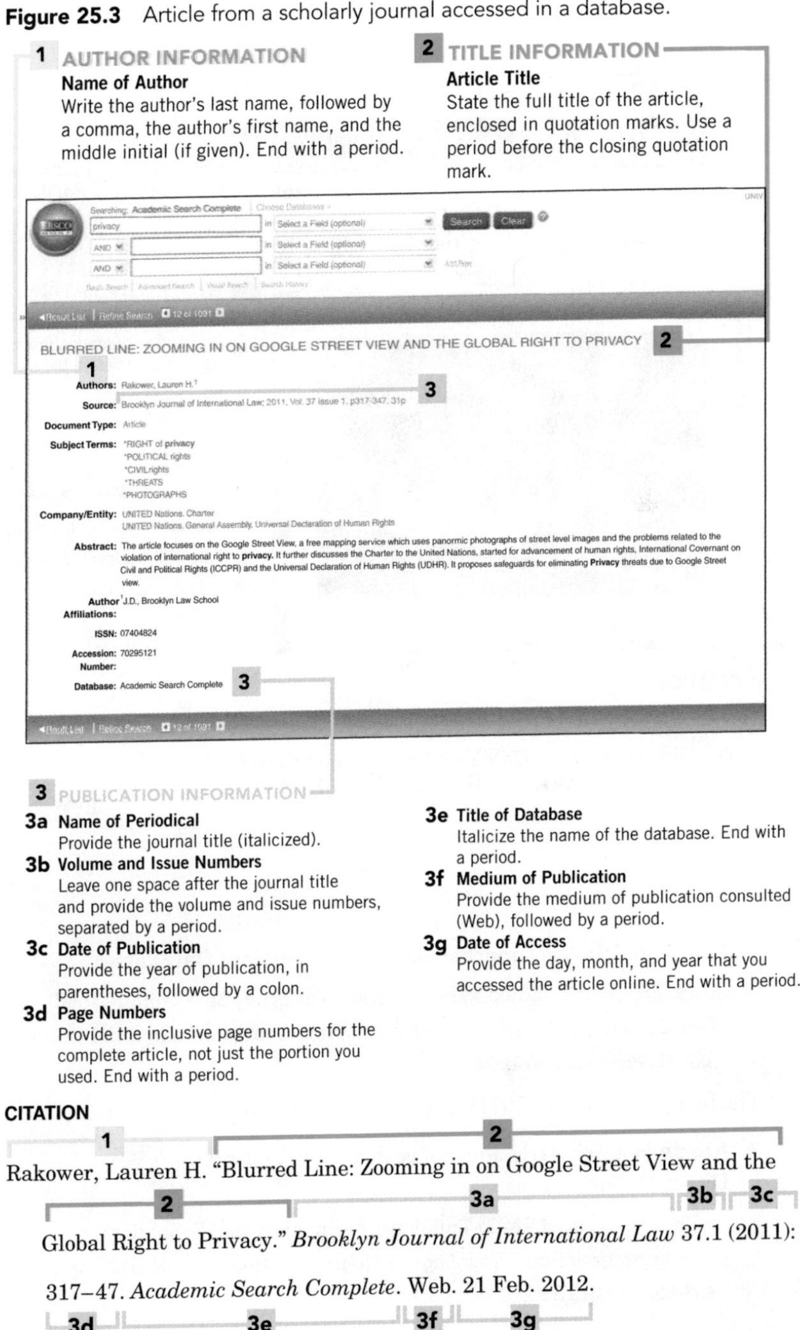
1 AUTHOR INFORMATION
Name of Author
Write the author's last name, followed by a comma, the author's first name, and the middle initial (if given). End with a period.
2 TITLE INFORMATION
Article Title
State the full title of the article, enclosed in quotation marks. Use a period before the closing quotation mark.
Searching: Academic Search Complete
privacy
Search
Clear
BLURRED LINE: ZOOMING IN ON GOOGLE STREET VIEW AND THE GLOBAL RIGHT TO PRIVACY
Authors: Rakower, Lauren H.
Source: Brooklyn Journal of International Law; 2011, Vol. 37 Issue 1, p317-347, 31p
Document Type: Article
Subject Terms: *RIGHT of privacy
*POLITICAL rights
*CIVIL rights
*THREATS
*PHOTOGRAPHS
Company/Entity: UNITED Nations. Charter
UNITED Nations. General Assembly. Universal Declaration of Human Rights
Abstract: The article focuses on the Google Street View, a free mapping service which uses panormic photographs of street level images and the problems related to the violation of international right to privacy. It further discusses the Charter to the United Nations, started for advancement of human rights, International Covernant on Civil and Political Rights (ICCPR) and the Universal Declaration of Human Rights (UDHR). It proposes safeguards for eliminating Privacy threats due to Google Street view.
Author Affiliations: J.D., Brooklyn Law School
ISSN: 07404824
Accession Number: 70295121
Database: Academic Search Complete
3 PUBLICATION INFORMATION
3a Name of Periodical
Provide the journal title (italicized).
3b Volume and Issue Numbers
Leave one space after the journal title and provide the volume and issue numbers, separated by a period.
3c Date of Publication
Provide the year of publication, in parentheses, followed by a colon.
3d Page Numbers
Provide the inclusive page numbers for the complete article, not just the portion you used. End with a period.
3e Title of Database
Italicize the name of the database. End with a period.
3f Medium of Publication
Provide the medium of publication consulted (Web), followed by a period.
3g Date of Access
Provide the day, month, and year that you accessed the article online. End with a period.
CITATION
Rakower, Lauren H. "Blurred Line: Zooming in on Google Street View and the Global Right to Privacy." *Brooklyn Journal of International Law* 37.1 (2011): 317–47. *Academic Search Complete*. Web. 21 Feb. 2012.

Figure 25.4 Article from periodical on the Web.

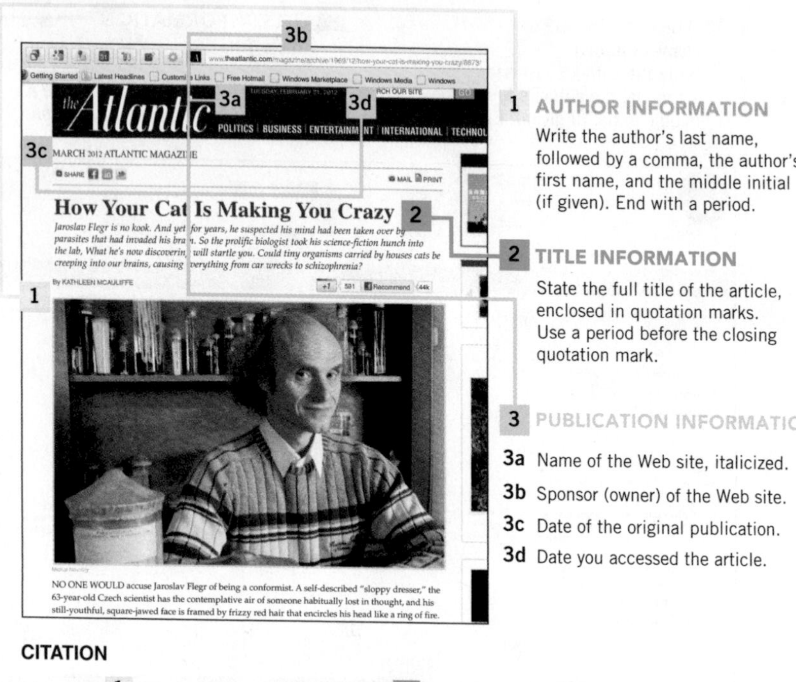

CITATION

1 2

McAuliffe, Kathleen. "How Your Cat Is Making You Crazy." *TheAtlantic.com*. The Atlantic, Mar. 2012. Web. 21 Feb. 2012.

3

2. Article in Scholarly Journal with a Print Version: Database

Williams, Bronwyn T. "Seeking New Worlds: The Study of Writing beyond Our Classrooms." *College Composition and Communication*. 62.1 (2010): 127–46. *Proquest*. Web. 24 Oct. 2011.

The final date (24 Oct. 2011) is the date you accessed the article on the Web.

3. Article in a Scholarly Journal with a Print Version: Direct Online Access

Hoge, Charles W., et al. "Mild Traumatic Brain Injury in U.S. Soldiers Returning from Iraq." *New England Journal of Medicine* 358.5 (2008): 453–63. Web. 10 Sept. 2008.

4. Article in a Scholarly Journal Published Only Online: Direct Online Access

Rutz, Paul X. "What a Painter of 'Historical Narrative' Can Tell Us about War Photography." *Kairos* 14.3 (2010). Web. 11 Nov. 2010.

Some periodicals appear only online and publish no print version.

5. Article in a Weekly or Biweekly Magazine: Print

Foroohar, Rana. "Why the World Isn't Getting Smaller." *Time* 27 June 2011: 20. Print.

If there is no author given, begin with the title of the article.

"The Price Is Wrong." *Economist* 2 Aug. 2003: 58–59. Print.

6. Article in a Weekly or Biweekly Magazine: Database

Foroohar, Rana. "Why the World Isn't Getting Smaller." *Time* 19 June 2011. *Academic Search Complete*. Web. 28 Aug. 2011.

7. Article in a Weekly or Biweekly Magazine: Direct Online Access

Foroohar, Rana. "Why the World Isn't Getting Smaller." *Time*. Time, 19 June 2011. Web. 27 Aug. 2011.

The name of the Web site is italicized. The sponsor (owner) of the Web site precedes the date of publication.

8. Article in a Monthly or Bimonthly Magazine: Print

Goetz, Thomas. "The Feedback Loop." *Wired* July 2011: 126–33. Print.

9. Article in a Monthly or Bimonthly Magazine: Database

Goetz, Thomas. "The Feedback Loop." *Wired* July 2011: 126–33. *ProQuest*. Web. 16 Sept. 2011.

10. Article in a Monthly or Bimonthly Magazine: Direct Online Access

Goetz, Thomas. "The Feedback Loop." *Wired*. Conde Nast, 19 June 2011. Web. 16 Sept. 2011.

11. Article Published Only Online: Direct Online Access

Ramirez, Eddy. "Comparing American Students with Those in China and India." *U.S. News and World Report*. U.S. News and World Report, 30 Jan. 2008. Web. 4 Mar. 2008.

Many periodicals have "extra" online content that doesn't appear in print. The article in example 11 is only online.

12. Article in a Newspaper: Print

Hesse, Monica. "Love among the Ruins." *Washington Post* 24 Apr. 2011: F1+. Print.

Omit *A, An,* or *The* as the first word in a newspaper title. Give the day, month, and year of the issue (and the edition, if applicable). If sections are designated, give the section letter as well as the page number. If an article runs on nonconsecutive pages, give the starting page number followed by a plus sign (for example, 1+ for an article that starts on page 1 and continues on a later page).

If no author is listed, begin with the title of the article.

"Prepping for Uranium Work." *Denver Post* 18 June 2011: B2. Print.

If the city of publication is not part of the title, put it in square brackets after the title, not italicized.

13. Article in a Newspaper with Print Version: Database

Hesse, Monica. "Falling in Love with St. Andrews, Scotland." *Washington Post* 24 Apr. 2011. *LexisNexis Academic*. Web. 3 Oct. 2011.

14. Article in a Newspaper with Print Version: Direct Online Access

Hesse, Monica. "Falling in Love with St. Andrews, Scotland." *Washington Post*. Washington Post, 22 Apr. 2011. Web. 3 Oct. 2011.

15. Article from a News Site Published Only Online: Direct Online Access

Katz, David. "What to Do about Flu? Get Vaccinated." *Huffington Post*. Huffington Post, 28 Oct. 2010. Web. 25 May 2012.

16. Editorial: Print

"Primary Considerations." Editorial. *Washington Post* 27 Jan. 2008: B6. Print.

If an author is listed, include her or his name before the title, then provide the title and information about the type of publication.

17. Editorial: Database

"Primary Considerations." Editorial. *Washington Post* 27 Jan. 2008. *LexisNexis Academic*. Web. 14 Feb. 2008.

18. Editorial: Direct Online Access

"Garbage In, Garbage Out." Editorial. *Los Angeles Times*. Los Angeles Times, 2 Feb. 2008. Web. 22 Mar. 2008.

19. Letter to the Editor: Print

Goldstein, Lester. "Roach Coaches: The Upside." Letter. *Sierra* May/June 2011: 2. Print.

If the letter has a title, include it, then identify it as "Letter," as in example 19. If there is no title, include just the type, as in example 20.

20. Letter to the Editor: Direct Online Access

Ennis, Heather B. Letter. *U.S. News and World Report*. U.S. News and World Report, 20 Dec. 2007. Web. 22 Dec. 2007.

21. Review: Print

Shenk, David. "Toolmaker, Brain Builder." Rev. of *Beyond Deep Blue: Building the Computer That Defeated the World Chess Champion*, by Feng-Hsiung Hsu. *American Scholar* 72 (2003): 150–52. Print.

The review in example 21 is of a book.

22. Review: Direct Online Access

Travers, Peter. Rev. of *Beginners*, dir. Mike Mills. *Rolling Stone*. Rolling Stone, 2 June 2011. Web. 25 Nov. 2011.

The review in example 22 is of a film.

23. Article in a Collection of Reprinted Articles: Print

Brumberg, Abraham. "Russia after Perestroika." *New York Review of Books* 27 June 1991: 53–62. Rpt. in *Russian and Soviet History*. Ed. Alexander Dallin. Vol. 14. New York: Garland, 1992. 300–20. Print.

Textbooks used in college writing courses often collect previously printed articles.

Wallace, David Foster. "Consider the Lobster." *Gourmet* Aug. 2004: 50–55. Rpt. in *Creating Nonfiction: A Guide and Anthology*. Becky Bradway and Doug Hesse. Boston: Bedford, 2009. 755–69. Print.

24. Article in a Looseleaf Collection of Reprinted Articles: Print

Hayden, Thomas. "The Age of Robots." *U.S. News and World Report* 23 Apr. 2001, 44+. Print. *Applied Science 2002*. Ed. Eleanor Goldstein. Boca Raton: SIRS, 2002. Art. 66.

Give the citation for the original publication first, followed by the citation for the collection.

25. Abstract in a Collection of Abstracts: Print

Marcus, Hazel R., and Shinobu Kitayamo. "Culture and the Self: Implications for Cognition, Emotion, and Motivation." *Psychological Review* 88 (1991): 224–53. Abstract. *Psychological Abstracts* 78 (1991): item 23878. Print.

If a reader could not know that the cited material is an abstract, write the word *Abstract,* not italicized, followed by a period. Give publication information about the collection of abstracts. For abstracts identified by item numbers rather than page numbers, use the word *item* before the item number.

26. Abstract: Database

Marcus, Hazel R., and Shinobu Kitayamo. "Culture and the Self: Implications for Cognition, Emotion, and Motivation." Abstract. *Psychological Abstracts* 78 (1991): item 23878. *PsycINFO*. Web. 10 Apr. 2004.

This entry is for the same abstract shown in item 25, but here it is accessed from a database.

BOOKS

You can read books these days in four different formats.

1. **Print.**
2. **Digital version through an e-book.** E-Books are electronic versions of books for digital readers like the Kindle, Nook, iPad, or so on.
3. **Digital version from a database.** Some books are available through library databases; in a sense, you're "checking out the books" online.
4. **Digital version through direct online access.** Versions of some older books, whose copyrights have expired because their authors died more than 70 years ago, are available directly on the Web. Portions of several more recent books are also available directly on the Web, through sites like Google Books. However, the section you might need for your research is frequently not available.

Figure 25.5 shows how to cite a single-author print book. Figure 25.6 (page 330) shows how to cite a digital version of a book accessed through a database. We provide examples of all formats in examples 27–30. The same principles apply to all books. We also note that there are audio versions of some books: recordings of an actor (or sometimes, the author) reading the book. We explain how to cite audio books in example 67.

27. Book by One Author: Print

Turkle, Sherry. *Alone Together: Why We Expect More from Technology and Less from Each Other.* New York: Basic, 2011. Print.

28. Book by One Author: E-Book

Turkle, Sherry. *Alone Together: Why We Expect More from Technology and Less from Each Other.* New York: Basic, 2011. Kindle file.

Figure 25.5 Single-author print book.

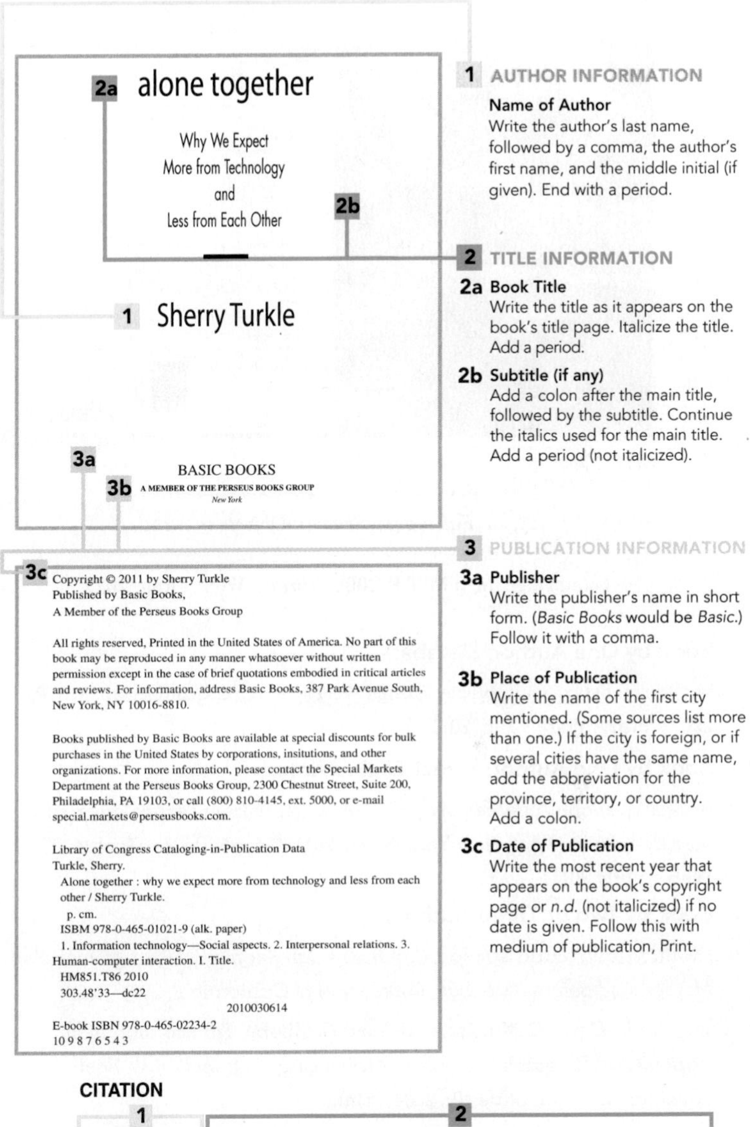

CITATION

1 2

Turkle, Sherry. *Alone Together: Why We Expect More from Technology and Less from Each Other*. New York: Basic, 2004. Print.

2 3

Figure 25.6 Digital version of a book accessed through a database.

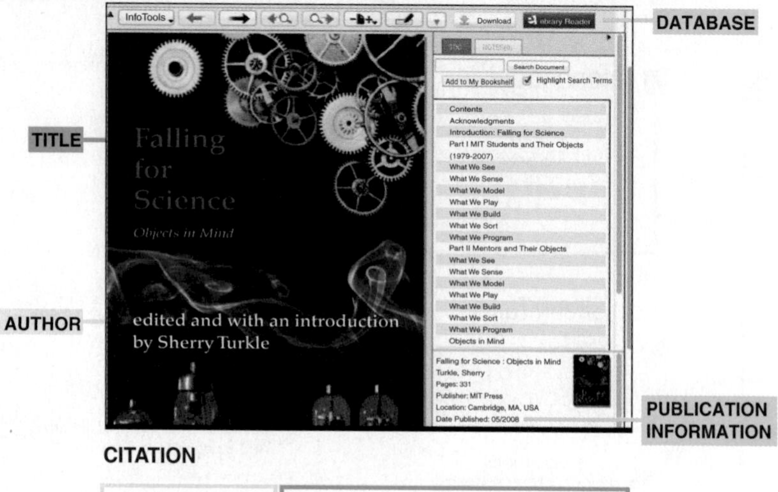

CITATION

Turkle, Sherry, ed. *Falling for Science: Objects in Mind.* Cambridge, MA: MIT P, 2008. *Ebrary*. Web. 3 Aug. 2012.

29. Book by One Author: Database

Turkle, Sherry. *Evocative Objects: Things We Think With*. Cambridge: MIT P, 2007. *Ebrary*. Web. 3 May 2011.

30. Book by One Author: Direct Online Access

Turkle, Sherry. *Alone Together: Why We Expect More from Technology and Less from Each Other*. New York: Basic, 2011. *Google Books*. Google, 2011. Web. 25 July 2011.

31. Book by Two or Three Authors

Edin, Kathryn, and Maria Kefalas. *Promises I Can Keep: Why Poor Women Put Motherhood before Marriage*. Berkeley: U of California P, 2005. Print.

Lynam, John K., Cyrus G. Ndiritu, and Adiel N. Mbabu. *Transformation of Agricultural Research Systems in Africa: Lessons from Kenya*. East Lansing: Michigan State UP, 2004. Print.

For e-books, adapt this model to example 28. For a book in a database, see example 29. For a book accessed directly online, see example 30.

32. Book by More Than Three Authors

Saul, Wendy, et al. *Beyond the Science Fair: Creating a Kids' Inquiry Conference*. Portsmouth: Heinemann, 2005. Print.

Give only the first author's name, followed by a comma and the phrase *et al.* (abbreviated from the Latin *et alii*, meaning "and others"), or list all names in full in the order in which they appear on the title page.

For e-books, adapt this model to example 28. For a book in a database, see example 29. For a book accessed directly online, see example 30.

33. Two or More Works by the Same Author(s)

Jenkins, Henry. *Convergence Culture: Where Old and New Media Collide*. New York: New York UP, 2006. Print.

---. *Fans, Bloggers, and Gamers: Exploring Participatory Culture*. New York: New York UP, 2006. Print.

Give author name(s) in the first entry only. In the second and subsequent entries, use three hyphens and a period to stand for exactly the same name(s). If the person served as editor or translator, put a comma and the appropriate abbreviation (*ed.* or *trans.*) following the three hyphens. Arrange the works in alphabetical (not chronological) order according to book title, ignoring labels such as *ed.* or *trans.*

For e-books, adapt this model to example 28. For a book in a database, see example 29. For a book accessed directly online, see example 30.

34. Book by a Group or Corporate Author

American Psychological Association. *Publication Manual of the American Psychological Association*. 6th ed. Washington: APA, 2010. Print.

Cite the full name of the corporate author first, omitting the first articles *A*, *An*, or *The*. When a corporate author is also the publisher, use a shortened form of the corporate name at the publisher position.

For e-books, adapt this model to example 28. For a book in a database, see example 29. For a book accessed directly online, see example 30.

35. Book with No Author Named

The Chicago Manual of Style. 16th ed. Chicago: U of Chicago P, 2010. Print.

If there is no author's name on the title page, begin the citation with the title. Alphabetize the entry according to the first significant word of the title (ignore *A, An*, or *The*).

For e-books, adapt this model to example 28. For a book in a database, see example 29. For a book accessed directly online, see example 30.

36. Book with an Author and an Editor

Stowe, Harriet Beecher. *Uncle Tom's Cabin*. Ed. Elizabeth Ammons. New York: Norton, 2010. Print.

If your paper refers to the work of the book's author, put the author's name first. If your paper refers to the work of the editor, put the editor's name first.

Ammons, Elizabeth, ed. *Uncle Tom's Cabin.* By Harriet Beecher Stowe. New York: Norton, 2010. Print.

For e-books, adapt this model to example 28. For a book in a database, see example 29. For a book accessed directly online, see example 30.

37. Translation

Nesbo, Jo. *The Leopard.* Trans. Don Bartlett. New York: Vintage, 2011.

For e-books, adapt this model to example 28. For a book in a database, see example 29. For a book accessed directly online, see example 30.

38. Work in Several Volumes or Parts

Chrisley, Ronald, ed. *Artificial Intelligence: Critical Concepts.* Vol. 1. London: Routledge, 2000. Print. 4 vols.

If you are citing only one volume, put the volume number before the publication information. If you wish, you can give the total number of volumes at the end of the entry. MLA recommends using arabic numerals, even if the source uses roman numerals (*Vol. 6* rather than *Vol. VI*).

For e-books, adapt this model to example 28. For a book in a database, see example 29. For a book accessed directly online, see example 30.

39. Anthology or Edited Book

Purdy, John L., and James Ruppert, eds. *Nothing but the Truth: An Anthology of Native American Literature.* Upper Saddle River: Prentice, 2001. Print.

Use this model if you are citing an entire anthology. In the example above, *ed.* stands for "editor," so use *eds.* when more than one editor is named.

For e-books, adapt this model to example 28. For a book in a database, see example 29. For a book accessed directly online, see example 30.

40. One Selection from an Anthology or an Edited Book

Trujillo, Laura. "Balancing Act." *Border-Line Personalities: A New Generation of Latinas Dish on Sex, Sass, and Cultural Shifting*. Ed. Robyn Moreno and Michelle Herrera Mulligan. New York: Harper, 2004. 61–72. Print.

Teasdale, Sara. "Driftwood." *Flame and Shadow*. Ed. A. Light. N.p., 1920. *Project Gutenberg*. 1 July 1996. Web. 18 Aug. 2008.

Give the author and title of the selection first and then the full title of the anthology. Information about the editor starts with *Ed.* (for "Edited by"), so don't use *Eds.* when there is more than one editor. Give the name(s) of the editor(s) in normal order rather than reversing first and last names. Give the page range of the selection at the end.

41. More Than One Selection from the Same Anthology or Edited Book

Bond, Ruskin. "The Night Train at Deoli." Chaudhuri 415–18.

Chaudhuri, Amit, ed. *The Vintage Book of Modern Indian Literature*. New York: Vintage, 2004. Print.

Vijayan, O.V. "The Rocks." Chaudhuri 291–96.

If you cite more than one selection from the same anthology, you can list the anthology as a separate entry with all of the publication information. Also list each selection from the anthology by author and title of the selection, but give only the name(s) of the editor(s) of the anthology and the page number(s) for each selection. Here, *ed.* stands for "editor," so it is correct to use *eds.* when more than one editor is named. List selections separately in alphabetical order by author's last name.

42. Article in a Reference Book

Burnbam, John C. "Freud, Sigmund." *The Encyclopedia of Psychiatry, Psychology, and Psychoanalysis*. Ed. Benjamin B. Wolman. New York: Holt, 1996. Print.

If the articles in the book are alphabetically arranged, you don't need to give volume and page numbers.

If no author is listed, begin with the title of the article.

"Ireland." *The New Encyclopaedia Britannica: Macropaedia*. 15th ed. 2002. Print.

If you're citing a widely used reference work, don't give full publication information. Instead, give only the edition and year of publication.

43. Article in a Reference Book: Database

"Lobster." *Encyclopaedia Britannica Online*. Encyclopaedia Britannica, 2011. Web. 29 June 2011.

44. Second or Later Edition

MLA Handbook for Writers of Research Papers. 7th ed. New York: MLA, 2009. Print.

If a book is not a first edition, the edition number is on the title page. Place the abbreviated information (*2nd ed., 3rd ed.*, etc.) between the title and the publication information. Give only the latest copyright date for the edition you are using.

For e-books, adapt this model to example 28. For a book in a database, see example 29. For a book accessed directly online, see example 30.

45. Introduction, Preface, Foreword, or Afterword

Hesse, Doug. Foreword. *The End of Composition Studies*. By David W. Smit. Carbondale: Southern Illinois UP, 2004. ix–xiii. Print.

Give first the name of the writer of the part you're citing and then the name of the cited part, capitalized but not underlined or in quotation marks. After the book title, put *By* and the book author's full name, if different from the writer of the cited material. If the writer of the cited material is the same as the book author, use only the last name after *By*. After the publication information, give inclusive page numbers for the cited part, using roman or arabic numerals as the source does. When the introduction, preface, foreword, or afterword has a title, include it in the citation before the section name, as in the following example:

Fox-Genovese, Elizabeth. "Mothers and Daughters: The Ties That Bind." Foreword. *Southern Mothers*. Ed. Nagueyalti Warren and Sally Wolff. Baton Rouge: Louisiana State UP, 1999. iv–xviii. Print.

For e-books, adapt this model to example 28. For a book in a database, see example 29. For a book accessed directly online, see example 30.

46. Unpublished Dissertation or Essay

Stuart, Gina Anne. "Exploring the Harry Potter Book Series: A Study of Adolescent Reading Motivation." Diss. Utah State U, 2006. Print.

Treat published dissertations as books.

For e-books, adapt this model to example 28. For a book in a database, see example 29. For a book accessed directly online, see example 30.

47. Reprint of an Older Book

Coover, Robert. *A Night at the Movies, Or, You Must Remember This.* 1987. Champaign: Dalkey Archive, 2007.

Republishing information can be found on the copyright page.

For e-books, adapt this model to example 28. For a book in a database, see example 29. For a book accessed directly online, see example 30.

48. Book in a Series or Scholarly Project

Ardell, Jean Hastings. *Breaking into Baseball: Women and the National Pastime*. Carbondale: Southern Illinois UP, 2005. Print. Writing Baseball Series.

49. Book with a Title within a Title

Lumiansky, Robert M., and Herschel Baker, eds. *Critical Approaches to Six Major English Works:* Beowulf *through* Paradise Lost. Philadelphia: U of Pennsylvania P, 1968. Print.

MLA prefers the previous example, in which the embedded title is neither italicized nor set within quotation marks. However, MLA also accepts a second style for handling embedded titles. In this style, set the normally independent titles within quotation marks and italicize them, as follows:

Lumiansky, Robert M., and Herschel Baker, eds. *Critical Approaches to Six Major English Works: "Beowulf" through "Paradise Lost."* Philadelphia: U of Pennsylvania P, 1968. Print.

Use whichever style your instructor prefers.

For e-books, adapt this model to example 28. For a book in a database, see example 29. For a book accessed directly online, see example 30.

50. Bible or Sacred Text

Bhagavad Gita. Trans. Juan Mascaro. Rev. ed. New York: Penguin, 2003. Print.

The Holy Bible: New International Version. New York: Harper, 1983. Print.

The Qur'an. Trans. M.A.S. Abdel Haleem. New York: Oxford UP, 2004. Print.

For e-books, adapt this model to example 28. For a book in a database, see example 29. For a book accessed directly online, see example 30.

51. Government Publication with No Author

United States. Cong. Senate. Select Committee on Intelligence. *Report on the U.S. Intelligence Community's Prewar Intelligence Assessment of Iraq*. 108th Cong., 1st sess. Washington: GPO, 2004. Print.

For government publications that name no author, start with the name of the government or government body. Then name the government agency. (*GPO* is a standard abbreviation for *Government Printing Office*, the publisher of most US government publications.) Then include the title, any series information, the publication date, and the medium of publication.

For e-books, adapt this model to example 28. For a book in a database, see example 29. For a book accessed directly online, see example 30.

52. Government Publication with Named Author

Wallace, David Rains. *Yellowstone: A Natural and Human History, Yellowstone National Park, Idaho, Montana, and Wyoming*. U.S. Interior Dept. National Park Service. Official National Park Handbook 150. Washington: GPO, 2001. Print.

MLA also permits an alternative format, with the government body first, then the title, then "By" followed by the author's name.

United States. Interior Dept. National Park Service. *Yellowstone: A Natural and Human History, Yellowstone National Park, Idaho, Montana, and Wyoming*. By David Rains Wallace. Official National Park Handbook 150. Washington: GPO, 2001. Print.

For e-books, adapt this model to example 28. For a book in a database, see example 29. For a book accessed directly online, see example 30.

53. Government Publication: Direct Online Access

Huff, C. Ronald. *Comparing the Criminal Behavior of Youth Gangs and At-Risk Youths*. United States Dept. of Justice. Natl. Inst. of Justice. Oct. 1998. Web. 5 Aug. 2008.

54. Published Proceedings of a Conference

Rocha, Luis Mateus, et al., eds. *Artificial Life X: Proceedings of the Tenth International Conference on the Simulation and Synthesis of Living Systems*. 3–7 June 2006, Bloomington, IN. Cambridge: MIT P, 2006. Print.

For e-books, adapt this model to example 28. For a book in a database, see example 29. For a book accessed directly online, see example 30.

IMAGES, AUDIO, FILM, AND VIDEO

55. Photograph, Painting, Drawing, Illustration, etc. (Original)

Mydans, Carl. *General Douglas MacArthur Landing at Luzon, 1945*. Gelatin silver print. Soho Triad Fine Art Gallery, New York. 21 Oct.–28 Nov. 1999.

Give the name of the image's maker, if known, the title or caption of the image, the type of image, where you viewed the image, and when. If the image has no title, provide a brief description.

56. Photograph, Painting, Drawing, Illustration, etc. in a Periodical: Print

Greene, Herb. *Grace Slick*. Photograph. *Rolling Stone* 30 Sept. 2004: 102. Print.

Include maker, title, and type as in 55, but include publication information as for a print article.

57. Photograph, Painting, Drawing, Illustration, etc. in a Periodical: Direct Online Access

Morris, Christopher. *Man in Camouflage*. Photograph. *Atlantic*. The Atlantic Monthly Group, July/Aug. 2011. Web. 5 Aug. 2011.

58. Photograph, Painting, Drawing, Illustration, etc. in a Book: Print

The World's Most Populous Countries. Illustration. *Maps of the Imagination: The Writer as Cartographer*. By Peter Turchi. San Antonio: Trinity UP, 2004. 116–17. Print.

59. Photograph, Painting, Drawing, Illustration, etc.: Direct Online Access

Bourke-White, Margaret. *Fort Peck Dam, Montana*. 1936. Gelatin silver print. *Metropolitan Museum of Art*. Web. 5 Aug. 2008.

Give information about the Web site, the medium of publication, and the access date.

van Gogh, Vincent. *The Starry Night*. 1889. Oil on canvas. *MOMA*. Museum of Modern Art. Web. 5 Dec. 2011.

60. Comic or Cartoon: Print

Sutton, Ward. "Ryan's a Late Adopter." Cartoon. *New Yorker* 2 May 2011: 64. Print.

61. Comic or Cartoon: Direct Online Access

Harris, Sidney. "We have lots of information technology." Cartoon. *New Yorker*. Conde Nast, 27 May 2002. Web. 9 Feb. 2007.

62. Slide Show: Direct Online Access

Erickson, Britta, narr. *Visionaries from the New China*. *Atlantic*. Atlantic Monthly Group, 18 June 2007. Web. 11 Sept. 2008.

63. Photo Essay: Direct Online Access

Nachtwey, James. "Crime in Middle America." *Time*. Time, 2 Dec. 2006. Web. 5 May 2007.

64. Image from a Social Networking Site

Gristellar, Ferdinand. *The Gateway Arch*. Photograph. *Ferdinand Gristellar*. Facebook, 7 Aug. 2009. Web. 3 Sept. 2009.

65. Image from a Service or Distributor

World Perspectives. *Launching of the Space Shuttle* Columbia, *Florida, USA, 1998*. Photograph. Getty Images #AT3775-001. Web. 3 Mar. 2011.

In this example, the photographer was listed as "World Perspectives." Include the name of the service or distributor, and the item number or other identifier, if any.

66. Map, Chart, or Other Graphic: Direct Online Access

"Hurricane Rita." Graphic. *New York Times Online*. New York Times, 24 Sept. 2005. Web. 24 Sept. 2005.

67. Audio Book

Turkle, Sherry. *Alone Together: Why We Expect More from Technology and Less from Each Other*. Narr. Laural Merlington. Tantor Media, 2011. CD.

68. Sound Recording: CD, DVD

Verdi, Giuseppe. *Requiem*. Chicago Symphony Orchestra and Chorus. Cond. Ricardo Muti. CSO Resound, 2010. CD.

Put first the name most relevant to what you discuss in your paper (performer, conductor, work performed). Include the recording's title, the medium for any recording other than a CD (*LP, Audiocassette*), the name of the issuer, and the year the work was issued.

69. Sound Recording: MP3

Radiohead. "Jigsaw Falling into Place." *In Rainbows*. Radiohead, 2007. MP3 file.

70. Sound Recording: Direct Online Access

Komunyakaa, Yusef. "My Father's Love Letters." *Poets.org Listening Booth*. Academy of American Poets, 5 May 1993. Web. 19 Aug. 2008.

71. Podcast: Direct Online Access

Blumberg, Alex, and Adam Davidson. "The Giant Pool of Money." Podcast. *This American Life*. 9 May 2008. Web. 19 Oct. 2009.

A podcast is an audio recording that is posted online. Thus, the publication medium is *Web*. Include as much of the following information as you can identify: author, title, sponsoring organization or Web site, date posted, and date accessed.

72. Film, Videotape, or DVD

It Happened One Night. Screenplay by Robert Riskin. Dir. and Prod. Frank Capra. Perf. Clark Gable and Claudette Colbert. 1934. Sony Pictures, 1999. DVD.

Give the title first, and include the director, the distributor, and the year. For films that were subsequently released on tape or DVD, provide the original release date of the movie *before* the type of medium. Other information (writer, producer, major actors) is optional but helpful. Put first names first.

73. Video or Film: Direct Online Access

For video downloads, include the download date and the source.

It Happened One Night. Screenplay by Robert Riskin. Dir. and Prod. Frank Capra. Perf. Clark Gable and Claudette Colbert. 1934. *Netflix*. Web. 15. Dec. 2011.

CNN. *Challenger Disaster Live on CNN*. *YouTube.com*. YouTube, 27 Jan. 2011. Web. 4 Mar. 2011.

Use this format for videos from YouTube and similar sites.

74. Broadcast Television or Radio Program

Include at least the title of the program (in italics), the network, the local station and its city, and the date of the broadcast.

Not for Ourselves Alone: The Story of Elizabeth Cady Stanton and Susan B. Anthony. By Ken Burns. Perf. Julie Harris, Ronnie Gilbert, and Sally Kellerman. Prod. Paul Barnes and Ken Burns. PBS. WNET, New York. 8 Nov. 1999. Television.

The Madeleine Brand Show. SCPR. KPCC, Pasadena. 20 June 2011. Radio.

For a series, also supply the title of the specific episode (in quotation marks) before the title of the program (italicized) and the title of the series (neither underlined nor in quotation marks).

"The Bruce-Partington Plans." *Sherlock Holmes*. RMPBS. KRMA, Denver. 30 June 2011. Television.

75. Television or Radio Program: Direct Online Access

"Bill Moyers." *The Daily Show*. Perf. Jon Stewart. Comedy Central. *Hulu.com*. Hulu, 1 June 2011. Web. 22 Sept. 2011.

"The Disappearing Incandescent Bulb." *The Madeleine Brand Show*. SCPR. KPCC, Pasadena. 20 June 2011. Web. 6 Oct. 2011. <http://www.scpr.org/programs/madeleine-brand/2011/06/20/the-disappearing-incandescent-bulb/>.

Because this source may be difficult to find, the URL is listed.

OTHER INTERNET SOURCES

This section shows models for other online sources. For such sources, provide as much of the following information as you can.

1. The author's name, if given.
2. In quotation marks, the title of a short work (Web page, brief document, essay, article, message, and so on); or italicized, the title of a book.
3. Publication information for any print version, if it exists.
4. The name of an editor, translator, or compiler, if any, with an abbreviation such as *Ed.*, *Trans.*, or *Comp.* before the name.
5. Publication information for the Web:
   a. The italicized title of the Internet site (scholarly project, database, online periodical, professional or personal Web site). If the site has no title, describe it: for example, *Home page*.
   b. The date of electronic publication (including a version number, if any) or posting or the most recent update.

c. The name of a sponsoring organization, if any.
d. The medium of publication: Web.
e. The date you accessed the material.
f. The URL in angle brackets (< >), only when the reader probably could not locate the source without it. If you must break a URL at the end of a line, break only after a slash and do not use a hyphen.

Figure 25.7 shows how to cite a page from a Web site. Figure 25.8 (page 342) shows how to cite a posting on a blog.

76. Entire Web Site

WebdelSol.Com. Ed. Michael Neff. 2011. Web. 4 Aug. 2011.

77. Home Page (Organization or Company)

Association for the Advancement of Artificial Intelligence. AAAI, n.d. Web. 17 Oct. 2011.

78. Personal Home Page

Hesse, Doug. Home page. Web. 1 Nov. 2011. <http://portfolio.du.edu/dhesse>.

Provide the URL if the page might be difficult to find.

79. Page from a Web Site

"Protecting Whales from Dangerous Sonar." *National Resources Defense Council.* NRDC, 9 Nov. 2005. Web. 12 Dec. 2005.

"Ethical and Social Implications of AI for Society." *Association for the Advancement of Artificial Intelligence.* AAAI, 3 May 2012. Web. 19 May 2012.

Provide as much information as you can, starting with the author, if available, and the title of the page, followed by the site information.

80. Academic Department Home Page

Writing. Dept. home page. Grand Valley State U. Web. 26 Feb. 2010.

81. Course Home Page

St. Germain, Sheryl. Myths and Fairytales: From *Inanna* to *Edward Scissorhands.* Course home page. Summer 2003. Dept. of English, Iowa State U. Web. 20 Feb. 2005. <http://www.public.iastate.edu/sgermain/531.homepage.html>.

82. Government or Institutional Web Site

Home Education and Private Tutoring. Pennsylvania Department of Education, 2005. Web. 5 Aug. 2008.

Figure 25.7 Page from a Web site.

1 TITLE

Title of the Work
State the full title of the work cited, enclosed in quotation marks. Use a period before the closing quotation mark.

2 PUBLICATION INFORMATION

2a Title of the Overall Web Site
Provide the title of the Web site (italicized), followed by a period.

2b Publisher or Sponsor of the Web Site
Leave one space after the title of the overall Web site and provide the publisher or sponsor of the Web site. If this information is not available, use *N.p.* End with a comma.

2c Date of Publication
Provide the available date (day, month, and year) of publication, followed by a period. If no date is available, use *n.d.*

2d Medium of Publication
Provide the medium of publication consulted (*Web*), followed by a period.

2e Date of Access
Provide the day, month, and year that you accessed the article online. End with a period.

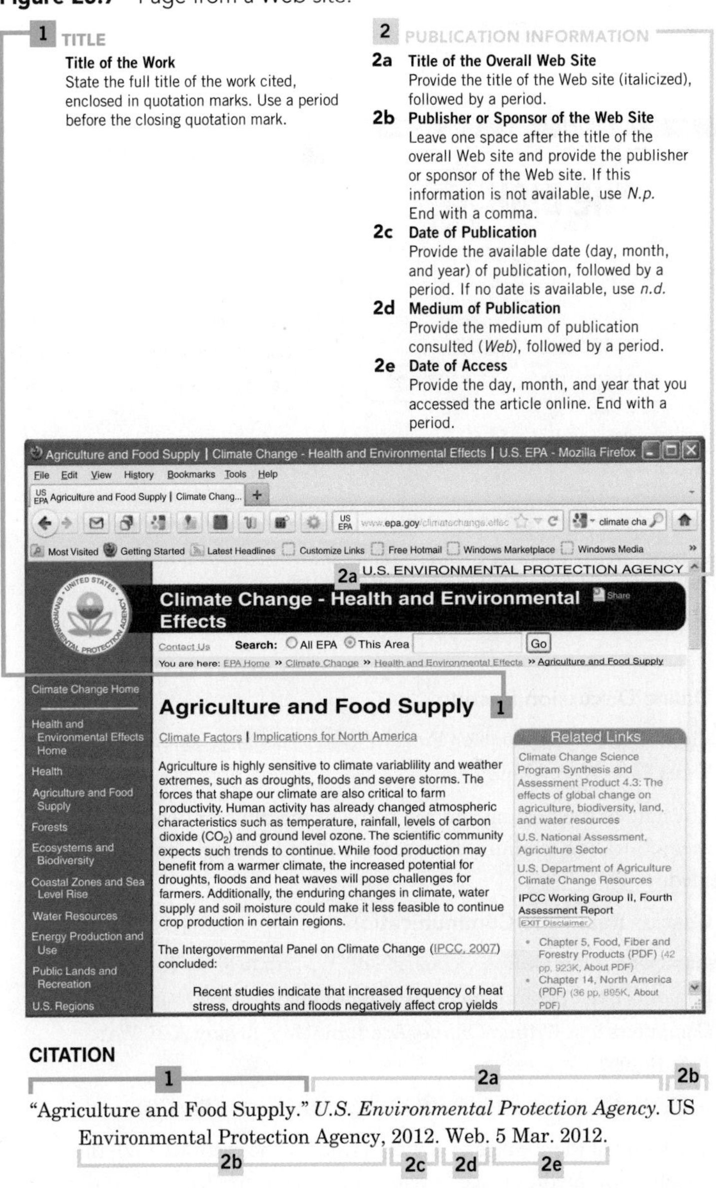

CITATION

[1] "Agriculture and Food Supply." [2a] *U.S. Environmental Protection Agency.* [2b] US Environmental Protection Agency, [2c] 2012. [2d] Web. [2e] 5 Mar. 2012.

Figure 25.8 Posting on a blog.

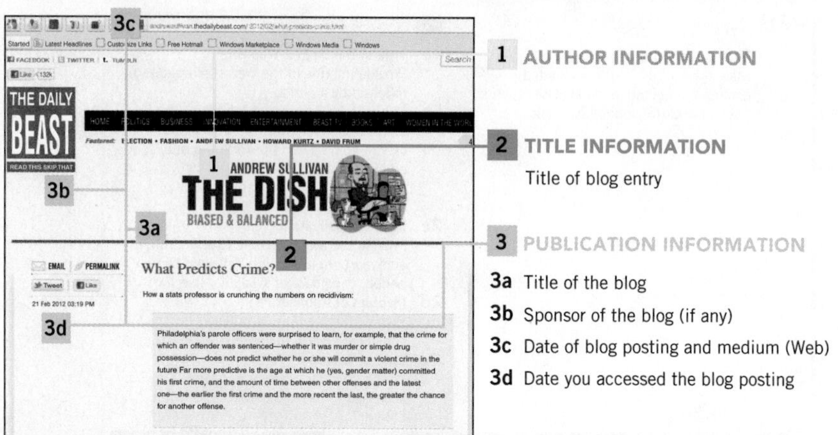

CITATION

1 2 3

Sullivan, Andrew. "What Predicts Crime?" *The Dish: Biased and Balanced.* The Daily Beast, 21 Feb. 2012. Web. 18 Mar. 2012.

3

83. Online Discussion Posting

Firrantello, Larry. "Van Gogh on Prozac." Online posting. 23 May 2005. *Salon Table Talk*. Web. 7 June 2005.

Give the date of the posting and the name of the bulletin board, if any. Then give the publication medium, the access date and, in angle brackets, the URL if needed.

84. Chat or Real-Time Communication

Berzsenyi, Christyne. Online discussion of "Writing to Meet Your Match: Rhetoric, Perceptions, and Self-Presentation for Four Online Daters." *Computers and Writing Online*. AcadianaMoo, 13 May 2007. Web. 13 May 2007.

Glenn, Maria. Chat. *Laurence Smith*. 9 Sept. 2010. Web. 9 Sept. 2010.

Give the name of the speaker or writer, a title for the event (if any), the forum, date, publication medium, access date, and URL if needed.

85. E-Mail Message

Martin, Tara. "Visit to Los Alamos." Message to David Sanz. 25 July 2010. E-mail.

Start with the name of the person who wrote the e-mail message. Give the title or subject line in quotation marks. Then describe the message, including the recipient's name. Add the date. Finally, write the medium of delivery (E-mail).

86. Posting on a Blog

Phillips, Matthew. "Need to Go to the ER? Not Until the Game's Over." *Freakonomics*. Freakonomics, LLC, 15 June 2011. Web. 14 Aug. 2011.

87. Wiki

"NASCAR Sprint Cup Series." *NASCAR Wiki*. Wikia, 11 Jan. 2011. Web. 6 Apr. 2011.

88. Posting on a Social Networking Site

Adler-Kassner, Linda. "Conversations toward Action." *Council of Writing Program Administrators*. Facebook, 5 Feb. 2010. Web. 6 May 2011.

OTHER PRINT, NONPRINT, AND ELECTRONIC SOURCES

89. Published or Unpublished Letter

Irvin, William. Letter to Lesley Osburn. 7 Dec. 2011. MS.

Williams, William Carlos. Letter to his son. 13 Mar. 1935. *Letters of the Century: America 1900–1999*. Ed. Lisa Grunwald and Stephen J. Adler. New York: Dial, 1999: 225–26. Print.

Begin the entry with the the author of the letter. Note the recipient, too. If the letter is published in a periodical, a book, or online, follow the appropriate citation format for these sources.

90. Microfiche Collection of Articles

Wenzell, Ron. "Businesses Prepare for a More Diverse Work Force." *St. Louis Post Dispatch* 3 Feb. 1990: 17. Microform. *NewsBank: Employment* 27 (1990): fiche 2, grid D12.

A microfiche is a transparent sheet of film (a *fiche*) with microscopic printing that needs to be read through a special magnifier. Each fiche holds several pages, with each page designated by a grid position. A long document may appear on more than one fiche.

91. Map or Chart

Colorado Front Range Mountain Bike Topo Map. Map. Nederland: Latitude 40, 2001. Print.

If you have accessed the map or chart online, follow example 66.

92. Report or Pamphlet

National Commission on Writing in America's Schools and Colleges. *The Neglected "R": The Need for a Writing Revolution.* New York: College Board, 2003. Print.

Use the format for books, to the extent possible, including whether you're citing a print or digital version.

93. Legal Source

Brown v. Board of Educ. 347 US 483-96. Supreme Court of the US. 1954. Print.

Include the name of the case, the number of the case (preceded by *No.*), the name of the court deciding the case, and the date of the decision. Legal sources can frequently be accessed through a database:

Brown v. Board of Educ. 347 US 483-96. Supreme Court of the US. 1954. *LexisNexis Academic*. Web. 25 Jan. 2010.

94. Interview

Friedman, Randi. Telephone interview. 30 Aug. 2008.

Winfrey, Oprah. "Ten Questions for Oprah Winfrey." By Richard Zoglin. *Time* 15 Dec. 2003: 8. Print.

Pope, Carl. Interview by Amy Standen. *Salon.com*. Salon Media Group, 29 Apr. 2002. Web. 27 Jan. 2005.

Note the type of interview, for example "Telephone" or "Personal" (face-to-face). For a published interview, give the name of the interviewed person first, identify the source as an interview, and then give details as for any published source: title; author (preceded by the word *By*); and publication details. Follow the citation format for a periodical, book, or Web source, as appropriate.

95. Lecture or Speech

Kennedy, John Fitzgerald. Greater Houston Ministerial Assn. Rice Hotel, Houston. 12 Sept. 1960. Speech.

Katz, Jennifer. "Spiral Galaxies." Astronomy 1000. University of Denver, Denver. 7 Feb. 2011. Lecture.

96. Live Performance (Play, Concert, Dance etc.)

All My Sons. By Arthur Miller. Dir. Calvin McLean. Center for the Performing Arts, Normal, IL. 27 Sept. 2005. Performance.

Nelson, Willie. Concert. Red Rocks Amphitheater, Denver. 22 June 2011. Performance.

97. Work of Art, Original

Cassatt, Mary. *La Toilette*. 1890. Oil on canvas. Art Institute of Chicago.

Fourquet, Léon. *The Man with the Broken Nose*. 1865. Marble. Musée Rodin, Paris.

98. Musical Score

Schubert, Franz. *Unfinished Symphony*. 1822. Print.

Italicize any musical work that has a title, such as an opera, a ballet, or a named symphony. Don't underline or put in quotation marks music identified only by form, number, and key, as follows.

Schubert, Franz. Symphony no. 8 in B minor. 1822. Print.

To cite a published score, use the following format.

Schubert, Franz. *Symphony in B Minor (Unfinished)*. 1822. Ed. Martin Cusid. New York: Norton, 1971. Print.

99. Advertisement

Southwest Airlines. Advertisement. ABC. 24 Aug. 2010. Television.

Canon Digital Cameras. Advertisement. *Time* 2 June 2003: 77. Print.

Samsung. Advertisement. *RollingStone*. Wenner Media, 8 Nov. 2005. Web. 11 Nov. 2005.

100. Video Game or Software

The Island: Castaway. N.p.: Awem Studio, 2010. Game.

"N.p." indicates that the place of publication is unknown.

101. Nonperiodical Publications on CD, DVD, or Magnetic Tape

Perl, Sondra. *Felt Sense: Guidelines for Composing*. Portsmouth: Boynton, 2004. CD.

Citations for publications on DVD, CD-ROM, or other recording formats follow guidelines for print publications, with two additions: list the publication medium (for example, *CD*), and give the vendor's name.

102. Materials on CD or DVD with a Print Version

"The Price Is Right." *Time* 20 Jan. 1992: 38. *Time Man of the Year*. CD-ROM. New York: Compact, 1993.

Information for the print version ends with the article's page number, 38. Following that comes the title of the CD-ROM (*Time Man of the Year*) and its publication information.

103. Materials on CD or DVD with No Print Version

"Artificial Intelligence." *Encarta 2003*. Redmond: Microsoft, 2003. CD-ROM.

Encarta 2003 is a CD-ROM encyclopedia with no print version.

104. PowerPoint or Similar Presentation

Delyser, Ariel. "Political Movements in the Philippines." University of Denver. 7 Feb. 2010. PowerPoint.

105. Work in More Than One Publication Medium

Shamoon, Linda, et al., eds. *Coming of Age: The Advanced Writing Curriculum. Coming of Age Course Descriptions*. Portsmouth: Boynton, 2000. Print, CD-ROM.

This book and CD-ROM come together. Each has its own title, but the publication information—Portsmouth: Boynton, 2000—applies to both.

25F What are MLA format guidelines for your research papers?

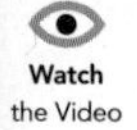
Watch the Video

Check whether your instructor has special instructions for the final draft of your research paper. If there are no special instructions, you can use the MLA STYLE guidelines here. The student paper in 25G was prepared according to these MLA guidelines.

25F.1 General formatting instructions—MLA

Use 8½-by-11-inch white paper. Double-space throughout. Use a one-inch margin on the left, right, top, and bottom. Don't justify the type.

Drop down ½ inch from the top edge of the paper to the name-and-page-number line described here. Then drop down another 1/2 inch to the first line, whether that is a heading, a title, or a line of the text of your paper. For an example, see page 351.

Paragraph indents in the body of the paper and indents in Notes and Works Cited are ½ inch, or about five characters. The indent in Microsoft Word is a hanging indent of 0.5 for "first line." The indent for a set-off quotation (see p. 352) is 1 inch, or about ten characters.

25F.2 Order of parts—MLA

Use this order for the parts of your paper: body of the paper; endnotes, if any (headed "Notes," without quotation marks); Works Cited list; attachments, if any (such as questionnaires, data sheets, or any other material your instructor tells you to include). Number all pages consecutively.

25F.3 Name-and-page-number header for all pages—MLA

Use a header consisting of a name-and-page-number line on every page of your paper, including the first, unless your instructor requires otherwise. Most word-processing programs have an "insert header" or "view header" function that automatically places a header ½ inch from the top edge of the page. In the header, type your last name (capitalize only the first letter), then leave a one-character space, and end with the page number. Align the header about an inch from the right edge of the paper; in most word-processing programs, this is a "flush right" setting.

25F.4 First page—MLA

MLA doesn't require a cover page but understands that some instructors do, in which case you should follow your instructor's prescribed format.

If your instructor does not require a cover page, use a four-line heading at the top of the first page. Drop down 1 inch from the top of the page. Start each line at the left margin, and include the following information.

Your name (first line)

Your instructor's name (second line)

Your course name and section (third line)

The date you hand in your paper (fourth line)

For the submission date, use either day-month-year form (26 Nov. 2012) or month-day-year style (Nov. 26, 2012).

On one double-spaced line below this heading, center the title of your paper. Don't underline the title or enclose it in quotation marks. On the line below the title, start your paper. As we noted earlier, double-space lines throughout your paper.

❶ **Capitalization Alerts:** (1) Use a capital letter for the first word of your title and the first word of a subtitle, if you include one. Start every NOUN, PRONOUN, VERB, ADVERB, ADJECTIVE, and SUBORDINATING CONJUNCTION with a capital letter. Capitalize the last word of your title, no matter what part of speech it is. In a hyphenated compound word (two or more words used together to express one idea), capitalize every word that you would normally capitalize: Father-in-Law.

(2) Don't capitalize an article (*a, an, the*) unless one of the preceding capitalization rules applies to it. Don't capitalize PREPOSITIONS, no matter how many letters they contain. Don't capitalize COORDINATING CONJUNCTIONS. Don't capitalize the word *to* used in an INFINITIVE. ●

25F.5 Notes—MLA

In MLA style, footnotes or endnotes serve two specific purposes: (1) for ideas and information that do not fit into your paper but are still worth relating; and (2) for bibliographic information that would intrude if you were to include it in your text.

TEXT OF PAPER

Eudora Welty's literary biography, *One Writer's Beginnings*, shows us how both the inner world of self and the outer world of family and place form a writer's imagination.[1]

CONTENT NOTE—MLA

1. Welty, who valued her privacy, resisted investigation of her life. However, at the age of seventy-four, she chose to present her own autobiographical reflections in a series of lectures at Harvard University.

TEXT OF PAPER

Barbara Randolph believes that enthusiasm is contagious (65).[1] Many psychologists have found that panic, fear, and rage spread more quickly in crowds than positive emotions do, however.

BIBLIOGRAPHIC NOTE—MLA

1. Others who agree with Randolph include Thurman 21, 84, 155; Kelley 421–25; and Brookes 65–76.

If you use a note in your paper (see p. 346), try to structure the sentence so that the note number falls at the end. The ideal place for a note number, which appears slightly raised above the line of words (called a "superscript number"), is after the sentence-ending punctuation. Don't leave a space before the number. Word processing programs have commands for inserting "references" such as notes, and you'll want to choose endnotes rather than footnotes. If you use the references feature to insert a note, the program will generally open a box in which you type the words of your note, the program then saves all your notes together, in order. If, instead, you use the "font" command, type the number on the line, highlight it, click on "superscript" in the font box, and then click "OK." Number the notes consecutively throughout the paper.

Place your notes on a separate page after the last page of the body of your paper and before the Works Cited list. Order them sequentially as they appear in the paper. Center the word *Notes* at the top of the page, using the same 1-inch margin; don't underline it or enclose it in quotation marks.

If you have notes that accompany tables or figures, treat them differently. Place table or figure notes below the table or illustration. Instead of note numbers, use raised lowercase letters: a, b, c.

25F.6 Works Cited list—MLA

The Works Cited list starts on a new page and has the same name-and-page-number heading as the previous pages. One inch below the top edge of the page, center the words "Works Cited." Don't underline them or put them in quotation marks.

Start the first entry in your list at the left margin one double space after the Works Cited heading. If an entry takes more than one line, indent each subsequent line after the first ½ inch. Double space all lines throughout.

25G A student's MLA-style research paper

MLA STYLE doesn't require an outline before a research paper. Nevertheless, many instructors want students to submit them. Most instructors prefer the standard traditional outline format that we discuss in section 5G. Unless you're told otherwise, use that format.

View the Model Document

Some instructors prefer what they consider a more contemporary outline format. Never use it unless it's explicitly assigned. It differs because it outlines the content of the INTRODUCTORY and CONCLUDING PARAGRAPHS, and full wording of the THESIS STATEMENT is placed in the outline of the introductory paragraph. We show an example of this type in the topic outline of Andrei Gurov's paper which appears next.

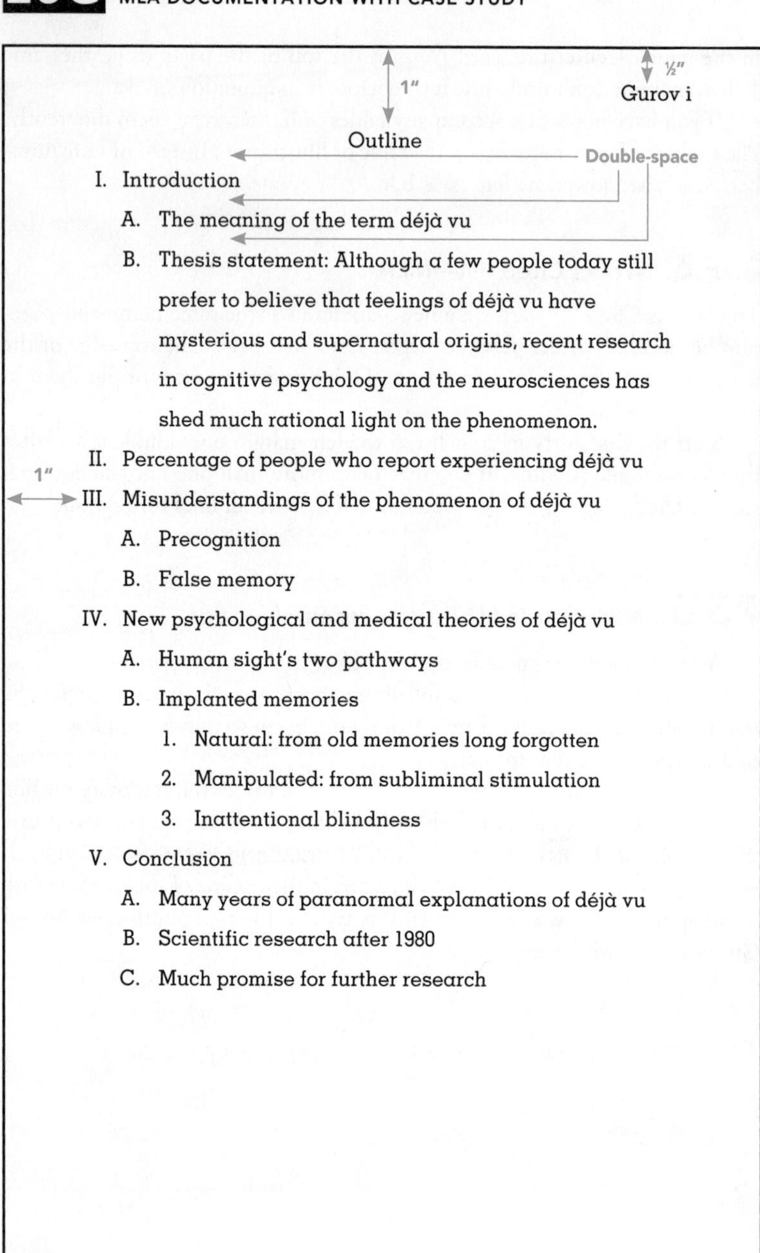

Gurov i

Outline

I. Introduction
   A. The meaning of the term déjà vu
   B. Thesis statement: Although a few people today still prefer to believe that feelings of déjà vu have mysterious and supernatural origins, recent research in cognitive psychology and the neurosciences has shed much rational light on the phenomenon.

II. Percentage of people who report experiencing déjà vu

III. Misunderstandings of the phenomenon of déjà vu
   A. Precognition
   B. False memory

IV. New psychological and medical theories of déjà vu
   A. Human sight's two pathways
   B. Implanted memories
      1. Natural: from old memories long forgotten
      2. Manipulated: from subliminal stimulation
      3. Inattentional blindness

V. Conclusion
   A. Many years of paranormal explanations of déjà vu
   B. Scientific research after 1980
   C. Much promise for further research

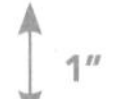

½"

Gurov 1

Andrei Gurov

Professor Ryan

English 101, Section A4

12 Dec. 2011

Student information appears top left, in four lines, double-spaced.

Déjà Vu: At Last a Subject for Serious Study

Center title one double space below information.

"Brain hiccup" might be another name for *déjà vu*, French for "already seen." During a moment of déjà vu, a person relives an event that in reality is happening for the first time. The hiccup metaphor seems apt because each modern scientific explanation of the déjà vu phenomenon involves a doubled event, as this paper will demonstrate. However, such modern scientific work was long in coming. In his article "The Déjà Vu Illusion," today's leading researcher in the field, Alan S. Brown at Southern Methodist University, states that "for over 170 years, this most puzzling of memory illusions has intrigued scholars" but was hampered when "during the behaviorist era . . . the plethora of parapsychological and psychodynamic interpretations" multiplied rapidly (256). Thus, notions of the supernatural and magic halted the scientific study of déjà vu for almost two centuries. By the first quarter of the twentieth century, it began again slowly. Although a few people today still prefer to believe that feelings of déjà vu have mysterious or supernatural origins, recent research in cognitive psychology and the neurosciences has shed much rational light on the phenomenon.

To capture interest, Andrei creates an unusual term and quotes a researcher.

Thesis statement presents the main idea.

continued >>

(Proportions shown in this paper are adjusted to fit space limitations of this book. Follow actual dimensions discussed in this book and your instructor's directions.)

Header includes student's last name and the page number.

Andrei summarizes one of three sources by Brown; a shortened title and page number show which.

Brackets mean Andrei inserted "studied" to make the sentence flow smoothly.

Andrei realizes instructor will know he wrote this sentence, which needs no documentation.

Block indent quotations of four lines or more. "[author's emphasis]" shows "THEN" was capitalized in original. Source had no pages.

Gurov 2

Some people report never having experienced déjà vu, and the percentages vary for the number of people who report having lived through at least one episode of it. In 2004, Brown reports that of the subjects he has interviewed, an average of 66 percent say that they have had one or more déjà vu experiences during their lives (*Experience* 33). However, in early 2005 in "Strangely Familiar," Uwe Wolfradt reports that "various studies indicate that from 50 to 90 percent of the people [studied] can recall having had at least one such déjà vu incident in their lives."

Perhaps part of the reason for this variation in the range of percentages stems from a general misunderstanding of the phrase *déjà vu*, even by some of the earlier scientific researchers twenty or more years ago. Indeed, in today's society, people throw around the term *déjà vu* without much thought. For example, it is fairly common for someone to see or hear about an event and then say, "Wow. This is déjà vu. I had a dream that this exact same thing happened." However, dreaming about an event ahead of time is a different phenomenon known as *precognition*, which relates to the paranormal experience of extrasensory perception. To date, precognition has never been scientifically demonstrated. As Johnson explains about dreams, however,

> . . . there is usually very little "data," evidence, or documentation to confirm that a Precognition has taken place. If a person learns about some disaster and THEN [author's emphasis] tells people that he/she has foreseen it the day before, that may or may not be true, because there is usually not corroborative confirmation of what the person claims.

continued >>

Gurov 3

Thus, precognition, a phenomenon talked about frequently but one that has never held up under scientific scrutiny, is definitely not the same as déjà vu.

False memory is another phenomenon mislabeled *déjà vu*. It happens when people are convinced that certain events took place in their lives, even though the events never happened. This occurs when people have strong memories of many unrelated occurrences that suddenly come together into a whole that's very close to the current experience. It seems like a déjà vu experience. This occurs from the

> converging elements of many different but related experiences. When this abstract representation, which has emerged strictly from the melding together of strongly associated elements, happens to correspond to the present experience, a déjà vu may be the outcome. (Brown, *Experience* 160)

Phrase introduces quotation.

All source information put in a parenthetical citation. Block quotation periods come before citation.

To illustrate lab-induced false memory, Brown in *The Déjà Vu Experience* cites investigations in which subjects are shown lists of words related to sleep; however, the word *sleep* itself is not on the list. In recalling the list of words, most subjects insist that the word *sleep* was indeed on the list, which means that the memory of a word that was never there is false memory. This is exactly what happens when well-intentioned eyewitnesses believe they recall certain criminal acts even though, in fact, they never saw or experienced the events at all (159).

Only page number goes in parentheses when author named in text.

In the last twenty years especially, new theories have come to the fore as a result of rigorous work from psychological and medical points of view. In *Experience*, Brown surveys the literature and concludes that this relatively young field

continued >>

Gurov 4

Transition paragraph introduces four new topics.

of investigation is dividing itself into four categories: (1) dual processing, (2) memory, (3) neurological, and (4) attentional. This paper briefly discusses the first and second as each relates to the third. Next, I discuss the fourth as it relates to the second.

Two related sources in one citation, separated by semicolon.

Discusses first topic from previous paragraph.

Citation shows paragraph summarizes several source pages.

Brain-based studies of the human sense of sight are one heavily researched theory of déjà vu that has been partially explained in the last two decades. Such studies focus on the dual pathways by which the sight of an event reaches the brain (Glenn; Carey F1). For example, the left hemisphere processes information from the right eye and the right hemisphere processes information from the left eye. The brain is incapable of storing data with respect to time and is only able to "see" events in relation to others. Each eye interprets data separately, at the same precise time. According to research, the human brain can perceive two visual stimuli at one instant as long as they are "seen" less than 25 milliseconds apart. Since the human brain is capable of interpreting both signals within this time, when events are perceived normally, they are seen and recognized by the brain as one single event (Weiten 69, 97–99, 211).

To develop topic sentence, Andrei summarizes Johnson's explanation.

Occasionally, however, the neurological impulses that carry data from each eye to the brain are delayed. As Johnson explains, the person might be fatigued or have had his or her attention seriously distracted (as when crossing the street at a dangerous intersection). As a result, one signal may reach the brain in under 25 milliseconds, while the other signal is slowed and reaches the brain slightly more than 25 milliseconds later. Even a few milliseconds' delay makes the second incoming signal arrive late—and, without fail, the brain interprets the stimuli as two separate events rather than one event. The

continued >>

Gurov 5

person thus has the sensation of having seen the event before because the brain has recognized the milliseconds-later event as a memory.

Implanted memories are another well-researched explanation for the déjà vu phenomenon. Examples of implanted memories originate in both the natural and the lab-induced experiences of people. For instance, perhaps a person walks into the kitchen of a new friend for the first time and, although the person has never been there before, the person feels certain that he or she has. With hypnosis and other techniques, researchers could uncover that the cupboards are almost exactly like those that the person had forgotten were in the kitchen of the person's grandparents' house and that the scent of baking apple pie is identical to the smell the person loved when walking into the grandparents' home during holidays (Carey F1). Colorado State University Professor Anne Cleary and her colleagues conducted an experiment in which students studied images of simple scenes and then were shown a second set of images. Some of the second set were made to resemble the original study images. Students tended to "remember" those scenes that had elements in common, even if they were not identical (1083).

Discusses second topic, memory, introduced above.

Specific example makes the point vividly.

Thomas McHugh, a researcher at MIT, believes he has even discovered the specific neurological "memory circuit" in the brain that is the source of this kind of déjà vu (Lemonick). This circuit allows people to complete memories with just a single cue. For example, you can remember much about a football game you saw even if someone just mentions the two teams involved. Sometimes, however, the circuit "misfires," and it signals that a

Develops third topic with research on memory.

Specific example clarifies the point.

continued >>

Gurov 6

new memory is actually part of the pattern of an old one. Researchers Akira O'Connor, Colin Lever, and Chris Moulin claim that the false sensations of memory differ from those of familiarity. They call the former "déjà vécue," and note serious cases in which people live much of their life in this state. It remains to be seen whether their distinction will be confirmed.

Andrei illustrates concept by summarizing Wolfradt's account of Jacoby's work.

Wolfradt describes a lab-induced experiment in which psychologist Larry L. Jacoby in 1989 manipulated a group of subjects so that he could implant a memory that would lead to a déjà vu experience for each of them. He arranged for his subjects to assemble in a room equipped with a screen in front. He flashed on the screen one word so quickly that no one was consciously aware they had seen the word. Jacoby was certain, however, that the visual centers of the brain of each subject had indeed "seen" the word. Later, when he flashed the word leaving it on the screen long enough for the subjects to consciously see it, everyone indicated they had seen the word somewhere before. All the subjects were firmly convinced that the first time they had seen the word, it absolutely was not on the screen at the front of the room they were in. Some became annoyed at being asked over and over. Since Jacoby's work, lab-induced memory research has become very popular in psychology. In fact, it has been given its own name: *priming*. Alan Brown and Elizabeth Marsh confirmed Jacoby's findings in three follow-up studies (38–41).

Andrei begins fourth topic introduced earlier.

Inattention, or what some researchers call "inattentional blindness," is also an extensively researched explanation for the déjà vu experience. Sometimes people can see objects without any impediment right before them but still not process

continued >>

Gurov 7

the objects because they're paying attention to something else (Brown, *Experience* 181). The distraction might be daydreaming, a sudden lowering of energy, or simply being drawn to another object in the environment. As David Glenn explains in "The Tease of Memory":

> Imagine that you drive through an unfamiliar town but pay little attention because you're talking on a cellphone [sic]. If you then drive back down the same streets a few moments later, this time focusing on the landscape, you might be prone to experience déjà vu. During your second pass, the visual information is consciously processed in the hippocampus [of the brain] but feels falsely "old" because the images from your earlier drive still linger in your short term memory.

The word "sic," in brackets, shows the source mistakenly made "cell phone" one word.

The busy lifestyle today would seem to lead to many distractions of perception and thus to frequent experiences of déjà vu; however, these are no more frequently reported than any other causes reported concerning déjà vu.

Andrei anticipates and answers a reader's possible question.

One compelling laboratory experiment studying inattention is described by Carey in "Déjà Vu: If It All Seems Familiar, There May Be a Reason." He recounts a test with many college students from Duke University in Durham, North Carolina. The students were asked to look at a group of photographs of the campus of Southern Methodist University in Dallas, Texas, that were flashed before them at a very quick speed. A small black or white cross was superimposed on each photograph, and the students were instructed to find the cross and focus on it (F6). Brown in *The Déjà Vu Experience* explains

In order to explain "inattention," Andrei summarizes an experiment at some length.

continued >>

Gurov 8

that the researchers assumed that the quick speed at which the photographs had been shown would result in no one's having noticed the background scenes. A week's time passed, and the same students were shown the pictures again, this time without the crosses. Almost all insisted that they had been to the college campus shown in the photos, which was physically impossible for that many students since they lived in Durham, North Carolina, and the college in the photographs was in Dallas, Texas (182–83). This means that the scenes in the photographs did indeed register in the visual memories of the students in spite of the quick speed and the distraction of looking only for the crosses.

Parenthetical citation shows pages summarized in this sentence.

The worlds of psychology and neurology have learned much since the age of paranormal interpretations of déjà vu experiences, starting around 1935. That is when rational science energetically began its disciplined investigations of brain-based origins of the déjà vu phenomenon. Concepts such as dual processing of sight, implanted memories, and inattentional blindness, among other theories, have gone far in opening the door to the possibilities of many more inventive theories to explain incidents of déjà vu. The leading researcher in the field today, Alan S. Brown, is among the strongest voices urging a vast expansion of investigations into this still relatively unexplored phenomenon. He is optimistic this will happen, given his whimsical remark to Carlin Flora of *Psychology Today:* "We are always fascinated when the brain goes haywire." Researchers conducting these studies might watch for the unsettling experiences of other investigators who "have had déjà vu about having déjà vu" (Phillips).

Concluding paragraph reviews theories that were presented in paper.

Two quotations, by Flora and Phillips, create a memorable ending.

continued >>

Gurov 9

Works Cited

Brown, Alan S. *The Déjà Vu Experience: Essays in Cognitive Psychology*. New York: Psychology, 2004. Print.

---. "The Déjà Vu Illusion." *Current Directions in Psychological Science* 13.6 (2004): 256–59. Print.

--- and Elizabeth J. Marsh. "Digging into Deja Vu: Recent Research on Possible Mechanisms." *The Psychology of Learning and Motivation: Advances in Research and Theory*. Ed. Brian H. Ross. Burlington: Academic P, 2010, 33–62. Web. 20 Nov. 2011.

Carey, Benedict. "Déjà Vu: If It All Seems Familiar, There May Be a Reason." *New York Times* 14 Sept. 2004: F1+. *LexisNexis*. Web. 11 Nov. 2011.

Flora, Carlin. "Giving Déjà Vu Its Due." *Psychology Today* Mar.–Apr. 2005: 27. *Academic Search Premier*. Web. 7 Nov. 2011.

Glenn, David. "The Tease of Memory." *Chronicle of Higher Education* 23 July 2004: A12. Print.

Johnson, C. "A Theory on the Déjà Vu Phenomenon." 8 Dec. 2001. Web. 20 Nov. 2011.

Lemonick, Michael D. "Explaining Déjà Vu." *Time* 20 Aug. 2007. *Academic Search Premier*. Web. 5 Dec. 2011.

O'Connor, Akira R., Colin Lever, and Chris J. A. Moulin. "Novel Insights into False Recollection: A Model of Deja Vecu." *Cognitive Neuropsychiatry* 15.1–3 (2010): 118–44. Web. 14 Nov. 2011.

Phillips, Helen. "Looks Familiar." *New Scientist* 201.2701 (28 Mar. 2009): 28–31. Web. 20 Nov. 2011.

Works Cited, centered, begins on a new page. While Andrei's Working Bibliography had twice as many sources, his final draft includes only those related to his thesis.

Sources are listed in alphabetical order and double-spaced throughout, using hanging indentations.

Final Works Cited list has thirteen sources, five popular and the rest scholarly, proportions typical of a first-year college-level research paper.

continued >>

Gurov 10

Thompson, Rebecca G., et al. "Persistent Déjà Vu: A Disorder of Memory." *International Journal of Geriatric Psychiatry* 19.9 (2004): 906–07. Print.

Weiten, Wayne. *Psychology: Themes and Variations*. Belmont: Wadsworth, 2005. Print.

Wolfradt, Uwe. "Strangely Familiar." *Scientific American Mind* 16.1 (2005): 32–37. *Academic Search Elite*. Web. 7 Nov. 2011.

26 APA Documentation with Case Study

Quick Points You will learn to

- Use APA in-text parenthetical documentation (see 26B and 26C).
- Use APA guidelines for a References list (see 26D and 26E).
- Format your paper according to APA guidelines (see 26I).

APA In-Text Citations Directory

APA References List Directory

26A What is APA documentation style?

The American Psychological Association (APA) sponsors the **APA style**, a DOCUMENTATION* system widely used in the social sciences. APA style has two equally important features that need to appear in research papers.

1. Within the body of your paper, you need to use IN-TEXT CITATIONS, in parentheses, to acknowledge your SOURCES as described in sections 26B and 26C.
2. At the end of the paper, provide a list of the sources you used—and only those sources. Title this list, which contains complete bibliographic information about each source, "References," as explained in sections 26D and 26E.

See 26I for a sample student paper in APA style.

26B What are APA in-text parenthetical citations?

APA style requires parenthetical documentation (also called in-text citations) that identify a source by the author's name and the copyright year. If there is no author, use a shortened version of the title. In addition, APA style requires page numbers for DIRECT QUOTATIONS, but it recommends using them also for PARAPHRASES and SUMMARIES. Some instructors expect you to give page references for paraphrases and summaries and others don't, so find out your instructor's preference to avoid any problems. Put page numbers in parentheses, using the abbreviation *p.* before a single page number and *pp.* when the material you're citing falls on more than one page. Separate the parts of a parenthetical citation with commas. End punctuation always follows the citation unless it's a long quotation set in block style in which case the citation comes after the end punctuation.

If you refer to a work more than once in a paragraph, APA style recommends giving the author's name and the date at the first mention and then using only the name after that. However, if you're citing two or more works by the same author, include the date in each citation to identify which work you're citing. When two or more sources have the same last name, keep them clearly separate by using both first and last names in the text or first initial(s) and last names in parentheses.

*Words printed in SMALL CAPITAL LETTERS are discussed elsewhere in the Terms Glossary at the back of the book.

26C What are APA examples for in-text citations?

This section shows how to cite various kinds of sources in the body of your paper. The directory at the beginning of this tab corresponds to the numbered examples in this section.

1. Paraphrased or Summarized Source

Modern technologies and social media tend to fragment individual identities (Conley, 2009).

Author name and date cited in parentheses.

Dalton Conley (2009) contends that modern technologies and social media fragment individual identities.

Author name cited in text; date cited in parentheses.

2. Source of a Short Quotation

Approaches adopted from business to treat students as consumers "do not necessarily yield improved outcomes in terms of student learning" (Arum & Roksa, 2011, p. 137).

Author names, date, and page reference cited in parentheses.

Arum & Roksa (2011) find that approaches adopted from business to treat students as consumers "do not necessarily yield improved outcomes in terms of student learning" (p. 137).

Author names cited in text, followed by the date cited in parentheses incorporated into the words introducing the quotation; page number in parentheses immediately following the quotation.

3. Source of a Long Quotation

When you use a quotation of forty or more words, set it off in block style indented ½ inch from the left margin. Don't use quotation marks. Place the parenthetical reference one space after the end punctuation of the quotation's last sentence.

Although some have called for regulating online games, others see such actions as unwarranted:

> Any activity when taken to excess can cause problems in a person's life, but it is unlikely that there would be legislation against, for example, people excessively reading or exercising. There is no argument that online gaming should be treated any differently. (Griffiths, 2010, pp. 38–39)

Author name, date, and page reference cited in parentheses following the end punctuation.

4. One Author

> One of his questions is, "What binds together a Mormon banker in Utah with his brother or other coreligionists in Illinois or Massachusetts?" (Coles, 1993, p. 2).

In a parenthetical reference in APA style, a comma and a space separate a name from a year and a year from a page reference.

5. Two Authors

If a work has two authors, give both names in each citation.

> One report describes 2,123 occurrences (Krait & Cooper, 2003).
>
> The results that Krait and Cooper (2003) report would not support the conclusions Davis and Sherman (1999) draw in their review of the literature.

When you write a parenthetical in-text citation naming two (or more) authors, use an ampersand (&) between the final two names (as in the first example). However, write out the word *and* for references you include in your own sentence (as in the second example).

6. Three, Four, or Five Authors

For three, four, or five authors, use all of the authors' last names in the first reference. In all subsequent references, use only the first author's last name followed by *et al.* (meaning "and others"). No period follows *et*, but one always follows *al.*

FIRST REFERENCE

> In one study, only 30% of the survey population could name the most commonly spoken languages in five Middle Eastern countries (Ludwig, Rodriquez, Novak, & Ehlers, 2008).

SUBSEQUENT REFERENCE

> Ludwig et al. (2008) found that most Americans could identify the language spoken in Saudi Arabia.

7. Six or More Authors

For six or more authors, name the first author followed by *et al.* in all in-text references, including the first.

These injuries can lead to an inability to perform athletically, in addition to initiating degenerative changes at the joint level (Mandelbaum et al., 2005).

8. Author(s) with Two or More Works in the Same Year

If you use more than one source written in the same year by the same author(s), alphabetize the works by title for the REFERENCES list, and assign letters in alphabetical order to each work: (2007a), (2007b), (2007c). Use the year–letter combination in parenthetical references. Note that a citation of two or more such works lists the year extensions in alphabetical order.

Most recently, Torrevillas (2007c) draws new conclusions from the results of eight experiments conducted with experienced readers (Torrevillas, 2007a, 2007b).

9. Two or More Authors with the Same Last Name

Include first initials for every in-text citation of authors who share a last name. Be sure to use the same initials appearing in your References list at the end of your paper. (In the second example, a parenthetical citation, the name order is alphabetical, as explained in item 12.)

R. A. Smith (2008) and C. Smith (1999) both confirm these results.

These results have been confirmed independently (C. Smith, 1999; R. A. Smith, 2008).

10. Group or Corporate Author

If you use a source in which the "author" is a corporation, agency, or group, an in-text reference gives that name as author. Use the full name in each citation, unless an abbreviated version of the name is likely to be familiar to your audience. In that case, use the full name and give its abbreviation in brackets at the first citation; then, use the abbreviation for subsequent citations.

Although the space shuttle program has ended, other programs will continue to send Americans into space (National Aeronautics and Space Administration [NASA], 2011).

In subsequent citations, use the abbreviated form alone.

11. Work Listed by Title

If no author is named, use a shortened form of the title for in-text citations. Ignoring *A, An,* or *The*, make the first word the one by which you alphabetize the title in your References list at the end of your paper. The following example refers to an article fully titled "Are You a Day or Night Person?"

> Scientists group people as "larks" or "owls" on the basis of whether individuals are more efficient in the morning or at night ("Are You," 1989).

12. Two or More Sources in One Reference

If more than one source has contributed to an idea or opinion in your paper, cite the sources alphabetically by author in one set of parentheses; separate each source of information with a semicolon, as in the following example.

> Conceptions of personal space vary among cultures (Morris, 1977; Worchel & Cooper, 1983).

13. Personal Communication, Including E-Mail and Other Nonretrievable Sources

Telephone calls, personal letters, interviews, and e-mail messages are "personal communications" that your readers can't access or retrieve. Acknowledge personal communications in parenthetical references, but never include them in your References list at the end of your paper.

> Recalling his first summer at camp, one person said, "The proximity of 12 other kids made me—an only child with older, quiet parents—frantic for eight weeks" (A. Weiss, personal communication, January 12, 2011).

14. Retrievable Online Sources

When you quote, paraphrase, or summarize an online source that is available to others, cite the author (if any) or title and the date as you would for a print source, and include the work in your References list.

> It is possible that similarity in personality is important in having a happy marriage (Luo & Clonen, 2005, p. 324).

15. Sources with No Page Numbers

If an online or other source doesn't provide page numbers, use the paragraph number, if available, preceded by the abbreviation *para.* It is rare, however, to number paragraphs. If you can't find a page or paragraph number, cite a heading if possible.

(Daniels, 2010, para. 4)

(Sanz, 2009, Introduction)

(Herring, 2011)

16. Source Lines for Graphics and Table Data

If you use a graphic from another source or create a table using data from another source, provide a note at the bottom of the table or graphic, crediting the original author and the copyright holder. Here are examples of two source notes, one for a graphic using data from an article, the other for a graphic reprinted from a book.

GRAPHIC USING DATA FROM AN ARTICLE

Note. The data in columns 1 and 2 are from "Advance Organizers in Advisory Reports: Selective Reading, Recall, and Perception" by L. Lagerwerf et al., 2008, *Written Communication, 25*(1), p. 68. Copyright 2008 by Sage Publications.

GRAPHIC FROM A BOOK

Note. From *Academically Adrift: Limited Learning on College Campuses* (p. 97), by R. Arum and J. Roksa, 2011, Chicago: University of Chicago Press. Copyright 2011 by The University of Chicago.

26D What are APA guidelines for a References list?

The **References** list at the end of your research paper provides complete bibliographic information for readers who may want to access the SOURCES you drew on to write your paper.

Include in the References list all the sources you quote, paraphrase, or summarize in your paper so that readers can find the same sources with reasonable effort. Never include in your References list any source that's not generally available to other people (see item 13 in 26C). Quick Box 26.1 provides general information about an APA References list, and section 26E gives many models for specific kinds of entries. See 26I for a sample of a student References list.

Quick Box 26.1

Guidelines for an APA-style References list

TITLE

The title is "References," centered, without quotation marks, italics, or underlining.

PLACEMENT OF LIST

Start a new page numbered sequentially with the rest of the paper, immediately after the body of the paper.

CONTENTS AND FORMAT

Include all quoted, paraphrased, or summarized sources in your paper that are not personal communications; however, if your instructor tells you also to include all the references you have simply consulted, please do so. Start each entry on a new line, and double-space all lines. Use a *hanging indent* style: The first line of each entry begins flush left at the margin, and all other lines are indented ½ inch.

Wolfe, C. R. (2011). Argumentation across the curriculum. *Written Communication, 28,* 193–218.

SPACING AFTER PUNCTUATION

APA calls for one space after commas, periods, question marks, and colons.

ARRANGEMENT OF ENTRIES

Alphabetize by the author's last name. If no author is named, alphabetize by the first significant word (ignore *A, An,* or *The*) in the title of the work.

AUTHORS' NAMES

Use last names, first initials, and middle initials, if any. Reverse the order for all authors' names, and use an ampersand (&) before the last author's name: Mills, J. F., & Holahan, R. H.

Give names in the order in which they appear on the work. Use a comma between each author's last name and first initial and after each complete name except the last. Use a period after the last author's name.

DATES

Date information follows the name information and is enclosed in parentheses. If date information falls at the end of your sentence, place a period followed by one space after the closing parenthesis.

For books, articles in journals that have volume numbers, and many other print and nonprint sources, the year of publication or production is

continued >>

Quick Box 26.1 (continued)

the date to use. For articles from most general-circulation magazines and newspapers, use the year followed by a comma and then the exact date that appears on the issue (month, month and day, or season, depending on the frequency of the publication). Capitalize any words in dates, and use no abbreviations.

CAPITALIZATION OF TITLES

For book, article, and chapter titles, capitalize the first word, the first word after a colon between a title and subtitle, and any proper nouns. For names of journals and proceedings of meetings, capitalize the first word; all NOUNS, VERBS, ADVERBS, and ADJECTIVES; and any other words four or more letters long.

FORMAT OF TITLES

Use no italics, quotation marks, or underlines for titles of shorter works (poems, short stories, essays, articles, Web pages). Italicize titles of longer works (books, newspapers, journals, or Web sites). If an italic typeface is unavailable, underline the title and the end punctuation using one unbroken line.

Do not drop any words (such as *A*, *An*, or *The*) from the titles of periodicals such as newspapers, magazines, and journals. See 26F for information on formatting the title of your own APA research paper.

ABBREVIATIONS OF MONTHS

Do not abbreviate the names of months in any context.

PAGE NUMBERS

Use all digits, omitting none. For references to books and newspapers only, use *p.* (for one page) and *pp.* (for more than one page) before page numbers. List all discontinuous pages, with numbers separated by commas: pp. 32, 44–45, 47–49, 53.

PUBLICATION INFORMATION

Publication information varies according to type of source. See 26E for how to cite articles from periodicals (both print or online), books (both print or digital), images and video, other Web sources, and miscellaneous sources.

26E What are APA examples for sources in a References list?

The directory at the beginning of this tab corresponds to the numbered examples in this section. For quick help deciding which example you should follow, see the decision flowchart in Figure 26.1. You can find other examples in the *Publication Manual of the American Psychological Association* (6th edition) or at the APA Web site, http://www.apastyle.org.

Figure 26.1 Decision-making flowchart for APA References citations.

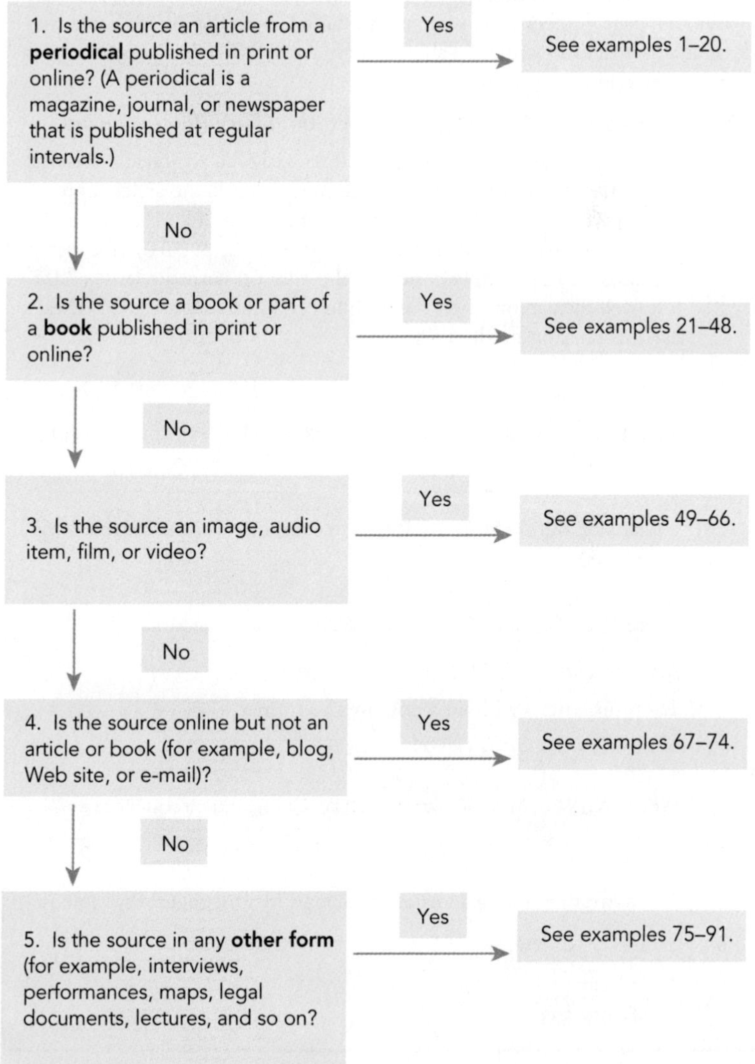

Quick Box 26.2 summarizes the basic entries for periodical entries. Variations on the basic entries follow the Quick Box.

Quick Box 26.2

Basic entries for periodical articles with and without DOIs—APA

Citations for periodical articles contain four major parts: author, date, title of article, and publication information (usually, the periodical title, volume number, page numbers, and sometimes a digital object identifier). Some citations also include information about the type of source in brackets; examples are reviews, motion pictures, and so on.

1. Articles with a DOI (Digital Object Identifier): Print or online

   A **DOI** is a numerical code sometimes assigned to journal articles. The DOI for an article will be the same even if the article appears in different versions including print and online. (To see where you can find an article's DOI, refer to Figure 26.2, p. 374.) If a source contains a DOI, simply conclude the citation with the letters "doi" followed by a colon, then the number. If a source has a DOI, always use this citation method.

   AUTHOR · DATE · ARTICLE TITLE · PUBLICATION INFORMATION · DOI

   Agliata, A. K., Tantelff-Dunn, S., & Renk, K. (2007). Interpretation of teasing during early adolescence. *Journal of Clinical Psychology, 63*(1), 23–30. doi: 10.1002/jclp.20302

2. Articles with no DOI: Print

   For print articles without a doi, use this format.

   AUTHOR · DATE · ARTICLE TITLE · PERIODICAL TITLE · VOLUME NUMBER · PAGE RANGE

   Wood, W., Witt, M. G., & Tam, L. (2005). Changing circumstances, disrupting habits. *Journal of Personality and Social Psychology, 88*, 918–933.

continued >>

Quick Box 26.2 (continued)

3. Articles with no DOI: Online

For online articles without a DOI, retrieval information begins with the words "Retrieved from," then the URL of the periodical's Web home page, and, occasionally, additional information. If you found the article through an online subscription database, do a Web search for the URL of the periodical's home page on the Web, and include the home page URL. If you can't find the periodical's Web home page, then name the database in your retrieval statement: for example, "Retrieved from Academic Search Premier database" (see example 20). If a URL must be divided on two or more lines, only break the address before slashes or punctuation marks.

Retrieval date: Include the date you retrieved the information only if the item does not have a publication date, is from an online reference book, or is likely to be changed in the future (such as a prepublication version of an article, a Web page, or a Wiki; see citation 72).

AUTHOR / DATE / ARTICLE TITLE

Eagleman, D. (2011, July/August). The brain on trial.

MAGAZINE TITLE / ONLINE RETRIEVAL INFORMATION

The Atlantic. Retrieved from http://www.theatlantic.com

Notice that the only punctuation in the URL is part of the address. Do not add a period after a URL.

PERIODICALS—APA REFERENCES

1. Article in a Journal with Continuous Pagination: Print

Williams, B. T. (2010). Seeking new worlds: The study of writing beyond our classrooms. *College Composition and Communication, 62*, 127–146.

Continuous pagination means that page numbers in each issue of a volume begin where the page numbers in the previous issue left off. So, for example, if issue one stopped at page 125, issue two would start at page 126. Just give the volume number, italicized after the journal title.

2. Article in a Journal with Continuous Pagination: Online, with DOI

Gurung, R., & Vespia, K. (2007). Looking good, teaching well? Linking liking, looks, and learning. *Teaching of Psychology, 34*, 5–10. doi: 10.1207/s15328023top3401_2

Figure 26.2 Journal article available in print and online, with a DOI.

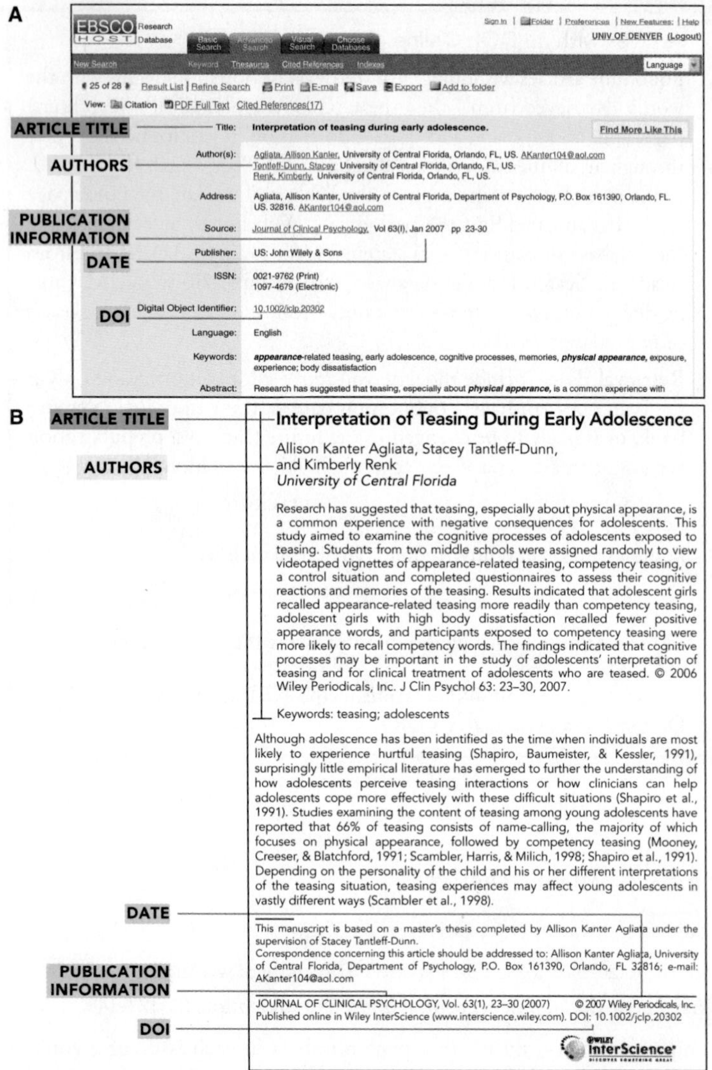

EBSCO HOST Research Database | Basic Search | Advanced Search | Visual Search | Choose Databases
Sign In | Folder | Preferences | New Features! | Help
UNIV OF DENVER (Logout)
New Search | Keyword | Thesaurus | Cited References | Indexes | Language
25 of 28 | Result List | Refine Search | Print | E-mail | Save | Export | Add to folder
View: Citation | PDF Full Text | Cited References(17)

Title:	**Interpretation of teasing during early adolescence.**
Author(s):	Agliata, Allison Kanter, University of Central Florida, Orlando, FL, US. AKanter104@aol.com Tantleff-Dunn, Stacey University of Central Florida, Orlando, FL, US. Renk, Kimberly, University of Central Florida, Orlando, FL, US.
Address:	Agliata, Allison Kanter, University of Central Florida, Department of Psychology, P.O. Box 161390, Orlando, FL. US. 32816. AKanter104@aol.com
Source:	Journal of Clinical Psychology, Vol 63(I), Jan 2007 pp 23-30
Publisher:	US: John Wiley & Sons
ISSN:	0021-9762 (Print) 1097-4679 (Electronic)
Digital Object Identifier:	10.1002/jclp.20302
Language:	English
Keywords:	***appearance***-related teasing, early adolescence, cognitive processes, memories, ***physical appearance***, exposure, experience; body dissatisfaction
Abstract:	Research has suggested that teasing, especially about ***physical apperance***, is a common experience with

Find More Like This

Interpretation of Teasing During Early Adolescence

Allison Kanter Agliata, Stacey Tantleff-Dunn, and Kimberly Renk
University of Central Florida

Research has suggested that teasing, especially about physical appearance, is a common experience with negative consequences for adolescents. This study aimed to examine the cognitive processes of adolescents exposed to teasing. Students from two middle schools were assigned randomly to view videotaped vignettes of appearance-related teasing, competency teasing, or a control situation and completed questionnaires to assess their cognitive reactions and memories of the teasing. Results indicated that adolescent girls recalled appearance-related teasing more readily than competency teasing, adolescent girls with high body dissatisfaction recalled fewer positive appearance words, and participants exposed to competency teasing were more likely to recall competency words. The findings indicated that cognitive processes may be important in the study of adolescents' interpretation of teasing and for clinical treatment of adolescents who are teased. © 2006 Wiley Periodicals, Inc. J Clin Psychol 63: 23–30, 2007.

Keywords: teasing; adolescents

Although adolescence has been identified as the time when individuals are most likely to experience hurtful teasing (Shapiro, Baumeister, & Kessler, 1991), surprisingly little empirical literature has emerged to further the understanding of how adolescents perceive teasing interactions or how clinicians can help adolescents cope more effectively with these difficult situations (Shapiro et al., 1991). Studies examining the content of teasing among young adolescents have reported that 66% of teasing consists of name-calling, the majority of which focuses on physical appearance, followed by competency teasing (Mooney, Creeser, & Blatchford, 1991; Scambler, Harris, & Milich, 1998; Shapiro et al., 1991). Depending on the personality of the child and his or her different interpretations of the teasing situation, teasing experiences may affect young adolescents in vastly different ways (Scambler et al., 1998).

This manuscript is based on a master's thesis completed by Allison Kanter Agliata under the supervision of Stacey Tantleff-Dunn.
Correspondence concerning this article should be addressed to: Allison Kanter Agliata, University of Central Florida, Department of Psychology, P.O. Box 161390, Orlando, FL 32816; e-mail: AKanter104@aol.com

JOURNAL OF CLINICAL PSYCHOLOGY, Vol. 63(1), 23–30 (2007) © 2007 Wiley Periodicals, Inc.
Published online in Wiley InterScience (www.interscience.wiley.com). DOI: 10.1002/jclp.20302

WILEY InterScience

CITATION

Agliata, A.K., Tantleff-Dunn, S., & Renk, K. (2007). Interpretation of teasing during early adolescence. *Journal of Clinical Psychology, 63*(1). 23–30. doi: 10.1002/jcpl.2302

3. Article in a Journal with Continuous Pagination: Online, No DOI

Pollard, R. (2002). Evidence of a reduced home field advantage when a team moves to a new stadium. *Journal of Sports Sciences, 20*, 969–974. Retrieved from http://www.tandf.co.uk/journals/risp

No retrieval date is included because the final version of the article is being referenced.

4. Article in a Journal That Pages Each Issue Separately: Print

Peters, B. (2011). Lessons about writing to learn from a university–high school partnership. *WPA: Writing Program Administration, 34*(2), 59–88.

Give the volume number, italicized with the journal title, followed by the issue number in parentheses (not italicized), and the page number(s).

5. Article in a Journal That Pages Each Issue Separately: Online, with No DOI

Peters, B. (2011). Lessons about writing to learn from a university–high school partnership. *WPA: Writing Program* Administration, 34(2). Retrieved from http://wpacouncil.org/journal/index.html

6. In-press Article: Online

George, S. (in press). How accurately should we estimate the anatomical source of exhaled nitric oxide? *Journal of Applied Physiology*. doi:10.1152/japplphysiol.00111.2008. Retrieved February, 2008 from http://jap.physiology.org/papbyrecent.shtml

In press means that an article has been accepted for publication but has not yet been published in its final form. Therefore, there is no publication date, so although the article has a DOI, it also has a "retrieved from" statement that includes a date, in case anything changes.

7. Article in a Weekly or Biweekly Magazine: Print

Foroohar, R. (2011, June 27). Why the world isn't getting smaller. *Time*, 20.

Give the year, month, and date. If no author is listed, begin with the title of the article.

The price is wrong. (2003, August 2). *The Economist, 368*, 58–59.

8. Article in a Weekly or Biweekly Magazine: Online

Foroohar, R. (2011, June 27). Why the world isn't getting smaller. *Time*. Retrieved from http://www.time.com/time/

9. Article in a Monthly or Bimonthly Periodical: Print

Goetz, T. (2011, July). The feedback loop. *Wired, 19*(7), 126–133.

Give the year and month(s). Insert the volume number, italicized with the periodical title. Put the issue number in parentheses; do not italicize it.

10. Article in a Newspaper: Print

Hesse, M. (2011, April 24). Love among the ruins. *The Washington Post*, p. F1.

Use the abbreviation *p.* (or *pp.* for more than one page) for newspapers. If no author is listed, begin with the title of the article.

Prepping for uranium work. (2011, June 18). *The Denver Post*, p. B2.

11. Article in a Newspaper: Online

Hesse, M. (2011, April 22). Falling in love with St. Andrews, Scotland. *The Washington Post*. Retrieved from http://www.washingtonpost.com/

Give the URL from the newspaper's Web site. Some newspapers publish only online. Treat them the same way, as follows:

Katz, D. (2010, October 28). What to do about flu? Get vaccinated. *Huffington Post*. Retrieved from http://www.huffingtonpost.com

12. Editorial: Print

Primary considerations. (2008, January 27). [Editorial]. *The Washington Post*, p. B6.

Include the type of writing in brackets immediately after the date. For example [Editorial] or [Review] or [Letter].

13. Editorial: Online

Primary considerations. (2008, January 27). [Editorial]. *The Washington Post*. Retrieved from http://www.washingtonpost.com

14. Letter to the Editor: Print

Goldstein, L. (2011, May/June). [Letter to the editor]. Roach coaches: The upside. *Sierra*, 2.

15. Letter to the Editor: Online

Ennis, H. B. (2007, December 22). [Letter to the editor]. *U.S. News and World Report*. Retrieved from http://www.usnews.com

16. Book Review: Print

Shenk, D. (2003, Spring). Toolmaker, brain builder. [Review of the book *Beyond Deep Blue: Building the computer that defeated the world chess champion* by Feng-Hsiung Hsu]. *The American Scholar, 72*, 150–152.

17. Movie Review: Online

Travers, P. (2011, June 2). [Review of the motion picture *Beginners*, directed by Mike Mills]. *RollingStone*. Retrieved from http://www.rollingstone.com

18. Article in a Looseleaf Collection of Reprinted Articles

Hayden, T. (2002). The age of robots. In E. Goldstein (Ed.), *Applied Science 2002. SIRS 2002*, Article 66. (Reprinted from *U.S. News & World Report*, pp. 44–50, 2001, April 23).

19. Online Magazine Content Not Found in Print Version

Shulman, M. (2008, January 3). 12 diseases that altered history. [Supplemental material]. *U.S. News & World Report*. Retrieved from http://health.usnews .com/

The bracketed phrase [Supplemental material] indicates that content appears in the online version of this source that does not appear in the print version.

20. Abstract from a Secondary Source: Online

Walther, J. B., Van Der Heide, B., Kim, S., Westerman, D., & Tong, S. (2008). The role of friends' appearance and behavior on evaluations of individuals on Facebook: Are we known by the company we keep? *Human Communication Research 34*(1), 28–49. Abstract retrieved from PsycINFO database.

BOOKS—APA REFERENCES

Quick Box 26.3 summarizes the basic entry for books, both print and electronic. Variations on the basic entries follow. Where to locate a book's citation information is shown in Figure 26.3 (page 379).

Quick Box 26.3

Basic entries for books—APA

All citations for books have four main parts: author, date, title, and publication information. For traditional print books, publication information includes place of publication and the name of the publisher. For electronic versions of books, publication information also includes retrieval information.

PLACE OF PUBLICATION

For U.S. publishers, give the city and state, using two-letter postal abbreviations listed in most dictionaries. For publishers in other countries, give

continued >>

Quick Box 26.3 (continued)

city and country spelled out. However, if the state or country is part of the publisher's name, omit it after the name of the city.

PUBLISHERS

Use a shortened version of the publisher's name except for an association, corporation, or university press. Drop *Co., Inc., Publishers,* and the like, but retain *Books* or *Press*.

AUTHOR DATE TITLE

Wood, G. S. (2011). *The idea of America: Reflections on the birth of the United States.* New York, NY: Penguin Press.

PUBLICATION INFORMATION

RETRIEVAL INFORMATION FOR ELECTRONIC BOOKS

If a book has a DOI (Document Object Identifier; see Quick Box 26.2 for an explanation), include that number after the title, preceded by doi and a colon. Most electronic books do not have a DOI. When there is no DOI, use "Retrieved from" followed by the URL where you accessed the book.

21. Book by One Author: Print

Turkle, S. (2011). *Alone together: Why we expect more from technology and less from each other.* New York, NY: Basic Books.

22. Book by One Author: Online

Turkle, S. (2007). *Evocative objects: Things we think with.* Retrieved from http://0-site.ebrary.com.bianca.penlib.du.edu/

Some books are increasingly available through library databases. APA does not include the name or location of the publisher in citations for online books.

23. Book by One Author: E-book or E-reader

Hertsgaard, M. (2011). *Hot: Living through the next fifty years on Earth.* [Kindle version]. Retrieved from http://amazon.com

The name of the version appears in brackets following the title, for example [Kindle version] or [Nook version]. "Retrieved from" precedes the URL of the site from which you downloaded the book.

24. Book by Two Authors

Edin, K., & Kefalas, M. (2005). *Promises I can keep: Why poor women put motherhood before marriage.* Berkeley, CA: University of California Press.

Figure 26.3 Citation information for a print book—APA.

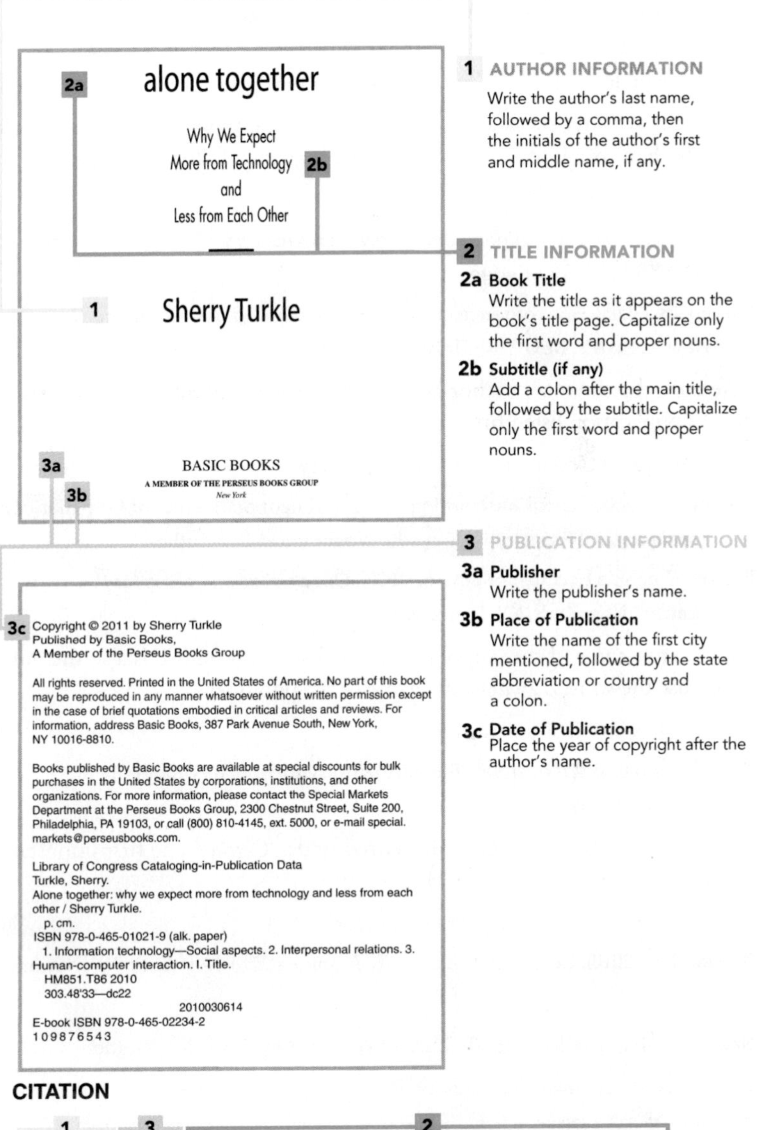

25. Book by Three or More Authors

Lynam, J. K., Ndiritu, C. G., & Mbabu, A. N. (2004). *Transformation of agricultural research systems in Africa: Lessons from Kenya.* East Lansing, MI: Michigan State University Press.

For a book by three to six authors, include all the authors' names. For a book by more than six authors, use only the first six names followed by *et al.*

26. Two or More Books by the Same Author(s)

Jenkins, H. (1992). *Textual poachers: Television fans and participatory culture.* New York, NY: Routledge.

Jenkins, H. (2006). *Convergence culture: Where old and new media collide.* New York, NY: New York University Press.

References by the same author are arranged chronologically, with the earlier date of publication listed first.

27. Book by a Group or Corporate Author

American Psychological Association. (2010). *Publication manual of the American Psychological Association* (6th ed.). Washington, DC: Author.

Boston Women's Health Collective. (1998). *Our bodies, ourselves for the new century.* New York, NY: Simon & Schuster.

Cite the full name of the corporate author first. If the author is also the publisher, use the word *Author* as the name of the publisher.

28. Book with No Author Named

The Chicago manual of style (16th ed.). (2010). Chicago, IL: University of Chicago Press.

Ignoring *The*, this would be alphabetized under *Chicago*, the first important word in the title.

29. Book with an Author and an Editor

Stowe, H. B. (2010). *Uncle Tom's cabin.* (E. Ammons, Ed.). New York, NY: Norton.

30. Translation

Nesbo, J. (2011). *The leopard.* (D. Bartlett, Trans.) New York, NY: Vintage.

31. Work in Several Volumes or Parts

Chrisley, R. (Ed.). (2000). *Artificial intelligence: Critical concepts* (Vols. 1–4). London, England: Routledge.

32. Anthology or Edited Book

Purdy, J. L., & Ruppert, J. (Eds.). (2001). *Nothing but the truth: An anthology of Native American literature.* Upper Saddle River, NJ: Prentice Hall.

33. One Selection in an Anthology or an Edited Book

Trujillo, L. (2004). Balancing act. In R. Moreno & M. H. Mulligan (Eds.), *Borderline personalities: A new generation of Latinas dish on sex, sass, and cultural shifting* (pp. 61–72). New York, NY: HarperCollins.

Give the author of the selection first. The word *In* introduces the larger work from which the selection is taken. To refer to an anthology, see the Chaudhuri citation in example 35.

34. Chapter from an Edited Book: Online

Gembris, H. (2006). The development of musical abilities. In R. Colwell (Ed). *MENC handbook of musical cognition and development*. New York, NY: Oxford University Press (pp.124–164). Retrieved from http://books.google.com/books/

35. Selection in a Work Already Listed in References

Bond, R. (2004). The night train at Deoli. In A. Chaudhuri (Ed.), *The Vintage book of modern Indian literature* (pp. 415–418). New York, NY: Vintage Books.

Chaudhuri, A. (Ed.). (2004). *The Vintage book of modern Indian literature*. New York, NY: Vintage Books.

Provide full information for the already cited anthology (first example), along with information about the individual selection. Put entries in alphabetical order.

36. Article in a Reference Book

Burnbam, J. C. (1996). Freud, Sigmund. In B. B. Wolman (Ed.), *The encyclopedia of psychiatry, psychology, and psychoanalysis* (p. 220). New York, NY: Holt.

If no author is listed, begin with the title of the article.

Ireland. (2002). In *The new encyclopaedia Britannica: Macropaedia* (15th ed., Vol. 21, pp. 997–1018). Chicago, IL: Encyclopaedia Britannica.

37. Second or Later Edition

Modern Language Association. (2009). *MLA handbook for writers of research papers* (7th ed.). New York, NY: Author.

Any edition number appears on the title page. Place it in parentheses after the title.

38. Introduction, Preface, Foreword, or Afterword

Hesse, D. (2004). Foreword. In D. Smit, *The end of composition studies* (pp. ix–xiii). Carbondale, IL: Southern Illinois University Press.

If you're citing an introduction, preface, foreword, or afterword, give its author's name first. After the year, give the name of the part cited. If the writer of the material you're citing isn't the author of the book, use the word *In* and the author's name before the title of the book.

39. Reprint of an Older Book

Coover, R. (2007). *A night at the movies, or, you must remember this.* Champaign, IL: Dalkey Archive, 2007. (Original work published 1987)

You can find republishing information on the copyright page.

40. Book in a Series

Ardell, J. H. (2005). *Breaking into baseball: Women and the national pastime.* Carbondale, IL: Southern Illinois University Press.

Give the title of the book but not of the whole series.

41. Book with a Title within a Title

Lumiansky, R. M., & Baker, H. (Eds.). (1968). *Critical approaches to six major English works:* Beowulf *through* Paradise Lost. Philadelphia, PA: University of Pennsylvania Press.

42. Government Publication: Print

U.S. Congress. House Subcommittee on Health and Environment of the Committee on Commerce. (1999). *The nursing home resident protection amendments of 1999* (99-0266-P). Washington, DC: U.S. Government Printing Office.

U.S. Senate Special Committee on Aging. (1998). *The risk of malnutrition in nursing homes* (98-0150-P). Washington, DC: U.S. Government Printing Office.

Use the complete name of a government agency as author when no specific person is named.

43. Government Publication: Online

United States. Federal Reserve Board. (1998, July 22). *Conduct of monetary policy; report of the Federal Reserve Board pursuant to the Full Employment and Balanced Growth Act of 1978;* July 21, 1998 report. Retrieved 3 December 1998 from the Federal Reserve Web site: http://www.federalreserve.gov/boarddocs/hh/1998/july/fullreport.htm

44. Published Proceedings of a Conference

Rocha, L., Yaeger, L., Bedau, M., Floreano, D., Goldstone, R., & Vespignani, A. (Eds.). (2006, June). *Artificial Life X: Proceedings of the Tenth International Conference on the Simulation and Synthesis of Living Systems.* Bloomington, IN. Cambridge, MA: MIT Press.

45. Thesis or Dissertation

Stuart, G. A. (2006). *Exploring the Harry Potter book series: A study of adolescent reading motivation.* Retrieved from ProQuest Digital Dissertations. (AAT 3246355)

The number in parentheses at the end is the accession number.

46. Entry from Encyclopedia: Online

Turing test. (2008). In *Encyclopaedia Britannica*. Retrieved February 9, 2008, from http://www.britannica.com/bps/topic/609757/Turing-test

Because the reference is to a work that may change, a retrieval date is included.

47. Entry from a Dictionary: Online

Asparagus. (n.d.). *Merriam-Webster's online dictionary*. Retrieved February 9, 2008, from http://dictionary.reference.com/

48. Entry from a Handbook: Online

Gembris, H. (2006). The development of musical abilities. In R. Colwell (Ed). *MENC handbook of musical cognition and development*. New York, NY: Oxford University Press (pp. 124–164). Retrieved from http://books.google.com/books/

IMAGES, AUDIO, FILM, AND VIDEO

49. Photograph, Painting, Drawing, Illustration, etc.: Original

Cassatt, Mary. (1890). *La toilette*. [Painting]. Art Institute of Chicago.

Fourquet, Léon. (1865). *The man with the broken nose.* [Sculpture]. Paris, France: Musée Rodin.

Mydans, C. (1999, October 21–November 28). *General Douglas MacArthur landing at Luzon, 1945* [Photograph]. New York, NY: Soho Triad Fine Art Gallery.

This form is for original works appearing in a gallery, museum, private collection, etc. The date in the third example shows that the work appeared only for a brief period, in this case at the Soho Triad Fine Art Gallery. Note that the medium of the work appears in brackets after its title.

50. Photograph, Painting, Drawing, Illustration, etc. in a Periodical: Print

Greene, H. *Grace Slick*. (2004, September 30). [Photograph]. *Rolling Stone*, 102.

51. Photograph, Painting, Drawing, Illustration, etc. in a Periodical: Online

Morris, C. (2011, July/August). *Man in camouflage*. [Photograph]. *The Atlantic*. Retrieved from http://theatlantic.com

52. Photograph, Painting, Drawing, Illustration, etc. in a Book: Print

The world's most populous countries. (2004). [Illustration]. In P. Turchi, *Maps of the imagination: The writer as cartographer* (pp. 116–117). San Antonio, TX: Trinity University Press.

Indicate the type of image in brackets following the title or, as in this example, the date.

53. Comic or Cartoon: Print

Sutton, W. (2011, May 2). Ryan's a Late Adopter. [Cartoon]. *The New Yorker, 87*(11), 64.

54. Comic or Cartoon: Online

Harris, S. (2002, May 27). We have lots of information technology. [Cartoon]. *The New Yorker*. Retrieved from http://www.newyorker.com

55. Photo Essay: Online

Nachtwey, J. (2006, December 2). *Crime in middle America.* [Photo essay]. *Time.* Retrieved from http:/www.time.com

56. Image from a Social Networking Site

Gristellar, F. (2009, August 7). *The Gateway Arch.* [Photograph]. Retrieved from https://www.facebook.com/qzprofile.php?id=7716zf92444

57. Image from a Service or Distributor

World Perspectives. (1998). *Launching of the Space Shuttle Columbia, Florida, USA, 1998.* [Photograph]. Retrieved from http://gettyimages.com #AT3775-001.

In this example, the photographer was listed as "World Perspectives." Include the name of the service or distributor (in this case Getty Images), and the item number or other identifier, if any.

58. Map, Chart, or Other Graphic: Online

Hurricane Rita. (2005, September 24) [Graphic]. *New York Times Online.* Retrieved from http://www.nytimes.com/packages/html/national /20050923_RITA_GRAPHIC/index.html

59. Audio Book

Turkle, S. (2011). *Alone together: Why we expect more from technology and less from each other.* [MP3-CD]. Old Saybrook, CT: Tantor Media.

60. Sound Recording

Verdi, G. (1874). Requiem. [Recorded by R. Muti (Conductor) and the Chicago Symphony Orchestra and Chorus]. On *Requiem* [CD]. Chicago, IL: CSO Resound. (2010)

Winehouse, A. (2007). Rehab. On *Back to Black* [MP3]. Universal Republic Records. Retrieved from http://amazon.com

List the composer, date, title of the section, performer (if different from the composer), title of the album or compilation and then publication or retrieval information.

61. Audio Podcast

Blumberg, A., & Davidson, D. (Producers). (2008, May 9). *The giant pool of money*. [Audio podcast]. Retrieved from http://thisamericanlife.org

62. Film, Videotape, or DVD

Capra, F. (Director/Producer). (1934). *It happened one night* [Motion Picture]. United States: Columbia Pictures.

Madden, J. (Director), Parfitt, D., Gigliotti, D., Weinstein, H., Zwick, E., & Norman, M. (Producers). (2003). *Shakespeare in love* [DVD]. United States: Miramax. (Original motion picture released 1998)

For video downloads, include the download date and the source.

Capra, F. (Director/Producer). (2010). *It happened one night* [Motion Picture]. United States: Columbia Pictures. Retrieved from Netflix. (Original motion picture released 1934)

63. Video: Online

CNN. (2011, January 27). *Challenger disaster live on CNN* [Video file]. Retrieved from http://www.youtube.com/watch?v=AfnvFnzs91s

Wesch, M. (2007, January 31). *Web 2.0 . . . the machine is us/ing us.* [Video file]. Retrieved from http://www.youtube.com/watch?v=6gmP4nk0EOE

Use this format for videos from YouTube and similar sites.

64. Broadcast Television or Radio Program, Single Event

Burns, K. (Writer/Producer), & Barnes, P. (Producer). (1999, November 8). *Not for ourselves alone: The story of Elizabeth Cady Stanton and Susan B. Anthony* [Television broadcast]. New York, NY: Public Broadcasting Service.

65. Episode from a Television or Radio Series

Doyle, A. C., & Hawkesworth, J. (Writers), & Gorrie, J. (Director). (2011, June 30). The Bruce-Partington plans. *Sherlock Holmes*. [Television broadcast]. KRMA, Denver, CO.

Brand, M. (Anchor). (2011, June 20). *The Madeleine Brand show* [Radio broadcast]. Pasadena, CA: KPCC.

66. Television or Radio Program: Online

Stewart, J. (Performer). (2011, June 1). Bill Moyers. *The Daily Show*. [Video file]. Retrieved from http://www.hulu.com

The disappearing incandescent bulb. (2011, June 20). *The Madeleine Brand Show*. [Radio recording]. KPCC, Pasadena, CA. Retrieved from http://www.scpr.org/programs/madeleine-brand/2011/06/20/the-disappearing-incandescent-bulb/

Give the name of the writer, director, or performer, if available; the date; the title of the episode; the title of the program or series; the type of recording; and retrieval information. Because the second source may be difficult to find, the URL is listed.

OTHER ONLINE SOURCES

If a Web source has a publication or posting date, the retrieval statement includes just the URL. If there is no publication date, include the date of retrieval.

ARTICLE TITLE — DATE

Think again: Men and women share cognitive skills. (2006).

PUBLICATION INFORMATION — RETRIEVAL INFORMATION

American Psychological Association. Retrieved from

URL

http://www.psychologymatters.org/thinkagain.html

Nonretrievable sources: If others can't access a source you have used, APA style says not to include it in your References list. Examples are personal communications such as e-mail or text messages. Instead, cite them in the text with a parenthetical notation saying it's a personal communication (see example 70). If you have a scholarly reason to cite a message from a newsgroup, forum, social networking group, or electronic mailing list that is available in an electronic archive, then see examples 69, 71, 72, 73, and 74.

67. Entire Web Site

Association for the Advancement of Artificial Intelligence. (2008, March). Retrieved March 17, 2008, from http://www.aaai.org

Neff, M. (Ed.). (2011). WebdelSol. Retrieved August 4, 2011, from http://webdelsol.com

Because material on a Web site may change, use a "retrieved from" date.

68. Page from a Web Site

Think again: Men and women share cognitive skills. (2006). American Psychological Association. Retrieved January 18, 2011, from http://www.psychologymatters.org/thinkagain.html

Pennsylvania Department of Education. (n.d). Home education and private tutoring. Retrieved March 4, 2011, from http://www.education.state.pa.us/portal/server.pt/community/home_education_and_private_tutoring/20311

In the second example, "n.d." indicates there was no date given. The retrieval information, however, contains a date.

69. Real-Time Online Communication

Berzsenyi, C. (2007, May 13). Writing to meet your match: Rhetoric, perceptions, and self-presentation for four online daters. *Computers and Writing Online*. [Synchronous discussion]. Retrieved from http://acadianamoo.org

If a chat, discussion, or synchronous (meaning available as it is happening) online-presentation can be retrieved by others, include it in your References list.

70. E-Mail Message

Because e-mails to individuals cannot be retrieved by others, they should not appear on the References list. Cite them in the body of your paper, as in this example:

> The wildfires threatened several of the laboratory facilities at Los Alamos (e-mail from T. Martin on June 20, 2011).

71. Posting on a Blog

Phillips, M. (2011, June 15). Need to go to the ER? Not until the game's over. [Web log post]. Retrieved from http://www.freakonomics.com/2011/06/15/need-to-go-to-the-er-not-until-the-games-over/

72. Wiki

NASCAR Sprint Cup series. (2011). [Wiki]. Retrieved April 6, 2011, from http://nascarwiki.com

Machine learning. (n.d.) Retrieved January 5, 2008, from Artificial Intelligence Wiki: http://www.ifi.unizh.ch/ailab/aiwiki/aiw.cgi

N.d. means "no date." Because a Wiki can change by its very nature, always include a retrieval date.

73. Posting on a Social Networking Site

Adler-Kassner, L. (2011, May 6). Conversations toward action. [Facebook group]. Retrieved from Council of Writing Program Administrators at https://www.facebook.com/groups/106575940874

Include the citation in your References list only if it is retrievable by others. If it's not, cite it only in the body of your paper, as in example 70.

74. Message on an Online Forum, Discussion Group, or Electronic Mailing List

Firrantello, L. (2005, May 23). Van Gogh on Prozac. *Salon Table Talk*. [Online forum posting]. Retrieved February 15, 2009, from http://www.salon.com

Boyle, F. (2002, October 11). Psyche: Cemi field theory: The hard problem made easy [Discussion group posting]. Retrieved from news://sci.psychology.consciousness

Haswell, R. (2005, October 17). A new graphic/text interface. [Electronic mailing list message]. Retrieved May 20, 2011, from http://lists.asu.edu/archives /wpa-l.html

APA advises using *electronic mailing list*, as Listserv is the name of specific software.

OTHER SOURCES

75. Letters

Williams, W. C. (1935). [Letter to his son]. In L. Grunwald & S. J. Adler (Eds.), *Letters of the century: America 1900–1999* (pp. 225–226). New York, NY: Dial Press.

In the APA system, unpublished letters are considered personal communications inaccessible to general readers, so they do not appear in the References list. They are cited only in the body of the paper (see example 70). Letters that have been published or can be retrieved by others are cited as shown in this example.

76. Map or Chart

Colorado Front Range Mountain Bike Topo Map [Map]. (2001). Nederland, CO: Latitude 40.

77. Report, Pamphlet, or Brochure

National Commission on Writing in America's Schools and Colleges. (2003). *The neglected "R": The need for a writing revolution* (Report No. 2). New York, NY: College Board.

U.S. Department of Agriculture. (2007). *Organic foods and labels* [Brochure]. Retrieved December 8, 2008, from http://www.ams.usda.gov/nop /Consumers/brochure.html

78. Legal Source

Brown v. Board of Educ., 347 U.S. 483 (1954).

Include the name of the case, the number of the case, the name of the court deciding the case (if other than the US Supreme Court), and the year of the decision.

79. Abstract Submitted for Meeting or Poster Session

Wang, H. (2007). Dust storms originating in the northern hemisphere of Mars. [Abstract]. AGU 2007 Fall Meeting. Retrieved from http://www.agu.org /meetings/fm07/?content=program

80. Advertisement

Swim at home. (2005). [Advertisement]. *The American Scholar 74*(2), 2.

Nikon D7000. (2010, November). [Advertisement]. Retrieved December 12, 2010, from http://rollingstone.com

Southwest Airlines. (2010, August 24). [Advertisement]. ABC television.

81. Computer Software or Video Game

The Island: Castaway. (2010). [Video game]. N.p: Awem Studio.

"N.p." indicates that the place of publication is unknown.

Guitar hero III: Legends of rock. (2007). [Video game]. Santa Monica, CA: Activision.

Provide an author name, if available. Standard software (Microsoft Word) and program languages (C++) don't need to be given in the References list.

82. Policy Brief

Haskins, R., Paxson, C., & Donahue, E. (2006). *Fighting obesity in the public schools.* Retrieved from http://www.brookings.edu/media/Files/rc /papers/2006/spring_childrenfamilies_haskins/20060314foc.pdf

83. Presentation Slides or Images

Alaska Conservation Solutions. (2006). Montana global warming [PowerPoint slides]. Retrieved from http://www.alaskaconservationsolutions.com/acs /presentations.html

Delyser, A. (2010, February 7). Political movements in the Philippines. [Prezi slides]. University of Denver.

84. Interview

In APA style, a personal interview is not included in the References list. Cite the interview in the text as a personal communication, as in the following example.

Randi Friedman (personal communication, June 30, 2010) endorses this view.

If the interview is published or can be retrieved by others, cite it as follows:

85. Lecture, Speech, or Address

Kennedy, J. F. (1960, September 12). Speech to the Greater Houston Ministerial Association, Rice Hotel, Houston, TX.

86. Live Performance

Miller, A. (Author), & McLean, C. (Director). (2005, September 27). *All my sons* [Theatrical performance]. Center for the Performing Arts, Normal, IL.

Nelson, W. (2011, June 22). *Country Throwdown Tour* [Concert]. Red Rocks Amphitheater, Denver, CO.

87. Microfiche Collection of Articles

Wenzell, R. (1990, February 3). Businesses prepare for a more diverse work force. [Microform]. *St. Louis Post Dispatch*, p. 17. *NewsBank: Employment* 27, fiche 2, grid D12.

A microfiche is a transparent sheet of film (a *fiche*) with microscopic printing that needs to be read through a special magnifier. Each fiche holds several pages, with each page designated by a grid position. A long document may appear on more than one fiche.

88. Musical Score

Schubert, F. (1971). *Symphony in B Minor (Unfinished).* M. Cusid (Ed.). [Musical score]. New York, NY: Norton. (Original work composed 1822)

89. Nonperiodical Publications on CD, DVD, or Magnetic Tape

Perl, S. (2004). *Felt Sense: Guidelines for Composing.* [CD]. Portsmouth, NH: Boynton.

90. Materials on CD or DVD with a Print Version

The price is right. (1992, January 20). *Time*, 38. In *Time Man of the Year*. [CD]. New York, NY: Compact.

Information for the print version ends with the article's page number, 38. Following that comes the title of the CD-ROM (*Time Man of the Year*) and its publication information.

91. Materials on CD or DVD with No Print Version

Artificial intelligence. (2003). *Encarta 2003*. [CD]. Redmond, WA: Microsoft.

Encarta 2003 is a CD-ROM encyclopedia with no print version. "Artificial Intelligence" is the title of an article in *Encarta 2003*.

26F What are APA guidelines for writing an abstract?

As the APA *Publication Manual* (2010) explains, "an abstract is a brief, comprehensive summary" (p. 25) of a longer piece of writing. The APA estimates that an **abstract** should be no longer than about 120 words. Your instructor may require that you include an abstract at the start of a paper; if you're not sure, ask. Make the abstract accurate, objective, and exact. For an example of an abstract, see the student paper in 26I.

26G What are APA guidelines for content notes?

Content notes (usually called footnotes) in APA-style papers add relevant information that cannot be worked effectively into a text discussion. Use consecutive arabic numerals for note numbers. Try to arrange your sentence so that the note number falls at the end. Use a numeral raised slightly above the line of words and immediately after the final punctuation mark. Footnotes may either appear at the bottom of the page they appear on or all together on a separate page following the References. See page 393 for instructions on formatting the Footnotes page.

26H What are APA format guidelines for research papers?

Ask whether your instructor has instructions for preparing a final draft. If not, you can use the APA guidelines here. For an illustration of these guidelines, see the student paper in 26I.

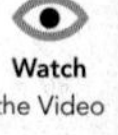

26H.1 General instructions—APA

Print on 8½-by-11-inch white paper and double space. Set at least a 1-inch margin on the left, and leave no less than 1 inch on the right and at the bottom.

Leave ½ inch from the top edge of the paper to the title-and-page-number line (also known as a running head). Leave another ½ inch (or 1 inch from the top edge of the paper) before the next line on the page, whether that's a heading (such as "Abstract" or "Notes") or a line of your paper.

Indent the first line of all paragraphs ½ inch, except in your abstract, the first line of which isn't indented. Do not justify the right margin. Indent footnotes ½ inch.

26H.2 Order of parts—APA

Number all pages consecutively. Use this order for the parts of your paper:

1. Title page
2. Abstract (if required)
3. Body of the paper
4. References
5. Appendixes, if any
6. Footnotes, if any
7. Attachments, if any (questionnaires, data sheets, or other material your instructor asks you to include)

26H.3 Title-and-page-number line (running head) for all pages—APA

Use a title-and-page-number line on all pages of your paper. Place it ½ inch from the top edge of the paper, typing the title (use a shortened version if necessary) and leaving a five-character space before the page number. Use all capital letters in your running head. End the title-and-page-number line 1 inch from the right edge of the paper. Ask whether your instructor wants you to include your last name in the running head. The "header" tool on a word processing program will help you create the title-and-page-number line easily. See the sample student paper on page 396.

26H.4 Title page—APA

Use a separate title page. Include your running head. Center your complete title vertically and horizontally on the page. (Don't italicize, underline, or enclose your title it in quotation marks.) On the next line, center your name, and below that center the course title and section, your professor's name, and the date. See the sample student paper on page 396.

Alerts: (1) Use the guidelines here for capitalizing the title of your own paper and for capitalizing titles you mention in the body of your paper (but not in the REFERENCES list; see Quick Box 26.1).

(2) Use a capital letter for the first word of your title and for the first word of a subtitle, if any. Start every NOUN, PRONOUN, VERB, ADVERB, and ADJECTIVE

with a capital letter. Capitalize each main word in a hyphenated compound word (two or more words used together to express one idea): *Father-in-Law, Self-Consciousness.*

(3) Do not capitalize ARTICLES (*a, an, the*) unless one of the other capitalization rules applies to them. Do not capitalize PREPOSITIONS and CONJUNCTIONS unless they're four or more letters long. Do not capitalize the word *to* used in an INFINITIVE.

(4) In your running head, capitalize all letters. ●

26H.5 Abstract—APA

See 26F for advice about the abstract of your paper. Type the abstract on a separate page, using the numeral 2 in the title-and-page-number line. Center the word *Abstract* 1 inch from the top of the paper. Do not italicize or underline it or enclose it in quotation marks. Double-space below this title, and then start your abstract, double-spacing it. Do not indent the first line.

26H.6 Set-off quotations—APA

Set off (display in block style) quotations of forty words or more. See 26C for a detailed explanation and example.

26H.7 References list—APA

Start a new page for your References list immediately after the end of the body of your paper. One inch from the top of the paper center the word *References.* Don't italicize, underline, or put it in quotation marks. Double-space below it. Start the first line of each entry at the left margin, and indent any subsequent lines five spaces or ½ inch from the left margin. Use this hanging indent style unless your instructor prefers a different one. Double-space within each entry and between entries.

26H.8 Footnotes—APA

Put any notes on a separate page after the last page of your References list and any Appendixes. Center the word *Footnotes* one inch from the top of the paper. Do not italicize or underline it or put it in quotation marks.

On the next line, indent ½ inch and begin the note. Raise the note number slightly (you can use the superscript feature in your word processing program), and then start the words of your note, leaving no space after the number. If the note is more than one typed line, do not indent any line after the first. Double-space throughout.

26I A student's APA-style research paper

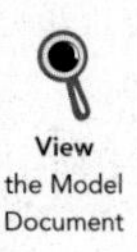
View the Model Document

Here is a student's research paper written according to APA STYLE. We first discuss the planning, researching, drafting, and revising that Leslie Palm did. We also include her final draft, including her title page, abstract, and References page.

> **Case Study**
>
> Leslie Palm was given this assignment for a research paper in an introductory sociology class: Write a research paper of 1,500 to 2,000 words about some aspect of contemporary gender roles. For guidance, refer to the *Simon and Schuster Handbook for Writers*, Chapters 21–24. Use APA documentation, explained in sections 26A–26E. Your topic, research question, and working bibliography are due in two weeks, and a draft of your paper is due two weeks later, both for peer review and instructor feedback. Your final draft is due one week after you receive comments on your first one.

When Leslie read her assignment, she was both pleased and intimidated by the amount of choice she had. She created a research checklist (Quick Box 21.3) and began a RESEARCH LOG, in which she listed several broad topics. These included women in sports, how men and women are portrayed in television shows, how boys and girls experience schooling, gender roles in the workplace, and many others. An avid video game player, Leslie had heard that women were attracted to different features of games than men, and she started pursing that topic. In the process, she started thinking about how other players, especially those multiple player online games, have responded to her. This eventually led to her RESEARCH QUESTION: "How are female characters in video games portrayed and treated?"

Leslie checked to see whether she could find enough credible sources to address this question. She accessed her college library's home page and searched the Academic Search Premier database, using combinations of KEYWORDS "gender," "video games," "female characters," "players," "physical characteristics," and so on. When the results turned up several dozen hits, she figured the topic and research question would work. She used NoodleBib software (21N) to gather the most promising sources into a WORKING BIBLIOGRAPHY, and she downloaded full-text versions of some of the articles and chapters. Leslie also did a general Internet search. Although this search yielded thousands of hits, many were off-topic, and still others, on evaluation, did not seem credible or sufficiently scholarly. However, she did find two sources that she added to her working bibliography.

She considered doing some field research, including e-mail interviews of several women gamers that she knew. Although she began that process, she realized that she didn't have enough time to do it well. She also checked with her professor, who preferred scholarly sources.

Leslie began reading her sources and taking CONTENT NOTES. She opened a document called "Women and Video Games Notes," inserted a heading for each source, and typed summaries or quotations from each source under its heading, along with her own thoughts about what the sources meant and how she might use them. Gradually, themes and issues began to emerge. Leslie opened a second document called "Women and Video Games Themes," in which she cut and pasted her content notes under topical headings. From this, she created a rough OUTLINE and began writing a draft. Her first rough draft allowed her to try out a thesis statement, check the logical arrangement of her material, and see whether she could synthesize her many sources.

That draft was almost 2,500 words. She asked a PEER RESPONSE GROUP which parts of the paper they found most interesting, and which topics she might cut. Leslie received helpful feedback, including that she was spending too much time describing individual games without analyzing them and that her topic about how young girls and boys learn to play, while interesting, was off-topic for this paper. Her instructor also pointed out these issues; in addition, she noted places where Leslie needed to do more research to back up some general claims.

Through a combination of cutting and adding, she produced a second draft. Using Chapter 26 of the *Simon and Schuster Handbook for Writers* as a guide, Leslie had to attend very closely to the details of correct PARENTHETICAL IN-TEXT CITATIONS (see 26B and 26C) within her paper and a correct REFERENCES list (see 26D and 26E) at the end. Because she'd used MLA DOCUMENTATION STYLE in other courses, she made sure not to confuse the two styles. Before doing her final editing and proofreading, Leslie wrote an abstract and made sure the format of the paper met APA standards.

Her final draft follows.

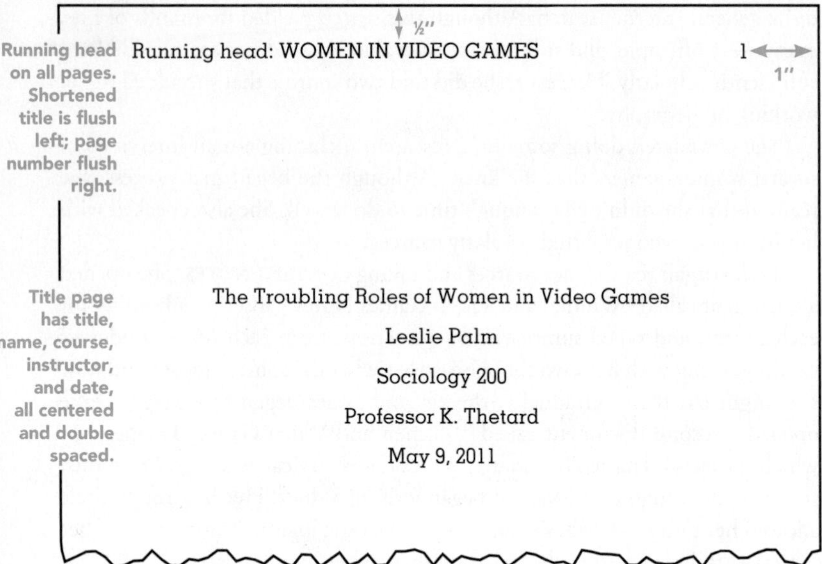

½"
Running head: WOMEN IN VIDEO GAMES
1
1"
The Troubling Roles of Women in Video Games
Leslie Palm
Sociology 200
Professor K. Thetard
May 9, 2011

Running head on all pages. Shortened title is flush left; page number flush right.

Title page has title, name, course, instructor, and date, all centered and double spaced.

½" 1"

WOMEN IN VIDEO GAMES 2

1"

Abstract, if required, goes on page 2.

Abstract

Despite the fact that 40% of video game players are women, female characters and players are treated in ways that are problematic. Video games often portray unrealistic physical characteristics of female characters, exaggerating certain body features. Many games portray women either as vulnerable "damsels in distress" or as sexually aggressive. Women game players often experience stereotyping or harassment. Recent games are changing the way they present female characters.

continued >>

The Depiction of Women in Video Games

Lady Reagan Cousland the First jogs across a virtual pastoral landscape with a two-handed battleax strapped across her shoulders. She is the Player Character in a play through of *Dragon Age: Origins*, a 2009 single-player role-play game, and she is trying to progress through the main quest. However, other characters taunt her. "I have never seen a woman Grey Warden before," says one skeptically. Lady rolls her eyes before sharply answering, "That's because women are too smart to join."

"So what does that make you?" asks the interrupter.

"Insane," she replies.

This exchange exemplifies how women have frequently been portrayed and treated in video games for over two decades. Gaming has long been inaccurately considered an activity pursued almost solely by reclusive males caricatured as "pale loners crouched in the dark among Mountain Dew bottles and pizza boxes" (Wong, 2010). Game producers have mostly catered to this stereotypical player, with discouraging results. Despite evidence that large numbers of women play video games, and despite some important changes, women game characters continue to be physically objectified, represented either as passive or sexually aggressive, and even harassed.

According to data from the Entertainment Software Association (2011), 67% of American households own a video game console of some variety—and 40% of all players are women. In fact, "Women over 18 years of age are one of the

If you have an abstract, begin body of paper on page 3; if not, on page 2.

Introductory paragraphs create interest with a scene.

In-text citation has name and date; source had no pages.

Thesis statement.

continued >>

Brackets show writer added language to make quotation fit sentence.

Page number in citation for direct quote.

industry's fastest growing demographics, [representing] a greater portion of the game-playing population (33 percent) than boys age 17 or younger (20 percent)" (Entertainment Software Association, 2011). And yet, studies show that both male and female gamers believe games to be a "particularly masculine pursuit" (Selwyn, 2007, p. 533).

Physical Characteristics of Female Characters

Paragraph develops first main point, in topic sentence.

The most obvious gender stereotyping in many games comes from the nature of the characters' bodies or avatars. A 2007 content analysis of images of video game characters from top-selling American gaming magazines showed that male characters (83%) are more likely than female characters (62%) to be portrayed as aggressive; however, female characters are more likely to be sexualized (60 vs. 1%) and scantily clad (39 vs. 1%) (Dill & Thill, 2007, pp. 851–864). Even female characters that are considered strong or dominant in personality (such as Morgainn in *Dragon Age: Origins* or Sheva in *Resident Evil 5*) routinely dress in tops that are essentially strips of fabric and skin-tight leather pants. In fact, the reward for beating *Resident Evil 5* is that you get to dress the avatar Sheva in a leopard-print bikini.

With author and date in sentence, only quoted page numbers go in citation.

In *Gender Inclusive Game Design*, Sherri Graner Ray (2003) outlined the physical traits seen between male and female avatars: females are characterized by "exaggerated sexual features such as large breasts set high on their torso, large buttocks, and a waist smaller than her head" (pp. 102–04). Dickerman, Christensen, and Kerl-McClain (2008) found similar qualities. Analyzing characters in 60 video games, Professors Edward Downs and Stacy Smith (2010) found that women were

continued >>

WOMEN IN VIDEO GAMES 5

more likely to be "hypersexualized" then men, depicted with unrealistic body proportions, inappropriate clothing, and other qualities (p. 728).

Even nonhuman females receive this treatment. Game designer Andrea Rubenstein (2007) questions why females of nonhuman races in the popular game *World of Warcraft* are so much smaller and more feminine than their male counterparts. Of one species she notes, "The male is massive: tall with unnaturally large muscles and equally large hooves. . . . It would not be unreasonable to expect the female of the species to be similar." Apparently in *World of Warcraft's* earliest designs, the genders were far more similar; however, when screened to a pool of test gamers, complaints that the females were "ugly" resulted in their being changed to their current form. One scholar notes, "Since gamers and the like have been used to video representations of scantily-clad females and steroid-enhanced males," it is understandable that they would design nonhuman races in a similar way (Bates, 2005, p. 13).

"Even . . . treatment" is an effective transition that continues point from previous paragraph.

Direct quotation embedded in a sentence.

Gender and Character Behavior

Second heading.

The personalities of the characters also demonstrate the gender bias in many games. Dietz's 1998 study of 33 games found that most did not portray women at all. Even ten years later, 86% of game characters were male (Downs & Smith, 2009). Only five of the games in Dietz's study portrayed women as heroes or action characters. The second most common portrayal in this study was as "victim or as the proverbial 'Damsel in Distress' " (Dietz, 1998, pp. 434–35). Examples of vulnerable women stretch from the 1980s to today, from Princess Peach (Nintendo's *Mario*) and Princess Zelda

Topic sentence states second point.

continued >>

(Nintendo's *The Legend of Zelda*) to Alice Wake (Remedy Entertainment's *Alan Wake*), Ashley Graham (Capcom's *Resident Evil 4*), and Alex Roivas (Nintendo's *Eternal Darkness: Sanity's Requiem*). The helpless woman, simply put, is a video game staple, as college students overwhelmingly recognized in one study (Ogletree & Drake, 2007).

Citation for source by 2 authors; no page number because not a direct quotation.

A different staple role gaining popularity is that of the aggressive but sexy woman who will seduce you at night and then shoot you in the morning. Bayonetta, Jill Valentine (in *Resident Evil 3* and *Resident Evil 5*) and, of course, Lara Croft of the *Tomb Raider* series are all examples of this archetype. There is some debate as to whether these examples are evidence of new female power and liberation or simply a new form of exploitation. Dill and Thill (2007) argue that an aggressive female is not necessarily a liberated one, and that "many of these images of aggressive female video game characters glamorize and sexualize aggression." Eugene Provenzo agrees, pointing out that the contradiction between "the seeming empowerment of women, while at the same time . . . they're really being exploited in terms of how they're shown, graphically" (Huntermann, 2000).

Paragraph introduces different aspect of second main point.

Ellipses show writer has cut language from quotation.

Lara Croft is perhaps the epitome of the energetic, aggressive character as an over-exaggerated sexual object. Lead graphic artist Toby Gard went through five designs before arriving at her final appearance, and he began with the desire to counter stereotypical female characters, which he describes as "either a bimbo or a dominatrix" (Yang, 2007). Gard's inspirations included Swedish pop artist Neneh Cherry and comic book character Tank Girl, both feminist icons. Croft's original

Specific example of female character.

continued >>

incarnation was as the South American woman Lara Cruz. Gard disavows accusations of sexism in the design, and insists that the character's iconic breasts were a programming accident that the rest of the team fought to keep (McLaughlin & Rus, 2008).

The Treatment of Women Gamers

Heading followed by topic sentence that introduces third main point.

Video game culture reinforces negative gender roles for female players. Many multiplayer games encourage players to use headsets and microphones, a gender-revealing practice that is intended for easy strategizing. However, it often leads to sexual harassment and lewd commentary that also carries over to message boards, comments sections, and internet forums. Technology blogger Kathy Sierra was forced to abandon her website after multiple misogynistic comments and e-mails. Ailin Graef, who has made millions in the 3D chat-platform Second Life, was "swarmed by flying pink penises" during an interview in that virtual world (McCabe, 2008).

Two examples illustrate harassment.

A study by psychologists at Nottingham Trent University in England determined that 70% of female players in massively-multiplayer online games chose to "construct male characters when given the option," presumably in an attempt to avoid such actions as female posters on gaming message boards being asked to post pictures of their breasts or "get the f*** off" (McCabe, 2008). Women gamers are considered so rare (which is surprising, given that they makes up 40% of players) that it's a common occurrence for male gamers to respond with a degree of shock any time a female shows up in game—even if that shock is complimentary or respectful. Sarah Rutledge, a 25-year-old female med student said of her gaming on *World of Warcraft*,

Paragraph provides more examples of women players' treatment.

continued >>

Because source was a personal interview and not retrievable by others, Leslie cites it only in text, not in References.

> On the one hand, you get a lot of help and attention from guys playing the game, which can be helpful. You get invitations to join groups. But it's clear this has less to do with my ability than the fact I'm that curious creature: a woman. (personal communication, April 29, 2011)

One team of researchers found significant differences between men and women game players in gaining positive affects from gaming. They found males more likely than females to develop leadership, teamwork, and communicative skills, and they suggest this demonstrates games' biases toward males (Thirunarayanon, Vilchez, Abreau, Ledesma, & Lopez, 2010, p. 324).

Heading precedes a topic sentence that complicates paper's thesis.

Gradual Changes in Gender Roles and Gaming

In recent years gender roles have somewhat shifted. Often role-playing games permit the user to choose various characteristics of the Player Character, including making her female. Aside from appearance and responses from Non-Player Characters, the gender rarely affects a character's actual skills or attributes. More games have been released with females as the sole protagonists, including *Silent Hill 3* (Heather Mason), *No One Lives Forever* (Cate Archer), *Mirror's Edge* (Faith), and *Heavenly Sword* (Nariko). Jade, the protagonist of *Beyond Good and Evil* (released in 2003), has been praised for being strong and confident without being overtly sexualized. So have characters like Alyx Vance (co-protagonist of 2004's *Half-Life 2*) and Chell (protagonist of *Portal*, 2007, and *Portal 2*, 2011).

Leslie includes characters' names in parentheses to provide more information.

Chell in particular was heralded as a massive step forward in gender dynamics. People were surprised that "as the

continued >>

player, you're never even aware that you're a woman until you catch a glimpse of yourself in the third person" (*iVirtua*, 2007). In this way, Chell echoes the "original" feminist character Samus Aran of Nintendo's 1986 *Metroid;* one only discovers that Aran is female when she removes her bulky robot-armor during the ending scene, after twenty-plus hours of first-person gameplay. *Portal*, despite being an indie game produced by students as their thesis, became a hit, was wildly acclaimed by critics, and won multiple awards.

Paragraph gives more detail for an example mentioned in previous sentence.

These developments don't satisfy all fans.. Some argue that a more all-inclusive focus actually threatens the quality of experience for stereotypically straight male gamers. Bioware, a Canada-based gaming company, came under fire during the releases of two major titles for featuring romance and dialogue options that cater not only to women, but to gays and lesbians. The release of *Dragon Age 2* in 2011 caused an uproar on its own message boards for allowing romantic options to be bisexual. One fan, "Bastal" (2011), protested that

Complicating information gives paper a richer texture.

> the overwhelming majority of RPG gamers are indeed straight and male. . . . That's not to say there isn't a significant number of women who play Dragon Age and that BioWare should forego the option of playing as a women altogether, but there should have been much more focus in on making sure us male gamers were happy.

Quotation longer than 40 words set off block style, no quotation marks. Reference information appears in the part of the sentence introducing quote. Online source had no pages.

He and others then go on to propose a mode, which, if activated, would force male Companions to flirt only with female PCs, and vice versa. However, such views disturb game

continued >>

creators like David Gaider (2010), who argued that people like Baltas are

> so used to being catered to that they see the lack of catering as an imbalance. . . . The person who says that the only way to please them is to restrict options for others is, if you ask me, the one who deserves it least.

Conclusion

"If we just continue to cater to existing (male) players, we're never going to grow," says Beth Llewellyn, senior director of corporate communications for Nintendow (Kerwick, 2007). Video game companies have begun producing a new generation of games that give women the opportunity to grab a laser gun or broadsword and duke it out in billion-dollar franchises like *Halo, Fallout, Mass Effect, World of Warcraft* and *Guild Wars*. However, depicting women more accurately and favorably in games reaches a goal more important than mere entertainment. "Video-simulated interfaces" are being used to train people for various professions (Terlecki et al., 2010, p. 30), and it is crucial that these environments are suitable for all. The promising news is that while there is still extensive gender stereotyping (in both the gaming and the real world), game makers are taking giant strides—in both boots and heels.

Leslie includes the speaker's credentials, for emphasis.

Sentence helps answer the "so what?" question.

Because there are more than 6 authors, Leslie uses the first author and "et al."

Memorable final image.

continued >>

WOMEN IN VIDEO GAMES 11

References

References begin on new page. "References" centered. Double-spaced and hanging indentations throughout.

Bastal. (2011, March 22). Bioware neglected their main demographic: The straight male gamer. [Online discussion posting]. Retrieved from http://social.bioware.com/forum/1/topic/304/index/6661775&lf=8 (Topic 304, Msg. 1)

Bates, M. (2005). *Implicit identity theory in the rhetoric of the massively multiplayer online role-playing game (MMORPG)*. (Doctoral Dissertation, Pennsylvania State University.) Available from ProQuest Dissertations and Theses database. (AAT 3172955)

Beasley, B., & Standley, T. C. (2002). Shirts vs. skirts: Clothing as an indicator of gender role stereotyping in video games. *Mass Communication & Society 5*, 279–93.

Journal article in print.

Dietz, T. L. (1998). An examination of violence and gender role portrayals in video games: Implications for gender socialization and aggressive behavior. *Sex Roles, 38*, 433–35.

Dickerman, C., Christensen, J., & Kerl-McClain, S. B. (2008). Big breasts and bad guys: Depictions of gender and race in video games. *Journal of Creativity in Mental Health, 3*(1), 20–29. doi: 10.1080/15401380801995076

Journal article online, with DOI.

Dill, K. E., & Thill, K. P. (2007, October 17). Video game characters and the socialization of gender roles: Young people's perceptions mirror sexist media depictions. *Sex Roles, 57*, 861–64.

Downs, E., & Smith, S. L. (2010): Keeping abreast of hypersexuality: A video game character content analysis. *Sex Roles, 62*, 721–733. doi: 10:1007/s11199-009-9637-1

continued >>

Video game. *Dragon Age: Origins.* (2009). [Video Game]. Edmonton, Canada: Bioware Studios.

Entertainment Software Association. (2011). *Essential facts about the computer and video game industry 2010: Sales, demographic and usage data.* Washington, DC: Author. Retrieved from http://www.theesa.com/

Comment in an online discussion. Gaider, D. (2011, April 2). Response: Bioware neglected their main demographic. [Online forum comment]. Retrieved from http://social.bioware.com/forum/1/topic/304/index/6661775&lf=8 (Topic 304, Msg. 2)

Huntemann, N. (Producer & Director). (2000). *Game over: Gender, race & violence in video games.* [Video]. USA: Media Education Foundation. Retrieved from http://www.mediaed.org/

iVirtua Editorial Team. (2007, December 9). Portal is a feminist masterpiece. London, England: iVirtua Media Group. Retrieved from http://www.ivirtuaforums.com/portal-is-a-feminist-masterpiece-great-read-media-studies-t14-61

Kerwick, M. (2007, May 13). Video games now starring strong female characters. *The Record.* Retrieved from http://www.popmatters.com/female-characters

Newspaper article available online. McCabe, J. (2008, March 6). Sexual harassment is rife online. No wonder women swap gender. *The Guardian*, p. G2. Retrieved from http://www.guardian.co.uk/

Ogletree, S. M., & Drake, R. (2007). College students' video game participation and perceptions: Gender differences and implications. *Sex Roles, 56*, 537–542. doi: 10.1007/s11199-007-9193-5

continued >>

WOMEN IN VIDEO GAMES 13

Ray, S. G. (2003). *Gender inclusive game design: Expanding the market*. Hingham, MA: Charles River Media.

Rubenstein, J. (2007, May 26). Idealizing fantasy bodies. *Iris Gaming Network*. Retrieved from http://theirisnetwork.org/

Terlecki, M., Brown, J., Harner-Steciw, L., Irvin-Hannum, J., Marchetto-Ryan, N., Ruhl, L., & Wiggins, J. (2011). Sex differences and similarities in video game experience, preferences, and self-efficacy: Implications for the gaming industry. *Current Psychology, 30*, 22–33. doi: 10.1007/s12144-010-9095-5

Thirunarayanon, M. O., Vilchez, M., Abreu, L., Ledesma, C., & Lopez, S. (2010). A survey of video game players in a public, urban research university. *Educational Media International, 47*, 311–327. doi: 10.1080/09523987-2010.535338

Wong, D. (2010, May 24). Five reasons it's still not cool to admit you're a gamer. *Cracked*. Retrieved from http://www.cracked.com/article_18571

Article from a Web site.

27 Chicago Manual (CM) and Council of Science Editors (CSE) Documentation

Quick Points You will learn to

➤ Understand CM-style documentation (see 27A).
➤ Use CM-style documentation for Bibliographic notes (see 27B).
➤ Understand CSE-style documentation (see 27C).
➤ Use CSE-style documentation for a References list (see 27D).

27A What is CM-style documentation?

Watch the Video

The Chicago Manual of Style (CM) endorses two styles of documentation. One, **CM style**, is an author–date style, similar to the APA STYLE of IN-TEXT CITATIONS (see Ch. 26), that includes a list of SOURCES usually titled "Works Cited" or "References."

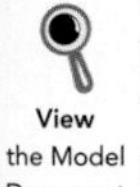
View the Model Document

The other CM style uses a **bibliographic note system**. This system gives information about each source in two places: (1) in a *footnote* (at the bottom of a page) or an *endnote* (in a separate page following your paper) and, (2) if required, in a BIBLIOGRAPHY that begins on a separate page. We present this style here because it's often used in such humanities courses as art, music, history, philosophy, and sometimes English. Within the bibliographic note system, there are two substyles: "full" and "short."

27A.1 The full bibliographic note system in CM style

The CM full bibliographic note system requires you to give complete information, in a footnote or an endnote, the first time you cite a source. Because you're giving full information, you don't need to include a bibliography page. If you cite a source a second time, you provide shortened information that includes the last name(s) of the author(s) and the key words in the work's title. The following example uses the full bibliographic note system.

TEXT

Ulrich points out that both Europeans and Native Americans told war stories, but with different details and different emphases.[3]

FULL FOOTNOTE (SAME PAGE) OR ENDNOTE (SEPARATE PAGE FOLLOWING TEXT)

3. Laurel Thatcher Ulrich, *The Age of Homespun: Objects and Stories in the Creation of an American Myth* (New York: Knopf, 2001), 269.

SECOND CITATION OF THIS SOURCE

6. Ulrich, *Age of Homespun*, 285.

27A.2 The short bibliographic note system, plus bibliography, in CM style

In the abbreviated bibliographic note system, even your first endnote or footnote provides only brief information about the source. You provide complete information in a bibliography, which appears as a separate page at the end of the paper. Following is an example of using the short bibliographic note system.

TEXT

Ulrich points out that both Europeans and Native Americans told war stories, but with different details and different emphases.[3]

ABBREVIATED FOOTNOTE (SAME PAGE) OR ENDNOTE (SEPARATE PAGE FOLLOWING TEXT)

3. Ulrich, *Age of Homespun*, 269.

BIBLIOGRAPHY (SEPARATE PAGE AT END OF THE PAPER)

Ulrich, Laurel Thatcher. *The Age of Homespun: Objects and Stories in the Creation of an American Myth*. New York: Knopf, 2001.

Alert: Ask your instructor which style he or she prefers. Remember that CM style requires a separate bibliography only when you use the short notes style, but your instructor may also prefer one with the full style. ●

Quick Box 27.1 provides guidelines for compiling CM-style bibliographic notes.

Quick Box 27.1

Guidelines for compiling CM-style bibliographic notes

TITLE AND PLACEMENT OF NOTES

If you're using endnotes, place them all on a separate page, before your bibliography. Center the heading "Notes" an inch from the top of the page, without using italics, underlining, or quotation marks. If you're using footnotes, place them at the bottom of the page on which the source needs to be credited. Never use a title above a note at the foot of the page. CM generally uses blank space (not a line) to divide the footnote(s) from the body text.

continued >>

Quick Box 27.1 (continued)

TITLE AND PLACEMENT OF BIBLIOGRAPHY

The abbreviated notes style requires a bibliography, which begins on a separate page at the end of the paper, following the endnotes page. An inch from the top of the page, center the heading "References" or "Works Cited" (either is acceptable in CM style). Don't underline or italicize the heading or put it in quotation marks.

FORMAT FOR ENDNOTES AND FOOTNOTES

Include an endnote or a footnote every time you use a source. Number notes sequentially throughout your paper whether you're using endnotes or footnotes. Use superscript (raised) arabic numerals for the footnote or endnote numbers in your paper. Position note numbers after any punctuation mark except the dash. The best position is at the end of a sentence, unless that position would be so far from the source material that it would be confusing. Don't use raised numbers in the endnote or footnote itself. Place the number, followed by a period, on the same line as the content of the note. Single-space both within each note and between notes. Indent each note's first line three-tenths of an inch (0.3" tab), which equals about three characters, but place subsequent lines flush left at the margin.

SPACING AFTER PUNCTUATION

A single space follows all punctuation, including the period.

AUTHORS' NAMES

In endnotes and footnotes, give the name in standard (first-name-first) order, with names and initials as given in the original source. Use the word *and* before the last author's name if your source has more than one author.

In the bibliography, invert the name: last name, first name. If a work has two or more authors, invert only the first author's name. If your source has up to ten authors, give all the authors' names. If your source has eleven or more authors, list only the first seven and use *et al.* for the rest.

CAPITALIZATION OF SOURCE TITLES

Capitalize the first and last words and all major words.

SPECIAL TREATMENT OF TITLES

Use italics for titles of long works (such as books or periodicals), and use quotation marks around the titles of shorter works (such as articles or stories). Omit *A*, *An*, and *The* from the titles of newspapers and periodicals. For an unfamiliar newspaper title, list the city (and state, in parentheses, if the city isn't well known): *Newark (NJ) Star-Ledger*, for example. Use postal abbreviations for states.

continued >>

Quick Box 27.1 (continued)

PUBLICATION INFORMATION

Enclose publication information in parentheses. Use a colon and one space after the city of publication. Give complete publishers' names or abbreviate them according to standard abbreviations in *Books in Print*. Omit *Co., Inc.*, and so on. Spell out *University* or abbreviate to *Univ.* Never use *U* alone. Spell out *Press;* never use *P* alone. Don't abbreviate publication months.

PAGE NUMBERS

For inclusive page numbers, give the full second number for 2 through 99. For 100 and beyond, give the full second number only if a shortened version would be ambiguous: 243–47, 202–6, 300–304. List all discontinuous page numbers. (See "First Endnote or Footnote: Book" toward the end of this box.) Use a comma to separate parenthetical publication information from the page numbers that follow it. Use the abbreviations *p.* and *pp.* with page numbers only for material from newspapers, for material from journals that do not use volume numbers, and to avoid ambiguity.

CONTENT NOTES

Try to avoid using content notes, which differ from citation notes by providing information or ideas, not just references. If you must use them, use footnotes, not endnotes, with symbols rather than numbers: an asterisk (*) for the first note on that page and a dagger (†) for a second note on that page.

FIRST ENDNOTE OR FOOTNOTE: BOOK

For books, include the author, title, publication information, and page numbers when applicable. Some notes also include information about publication type (see example 12, below).

1. Becky Bradway, *Pink Houses and Family Taverns* (Bloomington: University of Indiana Press, 2002), 23.

FIRST ENDNOTE OR FOOTNOTE: ARTICLE

For articles, include the author, article title, journal title, volume number, year, and page numbers.

1. D. D. Cochran, W. Daniel Hale, and Christine P. Hissam, "Personal Space Requirements in Indoor versus Outdoor Locations," *Journal of Psychology* 117 (1984): 132–33.

SECOND MENTION IN ENDNOTES OR FOOTNOTES

Second (or later) citations of the same source can be brief. See 27B, example 1.

27B What are CM examples for bibliographic notes?

The following directory corresponds to the sample bibliographic note forms that follow it. In a few cases, we give sample Bibliography forms as well. If you need a model that isn't here, consult *The Chicago Manual of Style*, 16th ed. (Chicago: University of Chicago Press, 2010).

Directory for CM Bibliographic Notes System

PERIODICALS

1. Article in a Scholarly Journal: Print

1. Bronwyn T. Williams. "Seeking New Worlds: The Study of Writing beyond Our Classrooms." *College Composition and Communication* 62, no. 1 (2010): 131. [full note]

2. Williams, "Seeking New Worlds," 131. [short note]

In a note, the author's name appears in regular order. Commas separate elements except for the page number, which follows a colon. In a full note, the volume number comes one space after the journal title. If there is an issue number, precede it with "no." (abbreviation of "number"). Provide both volume and issue number, if available.

Bibliography

Williams, Bronwyn T. "Seeking New Worlds: The Study of Writing beyond Our Classrooms," *College Composition and Communication* 62. no. 1 (2010): 127–46.

In the bibliography entry needed for the short note version, the author's name appears inverted, last name first. Periods separate the elements.

2. Article in Scholarly Journal: Online with a DOI

1. Regan Gurung and Kristin Vespia, "Looking Good, Teaching Well? Linking Liking, Looks, and Learning," *Teaching of Psychology* 34, no. 1 (2007): 7, doi: 10.1207/ s15328023top3401_2. [full note]

2. Gurung and Vespia, "Looking Good," 7. [short note]

Bibliography

Gurung, Regan, and Kristin Vespia. "Looking Good, Teaching Well? Linking Liking, Looks, and Learning." *Teaching of Psychology* 34, no. 1 (2007): 5–10. doi: 10.1207/ s15328023top3401_2.

For an explanation of Document Object Identifiers (DOI), see Quick Box 26.2.

3. Article in a Scholarly Journal: Online with a URL

1. Richard A. Bryant, "Disentangling Mild Traumatic Brain Injury and Stress Reactions," *New England Journal of Medicine* 358, no. 5 (2008): 527, http://www.nejm.org/doi/full/10.1056/NEJMe078235.

2. Bryant, "Disentangling," 527.

Bibliography

Bryant, Richard A. "Disentangling Mild Traumatic Brain Injury and Stress Reactions." *New England Journal of Medicine* 358, no. 5 (2008): 525–527. http://www.nejm.org/doi/full/10.1056/NEJMe078235

4. Article in a Scholarly Journal: From a Database

1. Bronwyn T. Williams, "Seeking New Worlds: The Study of Writing beyond Our Classrooms," *College Composition and Communication* 62, no.1 (2010): 143, Proquest.

Williams, "Seeking New Worlds," 143.

Bibliography

Williams, Bronwyn T. "Seeking New Worlds: The Study of Writing beyond Our Classrooms." *College Composition and Communication* 62, no. 1 (2010): 127–46. Proquest.

For articles from library or commercial databases, include as much information as possible about any print version. List the name of the database at the end of the entry (Proquest, in the preceding example). If the article has a stable URL (a unique URL that is permanently associated with it), provide it, as in the following example:

3. Michael Harker, "The Ethics of Argument: Rereading *Kairos* and Making Sense in a Timely Fashion," *College Composition and Communication* 59, no. 1 (2007): 77–97, http://www.jstor.org/stable/20456982.

5. Article in a Weekly or Biweekly Magazine: Print

1. Rana Foroohar, "Why the World Isn't Getting Smaller," *Time*, June 27, 2011, 20.

2. Foroohar, "Why the World," 20.

Bibliography

Foroohar, Rana. "Why the World Isn't Getting Smaller." *Time*. June 27, 2011, 20.

CM recommends citing magazine articles by the date only. If there is no author given, begin with the title of the article.

3. "The Price Is Wrong." *Economist*, August 2, 2008, 58–59.

6. Article in a Weekly or Biweekly Magazine: Online with a URL

1. Rana Foroohar, "Why the World Isn't Getting Smaller," *Time*, June 19, 2011, http://www.time.com/time/magazine/article/0,9171,2078119,00.html

2. Foroohar, "Why the World."

Bibliography

Foroohar, Rana. "Why the World Isn't Getting Smaller." *Time*, June 19, 2011. http://www.time.com/time/magazine/article/0,9171,2078119,00.html.

The online version of this article did not list page numbers.

7. Article in a Monthly or Bimonthly Magazine: Print

1. Thomas Goetz, "The Feedback Loop," *Wired*, July 2011, 127.

See examples 1–6 for short note and bibliography forms.

8. Article in a Monthly or Bimonthly Magazine: Online

1. Thomas Goetz, "Harnessing the Power of Feedback Loops," *Wired*, July 2011, http://www.wired.com/magazine/2011/06/ff_feedbackloop/.

See examples 1–6 for short note and bibliography forms.

9. Article in a Newspaper: Print

1. Monica Hesse, "Love Among the Ruins," *Washington Post*, April 24, 2011, F1.

In CM style, page numbers for newspapers are optional and usually not included, but we've shown how to include one if your instructor requires. If no author is listed, begin with the title of the article:

2. "Prepping for Uranium Work," *Denver Post*, June 18, 2011.

If the city of publication is not part of the title, put it in square brackets after the title, not italicized:

3. "Goose Lake Council to Consider Study Proposal," *The Observer* [DeWitt, IA], July 30, 2011.

See examples 1–6 for short note and bibliography forms.

10. Article in a Newspaper: Online

1. Monica Hesse, "Falling in Love with St. Andrews, Scotland," *Washington Post*, April 24, 2011, http://www.washingtonpost.com/lifestyle/travel/falling-in-love-with-st-andrews-scotland/2011/04/18/AFWZuoPE_story.html.

See examples 1–6 for short note and bibliography forms.

11. Editorials

1. "Primary Considerations," *Washington Post*, January 27, 2008: B6.

2. "Garbage In, Garbage Out," *Los Angeles Times*, February 2, 2008, http://www.latimes.com/news/printedition/la-ed-payroll2feb02,0,7684087.story.

Editorials are treated like any other newspaper article. If an author is listed, include her or his name before the title. See examples 1–6 for short note and bibliography forms.

12. Letter to the Editor: Print

1. Lester Goldstein, letter to the editor, *Sierra*, May/June 2011, 2.

CM style does not include any title that might be given for a letter to the editor. See examples 1–6 for short note and bibliography forms.

13. Letter to the Editor: Online

1. Heather B. Ennis, letter to the editor, *U.S. News and World Report*, 22 Dec. 2007, http://www.usnews.com/opinion/blogs/letters-to-the-editor/2007/12/20/sanctuaries-for-the-spirit.

See examples 1–6 for short note and bibliography forms.

14. Review

1. David Shenk, "Toolmaker, Brain Builder," review of *Beyond Deep Blue: Building the Computer That Defeated the World Chess Champion*, by Feng-Hsiung Hsu, *American Scholar* 72 (Spring 2003): 150–52.

2. Peter Travers, review of *Beginners*, directed by Mike Mills. *RollingStone*, June 2, 2011, http://www.rollingstone.com/movies/reviews/beginners-20110602.

Provide the name of the reviewer; title of the review, if any; the words "review of" followed by the name of the work reviewed; the name of the author, composer, director, etc.; then publication information. See examples 1–6 for short note and bibliography forms.

15. Article in a Looseleaf Collection of Reprinted Articles: Print

1. Thomas Hayden, "The Age of Robots," *US News and World Report,* April 23, 2001. Reprinted in *Applied Science 2002,* ed. Eleanor Goldstein (Boca Raton, FL: SIRS, 2002), art. 66.

Give the citation for the original publication first, followed by the citation for the collection. See examples 1–6 for short note and bibliography forms.

16. Abstract: Print

1. Hazel R. Marcus and Shinobu Kitayamo, "Culture and the Self: Implications for Cognition, Emotion, and Motivation," *Psychological Abstracts* 78 (1991), item 23878.

See examples 1–6 for short note and bibliography forms.

BOOKS

17. Book by One Author: Print

1. Sherry Turkle, *Alone Together: Why We Expect More from Technology and Less from Each Other* (New York: Basic Books, 2011), 43. [full note]

2. Turkle, *Alone Together,* 43. [short note]

Bibliography

Turkle, Sherry. *Alone Together: Why We Expect More from Technology and Less from Each Other.* New York: Basic Books, 2011.

18. Book by One Author: Downloaded from Library or Bookseller

1. Sherry Turkle, *Alone Together: Why We Expect More from Technology and Less from Each Other* (New York: Basic Books, 2011), Kindle edition, chap. 2. [full note]

2. Turkle, *Alone Together,* chap. 2. [short note]

Because books in electronic format often don't have stable page numbers, listing a chapter helps readers locate the citation.

Bibliography

Turkle, Sherry. *Alone Together: Why We Expect More from Technology and Less from Each Other.* New York: Basic Books, 2011. Kindle edition.

19. Book by One Author: Online

1. Sherry Turkle, *Alone Together: Why We Expect More from Technology and Less from Each Other* (New York: Basic Books, 2011), 43, http://books.google.com/. [full note]

2. Turkle, *Alone Together*, 43. [short note]

Bibliography

Turkle, Sherry. *Alone Together: Why We Expect More from Technology and Less from Each Other.* New York: Basic Books, 2011. http://books.google.com/.

20. Book by Two or Three Authors

1. Kathryn Edin and Maria Kefalas, *Promises I Can Keep: Why Poor Women Put Motherhood before Marriage* (Berkeley: University of California Press, 2005), 28.

2. Edin and Kefalas, *Promises*, 28.

Bibliography

Edin, Kathryn, and Maria Kefalas. *Promises I Can Keep: Why Poor Women Put Motherhood before Marriage.* Berkeley: University of California Press, 2005.

Include the names of two or three authors in notes. In the bibliography, invert the name of only the first author. For e-books, adapt this model to example 18. For a book accessed online, see example 19.

21. Book by More Than Three Authors

1. Wendy Saul et al., *Beyond the Science Fair: Creating a Kids' Inquiry Conference.* (Portsmouth: Heinemann, 2005), 74. [full note]

2. Saul et al., *Beyond the Science Fair*, 74. [short note]

Bibliography

Saul, Wendy, Donna Dieckman, Charles R. Pearce, and Donna Neutze. *Beyond the Science Fair: Creating a Kids' Inquiry Conference.* Portsmouth, NH: Heinemann, 2005.

In notes, give only the first author's name, followed by the phrase *et al.* (abbreviated from the Latin *et alii*, meaning "and others"). In the bibliography list all names in full in the order in which they appear on the title page. For e-books, adapt this model to example 18. For a book accessed online, see example 19.

22. Two or More Works by the Same Author(s)

Bibliography

Jenkins, Henry. *Convergence Culture: Where Old and New Media Collide.* New York: New York University Press, 2006.

---. *Fans, Bloggers, and Gamers: Exploring Participatory Culture.* New York: New York University Press, 2006.

Give author name(s) in the first entry only. In the second and subsequent entries, use three hyphens and a period to stand for exactly the same name(s). If the person served as editor or translator, put a comma and the appropriate abbreviation (*ed.* or *trans.*) following the three hyphens. Arrange the works in alphabetical (not chronological) order according to book title. For e-books, adapt this model to example 18. For a book accessed online, see example 19.

23. Book by a Group or Corporate Author

1. American Psychological Association, *Publication Manual of the American Psychological Association*, 6th ed. (Washington, DC: APA, 2010).

Cite the full name of the corporate author first, omitting the first articles *A*, *An*, or *The*. For e-books, adapt this model to example 18. For a book accessed online, see example 19. For short notes and bibliography forms, see examples 17–21.

24. Book with No Author Named

1. *The Chicago Manual of Style*, 16th ed. (Chicago: University of Chicago Press, 2010), 711.

If there is no author's name on the title page, begin the citation with the title. Alphabetize the entry according to the first significant word of the title (ignore *A, An*, or *The*).

For e-books, adapt this model to example 18. For a book accessed online, see example 19. For short notes and bibliography forms, see examples 17–21.

25. Book with an Author and an Editor

1. Harriet Beecher Stowe, *Uncle Tom's Cabin*, ed. Elizabeth Ammons (New York: Norton, 2010), 272.

2. Stowe, *Uncle Tom's Cabin*, 272.

Bibliography

Stowe, Harriet Beecher. *Uncle Tom's Cabin.* Edited by Elizabeth Ammons. New York: Norton, 2010.

If your paper refers to the work of the book's author, put the author's name first. If your paper refers to the work of the editor, put the editor's name first.

Ammons, Elizabeth, ed. *Uncle Tom's Cabin.* By Harriet Beecher Stowe. New York: Norton, 2010.

For e-books, adapt this model to example 18. For a book accessed directly online, see example 19.

26. Translation

1. Jo Nesbo, *The Leopard,* trans. Don Bartlett (New York: Vintage, 2011), 7.

For e-books, adapt this model to example 18. For a book accessed online, see example 19. For short notes and bibliography forms, see examples 17–21.

27. Work in Several Volumes or Parts

1. Ronald Chrisley, ed., *Artificial Intelligence: Critical Concepts* (London: Routledge, 2000), 4:25.

Bibliography

Chrisley, Ronald, ed. *Artificial Intelligence: Critical Concepts.* Vol. 4. London: Routledge, 2000.

If you are citing only one volume, put only that volume number before the publication information. For e-books, adapt this model to example 18. For a book accessed online, see example 19. For short notes and bibliography forms, see examples 17–21.

28. Anthology or Edited Book

1. John L. Purdy and James Ruppert, eds., *Nothing but the Truth: An Anthology of Native American Literature* (Upper Saddle River, NJ: Prentice, 2001), 12.

2. Purdy and Ruppert, *Nothing but the Truth,* 12.

Bibliography

Purdy, John L., and James Ruppert, eds. *Nothing but the Truth: An Anthology of Native American Literature.* Upper Saddle River, NJ: Prentice, 2001.

Use this model if you are citing an entire anthology. In the preceding example, *eds.* stands for "editors;" use *ed.* when only one editor is named. For e-books, adapt this model to example 18. For a book accessed directly online, see example 19.

29. One Selection from an Anthology or an Edited Book

1. Laura Trujillo, "Balancing Act," in *Border-Line Personalities: A New Generation of Latinas Dish on Sex, Sass, and Cultural Shifting*, ed. Robyn Moreno and Michelle Herrera Mulligan (New York: Harper, 2004), 62.

2. Trujillo, "Balancing Act," 62.

Bibliography

Trujillo, Laura. "Balancing Act." In *Border-Line Personalities: A New Generation of Latinas Dish on Sex, Sass, and Cultural Shifting*, edited by Robyn Moreno and Michelle Herrera Mulligan, 61–72. New York: Harper, 2004.

For e-books, adapt this model to example 18. For a book accessed directly online, see example 19.

30. More Than One Selection from the Same Anthology or Edited Book

Bibliography

Bond, Ruskin. "The Night Train at Deoli." In Chaudhuri, *Vintage Book*, 415–18.

Chaudhuri, Amit, ed. *The Vintage Book of Modern Indian Literature*. New York: Vintage, 2004.

Vijayan, O.V. "The Rocks." In Chaudhuri, *Vintage Book*, 291–96.

When you cite more than one selection from the same anthology, you can list the anthology as a separate entry with all of the publication information. Also list each selection from the anthology by author and title of the selection, but give only the name(s) of the editor(s) of the anthology, a short title, and the page number(s) for each selection. List selections separately in alphabetical order by author's last name. For e-books, adapt this model to example 18. For a book accessed online, see example 19. For short notes and bibliography forms, see examples 17–21.

31. Article in a Dictionary or Encyclopedia

1. *Encyclopaedia Britannica*, 15th ed., s.v. "Ireland."

If you're citing a widely used reference work, don't give full publication information. Instead, give only the edition and year of publication. In this case, *s.v.* means *sub vero* ("under the word"), which indicates looking up "Ireland" alphabetically in the source.

If the articles in the book are alphabetically arranged, you don't need to give volume and page numbers. If no author is listed, begin with the title of the article. For references with more substantial articles, cite them as you would chapters in a book:

1. Burnbam, John C. "Freud, Sigmund." *The Encyclopedia of Psychiatry, Psychology, and Psychoanalysis.* Ed. Benjamin B. Wolman. New York: Holt, 1996.

32. Article in a Reference Book: Database

1. Encyclopaedia Britannica Online, s.v. "Lobster," accessed June 29, 2011, http://www.britannica.com/EBchecked/topic/345506/lobster.

33. Second or Later Edition

1. *MLA Handbook for Writers of Research Papers*, 7th ed. (New York: MLA, 2009).

If a book is not a first edition, the edition number is on the title page. Place the abbreviated information (*2nd ed., 3rd ed.*, etc.) between the title and the publication information. Give only the latest copyright date for the edition you are using.

For e-books, adapt this model to example 18. For a book accessed online, see example 19. For short notes and bibliography forms, see examples 17–21.

34. Introduction, Preface, Foreword, or Afterword

1. Doug Hesse, foreword to *The End of Composition Studies*, by David W. Smit (Carbondale: Southern Illinois University Press, 2004), xi.

2. Hesse, foreword, xi.

Bibliography

Hesse, Doug. Foreword to *The End of Composition Studies*, by David W. Smit. ix–xiii. Carbondale: Southern Illinois UP, 2004.

Give first the name of the writer of the part you're citing and then the name of the cited part, without italics or quotation marks. When the introduction, preface, foreword, or afterword has a title, include it in the citation before the section name, as in the following example:

Fox-Genovese, Elizabeth. "Mothers and Daughters: The Ties That Bind." Foreword to *Southern Mothers*, iv–xviii. Edited by Nagueyalti Warren and Sally Wolff. Baton Rouge, LA: Louisiana State University Press, 1999.

For e-books, adapt this model to example 18. For a book accessed directly online, see example 19.

35. Unpublished Dissertation or Essay

1. Gina Anne Stuart, "Exploring the Harry Potter Book Series: A Study of Adolescent Reading Motivation," (PhD diss., Utah State University, 2006), ProQuest (AAT 3246355).

State the author's name first, then the title in quotation marks (not underlined), then a descriptive label (such as *Diss.* or *Unpublished essay*), followed by the degree-granting institution (for dissertations), and finally the date. Treat published dissertations as books. In the preceding example, "ProQuest" is the name of the database containing the dissertation, and the number in parentheses at the end is the accession number.

36. Reprint of an Older Book

1. Robert Coover, *A Night at the Movies, Or, You Must Remember This* (Champaign, IL: Dalkey Archive, 2007). First published 1987 by William Heinemann Ltd.

Republishing information can be found on the copyright page. For e-books, adapt this model to example 18. For a book accessed online, see example 19. For short notes and bibliography forms, see examples 17–21.

37. Book in a Series or Scholarly Project

1. Jean Hastings Ardell, *Breaking into Baseball: Women and the National Pastime*, Writing Baseball Series (Carbondale: Southern Illinois University Press, 2005).

For e-books, adapt this model to example 18. For a book accessed online, see example 19. For short notes and bibliography forms, see examples 17–21.

38. Book with a Title within a Title

1. Robert M. Lumiansky and Herschel Baker, eds, *Critical Approaches to Six Major English Works: "Beowulf" Through "Paradise Lost"* (Philadelphia: University of Pennsylvania Press, 1968).

Set the normally independent titles within quotation marks and italicize them. For e-books, adapt this model to example 18. For a book accessed online, see example 19. For short notes and bibliography forms, see examples 17–21.

39. Bible or Sacred Text

Bibliography

Bhagavad Gita. Translated by Juan Mascaro. Rev. ed. New York: Penguin, 2003.

The Holy Bible: New International Version. New York: Harper, 1983.

The Qur'an. Translated by M.A.S. Abdel Haleem. New York: Oxford University Press, 2004.

For e-books, adapt this model to example 18. For a book accessed online, see example 19. For short notes and bibliography forms, see examples 17–21.

40. Government Publication

Bibliography

US Senate. Select Committee on Intelligence. *Report on the U.S. Intelligence Community's Prewar Intelligence Assessment of Iraq.* 108th Cong., 1st sess. Washington, DC: Government Printing Office, 2004.

For government publications that name no author, start with the name of the government or government body. Then name the government agency. Then include the title, any series information, and publication information. If there is an author, begin with the author's name:

Wallace, David Rains. *Yellowstone: A Natural and Human History; Yellowstone National Park, Idaho, Montana, and Wyoming.* Interior Dept. National Park Service. Official National Park Handbook 150. Washington, DC: Government Printing Office, 2001.

41. Government Publication: Online

1. Ronald C. Huff, *Comparing the Criminal Behavior of Youth Gangs and At-Risk Youths* (United States. Dept. of Justice. Natl. Inst. of Justice. October, 1998), https://www.ncjrs.gov/txtfiles/172852.txt.

42. Published Proceedings of a Conference

1. Luis Mateus Rocha, ed., *Artificial Life X: Proceedings of the Tenth International Conference on the Simulation and Synthesis of Living Systems* (Cambridge, MA: MIT Press, 2006).

Treat published proceedings as you would chapters in a book.

IMAGES, AUDIO, FILM, AND VIDEO

The Chicago Manual of Style, 16th Edition, includes no examples of notes or bibliographic entries for photographs, illustrations, graphs or other images. When such materials are reproduced in a paper, CM recommends including a caption beneath the image, with source information included at the end of the caption. However, because student papers often refer to images as sources or discuss them as examples, we have provided some examples below, in CM style.

43. Photograph, Painting, Drawing, Illustration, etc. (Original)

1. Carl Mydans, *General Douglas MacArthur Landing at Luzon, 1945*, photograph displayed at Soho Triad Fine Art Gallery, New York (October 21–November 28, 1999).

2. Mydans, *General Douglas MacArthur*.

Bibliography

Mydans, Carl. *General Douglas MacArthur Landing at Luzon, 1945.* Photograph displayed at Soho Triad Fine Art Gallery, New York. October 21–November 28, 1999.

Give the name of the image's maker, if known, the title or caption of the image, the type of image, where you viewed the image, and when. If the image has no title, provide a brief description.

44. Photograph, Painting, Drawing, Illustration, etc. in a Periodical: Print

1. Herb Greene, *Grace Slick*, photograph, *Rolling Stone*, September 30, 2004: 102.

2. Greene, *Grace Slick*, 102.

Bibliography

Greene, Herb. *Grace Slick*. Photograph. *Rolling Stone* September 30, 2004: 102.

45. Photograph, Painting, Drawing, Illustration, etc. in a Periodical: Online

1. Christopher Morris, *Man in Camouflage*, photograph, *The Atlantic,* July/August 2011, http://www.theatlantic.com/magazine/archive/2011/07/invisible-inc/8523/

2. Morris, *Man in Camouflage*.

Bibliography

Morris, Christopher. *Man in Camouflage*. Photograph. *The Atlantic*. July/August 2011. http://www.theatlantic.com/magazine/archive/2011/07/invisible-inc/8523/.

46. Photograph, Painting, Drawing, Illustration, etc. in a Book: Print

Bibliography

"The World's Most Populous Countries." Illustration in *Maps of the Imagination: The Writer as Cartographer*, by Peter Turchi, 116–17. San Antonio, TX: Trinity University Press, 2004.

See 44 for example of notes.

47. Comic or Cartoon: Print

Bibliography

Sutton, Ward. "Ryan's a Late Adopter." Cartoon. *New Yorker*, May 2, 2011.

See 44 for example of notes.

48. Slide Show or Photo Essay: Online

Bibliography

Nachtwey, James. Crime in Middle America. *Time*, December 2, 2006. Accessed May 4, 2011, http://www.time.com/time/photogallery/0,29307,1947522,00.html.

See 44 for example of notes.

49. Image from a Service or Distributor

Bibliography

World Perspectives. *Launching of the Space Shuttle Columbia, Florida, USA, 1998.* Photograph. Accessed March 3, 2011, from http://gettyimages.com. Getty Images (#AT3775-001).

In this example, the photographer was listed as "World Perspectives." Include the name of the service or distributor, and the item number or other identifier, if any. See 44 for example of notes.

50. Online Map, Chart, or Other Graphic: Online

Bibliography

"Hurricane Rita." Graphic from *New York Times Online*, September 24, 2005. http://www.nytimes.com/packages/html/national/20050923_RITA_GRAPHIC/index.html.

See 44 for example of notes.

51. Audio Book

1. Sherry Turkle, *Alone Together: Why We Expect More from Technology and Less from Each Other*, read by Laural Merlington, Tantor Media, 2011, CD.

52. Sound Recording

Verdi, Giuseppe. *Requiem*. Chicago Symphony Orchestra and Chorus. Ricardo Muti. CSO Resound B003WL7EJE, 2010. 2 compact discs.

Put first the name most relevant to what you discuss in your paper (performer, conductor, work performed). Include the recording's title, other information (performer, composer, conductor), the name of the issuer, the date the work was issued, the medium, and any additional recording information.

Radiohead. "Jigsaw Falling into Place." From *In Rainbows*. Radiohead, 2007. MP3 file.

53. Sound Recording: Online

Komunyakaa, Yusef. "My Father's Love Letters." Performed by Yusef Komunyakaa. Internet Poetry Archive, University of North Carolina Press. http://www.ibiblio.org/ipa/audio/komunyakaa/my_father%27s_love_letters.mp3.

54. Podcast

Blumberg, Alex and Adam Davidson. "The Giant Pool of Money." *This American Life*. Podcast audio. May 9, 2008. http://www.thisamericanlife.org/radio-archives/episode/355/the-giant-pool-of-money.

55. Film, Videotape, or DVD

It Happened One Night. Directed and produced by Frank Capra. 1934; Culver City, CA: Sony Pictures, 1999. DVD.

Give the title first, and include the director, the distributor, and the year. For films that were subsequently released on tape or DVD, provide the original release date of the movie. Other information (writer, producer, major actors) is optional but helpful. Put first names first.

For video downloads, include the download date and the source.

It Happened One Night. Directed and produced by Frank Capra. 1934; Accessed December 15, 2010, from Netflix.

56. Video or Film: Online

"Challenger Disaster Live on CNN." YouTube video. Posted by CNN, January 27, 2011. http://www.youtube.com/watch?v=AfnvFnzs9ls.

57. Broadcast Television or Radio Program

Include at least the title of the program (in italics), the network, the local station and its city, and the date of the broadcast.

Not for Ourselves Alone: The Story of Elizabeth Cady Stanton and Susan B. Anthony. By Ken Burns. Perf. Julie Harris, Ronnie Gilbert, and Sally Kellerman. Prod. Paul Barnes and Ken Burns. PBS. WNET, New York. 8 Nov. 1999.

The Madeleine Brand Show. KPCC, Pasadena. 20 June 2011.

58. Television or Radio Program: Online

1. "Bill Moyers," *The Daily Show, with Jon Stewart,* Comedy Central, June 1, 2011, http://www.thedailyshow.com/watch/wed-june-22-2005/bill-moyers.

2. "The Disappearing Incandescent Bulb," *The Madeleine Brand Show,* KPCC, June 20, 2011, http://www.scpr.org/programs/madeleine-brand/2011/06/20/the-disappearing-incandescent-bulb/.

OTHER ONLINE SOURCES

59. Entire Web Site

WebdelSol.Com. Ed. Michael Neff. Accessed August 4, 2011. http://www.webdelsol.com.

Association for the Advancement of Artificial Intelligence. Accessed October 17, 2011. http://www.aaai.org/home.html.

60. Page from a Web Site

American Psychological Association. "Think Again: Men and Women Share Cognitive Skills." Last modified January 18, 2006. http://www.apa.org/research/action/share.aspx.

Provide as much information as you can, starting with the author, if available, and the title of the page, followed by the site information.

61. Online Discussion or Electronic Mailing List Posting

1. Richard Haswell to WPA-L mailing list, October 17, 2005, "A New Graphic/Text Interface," http://lists.asu.edu/archives/wpa-l.html.

62. Chat or Real-Time Communication

Bibliography

Berzsenyi, Christyne. Online discussion of "Writing to Meet Your Match: Rhetoric, Perceptions, and Self-Presentation for Four Online Daters." *Computers and Writing Online*. AcadianaMoo. May 13, 2007. Accessed March 3, 2012. http://acadianamoo.com.

Glenn, Maria. Chat. *Facebook*, September 9, 2010. Accessed September 9, 2010.

Give the name of the speaker or writer, a title for the event (if any), the forum, date, publication medium, access date, and URL if needed.

63. E-Mail Message

1. Tara Martin, "Visit to Los Alamos," e-mail message to author, July 25, 2010.

Bibliography

Martin, Tara. "Visit to Los Alamos." E-mail message to author. July 25, 2010.

64. Posting on a Blog

1. Matthew Phillips, "Need to Go to the ER? Not Until the Game's Over." *Freakonomics.com* (blog). June 15, 2011, http://www.freakonomics.com/2011/06/15/need-to-go-to-the-er-not-until-the-games-over/.

Bibliography

Freakonomics.com (blog), http://www.freakonomics.com/.

65. Wiki

1. *NASCAR Wiki*, s.v. "NASCAR Sprint Cup Series," last modified January 11, 2011, http://nascarwiki.com.

OTHER SOURCES

66. Published or Unpublished Letter

Irvin, William. William Irvin to Lesley Osburn, December 8, 2011.

Williams, William Carlos. William Carlos Williams to his son, March 13, 1935. In *Letters of the Century: America 1900–1999*, edited by Lisa Grunwald and Stephen J. Adler, 225–26. New York: Dial, 1999.

67. Microfiche Collection of Articles

Wenzell, Ron. "Businesses Prepare for a More Diverse Work Force." *St. Louis Post Dispatch*, February 3, 1990: 17. Microform. *NewsBank: Employment* 27 (1990): fiche 2, grid D12.

68. Map or Chart

Colorado Front Range Mountain Bike Topo Map. Nederland, CO: Latitude 40, 2001.

If you have accessed the map or chart online, please follow example 49.

69. Report or Pamphlet

National Commission on Writing in America's Schools and Colleges. *The Neglected "R": The Need for a Writing Revolution*. New York: College Board, 2003.

Use the format for books, to the extent possible, including whether you're citing a print or online version.

70. Legal Source

1. Brown v. Bd. of Education, 347 U.S. 483 (1954).

Include the name of the case, the number of the case (preceded by *No.*), the name of the court deciding the case, and the date of the decision. Legal sources can frequently be accessed through a database:

2. Brown v. Bd. of Education, 347 U.S. 483 (1954). LexisNexis Academic.

71. Interview

1. Randi Friedman, telephone interview by author, August 30, 2011.

2. Carl Pope, interview by Amy Standen, *Salon.com*, April 29, 2002, http://www.salon.com/people/interview/2002/04/29/carlpope.

Note the type of interview, for example "telephone" or "personal" (face-to-face). For a published interview, give the name of the interviewed person first, identify the source as an interview, and then give details as for any published source. Follow the citation format for a periodical, book, or online source, as appropriate.

72. Lecture or Speech

1. Jennifer Katz, "Spiral Galaxies" (lecture in Astronomy 1000, University of Denver, Denver, CO, February 7, 2011).

Bibliography

Katz, Jennifer. "Spiral Galaxies." Lecture in Astronomy 1000, University of Denver, Denver, CO, February 7, 2011.

King, Martin Luther. "I Have a Dream." Speech presented at the Lincoln Memorial, Washington, DC, August 28, 1963. MP3 on American Rhetoric Top 100 Speeches. http://www.americanrhetoric.com/speeches /mlkihaveadream.htm.

If citing only the original, the entry would end after "1963." This entry goes on to cite an online version.

73. Live Performance (Play, Concert, Dance etc.)

Miller, Arthur. *All My Sons.* Directed by Calvin McLean. Performed at the Center for the Performing Arts, Normal, IL, September 27, 2005.

Nelson, Willie. *Country Throwdown Tour.* Performed at Red Rocks Amphitheater, Denver, CO, June 22, 2011.

74. Published Musical Score

1. Franz Schubert, *Symphony in B Minor (Unfinished)*, ed. Martin Cusid. New York: Norton, 1971.

75. Advertisement

1. Southwest Airlines, advertisement, ABC television, August 24, 2010.

2. Canon Digital Cameras, advertisement, *Time,* June 2, 2003, 77.

3. Budget Truck Rental, advertisement, *Huffington Post,* August 2, 2011, http://www.huffingtonpost.com.

76. Video Game or Software

The Island: Castaway. Computer game. N.p: Awem Studio, 2010.

"N.p." indicates that the place of publication is unknown.

27C What is CSE-style documentation?

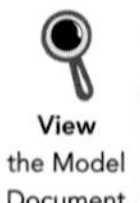

The Council of Science Editors, or CSE, produces a manual called *Scientific Style and Format* to guide publications in mathematics, the life sciences, and the physical sciences. The information in this chapter adheres to the style guidelines in the seventh edition of that manual. For up-to-date information, go to the organization's Web site at http://www.councilscienceeditors.org.

CSE has two components: (1) citations within the text, called "in-text references," tied to (2) a bibliography, called "end references," at the end of the text. However, CSE offers three different options for in-text references: the citation-sequence system, the name-year system, and the citation-name system. In this chapter we explain the citation-name system, which the CSE most strongly endorses.

In the citation-name system, the in-text references use numbers to refer to end references that are arranged alphabetically. In other words, first complete the list of end references, arranging them alphabetically by author. Then, number each reference; for example, if you were documenting references by Schmidt, Gonzalez, Adams, and Zurowski, in your end references, you would arrange them:

1. Adams . . .
2. Gonzalez . . .
3. Schmidt . . .
4. Zurowski . . .

Finally, use superscript (raised) numbers for source citations in your sentences that correspond to the numbered author names in the end references. (Numbers in parentheses are also acceptable.)

IN-TEXT REFERENCES—CITATION-NAME

Sybesma[2] insists that this behavior occurs periodically, but Crowder[1] claims never to have observed it.

END REFERENCES—CITATION-NAME

1. Crowder W. Seashore life between the tides. New York: Dodd, Mead; 1931. New York: Dover Reprint; 1975. 372 p.
2. Sybesma C. An introduction to biophysics. New York: Academic; 1977. 648 p.

Quick Box 27.3 gives guidelines for compiling a References list. Especially pay attention to the arrangement of entries in a citation-name system.

When you're citing more than one reference at a time, list each source number in numeric order, followed by a comma with no space. Use a hyphen to show the range of numbers in a continuous sequence, and put all in superscript: [2,5–7,9]

Quick Box 27.3

Guidelines for compiling a CSE-style Cited References list

TITLE

Use "Cited References" or "References" as the title (no underlining, no italics, no quotation marks).

PLACEMENT OF LIST

Begin the list on a separate page at the end of the research paper. Number the page sequentially with the rest of the paper.

CONTENT AND FORMAT OF CITED REFERENCES

Include all sources that you quote, paraphrase, or summarize in your paper. Center the title one inch from the top of the page. Start each entry on a new line. Put the number, followed by a period and a space, at the regular left margin. If an entry takes more than one line, indent the second and all other lines under the first word, not the number. Single-space each entry and double-space between entries.

SPACING AFTER PUNCTUATION

CSE style specifies no space after date, issue number, or volume number of a periodical, as shown in the models in 27D.

ARRANGEMENT OF ENTRIES

Sequence the entries in alphabetical order by author, then title, etc. Number the entries. Put the number, followed by a period and a space, at the regular left margin.

AUTHORS' NAMES

Reverse the order of each author's name, giving the last name first. For book citations, you can give first names or use only the initials of first and (when available) middle names; for journal citations, use only initials. However, CSE style recommends you use only initials. Don't use a period or a space between first and middle initials. Use a comma to separate the names of multiple authors identified by initials; however, if you use full first names, use a semicolon. Don't use *and* or *&* with authors' names. Place a period after the last author's name.

continued >>

Quick Box 27.3 (continued)

TREATMENT OF TITLES

Never underline or italicize titles or enclose them in quotation marks. Capitalize a title's first word and any proper nouns. Don't capitalize the first word of a subtitle unless it's a proper noun. Capitalize the titles of academic journals. If the title of a periodical is one word, give it in full; otherwise, abbreviate the title according to recommendations established by the *American National Standard for Abbreviations of Titles of Periodicals*. Capitalize a newspaper title's major words, giving the full title but omitting *A, An*, or *The* at the beginning.

PLACE OF PUBLICATION

Use a colon after the city of publication. If the city name could be unfamiliar to readers, add in parentheses the postal abbreviation for the US state or Canadian province. If the location of a foreign city will be unfamiliar to readers, add in parentheses the country name, abbreviating it according to International Organization for Standardization (ISO) standards. Find ISO country codes at http://www.iso.org.

PUBLISHER

Give the name of the publisher, without periods after initials, and use a semicolon after the publisher's name. Omit *The* at the beginning or *Co., Inc., Ltd.*, or *Press* at the end. However, for a university press, abbreviate *University* and *Press* as *Univ* and *Pr*, respectively, without periods.

PUBLICATION MONTH

Abbreviate all month names longer than three letters to their first three letters, but do not add a period.

PAGE NUMBERS

For inclusive page numbers, shorten the second number as much as possible, making sure that the number isn't ambiguous. For example, use 233–4 for 233 to 234; 233–44 for 233 to 244; and 233–304, not 233–04, for 233 to 304. Give the numbers of all discontinuous pages, separating successive numbers or ranges with a comma: 54–7, 60–6.

TOTAL PAGE NUMBERS

When citing an entire book, the last information unit gives the total number of book pages, followed by the abbreviation *p* and a period.

continued >>

Quick Box 27.3 (continued)

FORMAT FOR CITED REFERENCES ENTRIES: BOOKS

Citations for books usually list author(s), title, publication information, and pages (either total pages when citing an entire work or inclusive pages when citing part of a book). Each unit of information ends with a period. Some entries have additional information.

1. Primrose SB, Twyman RM, Old RW. Principles of gene manipulation. London: Blackwell; 2002. 390 p.

FORMAT FOR CITED REFERENCES ENTRIES: ARTICLES

Citations for articles usually list author(s), article title, and journal name and publication information, each section followed by a period. Abbreviate a journal's name only if it's standard in your scientific discipline. For example, *Exp Neurol* is the abbreviated form for *Experimental Neurology*. In the following example, the volume number is 184, and the issue number, in parentheses, is 1. Notice the lack of a space after the semicolon, before the parentheses, and after the colon. Some entries have additional information.

1. Ginis I, Rao MS. Toward cell replacement therapy: promises and caveats. Exp Neurol. 2003;184(1):61–77.

27D What are CSE examples for sources in a list of references?

The directory that follows corresponds to the sample references that follow it. If you need a model not included in this book, consult *Scientific Style and Format*, 7th ed. (2006).

Directory: CSE Style for a Cited References List

BOOKS AND PARTS OF BOOKS

1. Book by One Author

1. Hawking SW. Black holes and baby universes and other essays. New York: Bantam; 1993. 320 p.

Use one space but no punctuation between an author's last name and the initial of the first name. Don't put punctuation or a space between first and middle initials (*Hawking SW*). Do, however, use the hyphen in a hyphenated first and middle name (for example, *Gille J-C* represents *Jean-Charles Gille* in the next item).

2. Book by More Than One Author

1. Wegzyn S, Gille J-C, Vidal P. Developmental systems: at the crossroads of system theory, computer science, and genetic engineering. New York: Springer-Verlag; 1990. 595 p.

3. Book by a Group or Corporate Author

1. Chemical Rubber Company. Handbook of laboratory safety. 3rd ed. Boca Raton (FL): CRC; 1990. 1352 p.

4. Anthology or Edited Book

1. Heerrmann B, Hummel S, editors. Ancient DNA: recovery and analysis of genetic material from paleontological, archeological, museum, medical, and forensic specimens. New York: Springer-Verlag; 1994. 1020 p.

5. One Selection or Chapter in an Anthology or Edited Book

1. Basov NG, Feoktistov LP, Senatsky YV. Laser driver for inertial confinement fusion. In: Bureckner KA, editor. Research trends in physics: inertial confinement fusion. New York: American Institute of Physics; 1992. p. 24–37.

6. Translation

1. Magris C. A different sea. Spurr MS, translator. London: Harvill; 1993. 194 p. Translation of: Un mare differente.

7. Reprint of an Older Book

1. Carson R. The sea around us. New York: Oxford Univ Pr; 1951. New York: Oxford Univ Pr; 1991. 288 p.

8. All Volumes of a Multivolume Work

1. Crane FL, Moore DJ, Low HE, editors. Oxidoreduction at the plasma membrane: relation to growth and transport. Boca Raton (FL): CRC; 1991. 2 vol.

9. Unpublished Dissertation or Thesis

1. Baykul MC. Using ballistic electron emission microscopy to investigate the metal-vacuum interface [dissertation]. [Orem (UT)]: Polytechnic University; 1993. 111 p. Available from: UMI Dissertation Express, http://tls.il.proquest.com/hp/Products/DisExpress.html, Document 9332714.

10. Published Article from Conference Proceedings

1. Tsang CP, Bellgard MI. Sequence generation using a network of Boltzmann machines. In: Tsang CP, editor. Proceedings of the 4th Australian Joint Conference on Artificial Intelligence; 1990 Nov 8–11; Perth, AU. Singapore: World Scientific; 1990. p. 224–33.

PRINT ARTICLES FROM JOURNALS AND PERIODICALS

11. Article in a Journal

1. Ginis I, Rao MS. Toward cell replacement therapy: promises and caveats. Exp Neurol. 2003;184(1):61–77.

Give both the volume number and the issue number (here, *184* is the volume number and *1* is the issue number). Note that there is no space between the year and the volume, the volume and the issue, or the issue and the pages.

12. Journal Article on Discontinuous Pages

1. Richards FM. The protein folding problem. Sci Am. 1991;246(1):54–57, 60–66.

13. Article with No Identifiable Author

1. Cruelty to animals linked to murders of humans. AWIQ 1993 Aug;42(3):16.

14. Article with Author Affiliation

1. DeMoll E, Auffenberg T (Department of Microbiology, University of Kentucky). Purine metabolism in *Methanococcus vannielii*. J Bacteriol. 1993;175:5754–5761.

15. Entire Issue of a Journal

1. Whales in a modern world: a symposium held in London, November 1988. Mamm Rev. 1990 Jan;20(9).

The date of the symposium, November 1988, is part of the title of this issue.

16. Signed Newspaper Article

1. Kilborn PT. A health threat baffling for its lack of a pattern. New York Times (Final ed.). 2003 Jun 22;Sect. A:14 (col. 2).

Sect. stands for *section*. Note that there is no space between the date and the section.

17. Unsigned Newspaper Article

1. Supercomputing center to lead security effort. Pantagraph (Bloomington, IL) 2003 Jul 4; Sect. A:7.

18. Editorial or Review

CSE allows "notes" after the page number(s) that will help readers understand the nature of the reference.

1. Leshner AI. "Glocal" science advocacy [editorial]. Science. 2008;319(5865):877.
2. Myer A. Genomes evolve, but how? Nature. 2008;451(7180):771. Review of Lynch M, The Origins of Genome Architecture.

ELECTRONIC SOURCES ON THE INTERNET

In general, CSE style requires that you cite electronic sources by including the author's name, if available; the work's title; the type of medium, in brackets, such as [*Internet*] or [*electronic mail on the Internet*]; the title of the publication if there's a print version or, if not, the place of publication and the publishing organization; the date the original was published or placed on the Internet; the date you accessed the publication, preceded by the word *cited* enclosed in brackets; and the address of the source, if from the Internet or a database. Omit end punctuation after an Internet address.

19. Books on the Internet

1. Colwell R, editor. MENC handbook of musical cognition and development [Internet]. New York: Oxford University Press; c2006 [cited 2011 Feb 4]. Available from: http://books.google.com/books/

20. Articles with Print Versions on the Internet

1. Pollard R. Evidence of a reduced home field advantage when a team moves to a new stadium. J Sport Sci [Internet]. 2002 [cited 2010 Nov 5]; 20(12):969–974. Available from: http://0-find.galegroup.com.bianca.penlib.du.edu:80/itx/start.do?prodId=AONE

21. Articles Available Only on the Internet

1. Overbye D. Remembrance of things future: the mystery of time. The New York Times on the Web [Internet]. 2005 Jun 28 [cited 2009 Dec 11]. Available from: http://www.nytimes.com/2005/06/28/science/28time.html

22. Web Pages

Begin with author, if available; otherwise, begin with title.

1. Think again: men and women share cognitive skills [Internet]. Washington (DC): American Psychological Association; 2006 [cited 2011 Jan 17]. Available from: http://www.psychologymatters.org/thinkagain.html

2. Welcome to AAAI [Internet]. Menlo Park (CA): Association for the Advancement of Artificial Intelligence; c2008 [cited 2011 Mar 17]. Available from: http://www.aaai.org

23. Videos or Podcasts

1. Wesch M. Web 2.0 . . . the machine is us/ing us [Internet]. 2007 Jan 31 [cited 2010 Dec 14]. Available from: http://www.youtube.com /watch?v=6gmP4nk0EOE

OTHER SOURCES

24. Map

1. Russia and post-Soviet republics [political map]. Moscow: Mapping Production Association; 1992. Conical equidistant projection; 40 × 48 in., color, scale 1:8,000,000.

25. Unpublished Letter

1. Darwin C. [Letter to Mr. Clerke, 1861]. Located at: University of Iowa Library, Iowa City.

26. Video Recording

1. Nova—The elegant universe [DVD]. Boston: WGBH; 2004. 2 DVDs: 180 min., sound, color.

27. Slide Set

1. Human parasitology [slides]. Chicago: American Society of Clinical Pathologists; 1990. Color. Accompanied by: 1 guide.

28. Presentation Slides

1. Beaudoin E. Fruit fly larvae [PowerPoint slides]. Denver (CO): University of Denver; 2010 Oct 17. 49 slides.

PART

5

Understanding Grammar and Writing Correct Sentences

28 Parts of Speech and Sentence Structures

Quick Points You will learn to

- Identify the parts of speech (see 28A–28J).
- Identify the parts of sentences (see 28K).

PARTS OF SPEECH

28A Why learn the parts of speech?

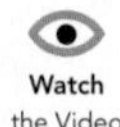

Learning the parts of speech helps you classify words according to their function in a sentence. To determine a word's part of speech, see how the word functions in a sentence. A word may have more than one function.

- We ate **fish**.

  Fish is a noun. It names a thing.

- We **fish** on weekends.

  Fish is a verb. It names an action.

28B What is a noun?

A **noun** names a person, place, thing, or idea: *student, college, textbook, education*. Quick Box 28.1 lists different kinds of nouns.

ESOL Tips: Here are some useful tips for working with NOUNS.*

- Nouns often appear with articles, other determiners, or limiting adjectives. See section 28F and Chapter 51.
- Words with these suffixes (word endings) are usually nouns: *-ness, -ence, -ance, -ty*, and *-ment*.

*Words printed in SMALL CAPITAL LETTERS are discussed elsewhere in the text and are defined in the Terms Glossary at the back of this book.

Quick Box 28.1

Nouns

PROPER	names specific people, places, or things (first letter is always capitalized)	*Bruno Mars, Paris, Toyota*
COMMON	names general groups, places, people, or things	*singer, city, automobile*
CONCRETE	names things experienced through the senses: sight, hearing, taste, smell, or touch	*landscape, pizza, thunder*
ABSTRACT	names a quality, state, or idea	*freedom, shyness*
COLLECTIVE	names groups	*family, team*
NONCOUNT OR MASS	names "uncountable" things	*water, time*
COUNT	names countable items	*lake, minute*

28C What is a pronoun?

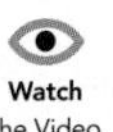

A **pronoun** takes the place of a NOUN. The words or word that a pronoun replaces is called the pronoun's ANTECEDENT. See Quick Box 28.2 for a list of different kinds of pronouns. For information on how to use pronouns correctly, see Chapters 30 and 31.

- **David** is an accountant.

  The noun *David* names a person.

- **He** is an accountant.

  The pronoun *he* refers to its antecedent, *David.*

- The finance committee needs to consult **him**.

  The pronoun *him* refers to its antecedent, *David.*

Quick Box 28.2

Pronouns

PERSONAL *I, you, its, her, they, ours,* etc.	refers to people or things	*I saw **her** take a book to **them**.*
RELATIVE *who, which, that, whom*	introduces certain NOUN CLAUSES and ADJECTIVE CLAUSES	*The book **that** I lost was valuable.*

continued >>

Quick Box 28.2 (continued)

INTERROGATIVE *which, who, whose,* and others	introduces a question	***Who*** *called?*
DEMONSTRATIVE *this, that, these, those*	points out the antecedent	*Whose books are* ***these?***
REFLEXIVE OR INTENSIVE *myself, themselves,* and other *-self* or *-selves* words	reflects back to the antecedent in the same sentence; intensifies the antecedent	*They claim to support* ***them-selves. I myself*** *doubt it.*
RECIPROCAL *each other, one another*	refers to individual parts of a plural antecedent	*We respect* ***each other.***
INDEFINITE *all, anyone, each,* and others	refers to nonspecific persons or things	***Everyone*** *is welcome here.*

● **EXERCISE 28-1** Underline and label all nouns (N) and pronouns (P). Refer to 28A through 28C for help.

EXAMPLE

My (P) mother (N) celebrated her (P) eightieth birthday (N) this summer (N) with her (P) family (N) and friends (N); she (P) greatly enjoyed the festivities (N).

1. More and more people live into their eighties and nineties because they get better health benefits and they take better care of themselves.
2. Many elderly people now live busy lives, continuing in businesses or volunteering at various agencies.
3. My mother, Elizabeth, for example, spends four hours each morning as a volunteer for the Red Cross, where she takes histories from blood donors.
4. My neighbors, George and Sandra, who are eighty-six years old, still own and run a card and candy shop.
5. Age has become no obstacle for active seniors as evidenced by the activities they pursue today. ●

28D What is a verb?

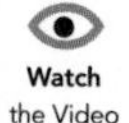

Main verbs express action, occurrence, or state of being. For information on how to use verbs correctly, see Chapter 29.

- You **danced.** [action]
- The audience **became** silent. [occurrence]
- Your dancing **was** awesome! [state of being]

Alert: If you're not sure whether a word is a verb, try substituting a different TENSE for the word. If the sentence still makes sense, the word is a verb.

NO He is a **changed** man. He is a **will change** man.

YES The man **changed** his mind. The man **will change** his mind.

EXERCISE 28-2 Underline all main verbs. Refer to 28D for help.

EXAMPLE

The study of bats produces some surprising information.

1. Most bats developed many years ago from a shrewlike mammal.
2. One thousand different types of bats exist.
3. Bats comprise almost one quarter of all mammal species.
4. The smallest bat in the world measures only one inch long, while the biggest is sixteen inches long.
5. Bats survive in widely varied surroundings, from deserts to cities.

28E What is a verbal?

Verbals are verb forms functioning as NOUNS, ADJECTIVES, or ADVERBS. Quick Box 28.3 lists the three different kinds of verbals.

Quick Box 28.3

Verbals and their functions

INFINITIVE *to* + verb	1. noun	***To eat*** *now is inconvenient.*
	2. adjective or adverb	*Still, we have far* ***to go***.
PAST PARTICIPLE *-ed* form of REGULAR VERB or equivalent in IRREGULAR VERB	adjective	***Boiled, filtered*** *water is safe.*
PRESENT PARTICIPLE *-ing* form of verb	1. noun (called a GERUND)	***Eating*** *in diners on the road is an adventure.*
	2. adjective	***Running*** *water may not be safe.*

ESOL Tip: For information about correctly using the verbals called *infinitives* and *gerunds* as objects, see Chapter 55.

28F What is an adjective?

Watch the Video

Adjectives describe or limit NOUNS, PRONOUNS, and word groups that function as nouns. For information on how to use adjectives correctly, see Chapter 32.

- I saw a **green** tree.

  Green describes the noun *tree*.

- It was **leafy**.

  Leafy describes the pronoun *it*.

- The flowering trees were **beautiful**.

  Beautiful describes the noun phrase *the flowering trees*.

ESOL Tip: You can identify some adjectives by their endings. Often, words with the SUFFIXES *-ful, -ish, -less*, and *-like* are adjectives.

Determiners, frequently called *limiting adjectives*, tell whether a noun is general (*a* tree) or specific (*the* tree). Determiners also tell which one (*this* tree), how many (*twelve* trees), whose (*our* tree), and similar information.

The determiners *a, an*, and *the* are almost always called **articles**. *The* is a **definite article**. Before a noun, *the* conveys that the noun refers to a specific item (*the* plan). *A* and *an* are **indefinite articles**. They convey that a noun refers to an item in a nonspecific or general way (*a* plan).

Alert: Use *a* before a word that starts with a consonant: *a carrot, a broken egg, a hip*. Use *an* before a word that starts with a vowel sound: *an honor, an old bag, an egg*.

ESOL Tip: For information about using articles with COUNT and NONCOUNT NOUNS, PROPER NOUNS, and GERUNDS, see Chapter 52.

Quick Box 28.4 lists kinds of determiners. Notice, however, that some words in Quick Box 28.4 function also as pronouns. To identify a word's part of speech, check to see how it functions in each particular sentence.

- **That** car belongs to Harold.

  That is a limiting adjective.

- **That** is Harold's car.

  That is a demonstrative pronoun.

Quick Box 28.4

Determiners (or limiting adjectives)

ARTICLES *a, an, the*	***The** news reporter used **a** cell phone to report **an** assignment.*
DEMONSTRATIVE *this, these, that, those*	***Those** students rent **that** house.*
INDEFINITE *any, each, few, other, some,* and others	***Few** films today have complex plots.*
INTERROGATIVE *what, which, whose*	***What** answer did you give?*
NUMERICAL *one, first, two, second,* and others	*The **fifth** question was tricky.*
POSSESSIVE *my, your, their,* and others	***My** violin is older than **your** cello.*
RELATIVE *what, which, whose, whatever,* etc.	*We do not know **which** road to take.*

28G What is an adverb?

Adverbs describe or limit VERBS, ADJECTIVES, other adverbs, and CLAUSES. For information on how to use adverbs correctly, see Chapter 32.

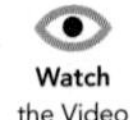

- Chefs plan meals **carefully**.

  Carefully describes the verb *plan.*

- Fruits offer **very** crucial vitamins.

  Very describes the adjective *crucial.*

- Those french fries are **too** heavily salted.

  Too describes the adverb *heavily.*

- **Fortunately**, people are learning that overuse of salt is harmful.

  Fortunately describes the rest of the sentence, an independent clause.

Descriptive adverbs show levels of intensity, usually by adding *more* (or *less*) and *most* (or *least*): *more* happily, *least* clearly (32C). Many descriptive adverbs are formed by adding *-ly* to adjectives: *sadly, loudly, normally.* But many adverbs do not end in *-ly: very, always, not, yesterday,* and *well* are a few. Some adjectives look like adverbs but are not: *brotherly, lonely, lovely.*

Relative adverbs are words such as *where, why,* and *when.* They are used to introduce adjective or noun clauses.

Conjunctive adverbs describe by creating logical connections to other words. Conjunctive adverbs can appear anywhere in a sentence.

- **However**, we consider Isaac Newton an even more important scientist.
- We consider Isaac Newton, **however**, an even more important scientist.
- We consider Isaac Newton an even more important scientist, **however**.

Quick Box 28.5 lists the kinds of relationships that conjunctive adverbs can show.

Quick Box 28.5

Conjunctive adverbs and relationships they express

Relationship	Words
ADDITION	*also, furthermore, moreover, besides*
CONTRAST	*however, still, nevertheless, conversely, nonetheless, instead, otherwise*
COMPARISON	*similarly, likewise*
RESULT OR SUMMARY	*therefore, thus, consequently, accordingly, hence, then*
TIME	*next, then, meanwhile, finally, subsequently*
EMPHASIS	*indeed, certainly*

● **EXERCISE 28-3** Underline and label all adjectives (ADJ) and adverbs (ADV). For help, consult 28E through 28G.

EXAMPLE

Young (ADV) families carefully (ADJ) looking for a good (ADJ) pet should consider domesticated (ADV) rats.

1. Rats are clean animals that easily bond to their human companions.
2. Two rats are better than one because they are gregarious animals who desperately need social interaction.
3. As intelligent animals, rats can be quickly trained to perform many tricks.
4. Humans consistently have been keeping rats as household pets for over 100 years.
5. Finally, they pose no more health risks than other pets. ●

28H What is a preposition?

Prepositions are words that convey relationships, usually of time or space. Common prepositions include *in, of, by, after, to, on, over*, and *since*. A preposition and the word or words it introduces form a PREPOSITIONAL PHRASE. For information about prepositions and commas, see 42K.2.

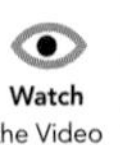
Watch the Video

- **In the fall**, we will hear a concert **by our favorite tenor**.
- **After the concert**, he will fly **to San Francisco**.

ESOL Tip: For a list of prepositions and their IDIOMS, see Chapter 54.

28I What is a conjunction?

A **conjunction** connects words, PHRASES, or CLAUSES. **Coordinating conjunctions** connect words, phrases, or clauses of equal rank. Quick Box 28.6 lists the coordinating conjunctions and the relationships they express.

- We hike **and** camp every summer.

  And joins two words.
- We hike along scenic trails **or** in the wilderness.

  Or joins two phrases.
- I love the outdoors, **but** my family does not.

  But joins two clauses.

Quick Box 28.6

Coordinating conjunctions and relationships they express

Relationship	Words	Relationship	Words
ADDITION	*and*	REASON OR CAUSE	*for*
CONTRAST	*but, yet*	CHOICE	*or*
RESULT OR EFFECT	*so*	NEGATIVE CHOICE	*nor*

Correlative conjunctions are two conjunctions used as pairs: *both . . . and; either . . . or; neither . . . nor; not only . . . but (also);* and *whether . . . or.*

- **Both** English **and** Spanish are spoken in many homes in the United States.
- **Not only** students **but also** businesspeople should study a second language.

Quick Box 28.7

Subordinating conjunctions and relationships they express

Relationship	Words
TIME	*after, before, once, since, until, when, whenever, while*
REASON OR CAUSE	*as, because, since*
RESULT OR EFFECT	*in order that, so, so that, that*
CONDITION	*if, even if, provided that, unless*
CONTRAST	*although, even though, though, whereas*
LOCATION	*where, wherever*
CHOICE	*than, whether*

Subordinating conjunctions introduce DEPENDENT CLAUSES, clauses of less importance than the INDEPENDENT CLAUSE in the sentence. Quick Box 28.7 lists the most common subordinating conjunctions. For information about how to use them correctly, see 38D through 38M.

- **Because** it snowed, school was canceled.
- Many people were happy **after** they heard the news.

28J What is an interjection?

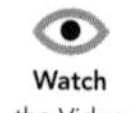

An **interjection** expresses strong or sudden emotion. Alone, an interjection is usually punctuated with an exclamation point (!). As part of a sentence, an interjection is usually set off by one or more commas.

- **Hooray!** I won the race.
- **Oh**, my friends missed seeing the finish.

● **EXERCISE 28-4** Identify the part of speech of each numbered and underlined word. Choose from noun, pronoun, verb, adjective, adverb, preposition, coordinating conjunction, correlative conjunction, and subordinating conjunction. For help, consult 28B through 28I.

The Mason-Dixon line primarily (1) marks the boundary (2) between Pennsylvania and Maryland. It was surveyed in the eighteenth (3) century by Charles Mason and Jeremiah Dixon, who had previously (4) worked together on a scientific (5) expedition to South Africa.

In 1760, the Calverts of Maryland and the Penns of Pennsylvania [6]hired Mason and Dixon to settle a [7]boundary dispute between their parcels [8]of land. Mason and Dixon [9]marked their line every [10]five miles using [11]stones shipped from England, which are called crownstones. These markers were decorated with two coats-of-arms and can still be found scattered [12]throughout this part of the country.

[13]Even though Mason [14]and Dixon were British, [15]they had very different backgrounds. Mason was the son of a baker and trained in astronomy. Dixon was a Quaker, and [16]he specialized in surveying.

The line they drew in America eventually [17]became a [18]symbolic division [19]between free states and slave states [20]until the end of the Civil War. [21]Because of the line's importance, [22]it has been the focus of [23]both literature and music, such as the [24]song "Sailing to Philadelphia" by Mark Knopfler. ●

SENTENCE STRUCTURES

28K How is a sentence defined?

On a strictly mechanical level, a **sentence** starts with a capital letter and finishes with a period, question mark, or exclamation point. Grammatically, a sentence consists of an INDEPENDENT CLAUSE: *Boxing is dangerous.* From the perspective of its purpose, a sentence is defined as listed in Quick Box 28.8 on page 450.

28L What are a subject and a predicate in a sentence?

The **subject** and **predicate** of a sentence are its two essential parts. Without both, a group of words isn't a sentence. Quick Box 28.9 (page 450) shows the sentence pattern with both. Terms used in the Quick Box are defined after it.

Quick Box 28.8

Sentences and their purposes

- A **declarative sentence** makes a statement:
  - Boxing is dangerous.
- An **interrogative sentence** asks a question:
  - Is boxing dangerous?
- An **imperative sentence** gives a command:
  - Be careful when you box.
- An **exclamatory sentence** expresses strong feeling:
  - How I love boxing!

Quick Box 28.9

Sentence pattern I: Subjects and predicates

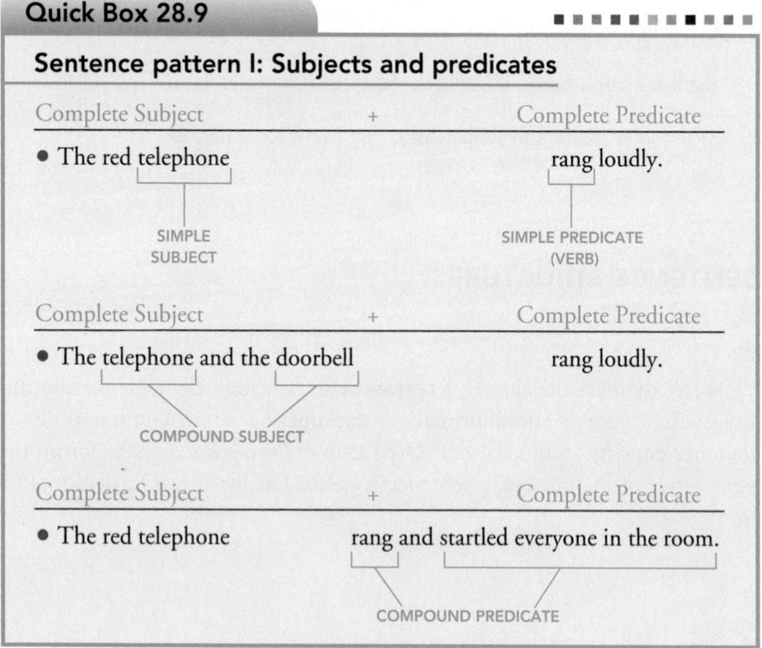

Complete Subject + Complete Predicate
The red telephone rang loudly.
SIMPLE SUBJECT
SIMPLE PREDICATE (VERB)
Complete Subject + Complete Predicate
The telephone and the doorbell rang loudly.
COMPOUND SUBJECT
Complete Subject + Complete Predicate
The red telephone rang and startled everyone in the room.
COMPOUND PREDICATE

The **simple subject** is the word or group of words that acts, is described, or is acted on.

- The **telephone** rang.
- The **telephone** is red.
- The **telephone** was being connected.

The **complete subject** is the simple subject and its MODIFIERS.

- **The red telephone** rang.

A complete **compound subject** consists of two or more NOUNS or PRONOUNS and their modifiers.

- **The telephone and the doorbell** rang.

The **predicate** contains the VERB in the sentence. The predicate tells what the subject does, experiences, or what is being done to it.

- The telephone **rang**.
- The telephone **is** red.
- The telephone **was being connected**.

A **simple predicate** contains only the verb.

- The lawyer **listened**.

A **complete predicate** contains the verb and its modifiers.

- The lawyer **listened carefully**.

A **compound predicate** contains two or more verbs.

- The lawyer **listened and waited**.

ESOL Tips: (1) The subject of a declarative sentence usually comes before the predicate, but there are exceptions (37O). In sentences that ask a question, part of the predicate usually comes before the subject. For more information about word order in English sentences, see Chapter 53. (2) In English, don't add a PERSONAL PRONOUN to repeat the stated noun.

NO My **grandfather he** lived to be eighty-seven.

YES My **grandfather** lived to be eighty-seven.

NO **Winter storms** that bring ice, **they** cause traffic problems.

YES **Winter storms** that bring ice cause traffic problems.

EXERCISE 28-5 Use a slash to separate the complete subject from the complete predicate.

EXAMPLE

The Hollywood Sign is a famous American landmark.
The Hollywood Sign / is a famous American landmark.

1. The well-known sign was first built in 1923.
2. Originally, it spelled out the word "Hollywoodland."
3. The Hollywood Chamber of Commerce removed the word "land" from the sign in 1949.
4. The sign's caretaker, Albert Kothe, destroyed the letter "H" by crashing his car into it.
5. Excited visitors still flock to Mount Lee to see this cultural icon. ●

28M What are direct and indirect objects?

A **direct object** is a noun, pronoun, or group of words that completes the meaning of a TRANSITIVE VERB. To find a direct object, ask *whom?* or *what?* after the verb.

An **indirect object** tells *to whom* or *for whom* the action of a verb is directed. To find an indirect object, ask ***to** whom? **for** whom? **to** what?* or ***for** what?* after the verb.

Direct objects and indirect objects always fall in the PREDICATE of a sentence. Quick Box 28.10 shows how direct and indirect objects function.

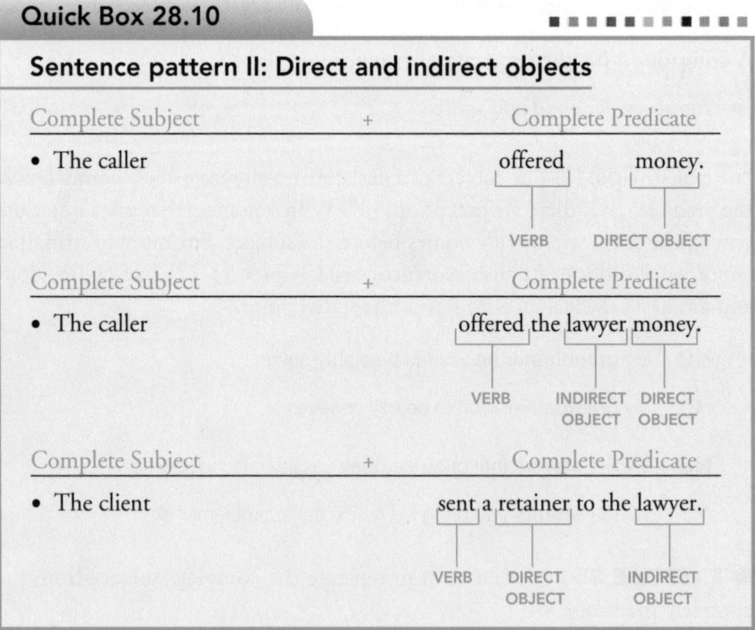

ESOL Tips: (1) In sentences with indirect objects that follow the word *to* or *for*, always put the direct object before the indirect object.

NO Will you please give **to John** this letter?

YES Will you please give this letter **to John?**

(2) When a PRONOUN is used as an indirect object, some verbs require *to* or *for* before the pronoun, and others do not. Consult the *Dictionary of American English* (Heinle and Heinle) about each verb when you're unsure.

NO Please explain **me** the rule.

The verb *explain* requires *to* before an indirect object.

YES Please explain the rule **to me**.

YES Please give **me** that book. Please give that book **to me**.

Give uses both patterns.

(3) When both the direct object and the indirect object are pronouns, put the direct object first and use *to* with the indirect object.

NO He gave **me it**.

YES He gave **it to me**.

YES Please give **me the letter**.

(4) Even if a verb does not require *to* before an indirect object, you may use *to* if you prefer. If you do use *to*, be sure to put the direct object before the indirect object.

YES Our daughter sent **our son** a gift.

YES Our daughter sent a gift **to our son**.

EXERCISE 28-6 Draw a single line under all direct objects and a double line under all indirect objects. For help, consult 28M.

EXAMPLE

Toni Morrison's award-winning novels give readers the gifts of wisdom, inspiration, and pleasure.

1. Literary critics gave high praise to Toni Morrison for her first novel, *The Bluest Eye*, but the general public showed little interest.
2. *Song of Solomon* won Morrison the National Book Critics Circle Award in 1977, and *Beloved* won her the Pulitzer Prize in 1988.
3. A literary panel awarded Toni Morrison the 1993 Nobel Prize in Literature, the highest honor a writer can receive.

4. Her 1998 novel, *Paradise*, traces for readers the tragic lives of a rejected group of former slaves.
5. Twenty-five years after *The Bluest Eye* was published, Oprah Winfrey selected it for her reader's list, and it immediately became a bestseller. ●

28N What are complements, modifiers, and appositives?

COMPLEMENTS

A **complement** renames or describes a subject or an object in the predicate.

A **subject complement** is a NOUN, PRONOUN, or ADJECTIVE that follows a LINKING VERB. An **object complement** follows a DIRECT OBJECT and either describes or renames the direct object. Quick Box 28.11 shows how subject and object complements function in a sentence.

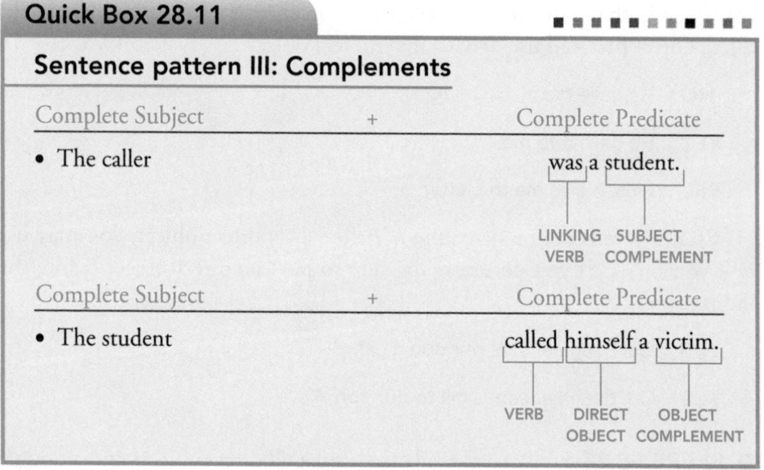

Quick Box 28.11
Sentence pattern III: Complements
Complete Subject + Complete Predicate
• The caller
was a student.
LINKING VERB
SUBJECT COMPLEMENT
Complete Subject + Complete Predicate
• The student
called himself a victim.
VERB
DIRECT OBJECT
OBJECT COMPLEMENT

● **EXERCISE 28-7** Underline all complements, and identify each as a subject complement (SUB) or an object complement (OB).

1. Graphology is the study of handwriting.
2. Some scientists and psychologists call graphology a pseudoscience.
3. According to supporters of graphology, it is useful in law, business, and medicine.
4. Trained, professional graphologists are often consultants in legal cases.
5. For example, graphologists consider small letters evidence of shyness. ●

MODIFIERS

A **modifier** is a word or group of words that describes or limits other words. Modifiers appear in the subject or the predicate of a sentence.

- The **large red** telephone rang **loudly**.

  The adjectives *large* and *red* modify the noun *telephone*. The adverb *loudly* modifies the verb *rang*.

- The person **on the telephone** was **extremely** upset.

  The prepositional phrase *on the telephone* modifies the noun *person;* the adverb *extremely* modifies the adjective *upset*.

- **Because the lawyer's voice was calm**, the caller felt reassured.

  The adverb clause *because the lawyer's voice was calm* modifies the independent clause *the caller felt reassured*.

APPOSITIVES

An **appositive** renames the noun or pronoun preceding it.

- The student's story, **a tale of broken promises**, was complicated.

  The appositive *a tale of broken promises* renames the noun *story*.

- The lawyer consulted an expert, **her law professor**.

  The appositive *her law professor* renames the noun *expert*.

- The student, **Joe Jones**, asked to speak to his lawyer.

  The appositive *Joe Jones* renames the noun *student*.

Alert: For more about appositives and NONRESTRICTIVE ELEMENTS, see 42F. ●

28O What is a phrase?

A **phrase** is a group of words that does not contain both a SUBJECT and a PREDICATE and therefore cannot stand alone as an independent unit.

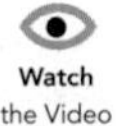

NOUN PHRASE

A **noun phrase** functions as a noun in a sentence.

- The **modern census** dates back to the seventeenth century.

VERB PHRASE

A **verb phrase** functions as a verb in a sentence.

- Two military censuses **are mentioned** in the Bible.

PREPOSITIONAL PHRASE

A **prepositional phrase** always starts with a preposition and functions as a modifier.

- William the Conqueror conducted a census **of landowners in 1086**.

  Two prepositional phrases come in a row, beginning with *of* and *in*.

ABSOLUTE PHRASE

An **absolute phrase** is a noun phrase that modifies the entire sentence.

- **Censuses being the fashion**, Quebec and Nova Scotia took sixteen counts between 1665 and 1754.
- Eighteenth-century Sweden and Denmark had complete records of their populations, **each adult and child having been counted**.

VERBAL PHRASE

A **verbal phrase** contains a verb form that functions as a noun or an adjective. They include INFINITIVES, present participles, past participles, and gerunds.

- In 1624, Virginia began **to count its citizens** in a census.

  To count its citizens is an infinitive phrase functioning as a direct object.

- **Amazed by some people's answers**, census takers always listen carefully.

  Amazed by some people's answers is a past participial phrase.

- **Going from door to door**, census takers interview millions of people.

  Going from door to door is a present participial phrase.

- **Going from door to door** takes many hours.

  The gerund phrase functions as the subject.

GERUND PHRASE

Although both **gerund phrases** and **present-tense participial phrases** use the *-ing* form of the verb, a gerund phrase functions only as a noun, whereas a participial phrase functions only as a modifier.

- **Including everyone in the census** mattered.

  This is a gerund phrase because it functions as a noun, the subject of the sentence.

- **Including everyone in the census**, Abby worked carefully.

  This is a present participial phrase because it functions as a modifier describing Abby.

● **EXERCISE 28-8** Combine each set of sentences into a single sentence by converting one sentence into a phrase—a noun phrase, a verb phrase, prepositional phrase, absolute phrase, verbal phrase, or gerund phrase. You can omit, add, or change words. Identify which type of phrase you created.

EXAMPLE

The key grip is an important person in the making of a film. The key grip is the chief rigging technician on the movie set.

Serving as the chief rigging technician on a movie set, the key grip is an important person in the making of a film. (verbal phrase)

1. They key grip is the head of the grip department. Grips provide support to the camera department.
2. Grips work with such camera equipment as tripods, dollies, and cranes. Grips have to set up this equipment in a variety of settings during the making of a feature film.
3. Grips are also responsible for safety on the movie set. They have to watch over potentially dangerous equipment like ladders, stands, and scaffolds.
4. The "best boy grip" is the assistant to the key grip. The "best boy electric" is the assistant to the gaffer, who is the head electrician.
5. Electricians handle all of the lights on a movie set. Grips are in charge of all of the nonelectrical equipment related to light.
6. Sometimes grips are needed to reduce sunlight. They can do this by installing black fabric over windows and other openings.
7. The use of grips dates back to circuses and vaudeville. Early grips held on to hand-cranked cameras to reduce movement. ●

28P What is a clause?

A **clause** is a group of words with both a SUBJECT and a PREDICATE. Clauses are either *independent* (*main*) *clauses*, or *dependent* (*subordinate*) *clauses*.

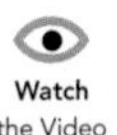

Watch the Video

INDEPENDENT CLAUSES

An **independent clause** contains a subject and a predicate and can stand alone as a sentence. Quick Box 28.12 (page 458) shows the basic pattern.

DEPENDENT CLAUSES

A **dependent clause** contains a subject and a predicate but can't stand alone as a sentence. Dependent clauses are either adverb clauses or adjective clauses.

Quick Box 28.12

Sentence pattern IV: Independent clauses

Independent Clause		
Complete Subject	+	Complete Predicate
• The telephone		rang.

ADVERB CLAUSES

An **adverb clause** starts with a subordinating conjunction, such as *although*, *because*, *when*, or *until*. Adverb clauses usually answer some question about the independent clause: How? Why? When?

- **When the bond issue passes**, the city will install sewers.

  The adverb clause modifies the verb phrase *will install;* it explains when.
- They are drawing up plans **as quickly as they can**.

  The adverb clause modifies the verb phrase *drawing up;* it explains how.
- **Because homeowners know the flooding will end**, they feel relief.

  The adverb clause modifies the entire independent clause; it explains why.

Alert: When you write an adverb clause before an independent clause, separate the clauses with a comma; see 42C. ●

ADJECTIVE CLAUSES

An **adjective clause**, also called a *relative clause*, starts with a **relative pronoun**, such as *who, which*, or *that* or a RELATIVE ADVERB, such as *when* or *where*. An adjective clause modifies the noun or pronoun that it follows. Quick Box 28.13 shows how adverb and adjective clauses function in sentences.

- The car **that Jack bought** is practical.
- The day **when I can buy my own car** is getting closer.

Use *who, whom, whoever, whomever*, and *whose* when an adjective clause refers to a person or to an animal with a name.

- The Smythes, **who collect cars**, are wealthy.
- Their dog Bowser, **whom they spoil**, has his own car.

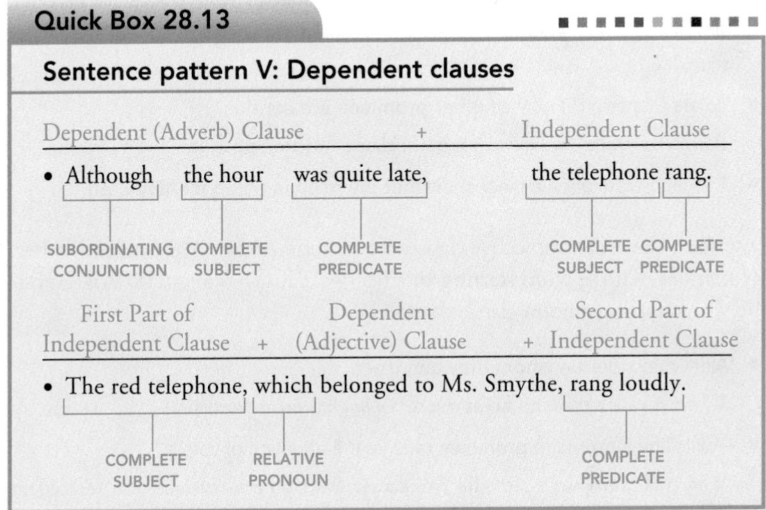

Quick Box 28.13
Sentence pattern V: Dependent clauses
Dependent (Adverb) Clause + Independent Clause
• Although the hour was quite late, the telephone rang.
SUBORDINATING CONJUNCTION
COMPLETE SUBJECT
COMPLETE PREDICATE
COMPLETE SUBJECT
COMPLETE PREDICATE
First Part of Independent Clause + Dependent (Adjective) Clause + Second Part of Independent Clause
• The red telephone, which belonged to Ms. Smythe, rang loudly.
COMPLETE SUBJECT
RELATIVE PRONOUN
COMPLETE PREDICATE

Use *which* or *that* when an adjective clause refers to a thing or to an animal that isn't a pet. Sometimes, writers omit *that* from an adjective clause. For help in choosing between *that* or *which*, see Quick Box 30.4 in section 30S.

EXERCISE 28-9 Underline the dependent clause in each sentence, and label it an adjectival (ADJ) or an adverbial (ADV) clause. For help, consult 28P.

EXAMPLE

ADV

The Stanley Hotel, which is located in Estes Park, Colorado, was built in 1909.

1. The Stanley Hotel is famous because it inspired Stephen King's novel *The Shining*.
2. Although based on King's book, the movie *The Shining* was filmed in England.
3. F. O. Stanley moved to Estes Park when he was diagnosed with tuberculosis.
4. He then built the hotel that now bears his name.
5. Visitors who believe the hotel is haunted claim to see Stanley's ghost in the lobby.

NOUN CLAUSES

Noun clauses function as nouns. Noun clauses can begin with many of the same words that begin adjective clauses: *that, who, which*, and their derivatives, as well as *when, where, whether, why*, and *how*.

- **What politicians promise** is not always dependable.

  What politicians promise is a noun clause functioning as the subject of the sentence.

- Voters often don't know **whether promises are serious**.

  Whether promises are serious is a noun clause functioning as the direct object.

- The electorate often cannot know **that the truth is being manipulated**.

Noun clauses and adjective clauses are sometimes confused with each other. Remember that the word starting an adjective clause has an ANTECEDENT, but the word starting a noun clause doesn't.

- Alert voters decide **whom they can trust**.

  Whom they can trust is a noun clause; *whom* has no antecedent.

- Politicians **who make promises** receive the attention of voters.

  Who make promises is an adjective clause describing *politicians*, the antecedent of *who*.

ESOL Tip: Noun clauses in INDIRECT QUESTIONS are phrased as statements, not questions: *Kara asked why we needed the purple dye*. Don't phrase a noun clause this way: *Kara asked why* did [or do] *we need the purple dye?*

ELLIPTICAL CLAUSES

An elliptical clause omits one or more words that are easily inferred from the context. To check for correctness, insert the word or words you omitted and look for grammatical accuracy.

- Engineering is one of the majors **[that] she considered**.
- She decided **[that] she would rather major in management**.
- **After [he takes] a refresher course**, he will be eligible for a raise.
- She is taller than I [am].

EXERCISE 28-10 Use subordinate conjunctions and relative pronouns from the following list to combine each pair of sentences. You may use words more than once, but try to use as many different ones as possible. Some sentence pairs may be combined in several ways. Create at least one elliptical construction.

since	which	if	after	when	as
although	so that	unless	because	even though	that

EXAMPLE

Bluegrass music is associated with American South. It has roots in Irish and Scottish folk music.

Even though it has roots in Irish and Scottish folk music, bluegrass is associated with the American South.

1. Certain aspects of jazz seem to have influenced bluegrass. It involves players of an instrumental ensemble improvising around a standard melody.
2. However, the instruments used in jazz are very different than those played in bluegrass. This style of music usually uses a banjo, fiddle, mandolin, and dobro.
3. The singing in bluegrass involves tight harmonies and a tenor lead singer. People who listen closely to the vocal arrangements can hear this.
4. Bill Monroe, the founder of bluegrass, added banjo player Earl Scruggs to his band, the Blue Grass Boys. This allowed him to produce a fuller sound.
5. The Blue Grass Boys went into the studio in 1945 to record some songs for Columbia Records. They hit the charts with "Kentucky Waltz" and "Footprints in the Snow."
6. They began touring America with their own large circus tent. They then became one of the most popular acts in country music.
7. Lester Flatt and Earl Scruggs left Bill Monroe's band. They formed their own group called the Foggy Mountain Boys.
8. A famous Flatt & Scruggs song is considered one of the most popular and difficult to play on the banjo. This song is called "Foggy Mountain Breakdown."
9. Most banjo players cannot play "Foggy Mountain Breakdown" at the same speed that Earl Scruggs plays it. Very skilled players can.
10. Bluegrass must continue to attract new and young fans. Otherwise, it will fade into obscurity. ●

28Q What are the four sentence types?

English uses four SENTENCE types: simple, compound, complex, and compound complex. A **simple sentence** consists of one INDEPENDENT CLAUSE and no DEPENDENT CLAUSES.

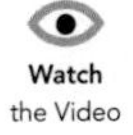
Watch the Video

- Charlie Chaplin was born in London on April 16, 1889.

A **compound sentence** consists of two or more independent clauses. These clauses may be connected by a COORDINATING CONJUNCTION, a semicolon alone, or a semicolon and a CONJUNCTIVE ADVERB.

- His father died early, **and** his mother spent time in mental hospitals.
- Many people enjoy Chaplin films**;** others do not.
- Many people enjoy Chaplin films**; however**, others do not.

A **complex sentence** is composed of one independent clause and one or more dependent clauses. (Dependent clauses are boldfaced.)

- **When times were bad**, Chaplin lived in the streets.
- **When Chaplin performed with a troupe that was touring the United States**, he was hired by Mack Sennett, **who owned the Keystone Company**.

A **compound-complex sentence** joins a compound sentence and a complex sentence. It contains two or more independent clauses and one or more dependent clauses. (Dependent clauses are boldfaced.)

- Chaplin's comedies were very successful, and he became rich **because he was enormously popular for playing the Little Tramp, who was loved for his tiny mustache, baggy trousers, big shoes, and trick derby**.
- **When studios could no longer afford him**, Chaplin co-founded United Artists, and then he produced and distributed his own films.

Alerts: (1) Use a comma before a coordinating conjunction connecting two independent clauses; see 42B. ●

● **EXERCISE 28-11** Decide whether each of the following sentences is simple, compound, complex, or compound-complex.

EXAMPLE

Air Force One is a term used to describe a technologically advanced aircraft used by the President of the United States. (simple)

1. Technically, Air Force One is the call name of any Air Force airplane carrying the President, but it usually refers to a specific airplane made by Boeing.
2. Because the aircraft is capable of being refueled in midair, Air Force One has unlimited range.
3. The onboard electronics are well protected, and they include the most advanced communications technology because the airplane often functions as a mobile command center.
4. The airplane provides 4,000 square feet of floor space and three levels, and it includes a large office and conference room.
5. Because the plane contains a fully operational medical center suite, Air Force One can provide essential medical care to the President.
6. The plane's two food galleys can feed up to 100 people at a time.

7. In order to accommodate the President's companions, the airplane includes rooms and services for advisors, Secret Service officers, members of the press, and other guests.
8. Even though Theodore Roosevelt was the first President to fly in an airplane in 1910, the call sign "Air Force One" was not created until 1953, when President Eisenhower flew in commercial air space.
9. The name "Marine One" usually refers to a helicopter carrying the U.S. President, and a helicopter carrying the Vice President is called "Marine Two."
10. Any aircraft of the United States Navy carrying the President is designated as "Navy One." ●

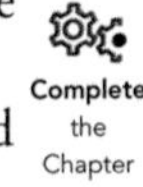

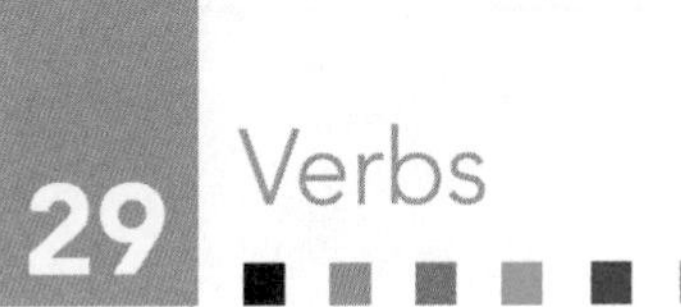

29 Verbs

Quick Points You will learn to

- ➤ Explain the functions and forms of verbs (see 29A–29F).
- ➤ Use verb tenses to express time (see 29G–29K).

29A What do verbs do?

A **verb** expresses an action, an occurrence, or a state of being.

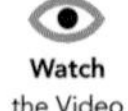

- Many people **overeat** on Thanksgiving.
- Mother's Day **fell** early this year.
- Memorial Day **is** tomorrow.

Verbs also reveal when something occurs—in the present, the past, or the future. See Quick Box 29.1 and Quick Box 29.2 (page 464).

LINKING VERBS

Linking verbs are main verbs that indicate a state of being or a condition. A linking verb is like an equal sign between a subject and its SUBJECT COMPLEMENT. Quick Box 29.3 on page 465 shows how linking verbs function.

Quick Box 29.1

Information that verbs convey

PERSON	First person (the speaker: ***I*** *dance*), second person (the one spoken to: ***you*** *dance*), or third person (the one spoken about: ***the man*** *dances*).
NUMBER	Singular (*he* ***dances***) or plural (*they* ***dance***).
TENSE	Past (*we* ***danced***), present (*we* ***dance***), or future (*we* ***will dance***); see 29G through 29K.
MOOD	Moods are indicative (*we dance*), imperative (commands and polite requests: *dance*), or conditional (speculation, wishes: *if we were dancing* . . .); see 29L and 29M.
VOICE	Active voice or passive voice; see 29N through 29P.

Quick Box 29.2

Types of verbs

MAIN VERB	The word in a PREDICATE that says something about the SUBJECT: *She* ***danced*** *for the group.*
AUXILIARY VERB	A verb that helps a main verb convey information about TENSE, MOOD, or VOICE (29E). The verbs *be, do*, and *have* can be auxiliary verbs or main verbs. The verbs *can, could, may, might, should, would, must,* and others are MODAL AUXILIARY VERBS. They add shades of meaning such as ability or possibility to verbs: *She* ***might dance.***
LINKING VERB	The verb that links a subject to a COMPLEMENT. *She* ***was*** *happy dancing. Be* is the most common linking verb; sometimes sense verbs (*smell, taste*) or verbs of perception (*seem, feel*) function as linking verbs. See also Quick Box 29.3.
TRANSITIVE VERB	The verb followed by a DIRECT OBJECT that completes the verb's message: *They* ***sent*** *her a fan letter.*
INTRANSITIVE VERB	A verb that requires no direct object: *Earlier she* ***danced.***

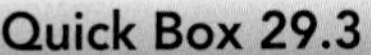

Linking verbs

- Linking verbs may be forms of the verb *be* (*am, is, was, were*).

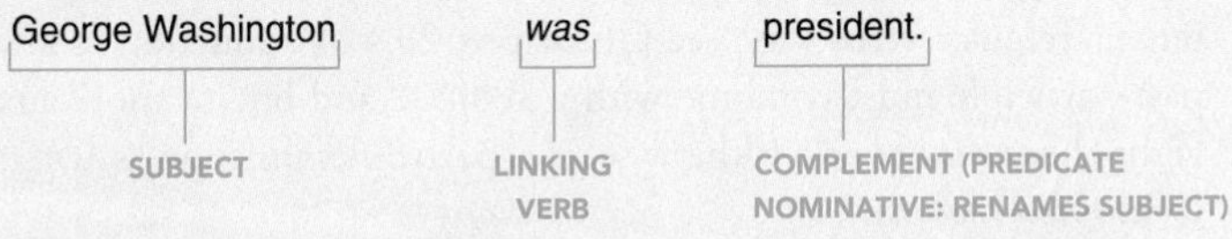

- Linking verbs may deal with the senses (*look, smell, taste, sound, feel*).

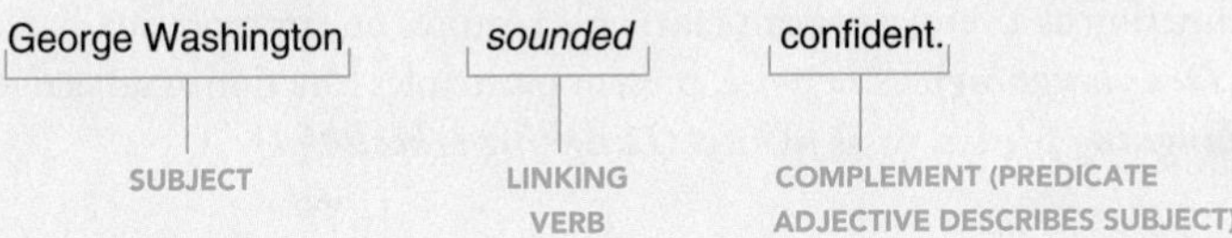

- Linking verbs can be verbs that convey a sense of existing or becoming—*appear, seem, become, get, grow, turn, remain, stay*, and *prove*, for example.

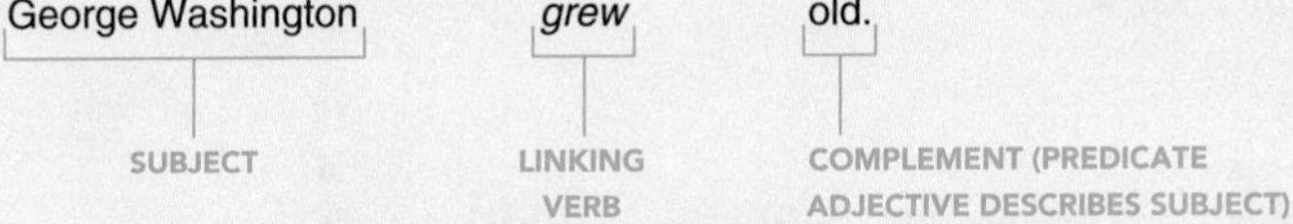

- To test whether a verb other than a form of *be* is as a linking verb, substitute *was* (for a singular subject) or *were* (for a plural subject) for the original verb. If the sentence makes sense, the original verb is a linking verb.

  NO Washington *grew* a beard → Washington *was* a beard.

  YES Washington *grew* old → Washington *was* old.

  Grew is a linking verb.

VERB FORMS

29B What are the forms of main verbs?

A MAIN VERB names an action (*People **dance***), an occurrence (*They **grow** tired*), or a state of being (*It **will be** hot later*). Main verbs have four forms.

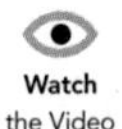

- The **simple form** conveys an action, occurrence, or state of being taking place in the present (*I **laugh***) or, with an AUXILIARY VERB, in the future (*I **will laugh***).

- The **past-tense form** conveys an action, occurrence, or state completed in the past (*I **laughed***). REGULAR VERBS add *-ed* or *-d* to the simple form. IRREGULAR VERBS vary (see Quick Box 29.4 [page 468] for a list of common irregular verbs).
- The **past participle form** in regular verbs uses the same form as the past tense. Irregular verbs vary; see Quick Box 29.4. To function as a verb, a past participle must combine with a SUBJECT and one or more auxiliary verbs (*I **have laughed***). Otherwise, past participles function as ADJECTIVES (***crumbled** cookies*).
- The **present participle form** adds *-ing* to the simple form (***laughing***). To function as a verb, a present participle requires one or more auxiliary verbs (*I **was laughing***). Otherwise, present participles function as adjectives (*my **laughing** friends*) or as NOUNS (***Laughing** is healthful*).

ESOL Tip: When verbs function as other parts of speech, they're called VERBALS. Verbals are INFINITIVES, PARTICIPLES, or GERUNDS. For information about using gerunds and infinitives as OBJECTS after certain verbs, see Chapter 55. ●

29C What is the -s, or -es, form of a verb?

The *-s* form of a verb is the third-person singular in the PRESENT TENSE. The ending *-s* (or *-es*) is added to the verb's SIMPLE FORM (*smell* becomes *smells*, as in *The bread **smells** delicious*).

Be and *have* are irregular verbs. For the third-person singular, present tense, *be* uses *is* and *have* uses *has*.

- The cheesecake **is** popular.
- The éclair **has** chocolate icing.

Even if you drop the *-s* ending in speech, always use it in writing.

- He **is** [not *be*] hungry.
- The bakery **has** [not *have*] fresh bread.

● **EXERCISE 29-1** Rewrite each sentence, changing the subjects to the word or words given in parentheses. Change the form of the verbs shown in italics to match the new subject. Keep all sentences in the present tense. For help, consult 29C.

EXAMPLE

The Oregon giant earthworm *escapes* all attempts at detection. (Oregon giant earthworms)

Oregon giant earthworms escape all attempts at detection.

1. Before declaring the Oregon giant earthworm a protected species, U.S. government agencies *require* concrete proof that it *is* not extinct. (a government agency) (they)
2. A scientist who *finds* one alive will demonstrate that Oregon giant earthworms *do* still exist, despite no one's having seen any for over twenty years. (Scientists) (the Oregon giant earthworm)
3. Last seen in the Willamette Valley near Portland, Oregon, the earthworms *are* white, and they *smell* like lilies. (the earthworm) (it)
4. Oregon giant earthworms *grow* up to three feet long. (The Oregon giant earthworm)
5. A clump of soil with a strange shape *indicates* that the giant creatures *continue* to live, but to demonstrate that they *are* not extinct, only a real specimen will do. (clumps of soil) (creature) (it) ●

29D What is the difference between regular and irregular verbs?

A **regular verb** forms its PAST TENSE and PAST PARTICIPLE by adding *-ed* or *-d* to the SIMPLE FORM: *type, typed; cook, cooked; work, worked; taste, tasted.*

In informal speech, some people skip over the *-ed* sound. In ACADEMIC WRITING, however, be sure to use it.

NO The cake was **suppose** to be ready.

YES The cake was **supposed** to be ready.

NO We **use** to bake.

YES We **used** to bake.

Irregular verbs don't consistently add *-d* or *-ed* endings to the simple verb to form the past tense and past participle. Unfortunately, a verb's simple form doesn't offer any indication whether the verb is regular or irregular. Quick Box 29.4 (page 468) lists the most frequently used irregular verbs.

Alert: For information about changing *y* to *i*, or doubling a final consonant before adding the *-ed* ending, see 49D. ●

Quick Box 29.4

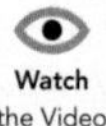
Watch the Video

Common irregular verbs

Simple Form	Past Tense	Past Participle
arise	arose	arisen
awake	awoke *or* awaked	awaked *or* awoken
be (is, am, are)	was, were	been
beat	beat	beaten
become	became	become
begin	began	begun
bend	bent	bent
bite	bit	bitten *or* bit
blow	blew	blown
break	broke	broken
bring	brought	brought
build	built	built
burst	burst	burst
buy	bought	bought
catch	caught	caught
choose	chose	chosen
cling	clung	clung
come	came	come
cost	cost	cost
cut	cut	cut
deal	dealt	dealt
dig	dug	dug
dive	dived *or* dove	dived
do	did	done
draw	drew	drawn
drink	drank	drunk
drive	drove	driven
eat	ate	eaten
fall	fell	fallen
fight	fought	fought
find	found	found
fly	flew	flown
forget	forgot	forgotten *or* forgot
freeze	froze	frozen

continued >>

Quick Box 29.4 (continued)

Simple Form	Past Tense	Past Participle
get	got	got *or* gotten
give	gave	given
go	went	gone
grow	grew	grown
hang ("to suspend")*	hung	hung
have	had	had
hear	heard	heard
hide	hid	hidden
hurt	hurt	hurt
keep	kept	kept
know	knew	known
lay	laid	laid
lead	led	led
lend	lent	lent
let	let	let
lie	lay	lain
light	lighted *or* lit	lighted *or* lit
lose	lost	lost
make	made	made
mean	meant	meant
prove	proved	proved *or* proven
read	read	read
ride	rode	ridden
ring	rang	rung
rise	rose	risen
run	ran	run
say	said	said
see	saw	seen
seek	sought	sought
send	sent	sent
set	set	set
shake	shook	shaken
shoot	shot	shot

*When it means "to execute by hanging," *hang* is a regular verb: *In wartime, some armies routinely **hanged** deserters.*

continued >>

Quick Box 29.4 (continued)

Simple Form	Past Tense	Past Participle
show	showed	shown *or* showed
shrink	shrank	shrunk
sing	sang	sung
sink	sank *or* sunk	sunk
sit	sat	sat
slay	slew	slain
sleep	slept	slept
speak	spoke	spoken
spin	spun	spun
spring	sprang *or* sprung	sprung
stand	stood	stood
steal	stole	stolen
sting	stung	stung
stink	stank *or* stunk	stunk
strike	struck	struck
swear	swore	sworn
swim	swam	swum
swing	swung	swung
take	took	taken
teach	taught	taught
throw	threw	thrown
wake	woke *or* waked	woken *or* waked
wear	wore	worn
wring	wrung	wrung
write	wrote	written

● **EXERCISE 29-2** Write the correct past-tense form of the regular verbs given in parentheses. For help, consult 29D.

EXAMPLE

Native North Americans (invent) invented the game of lacrosse.

(1) Ancient lacrosse games (involve) ____________ up to 1,000 men and (last) ____________ the entire day. (2) Native Americans (play) ____________ the game using balls they (create) ____________ out of deerskin and wood.

(3) Lacrosse (serve) ____________ many purposes in tribal life as warriors (train) ____________ for battle and (resolve) ____________ conflicts. (4) French missionaries eventually (name) ____________ the game "la crosse," perhaps referring to the staffs Jesuit bishops (use) ____________. (5) Lacrosse (resemble) ____________ the Irish sport hurling, so when Irish immigrants (arrive) ____________ in America in the 19th century, they (help) ____________ to make the game more popular. ●

● **EXERCISE 29-3** Write the correct past-tense form of the irregular verbs given in parentheses. For help, consult Quick Box 29.4 in 29D.

EXAMPLE

In August 1969, the Woodstock music festival (begin) began as thousands of fans (drive) drove to upstate New York for three days of music.

(1) The official name of the festival (is) ____________ the Woodstock Music and Art Fair. (2) It (draw) ____________ nearly half a million people to Max Yasgur's farm, which (stand) ____________ in the small town of Bethel, New York. (3) The concert (have) ____________ to move to Bethel at the last minute after residents of the town of Woodstock (forbid) ____________ organizers to hold the festival in their town. (4) Those who (come) ____________ to hear music were not disappointed, since several well known artists (sing) ____________ to the large crowd. (5) Performers such as Jimi Hendrix, Santana, and Janis Joplin (lend) ____________ their talents to the festival. (6) Even though rain clouds occasionally (cast) ____________ a shadow on the events, most people (stick) ____________ it out the entire three days. (7) According to some reports, two women (give) ____________ birth during the festival. (8) Because of the relatively peaceful atmosphere, many people (see) ____________ the event as a symbol of countercultural ideals. (9) Filmmaker Michael Wadleigh (strive) ____________ to capture that atmosphere in the film *Woodstock*, which he (shoot) ____________ and edited with the help of a young Martin Scorsese. (10) The festival also (lead) ____________ to a song written by Joni Mitchell called "Woodstock." (11) That song (become) ____________ a hit for Crosby, Stills, Nash, and Young, which (make) ____________ its debut as a group at Woodstock. (12) Although organizers (try) ____________ to turn a profit with the event, they (lose) ____________ money because many attendees did not purchase tickets. ●

29E What are auxiliary verbs?

Listen to the Podcast

Auxiliary verbs, also called *helping verbs*, combine with MAIN VERBS to make VERB PHRASES. Quick Box 29.5 shows how auxiliary verbs work.

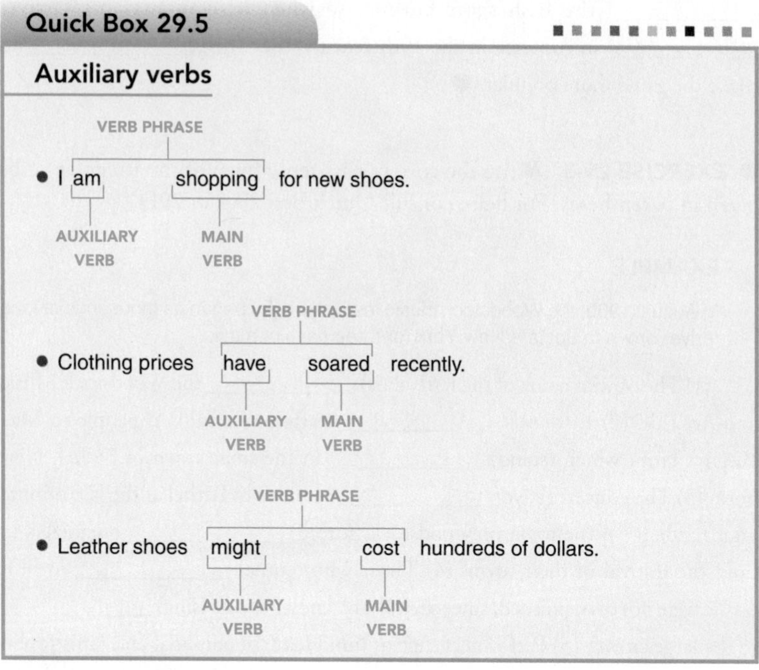

USING *BE, DO, HAVE*

The three most common auxiliary verbs, *be, do*, and *have*, can also be main verbs. Their forms vary widely, as Quick Boxes 29.6 and 29.7 show.

ESOL Tip: When *be, do*, and *have* function as auxiliary verbs for a third-person singular subject, don't add *-s* to the main verb.

NO **Does** the library **closes** at 6:00?

YES **Does** the library **close** at 6:00?

MODAL AUXILIARY VERBS

Can, could, shall, should, will, would, may, might, and *must* are **modal auxiliary verbs**, which show the speaker's MOOD toward the VERB. They never change form.

- Exercise **can lengthen** lives. [possibility]
- She **can jog** for five miles. [ability]

Quick Box 29.6

Forms of the verb *be*

SIMPLE FORM	he
-s FORM	is
PAST TENSE	was, were
PRESENT PARTICIPLE	being
PAST PARTICIPLE	been

Person	**Present Tense**	**Past Tense**
I	am	was
you (singular)	are	were
he, she, it	is	was
we	are	were
you (plural)	are	were
they	are	were

Quick Box 29.7

Forms of the verbs *do* and *have*

SIMPLE FORM	do	have
-s FORM	does	has
PAST TENSE	did	had
PRESENT PARTICIPLE	doing	having
PAST PARTICIPLE	done	had

- You **must** jog regularly. [necessity, obligation]
- People **should protect** their bodies. [advisability]
- **May** I **exercise?** [permission]

ESOL Tip: For more about modal auxiliary verbs and the meanings they communicate, see Chapter 56.

● **EXERCISE 29-4** Using the auxiliary verbs in the following list, fill in the blanks in the following passage. Use each auxiliary word only once, even if a listed word can fit into more than one blank. For help, consult 29E.

are have may will might can has

EXAMPLE

Completing a marathon can be the highlight of a runner's life.

(1) The marathon ____________ been a challenging and important athletic event since the 19th century. (2) Athletes who ____________ training for a marathon ____________ use one of the many online training guides. (3) Running with a partner or friend ____________ boost confidence and motivation. (4) Beginning runners ____________ find the first few weeks difficult but ____________ soon see dramatic improvement in their performance. (5) Those who ____________ successfully finished the race often want to repeat the experience. ●

29F What are intransitive and transitive verbs?

An **intransitive verb** requires no object to complete the verb's meaning: *I sing.* A **transitive verb** needs an object to complete the verb's meaning: *I need a guitar.* Many verbs can be transitive or intransitive, whereas others are only transitive: *need, have, like.* Only transitive verbs function in the PASSIVE VOICE.

The verbs *lie* and *lay* are often confused. *Lie* is intransitive and means "to recline, to rest." *Lay* is transitive and means "to put something down." In Quick Box 29.8, the word *lay* is both the past tense of *lie* and the present-tense simple form of *lay*. That makes things difficult, so our best advice is to memorize them.

Two other verb pairs tend to confuse people because of their intransitive and transitive forms: *raise* and *rise* and *set* and *sit*. *Raise* and *set* are transitive; they must be followed by an object. *Rise* and *sit* are intransitive; they cannot be followed by an object.

● **EXERCISE 29-5** Underline the correct word of each pair in parentheses. For help, consult 29F.

EXAMPLE

During the summer, Caroline enjoys (lying/laying) on the beach.

(1) One day, after (setting/sitting) her chair on the sand, Caroline (lay/laid) her blanket near her umbrella. (2) Worried about getting a sunburn, she (raised/rose) her umbrella and (lay/laid) under it. (3) After a brief nap, Caroline began (rising/raising) to her feet when she realized she had forgotten where she had (lain/laid) her cooler. (4) She soon found it (lying/laying) near her car, just where she had (sat/set) it earlier. (5) She decided to pick it up and (lie/lay) it down near where her blanket (lies/lays). ●

Quick Box 29.8

Listen to the Podcast

Using *lie* and *lay*

	lie	**lay**
SIMPLE FORM	lie	lay
-*s* FORM	lies	lays
PAST TENSE	lay	laid
PRESENT PARTICIPLE	lying	laying
PAST PARTICIPLE	lain	laid

INTRANSITIVE FORMS

PRESENT TENSE The hikers **lie** down to rest.

PAST TENSE The hikers **lay** down to rest.

TRANSITIVE FORMS

PRESENT TENSE The hikers **lay** their backpacks on a rock.
Backpacks is a direct object.

PAST TENSE The hikers **laid** their backpacks on a rock.
Backpacks is a direct object.

VERB TENSE

29G What is verb tense?

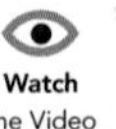
Watch the Video

Verb **tense** conveys time by changing form. The three **simple tenses** in English divide time into present, past, and future. The simple **present tense** describes what happens regularly or what is consistently or generally true. The simple **past tense** indicates an action completed or a condition ended. The simple **future tense** indicates action to be taken or a condition not yet experienced.

- Rick **wants** to speak Spanish fluently. [simple present tense]
- Rick **wanted** to improve rapidly. [simple past tense]
- Rick **will want** to progress even further next year. [simple future tense]

The three PERFECT TENSES show more complex time relationships. For information on using the perfect tenses, see section 29I.

The three simple tenses and the three perfect tenses also have PROGRESSIVE FORMS. These forms indicate that the verb describes what is ongoing or continuing. For information on using progressive forms, see section 29J. Quick Box 29.9 (page 476) summarizes verb tenses and progressive forms.

Quick Box 29.9

Simple, perfect, and progressive tenses

SIMPLE TENSES

	Regular Verb	Irregular Verb	Progressive Form
PRESENT	I talk	I eat	I am talking; I am eating
PAST	I talked	I ate	I was talking; I was eating
FUTURE	I will talk	I will eat	I will be talking; I will be eating

PERFECT TENSES

	Regular Verb	Irregular Verb	Progressive Form
PRESENT PERFECT	I have talked	I have eaten	I have been talking; I have been eating
PAST PERFECT	I had talked	I had eaten	I had been talking; I had been eating
FUTURE PERFECT	I will have talked	I will have eaten	I will have been talking; I will have been eating

ESOL Tip: As Quick Box 29.9 shows, auxiliary verbs are necessary in the formation of most tenses, so never omit them.

NO I **talking** to you.

YES I **am talking** to you.

29H How do I use the simple present tense?

The **simple present tense** uses the SIMPLE FORM of the verb (see 29B). It describes what happens regularly, or what is generally or consistently true. Also, it can convey a specific future occurrence with verbs like *start, stop, begin, end, arrive*, and *graduate*.

- Calculus class **meets** every morning. [regularly occurring action]
- Mastering calculus **takes** time. [general truth]
- The course **ends** in eight weeks. [specific future event]

Alert: For a work of literature, always use the present tense.

- In Shakespeare's *Othello*, Iago **manipulates** Othello, who **loves** his wife.

29I How do I form and use the perfect tenses?

The **perfect tenses** describe actions or occurrences that affect the present or some other specified time. The perfect tenses are composed of an AUXILIARY VERB and a main verb's PAST PARTICIPLE (29B).

For the **present perfect tense** (see Quick Box 29.9), use *has* only for the third-person singular subjects and *have* for all other subjects. For the **past perfect**, use *had* with the past participle. For the **future perfect**, use *will have* with the past participle.

PRESENT PERFECT	America **has offered** help.
PRESENT PERFECT	The earthquake **has created** terrible hardship.
PAST PERFECT	After the tornado **had passed**, the heavy rain started.
	The tornado occurred before the rain, so the earlier event uses *had*.
FUTURE PERFECT	Our chickens' egg production **will have reached** five hundred per day by next year.
	The event will occur before a specified time.

29J How do I form and use progressive forms?

Progressive forms describe an ongoing event, action, or condition. They also express habitual or recurring actions or conditions. All progressive tenses use a form of the verb *be* plus the present participle of the main verb. The **present progressive** use a form of *be* to agree with its subject in person and number; the **present perfect progressive** uses a form of *be* to agree with its subject in number.

PRESENT PROGRESSIVE	The smog **is stinging** everyone's eyes.
PAST PROGRESSIVE	Eye drops **were selling** well last week.
FUTURE PROGRESSIVE	We **will be buying** more eye drops than usual this month.
	Recurring event that will take place in the future.
PRESENT PERFECT PROGRESSIVE	Scientists **have been warning** us about air pollution for years.
PAST PERFECT PROGRESSIVE	We **had been ordering** three cases of eye drops a month until the smog worsened.
FUTURE PERFECT PROGRESSIVE	By May, we **will have been selling** eye drops for eight months.

● **EXERCISE 29-6** Underline the correct verb in each pair of parentheses. If more than one answer is possible, be prepared to explain the differences in meaning between the two choices. For help, consult 29G through 29J.

EXAMPLE

According to an article in *National Geographic News*, weird plants (are taking root, would have taken root) in ordinary backyards.

1. Some, smelling like spoiled meat, (will have ruined, are ruining) people's appetites.
2. Stalks similar to male anatomy (typify, are typifying) other examples.
3. *Shockingly large*, *black*, *carnivorous*, and *volatile* (describe, is describing) additional unusual plants.
4. Indeed, many unusual plants (live, lived) in places the world over today.
5. Many people now (are planting, planted) these weird items in their backyards.
6. In 1999, in East Lothian, Scotland, Diane Halligan (founded, had founded) The Weird and Wonderful Plant Company because she (was, is) disappointed with the plant selection at her local garden centers.
7. Halligan (chose, is choosing) to open an extraordinary plant store because she (wanted, is wanting) to provide a source of unusual plants for others as well as herself.
8. Marty Harper in Staunton, Virginia, like Halligan in Scotland, (contends, are contending) that his company (fills, would have filled) a niche for himself and others.
9. Harper, after much study on the subject of strange plants, (is indicating, indicates) that Madagascar holds the record for the most weird plants on the planet.
10. Isolated from the rest of the world, Madagascar (has provided, will have provided) a haven for unusual plants to develop undisturbed.
11. *Rafflesia arnoldii* (is, are) the oddest plant Harper (has encountered, will have encountered).
12. Harper, in an interview with *National Geographic*'s John Roach, (reveals, is revealing) that *Rafflesia arnoldii*, a parasitic plant, (has, have) the world's largest bloom, stinks, and (held, holds) in its center six or seven quarts of water.
13. According to Harper, procreation (remains, has remained) the primary reason for the development of the ostensibly outlandish shapes, sizes, odors, and actions of these unusual plants the world over.

14. Douglas Justice, another weird-plant aficionado like Halligan and Harper, (says, is saying) he (wonders, is wondering) what (motivates, motivated) people to choose the odd plants.
15. Harper, however, (exclaims, is exclaiming), "Such plants (make, were making) me smile." ●

29K How do I use tense sequences accurately?

Verb **tense sequences** deliver messages about actions, occurrences, or states that occur at different times. Quick Box 29.10 shows how tenses in the same sentence can vary depending on the timing of actions (or occurrences or states).

Quick Box 29.10

Tense sequences

If your independent clause contains a simple-present-tense verb, then in your dependent clause you can

- use PRESENT TENSE to show same-time action:
  - I **avoid** shellfish because I **am** allergic to it.
- use PAST TENSE to show earlier action:
  - I **am** sure that I **deposited** the check.
- use the PRESENT PERFECT TENSE to show (1) a period of time extending from some point in the past to the present or (2) an indefinite past time:
  - They **claim** that they **have visited** the planet Venus.
  - I **believe** that I **have seen** that movie before.
- use the FUTURE TENSE for action to come:
  - The book **is** open because I **will be reading** it later.

If your independent clause contains a past-tense verb, then in your dependent clause you can

- use the past tense to show another completed past action:
  - I **closed** the door when you **told** me to.
- use the PAST PERFECT TENSE to show earlier action:
  - The sprinter **knew** that she **had broken** the record.
- use the present tense to state a general truth:
  - Christopher Columbus **determined** that the world **is** round.

continued >>

Quick Box 29.10 (continued)

If your independent clause contains a present-perfect-tense or past-perfect-tense verb, then in your dependent clause you can

- use the past tense:
  - The bread **has become** moldy since I **purchased** it.
  - Sugar prices **had** fallen before artificial sweeteners first appeared.

If your independent clause contains a future-tense verb, then in your dependent clause you can

- use the present tense to show action happening at the same time:
  - You **will be** rich if you **win** the prize.
- use the past tense to show earlier action:
  - You **will win** the prize if you **remembered** to mail the entry form.

TENSE SEQUENCES

- use the present perfect tense to show future action earlier than the action of the independent-clause verb:
  - The river **will flood** again next year unless we **have built** a better dam by then.

If your independent clause contains a future-perfect-tense verb, then in your dependent clause you can

- use either the present tense or the present perfect tense:
  - Dr. Chu **will have delivered** five thousand babies before she **retires**.
  - Dr. Chu **will have delivered** five thousand babies before she **has retired**.

Alert: Never use a future-tense verb in a dependent clause when the verb in the independent clause is in the future tense. Instead, use a present-tense verb or present-perfect-tense verb in the dependent clause.

NO The river **will flood** us unless we **will prepare** our defense.

YES The river **will flood** us unless we **prepare** our defense.

YES The river **will flood** us unless we **have prepared** our defense. ●

Tense sequences may include INFINITIVES and PARTICIPLES. To name or describe an activity or occurrence coming either at the same time as the time expressed in the MAIN VERB or after, use the **present infinitive.**

- I **hope to buy** a used car.

  To buy comes in the future. *Hope* is the main verb, and its action is now.

- **I hoped to buy** a used car.

  Hoped is the main verb, and its action is over.

- **I had hoped to buy** a used car.

  Had hoped is the main verb, and its action is over.

The PRESENT PARTICIPLE can show action happening at the same time.

- **Driving** his new car, the man **smiled**.

  The driving and the smiling happened at the same time.

To describe an action that occurs before the action in the main verb, use the perfect infinitive (*to have gone, to have smiled*), the PAST PARTICIPLE, or the present perfect participle (*having gone, having smiled*).

- Candida **claimed to have written** fifty short stories in college.

  Claimed is the main verb, and *to have written* happened first.

- **Pleased** with the short story, Candida **mailed** it to several magazines.

  Mailed is the main verb, and *pleased* happened first.

- **Having sold** one short story, Candida **invested** in a new computer.

  Invested is the main verb, and *having sold* happened first.

● **EXERCISE 29-7** Underline the correct verb in each pair of parentheses that best suits the sequence of tenses. Be ready to explain your choices. For help, consult 29K.

EXAMPLE

When he (is, was) seven years old, Yo-Yo Ma, possibly the world's greatest living cellist, (moves, moved) to the United States with his family.

1. Yo-Yo Ma, who (had been born, was born) in France to Chinese parents, (lived, lives) in Boston, Massachusetts, today and (toured, tours) as one of the world's greatest cellists.
2. Years from now, after Mr. Ma has given his last concert, music lovers still (treasure, will treasure) his many fine recordings.
3. Mr. Ma's older sister, Dr. Yeou-Cheng Ma, was nearly the person with the concert career. She had been training to become a concert violinist when her brother's musical genius (began, had begun) to be noticed.
4. Even though Dr. Ma eventually (becomes, became) a physician, she still (had been playing, plays) the violin.
5. The family interest in music (continues, was continuing), for Mr. Ma's children (take, had taken) piano lessons.

6. Although most people today (knew, know) Mr. Ma as a brilliant cellist, he (was making, has made) films as well.
7. One year, while he (had been traveling, was traveling) in the Kalahari Desert, he (films, filmed) dances of southern Africa's Bush people.
8. Mr. Ma first (becomes, became) interested in the Kalahari people when he (had studied, studied) anthropology as an undergraduate at Harvard University.
9. When he shows visitors around Boston now, Mr. Ma has been known to point out the Harvard University library where, he claims, he (fell asleep, was falling asleep) in the stacks when he (had been, was) a student.
10. Indicating another building, Mr. Ma admits that in one of its classrooms he almost (failed, had failed) German.●

MOOD

29L What is "mood" in verbs?

Mood in verbs conveys an attitude toward the action. English has three moods: *indicative, imperative*, and *subjunctive*. Use the **indicative mood** to make statements about real things, about highly likely things, and for questions about fact.

INDICATIVE The door to the tutoring center opened. [real]
She seemed to be looking for someone. [highly likely]
Do you want to see a tutor? [question about a fact]

The **imperative mood** expresses commands and direct requests. Often, the subject is omitted in an imperative sentence but is nevertheless implied to be either *you* or one of the indefinite pronouns such as *anybody, somebody*, or *everybody*.

Alert: Use an exclamation point after a strong command; use a period after a mild command or a request (see 41A, 41E).●

IMPERATIVE Please shut the door.
Watch out! That screw is loose.

The **subjunctive mood** expresses speculation, other unreal conditions, conjectures, wishes, recommendations, indirect requests, and demands. Often, the words that signal the subjunctive mood are *if, as if, as though*, and *unless*.

SUBJUNCTIVE If I **were** you, I would ask for a tutor.
He requested that he **be** given a leave of absence.

29M What are subjunctive forms?

For the **present subjunctive**, always use the SIMPLE FORM of the verb for all PERSONS and NUMBERS.

- The prosecutor asks that she **testify** [not *testifies*] again.
- It is important that they **be** [not *are*] allowed to testify.

For the **past subjunctive**, use the simple past tense: *I wish that I **had** a car*. The one exception is for the past subjunctive of *be:* Use *were* for all forms.

- I wish that I **were** [not *was*] leaving on vacation today.
- They asked if she **were** [not *was*] leaving on vacation today.

USING THE SUBJUNCTIVE IN *IF, AS IF, AS THOUGH,* AND *UNLESS* CLAUSES

In dependent clauses introduced by *if, as if, as though*, and *unless*, the subjunctive describes speculations, conditions contrary to fact or highly unlikely.

- If it **were** [not *was*] to rain, attendance at the race would be disappointing.
  The subjunctive *were* indicates speculation.
- The runner looked as if he **were** [not *was*] winded, but he said he wasn't.
  The subjunctive *were* indicates a condition contrary to fact.
- Unless rain **were** [not *was*] to create floods, the race will be held this Sunday.
  Floods are highly unlikely.

Not every clause introduced by *if, unless, as if,* or *as though* requires the subjunctive. Use the subjunctive only when the dependent clause describes speculation or a condition contrary to fact.

INDICATIVE If she **is** going to leave late, I **will** drive her to the race.
Her leaving late is highly likely.

SUBJUNCTIVE If she **were** going to leave late, I **would** drive her.
Her leaving late is a speculation.

USING THE SUBJUNCTIVE IN *THAT* CLAUSES

The subjunctive conveys wishes, requests, demands, or recommendations in *that* clauses.

- I wish that this race **were** [not *was*] over.
- He wishes that he **had seen** [not *saw*] the race.
- The judges demand that the doctor **examine** [not *examines*] the runners.

Also, MODAL AUXILIARY VERBS *would, could, might,* and *should* can convey speculations and conditions contrary to fact.

- If the runner **were** [not *was*] faster, we **would** see a better race.

The issue here is that when an INDEPENDENT CLAUSE expresses a conditional statement using a modal auxiliary verb, you want to be sure that in the DEPENDENT CLAUSE you don't use another modal auxiliary verb.

NO If I **would have trained** for the race, I **might have** won.

YES If I **had trained** for the race, I **might have** won.

● **EXERCISE 29-8** Fill in each blank with the correct form of the verb given in parentheses. For help, consult 29L and 29M.

EXAMPLE

Imagining the possibility of brain transplants requires that we (to be) be open-minded.

(1) If almost any organ other than the brain (to be) ____________ the candidate for a swap, we would probably give our consent. (2) If the brain (to be) ____________ to hold whatever impulses form our personalities, few people would want to risk a transplant. (3) Many popular movies have asked that we (to suspend) ____________ disbelief and imagine the consequences should a personality actually (to be) ____________ transferred to another body. (4) In real life, however, the complexities of a successful brain transplant require that not-yet-developed surgical techniques (to be) ____________ used. (5) For example, it would be essential that during the actual transplant each one of the 500 trillion nerve connections within the brain (to continue) ____________ to function as though the brain (to be) ____________ lying undisturbed in a living human body. ●

VOICE

29N What is "voice" in verbs?

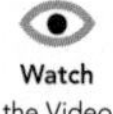
Watch the Video

Voice in a verb tells whether a subject acts or is acted on. A subject with an **active voice** verb performs the action.

- Most clams **live** in saltwater.
- They **burrow** into the sandy bottoms of shallow waters.

A subject with a **passive voice** verb receives the action indicated by the verb. Verbs in the passive voice use forms of *be, have,* and *will* as AUXILIARY VERBS with the PAST PARTICIPLE of the MAIN VERB.

- Clams **are considered** a delicacy by many people.
- Some types of clams **are** highly **valued** by seashell collectors.

29O How do I write in the active, not passive, voice?

Because the ACTIVE VOICE emphasizes the doer of an action, active constructions are more concise and dramatic (see 40C). Most sentences in the PASSIVE VOICE can be converted to active voice.

PASSIVE African tribal masks are often imitated by Western sculptors.

ACTIVE Western sculptors often imitate African tribal masks.

29P What are proper uses of the passive voice?

While the active voice is often better, sometimes you need to use the passive voice.

When the doer of an action is unknown or unimportant, writers use the passive voice.

- The lock **was broken** sometime after four o'clock.
- In 1899, the year I was born, a peace conference **was held** at The Hague.

—E. B. White, "Unity"

If you want to focus on events in a narrative, use the passive voice. Conversely, if you want to emphasize the people making the discoveries, use the active voice.

ACTIVE Joseph Priestley **discovered** oxygen in 1774.

PASSIVE Oxygen **was discovered** in 1774 by Joseph Priestley.

ACTIVE The postal clerk **sent** the unsigned letter before I **could retrieve** it from the mailroom.

The emphasis is on the doers of the action, *the postal clerk* and *I*, rather than on the events, *sent* and *could retrieve.*

PASSIVE The unsigned letter **was sent** before it **could be retrieved** from the postal clerk.

The emphasis is on the events, *was sent* and *could be retrieved*, not on the doers of the action.

EXERCISE 29-9 First, determine which sentences are in the active voice and which the passive voice. Second, rewrite each sentence in the other voice, and then decide which voice better suits the meaning. Be ready to explain your choice.

EXAMPLE

When Alfred Nobel wrote his last will in 1895, he created the Nobel Prizes. (*active; change to passive*)

The Nobel Prizes were created by Alfred Nobel, when he wrote his last will in 1895.

1. An enormous fortune was earned by Nobel when he invented dynamite in the 1860s. (*passive; change to active*)
2. An avid inventor, Nobel held over 300 patents. (*active; change to passive*)
3. *Nemesis*, a four-act play, was written by Nobel shortly before his death.
4. Beginning in 1901, the Nobel Prizes have honored people who work in physics, literature, chemistry, and world peace. (*active; change to passive*)
5. The list of categories for the Nobel Prize does not include mathematics. (*active; change to passive*) ●

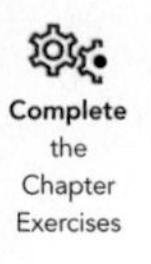
Complete the Chapter Exercises

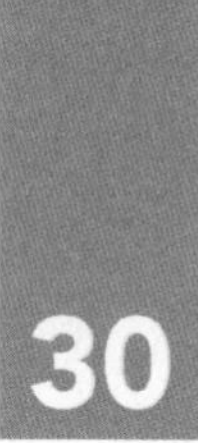

30 Pronouns: Case and Reference

Quick Points You will learn to

- Use the proper pronoun case (see 30A–30K).
- Use pronouns with clear reference (see 30L–30S).

PRONOUN CASE

30A What does "case" mean?

Watch the Video

Case shows the relationship (subject, object, possession) of nouns and pronouns to other words in a sentence. Pronouns use different forms in different cases (**subjective**, **objective**, **possessive**). Nouns change form only in the possessive case. (For use of the apostrophe in the possessive, see Chapter 45.)

30B What are personal pronouns?

Personal pronouns refer to persons or things. Quick Box 30.1 shows the case forms of personal pronouns in both the singular and the plural.

Quick Box 30.1

Case forms of personal pronouns

	Subjective	Objective	Possessive
SINGULAR	I, you, he, she, it	me, you, him, her, it	my, mine, your, yours, his, her, hers, its
PLURAL	we, you, they	us, you, them	our, ours, your, yours, their, theirs

Many difficult questions about pronoun case concern *who/whom* and *whoever/whomever*. For a discussion of how to choose between them, see 30G.

30C How do pronouns work in case?

In the subjective case, pronouns function as SUBJECTS.

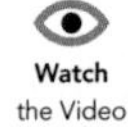

- **He** proposed!
- **He** and **I** wanted an inexpensive wedding.
- **We** googled several wedding performers.
- John and **I** found an affordable one-woman band.

  I is part of the compound subject *John and I*.

In the objective case, pronouns function as OBJECTS.

- We saw **her** perform in a city park.
- She noticed John and **me** immediately.
- We showed **her** our budget.
- She enjoyed auditioning for **him** and **me**.

  Him and me is the compound object of the preposition *for*.

In the possessive case, nouns and pronouns usually indicate ownership or imply a relationship.

- The **musician's contract** was very fair.

  The possessive noun *musician's* implies a type of ownership.

- **Her contract** was very fair.

  The possessive pronoun *her* implies a type of ownership.

- The **musicians' problems** stem from playing cheap instruments.

  The possessive noun *musicians'* implies a type of relationship.

- **Their problems** stem from playing with cheap instruments.

  The possessive pronoun *their* implies a type of relationship.

Sometimes, however, the notion of "ownership" is stretched in possessive constructions. In such cases, use either the possessive with an apostrophe, or use an "of the" phrase.

- The **musician's arrival** was eagerly anticipated.
- The **arrival of the musician** was eagerly anticipated.
- The **musician's performance** was thrilling.
- The **performance of the musician** was thrilling.

Alert: Never use an apostrophe in personal pronouns: *ours, yours, its, his, hers, theirs* (45C). ●

30D Which case is correct when *and* connects pronouns?

When *and* connects pronouns, or nouns and pronouns, the result is a compound construction. Compounding, which means "putting parts together in a whole," has no effect on case. Always use pronouns in the subjective case when they serve as the subjects of a sentence; also, always use pronouns in the objective case when they serve as objects in a sentence. Never mix cases.

COMPOUND PRONOUN SUBJECT	**He and I** saw the solar eclipse.
COMPOUND PRONOUN OBJECT	That eclipse astonished **him and me**.

When you're unsure of the case of a pronoun, use the "Troyka test for case" in Quick Box 30.2. In this four-step test, you drop some of the words from your sentence so that you can tell which case sounds correct.

When pronouns are in a PREPOSITIONAL PHRASE, they are always in the objective case. (That is, a pronoun is always the OBJECT of the preposition.) This rule holds whether the pronouns are singular or plural.

NO Ms. Lester gave an assignment ***to*** **Sam and I**.

YES Ms. Lester gave an assignment ***to*** **Sam and me**.

Be especially careful when pronouns follow the preposition *between*.

NO The dispute is ***between*** **Thomas and I**.

The prepositional phrase, which starts with the preposition *between*, cannot use the subjective-case pronoun *I*.

YES The dispute is ***between*** **Thomas and me**.

The prepositional phrase, which starts with the preposition *between*, calls for the objective-case pronoun *me*.

Quick Box 30.2

Listen to the Podcast

Troyka test for case

SUBJECTIVE CASE

STEP 1: Write the sentence twice, once using the subjective case, and once using the objective case.

STEP 2: Cross out enough words to isolate the element you are questioning.

~~Janet and~~ **me** learned about the moon.

~~Janet and~~ **I** learned about the moon.

STEP 3: Omit the crossed-out words and read each sentence aloud to determine which one sounds right.

NO **Me** learned about the moon.

YES **I** learned about the moon.

STEP 4: Select the correct version, and restore the words you crossed out.

Janet and I learned about the moon.

OBJECTIVE CASE

STEP 1: Write the sentence twice, once using the subjective case, and once using the objective case.

STEP 2: Cross out enough words to isolate the element you are questioning.

The astronomer taught ~~Janet and~~ **I** about the moon.

The astronomer taught ~~Janet and~~ **me** about the moon.

STEP 3: Omit the crossed-out words and read each sentence aloud to determine which one sounds right.

NO The astronomer taught **I** about the moon.

YES The astronomer taught **me** about the moon.

STEP 4: Select the correct version, and restore the words you crossed out.

The astronomer taught **Janet and me** about the moon.

● **EXERCISE 30-1** Underline the correct pronoun of each pair in parentheses of each pair in parentheses. For help, consult 30C and 30D.

EXAMPLE

Bill and (I, me) noticed two young swimmers being pulled out to sea.

(1) The two teenagers caught in the rip current waved and hollered at Bill and (I, me). (2) The harder (they, them) both swam toward shore, the further away the undercurrent pulled them from the beach. (3) The yellow banners had warned Bill and (I, me) that a dangerous rip current ran beneath the water. (4) I yelled at Bill, "Between you and (I, me), (we, us) have to save them!" (5) (He and I, Him and me) both ran and dove into the crashing waves. (6) As former lifeguards, Bill and (I, me) knew what to do. (7) (We, Us) two remembered that the rule for surviving a rip current is to swim across the current. (8) Only when swimmers are safely away from the current should (they, them) swim toward shore. (9) I reached the teenage girl, who cried, "My boyfriend and (I, me) are drowning." (10) Bill rescued the frightened teenage boy, and when they were safely on shore, the boy looked at (he and I, him and me) and gasped, "Thanks. The two of (we, us) know you saved our lives." ●

30E How do I match cases with appositives?

Match an APPOSITIVE to the same case as the word or words it renames. Whenever you're unsure about case, use the "Troyka test for case" in Quick Box 30.2 to get your answer.

- **We** [not *Us*] tennis players practice hard.

  The subjective pronoun *we* renames the subject *tennis players*.

- The winners **she and I** [not *her and me*] advanced to the finals.

  The subjective pronouns *she and I* rename the subject *winners*.

- The coach trains **us** [not *we*] tennis players to practice hard.

  The objective pronoun *us* renames the object *tennis players*.

- The crowd cheered the winners, **her and me** [not *she and I*].

  The objective pronouns *her and me* rename the object *winners*.

30F How does case work after linking verbs?

A pronoun that follows a LINKING VERB either renames the SUBJECT or shows possession. When the pronoun following the linking verb renames, use the subjective case. When the pronoun shows possession, use the possessive case. If you're unsure, use the "Troyka test for case" in Quick Box 30.2.

- The contest winner was **she**.
- The contest winners were **she** and **I**.
- The prize is **hers**.
- The prize is **ours**.

EXERCISE 30-2 Underline the correct pronoun of each pair in parentheses.

EXAMPLE

Last summer, my dad and (I, me) decided to take a road trip across the United States, something (we, us) have wanted to do since I was young.

1. Since (we, us) lived in California, (we, us) decided that a cross-country trip to New York City would be the most fun for (we, us).
2. (We, Us), my father and (I, me), collected road maps and learned that (we, us) would be taking even-numbered highways since they usually travel east/west.
3. My cousins live in Arizona, so (we, us) stayed with (they, them), and (they, them) showed us the Grand Canyon.
4. I think the Grand Canyon was more fun for (we, us) because (they, them) had seen it many times before.
5. After a conversation between (me, I) and my dad, (us, we) decided that we would like to see the St. Louis Arch next.
6. The famous Gateway Arch is interesting to (him and me, he and I) because it was designed by Finnish-American architect Eero Saarinen, and my father and (me, I) have relatives in Finland.
7. The next adventure for (we, us) travelers was driving through the Great Smoky Mountains in Tennessee.
8. My father and (me, I) learned that the mountains are called "smoky" because (they, them) are often covered in a natural fog that makes (they, them) look smoky.
9. Our next stop was in Washington, DC, where my brother and his family live. It was nice for (we, us) brothers to have some time to visit because (we, us) had not seen each other in a long time.
10. My father and (me, I) then drove the rest of the way to New York City. We flipped a coin to see who would get to drive the car when we arrived in the city. The winner was (me, I).

30G When should I use *who, whoever, whom,* and *whomever?*

Listen to the Podcast

Who and *whoever* are in the SUBJECTIVE CASE and function as subjects. *Whom* and *whomever* are in the OBJECTIVE CASE and function as objects.

Whenever you're unsure of whether to use *who* or *whoever* or to use *whom* or *whomever*, apply the "Troyka test for case" in Quick Box 30.2. If you see *who* or *whoever*, test by temporarily substituting *he, she*, or *they*. If you see *whom* or *whomever*, test by temporarily substituting *him, her*, or *them*.

- **Who/Whom** is coming to your party?
  He/She is coming to your party, so *who* is correct.

- Will you let **whoever/whomever** into the house?
  You will let *him/her* into the house, so *whomever* is correct.

In sentences with more than one clause, isolate the clause with the pronoun (shown in **boldface**), and apply the test.

- Give the package to **whoever/whomever is at the door**.
  He is at the door, so *whoever* is correct.

- Invite those guests **who/whom you can trust**.
  You believe you can trust *them*, so *whom is* correct.

- I will invite **whoever/whomever I wish to come**.
  I wish *them* to come, so *whomever* is correct.

- I will invite **whoever/whomever pleases me**.
  He pleases me so *whoever* is correct.

- I will not invite strangers **who/whom show up at the house**.
  They show up at the house, so *who* is correct.

- Don't tweet people **who/whom I did not invite**.
  I did not invite *them*, so *whom* is correct.

- If uninvited guests arrive, I will tell the police **who/whom they are**.
  They are *they* (not *them*), so *who* is correct.

Remember that *who* and *whoever* can function only as subjects or subject complements in clauses. If the person(s) you refer to perform some action or are linked to a subject, *who/whoever* is correct.

EXERCISE 30-3 Underline the correct pronoun of each pair in parentheses. For help, consult 30G.

EXAMPLE

Women (<u>who</u>, whom) both hold jobs outside the home and are mothers serve a "double shift."

(1) Women (who, whom) raise families do as much work at home as at their jobs. (2) In North American society, it is still mainly women (who, whom) cook dinner, clean the house, check the children's homework, read to them, and put them to bed. (3) Nevertheless, self-esteem runs high, some researchers have found, in many women on (who, whom) families depend for both wage earning and child rearing. (4) Compared with women (who, whom) pursue careers but have no children, those (who, whom) handle a double shift experience less anxiety and depression, according to the research. (5) Perhaps the reason for this finding is that those for (who, whom) the extra paycheck helps pay the bills feel pride and accomplishment when they rise to the challenge. (6) However, other studies note that women (who, whom) have both jobs and children experience tremendous stress. (7) Those (who, whom) feel unable both to support and to nurture their children despite their maximum efforts are the women for (who, whom) the dual responsibility is an almost unbearable burden. ●

30H What pronoun case comes after *than* or *as*?

When *than* or *as* is part of a sentence of comparison, the sentence sometimes doesn't include words to complete the comparison outright. Rather, by omitting certain words, the sentence implies the comparison. For example, *My two-month-old Saint Bernard is larger* ***than*** *most full-grown dogs [are]* doesn't need the final word *are.*

When a pronoun follows *than* or *as*, the meaning of the sentence depends entirely on whether the pronoun is in the subjective case or the objective case. Here are two sentences that convey two very different messages, depending on whether the subjective case (*I*) or the objective case (*me*) is used.

1. My sister loved that dog more ***than*** **I**.
2. My sister loved that dog more ***than*** **me**.

In sentence 1, because *I* is in the subjective case, the sentence means *My sister loved that dog more than* ***I*** *[loved it].* In sentence 2, because *me* is in the objective case, the sentence means *My sister loved that dog more than [she loved]* ***me.*** In both situations, you can check whether you're using the correct case by supplying the implied words to see if they make sense.

30I How do pronouns work before infinitives?

Most INFINITIVES consist of the SIMPLE FORMS of verbs that follow *to:* for example, *to laugh, to sing, to jump, to dance.* (A few exceptions occur when the *to* is optional: *My aunt helped the elderly man [to] cross the street;* and when the *to* is awkward: *My aunt watched the elderly man [to] get on the bus.*) For both the SUBJECTS of infinitives and the OBJECTS of infinitives, use the objective case.

- Our tennis coach expects **me** ***to serve***.
- Our tennis coach expects **him** ***to beat*** **me**.
- Our tennis coach expects **us** ***to beat*** **them**.

30J How do pronouns work with *-ing* words?

When a verb's *-ing* form functions as a NOUN, it's called a GERUND: *Brisk **walking** is excellent exercise.* When a noun or PRONOUN comes before a gerund, the POSSESSIVE CASE is required: ***His** brisk **walking** built up his stamina.* In contrast, when a verb's *-ing* form functions as a MODIFIER, it requires the subjective case for the pronoun, not the possessive case: ***He**, **walking** briskly, caught up to me.*

Here are two sentences that convey different messages, depending entirely on whether a possessive comes before the *-ing* word.

1. The detective noticed the **man** ***staggering***.
2. The detective noticed the **man's** ***staggering***.

Sentence 1 means that the detective noticed the *man;* sentence 2 means that the detective noticed the *staggering*. The same distinction applies to pronouns: When *the man* is replaced by *him* or *the man's* by *his*, the meaning is the same as in sentences 1 and 2.

1. The detective noticed **him** ***staggering***.
2. The detective noticed **his** ***staggering***.

Use these distinctions in ACADEMIC WRITING even if you don't in speech.

EXERCISE 30-4 Underline the correct pronoun of each pair in parentheses. For help, consult 30H through 30J.

EXAMPLE

Ricky Jay holds the world's record for card throwing; no one can throw a playing card faster than (he/him).

(1) Many magicians agree that no one is better at sleight-of-hand magic than (he/him). (2) Younger magicians often say that Ricky Jay influenced (their/them) to become professional performers. (3) In addition to (him/his) being a respected sleight-of-hand artist, Jay is also a scholar and historian. (4) His interest in strange performers led (him/he) to write *Learned Pigs and Fireproof Women*, which discusses unusual acts and begins with (him/his) explaining their appeal to audiences. (5) Jay's acting career has involved (his/him) performing in several different movies

and TV shows. (6) In the James Bond film *Tomorrow Never Dies*, few could have played a villain as well as (he/him). (7) Other roles include (him/his) narrating the introduction to the movie *Magnolia*. (8) Overall, few performers have had such as varied and interesting career as (him/he). ●

30K What case should I use for *-self* pronouns?

Two types of pronouns end in *-self:* reflexive pronouns and intensive pronouns.

A **reflexive pronoun** is used as an object that refers to the same person or thing as the subject.

- The **detective** disguised ***himself***.

  The reflexive pronoun *himself* refers to the subject *detective*.

- **We** purchased his disguise **ourselves**.

  The reflexive pronoun *ourselves* refers to the subject *we*.

Never use a reflexive pronoun to replace a personal pronoun in the subjective case even if you believe it sounds "lofty."

NO My teammates and **myself** will vote for a team captain.

YES My teammates and **I** will vote for a team captain.

NO That decision is up to my teammates and **myself**.

YES That decision is up to my teammates and **me**.

Intensive pronouns are used to emphasize preceding nouns or pronouns.

- The detective felt that **his career *itself*** was at risk.

  Itself emphasizes the previous noun *career*.

- He phoned his **attorney *himself***.

  Himself emphasizes the previous noun *he*.

PRONOUN REFERENCE

30L What is pronoun reference?

The word or group of words that a pronoun refers to is called its **antecedent**. To be clear to your readers, be sure your pronouns refer clearly to their antecedents.

> I knew a **woman**, lovely in **her** bones / When small **birds** sighed, **she** would sigh back at **them**.
>
> —Theodore Roethke, "I Knew a Woman"

30M What makes pronoun reference clear?

Pronoun reference is clear when your readers know immediately to whom or what each pronoun refers. Quick Box 30.3 lists guidelines for using pronouns clearly, and the section in parentheses is where each is explained.

Quick Box 30.3

Guidelines for clear pronoun reference

- Place pronouns close to their ANTECEDENTS (30N).
- Make a pronoun refer to a specific antecedent (30N).
- Do not overuse *it* (30Q).
- Reserve *you* only for DIRECT ADDRESS (30R).
- Use *that, which,* and *who* correctly (30S).

30N How can I avoid unclear pronoun reference?

Watch the Video

Every pronoun needs to refer to a specific, nearby ANTECEDENT. If the same pronoun in your writing has to refer to more than one antecedent, replace some pronouns with their antecedents.

NO In 1911, **Roald Amundsen** reached the South Pole just thirty-five days before **Robert F. Scott** arrived. **He** [who? Amundsen or Scott?] had told people that **he** [who? Amundsen or Scott?] was going to sail for the Arctic, but **he** [who? Amundsen or Scott?] was concealing **his** [whose? Amundsen's or Scott's?] plan. Soon, **he** [who? Amundsen or Scott?] turned south for the Antarctic.

YES In 1911, **Roald Amundsen** reached the South Pole just thirty-five days before **Robert F. Scott** arrived. **Amundsen** had told people that **he** was going to sail for the Arctic, but **he** was concealing **his** plan. Soon, **Amundsen** turned south for the Antarctic.

Alert: Be careful with the VERBS *said* and *told* in sentences that contain pronoun reference. To maintain clarity, use quotation marks and slightly reword each sentence to make the meaning clear.

NO **Her** mother told **her she** was going to visit **her** grandmother.

YES **Her** mother told **her**, "**You** are going to visit your grandmother."

YES **Her** mother told **her**, "**I** am going to visit your grandmother."

Further, if too much material comes between a pronoun and its antecedent, readers can lose track of the meaning.

- Alfred Wegener, a German meteorologist and professor of geophysics at the University of Graz in Austria, was the first to suggest that all the continents on earth were originally part of one large landmass. According to this theory, the supercontinent broke up long ago and the fragments drifted apart. Wegener He named this supercontinent Pangaea.

  Wegener, the antecedent of *he*, may be too distant for some readers. Remember to keep your pronouns and their antecedents close.

When you start a new paragraph, be cautious about beginning it with a pronoun whose antecedent is in a prior paragraph. You're better off repeating the word.

ESOL Tip: Many languages omit pronoun subjects because the verb contains subject information. In English, use the pronoun as a subject. For example, never omit *it* in the following: *Political science is an important academic subject.* ***It*** *is studied all over the world.*

EXERCISE 30-5 Revise so that each pronoun refers clearly to its antecedent. Either replace pronouns with nouns or restructure the material to clarify pronoun reference. For help, consult 30N.

EXAMPLE

People who return to work after years away from the corporate world often discover that business practices have changed. They may find fiercer competition in the workplace, but they may also discover that they are more flexible than before.

Here is one possible revision: *People who return to work after years away from the corporate world often discover that business practices have changed. Those people may find fiercer competition in the workplace, but they may also discover that business practices are more flexible than before.*

Most companies used to frown on employees who became involved in office romances. They often considered them to be using company time for their own enjoyment. Now, however, managers realize that happy employees are productive employees. With more women than ever before in the workforce and with people working longer hours, they have begun to see that male and female employees want and need to socialize. They are also dropping their opposition to having married couples on the payroll. They no longer automatically believe that they will bring family matters into the workplace or stick up for each other at the company's expense.

One departmental manager had doubts when a systems analyst for research named Laura announced that she had become engaged to Peter, who worked as a technician in the same department. She told her that either one or the other might have to transfer out of the research department. After listening to her plea that they be allowed to work together on a trial basis, the manager reconsidered. She decided to give Laura and Peter a chance to prove that their relationship would not affect their work. The decision paid off. They demonstrated that they could work as an effective research team, right through their engagement and subsequent marriage. Two years later, when Laura was promoted to assistant manager for product development and after he asked to move also, she enthusiastically recommended that Peter follow Laura to her new department. ●

30O How do pronouns work with *it, that, this,* and *which?*

Watch the Video

When you use *it, that, this,* and *which,* be sure that your readers can easily and unmistakably understand each word refers to.

NO Comets usually fly by the earth at 100,000 mph, whereas asteroids sometimes collide with the earth. **This** interests scientists.

Does *this* refer to the speed of the comets, to comets flying by the earth, or to asteroids colliding with the earth?

YES Comets usually fly by the earth at 100,000 mph, whereas asteroids sometimes collide with the earth. **This difference** interests scientists.

Adding a noun after *this* or *that* clarifies the meaning.

NO I told my friends that I was going to major in geology, **which** made my parents happy.

Does *which* refer to telling your friends or to majoring in geology?

YES My parents were happy **because I discussed my major with my friends**.

YES My parents were happy **because I chose to major in geology**.

Also, the title of any piece of writing stands alone. Therefore, in your first paragraph, never refer to your title with *this* or *that.* For example, if an essay's title is "Geophysics as a Major," the following holds for the first sentence:

NO **This subject** unites the sciences of physics, biology, and paleontology.

YES **Geophysics** unites the sciences of physics, biology, and paleontology.

30P How do I use *they* and *it* precisely?

The expression *they say* forces your readers to infer precisely who is saying. Your credibility as a writer depends on your mentioning a source precisely.

NO **They say** that earthquakes are becoming more frequent.

They doesn't identify the authority who made the statement.

YES **Seismologists** say that earthquakes are becoming more frequent.

The expressions *it said* and *it is said that* reflect imprecise thinking. Also, they're wordy. Revising such expressions improves your writing.

NO **It said** in the newspaper that California has minor earthquakes almost daily.

YES **The newspaper reported** that California has minor earthquakes almost daily.

30Q How do I use *it* to suit the situation?

The word *it* has three different uses in English. Here are examples of correct uses of *it*.

1. PERSONAL PRONOUN: Ryan wants to visit the 18-inch Schmidt telescope, but **it** is on Mount Palomar.
2. EXPLETIVE (sometimes called a *subject filler*, it delays the subject): **It** is interesting to observe the stars.
3. IDIOMATIC EXPRESSION (words that depart from normal use, such as using *it* as the sentence subject when writing about weather, time, distance, and environmental conditions): **It** is sunny. **It** is midnight. **It** is not far to the hotel. **It** is very hilly.

All three uses listed above are correct, but avoid combining them in the same sentence. The result can be an unclear and confusing sentence.

NO Because our car was overheating, **it** came as no surprise that **it** broke down just as **it** began to rain.

It is overused here, even though all three uses—2, 1, and 3 on the preceding list, respectively—are acceptable.

YES **It** came as no surprise that our overheating car broke down just as the rain began.

ESOL Tip: In some languages, *it* is not an expletive. In English, it is.

NO Is a lovely day.

YES **It** is a lovely day.

30R When should I use *you* for direct address?

Reserve *you* for **direct address**, writing that addresses the reader directly. For example, we use *you* in this handbook to address you, the student. *You* is not a suitable substitute for specific words that refer to people, situations, or occurrences.

NO Prison uprisings often happen **when you allow** overcrowding.
The reader, *you*, did not allow the overcrowding.

YES Prison uprisings often happen **when prisons are** overcrowded.

NO In Russia, **you** often have to stand in long lines to buy groceries.
Do *you*, the reader, plan to do your grocery shopping in Russia?

YES **Russian shoppers** often stand in long lines to buy groceries.

EXERCISE 30-6 Revise these sentences so that all pronoun references are clear. If a sentence is correct, circle its number. For help, consult 30O through 30R.

EXAMPLE

They say that reaching the summit of Mount Everest is easiest in the month of May.

Experienced climbers say that reaching the summit of Mount Everest is easiest in the month of May. [Revision eliminates imprecise use of *they*, see section 30P.]

1. Climbing Mount Everest is more expensive than you realize.
2. In addition to training, they need to raise as much as $60,000 for the expedition.
3. By contacting the Nepalese embassy in Washington, DC, you can secure the help of Sherpa guides.
4. The government of Nepal requires permits, copies of passports, and letters of recommendation for each climbing team.
5. Climbers will need to pack oxygen bottles, a first aid kit, medications, a satellite phone, walkie-talkies, and a laptop computer. This will ensure a climber's safety.
6. Climbers often use yaks because they are stronger than you and can carry more equipment.

7. They do not offer direct flights, so climbers from America usually need a couple of days to get to Katmandu, Nepal.
8. Once atop the mountain, you should prepare for the descent, which is just as dangerous as the ascent. ●

30S When should I use *that, which,* and *who?*

To use the pronouns *that* and *which* correctly, you want to check the context of the sentence you're writing. *Which* and *that* refer to animals and things. Only sometimes do they refer to anonymous or collective groups of people. Quick Box 30.4 shows how to choose between *that* and *which*. For information about the role of commas with *that* and *which*, see 42F.

Who refers to people and to animals mentioned by name.

- **John Polanyi, who** was awarded the Nobel Prize in Chemistry, speaks passionately in favor of nuclear disarmament.
- **Lassie, who** was known for her intelligence and courage, was actually played by a series of male collies.

Quick Box 30.4

Choosing between *that* and *which*

Choice: Some instructors and style guides use either *that* or *which* to introduce a **restrictive clause** (a DEPENDENT CLAUSE that is essential to the meaning of the sentence). Others may advise you to use only *that* so that your writing distinguishes clearly between restrictive and **nonrestrictive clauses**. Whichever style you use, be consistent in each piece of writing:

- The zoos ***that*** (or ***which***) **most children like** display newborn and baby animals.

  The words *most children like* are essential for delivering the meaning that children prefer zoos with certain features and make up a restrictive clause.

No choice: You are required to use *which* to introduce a nonrestrictive clause (a dependent clause that isn't essential to the meaning of the sentence or part of the sentence).

- Zoos, **which most children like**, attract more visitors if they display newborn and baby animals.

  The words *most children like* are not essential to the meaning of the sentence and make up a nonrestrictive clause.

Many professional writers reserve *which* for nonrestrictive clauses and *that* for restrictive clauses. Other writers use *that* and *which* interchangeably for restrictive clauses. For ACADEMIC WRITING, your instructor might expect you to maintain the distinction.

Alert: Use commas before and after a nonrestrictive clause. Don't use commas before and after a restrictive clause; see 42K.4. ●

● **EXERCISE 30-7** Fill in the blanks with *that, which,* or *who*. For help, consult 30S.

EXAMPLE

Antigua, which is an island in the West Indies, is a popular destination for European and American tourists.

1. Those ____________ like to travel to Antigua may enjoy online gambling, ____________ is legal on the island.
2. The sport ____________ is most popular in Antigua is cricket.
3. Celebrities ____________ own homes on the island include Oprah Winfrey, Eric Clapton, and Jamaica Kincaid.
4. The main airport, ____________ is named after Prime Minister V. C. Bird, is located in the capital, St. John's.
5. The cruise ships ____________ travel to Antigua often stop at St. John's, ____________ became the seat of government in 1981. ●

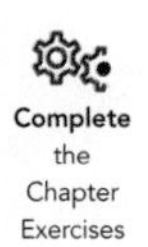
Complete the Chapter Exercises

31 Agreement

Quick Points You will learn to

- ➤ Match subjects and verbs in person and number (see 31A–31N).
- ➤ Match pronouns to the nouns to which they refer (see 31O–31T).

31A What is agreement?

Grammatical **agreement** links related grammatical forms. Specifically, you need to match subjects and verbs (see 31B through 31N) and pronouns and antecedents (see 31O through 31T).

SUBJECT–VERB AGREEMENT

31B What is subject–verb agreement?

Subject–verb agreement matches a SUBJECT to its VERB match in NUMBER (singular or plural) and PERSON (first, second, or third person). Quick Box 31.1 presents these major concepts in grammatical agreement.

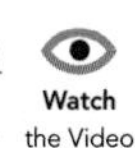

- The **firefly glows**.

  Firefly, a singular subject in the third person, matches *glows*, a singular verb in the third person.

- **Fireflies glow**.

  Fireflies, a plural subject in the third person, matches *glow*, a plural verb in the third person.

Quick Box 31.1

Grammatical agreement: first, second and third person

- **Number** refers to *singular* (one) and *plural* (more than one).
- The **first person** is the speaker or writer. *I* (singular) and *we* (plural) are the only subjects that occur in the first person.

  SINGULAR **I see** a field of fireflies.

  PLURAL **We see** a field of fireflies.

- The **second person** is the person spoken or written to. *You* (for both singular and plural) is the only subject that occurs in the second person.

  SINGULAR **You see** a shower of sparks.

  PLURAL **You see** a shower of sparks.

- The **third person** is the person or thing being spoken or written about. *He, she, it* (singular) and *they* (plural) are the third-person subject forms. Most rules for subject–verb agreement involve the third person.

  SINGULAR The **scientist sees** a cloud of cosmic dust.

  PLURAL The **scientists see** a cloud of cosmic dust.

31C Why is a final -s or -es in a subject or verb so important?

SUBJECT–VERB AGREEMENT often involves a final *s* (*or es* for words that end in *-s*). For verbs in the present tense, you form the SIMPLE FORM of third-person singular by adding *-s* or *-es: laugh, laughs; kiss, kis**ses***. Major exceptions are the verbs *be* (*is*), *have* (*has*), and *do* (*does*) (see 38C).

- That **student agrees** that **young teenagers watch** too much television.
- Those **young teenagers are** taking valuable time away from studying.
- That **student has** a part-time job for ten hours a week.
- Still, that **student does** well in college.

To make a subject plural, you add *-s* or *-es* to its end: *lip, lips; guess, gues**ses***. Exceptions include most pronouns (*they, it*) and a few nouns that for singular and plural either don't change (*deer, deer*) or change internally (*mouse, mice*). Quick Box 31.2 shows you the basic pattern for agreement using *-s* or *-es*.

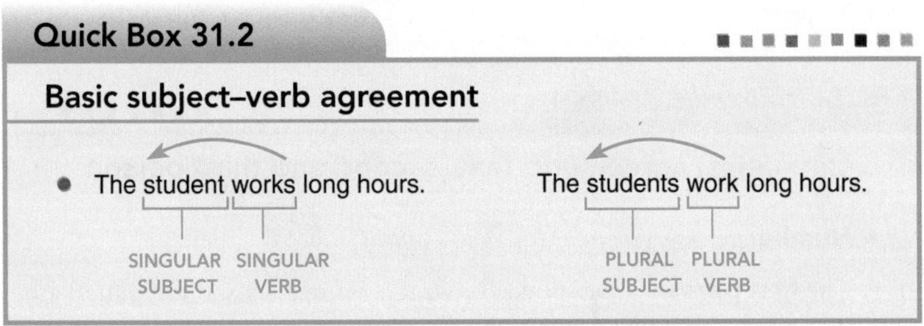

Alert: When you use an AUXILIARY VERB with a main verb, never add *-s* or *-es* to the main verb: *The coach **can walk*** [not *can walks*] *to campus. The coach **does like*** [not *does likes*] *his job.*

EXERCISE 31-1 Use the subject and verb in each set to write two complete sentences—one with a singular subject and one with a plural subject. Keep all verbs in the present tense. For help, consult 31C.

EXAMPLE

bird, sing

SINGULAR SUBJECT: When a *bird sings*, you will know spring is here.

PLURAL SUBJECT: When *birds sing*, you will know spring is here.

1. chair, rock
2. leaf, fall
3. river, flow
4. clock, tick
5. singer, sing
6. girl, laugh
7. hand, grab
8. loaf, rise ●

31D Can I ignore words between a subject and its verb?

You can ignore all words between a subject and its verb. Focus strictly on the subject and its verb. Quick Box 31.3 shows you this pattern.

NO **Winners** of the state contest **goes** to the national finals.

Winners is the subject; the verb must agree with it. Ignore the words *of the state contest.*

YES **Winners** of the state contest **go** to the national finals.

The subject *one of the . . .* requires a singular verb to agree with *one.* Ignore the plural noun that comes after *of the.* (For information on the phrase *one of the . . . who,* see 31L.)

NO **One** of the problems **are** the funds needed for travel expenses.

YES **One** of the problems **is** the funds needed for travel expenses.

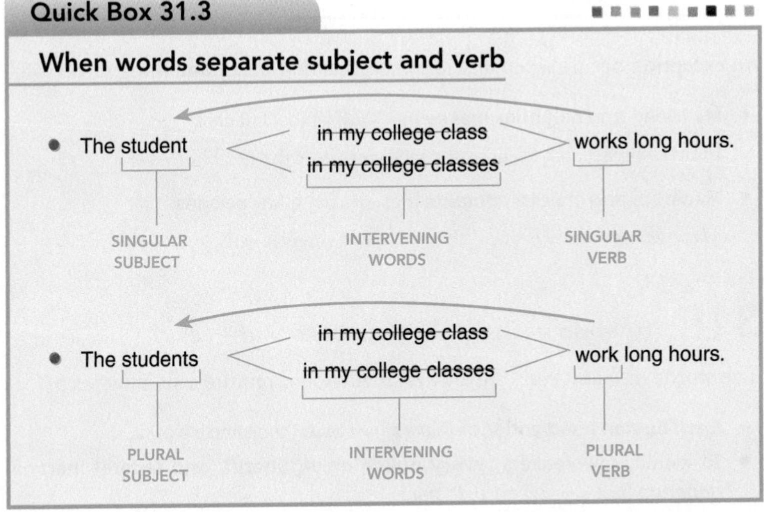

Similarly, eliminate all word groups between the subject and the verb, starting with *including, together with, along with, accompanied by, in addition to, except*, and *as well as*.

NO The **moon**, *as well as* the planet Venus, **are** visible in the night sky.
Moon is the subject. The verb must agree only with it.

YES The **moon**, as well as the planet Venus, **is** visible in the night sky.

31E How do verbs work when subjects are connected by *and*?

Use a plural verb with a COMPOUND SUBJECT joined by *and*. Quick Box 31.4 shows you this pattern. (For related material on PRONOUNS and ANTECEDENTS, see 31P.)

- **The Cascade Diner *and* Joe's Diner *have*** [not *has*] salmon today.
  These are two different diners.

Quick Box 31.4

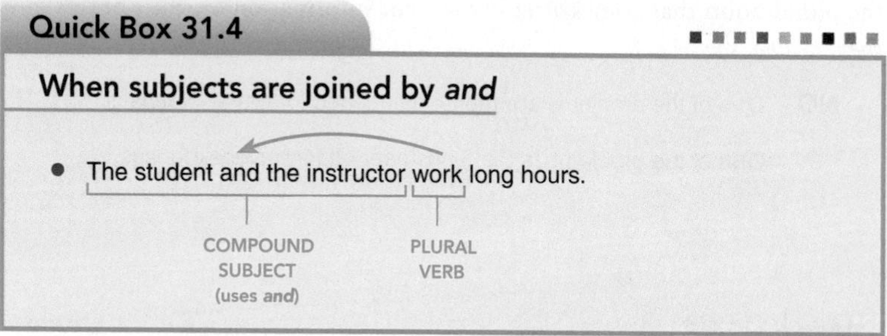

When subjects are joined by *and*
• The student and the instructor work long hours.
COMPOUND SUBJECT (uses *and*)
PLURAL VERB

An exception occurs when *and* joins subjects that mean one thing or person.

- **My friend *and* neighbor *makes*** [not *make*] excellent chili.
  In this sentence, the friend is the same person as the neighbor.
- **Macaroni *and* cheese *contains*** [not *contain*] many calories.
  Macaroni and cheese is one dish so it takes a singular verb.

31F How do verbs work with *each* and *every*?

The words *each* and *every* are always singular and require a singular verb.

- ***Each* human hand and foot *makes*** [not *make*] a distinctive print.
- To identify lawbreakers, ***every* police chief, sheriff, and federal marshal *depends*** [not *depend*] on such prints.

Alert: Don't use *each* or *every* at the same time: ***Each*** [not *Each and every*] *robber has been caught.* (For more information about pronoun agreement for *each* and *every*, see 31I, 31P, and 31R.) ●

31G How do verbs work when subjects are connected by *or*?

When SUBJECTS are joined by *or*—or by the sets *either . . . or, neither . . . nor, not only . . . but (also)*—the verb agrees only with its closest subject. Quick Box 31.5 shows this pattern with *either . . . or*. (For related material on pronouns and antecedents, see 31Q.)

- ***Neither*** ~~spiders~~ ***nor*** **flies upset** *me.*
- ***Not only*** ~~spiders~~ ***but also*** ~~all other~~ **arachnids have** four pairs of legs.
- ~~A meal of six clam fritters, two blue crabs,~~ ***or*** ~~a steamed~~ **lobster sounds** good.

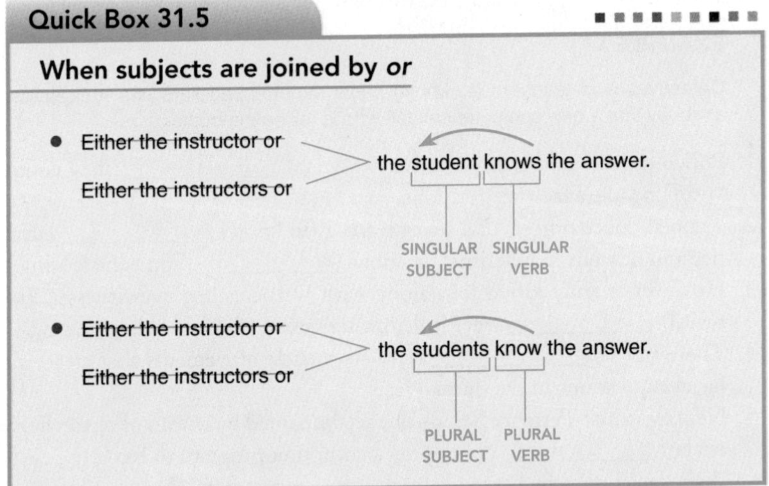

Quick Box 31.5
When subjects are joined by *or*
Either the instructor or
Either the instructors or
the student knows the answer.
SINGULAR SUBJECT
SINGULAR VERB
Either the instructor or
Either the instructors or
the students know the answer.
PLURAL SUBJECT
PLURAL VERB

31H How do verbs work with inverted word order?

In English sentences, the SUBJECT normally comes before its VERB: *Astronomy is interesting.* **Inverted word order** reverses the typical subject-verb pattern by putting the verb first. Most questions use inverted word order: *Is astronomy interesting?* In inverted word order, find the subject first and then check whether its verb agrees with it.

- Into deep space **shoot** probing **satellites.**

  The plural verb *shoot* agrees with the inverted plural subject *satellites.*

- On the television screen **is** an **image** of Saturn.

  The singular verb *is* agrees with the inverted singular subject *image.*

Alert: When *there* precedes the verb, see whether the subject is singular or plural, and then choose the form of *be* to agree with the subject. If *it* precedes the verb, use the singular form of *be* (*is, was*) whether the subject is singular or plural. ●

- **There *are*** nine **planets** in our solar system.
- **There *is*** probably no **life** on eight of them.
- **It *is*** astronomers who explore this theory daily.

  The verb *is* agrees with *it*, not with *astronomers.*

● **EXERCISE 31-2** Supply the correct present-tense form of the verb in parentheses. For help, consult 31C through 31H.

EXAMPLE

Detectives and teachers (to know) know experienced liars can fool almost anybody, but a new computer can tell who is telling the truth.

1. Police officers and teachers often (to wish) ____________ they could "read" people's facial expressions.
2. Trained police officers or a smart teacher (to know) ____________ facial tics and nervous mannerisms (to show) ____________ someone is lying.
3. However, a truly gifted liar, along with well-coached eyewitnesses, (to reveal) ____________ very little through expressions or behavior.
4. There (to be) ____________ forty-six muscle movements that create all facial expressions in the human face.
5. Neuroscientist Terrence Seinowski, accompanied by a team of researchers, (to be) ____________ developing a computer program to recognize even slight facial movements made by the most expert liars. ●

31I How do verbs work with indefinite pronouns?

Listen to the Podcast

Indefinite pronouns usually refer to nonspecific persons, things, quantities, or ideas. While most indefinite pronouns are singular, some are always plural, and a few can be singular *or* plural. Quick Box 31.6 lists indefinite pronouns according to what verb form they require. (For related material on pronouns and antecedents, see 31O–31R.)

Quick Box 31.6

Common indefinite pronouns

ALWAYS PLURAL

both	many

ALWAYS SINGULAR

another	every	no one
anybody	everybody	nothing
anyone	everyone	one
anything	everything	somebody
each	neither	someone
either	nobody	something

SINGULAR OR PLURAL, DEPENDING ON CONTEXT

all	more	none
any	most	Some

SINGULAR INDEFINITE PRONOUNS

- **Everything** about that intersection **is** dangerous.
- But whenever **anyone says** anything, **nothing is** done.
- **Each** of us **has** [not *have*] to shovel snow; **each is** [not *are*] expected to help.
- **Every** snowstorm of the past two years **has** [not *have*] been severe.
- **Every** one of them **has** [not *have*] caused massive traffic jams.

SINGULAR OR PLURAL INDEFINITE PRONOUNS (DEPENDING ON MEANING)

- **Some** of our streams **are** polluted.

  Some refers to the plural noun *streams*, so the plural verb *are* is correct.
- **Some** pollution **is** reversible, but **all** of it **threatens** the environment.

  Some and *all* refer to the singular noun *pollution*, so the singular verbs *is* and *threatens* are correct.
- **All** that environmentalists ask **is** to give nature a chance.

  All here means "the only thing," so the singular verb *is* is correct.
- Winter has driven the birds south; **all have** left.

  All refers to the plural noun *birds*, so the plural verb *have* is correct.

! Alerts: (1) Use *this, that, these,* and *those* to agree with *kind* and *type. This* and *that* are singular, as are *kind* and *type; these* and *those* are plural, as are *kinds* and *types:* **This** [not *These*] **kind** of rainwear is waterproof. **These** [not *This*] **kinds** of sweaters keep me warm. (2) Rules for indefinite pronouns can conflict with methods of avoiding SEXIST LANGUAGE. For suggestions, see 31S. ●

31J How do verbs work with collective nouns?

Listen to the Podcast

A **collective noun** names a group of people or things: *family, audience, class, number, committee, team, group,* and the like. When the group acts as one unit, use a singular verb. When members of the group act individually, use a plural verb.

- The senior **class** nervously ***awaits*** final exams.

  The *class* is acting as a single unit, so the verb is singular.

- The senior **class** ***were fitted*** for their graduation robes today

  The class members were fitted as individuals, so the verb is plural.

31K Does a linking verb agree with the subject complement?

Although a LINKING VERB joins a SUBJECT to its SUBJECT COMPLEMENT, the linking verb agrees with the subject, not with the subject complement.

NO The worst **part** of owning a car ***are*** the bills.

The subject is the singular *part,* so the plural verb *are* is wrong.

YES The worst **part** of owning a car ***is*** the bills.

The singular subject *part* agrees with the singular verb *is.*

31L What verbs agree with *who, which,* and *that*?

If the ANTECEDENT of *who, which,* or *that* is singular, use a singular verb. If the antecedent is plural, use a plural verb.

- The scientist will share the prize with the **researchers *who* work** with her.

  Who refers to *researchers,* so the plural verb *work* is used.

- George Jones is the **student *who* works** in the science lab.

  Who refers to *student,* so the singular verb *works* is used.

The phrases *one of the* and *the only one of the* immediately before *who, which*, or *that* require different verbs. *Who, which*, or *that* refers to the plural NOUN immediately following *one of the*, so the verb must be plural. Although *the only one of* is also followed by a plural word, *who, which*, or *that* must be singular to agree with the singular *one*.

- Tracy is ***one of the*** students ***who* talk** in class.

  Who refers to *students*, a plural antecedent, so the verb *talk* is plural.

- Jim is ***the only one of the*** students ***who* talks** in class.

  Who refers to *one*, a singular antecedent, so the verb *talks* is singular.

● **EXERCISE 31-3** Supply the correct present-tense form of the verb in parentheses.

EXAMPLE

Anyone who goes to the theme park Dollywood (to know) knows that it is located in Tennessee.

1. Each of the park's guests (to enjoy) thrill rides, music, and dinner theaters.
2. The cast of the Showtreet Palace Theater (to perform) shows for tourists.
3. Kidsfest is one of the festivals that (to attract) visitors each year.
4. For some people, the best reason for visiting Dollywood (to be) the rides.
5. All of the rides (to run) all day long, and no one (to seem) to mind waiting in line to ride them. ●

31M How do verbs work with amounts, fields of study, and other special nouns?

AMOUNTS

SUBJECTS that refer to time, sums of money, distance, or measurement are singular. They take singular verbs.

- **Two hours *is*** not enough time to finish. [time]
- **Three hundred dollars *is*** what we must pay. [sum of money]
- **Two miles *is*** a short sprint for some serious joggers. [distance]
- **Three-quarters of an inch *is*** needed for a perfect fit. [measurement]

FIELDS OF STUDY

The name for a field of study is singular even if it appears to be plural: *economics, mathematics, physics*, and *statistics*.

- ***Statistics* is** required of science majors.

  Statistics is a course of study, so the singular verb *is* is correct.

- ***Statistics* show** that a teacher shortage is coming.

  Statistics means *projections* here, so the plural verb *show* is correct.

SPECIAL NOUNS

Athletics, news, ethics, and *measles* are singular despite their plural appearance. Also, *United States of America* is singular: However, *politics* and *sports* take singular or plural verbs, depending on the meaning of the sentence.

- The ***news* gets** better each day.

  News is a singular noun, so the singular verb *gets* is correct.

- ***Sports* is** a good way to build physical stamina.

  Sports is one general activity, so the singular verb *is* is correct.

- Three ***sports* are** offered at the recreation center.

  Sports are separate activities, so the plural verb *are* is correct.

Jeans, pants, scissors, clippers, tweezers, eyeglasses, thanks, and *riches* are some words that require a plural verb, even though they refer to one thing. However, if you use *pair* with *jeans, pants, scissors, clippers, tweezers,* or *eyeglasses,* use a singular verb for agreement.

- These ***slacks* need** pressing.
- This ***pair*** of slacks **needs** pressing.

  Series and *means* can be singular or plural, according to their meaning.

- Two new TV ***series* are** big hits.

  Series refers to two individual items, so the plural verb *are* is correct.

- A ***series*** of disasters **is** plaguing our production.

  Series refers to a single group of disasters, so the singular verb *is* is correct.

31N How do verbs work with titles, company names, and words as themselves?

TITLES

A title itself refers to one work or entity, so a singular verb is correct.

- ***Breathing Lessons*** by Anne Tyler **is** a prize-winning novel.

COMPANY NAMES

A company should be treated as a singular unit, requiring a singular verb.

- ***Cohn Brothers* boxes** and **delivers** fine art.

WORDS AS THEMSELVES

Whenever you write about words as themselves to call attention to those words, use a singular verb, even if more than one word is involved.

- ***We* implies** that everyone is included.
- ***Protective reaction strikes* was** a euphemism for *bombing.*

EXERCISE 31-4 Supply the correct present-tense form of the verb in parentheses. For help, consult 31I through 31N.

EXAMPLE

The movie *Wordplay* is about those who (to enjoy) enjoy solving crossword puzzles.

1. When the movie plays at theaters, the audience often (to consist) ____________ of different ages and types of people.
2. For fans of crossword puzzles, the major attraction (to be) ____________ the challenges they present.
3. Every creator of puzzles (to know) ____________ that in the most successful puzzles all of the clues (to be) ____________ interesting.
4. *Setters* (to be) ____________ is a term used by crossword puzzle fans to describe someone who creates puzzles.
5. These fans, which (to include) ____________ celebrities like Jon Stewart, consider the Sunday puzzle in the *New York Times* one of the most difficult.

EXERCISE 31-5 This exercise covers all of subject-verb agreement (see 31B through 31N). Supply the correct form of the verb in parentheses.

EXAMPLE

Recent research suggests that high levels of social status (to bring) bring high levels of stress.

1. Most people (to believe) ____________ that poor people obviously suffer considerably more from stress than do very wealthy people.
2. They understand that meeting basic needs like food and shelter (to generate) ____________ huge amounts of stress.
3. A steady income and a large saving account clearly (to reduce) ________ stress levels and (to have) ______ mental and physical health benefits.
4. However, these benefits (to be) __________ true only to a certain point.
5. Research by sociologist Scott Schieman shows that people at the highest levels of society actually (to have) ______ high levels of stress.
6. There (to be) ______ many possible reasons for this effect.

7. One reason (to suggest) ________ that success makes people who are driven to succeed work even harder, creating a vicious cycle for them.
8. Another reason, which (to view) _______ an apparent perk of high status as an actual disadvantage, (to say) _____ that having authority over others (to result) _______ in people continually getting involved in conflict.
9. Statistics (to show) ______ that young professionals who (to be) _____ used to technological interruptions in demanding work settings may deal with stress better than older ones.
10. Even if it brings high stress, most of us (to prefer) _______ having high status over having low. ●

PRONOUN–ANTECEDENT AGREEMENT

31O What is pronoun–antecedent agreement?

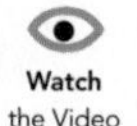

Pronoun–antecedent agreement means that a PRONOUN matches its ANTECEDENT in NUMBER (singular or plural) and PERSON (first, second, or third person). Quick Box 31.7 shows you how to visualize this pattern of grammatical agreement. You might also want to consult Quick Box 31.1 in 31B for explanations and examples of the concepts *number* and *person*.

- The **firefly** glows when **it** emerges from **its** nest at night.

  The singular pronouns *it* and *its* match their singular antecedent, *firefly*.
- **Fireflies** glow when **they** emerge from **their** nests at night.

  The plural pronouns *they* and *their* match their plural antecedent, *fireflies*.

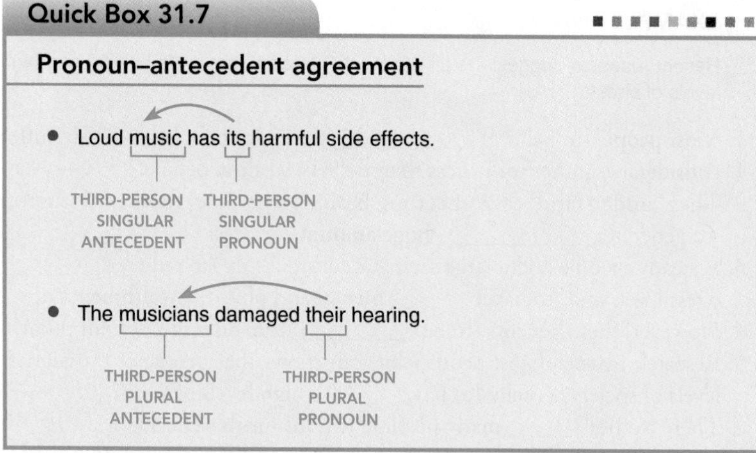

Quick Box 31.7
Pronoun–antecedent agreement
Loud music has its harmful side effects.
THIRD-PERSON SINGULAR ANTECEDENT
THIRD-PERSON SINGULAR PRONOUN
The musicians damaged their hearing.
THIRD-PERSON PLURAL ANTECEDENT
THIRD-PERSON PLURAL PRONOUN

31P How do pronouns work when *and* connects antecedents?

When *and* connects two or more ANTECEDENTS, they require a plural pronoun. This rule applies even if each separate antecedent is singular. (For related material on subjects and verbs, see 31E.)

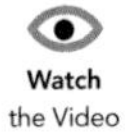

- The **Cascade Diner** *and* **Joe's Diner** have closed **their** doors.

  Two separate diners require a plural pronoun reference.

When *and* joins singular nouns that nevertheless refer to a single person or thing, use a singular pronoun.

- **My friend *and* neighbor** makes **his** [not *their*] excellent chili every Saturday.

  The friend is the same person as the neighbor, so the singular *his* (or *her*) is correct. If these were two separate persons, *their* would be correct.

EACH, EVERY

The words *each* and *every* are singular, even when they refer to two or more antecedents joined by *and*. The same rule applies when *each* or *every* is used alone (see 31I). (For related material on subjects and verbs, see 31F.)

- ***Each* human hand *and* foot** leaves **its** [not *their*] distinctive print.

The rule still applies when the construction *one of the* follows *each* or *every*.

- ***Each one of the* robbers** left **her** [not *their*] fingerprints at the scene.

31Q How do pronouns work when *or* connects antecedents?

When *or*, *nor*, or *but* join ANTECEDENTS, the pronoun agrees only with the nearest antecedent, whether singular or plural. Quick Box 31.8 (page 516) shows you this pattern. (For related material on subjects and verbs, see 31G.)

- When a diner closes, either local mice or **the owner's cat** gets **itself** a meal.
- When a diner closes, either the owner's cat or **local mice** get **themselves** a meal.

31R How do pronouns work when antecedents are indefinite pronouns?

INDEFINITE PRONOUNS usually refer to nonspecific persons, things, quantities, or ideas. But in a sentence, context clarifies an indefinite pronoun's meaning, even if the pronoun has no specific antecedent. Most indefinite pronouns are

Quick Box 31.8

When antecedents are joined by *or*

- Either the loudspeakers or the microphone needs its electric cord repaired.

  SINGULAR ANTECEDENT — SINGULAR PRONOUN

- Either the microphone or the loudspeakers needs their electric cords repaired.

  PLURAL ANTECEDENT — PLURAL PRONOUN

singular. Two indefinite pronouns, *both* and *many*, are plural. A few indefinite pronouns can be singular or plural, depending on the meaning of the sentence.

For a list of indefinite pronouns, see Quick Box 31.6 in 31I. For more information about avoiding sexist language, especially with indefinite pronouns, see 31S. (For related material on subjects and verbs, see 31I.)

SINGULAR INDEFINITE PRONOUNS

- **Everyone** hopes to get **his or her** [not *their*] degree within a year.
- **Anybody** wanting to wear a cap and gown at graduation must have **his or her** [not *their*] measurements taken.
- **Each** of the students handed in **his or her** [not *their*] final term paper.

Alert: The use of *their* as a singular indefinite pronoun is becoming more common, even in many respectable publications. Although this usage may become standard in the future, we recommend that you avoid it.

SINGULAR *OR* PLURAL INDEFINITE PRONOUNS

- When winter break arrives for students, **most** leave **their** dormitories.

  Most refers to *students*, so the plural pronoun *their* is correct.

- As for the luggage, **most** is already on **its** way to the airport.

  Most refers to *luggage*, so the singular pronoun *its* is correct.

- **None** thinks that **he or she** will miss graduation.

  None is singular here, so the singular pronoun phrase *he or she* is correct.

- **None** of the students has paid **his or her** [not *their*] graduation fee yet.

  None is singular here, so the singular pronoun phrase *his or her* is correct.

- **None** are so proud as **they** who graduate.

  None is plural here, so the plural pronoun *they* is correct.

31S How do I use nonsexist pronouns?

A word is **nonsexist** when it carries neither male nor female gender. Each PRONOUN in English carries one of three genders: male (*he, him, his*); female (*she, her, hers*); or neutral (*you, your, yours, we, our, ours, them, they, their, theirs, it, its*). Usage today favors nonsexist word choices. You therefore want to use gender-free pronouns whenever possible. Quick Box 31.9 shows three ways to avoid using masculine pronouns when referring to males and females together.

Questions often arise concerning the use of *he or she* and *his or her*. In general, writers find these gender-free pronoun constructions awkward. To avoid them, many writers make the antecedents plural. Doing this becomes problematic when the subject is a SINGULAR INDEFINITE PRONOUN (see Quick Box 31.6 in section 31I). In the popular press (such as newspapers and magazines), the use of the plural pronoun *they* or *them* with a singular antecedent has been gaining favor. In ACADEMIC WRITING, however, it is better for you not to follow the practice of the popular press. Language practice changes, however, so what we say here is our best advice as we write this book.

Quick Box 31.9

Avoiding the masculine pronoun when referring to males and females together

- **Solution 1:** Use a pair of pronouns—as in the phrase *he or she*. However, avoid using a pair more than once in a sentence or in many sentences in a row. A *he or she* construction acts as a singular pronoun.
  - **Everyone** hopes that **he or she** will win a scholarship.
  - A **doctor** usually has time to keep up to date only in **his or her** specialty.
- **Solution 2:** Revise into the plural.
  - **Many students** hope that **they** will win a scholarship.
  - **Most doctors** have time to keep up to date only in **their** specialties.
- **Solution 3:** Recast the sentence.
  - Everyone hopes to win a scholarship.
  - Few specialists have time for general reading.

31T How do pronouns work when antecedents are collective nouns?

A COLLECTIVE NOUN names a group of people or things, such as *family, group, audience, class, number, committee*, and *team*. When the group acts as one unit, use a singular pronoun to refer to it. When the group's members act individually, use a plural pronoun. If the sentence is awkward, substitute a plural noun for the collective noun. (For related material on subjects and verbs, see 31J.)

- The **audience** cheered as **it** stood to applaud the performers.

  The *audience* acted as one unit, so the singular pronoun *it* is correct.

- The **audience** put on **their** coats and walked out.

  The members of the audience acted as individuals, so all actions become plural; therefore, the plural pronoun *their* is correct.

- The **family** spends **its** vacation in Rockport, Maine.

  All the family members went to one place together.

If instead you wrote *The family spend their vacations in Maine, Hawaii, and Rome*, that might mean that each family member is going to a different place. You may prefer to revise that awkward sentence and use a plural noun phrase instead of a collective noun.

- The **family members** spend **their** vacations in Maine, Hawaii, and Rome.

● **EXERCISE 31-6** Underline the correct pronoun in parentheses. For help, consult 31O through 31T.

EXAMPLE

Many wonder where inventors like Benjamin Franklin get (his or her, <u>their</u>) creative energy.

1. Many so-called Founding Fathers are famous one or two of (his, his or her, their) accomplishments, but anyone who knows (his, her, his or her, their) history knows that Franklin is known for many things, including (his, her, his or her, their) inventions.
2. The armonica is not one of his well known inventions, but (its, their) design is ingenious.
3. Also called the glass harmonica, the armonica required a person to place (himself, herself, himself or herself) in front of the instrument and to rotate (its, their) glass bowls.
4. The lightning rod and the Franklin stove established his reputation as an inventor, but (it, they) remained in public domain because Franklin refused to secure patents for his inventions.

5. An inventor like Franklin does not limit (his, her, his or her, their) imagination to one field of science.
6. (He, She, He or she, They) can instead pursue many questions and the challenges (they, it) pose.
7. All scientists who study electricity should know that Ben Franklin provided the names (he, she, he or she, they) still use today for positive and negative electrons.
8. Franklin also named the Gulf Stream and mapped (their, its) current.
9. Franklin formed the first public lending library in America, which allowed people to borrow (its, their) books and read them at (his, her, his or her, their) leisure.
10. His public service record also includes the reform of the postal system and the establishment of The Academy and College of Philadelphia, which later merged (their, its) students with those of the State of Pennsylvania to become the University of Pennsylvania. ●

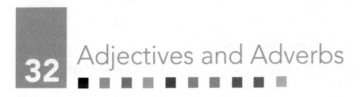

32 Adjectives and Adverbs

Quick Points You will learn to

- Distinguish between adjectives and adverbs (see 32A).
- Use adjectives and adverbs correctly (see 32B–32F).

32A What are the differences between adjectives and adverbs?

Although ADJECTIVES and ADVERBS both serve as modifiers—as words that describe other words—adjectives modify nouns and pronouns; adverbs modify verbs, adjectives, or other adverbs.

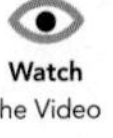

ADJECTIVE The **brisk** *wind* blew.

The adjective *brisk* modifies the noun *wind*.

ADVERB The wind *blew* **briskly**.

The adverb *briskly* modifies the verb *blew*.

Many adverbs simply add *-ly* to an adjective (*eat swiftly, eat frequently, eat loudly*); others do not (*eat fast, eat often, eat well*). Not all words with an *-ly* ending are adverbs; some adjectives also end in *-ly* (*friendly dog*).

ESOL Tips: (1) In English, the adjective is always singular, even if its noun is plural: *The* ***hot*** [not *hots*] *drinks warmed us up*. (2) Word order in English restricts the placement of adjectives and adverbs: *Thomas closed* [don't place the adverb *carefully* here] *the window* ***carefully*** (see 54B and 54C).

EXERCISE 32-1 Underline and label all adjectives (ADJ) and adverbs (ADV). Then, draw an arrow from each adjective and adverb to the word or words it modifies. Ignore *a, an,* and *the* as adjectives. For help, consult 32A.

EXAMPLE

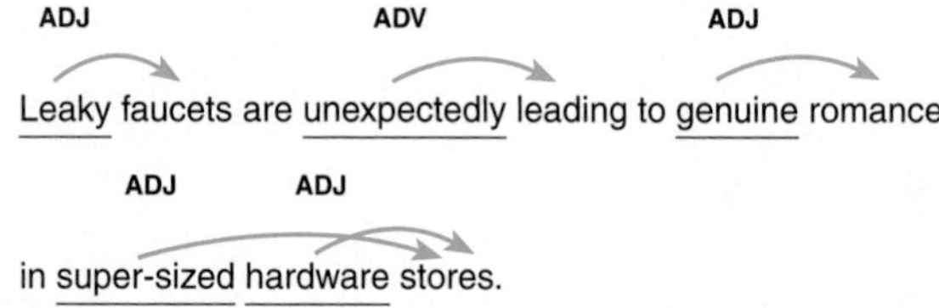

1. Today's singles carefully look for possible mates at discount home improvement stores across the country.
2. Understandably, many people find these stores a healthy alternative to dark bars and blind dates.
3. Recently, an employee in the flooring department quietly confided that the best nights for singles are Wednesdays and Thursdays, while weekends generally attract families.
4. A young single mom returns home excitedly because a quick trip to the lumber department for a new door resulted in a date for Saturday night.
5. A lonely widower in his fifties jokingly says he wishes he had developed earlier an interest in wallpapering and gardening.

32B When should I use adverbs—not adjectives—as modifiers?

Use only adverbs, not adjectives, to MODIFY verbs, adjectives, and other adverbs.

NO The candidate inspired us **great**.

Adjective *great* cannot modify verb *inspired*.

YES The candidate inspired us **greatly**.
Adverb *greatly* can modify verb *inspired*.

NO The candidate felt **unusual** energetic.
Adjective *unusual* cannot modify adjective *energetic*.

YES The candidate felt **unusually** energetic.
Adverb *unusually* can modify adjective *energetic*.

NO The candidate spoke **exceptional** forcefully.
Adjective *exceptional* cannot modify adverb *forcefully*.

YES The candidate spoke **exceptionally** forcefully.
Adverb *exceptionally* modifies adverb *forcefully*.

32C What is wrong with double negatives?

A **double negative** uses two negative MODIFIERS when only one is clearly needed. Negative modifiers include *no, never, not, none, nothing, hardly, scarcely*, and *barely*.

Watch the Video

NO The factory workers will **never** vote for **no** strike.

YES The factory workers will **never** vote for **a** strike.

NO The union members did **not** have **no** money in reserve.

YES The union members did **not** have **any** money in reserve.

YES The union members had **no** money in reserve.

All verbs ending in *-n't* (*isn't, didn't, hasn't*) are also negatives (see 27D). When you use *-n't* contractions in sentences, don't add a second negative.

NO He **didn't** hear **nothing**.

YES He **didn't** hear **anything**.

NO They **haven't** had **no** meetings.

YES They **haven't** had **any** meetings.

Likewise, be careful to use the word *nor* only with *neither*.

NO Stewart **didn't** eat dinner **nor** watch television last night.

YES Stewart **didn't** eat dinner **or** watch television last night.

YES Stewart **neither** ate dinner **nor** watched television last night.

32D Do adjectives or adverbs come after linking verbs?

LINKING VERBS connect a SUBJECT to a COMPLEMENT. Always use an adjective, not an adverb, as the complement.

- The *guests looked* **happy**.

  The verb *looked* links subject *guests* to the adjective *happy*.

The words *look, feel, smell, taste, sound*, and *grow* may be linking verbs or action verbs. Use an adjective complement after a linking verb.

- Zora *looks* **happy**.

  Looks functions as a linking verb, so the adjective *happy* is correct.

- Zora *looks* **happily** at the sunset.

  Looks doesn't function as a linking verb, so the adverb *happily* is correct.

BAD, BADLY

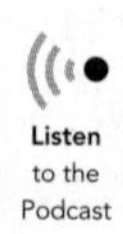
Listen to the Podcast

Be alert to accepted academic usage of the words *bad* (adjective) and *badly* (adverb) after linking verbs.

NO The students felt **badly**.

This means the students used their sense of touch badly.

YES The student felt **bad**.

This means the student had a bad feeling about something.

NO The food smelled **badly**.

This means the food had a bad ability to smell.

YES The food smelled **bad**.

This means the food had a bad smell to it.

GOOD, WELL

The word *well* is used as adjective to refer only to health. Otherwise, *well* is an adverb.

- Evander seems **well**.

  The adjective *well* describes how Evander's health seems to be.

- Evander writes **well**.

  The adverb *well* describes the verb *writes*.

Use *good* as an adjective, except when you refer to health.

NO She sings **good**.

The adjective *good* cannot describe the verb *sings*.

YES She sings **well**.

The adverb *well* describes the verb *sings*.

● **EXERCISE 32-2** Underline the correct uses of negatives, adjectives, and adverbs by selecting between the choices in parentheses.

EXAMPLE

The Concert for Bangladesh (famous, famously) occurred on August 1st, 1971, and included two (large, largely) shows performed (energetic, energetically) at Madison Square Garden.

1. The concert did a (good, well) job raising awareness of the refugees who were treated (bad, badly) during the Bangladesh Liberation War and who also suffered (great, greatly) from a massive cyclone that hit the area in 1970.
2. The (high, highly) anticipated concert included several (famous, famously) musicians, who played (good, well) for the audience.
3. Members of the audience didn't (ever, never) expect to see George Harrison, who had not performed since the Beatles broke up, but he looked (happily, happy) as he played some of his (great, greatly) songs.
4. Another (notable, notably) important appearance was that of Bob Dylan, who appeared (rare, rarely) in public in the early 1970s, but he neither disappointed (nor, or) frustrated the crowd when he took the stage.
5. Many people consider this (massively, massive) show to be one of the first benefit concerts that are now more (common, commonly), and its roster of rock stars (easy, easily) makes it an important event. ●

32E What are comparative and superlative forms?

Comparison refers to a change in the form of modifiers (adjectives and adverbs) to indicate degrees of quality or intensity. When you compare two people or things, use the **comparative** form. When you compare three or more, use the **superlative** form.

Listen to the Podcast

REGULAR FORMS OF COMPARISON

Most adjectives and adverbs show comparison in one of two ways: either by adding *-er* or *-est* endings or by adding the words *more, most, less*, and *least* (see Quick Box 32.1 on page 524). The number of syllables in the modifier often determines which form to use.

Quick Box 32.1

Regular forms of comparison for adjectives and adverbs

POSITIVE Use when nothing is being compared.

COMPARATIVE Use when two things are being compared. Add the ending *-er* or the word *more* or *less.*

SUPERLATIVE Use to compare three or more things. Add the ending *-est* or the word *most* or *least.*

Positive [1]	Comparative [2]	Superlative [3+]
green	greener	greenest
happy	happier	happiest
selfish	less selfish	least selfish
beautiful	more beautiful	most beautiful

- **One-syllable words** usually take *-er* and *-est* endings: *large, larger, largest* (adjectives); *far, farther, farthest* (adverbs).
- **Adjectives of two syllables** vary. If the word ends in *-y*, change the *y* to *i* and add *-er, -est* endings: *pretty, prettier, prettiest.* Otherwise, some two-syllable adjectives take *-er, -est* endings: *yellow, yellower, yellowest.* Others take *more, most* and *less, least: tangled, more tangled, most tangled; less tangled, least tangled.*
- **Adverbs of two syllables** use *more, most* and *less, least: quickly, more quickly, most quickly; less quickly, least quickly.*
- **Three-syllable words** use *more, most* and *less, least: exotic, more/most exotic, less/least exotic* (adjective); *busily, more/most busily, less/least busily* (adverb).

! **Alert:** Be careful not to use a double comparative or double superlative. Use either the *-er* and *-est* endings or *more, most* or *less, least.*

- He was **younger** [not *more younger*] than his brother.
- Her music was the **loudest** [not *most loudest*] on the stereo.

IRREGULAR FORMS OF COMPARISON

Quick Box 32.2 lists *irregular* modifiers. We suggest that you memorize these for easy recall.

Quick Box 32.2

Irregular forms of comparison for adjectives and adverbs

Positive [1]	Comparative [2]	Superlative [3+]
good (*adjective*)	better	best
well (*adjective* and *adverb*)	better	best
bad (*adjective*)	worse	worst
badly (*adverb*)	worse	worst
many	more	most
much	more	most
some	more	most
little*	less	least

*When you're using *little* for items that can be counted (e.g., pickles), use the regular forms *little, littler, littlest.*

Alerts: (1) *Less* and *fewer* aren't interchangeable. Use *less* with NONCOUNT NOUNS, either items or values: *The sugar substitute has less* ***aftertaste***. Use *fewer* with numbers or COUNT NOUNS: *The sugar substitute has fewer* ***calories***. (2) Don't use *more, most* or *less, least* with absolute adjectives, adjectives that indicate a noncomparable quality or state, such as *unique* or *perfect*. Something either *is*, or *is not*, one of a kind. Degrees of intensity don't apply: *This teapot is* ***unique*** [not *the most unique*]; *The artisanship is* ***perfect*** [not *the most perfect*]. ●

● **EXERCISE 32-3** Complete the chart that follows. Then, write a sentence for each word in the completed chart.

EXAMPLE

Tall, taller, tallest

The *tall* tree became *taller* over the years, but it was never the *tallest* in the forest.

Positive	Comparative	Superlative
______	bigger	______
slow	______	______
______	more comfortable	______
______	______	most attractive
lucky	______	______
______	______	happiest ●

32F Why avoid a long string of nouns as modifiers?

NOUNS sometimes MODIFY other nouns: *truck driver, train track, security system.* Usually, these combinations don't trouble readers. However, when you string together too many nouns in a row as modifiers, you challenge readers to distinguish the modifying nouns from the nouns being modified. You can revise such sentences in several ways.

REWRITE THE SENTENCE

NO The traffic accident vehicle description form instructions are clear.

YES The form for describing vehicles in traffic accidents has clear instructions.

CHANGE ONE NOUN TO A POSSESSIVE AND ANOTHER TO AN ADJECTIVE

NO He will take the **United States Navy examination** for **navy engineer training**.

YES He will take the *United States* ***Navy's*** *examination* for ***naval*** *engineer training.*

CHANGE ONE NOUN TO A PREPOSITIONAL PHRASE

NO Our **student adviser training program** has won many awards.

YES Our *training program* ***for student advisers*** has won many awards.

This revision requires a change from singular *adviser* to plural *advisers.*

● **EXERCISE 32-4** Underline the better choice in parentheses. For help, consult this entire chapter.

EXAMPLE

Alexis, a huge and powerful six-year-old Siberian tiger, (curious, curiously) explores her new zoo home together with five other tigers.

1. The new tiger home at the world-famous Bronx Zoo is a (special, specially) designed habitat, planted with (dense, denser) undergrowth so that it (close, closely) imitates the tigers' natural wilderness.
2. Like tigers in the wild, the six tigers in this habitat, which (more, many) experts consider the (more authentic, most authentic) of all artificial tiger environments in the world, will face some of the physical challenges and sensory experiences that keep them happy and (healthy, healthier).
3. Research shows that tigers feel (bad, badly) and fail to thrive in zoos without enrichment features placed in (good, well) locations to inspire tigers to stalk (stealthy, stealthily) through underbrush, loll (lazy, lazily) on heated rocks, or tug (vigorous, vigorously) on massive pull toys.

4. Wildlife zoologists think that the new Tiger Mountain exhibit will also serve zoo visitors (good, well) by allowing them to observe and admire the amazing strength, agility, and intelligence of a (rapid, rapidly) dwindling species.
5. Today, (fewer, less) than 5,000 Siberian tigers remain in the wild, which makes it imperative for zoos to raise people's awareness of the (great, greatest) need to prevent the extinction of these big cats that are considered among the (more, most) powerful, beautiful animals in the world. ●

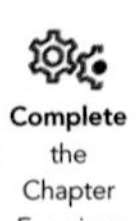
Complete the Chapter Exercises

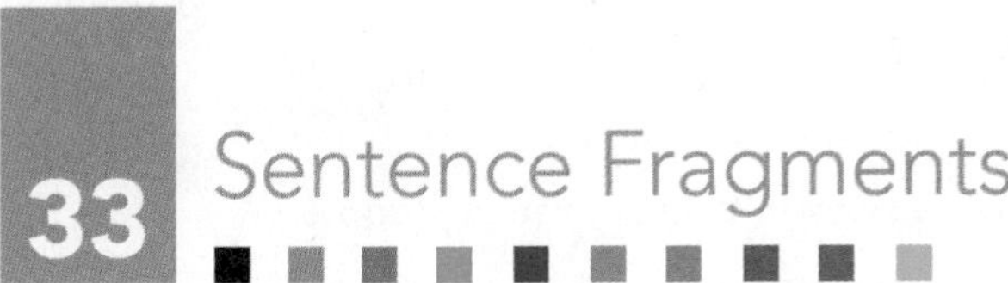

33 Sentence Fragments

Quick Points You will learn to

- Identify sentence fragments (see 33A–33B).
- Correct sentence fragments (see 33C–33G).
- Use intentional sentence fragments only when appropriate (see 33H).

33A What is a sentence fragment?

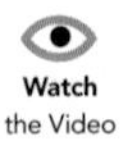
Watch the Video

A **sentence fragment** begins with a capital letter and ends with a period (or question mark or exclamation point), but it doesn't contain an INDEPENDENT CLAUSE. Fragments are merely unattached PHRASES or DEPENDENT CLAUSES.

FRAGMENT The rock star with many fans. [no verb]

CORRECT The rock star with many fans toured on a special bus.

FRAGMENT Traveled across the USA. [no subject]

CORRECT The rock star's bus traveled across the USA.

FRAGMENT Through the night. [a phrase without a verb or subject]

CORRECT The rock star's bus traveled through the night.

FRAGMENT Because the bus rolled along smoothly. [dependent clause starting with subordinating conjunction because]

CORRECT Because the bus rolled along smoothly, the rock star slept soundly.

FRAGMENT Which allowed him to wake up refreshed. [dependent clause starting with relative pronoun which]

CORRECT The rock star slept soundly on the bus, which allowed him to wake up refreshed.

To learn to recognize sentence fragments, see 33B; to learn several ways to correct sentence fragments, see 33C through 33F.

The time for correcting fragments is not during DRAFTING. Instead, if you suspect you've written a sentence fragment, simply underline or highlight it and move on. Then during REVISING or EDITING, you can easily find it to check and correct.

33B How can I recognize a sentence fragment?

Quick Box 33.1 shows you how to recognize a sentence fragment. Following this Quick Box, we show how to correct each type of sentence fragment in 33C, 33D, and 33E.

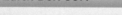

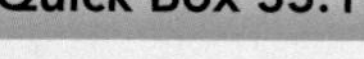

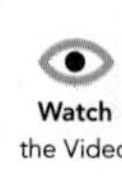

How to recognize four types of sentence fragments

1. If a word group starts with a SUBORDINATING CONJUNCTION, such as *when*, without being joined to a complete sentence, it's a sentence fragment (see 33C).

   FRAGMENT **When winter comes early.**

   CORRECT **When winter comes early,** ice often traps whales in the Arctic Ocean.

   CORRECT **Winter comes early.**

2. If a word group includes no VERB and ends with a period, it's a sentence fragment (see 33D).

   FRAGMENT **Whales in the Arctic Ocean.**

   CORRECT Whales **live** in the Arctic Ocean.

   Note that a VERBAL (the ones ending in *-ing* or *-ed*) is not a verb unless it teams up with an AUXILIARY VERB, such as *is* or *are* (see 33D). Verbals beginning with *to*, called INFINITIVES, remain as verbals. Auxiliary verbs have no effect on them.

continued >>

Quick Box 33.1 (continued)

FRAGMENT **Whales living in the Arctic Ocean.**

CORRECT Whales **are living** in the Arctic Ocean.

3. If a word group lacks a SUBJECT and ends with a period, it's a sentence fragment (see 33E).

FRAGMENT **Were trapped by the solid ice.**

CORRECT The whales **were trapped by the solid ice.**

4. If a word group is the second half of a COMPOUND PREDICATE and stands alone ending in a period, it's a sentence fragment. Compound predicates always start with one of the seven COORDINATING CONJUNCTIONS (*and, but, so, yet, for, or, nor;* see 33F).

FRAGMENT The whales panicked in the confines of the ice. **And thrashed about, bumping into each other.**

CORRECT The whales panicked in the confines of the ice **and thrashed about, bumping into each other.**

● **EXERCISE 33-1** Identify each word group as either a complete sentence or a fragment. If the word group is a sentence, circle its number. If it's a fragment, tell why it's incomplete. For help, see Quick Box 33.1.

EXAMPLE

Although having a five-year-old Twinkie might not seem desirable.

[Fragment. Starts with a subordinating conjunction (although) and lacks an independent clause to complete the thought.]

1. Because scientists are working on making foods "indestructible."
2. New preservation technologies responsible for bread puddings that can last four years.
3. Success with current experiments might mean people having to buy groceries only once a month.
4. That people on limited budgets won't have to throw away as much food.
5. Solves three challenges in making food last longer: controlling moisture, exposure to air, and bacteria and molds.
6. "Super sandwiches" packaged with chemicals that absorb oxygen can last three to five years.
7. To control bacteria, sterilizing food in a pouch subjected to pressures of 87,000 pounds per square inch.

8. Because of their tough protein fibers, meat products stand up particularly well to new preserving techniques.
9. Although victims of disasters like earthquakes, floods, and fires benefit from foods that can be stockpiled.
10. Stores with less need of refrigeration. ●

33C How can I correct a fragment that starts with a subordinating word?

First, you want to become entirely familiar with the list of SUBORDINATING CONJUNCTIONS (complete list appears in section 28I). If a word group starts with a subordinating conjunction without being joined to a complete sentence, it's a sentence fragment.

FRAGMENT **Because the ship had to cut through the ice.**

CORRECT **Because the ship had to cut through the ice**, the rescue effort took time.

The sentence fragment starts with the subordinating conjunction *because* and ends in a period, so it's a word group, not a complete sentence. Attaching the fragment to the start of an added complete sentence corrects the error.

CORRECT The rescue effort took time **because the ship had to cut through the ice**.

Attaching the fragment to the end of an added complete sentence corrects the error.

CORRECT **The ship had to cut through the ice.**

Dropping the subordinating conjunction *because* from the fragment corrects the error.

FRAGMENT **Although the ice was twelve inches thick.**

CORRECT **Although the ice was twelve inches thick**, the Russian icebreaker moved quickly.

CORRECT The Russian icebreaker moved quickly, **although the ice was twelve inches thick.**

The fragment starts with the subordinating conjunction *although* and ends in a period, so it's just a word group. Attaching the fragment to a complete sentence corrects the error.

CORRECT **The ice was twelve inches thick.**

Dropping the subordinating conjunction *although* eliminates the fragment.

Unless they start a question, the subordinating words *who* or *which* create a special type of sentence fragment.

FRAGMENT **Who thought the whales might panic from fear of the ship's noise.**

CORRECT The ship's loud motor worried the crew, **who thought the whales might panic from fear of the ship's noise**.

Attaching the *who* fragment at the end of the complete sentence where it makes sense corrects the error.

FRAGMENT **Which sent booming sound waves through the water.**

CORRECT The ship's loud motor, **which sent booming sound waves through the water**, worried the crew.

Placing the *which* fragment in the middle of the complete sentence where it makes sense corrects the error.

CORRECT The ship's loud motor, **which sent booming sound waves through the water**, worried the crew, **who thought the whales might panic from fear of the ship's noise**.

Combining both the *who* and *which* sentence fragments with the complete sentence creates a richly textured message.

33D How can I correct a fragment that lacks a verb?

If a word group includes no VERB and ends with a period, it's a sentence fragment. In looking for a verb, don't mistake a verbal for a complete verb. Verbals ending in *-ing* or *-ed* become verbs only when teamed up with an AUXILIARY VERB. Verbals beginning with *to*, called INFINITIVES, remain as verbals; auxiliary verbs have no effect on them.

FRAGMENT The sailors **debating** whether **to play** classical music over the ship's sound system.

CORRECT The sailors **were debating** whether **to play** classical music over the ship's sound system.

Adding the auxiliary verb *were* to *debating* creates a complete verb, which corrects the error.

FRAGMENT The ship's crew **working** against time **to outrun** the hungry polar bears near the whales.

CORRECT The ship's crew **was working** against time **to outrun** the hungry polar bears near the whales.

Adding the auxiliary verb *were* to *working* creates a complete verb, which corrects the error.

An APPOSITIVE is a descriptive word group that lacks a verb, so it can't stand alone as a sentence. An appositive needs to be placed within a sentence immediately next to what it describes.

FRAGMENT **With their powerful sense of smell**. The polar bears ran toward nearby openings in the ice.

CORRECT **With their powerful sense of smell**, the polar bears ran toward nearby openings in the ice.

CORRECT The polar bears, **with their powerful sense of smell**, ran toward nearby openings in the ice.

The appositive placed immediately next to "the polar bears" within the sentence corrects the error.

FRAGMENT **An enormously powerful icebreaker.** The ship arrived to free the whales.

CORRECT **An enormously powerful icebreaker**, the ship arrived to free the whales.

CORRECT The ship, **an enormously powerful icebreaker**, arrived to free the whales.

The appositive placed immediately next to "the ship" within the sentence corrects the error.

If a TRANSITIONAL EXPRESSION (complete list in 6G) starts a word group that lacks a verb, it's a sentence fragment.

FRAGMENT **Therefore**, the hungry polar bears.

CORRECT **Therefore, the polar bears were hungry.**

CORRECT **Therefore, the hungry polar bears** knew they might soon have a feast.

The sentence fragment revised into a complete sentence or attached to a nearby sentence corrects the error.

FRAGMENT **For example, Bach's sonatas for flute.**

CORRECT The ship's crew chose **Bach's sonatas for flute**.

CORRECT The crew wanted to play high-pitched music, **for example Bach's sonatas for flute**.

The sentence fragment revised into a complete sentence or attached to a nearby sentence corrects the error.

33E How can I correct a fragment that lacks a subject?

If a word group lacks a SUBJECT and ends with a period, it's a sentence fragment.

FRAGMENT **Had heard recordings of the high-pitched calls whales make.**

CORRECT Some crew members **had heard recordings of the high-pitched calls whales make**.

Inserting the subject *Some crew members* at the start of the fragment corrects the error.

FRAGMENT **Allowed some local inhabitants to take a few whales for much-needed food.**

CORRECT The icebreaker's captain **allowed some local inhabitants to take a few whales for much-needed food**.

Inserting the subject *The icebreaker's captain* at the start of the fragment corrects the error.

33F How can I correct a fragment that's a part of a compound predicate?

Many types of COMPOUND PREDICATES occur in sentences. One type contains two or more verbs connected by a COORDINATING CONJUNCTION (*and, but, for, or, nor, yet, so*). When a compound predicate isn't attached to the end of its companion sentence, it is a sentence fragment.

FRAGMENT With a flute concerto playing loudly on its speakers, the ship finally reached the whales. **And led them to freedom**.

CORRECT With a flute concerto playing loudly on its speakers, the ship finally reached the whales **and led them to freedom**.

Joining the compound predicate to the end of the complete sentence corrects the error.

CORRECT With a flute concerto playing loudly on its speakers, the ship finally reached the whales. **The ship led them to freedom**.

Dropping *and* and inserting a subject "the ship" corrects the error.

FRAGMENT The international media wrote about the amazing rescue of the trapped whales. **And the story spread throughout the world**.

CORRECT The international media wrote about the amazing rescue of the trapped whales, **and the story spread throughout the world**.

Joining the compound predicate to the end of the complete sentence corrects the error.

CORRECT The international media wrote about the amazing rescue of the trapped whales. **The story spread throughout the world.**

Dropping *and* and inserting a subject "the story" corrects the error.

● **EXERCISE 33-2** Find and correct any sentence fragments. If a sentence is correct, circle its number. For help, consult 33A through 33F.

EXAMPLE

Even though lice are a common problem for young children.

Correct: Lice are a common problem for young children.

1. Even though lice are not dangerous and do not spread disease, parents tend to worry about their children. Who have been infected with this parasite.
2. Although good hygiene is important, it does not prevent lice infestation. Which can occur on clean, healthy scalps.
3. Spread only through direct contact. Lice are unable to fly or jump.
4. Evidence of lice has been found on ancient Egyptian mummies, which suggests that lice have been annoying humans for a long time.
5. While lice can spread among humans who share combs or pillows or hats. Lice cannot be spread from pets to humans.
6. Doctors may prescribe special shampoos and soaps. To help get rid of the lice on a child's head.
7. Because lice do not like heat, experts recommend putting infected sheets and stuffed animals and pillows in a dryer for thirty minutes.
8. Just one is called a *louse*, and a louse egg is called a *nit*. Which is where we get the words *lousy* and *nit-pick*.
9. Using a hair dryer after applying a scalp treatment can be dangerous. Because some treatments contain flammable ingredients.
10. Although lice cannot live for more than twenty-four hours without human contact. ●

● **EXERCISE 33-3** Go back to Exercise 33-1 and revise the sentence fragments into complete sentences. In some cases, you may be able to combine two fragments into one complete sentence. ●

33G How can I correct a list that is a fragment?

Two special fragment problems involve lists and examples. Lists and examples must be part of a complete sentence, unless they are formatted as a column.

You can correct a list fragment by attaching it to the preceding independent clause using a colon or a dash. You can correct an example fragment by attaching it to an independent clause (with or without punctuation, depending on the meaning) or by rewriting it as a complete sentence.

FRAGMENT You have a choice of desserts. **Carrot cake, chocolate silk pie, apple pie, or peppermint ice cream**.

The list cannot stand on its own as a sentence.

CORRECT You have a choice of desserts: carrot cake, chocolate silk pie, apple pie, or peppermint ice cream.

CORRECT You have a choice of desserts—carrot cake, chocolate silk pie, apple pie, or peppermint ice cream.

FRAGMENT Several good places offer brunch. **For example, the restaurants Sign of the Dove and Blue Yonder**.

Examples can't stand on their own as a sentence.

CORRECT Several good places offer brunch—**for example**, the restaurants Sign of the Dove and Blue Yonder.

CORRECT Several good places offer brunch. **Two examples are** the restaurants Sign of the Dove and Blue Yonder.

33H How can I recognize intentional fragments?

Professional writers sometimes intentionally use fragments for emphasis and effect.

> But in the main, I feel like a brown bag of miscellany propped against a wall. Pour out the contents, and there is discovered a jumble of small things priceless and worthless. **A first-water diamond, an empty spool, bits of broken glass, lengths of string, a key to a door long since crumbled away, a rusty knife-blade, old shoes saved for a road that never was and never will be, a nail bent under the weight of things too heavy for any nail, a dried flower or two still a little fragrant.**
>
> —Zora Neale Hurston, *How It Feels to Be Colored Me*

Today, such fragments are also common in popular magazines and advertisements. A writer's ability to judge the difference between acceptable and unacceptable sentence fragments comes from much experience writing and from reading the works of skilled writers. Some instructors consider a sentence fragment an error; other teachers occasionally accept well-placed intentional fragments after a student has shown the consistent ability to write well-constructed complete sentences. Therefore, if you'd like to use a fragment for emphasis and effect, we advise that you either ask for your teacher's permission ahead of time or write a footnote to your essay that says you're using a sentence fragment intentionally and why.

● **EXERCISE 33-4** Revise this paragraph to eliminate all sentence fragments. In some cases, you can combine word groups to create complete sentences; in other cases, you must supply missing elements to rewrite. Some sentences may not require revision. In your final version, check not only the individual sentences but also the clarity of the whole paragraph. For help, consult 33B through 33F.

EXAMPLE

Although the subject of many amusing anecdotes. Diogenes remains an influential figure in Greek philosophy.

Correct: Although the subject of many amusing anecdotes, Diogenes remains an influential figure in Greek philosophy.

(1) Throughout his career as a philosopher and Cynic, Diogenes cultivated a following. That included the likes of Aristotle and Alexander the Great. (2) Diogenes was an important member of the Cynics, a group of people who rejected conventional life. The word *Cynic* comes from the Greek word for dog. (3) Diogenes lived like a beggar and slept in a tub. Which he carried around with him wherever he went. (4) He rejected the pursuit of wealth and once destroyed his wooden bowl. Because he saw a peasant boy drinking water with his hands. (5) Although none of his writings have survived, Diogenes produced dialogues and a play. That allegedly describes a social utopia in which people live unconventional lives. (6) Since he often walked around Athens in broad daylight with a lamp looking for an honest man. (7) When Plato defined *man* as a featherless biped, Diogenes plucked a chicken and said, "Here is Plato's man." (8) According to legend, Diogenes was once sunbathing when he was approached by Alexander the Great. Who was a fan of the eccentric Cynic. (9) Alexander asked if he could do anything for Diogenes. Which the philosopher answered by saying, "Don't block my sunlight." (10) Because Diogenes is a strange and interesting character. He has inspired works by such writers and artists as William Blake, Anton Chekhov, and Rabelais. ●

● **EXERCISE 33-5** Revise this paragraph to eliminate all sentence fragments. In some cases, you can combine word groups to create complete sentences; in other cases, you must supply missing elements to revise word groups. Some sentences may not require revision. In your final version, check not only the individual sentences but also the clarity of the whole paragraph. Refer to 33A through 33E for help.

(1) The English games cricket and rounders. (2) Are the forerunners of the American game baseball. (3) Which became popular in America in the nineteenth century. (4) According to the *New York Morning News*, in an article

from 1845. (5) Members of the New York Knickerbockers Club played the first reported baseball game. (6) Taking place at Elysian Fields in Hoboken, New Jersey. (7) Creating one of baseball's first teams, and writing "20 Original Rules of Baseball." (8) Alexander Cartwright is often called The Father of Baseball. (9) By scholars and historians of the game. (10) His new rules, which became known as Knickerbocker Rules. (11) Changed baseball in a number of ways. (12) Such as giving each batter three strikes and each inning three outs. (13) The first game, therefore. (14) That used the Knickerbocker Rules was played on June 19, 1846, in New Jersey. (15) Acting as umpire for this game. (16) Cartwright charged six-cent fines for swearing. (17) The Knickerbockers lost this game by 22 points to a team. (18) That was known as "The New York Nine." ●

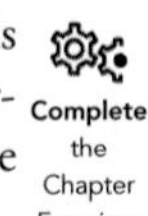

34 Comma Splices and Run-On Sentences

Quick Points You will learn to

- Identify comma splices and run-on sentences (see 34A–34B).
- Correct comma splices and run-on sentences (see 34C–34G).

34A What are comma splices and run-on sentences?

A **comma splice**, also called a *comma fault*, occurs when a comma, rather than a period, is used incorrectly between two or more complete sentences.

A **run-on sentence**, also called a *fused sentence* or a *run-together sentence*, occurs when two complete sentences run into each other without any punctuation. Comma splices and run-on sentences create confusion because readers can't tell where one thought ends and another begins.

COMMA SPLICE The icebergs broke off from the **glacier, they** drifted into the sea.

RUN-ON SENTENCE The icebergs broke off from the **glacier they** drifted into the sea.

CORRECT The icebergs broke off from the **glacier. They** drifted into the sea.

There is one exception. A comma is correct between two independent clauses if the comma is followed by one of the seven coordinating conjunctions: *and, but, for, or, nor, yet, so*. See Chapter 42.

CORRECT The icebergs broke off from the glacier, **and** they drifted into the sea.

Alert: Occasionally, when your meaning suggests it, you can use a colon or a dash to join two independent clauses. ●

During DRAFTING, if you suspect that you've written a comma splice or a run-on sentence, simply underline or highlight it in boldface or italics, and move on. Later, you can easily find it to check and correct during REVISING and EDITING.

34B How can I recognize comma splices and run-on sentences?

When you know how to recognize an INDEPENDENT CLAUSE, you'll know how to recognize COMMA SPLICES and RUN-ON SENTENCES. An independent clause contains a SUBJECT and a PREDICATE and can stand alone as a complete sentence. Also, an independent clause doesn't begin with a SUBORDINATING CONJUNCTION or a RELATIVE PRONOUN, words that create dependence.

Interestingly, almost all comma splices and run-on sentences are caused by only four patterns. If you become familiar with these four patterns, listed in Quick Box 34.1, you'll more easily locate them in your writing.

Alert: To proofread for comma splices, cover all words on one side of the comma and see if the words remaining form an independent clause. If they do, next cover all words you left uncovered, on the other side of the comma. If the second side of the comma is also an independent clause, you're looking at a comma splice. (This technique doesn't work for run-on sentences because a comma isn't present.) ●

Experienced writers sometimes use a comma to join very short independent clauses, especially if one independent clause is negative and the other is positive: *Mosquitoes don't **bite, they** stab*. In ACADEMIC WRITING, you'll be safe if you use a period or a semicolon, if the two independent clauses are closely related in meaning: *Mosquitoes don't **bite; they** stab*.

Quick Box 34.1

Detecting comma splices and run-on sentences

Watch the Video

- Watch out for a PERSONAL PRONOUN starting the second independent clause.

NO The physicist Marie Curie discovered **radium, she** won two Nobel Prizes.

YES The physicist Marie Curie discovered **radium. She** won two Nobel Prizes.

- Watch out for a CONJUNCTIVE ADVERB (such as *furthermore, however, similarly, therefore,* and *then;* see Quick Box 28.5, section 28G, for a complete list) starting the second independent clause.

NO Marie Curie and her husband, Pierre, worked together at **first, however**, he died tragically at age forty-seven.

YES Marie Curie and her husband, Pierre, worked together at **first. However**, he died tragically at age forty-seven.

- Watch out for a TRANSITIONAL EXPRESSION (such as *in addition, for example, in contrast, of course,* and *meanwhile;* see Quick Box 6.4, section 6G.1, for a complete list) starting the second independent clause.

NO Marie Curie and her husband won a Nobel Prize for the discovery of **radium, in addition, Marie** herself won another Nobel Prize for her work on the atomic weight of radium.

YES Marie Curie and her husband won a Nobel Prize for the discovery of **radium; in addition, Marie** herself won another Nobel Prize for her work on the atomic weight of radium.

- Watch out for a second independent clause that explains, contrasts with, or gives an example of what's said in the first independent clause.

NO Marie Curie died of leukemia in **1934, exposure** to radioactivity killed her.

YES Marie Curie died of leukemia in **1934. Exposure** to radioactivity killed her.

34C How do I use a period to correct comma splices and run-on sentences?

You can use a period to correct comma splices and run-on sentences by placing the period between the two sentences.

COMMA SPLICE	A shark is all **cartilage, it** has no bones in its body.
RUN-ON SENTENCE	A shark is all **cartilage it** has no bones in its body.
CORRECT	A shark is all **cartilage. It** has no bones in its body.
COMMA SPLICE	Sharks can smell blood from a quarter mile **away, they** then swim toward the source like a guided missile.
RUN-ON SENTENCE	Sharks can smell blood from a quarter mile **away they** then swim toward the source like a guided missile.
CORRECT	Sharks can smell blood from a quarter mile **away. They** then swim toward the source like a guided missile.

34D How do I use a semicolon to correct comma splices and run-on sentences?

You can use a semicolon to correct comma splices and run-on sentences by placing the semicolon between the two sentences. Use a semicolon only when the separate sentences are closely related in meaning.

COMMA SPLICE	The great white shark supposedly eats **humans, research** shows that most white sharks spit them out after one bite.
RUN-ON SENTENCE	The great white shark supposedly eats **humans research** shows that most white sharks spit them out after one bite.
CORRECT	The great white shark supposedly eats **humans; research** shows that most white sharks spit them out after one bite.

34E How do I use a comma and a coordinating conjunction to correct comma splices and run-on sentences?

Watch the Video

You can correct a comma splice or a run-on sentence by inserting a comma followed by a coordinating conjunction (*and, but, for, or, nor, yet, so*) between the two independent clauses (42B).

When you use a coordinating conjunction, be sure that your choice fits the meaning of the material. *And* signals addition; *but* and *yet* signal contrast; *for* and *so* signal cause; and *or* and *nor* signal alternatives.

COMMA SPLICE	All living creatures send weak electrical charges in **water, a shark** skin can detect these signals.
RUN-ON SENTENCE	All living creatures send weak electrical charges in **water a shark** can detect these signals.
CORRECT	All living creatures send weak electrical charges in **water,** and **a shark** can detect these signals.

● **EXERCISE 34-1** Revise the comma splices and run-on sentences by using a period, a semicolon, or a comma and coordinating conjunction.

EXAMPLE

Near the town of Bluffdale, Utah, in a desert valley by the Wasatch Range, is a massive building five times the size of the U.S. Capitol it will soon be filled with computers and intelligence experts.

Revised: Near the town of Bluffdale, Utah, in a desert valley by the Wasatch Range, is a massive building five times the size of the U.S. Capitol. It will soon be filled with computers and intelligence experts.

1. The Utah Data Center will store vast amounts of emails, cell phone calls, Internet searches, and other personal data, for example, agents will be able to track down everything from parking receipts to plane ticket information.
2. However, this $2 billion complex is designed to do more than serve as a warehouse of digital data breaking codes will be one of its major efforts.
3. The National Security agency is in charge of the Utah Data Center and will handle the data analysis, code breaking, and recommendations for action information gathered may prevent criminal or terrorist actions, increasing American security.
4. Some people worry that the center may exceed traditional security practices, it will have the capacity and even the mission to collect and analyze billions of messages from American citizens, storing trillions of pieces of data.
5. In an age where personal computers can routinely store as much as one or two terabytes of data, the capacity of the new data center is staggering, able to hold over a yottabyte equal to over 500 quintillion pages of text, a yottabyte is more than the total amount of human knowledge ever created. ●

34F How do I use clauses to correct comma splices and run-on sentences?

You can correct a comma splice or run-on sentence by revising one of the two independent clauses into a dependent clause when one idea can logically be subordinated to the other. Also, be careful never to end the dependent clause with a period or semicolon. If you do, you've created a SENTENCE FRAGMENT.

CREATE DEPENDENT CLAUSES WITH SUBORDINATING CONJUNCTIONS

One way to create a dependent clause is to insert a SUBORDINATING CONJUNCTION (such as *because, although, when,* and *if*—see Quick Box 28.7, section 28I, for a complete list). Always choose a subordinating conjunction that fits the meaning of each particular sentence. Dependent clauses that begin with a subordinating conjunction are called ADVERB CLAUSES.

COMMA SPLICE Homer and Langley Collyer had packed their house from top to bottom with **junk, police** could not open the front door to investigate a reported smell.

RUN-ON SENTENCE Homer and Langley Collyer had packed their house from top to bottom with **junk police** could not open the front door to investigate a reported smell.

CORRECT **Because** Homer and Langley Collyer had packed their house from top to bottom with **junk, police** could not open the front door to investigate a reported smell.

Because starts a dependent clause that is joined by a comma with the independent clause starting with *police.*

COMMA SPLICE Old newspapers and car parts filled every room to the **ceiling, enough** space remained for fourteen pianos.

RUN-ON SENTENCE Old newspapers and car parts filled every room to the **ceiling enough** space remained for fourteen pianos.

CORRECT **Although** old newspapers and car parts filled every room to the **ceiling, enough** space remained for fourteen pianos.

The subordinating conjunction *although* starts a dependent clause that is joined by a comma with the independent clause starting with *enough.*

Alert: Place a comma between an introductory dependent clause and the independent clause that follows (see 42C). ●

CREATE DEPENDENT CLAUSES WITH RELATIVE PRONOUNS

You can create a dependent clause with a RELATIVE PRONOUN (*who, whom, whose, which, that*). Dependent clauses with a relative pronoun are called ADJECTIVE CLAUSES.

COMMA SPLICE The Collyers had been crushed under a pile of **debris, the debris** had toppled onto the men.

RUN-ON SENTENCE The Collyers had been crushed under a pile of **debris the debris** toppled onto the men.

CORRECT The Collyers had been crushed under a pile of **debris *that* had toppled** onto the men.

The relative pronoun *that* starts a dependent clause and is joined with the independent clause starting with *The Collyers*, after deletion of *the debris*.

Alert: Sometimes you need commas to set off an adjective clause from the rest of the sentence. This happens only when the adjective is NONRESTRICTIVE (nonessential), so check carefully (see 42F). ●

● **EXERCISE 34-2** Working individually or with your peer-response group, identify and then revise the comma splices and run-on sentences. Circle the numbers of correct sentences.

EXAMPLE

COMMA SPLICE Basketball was invented in 1891, today, it is one of the world's most popular sports.

RUN-ON SENTENCE Basketball was invented in 1891 today, it is one of the world's most popular sports.

CORRECT Basketball was invented in 1891; today, it is one of the world's most popular sports.

1. James Naismith, a physical education professor at what is known today as Springfield College, needed an indoor sport for his students to play on rainy days, he invented basketball.
2. At first, he didn't use a net he used a peach basket.
3. Dribbling, the act of bouncing the ball between passes and shots, did not become common in basketball until much later, originally, players merely carried the ball.
4. Backboards were also not introduced until later, this kept fans from being able to interfere with the action.
5. Without balls made specifically for the sport, early basketball players had to use soccer balls in the 1950s, Tony Hinkle introduced the now famous orange balls that are easier for players and spectators to see.
6. The first official basketball game was played in 1892 in Albany, New York, only one point was scored.
7. Founded in 1946, the National Basketball Association (NBA) began with the help of owners of ice hockey arenas, many consider the game between the Toronto Huskies and the New York Knickerbockers in 1946 as the first official NBA game.
8. Although a three-point rule was first used in 1933, the NBA did not officially add the rule until 1979, the year that Larry Bird and Magic Johnson began playing professionally.

9. On March 2nd, 1962, in Hershey, Pennsylvania, Wilt Chamberlain, playing for the Philadelphia Warriors, scored a record 100 points in one game his average for the season was 50.4 points per game.
10. Now a worldwide sport, basketball debuted in the Olympics in 1936, the United States defeated Canada in a game played outdoors. ●

34G How do I use adverbs and transitions to correct comma splices and run-on sentences?

CONJUNCTIVE ADVERBS and other TRANSITIONAL EXPRESSIONS link ideas between sentences. When these words fall between sentences, a period or semicolon must immediately precede them, and a comma usually follows them.

Conjunctive adverbs include such words as *however, therefore, hence, next, then, thus, furthermore*, and *nevertheless* (see Quick Box 28.5, section 28G, for a complete list). Be careful to remember that conjunctive adverbs are not COORDINATING CONJUNCTIONS (*and, but*, and so on; see 34C.3).

COMMA SPLICE Hannibal wanted to conquer Rome, **hence**, he crossed the Alps.

RUN-ON SENTENCE Hannibal wanted to conquer Rome **hence**, he crossed the Alps.

CORRECT Hannibal wanted to conquer Rome. **Hence**, he crossed the Alps.

CORRECT Hannibal wanted to conquer Rome; **hence**, he crossed the Alps.

Transitional expressions include *for example, for instance, in addition, in fact, of course*, and *on the one hand/on the other hand* (see Quick Box 6.4, section 6G, for a complete list).

COMMA SPLICE Hannibal enjoyed much public acclaim, **for** example, he achieved both military and political success.

RUN-ON SENTENCE Hannibal enjoyed much public acclaim **for** example, he achieved both military and political success.

CORRECT Hannibal enjoyed much public acclaim. **For** example, he achieved both military and political success.

CORRECT Hannibal enjoyed much public acclaim; **for** example, he achieved both military and political success.

! Alert: A conjunctive adverb or a transitional expression is usually followed by a comma when it starts a sentence (see 42C). ●

EXERCISE 34-3 Revise comma splices or run-on sentences caused by incorrectly punctuated conjunctive adverbs or other transitional expressions. If a sentence is correct, circle its number.

however	therefore	also	next	then	thus
furthermore	nevertheless	indeed	for example		

EXAMPLE

Las Vegas is a large and popular city in Nevada known for entertainment and gambling, nevertheless, it was once a small, desert city.

Corrected: Las Vegas is a large and popular city in Nevada known for entertainment and gambling. Nevertheless, it was once a small, desert city.

1. When Las Vegas was first counted by the U.S. Census in 1910, it was a tiny town, indeed, the entire county only had 3,000 people.
2. Only a hundred years later, however, the population had ballooned to over half a million people.
3. Las Vegas remained a small railroad town for the first couple of decades of the twentieth century, then, when the nearby Hoover Dam was built in 1935, Las Vegas began to grow.
4. Other factors contributed to the growth of Las Vegas, for example, gambling was legalized in 1931 and many scientists moved there during World War II to work on the Manhattan Project.
5. Las Vegas is now famous for its gambling, therefore, it is sometimes known as "Sin City."

EXERCISE 34-4 Revise all comma splices and run-on sentences, using as many different methods of correction as you can.

(1) Energy psychology represents fairly new methods joining Eastern lines of thought to the mind and body and Western psychology and psychotherapy, according to an article by Leonard Holmes, PhD, proponents of energy psychology contend that striking acupuncture points and at the same time recalling an anxiety-producing incident can alleviate anxiety and phobias. (2) Holmes inquires whether this idea is true in fact, he goes on to question the connection the acupuncture points have to anxiety. (3) In the early 1980s, Roger Callahan, PhD, popularized procedures utilizing energy psychology, he called the procedures "The Callahan Technique" or "Thought Field Therapy." (4) In the beginning, Callahan's training programs were costly, generally hundreds of dollars, now, on the other hand, they are moderately priced. (5) Other therapists such as clinical psychologist David Feinstein, PhD, have joined the ranks promoting energy psychology, interestingly, Feinstein sells an interactive CD-ROM that presents guidance

in energy psychology/psychotherapy. (6) A qualified therapist can use the CD-ROM laypersons should not experiment with the contents of the CD-ROM. (7) Today, proponents of energy psychology contend it results in the successful handling of problems such as trauma, abuse, depression, and addictive cravings, other uses for energy psychology, or "Emotional Freedom Techniques" (EFT), as Gary Craig calls them on his Web site, include treatment for medical conditions such as headaches and breathing difficulties. (8) Craig, not a licensed health professional, contends the "missing piece to the healing puzzle" is EFT he quotes from supposedly scientific clinical trials indicating that patients have seen dramatic results in their conditions because of EFT. (9) Holmes thinks energy psychotherapy is still too early in its development to be widely applied he cautions the general public to avoid trying it on their own. (10) Holmes advises extreme caution for psychologists about continuing to use EFT more needs to be known from research. ●

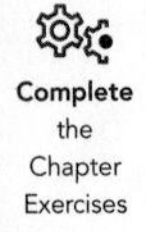
Complete the Chapter Exercises

35 Misplaced and Dangling Modifiers

Quick Points You will learn to

- Place modifiers carefully so that your intended meaning is clear (see 35A–35E).

MISPLACED MODIFIERS

35A What is a misplaced modifier?

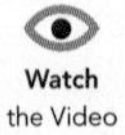
Watch the Video

A MODIFIER is a word or group of words that describes or limits another word or group of words. A **misplaced modifier** is positioned incorrectly in a sentence, which means that it describes another word and changes the writer's meaning. Always place a modifier as close as possible to what it describes.

AVOIDING SQUINTING MODIFIERS

A misplaced **squinting modifier** can modify both the words before it and after it. Position your modifiers to communicate the meaning you intend.

NO The speaker addressing us loudly condemned unions.

Which happened loudly, addressing or condemning?

YES Addressing us loudly, the speaker condemned unions.

YES The speaker addressing us condemned unions loudly.

PLACING LIMITING WORDS CAREFULLY

Words such as *only, not only, just, not just, almost, hardly, nearly, even, exactly, merely, scarcely,* and *simply* can change the meaning of a sentence according to their placement. Note how placement of *only* changes the meaning of this sentence: *Professional coaches say that high salaries motivate players.*

- **Only** professional coaches say that high salaries motivate players.
  No one else says this.
- Professional coaches **only** say that high salaries motivate players.
  The coaches probably do not mean what they say.
- Professional coaches say **only** that high salaries motivate players.
  The coaches say nothing else.
- Professional coaches say that **only** high salaries motivate players.
  Nothing except high salaries motivates players.
- Professional coaches say that high salaries **only** motivate players.
  High salaries do nothing other than motivate players.
- Professional coaches say that high salaries motivate **only** players.
  High salaries motivate the players but no one else.

35B How can I avoid split infinitives?

An INFINITIVE is a verb preceded by the word *to:* I want *to design* boldly. A **split infinitive** occurs when words are placed between *to* and its verb: I want *to boldly design*. Often, the effect is awkward.

NO The student tried **to in some way pacify** his instructor.

In some way is misplaced because it splits *to pacify*.

YES The student tried **to pacify** his instructor in some way.

YES In some way, the student tried **to pacify** his instructor.

Sometimes a split infinitive can actually achieve clarity or emphasis. Consider how the meaning changes in the sentence below, depending on whether the infinitive is split.

- She wanted *to more than double* her earnings.
- She wanted *to double more than* her earnings.

When you create clarity or achieve emphasis by splitting your infinitive, split freely.

35C How can I avoid other splits in my sentences?

Separation of closely related sentence elements, such as a subject and its verb or a verb and its object, causes your readers to lose meaningful connections between these words.

NO The announcer of Orson Wells's radio drama "War of the Worlds," because the script opened with a graphic descriptions of emergency broadcasts, convinced many people that the Earth was being invaded by Martians.

Readers lose the connection between the subject *announcer* and its verb *convinced.*

YES Because the script opened with graphic descriptions of emergency broadcasts, the announcer of Orson Wells's radio drama "War of the Worlds" convinced many people that the Earth was being invaded by Martians.

Readers easily grasp the connection between subject *announcer* and verb *convinced.*

NO Many churches **held** for their frightened communities **"end of the world" prayer services**.

Readers lose the connection between verb *held* and object *prayer services.*

YES Many churches **held "end of the world" prayer services** for their frightened communities.

Readers easily grasp the connection between verb *held* and object *prayer services.*

● **EXERCISE 35-1** Revise these ten sentences to correct misplaced modifiers, split infinitives, and other splits. If a sentence is correct, circle its number. For help, consult 35A through 35C.

EXAMPLE

The city of Deadwood is known for its many notorious residents made popular by a TV show including Wild Bill Hickok and Calamity Jane.

Made popular by a TV show, the city of Deadwood is known for its many notorious residents, including Wild Bill Hickok and Calamity Jane.

1. Deadwood, because of its location near the Deadwood Gulch and the Black Hills of South Dakota, was named for the dead trees found in that canyon.
2. The city's founding, during a gold rush that attracted a quarter of a million miners to the area, was in 1876.
3. The main source of revenue for the city was gambling, which was outlawed in 1905 but reinstated in 1989.
4. Today, tourists who visit Deadwood often gamble and enjoy the historical reenactments of the town's famous events.
5. Deadwood nearly was the home to a dozen of famous characters from the Old West.
6. Serving as the sheriff of Hays City and Abilene, Wild Bill Hickok worked to with an iron fist tame the lawless towns of the frontier.
7. Hickok moved to Deadwood after he without much success performed in a Wild West show.
8. During a poker game at Nuttall & Mann's saloon, Jack McCall shot for unknown reasons Will Bill.
9. The cards Hickok was holding included a pair of black aces, a pair of black eights, and an unknown fifth card now known as the dead man's hand.
10. The legends of Deadwood and Wild Bill in the stories of fiction writers and TV shows continue to grow. ●

● **EXERCISE 35-2** Using each list of words and phrases, create all the possible logical sentences. Insert commas as needed. Explain differences in meaning among the alternatives you create. For help, consult 35A through 35C.

EXAMPLE exchange students
learned to speak French
while in Paris
last summer

A. Last summer,/exchange students/learned to speak French/while in Paris.
B. While in Paris,/exchange students/learned to speak French/last summer.
C. Exchange students/learned to speak French/while in Paris/last summer.
D. Exchange students/learned to speak French/last summer/while in Paris.

1. chicken soup
   according to folklore
   helps
   cure colds
2. tadpoles
   instinctively
   swim
   toward
   their genetic relatives
3. the young driver
   while driving
   in the snow
   skidded carelessly
4. climbed
   the limber teenager
   a tall palm tree
   to pick a ripe coconut
   quickly
5. and cause mini-avalanches
   ski patrollers
   set explosives
   often
   to prevent
   big avalanches ●

DANGLING MODIFIERS

35D How can I avoid dangling modifiers?

A **dangling modifier** describes or limits a word or words that never actually appear in the sentence. To correct a dangling modifier, state clearly your intended SUBJECT in the sentence.

NO **Approaching the island, a mountainous wall** was foreboding.

This sentence suggests that the mountainous wall was approaching the island.

YES Approaching the island, **we** saw a foreboding mountainous wall.

YES As we approached the island, **we** saw a foreboding mountainous wall.

Both revised sentences include the subject *we*.

NO To allay our fears, our ship swerved around the island.

This sentence suggests that our ship allayed our fears.

YES To allay our fears, the pilot swerved our ship around the island.

A major cause of dangling and misplaced modifiers is the unnecessary use of the PASSIVE VOICE. Whenever possible, use the ACTIVE VOICE.

NO **To earn money, tutoring services** are offered by Marlin.

Tutoring services cannot earn money; *are offered* is passive voice.

YES **To earn money, Marlin** offers tutoring services.

● **EXERCISE 35-3** Identify and correct any dangling modifiers in these sentences. If a sentence is correct, circle its number. For help, consult 35D.

EXAMPLE

To understand what happened to Krakatoa, the volcano and its history must be studied.

Corrected: To understand what happened to Krakatoa, one must study the volcano and its history.

1. In 1883, massive destruction was caused by the eruption of the volcano Krakatoa, an event recently examined in the book *Krakatoa: The Day the World Exploded.*
2. Exploding with a force 13,000 times stronger than the bomb dropped on Hiroshima, people thousands of miles away heard the eruption.
3. The loudest sound historically reported was generated by the explosion, with devastating tsunamis soon following.
4. Ejecting tons of debris into the air, the volcano destroyed or damaged hundreds of nearby villages.
5. Beginning to erupt around late July, larger eruptions didn't start until the middle of August.
6. Reaching over 100 feet in height and traveling at devastating speeds, major destruction was caused on the coastlines of Sumatra.
7. Lasting much longer than expected, people in nearby areas felt aftershocks until February of 1884.
8. To understand the magnitude of this volcanic eruption, changes in weather patterns were studied by scientists.
9. Darkening the sky for days afterwards and producing unusual sunsets, the ash and gases from the volcano temporarily lowered the average temperature of the earth.
10. Affecting the art of its time, the background of Edvard Munch's famous painting *The Scream* was inspired by Krakatoan sunsets. ●

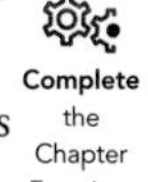

Complete the Chapter Exercises

35E How can I proofread successfully for misplaced and dangling modifiers?

Sentence errors like MISPLACED MODIFIERS and DANGLING MODIFIERS are hard to spot because of the way the human brain works. Writers know what they mean to say when they write. When they PROOFREAD, however, they often misread what they've written for what they intended to write. The mind unconsciously adjusts for the error. In contrast, readers see only what's on the paper or screen. We suggest that you read your writing aloud, or have someone else read it to you, to proofread it for these kinds of problems.

36 Shifting and Mixed Sentences

Quick Points You will learn to

➤ Write sentences that have consistent grammatical forms (see 36A–36J).

SHIFTING SENTENCES

36A What is a shifting sentence?

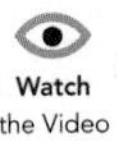

A **shift** within a sentence—or between sentences—is an unnecessary, often confusing, change in PERSON, NUMBER, SUBJECT, VOICE, TENSE, MOOD or DIRECT or INDIRECT DISCOURSE. When you begin writing in THIRD PERSON, for example, you challenge your readers if you switch to SECOND PERSON.

You can avoid writing shifting sentences and paragraphs by remaining consistent in your grammatical forms.

36B How can I avoid shifts in person and number?

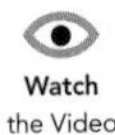

Person indicates who or what performs or receives action. FIRST PERSON (*I, we*) is the writer or speaker; SECOND PERSON (*you*) is someone written or spoken to; THIRD PERSON (*he, she it, they*) is someone or something written or spoken about. Shifts in person often challenge your readers to clarify your meaning.

NO I enjoy reading financial forecasts, but **you** wonder which are accurate.

First person *I* shifts unnecessarily to second person *you.*

YES I enjoy reading financial forecasts, but **I** wonder which are accurate.

NUMBER means *singular* (one) or *plural* (more than one). Be alert for needless shifts from one number to the other number.

NO Because **people** are living longer, **an employee** now retires later.

The plural *people* needlessly shifts to the singular *employee.*

YES Because **people** are living longer, **employees** now retire later.

In ACADEMIC WRITING, reserve *you* for addressing the reader directly. Use the third person for general statements.

NO **I** like my job in personnel because **you** get to interview job applicants.

The shift from first person *I* to second person *you* is misleading.

YES **I** like my job in personnel because **I** get to interview job applicants.

NO When **politicians** accept bribes, **you're** violating an oath of office.

The shift from third person *politicians* to second person *you* is misleading.

YES When **politicians** accept bribes, **they're** violating an oath of office.

Be careful with singular words (often NOUNS) used in a general sense, such as *employee, student, consumer, neighbor, someone*. These third person singular words require third person singular pronoun references: *he*, *she*, and *it*. Because *they* is a plural pronoun, the word *they* cannot refer to a singular noun.

NO When **an employee** is treated with respect, **they** are more motivated to do a good job.

The plural pronoun *they* cannot refer to the singular *an employee.*

YES When **an employee** is treated with respect, **he or she** is more motivated to do a good job.

YES When **employees** are treated with respect, **they** are more motivated to do a good job.

YES **An employee** who is treated with respect is more motivated to do a good job.

YES **Employees** who are treated with respect are more motivated to do a good job.

Alert: With INDEFINITE PRONOUNS (such as *someone, everyone*, or *anyone*), choose GENDER-NEUTRAL LANGUAGE. For advice, see 31S. ●

● **EXERCISE 36-1** Eliminate shifts in person and number between, as well as within, sentences. Some sentences may not need revision. For help, consult 36B.

(1) First-time visitors to the Mall of America may be overwhelmed by its size, but you will also see its helpful design. (2) A shopper will notice that the mall is divided into architecturally distinct areas so they won't get lost. (3) The four sides of the mall have different themes and matching décor, so it is easy to navigate. (4) The architects named the four sides the North Garden, South Avenue, East Broadway, and West Market. (5) He or she also called the fourth floor's collection of nightclubs the Upper East Side to reflect an urban environment. (6) In spite of skeptics who thought the mall would never make money, it has been consistently successful in

renting its retail space and attracting shoppers. (7) The amusement park in the middle of the mall remains an important draw for families and children, and they have roller coasters and water rides. (8) Couples can enjoy fine dining and high-end shopping, and you can even get married in the mall's wedding chapel. ●

36C How can I avoid shifts in subject and voice?

A SHIFT in SUBJECT is rarely justified when it is accompanied by a shift in VOICE. The voice of a sentence is either *active* (*People expect changes*) or *passive* (*Changes are expected*). Some subject shifts, however, are justified by the meaning of a passage: for example, *People look forward to the future, but the future holds many secrets.*

NO Most **people expect** major improvements in the future, but some **hardships are** also **anticipated**.

Both the subject (*people* to *hardships*) and the voice (active to passive) shift.

YES Most **people expect** major improvements in the future, but **they** also **anticipate** some hardships.

YES Most **people expect** major improvements in the future but also **anticipate** some hardships.

36D How can I avoid shifts in tense and mood?

TENSE refers to the time (past, present, future) in which the action of a VERB takes place. *We **will go** shopping after we **finish** lunch.* An unnecessary tense SHIFT within or between sentences can make the statement confusing or illogical.

NO A campaign to clean up films in the United States **began** in the 1920s as various groups **try** to ban sex and violence from movies.

The tense shifts from the past *began* to the present *try*.

YES A campaign to clean up films in the United States **began** in the 1920s as various groups **tried** to ban sex and violence from movies.

NO Film producers and distributors **created** the Production Code in the 1930s. Films that **fail** to get the board's seal of approval **do not receive** wide distribution.

This shift occurs between sentences—the past tense *created* shifts to the present tense *fail* and *do not receive*.

YES Film producers and distributors **created** the Production Code in the 1930s. Films that **failed** to get the board's seal of approval **did not receive** wide distribution.

MOOD indicates whether a sentence is a statement or a question (INDICATIVE MOOD), a command or request (IMPERATIVE MOOD), or a conditional or other-than-real statement (SUBJUNCTIVE MOOD). A shift in mood creates an awkward construction and can cause confusion.

NO The Production Code included guidelines on violence: **Do not show** details of brutal murders, and films **should not show** how to commit crimes.

The verbs shift from the imperative mood *do not show* to the indicative mood *films should not show.*

YES The Production Code included guidelines on violence: **Do not show** details of brutal murders, and **do not show** how to commit crimes.

This revision uses the imperative mood for both guidelines.

YES The Production Code included guidelines on violence: Films **were not to show** the details of brutal murders or ways to commit crimes.

NO The code's writers worried that **if a crime were** accurately **depicted** in a movie, **copycat crimes will follow**.

The sentence shifts from the subjunctive mood *if a crime were depicted* to the indicative mood *copycat crimes will follow.*

YES The code's writers worried that **if a crime were** accurately **depicted** in a movie, **copycat crimes would follow**.

36E How can I avoid shifts between indirect and direct discourse?

Indirect discourse is not enclosed in quotation marks because it reports, rather than quotes, something that someone said. In contrast, **direct discourse** is enclosed in quotation marks because it quotes exactly the words that someone said. Do not write sentences that mix indirect and direct discourse. Such SHIFTS confuse readers, who can't tell what was said and what is being merely reported.

NO She asked me **was I going out**.

This sentence shifts from indirect to direct discourse. Direct discourse requires quotation marks and changes in language.

YES She asked me **whether I was going out**.

This revision uses indirect discourse consistently.

YES She asked me **if I was going out**.

This revision uses indirect discourse consistently.

YES She asked me, **"Are you going out?"**

This revision uses direct discourse with quotation marks. It makes the changes in language (such as INVERTED ORDER and verb TENSE) that accompany direct discourse.

Whenever you change from direct discourse to indirect discourse (when you decide to paraphrase rather than quote someone directly, for example), you need to make changes in TENSE and in other grammatical features for your writing to make sense. Simply removing quotation marks is not enough.

● **EXERCISE 36-2** Revise these sentences to eliminate incorrect shifts within sentences. Some sentences can be revised in several ways. For help, consult 36B through 36E.

EXAMPLE

In 1942, the U.S. government is faced with arresting five million people for not paying their federal income taxes.

In 1942, the U.S. government *was* faced with arresting five million people for not paying their federal income taxes.

1. Congress needed money to pay for U.S. participation in World War II, so a new tax system was proposed.
2. Tax payments were due on March 15, not April 15 as it is today.
3. For the first time, Congress taxed millions of lower-income citizens. Most people do not save enough to pay the amount of taxes due.
4. When a scientific poll showed lawmakers that only one in seven Americans had saved enough money, he became worried. ●

● **EXERCISE 36-3** Revise this paragraph to eliminate incorrect shifts between sentences and within sentences. For help, consult 36B through 36E.

(1) According to sociologists, people experience role conflict when we find ourselves trying to juggle too many different social roles. (2) When people reach overload, he or she decided, "to cut back somewhere." (3) For example, a well-known politician might decide not to run for reelection because family life would be interfered with by the demands of the campaign. (4) In other cases, you may delay having children so they can achieve early career success. (5) A person might say to themselves that I can't do this right now and focus instead on career goals. (6) In yet another example, a plant manager might enjoy social interaction with employees but consequently find themselves unable to evaluate him or her objectively. (7) In short, sociologists find that although not all role conflicts cause problems, great hardships are suffered by some individuals faced with handling difficult balancing acts. (8) People can minimize role conflicts, however, if we learn

to compartmentalize our lives. (9) A good example of this is people saying that I'm going to stop thinking about my job before I head home to my family. ●

MIXED SENTENCES

36F What is a mixed sentence?

A **mixed sentence** begins a sentence with one kind of construction (such as a PHRASE) and then switches to another (such as a PREDICATE). This scrambling of sentence parts dilutes your meaning. To avoid this error, match your opening (often your SUBJECT) to what follows both logically and grammatically.

NO When we lost first prize motivated us to train harder.

The PREDICATE of the sentence *motivated us to train harder* has no subject.

YES When we lost first prize, we became motivated to train harder.

YES Losing first prize motivated us to train harder.

NO Because early television included news programs became popular with the public.

The start of this sentence sets up a reason that doesn't match the rest of the sentence.

YES Early television included news programs, which became popular with the public.

NO Because of my damage to a library book is why they fined me heavily.

A prepositional phrase such as *because of my damage* can't be the subject of a sentence.

YES Because I damaged a book, the library fined me heavily.

YES Because of the damage to my library book, I was fined heavily.

The phrase *the fact that* lacks CONCISENESS, and it also tends to cause a mixed sentence.

NO The fact that quiz show scandals in the 1950s prompted the networks to produce even more news shows.

YES The fact is that quiz show scandals in the 1950s prompted the networks to produce even more news shows.

Adding *is* clarifies the meaning.

YES Quiz show scandals in the 1950s prompted the networks to produce even more news shows.

Dropping *the fact that* clarifies the meaning.

36G How can I correct a mixed sentence due to faulty predication?

Faulty predication, sometimes called *illogical predication*, occurs when a SUBJECT and its PREDICATE don't make sense together.

NO The purpose of television was invented to entertain people.

A *purpose* cannot be *invented.*

YES The purpose of television was to entertain people.

YES Television was invented to entertain people.

Faulty predication often results from a lost connection between a subject and its SUBJECT COMPLEMENT.

NO Walter Cronkite's outstanding **characteristic** as a newscaster **was credible**.

Cronkite may be credible but not his *characteristic.*

YES Walter Cronkite's outstanding **characteristic** as a newscaster **was credibility**.

When *credibility* replaces *credible,* the sentence is correct.

YES Walter Cronkite was credible as a newscaster.

Credible is correct when *Walter Cronkite* becomes the subject.

In ACADEMIC WRITING, avoid nonstandard constructions such as *is when* and *is where*. Often they lead to faulty predication.

NO A disaster **is when** TV news shows get some of their highest ratings.

YES TV news shows get some of their highest ratings during a disaster.

In academic writing, avoid constructions such as *the reason . . . is because.* Using both *reason* and *because* says the same thing twice.

NO One **reason** that TV news captured national attention in the 1960s **is because** it covered the Vietnam War thoroughly.

YES One **reason** TV news captured national attention in the 1960s **is that** it covered the Vietnam War thoroughly.

YES TV news captured national attention in the 1960s **because** it covered the Vietnam War thoroughly.

● **EXERCISE 36-4** Revise the mixed sentences so that the beginning of each sentence fits logically with its end. If a sentence is correct, circle its number. For help, consult 36F and 36G.

EXAMPLE

The reason a newborn baby may stare at her hands or feet is because she can only focus on nearby objects.

A newborn baby may stare at her hands or feet because she can only focus on nearby objects.

1. By showing babies plain, black-and-white images will help them learn to recognize shapes and focus their vision.
2. Even though babies can see their parents' faces will not respond with a smile until they are a few weeks old.
3. Babies may gaze intently into a small, unbreakable mirror attached to the inside of their cribs.
4. While following an object with her eyes is when eye coordination develops.
5. Because of a newborn's limited ability to see color forces him to focus only on bright colors.
6. The reason babies occasionally cross their eyes is because they are perfecting their tracking skills.
7. Whether a light sleeper or a heavy sleeper, a typical baby does not need complete silence in order to rest well.
8. The fact that newborns can vary dramatically in their sensitivity to sounds and ability to sleep in noisy environments.
9. The reason that a two-month-old baby turns her head toward her parents' voice is because she is beginning to recognize familiar sounds.
10. Through changing his facial expression indicates he may find a particular sound soothing or comforting. ●

36H What are correct elliptical constructions?

An **elliptical construction** deliberately leaves out one or more words in a sentence for CONCISENESS.

- Victor has his book and Joan's.

This means *Victor has his book and Joan's book*. The second *book* is left out deliberately.

Your elliptical constructions are correct when your discarded words are identical to words that are already in your sentence. The sample sentence above has an incorrect elliptical construction if the writer means that *Victor has his book, and Joan has her book*.

NO During the 1920s, cornetist Manuel Perez **was leading** one jazz group, and Tommy and Jimmy Dorsey another.

The words *was leading* cannot take the place of *were leading*, which is required after *Tommy and Jimmy Dorsey*.

YES During the 1920s, cornetist Manuel Perez **was leading** one jazz group, and Tommy and Jimmy Dorsey **were leading** another.

YES During the 1920s, cornetist Manuel Perez **led** one jazz group, and Tommy and Jimmy Dorsey another.

Led is correct with both *Manuel Perez* and *Tommy and Jimmy Dorsey*, so *led* can be omitted after *Dorsey*.

36I What are correct comparisons?

When you write a sentence in which you want to compare two or more things, make sure that no important words are omitted.

NO Individuals driven to achieve make **better** business executives.

Better is a word of comparison (see 32E), but no comparison is stated.

YES Individuals driven to achieve make **better** business executives **than do people not interested in personal accomplishments**.

NO Most personnel officers value high achievers **more than risk takers**.

More is a word of comparison, but it's unclear whether the sentence means that *personnel officers* or *risk takers* value achievers more.

YES Most personnel officers value high achievers **more than they value** risk takers.

YES Most personnel officers value high achievers **more than** risk takers **do**.

36J How can I proofread successfully for little words I forget to use?

If you unintentionally omit little words, such as articles, conjunctions, and prepositions, read your writing aloud or ask someone else to.

NO On May 2, 1808, citizens Madrid rioted against French soldiers and were shot.

YES On May 2, 1808, citizens **of** Madrid rioted against French soldiers and were shot.

NO The Spanish painter Francisco Goya recorded both the riot the execution in a pair of pictures painted 1814.

YES The Spanish painter Francisco Goya recorded both the riot **and** the execution in a pair of pictures painted **in** 1814.

● **EXERCISE 36-5** Revise these sentences to correct elliptical constructions, to complete comparisons, or to insert any missing words.

1. Champagne is a kind of sparkling wine grown in Champagne region France.
2. To be considered champagne, a sparkling wine must meet several conditions described French law.
3. The location of the vineyard is one requirement, and type of grapes another.
4. Most champagne producers agree that the Chardonnay and Pinot Noir grapes make champagne taste better.
5. When owners celebrate the launch of a new ship, they use bottles of champagne more often. ●

Complete the Chapter Exercises

PART

6

Writing Effectively, Writing with Style

37 Style, Tone, and the Effects of Words

Quick Points You will learn to

- Create an effective style and tone in writing (see 37A–37E).
- Use word choices that affect clarity, style, and tone (see 37F–37I).
- Avoid certain types of language (see 37J).

37A What are style and tone in writing?

Style and **tone** both refer to *how* you say something, in contrast with *what* you're saying. Consider the familiar instruction to airline passengers:

> "In preparation for landing, please return your seatbacks and tray tables to their fully upright and locked positions."

Flight attendants could provide the same directions in a different style:

> "Hey, we're landing. Put your seatbacks up, and while you're at it, put your tray tables up, too."

They could even say:

> "Our landing preparations oblige us to request your kind participation in the restoration of all seatbacks and tray tables to vertical modes."

The directions are the same, and all three examples are grammatically correct. However, you get a very different sense of the style and tone in each case. The first is polite and direct, the second is casual and chatty, and the third is pretentious and bureaucratic.

Neither style nor tone are rule bound, the way that grammar is. Writers have choices, and the kinds of words they choose and kinds of sentences they write affect style and tone. Of course, certain styles are appropriate for certain writing situations, and almost all situations require standard edited English.

37B What is standard edited English?

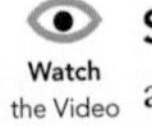
Watch the Video

Standard edited English reflects the kind of written language expected in academic, business, and serious public writings. These standards apply in magazines such as *The Atlantic* and *Time;* in newspapers such as the *Washington*

Post and the *Wall Street Journal;* and in most nonfiction books. Standard edited English conforms to the widely established rules of grammar, sentence structure, punctuation, and spelling we cover in this handbook.

Although English has become the primary global language for business and other uses, it has many varieties. For example, American English differs from British English in terms of spellings ("color" v. "colour") or vocabulary ("truck" v. "lorry"). Even within the United States there are regional and cultural differences. Regional languages, also called **dialects**, are specific to certain geographical areas. For example, a *dragonfly* is a *snake feeder* in parts of Delaware, a *darning needle* in parts of Michigan, and a *snake doctor* or an *ear sewer* in parts of the southern United States. Depending on where you live, soft drinks are known as "soda," "pop," or "Coke."

It's important to realize that people who use regional or cultural variations communicate clearly to other members of their group. There's nothing essentially "wrong" with those dialects, then—except when their speakers and writers want to communicate with wider audiences. In academic, business, and civic situations, individuals clearly benefit from "code switching" to standard edited English, even if they continue using home languages in personal situations. It's no different from needing to switch from the casual language of Facebook to the more formal language of a job application letter. You need to use standard edited English for academic writing.

37C How can I write with style?

Writing with style comes with lots of practice and revision. It rarely shows up on most first drafts. Experimenting with different sentence structures and word choices, then thinking carefully about their effects, helps you create an effective style. Quick Box 37.1 gives several tips.

Quick Box 37.1

How to create a good writing style

- Use standard edited English (see 37B).
- Choose the right level of formality, personality and voice, and creativity for each writing situation (see 37D).
- Choose an appropriate tone (see 37E).
- Use exact diction and specific words (see 37F and 37G).

continued >>

Quick Box 37.1 (continued)

- Use figurative language (see 37H).
- Use gender-neutral language (see 37I).
- Avoid manipulative language, clichés, euphemisms, jargon, and bureaucratic language (see 37J).
- Try out different sentence types to maintain readers' interest (see 38A, 38N, 38R).
- Use sentence coordination and subordination to vary the pace (see 38D–38M).
- Vary sentence length to keep your readers' attention (see 38C).
- Employ the gracefulness of parallelism in sentences and larger sections for the pleasure of your readers (see Chapter 39).

37D What defines style and tone in writing?

Style and tone operate together through a combination of varying levels of formality, voice, and creativity, as we lay out in Quick Box 37.2.

Quick Box 37.2

Elements and levels of style

Elements	Levels		
Formality	Informal	Semiformal	Formal
Voice	Intimate	Familiar/Polite	Impersonal
Surprise or creativity	Low (transparent)	Medium (translucent)	High (artistic)

The **level of formality** in writing can be roughly divided into three categories. Formal writing belongs in the structures and language of ceremonies, contracts, policies, or some literary writing. "Formal writing," by the way, doesn't mean dull and drab. **Informal writing** is casual, colloquial, and sometimes playful, usually found in text messages or social networks. Semiformal writing, which sits between these poles, is found in academic writing, as well as in much business and public writing. Its style is clear and efficient, and its tone is reasonable and evenhanded.

Generally, when you write for an audience about whom you know little, use a semiformal to formal style and tone. If informal writings are T-shirts and jeans, and formal writings are tuxedos and evening gowns, then semiformal writings are business-casual attire. Here are examples of writing in the three levels of formality.

INFORMAL	It's totally sweet how gas makes stars.
SEMIFORMAL	Gas clouds slowly transform into stars.
FORMAL	The condensations of gas spun their slow gravitational pirouettes, slowly transmogrifying gas cloud into star.

—Carl Sagan, "Starfolk: A Fable"

VOICE or **personality** refers to how much the writer calls attention to him- or herself, how much the writing conveys the presence of an individual person and, if so, what kind of person he or she seems to be. An intimate voice treats the reader as a close friend. A familiar or polite voice includes only experiences or personal thoughts that you might share in a professional relationship with an instructor, supervisor, or colleague. In such writing, the reader can glimpse the writer behind the language, but the emphasis is on content. An impersonal voice reveals nothing about the writer, so that the content is all that the reader notices.

Look at the following paragraph.

> I would be willing to bet serious money that right now in your kitchen you have olive oil, garlic, pasta, parmesan cheese, and dried basil (maybe even fresh basil!). Nothing exotic there, right? They're ingredients we take for granted. But their appearance in our kitchens is a relatively recent phenomenon. Believe me, those big-flavor items did not come over on the Mayflower. It took generations, even centuries, for Americans to expand their culinary horizons to the point where just about everybody cooks Italian and orders Chinese take-out. Heck, the supermarket in my little Connecticut hometown even has a sushi bar.
>
> —Thomas J. Craughwell, "If Only the Pilgrims Had Been Italian"

Several words and phrases in the passage create an intimate and informal voice, including "I would be willing to bet serious money," "believe me," and "heck." This is the voice of someone casual and confident enough to refer inclusively to "we" and use a chatty sentence fragment ("Nothing exotic there, right?") as if we're friends sitting in a coffee shop.

However, with a little revision, we can reduce the sound of the author's voice:

> Most kitchens have olive oil, garlic, pasta, parmesan cheese, and dried or fresh basil. Although these are ingredients people take for granted, they appeared in kitchens relatively recently. They did not come over on the Mayflower. It took generations, even centuries, for Americans to expand their culinary horizons to the point where just about everybody cooks Italian and orders Chinese take-out. Even a small town supermarket may have a sushi bar.

Writers can get carried away with voice, creating one that is too friendly, self-important, or even annoying: A strong voice is inappropriate in some writing situations, including some academic writing and most business writing.

INTIMATE	Ever since I was a kid, TV shows with stupid characters bugged me. Do you maybe think it's because I've screwed up so much myself that I hate having my nose rubbed in it?
FAMILIAR/POLITE	I am frequently embarrassed by certain characters' actions on television shows.
IMPERSONAL	Characters' actions on television shows occasionally prove a source of embarrassment to certain viewers.

Creativity refers to the "surprise" element in writing, the degree to which readers notice the language itself rather than the content the language conveys. Consider, for example, the difference between "The room was red" and "The room was the color of a Daytona Beach sunburn." Figurative language (see 37C) creates surprise or calls attention to language. Writing that has a low level of surprises is *transparent*, like a clear window; readers scarcely notice its language. Writing with a medium level of surprises is *translucent*, like a lightly colored pane of glass; readers occasionally notice and appreciate the language, but content is primary. If a piece of writing is consistently surprising, it is *artistic*, like a stained glass window; the language frequently demands attention to itself.

TRANSPARENT	The acting in the film was unsuccessful, and the plot was dull.
TRANSLUCENT	The acting in the film was dismal, the plot a test of endurance.
ARTISTIC	Watching the acting and enduring the plot was like eating pizza that lacked a crust: frustrating, unsatisfying, and making you wish you hadn't taken a bite.

Of course, "artistic" does not necessarily mean better; extensive creativity is inappropriate in many writing situations. If you're writing instructions, science reports, or business projects, for example, you don't want language that calls attention to itself. A translucent or transparent style, however, will serve you well in most academic situations.

● **EXERCISE 37-1** Working individually or in a group, describe the style of each of the following paragraphs in terms of formality, voice, and surpise.

1. Google has yet to hit upon a strategy that combines the innovation it is known for with an appeal to the self-interest that is the currency of the capital's power brokers. One reason AT&T and Microsoft have succeeded in stoking antitrust interest against Google—quite ironic, given that both companies

have been subject to large government antitrust actions—is that they're better versed in the fine points of lobbying. Both companies, for example, hold sway over many lawmakers by frequently reminding them how many employees live in their districts ("jobs" is a metric lawmakers respond to).

—Joshua Green, "Google's Tar Pit"

2. Prices are rising for the black sludge that helps make the world's gears turn. If you think we're talking about oil, think again. Petroleum prices have tumbled from their record highs. No sooner was there relief at the pump, however, than came a squeeze at the pot. That jolt of coffee that a majority of American adults enjoy on a daily basis has gotten more expensive and could go even higher this year. . . .

—*New York Times*, "Joe Economics"

3. In addition to participating in the promulgation of Treasury (Tax) Regulations, the IRS publishes a regular series of other forms of official tax guidance, including revenue rulings, revenue procedures, notices, and announcements. See Understanding IRS Guidance—A Brief Primer for more information about official IRS guidance versus non-precedential rulings or advice.

—Internal Revenue Service, "Tax Code, Regulations, and Official Guidance"

4. Studies of home-based telework by women yield mixed results regarding the usefulness of telework in facilitating work–life balance. Most research on the social impacts of home-based telework focuses on workers—employees or self-employed—who deliberately choose that alternative work arrangement. Labour force analysts, however, predict an increase in employer-initiated teleworking. As a case study of the workforce of one large, financial-sector firm in Canada, this article considers the conditions of employment of involuntary teleworkers, those required by their employer to work full-time from a home office. In-depth interviews were conducted with a sample of 18 female teleworkers working for the case study firm in a professional occupation.

—Laura C. Johnson, Jean Andrey, and Susan M. Shaw, "Mr. Dithers Comes to Dinner"

5. I remember vividly the moment that I entered the world of literacy, education, institutional "correctness," and, consequently, identity. I was demonstrating to my older sister how I wrote my name. The memory comes after I had been literally taught how to do it—which strokes of the pencil to use to create the symbols that equate to my name.

—Elise Geraghty, "In the Name of the Father" ●

● **EXERCISE 37-2** Select one of the paragraphs in Exercise 37-1. Revise that paragraph to create a very different voice for it. ●

37E What is tone in writing?

Tone in writing operates like tone of voice, except that you can't rely on facial expressions and voice intonations to communicate your message. Your choice of words determines how your readers "hear" you, and we list several different tones and examples in Quick Box 37.3.

Achieving the tone you want calls for experimenting with different words with similar meanings. If you consult a thesaurus, be sure to check the definition of any synonym that's new to you. Lynn once had an excellent student who used the word "profound" instead of "deep," without looking it up in a dictionary. The result was this sentence: "The trenches beneath some parts of that sea were dangerously profound." That misuse ruined an otherwise intelligent passage.

As with style, appropriate tone results from trying options. Quick Box 37.4 offers you some suggestions.

Quick Box 37.3

Some examples of desirable and undesirable tone

SERIOUS	It is important to respect the rights of all individuals participating in the meeting.
LIGHT OR BREEZY	Be nice to all the folks at the meeting, OK?
SARCASTIC	I suppose we'll all live happily ever after if we just smile and have tea and cupcakes.
MEAN	Respect others or suffer the consequences.
CONDESCENDING	Now, everyone, I know it's asking a lot of your little brains to understand, but please play nice with each other during our meeting today.
PRETENTIOUS	The degree of niceness displayed by meeting participants to one another, especially regarding each individual's rights, must be high in order to create optimal outcomes.
WHINING	It's so hard when we don't respect each other, so can't we please, for just this once and just for me, have a polite meeting?

Quick Box 37.4

How to use appropriate tone in writing

- Reserve a highly informal tone for conversational writing.
- Use a semiformal tone in your academic writing and when you write for supervisors, professionals, and other people you know only from a distance.
- Choose a tone that suits your topic and your readers.
- Whatever tone you choose, be consistent throughout a piece of writing.

● **EXERCISE 37-3** Revise each of the sentences to create a very different tone. The sentences in Quick Box 37.3 provide some examples. For a further challenge, see how many different tones you can create.

1. Many Americans spend much of their leisure time watching professional sports.
2. If you want to waste your money buying organic foods, who am I to stop you?
3. When considering the purchase of clothing in order to possess a serviceable wardrobe, it is imperative to select items in which the color combinations are harmonious and pleasing. ●

37F How can using exact diction enhance my writing?

Diction refers to your word choices. Your best chance of delivering your intended message is to choose words that fit your meaning exactly. To choose words exactly—that is, to have good diction—be alert to the concepts of DENOTATION and CONNOTATION.

37F.1 What is denotation in words?

The **denotation** of a word is its exact, literal meaning found in a reliable dictionary.

- An unabridged dictionary contains the most extensive, complete, and scholarly entries. *Unabridged* means "not shortened." The most comprehensive, authoritative unabridged dictionary of English is the *Oxford English Dictionary* (OED), which traces each word's history and gives quotations to illustrate changes in meaning and spelling over the life of the word.

- An abridged dictionary contains most commonly used words. *Abridged* means "shortened." Abridged dictionaries that serve the needs of most college students are "college editions." Typical of these are *Merriam-Webster's Collegiate Dictionary* (available online and in print) and *The New American Webster Handy College Dictionary*.
- A specialized dictionary focuses on a single area of language. You can find dictionaries of **slang** (for example, *Dictionary of Slang and Unconventional English*); word origins (for example, *Dictionary of Word and Phrase Origins*); synonyms (for example, *Roget's 21st Century Thesaurus*); **usage** (for example, *Garner's Modern American Usage*); idioms (for example, *A Dictionary of American Idioms*); regionalisms (for example, *Dictionary of American Regional English*); and many others.

ESOL Tip: *The Oxford Dictionary of American English* is particularly useful for students who speak English as a second (or third) language.

37F.2 What is connotation in words?

Connotation refers to ideas associated with a word. For example, *home* usually evokes more emotion than its denotation "a dwelling place" or its synonym *house*. *Home* carries the connotation, for some, of the pleasures of warmth, security, and love of family. For others, however, *home* may carry unpleasant connotations, such as abusive experiences.

USING A THESAURUS

In distinguishing among SYNONYMS—words close in meaning to each other—a thesaurus demonstrates connotation in operation. As you use a thesaurus, remain alert to the subtle differences of meaning. For instance, using *notorious* to describe a person famous for praiseworthy achievements is wrong. Although *notorious* means "well-known" and "publicly discussed"—which is true of famous people—the connotation of the word is "unfavorably known or talked about." George Washington is famous, not notorious. Adolf Hitler, by contrast, is notorious.

Alert: Most word-processing programs include a thesaurus. But be cautious in using it. Unless you know the exact meaning and part of speech of a synonym, you may choose a wrong word or create a grammatical error. For example, one thesaurus offers these synonyms for *deep* in the sense of "low (down, inside)": *low, below, beneath*, and *subterranean*. None of these could replace *deep* in a sentence such as *The crater is too deep* [not *too low, too below, too beneath*, or *too subterranean*] *to be filled with sand or rocks.*

● **EXERCISE 37-4** Working individually or with a group, look at each list of words and divide the words among three headings: "Positive" (good connotations); "Negative" (bad connotations); and "Neutral" (no connotations). If you think that a word belongs under more than one heading, you can assign it more than once, but be ready to explain your thinking. For help, consult a good dictionary.

EXAMPLE

assertive, pushy, firm, forceful, confident

Positive: assertive, confident; *Negative:* pushy, forceful; *Neutral:* firm

1. old, decrepit, elderly, mature, over the hill, venerable, veteran, antique, experienced
2. resting, inactive, unproductive, downtime, recess, quietude, standstill, vacation, interval
3. smart, know-it-all, brilliant, eggheaded, brainy, sharp, ingenious, keen, clever, intelligent
4. weird, unique, peculiar, strange, eccentric, inscrutable, peculiar, kooky, singular, one-of-a-kind, distinctive
5. smell, aroma, stench, fragrance, scent, whiff, bouquet, odor ●

37G How can using specific words enhance my writing?

Specific words identify individual items in a group (*snap peas, sweet corn*). General words relate to an overall group (*food*). Concrete words identify what can be perceived by the senses, by being seen, heard, tasted, felt, smelled (*warm, juicy cherry pie*), and convey specific images and details. Abstract words denote qualities (*nice*), concepts (*speed*), relationships (*friends*), acts (*cooking*), conditions (*bad weather*), and ideas (*justice*) and are more general.

Usually, specific and concrete words bring life to general and abstract words. Therefore, whenever you use general and abstract words, try to supply enough specific, concrete details and examples to illustrate them. Here are sentences with general words that come to life when revised with specific words.

GENERAL His car gets good gas mileage.

SPECIFIC His Miser gets about 35 mpg on the highway and 30 mpg in the city.

GENERAL Her car is comfortable and easy to drive.

SPECIFIC When she drives her new Cushia on a five-hour trip, she arrives refreshed and does not need a long nap to recover, as she did when she drove her ten-year-old Beater.

What separates most good writing from bad is the writer's ability to move back and forth between the general and the specific. Consider these sentences that effectively use a combination of general and specific words:

- The carnival at night [GENERAL], a shimmering glow of blue, red, and neon lights [CONCRETE], was amazing [ABSTRACT]. The Pikes Peak Plummet [SPECIFIC], a hundred foot tower of black metal and chrome [CONCRETE], hurled twenty riders down a sixty-degree slope [CONCRETE]. The Whirlpool [SPECIFIC] spun screaming teens [CONCRETE] in an open cylinder [GENERAL], bathing them in fluorescent strobe lights [CONCRETE].

● **EXERCISE 37-5** Revise this paragraph by providing specific and concrete words and phrases to explain and enliven the ideas presented here in general and abstract language. You may revise the sentences to accommodate your changes.

> A while ago, I visited a nice restaurant. It was located in a good neighborhood, and it was easy to find. The inside of the restaurant was pretty. There were a lot of decorations, which gave it character. The menu was creative and interesting. The food was delivered quickly, and the service was friendly. I enjoyed eating the meal. The appetizers were delicious and refreshing. The price of the meal was reasonable considering how much food I ordered. ●

37H What is figurative language?

Figurative language makes comparisons and connections that draw on one idea or image to enhance another. Quick Box 37.5 explains the different types of figurative language and describes one type you should avoid, the **mixed metaphor**.

Quick Box 37.5

Types of figurative language

- **Analogy:** Comparing similar traits shared by dissimilar things or ideas. Its length can vary from one sentence (which often takes the form of a simile or metaphor) to a paragraph.
  - A **cheetah sprinting across the dry plains** after its prey, the **base runner dashed** for home plate, cleats kicking up dust.

continued >>

Quick Box 37.5 (continued)

- **Irony:** Using words to suggest the opposite of their usual sense.
  - Told that a minor repair on her home would cost $2,000 and take two weeks, she said, **"Oh, how nice!"**
- **Metaphor:** Comparing otherwise dissimilar things. A metaphor doesn't use the word *like* or *as* to make a comparison. (See below about not using mixed metaphors.)
  - Rush-hour **traffic** in the city **bled out through major arteries** to the suburbs.
- **Personification:** Assigning a human trait to something not human.
  - The **book begged** to be read.
- **Overstatement** (also called *hyperbole*): Exaggerating deliberately for emphasis.
  - If this paper is late, the professor will **kill** me.
- **Simile:** Comparing dissimilar things. A simile uses the word *like* or *as*.
  - Langston Hughes observes that a deferred **dream dries up "like a raisin in the sun."**
- **Understatement:** Emphasizing by using deliberate restraint.
  - It feels **warm** when the temperature reaches **105 degrees**.
- **Mixed metaphor:** Combining two or more inconsistent images in one sentence or expression. Never use a mixed metaphor.

NO The violence of the hurricane reminded me of a train ride.
A train ride is not violent, stormy, or destructive.

YES The violence of the hurricane reminded me of a train's crashing into a huge tractor trailer.

● **EXERCISE 37-6** Working individually or with a group, identify each type of figurative language or figure of speech. Also revise any mixed metaphors.

1. Exercise for the body is like education for the mind.
2. Waking up in the morning to exercise can be as hard as starting a car with a dead battery.
3. Exercise is the key ingredient in the recipe for a healthy life.
4. When I started my diet, I was dying of hunger!
5. When you exercise, pull out all the stops so you that you can put the pedal to the metal.
6. That last mile of my run punished me without mercy.
7. Exercising a muscle is like practicing an instrument.

8. "Oh, I feel absolutely great," she gasped after finishing a long run.
9. If the body is a temple, then regular exercise keeps the temple clean and strong.
10. Nothing good can happen in your life unless you exercise. ●

37l What is gender-neutral language?

Watch the Video

Gender-neutral language, also called *gender-free* or *nonsexist language*, uses terms that don't draw unnecessary attention to whether the person is male or female (for example, in replacing *policeman* with *police officer* or *doctors' wives* with *doctors' spouses*).

Sexist language assigns roles or characteristics to people based on their sex and discriminates against both men and women. For example, it assumes that nurses and homemakers are female by calling them "she," and that surgeons and stockbrokers are male by calling them "he." One common instance of sexist language occurs when writers us the pronoun *he* for anyone whose sex is unknown or irrelevant. Using masculine pronouns to represent all people distorts reality.

Nearly all businesses and professional organizations use gender-neutral language in written communications. This sound business practice promotes accuracy and fairness and includes all potential clients.

Gender-neutral language rejects demeaning **stereotypes** or outdated assumptions, such as "women are bad drivers" and "real men don't cry." In academic writing, treat both sexes equally. For example if you describe a woman by her looks, clothes, or age, do the same for a man in that context. Refer to names and titles in the same way for both men and women. Quick Box 37.6 offers you guidelines.

Quick Box 37.6

How to avoid sexist language

- Avoid using only the masculine pronoun to refer to males and females together. The *he or she* and *his or hers* phrases act as singular PRONOUNS that require singular VERBS. Avoid using *he or she* constructions more than once in a sentence or in consecutive sentences. Try switching to plural or omitting the gender-specific pronoun.

  NO A **doctor** has little time to read outside **his** specialty.

  YES A **doctor** has little time to read outside **his or her** specialty.

continued >>

Quick Box 37.6 (continued)

NO A successful **stockbroker** knows **he** has to work long hours.
YES Successful **stockbrokers** know **they** have to work long hours.

NO **Everyone** hopes that **he or she** will win the scholarship.
YES **Everyone** hopes to win the scholarship.

- Avoid using *man* when referring to both men and women.

NO **Man** is a social animal.
YES **People** are social animals.

NO The history of **mankind** is predominately violent.
YES **Human** history is predominately violent.

NO Dogs are **men's** best friends.
YES Dogs are **people's** best friends.

- Avoid stereotyping jobs and roles by **gender** when referring to both men and women.

NO	YES
chairman	chair, chairperson
policeman	police officer
businessman	businessperson, business executive
statesman	statesperson, diplomat
teacher . . . she	teachers . . . they
principal . . . he	principals . . . they

- Avoid expressions that seem to exclude one sex.

NO	YES
the common man	the average person
man-sized sandwich	huge sandwich
old wives' tale	superstition

- Avoid using demeaning and patronizing labels.

NO	YES
male nurse	nurse
gal Friday	assistant
coed	student
My girl can help.	My secretary can help. (*Or, better still:* Ida Morea can help.)

● **EXERCISE 37-7** Working individually or with a group, revise these sentences by changing sexist language to gender-neutral language. For help, consult 37I.

1. Dogs were one of the first animals to be domesticated by mankind.
2. Traditionally, certain breeds of dogs have helped men in their work.
3. On their long shifts, firemen often kept Dalmatians as mascots and companions, whereas policemen preferred highly intelligent and easily trained German shepherds.
4. Another breed, the Newfoundland, accompanied many fishermen on their ocean voyages, and the Newfoundland has been credited with rescuing many a man overboard.
5. Breeds known as hunting dogs have served as the helpers and companions of sportsmen.
6. Maids and cleaning women didn't need dogs, so no breed of dog is associated with women's work.
7. Another group that dogs have not helped is postmen.
8. Everyone who owns a dog should be sure to spend some time exercising his dog and making sure his dog is in good health.
9. No man-made inventions, such as televisions or computers, can take the place of having a dog.
10. Now even though most dogs do not work, they are still man's best friend. ●

Alert: Increasingly, you see "they" or "their" used as a singular pronoun, as in "Someone tripped and broke their nose." The English language continually changes, and perhaps in a few years this growing usage will become perfectly acceptable because it fills a need: English lacks a gender-neutral singular pronoun. However, such usage is still considered nonstandard in most academic and professional settings. ●

37J What other types of language do I want to avoid?

In addition to avoiding sexist language, you need also to avoid several other kinds of language. We summarize this advice in Quick Box 37.7.

37J.1 Clichés

A **cliché** is an expression that has become worn out from overuse. Examples of clichés are *cheap as dirt*, *dead as a doornail*, and *straight as an arrow*. If you've heard certain expressions repeatedly, so has your reader. Try substituting your own fresh wording.

Quick Box 37.7

Language to avoid in academic writing

- Never use **slanted language**, also called *loaded language;* readers feel manipulated by the overly emotional TONE and DICTION.

  NO Our senator is a deceitful, crooked thug.

  YES Our senator lies to the public and demands bribes.

  NO Why do labs hire monsters to maim helpless kittens and puppies?

  YES Why do labs employ technicians who harm kittens and puppies?

- Never use pretentious language; readers realize you're showing off.

  NO As I alighted from my vehicle, my clothing became besmirched with filth.

  YES My coat got muddy as I got out of my car.

  NO He has a penchant for ostentatiously flaunting recently acquired haberdashery accoutrements.

  YES He tends to show off his new clothes shamelessly.

- Never use sarcastic language; readers realize you're being nasty.

  NO He was a regular Albert Einstein with my questions.

  This is sarcastic if you mean the opposite.

  YES He had trouble understanding my questions.

- Never use **colloquial language;** readers sense you're being overly casual and conversational.

  NO Christina tanked chemistry.

  YES Christina failed chemistry.

- Never use nonstandard English.
- Never use SEXIST LANGUAGE or STEREOTYPES (see 37I).
- Never use CLICHÉS (see 37J.1).
- Never use unnecessary JARGON (see 37J.2).
- Never use EUPHEMISMS, also called *doublespeak;* readers realize you're hiding the truth (more in 37J.3).
- Never use BUREAUCRATIC LANGUAGE (see 37J.4).

Interestingly, however, English is full of idioms that aren't clichés, phrases like *by and large* or and *from place to place*. You can use them freely. If you're not sure of how to tell the difference between a cliché and a common word group, remember that a cliché often—but not always—contains an image (*busy as a bee* and *strong as an ox*).

● **EXERCISE 37-8** Working individually or with a group, revise these clichés. Use the idea in each cliché to write a sentence of your own in plain, clear English.

1. The Raging Manatees softball players came to grips with the fact that their upcoming game would be a tough row to hoe.
2. The bottom line was that their worthy opponents, the Fierce Sunflowers, took no prisoners.
3. Still, the Manatees knew that they had to play like there was no tomorrow, because taking it one game at time would be the key to success.
4. Snatching victory from the jaws of defeat depended on remembering that their opponents still put on uniforms one leg at a time.
5. Although the effort would be Herculean, at the end of the day, the Manatees knew they could make the best of a bad situation. After all, the bigger they are, the harder they fall. ●

37J.2 Jargon

Jargon is the specialized vocabulary of a particular group, whether in academic disciplines, certain industries, hobbies, sports, and so on. Jargon uses words that people outside that group might not understand.

Reserve jargon for a specialist AUDIENCE. For example, a football fan easily understands a sportswriter's use of words such as *punt* and *safety*, but they are jargon words to people unfamiliar with American-style football. When you must use jargon for a nonspecialist audience, be sure to explain any special meanings.

The following example from a college textbook uses appropriate specialized language. The authors can assume that students know the meaning of *eutrophicates, terrestrial*, and *eutrophic.*

> As the lake eutrophicates, it gradually fills until the entire lake will be converted into a terrestrial community. Eutrophic changes (or eutrophication) are the nutritional enrichment of the water, promoting the growth of aquatic plants.
>
> —Davis and Solomon, *The World of Biology*

37J.3 Euphemisms

A **euphemism** is a more pleasing way of stating something that people find unpleasant. Sometimes, good manners dictate that we use euphemisms like *passed away* instead of *died.*

At other times, however, euphemisms drain truth from your writing. Unnecessary euphemisms might describe socially unacceptable behavior (for example, *Lee has an artfully vivid imagination* instead of *Lee lies*) or try to hide facts (for example, *He is between jobs* instead of *He's unemployed*). Avoid unnecessary euphemisms.

NO Our company will **downsize** to meet efficiency standards.

YES Our company has to cut jobs to maintain our profits.

NO We consider our hostages as **foreign guests** guarded by **hosts**.

YES We consider our hostages as enemies to be guarded closely.

37J.4 Bureaucratic language

Bureaucratic language uses words that are stuffy, overblown, and unnecessarily complex. This kind of language complicates the message and makes readers feel left out.

NO Given the certitude of deleterious outcomes from the implementation of pending policy changes, it shall be incumbent upon us to remedy negative consequences with positive alternatives as yet to be determined. In the event that said outcomes are to be derived and agreed upon by all constituencies having stake in their deployment, a directive shall be issued to each and every stakeholder for the purpose of responding to anticipated negative policy change outcome eventualities.

—from a corporate human resources manual

We would like to give a YES alternative for this example but regret that we can't understand enough of it to do so. If you, gentle reader, can, please contact us at doug.hesse@gmail.com or 2LTROYKA@gmail.com.

● **EXERCISE 37-9** Working individually or with a group, revise these examples of pretentious language, jargon, euphemisms, and bureaucratic language. For help, consult 37J.

1. Allow me to express my humble gratitude to you two benefactors for your generous pledge of indispensable support on behalf of the activities of our Bay City's youngsters.
2. No lateral transfer applications will be processed before an employee's six-month probation period terminates.
3. She gave up the ghost shortly after her husband kicked the bucket.
4. Creating nouns in positions meant for verbs is to utter ostentatious verbalizations that will lead inexorably to further obfuscations of meaning.
5. After his operation, he would list to port when he stood up and list to starboard when he sat down.

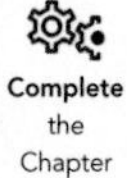
Complete the Chapter Exercises

6. The precious youths were joy riding in a temporarily displaced vehicle.
7. The forwarding of all electronic communiqués must be approved by a staff member in the upper echelon.
8. Coming to a parting of the ways is not as easy as pie. ●

38 Sentence Variety and Style

Quick Points You will learn to

- Use a variety of sentence patterns to give interest to your writing (see 38A, 38L–38P).
- Use variety and emphasis in your sentences (see 38B–38K).

38A How do sentences affect style?

Sentences affect style through their length (see 38C), structures like COORDINATION and SUBORDINATION (see 38K), and types. The main sentence types in English are SIMPLE, COMPOUND, COMPLEX, and COMPOUND-COMPLEX (see 28Q). A flurry of short, simple sentences creates a blunt style but loses readers' interest. A series of long compound, complex, or compound-complex sentences creates a lofty or stuffy style but sacrifices clarity. You can see the difference in the two versions of the same piece below.

1. Short, simple sentences

> The most worshipped and praised of all ancient sewers was Rome's Cloaca Maxima. It resided within the shrine of the goddess Cloacina. Warriors came here to purge themselves after battle. Young couples purified themselves here before marriage. The lovely Cloacina was an emanation of Venus. Her statue overlooked the imperial city's sewer pipes. The pipes transported 100,000 pounds of ancient *excrementum* [human waste] a day. It was built in the sixth century B.C. by the two Tarquins. It was hailed as one of the three marvels of Rome. The Cloaca became one of the city's great tourist traps. Agrippa rode a boat through it. Nero washed his hands in it.

2. Longer, compound and complex sentences

> The most worshipped and praised of all ancient sewers was Rome's Cloaca Maxima, whose spirit resided within the shrine of the goddess Cloacina, where warriors came to purge themselves after battle and young couples purified themselves before marriage. The lovely Cloacina was an emanation of Venus, and her statue overlooked the imperial city's sewer pipes as they transported 100,000 pounds of ancient *excrementum* [human waste] a day. Built in the sixth century B.C. by the two Tarquins, hailed as one of the three marvels of Rome, the Cloaca became one of the city's great tourist traps. Agrippa rode a boat through it. Nero washed his hands in it.
>
> —Frederick Kaufman, "Wasteland"

The second version was published in *Harper's Magazine*, which is aimed at a well-educated general AUDIENCE. Even that version ends with two simple sentences, a refreshing break after the longer ones. In fact, effective and stylistically interesting writing often contains a VARIETY of styles.

38B What are variety and emphasis in writing?

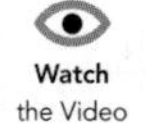

When you write sentences of different lengths and types, you create sentence variety. Along with sentence variety, emphasis adds weight to important ideas.

Using techniques of variety and emphasis adds style and clarity to your writing. As you revise, apply the principles of variety and emphasis.

38C How do different sentence lengths create variety and emphasis?

To emphasize one idea among many others, you can express it in a sentence noticeably different in length from the sentences surrounding it. In the following example, a four-word sentence between two longer sentences carries the key message of the passage (**boldface** added).

> Today is one of those excellent January partly cloudies in which light chooses an unexpected landscape to trick out in gilt, and then shadow sweeps it away. **You know you're alive**. You take huge steps, trying to feel the planet's roundness arc between your feet.
>
> —Annie Dillard, *Pilgrim at Tinker Creek*

Sometimes a string of short sentences creates impact and emphasis. Yet, at other times, a string of short sentences can be dull to read.

● **EXERCISE 38-1** The following paragraph is dull because it has only short sentences. Combine some of the sentences to make a paragraph that has a variety of sentence lengths.

> There is a problem. It is widely known as sick-building syndrome. It comes from indoor air pollution. It causes office workers to suffer. They have trouble breathing. They have painful rashes. Their heads ache. Their eyes burn. ●

Similarly, a string of COMPOUND SENTENCES can be monotonous to read and may fail to communicate relationships among ideas.

● **EXERCISE 38-2** The following paragraph is dull because it has only compound sentences. Revise it to provide more variety.

> Science fiction writers are often thinkers, **and** they are often dreamers, **and** they let their imaginations wander. Jules Verne was such a writer, **and** he predicted spaceships, **and** he forecast atomic submarines, **but** most people did not believe airplanes were possible. ●

38D What are coordination and subordination?

Watch the Video

Coordination is an arrangement of ideas of approximately equal importance. **Subordination**, by contrast, arranges ideas of unequal importance. Using these arrangements effectively creates variety and emphasis in your writing. We explain these further in 38E and 38H, but here's an example.

TWO SENTENCES	The sky grew cloudy. The wind howled.
USING COORDINATION	The sky grew cloudy, and the wind howled.
USING SUBORDINATION 1	As the sky grew cloudy, the wind howled.
	Here, the *wind* receives the focus.
USING SUBORDINATION 2	As the wind howled, the sky grew cloudy.
	Here the *sky* receives the focus.

38E What is coordination of sentences?

COORDINATION of sentences is an arrangement of equivalent or balanced ideas in two or more INDEPENDENT CLAUSES. Coordination produces harmony by bringing related elements together. Whenever you use the device of coordination of sentences, be sure that it communicates the meaning you intend.

- The sky turned **brighter, and** people emerged happily from buildings.
- The sky turned **brighter;** people emerged happily from buildings.

38F What is the structure of a coordinate sentence?

A **coordinate sentence**, also called a *compound sentence* (28Q), consists of two or more INDEPENDENT CLAUSES joined either by a semicolon or by a comma and a COORDINATING CONJUNCTION. Here is the pattern for coordination of sentences.

Independent clause { **, and** / **, but** / **, for** / **, or** / **, nor** / **, yet** / **, so** / **;** } independent clause.

38G What meaning does each coordinating conjunction convey?

When you use a **coordinating conjunction**, be sure that its meaning expresses the relationship between the equivalent ideas that you intend.

- **and** means addition
- **but** and **yet** mean contrast
- **for** means reason or choice
- **or** means choice
- **nor** means negative choice
- **so** means result or effect

Alert: Always use a comma before a coordinating conjunction that joins two INDEPENDENT CLAUSES (42B).●

38H How can I use coordination effectively?

COORDINATION is effective when each INDEPENDENT CLAUSE is related or equivalent. If they aren't, the result is an illogical pairing of unrelated ideas.

NO Computers came into common use in the 1970s, and they sometimes make costly errors.

The two ideas ideas are not related or equivalent.

YES Computers came into common use in the 1970s, and now they are indispensable business tools.

Coordination also succeeds when it's not overused. Simply bundling sentences together with COORDINATING CONJUNCTIONS overburdens readers.

NO Dinosaurs could have disappeared for many reasons, **and** one theory holds that a sudden shower of meteors and asteroids hit the earth, **so** the impact created a huge dust cloud that caused a false winter. The winter lasted for years, **and** the dinosaurs died.

YES Dinosaurs could have disappeared for many reasons. One theory holds that a sudden shower of meteors and asteroids hit the earth. The impact created a huge dust cloud that caused a false winter. The winter lasted for years, killing the dinosaurs.

● **EXERCISE 38-3** Working individually or with a group, revise these sentences to eliminate illogical or overused coordination. If you think a sentence needs no revision, explain why.

EXAMPLE

The ratel is an animal often called a "honey badger," and it's actually more closely related to a weasel than a badger.

The ratel is an animal often called a "honey badger," **but** it's actually more closely related to a weasel than a badger.

1. The honey badger is a difficult opponent for predators, and it has thick, loose skin that protects it from injury, and it is able to fight fiercely with its strong claws.
2. Honey badgers are known to be fearless fighters, but they can often survive bites from venomous snakes.
3. They are skilled at digging their own burrows, but these holes usually only have one passage and are not very large.
4. Primarily carnivorous, honey badgers hunt rodents, snakes, and even tortoises, so at times they also eat vegetables, roots, and berries.
5. Honey badgers are difficult to kill and are expert burrowers, but they are a common nuisance to farmers and ranchers. ●

38l What is subordination in sentences?

SUBORDINATION is an arrangement of ideas of unequal importance within a sentence. Subordination is effective when you place the more important idea in an INDEPENDENT CLAUSE and the less important, subordinate idea in a DEPENDENT CLAUSE. Let your own judgment decide which of your ideas is most important, and subordinate other ideas to it.

INDEPENDENT CLAUSE — DEPENDENT CLAUSE

- Two cowboys fought a dangerous Colorado snowstorm **while they were looking for cattle.** **When they came to a canyon**, they saw outlines of buildings through the blizzard.

DEPENDENT CLAUSE — INDEPENDENT CLAUSE

The passage below conveys the same message without subordination.

- Two cowboys fought a dangerous Colorado snowstorm. They were looking for cattle. They came to a canyon. They saw outlines of buildings through the blizzard.

38J What is the structure of a subordinate sentence?

A subordinate sentence starts the DEPENDENT CLAUSE with either a SUBORDINATING CONJUNCTION or a RELATIVE PRONOUN.

If they are very lucky, the passengers may glimpse dolphins near the ship.

—Elizabeth Gray, student

Pandas are solitary animals, **which** means they are difficult to protect from extinction.

—Jose Santos, student

For patterns of subordination, see Quick Box 38.1. Dependent clauses are either ADVERB CLAUSES or ADJECTIVE CLAUSES. An adverb clause starts with a subordinating conjunction. An adjective clause starts with a relative pronoun.

Quick Box 38.1

Subordination

SENTENCES WITH ADVERB CLAUSES

- **Adverb clause**, independent clause.
  - **After the sky grew dark**, the wind died suddenly.
- Independent clause, **adverb clause**.
  - Birds stopped singing, **as they do during an eclipse**.
- Independent clause **adverb clause**.
  - The stores closed **before the storm began**.

continued >>

Quick Box 38.1 (continued)

SENTENCES WITH ADJECTIVE CLAUSES

- Independent clause **restrictive (essential)* adjective clause**.
  - Forecasts warned of a storm **that might bring a ten-inch snowfall**.
- Independent clause, **nonrestrictive (nonessential)* adjective clause**.
  - Spring is the season for tornadoes, **which may have wind speeds over 220 miles an hour**.
- Beginning of independent clause **restrictive (essential)* adjective clause** end of independent clause.
  - Anyone **who lives through a tornado** remembers its power.
- Beginning of independent clause, **nonrestrictive (nonessential)* adjective clause**, end of independent clause.
  - The sky, **which had been clear**, turned greenish black.

*For an explanation of RESTRICTIVE and NONRESTRICTIVE ELEMENTS, see section 42F.

38K What meaning does each subordinating conjunction convey?

When you choose a SUBORDINATING CONJUNCTION, be sure that its meaning expresses the relationship between the ideas that you want to convey. Quick Box 38.2 lists subordinating conjunctions according to their different meanings.

Quick Box 38.2

Subordinating conjunctions and their meanings

TIME

after, before, once, since, until, when, whenever, while

- **After** you have handed in your report, you cannot revise it.

REASON OR CAUSE

as, because, since

- **Because** you have handed in your report, you cannot revise it.

PURPOSE OR RESULT

in order that, so that, that

- I want to read your report **so that** I can evaluate it.

continued >>

Quick Box 38.2 (continued)

CONDITION

even if, if, provided that, unless

- **Unless** you have handed in your report, you can revise it.

CONTRAST

although, even though, though, whereas, while

- **Although** you have handed in your report, you can ask to revise it.

CHOICE

than, whether

- You took more time to revise **than** I did before the lab report deadline.

PLACE OR LOCATION

where, wherever

- **Wherever** you say, I'll come to hand in my report.

EXERCISE 38-4 Working individually or with a group, combine each pair of sentences, using an adverb clause to subordinate one idea. Then, revise each sentence so that the adverb clause becomes the independent clause.

EXAMPLE

The U.S. Mint produces new coins. The U.S. Bureau of Engraving and Printing makes $1, $5, $10, $20, $50, and $100 bills.

a. While the U.S. Mint produces new coins, the U.S. Bureau of Engraving and Printing makes $1, $5, $10, $20, $50, and $100 bills.

b. While the U.S. Bureau of Engraving and Printing makes $1, $5, $10, $20, $50, and $100 bills, the U.S. Mint produces new coins.

1. The U.S. Mint can produce more than 50 million coins a day. The U.S. Bureau of Engraving and Printing can produce 20 million notes a day.
2. The Federal Reserve Banks are responsible for both destroying old money and ordering new coins and notes. They must keep the right amount of money in circulation.
3. Coins can stay in circulation for decades. People let them accumulate in jars and drawers in their homes.
4. A $1 bill lasts about fifteen to eighteen months. It reaches its average life span.
5. The U.S. Federal Reserve Banks destroy dirty, worn, and torn bills. The Federal Reserve Banks are destroying more than $40 billion worth of money a year.

● **EXERCISE 38-5** Working individually or with a group, combine each pair of sentences, using an adjective clause to subordinate one idea to the other. Then, revise each sentence so that the adjective clause becomes the independent clause. Use the relative pronoun given in parentheses. For help, consult sections 38I through 38K, especially Quick Box 38.1.

EXAMPLE

Aristides was an ancient Greek politician famous for his honesty and judgment. He was known as Aristides the Just. (who)

a. Aristides, *who* was an ancient Greek politician famous for his honesty and judgment, was known as Aristides the Just.

b. Aristides, *who* was known as Aristides the Just, was an ancient Greek politician famous for his honesty and judgment.

1. An ancient Greek law allowed voters to banish politicians from their city. It asked citizens to write the name of an unpopular politician on their ballots. (that)
2. A voter was filling out a ballot when Aristides the Just walked by. The voter needed help in spelling *Aristides*. (who)
3. Aristides knew the voter did not recognize him. He asked why the voter wanted to banish that particular politician. (who)
4. The voter said he resented hearing someone called "the Just" all the time. He handed Aristides his ballot. (who)
5. Aristides' reaction demonstrated that the nickname "the Just" was well deserved. His reaction was to write his own name on the voter's ballot even though that person's vote helped banish Aristides. (which) ●

38L How can I use subordination effectively?

Effective SUBORDINATING CONJUNCTIONS communicate a logical relationship between the INDEPENDENT CLAUSE and the DEPENDENT CLAUSE. See Quick Box 38.2 for a list of subordinating conjunctions and their meanings.

NO **Because** he was injured in the sixth inning, he remained in the game.

Because is illogical here; it says that his injury caused him to remain.

YES **Although** he was injured in the sixth inning, he remained in the game.

Although is logical here; it says that he remained despite his injury.

Subordination is also effective when you avoid overusing it and crowding too many ideas together in one sentence. If you write a sentence with two or more dependent clauses, check that your message is clear.

NO A new technique for eye surgery, **which is supposed to correct nearsightedness, which previously could be corrected only by glasses**, has been developed, **although many eye doctors do not approve of the new technique because it can create unstable vision, which includes intense glare from headlights on cars and many other light sources**.

The base sentence *A new technique for eye surgery has been developed* is lost among five dependent clauses.

YES A new technique for eye surgery, **which is supposed to correct nearsightedness**, has been developed. Previously, only glasses could correct nearsightedness. Many doctors do not approve of the new technique **because it can create unstable vision**. The problems include intense glare from car headlights and many other sources of light.

This revision breaks one long sentence into four sentences, which clarifies the relationships among the ideas. Two dependent clauses remain, which balance well with the other sentence constructions. Some words have been moved to new positions.

ESOL Tip: If readers advise that your sentences are too complex, limit the number of words in each sentence. Many ESOL instructors recommend that you revise any sentence that contains more than three clauses in any combination. ●

● **EXERCISE 38-6** Working individually or with a group, correct illogical or excessive subordination in this paragraph. As you revise according to the message you want to deliver, use some dependent clauses as well as some short sentences.

Although many people in the United States consider the hot dog an American invention, it actually originated in Germany in 1852 when butchers in Frankfurt, Germany, stuffed meat into a long casing, which, in honor of the town, they called a "frankfurter." Because one butcher noticed that the frankfurter resembled the shape of his dog, a dachshund, he decided to name the meat roll a "dachshund sausage," a name which caught on in Germany. When Germans brought dachshund sausages to the United States, peddlers sold them on the streets, although the dachshund sausages were so hot that people often burned their fingers because they had trouble holding the meat. When one clever peddler put the sausage in a bun, a *New York Times* cartoonist decided to draw a picture of hot dachshund sausages in buns, although he called them "hot dogs" because he didn't know how to spell *dachshund*. ●

38M How can I effectively use coordination and subordination together?

Your writing style improves when you combine a variety of sentence types, using COORDINATION and SUBORDINATION to improve the flow of ideas. This paragraph demonstrates a good balance of coordination and subordination.

> When I was growing up, I lived on a farm just across the field from my grandmother. My parents were busy trying to raise six children and to establish their struggling dairy farm. It was nice to have Grandma so close. While my parents were providing the necessities of life, my patient grandmother gave her time to her shy, young granddaughter. I always enjoyed going with Grandma and collecting the eggs that her chickens had just laid. Usually, she knew which chickens would peck, and she was careful to let me gather the eggs from the less hostile ones.
>
> —Patricia Mapes, student

When you use both coordination and subordination, never use both a COORDINATE CONJUNCTION and a SUBORDINATE CONJUNCTION to express one relationship in one sentence.

NO **Although** the story was well written, **but** it was too illogical.

Select either *although* or *but* to express the contrast, not both.

YES **Although** the story was well written, it was too illogical.

YES The story was well written, **but** it was too illogical.

● **EXERCISE 38-7** Working individually or in a group, use subordination and coordination to combine these sets of short, choppy sentences. For help, consult all sections of this chapter.

EXAMPLE

Owls cannot digest the bones and fur of the mice and birds they eat. They cough up a furry pellet every day.

Because owls cannot digest the bones and fur of the mice and birds they *eat, they* cough up a furry pellet every day.

1. Owl pellets are a rich teaching tool in biology classrooms around the country. The pellets provide an alternative to dissecting frogs and other animals.
2. Inside the pellet are the remains of the owl's nightly meal. They include beautifully cleaned hummingbird skulls, rat skeletons, and lots of bird feathers.
3. The owl-pellet market has been cornered by companies in New York, California, and Washington. These companies distribute pellets to thousands of biology classrooms all over the world.

4. Company workers scour barns and the ground under trees where owls nest to pick up the pellets. The pellets sell for $1 each.
5. The owl-pellet business may have a short future. The rural areas of the United States are vanishing. Old barns are being bulldozed. All the barns are torn down. The owls will be gone, too. ●

38N How do occasional questions, commands, or exclamations create variety and emphasis?

Most English sentences are DECLARATIVE—they make statements; they declare. For emphasis and variety, consider three other types of sentences you can choose.

An INTERROGATIVE sentence poses a question. Occasional questions, appropriately placed, tend to involve readers. An IMPERATIVE sentence issues a command. Occasional mild commands, appropriately used, gently urge readers to think along with you. An EXCLAMATORY sentence expresses strong or sudden emotion. Use exclamatory sentences sparingly in ACADEMIC WRITING.

Alert: A declarative statement ends with a period (see Chapter 41)—or semicolon (see Chapter 43) or colon (see Chapter 44). A mild command ends with a period. A strong command and an exclamation end with an exclamation point (see Chapter 41). ●

Here's a paragraph with declarative, interrogative, and imperative sentences.

> Imagine what people ate during the winter as little as seventy-five years ago. They ate food that was local, long-lasting, and dull, like acorn squash, turnips, and cabbage. Walk into an American supermarket in February and the world lies before you: grapes, melons, artichokes, fennel, lettuce, peppers, pistachios, dates, even strawberries, to say nothing of ice cream. Have you ever considered what a triumph of civilization it is to be able to buy a pound of chicken livers? If you lived on a farm and had to kill a chicken when you wanted to eat one, you wouldn't ever accumulate a pound of chicken livers.
>
> —Phyllis Rose, "Shopping and Other Spiritual Adventures in America Today"

38O What are cumulative and periodic sentences?

In an **cumulative sentence**, the most common in English, information accumulates after an opening SUBJECT and VERB. To build suspense into your writing, you might occasionally use a **periodic sentence**. A periodic sentence reserves its main idea—its punch—until the end of the sentence. When you overuse them, however, periodic sentences lose their punch.

CUMULATIVE A car hit a shoulder and turned over at midnight last night on the road from Las Vegas to Death Valley Junction.

PERIODIC At midnight last night, on the road from Las Vegas to Death Valley Junction, a car hit a shoulder and turned over.

—Joan Didion, "On Morality"

You can build both cumulative and periodic sentences to dramatic—and sometimes excessive—lengths.

EXAMPLE: How cumulative sentences can grow

1. The downtown bustled with new construction.
2. **The downtown bustled with new construction**, as buildings shot up everywhere, transforming the skyline.
3. **The downtown bustled with new constructio**n, as buildings shot up everywhere, each a mixture of glass and steel, in colors from rust red to ice blue, transforming the skyline from a shy set of bumps to a bold display of mountains

EXAMPLE: How periodic sentences can grow

1. Marla accepted the job offer.
2. With some reservations about the salary offer and location, **Marla accepted the job offer**.
3. After a day of agonizing and a night without sleep, still having some reservations about the salary offer and location, especially with the company being in an unappealing city more than 400 miles from her fiancé, **Marla accepted the job offer**.

38P How can modifiers create variety and emphasis?

MODIFIERS can add richness to your writing and create a pleasing mixture of variety and emphasis. The longer cumulative and periodic sentence examples in section 38O illustrate the use of modifiers. Your choice of where to place modifiers depends on the focus you want each sentence to communicate, either on its own or in concert with its surrounding sentences. Place modifiers carefully to avoid the error known as a MISPLACED MODIFIER.

NO (MISPLACED MODIFIER) A huge, hairy, grunting thing, I agreed that the bull was scary.

YES A huge, hairy, grunting thing, the bull was scary, I agreed.

In the No example, it sounds like the writer, I, was huge, hairy, and grunting!

BASIC SENTENCE	The river rose.
ADJECTIVE	The **swollen** river rose.
ADVERB	The river rose **dangerously**.
PREPOSITIONAL PHRASE	The river rose **above its banks**.
PARTICIPIAL PHRASE	**Swelled by melting snow,** the river rose.
ABSOLUTE PHRASE	**Uprooted trees swirling away in the current,** the river rose.
ADVERB CLAUSE	**Because the snows had been heavy that winter,** the river rose.
ADJECTIVE CLAUSE	The river, **which runs through vital farmland,** rose.

● **EXERCISE 38-8** Working individually or with a group, expand each sentence by adding each kind of modifier illustrated in section 38P.

1. I bought a ball.
2. We found the park.
3. The children arrived.
4. The sun shone.
5. We played the game. ●

38Q How does repetition affect style?

You can repeat words that express a main idea to create a rhythm that draws attention to the main idea. PARALLELISM (Chapter 39), another kind of repetition, repeats grammatical structures as well as words. Here's an example that uses deliberate repetition along with a variety of sentence lengths to deliver its meaning.

> All traces of life, of natural expression, were gone from him. His face was like a human skull, a death's head, spouting **blood**. The eyes were filled with **blood**, the nose streamed with **blood**, the mouth gaped **blood**.
>
> —William Hazlitt, "The Fight"

At the same time, don't confuse deliberate repetition with a lack of vocabulary variety.

NO An insurance agent can be an excellent adviser when you want to buy a car. An insurance agent has complete records on most cars. An insurance agent knows which car models are prone to accidents. An insurance agent can tell you which car models are expensive to repair if they are in a collision. An insurance agent can tell you which models are most likely to be stolen.

Synonyms for *insurance agent, car,* and *model* should be used. Also, the sentence structure here lacks variety.

YES If you are thinking of buying a new car, an insurance agent, who usually has complete records on most cars, can be an excellent adviser. Any professional insurance broker knows which automobile models are prone to have accidents. Did you know that some cars suffer more damage than others in a collision? If you want to know which vehicles crumple more than others and which are the most expensive to repair, ask an insurance agent. Similarly, some car models are more likely to be stolen, so find out from the person who specializes in dealing with car insurance claims.

38R How else can I create variety and emphasis?

CHANGING WORD ORDER

Standard word order in English places the SUBJECT before the VERB.

- The **mayor** ***walked*** into the room.

  Mayor, the subject, comes before the verb *walked*.

Inverted order, which places the verb before the subject, creates emphasis.

- Into the room ***walked*** the **mayor**.

  Mayor, the subject, comes after the verb *walked*.

CHANGING A SENTENCE'S SUBJECT

The subject of a sentence establishes the focus for that sentence. To create the emphasis you want, you can vary each sentence's subject. Notice how the focus changes in each sentence below according to the subject (and its corresponding verb).

- **Our study showed** that 25 percent of college freshmen gain weight.

  Focus is on the study.

- **College freshmen gain weight** 25 percent of the time, our study shows.

  Focus is on the freshmen.

- **Weight gain hits** 25 percent of college freshmen, our study shows.

  Focus is on weight gain.

- **Twenty-five percent of college freshmen** gain weight, our study shows.

  Focus is on the percentage of students.

● **EXERCISE 38-9** Working individually or with a group, revise the sentences in each paragraph to change the passage's style. For help, consult the advice in all sections of this chapter.

1. Thirst is the body's way of surviving. Every cell in the body needs water. People can die by losing as little as 15 to 20 percent of their water requirements. Blood contains 83 percent water. Blood provides indispensable nutrients for the cells. Blood carries water to the cells. Blood carries waste away from the cells. Insufficient water means cells cannot be fueled or cleaned. The body becomes sluggish. The body can survive eleven days without water. Bodily functions are seriously disrupted by a lack of water for more than one day. The body loses water. The blood thickens. The heart must pump harder. Thickened blood is harder to pump through the heart. Some drinks replace the body's need for fluids. Alcohol or caffeine in drinks leads to dehydration. People know they should drink water often. They can become moderately dehydrated before they even begin to develop a thirst.

2. June is the wet season in Ghana. Here in Accra, the capital, the morning rain has ceased. The sun heats the humid air. Pillars of black smoke begin to rise above the vast Agbobgloshie Market. I follow one plume toward its source. I pass lettuce and plantain vendors. I pass stalls of used tires. I walk through a clanging scrap market. In the market hunched men bash on old alternators and engine blocks.

—Based on a paragraph by Chris Carroll in "High Tech Trash"

3. Because of the development of new economies around the world, with resulting demands for new construction and goods, especially in places like China, there is a high demand for steel, and a new breed of American entrepreneurs is making money in meeting this opportunity. For much of industrial history, steel was made from iron ore and coke, a process that resulted in what might be called "new steel." However, it has now become even more profitable to make recycled steel, melting down junk and recasting it, a process made possible because steel, unlike paper and plastic, can be recycled indefinitely. Because the process saves energy and helps the environment by saving on the amount of ore that has to be mined, manufacturing recycled steel has benefits beyond profitability. ●

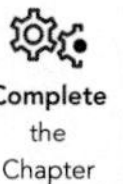

Complete the Chapter Exercises

39 Parallelism

Quick Points You will learn to

➤ Use parallel structures to give rhythm and grace to your writing (see 39A–39E).

39A What is parallelism?

When words, PHRASES, or CLAUSES within a sentence match in grammatical form, the result is **parallelism**. Parallelism can emphasize information or stress ideas in your writing.

- I came; I saw; I conquered

You gain several advantages in using parallel structures:

- You can express ideas of equal weight in your writing.
- You can emphasize important information or ideas.
- You can add rhythm and grace to your writing style.

Many writers attend to parallelism when they are REVISING. If you think while you're DRAFTING that your parallelism is faulty or that you can enhance your style by using parallelism, underline or highlight the material and keep moving forward. When you revise, you can return to the places you've marked.

Using COORDINATION, a **balanced sentence** delivers contrast, usually between two INDEPENDENT CLAUSES. Often, one clause is positive, the other negative.

> By night, the litter and desperation disappeared as the city's glittering lights came on; by day, the filth and despair reappeared as the sun rose.
>
> —Jennifer Kirk, student

Alert: In ACADEMIC WRITING, to avoid appearing to make the error of a COMMA SPLICE, use a semicolon (or revise in some other way), as in the following sentence.

- Mosquitoes don't bite; they stab. ●

39B How do words, phrases, and clauses work in parallel form?

When you put words, PHRASES, and CLAUSES into parallel form, you enhance your writing style with balance and grace.

PARALLEL WORDS — Recommended exercise includes running, swimming, and cycling.

PARALLEL PHRASES — Exercise helps people maintain healthy bodies and handle mental pressures.

PARALLEL CLAUSES — Many people exercise because they want to look healthy, because they need to increase stamina, and because they hope to live longer.

39C How does parallelism deliver impact?

Deliberate, rhythmic repetition of parallel forms creates balance, reinforcing the impact of a message.

> Go back to Mississippi, go back to Alabama, go back to South Carolina, go back to Georgia, go back to Louisiana, go back to the slums and ghettos of our northern cities, knowing that somehow this situation can and will be changed.
>
> —Martin Luther King Jr., "I Have a Dream"

If King had not used PARALLELISM, his message would have made less of an impact on his listeners. His structures reinforce the power of his message. A sentence without parallelism might have carried his message, but with far less effect: *Return to your homes in Mississippi, Alabama, South Carolina, Georgia, Louisiana, or the northern cities, and know that the situation will be changed.*

Here's a longer passage in which parallel structures, concepts, and rhythms operate. Together, they echo the intensity of the writer's message.

> The strongest reason why we ask for woman a voice in the government under which she lives; in the religion she is asked to believe; equality in social life, where she is the chief factor; a place in the trades and professions, where she may earn her bread, is **because** of her birthright to self-sovereignty; **because**, as an individual, she must rely on herself. No matter how much women prefer **to lean**, **to be** protected and supported, nor how much men desire **to have** them do so, they must make the voyage of life alone, and for safety in an emergency they must know something of the laws of navigation. To guide our own craft, we must be captain, pilot, engineer; with chart and compass to stand at the

wheel; to watch the wind and waves and know when to take in the sail, and to read the signs in the firmament over all.

—Elizabeth Cady Stanton, "Address for the Hearing of the Woman Suffrage Association"

● **EXERCISE 39-1** Working individually or with a group, highlight all parallel elements of the preceding Elizabeth Cady Stanton passage in addition to those shown in boldface. ●

39D How can I avoid faulty parallelism?

Faulty parallelism occurs when you join nonmatching grammatical forms.

PARALLELISM WITH COORDINATING CONJUNCTIONS

The coordinating conjunctions are *and, but, for, or, nor, yet,* and *so*. To avoid faulty parallelism, write the words that accompany coordinating conjunctions in matching grammatical forms.

NO **Love *and* being married** go together.

YES **Love *and* marriage** go together.

YES **Being in love *and* being married** go together.

PARALLELISM WITH CORRELATIVE CONJUNCTIONS

Correlative conjunctions are paired words such as *not only . . . but (also), either . . . or*, and *both . . . and*. To avoid faulty parallelism, write the words joined by correlative conjunctions in matching grammatical forms.

NO *Either* you must attend classes *or* will be failing the course.

YES *Either* you attend classes *or* fail the course.

PARALLELISM WITH *THAN* AND *AS*

To avoid faulty parallelism when you use *than* and *as* for comparisons, write the elements of comparison in matching grammatical forms.

NO **Having a solid marriage** can be more satisfying ***than* the acquisition of wealth.**

YES **Having a solid marriage** can be more satisfying ***than* acquiring wealth.**

YES **A solid marriage** can be more satisfying ***than*** **wealth.**

PARALLELISM WITH FUNCTION WORDS

Function words include ARTICLES (*the, a, an*); the *to* of the INFINITIVE (*to* love); PREPOSITIONS (for example, *of, in, about*); and sometimes RELATIVE PRONOUNS. When you use parallel structures, be consistent about either repeating or omitting a function word. Generally, repeat function words when the repetition clarifies your meaning or highlights the parallelism.

NO **To assign** unanswered letters their proper weight, **free** us from the expectations of others, **to give** us back to ourselves—here lies the great, the singular power of self-respect.

YES **To assign** unanswered letters their proper weight, **to free** us from the expectations of others, **to give** us back to ourselves—here lies the great, the singular power of self-respect.

—Joan Didion, "On Self-Respect"

I have in my own life a precious friend, a woman of 65 **who has** lived very hard, **who is** wise, **who listens** well, **who has been** where I am and can help me understand it, and **who represents** not only an ultimate ideal mother to me but also the person I'd like to be when I grow up.

—Judith Viorst, "Friends, Good Friends—and Such Good Friends"

We looked into the bus, which **was** painted blue with orange daisies, **had** picnic benches instead of seats, and **showed** yellow curtains billowing out its windows.

—Kerrie Falk, student

● **EXERCISE 39-2** Working individually or with a group, revise these sentences by putting appropriate information in parallel structures. For help, consult sections 39A through 39E.

EXAMPLE

Difficult bosses affect not only their employees' performances but their private lives are affected as well.

Difficult bosses affect not only their employees' performances *but their private lives as well.*

1. According to the psychologist Harry Levinson, the five main types of bad boss are the workaholic, the kind of person you would describe as bullying, a person who communicates badly, the jellyfish type, and someone who insists on perfection.
2. As a way of getting ahead, to keep their self-respect, and for survival purposes, wise employees handle problem bosses with a variety of strategies.
3. To cope with a bad-tempered employer, workers can both stand up for themselves and reasoning with a bullying boss.

4. Often, bad bosses communicate poorly or fail to calculate the impact of their personality on others; being a careful listener and sensitivity to others' responses are qualities that good bosses possess.
5. Employees who take the trouble to understand what makes their bosses tick, engage in some self-analysis, and staying flexible are better prepared to cope with a difficult job environment than suffering in silence like some employees. ●

● **EXERCISE 39-3** Working individually or with a group, combine the sentences in each numbered item, using techniques of parallelism. For help, consult sections 39A through 39E.

EXAMPLE

College scholarships are awarded not only for academic and athletic ability, but there are also scholarships that recognize unusual talents. Other scholarships even award accidents of birth, like left-handedness.

College scholarships are awarded not only for academic and athletic ability *but also for unusual talents and even for accidents of birth, like left-handedness*.

1. A married couple met at Juniata College in Huntingdon, Pennsylvania. They are both left-handed, and they have set up a scholarship for needy left-handed students attending Juniata.
2. Writers who specialize in humor bankroll a student humor writer at the University of Southern California in Los Angeles. A horse-racing association sponsors a student sportswriter. The student must attend Vanderbilt University in Nashville, Tennessee.
3. The Rochester Institute of Technology in New York State chose 150 students born on June 12, 1979. Each one received a grant of $1,500 per year. These awards were given to select students to honor the school's 150th anniversary, which was celebrated on June 12, 1979.
4. The College of Wooster in Ohio grants generous scholarships to students if they play the bagpipes, a musical instrument native to Scotland. Students playing the traditional Scottish drums and those who excel in Scottish folk dancing also qualify.
5. In return for their scholarships, Wooster's bagpipers must pipe for the school's football team. The terms of the scholarships also require the drummers to drum for the team. The dancers have to cheer the athletes from the sidelines. ●

● **EXERCISE 39-4** Working individually or with a group, underline the parallel elements in these passages. Next, imitate the parallelism in the examples, using a different topic of your choice for each.

A. Even though large tracts of Europe and many old and famous States have fallen or may fall into the grip of the Gestapo and all the odious apparatus of Nazi rule, we shall not flag or fail. We shall go on to the end. We shall fight in France, we shall fight on the seas and oceans, we shall fight with growing confidence and growing strength in the air, we shall defend our island, whatever the cost may be. We shall fight on the beaches, we shall fight on the landing grounds, we shall fight in the fields and in the streets, we shall fight in the hills; we shall never surrender, and if, which I do not for a moment believe, this island or a large part of it were subjugated and starving, then our Empire beyond the seas, armed and guarded by the British Fleet, would carry on the struggle, until, in God's good time, the new world, with all its power and might, steps forth to the rescue and the liberation of the old.

—Winston Churchill

B. Our religion is the traditions of our ancestors—the dreams of our old men, given them in solemn hours of the night by the Great Spirit; and the visions of our sachems, and is written in the hearts of our people.

Our dead never forget this beautiful world that gave them being. They still love its verdant valleys, its murmuring rivers, its magnificent mountains, sequestered vales and verdant lined lakes and bays, and ever yearn in tender fond affection over the lonely hearted living, and often return from the happy hunting ground to visit, guide, console, and comfort them.

It matters little where we pass the remnant of our days. They will not be many. The Indian's night promises to be dark. Not a single star of hope hovers above his horizon. Sad-voiced winds moan in the distance. Grim fate seems to be on the Red Man's trail, and wherever he will hear the approaching footsteps of his fell destroyer and prepare stolidly to meet his doom, as does the wounded doe that hears the approaching footsteps of the hunter.

—Oration attributed to Chief Seattle ●

39E How does parallelism work in outlines and lists?

All items in formal OUTLINES and lists must be parallel in grammar and structure. (For more about outline format and outline development, see section 5G.)

OUTLINES

NO Reducing Traffic Fatalities

I. Stricter laws
   A. Top speed should be 55 mph on highways.
   B. Higher fines
   C. Requiring jail sentences for repeat offenders

II. The use of safety devices should be mandated by law.

YES Reducing Traffic Fatalities

I. Passing stricter speed laws
   A. Making 55 mph the top speed on highways
   B. Raising fines for speeding
   C. Requiring jail sentences for repeat offenders
II. Mandating by law the use of safety devices

LISTS

NO Workaholics share these characteristics:
1. They are intense and driven.
2. Strong self-doubters
3. Labor is preferred to leisure by workaholics.

YES Workaholics share these characteristics:
1. They are intense and driven.
2. They have strong self-doubts.
3. They prefer labor to leisure.

● **EXERCISE 39-5** Working individually or with a group, revise this outline so that all lines are complete sentences in parallel form. For help, consult sections 5G and 39E.

IMPROVING HEALTH

I. Exercise
   A. Aerobics
   B. Stretching and strength training
   C. Vary routine
II. Better Eating Habits
   A. Healthy food
   B. Eat less
   C. Eat more often ●

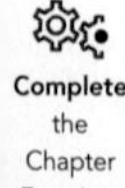

Complete the Chapter Exercises

40 Conciseness

Quick Points You will learn to

➤ Write concisely (40A–40E).

40A What is conciseness?

Clear writing requires **conciseness**—sentences that are direct and to the point. By contrast, **wordiness** means you are padding sentences with words and phrases that increase the word count but contribute no meaning. As you're REVISING, look for ways to make your sentences more concise.

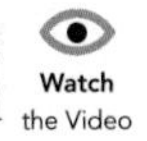

WORDY ~~As a matter of fact,~~ T local the television station ~~which is in the local area~~ wins ~~a great~~ many awards ~~in the final analysis~~ because of its ~~type of~~ coverage of ~~all kinds of~~ controversial issues.

CONCISE The local television station wins many awards for its coverage of controversial issues.

40B What common expressions are not concise?

Many common expressions we use in informal speech are not concise. Quick Box 40.1 lists some and shows you how to eliminate them.

Quick Box 40.1

Cutting unnecessary words and phrases

Empty Word or Phrase	Wordy Example Revised
as a matter of fact	Many marriages~~, as a matter of fact,~~ end in divorce.
at the present time	The revised proposal for outdoor lighting angers many villagers now ~~at the present time~~.

continued >>

Quick Box 40.1 (continued)

Empty Word or Phrase	Wordy Example Revised
because of the fact that, in light of the fact that, due to the fact that	Because ~~of the fact that~~ the museum has a special exhibit, it stays open late.
by means of	We traveled by ~~means of a~~ car.
factor	The project's final cost was ~~the~~ essential ~~factor~~ to consider.
for the purpose of	Work crews arrived ~~for the purpose of~~ to fixing the potholes.
have a tendency to	The team ~~has a tendency~~ tends to lose home games.
in a very real sense	~~In a very real sense,~~ A all firefighters are heroes.
in the case of	~~In the case of~~ T the election~~, it~~ will be close.
in the event that	~~In the event that~~ If you're late, I will buy our tickets.
in the final analysis	~~In the final analysis,~~ N no two eyewitnesses agreed on what they saw.
in the process of	We are ~~in the process of~~ reviewing the proposal.
it seems that	~~It seems that~~ T the union went on strike over health benefits.
manner	The child spoke reluctantly. ~~in a reluctant manner.~~
nature	The movie review was ~~of a~~ sarcastic ~~nature~~.
that exists	The crime rate ~~that exists~~ is unacceptable.
the point I am trying to make	~~The point I am trying to make is~~ T television reporters invade our privacy.
type of, kind of	Gordon took a relaxing ~~type of~~ vacation.
What I mean to say is	~~What I mean to say is~~ I love you.

● **EXERCISE 40-1** Working individually or with a group, revise this paragraph in two steps. First, underline all words that interfere with conciseness. Second, revise each sentence to make it more concise. (You'll need to drop words and replace or rearrange others.)

EXAMPLE

Because of the fact that a new building in Dubai was recently declared the "Tallest Building in the World," some people have a tendency to wonder how such a title is granted.

1. Because <u>of the fact that</u> a new building in Dubai was recently declared the "Tallest Building in the World," some people <u>have a tendency to</u> wonder who grants such a title.
2. Because a new building in Dubai was recently declared the "Tallest Building in the World," some wonder who grants such a title.

1. Tall buildings that exist are measured by a group known as The Council on Tall Buildings and Urban Habitat.
2. This group, as a matter of fact, was founded in 1969 and is responsible for determining which building is the tallest.
3. Due to the fact that buildings serve many purposes, it seems that there is debate on which buildings deserve consideration.
4. I am trying to make the point that The Council on Tall Buildings and Urban Habitat must distinguish between buildings and towers.
5. To be considered, a building has to be the kind of structure that has usable floor area.
6. In the event that a structure has no usable floor area, it is designated a tower.
7. Height is determined by means of measuring from the lowest pedestrian entrance to the highest point of the building.
8. There are debates that exist over the definitions used by the Council on Tall Buildings.
9. For example, in the event that a building has not opened yet, it cannot be considered.
10. Another debate and matter of controversy is whether a building's antenna is an essential factor in determining its height. ●

40C What sentence structures usually work against conciseness?

Two sentence structures, although appropriate in some contexts, often work against CONCISENESS: EXPLETIVE constructions and the PASSIVE VOICE.

AVOIDING EXPLETIVE CONSTRUCTIONS

An **expletive construction** starts with *it* or *there* followed by a form of the VERB *be*. When you cut the expletive and revise, the sentence is more concise.

- ~~It is necessary for s~~Students ~~to~~ must fill in both questionnaires.
- ~~There are e~~Eight instructors ~~who~~ teach in the Computer Science Department.

ESOL Tips: (1) *It* in an expletive construction is not a PRONOUN referring to an ANTECEDENT. When expletive *it* occupies the subject position, the actual subject comes after the expletive: *It was the students who asked the question. Students* is the subject, not *it.* (2) *There* in an expletive construction does not indicate place. Although expletive *there* occupies the subject position, the actual subject comes after the expletive: *There were many students present. Students* is the subject, not *there.*

AVOIDING THE PASSIVE VOICE

In general, the passive voice is less concise and less lively than the ACTIVE VOICE. In the active voice, the subject performs the action named by the verb.

ACTIVE Professor Higgins teaches public speaking.

Professor Higgins, the subject, performs the action *teaches.*

In the passive voice, the subject receives the action named by the verb.

PASSIVE Public speaking is taught by Professor Higgins.

Public speaking, the subject, receives the action *taught.*

Unless your meaning justifies using the passive voice, choose the active voice. (For more information, see sections 29N through 29P.)

PASSIVE Volunteer work was done by students for credit in sociology.

The passive phrase *was done by students* is unnecessary for the intended meaning. *Students,* not *volunteer work,* are doing the action and should get the action of the verb.

ACTIVE **The students did** volunteer work for credit in sociology.

ACTIVE **Volunteer work earned** students credit in sociology.

Since the verb has changed to *earned, volunteer work* performs the action of the verb.

The passive voice often creates wordy, overblown sentences, suggesting that a writer hasn't carefully revised.

NO One very important quality that can be developed during a first job is self-reliance. This strength was gained by me when I was allowed by my supervisor to set up and conduct a survey project on my own.

YES Many develop the important quality of self-reliance during their first job. I gained this strength when my supervisor allowed me to set up and conduct my own survey project.

YES During their first job, many people develop self-reliance, as I did when my supervisor let me set up and conduct my own survey project.

If you're writing on a computer, you may find it helpful to use the word processing application's "Search" or "Find" feature to locate the words "was, is, be, were, and been" when you revise. This trick can help you find possible uses of passive voice and judge whether or not they need revision.

40D How else can I revise for conciseness?

Four other techniques can help you achieve CONCISENESS: eliminating unplanned repetition (40D.1); combining sentences (40D.2); shortening CLAUSES (40D.3); and shortening PHRASES and cutting words (40D.4).

40D.1 Eliminating unplanned repetition

Unplanned repetition delivers the same message more than once, usually in slightly different words. Unplanned repetition, or redundancy, unnecessarily burdens readers. The opposite—planned repetition—can create a powerful rhythmic effect (see 39E). As you revise, check that every word is necessary for delivering your message.

NO Bringing **the project** to **final completion** three weeks early, the supervisor of **the project** earned our **respectful regard**.

Completion implies *bringing to final; project* is used twice in one sentence; and *regard* implies *respect.*

YES Completing the project three weeks early, the supervisor earned our respect.

Eighteen words are reduced to eleven.

NO **Astonished**, the architect **circled around** the building **in amazement**.

Circled means "went around," and *astonished* and *in amazement* have the same meaning.

YES **Astonished**, the architect **circled** the building.

Nine words are reduced to six.

YES The architect **circled** the building **in amazement**.

Nine words are reduced to seven.

ESOL Tip: In all languages, words can carry an implied message. In English, some implied meanings can cause redundancy in writing. For example, *I wrote my blog by computer* is redundant. In English, *to write a blog* implies *by computer*. As you become more familiar with American English, you'll begin to notice such redundancies.

40D.2 Combining sentences

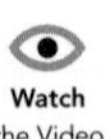
Watch the Video

Sometimes you can fit information from several sentences into one sentence. (For more about combining sentences, see Chapter 38, particularly sections 38C, 38E, 38J, and 38M.)

TWO SENTENCES The *Titanic* hit an iceberg and sank. Seventy-three years later, a team of French and American scientists located the ship's resting site.

SENTENCES COMBINED Seventy-three years after the *Titanic* hit an iceberg and sank, a team of French and American scientists located the ship's resting site.

TWO SENTENCES Cameras revealed that the stern of the ship was missing and showed external damage to the ship's hull. Otherwise, the *Titanic* was in excellent condition.

SENTENCES COMBINED Aside from a missing stern and external damage to the ship's hull, the *Titanic* was in excellent condition.

40D.3 Shortening clauses

Look at clauses to see if you can more concisely convey the same information. For example, sometimes you can cut a RELATIVE PRONOUN and its verb.

WORDY The *Titanic*, **which was** a huge ocean liner, sank in 1912.

CONCISE The Titanic, a huge ocean liner, sank in 1912.

Sometimes you can reduce a clause to a word.

WORDY The scientists held a memorial service for the passengers and crew **who had drowned**.

CONCISE The scientists held a memorial service for the **drowned** passengers and crew.

An ELLIPTICAL CONSTRUCTION (see sections 28P and 36H) can shorten a clause. If you use this device, be sure that omitted words are implied clearly.

WORDY **When they were** confronted with disaster, some passengers behaved heroically, **while** others **behaved** selfishly.

CONCISE Confronted with disaster, some passengers behaved heroically, others selfishly.

40D.4 Shortening phrases and cutting words

Sometimes you can reduce a phrase or redundant word pair to a single word. Redundant word pairs and phrases include *each and every, one and only, forever and ever, final and conclusive, perfectly clear, few* (or *many*) *in number, consensus of opinion*, and *reason . . . is because*.

NO **Each and every** person was hungry after the movie.

YES **Every** person was hungry after the movie.

YES **Each** person was hungry after the movie.

NO The **consensus of opinion** was that the movie was dull.

YES The **consensus** was that the movie was dull.

YES **Everyone agreed** that the movie was dull.

WORDY More than fifteen hundred **travelers on that voyage** died in the shipwreck.

CONCISE More than fifteen hundred **passengers** died in the shipwreck.

Sometimes you can rearrange words so that others can be deleted.

WORDY Objects **found** inside the ship included **unbroken** bottles of wine and expensive **undamaged** china.

CONCISE **Undamaged** objects inside the ship included bottles of wine and expensive china.

40E How do verbs affect conciseness?

Action verbs are strong verbs. *Be* and *have* are verbs that can lead to wordy sentences. Action verbs can increase the impact of your writing and reduce the number of words in your sentences. You can often use strong verbs to reduce PHRASES and to replace NOUNS.

WEAK VERB The plan before the city council **has to do with** tax rebates.

STRONG VERB The plan before the city council **proposes** tax rebates.

WEAK VERBS The board members **were of the opinion** that the changes in the rules **were changes they would not accept**.

STRONG VERBS The board members **said** that **they would reject** the changes in the rules.

REPLACING A PHRASE WITH A VERB

Phrases such as *be aware of, be capable of, be supportive of* can often be replaced with one-word verbs.

- I **envy** [not *am envious of*] your mathematical ability.
- I **appreciate** [not *am appreciative of*] your modesty.
- Your skill **illustrates** [not *is illustrative of*] how hard you studied.

REVISING NOUNS INTO VERBS

Many nouns ending with *-ance, -ment*, and *-tion* (*toler**ance***, *enforce**ment***, *narra**tion***) are derived from verbs. Use of the vibrant verb will make your writing more concise.

NO The **accumulation of** paper lasted thirty years.

YES The paper **accumulated** for thirty years.

NO We **arranged for the establishment of** a student advisory committee.

YES We **established** a student advisory committee.

NO The building **had the appearance of** having been neglected.

YES The building **appeared** to have been neglected.

● **EXERCISE 40-2** Working individually or with a group, combine each set of sentences to eliminate wordy constructions.

EXAMPLE

Original: The Brooklyn Bridge was completed in 1883. It is one of the oldest suspension bridges in the United States

Revised: Completed in 1883, the Brooklyn Bridge is one of the oldest suspension bridges in the United States

1. The Brooklyn Bridge spans the East River. It connects Manhattan and Brooklyn. The span of the bridge is 1,595 feet.
2. When the Brooklyn Bridge opened, it was the longest suspension bridge in the world. It was the longest suspension bridge until 1903. In 1903, the Williamsburg Bridge became the longest suspension bridge in the world.
3. The original designer of the bridge was John Augustus Roebling. He was a German immigrant. He injured his foot then died from an infection. Before he died, he turned over control of construction to his son. His son's name was Washington Roebling.
4. Emily Warren Roebling supervised most of the building of the Brooklyn Bridge. Her husband, Washington Roebling, was unable to oversee construction. He had to stop working after suffering an illness.
5. Emily Warren Roebling spent fourteen years helping her husband oversee the building of the bridge. Her husband was sick. She had to learn

important things. She learned about stress analysis, cable construction, and catenary curves.

6. The bridge opened in May of 1883. Its opening was attended by several thousand people. The current president, Chester A. Arthur, attended the opening.
7. Some people were concerned about the bridge. They worried about the bridge's stability. P.T. Barnum was the founder of a famous circus. He led a parade of elephants over the bridge. There were 21 elephants in the parade.
8. The bridge celebrated its 100th anniversary in 1983. The president of the United States at that time was Ronald Reagan. He led a parade of cars across the bridge during the celebration.
9. Ken Burns is a filmmaker. In 1981, he made a documentary about the Brooklyn Bridge. Ken Burns has also directed documentaries about baseball and jazz and the Civil War.
10. The bridge has six lanes of automobile traffic. The bridge also allows for pedestrians to cross. Pedestrians can cross on a wide pedestrian walkway open to people who are walking. ●

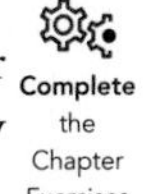

PART

7

Using Punctuation and Mechanics

41 Periods, Question Marks, and Exclamation Points

Quick Points You will learn to

➤ Use periods, question marks, and exclamation points correctly (see 41A–41F).

Periods, question marks, and exclamation points are collectively called *end punctuation* because they occur at the ends of sentences.

- I love you**.** Do you love me**?** I love you**!**

PERIODS

41A When does a period end a sentence?

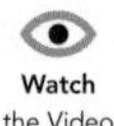
Watch the Video

A period ends a statement, a mild command, or an INDIRECT QUESTION.* Never use a period to end a DIRECT QUESTION, a strong command, or an emphatic declaration.

END OF A STATEMENT

- A journey of a thousand miles must begin with a single step.

—Lao-tsu, *The Way of Lao-tsu*

MILD COMMAND

- Put a gram of boldness into everything you do.

—Baltasar Gracian

INDIRECT QUESTION

- I asked if they wanted to climb Mt. Ross.

  If this statement were a direct question, it would end with a question mark: *I asked, "Do you want to climb Mt. Ross?"*

---

*Words printed in SMALL CAPITAL LETTERS are discussed elsewhere in the text and are defined in the Terms Glossary at the back of this book.

41B How do I use periods with abbreviations?

Most abbreviations (*Dr., Mr., Ms., Jr., Fri., St., a.m., p.m.*) call for periods; a few don't. (For more about abbreviations, see 48I through 48L.)

Alert: In ACADEMIC WRITING, spell out—don't abbreviate—the word *professor.* ●

Abbreviations without periods include the postal codes for states (for example, IL, CO) and the names of some organizations and government agencies (for example, CBS and NASA).

- **Ms**. Yuan, who works at **NASA**, lectured to **Dr**. Garcia's physics class at 9:30 **a.m**.

Alert: At the end of a sentence, a single period marks both the abbreviation and the end of the sentence. However, a question mark or exclamation point follows an abbreviation period at the end of a sentence.

- The phone rang at 4:00 **a.m**.
- It's upsetting to answer a wrong-number call at 4:00 **a.m.!**
- Who would call at 4:00 **a.m.?** ●

QUESTION MARKS

41C When do I use a question mark?

A question mark ends a **direct question**, one that quotes exact words. (A period ends an **indirect question**, which tells of a question.)

- How many attempts have been made to climb Mt. Everest?

  An indirect question would end with a period: *She wants to know how many attempts have been made to climb Mt. Everest.*

Alert: Never use a question mark with a period, comma, semicolon, or colon.

NO She asked, "How are you**?.**"

YES She asked, "How are you**?**" ●

Use a question mark after each question in a series whether or not you choose to capitalize the first word. (Do capitalize the first word when a question forms a complete sentence.)

- Whose rights does voter fraud violate**?** Mine**?** Yours**?** Or everyone's**?**

A polite command or request can be followed by either a period or a question mark. Choose consistently within each piece of your writing.

- Would you please send me a copy**.**

or

- Would you please send me a copy**?**

41D When can I use a question mark in parentheses?

Use a question mark within parentheses only when a preceding date or other numerical information is unknown.

- Chaucer was born in 1340 (?) in London.

The word *about* is often more graceful: *Chaucer was born* ***about*** *1340.*

Also, use precise wording, not (?), to show IRONY or sarcasm.

NO My algebra class is a pleasant **(?)** experience.

YES My algebra class is as pleasant as a root canal.

EXCLAMATION POINTS

41E When do I use an exclamation point?

An exclamation point ends a strong command (*Look out behind you! Tell me the truth now!*) or an emphatic declaration (*There's been an accident! Hail to the Chief!*)

Alert: Never combine an exclamation point with a period, comma, semicolon, or colon.

NO "There's been an accident**!,**" she shouted.

YES "There's been an accident**!**" she shouted.

YES "There's been an accident," she shouted.

Use this form if you prefer not to use an exclamation point. ●

41F What is considered overuse of exclamation points?

In ACADEMIC WRITING, use words, not exclamation points, to communicate the intensity of your message. Use this mark sparingly.

When we were in Nepal, we tried each day to see Mt. Everest. But each day we failed. **Clouds defeated us!** The summit never emerged from a heavy overcast.

Also, using exclamation points too frequently suggests an exaggerated sense of urgency.

NO Mountain climbing can be dangerous. You must know correct procedures! You must have the proper equipment! Otherwise, you could die!

YES Mountain climbing can be dangerous. You must know correct procedures**.** You must have the proper equipment**.** Otherwise, you could die**!**

Use precise wording, not (!), to show amazement or sarcasm.

NO At 29,035 feet **(!)**, Mt. Everest is the world's highest mountain. Yet, Chris **(!)** wants to climb it.

YES At **a majestic** 29,035 feet, Mt. Everest is the world's highest mountain. Yet, Chris, **amazingly,** wants to climb it.

● EXERCISE 41-1 Insert any needed periods, question marks, and exclamation points and delete any unneeded ones. For help, consult all sections of this chapter.

EXAMPLE

Dr Madan Kataria, who calls himself the Giggling Guru (!), established the world's first laughter club in 1995.

Dr**.** Madan Kataria, who calls himself the Giggling Guru**,** established the world's first laughter club in 1995.

1. More than 1,000 (?) laughter clubs exist throughout the world, each seeking to promote health by reducing stress and strengthening the immune system!
2. Dr Madan Kataria, a physician in Bombay, India, developed a yoga-like (!) strategy based on group (!) laughter and then set up laughter clubs.
3. Laughter clubs say, "Yes!" when asked, "Is laughter the best medicine."
4. The clubs' activities include breathing and stretching exercises and playful (?) behaviors, such as performing the opera laugh (!), the chicken laugh (!), and the "Ho-Ho, Ha-Ha" (?) exercise.
5. According to the German psychologist Dr Michael Titze, "In the 1950s people used to laugh eighteen minutes a day (!), but today we laugh not more than six (?) minutes per day, despite huge rises in the standard of living." ●

● EXERCISE 41-2 Insert needed periods, question marks, and exclamation points. For help, consult all sections of this chapter.

Complete the Chapter Exercises

Weather experts refer to a rise in surface temperature of the Pacific Ocean as El Niño, but La Niña refers to a drop in ocean temperature What effects can these changes cause In the spring of 1998, the cold water of La Niña surfaced quickly and produced chaotic and destructive weather In the American Northeast, rainfall amounts for June were three times above normal But no one expected the strangest consequence: snow in June Can you imagine waking up on an early summer morning in New England to snow Throughout the summer, most New England states failed to experience a single heat wave, which requires more than three days of 90 degree weather During that winter, the Great Lakes experienced record warmth, but California suffered from disastrously cold air A citrus freeze caused $600 million of damage That's more than half a billion dollars. ●

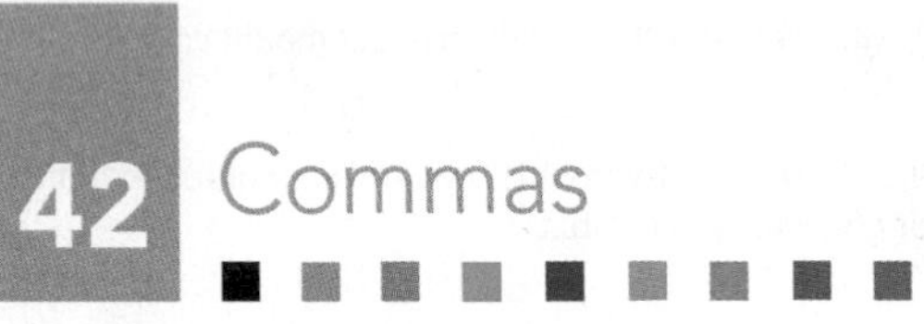

42 Commas

Quick Points You will learn to

➤ Use commas correctly (see 42A–42L).

42A What is the role of the comma?

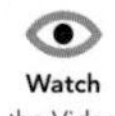
Watch the Video

The most frequently used mark of punctuation, a comma separates items of thought within a sentence. Quick Box 42.1 shows most uses of the comma. For a fuller explanation, check the sections indicated in parentheses.

Quick Box 42.1

Key uses of commas

COMMAS WITH COORDINATING CONJUNCTIONS LINKING INDEPENDENT CLAUSES (42B)

- Most people throw postcards out**, but** some are quite valuable.

COMMAS AFTER INTRODUCTORY ELEMENTS (42C)

- **Although most postcards cost only a quarter,** one recently sold for thousands of dollars.
- **On postcard racks,** several designs are usually available.
- **For example,** animals are timeless favorites.
- **However,** most cards show local landmarks.

continued >>

Quick Box 42.1 (continued)

COMMAS WITH ITEMS IN A SERIES (42D)

- **Places, paintings, and people** appear on postcards.
- **Places, paintings, people, animals** occupy dozens of display racks.

COMMAS WITH COORDINATE ADJECTIVES (42E)

- Some postcards feature **appealing, dramatic** scenes.

NO COMMAS WITH CUMULATIVE ADJECTIVES (42E)

- Other postcards feature **famous historical** scenes.

COMMAS WITH NONRESTRICTIVE ELEMENTS (42F)

- **Four years after the first postcard appeared,** the U.S. government began to issue prestamped postcards.
- The Golden Age of postcards**, which lasted from about 1900 to 1929,** yielded many especially valuable cards.
- Collectors swarm postcard shows**,** which draw national attention.

NO COMMAS WITH RESTRICTIVE ELEMENTS (42F)

- Collectors **who attend these shows** may specialize in a particular kind of postcard.

COMMAS WITH QUOTED WORDS (42H)

- One collector told me**,** "Hitting a show is like digging for gold."
- "I always expect to find a priceless postcard**,**" he said.
- "Everyone there**,**" he joked**,** "believes a million-dollar card is hidden in the next stack."

42B How do commas work with coordinating conjunctions?

Never use a comma when a coordinating conjunction links only two words, two PHRASES, or two DEPENDENT CLAUSES.

NO Habitat for Humanity depends on volunteers for **labor, and donations** to help with its construction projects.

Labor and *donations* are two words; the conjunction explains their relationship. No comma is needed.

YES Habitat for Humanity depends on volunteers for **labor and donations** to help with its construction projects.

NO Each language has **a beauty of its own, and forms of expression** that are duplicated nowhere else.

A *beauty of its own* and *forms of expression* are only two phrases.

YES Each language has **a beauty of its own and forms of expression** that are duplicated nowhere else.

—Margaret Mead, "Unispeak"

Do use a comma when a coordinating conjunction links two or more INDEPENDENT CLAUSES. Place the comma before the coordinating conjunction.

- The sky turned dark gray**, and** the wind died suddenly.
- The November morning had just begun**, but** it looked like dusk.
- Shopkeepers closed their stores early**, for** they wanted to get home.
- Soon high winds would start**, or** thick snow would begin silently.
- Farmers could not continue harvesting**, nor** could they round up their animals in distant fields.
- Drivers tried to reach safety**, yet** some unlucky ones were stranded.
- The firehouse whistle blew twice**, so** we knew a blizzard was closing in.

Exceptions

- Two short contrasting independent clauses are often linked by a comma with no coordinating conjunction: *Rex barks, he doesn't bite*. For ACADEMIC WRITING, however, your instructor may prefer a period or a semicolon (see Ch. 43) to a comma.
- When one or both independent clauses linked by a coordinating conjunction contain other commas, dropping the coordinating conjunction and using a semicolon instead of the comma clarifies meaning.
    - With temperatures below freezing**,** the snow did not melt**;** ~~and~~ **people** wondered, gazing at the white landscape, when they would see grass again.

Alerts: (1) Never put a comma *after* a coordinating conjunction that joins independent clauses.

NO A house is renovated in two weeks **but,** a loft takes a week.

YES A house is renovated in two weeks**, but** a loft takes a week.

(2) Never use a comma alone between independent clauses, or you'll create the error known as a COMMA SPLICE (see Chapter 34).

NO Five inches of snow fell in two hours**,** driving was hazardous.

YES Five inches of snow fell in two hours**, and** driving was hazardous. ●

● **EXERCISE 42-1** Working individually or in a group, combine each pair of sentences using the coordinating conjunction shown in parentheses. Rearrange words when necessary.

EXAMPLE

Esperanto is a language invented by L. L. Zamenhof in 1887. It is now the most widely spoken artificial language. (and)

Esperanto is a language invented by L. L. Zamenhof in 1887, and it is now the most widely spoken artificial language.

for and nor but or yet so

1. Zamenhof believed that his invention would foster world peace. He believed that if people spoke a common language wars would cease. (for)
2. No country recognizes Esperanto as an official language. It is spoken by many people in at least 115 countries. (but)
3. Published in Warsaw, the first book of Esperanto grammar appeared in 1887. The first world congress of Esperanto speakers was held in France in 1905. (and)
4. Before World War II, Hitler denounced Esperanto. Its creator was Jewish. (for)
5. Stalin also attacked Esperanto and would not grant it official status. He would not allow its use in the Soviet Union. (nor)
6. The U.S. military has used Esperanto in training exercises. Soldiers can practice communicating in a foreign language. (so)
7. Similar to English, Esperanto uses 23 consonants and 5 vowels. It also uses 2 semivowels. (yet)
8. Most speakers of Esperanto have to learn the language through their own study. They learn in courses taught by volunteers. (or)
9. Esperanto has made its way into popular culture in movies, music, and literature. There is even a 1965 movie starring William Shatner in which all the dialogue is in Esperanto. (and)
10. If you want to learn Esperanto, it can be difficult to find support. There are Esperanto clubs in over 50 U.S. cities and many universities. (but) ●

42C How do commas work with introductory clauses, phrases, and words?

A comma follows any introductory word, PHRASE, or CLAUSE that precedes an INDEPENDENT CLAUSE.

- **Predictably,** many dieters say sugar craving is their worst problem.
- **Before 1700,** sugar refineries appeared in London and New York.
- **Beginning in infancy,** we develop lifelong tastes for sweet foods.

- **Sweets being a temptation for many adults,** most parents avoid commercial baby foods that contain sugar.
- **Although fructose comes from fruit,** it's still sugar.
- **Nevertheless,** many people think fructose isn't harmful.
- **To satisfy a craving for ice cream,** even timid people sometimes brave midnight streets.

EXCEPTION

Some writers omit the comma after a short, unmistakably clear introductory element. In ACADEMIC WRITING, however, you'll never be wrong if you use the comma.

YES In 1992**,** the Americans with Disabilities Act was passed.

YES In 1992 the Americans with Disabilities Act was passed.

Place a comma after an introductory **interjection**, a word that conveys strong, sudden emotion: ***Oh***, *are you allergic to cats?* ***Well***, *you can't stop sneezing.*

! Alert: Use a comma before and after a sentence MODIFIER in the middle of a sentence. When the sentence MODIFIER starts a sentence, follow it with a comma. When the sentence MODIFIER ends a sentence, put a comma before it.

- **By the way,** the parade begins at noon.
- The parade**, by the way,** begins at noon.
- The parade begins at noon**, by the way**.

- **However,** our float isn't finished.
- Our float**, however,** isn't finished.
- Our float isn't finished**, however**. ●

● **EXERCISE 42-2** Working individually or with a group, combine each set of sentences into one sentence according to the direction in parentheses. Use a comma after the introductory element. You can add, delete, and rearrange words as needed. For help, consult 42C.

EXAMPLE

People have known that humor is good for them. They have known this for a long time. (Begin with *for a long time.*)

For a long time, people have known that humor is good for them.

1. People laugh. Scientists study them to find out what actually happens. (Begin with *when.*)
2. Scientists track our physiological reactions. They discover the chemicals we produce while we are laughing. (Begin with *in fact.*)

3. Our brains use dopamine when we laugh. Dopamine is a chemical we produce that makes us feel good. (Begin with *produced.*)
4. We sometimes activate our tear ducts by laughing. That reduces stress. (Begin with *interestingly.*)
5. Scientists tested people's saliva immediately after they laughed. Scientists concluded that immune systems may benefit from laughter. (Begin with *immediately.*)
6. Blood pressure and heart rates tend to go below baseline after we laugh. People should be happy about this effect because that's what happens after we exercise well. (Begin with *although.*)
7. Laughter causes the inner lining of our blood vessels to expand. This expansion produces good chemicals in our bodies. (Begin with *in addition.*)
8. One of these good chemicals is nitric oxide. It reduces inflammation and clotting. (Begin with *in the human body.*)
9. Laughter may even help with pain management. Laughter seems to have an analgesic effect. (Begin with *seeming.*)
10. Humor has so many physical benefits, and it makes us feel better. Try to enjoy a few laughs every day. (Begin with *because.*) ●

42D How do commas work with items in a series?

Listen to the Podcast

A series is a group of three or more elements—words, PHRASES, or CLAUSES—that match in grammatical form and are of equal importance in a sentence.

Marriage requires **sexual, financial, and emotional** discipline.

—Anne Roiphe, "Why Marriages Fail"

Culture is a way of **thinking, feeling, believing**.

—Clyde Kluckhohn, *Mirror for Man*

My love of flying stems from my days of ice **skates, of swings, and of bicycles**.

—Tresa Wiggins, student

We have been taught **that children develop by ages and stages, that the steps are pretty much the same for everybody, and that to grow out of the limited behavior of childhood, we must climb them all**.

—Gail Sheehy, *Passages*

Some publications omit the comma before *and* in a series. Check with your instructor about his or her preference.

NO The sweater comes in **blue, green, pink and black**.

Do the sweaters come in three or four colors?

YES The sweater comes in **blue, green, pink, and black**.

The comma before *and* indicates in four colors.

At all times, however, follow the "toast, juice, and ham and eggs" rule. That is, when one of the items in a series contains *and*, don't use a comma in that item.

When items in a series contain commas or other punctuation, separate them with SEMICOLONS instead of commas (see 43E).

If it's a bakery**,** they have to sell cake**;** if it's a photography shop**,** they have to develop film**;** and if it's a dry-goods store**,** they have to sell warm underwear.

—Art Buchwald, "Birth Control for Banks"

With three or more numbered or lettered items in a series, use commas (or semicolons if the items themselves contain commas) to separate them.

- To file your insurance claim, please enclose (1) a letter requesting payment**,** (2) a police report about the robbery**, and** (3) proof of purchase of the items you say are missing.

Alert: In a series, never use a comma before the first item or after the last item, unless a different rule makes it necessary.

NO **Artists, writers, and poets, have engaged** in daydreaming.

YES Artists, writers, and poets have engaged in daydreaming.

NO Such dreamers include**,** Miró, Debussy, Dostoevsky, and Dickinson.

YES Such dreamers include Miró, Debussy, Dostoevsky, and Dickinson.

YES Such dreamers include**, of course,** Miró, Debussy, Dostoevsky, and Dickinson.

As a sentence modifier, *of course* is set off from the rest of the sentence by commas before and after it (see 42C).

EXERCISE 42-3 Insert commas to separate the items in a series. If a sentence needs no commas, explain why.

EXAMPLE

Many punk and rock bands, such as Ramones The Talking Heads and Blondie, got their start in a famous club called CBGB.

Many punk and rock bands, such as Ramones**,** The Talking Heads**,** and Blondie, got their start in a famous club called CBGB.

1. Even though the club became famous for punk music, it was originally built for musicians who played country bluegrass and blues.

2. Founded in 1973 by Hilly Kristal, CBGB, located in the Bowery in New York City, is sometimes called "CBs" or "CBGBs."
3. Famous performances by singer Patti Smith the band Television and the British band The Police made CBGB an important place in the history of punk music.
4. The club has become part of popular American culture, making appearances in the TV show *The Simpsons* the Broadway show *Rent* and in the video game *Guitar Hero: Warriors of Rock*.
5. Legal battles financial troubles and political conflicts caused CBGB to close its doors in 2006, after a tribute concert featuring appearances by members of the Red Hot Chili Peppers and the band Television. ●

42E How do commas work with coordinate adjectives?

Listen to the Podcast

Coordinate adjectives are two or more ADJECTIVES of equal weight that describe—that is, modify—a NOUN. In contrast, **cumulative adjectives** build meaning from word to word, as they move toward the noun. The key to applying this rule is recognizing when adjectives are coordinate and when they aren't. Quick Box 42.2 tells you how.

Quick Box 42.2

Tests for coordinate and cumulative adjectives

If either one of these tests works, the adjectives are coordinate and require a comma between them.

- Can the order of the adjectives be reversed without changing the meaning or creating nonsense? If yes, use a comma.

NO The concert featured **new several** bands.
New several makes no sense.

YES The **huge, restless** crowd waited for the concert to begin.
Restless, huge still carries the same meaning, so these are coordinate adjectives.

- Can *and* be sensibly inserted between the adjectives? If yes, use a comma.

NO The concert featured **several and new** bands.
Several and new makes no sense.

YES The **huge and restless** crowd waited.
Modifier *huge and restless* makes sense, so these are coordinate adjectives.

- Fans cheered as the **pulsating, rhythmic** music filled the stadium.

  Pulsating and *rhythmic* are coordinate adjectives.

- Each band had a **distinctive musical** style.

  Distinctive and *musical* aren't coordinate adjectives.

Alert: Don't put a comma after a final coordinate adjective.

NO Hundreds of **roaring, cheering, yelling, fans** filled the stadium.

YES Hundreds of **roaring, cheering, yelling fans** filled the stadium.

EXERCISE 42-4 Insert commas to separate coordinate adjectives. If a sentence needs no commas, explain why. For help, consult 42E.

EXAMPLE

A scruffy beloved animal named Owney served as the unofficial mascot of the U.S. Railway Mail Service for nine years in the late 19th century.

A scruffy, beloved animal named Owney served as the unofficial mascot of the U.S. Railway Mail Service for nine years in the late 19th century.

1. Owney was a brown terrier-mix dog.
2. The myth was that he showed up as a skinny hungry stray one cold winter night in Albany, New York.
3. Owney began riding trains across the United States, where his fame earned him numerous shiny medals, so many that Postmaster General John Wanamaker gave him a harness to carry them all.
4. By 1897, the old sick dog had become somewhat mean, and he had to be put down after attacking a mail clerk.
5. Sad grateful postal workers raised money to have Owney's body preserved by taxidermy, and it still remains in the U.S. Postal museum.

42F How do commas work with nonrestrictive elements?

A **restrictive element** pinpoints, narrows, or restricts the meaning of its ANTECEDENT to a particular person or class: *Don't eat tomatoes **that are canned**.* A **nonrestrictive element** describes but does not pinpoint, narrow, or restrict the meaning of its antecedent: *Berries, **which sweeten your breakfast**, are highly nutritious.*

Use commas to separate nonrestrictive elements from the rest of a sentence. Do not use commas to separate restrictive elements from their antecedents. Simply stated:

- Restrictive element—do not use commas.
- Nonrestrictive element—use commas.

NO Someone**, named Princess,** canceled the concert.

Named Princess narrows who *someone* is to Princess; it is restrictive. Commas are unnecessary.

YES Someone **named Princess** canceled the concert.

A restrictive, pinpointing element requires no comma.

NO Princess **who writes all her material** is suing her promoter.

Who writes all her material is descriptive and does not pinpoint Princess; it is nonrestrictive. Commas are required.

YES Princess**, who writes all her material,** is suing her promoter.

A nonrestrictive element needs to be set off by commas.

NO Princess started playing on a piano**, that was out of tune**.

That was out of tune is restrictive because it identifies the piano. No comma is necessary.

YES Princess started playing on a piano **that was out of tune**.

A restrictive, pinpointing clause requires no comma.

NO **A prolific artist** Princess is on her way to fame and fortune.

A prolific artist is a descriptive, nonrestrictive element, so it requires a comma.

YES **A prolific artist,** Princess is on her way to fame and fortune.

A nonrestrictive element requires a comma.

● **EXERCISE 42-5** Using your knowledge of restrictive and nonrestrictive elements, insert commas as needed. If a sentence is correct, explain why. For help, consult 42F.

EXAMPLE

During the summer when butterflies are most active gardeners can attract them by planting the right flowers.

During the summer**,** when butterflies are most active**,** gardeners can attract them by planting the right flowers.

1. In spring as birds and bees look for water and food certain plants and trees provide those needs and thus attract the greatest number of airborne visitors.
2. Gardeners who learn to attract birds may find they have fewer problems with insects and other unwelcome pests.
3. During suburban sprawl when cities eat up more and more land birds have to adapt by putting their nests in buildings.

4. Birds are attracted to pines and evergreens where they can find food and shelter.
5. Hungry birds who are not picky will enjoy a feeder stocked with black oil sunflower seeds.
6. Birds also need to eat insects which provide a higher protein content than seeds.
7. Some common plants such as butterfly weed and lantana are ideal for attracting butterflies.
8. Because they have the nectar that butterflies want these plants enhance any butterfly garden.
9. As butterflies pass by a garden looking for bright colors and strong fragrances they will notice flowers planted in large clumps.
10. Gardens that are favorable to birds and butterflies will also invite honeybees and other pollinators. ●

42G How do commas set off parenthetical expressions, contrasts, words of direct address, and tag sentences?

When you use parenthetical expressions, contrasts, direct address, or tag sentences, you insert information that is not essential to the principal message of your sentence. Set off such information with commas.

Parenthetical expressions are "asides."

- American farmers **(according to U.S. government figures)** export more wheat than they sell at home.
- A major drought**, sad to say,** wiped out this year's wheat crop.

Use commas to set off expressions of contrast, which state what is *not* the case.

- Feeding the world's population is a serious**, though not impossible,** problem.
- We must battle world hunger continuously**, not only as famine strikes**.

Use commas to set off words of direct address, which name the person or group being spoken to (addressed).

- Join me**, brothers and sisters,** to end hunger.
- Your contribution to the Relief Fund**, Steve,** will help us greatly.

A **tag sentence** ends with a "tag," an attached phrase or question. Set off a tag with a comma. When the tag is a question, the sentence ends with a question mark.

- People will give blood regularly**, I hope**.
- The response to the blood drive was impressive**, wasn't it?**
- The drought the ended**, hasn't it?**

● **EXERCISE 42-6** Add commas to set off any parenthetical or contrasting elements, words of direct address, and tag sentences. Adjust end punctuation as necessary. For help, consult 42G.

EXAMPLE

Writer's block it seems to me is a misunderstood phenomenon.

Writer's block**,** *it seems to me***,** is a misunderstood phenomenon.

1. An inability to write some say stems from lack of discipline and a tendency to procrastinate.
2. In other words the only way to overcome writer's block is to exert more willpower.
3. But writer's block is a complex psychological event that happens to conscientious people not just procrastinators.
4. Such people strangely enough are often unconsciously rebelling against their own self-tyranny and rigid standards of perfection.
5. If I told you my fellow writer that all it takes to start writing again is to quit punishing yourself, you would think I was crazy wouldn't you? ●

42H How do commas work with quoted words?

Use commas to set off expressions (such as *he wrote* or *she proclaimed*) that accompany DIRECT DISCOURSE.

- Speaking of ideal love, the poet William Blake wrote**,** "Love seeketh not itself to please."
- "My love is a fever**,**" said William Shakespeare about love's passion.
- "I love no love**,**" proclaimed the poet Mary Coleridge**,** "but thee."

EXCEPTION

When the quoted words are blended into the grammatical structure of your sentence, don't use commas to set them off. These are instances of **indirect quotation** or INDIRECT DISCOURSE, usually occurring with *as* and *that.*

- The duke describes the duchess **as** "too soon made glad."
- The duchess insists **that** "appearing glad often is but a deception."

Alert: When the quoted words end with an exclamation point or a question mark, retain that original punctuation, even if explanatory words follow.

QUOTED WORDS *"O Romeo! Romeo!"*

NO "O Romeo! Romeo**!,**" whispered Juliet from her window.

NO "O Romeo! Romeo," whispered Juliet from her window.

YES "O Romeo! Romeo**!**" whispered Juliet from her window.

QUOTED WORDS *"Wherefore art thou Romeo?"*

NO "Wherefore art thou Romeo?," Juliet urgently asked.

NO "Wherefore art thou Romeo," Juliet urgently asked.

YES "Wherefore art thou Romeo**?**" Juliet urgently asked. ●

● **EXERCISE 42-7** Punctuate the following dialogue correctly. If a sentence is correct, explain why.

EXAMPLE

NO "I'm bored!," cried the little girl.

YES "I'm bored!" cried the little girl.

1. "Well, then" the girl's father replied "what would you like to do?"
2. The girl responded by saying that the park "sounds like a lot of fun."
3. "Have you finished your homework?," asked the father.
4. The little girl said "I don't have any homework to do. I finished it yesterday."
5. "Then let's go to the park!," announced the father. ●

42l How do commas work in dates, names, addresses, correspondence, and numbers?

When you write dates, names, addresses, correspondence, and numbers, use commas according to accepted practice. Quick Boxes 42.3 through 42.6 provide some guidelines.

Quick Box 42.3

Commas with dates

- Use a comma between the date and the year: ***July 20, 1969***.
- Use a comma between the day and the date: ***Sunday, July 20***.
- Within a sentence, use a comma on both sides of the year in a full date: *Americans sat near a TV set on July **20, 1969,** to watch the lunar landing.*
- Never use a comma when only the month and year, or the month and day, are given. Also, never use a comma between the season and year.

  YES People knew that one day in **July 1969** would change the world.

  YES News coverage was especially heavy on **July 21**.

  YES In **summer 1969** a man walked on the moon.
- Never use a comma in an inverted date, a form used in the U.S. military and throughout the world except in the United States.

  YES People stayed near their televisions on **20 July 1969** to watch the lunar landing.

Quick Box 42.4

Commas with names, places, and addresses

- When an abbreviated academic degree (*MD, PhD*) comes after a person's name, use a comma between the name and the title (*Angie Eng, MD*), and also after the title if other words follow in the sentence: *The jury listened closely to the expert testimony of **Angie Eng, MD, last week**.*
- When an indicator of birth order or succession (*Jr., Sr., III, IV*) follows a name, never use a comma: *Martin Luther **King Jr**.* or *Henry **Ford II***
- When you invert a person's name, use a comma to separate the last name from the first: ***Troyka, David***
- When city and state names are written together, use a comma to separate them: ***Philadelphia, Pennsylvania***. If the city and state fall within a sentence, use a comma after the state as well: *My family settled in **Philadelphia, Pennsylvania,** before I was born.*
- When a complete address is part of a sentence, use a comma to separate all the items, except the state and ZIP code: *I wrote to **Shelly Kupperman, 1001 Rule Road, Upper Saddle River, NJ 07458,** for more information about the comma.*

Quick Box 42.5

Commas in correspondence

- For the opening of an informal letter, use a comma: **Dear Betty,**
- For the opening of a business or formal letter, use a colon:

  Dear Ms. Kiviat:
- For the close of a letter, use a comma:

  Sincerely yours, **Best regards,** **Love,**

Quick Box 42.6

Commas with numbers

- Counting from right to left, put a comma after every three digits in numbers with more than four digits.

  72,867 156,567,066
- A comma is optional in most four-digit numbers. Be consistent within each piece of writing.

$1776	$1,776
1776 miles	1,776 miles
1776 potatoes	1,776 potatoes
- Never use a comma in a four-digit year: **1990** (*Note:* If the year has five digits or more, do use a comma: **25,000 BC**.)
- Never use a comma in an address of four digits or more: ***12161 Dean Drive***
- Never use a comma in a page number of four digits or more: ***see page 1338***
- Use a comma to separate related measurements written as words: ***five feet, four inches***
- Use a comma to separate a scene from an act in a play: ***act II, scene iv*** (or ***act 2, scene 4***)
- Use a comma to separate references to a page and a line: ***page 10, line 6***

● **EXERCISE 42-8** Insert commas where they are needed. For help, consult 42I.

EXAMPLE

On June 1 1984 the small German-French production company released a feature film called *Paris Texas.*

On June 1**,** 1984**,** the small German-French production company released a feature film called *Paris***,** *Texas.*

1. Made by the noted German director Wim Wenders, *Paris Texas* was set in an actual town in Lamar County Texas with a population of 24699.
2. The movie's title was clearly intended to play off the slightly more famous Paris in France.
3. The custom of naming little towns in the United States after cosmopolitan urban centers in the Old World has resulted in such places as Athens Georgia and St. Petersburg Florida.
4. As of December 1 2005 the American St. Petersburg was estimated to have nearly 250000 citizens and the American Athens nearly 109000.
5. By comparison, St. Petersburg Russia and Athens Greece were estimated to have populations of 4 million and 1 million, respectively. ●

42J How do commas clarify meaning?

A comma is sometimes needed to clarify the meaning of a sentence, even when no rule calls for one. You may prefer to revise your sentence to prevent misreading.

NO Of the gymnastic team's twenty five were injured.

YES Of the gymnastic team's **twenty, five** were injured.

YES Of **twenty on** the gymnastic team, five were injured. [preferred]

NO Those who can practice many hours a day.

YES **Those who can,** practice many hours a day.

YES **They** practice many hours a day **when they can**. [preferred]

NO George dressed and performed for the sellout crowd.

YES **George dressed,** and performed for the sellout crowd.

YES **After** George dressed**, he** performed for the sellout crowd. [preferred]

● **EXERCISE 42-9** Working individually or with a group, insert commas to prevent misreading.

EXAMPLE

NO Of all the parts of the human body teeth tend to last the longest.

YES Of all the parts of the human body**,** teeth tend to last the longest.

1. Humans like some other animals have two sets of teeth over a lifetime.
2. Sharks known for having deadly bites develop several sets of teeth throughout their lives.
3. Adult humans typically have 32 teeth 12 more than they had as children.
4. For children eruptions of teeth, also called teething, can be painful.
5. People who brush their teeth develop healthy gums and mouths. ●

42K How can I avoid misusing commas?

Most misuses of the comma are overuses—inserting unnecessary commas. This section summarizes the Alert notes in this chapter and lists other frequent misuses of the comma.

When advice against overusing a comma clashes with a rule requiring one, follow the rule that requires the comma.

- The town of Kitty Hawk, North Carolina, attracts thousands of tourists each year.

  While commas don't normally separate subject from verb, the comma is required here because of the rule that calls for a comma when the name of a state follows the name of a city within a sentence (see 42I).

42K.1 Commas with coordinating conjunctions

Never use a comma after a COORDINATING CONJUNCTION that joins two INDEPENDENT CLAUSES, unless another rule makes it necessary (see 42B). Also, don't use a comma to separate two items joined with a coordinating conjunction—there must be at least three (see 42D).

NO The sky was dark gray **and,** it looked like dusk.

YES The sky was dark gray**, and** it looked like dusk.

NO **The moon, and the stars** were shining last night.

YES **The moon and the stars** were shining last night.

42K.2 Commas with subordinating conjunctions and prepositions

Never put a comma after a SUBORDINATING CONJUNCTION or a PREPOSITION, unless another rule makes it necessary.

NO **Although,** the storm brought high winds, it did no damage.

YES **Although the storm brought high winds,** it did no damage.

The comma follows the full introductory subordinate clause, not the subordinate conjunction that begins it.

NO The storm did no damage **although,** it brought high winds.

YES The storm did no damage **although it brought high winds.**

No comma is required after a subordinating conjunction.

NO People expected worse **between,** the high winds and the heavy downpour.

YES People expected worse **between the high winds and the heavy downpour**.

Don't separate prepositions from their objects with commas.

42K.3 Commas in a series

Never use a comma before the first, or after the last, item in a series, unless another rule makes it necessary (see 42D).

NO The gymnasium was decorated **with, red, white, and blue** ribbons for the Fourth of July.

NO The gymnasium was decorated with **red, white, and blue, ribbons** for the Fourth of July.

YES The gymnasium was decorated with **red, white, and blue** ribbons for the Fourth of July.

Never put a comma between a final COORDINATE ADJECTIVE and the NOUN that the adjectives modify. Also, don't use a comma between adjectives that are not coordinate (see 42E).

NO He wore an **old, baggy, sweater**.

YES He wore an **old, baggy sweater**. [coordinate adjectives]

NO He has **several, new sweaters**.

YES He has **several new sweaters**. [noncoordinate, or cumulative, adjectives]

42K.4 Commas with restrictive elements

Never use a comma to set off a RESTRICTIVE (limiting) element from the rest of a sentence (see 42F).

NO **Vegetables, stir-fried in a wok,** are crisp and flavorful.

Stir-fried in a wok is limiting, so commas aren't required.

YES **Vegetables stir-fried in a wok** are crisp and flavorful.

42K.5 Commas with quotations

Use commas only with DIRECT DISCOURSE, never with INDIRECT DISCOURSE.

NO Jon said **that, he likes** stir-fried vegetables.

YES Jon said **that he likes** stir-fried vegetables.

YES **Jon said, "I like** stir-fried vegetables."

42K.6 Commas that separate a subject from its verb or a verb from its object*

A comma is distracting between these elements, but in some cases another comma rule might supersede this guideline (as in the first example in section 42K).

NO **The brothers Wright, made** their first successful airplane flights on December 17, 1903.

As a rule, a comma doesn't separate a subject from its verb.

YES **The brothers Wright made** their first successful airplane flights on December 17, 1903.

NO These inventors enthusiastically **tackled, the problems** of powered flight and aerodynamics.

As a rule, a comma doesn't separate a verb from its object.

YES These inventors enthusiastically **tackled the problems** of powered flight and aerodynamics.

● **EXERCISE 42-10** Some commas have been deliberately misused in these sentences. Delete misused commas. If a sentence is correct, explain why.

EXAMPLE

NO Alchemy was an important philosophical and scientific tradition, that led to the development of chemistry and medicine.

---

*Preposition/object is covered in 42K.2.

YES Alchemy was an important philosophical and scientific tradition that led to the development of chemistry and medicine.

1. One of the goals of alchemy was the development, of the philosopher's stone.
2. In addition to turning base metals into the gold, the philosopher's stone, was supposed to grant immortality or eternal youth.
3. According to other legends, the philosopher's stone also, cured illnesses, revived dead plants, and created clones.
4. The fantastic claims about the philosopher's stone and mentions of it in historical writings, can be traced as far back as the fourth century.
5. Because, alchemists were attempting to turn metals into gold, they developed some laboratory techniques that are still used in chemistry.
6. Alchemy also helped develop important ideas, that are used in modern medicine, such as the dangers of heavy metal poisoning.
7. Robert Boyle, considered to be a founder of modern chemistry, began his work, as an alchemist.
8. The famous, important, scientist Isaac Newton wrote more about his work in alchemy than he did about optics or physics.
9. The origins of European alchemy, date back to ancient Greece and Egypt.
10. Unlike modern science, alchemy also relied upon, religion, mythology, ancient wisdom, and the occult. ●

42L How can I avoid comma errors?

You can avoid most comma errors with these two bits of advice:

- As you write or reread what you've written, never insert a comma simply because you happen to pause to think or take a breath before moving on. Pausing isn't a reliable guide to comma usage. Throughout the United States and the world, people's breathing rhythms, accents, and thinking patterns vary greatly.

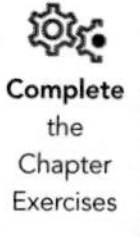

- As you're writing, if you're unsure about a comma, insert a circled comma. When you're EDITING, check this handbook for the rule that applies.

43 Semicolons

Quick Points You will learn to

➤ Use semicolons correctly (see 43A–43E).

43A What are the uses of a semicolon?

A semicolon marks within a sentence a distinction that ranks stronger than a comma but less than a period. Quick Box 43.1 shows different patterns for using semicolons.

Quick Box 43.1

Semicolon patterns

- Independent clause; independent clause (see 43B).
- Independent clause; conjunctive adverb, independent clause (see 43C).
- Independent clause; transitional expression, independent clause (see 43C).
- Independent clause, one that contains a comma; coordinating conjunction followed by independent clause (see 43D).
- Independent clause; coordinating conjunction followed by independent clause, one that contains a comma (see 43D).
- Independent clause, one that contains a comma; coordinating conjunction followed by independent clause, one that contains a comma (see 43D).
- Independent clause containing a series of items, any of which contains a comma; another item in the series; and another item in the series (see 43E).

43B When can I use a semicolon, instead of a period, between independent clauses?

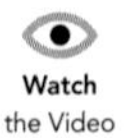

Decide whether a period (full separation) or a semicolon (partial separation) better distinguishes your closely related complete sentences (or INDEPENDENT CLAUSES). Be sure that a grammatically complete thought precedes your period or semicolon.

- Ours is my spouse's second marriage. For me, it's the first, last, and only.

  The emphasis and contrast in the second sentence rate a period.

  This is my husband's second marriage**;** it's the first for me.

  —Ruth Sidel, "Marion Deluca"

Alert: Never use a comma alone between independent clauses; else, you'll create the error known as a COMMA SPLICE (Chapter 34). ●

43C When else can I use a semicolon between independent clauses?

When the second of a set of independent clauses closely related in meaning starts with a CONJUNCTIVE ADVERB or with a TRANSITIONAL EXPRESSION, you can choose to separate the clauses with a semicolon instead of a period. Also, insert a comma following a conjunctive adverb or transitional expression that starts an independent clause. Although some professional writers today omit the comma after short words (*then, next, soon*), the rule remains for most ACADEMIC WRITING.

- The average annual rainfall in Death Valley is about two inches**; nevertheless,** hundreds of plant and animal species survive and even thrive there.
- Photographers have spent years recording desert life cycles**; as a result,** we can watch bare sand flower after a spring storm.

Alert: Never use only a comma between independent clauses that are connected by a conjunctive adverb or word of transition—this rule will prevent you from creating the error known as a COMMA SPLICE. ●

43D How do semicolons work with coordinating conjunctions?

Typically, a comma separates two INDEPENDENT CLAUSES linked by a SUBORDINATING CONJUNCTION (see 42B). However, when one or more of the independent clauses already contain a comma, link the independent clauses with a semicolon. This can help your reader see the relationship between the ideas more clearly. Quick Box 43.1 shows the various combinations of this pattern.

When the peacock has presented his back, the spectator will usually begin to walk around him to get a front view**; but** the peacock will continue to turn so that no front view is possible.

—Flannery O'Connor, "The King of the Birds"

Our Constitution is in actual operation; everything appears to promise that it will last**; but** in this world, nothing is certain but death and taxes.

—Benjamin Franklin, in a 1789 letter

For anything worth having, one must pay the price**; and** the price is always work, patience, love, self-sacrifice.

—John Burroughs

43E When should I use semicolons between items in a series?

When a sentence contains a series of items that are long or that already contain one or more commas, separate the items with semicolons. Punctuating this way groups the elements so that your reader can see where one item ends and the next begins.

- The assistant chefs chopped onions, green peppers, and parsley**;** sliced chicken and duck breasts into strips**;** started a broth simmering**; and** filled a large, shallow copper pan with oil.

43F How do I avoid misusing the semicolon?

DON'T USE A SEMICOLON AFTER AN INTRODUCTORY PHRASE

If you use a semicolon after an introductory phrase, you create the error known as a sentence fragment (see Chapter 33).

NO **Open until midnight;** the computer lab is well used.

The semicolon suggests that *open until midnight* is an independent clause.

YES **Open until midnight,** the computer lab is well used.

DON'T USE A SEMICOLON WITH A DEPENDENT CLAUSE

If you use a semicolon with a DEPENDENT CLAUSE, you create a fragment.

NO **Although the new dorms have computer facilities;** many students still prefer to go to the computer lab.

The semicolon suggests that an independent clause precedes it.

YES **Although the new dorms have computer facilities,** many students still prefer to go to the computer lab.

USE A COLON, NOT A SEMICOLON TO INTRODUCE A LIST

When the words that introduce a list form an independent clause, use a colon, never a semicolon (44B).

NO **The newscast featured three major stories;** the latest pictures of Uranus, a speech by the president, and dangerous brush fires in Nevada.

The newscast featured three major stories is an independent clause, so the punctuation before the list should be a colon, not a semicolon.

YES **The newscast featured three major stories:** the latest pictures of Uranus, a speech by the president, and dangerous brush fires in Nevada.

● **EXERCISE 43-1** Insert semicolons as needed in these items. Also, fix any incorrectly used semicolons. If a sentence is correct, explain why. For help, consult all sections of this chapter.

EXAMPLE

Bicycle racing is as popular in Europe as baseball or basketball is in the United States, it is even more heavily commercialized.

Bicycle racing is as popular in Europe as baseball or basketball is in the United States; it is even more heavily commercialized.

1. The Tour de France is the world's best-known bicycle race, the 94-year-old Giro d'Italia runs a close second.
2. Both are grueling, three-week-long events that require cyclists to cover over 2,000 miles of difficult, mountainous terrain, and both are eagerly anticipated, draw enormous crowds along their routes, and receive extensive media coverage.
3. That media attention leads to marketing opportunities for the events' sponsors; which place ads along the race's route, in the nearby towns, and on the cyclists themselves.
4. Martin Hvastija, a participant in the 2003 Giro d'Italia, had no chance of winning the race, nevertheless, he drew extensive media attention for his sponsors.
5. His method was simple; he managed to ride out in front of the field for a few brief miles.
6. Although he had no chance of winning the race; newscasters beamed his image around the world during the short time he was a front-runner, during the same period; showing the world the brightly colored advertising logos on his jersey.
7. In addition to sponsoring individual athletes, corporations plaster ads all over the towns that the race goes through, they toss samples, coupons, and gadgets to spectators from promotional vehicles that ride the route an hour ahead of the cyclists, and they run ads during TV and radio coverage of the race.

8. In 2003, the organizers of the Giro took in over $8 million in fees from advertisers and $12 million in broadcast rights from the Italian state-owned TV network, RAI, however, these figures were down a bit from the previous year.
9. An additional source of revenues for race organizers is fees from the towns where the race starts and ends each day, as a result, organizers determine the actual course according to which cities are willing to pay the $120,000 charge.
10. Media watchers think the Giro d'Italia could become even more profitable and popular, especially among young adults, but only if it took a cue from the Tour de France by encouraging; more international press coverage, more star riders, and even heavier corporate sponsorship. ●

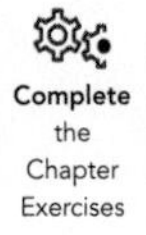
Complete the Chapter Exercises

● **EXERCISE 43-2** Combine each set of sentences into one sentence so that it contains two independent clauses. Use a semicolon correctly between the two clauses. You may add, omit, revise, and rearrange words. Try to use all the patterns in this chapter, and explain the reasoning behind your decisions. More than one revision may be correct. For help, consult all sections of this chapter.

EXAMPLE

Although not as well known as Thomas Edison, the inventor Nikola Tesla was a revolutionary and important scientist. One biographer calls him "the man who invented the twentieth century."

Although not as well known as Thomas Edison, the inventor Nikola Tesla was a revolutionary scientist; one biographer calls him "the man who invented the twentieth century."

1. Tesla was born in what is now Croatia and studied at the Technical University at Graz, Austria. He excelled in physics, mechanical engineering, and electrical engineering.
2. Tesla's accomplishments include inventing alternating current. He also contributed to the fields of robotics, computer science, and wireless technology. And he helped increase knowledge of nuclear physics, ballistics, and electromagnetism.
3. The Italian inventor Guglielmo Marconi and Tesla both claimed to have invented the radio. However, the U.S. Supreme Court, in 1943, upheld Tesla's radio patent and officially credited him as the device's inventor.
4. In 1901, Tesla began construction of a tower that he claimed would create a global network of wireless communication and be able to control the weather. Unfortunately, Tesla soon lost funding and never finished the project.
5. At his lab in Colorado Springs, he was able to produce artificial lightning. This scene was vividly portrayed in the 2006 film *The Prestige*. ●

44 Colons

Quick Points You will learn to

➤ Use colons correctly (see 44A–44E).

44A What are the uses of a colon?

A colon anticipates a list, an APPOSITIVE, or a QUOTATION after an INDEPENDENT CLAUSE. Quick Box 44.1 shows different patterns for using a colon.

Quick Box 44.1

Colon patterns

- Independent clause**:** list (see 44B).
- Independent clause**:** appositive (see 44B).
- Independent clause**:** "Quoted words" (see 44B).
- Independent clause**:** Independent clause that explains or summarizes the prior independent clause (see 44B).

44B When can a colon introduce a list, an appositive, or a quotation?

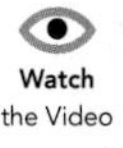

When a complete sentence—that is, an INDEPENDENT CLAUSE—introduces a list, an APPOSITIVE, or a QUOTATION, place a colon before the words being introduced. These words don't have to form an independent clause themselves, but a complete sentence before the colon is essential.

INTRODUCING LISTED ITEMS

When a complete sentence introduces a list, a colon is required, as demonstrated in the following example.

- **If you really want to lose weight, you must do three things:** eat smaller portions, exercise, and drink lots of water.

  An independent clause precedes the list, so a colon is correct.

When the lead-in words at the end of an independent clause are *such as, including, like*, or *consists of*, never use a colon. If the lead-in words at the end of an independent clause are *the following* or *as follows*, do use a colon.

- **The students demanded improvements *such as*** an expanded menu in the cafeteria, improved janitorial services, and more up-to-date textbooks.
- **The students demanded *the following:*** an expanded menu in the cafeteria, improved janitorial services, and more up-to-date textbooks.

INTRODUCING APPOSITIVES

An APPOSITIVE is a word or words that rename a NOUN or PRONOUN. When an appositive is introduced by an independent clause, use a colon.

- **Only cats are likely to approve of one old-fashioned remedy for cuts:** a lotion of catnip, butter, and sugar.

  An independent clause comes before the appositive: *a lotion of catnip, butter, and sugar* renames *old-fashioned remedy*.

INTRODUCING QUOTATIONS

When an independent clause introduces a quotation, use a colon after it. (If the words introducing a quotation don't form an independent clause, use a comma.)

- **The little boy in *E.T.* did say something neat:** "How do you explain school to a higher intelligence?"

  The required independent clause comes before the quotation.

—George F. Will, "Well, I Don't Love You, E.T."

44C When can I use a colon between two independent clauses?

Quick Box 44.1 shows the pattern for using a colon before a second INDEPENDENT CLAUSE that explains or summarizes a first independent clause. The first word after a colon may be capitalized for emphasis: *I'll say it once again: Snakes are lovable. I'll say it again: snakes are lovable*. Either option is correct.

44D What standard formats require a colon?

A variety of standard formats in American English require a colon. Also, colons are used in many DOCUMENTATION STYLES, as shown in Chapters 25, 26, and 27.

TITLE AND SUBTITLE

A Brief History of Time: From the Big Bang to Black Holes

HOURS, MINUTES, AND SECONDS

The plane took off at 7:15 p.m.

The runner passed the halfway point at 1:23:02.

Alert: In the military, hours and minutes are written without colons: *We meet at 0430, not at 0930.* ●

REFERENCES TO BIBLE CHAPTERS AND VERSES

Psalms 23:1–3

Luke 3:13

MEMOS

Date: January 9, 2012

To: Dean Kristen Olivero

From: Professor Daniel Black

Re: Student Work-Study Program

SALUTATION IN A BUSINESS LETTER

Dear Dr. Jewell:

44E When is a colon wrong?

INDEPENDENT CLAUSES

A colon introduces a list, an APPOSITIVE, or a QUOTATION only after an INDEPENDENT CLAUSE. Similarly, a colon can be used between two independent clauses when the second summarizes or explains the first.

NO The cook bought: eggs, milk, cheese, and bread.

The cook bought isn't an independent clause.

YES The cook bought eggs, milk, cheese, and bread.

A colon never follows a PHRASE or DEPENDENT CLAUSE. It follows an INDEPENDENT CLAUSE.

NO Day after day: the drought dragged on.

Day after day is a phrase, not an independent clause.

YES Day after day, the drought dragged on.

NO After the drought ended: the farmers celebrated.

After the drought ended is a dependent clause, not an independent clause.

YES After the drought ended, the farmers celebrated.

LEAD-IN WORDS

Never use a colon after the lead-in words *such as, including, like,* and *consists of.*

NO The health board discussed many problems **such as:** poor water quality, aging sewage treatment systems, and the lack of alternative water supplies.

YES The health board discussed poor water quality, aging sewage treatment systems, and the lack of alternative water supplies.

This revision requires no colon.

YES The health board discussed many problems**, such as** poor water quality, an aging sewage treatment system, and the lack of alternative water supplies.

A comma, not a colon, is correct before *such as.*

YES The health board discussed many problems**:** poor water quality, aging sewage treatment systems, and the lack of alternative water supplies.

The colon after the independent clause introduces a list.

● **EXERCISE 44-1** Insert colons where needed and delete any not needed. If a sentence is correct, explain why.

EXAMPLE

NO After months of work, Carlos was finally ready to mail his college applications to the following schools, Valley College, East California University, and Blakeville College.

YES After months of work, Carlos was finally ready to mail his college applications to the following schools: Valley College, East California University, and Blakeville College.

1. To prepare for the application process, Carlos read the book *Expanding Your Options, A Guide to Writing a Successful College Application.*
2. Date 2 March 2012
To Office of Admissions
To whom it may concern
3. Since the post office closed at 530, Carlos had to rush to meet the application deadline.
4. To represent himself effectively, Carlos wrote his application letter about his many successes, such as: his high grade point average, his work as the high school newspaper editor, and his community service.
5. After his application was completed and in the mail: he started to look forward to hearing back from the colleges.
6. He decided not to worry when he remembered the words of his favorite Bible quote from Matthew 6,34.

7. He also remembered the encouraging words from his guidance counselor: "Don't worry, Carlos. Something will work out for you."
8. He hoped that he would be accepted to his first choice, Valley College.
9. Valley College was his first choice because it offered: beautiful scenery, a diverse student body, and a small teacher-student ratio.
10. However: Valley College is very selective and admits only a small percentage of applicants. ●

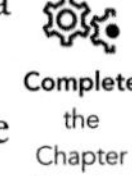
Complete the Chapter Exercises

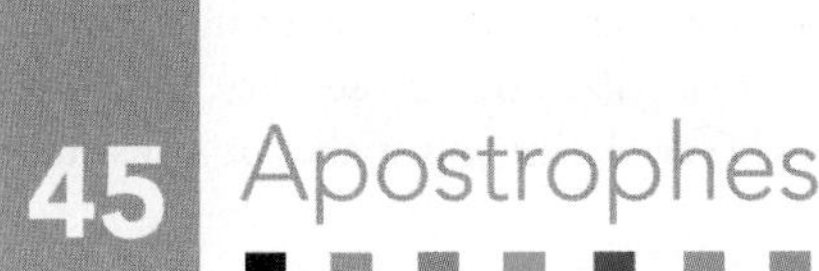

45 Apostrophes

Quick Points You will learn to

➤ Use apostrophes correctly (see 45A–45G).

45A What is the role of the apostrophe?

The apostrophe plays four roles: It creates the POSSESSIVE CASE of NOUNS (see 45B), forms the possessive case of INDEFINITE PRONOUNS (see 45E), stands for one or more omitted letters (a CONTRACTION; see 45D), and helps form plurals of letters and numerals (see 45F).

In contrast, here are two roles the apostrophe doesn't play: It doesn't form the plurals of nouns, and it doesn't form the plural of PERSONAL PRONOUNS in the possessive case.

45B How do I use an apostrophe to show a possessive noun?

An apostrophe works with a NOUN to form the POSSESSIVE CASE, which shows ownership or a close relationship.

Watch the Video

OWNERSHIP The **writer's** pen ran out of ink.

CLOSE RELATIONSHIP The **novel's** plot is complicated.

Possession in nouns can be communicated in two ways: by a PHRASE starting with *of* (*comments **of** the instructor; comments **of** Professor Furman*) or by an apostrophe and the letter *s* (*the instructor's comments; Professor Furman's comments*). Here's a list of specific rules governing the usage of *'s*.

- **Add *'s* to nouns not ending in *-s:***
  - She felt a **parent's** joy.

    Parent is a singular noun not ending in *-s*.
  - We care about our **children's** education.

    Children is a plural noun not ending in *-s*.
- **Add *'s* to singular nouns ending in *-s:*** You can add either *'s* or the apostrophe alone to show possession when a singular noun ends in *-s*. In this handbook, we use *'s* to clearly mark singular-noun possessives, no matter what letter ends the noun. Whichever choice you make, be consistent within each piece of writing.
  - The **bus's** (or **bus'**) air conditioning is out of order.
  - **Chris's** (or **Chris'**) ordeal ended.

  If you encounter a tongue-twisting pronunciation (*Moses's story*), you may decide not to add the additional *-s* (*Moses' story*). Do remember, however, to be consistent within each piece of writing.
- **Add only an apostrophe to a plural noun ending in *-s:***
  - The two **boys'** statements helped solve the crime.
  - The **workers'** contract permits three **months'** maternity leave.
- **Add *'s* to the last word in compound words and phrases:**
  - His **mother-in-law's** corporation has bought out a competitor.
  - The **attorney general's** investigation led to several arrests.
- **Add *'s* to each noun in individual possession:**
  - **Shirley's** and **Kayla's** houses are next to each other.

    Shirley and Kayla each own a house; they don't own the houses jointly.
- **Add *'s* to only the last noun in joint or group possession:**
  - **Kareem and Brina's** house has a screened porch.

    Kareem and Brina own one house.
  - **Pat and Justin's** houses always have nice lawns.

    Pat and Justin jointly own more than one house.

45C How do I use an apostrophe with possessive pronouns?

When a POSSESSIVE PRONOUN ends with *-s* (*hers, his, its, ours, yours*, and *theirs*), never add an apostrophe. Following is a list of PERSONAL PRONOUNS and their possessive forms. None of these possessive forms use *'s*.

Personal Pronouns	Possessive Forms	Personal Pronouns	Possessive Forms
I	my, mine	it	its
you	your, yours	we	our, ours
he	his	they	their, theirs
she	her, hers	who	whose

45D How do I use an apostrophe with contractions?

In a **contraction**, an apostrophe takes the place of one or more omitted letters. Be careful not to confuse a contraction with a POSSESSIVE PRONOUN. Doing so is a common spelling error, which many people—including employers—consider unprofessional. Whether or not that's fair, it's usually true.

Listen to the Podcast

it's (contraction for *it is*) **its** (possessive pronoun)
they're (contraction for *they are*) **their** (possessive pronoun)
who's (contraction for *who is*) **whose** (possessive form of *who*)
you're (contraction for *you are*) **your** (possessive pronoun)

NO The government has to balance **it's** budget.

YES The government has to balance **its** budget.

NO The professor **who's** class was canceled is ill.

YES The professor **whose** class was canceled is ill.

Remember that many instructors think contractions aren't appropriate in ACADEMIC WRITING. Nevertheless, the *MLA Handbook* accepts contractions, including *'90s* for *the 1990s*. In this handbook, we use contractions because we're addressing you, the student. We suggest, however, that before you use contractions in your academic writing, you check with your instructor. Here's a list of common contractions.

COMMON CONTRACTIONS

aren't = *are not*	isn't = *is not*	we're = *we are*
can't = *cannot*	it's = *it is*	weren't = *were not*
didn't = *did not*	let's = *let us*	we've = *we have*
don't = *do not*	she's = *she is*	who's = *who is*
he's = *he is*	there's = *there is*	won't = *will not*
I'd = *I would, I had*	they're = *they are*	you're = *you are*
I'm = *I am*	wasn't = *was not*	

Alert: One contraction required in all writing is *o'clock* (which means *of the clock*, an expression used long ago). ●

45E How do I use an apostrophe with possessive indefinite pronouns?

An apostrophe works with an INDEFINITE PRONOUN (see list in Quick Box 31.6 in 31I) to form the POSSESSIVE CASE, which shows ownership or a close relationship.

OWNERSHIP	**Everyone's** dinner is ready.
CLOSE RELATIONSHIP	**Something's** aroma is appealing.

Possession in indefinite pronouns can be communicated in two ways: by a PHRASE starting with *of* (*comments **of** everyone*) or by an apostrophe and the letter *s* (*everyone**'s** comments*).

45F How do I form the plural of miscellaneous elements?

Until recently, the plural of elements such as letters meant as letters, words meant as words, numerals, and symbols could be formed by adding either *'s* or *s*. Current MLA guidelines endorse the use of *s* only, with the exception of adding *'s* to letters meant as letters. MLA recommends using italics for letters meant as letters and words meant as words. The following examples reflect MLA practices.

PLURAL OF LETTERS MEANT AS LETTERS	Printing ***W's*** confuses young children.
PLURAL OF LETTERS MEANT AS WORDS	He earned all **Bs** in his courses.
PLURAL OF WORDS MEANT AS WORDS	Too many ***ifs*** in a contract make me suspicious.
PLURAL OF NUMBERS	Her e-mail address contains many **7s.**

PLURAL OF YEARS I remember the **1990s** well.

PLURAL OF SYMBOLS What do those **&s** mean?

45G When is an apostrophe wrong?

If you're a writer who makes apostrophe errors repeatedly, memorize the rules you need. Then you won't be annoyed by "that crooked little mark," a nickname popular with students who wish the apostrophe would go away. Quick Box 45.1 lists the major apostrophe errors.

Quick Box 45.1

Leading apostrophe errors

- Never use an apostrophe with a PRESENT-TENSE verb.
  - Exercise **plays** [not **play's**] an important role in how long we live.
- Always use an apostrophe after the *-s* in a POSSESSIVE plural of a noun.
  - **Patients'** [not **Patients**] questions seek detailed answers.
- Never add an apostrophe at the end of a nonpossessive noun ending in *-s*.
  - Medical **studies** [not **studies'** or **study's**] show this to be true.
- Never use an apostrophe to form a nonpossessive plural.
  - **Teams** [not **Team's**] of doctors have studied the effects of cholesterol.

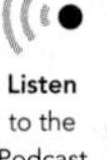
Listen to the Podcast

EXERCISE 45-1 Rewrite these sentences to insert *'s* or an apostrophe alone to make the words in parentheses show possession. (Delete the parentheses.) For help, consult 45B and 45E.

EXAMPLE

All boxes, cans, and bottles on a (supermarket) shelves are designed to appeal to (people) emotions.

All boxes, cans, and bottles on a *supermarket's* shelves are designed to appeal to *people's* emotions.

1. A (product) manufacturer designs packaging to appeal to (consumers) emotions through color and design.
2. Marketing specialists know that (people) beliefs about a (product) quality are influenced by their emotional response to the design of its package.

3. Circles and ovals appearing on a (box) design supposedly increase a (product user) feelings of comfort, while bold patterns and colors attract a (shopper) attention.
4. Using circles and bold designs in (Arm & Hammer) and (Tide) packaging produces both effects in consumers.
5. (Heinz) ketchup bottle and (Coca-Cola) famous logo achieve the same effects by combining a bright color with an old-fashioned, "comfortable" design.
6. Often, a (company) marketing consultants will custom-design products to appeal to the supposedly "typical" (adult female) emotions or to (adult males), (children), or (teenagers) feelings.
7. One of the (marketing business) leading consultants, Stan Gross, tests (consumers) reactions to (companies) products and their packages by asking consumers to associate products with well-known personalities.
8. Thus, (test takers) responses to (Gross) questions might reveal that a particular brand of laundry detergent has (Russell Crowe) toughness, (Oprah Winfrey) determination, or (someone else) sparkling personality.
9. Manufacturing (companies) products are not the only ones relying on (Gross) and other corporate (image makers) advice.
10. (Sports teams) owners also use marketing specialists to design their (teams) images, as anyone who has seen the angry bull logo of the Chicago Bulls basketball team will agree. ●

Complete the Chapter Exercises

● **EXERCISE 45-2** Rewrite these sentences so that each has a possessive noun. For help, consult 45B and 45E.

EXAMPLE

The light of a firefly gives off no heat.

A *firefly's* light gives off no heat.

1. The scientific name of a firefly is *lampyridae*, but nicknames of the bug include *glowworm* and *lightning bug*.
2. More than two thousand species of fireflies can be found throughout the temperate climates of the world.
3. The light of a firefly is caused by a chemical reaction in the organs of the abdomen.
4. Fireflies played a role in the mythology of ancient Mayans and were often compared to the light of a star.
5. Although it may be in the interest of nobody to know, fireflies are not flies at all; they are, according to the classifications of scientists, beetles. ●

46 Quotation Marks

Quick Points You will learn to

➤ Use quotation marks correctly (see 46A–46I).

46A What is the role of quotation marks?

Quotation marks are most often used to enclose **direct quotations**—a speaker or writer's exact words. In addition, quotation marks enclose titles, and they alert readers to words you single out for consideration.

Double quotation marks open and close the entire quotation. Single quotation marks signal quotations within quotations: *Ray said, "I heard a man shout 'Help me,' but I couldn't respond."* Quotation marks operate only in pairs: to open and to close. Be sure to close all quotation marks you open.

Throughout this book, we use MLA STYLE to format examples. Other documentation styles require different formats. For MLA style, see Chapter 25; for APA STYLE, see Chapter 26.

46B How do I use quotation marks with short direct quotations?

Use double quotation marks to start and finish a **short quotation**, which, in MLA STYLE, means a quotation fewer than four typed lines. Offer DOCUMENTATION information after a short quotation, before the sentence's period.

SHORT QUOTATIONS

Remarked director Fritz Lang of his masterpiece *Siegfried*, "Nothing in this film is accidental" (228).

A recent survey of leading employers found that almost all professional employees "are expected to write competently on the job" (11).

46C Are quotation marks used with long quotations?

No. In MLA STYLE, a quotation is *long* if it occupies four or more typed lines. Instead of using quotation marks with a **long quotation**, indent all its lines as a block (that is, the quotation is "set off" or "displayed"). Give DOCUMENTATION information after the period that ends the quotation.

LONG QUOTATIONS

Gardner uses criteria by which to judge whether an ability deserves to be categorized as an "intelligence." Each must confer

> a set of skills of problem solving—enabling the individual to resolve genuine problems or difficulties [author's emphasis] that he or she encounters and laying the groundwork for the acquisition of new knowledge. (*Frames* 60–61)

In the Gardner example above, note that a capital letter is *not* used to start the quotation. The lead-in words (*Each must confer*) form an incomplete sentence, so they need the quotation to complete the sentence.

Goleman also emphasizes a close interaction of the emotional and rational states with the other intelligences that Gardner has identified:

> These two minds, the emotional and the rational, operate in tight harmony for the most part, intertwining their very different ways of knowing to guide us through the world. Ordinarily there is a balance between emotional and rational minds, with emotion feeding into and informing the operations of the rational mind, and the rational mind refining and sometimes vetoing the inputs of the emotions. (9)

In the Goleman example above, note that a capital letter starts the quotation because the lead-in words are a complete sentence. (A colon can also end the lead-in sentence because it's preceded by an independent clause; see 44B.)

Alert: Whether a quotation is one word or occupies many lines, always document its SOURCE. Also, when you quote material, be very careful to record the words exactly as they appear in the original. ●

46D How do I use quotation marks for quotations within quotations?

Watch the Video

MLA STYLE uses different formats for short and long quotations of prose that contain quotes within them. Quotes within short quotations take single quotation marks, while double quotes enclose the entire quotation. Give documentation information after the entire quotation, before the sentence's ending period. For other documentation styles, check each style's manual.

Quotes within longer quotations—four or more lines set off in a block—use double and single quotation marks exactly as the original source does. Give documentation information after the long quotation following the closing punctuation.

SHORT QUOTATIONS: USE SINGLE WITHIN DOUBLE QUOTATION MARKS (MLA STYLE)

With short quotations, the double quotation marks show the beginning and end of words taken from the source; the single quotation marks replace double marks used in the source.

ORIGINAL SOURCE

Most scientists concede that they don't really know what "intelligence" is. Whatever it might be, paper and pencil tests aren't the tenth of it.

—Brent Staples, "The IQ Cult," p. 293

STUDENT'S USE OF THE SOURCE

Brent Staples argues in his essay about IQ as an object of reverence: "Most scientists concede that they don't really know what 'intelligence' is. Whatever it might be, paper and pencil tests aren't the tenth of it" (293).

LONG QUOTATIONS: USE QUOTATION MARKS AS IN SOURCE

Since long quotations are set off (displayed) without being enclosed in quotation marks, show any double and single quotation marks exactly as the source does.

46E How do I use quotation marks for quotations of poetry and dialogue?

POETRY (MLA STYLE)

A *short* poetry quotation includes three lines or fewer of a poem. As with prose quotations (see 46D), double quotation marks enclose the material. If the poetry lines contain double quotation marks, change them to single quotation marks. To show a break between lines of poetry, use a slash (/) with one space on each side. Give DOCUMENTATION information after a short poetry quotation, before the period that ends the sentence (see also 47E).

- As Auden wittily defined personal space, "some thirty inches from my nose / The frontier of my person goes" (*Complete* 205).

A quotation of poetry is *long* if it includes more than three lines of a poem. As with prose quotations (see 46D), indent all lines as a block, without quotation marks. Start new lines exactly as your source does. Give documentation information after the quotation and after the period that ends the quotation.

Alert: When you quote poetry, follow the capitalization of your source. ●

DIALOGUE (MLA AND APA STYLES)

Dialogue, also called DIRECT DISCOURSE, presents a speaker's exact words. Enclose dialogue in quotation marks. In contrast, INDIRECT DISCOURSE reports what a speaker said and requires no quotation marks. Additionally, PRONOUN use and VERB TENSES also differ for these two types of discourse.

DIRECT DISCOURSE	The mayor said, **"I** intend to veto that bill."
INDIRECT DISCOURSE	The mayor said **that he intended** to veto that bill.

Use double quotation marks at the beginning and end of a speaker's words. This tells your reader which words are the speaker's. Also, start a new paragraph each time the speaker changes.

> "I don't know how you can see to drive," she said.
>
> "Maybe you should put on your glasses."
>
> "Putting on my glasses would help you to see?"
>
> "Not me; you," Macon said. "You're focused on the windshield instead of the road."
>
> —Anne Tyler, *The Accidental Tourist*

In American English, if two or more paragraphs present a single speaker's words, start each new paragraph with double quotation marks, but save the closing double quotation marks until the end of the last quoted paragraph.

● **EXERCISE 46-1** Working individually or with a group, decide whether each sentence that follows is direct or indirect discourse and then rewrite each sentence in the other form. Make any changes needed for grammatical correctness. With direct discourse, put the speaker's words wherever you think they belong in the sentence.

EXAMPLE

Dr. Sanchez explained to Mary that washing her hands in an important part of hygiene.

Dr. Sanchez explained, "Washing your hands is an important part of hygiene."

1. Mary asked, "If my hands aren't dirty, why is it so important to wash them?"
2. Dr. Sanchez replied that many diseases are spread because of inadequately washed and infected hands.
3. The Centers for Disease Control, explained Dr. Sanchez, argues that hand washing may seem trivial but it is a vital part of public health.

4. Mary asked, "Is it ok to use alcohol-based hand sanitizers instead of soap and water?"
5. Dr. Sanchez replied that soap and clean water are best, but a sanitizer with at least 60% alcohol is also very effective. ●

46F How do I use quotation marks with titles of short works?

Titles of certain short works are enclosed in quotation marks (other works, usually longer, need italics; see 48G). Short works include short stories, essays, poems, articles from periodicals, pamphlets, brochures, songs, and individual episodes of a series on television or radio.

- What is the rhyme scheme of Poe's poem "The Raven"?
- Have you read "The Lottery"? [short story]
- The best source I found is "The Myth of Political Consultants." [magazine article]
- Rand's essay "Apollo II" offers an eyewitness account of the launch.

Titles of some other works are neither enclosed in quotation marks nor written in italics. For guidelines, see Quick Box 48.1 in 48E and Quick Box 48.2 in 48G.

Alert: Unless the title of a paper you wrote quotes someone, don't enclose it in quotation marks. ●

● **EXERCISE 46-2** Working individually or with a group, correct any misuses of quotation marks. For help, consult 46F.

1. The song America the Beautiful by Katharine Lee Bates celebrates the natural beauty and the ideals that many people associate with the United States.
2. Ralph Waldo Emerson's essay The American Scholar praises the ideals of independence and self-reliance in American education and was first heard as an oration delivered to the "Phi Beta Kappa Society."
3. However, not only the ideals, but also the harsh realities of life in America for Filipino immigrants form the basis of Carlos Bulosan's autobiography, America Is in the Heart.
4. A film that honestly and poignantly reveals the realities facing a family of Irish immigrants in New York City and their hopes for a better life is In America.
5. The poet Langston Hughes in his poem Let America Be America Again is fierce in his criticism of the way poor people and minorities are often treated in the United States. ●

46G How do I use quotation marks for words used as words?

Choose consistently either quotation marks or italics to refer to a word as a word.

NO Many people confuse affect and effect.

YES Many people confuse "affect" and "effect."

YES Many people confuse *affect* and *effect*.

Always put quotation marks around the English translation of a word or PHRASE. Also, use italics for the word or phrase in the other language.

- My grandfather usually ended arguments with *de gustibus non disputandum est* ("there is no disputing about tastes").

Many writers use quotation marks around words or phrases meant ironically or in other nonliteral ways.

- The proposed tax "reform" is actually a tax increase.

You can place quotation marks around technical terms—but only the first time they appear. Once you use and define the term, you no longer need quotation marks.

- "Plagiarism"—the undocumented use of another person's words or ideas—can result in expulsion. Plagiarism is a serious offense.

If you use a slang term in ACADEMIC WRITING, use quotation marks. However, when possible, revise your slang with language appropriate to academic writing.

- They "eat like birds" in public, but they "stuff their faces" in private.
- They **nibble** in public, but they **gorge themselves** in private.

A nickname doesn't call for quotation marks, unless you use the nickname along with the full name. When a person's nickname is widely known, you don't have to give both the nickname and the full name. For example, use *Representative Gabrielle Giffords* or *Representative Gabby Giffords*, whichever is appropriate in context. Because she's well known, don't use *Representative Gabrielle "Gabby" Giffords.*

● **EXERCISE 46-3** Working individually or with a group, correct any misuses of quotation marks. If you think a sentence is correct, explain why. For help, consult 46G.

EXAMPLE

The word asyndeton simply means that a conjunction has been omitted, as when Shakespeare writes, A woman mov'd is like a fountain troubled, / Muddy, ill seeming, thick, bereft of beauty.

The word "asyndeton" simply means that a conjunction has been omitted, as when Shakespeare writes, "A woman mov'd is like a fountain troubled, / Muddy, ill seeming, thick, bereft of beauty."

1. Shakespeare's phrases such as the sound and the fury from *Macbeth* and pale fire from *The Tempest* have been used by authors such as William Faulkner and Vladimir Nabokov as titles for their books.
2. Shakespeare's understanding of human nature was "profound" and helped him become a "prolific" writer.
3. Many words used commonly today, such as "addiction" and "alligator," were first used in print by Shakespeare.
4. To understand the difference between the words sanguinary and *sanguine* is important for a reader of Shakespeare because the former means bloody and the latter means optimistic.
5. In the play *Romeo and Juliet*, one of Shakespeare's most famous quotations is What's in a name? That which we call a rose / By any other name would smell as sweet. ●

46H How do I use quotation marks with other punctuation?

COMMAS AND PERIODS WITH QUOTATION MARKS

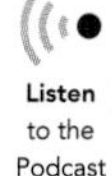
Listen to the Podcast

An appropriate comma or period is always placed *inside* the closing quotation mark.

- Jessica enjoyed F. Scott Fitzgerald's story "The Freshest Boy," so she was eager to read his novels.
- Max said, "Don't stand so far away from me."
- Edward T. Hall coined the word "proxemia."

SEMICOLONS AND COLONS WITH QUOTATION MARKS

A semicolon or colon is placed *outside* the closing quotation mark, unless it is part of the quotation.

- Computers offer businesses "opportunities that never existed before"; some workers disagree. [semicolon after closing quotation mark]
- We have to know each culture's standard for "how close is close": No one wants to offend. [colon after closing quotation mark]

QUESTION MARKS, EXCLAMATION POINTS, AND DASHES WITH QUOTATION MARKS

If the punctuation marks belong to the words enclosed in quotation marks, put them inside the quotation marks.

- "Did I Hear You Call My Name**?**" was the winning song.
- "I've won the lottery**!**" Arielle shouted.
- "Who's there? Why don't you ans**—**"

If a question mark, an exclamation point, or a dash doesn't belong to the material being quoted, put the punctuation outside the quotation marks.

- Have you read Nikki Giovanni's poem "Knoxville, Tennessee"**?**
- If only I could write a story like David Wallace's "Girl with Curious Hair"**!**
- Weak excuses—a classic is "My dog ate my homework"—never convince.

When you use quotation marks and want to know how they work with capital letters, see 48D; with brackets, 47C; with ellipsis points, 47D; and with the slash, 47E.

46I When are quotation marks wrong?

Never enclose a word in quotation marks simply for intensity or sarcasm.

NO I'm "very" happy about the news.

YES I'm very happy about the news.

Never enclose the title of your paper in quotation marks (or underline it). However, if the title of your paper contains another title that requires quotation marks, use those marks only for the included title.

NO "The Elderly in Nursing Homes: A Case Study"

YES The Elderly in Nursing Homes: A Case Study

NO Character Development in Shirley Jackson's Story The Lottery

YES Character Development in Shirley Jackson's Story "The Lottery"

● **EXERCISE 46-4** Correct any errors in the use of quotation marks and other punctuation with quotation marks. If you think a sentence is correct, explain why.

1. Mark Twain's observation "—Facts are stubborn things, but statistics are more pliable.—" is an interesting critique of news media.
2. Twain valued travel and said that it "liberates the vandal." He argues that you cannot become: "bigoted, opinionated, stubborn, narrow-minded"

if you travel. Someone who refuses to travel is, "stuck in one place" and thinks that" God made the world" for his "comfort and satisfaction."

3. In a poem called Genius, Mark Twain says that: Genius, like gold and precious stones / is chiefly prized because of its rarity.
4. Was it Shakespeare or Twain who wrote, "The course of true love never did run smooth?"
5. In a speech offering advice to young people, Twain said, "Be respectful to your superiors, if you have any". ●

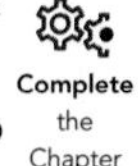

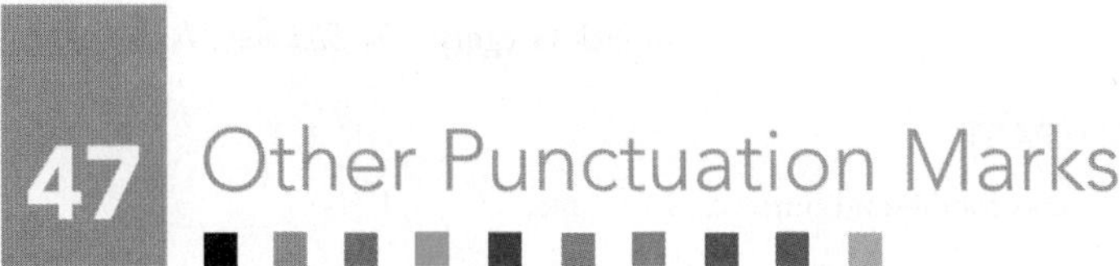

47 Other Punctuation Marks

Quick Points You will learn to

➤ Use dashes, parentheses, brackets, ellipses, and slashes correctly (see 47A–47I).

While dashes, parentheses, brackets, ellipsis points, slashes, and hyphens are not used frequently, each serves a purpose(s) and gives you further opportunities for writing precision and style.

DASH

47A When can I use a dash in my writing?

The dash, typed as two unspaced hyphens, interrupts a thought within a sentence—in the middle or at the end—for special emphasis or commentary. If you handwrite a dash, make it about twice as long as a hyphen.

USING DASHES FOR SPECIAL EMPHASIS

To emphasize an example, a definition, an appositive, or a contrast, you can use a dash or dashes. A dash tells your readers to take note, something special is coming. Use dashes sparingly so that you don't dilute their impact.

EXAMPLE

The caretakers—those who are helpers, nurturers, teachers, mothers—are still systematically devalued.

—Ellen Goodman, "Just Woman's Work?"

DEFINITION

Although the emphasis at the school was mainly language—speaking, reading, writing—the lessons always began with an exercise in politeness.

—Jade Snow Wong, *Fifth Chinese Daughter*

APPOSITIVE

Two of the strongest animals in the jungle are vegetarians—the elephant and the gorilla.

—Dick Gregory, *The Shadow That Scares Me*

CONTRAST

Fire cooks food—and burns down forests.

—Smokey the Bear

Place what you emphasize with dashes next to or nearby the material it refers to so that what you want to accomplish with your emphasis is not lost.

NO The current **argument is**—one that faculty, students, and coaches debate fiercely—whether to hold athletes to the same academic standards as others face.

YES The current **argument**—one that faculty, students, and coaches debate fiercely—**is** whether to hold athletes to the same academic standards as others face.

USING DASHES TO EMPHASIZE AN ASIDE

An aside, a writer's commentary often expressing personal views, is generally inappropriate for academic writing. Before you insert an aside, carefully consider both your writing purpose and your audience.

Television showed us the war. It showed us the war in a way that was—if you chose to watch television, at least—unavoidable.

—Nora Ephron, *Scribble Scribble*

Alerts: (1) If the words within a pair of dashes require a question mark or an exclamation point, place it before the second dash.

- A first date—do you remember**?**—stays in the memory forever.

(2) Never use commas, semicolons, or periods next to dashes. If such a need arises, revise your writing.

(3) Never enclose quotation marks in dashes except when the meaning requires them. These two examples show that, when required, the dash stops before or after the quotation marks; the two punctuation marks do not overlap.

- Many of George Orwell's essays—"A Hanging," for example—draw on his experiences as a civil servant.
- "Shooting an Elephant"—another Orwell essay—appears in many anthologies. ●

● **EXERCISE 47-1** Write a sentence about each topic, shown in italics. Use dashes to set off what is asked for, shown in roman, in each sentence. For help, consult 47A.

EXAMPLE

punctuation mark, an aside

Sometimes I get confused—but what's new?—about the difference between a colon and a semicolon.

1. *ice cream flavor*, an aside
2. *a shape*, a definition
3. *sport*, an appositive
4. *public transportation*, an example
5. *occupation*, a contrast
6. *musical instrument*, a definition
7. *TV show*, an aside
8. *American president*, an example
9. *country*, an appositive
10. *animal*, a contrast ●

PARENTHESES

47B When can I use parentheses in my writing?

Parentheses enclose material which (unlike dashes, 47A) connects the inserts they enclose loosely, not emphatically, to your sentence. Use parentheses sparingly. Overusing them causes your writing to lurch, not flow.

USING PARENTHESES TO ENCLOSE INTERRUPTING WORDS

EXPLANATION

After they've finished with the pantry, the medicine cabinet, and the attic, they will throw out the red geranium (too many leaves), sell the dog (too many fleas), and send the children off to boarding school (too many scuffmarks on the hardwood floors).

—Suzanne Britt, "Neat People vs. Sloppy People"

EXAMPLE

Though other cities (Dresden, for instance) had been utterly destroyed in World War II, never before had a single weapon been responsible for such destruction.

—Laurence Behrens and Leonard J. Rosen, *Writing and Reading Across the Curriculum*

ASIDE

The older girls (non-graduates, of course) were assigned the task of making refreshments for the night's festivities.

—Maya Angelou, *I Know Why the Caged Bird Sings*

The sheer decibel level of the noise around us is not enough to make us cranky, irritable, or aggressive. (It can, however, affect our mental and physical health, which is another matter.)

—Carol Tavris, *Anger: The Misunderstood Emotion*

USING PARENTHESES FOR LISTED ITEMS AND ALTERNATIVE NUMBERS

Parentheses enclose the numbers (or letters) of listed items within a sentence. A displayed list uses periods, not parentheses, to enclose items.

- The topics to be discussed are **(1)** *membership,* **(2)** *fundraising, and* **(3)** *networking.*

Alerts: For listed items that fall within a sentence, (1) use a colon before a list only if an INDEPENDENT CLAUSE comes before the list, and (2) use commas or semicolons to separate three or more items, but be consistent within a piece of writing. If, however, any item contains punctuation itself, use a semicolon to separate the items. ●

In legal writing and in some BUSINESS WRITING, you can use parentheses to enclose a numeral that repeats a spelled-out number.

- The monthly rent is three hundred fifty dollars **($350)**.
- Your order of fifteen **(15)** gross was shipped today.

In ACADEMIC WRITING, especially in subjects in which the use of figures or measurements is frequent, enclose alternative or comparative forms of the same number in parentheses: *2 mi (3.2 km)*.

USING OTHER PUNCTUATION WITH PARENTHESES

A parenthetical complete sentence inserted within the body of another sentence does not start with a capital letter or end with a period. (It would, however, end with a question mark or exclamation point if one is required.) A complete parenthetical sentence standing alone follows regular rules of punctuation, as the previous sentence highlights.

NO If you decide to join us (We hope you do.), bring your dog also.

YES If you decide to join us (we hope you do), bring your dog also.

YES If you decide to join us, bring your dog also. (We hope you do.)

YES Your dog (isn't Rex his name?) will delight all my other guests.

As in the preceding examples, place a required comma outside your closing parenthesis unless you're using commas to set off a numbered list.

Place parentheses around quotation marks that come before or after any quoted words.

NO Alberta Hunter "(Down Hearted Blues)" is known for singing jazz.

YES Alberta Hunter ("Down Hearted Blues") is known for singing jazz.

BRACKETS

47C When do I need to use brackets in my writing?

Use brackets to feature an insert, such as an additional word or a brief definition, added by you to material which you are quoting.

ADJUSTING A QUOTATION WITH BRACKETS

When you use a quotation, you might need to change the form of a word (a verb's tense, for example), add a brief definition, or fit the quotation into the grammatical structure of your sentence. In such cases, enclose the material you have inserted into the quotation in brackets.

ORIGINAL SOURCE

Current research shows that successful learning takes place in an active environment.

—Deborah Moore, "Facilities and Learning Styles," p. 22

QUOTATION WITH BRACKETS

Deborah Moore supports a student-centered curriculum and agrees with "current research [that] shows that successful learning takes place in an active environment" (22).

ORIGINAL SOURCE

The logic of the mind is *associative;* it takes elements that symbolize a reality, or trigger a memory of it, to be the same as that reality.

—Daniel Goleman, *Emotional Intelligence*, p. 294

QUOTATION WITH BRACKETS

The kinds of intelligence are based in the way the mind functions: "The logic of the mind is *associative* **[one idea connects with another]**; it takes elements that symbolize a reality, or trigger a memory of it, to be the same as that reality" (Goleman 294).

USING BRACKETS TO POINT OUT AN ERROR IN A SOURCE OR TO ADD INFORMATION WITHIN PARENTHESES

In words you want to quote, sometimes page-makeup technicians or authors make a mistake without realizing it—a wrong date, a misspelled word, or an error of fact. You fix that mistake by putting your correction in brackets. This tells your readers that the error was in the original work and not made by you.

USING [SIC] TO SHOW A SOURCE'S ERROR

Insert *sic* (without italics), enclosed in brackets, in your MLA-style essays and research papers to show your readers that you've quoted an error accurately. *Sic* is a Latin word that means "so," or "thus," which says "It is so (or thus) in the original."

USE FOR ERROR

- A journalist wrote, "The judge accepted an [sic] plea of not guilty."

USE FOR MISSPELLING

- The building inspector condemned our structure in no uncertain terms: "There [sic] building is uninhabitable," he wrote.

USING BRACKETS WITHIN PARENTHESES

Use brackets to insert information within parentheses.

- That expression **(first used in *A Fable for Critics* [1848] by James R. Lowell)** was popularized in the early twentieth century by Ella Wheeler Wilcox.

ELLIPSIS POINTS

47D How do I use ellipsis points in my writing?

The word *ellipsis* means "omission." Ellipsis points in writing are a series of three spaced dots (use the period key on the keyboard). Use ellipsis points to indicate you've intentionally omitted words—even a sentence or more—from the source you're quoting. These rules apply to both prose and poetry.

47D.1 Using ellipsis points with prose

ORIGINAL SOURCE

These two minds, the emotional and the rational, operate in tight harmony for the most part, intertwining their very different ways of knowing to guide us through the world. Ordinarily, there is a balance between emotional and rational minds, with emotion feeding into and informing the operations of the rational mind, and the rational mind refining and sometimes vetoing the inputs of the emotions. Still, the emotional and rational minds are semi-independent faculties, each, as we shall see, reflecting the operation of distinct, but interconnected, circuitry in the brain.

—Daniel Goleman, *Emotional Intelligence*, p. 9

QUOTATION OF SELECTED WORDS, NO ELLIPSIS NEEDED

Goleman explains that the "two minds, the emotional and the rational" usually provide "a balance" in our daily observations and decision making (9).

QUOTATION WITH ELLIPSIS MID-SENTENCE

Goleman emphasizes the connections between parts of the mind: "Still, the emotional and rational minds are semi-independent faculties, each **. . .** reflecting the operation of distinct, but interconnected, circuitry in the brain" (9).

QUOTATION WITH ELLIPSIS AND PARENTHETICAL REFERENCE

Goleman emphasizes that the "two minds, the emotional and the rational, operate in tight harmony for the most part **. . .** " (9).

Note: In MLA style, place a sentence-ending period after the parenthetical reference.

QUOTATION WITH ELLIPSIS ENDING THE SENTENCE

On page 9, Goleman states: "These two minds, the emotional and the rational, operate in tight harmony for the most part. . . ."

Note: In MLA style, when all documentation information is written into a sentence—that is, not placed in parentheses at the end of the sentence—there's no space between the sentence-ending period and an ellipsis.

QUOTATION WITH SENTENCE OMITTED

Goleman explains: "These two minds, the emotional and the rational, operate in tight harmony for the most part, intertwining their very different ways of knowing to guide us through the world. . . . Still, the emotional and rational minds are semi-independent faculties" (9).

QUOTATION WITH WORDS OMITTED FROM THE MIDDLE OF ONE SENTENCE TO THE MIDDLE OF ANOTHER

Goleman states: "Ordinarily, there is a balance between emotional and rational minds . . . reflecting the operation of distinct, but interconnected, circuitry in the brain" (9).

QUOTATION WITH WORDS OMITTED FROM THE BEGINNING OF A SENTENCE AND FROM THE MIDDLE OF ONE SENTENCE TO A COMPLETE OTHER SENTENCE

Goleman explains: ". . . there is a balance between emotional and rational minds. . . . Still, the emotional and rational minds are semi-independent faculties, each, as we shall see, reflecting the operation of distinct, but interconnected, circuitry in the brain" (9).

When you omit words from a quotation, you also omit punctuation related to those words, unless it's needed for the sentence to be correct.

Goleman explains: "These two minds . . . operate in tight harmony" (9).

Comma in original source omitted after *minds*.

Goleman explains that the emotional and rational minds work together while, "still, . . . each, as we shall see, [reflects] the operation of distinct, but interconnected, circuitry in the brain" (9).

Comma kept after *still* because it's an introductory word; *still* changed to begin with lowercase letter because it's now in the middle of the sentence; form of *reflecting* changed to improve the sense of sentence.

47D.2 Using ellipsis points with poetry

When you omit one or more words from a line of poetry, follow the rules stated above for prose. However, when you omit a full line or more from poetry, use a full line of spaced dots.

ORIGINAL SOURCE

LITTLE BOY BLUE
Little boy blue, come blow your horn,
The sheep's in the meadow, the cow's in the corn
Where is the little boy who looks after the sheep?
He's under the haystack, fast asleep.

QUOTATION WITH LINES OMITTED

LITTLE BOY BLUE
Little boy blue, come blow your horn,

. . . .

Where is the little boy who looks after the sheep?
He's under the haystack, fast asleep.

SLASH

47E When can I use a slash in my writing?

The slash (/), also called a *virgule* or *solidus*, is a diagonal line that separates or joins words in special circumstances.

USING A SLASH TO SEPARATE QUOTED LINES OF POETRY

To quote more than three lines of a poem, follow the rules in 46E. To quote three lines or fewer, enclose them in quotation marks and run them into your sentence—and use a slash to divide one line from the next. Leave a space on each side of the slash.

- One of my mottoes comes from the beginning of Anne Sexton's poem "Words": "Be careful of words, / even the miraculous ones."

Capitalize and punctuate each line of poetry as in the original—but even if the quoted line of poetry doesn't have a period, use one to end your sentence. If your quotation ends before the line of poetry ends, use ellipsis points (see 47D).

USING A SLASH FOR NUMERICAL FRACTIONS IN MANUSCRIPTS

To type numerical fractions, use a slash (with no space before or after the slash) to separate the numerator and denominator. In mixed numbers—that is, whole numbers with fractions—leave a space between the whole number and its fraction: 1 2/3, 3 7/8. Do not use a hyphen. (For information about using spelled-out and numerical forms of numbers, see 48M through 48O.)

USING A SLASH FOR *AND/OR*

When writing in the humanities, try not to signal alternatives with a slash, such as *and/or*. Where such combinations are acceptable, separate the words with a slash. Leave no space before or after the slash. In the humanities, listing both alternatives is usually better than separating choices with a slash.

NO The best quality of reproduction comes from 35 mm slides/direct-positive films.

YES The best quality of reproduction comes from 35 mm slides **or** direct-positive films.

NO Each student must locate his/her own source material.

YES Each student must locate his **or** her own source material.

● **EXERCISE 47-2** Supply needed dashes, parentheses, brackets, ellipsis points, and slashes. If a sentence is correct as written, circle its number. In some sentences, when you can use either dashes or parentheses, explain your choice.

EXAMPLE

There have been several famous entertainers Hedy Lamarr, Skunk Baxter, Brian May who are also accomplished scientists.

There have been several famous entertainers—Hedy Lamarr, Skunk Baxter, Brian May—who are also accomplished scientists.

1. Brian May is famous for being the guitar player for the rock band Queen one of my favorite bands of all time, but he also has a Ph.D. in astrophysics.
2. Besides being the guitarist, he also wrote one of Queen's biggest hits ("We Will Rock You" (1977)).
3. May wrote the lyrics for this famous rock anthem that includes the two lines, "Gonna take on the world some day, You got blood on your face."
4. After May earned his Ph.D. in astrophysics in 2008, another astronomer joked, "I don't know any scientists who look as much like Isaac Neuton (sic) as you do."
5. Of all the early Hollywood actresses, Lana Turner, Judy Garland, Ava Gardner, Hedy Lamarr may have been one of the most famous.

6. But Lamarr also invented a frequency-hopping system that is still used in the following modern devices: 1 wireless telephones 2 Bluetooth technology and 3 Wi-Fi networks.
7. Skunk Baxter is a guitar player known for his work with Steely Dan, "Rikki Don't Lose That Number" and "Reeling in the Years," and The Doobie Brothers, "Takin' It to the Street" and "What a Fool Believes."
8. In describing his decision to make a career change, Baxter said, "After we the band The Doobie Brothers had been together for so many years, many of the members diverged to their own musical directions."
9. Having some connections in the military, his next-door neighbor was a missile designer, Baxter began experimenting with new designs for data-compression algorithms.
10. This long-haired rock star—can you imagine?—was even granted high-level government security clearance by the U.S. Department of Defense. ●

● **EXERCISE 47-3** Follow the directions for each item. For help, consult all sections of this chapter.

EXAMPLE

Write a sentence that uses dashes and includes a definition.

I like to study Romance languages—languages derived from Latin.

1. Write a sentence that contains a numbered list.
2. Write a sentence that uses parentheses to set off a definition.
3. Quote a passage from the poem below that omits an entire line.
4. Write a sentence that quotes two lines from the poem below, and use a slash to separate the two lines.
5. Quote any part of the poem below and uses ellipsis points to omit word(s) from the poem.

Little Lamb, who made thee?
    Dost thou know who made thee?
Gave thee life, and bid thee feed
By the stream and o'er the mead;
Gave thee clothing of delight,
Softest clothing, woolly, bright;
Gave thee such a tender voice,
Making all the vales rejoice?
    Little Lamb, who made thee?
    Dost thou know who made thee?
        —William Blake ●

HYPHEN

47F When do I need a hyphen in my writing?

A hyphen serves to divide words at the end of a line, to combine words into compounds, and to communicate numbers.

47G When do I use a hyphen at the end of a line?

Listen to the Podcast

Set the default on your word processing program to avoid hyphenation. If you must divide a word, keep in mind the following procedures: (1) wherever possible, avoid dividing words with hyphens at the end of a line; (2) if a division is necessary, divide longer words by syllable and between consonants if possible (*omit-ting, ful-ness, sep-arate*); (3) never divide for one or two letters or for any one-syllable words (like *wealth* or *screamed*); (4) don't divide the last word on the first line of a paper, the last word in a paragraph, or the last word on a page.

47H How do I use a hyphen with prefixes and suffixes?

Prefixes are syllables in front of a **root**—a word's core, which carries the origin or meaning. Prefixes modify meanings. **Suffixes** also have modifying power, but they follow roots. Some prefixes and suffixes are attached to root words with hyphens, but others are not. Quick Box 47.1 shows you how to decide.

Quick Box 47.1

Hyphens with prefixes and suffixes

- Use hyphens after the prefixes *all-*, *ex-*, *quasi-*, and *self-*.

  YES all-inclusive self-reliant

- Never use a hyphen when *self* is a root word, not a prefix.

  NO self-ishness self-less

  YES selfishness selfless

- Use a hyphen to avoid a distracting string of letters.

  NO anti**i**ntellectual be**lll**ike pr**oo**utsourcing

  YES anti**-i**ntellectual bel**l-l**ike pr**o-o**utsourcing

continued >>

Quick Box 47.1 (continued)

- Use a hyphen to add a prefix or suffix to a numeral or a word that starts with a capital letter.

NO	post1950	proAmerican	Rembrandtlike
YES	post-1950	pro-American	Rembrandt-like

- Use a hyphen before the suffix *-elect*.

NO presidentelect

YES president-elect

- Use a hyphen to prevent confusion in meaning or pronunciation.

YES	re-dress (means *dress again*)	redress (means *set right*)
YES	un-ionize (means *remove the ions*)	unionize (means *form a union*)

- Use a hyphen when two or more prefixes apply to one root word.

YES pre- and post-Renaissance

47I How do I use hyphens with compound words?

A COMPOUND WORD puts two or more words together to express one concept. Compound words come in three forms: an open-compound word, as in *night shift;* hyphenated words, as in *tractor-trailer;* and a closed-compound word, as in *handbook*. Quick Box 47.2 lists basic guidelines for positioning hyphens in compound words.

Quick Box 47.2

Hyphens with compound words

- Divide a compound word already containing a hyphen only after that hyphen, if possible. Also, divide a closed-compound word only between the two complete words, if possible.

NO	self-con-scious	sis-ter-in-law	mas-terpiece
YES	self-conscious	sister-in-law	master-piece

continued >>

Quick Box 47.2 (continued)

- Use a hyphen between a prefix and an open-compound word.

  NO antigun control [*gun control* is an open-compound word]

  YES anti-gun control

- Use a hyphen for most compound words that precede a noun but not for most compound words that follow a noun.

  YES well-researched report report is well researched

- Use hyphens when a compound modifier includes a series.

  YES two-, three-, or four-year program

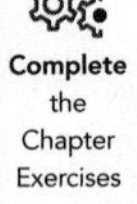

Complete the Chapter Exercises

- Never use a hyphen when a compound modifier starts with an *-ly* adverb.

  NO happily-married couple loosely-tied package

  YES happily married couple loosely tied package

- Use a hyphen with most COMPARATIVE (*-er*) and SUPERLATIVE (*-est*) compound forms, but not when the compound modifier includes *more/most* or *less/least*.

  NO better fitting shoe

  YES better-fitting shoe

  NO least-significant factors

  YES least significant factors

- Never use a hyphen when a compound modifier is a foreign phrase.

  YES *post hoc* fallacies

- Never use a hyphen with a possessive compound.

  NO a full-week's work eight-hours' pay

  YES a full week's work eight hours' pay

48 Capitals, Italics, Abbreviations, and Numbers

Quick Points You will learn to

- Use capital letters correctly (see 48A–48E).
- Use italics (underlining) correctly (see 48F–48H).
- Use abbreviations correctly (see 48I–48L).
- Use spelled out numbers and numerals correctly (see 48M–48N).

CAPITALS

48A When do I capitalize a "first" word?

FIRST WORD IN A SENTENCE

Always capitalize the first letter of the first word in a sentence.

- **F**our inches of snow fell last winter.

A SERIES OF QUESTIONS

If a series of questions imply, but are not themselves, complete sentences, you can choose capitals or not. Simply be consistent in each piece of writing.

- Whose rights does voter fraud deny? **M**ine? **Y**ours? **O**r everyone's?
- Whose rights does voter fraud deny? **m**ine? **y**ours? **o**r everyone's?

SMALL WORDS IN TITLES OR HEADINGS

Capitalize the first word and all principal words of titles or headings. Do not capitalize ARTICLES, PREPOSITIONS, or CONJUNCTIONS in titles or headings unless one begins the title: *The Man without a Country.*

Capitalize the pronoun *I* and the interjection *O* (not *oh*) wherever these appear in a sentence: *Captain, O captain, I will follow you.*

AFTER A COLON

When a complete sentence follows a colon, choose consistently either a capital or lowercase letter in each piece of writing. If what follows your colon is not a complete sentence, don't capitalize the first word.

- The question remains: **W**hat will the jury decide?
- The question remains: **w**hat will the jury decide?
- The jury is considering all the evidence: **m**otive, means, opportunity.

Alert: A colon can follow only a complete sentence (see 44A). ●

FORMAL OUTLINE

In a formal outline, start each item with a capital letter. Use a period only when the item is a complete sentence.

48B When do I use capitals with listed items?

A LIST WITHIN A SENTENCE

When a sentence itemizes other sentences, capitalize and punctuate the items as complete sentences: *The bank robbers made demands: (1)* ***T****hey want money. (2)* ***T****hey want hostages. (3)* ***T****hey want transportation.* When the items are not complete sentences, use commas between them unless the items contain commas. When they do, use semicolons between items. Use the word *and* before the last item if there are three or more nonsentence items.

YES The reasons for the delay were (1) **b**ad weather, (2) **p**oor scheduling**, and** (3) **e**quipment failure.

YES The reasons for the delay were (1) **b**ad weather, which had been predicted**;** (2) **p**oor scheduling, which is the airline's responsibility**; and** (3) **e**quipment failure, which no one can predict.

A DISPLAYED LIST

In a displayed list, each item starts on a new line. If the items are sentences, capitalize and punctuate the items as sentences. If the items are not sentences, choose a capital letter or not and punctuate appropriately. Simply be consistent in each piece of writing.

YES We found three reasons for the delay:

1. **B**ad weather held up delivery of materials.
2. **P**oor scheduling created confusion.
3. **I**mproper machine maintenance caused an equipment failure.

YES The reasons for the delay were

1. **b**ad weather,
2. **p**oor scheduling**, and**
3. **e**quipment failure.

Alerts: (1) If a complete sentence leads into a displayed list, you can end the sentence with a colon. However, if an incomplete sentence leads into a displayed list, use no punctuation. (2) Use PARALLELISM in a list. For example, if one item is a sentence, use sentences for all the items (see 39E); or if one item starts with a VERB, start all items with a verb in the same TENSE; and so on. ●

48C When do I use capitals with sentences in parentheses?

When you write a complete sentence within parentheses that falls within another sentence, don't start with a capital or end with a period—but do use a question mark or exclamation point, if needed. When you write a sentence within parentheses that doesn't fall within another sentence, capitalize and punctuate it as a complete sentence.

> I did not know . . . they called it the Cuban Missile Crisis. But I remember Castro. **(W**e called him Castor Oil and were awed by his beard**.)** We might not have worried so much **(w**hat would the communists want with our small New Hampshire town**?)** except we lived 10 miles from a U.S. air base.
>
> —Joyce Maynard, "An 18-Year-Old Looks Back on Life"

48D When do I use capitals with quotations?

If a quotation within your sentence is itself not a complete sentence, never capitalize the first quoted word. If the quotation you have used in your sentence is itself a complete sentence always capitalize the first word.

- Mrs. Enriquez says that students who are learning a new language should visit that country and "**a**bsorb a good accent with the food."
- Talking about students who live in a new country Mrs. Enriquez says, "**T**hey'll absorb a good accent with the food."

In DIRECT DISCOURSE, introduced with verbs like *said, asked*, and others (see 18K) followed by a comma, capitalize the first letter of a quoted sentence. Don't capitalize partial quotes situated within a sentence, or the first word of a quoted sentence, which resumes after your commentary.

- Snooki said, "**I**taly was awesome! **T**he pasta totally rocked."

  Quoted complete sentences always begin with capital letters.

- Snooki said that Italy was "**a**wesome," and that its pasta "**r**ocked."

  Partial quotations situated within a sentence need no capitals.

- "**I**taly and its pasta," snickered Snooki, "**t**otally rocked."

  There is no need to capitalize *totally;* it simply continues the quote.

48E When do I capitalize nouns and adjectives?

Capitalize **proper nouns** and ADJECTIVES formed from them to assign specificity: *We lease space in the building. We lease space in the **F**latiron **B**uilding. He studies at a college in Boston. He studies at **B**oston **C**ollege.*

Nouns and adjectives which are now COMMON lose capitals: *My in-laws purchased this **c**hina. I devour **f**rench fries daily.*

Should you notice capitalized words (like Company or Faculty) in professional writing which contradict our rules, remember that all writing is addressed to a specific AUDIENCE to achieve a specific PURPOSE. The context may favor capitalization of these words. Quick Box 48.1 models capitalization.

Quick Box 48.1

Capitalization

	Capitals	**Lowercase Letters**
NAMES	Mother Teresa (*also, used as names:* Mother, Dad, Mom, Pa) Doc Holliday	my mother [relationship] the doctor [role]
TITLES	President Truman	the president
	Democrat [party member]	a democrat [believer in democracy]
	Representative Harold Ford	the congressional representative
	Senator Jon Kyl	a senator
	Queen Elizabeth II	the queen
GROUPS OF PEOPLE	Caucasian [race]	white, black [*also* White, Black]
	African American, Hispanic [ethnic group]	
	Irish, Korean, Canadian [nationality]	
	Jewish, Catholic, Protestant, Buddhist [religious affiliation]	
ORGANIZATIONS	Congress	the legislative branch of the U.S. government
	the Ohio State Supreme Court	the state supreme court
	the Republican Party	the party
	Wink Inc.	the company
	Chicago Cubs	a baseball team

continued >>

Quick Box 48.1 (continued)

	Capitals	Lowercase Letters
	American Medical Association	a professional group
	Sigma Chi	a fraternity
	Alcoholics Anonymous	a self-help group
PLACES	Los Angeles	the city
	the South [region]	turn south [direction]
	the West Coast	the U.S. states along the western seaboard
	Main Street	the street
	Atlantic Ocean	the ocean
	the Black Hills	the hills
BUILDINGS	the Capitol [in Washington, DC]	the state capitol
	Ace High School	a high school
	Front Road Café	a restaurant
	Highland Hospital	a hospital
SCIENTIFIC TERMS	Earth [as one of nine planets]	the earth [otherwise]
	the Milky Way, the Galaxy [as name]	our galaxy, the moon, the sun
	Streptococcus aureus	a streptococcal infection
	Gresham's law	the theory of relativity
LANGUAGES, SCHOOL COURSES	Spanish, Chinese	
	Chemistry 342	a chemistry course
	History 111	my history class
	Introduction to Photography	a photography course
NAMES OF SPECIFIC THINGS	Black Parrot tulip	a climbing rose
	Purdue University	the university
	Heinz ketchup	ketchup, sauce
	a Toyota Camry	a car
	Twelfth Dynasty	the dynasty
	the *Boston Globe*	a newspaper
TIMES, SEASONS, HOLIDAYS	Monday, Fri.	today
	September, February	a month
	the Roaring Twenties	the decade
	the Christmas season	spring, summer, autumn, winter, the fall semester

continued >>

Quick Box 48.1 (continued)

	Capitals	Lowercase Letters
	Kwanzaa, New Year's Day	a feast day, the holiday
	Passover, Ramadan	a religious holiday or observance
HISTORICAL EVENTS AND DOCUMENTS	World War II	the war
	Battle of the Bulge	the battle
	the Great Depression (of the 1930s)	the depression [any serious economic downturn]
	the Reformation	the eighteenth century
	Paleozoic	an era or age, prehistory
	the Bill of Rights	fifth-century manuscripts
RELIGIOUS TERMS	Athena, God	a goddess, a god
	Islam	a religion
	the Torah, the Koran (or Qur'an)	a holy book
	the Bible	biblical
LETTER PARTS	Dear Ms. Schultz:	
	Sincerely,	
	Yours truly,	
PUBLISHED AND RELEASED MATERIAL	"The Lottery"	[Capitalize first letter of first word and all other major words]
	A History of the United States to 1877	
	Jazz on Ice	the show, a performance
	Nixon Papers	the archives
	Mass in B Minor	the B minor mass
ACRONYMS AND INITIALISMS	NASA, NATO, UCLA, AFL-CIO, DNA	
COMPUTER TERMS	Gateway, Dell	a computer company
	Microsoft Word	computer software
	Firefox	a browser
	the Internet	a computer network
	World Wide Web, the Web	www
	Web site, Web page	a home page, a link
PROPER ADJECTIVES	Victorian	southern
	Midwestern	transatlantic
	Indo-European	alpine

● **EXERCISE 48-1** Individually or with a group, add capital letters as needed. See 48A through 48E for help.

1. The state of california is best known as the golden state, but other nicknames include the land of milk and honey, the el dorado state, and the grape state.
2. Most people think of san Francisco as northern california, but the city of Eureka, from the greek word meaning "I have found it," is 280 miles north of san Francisco, and the state line is another 90 miles north of eureka.
3. South of san Francisco on the california coast is santa Barbara, which hosts the annual Dickens Universe, a weeklong series of studies and celebrations of the famous writer charles dickens.
4. The highest point in the contiguous United States is mt. Whitney at 14,495 feet high, and the lowest place in the contiguous United States is bad Water in death valley at 282 feet below sea level, both located in california.
5. Having approximately 500,000 detectable seismic tremors per year, california rocks, literally.
6. Because the tehema county fairgrounds are located in red bluff, california hosts the largest three-day rodeo in the united States.
7. Numerous songs have been written about california, including "california girls" by the beach boys and the theme of the tv show *the beverly hillbillies.*
8. san Bernardino county with almost three million acres is the largest county in the united states.
9. Hollywood and movie stars are what many people associate california with, and well they might because two of California's governors, ronald reagan and arnold schwarzenegger, were actors before they became governors.
10. When told all these fantastic facts about california, a stereotypical valley girl would respond, "whatever." ●

ITALICS

48F What are italics?

Italic typeface slants to the right (*like this*); roman typeface does not (like this). MLA STYLE requires italics, not underlining, in all documents.

ROMAN your writing
ITALICS *your writing*

48G How do I choose between using italics and quotation marks?

As a rule, use italics for titles of long works (*Juno*, a movie) or for works that contain subsections (*Masterpiece Theater*, a television show). Generally, use quotation marks for titles of shorter works ("One and Only," a song) and for titles of subsections within longer works such as books (Chapter 1, "Loomings"). Quick Box 48.2 models usage in italics.

Quick Box 48.2

Italics, quotation marks, or nothing

Italics	Quotation Marks or Nothing
TITLES AND NAMES	
Sense and Sensibility [a novel]	title of student essay
Death of a Salesman [a play]	act 2 [part of a play]
A Beautiful Mind [a film]	the Epilogue [a part of a film or book]
Collected Works of O. Henry [a book]	"The Last Leaf" [a story in a book]
Simon & Schuster Handbook for Writers [a textbook]	"Agreement" [a chapter in a book]
The Prose Reader [a collection of essays]	"Putting in a Good Word for Guilt" [an essay]
Iliad [a book-length poem]	"Nothing Gold Can Stay" [a short poem]
Scientific American [a magazine]	"The Molecules of Life" [an article in a magazine]
Symphonie Fantastique [a long musical work]	Violin Concerto No. 2 in B-flat Minor [a musical work identified by form, number, and key—neither quotation marks nor italics]
U2 18 Singles [an album]	"With or Without You" [a song]
Lost [a television series]	"Something Nice Back Home" [an episode of a television series]
Kids Count [a Web site title]	Excel [a software program]

continued >>

Quick Box 48.2 (continued)

Italics	Quotation Marks or Nothing
the *Los Angeles Times* [a newspaper]*	
OTHER WORDS	
semper fidelis [words in a language other than English]	burrito, chutzpah [widely understood non-English words]
What does *our* imply? [a word meant as a word]	
the *abc*'s; the letter *x* [letters meant as letters]	6s and 7s; & [numerals and symbols]

*When *The* is part of a newspaper's title, don't capitalize or italicize it in MLA-style or CM-style documentation. In APA-style and CSE-style documentation, capitalize and italicize *The*.

48H Can I use italics for special emphasis?

Some professional writers, especially writers of self-help material, occasionally use italics to clarify or stress points. In ACADEMIC WRITING, however, you're expected to convey special emphasis with your choice of words and sentence structure, not with italics (or underlining). If your message absolutely calls for it, use italics sparingly—when you're sure nothing else will do.

> Many people we *think* are powerful turn out on closer examination to be merely frightened and anxious.
>
> —Michael Korda, *Power!*

● **EXERCISE 48-2** Edit these sentences for correct use of italics (or underlining), quotation marks, and capitals.

1. While waiting for my Dentist to call my name, I flipped through a copy of a magazine called "Entertainment Digest."
2. I enjoyed reading the Magazine because it included several interesting articles: Movie reviews, recipes, and tips for Spring cleaning.
3. I read a review of the movie "Night comes calling," which I learned is an adaptation of english writer Hugo Barrington's short story *Adventures in the Fog*.

4. I asked the Receptionist if I could keep the magazine because a few of the articles might help me in my Spanish and Economics classes.
5. For example, there was an article on a composer who wrote an Opera about *The Spanish Civil War.* ●

ABBREVIATIONS

481 What are standard practices for using abbreviations?

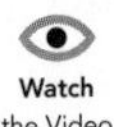
Watch the Video

Some abbreviations are standard in writing (*Mr.*, not *Mister*, in a name; *St.* Louis, the city, not *Saint* Louis). In some situations, you may have a choice whether to abbreviate or spell out a word. Choose what seems suited to your writing PURPOSE and your AUDIENCE, and be consistent within each piece of writing.

NO The great painter Vincent Van Gogh was **b.** in Holland in 1853, but he lived most of his life and died in **Fr.**

YES The great painter Vincent Van Gogh was **born** in Holland in 1853, but he lived most of his life and died in **France**.

NO Our field hockey team left after Casey's **psych** class on **Tues.**, **Oct**. 10, but the flight had to make an unexpected stop (in **Chi**.) before reaching **L.A**.

YES Our field hockey team left after Casey's **psychology** class on **Tuesday**, **October** 10, but the flight had to make an unexpected stop (in **Chicago**) before reaching **Los Angeles**.

NO Please confirm in writing your order for one **doz**. helmets in **lg** and **x-lg**.

YES Please confirm in writing your order for one **dozen** helmets in **large** and **extra large**.

Alerts: (1) Many abbreviations call for periods (*Mrs., Ms., Dr.*), but the practice is changing. The trend today is to drop the periods (*PS*, not *P.S.; MD*, not *M.D.; US*, not *U.S.*), yet firm rules are still evolving.

(2) Acronyms (pronounceable words formed from the initials of a name) generally have no periods: *NASA* (National Aeronautics and Space Administration) and *AIDS* (*a*cquired *i*mmune *d*eficiency *s*yndrome).

(3) Initialisms (names spoken as separate letters) usually have no periods (*IBM, ASPCA, UN*).

(4) U.S. Postal abbreviations for states have no periods (48K).

(5) When the final period of an abbreviation falls at the end of a sentence, that period serves also to end the sentence. ●

48J How do I use abbreviations with months, time, eras, and symbols?

MONTHS

According to MLA STYLE, abbreviations for months belong only in "Works Cited" lists, tables, charts, and the like. Write out the full spelling, never the abbreviation, in your ACADEMIC WRITING.

TIMES

Use the abbreviations *a.m.* and *p.m.* only with exact times: *7:15 a.m.; 3:47 p.m.* MLA style calls for the use of lowercase letters.

Alert: Never use *a.m.* and *p.m.* in place of *morning, evening,* and *night.*

NO My hardest final exam is in the **a.m**. tomorrow, but by early **p.m**., I'll be ready to study for the rest of my finals.

YES My hardest final exam is in the **morning** tomorrow, but by early **evening**, I'll be ready to study for the rest of my finals. ●

ERAS

In MLA style, use capital letters, without periods, in abbreviations for eras. Some writers prefer *CE* ("common era") to *AD* (Latin for *anno Domini*, "in the year of our Lord") as the more inclusive term. In addition, many writers prefer *BCE* ("before the common era") to *BC* ("before Christ").

When writing the abbreviations for eras, place *AD* before the year (*AD 476*) and all the others after the year (*29 BC; 165 BCE; 1100 CE*).

SYMBOLS

In MLA style, decide whether to use symbols or spelled-out words according to your topic and the focus of your document (see also 48M). However, only use a freestanding symbol, such as *$, %,* or *¢* with a numeral. With many exceptions, spell both the symbol and the numeral accompanying it (*twenty centimeters*), unless the number is more than one or two words (*345 centimeters,* not *three hundred forty-five centimeters*).

The exceptions include *$18; 7 lbs.; 24 KB; 6:34 a.m.; 5"; 32°;* and numbers in addresses, dates, page references, and decimal fractions (*8.3*). In writing about money, the form *$25 million* is an acceptable combination of symbol, numeral, and spelled-out word.

In confined spaces, such as charts and tables, use symbols with numerals (2¢). In documents that focus on technical matters, use numerals but spell out the unit of measurement (*2,500 pounds*)—in MLA style. Guidelines in other documentation styles differ, so you need to check each style's manual.

48K How do I use abbreviations for other elements?

TITLES

Use either a title of address before a name (***Dr.** Daniel Klausner*) or an academic degree after a name (*Daniel Klausner, **PhD***), not both. However, because *Jr., Sr., II, III,* and so forth are part of a name, you can use both titles of address and academic degrees: ***Dr.** Martin Luther King **Jr.**; John Jay **II, MD**.*

! Alerts: (1) Insert a comma both before and after an academic degree that follows a person's name, unless it falls at the end of a sentence: *Joshua Coleman, **LLD**, is our guest speaker,* or *Our guest speaker is Joshua Coleman, **LLD**.* (2) Never put a comma before an abbreviation that is part of a given name: *Steven Elliott **Sr.,** Douglas Young **III**.* ●

NAMES AND TERMS

If you use a term frequently in a piece of writing, follow these guidelines: The first time you use the term, spell it out completely and then put its abbreviation in parentheses immediately after. In later references, use the abbreviation alone.

- Spain voted to continue as a member of the **North Atlantic Treaty Organization** (**NATO**), to the surprise of other **NATO** members.

Use the abbreviation *U.S.* as a modifier before a noun (*the **U.S.** ski team*), but spell *United States* when you use it as a noun (*the ski team of the **United States***).

ADDRESSES

If you include a full address in a piece of writing, use the two-letter postal abbreviation for the state name. For any other combination of a city and a state, or a state by itself, spell out the state name; never abbreviate it.

! Alert: When you write the names of a U.S. city and state within a sentence, use a comma before and after the state.

NO Portland, Oregon is much larger than Portland, Maine.

YES Portland, Oregon, is much larger than Portland, Maine.

If you include a ZIP code, however, don't use a comma after the state. Do place the comma after the ZIP code. ●

SCHOLARLY WRITING (MLA STYLE)

MLA style permits abbreviations for the scholarly terms listed in Quick Box 48.3. Never use them in the body of your ACADEMIC WRITING. Reserve them for your "Works Cited" lists and for any notes you might write in a separate list at the end of your research paper.

Quick Box 48.3

Major scholarly abbreviations—MLA style

anon.	anonymous	**i.e.**	that is
b.	born	**ms., mss.**	manuscript, manuscripts
c. *or* ©	copyright	**NB**	note well (*nota bene*)
c. *or* **ca.**	circa *or* about [with dates]	**n.d.**	no date (of publication)
cf.	compare	**p., pp.**	page, pages
col., cols.	column, columns	**par.**	paragraph
d.	died	**pref.**	preface, preface by
ed., eds.	edition, edited by, editor(s)	**rept.**	report, reported by
		rev.	review, reviewed by; revised, revised by
e.g.	for example		
esp.	especially	**sec., secs.**	section, sections
et al.	and others	**v.** *or* **vs.**	versus [*v.* in legal cases]
ff.	following pages, following lines, folios	**vol., vols.**	volume, volumes

48L When can I use *etc.*?

Avoid *etc.*, Latin for "and the rest," in ACADEMIC WRITING. Instead, use substitutes such as *and the like, and so on*—or better yet, use a more concrete description. If you do use *etc.*, use a *single period* after it even at the end of a sentence. Follow the single period with a comma if *etc.* comes before the end.

NO For the picnic, we bought paper plates, plastic forks, **etc..**

YES For the picnic, we bought paper plates, plastic forks, and **other disposable items.**

Alert: If you do write *etc.*, always put a comma after the period if the abbreviation falls in the middle of a sentence. ●

● **EXERCISE 48-3** Working individually or with a group, revise these sentences for correct use of abbreviations. For help, consult 48I through 48L.

1. Originally named the Geo. S. Parker Company, located in Salem, Mass., the toy co. changed its name to Parker Bros. when Chas. joined the business in 1888.

2. Sev. of their games have become quite famous, esp. Monopoly and Clue, both of which were released in the 20th cent.
3. The obj. of the game Monopoly (meaning "dominating the mkt.") is to get the most $ by purchasing, renting, & selling real est.
4. Clue, another pop. brd. game, is a murder mys. in which players move from 1 rm. to another, making accusations to reveal the i.d. of the murderer, the weapon used, and the room where the crime took place.
5. On a cold day in Jan., when the snow is 3 ft. deep and it's dark by early eve., passing the hrs. with your fam. and friends playing a board game is great fun. ●

NUMBERS

48M When do I use spelled-out numbers?

Watch the Video

Your decision to write a number as a word or as a figure depends on what you're referring to and how often numbers occur in your piece of writing. The guidelines we give in this handbook are for MLA STYLE, which focuses on writing in the humanities. For other disciplines, consult their style manuals.

When you use numbers to refer to more than one category, reserve figures for some categories of numbers and spelled-out words for other categories. Never mix spelled-out numbers and figures for a particular category.

NO In **four** days, bids increased from **five** to **eight** to **17** to **233**.

YES In **four** days, bids increased from **5** to **8** to **17** to **233**.

Numbers referring to bids are written as numerals, while *four* is spelled out because it refers to a different category: days.

Alert: For two-word numbers, use a hyphen between the spelled-out words, starting with *twenty-one* and continuing through *ninety-nine*. ●

If you use numbers infrequently in a document, spell out all numbers that call for no more than two words: *fifty-two cards, twelve hundred students*. If you use specific numbers often in a document (temperatures when writing about climate, percentages in an economics essay, or other specific measurements of time, distance, and other quantities), use figures: *36 inches, 11 nanoseconds*. In an approximation, spell out the numbers: *About twelve inches of snow fell*.

In the humanities, the names of centuries are always spelled out: *the eighteenth century*.

When you write for courses in the humanities, never start a sentence with a figure. Spell the number, or revise the sentence so that the number doesn't fall at the beginning. For practices in other disciplines, consult their manuals.

NO **$375 dollars** for each credit is the tuition rate for nonresidents.

YES **Three hundred seventy-five dollars** for each credit is the tuition rate for nonresidents.

YES The tuition rate for nonresidents is **$375** for each credit.

48N What are standard practices for writing numbers?

Quick Box 48.4 shows standard practices for writing numbers. Consider it a basic guide, and rely on the manual of each documentation style for answers to other questions you may have.

Quick Box 48.4

Specific numbers in writing

DATES	August 6, 1941 1732–1845 from 34 BC TO AD 230 (*or* 34 BCE to 230 CE)
ADDRESSES	10 Downing Street 237 North 8th Street Export Falls, MN 92025
TIMES	8:09 a.m., 6:00 p.m. six o'clock (*not* 6 o'clock) four in the afternoon *or* 4 p.m. (*not* four p.m.)
DECIMALS AND FRACTIONS	0.01 98.6 3.1416 7/8 12 1/4 a sixth three-quarters (*not* 3-quarters) one-half
CHAPTERS AND PAGES	Chapter 27, page 2 p. 1023 *or* pp. 660–62 (MLA style)
SCORES AND STATISTICS	a 6–0 score 29% (or twenty-nine percent) a 5 to 1 ratio (*and* a ratio of 5:1) a one percent change (*and* at the 1 percent level)

continued >>

Quick Box 48.4 (continued)

IDENTIFICATION NUMBERS	94.4 on the FM dial please call (012) 345–6789
MEASUREMENTS	67.8 miles per hour 2 level teaspoons a 700-word essay 8-by-10-inch photograph 2 feet 1.5 gallons 14 liters
ACT, SCENE, AND LINE	act 2, scene 2 (*or* act II, scene ii) lines 75–79
TEMPERATURES	40°F *or* –5°F 20° Celsius
MONEY	$1.2 billion $3.41 25¢ (*or* twenty-five cents) $10,000

EXERCISE 48-4 Revise these sentences so that the numbers are in correct form, either spelled out or as figures.

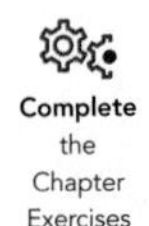
Complete the Chapter Exercises

1. The 102-story Empire State building, which is one thousand two hundred and fifty feet tall, is struck by lightning on an average of five hundred times a year.
2. If you have three quarters, four dimes, and 4 pennies, you have $1 and nineteen cents, but you still can't make even change for a dollar.
3. Lake Tahoe is the second deepest lake in the United States with a maximum depth of five hundred and one meters (1,645 ft).
4. 37 percent of Americans have passports, which means that nearly 2 out of 3 U.S. citizens cannot fly to Canada.
5. On March 2nd, nineteen sixty two, Wilt Chamberlain, playing basketball for the Philadelphia Warriors, scored 100 points.
6. Some people trace the origin of the knock-knock joke back to act two, scene three of Shakespeare's sixteen-eleven play *Macbeth*.
7. If you place a vertical stick in the ground on the Equator, it will cast no shadow at 12 o'clock p.m. on March twenty first.
8. Bamboo plants can grow up to one hundred centimeters every 24 hours, and they grow best in warm climates, but some species can survive in temperatures as low as twenty degrees below zero Fahrenheit.

9. The Boston Marathon, which began in 1897, is the world's oldest annual marathon and is held the 3rd Monday of every April.
10. 500,000 spectators watch the Boston Marathon every year as an average of twenty thousand runners each try to complete the twenty six point two mile run. ●

49 Spelling

Quick Points You will learn to

- Use spelling rules to improve your spelling (see 49C–49E).
- Distinguish between homonyms and other easily confused words (see 49F).

49A What makes a good speller?

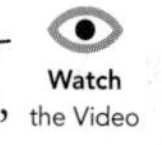

You may be surprised to learn that many fine writers do not consider themselves good spellers. They do understand, however, two features of spelling, which may help you if you believe you struggle with precise spelling.

First, precise spelling matters only in final drafts. The best time to check the spelling of words you doubt is as you're EDITING. Second, check the spelling of those words you doubt by consulting a dictionary. If you're unsure of the first few letters, then think of and find a synonym for your word in a thesaurus. Perhaps you'll see your word there—or an even sharper, clearer word.

Remember, a spell-check program in a word processor does not alert you to an error if you write another legitimate word. For example, if you write ***a****ffect* when you mean ***e****ffect*, or *f****ro****m* when you mean *f****or****m*, spell-checks detect no error; alert readers do. To avoid noticeable spelling errors, rely on some helpful hints below.

49B How can I proofread for errors in spelling and hyphen use?

Many spelling errors are the result of illegible handwriting, slips of the pen, or typographical mistakes. Catching these "typos" requires especially careful proofreading, using the techniques in Quick Box 49.1 (page 694).

Quick Box 49.1

Proofreading for errors in spelling

- Slow down your reading speed to allow yourself to concentrate on the individual letters of words rather than on the meaning of the words.
- Stay within your "visual span," the number of letters you can identify with a single glance (for most people, about six letters).
- Put a ruler or large index card under each line as you proofread, to focus your vision and concentration.
- Read each paragraph in reverse, from the last sentence to the first. This allows you to focus on spelling instead of meaning.

49C How are plurals spelled?

Watch the Video

The most common plural form adds *-s* or *-es* at the end of the word. The following list covers all variations of creating plurals.

- **Adding *-s* or *-es*:** Plurals of most words are formed by adding *-s: leg, leg**s**; shoe, shoe**s**; stomach, stomach**s***. Words ending in *-s, -sh, -x, -z,* or "soft" *-ch* (as in *beach*) are formed by adding *-es* to the singular: *lens, lens**es**; tax, tax**es**; beach, beach**es***.
- **Words ending in *-o*:** Add *-s* if the *-o* is preceded by a vowel: *radio, radio**s**; cameo, cameo**s***. Add *-es* if the *-o* is preceded by a consonant: *potato, potato**es***. With a few words, you can choose the *-s* or *-es* plural form, but current practice generally supports adding *-es: cargo, cargo**es**; zero, zero**s*** or *zero**es***.
- **Words ending in *-f* or *-fe*:** Some words ending in *-f* and *-fe* are made plural by adding *-s: belief, belief**s***. Others require changing *-f* or *-fe* to *-ves: life, li**ves**; leaf, lea**ves***. Words ending in *-ff* or *-ffe* simply add *-s: staff, staff**s**; giraffe, giraffe**s***.
- **Compound words:** For most compound words, add *-s* or *-es* at the end of the last word: *checkbook**s**, player-coach**es***. In a few cases, the first word is made plural: *sister-in-law, sister**s**-in-law; mile**s** per hour*. (For information about hyphens in compound words, see 49G.)
- **Internal changes and endings other than *-s*:** A few words change internally or add endings other than *-s* to become plural: *foot, f**ee**t; man, m**e**n; crisis, cris**e**s; child, child**ren***.
- **Foreign words:** The best advice is to check your dictionary. Many Latin words ending in *-um* form the plural by changing *-um* to *-a: curricul**um***,

curricula; datum, data; medium, media. Also, Latin words that end in *-us* usually form the plural by changing *-us* to *-i: alumnus, alumni; syllabus, syllabi.* In addition, Greek words that end in *-on* usually form the plural by changing *-on* to *-a: criterion, criteria; phenomenon, phenomena.*

- **One-form words:** Some words have the same form in both the singular and the plural: nine *deer*, many *fish*, four *elk*.

EXERCISE 49-1 Write the correct plural form of these words. For help, consult 49C.

1. yourself
2. sheep
3. photo
4. woman
5. appendix
6. millennium
7. lamp
8. runner-up
9. criterion
10. lunch
11. echo
12. syllabus
13. wife
14. get-together
15. crisis

49D How are suffixes spelled?

A SUFFIX is an ending added to a word that changes the word's meaning or its grammatical function. For example, adding the suffix *-able* to the VERB *depend* creates the ADJECTIVE *dependable*.

Watch the Video

- ***-y* words:** If the letter before a final *-y* is a consonant, change the *-y* to *-i* and add the suffix: *try, **tries**, **tried**.* Keep the *-y* when the suffix begins with *-i* (*apply, app**lying***). If the letter before the final *-y* is a vowel, keep the final *-y: employ, employ**ed**, employ**ing**.* These rules don't apply to IRREGULAR VERBS (see Quick Box 29.4 in section 29D).
- ***-e* words:** Drop a final *-e* when the suffix begins with a vowel, unless doing this would cause confusion: for example, *be* + *ing* can't be written *bing*, but *require* does become *requiring; like* does become *liking*. Keep the final *-e* when the suffix begins with a consonant: *require, require**ment**; like, like**ly**.* Exceptions include *argue, argu**ment**; judge, jud**gment**; true, tru**ly**.*
- **Words that double a final letter:** If the final letter is a consonant, double it *only* if it passes three tests: (1) Its last two letters are a vowel followed by a consonant; (2) it has one syllable or is accented on the last syllable; (3) the suffix begins with a vowel: *drop, drop**ped**; begin, begin**ning**; forget, forget**table**.*
- ***-cede, -ceed, -sede* words:** Only one word in the English language ends in *-sede: super**sede**.* Only three words end in *-ceed: ex**ceed**, pro**ceed**, suc**ceed**.* All other words with endings that sound like "seed" end in *-cede: con**cede**, inter**cede**, pre**cede**.*

- ***-ally* and *-ly* words:** The suffixes *-ally* and *-ly* turn words into adverbs. For words ending in *-ic*, add *-ally: logic**ally**, statistic**ally***. Otherwise, add *-ly: quick**ly**, sharp**ly***.
- ***-ance, -ence*, and *-ible, -able:*** No consistent rules govern words with these suffixes. When in doubt, look up the word.

49E What is the *ie, ei* rule?

The famous rhymed rule for using *ie* and *ei* is usually true:

> *I* before *e* [bel**ie**ve, f**ie**ld, gr**ie**f],
> Except after *c* [c**ei**ling, conc**ei**t],
> Or when sounded like "ay"—
> As in n*ei*ghbor and w*ei*gh [**ei**ght, v**ei**n].

You may want to memorize (sorry!) several exceptions to this rule.

- ***ie:*** consc**ie**nce, financ**ie**r, sc**ie**nce, spec**ie**s
- ***ei:*** **ei**ther, n**ei**ther, l**ei**sure, s**ei**ze, counterf**ei**t, for**ei**gn, forf**ei**t, sl**ei**ght (as in *sleight of hand*), w**ei**rd

● **EXERCISE 49-2** Follow the directions for each group of words. For help, consult 49D and 49E.

1. Add *-able* or *-ible:* (a) profit; (b) reproduce; (c) control; (d) coerce; (e) recognize.
2. Add *-ance* or *-ence:* (a) luxuri_____; (b) prud_____; (c) devi_____; (d) resist_____; (e) independ_____.
3. Drop the final *-e* as needed: (a) true + ly; (b) joke + ing; (c) fortunate + ly; (d) appease + ing; (e) appease + ment.
4. Change the final *-y* to *-i* as needed: (a) happy + ness; (b) pry + ed; (c) pry + ing; (d) dry + ly; (e) beautify + ing.
5. Double the final consonant as needed: (a) commit + ed; (b) commit + ment; (c) drop + ed; (d) occur + ed; (e) regret + ful.
6. Insert *ie* or *ei* correctly: (a) rel_____f; (b) ach_____ve; (c) w_____rd; (d) n_____ce; (e) dec_____ve. ●

49F Why are commonly confused words and homonyms misspelled?

English is rich with **homonyms**—words that sound alike but have different meanings and spellings: *hear, here; to, too, two; elicit, illicit; accept, except.*

In addition, "swallowed pronunciation," which occurs when speakers blur word endings, often causes misspellings and other errors: *use* and *used; prejudice* and *prejudiced. Should of* is always incorrect, but it sounds like *should've*, a CONTRACTION for *should have*.

For more information about word usage that affects spelling, see the Usage Glossary in the back of the book. Quick Box 49.2 lists homonyms and other words that can be confused and lead to misspellings.

Quick Box 49.2

Homonyms and other frequently confused words

- ACCEPT — to receive
  EXCEPT — with the exclusion of
- ADVICE — recommendation
  ADVISE — to recommend
- AFFECT — to influence [VERB]; emotion [NOUN]
  EFFECT — result [NOUN]; to bring about or cause [VERB]
- AISLE — space between rows
  ISLE — island
- ALLUDE — to make indirect reference to
  ELUDE — to avoid
- ALLUSION — indirect reference
  ILLUSION — false idea, misleading appearance
- ALREADY — by this time
  ALL READY — fully prepared
- ALTAR — sacred platform or place
  ALTER — to change
- ALTOGETHER — thoroughly
  ALL TOGETHER — everyone or everything in one place
- ARE — PLURAL form of *to be*
  HOUR — sixty minutes
  OUR — plural form of *my*
- ASCENT — the act of rising or climbing
  ASSENT — consent [NOUN]; to consent [VERB]
- ASSISTANCE — help
  ASSISTANTS — helpers
- BARE — nude, unadorned
  BEAR — to carry; an animal

continued >>

Quick Box 49.2 (continued)

• BOARD	piece of wood
BORED	uninterested
• BRAKE	device for stopping
BREAK	to destroy, make into pieces
• BREATH	air taken in
BREATHE	to take in air
• BUY	to purchase
BY	next to, through the agency of
• CAPITAL	major city; money
CAPITOL	government building
• CHOOSE	to pick
CHOSE	PAST TENSE of *choose*
• CITE	to point out
SIGHT	vision
SITE	a place
• CLOTHES	garments
CLOTHS	pieces of fabric
• COARSE	rough
COURSE	path; series of lectures
• COMPLEMENT	something that completes
COMPLIMENT	praise, flattery
• CONSCIENCE	sense of morality
CONSCIOUS	awake, aware
• COUNCIL	governing body
COUNSEL	advice [NOUN]; to advise [VERB]
• DAIRY	place associated with milk production
DIARY	personal journal
• DESCENT	downward movement
DISSENT	disagreement
• DESERT	to abandon [VERB]; dry, usually sandy area [NOUN]
DESSERT	final, sweet course in a meal
• DEVICE	a plan; an implement
DEVISE	to create

continued >>

Quick Box 49.2 (continued)

• DIE	to lose life (dying) [VERB]; one of a pair of dice [NOUN]
DYE	to change the color of something (dyeing)
• DOMINANT	commanding, controlling
DOMINATE	to control
• ELICIT	to draw out
ILLICIT	illegal
• EMINENT	prominent
IMMANENT	living within; inherent
IMMINENT	about to happen
• ENVELOP	to surround
ENVELOPE	container for a letter or other papers
• FAIR	light-skinned; just, honest
FARE	money for transportation; food
• FORMALLY	conventionally, with ceremony
FORMERLY	previously
• FORTH	forward
FOURTH	number four in a series
• GORILLA	animal in ape family
GUERRILLA	fighter conducting surprise attacks
• HEAR	to sense sound by ear
HERE	in this place
• HOLE	opening
WHOLE	complete; an entire thing
• HUMAN	relating to the species *Homo sapiens*
HUMANE	compassionate
• INSURE	to buy or give insurance
ENSURE	to guarantee, protect
• ITS	POSSESSIVE form of *it*
IT'S	CONTRACTION for *it is*
• KNOW	to comprehend
NO	negative
• LATER	after a time
LATTER	second one of two things

continued >>

Quick Box 49.2 (continued)

• LEAD	a heavy metal [NOUN]; to guide [VERB]
LED	past tense of *lead*
• LIGHTNING	storm-related electricity
LIGHTENING	making lighter
• LOOSE	unbound, not tightly fastened
LOSE	to misplace
• MAYBE	perhaps [ADVERB]
MAY BE	might be [VERB]
• MEAT	animal flesh
MEET	to encounter
• MINER	a person who works in a mine
MINOR	underage; less important
• MORAL	distinguishing right from wrong; the lesson of a fable, story, or event
MORALE	attitude or outlook, usually of a group
• OF	PREPOSITION indicating origin
OFF	away from; not on
• PASSED	past tense of *pass*
PAST	at a previous time
• PATIENCE	forbearance
PATIENTS	people under medical care
• PEACE	absence of fighting
PIECE	part of a whole; musical arrangement
• PERSONAL	intimate
PERSONNEL	employees
• PLAIN	simple, unadorned
PLANE	to shave wood; aircraft
• PRECEDE	to come before
PROCEED	to continue
• PRESENCE	being at hand; attendance at a place or in something
PRESENTS	gifts
• PRINCIPAL	foremost [ADJECTIVE]; school head [NOUN]
PRINCIPLE	moral conviction, basic truth

continued >>

Quick Box 49.2 (continued)

• QUIET	silent, calm
QUITE	very
• RAIN	water that falls to earth [NOUN]; to fall like rain [VERB]
REIGN	to rule
REIN	strap to guide or control an animal [NOUN]; to guide or control [VERB]
• RAISE	to lift up
RAZE	to tear down
• RESPECTFULLY	with respect
RESPECTIVELY	in that order
• RIGHT	correct; opposite of *left*
RITE	ritual
WRITE	to put words on paper
• ROAD	path
RODE	past tense of *ride*
• SCENE	place of an action; segment of a play
SEEN	viewed
• SENSE	perception, understanding
SINCE	measurement of past time; because
• STATIONARY	standing still
STATIONERY	writing paper
• THAN	in comparison with; besides
THEN	at that time; next; therefore
• THEIR	possessive form of *they*
THERE	in that place
THEY'RE	contraction of *they are*
• THROUGH	finished; into and out of
THREW	past tense of *throw*
THOROUGH	complete
• TO	toward
TOO	also; indicates degree (*too much*)
TWO	number following *one*
• WAIST	midsection of the body
WASTE	discarded material [NOUN]; to squander, to fail to use up [VERB]

continued >>

Quick Box 49.2 (continued)

• WEAK	not strong
WEEK	seven days
• WEATHER	climatic condition
WHETHER	if, when alternatives are expressed or implied
• WHERE	in which place
WERE	past tense of *be*
• WHICH	one of a group
WITCH	female sorcerer
• WHOSE	possessive form of *who*
WHO'S	contraction for *who is*
• YOUR	possessive form of *you*
YOU'RE	contraction for *you are*
YORE	long past

● **EXERCISE 49-3** Circle the correct homonym or commonly confused word of each group in parentheses.

If (your, you're) an adult in 2012, (its, it's) three times more likely that you will live alone than you would (have, of) if you'd been an adult in 1950. (Know, No) longer is getting married (right, write, rite) out of high school or college considered a normal (right, write, rite) of passage. In the (passed, past), the (sight, cite, site) of a thirty-year-old living by him- or herself would have been (seen, scene) (by, buy, bye) many as (quite, quiet) disturbing. Even recently, the book *The Lonely American* (raised, razed) the concern that (maybe, may be) living alone would (lead, led) to (later, latter) depression. However, (to, two, too) (choose, chose) to live alone is no longer viewed as a (rode, road) to unhappiness. In fact, evidence shows that people who live alone tend to compensate by being socially active. (Weather, Whether) you feel lonely is less a matter of your circumstances (then, than) a matter of your activities. Sociologist Eric Klinenberg conveys the (sense, since) that (excepting, accepting) (whose, who's) happy simply on the basis of (their, there) living arrangements is (altogether, all together) a (waste, waist) of time. ●

49G What are compound words?

A **compound word** puts together two or more words to express one concept.

Complete the Chapter Exercises

Open compound words remain as separate words, such as *decision making, problem solving*, and *editor in chief.*

Hyphenated compound words use a hyphen between the words, such as *trade-in, fuel-efficient*, and *tax-sheltered.* For punctuation advice about hyphens, see 47I.

Closed compound words appear as one word, such as *proofread, citywide*, and *workweek.*

Single-word compounds usually start as open (two-word) compounds and then become hyphenated compounds before ending up as closed compounds. To check whether a compound term consists of closed, hyphenated, or open words, consult an up-to-date dictionary.

PART

8

Writing When English Is Not Your First Language

A Message to Multilingual Writers

Depending on how, when, and where you began learning English, you might feel very comfortable with spoken English but not written American English. Or you might understand English grammar quite well, but you might struggle with idioms, slang, and sentence structure. You might be an international student just learning the expectations of ACADEMIC WRITING* in American English, or you might be a bilingual student who went to high school in the United States. You might be an adult returning to school encountering academic writing for the first time, or you might be a student who received an advanced degree in another country but must now master written American English.

Learning to write American English is like learning to play a musical instrument. Few people can play fluently without first making many errors. If you become frustrated about the errors that you make in written English, we encourage you to realize that such mistakes show you're moving normally through the stages of second-language development. As with your progress in speaking, listening, and reading in a new language, absorbing the rules of American English grammar takes time.

What can help you advance as quickly as possible? If you attended school elsewhere before coming to the United States, we recommend that you recall how you were taught to present ideas in your written native language. Chances are you encountered quite a different system, especially when presenting information or making an argument. Compare your native system to how writing American English works. Becoming conscious of the similarities and differences can help you understand typical writing strategies in American English.

For example, most college essays and research papers in the United States use a direct tone and straightforward structure. Typically, the THESIS STATEMENT (the central message of the piece of writing) is expected at the end of the first paragraph; in a longer piece of writing, at the end of the second paragraph. Each paragraph that follows, known as a BODY PARAGRAPH, relates in content directly to the essay's thesis statement. Each body paragraph usually starts with a TOPIC SENTENCE that contains the main point of that paragraph. The rest of each body paragraph supports the main point made in the topic sentence. The final paragraph of an essay brings the content to a reasonable conclusion that grows from what has been written in the prior paragraphs.

We urge you always to honor your culture's writing traditions and structures. They reflect the richness of your heritage. We suggest that you look for possible interesting ways to blend the traditions and structures of writing in

* Words printed in SMALL CAPITAL LETTERS are discussed elsewhere in the text and are defined in the Terms Glossary at the back of this book.

your first language with the conventions of academic writing in the United States. We suggest, too, that you get to know *The American Heritage English as a Second Language Dictionary* because it includes many English idioms as well as sample sentences and phrases. If your college library doesn't own a few copies, ask your professor to request that the reference librarian purchase some for students like you to consult.

Our *Simon & Schuster Handbook* offers four special features we've designed specifically for you as a multilingual learner. Chapters 28 through 49 focus on the most challenging grammar issues that you face as you learn to write English. The chapters in the "ESOL" section that follow this letter address major grammar issues that often trouble multilingual writers. Also, in various chapters throughout the book, ESOL Tips offer you specific helpful hints about non-U.S. cultural references and grammar issues. As important, in Chapter 50 we've provided an "English Errors Transferred from Other Languages" chart in which you'll find information about trouble spots that commonly occur when speakers of selected non-English languages speak, read, or write English.

We greatly enjoy discovering the rich variations in the writing traditions of our students from many cultures of the world. As responsible U.S. writing teachers, however, we must explain what you need to do as writers in the United States. If you were in one of our classes, we would say "Welcome!" and ask you to teach us about writing in your native language. Using your knowledge of writing in your first language, we want to help you learn how to approach writing effectively in American English. You bring a richness of experience in communicating in more than one language that most U.S. students have never had, and we hope you're always proud of that experience.

Lynn Quitman Troyka
Doug Hesse

50 Multilingual Students Writing in U.S. Colleges and Universities

Quick Points You will learn to

➤ Use the skills needed by multilingual writing students (see 50A–50E).

50A What do U.S. writing instructors expect in student writing?

Your past writing experiences influence the way you approach writing assignments. In the next passage, a bilingual student illustrates how her past experiences influenced her interpretation of writing assignments in the United States. (Note: The original draft has been edited to improve readability.)

> When I studied in the United States, I felt puzzled with different types of writing assignments. When I wrote my first term paper, I did not know what my professor did expect from me and how to construct my paper. My previous training in my first and second language writing taught me little about how to handle American English writing assignments. Because language teaching in my country is exam-oriented, I learned to write in Chinese and in English in the same way. I read a sample paper, analyzed its content and structure, and tried to apply its strengths to my own writing. Writing was not a creative process to express myself but something that was to be copied for the purpose of taking exams. As a result, when I didn't have a sample for my assignments, I really didn't know how to start.

If you're like this student, you may have difficulty understanding what your instructor expects you to do with a specific writing assignment. Your instructor might expect you to present a clear position on a topic; or to use examples from your personal experience to support your ideas; or to use quotations and comment on specific ideas from an assigned reading or an outside source; or all three. You can't expect yourself to guess what's needed, so never hesitate to ask your instructor questions about the assignment so that you understand exactly what he or she expects.

If your instructor asks students to write about a topic that relates to aspects of American culture with which you're not familiar, talk to him or her about the situation. Ask for guidance in how to find more information about the topic. Conversely, if you're writing about your own culture, keep in mind that your instructor and classmates may not know very much about it. This means you need to explain information and ideas for them in more detail than you would if you were writing for people who share your background. Here's how one student explains that experience.

> If I were writing in Chinese to Chinese readers and wanted to draw on a story in Chinese history as evidence, I would simply mention the name of the historic event or briefly introduce the story. However, when I am writing in American English to tell the readers the same story, I need to tell the story in detail. Otherwise, the U.S. readers would surely get lost.

50B What do U.S. instructors expect for analysis of readings?

When you write a paper based on a reading or on sources you have found for a research project, your teacher wants you to connect these sources to your own ideas after you read and analyze the material. Chapter 20 gives detailed advice about this type of writing. You need to refer to specific ideas and sentences in the material you are writing about, but you cannot rely too heavily on the author's wording and sentence structure; you need to use your own words and sentences by quoting, paraphrasing, or summarizing (see Ch. 18). In U.S. colleges and universities, if you use another author's words, sentence structure, or ideas, you must give the author credit. You do this by using DOCUMENTATION—and quotation marks when you use the exact words. If you don't, it's considered to be a serious offense called PLAGIARISM, which is the same as stealing something that belongs to someone else.

In contrast, using an author's wording in some cultures is not a problem. It may even be seen as a way of complimenting the author. Chapter 19 of this handbook provides detailed information about how to avoid getting into serious legal and academic trouble by engaging in plagiarism. Chapters 25–27 provide examples of four different documentation styles that you might use in your academic writing in the United States. Always ask your instructor if you're uncertain which style to follow.

Documenting sources helps your writing in two ways. By showing your honesty, documentation helps to develop your credibility as a writer. This improves your ethical stance, called *ethos* in Latin (see 3B). Also, giving credit to the original authors shows that you have done the necessary background work to find out what other people have said on a topic.

50C What kind of dictionary can help me the most?

As we suggest in our letter to ESOL students before this chapter, *The American Heritage English as a Second Language Dictionary* is an excellent resource. As important, we urge you to resist any dictionary that only translates words between your native language and English. Such a word-by-word system can't give you the ideas behind the English words. Instead, use an English-English dictionary (sometimes called a "Learner's Dictionary"), one written for non-native learners of English. Be careful of online translation programs such as GoogleTranslate because they often don't present the correct meaning.

50D How do I work with peer response groups, if required?

If your writing instructors expect you to participate in peer response groups (also called "peer review groups" or "peer editing"), refer to Chapter 9 in this handbook for explicit directions. Such activities might be new to you. Here are some strategies specifically for ESOL students to help make this experience more pleasant and useful.

- **If you need to comment on another's writing, word your statements or questions carefully:** For example, asking "How does this idea support your topic or relate back to your topic sentence or thesis statement?" sounds more polite and tactful than, "I don't see how this idea supports your topic."
- **Use modals auxiliary verbs to "hedge" your suggestions**. In English, modal auxiliary verbs often "soften" a statement. For example, "seem" in this statement makes it more polite: "This support does not seem to relate to your topic." It's nicer than "This support has no relation to your topic."
- If your writing instructors make comments on drafts of your essays, they expect to see suitable changes in your final essay based on their comments. Therefore, if you're unsure about what an instructor's comment means, never hesitate to ask for an interpretation—either from your instructor or from a tutor in the writing center.

50E What English errors come from other languages?

ENGLISH ERRORS TRANSFERRED FROM OTHER LANGUAGES

Languages	Error Topic	Sample Errors	Corrected Errors
	Singulars and Plurals (Ch. 52)		
Chinese, Japanese, Korean, Thai	no (or optional) plural forms of nouns, including numbers	**NO** She wrote many good **essay**. **NO** She typed two **paper**.	**YES** She wrote many good **essays**. **YES** She typed two **papers**.

continued >>

Languages	Error Topic	Sample Errors	Corrected Errors
Hebrew, Italian, Japanese, Spanish	use of plural with embedded plurals	**NO** We cared for five **childrens**.	**YES** We cared for five **children**.
Italian, Spanish	adjectives carry plural	**NO** They are **Americans** students.	**YES** They are **American** students.
Articles (Ch. 53)			
Chinese, Japanese, Hindi, Korean, Russian, Swahili, Thai, Turkish, Urdu	no article (*a, an, the*) but can depend on whether article is definite/indefinite	**NO** He ate sandwich.	**YES** He ate **a** sandwich.
Word Order (Ch. 54)			
Arabic, Hebrew, Russian, Spanish, Tagalog	verb before subject	**NO Questioned Avi** the teenagers.	**YES Avi questioned** the teenagers.
Chinese, Japanese, Hindi, Thai	inverted word order confused in questions	**NO The book was it** heavy?	**YES Was the book** heavy?
Chinese, Japanese, Russian, Thai	sentence adverb misplaced	**NO** We will go home **possibly** now.	**YES Possibly**, we will go home now.
Gerunds, Infinitives, and Participles (Ch. 56)			
French, German, Greek, Hindi, Russian, Urdu	no progressive forms or overuse of progressive forms with infinitive	**NO** They **talk** while she **talk**. **NO** They **are wanting** to talk now.	**YES:** They **are talking** while she **is talking**. **YES** They **want** to talk now.
Arabic, Chinese, Farsi, Russian	omit forms of *be*	**NO** She happy. **NO** She **talk** loudly.	**YES** She **is** happy. **YES** She **talks** loudly.
Chinese, Japanese, Korean, Russian, Thai	no verb ending changes for person & number	**NO** He **laugh** yesterday.	**YES** He **laughed** yesterday.
Arabic, Chinese, Farsi, French, Thai, Vietnamese	no or nonstandard verb-tense markers	**NO** They **has arrived** yesterday.	**YES** They **arrived** yesterday.
Japanese, Korean, Russian, Thai, Vietnamese	nonstandard passives	**NO** A car accident **was happened**.	**YES** A car accident **was caused by the icy roads**.

51 Handling Sentence-Level Issues in English

Quick Points You will learn to

➤ Recognize sentence-level errors in English (see 51A–51K).

51A How can I improve the grammar and vocabulary in my writing?

The best way to improve your English-language writing, including your grammar and vocabulary, is by writing. Many students also find it helpful to read as much as they can in English to see how other authors organize their writing, use vocabulary, and structure their sentences. Improving your writing in a second language—or a first language, for that matter—takes time. You will probably find that your ability to communicate with readers improves dramatically if you work on the ideas outlined in the previous chapter. Sometimes, though, readers may find it hard to understand your ideas because of grammar or word choice problems. We have designed this chapter to help you improve in these areas.

51B How can I improve my sentence structure?

Sometimes students write sentences that are hard to understand because of problems with overall sentence structure or length. For example:

> **NO** When the school started, my first English class was English 1020 as a grammar class, I started learning the basics of grammar, and at the same time the basic of writing, I worked hard in that class, taking by the teacher advice, try to memorize a lot of grammar rules and at the same time memorize some words I could use them to make an essay point.

To correct the structural and length errors, the student needs to break the sentence into several shorter sentences (see Chapter 34), to revise her sentences so that they clearly connect to each other, and to work on her verb tenses. She might need to ask for extra help at the writing center or from her instructor.

> **YES** When school started, my first English class, English 1020, was a grammar class, where I started learning the basics of grammar. At the same time, I learned the basics of writing. I worked hard in that class, taking the teacher's advice and memorizing a lot of grammar rules. In addition, I memorized some words I could use in my essays to make my points.

● **EXERCISE 51-1** Many different revisions of the previous example of a student's uncorrected paragraph are possible. Write a different revision of that student's paragraph. ●

● **EXERCISE 51-2** A student wrote the following passage about his experiences learning English. Rewrite the passage, improving the student's sentence structure and punctuation. In your revision of this passage, correct any errors that you see in grammar or spelling. Afterward, compare your revision with a classmate's. Then examine a piece of your own writing to see if you need to revise any of your sentences because of problems with sentence structure. (While you are doing this, if you have any questions about correct word order in English, see Chapter 54.)

> I went to school in my country since I was three years old, I was in Arabic and French school, and that's was my dad choice because his second language is French. So my second language at that time was French. In my elementary school I started to learn how to make an essay in French and Arabic. I learned the rules and it is too deferent from English. But later on when I was in my high school I had two choices between English class and science class so I choose the science because that's was my major. After I graduate I went to American university and I start studying English and my first class was remedial English for people doesn't know anything about this language. I went to this class about two months and then I have moved to a new place and I start from the beginning as an ESL student. ●

51C How can I improve my word choice (vocabulary)?

An important aspect of writing in a second language is having enough vocabulary to express your ideas. Many students enjoy learning more and more words to be able to communicate precise meanings. Experiment in your writing with new words that you hear and read in other contexts. Keep lists of new words, and try to add a few new words each day.

51D How can I find and correct errors in my own writing?

Some multilingual writers find it easiest to find and correct their grammar errors by reading their writing aloud and listening for mistakes. This method is often preferred by students who feel their spoken English is better than their written English. Other writers like to ask a friend who is a native speaker of English to check their writing. Still other multilingual writers prefer to circle each place where they think they've made an error and then use their handbook to check themselves.

You might also keep a list of the types of grammar errors you make so that you can become especially sensitive to errors when proofreading. The best system is to make a master list of the errors in categories so that you can check efficiently. Section 51J provides an example of how to track your errors.

51E How can I correct verb errors in my writing?

51E.1 Verb Tense Errors

Many multilingual writers consider verb-form errors the most difficult to correct. They want to be sure that their verb forms express the appropriate time frame for the event or situation they're describing. For a detailed discussion of verb forms, see 29B–29F.

● **EXERCISE 51-3** Read the following passage in which a student describes his experiences as an international traveler. The student's instructor has underlined errors related to time frames expressed by the verbs. Correct the underlined verbs, changing them to the correct time frames.

My earliest memory of traveling was going to the Post Office with my dad to apply for a passport. I must have been eight or nine years old, and I flinched when the man <u>takes</u> my picture.

After I got my passport, we <u>plan</u> a trip to Europe. We visited France, Spain, and Portugal, then <u>cross</u> the Channel into Great Britain. I loved seeing the famous sights in England. I <u>am</u> excited to see Great Ben, and I even <u>have</u> a picture taken with me and a Royal Guard in front of Buckingham Palace. I <u>try</u> everything to make him smile, but he <u>keeps</u> his face cold as stone.

When I was a few years older, I <u>travel</u> to Germany as an exchange student. I had been studying the Reformation, so I <u>want</u> to see the famous Wittenberg church where Martin Luther <u>nails</u> his ninety-five theses to a door. During that trip, I also enjoy some leisure time at the very popular Oktoberfest, where I drink beer and enjoy the music. ●

If you struggle with errors in verb tense in your writing, try reading through your draft once and circling all the verbs. Then check each one in isolation.

51E.2 Verbal Errors

Some students are troubled by the distinction between a VERB and a VERBAL. A verbal is not a verb, but rather it's a verb form whose function has shifted to another part of speech. Three verbal forms are the participle (ADJECTIVE), the gerund (NOUN), and the infinitive (ADJECTIVE, NOUN, or ADVERB).

PARTICIPLE (ADJECTIVE): Our **shedding** elms do not look healthy.

PARTICIPLE (ADJECTIVE) Our **shedded** elms were cut down right away.

GERUND (NOUN): A rapid **shedding** of leaves usually indicates elm disease.

INFINITIVE (NOUN): Our elms were beginning **to shed** their leaves rapidly.

INFINITIVE (ADJECTIVE): Our trees with Dutch elm disease gave us no time **to waste**.

INFINITIVE (ADVERB): We cut our diseased trees **to maintain** the health of other trees.

Verbals used in sentences without AUXILIARY VERBS create SENTENCE FRAGMENTS.

NO Our elm trees **to maintain** their health.

YES Our elm trees have **to maintain** their health.

The auxiliary verb *have* completes the sentence.

NO Cutting down diseased elms **recommended**.

YES Cutting down diseased elms ***is* recommended**.

The auxiliary verb *is* completes the sentence.

NO Urban landscapers **hired** to protect city parks.

NO Urban landscapers **being hired** to protect city parks.

YES Urban landscapers ***are* being hired** to protect city parks.

The auxiliary verb *are* completes the sentence.

● **EXERCISE 51-4** Working individually or with a group, rewrite the following paragraph to eliminate the misuse of verbals as verbs. (Some sentences are correct.) You may add, change, or rearrange words.

Many embarrassing errors made by multinational corporations when translating U.S. brands or slogans abroad. For example, when Pepsi entered the Chinese market some years back, it translated the slogan, "Pepsi Brings You Back to Life," which means in Chinese, "Pepsi Brings Your Ancestors Back from the Grave." Braniff Airlines interested to tell passengers about the comfort of its seats by using the slogan "Fly in Leather." However, in Spanish, this slogan was translated into "Fly Naked." In Italy, a campaign by "Schweppes Tonic Water" aiming to quench customers' thirst. Understandably, Italians not rushing to buy what translate to "Schweppes Toilet Water." Advertisers outside the United States must remember that language, after all, is a primary tool that used to generate both customer interest and corporate profits. ●

51F How can I correct my errors in subject–verb agreement?

Subject–verb agreement means that a subject (a noun or a pronoun) and its verb must agree in number and in person. In the following two sentences, notice the difference in the way the subjects and the verbs that describe their actions agree: *Carolina runs charity marathons. They give her a sense of accomplishment.*

For more information about subject–verb agreement, review Chapter 31. To help you put subject-verb agreement rules into practice, try the next exercise.

● **EXERCISE 51-5** Examine the following student's description. The student's instructor has underlined verbs that do not agree with their subjects. Correct the underlined verb forms, changing them to agree with their subjects.

My goal <u>have</u> always been to learn how to enjoy travelling to different countries, which all <u>has</u> their own unique cultures. When I travel to unfamiliar places, I like to eat unusual dishes, even if they <u>appears</u> unusual at first. A tourist, even a seasoned one, <u>are</u> there to experience new things. And being willing to try new things <u>make</u> the journey more fulfilling. ●

51G How can I correct my singular/plural errors?

In English, if you're referring to more than one noun that is a count noun, you must make that noun plural, often by adding an *-s* ending. If you would like more information on this topic, see Chapter 52. To help you recognize when necessary plural forms are missing, try the next exercise.

● **EXERCISE 51-6** In the following passage, a student's instructor has underlined only the first two nouns that need to be plural. Read the passage, correct the two underlined nouns, and then find and correct the other nouns in the passage that need to be plural.

> Every country has its own <u>custom</u>. When traveling, it's important to remember that your way of doing <u>thing</u> may not be the same in other country. For example, in some places, it is common for customer to barter for a price on item for sale. Also, American generally shake hand when greeting one another, but in some places, it is common for friend to kiss. ●

Examine a piece of your own writing and make sure that you have used plural words correctly.

51H How can I correct my preposition errors?

Prepositions are words such as *in, on, for, over,* and *about,* which usually show where, how, or when. For example, in the sentence *She received flowers from her friend for her birthday,* the prepositions are *from* and *for.* Unlike some other languages, English has many prepositions, and knowing which one to use can be very difficult. You can find information about using prepositions in section 28H and in Chapter 55.

● **EXERCISE 51-7** In the following passage, the student's instructor has underlined problems with preposition use. Try to correct the preposition errors. In some cases, more than one answer may be correct. If you can't find the information you need from Chapter 55 or in a dictionary, you might ask a native English speaker for help.

> I've always wanted to learn languages other than my native language. I started taking English and French lessons <u>of</u> school and I liked the idea of becoming fluent <u>for</u> at least one language. I thought English would help me a lot <u>to</u> the future because it could help me communicate <u>to</u> people from all over the world. ●

If prepositions are something you struggle with in your own writing, ask an instructor or a native speaker of English to underline the errors in preposition usage in a piece of writing that you have done. Then go through your writing and correct the errors that have been underlined.

51I What other kinds of errors might I make?

Depending on your language background and your prior experience with writing in English (see 50E), you may make errors related to the use of articles (*a, an, the*), word order (where to place adjectives and adverbs in sentences), and various verb forms and noun forms (for example, problems with noncount nouns and helping verbs). For example, the next sentence has a problem with one article and the order of an adjective: *The New York City is a place exciting*. The corrected sentence is *New York City is an exciting place*. Chapters 52 through 57 address grammar errors that are often made by multilingual writers.

51J How can I keep track of my most common errors?

One way of becoming more aware of the types of errors you make is to keep track of the errors you often make in the papers you write. You can ask your instructor or a tutor to help you identify such errors, and you can make a list of them that you update regularly. Remember the passage from Exercise 51-3 about a student's travel experiences? After the student examined the teacher's comments on his paper, he made a list of his errors and included a correction and a note about the error type for each. Upon reviewing this list (see Figure 51.1), the student writer realized that many of his errors related to verb form.

Figure 51.1 A list of errors.

Specific Error	Correction	Type of Error
when the man takes	took	verb form
we plan a trip	planned	verb form
then cross the Channel	crossed	verb form
I am excited	was	verb form
I even have	had	verb form
I try everything	tried	verb form
he keeps his face	kept	verb form
I travel to Germany	traveled	verb form
I want to see	wanted	verb form
where Martin Luther nails	nailed	verb form
I also enjoy	enjoyed	verb form
where I drink beer	drank	verb form
and enjoy the music	enjoyed	verb form

● **EXERCISE 51-8** Using one or more pieces of your writing, make an error list similar to the previous one. (You could make this list on a sheet of paper or in an electronic file.) Examine the list. What are the most common types of errors that you make? Once you have identified your common error types, refer to the relevant proofreading exercises in this chapter and to the relevant ones in Chapters 52 through 57. Also, remember to keep your common errors in mind when you proofread your future writing assignments. You might even keep a master checklist that you can return to when you proofread your writing. ●

51K How can I improve my proofreading skills?

The most effective way to improve your proofreading skills is to practice frequently. Proofread your own writing and, after you have done so, ask your instructor, a tutor, or a friend who is a native English speaker to point out the location of errors that you did not see on your own. When you know which errors you've made, try to correct the errors without help. Finally, have your instructor or tutor check your corrections.

Another effective way to improve your proofreading skills is to exchange your writing with a partner. You can check for errors in his or her writing and he or she can check for errors in yours. You might find that, at first, it is easier to find errors if you look for one kind of error at a time. Try Exercises 51-9 and 51-10 for more proofreading practice.

● **EXERCISE 51-9** After you read the following passage, rewrite it, correcting the linguistic errors you find.

> I've always faced some problem in writing in English as it took me some time to get used to it. Facing these complexities encourage me to developed my skills in English writing. My first class in English was about grammar, spelling, and writing. I realize later that grammar is hard to learn, so I knew I have to put in a lot of effort to understand it perfectly and use it properly. I also had some difficulties for vocabulary, as it was hard to understand the meaning of some word.
>
> Another thing that helped me with my English was when my mother enroll me in an English learning center that specialize in teach writing skills. After a month of taking classes, my teacher saw some improvement in my grammar and vocabulary. To test me, she asked me to write an essay on how to be successful. I was really excite of it and started write it immediately. After I finish my essay and my teacher check it, my teacher suggested that I take a few more classes for her. She taught me how to organized my ideas. After finishing these classes I realize that my writing was getting much better with time. ●

● **EXERCISE 51-10** In the following paragraph, a student describes the study of English at private schools in Japan. After you read the paragraph, rewrite it, correcting the errors that you find.

Recently, the number of private language schools are increased in Japan. These schools put special emphasize on oral communication skills. In them, student takes not only grammars and reading classes, which help them pass school examinations, but also speaking, listening classes. They can also study English for six year, which is same period as in public schools. Some of the teacher in these school are native speaker of English. Since these teachers do not use Japanese in the class, the students have to use the English to participate it. They have the opportunity to use the English in their class more than public school students. It is said that the students who took English in private schools can speak English better than those student who go to public schools. ●

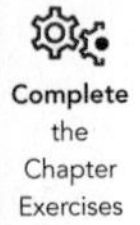

Complete the Chapter Exercises

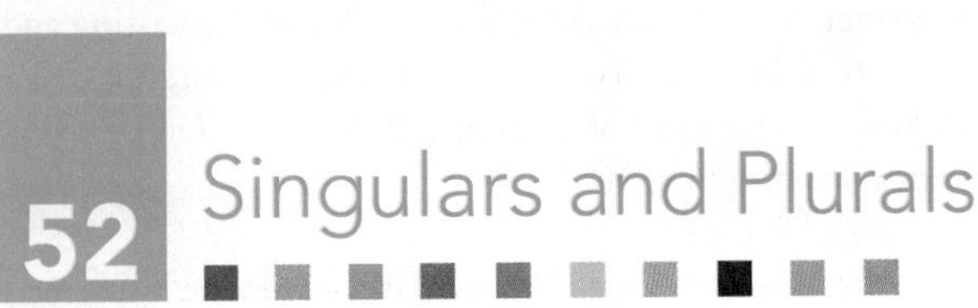

52 Singulars and Plurals

Quick Points You will learn to

- Distinguish between count and noncount nouns (see 52A).
- Use the proper determiners with singular and plural nouns (see 52B).

52A What are count and noncount nouns?

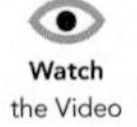

Watch the Video

Count nouns name items that can be counted: *a radio* or *radios, a street* or *streets, an idea* or *ideas, a fingernail* or *fingernails*. Count nouns can be SINGULAR or PLURAL.

Noncount nouns name things that are thought of as a whole and not split into separate, countable parts: *rice, knowledge, traffic*. There are two important rules to remember about noncount nouns: (1) They're never preceded by *a* or *an*, and (2) they are never plural.

Here are several categories of noncount nouns, with examples in each category:

GROUPS OF SIMILAR ITEMS	clothing, equipment, furniture, jewelry, junk, luggage, mail, money, stuff, traffic, vocabulary
ABSTRACTIONS	advice, equality, fun, health, ignorance, information, knowledge, news, peace, pollution, respect
LIQUIDS	blood, coffee, gasoline, water
GASES	air, helium, oxygen, smog, smoke, steam
MATERIALS	aluminum, cloth, cotton, ice, wood
FOOD	beef, bread, butter, macaroni, meat, pork
PARTICLES OR GRAINS	dirt, dust, hair, rice, salt, wheat
SPORTS, GAMES, ACTIVITIES	chess, homework, housework, reading, sailing, soccer
LANGUAGES	Arabic, Chinese, Japanese, Spanish
FIELDS OF STUDY	biology, computer science, history, literature, math
EVENTS IN NATURE	electricity, heat, humidity, moonlight, rain, snow, sunshine, thunder, weather

Some nouns can be countable or uncountable, depending on their meaning in a sentence. Most of these nouns name things that can be meant either individually or as "wholes" made up of individual parts.

COUNT You have **a hair** on your sleeve.

In this sentence, *hair* is meant as an individual, countable item.

NONCOUNT Kioko has black **hair**.

In this sentence, all the strands of *hair* are referred to as a whole.

COUNT **The rains** were late last year.

In this sentence, *rains* is meant as individual, countable occurrences of rain.

NONCOUNT **The rain** is soaking the garden.

In this sentence, all the particles of *rain* are referred to as a whole.

When you are editing your writing (see 5K), be sure that you have not added a plural *-s* to any noncount nouns, for they are always singular in form.

Alert: Be sure to use a singular verb with any noncount noun that functions as a SUBJECT in a CLAUSE. ●

To check whether a noun is count or noncount, look it up in a dictionary such as the *Dictionary of American English* (Heinle and Heinle). In this dictionary, count nouns are indicated by [C], and noncount nouns are indicated by [U] (for "uncountable"). Nouns that have both count and noncount meanings are marked [C;U].

52B How do I use determiners with singular and plural nouns?

DETERMINERS, also called *expressions of quantity*, are used to tell how much or how many with reference to NOUNS. Other names for determiners include *limiting adjectives, noun markers*, and ARTICLES. (For information about articles—the words *a, an*, and *the*—see Chapter 53.)

Choosing the right determiner with a noun can depend on whether the noun is NONCOUNT or COUNT (see 52A). For count nouns, you must also decide whether the noun is singular or plural. Quick Box 52.1 lists many determiners and the kinds of nouns that they can accompany.

Quick Box 52.1

Determiners to use with count and noncount nouns

GROUP 1: DETERMINERS FOR SINGULAR COUNT NOUNS

With every singular count noun, always use one of the determiners listed in Group 1.

a, an, the	**a house**	**an egg**	**the car**
one, any, some, every, each, either, neither, another, the other	**any house**	**each egg**	**another car**
my, our, your, his, her, its, their, nouns with *'s* or *s'*	**your house**	**its egg**	**Connie's car**
this, that	**this house**	**that egg**	**this car**
one, no, the first, the second, etc.	**one house**	**no egg**	**the fifth car**

continued >>

Quick Box 52.1 (continued)

GROUP 2: DETERMINERS FOR PLURAL COUNT NOUNS

All the determiners listed in Group 2 can be used with plural count nouns. Plural count nouns can also be used without determiners, as discussed in section 52B.

the	**the bicycles**	**the rooms**	**the idea**
some, any, both, many, more, most, few, fewer, the fewest, a lot of, a number of, other, several, all, all the	**some bicycles**	**many rooms**	**all ideas**
my, our, your, his, her, its, their, nouns with *'s* or *s'*	**our bicycles**	**her rooms**	**student's ideas**
these, those	**these bicycles**	**those rooms**	**these ideas**
no, two, three, etc.; *the first, the second, the third,* etc.	**no bicycles**	**four rooms**	**the first ideas**

GROUP 3: DETERMINERS FOR NONCOUNT NOUNS

All the determiners listed in Group 3 can be used with noncount nouns (always singular). Noncount nouns can also be used without determiners.

the	**the rice**	**the rain**	**the pride**
some, any, much, more, most, other, the other, little, less, the least, enough, all, all the, a lot of	**enough rice**	**a lot of rain**	**more pride**
my, our, your, his, her, its, their, nouns with *'s* or *s'*	**their rice**	**India's rain**	**your pride**
this, that	**this rice**	**that rain**	**this pride**
no, the first, the second, the third, etc.	**no rice**	**the first rain**	**no pride**

Alert: The phrases *a few* and *a little* convey the meaning "some": *I have* **a few** *rare books* means "I have *some* rare books." *They are worth* **a little** *money* means "They are worth *some* money."

Without the word *a*, the words *few* and *little* convey the meaning "almost none": *I have* **few** [or *very few*] *books* means "I have *almost no* books." *They are worth* **little** *money* means "They are worth *almost no* money." ●

52C How do I use *one of*, nouns as adjectives, and *states* in names or titles?

ONE OF CONSTRUCTIONS

One of constructions include *one of the* and a NOUN or *one of* followed by a DETERMINER–noun combination (*one of my hats, one of those ideas*). Always use a plural noun as the OBJECT when you use *one of the* with a noun or *one of* with an adjective–noun combination.

NO *One of the* **reason** to live here is the beach.

YES *One of the* **reasons** to live here is the beach.

NO *One of her best* **friend** has moved away.

YES *One of her best* **friends** has moved away.

The VERB in these constructions is always singular because it agrees with the singular *one*, not with the plural noun: **One** *of the most important inventions of the twentieth century* **is** [not *are*] *television*.

For advice about verb forms that go with *one of the . . . who* constructions, see 31L.

NOUNS USED AS ADJECTIVES

ADJECTIVES in English do not have plural forms. When you use an adjective with a PLURAL NOUN, make the noun plural but not the adjective: *the* **green** [not *greens*] *leaves*. Be especially careful when you use a word as a MODIFIER that can also function as a noun.

- The bird's wingspan is ten inches.

  Inches is functioning as a noun.

- The bird has a ten-inch wingspan.

  Inch is functioning as a modifier.

Do not add *-s* (or *-es*) to the adjective even when it is modifying a plural noun or pronoun.

NO Many **Americans** students are basketball fans.

YES Many **American** students are basketball fans.

NAMES OR TITLES THAT INCLUDE THE WORD *STATES*

States is a plural word. However, names such as *United States* or *Organization of American States* refer to singular things—one country and one organization, even though made up of many states. When *states* is part of a name or title referring to one thing, the name is a SINGULAR NOUN and therefore requires a SINGULAR VERB.

NO The **United States have** a large entertainment industry.

NO The **United State has** a large entertainment industry.

YES The **United States has** a large entertainment industry.

52D How do I use nouns with irregular plurals?

Some English nouns have irregularly spelled plurals. In addition to those discussed in section 49C, here are others that often cause difficulties.

PLURALS OF FOREIGN NOUNS AND OTHER IRREGULAR NOUNS

Whenever you are unsure whether a noun is plural, look it up in a dictionary. If no plural is given for a singular noun, add *-s* to form the plural.

Many nouns from other languages that are used unchanged in English have only one plural. If two plurals are listed in the dictionary, look carefully for differences in meaning. Some words, for example, keep the plural form from the original language for scientific usage and have another, English-form plural for nonscientific contexts: *formula, formulae, formulas; appendix, appendices, appendixes; index, indices, indexes; medium, media, mediums; cactus, cacti, cactuses; fungus, fungi, funguses.*

Words from Latin that end in *-is* in their singular form become plural by substituting *-es: parenthesis, parentheses; thesis, theses; oasis, oases.*

OTHER WORDS

Medical terms for diseases involving an inflammation end in *-itis: tonsillitis, appendicitis.* They are always singular.

The word *news,* although it ends in *s,* is always singular: *The* **news is** *encouraging.* The words *people, police,* and *clergy* are always plural even though they do not end in *s: The* **police are** *prepared.*

● **EXERCISE 52-1** Consulting all sections of this chapter, select the correct choice from the words in parentheses and write it in the blank.

Complete the Chapter Exercises

EXAMPLE

It can be tricky to bake (bread, breads) <u>bread</u> in Denver, Colorado, because of that city's high (elevation, elevations) <u>elevation</u>.

1. Denver has an elevation of 5,280 (foot, feet) __________, and changes must therefore be made to baking (recipe, recipes) __________.
2. The 5,280-(foot, feet) __________ elevation lowers the boiling point of (water, waters) __________.
3. The leading (American, Americans) __________ expert in high-altitude baking recommends adding more (flour, flours) __________ to bread recipes.
4. If your recipe includes different kinds of (liquid, liquids) __________, the expert recommends adding additional (liquid, liquid) __________ to combat dryness.
5. One of the (effect, effects) __________ of the high altitude is that the crust of a loaf of (bread, breads) __________ will cook faster. ●

53 Articles

Quick Points You will learn to

➤ Use articles correctly (see 53A–53C).

53A How do I use *a, an,* or *the* with singular count nouns?

Watch the Video

The words *a* and *an* are called INDEFINITE ARTICLES. The word *the* is called the DEFINITE ARTICLE. Articles are one type of DETERMINER. (For more on determiners, see 28F; for other determiners, see Quick Box 52.1 in 52B.) Articles signal that a NOUN will follow and that any MODIFIERS between the article and the noun refer to that noun.

a chair	**the** computer
a brown chair	**the** teacher's computer
a cold, metal chair	**the** lightning-fast computer

Every time you use a singular count noun, a COMMON NOUN that names one countable item, the noun requires some kind of determiner; see Group 1 in Quick Box 52.1 (in 52B) for a list. To choose between *a* or *an* and *the*, you need to determine whether the noun is **specific** or nonspecific. A noun is considered *specific* when anyone who reads your writing can understand exactly and specifically to what item the noun is referring. If the noun refers to any of a number of identical items, it is *nonspecific*.

For nonspecific singular count nouns, use *a* (or *an*). When the singular noun is specific, use *the* or some other determiner. Quick Box 53.1 can help you decide when a singular count noun is specific and therefore requires *the*.

Quick Box 53.1

When a singular count noun is specific and requires *the*

- **Rule 1: A noun is specific and requires *the* when it names something unique or generally and unambiguously known.**
    - **The sun** has risen above **the horizon**.

      Because there is only one *sun* and only one *horizon*, these nouns are specific in the context of this sentence.

- **Rule 2: A noun is specific and requires *the* when it names something used in a representative or abstract sense.**
    - Benjamin Franklin favored **the turkey** as **the national bird** of the United States.

      Because *turkey* and *national bird* are representative references rather than references to a particular turkey or bird, they are specific nouns in the context of this sentence.

- **Rule 3: A noun is specific and requires *the* when it names something defined elsewhere in the same sentence or in an earlier sentence.**
    - **The ship *Savannah*** was the first steam vessel to cross the Atlantic Ocean.

      Savannah names a specific ship.

    - **The carpet in my bedroom** is new.

      In my bedroom defines exactly which carpet is meant, so *carpet* is a specific noun in this context.

    - I have **a computer** in my office. **The computer** is often broken.

      Computer is not specific in the first sentence, so it uses *a*. In the second sentence, *computer* has been made specific by the first sentence, so it uses *the*.

continued >>

Quick Box 53.1 (continued)

- **Rule 4: A noun is specific and requires *the* when it names something that can be inferred from the context.**
  - Monday, I had to call the technician to fix my computer again.

    A technician would be any of a number of individuals; *the technician* implies the same person has been called before, and so it is specific in this context.

Alert: Use *an* before words that begin with a vowel sound. Use *a* before words that begin with a consonant sound. Go by the sound, not the spelling. For example, words that begin with *h* or *u* can have either a vowel or a consonant sound. Make the choice based on the sound of the first word after the article, even if that word is not the noun.

an idea **a g**ood idea

an umbrella **a u**seless umbrella

an honor **a history book** ●

One common exception affects Rule 3 in Quick Box 53.1. A noun may still require *a* (or *an*) after the first use if more information is added between the article and the noun: *I bought **a sweater** today. It was **a*** (not *the*) ***red sweater***. (Your audience has been introduced to *a sweater* but not *a red sweater*, so *red sweater* is not yet specific in this context and cannot take *the*.) Other information may make the noun specific so that *the* is correct. For example, *It was **the red sweater that I saw in the store yesterday*** uses *the* because the *that* CLAUSE makes specific which red sweater the writer means.

53B How do I use articles with plural nouns and with noncount nouns?

With plural nouns and NONCOUNT NOUNS, you must decide whether to use *the* or to use no article at all. (For guidelines about using DETERMINERS other than articles with nouns, see Quick Box 52.1 in 52B.) What you learned in 53A about NONSPECIFIC and SPECIFIC NOUNS can help you choose between using *the* or using no article. Quick Box 53.1 in 53A explains when a singular count noun's meaning is specific and calls for *the*. Plural nouns and noncount nouns with specific meanings usually use *the* in the same circumstances. However, a plural noun or a noncount noun with a general or nonspecific meaning usually does not use *the*.

- Geraldo grows **flowers** but not **vegetables** in his garden. He is thinking about planting **corn** sometime. [three nonspecific nouns]

PLURAL NOUNS

A plural noun's meaning may be specific because it is widely known.

- **The oceans** are being damaged by pollution.

  Because there is only one possible meaning for *oceans*—the oceans on the earth—it is correct to use *the*. This example is related to Rule 1 in Quick Box 53.1.

A plural noun's meaning may also be made specific by a word, PHRASE, or CLAUSE in the same sentence.

- Geraldo sold **the daisies from last year's garden** to the florist.

  Because the phrase *from last year's garden* makes *daisies* specific, *the* is correct. This example is related to Rule 3 in Quick Box 53.1.

A plural noun's meaning usually becomes specific by its use in an earlier sentence.

- Geraldo planted **tulips** this year. **The tulips** will bloom in April.

  Tulips is used in a general sense in the first sentence, without *the*. Because the first sentence makes *tulips* specific, *the tulips* is correct in the second sentence. This example is related to Rule 3 in Quick Box 53.1.

A plural noun's meaning may be made specific by the context.

- Geraldo fertilized **the bulbs** when he planted them last October.

  In the context of the sentences about tulips, *bulbs* is understood as a synonym for *tulips*, which makes it specific and calls for *the*. This example is related to Rule 4 in Quick Box 53.1.

NONCOUNT NOUNS

Noncount nouns are always singular in form (see 52A). Like plural nouns, noncount nouns use either *the* or no article. When a noncount noun's meaning is specific, use *the* before it. If its meaning is general or nonspecific, do not use *the*.

- Kalinda served us **rice**. She flavored **the rice** with curry.

  Rice is a noncount noun. By the second sentence, *rice* has become specific, so *the* is used. This example is related to Rule 3 in Quick Box 53.1.

- Kalinda served us **the rice that she had flavored with curry**.

  Rice is a noncount noun. *Rice* is made specific by the clause *that she had flavored with curry*, so *the* is used. This example is related to Rule 3 in Quick Box 53.1.

GENERALIZATIONS WITH PLURAL OR NONCOUNT NOUNS

Rule 2 in Quick Box 53.1 tells you to use *the* with singular count nouns that carry general meaning. With GENERALIZATIONS using plural or noncount nouns, omit *the*.

NO **The tulips** are **the flowers** that grow from **the bulbs**.

YES **Tulips** are **flowers** that grow from **bulbs**.

NO **The dogs** require more care than **the cats** do.

YES **Dogs** require more care than **cats** do.

53C How do I use *the* with proper nouns and with gerunds?

PROPER NOUNS

PROPER NOUNS name specific people, places, or things (see 28B). Most proper nouns do not require ARTICLES: *We visited **Lake Mead** with **Asha** and **Larry**.* As shown in Quick Box 53.2, however, certain types of proper nouns do require *the*.

Quick Box 53.2

Proper nouns that use *the*

- **Nouns with the pattern *the . . . of . . .***
  - **the** United States **of** America
  - **the** Republic **of** Mexico
  - **the** Fourth **of** July
  - **the** University **of** Paris
- **Plural proper nouns**
  - **the** United Arab Emirates
  - **the** Johnsons
  - **the** Rocky Mountains [*but* Mount Fuji]
  - **the** Chicago Bulls
  - **the** Falkland Islands [*but* Long Island]
  - **the** Great Lakes [*but* Lake Superior]
- **Collective proper nouns (nouns that name a group)**
  - **the** Modern Language Association
  - **the** Society of Friends

continued >>

Quick Box 53.2 (continued)

- **Some (but not all) geographical features**
  the Amazon **the** Gobi Desert **the** Indian Ocean
- **Three countries**
  the Congo **the** Sudan **the** Netherlands

GERUNDS

GERUNDS are PRESENT PARTICIPLES (the *-ing* form of VERBS) used as nouns: ***Skating** is challenging*. Gerunds are usually not preceded by *the*.

NO **The constructing** new bridges is necessary to improve traffic flow.

YES **Constructing** new bridges is necessary to improve traffic flow.

Use *the* before a gerund when two conditions are met: (1) The gerund is used in a specific sense (see 53A), and (2) the gerund does not have a DIRECT OBJECT.

NO **The designing fabric** is a fine art.

Fabric is a direct object of *designing*, so *the* should not be used.

YES **Designing** fabric is a fine art.

Designing is a gerund, so *the* is not used.

YES **The designing of** fabric is a fine art.

The is used because *fabric* is the object of the preposition *of* and *designing* is meant in a specific sense.

● **EXERCISE 53-1** Consulting all sections of this chapter, decide which of the words in parentheses is correct and write it in the blank. If no article is needed, leave the blank empty.

Complete the Chapter Exercises

EXAMPLE

In (a, an, the) ____ United States of America, (a, an, the) ____ highways are labeled with (a, an, the) ____ number that indicates (a, an, the) ____ highway's direction.

In (a, an, the) the United States of America, (a, an, the) [no article] highways are labeled with (a, an, the) a number that indicates the highway's direction.

1. If (a, an, the) ____ highway runs north and south, then it is designated with (a, an, the) ____ odd number, but (a, an, the) ____ highways that run east and west are given (a, an, the) ____ even number.

2. For example, (a, an, the) ____ highway that runs north and south along (a, an, the) ____ coast of California is called (a, an, the) ____ Highway 1.
3. (A, An, The) ____ interstate highway that runs east-to-west is given (a, an, the) ____ low even number if it is in (a, an, the) ____ southern U.S., such as (a, an, the) ____ Interstate 10.
4. (A, An, The) ____ three-digit freeway usually encircles (a, an, the) ____ major city.
5. One of (a, an, the) ____ America's most famous highways is (a, an, the) ____ Route 66, which is (a, an, the) ____ road that runs from Los Angeles to Chicago. ●

54 Word Order

Quick Points You will learn to

- Use appropriate English word order (see 54A).
- Place adjectives and adverbs in the proper places in sentences (see 54B–54C).

54A How do I understand standard and inverted word order in sentences?

In STANDARD WORD ORDER, the most common pattern for DECLARATIVE SENTENCES in English, the SUBJECT comes before the VERB. (To understand these concepts more fully, review 28L through 28P.)

SUBJECT ↓ VERB ↓

- That book was heavy.

With INVERTED WORD ORDER, the MAIN VERB or an AUXILIARY VERB comes before the subject. The most common use of inverted word order in English is in forming DIRECT QUESTIONS. Questions that can be answered with a yes or no begin with a form of *be* used as a main verb, with an auxiliary verb (*be, do, have*), or with a MODAL AUXILIARY (*can, should, will*, and others; see Chapter 57).

QUESTIONS THAT CAN BE ANSWERED WITH A YES OR NO

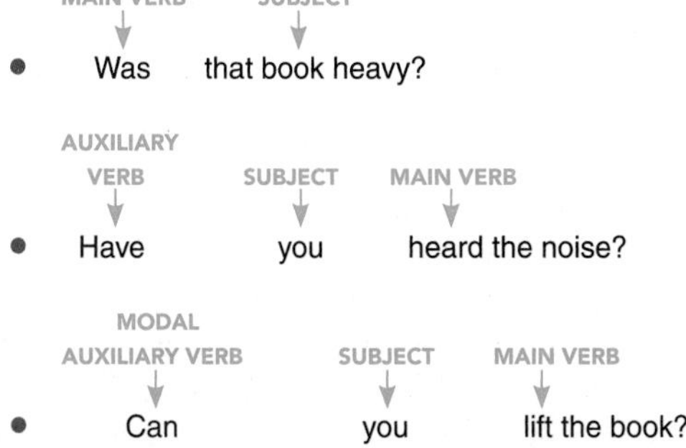

To form a yes-or-no question with a verb other than *be* as the main verb and when there is no auxiliary or modal as part of a VERB PHRASE, use the appropriate form of the auxiliary verb *do*.

AUXILIARY VERB — SUBJECT — MAIN VERB

- Do you want me to put the book away?

A question that begins with a question-forming word such as *why, when, where*, or *how* cannot be answered with a yes or no: ***Why** did the book fall?* Some kind of information must be provided to answer such a question; the answer cannot be simply yes or no because the question is not "*Did* the book fall?" Information on *why* it fell is needed: for example, *It was too heavy for me*.

INFORMATION QUESTIONS: INVERTED ORDER

Most information questions follow the same rules of inverted word order as yes-or-no questions.

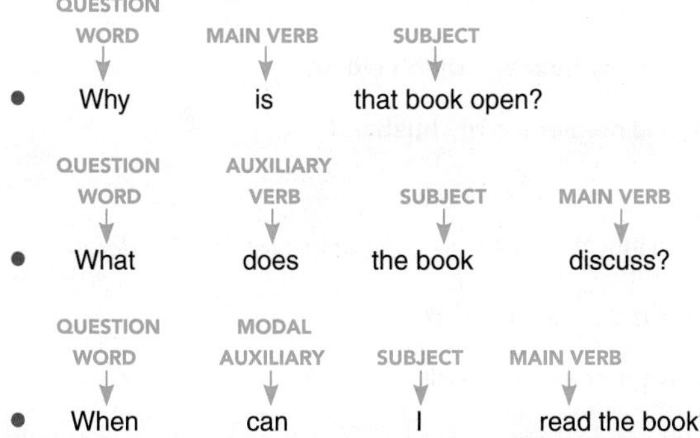

INFORMATION QUESTIONS: STANDARD ORDER

When *who* or *what* functions as the subject in a question, use standard word order.

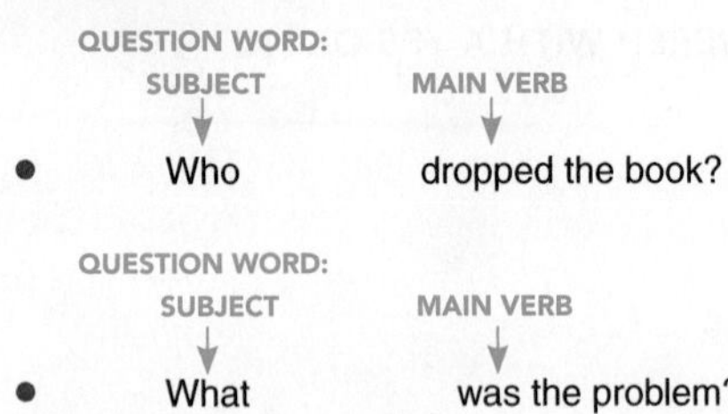

Alert: When a question has more than one auxiliary verb, put the subject after the first auxiliary verb.

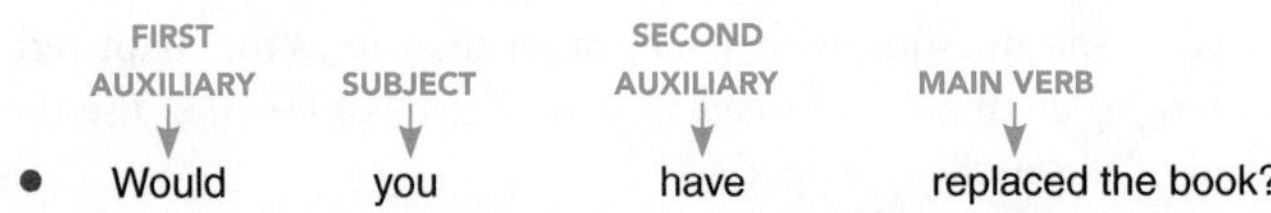

The same rules apply to emphatic exclamations: ***Was** that book heavy!* ***Did** she enjoy that book!* ●

NEGATIVES

When you use negatives such as *never, hardly ever, seldom, rarely, not only*, or *nor* to start a CLAUSE, use inverted order. These sentence pairs show the differences, first in standard order and then in inverted order.

- **I have never seen** a more exciting movie. [standard order]
- **Never have I seen** a more exciting movie. [inverted order]
- **She is not only** a talented artist **but also** an excellent musician.
- **Not only is she** a talented artist, **but she is also** an excellent musician.
- I didn't like the book, and **my husband didn't either**.
- I didn't like the book, and **neither did my husband**.

Alerts: (1) With INDIRECT QUESTIONS, use standard word order.

NO She asked **how did I drop** the book.

YES She asked **how I dropped** the book.

(2) Word order deliberately inverted can be effective, when used sparingly, to create emphasis in a sentence that is neither a question nor an exclamation (also see 38R). ●

54B How can I understand the placement of adjectives?

ADJECTIVES modify—describe or limit—NOUNS, PRONOUNS, and word groups that function as nouns (see 28F). In English, an adjective comes directly before the noun it describes. However, when more than one adjective describes the same noun, several sequences may be possible. Quick Box 54.1 shows the most common order for positioning several adjectives.

Quick Box 54.1

Word order: cumulative adjectives

1. **Determiners, if any:** *a, an, the, my, your, this, that, these, those,* and so on
2. **Expressions of order, including ordinal numbers, if any:** *first, second, third, next, last, final,* and so on
3. **Expressions of quantity, including cardinal (counting) numbers, if any:** *one, two, few, each, every, some,* and so on
4. **Adjectives of judgment or opinion, if any:** *pretty, happy, ugly, sad, interesting, boring,* and so on
5. **Adjectives of size or shape, if any:** *big, small, short, round, square,* and so on
6. **Adjectives of age or condition, if any:** *new, young, broken, dirty, shiny,* and so on
7. **Adjectives of color, if any:** *red, green, blue,* and so on
8. **Adjectives that can also be used as nouns, if any:** *French, Protestant, metal, cotton,* and so on
9. **The noun**

1	2	3	4	5	6	7	8	9
a		few		tiny		red		ants
the	last	six					Thai	carvings
my			fine		old		oak	table

54C How can I understand the placement of adverbs?

ADVERBS modify—describe or limit—VERBS, ADJECTIVES, other adverbs, or entire sentences (see 28G). Adverbs may be positioned first, in the middle, or last in CLAUSES. Quick Box 54.2 (page 736) summarizes adverb types, what they tell about the words they modify, and where each type can be placed.

Quick Box 54.2

Word order: positioning adverbs

ADVERBS OF MANNER	• describe *how* something is done • are usually in middle or last position	Nick **carefully** groomed the dog. Nick groomed the dog **carefully**.
ADVERBS OF TIME	• describe *when* or *how long* about an event • are usually in first or last position • include *just, still, already*, and similar adverbs, which are usually in middle position	**First**, he shampooed the dog. He shampooed the dog **first**. He had **already** brushed the dog's coat.
ADVERBS OF FREQUENCY	• describe *how often* an event takes place • are usually in middle position • are in first position when they modify an entire sentence (see "Sentence Adverbs" below)	Nick has **never** been bitten by a dog. **Occasionally**, he is scratched while shampooing a cat.
ADVERBS OF DEGREE OR EMPHASIS	• describe *how much* or *to what extent* about other modifiers • are directly before the word they modify • include *only*, which is easy to misplace (see 35A)	Nick is **extremely** calm around animals. [*Extremely* modifies *calm*.]
SENTENCE ADVERBS	• modify the entire sentence rather than just one word or a few words • include transitional words and expressions (see 6G.1), as well as such expressions as *maybe, probably, possibly, fortunately, unfortunately*, and *incredibly* • are in first position	**Incredibly**, he was once asked to groom a rat.

Alert: Do not let an adverb separate a verb from its DIRECT OBJECT or INDIRECT OBJECT.

EXERCISE 54-1 Consulting all sections of this chapter, find and correct any errors in word order.

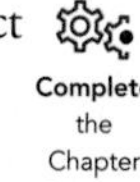

1. I was looking for a new interesting book, so I walked to the library.
2. Quietly, I asked the librarian where I could find biographies, and he pointed quickly his finger to a shelf.
3. I asked him, "You do have a biography of Emmy Noether?"
4. The librarian, who extremely was helpful, looked on a white old computer for me and said, "Yes."
5. "Where I can check it out?" I asked, excited to find finally a new book.

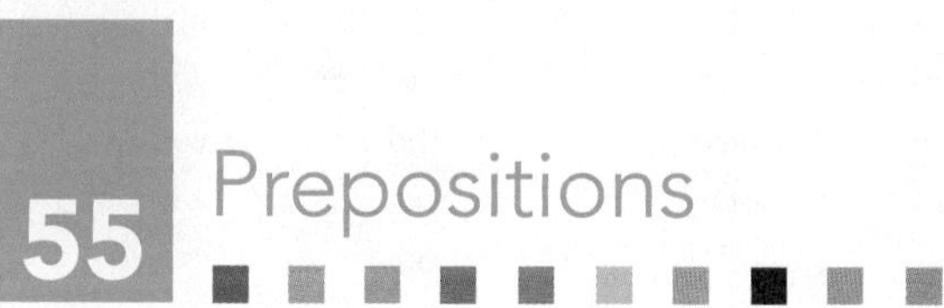

55 Prepositions

Quick Points You will learn to

- Use *in*, *at*, and *on* to show time and place (see 55B).
- Use prepositions correctly (see 55C–55E).

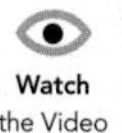

PREPOSITIONS function with other words in PREPOSITIONAL PHRASES (28O). Prepositional phrases usually indicate *where* (direction or location), *how* (by what means or in what way), or *when* (at what time or how long) about the words they modify.

This chapter can help you with several uses of prepositions, which function in combination with other words in ways that are often idiomatic—that is, peculiar to the language. The meaning of an **idiom** differs from the literal meaning of each individual word. For example, the word *break* usually refers to shattering, but the sentence *Yao-Ming* ***broke into*** *a smile* means that a smile appeared on Yao-Ming's face. Knowing which preposition to use in a specific context takes much experience in reading, listening to, and speaking the language. A dictionary like the *Dictionary of American English* (Heinle and Heinle) can be especially helpful when you need to find the correct preposition to use in cases not covered by this chapter.

55A How can I recognize prepositions?

Quick Box 55.1 lists many common prepositions.

Quick Box 55.1

Common prepositions

about	below	in	opposite	toward
above	beside	in front of	out	under
across	between	inside	outside	underneath
after	beyond	instead of	over	unlike
against	but	into	past	until
along	by	like	plus	up
among	concerning	near	regarding	with
around	despite	next	round	within
as	down	of	since	without
at	during	off	through	
because of	except	on	throughout	
before	for	onto	till	
behind	from	on top of	to	

55B How do I use prepositions with expressions of time and place?

Quick Box 55.2 shows how to use the prepositions *in, at,* and *on* to deliver some common kinds of information about time and place. Quick Box 55.2, however, does not cover every preposition that indicates time or place, nor does it cover all uses of *in, at,* and *on.* Also, the Quick Box does not include expressions that operate outside the general rules. (Both these sentences are correct: *You ride* ***in*** *the car* and *You ride* ***on*** *the bus.*)

Quick Box 55.2

Using *in*, *at*, and *on* to show time and place

TIME

- ***in* a year or a month** (*during* is also correct but less common)

  in 1995 **in** May

- ***in* a period of time**

  in a few months (seconds, days, years)

- ***in* a period of the day**

  in the morning (afternoon, evening)

  in the daytime (morning, evening) *but* **at** night

- ***at* a specific time or period of time**

  at noon **at** 2:00 **at** dawn **at** nightfall

  at takeoff (the time a plane leaves)

  at breakfast (the time a specific meal takes place)

- ***on* a specific day**

  on Friday **on** my birthday

PLACE

- ***in* a location surrounded by something else**

  in the province of Alberta **in** the kitchen

  in Utah **in** the apartment

  in downtown Bombay **in** the bathtub

- ***at* a specific location**

  at your house **at** the bank

  at the corner of Third Avenue and Main Street

- ***on* a surface**

  on page 20

  on the second floor *but* **in** the attic *or* **in** the basement

  on Washington Street

  on the mezzanine

  on the highway

55C How do I use prepositions in phrasal verbs?

Phrasal verbs, also called *two-word verbs* and *three-word verbs*, are VERBS that combine with PREPOSITIONS to deliver their meaning. In some phrasal verbs, the verb and the preposition should not be separated by other words: ***Look at*** *the moon* [not ***Look*** *the moon* ***at***]. In separable phrasal verbs, other words in the sentence can separate the verb and the preposition without interfering with meaning: ***I threw away*** *my homework* is as correct as ***I threw*** *my homework* ***away***.

Here is a list of some common phrasal verbs. The ones that cannot be separated are marked with an asterisk (*).

SELECTED PHRASAL VERBS

ask out	get along with*	look into
break down	get back	look out for*
bring about	get off	look over
call back	go over*	make up
drop off	hand in	run across*
figure out	keep up with*	speak to*
fill out	leave out	speak with*
fill up	look after*	throw away
find out	look around	throw out

Position a PRONOUN OBJECT between the words of a separable phrasal verb: *I threw* ***it*** *away*. Also, you can position an object PHRASE of several words between the parts of a separable phrasal verb: *I threw* ***my research paper*** *away*. However, when the object is a CLAUSE, do not let it separate the parts of the phrasal verb: *I threw away* ***all the papers that I wrote last year***.

Many phrasal verbs are informal and are used more in speaking than in writing. For ACADEMIC WRITING, a more formal verb is usually more appropriate than a phrasal verb. In a research paper, for example, *propose* or *suggest* might be a better choice than *come up with*. For academic writing, acceptable phrasal verbs include *believe in, benefit from, concentrate on, consist of, depend on, dream of* (or *dream about*), *insist on, participate in, prepare for*, and *stare at*. None of these phrasal verbs can be separated.

● **EXERCISE 55-1** Consulting the preceding sections of this chapter and using the list of phrasal verbs in 55C, write a one- or two-paragraph description of a typical day at work or school in which you use at least five phrasal verbs. After checking a dictionary, revise your writing, substituting for the phrasal verbs any more formal verbs that might be more appropriate for academic writing. ●

55D How do I use prepositions with past participles?

PAST PARTICIPLES are verb forms that function as ADJECTIVES (56F). Past participles end in either *-ed* or *-d*, or in an equivalent irregular form (29D). When past participles follow the LINKING VERB *be*, it is easy to confuse them with PASSIVE verbs (29N), which have the same endings. Passive verbs describe actions. Past participles, because they act as adjectives, modify NOUNS and PRONOUNS and often describe situations and conditions. Passive verbs follow the pattern *be* + past participle + *by: The child **was frightened by** a snake.* An expression containing a past participle, however, can use either *be* or another linking verb, and it can be followed by either *by* or a different preposition.

- The child **seemed frightened by** snakes.
- The child **is frightened of** all snakes.

Here is a list of expressions containing past participles and the prepositions that often follow them. Look in a dictionary for others. (See 56B on using GERUNDS after some of these expressions.)

SELECTED PAST PARTICIPLE PHRASES + PREPOSITIONS

be accustomed to
be acquainted with
be composed of
be concerned/worried about
be disappointed with (*or* in someone)
be discriminated against
be divorced from
be excited about
be finished/done with
be interested in
be known for
be located in
be made of (*or* from)
be married to
be pleased/satisfied with
be prepared for
be tired of (*or* from)

55E How do I use prepositions in expressions?

In many common expressions, different PREPOSITIONS convey great differences in meaning. For example, four prepositions can be used with the verb *agree* to create five different meanings.

Complete the Chapter Exercises

agree to means "to give consent": *I cannot **agree to** my buying you a new car.*

agree about means "to arrive at a satisfactory understanding": *We certainly **agree about** your needing a car.*

agree on means "to concur": *You and the seller must **agree on** a price for the car.*

agree with means "to have the same opinion": *I **agree with** you that you need a car.*

agree with also means "to be suitable or healthful": *The idea of having such a major expense does not **agree with** me.*

You can find entire books filled with English expressions that include prepositions. The following list shows a few that you're likely to use often.

SELECTED EXPRESSIONS WITH PREPOSITIONS

ability in
access to
accustomed to
afraid of
angry with *or* at
authority on
aware of
based on
capable of
certain of
confidence in
dependent on
different from
faith in
familiar with
famous for
frightened by
happy with
in charge of
independent of
in favor of
influence on *or* over
interested in
involved in [*something*]
involved with *someone*
knowledge of
made of
married to
opposed to
patient with
proud of
reason for
related to
suspicious of
time for
tired of

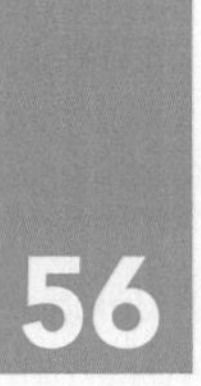

56 Gerunds, Infinitives, and Participles

Quick Points You will learn to

➤ Use gerunds and infinitives correctly (see 56A–56E).

PARTICIPLES are verb forms (see 29B). A verb's *-ing* form is its PRESENT PARTICIPLE. The *-ed* form of a regular verb is its PAST PARTICIPLE; IRREGULAR VERBS form their past participles in various ways (for example, *bend, bent; eat, eaten; think, thought*—for a complete list, see Quick Box 29.4 in 29D). Participles can function as ADJECTIVES (*a **smiling** face, a **closed** book*).

A verb's *-ing* form can also function as a NOUN (***Sneezing** spreads colds*), which is called a **gerund**. Another verb form, the **infinitive,** can also function as a noun. An infinitive is a verb's SIMPLE or base FORM, usually preceded by the word *to* (*We want everyone **to smile***). Verb forms—participles, gerunds, and infinitives—functioning as nouns or MODIFIERS are called VERBALS, as explained in 28E. This chapter can help you make the right choices among verbals.

56A How can I use gerunds and infinitives as subjects?

Gerunds are used more commonly than infinitives as subjects. Sometimes, however, either is acceptable.

- **Choosing** the right health club is important.
- **To choose** the right health club is important.

Alert: When a gerund or an infinitive is used alone as a subject, it is SINGULAR and requires a singular verb. When two or more gerunds or infinitives create a COMPOUND SUBJECT, they require a plural verb. (See 28L and 31E.)●

56B When do I use a gerund, not an infinitive, as an object?

Some VERBS must be followed by GERUNDS used as DIRECT OBJECTS. Other verbs must be followed by INFINITIVES. Still other verbs can be followed by either a gerund or an infinitive. (A few verbs can change meaning depending on whether they are followed by a gerund or an infinitive; see 56D.) Quick Box 56.1 (page 744) lists common verbs that must be followed by gerunds, not infinitives.

- Yuri **considered *calling*** [not *to call*] the mayor.
- He **was having trouble *getting*** [not *to get*] a work permit.
- Yuri's boss **recommended *taking*** [not *to take*] an interpreter to the permit agency.

Quick Box 56.1

Verbs and expressions that must be followed by gerunds

admit	dislike	object to
anticipate	enjoy	postpone
appreciate	escape	practice
avoid	finish	put off
consider	give up	quit
consist of	imagine	recall
contemplate	include	resist
delay	mention	risk
deny	mind	suggest
discuss	miss	tolerate

GERUND AFTER *GO*

The word *go* is usually followed by an infinitive: *We can* ***go to see*** [not *go seeing*] *a movie tonight.* Sometimes, however, *go* is followed by a gerund in phrases such as *go swimming, go fishing, go shopping*, and *go driving: I will* ***go shopping*** [not *go to shop*] *after work.*

GERUND AFTER *BE* + COMPLEMENT + PREPOSITION

Many common expressions use a form of the verb *be* plus a COMPLEMENT plus a PREPOSITION. In such expressions, use a gerund, not an infinitive, after the preposition. Here is a list of some of the most frequently used expressions in this pattern.

SELECTED EXPRESSIONS USING *BE* + COMPLEMENT + PREPOSITION

be (get) accustomed to	be interested in
be angry about	be prepared for
be bored with	be responsible for
be capable of	be tired of
be committed to	be (get) used to
be excited about	be worried about

- We **are excited about** ***voting*** [not *to vote*] in the next presidential election.
- Who **will be responsible for** ***locating*** [not *to locate*] our polling place?

Alert: Always use a gerund, not an infinitive, as the object of a preposition. Be especially careful when the word *to* is functioning as a preposition in a PHRASAL VERB (see 55C): *We are committed **to changing*** [not *to change*] *the rules.*

56C When do I use an infinitive, not a gerund, as an object?

Quick Box 56.2 lists selected common verbs and expressions that must be followed by INFINITIVES, not GERUNDS, as OBJECTS.

- She **wanted *to go*** [not *wanted going*] to the lecture.
- Only three people **decided *to question*** [not *decided questioning*] the speaker.

Quick Box 56.2

Verbs and expressions that must be followed by infinitives

agree	decline	like	promise
arrange	demand	manage	refuse
ask	deserve	mean	wait
attempt	expect	need	want
beg	hesitate	offer	
claim	hope	plan	
decide	learn	pretend	

INFINITIVE AFTER *BE* + COMPLEMENT

Gerunds are common in constructions that use a form of the verb *be* plus a COMPLEMENT and a PREPOSITION (see 56B). However, use an infinitive, not a gerund, when *be* plus a complement is not followed by a preposition.

- We **are eager *to go*** [not *going*] camping.
- I **am ready *to sleep*** [not *sleeping*] in a tent.

INFINITIVE TO INDICATE PURPOSE

Use an infinitive in expressions that indicate purpose: *I read a book **to learn** more about Mayan culture.* This sentence means "I read a book for the purpose of learning more about Mayan culture." *To learn* delivers the idea of purpose more concisely (see Chapter 40) than expressions such as *so that I can* or *in order to.*

INFINITIVE WITH *THE FIRST, THE LAST, THE ONE*

Use an infinitive after the expressions *the first, the last,* and *the one: Nina is the first* ***to arrive*** [not *arriving*] *and the last* ***to leave*** [not *leaving*] *every day. She's always the one* ***to do*** *the most.*

UNMARKED INFINITIVES

Infinitives used without the word *to* are called **unmarked infinitives**, or sometimes *bare infinitives.* An unmarked infinitive may be hard to recognize because it is not preceded by *to.* Some common verbs followed by unmarked infinitives are *feel, have, hear, let, listen to, look at, make* (meaning "compel"), *notice, see,* and *watch.*

- Please let me **take** [not *to take*] you to lunch. [unmarked infinitive]
- I want **to take** you to lunch. [marked infinitive]
- I can have Kara **drive** [not *to drive*] us. [unmarked infinitive]
- I will ask Kara **to drive** us. [marked infinitive]

The verb *help* can be followed by a marked or an unmarked infinitive. Either is correct: *Help me* ***put*** [or ***to put***] *this box in the car.*

Alert: Be careful to use parallel structure (see Chapter 39) correctly when you use two or more gerunds or infinitives after verbs. If two or more verbal objects follow one verb, put the verbals into the same form.

NO We went **sailing** and **to scuba dive**.

YES We went **sailing** and **scuba diving**.

NO We heard the wind **blow** and the waves **crashing**.

YES We heard the wind **blow** and the waves **crash**.

YES We heard the wind **blowing** and the waves **crashing**.

Conversely, if you are using verbal objects with COMPOUND PREDICATES, be sure to use the kind of verbal that each verb requires.

NO We enjoyed **scuba diving** but do not plan **sailing** again.

Enjoyed requires a gerund object, and *plan* requires an infinitive object; see Quick Boxes 56.1 and 56.2 in this chapter.

YES We enjoyed **scuba diving** but do not plan **to sail** again. ●

56D How does meaning change when certain verbs are followed by a gerund or an infinitive?

WITH *STOP*

The VERB *stop* followed by a GERUND means "finish, quit." *Stop* followed by an INFINITIVE means "interrupt one activity to begin another."

- We **stopped** ***eating***.

  We finished our meal.

- We **stopped** ***to eat***.

  We stopped another activity, such as driving, to eat.

WITH *REMEMBER* AND *FORGET*

The verb *remember* followed by an infinitive means "not to forget to do something": *I must* ***remember to talk*** *with Isa. Remember* followed by a gerund means "recall a memory": *I* ***remember talking*** *in my sleep last night.*

The verb *forget* followed by an infinitive means "fail to do something": *If you* ***forget to put*** *a stamp on that letter, it will be returned. Forget* followed by a gerund means "do something and not recall it": *I* ***forget having put*** *the stamps in the refrigerator.*

WITH *TRY*

The verb *try* followed by an infinitive means "make an effort": *I* ***tried to find*** *your jacket.* Followed by a gerund, *try* means "experiment with": *I* ***tried jogging*** *but found it too difficult.*

56E Why is the meaning unchanged whether a gerund or an infinitive follows sense verbs?

Sense VERBS include words such as *see, notice, hear, observe, watch, feel, listen to*, and *look at*. The meaning of these verbs is usually not affected by whether a GERUND or an INFINITIVE follows as the OBJECT. *I* ***saw*** *the water* ***rise*** and *I* ***saw*** *the water* ***rising*** both have the same meaning in American English.

● **EXERCISE 56-1** Write the correct form of the verbal object (either a gerund or an infinitive) for each verb in parentheses.

EXAMPLE

(Build) __________ a campfire can be challenging.

Building a campfire can be challenging.

1. While camping outside, people often want (build) _________ a fire for warmth or for cooking food.
2. If you have ever attempted (light) _________ a fire, you know that you need a reliable ignition source, such as sturdy matches or a good lighter.
3. You will be capable of (create) _________ a decent campfire if you use dry wood.
4. For the sake of safety, do not let the fire (spread) _________ outside the fire pit.
5. When you are finished, you need (extinguish) _________ the fire completely. ●

56F How do I choose between *-ing* and *-ed* forms for adjectives?

Deciding whether to use the *-ing* form (PRESENT PARTICIPLE) or the *-ed* form (PAST PARTICIPLE of a regular VERB) as an ADJECTIVE in a specific sentence can be difficult. For example, *I am* ***amused*** and *I am* ***amusing*** are both correct in English, but their meanings are very different. To make the right choice, decide whether the modified NOUN or PRONOUN is *causing* or if it is *experiencing* what the participle describes.

Use a present participle (*-ing*) to modify a noun or pronoun that is the agent or the cause of the action.

- Micah described your **interesting** plan.

  The noun *plan* causes what its modifier describes—interest; so *interesting* is correct.

- I find your plan **exciting**.

  The noun *plan* causes what its modifier describes—excitement; so *exciting* is correct.

Use a past participle (*-ed* in regular verbs) to modify a noun or pronoun that experiences or receives whatever the modifier describes.

- An **interested** committee wants to hear your plan.

  The noun *committee* experiences what its modifier describes—interest; so *interested* is correct.

- **Excited** by your plan, they called a board meeting.

  The pronoun *they* experiences what its modifier describes—excitement; so *excited* is correct.

Here are frequently used participles that convey very different meanings, depending on whether the *-ed* or the *-ing* form is used.

amused, amusing	frightened, frightening
annoyed, annoying	insulted, insulting
appalled, appalling	offended, offending
bored, boring	overwhelmed, overwhelming
confused, confusing	pleased, pleasing
depressed, depressing	reassured, reassuring
disgusted, disgusting	satisfied, satisfying
fascinated, fascinating	shocked, shocking

● **EXERCISE 56-2** Choose the correct participle from each pair in parentheses. For help, consult 56F.

Complete the Chapter Exercises

EXAMPLE

It can be a (satisfied, satisfying) satisfying experience to learn about the lives of artists.

1. The artist Frida Kahlo led an (interested, interesting) ______________ life.
2. When Kahlo was eighteen, (horrified, horrifying) ______________ observers saw her (injured, injuring) ______________ in a streetcar accident.
3. A (disappointed, disappointing) ______________ Kahlo had to abandon her plan to study medicine.
4. Instead, she began to create paintings filled with (disturbed, disturbing) ______________ images.
5. Some art critics consider Kahlo's paintings to be (fascinated, fascinating) ______________ works of art, though many people find them (overwhelmed, overwhelming) ______________. ●

57 Modal Auxiliary Verbs

Quick Points You will learn to

➤ Use modal auxiliary verbs to help main verbs convey information (see 57A–57C)

AUXILIARY VERBS are known as *helping verbs* because adding an auxiliary verb to a MAIN VERB helps the main verb convey additional information (see 29E). For example, the auxiliary verb *do* is important in turning sentences into questions. *You have to sleep* becomes a question when *do* is added: *Do you have to sleep?* The most common auxiliary verbs are forms of *be, have*, and *do*. Quick Boxes 29.6 and 29.7 in section 29E list the forms of these three verbs.

MODAL AUXILIARY VERBS are one type of auxiliary verb. They include *can, could, may, might, should, had better, must, will, would*, and others discussed in this chapter. Modals differ from *be, have*, and *do* used as auxiliary verbs in the specific ways discussed in Quick Box 57.1.

Quick Box 57.1

Modals versus other auxiliary verbs

- Modals in the present future are always followed by the SIMPLE FORM of a main verb: *I **might go** tomorrow.*
- One-word modals have no *-s* ending in the THIRD-PERSON SINGULAR: *She **could** go with me; he **could** go with me; they **could** go with me.* (The two-word modal *have to* changes form to agree with its subject: *I **have to** leave; she **has to** leave.*) Auxiliary verbs other than modals usually change form for third-person singular: *I **do** want to go; he **does** want to go.*
- Some modals change form in the past. Others (*should, would, must*, which convey probability, and *ought to*) use *have* + a PAST PARTICIPLE. *I **can do** it* becomes *I **could do** it* in PAST-TENSE CLAUSES about ability. *I **could do** it* becomes *I **could have done** it* in clauses about possibility.
- Modals convey meaning about ability, necessity, advisability, possibility, and other conditions: For example, *I can go* means "I am able to go." Modals do not describe actual occurrences.

57A How do I convey ability, necessity, advisability, possibility, and probability with modals?

CONVEYING ABILITY

The modal *can* conveys ability now (in the present), and *could* conveys ability before (in the past). These words deliver the meaning "able to." For the future, use *will be able to.*

- We **can** work late tonight.

  Can conveys present ability.

- I **could** work late last night, too.

  Could conveys past ability.

- I **will be able to** work late next Monday.

  Will be able is the future tense; *will* here is not a modal.

Adding *not* between a modal and the MAIN VERB makes the CLAUSE negative: *We **cannot** work late tonight; I **could not** work late last night; I **will not be able to** work late next Monday.*

Alert: You will often see negative forms of modals turned into CONTRACTIONS: *can't, couldn't, won't, wouldn't,* and others. Because contractions are considered informal usage by some instructors, you will never be wrong if you avoid them in ACADEMIC WRITING, except when you are reproducing spoken words. ●

CONVEYING NECESSITY

The modals *must* and *have to* convey a need to do something. Both *must* and *have to* are followed by the simple form of the main verb. In the present tense, *have to* changes form to agree with its subject.

- You **must** leave before midnight.
- She **has to** leave when I leave.

In the past tense, *must* is never used to express necessity. Instead, use *had to.*

PRESENT TENSE We **must** study today. We **have to** study today.

PAST TENSE We **had to** [not *must*] take a test yesterday.

The negative forms of *must* and *have to* also have different meanings. *Must not* conveys that something is forbidden; *do not have to* conveys that something is not necessary.

- You **must not** sit there.

  Sitting there is forbidden.

- You **do not have to** sit there.

  Sitting there is not necessary.

CONVEYING ADVISABILITY OR THE NOTION OF A GOOD IDEA

The modals *should* and *ought to* express the idea that doing the action of the main verb is advisable or is a good idea.

- You **should** go to class tomorrow morning.

In the past tense, *should* and *ought to* convey regret or knowing something through hindsight. They mean that good advice was not taken.

- You **should have** gone to class yesterday.
- I **ought to have** called my sister yesterday.

The modal *had better* delivers the meaning of good advice or warning or threat. It does not change form for tense.

- You **had better** see the doctor before your cough gets worse.

Need to is often used to express strong advice, too. Its past-tense form is *needed to*.

- You **need to** take better care of yourself. You **needed to** listen.

CONVEYING POSSIBILITY

The modals *may, might*, and *could* can be used to convey an idea of possibility or likelihood.

- We **may** become hungry before long.
- We **could** eat lunch at the diner next door.

For the past-tense form, use *may, might*, and *could*, followed by *have* and the past participle of the main verb.

- I **could have studied** French in high school, but I studied Spanish instead.

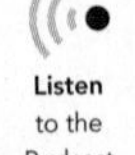
Listen to the Podcast

CONVEYING PROBABILITY

In addition to conveying the idea of necessity, the modal *must* can also convey probability or likelihood. It means that a well-informed guess is being made.

- Marisa **must** be a talented actress. She has been chosen to play the lead role in the school play.

When *must* conveys probability, the past tense is *must have* plus the past participle of the main verb.

- I did not see Boris at the party; he **must have left** early.

● **EXERCISE 57-1** Fill in each blank with the past-tense modal auxiliary that expresses the meaning given in parentheses.

EXAMPLE

Last week, I (necessity) had to go on a business trip and leave my dog with my friend.

1. My friend said that he (ability) _________ watch my dog, Patches, for me while I was gone.
2. My friend (possibility) _________ said "No," but he generously agreed to help me.
3. He (probability) _________ taken good care of my dog because Patches seemed happy.
4. I (advisability) _________ packed more food for my dog because my friend had to buy some dog food with his own money.
5. When I returned from my trip, I (necessity) _________ send my friend a thank-you note. ●

57B How do I convey preferences, plans, and past habits with modals?

CONVEYING PREFERENCES

The modal *would rather* expresses a preference. *Would rather*, the PRESENT TENSE, is used with the SIMPLE FORM of the MAIN VERB, and *would rather have*, the PAST TENSE, is used with the PAST PARTICIPLE of the main verb.

- We **would rather see** a comedy than a mystery.
- Carlos **would rather have stayed** home last night.

CONVEYING PLAN OR OBLIGATION

A form of *be* followed by *supposed to* and the simple form of a main verb delivers a meaning of something planned or of an obligation.

- I **was supposed to meet** them at the bus stop.

CONVEYING PAST HABIT

The modals *used to* and *would* express the idea that something happened repeatedly in the past.

- I **used to** hate going to the dentist.
- I **would** dread every single visit.

Alert: Both *used to* and *would* can be used to express repeated actions in the past, but *would* cannot be used for a situation that lasted for a period of time in the past.

NO I **would** live in Arizona.

YES I **used to** live in Arizona.

57C How can I recognize modals in the passive voice?

Modals use the ACTIVE VOICE, as shown in sections sections 57A and 57B. In the active voice, the subject does the action expressed in the MAIN VERB (see 29N and 29O).

Modals can also use the PASSIVE VOICE (29P). In the passive voice, the doer of the main verb's action is either unexpressed or is expressed as an OBJECT in a PREPOSITIONAL PHRASE starting with the word *by*.

PASSIVE The waterfront **can be seen** from my window.
ACTIVE **I can see** the waterfront from my window.

PASSIVE The tax form **must be signed** by the person who fills it out.
ACTIVE The person who fills out the tax form **must sign** it.

EXERCISE 57-2 Select the correct choice from the words in parentheses and write it in the blank. For help, consult 57A through 57C.

EXAMPLE

When I was younger, I (would, used to) used to love to go bicycle riding.

1. You (ought to have, ought have) ____________ called yesterday as you had promised you would.
2. Judging by the size of the puddles in the street outside, it (must be rained, must have rained) ____________ all night long.
3. Ingrid (must not have, might not have been) ____________ as early for the interview as she claims she was.
4. After all the studying he did, Pedro (should have, should have been) ____________ less frightened by the exam.
5. I have to go home early today, although I really (cannot, should not) ____________ leave before the end of the day because of all the work I have to do.

● **EXERCISE 57-3** Select the correct choice from the words in parentheses and write it in the blank. For help, consult 57A through 57C.

Complete the Chapter Exercises

EXAMPLE

We (must have, must) <u>must</u> study this afternoon.

1. Unfortunately, I (should not, cannot) ________________ go to the movies with you because I have to take care of my brother tonight.
2. Juan (would have, would have been) ________________ nominated class valedictorian if he had not moved to another city.
3. You (ought not have, ought not to have) ________________ arrived while the meeting was still in progress.
4. Louise (must be, must have been) ________________ sick to miss the party last week.
5. Had you not called in advance, you (may not have, may not have been) ________________ aware of the traffic on the expressway. ●

PART

9

Specific Writing Situations

58 An Overview of Writing Across the Curriculum

Quick Points You will learn to

- Adapt your writing to various college courses (see 58A).
- Use cue words to tell what your college writing needs to accomplish (see 58B).

58A What is writing across the curriculum?

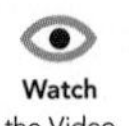

Writing across the curriculum refers to the writing you do in college courses beyond first-year composition. (A related term is "writing in the disciplines," which usually refers to writing that is specific to individual majors.) Many features are common to good writing across disciplines, but there are also important differences. A chemistry lab report, for example, differs from a history paper. Quick Box 58.1 summarizes different types of writing across the curriculum.

Quick Box 58.1

Comparing the disciplines

Discipline	Types of Assignments	Primary sources	Secondary sources	Usual documentation styles
HUMANITIES history, languages, literature, philosophy, art, music, theater	essays, response statements, reviews, analyses, original works such as stories, poems, autobiographies	literary works, manuscripts, paintings and sculptures, historical documents, films, plays, photographs, artifacts from popular culture	reviews, journal articles, research papers, books	MLA, CM
SOCIAL SCIENCES psychology, sociology, anthropology, education	research reports, case studies, reviews of the literature, analyses	surveys, interviews, observations, experiments, tests and measures	journal articles, scholarly books, literature reviews	APA

continued >>

Quick Box 58.1 (continued)

Discipline	Types of Assignments	Primary sources	Secondary sources	Usual documentation styles
NATURAL SCIENCES biology, chemistry, physics, mathematics	reports, research proposals and reports, science reviews	experiments, field notes, direct observations, measurements	journal articles, research papers, books	often CSE but varies by discipline

58B What do I need to know about audience and purpose across the curriculum?

Unless an instructor or assignment tells you otherwise, the audience for academic writing consists of scholars, professors, and students in particular fields. As a result, you need to follow the conventions (including format and organization, types of evidence, tone and style, and documentation style) that are expected in each discipline. It's useful to study examples of the kinds of writing you've been asked to produce.

Purposes can vary widely. Some tasks mainly require explaining information, while others require making an argument. Most assignments contain **cue words** that tell what your writing needs to accomplish. Quick Box 58.2 presents some common cue words.

Quick Box 58.2

Some common cue words

Cue Word	Meaning
ANALYZE	Separate into parts and discuss each, often including how it contributes to a meaning or implication.
CLASSIFY	Arrange in groups based on shared characteristics or functions.
CRITIQUE	Give your evaluation and support your reasons for it.
COMPARE	Show similarities and differences.

continued >>

Quick Box 58.2 (continued)

Cue Word	Meaning
DEFINE	Tell what something is to differentiate it from similar things.
DISCUSS	Explain and comment on, in an organized way, the various issues or elements involved.
EXPLAIN	Make clear a complex thing or process that needs to be illuminated or interpreted.
INTERPRET	Explain the meaning or significance of something.
REVIEW	Evaluate or summarize critically.
SUMMARIZE	Lay out the major points of something.
SUPPORT	Argue in favor of something.

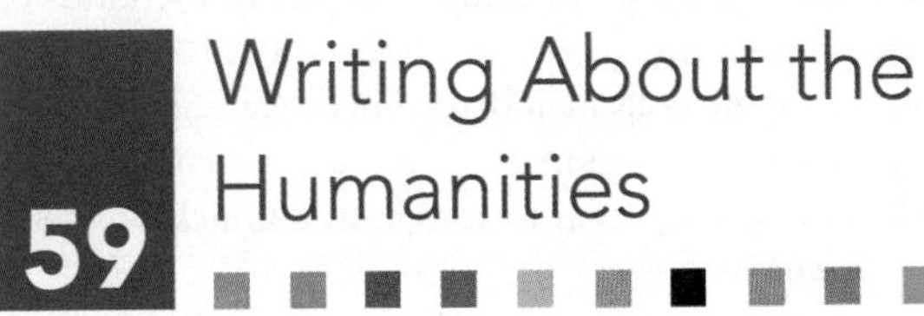

59 Writing About the Humanities

Quick Points You will learn to

- Understand the different types of humanities papers (see 59B).
- Understand different types of literature papers and identify major elements to analyze (see 59E–59F).

59A What are the humanities?

The humanities seek to represent and understand human experience, creativity, thought, and values. These disciplines usually include literature, languages, philosophy, and history; some colleges treat the fine arts (music, art, dance, theater, and creative writing) as part of the humanities.

59B What types of papers do I write in the humanities?

Writing in the humanities covers many types and purposes.

59B.1 Summaries

Occasionally your instructor will request an objective summary of a text; you might need to tell the plot of a novel or present the main points of an article (see 29B). Generally, however, a summary is a means to a greater end. For example, writing an interpretation often requires you to summarize parts of the source so that your points about it are clear.

59B.2 Syntheses

SYNTHESIS relates several texts, ideas, or pieces of information to one another (see 18F). For example, you might read several accounts of the events leading up to the Civil War and then write a synthesis that explains what caused that war.

59B.3 Responses

In a response, you give your personal reaction to a work, supported by explanations of your reasoning (see 20C). For example, do you think Hamlet's behavior makes sense? Do you agree with Peter Singer's philosophical arguments against using animals in scientific experiments? Clarify whether your instructor wants you to justify a response with references to a text.

59B.4 Interpretations

An interpretation explains the meaning or significance of a particular text, event, or work of art (Quick Box 59.1). For example, what does Plato's *Republic* suggest about the nature of a good society? What was the significance of the 9/11 tragedy for Americans' sense of security? Your reply isn't right or wrong; rather, you present your point of view and explain your reasoning. The quality of your reasoning determines how successfully you convey your point.

59B.5 Narratives

A narrative constructs a coherent story from separate facts or events. In a history class, for example, you might examine news events, laws, diaries and journals, and related materials to create a chronological version of what happened. You might interview people or others who knew them, read their letters or other writings, and consult related SOURCES, all to form a coherent story of their lives. Some writing assignments in the humanities may ask you to write about your memories or experiences. Chapter 10 provides detailed advice.

59B.6 Textual analyses

The humanities use a number of **analytical frameworks**, or systematic ways of investigating a work. Quick Box 59.1 summarizes several of them.

Quick Box 59.1

Selected analytical frameworks used in the humanities

RHETORICAL	Explores how and why people use LOGICAL, EMOTIONAL, and ETHICAL APPEALS to create desired effects on specific audiences, in specific situations (see 14C).
CULTURAL OR NEW HISTORICAL	Explores how social, economic, and cultural forces influence ideas, texts, art, laws, customs, and so on. Also explores how individual texts or events provide broader understandings of the past or present.
DECONSTRUCTIONIST	Assumes that the meaning of any given text is not stable or "in" the work. Rather, meaning always depends on contexts and the interests of the people in power. The goal of deconstruction is to produce multiple possible meanings of a work, often to undermine traditional interpretations.
FEMINIST	Focuses on how women are presented and treated, concentrating especially on power relationships between men and women.
FORMALIST	Centers on matters of structure, form, and traditional literary devices (plot, rhythm, imagery, symbolism, and others; see Quick Box 59.2).
MARXIST	Assumes that the most important forces in human experience are economic and material ones. Focuses on power differences between economic classes of people and the effects of those differences.
READER-RESPONSE	Emphasizes how the individual reader determines meaning. The reader's personal history, values, experiences, relationships, and previous reading all contribute to how he or she interprets a particular work or event.

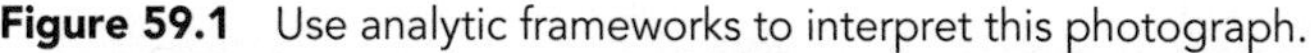

Figure 59.1 Use analytic frameworks to interpret this photograph.

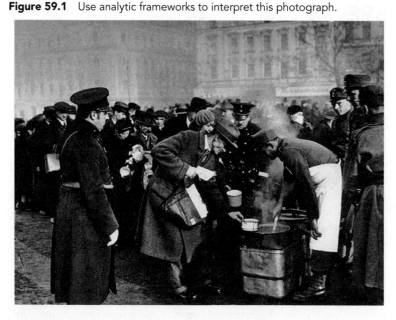

59C Which documentation style do I use in writing about the humanities?

Most fields in the humanities use the Modern Language Association (MLA) documentation style, which we explain and illustrate in Chapter 25. Some disciplines in the humanities use *Chicago Manual* (CM) style, as we explain in Chapter 27.

59D How do I write about literature?

Literature encompasses fiction (novels and stories), drama (plays, scripts, and some films), and poetry (poems and lyrics), as well as nonfiction with artistic qualities (memoirs, personal essays, and so on). Since ancient times, literature has represented human experience, entertained readers, and enlarged their perspectives about themselves, others, and different ways of living.

Writing effective papers about literature involves more than summarizing the plot. It involves CRITICAL THINKING and SYNTHESIS. In such papers, you state a CLAIM (an observation or a position about the work of literature) and convince your readers that your thesis is reasonable. For support, you make direct references to the work itself, by summarizing, paraphrasing, and quoting specific passages (see Ch. 18) and by explaining precisely *why* and *how* the selected passages support your interpretation.

59E How do I write different types of papers about literature?

When you read a literary work closely, look for details or passages that relate to your thesis. Mark up the text as you read by selectively underlining passages or by writing notes, comments, or questions in the margin.

59E.1 Writing a personal response

A personal response paper explains your reaction to a literary work or some aspect of it. You might write about why you did or did not enjoy reading a particular work, discuss whether situations in the work are similar to your personal experiences, explain why you agree or disagree with the author's point of view, or so on. For example, how do you react if a likable character breaks the law? As with all effective papers about literature, you need to explain your response by discussing specific elements of the text.

59E.2 Writing an interpretation

An interpretation explains the message or viewpoint that you think the work conveys. Most works of literature are open to more than one interpretation. Your task, then, is not to discover a single "right answer." Instead, your task is to determine a possible interpretation and provide an argument that supports it. The questions in Quick Box 59.2 (referring to the complete poem on pages 767–768) can help you write an effective interpretation paper.

Quick Box 59.2

Questions for an interpretation paper

1. What is a central theme of the work? For example, in the poem "Sympathy," a central theme might be despair. (The poem appears in 59H.)
2. How do particular parts of the work relate to the theme? In "Sympathy," the bird flying againt the cage shows despair.
3. If patterns exist in the work, what might they mean? Patterns include repeated images, situations, and words. In "Sympathy," the phrase "I know why the caged bird . . ." forms a pattern.
4. What meaning does the author create through the elements listed in Quick Box 59.3?
5. Why might the work end as it does?

59E.3 Writing a formal analysis

A formal analysis explains how elements of a literary work function to create meaning or effect. Your instructor may ask you to concentrate on one element or to discuss how a writer develops a theme through several elements. The paper by student Sara Kho (see 59H) is an example of an interpretation based on a formal analysis. Quick Box 59.3 describes some of the major literary elements you might use in formal analyses.

Quick Box 59.3

Major elements to analyze in literary works

PLOT	Events and their sequence
THEME	Central idea or message
STRUCTURE	Organization and relationship of parts to each other and to the whole
CHARACTERIZATION	Traits, thoughts, and actions of the people in the work
SETTING	Time and place of the action
POINT OF VIEW	Perspective or position from which a narrator or a main character presents the material
STYLE	How words and sentence structure present the material
IMAGERY	Descriptive language that creates mental pictures for the reader
TONE	Author's attitude toward the subject of the work—and sometimes toward the reader—as expressed through choice of words, imagery, and point of view
FIGURES OF SPEECH	Unusual use or combination of words, such as METAPHOR or SIMILE, for enhanced vividness or effect
SYMBOLISM	The use of a specific object or event to represent a deeper, often abstract, meaning or idea
RHYTHM	Beat, meter
RHYME	Repetition of similar sounds for their auditory effect

59E.4 Writing a cultural analysis

A cultural analysis relates a literary work to broader historical, social, cultural, or political situations. Quick Box 59.4 lists some common topics for cultural analysis.

Quick Box 59.4

Major topics for cultural analyses

GENDER	How does a work portray women or men and define or challenge their roles in society?
CLASS	How does a work portray relationships among the upper, middle, and lower classes? How do characters' actions or perspectives result from their wealth and power—or from their poverty and powerlessness?
RACE AND ETHNICITY	How does a work portray the influences of race and ethnicity on the characters' actions, status, and values?
HISTORY	How does a work reflect—or challenge—past events and values in a society?
AUTOBIOGRAPHY	How did the writer's life experiences influence his or her work?
GENRE	How is the work similar to or different from other works of its type (for example, plays, sonnets, mysteries, comic novels, memoirs)?

59F What special rules apply to writing about literature?

59F.1 Using correct verb tenses

Watch the Video

Always use the PRESENT TENSE when you describe or discuss a literary work or any of its elements: *Walter* [a character] ***makes*** *a difficult decision when he* ***turns down*** *Linder's offer to buy the house.* In addition, always use the present tense for discussing what an author has done in a specific work: *Lorraine Hansberry, author of* A Raisin in the Sun, ***explores*** *not only powerful racial issues but also common family dynamics.* Always use a PAST-TENSE VERB to discuss historical events or biographical information: *Lorraine Hansberry's* A Raisin in the Sun ***was*** *the first play by an African American woman to be produced on Broadway.*

59F.2 Using your own ideas and using secondary sources

Some assignments call only for your own ideas about a literary work. Other assignments call for you to use SECONDARY SOURCES, in which experts discuss the literary text or other material related to your topic. You can locate secondary sources by using the research process explained in Chapter 22.

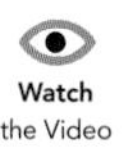
Watch the Video

59G How do I use documentation in writing about literature?

Documenting primary sources tells your readers exactly where to find the specific passages in the literary work you're quoting or summarizing. Documenting secondary sources credits the authors of those works and avoids PLAGIARISM. Unless your instructor requests another documentation style, use MLA STYLE (Ch. 25) for writing about literature.

59H A student's essay about literature

59H.1 Working on the assignment

Sara Kho, a student in first-year English, fulfilled an assignment to write an interpretation of Paul Laurence Dunbar's poem "Sympathy." In the process of drafting her paper, Sara realized that the images and the order in which they appeared are vital to understanding the poem.

59H.2 Learning about the poet, Paul Laurence Dunbar

Paul Laurence Dunbar was perhaps the first African American poet to receive wide critical acclaim. He was born in 1872, in Dayton, Ohio, to a mother who was a former slave and a father who had escaped slavery to fight in the Civil War. Supporters of his work included the Wright brothers (with whom he attended Dayton Central High) and the famous abolitionist Frederick Douglass. He worked briefly at the Library of Congress and read in various cities in the United States and in England. After producing twelve books of poetry, four books of short stories, a play, and five novels, he died in 1906, at the age of only 33.

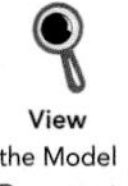
View the Model Document

SYMPATHY

Paul Laurence Dunbar

I know what the caged bird feels, alas!
When the sun is bright on the upland slopes;
When the wind stirs soft through the springing grass,
And the river flows like a stream of glass;
When the first bird sings and the first bud opes,

And the faint perfume from its chalice steals—
I know what the caged bird feels!

I know why the caged bird beats his wing
Till its blood is red on the cruel bars;
For he must fly back to his perch and cling
When he fain would be on the bough a-swing;
And a pain still throbs in the old, old scars
And they pulse again with a keener sting—
I know why he beats his wing!

I know why the caged bird sings, ah me,
When his wing is bruised and his bosom sore,—
When he beats his bars and he would be free;
It is not a carol of joy or glee,
But a prayer that he sends from his heart's deep core,
But a plea, that upward to Heaven he flings—
I know why the caged bird sings!

Student's essay about literature

Kho 1

Sara Kho
Professor Parrish
English 100
4 Mar. 2012

Images, Progression, and Meaning in "Sympathy"

How can a writer artfully convey the despair of not having freedom? Paul Laurence Dunbar faces that challenge in his poem "Sympathy," which uses the central image of a bird in a cage. By choosing a creature that did nothing to deserve its imprisonment, Dunbar invites readers to empathize with anyone who has experienced a similar fate. The poem artfully

continued >>

Kho 2

builds its message through precise images and a meaningful procession of ideas.

"Sympathy" appears in three seven-line stanzas that closely match each other. The rhyme scheme in each is ABAABCC, and the first and seventh lines of each stanza begin with "I know what" or "I know why." Those lines, in fact, are nearly identical, and the result is a tightly compressed, even repetitive poem that makes readers pay close attention to any changes. Those changes create a dramatic progression in the poem.

The imagery in the first stanza focuses on the world beyond the cage. It's a world of strong visual senses, the sun "bright upon the upland slopes" (line 2) and the river flowing "like a stream of glass" (4). But Dunbar also invokes smell, with the flower's perfume, and he invokes sounds, including the wind softly stirring the grass (3) and a bird singing (5). (In the third stanza, that singing becomes a key idea—and a much different one.) References to the sun on the hills and to the "first bird" and "first bud" suggest dawn and possibilities, with potential that is almost holy. After all, the flower bud is a "chalice," a sacred vessel holding communion wine (6). However, the caged bird is removed from this world, and while the poet says, "I know what the caged bird feels" (7), he does not specifically name or describe that feeling. Instead, we are left to draw our own conclusions, comparing the limits of the cage to the possibilities of nature.

The imagery in the second stanza is much harsher and more concrete. Instead of the internal state of the bird's feeling, the poet describes an external, physical action, the bird's wings

continued >>

Kho 3

beating against the cage "Till its blood is red on the cruel bars" (9). Clearly this is a futile, painful, and ongoing action. The bird's "pain still throbs" (12), even "When his wing is bruised and his bosom sore" (16). Yet the bird persists, desperately longing to fly from branch to branch rather than to sit on a single artificial perch, in a cage that denies flight to a creature whose nature is to fly.

The brutal images of the second stanza give way to the surprising insights of the third one, which also have a physical action but of a different sort. We generally think of bird songs as pretty sounds, conveying happiness. However, "Sympathy" makes them "not a carol of joy or glee" (18) but, rather, something mournful and somber. The song is an extension of and accompaniment to the self-torture of wings beating against the cage. By calling that song a "prayer" and a "plea" (20), the poet transforms the bird from a mere animal behaving instinctively to a being with consciousness performing intentionally, calling to heaven. By separating one of heaven's creatures from nature, whoever has imprisoned the bird has violated not only its freedom but also the divine order. Further, it makes listening to and enjoying the bird's song almost a perverse act, since the bird sings out of torment. The poem's progression from feeling to beating to singing, then, traces a progression from instinct to action to hope.

Of course, the poem is about more than birds in cages. The key refrain is "I know why," which emphasizes the poet's clear identification with the bird. He can know why the bird feels, acts, and prays because he experiences the same loss of

continued >>

Kho 4

freedom; he feels, acts, and prays for similar reasons. Given Dunbar's autobiography, it's obvious to see this poem as commenting directly on the treatment of African Americans in the nineteenth century, even after the Civil War, as attitudes and events continued to restrict former slaves. The images powerfully support that interpretation.

However, Dunbar carefully doesn't restrict the poem only to people in one time and situation. By choosing the common image of a bird in a cage, he invites readers to identify with anyone, in any place and time, who has lost his or her freedom, for reasons beyond their control. Some of those people—and readers may be among them—may be physically separated from the world, but for others, the "imprisonment" may be more emotional or metaphorical. Dunbar, finally, was free to write and publish this poem, but that didn't diminish his sympathy with the caged bird—or our own sympathy with him.

Kho 5

Work Cited

Dunbar, Paul Laurence. "Sympathy." *The Collected Poetry of Paul Laurence Dunbar*. Ed. Joanne M. Braxton. Charlottesville: UP of Virginia, 1993. 102. Print.

60 Writing in the Social and Natural Sciences

Quick Points You will learn to

- Understand different types of papers in the social sciences (see 60B).
- Understand different types of papers in the natural sciences (see 60E).

60A What are the social sciences?

The social sciences, which focus on people as individuals and in groups, include disciplines like economics, education, geography, political science, psychology, and sociology. In the social sciences, PRIMARY SOURCES include surveys and questionnaires, observations, interviews, and experiments. To prepare a questionnaire, use the guidelines in Quick Box 21.4 on page 262. For advice on collecting information through observation, see 21L, where we also explain interviewing strategies, especially in Quick Box 21.5.

The social sciences sometimes use data from experiments as a source. For example, if you want to learn how people react in a particular situation, you can set up that situation artificially and bring individuals (known as "subjects") into it to observe their behavior. With all methods of inquiry in the social sciences, you are required to treat subjects fairly and honestly, not in ways that could harm their body, mind, or reputation.

60B What are different types of papers in the social sciences?

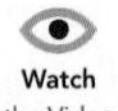

Instructors will sometimes assign the same kinds of writing in the social sciences as in the humanities (see 58C). Four additional types of papers are case studies, ethnographies, research reports, and research papers (or reviews of the literature).

60B.1 Case studies

A **case study** is an intensive study of one group or individual. Case studies are important in psychology, social work, education, medicine, and similar fields in which it's useful to form a comprehensive portrait of people. A case study is usually presented in a relatively fixed format, but the specific parts and their order vary. Most case studies contain the following components:

1. Basic identifying information about the individual or group
2. A history of the individual or group
3. Observations of the individual's or group's behavior
4. Conclusions and perhaps recommendations as a result of the observations

60B.2 Ethnographies

Ethnographies are comprehensive descriptions and interpretations of people interacting in a particular situation. Ethnographies commonly are written in education or the social sciences, with anthropology and sociology being prime examples. A sociologist might compose an ethnography of a classroom, for instance, to understand the interactions and relationships among students. The level of details needed in ethnographies has been described by anthropologist Clifford Geertz as "thick description." The more notes you take during observations, the better, because you can't be sure which ones will be important until you analyze and reflect on the information.

60B.3 Research reports

Research reports explain your own original research based on primary sources. Those sources may be interviews, questionnaires, observations, or experiments. Research reports in the social sciences often follow a prescribed format:

1. Statement of the problem
2. Background, sometimes including a review of the literature
3. Methodology
4. Results
5. Discussion of findings

60B.4 Research papers (or reviews of the literature)

More often for students, social science research requires you to summarize, analyze, and synthesize SECONDARY SOURCES. These sources are usually articles and books that report or discuss the findings of other people's primary research. To prepare a review of the literature, comprehensively gather and analyze the sources that have been published on a specific topic. *Literature* in this sense simply means "the body of work on a subject." Sometimes a review of the literature is a part of a longer paper, usually in the "background" section of a research report. Other times the entire paper might be an extensive review of the literature.

60C What documentation style do I use in the social sciences?

The most commonly used DOCUMENTATION STYLE in the social sciences is that of the American Psychological Association (APA). We describe APA documentation style and provide a sample student paper in Chapter 26. *Chicago Manual* (CM) documentation style is sometimes used in the social sciences (see Chapter 27).

60D What are the natural sciences?

The natural sciences include disciplines such as astronomy, biology, chemistry, geology, and physics. The sciences seek to describe and explain natural phenomena. The *scientific method*, commonly used in the sciences to make discoveries, is a procedure for gathering information related to a specific hypothesis. Quick Box 60.1 gives guidelines for using this method.

Quick Box 60.1

Guidelines for using the scientific method

1. Formulate a tentative explanation (a *hypothesis*) for a scientific phenomenon.
2. Read and summarize previously published information related to your hypothesis.
3. Plan a method of investigation to test your hypothesis.
4. Experiment, following exactly the investigative procedures you have outlined.
5. Observe closely the results of the experiment, and write notes carefully.
6. Analyze the results. Do they confirm the hypothesis?
7. Write a report of your research. At the end, you can suggest additional hypotheses that might be investigated.

60E How do I write different types of papers in the natural sciences?

Two major types of papers in the sciences are reports and reviews.

60E.1 Science reports

Science reports tell about observations and experiments. When they describe laboratory experiments, they're usually called lab reports. Formal reports feature the eight elements identified in Quick Box 60.2. Less formal reports, which are sometimes assigned in introductory college courses, might not include an abstract or a review of the literature. Ask your instructor which sections to include in your report.

Quick Box 60.2

Parts of a science report

1. **Title.** Precisely describes your report's topic.
2. **Abstract.** Provides a short overview of the report to help readers decide whether or not your research is of interest to them.
3. **Introduction.** States the purpose behind your research and presents the hypothesis. Any needed background information and a review of the literature appear here.
4. **Methods and materials.** Describes the equipment, material, and procedures used.
5. **Results.** Provides the information obtained from your efforts. Charts, graphs, and tables help present the data in a way that is easy for readers to grasp.
6. **Discussion.** Presents your interpretation and evaluation of the results. Did your efforts support your hypothesis? If not, can you suggest why not? Use concrete evidence in discussing your results.
7. **Conclusion.** Lists conclusions about the hypothesis and the outcomes of your efforts, paying particular attention to any theoretical implications that can be drawn from your work. Be specific in suggesting further research.
8. **List of references.** Presents references cited in the review of the literature, if any. Its format conforms to the requirements of the DOCUMENTATION STYLE in the particular science that is your subject.

60E.2 Science reviews

A science review discusses published information on a scientific topic. The purpose of the review is to synthesize for readers all the current knowledge about the issue. Sometimes, science reviews go a step further to present a new interpretation of previously published material; in such a review, the writer presents EVIDENCE to persuade readers that the new interpretation is valid.

If you're required to write a science review, you want to

1. choose a very limited scientific issue;
2. use information that is current—the more recently published the articles, books, and journals you consult, the better;
3. accurately paraphrase and summarize material (see Ch. 18); and
4. document your sources.

If your review runs longer than two or three pages, you might want to use headings to help readers understand your paper's organization and idea progression.

60F Which documentation style do I use in the natural sciences?

Documentation styles differ among the various sciences. A common style is that of the Council of Science Editors (CSE), described in Chapter 27.

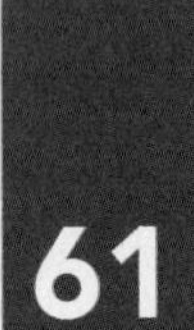

61 Writing Under Pressure

Quick Points You will learn to

➤ Identify skills that will help you write essay exams (see 61B).

61A When will I need to write under pressure?

All writers, student and professional, sometimes have to produce effective writing in a short time. Obvious examples are essay exams. Writers in the workplace frequently have to generate correspondence or reports in strict time limits.

61B How do I prepare for essay exams?

Begin preparing for exams well before the day of the test. Attend class diligently and take good notes. Be an active reader (see 3E).

Perhaps the best preparation comes from writing practice exams under time limits. Your instructors may offer questions from previous years or provide new questions to guide your studying. Alternatively, you may generate your own exam questions using cue words and key content words drawn from course material. Finally, ask your instructor whether an exam is "open book" so that you'll know if you can use books or notes during the test.

Because essay exams have firm time limits, you need to go through all of the steps in the WRITING PROCESS (see Ch. 5), but at high speed. Following are useful strategies.

- **Relax.** Never begin writing immediately. Instead, take a deep breath and let it out slowly to relax and focus your thoughts.
- **Read.** Read the test from beginning to end without skimming, so that you understand the questions completely. If you have a choice among topics, and equal credit is given to each, select the topics you know the most about.
- **Plan your time.** If the instructor indicates what percentage of your grade each question will affect, allot your time to your greatest advantage. Make sure to allow time for planning, DRAFTING, and proofreading.
- **Underline cue words.** These words tell you what you need to do in your essay. Quick Box 58.1, in section 58B, lists some common cue words with their meanings. Look for words such as *analyze, classify*, and *criticize*. An essay question might read like this:

    - **Analyze** Socrates' discussion of "good life" and "good death."

    Separate the concepts of "good life" and "good death" into parts and discuss each part.

- **Circle key content words.** Look for the keywords or major terms in a statement or question. An essay question might ask:

    - Review the effectiveness of **labor unions** in the **U.S. economy**.

    The key content words are *labor unions* and *U.S. economy.*

- **Use your time fully.** The best writers use every second available to write and polish. (Trust us, we've been in that spot often and have never regretted working right up to the time limit.)

62 Making Presentations

Quick Points You will learn to

- Adjust your presentation to fit your audience and purpose (see 62A–62C).
- Organize your presentation (see 62D).
- Use multimedia in your presentation (see 62E).

62A What are presentations?

Presentations—speeches often supported with multimedia tools—are common not only in college but also in work and public settings. Preparing a presentation and drafting a paper involve similar processes (see Ch. 5). This chapter provides additional advice.

62B How does my situation focus my presentation?

You need to adjust presentations to fit PURPOSES, AUDIENCES, roles, and any special considerations. Consider three different situations.

- You want to address a group of students to inform them about a film club you're starting.
- You need to persuade a management group at work to adopt a new set of procedures for making purchasing decisions.
- You plan to give a toast at a friend's wedding to express your feelings and to entertain the wedding guests.

Different approaches will be successful in each instance because your purpose and audience are different.

62C How do I adapt my message to my audience?

Adapting your presentation to your listeners means holding their interest and being responsive to their viewpoints. Consult the strategies for analyzing AUDIENCES in Quick Box 4.5 on page 54. Quick Box 62.1 suggests how to adapt your message to three types of audience.

Quick Box 62.1

Adapting a presentation to your audience

UNINFORMED AUDIENCE	Start with the basics and then move to a few new ideas. Define new terms and concepts and avoid unnecessary technical terms. Use visual aids and give examples. Repeat key ideas—but not too often.
INFORMED AUDIENCE	Never give more than a quick overview of the basics. Devote most of your time to new ideas and concepts.
MIXED AUDIENCE	In your introduction, acknowledge the more informed audience members who are present. Explain that you're going to review the basic concepts briefly so that everyone can build from the same knowledge base. Move as soon as possible toward more complex concepts.

62D How do I organize my presentation?

A presentation has three parts: introduction, body, and conclusion.

62D.1 Introducing yourself and your topic

All audience members want to know three things about a speaker: Who are you? What are you going to talk about? Why should I listen? To respond effectively to these unasked questions, try these suggestions.

- Grab your audience's attention with an interesting question, quotation, or statistic; a bit of background information; a compliment; or an anecdote. If necessary to establish your credibility—even if someone has introduced you—briefly and humbly mention your qualifications as a speaker about your topic.
- Give your audience a road map of your talk: Tell where you're starting, where you're going, and how you intend to get there. Your listeners need to know that you won't waste their time.

62D.2 Following your road map

Listening to a presentation is very different from reading an essay. Audiences generally need help following the speaker's line of reasoning. Here are some strategies to keep your listeners' minds from wandering.

- Signal clearly where you are on your road map by using cue word transitions such as *first, second*, and *third; subsequently, therefore*, and *furthermore;* or *before, then*, and *next.*
- Define unfamiliar terms and concepts and follow up with strong, memorable examples.
- Occasionally tell the audience what you consider significant, memorable, or especially relevant and why. Do so sparingly, at key points.
- Provide occasional summaries at points of transition. Recap what you've covered and say how it relates to what's coming next.

62D.3 Wrapping up your presentation

Try ending with these suggestions.

- Never let your voice volume fall or your clarity of pronunciation falter because the end is in sight.
- Don't introduce new ideas at the last minute.
- Signal that you are wrapping up your presentation using verbal cues, such as "In conclusion" and "Finally." When you say "finally," mean it!
- Make a dramatic, decisive statement; cite a memorable quotation; or issue a challenge. Allow a few seconds of silence, and then say "thank you." Use body language, such as stepping slightly back from the podium, and then sit down.

62E How do I use multimedia in presentations?

Multimedia elements such as visual aids, sound, and video can reinforce key ideas in your presentation by providing illustrations or concrete images for the audience.

62E.1 Using traditional visual aids

Here are various types of visual aids and their uses. When using them, always make text or graphics large enough to be read easily at a distance.

- **Posters** can dramatize a point, often with color or images. Make sure a poster is large enough for everyone in your audience to see it.
- **Dry-erase boards** are preferable to chalkboards because colors on them are visually appealing. Use them to roughly sketch an illustration or to emphasize a technical word.

- **Handouts** are useful when the topic calls for a longer text or when you want to give your audience something to refer to later. Short, simple handouts work best during a presentation. Always include DOCUMENTATION information for any SOURCES you used. A strategic handout can be a useful backup just in case other technologies are missing or broken. Remember to wait until everyone has one before you begin speaking about it.

62E.2 Using presentation software

PowerPoint, the most widely used presentation software, can create digital slides. (A similar program, "Impress," is free from www.openoffice.org.) These slides can contain words, images, or combinations of both. To project your slides during a presentation, you need an LCD projector connected to your computer and a separate screen. See Figure 62.1.

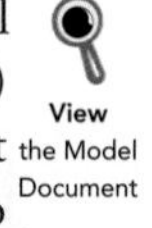

Never present so much information that your audience spends more time reading than to listening to you. Also, never simply read large amounts of text from your slides; your audience will quickly—and rightfully—become bored. People have coined the phrase "death by PowerPoint" in despair at presenters who simply repeat what's written on slides. For advice on designing presentation slides, see Quick Box 62.2 (page 782).

Figure 62.1 A sample PowerPoint slide.

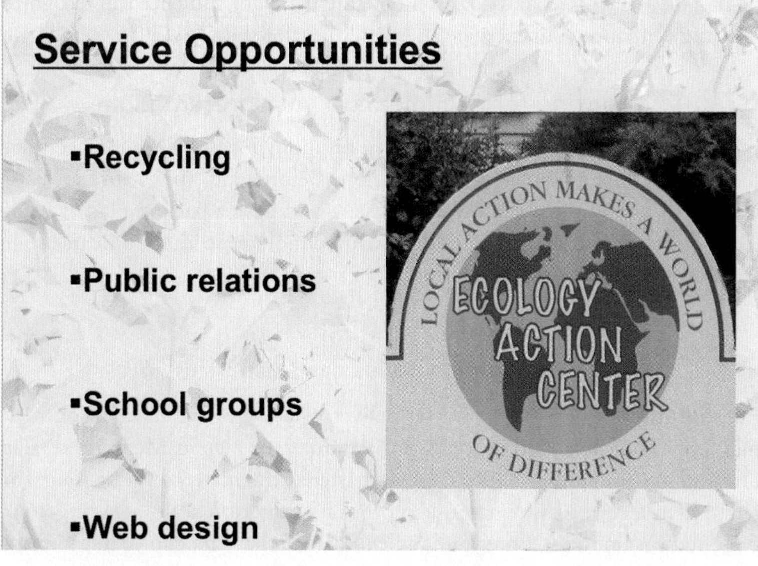
Service Opportunities
▪Recycling
▪Public relations
▪School groups
▪Web design
LOCAL ACTION MAKES A WORLD OF DIFFERENCE
ECOLOGY ACTION CENTER

Quick Box 62.2

Guidelines for designing PowerPoint or similar presentation slides

- **Keep slides simple.** Use only a few very short lines of text on each slide. An old rule is "six by six": no more than six lines, each with no more than six words.
- **Keep slides readable.** Make sure words and images are large enough to be read by everyone. Contrast is important. Use black text (or very dark colors) on a white background, or use white text on a very dark background.
- **Keep slides interesting.** A single well-chosen image can enhance a slide. Sometimes, in fact, a slide that consists only of an image (a photograph, a chart, or other graphic) can be quite effective.
- **Keep slides few.** It's far more effective to have 5 well-chosen and designed slides for a short talk than it is to have 20.

62E.3 Using sound or video clips

A brief sound file (for example, a few sentences from a speech) or a video clip (perhaps 20 to 30 seconds of footage) can occasionally help you illustrate a point. Keep them brief and be absolutely sure that your audience will recognize how they enhance your message and aren't just for show.

62E.4 Planning for multimedia in your presentation

Few things are more frustrating for you or annoying to your audience than technical problems during a presentation. Beforehand, make sure all your visual aids and multimedia will work well—and have a backup plan at hand in case they fail. Rehearse carefully with technology so that you can use it seamlessly during your presentation.

62F What presentation styles can I use?

Presentation style is the way you deliver what you have to say. You may memorize your talk, read it, speak without notes, or map it. Memorized talks often sound unnatural. Unless you've mastered the material well enough to recite it in a relaxed way, choose another presentation style. Reading your presentation aloud can bore your audience. If you have no choice but to read, avoid speaking in a monotone. Vary your pace and pitch. In general, avoid speaking without notes until you have considerable experience giving speeches, unless otherwise instructed by your professor or supervisor.

We recommend mapping your presentation. Mapping means creating a brief outline of your presentation's main points and examples, then using that outline to cue yourself.

Your body language can either add to or detract from your message. Eye contact is your most important nonverbal communication tool because it communicates confidence and shows respect for your listeners. Smile or nod at your audience as you begin. If you use a podium, stand squarely behind it before you begin speaking. When gestures aren't needed, rest your hands on the podium—don't scratch your head, dust your clothing, or fidget.

62G How do I make a collaborative presentation?

Group presentations are common in academic and business settings. Here are some guidelines to follow.

- Make sure, when choosing a topic or a position about an issue, that most members of the group are familiar with the subject.
- Lay out clearly each member's responsibilities for preparing the presentation.
- Agree on firm time limits for each person, if all members of the group are expected to speak for an equal amount of time. If there is no such requirement, people who enjoy public speaking can take more responsibility for delivery, and others can do more of the preparatory work or contribute in other ways.
- Allow enough time for practice. Plan at least two complete run-throughs of your presentation, using multimedia elements if you have them. Though each member can practice his or her own part alone, schedule practice sessions for the entire presentation as a group.
- As you practice your presentation, have different group members watch in order to make suggestions.

63 Writing for Digital Environments

Quick Points You will learn to

- Understand how to write for blogs and wikis (see 63B–63C).
- Understand how to create video and sound recordings and to produce Web sites (see 63D–63F).
- Understand good manners and privacy online (see 63G–63H).

63A What is writing for digital environments?

Writing for digital environments means producing texts that can best—or perhaps that can only—be read through computers, generally online. Examples include blogs, wikis, videos, podcasts, photo essays, Web pages, and social media. Digital composing (sometimes called "multimodal writing") opens possibilities that are difficult or impossible in traditional print papers. Digital environments

- Allow writers easily to incorporate images without the expense of printing.
- Allow writers to create or incorporate sound or visual recordings.
- Allow links to other sources available online.
- Allow instant publication to readers far and wide.
- Allow interactions, so that readers can share comments or writers can collaborate in different times and places.

Digital environments can also present challenges or complications by

- Requiring so much time and energy for design that they take attention away from writing.
- Raising copyright or ownership concerns by circulating found images without permission.
- Permitting people to post inappropriate comments on other peoples' work.
- Allowing work to be made public that isn't of the highest quality.

63B How do I write in a blog?

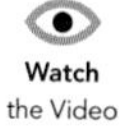

A Web log, or **blog**, is a Web site that displays a series of posts, or items. Posts are usually diary-like entries or observations but may also be images, videos, audio files, and links. Blogs generally focus on a particular topic.

Most have a similar design. The main content, a post about a particular topic, is in the center of the screen. The most recent post appears at the top of a page, followed by previous ones as a reader scrolls down. Many blogs contain a comment feature. Some blogs also have links to other blogs that focus on similar topics. Figure 63.1 shows a typical blog design.

Some instructors have students keep blogs as a course requirement. This follows the tradition of having students write journals as a regular way of writing about course content. The twist is that others can easily read and comment on each person's postings. If you're assigned to produce a course blog, your instructor will provide specific directions.

If you'd like to create your own blog, decide on a type and purpose, and imagine an AUDIENCE who cares about your perspective. You might participate in blogs and network with others, eventually gaining the attention of people who are interested in your ideas or experiences. Most important, have something interesting to say. Easily available software allows you to

Figure 63.1 Typical blog design.

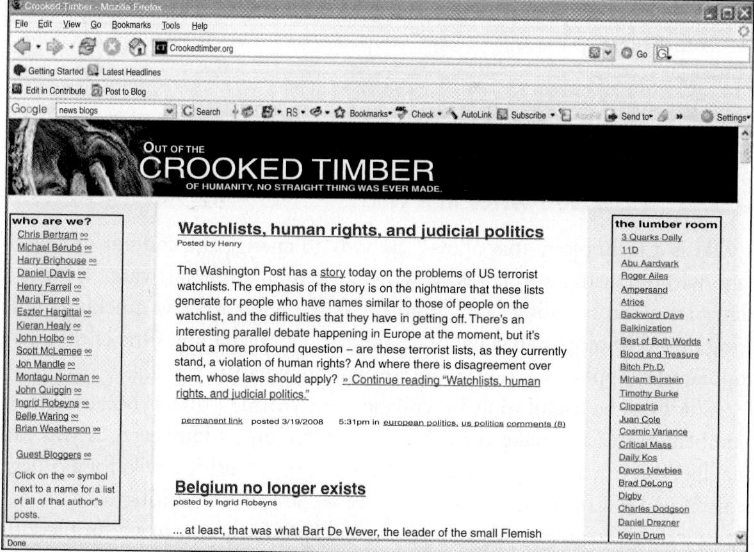

start blogging almost immediately with little worry or knowledge. For example, Blogger is a popular online community that gets you started with only a few mouse clicks. Quick Box 63.1 contains guidelines for writing in a blog.

Quick Box 63.1

Guidelines for writing in a blog

- **Pick a unique title for your blog.** People and Internet search engines will recognize your blog if it has a good title.
- **Decide whether to use your own name or a made-up username.** You can protect your privacy to some degree if you have a pseudonym (literally, a "false name") or username. Especially if you're writing about controversial topics or taking controversial positions, you might not want employers, instructors, or even relatives to know your identity. Of course, an anonymous username doesn't give you license to be irresponsible or unethical. On the other hand, the advantage of your real name is that you get credit (and, we suppose, blame) for your writings. Think carefully about this decision.
- **Link, show, and share.** Include links in your posts to other, similar posts or items from the Web. Post images, videos, or audio files, but do respect copyrights. Share your posts and blog by participating on other blogs.

63C How do I write in a wiki?

A **wiki** is a technology that allows anybody to change the content of a Web page without using special Web writing or uploading software. *Wiki* is a Hawaiian word meaning "fast," and the name refers to how quickly people using this technology can collaborate and revise information. One of the more popular wiki applications is the online encyclopedia, Wikipedia.

Wikis can be useful tools for collaborative writing projects because group members can easily make contributions and changes. However, as you can imagine, this can also lead to complications. If you're using a wiki for a college project, you'll want to review strategies in section 9B for writing with others. If you want to create a new wiki, setting one up is fairly easy using simple software like Pbwiki (http://pbwiki.com/education.wiki). Quick Box 63.2 offers guidelines for writing in a wiki.

Quick Box 63.2

Guidelines for writing in a wiki

- **Revise with respect for others.** Consider ways to preserve what the person before you has written. Instead of deleting material, you might add qualifications, for example, words like "possibly" or phrases such as "in some cases" or "some have argued." You might add a section entitled "opposing arguments" (see 13G) that suggests an alternative viewpoint.
- **Cite your sources.** Whenever possible, cite your sources, and in some cases, find corroborating sources. Any addition to a wiki entry that contains references to reputable sources is less likely to be deleted or revised later, making your influence more lasting.
- **Post images, videos, and audio files.** Include links and references from other sources on the Web, but in every case, respect copyrights.

63D How do I use photographs?

Digital cameras and the Internet have made it cheap and easy to circulate pictures. Our culture has become visually oriented, and pictures can often enhance digital documents. We explain how to find, make, adjust, and place photographs in 7E.

63E How do I create video and sound recordings?

As you probably know from YouTube, online videos can be a great source of entertainment (or, depending on your point of view, a great waste of time). However, videos and sound recordings (such as radio essays or **podcasts**) can also be effective ways to deliver information or even make arguments. Videos often present complicated how-to directions more effectively than can words alone. Documentaries (think of versions of Ken Burns' famous series on the Civil War or jazz) vividly convey people and events.

Watch the Video

Despite their advantages, video and sound projects can take considerable time and expertise to do well. Just like written texts, they require planning, drafting, and revising, using technologies. Quick Box 63.3 (page 788) offers guidelines.

Figure 63.2 (page 789) shows the opening to a documentary video that student Siena Pinney created about a forest fire.

Quick Box 63.3

Guidelines for producing sound and video recordings

- **Plan your recording**. A good video or podcast has a beginning, middle, and end. Decide what elements you need to record for each.
- **Create and practice a script**. If your project has a narrator (and most projects do), write a script that contains what you plan to say, what will be on camera when you say it, and what music or sound effects you'll need. Practice the script before you record.
- **Create a storyboard for visual projects**. A storyboard is a series of rough sketches (you can use stick people, for example) that show the major scenes or elements in your video. It helps you plan the sequence and keep track of what shots you need to make.
- **Arrange to interview and record people** who will appear in your recording. Have anyone appearing in your work sign a release, a form that gives you permission to circulate their voice and images.
- **Find an appropriate place to record**. Unless you're trying to capture a real atmosphere (such as the crowd at a ball game or a protest), find a quiet place with good acoustics.
- **Use the best equipment available**. A dedicated video camera will generally produce better quality than a regular digital camera that has video capacity, for example. A dedicated microphone will work much better than a laptop's built-in microphone. Your college may have equipment for checking out.
- **Edit what you've recorded or shot**. The real work of producing an effective recording comes in editing the raw footage. You'll need to shorten some elements, move some around, and add transitions. You may even need to shoot new material in the middle of the process. Learn how to use free or cheap sound editing programs like Audacity (audacity.sourceforge.net/) or video editing programs like MovieMaker or iMovie.

Figure 63.2 Opening shot of documentary video.

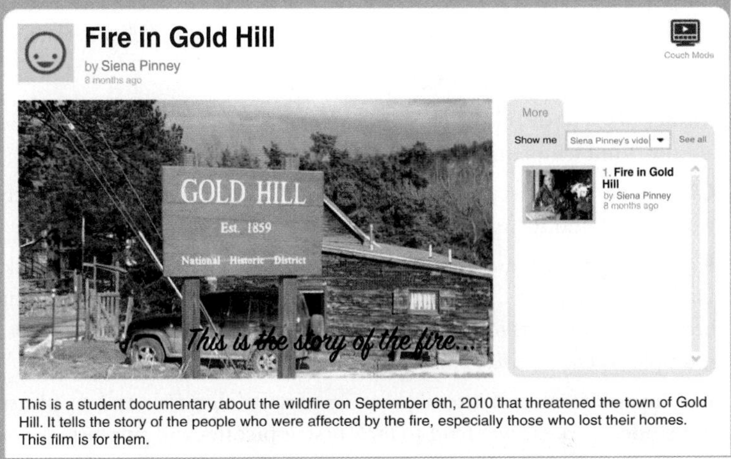
Fire in Gold Hill
by Siena Pinney
8 months ago
Couch Mode
GOLD HILL
Est. 1859
National Historic District
This is the story of the fire...
More
Show me
Siena Pinney's video
See all
1. Fire in Gold Hill
by Siena Pinney
8 months ago
This is a student documentary about the wildfire on September 6th, 2010 that threatened the town of Gold Hill. It tells the story of the people who were affected by the fire, especially those who lost their homes. This film is for them.

63F How do I produce Web sites?

The Web writing process has five parts: (1) writing the content, (2) creating the structure of the content, (3) laying out the material on the screen, (4) checking whether the Web material is usable, and (5) loading the Web site on a **server**, a computer that is always online and available to Internet users.

63F.1 Creating a structure for a Web site

Almost all Web sites have a **home page**, a page that introduces the site and provides links to other pages. The home page functions like a table of contents or an entryway to a building. It needs to be appealing and give visitors clear directions for navigating. Here are some guidelines for creating a site's structure.

- Determine all the pages your site might contain and whether these pages need to be grouped into categories (groups of pages all on the same topic).
- Generate a list of categories.
- Plan **hyperlinks**, which are direct electronic connections between two pages.

63F.2 Choosing a template or designing a site

Unless you have considerable time, expertise, and the need for a unique Web site, we recommend using one of thousands of templates available online. A template (sometimes called a "theme") has predesigned places for titles, menus, texts, images, and so on. Once you selected a template, you paste your own materials into those places. Sites like Wordpress or Blogger provide free templates.

Here's some general advice about choosing and using a Web template.

- **Apply good design principles** (see Ch. 7).
- **Model after desirable Web sites.** Choose sites that have designs you admire. Find templates that have most of their qualities.
- **Choose an appropriate title.** Make sure your page tells readers exactly what they'll find there.
- **Keep backgrounds and texts simple.** Strive for a clean, uncluttered look. Dark text on a plain light background is easiest to read, with white being best. SANS SERIF fonts tend to be easiest to read on computer screens. Avoid multiple typefaces, sizes, colors, and busy backgrounds.
- **Use images to attract attention to important elements and to please the reader.** Readers will tend to look first at pictures and graphics.
- **Provide identifying information.** Generally, the bottom of a page includes the date the page is updated, along with your contact information.

63F.3 Incorporating photos into Web pages

Keep in mind that photographs can take a long time to download unless you reduce the size of the file through the picture editor in Microsoft Word or use a program like Photoshop.

63F.4 Editing and testing usability

Before you upload your Web page to a server, edit and proofread it as carefully as you would a print document. Use the checklist in Quick Box 63.4.

Quick Box 63.4

Editing checklist for a Web site

- **Are any images broken?** Broken images show up as small icons instead of the pictures you want. The usual cause of broken images is mistyping the file name or failing to upload the image.
- **Do all the links work?** Missing, mistyped, or mislabeled files can cause broken links.
- **Is the Web site user-friendly?** Ask your friends, classmates, or colleagues to report anything unclear, inappropriate, or unattractive.

63F.5 Displaying a Web page

To display your finished Web page, you need space on a Web server, a centralized computer that is always online. Your college may offer Web space to its students, and services like WordPress and others offer free Web space. Your provider can explain how to upload content.

63G What is netiquette?

Netiquette, a word coined from *Net* and *etiquette*, demands that you use good manners as you write online or send e-mails. Unfortunately, blogs, discussion boards, and online comment sections are full of name-calling, personal attacks, and outlandish claims with no support, often unrelated to the topic at hand. Avoid being a troll (someone who posts irresponsibly), and avoid flaming (the sending of irresponsible messages). Avoid using ALL CAPS, which is both hard to read and taken as the equivalent of shouting, and also avoid writing in all lowercase letters, which can be taken as lazy or too cute.

When sending e-mails, use gender-neutral language. Always address business recipients or instructors by their full names, including any title such as *Ms.*, *Mr.*, or *Dr.* Also, use titles and last names, especially when you're communicating with people you've never met or corresponded with before. After you get to know people well, you might decide to lower your LEVEL OF FORMALITY. We suggest waiting until after those to whom you're writing begin to end their messages with their first names, especially when those people hold positions higher than yours.

63H What do I need to know about social networking?

Social networking platforms like Facebook or Twitter allow you to share material with others. Groups and organizations have set up social networking pages to publicize themselves, and some instructors have even developed pages for their courses.

As you use social networking, assume two things: (1) Nothing online is really private, and (2) Everything online is permanent. Even if you make everything private and visible only to approved friends, a stranger could easily end up viewing material you wouldn't want them to see. People have lost job opportunities because of what employers have found about them online. Only post things that you're confident represent you well, even to unforeseen readers. Don't be afraid to use and enjoy these powerful sites. We do! Just be sensible and aware.

Figure 63.3 Example of a social networking site.

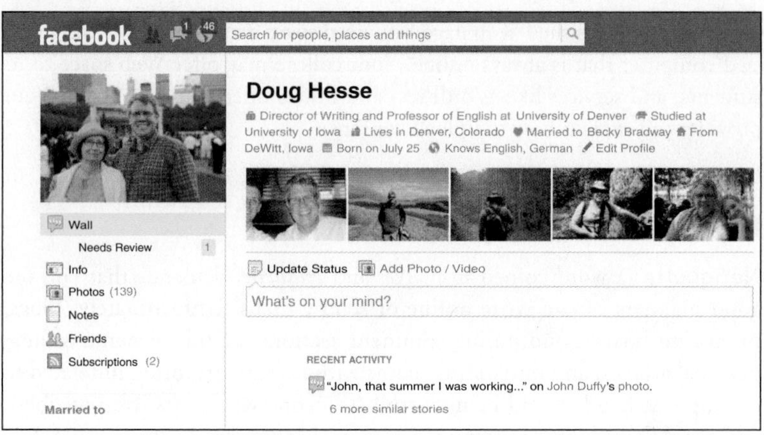

64 Writing for Work

Quick Points You will learn to

- Identify features of types of workplace writing (see 64B–64G).
- Create résumés and application letters (see 64H–64I).

64A Who writes in the workplace, and why?

If you're working, chances are good that you're writing. Writing infuses most workplaces, from corporate offices and health-care facilities to farms and factories. Even people who work independently (such as consultants, therapists, artists, and craftspeople) keep records, correspond with customers, and advertise their services. This chapter offers guidance for several common work-related writing tasks.

64B What are important features of work-related correspondence?

Correspondence is the general name for written communications, such as e-mails, memos, and letters, that you send to specific individuals. Your goal is to communicate plans, procedures, or purchases; share or ask for information; request specific actions; or influence decisions.

Work-related correspondence needs to appear professional, focused, and well informed. Avoid slang, abbreviations, informal words, or informal expressions. Use STANDARD EDITED ENGLISH grammar, spelling, and punctuation. Remember, too, that even casually written messages can have contractual significance or serve as evidence in court. Quick Box 64.1 provides general guidelines for writing work-related correspondence.

ESOL Tip: In some cultures, work-related correspondence is often sprinkled with elaborate language, many descriptive details, and even metaphors. Most American organizations, however, prefer correspondence that is clear and gets to the point quickly.

Quick Box 64.1

Guidelines for work-related correspondence

- Address the recipient by name.
- Use GENDER-NEUTRAL LANGUAGE.
- Announce the PURPOSE of your communication at the outset.
- Be clear, concise, and specific.
- Be honest, positive, and natural, using a personal touch.
- Never spread gossip, personal opinion, put-downs, jokes, or chain letters.
- Edit ruthlessly for CONCISENESS and correctness.

64C How do I write work-related e-mail?

Business e-mail has formal purposes and AUDIENCES and should be free of slang or abbreviations like LOL (laughing out loud) or BTW (by the way).

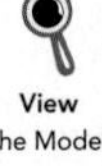
View the Model Document

The "cc" or "Copies" space is for the e-mail addresses of other people who need to see your message, even when they aren't expected to respond. When

Figure 64.1 A professional e-mail.

To: sherrel. ampadu@jpltech.com
From: Chris Malinowitz <cmalinowitz@chateauby.com>
Subject: Confirming Meeting Arrangements
Cc: dmclusky@chateauby.com
Bcc:
Attached: C:\Documents and Settings\Desktop\Chateau Menus.doc

Dear Ms. Ampadu:

I am writing to confirm the final arrangements for your business meeting on June 17, 2012, at our conference center.

As you directed, we will set the room in ten round tables, each seating six. We will provide a podium and microphone, an LCD projector and screen, and a white board with markers. I understand that you will be bringing your own laptop. Our technician can help you set up.

You indicated that you would like to provide lunch and refreshments at two breaks. Attached please find our menus. You will need to make your lunch selections at least 48 hours in advance.

If you have any questions or wish to make any changes, I would be pleased to accommodate your needs. Thank you for choosing The Chateau at Brickyard.

Sincerely,

Chris Malinowitz
Catering Director, The Chateau at Brickyard

you use the "Bcc" (blind copy) space, you're sending a copy to someone without your primary recipients' knowing about it. Often, it's rude to send blind copies, but you might choose to blind-copy a long list of e-mail addresses so your recipients don't have to scroll through lots of names.

For the body of your e-mail, single-space the text, and double-space between paragraphs. Start paragraphs flush left at the margin. When you need to include a separate document with your e-mail, such as a report, compose it as a separate document in your word processing program, and attach it to your e-mail. Figure 64.1 is an example of a professional e-mail.

Know your workplace's policy covering issues such as use of business e-mail accounts for personal purposes and any legal responsibilities concerning your e-mail. Increasingly, businesses monitor their employees' e-mail.

Quick Box 64.2 summarizes some key points about writing business e-mail.

Quick Box 64.2

Guidelines for writing business e-mail

- Write a specific, not general, topic on the Subject line.
- Start your e-mail with a sentence that tells what your message is about.
- Put the details of your message in the second paragraph. Supply any background information that your recipients may need.
- Conclude your e-mail by asking for certain information or a specific action, if such is needed, or by restating your reason for writing.
- Follow netiquette (see 63G).
- Keep your message brief and your paragraphs short.
- Be cautious about what you say in a business e-mail, which could be forwarded to others without your permission.
- Forward an e-mail message only if you've asked the original sender for permission.
- At the end of your message, before your full name and position, use a commonly accepted complimentary closing, such as *Sincerely, Cordially,* or *Regards.*

64D How do I format and write memos?

Memos are usually exchanged internally (within an organization or business). Today e-mail takes the place of most memos, unless the correspondence requires a physical record or signature. The guidelines for writing e-mail (see 64C) also pertain to memos.

View the Model Document

The standard format of a memo includes two major parts: the headings and the body.

To: [Name your audience—a specific person or group.]
From: [Give your name and your title, if any.]
Date: [Give the date on which you write the memo.]
Re: [State your subject as specifically as possible in the "Subject" or "Re" line.]

Here are some guidelines for preparing a memo.

- **Introduction:** State your purpose for writing and why your memo is worth your reader's attention. Either here or at the conclusion, mention whether the recipient needs to take action.

- **Body:** Present the essential information on your topic. If you write more than three or four paragraphs, use headings to divide the information into subtopics (see 7D).
- **Conclusion:** End with a one- to two-sentence summary, a specific recommendation, or what action is needed and by when. Finish with a "thank you" line.

64E How do I format business letters?

View the Model Document

E-mail has generally taken the place of business letters; however, letters are sometimes still used for formal correspondence or when you want to establish a physical record of your communications. Cover letters (also called "letters of transmittal") accompany résumés, packages, reports, or other documents. Here are guidelines for the format and content of your business letters.

- **Paper:** Use 8½-by-11-inch paper. The most suitable color is white. Fold your business letters horizontally into thirds to fit into a standard number 10 business envelope (9½ by 4 inches).
- **Letterhead:** Use the official letterhead stationery (name, address, and logo, if any) of the business where you're employed. If no letterhead exists, center your full name, address, and phone number at the top of the page, and use a larger font than for the content of your letter. Keep it simple.
- **Format:** Without indents, use single spacing within paragraphs and double spacing between paragraphs, which is called **block style**. Figure 64.2 shows a job application letter in business format.
- **Recipient's name:** Use the full name of your recipient whenever possible. If you can't locate a name, either through a phone call to a central switchboard or on the Internet, use a specific category—for example, "Dear Billing Department," placing the key word "Billing" first (not "Department of Billing"). Always use gender-neutral language.

64F How do I write business reports?

Reports inform others inside or outside the workplace. Internal reports are designed to convey information to others in your workplace. They serve various purposes. For example, if you attend a professional meeting, you might provide a report of what you learned for your supervisor and colleagues who weren't there. If you have conducted extensive consumer research telephone interviews with potential customers, you might summarize and analyze your findings in a report. Being clear and concise are vital.

External reports inform audiences beyond the workplace. Generally, they have a secondary function of creating a good impression of the organization.

Figure 64.2 Sample job application letter.

Monica A. Schickel
1817 Drevin Avenue
Denver, CO 80208

Cell phone: (303) 555-7722
E-mail: mnsschl@wordnet.com
Professional portfolio: www.schickelgraphics.net

May 3, 2012

Jaime Cisneros
Publications Director
R.L. Smith Consulting
2000 Wabash Avenue
Chicago, IL 60601

Dear Mr. Cisneros:

Please consider my application for the graphic designer position currently being advertised on your company's Web site. I believe that my professional experiences, education, and skills prepare me well for this opportunity.

I am currently completing a paid internship at Westword, a weekly features and entertainment magazine in Denver, CO, where I have worked as an effective member of a creative team. My responsibilities have included designing advertisements, laying out sections, and editing photographs. Other related experience includes commissions as an illustrator and photographer. My professional portfolio demonstrates the range and quality of my work. As the enclosed résumé notes, I have additional experience in business environments.

Next month I will earn a BA in graphic design from The University of Denver, where my course of study has included extensive work in graphic design, photography, drawing, and illustration. Simultaneously, I will complete a minor in digital media studies that has included courses in Web design, video editing, and sound editing. I have expertise in all the standard software applications that would be relevant to your position.

I would be pleased to provide further information and to interview at your convenience. The opportunities at R.L. Smith closely match my background and goals, and the prospect of joining your team in Chicago is exciting. I look forward to discussing how I can contribute to your publications department.

Sincerely,

Monica A. Schickel
Monica A. Schickel

Common examples are annual reports, in which companies summarize their accomplishments during the previous year. However, other kinds of external reports are also common. For example, a school principal may write a report to parents that explain students' results on a statewide achievement test. Figure 64.3 (page 798) shows a section of one company's report. Document

Figure 64.3 A company's external report.

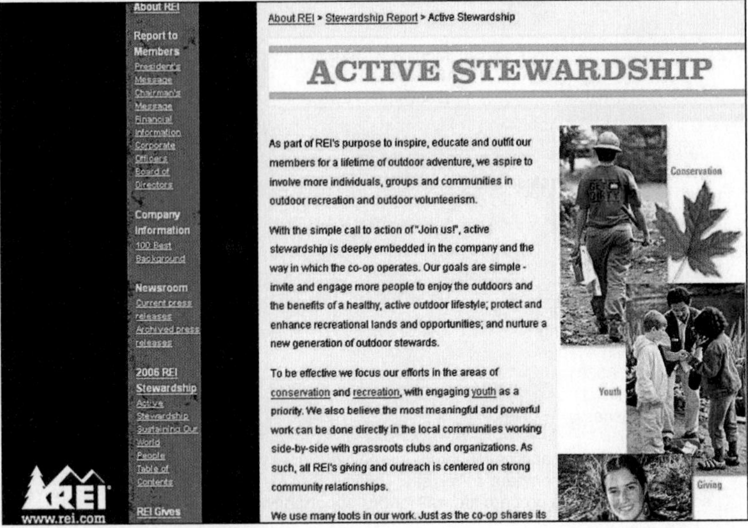

About REI

Report to Members
President's Message
Chairman's Message
Financial Information
Corporate Officers
Board of Directors

Company Information
100 Best
Background

Newsroom
Current press releases
Archived press releases

2006 REI Stewardship
Active Stewardship
Sustaining Our World
People
Table of Contents

REI Gives

REI
www.rei.com

About REI > Stewardship Report > Active Stewardship

ACTIVE STEWARDSHIP

As part of REI's purpose to inspire, educate and outfit our members for a lifetime of outdoor adventure, we aspire to involve more individuals, groups and communities in outdoor recreation and outdoor volunteerism.

With the simple call to action of "Join us!", active stewardship is deeply embedded in the company and the way in which the co-op operates. Our goals are simple - invite and engage more people to enjoy the outdoors and the benefits of a healthy, active outdoor lifestyle; protect and enhance recreational lands and opportunities; and nurture a new generation of outdoor stewards.

To be effective we focus our efforts in the areas of conservation and recreation, with engaging youth as a priority. We also believe the most meaningful and powerful work can be done directly in the local communities working side-by-side with grassroots clubs and organizations. As such, all REI's giving and outreach is centered on strong community relationships.

We use many tools in our work. Just as the co-op shares its

design, whether in print or on the computer screen, is important (see Ch. 7). Notice how the report in Figure 64.3 uses images and color.

64G How do I write business proposals?

We provide some detailed advice for writing proposals in Chapter 16. Business proposals are specialized versions of the larger category. They persuade readers to follow a plan, choose a product or service, or implement an idea. A marketing specialist might propose a new product line. A leader of a not-for-profit organization might propose a way to increase funding. Here are some specific guidelines for preparing a business proposal.

INTRODUCTION Explain the project's purpose and scope. Describe the problem that the project seeks to solve, and lay out your solution. Include dates for beginning and completing the work. Project the outcomes and the costs. Be accurate and precise.

BODY What is the product or service? What resources are needed? What are the phases of the project? Precisely how is each phase to be completed? What is the timeline? How will the project be evaluated?

CONCLUSION Summarize the benefits of this proposal. Thank readers for their time. Offer to provide further information.

64H How do I write a résumé?

A résumé details your accomplishments and employment history. Its purpose is to help a potential employer determine whether you'll be a suitable candidate. To make a favorable impression, follow the guidelines for writing a résumé in Quick Box 64.3. Today, many employers have applicants upload their résumés to an employment Web site or send them as an e-mail attachment. Sometimes employers use software to scan electronic résumés, looking for keywords. Figure 64.4 (page 801) presents a sample résumé.

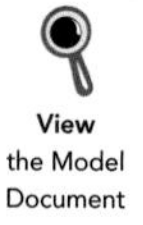
View the Model Document

Quick Box 64.3

Guidelines for writing a traditional, scannable, or plain-text résumé

- At the beginning, include your name, address, e-mail address, and telephone number.
- Make the résumé easy to read. Label the sections clearly, and target the résumé to the position you want. Help employers see your most significant attributes quickly and easily.
- Adjust your résumé to fit your purpose. For example, if you're applying for a job as a computer programmer, you'll want to emphasize different facts than you would if you were applying for a job selling computers in an electronics store.
- Use headings to separate blocks of information. Include the following headings, as appropriate: "Position Desired" or "Career Objective"; "Education"; "Experience"; "Licenses and Certifications"; "Related Experience"; "Honors and Awards"; "Publications and Presentations"; "Activities and Interests"; and "Special Abilities, Skills, and Knowledge."
- When you list your work experience, place your most recent job first; when listing education, place your most recent degrees, certificates, or enrollments first.
- Write telegraphically. Start with verb phrases, not with the word *I*, and omit *a*, *an*, and *the*.
- Include only relevant information.
- Tell the truth. An employer who discovers you lied will likely fire you.
- Include references, or state that you can provide them on request.
- Try to fit all of the information on one page. If you need a second page, make sure the most important information is on the first page.

continued >>

Quick Box 64.3 (continued)

- Proofread carefully; even one spelling error or one formatting error can eliminate you from consideration.
- For print résumés, use high-quality paper that is white or off-white.
- Scannable résumés are designed to be scanned by machines that digitize their content. Sophisticated software then searches the database to match key terms to position requirements. As a result, scannable résumés need to be simpler: don't use columns, different fonts, lines or other graphics, or bold or italic fonts. Choose a clean sans serif font such as Arial or Geneva in a 10–12 point size. Include keywords that the computer can match to the job. Here is the keyword list Monica Schickel created for the scannable version of the resume in Figure 64.4:

  KEYWORDS

  Publications experience, graphic design, editing, photography, supervisor, editing, customer service, digital media, excellent Spanish, Adobe Creative Suite, Photoshop, InDesign, Quark, CSS, Dreamweaver, Web design, illustrator, proofread, Excel, Access, Publisher, newspaper, layout, sales, willing to relocate
- Plain-text résumés can be pasted directly into e-mails or into application databases. Use the same standards as for scannable resumes. Start every line of text at the left margin.

64l How do I write a job application letter?

View the Model Document

A job application letter always needs to accompany your résumé. Avoid repeating what's already on the résumé. Instead, connect the company's expectations to your experience by emphasizing how your background has prepared you for the position. Your job application letter, more than your résumé, reflects your energy and personality. Today, many employers have applicants upload letters to an application Web site, send them as e-mail attachments, or even send them as e-mails themselves. See Figure 64.2 for a sample letter and Quick Box 64.4 (page 802) for guidelines.

ESOL Tip: In some cultures, job applications may include personal information, such as an applicant's age, marital status, number of children, religion, or political beliefs. In North America, however, this is not standard practice. Such personal information does not help an employer determine how well you can perform a particular job, so avoid including it in your application.

Figure 64.4 A sample résumé.

MONICA A. SCHICKEL

1817 Drevin Avenue
Denver, CO 80208
Cell phone: (303) 555-7722
E-mail: mnsschl@wordnet.com
Professional portfolio: www.schickelgraphics.net

OBJECTIVE: Entry level position as a graphic designer or publications assistant

EXPERIENCE

9/12 – present **Publications Intern** (half-time; paid), *Westword* (Denver, CO)
- Design advertisements
- Prepare photographs for publications
- Lay out the "Tempo" section
- Fact-check, edit, and proofread articles

6/10 - 8/12 **Customer Service Representative,** Wells Fargo Bank (Aurora CO).
- Sold accounts to customers; made all sales goals
- Created promotional posters

4/07 - 8/09 **Evening Assistant Manager,** McDonalds Restaurant (Longmont, CO).
- Supervised 7 cooks and counter workers
- Assured food and service quality

EDUCATION

8/11 – present Bachelor of Arts, The University of Denver, expected June 2013
Major: Graphic Arts; Minor: Digital Media Studies

8/09 – 5/11 AA General Education, Front Range Community College, May 2011

SKILLS AND SELECTED EXPERIENCES

- Expert in complete Adobe Creative Suite
- Expert in complete Microsoft Office Suite
- Excellent Spanish language skills
- Illustrator and photographer; have completed several commissions (see portfolio, above)
- Vice President, Student Residence Halls Association
- Cartoonist and Designer, *The DU Clarion* (campus newspaper)
- Excellent customer service skills

REFERENCES: Available on request

Quick Box 64.4

Guidelines for writing a job application letter

- Use one page only.
- Overall, think of your letter as a polite sales pitch about yourself and what benefits you can bring to the company. Don't be shy, but don't exaggerate.
- Use the same name, content, and format guidelines as for a business letter (see 64E).
- Address the letter to a specific person. If you can't discover a name, use a gender-neutral title such as "Dear Personnel Director."
  1. Telephone or send an e-mail to the company to which you're sending a letter or e-mail. State your reason for making contact, and ask for the name of the person to whom you need to address your letter.
  2. Address men as "Mr." and women as "Ms.," unless you're specifically told to use "Miss" or "Mrs." If your recipient goes by another title, such as "Dr." or "Professor," use it.
  3. If you can't identify a proper name and need to use a title alone, keep the title generic and gender-neutral.

     NO Dear Sir: [sexist] Dear Sir or Madam: [sexist for both genders]

     YES Dear Human Resources Officer: Dear Sales Manager:

- Open your letter by identifying the position for which you're applying.
- Mention your qualifications and explain how your background will meet the job requirements.
- Make clear that you're familiar with the company or organization; your research will impress the employer.
- End by being specific about what you can do for the company. If the job will be your first, give your key attributes—but make sure they're relevant. For instance, you might state that you're punctual, self-disciplined, eager to learn, and hardworking.
- State when you're available for an interview and how the potential employer can reach you.
- Edit and proofread the letter carefully. If you have to hand-correct even one error, print the letter again.

USAGE GLOSSARY

This usage glossary explains the customary manner of using particular words and PHRASES. As used here, *informal* and *colloquial* indicate that words or phrases occur commonly in speech but should be avoided in ACADEMIC WRITING. *Nonstandard* indicates that words or phrases should not be used in either standard spoken English or writing.

All grammatical terms mentioned here are defined in the Terms Glossary at the back of the book. Also consult the commonly confused words listed in Quick Box 49.2.

a, an Use *a* before words that begin with a consonant (*a dog, a grade, a hole*) or a consonant sound (*a one-day sale, a European*). Use *an* before words or acronyms that begin with a vowel sound or a silent *h* (*an owl, an hour, an MRI*). American English uses *a*, not *an*, before words starting with a pronounced *h*: *a* [*not* an] *historical event.*

accept, except The verb *accept* means "agree to, receive." As a preposition, *except* means "leaving out." As a verb, *except* means "exclude, leave out."

> The workers were ready to **accept** [verb] management's offer **except** [preposition] for one detail: They wanted the no-smoking rule **excepted** [verb] from the contract.

advice, advise *Advice*, a noun, means "recommendation." *Advise*, a verb, means "recommend, give advice."

> I **advise** [verb] you to follow your car mechanic's **advice** [noun].

affect, effect As a verb, *affect* means "cause a change in, influence." (*Affect* also functions as a noun in the discipline of psychology.) As a noun, *effect* means "result or conclusion"; as a verb, it means "bring about."

> Loud music **affects** people's hearing for life, so some bands have **effected** changes to lower the volume. Many fans, however, don't care about the harmful **effects** of high decibel levels.

aggravate, irritate *Aggravate* is used colloquially to mean "irritate." In formal writing, use *aggravate* to mean "intensify, make worse." Use *irritate* to mean "annoy, make impatient."

> The coach was **irritated** by her assistant's impatience, which **aggravated** the team's inability to concentrate.

ain't *Ain't* is a nonstandard contraction. Use *am not, is not*, or *are not* instead.

all right *All right* should be written as two words, never one (*not* alright).

allusion, illusion An *allusion* is an indirect reference to something. An *illusion* is a false impression or idea.

> The applicant's casual **allusions** to many European tourist attractions created the **illusion** that he had seen them himself.

a lot *A lot* is informal for *a great deal* or *a great many;* avoid it in academic writing. Write it as two words (*not* alot) when you do use it.

a.m., p.m. These abbreviations may also be written as A.M., P.M. Use them only with numbers, not as substitutes for *morning, afternoon*, or *evening.*

> We will arrive **in the afternoon** [*not* in the p.m.], and we have to leave no later than **8:00 a.m**.

among, amongst, between Use *among* for three or more items and *between* for two items. American English prefers *among* to *amongst.*

> My three roommates discussed **among** [*not* between *or* amongst] themselves the choice **between** staying in school and getting full-time jobs.

amount, number Use *amount* for uncountable things (*wealth, work, corn, happiness*). Use *number* for countable items.

> The **amount** of rice to cook depends on the **number** of dinner guests.

an See *a, an.*

and/or This term is appropriate in business and legal writing when either or both of two items can apply: *The process is quicker if you have a wireless connection and/or a fax machine.* In the humanities, writers usually express the alternatives in words: *This process is quicker if you have a wireless connection, a fax machine, or both.*

anyplace *Anyplace* is informal. Use *any place* or *anywhere* instead.

anyways, anywheres *Anyways* and *anywheres* are nonstandard. Use *anyway* and *anywhere* instead.

apt, likely, liable *Apt* and *likely* are used interchangeably. Strictly, *apt* indicates a tendency or inclination. *Likely* indicates a reasonable expectation or greater certainty than *apt. Liable* denotes legal responsibility or implies unpleasant consequences.

> Alan is **apt** to leave early on Friday. I will **likely** go with him to the party. Maggy and Gabriel are **liable** to be angry if we do not show up.

as, as if, as though, like Use *as, as if,* or *as though*, but not *like*, to introduce clauses.

> This hamburger tastes good, **as** [*not* like] a hamburger should. It tastes **as if** [*or* as though *but not* like] it were barbequed over charcoal.

Both *as* and *like* can function as prepositions in comparisons. Use *as* to indicate equivalence between two nouns or pronouns. Use *like* to indicate similarity but not equivalence.

> Beryl acted **as** [*not* like] the moderator in our panel.
>
> Mexico, **like** [*not* as] Argentina, belongs to the United Nations.

assure, ensure, insure *Assure* means "promise, convince." *Ensure* and *insure* both mean "make certain or secure," but *insure* is reserved for financial or legal certainty, as in insurance.

> The agent **assured** me that he could **insure** my roller blades but that only I could **ensure** that my elbows and knees would outlast the skates.

as to *As to* is nonstandard. Use *about* instead.

awful, awfully Do not use *awful* or *awfully* in place of *terribly, extremely*, or *very*.

a while, awhile As two words, *a while* (an article and a noun) can function as a subject or object. As one word, *awhile* is an adverb; it modifies verbs. In a prepositional phrase, the correct form is *a while: for a while, in a while, after a while.*

> The seals basked **awhile** in the sun after they had played for **a while** in the sea.

backup, back up As a noun, *backup* is a copy of electronic data. *Backup* can also be used as an adjective to mean "alternative." *Back up* is a verb phrase.

> Many people recommend that you **back up** even your **backup** files.

bad, badly *Bad* is an adjective; use it after linking verbs. (Remember that verbs like *feel* and *smell* can function as either linking verbs or action verbs.) *Badly* is an adverb and is nonstandard after linking verbs (see 32D).

> Farmers feel **bad** because a **bad** drought has **badly** damaged the crops.

beside, besides *Beside* is a preposition meaning "next to, by the side of."

> She stood **beside** the new car, insisting that she would drive.

As a preposition, *besides* means "other than, in addition to."

> No one **besides** her had a driver's license.

As an adverb, *besides* means "also, moreover."

> **Besides**, she owned the car.

better, had better Used in place of *had better, better* is informal.

> We **had better** [*not* We better] be careful.

between See *among, amongst, between.*

bring, take Use *bring* to indicate movement from a distant place to a near place or to the speaker. Use *take* to indicate movement from a near place or from the speaker to a distant place.

> If you **bring** a leash to my house, you can **take** the dog to the vet.

but, however, yet Use *but, however*, or *yet* alone, not in combination with each other.

> The economy is strong, **but** [*not* but yet *or* but however] unemployment is high.

can, may *Can* signifies ability or capacity; *may* requests or grants permission. In negations, however, *can* is acceptable in place of *may.*

> When you **can** get here on time, you **may** be excused early.

can't hardly, can't scarcely These double negatives are nonstandard (see 32C).

censor, censure The verb *censor* means "delete objectionable material, judge." The verb *censure* means "condemn or reprimand officially."

> The town council **censured** the mayor for trying to **censor** a report.

chairman, chairperson, chair Many prefer the gender-neutral terms *chairperson* and *chair* to *chairman; chair* is more common than *chairperson.*

complement, compliment Each term functions as both a noun and a verb. As a noun, *complement* means "something that goes well with or completes." As a noun, *compliment* means "praise, flattery." As a verb, *complement* means "bring to perfection, go well with; complete." As a verb, *compliment* means "praise, flatter."

> The president's **compliment** was a fine **complement** to our celebration.
>
> When the president **complimented** us, her praise **complemented** our joy.

comprise, include See *include, comprise.*

conscience, conscious The noun *conscience* means "a sense of right and wrong." The adjective *conscious* means "aware or awake."

> To live happily, be **conscious** of what your **conscience** tells you.

continual(ly), continuous(ly) *Continual* means "occurring again and again." *Continuous* means "occurring without interruption."

> Intravenous fluids were given **continuously** for three days after surgery, so nurses were **continually** hooking up new bottles of saline solution.

could care less *Could care less* is nonstandard; use *couldn't care less* instead.

could of *Could of* is nonstandard; use *could have* instead.

couple, a couple of These terms are informal. Use *a few* or *several* instead.

> Rest for **a few** [*not* a couple *or* a couple of] minutes.

criteria, criterion A *criterion* is "a standard of judgment." *Criteria* is the plural form of *criterion.*

> Although charisma is an important **criterion** for political candidates to meet, voters must also consider other **criteria**.

data This is the plural of *datum*, a rarely used word. Informally, *data* is commonly used as a singular noun requiring a singular verb. In academic or professional writing, it is more acceptable to treat *data* as plural.

> The researchers' **data** suggest that some people become addicted to e-mail.

different from, different than *Different from* is preferred for formal writing, although *different than* is common in speech.

> Please advise the council if your research produces data **different from** past results.

don't *Don't* is a contraction for *do not* but not for *does not* (use *doesn't*).

> She **doesn't** [*not* She don't] like crowds.

effect See *affect, effect.*

elicit, illicit The verb *elicit* means "draw forth or bring out." The adjective *illicit* means "illegal."

> The government's **illicit** conduct **elicited** mass protest.

emigrate (from), immigrate (to) *Emigrate* means "leave one country to live in another." *Immigrate* means "enter a country to live there."

> My great-grandmother **emigrated** from the Ukraine in 1890. After a brief stay in Germany, she **immigrated** to Canada in 1892.

ensure See *assure, ensure, insure.*

etc. *Etc.* is the abbreviation for the Latin *et cetera*, meaning "and the rest." For writing in the humanities, avoid using *etc.* outside parentheses. Acceptable substitutes are *and the like, and so on*, and *and so forth.*

everyday, every day The adjective *everyday* means "daily." *Every day* is an adjective-noun combination that can function as a subject or an object.

> Being late for work has become an **everyday** occurrence. **Every day** that I am late brings me closer to being fired.

everywheres Nonstandard for *everywhere.*

except See *accept, except.*

explicit, implicit *Explicit* means "directly stated or expressed." *Implicit* means "implied, suggested."

> The warning on cigarette packs is **explicit:** "Smoking is dangerous to health." The **implicit** message is "Don't smoke."

fewer, less Use *fewer* for anything that can be counted (with count nouns): *fewer dollars, fewer fleas, fewer haircuts.* Use *less* with collective or other noncount nouns: *less money, less scratching, less hair.*

finalize Academic audiences prefer *complete* or *make final* instead of *finalize.*

> After intense negotiations, the two nations **completed** [*not* finalized] a treaty.

former, latter When two items are referred to, *former* signifies the first one and *latter* signifies the second. Avoid using *former* and *latter* in a context with more than two items.

> Brazil and Ecuador are South American countries. Portuguese is the most common language in the **former**, Spanish in the **latter**.

go, say *Go* is nonstandard when used for forms of *say.*

> After he stepped on my hand, he **said** [*not* he goes], "Your hand was in my way."

gone, went *Gone* is the past participle of *go; went* is the past tense of *go.*

> They **went** [*not* gone] to the concert after Ira **had gone** [*not* had went] home.

good and This phrase is an informal intensifier; omit it from writing.

> They were **exhausted** [*not* good and tired].

good, well *Good* is an adjective. Using it as an adverb is nonstandard. *Well* is the equivalent adverb.

> **Good** maintenance helps cars run **well.**

hardly See *can't hardly, can't scarcely.*

have, of Use *have*, not *of*, after such verbs as *could, should, would, might*, and *must*.

> You **should have** [*not* should of] called first.

have got, have to, have got to Avoid using *have got* when *have* alone delivers your meaning.

> I **have** [*not* have got] two more sources to read.

Avoid using *have to* or *have got to* for *must*.

> I **must** [*not* have got to] finish this assignment today.

he/she, s/he, his, her To avoid sexist language, use *he or she* or *his or her*. A less wordy solution is to use plural pronouns and antecedents.

> Every mourner bowed **his or her** head [*not* his head *or* their head].
>
> The **mourners** bowed **their** heads.

humanity, humankind, humans, mankind To avoid sexist language, use *humanity, humankind*, or *humans* instead of *mankind*.

> Some people think computers have influenced **humanity** more than any other twentieth-century invention.

i.e. This abbreviation refers to the Latin term *id est*. In formal writing, use the English translation *that is*.

if, whether At the start of a noun clause, use either *if* or *whether*.

> I don't know **if** [*or* whether] I want to dance with you.

In conditional clauses, use *whether* (*or* whether or not) when alternatives are expressed or implied.

> I will dance with you **whether or not** I like the music. I will dance with you **whether** the next song is fast or slow.

In a conditional clause that does not express or imply alternatives, use *if*.

> **If** you promise not to step on my feet, I will dance with you.

illicit See *elicit, illicit.*

illusion See *allusion, illusion.*

immigrate See *emigrate, immigrate.*

imply, infer *Imply* means "hint at or suggest." *Infer* means "draw a conclusion." A writer or speaker implies; a reader or listener infers.

> When the governor **implied** that she would not seek reelection, reporters **inferred** that she was planning to run for vice president.

include, comprise The verb *include* means "contain or regard as part of a whole." The verb *comprise* means "to be composed of."

inside of, outside of These phrases are nonstandard when used to mean *inside* or *outside.*

> She waited **outside** [*not* outside of] the dormitory.

In time references, avoid using *inside of* to mean "in less than."

I changed clothes **in less than** [*not* inside of] ten minutes.

insure See *assure, ensure, insure.*

irregardless *Irregardless* is nonstandard. Use *regardless* instead.

is when, is where Avoid these constructions in giving definitions.

Defensive driving **requires that** [*not* is when] drivers stay alert.

its, it's *Its* is a possessive pronoun. *It's* is a contraction of *it is.*

The dog buried **its** bone.

It's a hot day.

kind, sort Use *this* or *that* with these singular nouns; use *these* or *those* with the plural nouns *kinds* and *sorts.* Also, do not use *a* or *an* after *kind of* or *sort of.*

Drink **these kinds of** fluids [*not* this kind of fluids] on **this sort of** [*not* this sort of a] day.

kind of, sort of These phrases are colloquial adverbs. In formal writing, use *somewhat* instead.

The campers were **somewhat** [*not* kind of] dehydrated after the hike.

lay, lie *Lay* (*laid, laid, laying*) means "place or put something, usually on something else" and needs a direct object. *Lie* (*lay, lain, lying*), meaning "recline," does not take a direct object (see 28M). Substituting *lay* for *lie* is nonstandard.

Lay [*not* Lie] the blanket down, and then **lay** the babies on it so they can **lie** [*not* lay] in the shade.

leave, let *Leave* means "depart"; *let* means "allow, permit." *Leave* is nonstandard for *let.*

Let [*not* Leave] me use your car tonight.

less See *fewer, less.*

lie See *lay, lie.*

like See *as, as if, as though, like.*

likely See *apt, likely, liable.*

lots, lots of, a lot of These are colloquial usages. Use *many, much,* or *a great deal* instead.

mankind See *humanity, humankind, humans, mankind.*

may See *can, may.*

maybe, may be *Maybe* is an adverb; *may be* is a verb phrase.

Maybe [adverb] we can win, but our team **may be** [verb phrase] too tired.

may of, might of *May of* and *might of* are nonstandard. Use *may have* and *might have* instead.

media This word is the plural of *medium*, yet colloquial usage now pairs it with a singular verb.

> The **media** saturates us with information about every fire.

morale, moral *Morale* is a noun meaning "a mental state relating to courage, confidence, or enthusiasm." As a noun, *moral* means an "ethical lesson implied or taught by a story or event"; as an adjective, *moral* means "ethical."

> One **moral** to draw from corporate downsizings is that overstressed employees suffer from low **morale**. Unhappy employees with otherwise high **moral** standards may steal from their employers.

most *Most* is nonstandard for *almost: Almost* [*not* Most] *all the dancers agree. Most* is correct as the superlative form of an adjective (*some, more, most*): *Most dancers agree*. It also makes the superlative form of adverbs and some adjectives: *most suddenly, most important.*

Ms. *Ms.* is a women's title free of reference to marital status, equivalent to *Mr.* for men. For a woman who does not use *Dr.* or another title, use *Ms.* unless she requests *Miss* or *Mrs.*

must of *Must of* is nonstandard. Use *must have* instead.

nowheres Nonstandard for *nowhere.*

number See *amount, number.*

of Use *have* instead of *of* after the following verbs: *could, may, might, must, should*, and *would.*

OK, O.K., okay All three forms are acceptable in informal writing. In academic writing, try to express meaning more specifically.

> The weather was **suitable** [*not* OK] for the picnic.

outside of See *inside of, outside of.*

plus *Plus* is nonstandard as a substitute for *and, also, in addition*, or *moreover.*

> The band will give three concerts in Hungary, **and** [*not* plus] it will tour Poland for a month. **Also** [*not* Plus], it may perform once in Vienna.

precede, proceed *Precede* means "go before." *Proceed* means "advance, go on; undertake; carry on."

> **Preceded** by elephants and tigers, the clowns **proceeded** into the tent.

pretty *Pretty* is an informal qualifying word; in academic writing, use *rather, quite, somewhat*, or *very.*

> The flu epidemic was **quite** [*not* pretty] severe.

principal, principle *Principle* means "a basic truth or rule." As a noun, *principal* means "chief person; main or original amount"; as an adjective, *principal* means "most important."

> During the assembly, the **principal** said, "A **principal** value in this society is the **principle** of free speech."

proceed See *precede, proceed.*

quotation, quote *Quotation* is a noun; *quote* is a verb. Do not use *quote* as a noun.

> The newspaper **quoted** the attorney general, and the **quotations** [*not* quotes] quickly showed up in public health messages.

raise, rise *Raise* (*raised, raised, raising*) means "lift" and needs a direct object. *Rise* (*rose, risen, rising*) means "go upward" and does not take a direct object (see 28M). Using these verbs interchangeably is nonstandard.

> If the citizens **rise** [*not* raise] up in protest, they may **raise** the flag of liberty.

real, really *Real* is nonstandard as an intensifier, and *really* is almost always unnecessary; leave it out.

reason is because This phrase is redundant; use *reason is that* instead.

> One **reason** we moved **is that** [*not* is because] we changed jobs.

regardless See *irregardless.*

respective, respectively The adjective *respective* relates the noun it modifies to two or more individual persons or things. The adverb *respectively* refers to a second set of items in a sequence established by a preceding set of items.

> After the fire drill, Dr. Pan and Dr. Moll returned to their **respective** offices [that is, each to his or her office] on the second and third floors, **respectively**. [Dr. Pan has an office on the second floor; Dr. Moll has an office on the third floor.]

right *Right* is a colloquial intensifier; use *quite, very, extremely,* or a similar word for most purposes.

> You did **very** [*not* right] well on the quiz.

rise See *raise, rise.*

scarcely See *can't hardly, can't scarcely.*

seen The past participle of *see* (*see, saw, seen, seeing*), *seen* is a nonstandard substitute for the past-tense form, *saw*. As a verb, *seen* must be used with an auxiliary verb.

> Last night, I **saw** [*not* seen] the show that you **had seen** in Florida.

set, sit *Set* (*set, set, setting*) means "put in place, position, put down" and must have a direct object. *Sit* (*sat, sat, sitting*) means "be seated" and does not take a direct object (see 28M). Using these verbs interchangeably is nonstandard.

> Susan **set** [*not* sat] the sandwiches beside the salad, made Spot **sit** [*not* set] down, and then **sat** [*not* set] on the sofa.

should of *Should of* is nonstandard. Use *should have* instead.

sit See *set, sit.*

sometime, sometimes, some time The adverb *sometime* means "at an unspecified time." The adverb *sometimes* means "now and then." *Some time* is an adjective–noun combination meaning "an amount or span of time."

> **Sometime** next year we have to take qualifying exams. I **sometimes** worry about finding **some time** to study for them.

sort of See *kind of, sort of*.

such *Such* is an informal intensifier; avoid it in academic writing unless it precedes a noun introducing a *that* clause.

> The play got **terrible** [*not* such terrible] reviews. It was **such** a dull drama **that** it closed after one performance.

supposed to, used to The final *d* is essential in both phrases.

> We were **supposed to** [*not* suppose to] leave early. I **used to** [*not* use to] wake up as soon as the alarm rang.

sure *Sure* is nonstandard as a substitute for *surely* or *certainly*.

> I was **certainly** [*not* sure] surprised at the results.

sure and, try and Both phrases are nonstandard. Use *sure to* and *try to* instead.

than, then *Than* indicates comparison; *then* relates to time.

> Please put on your gloves, and **then** put on your hat. It is colder outside **than** inside.

that there, them there, this here, these here These phrases are nonstandard. Use *that, them, this*, and *these*, respectively.

that, which Use *that* with restrictive (essential) clauses only. *Which* can be used with both restrictive and nonrestrictive clauses; many writers, however, use *which* only for nonrestrictive clauses and *that* for all restrictive clauses (see 42F).

> The house **that** [*or* which] Jack built is on Beanstalk Street, **which** [*not* that] runs past the reservoir.

their, there, they're *Their* is a possessive. *There* means "in that place" or is part of an expletive construction (see 40C). *They're* is a contraction of *they are*.

> **They're** going to **their** accounting class in the building **there** behind the library. **There** are twelve sections of Accounting 101.

theirself, theirselves, themself These are nonstandard. Use *themselves* instead.

them Use *them* as an object pronoun only. Do not use *them* in place of the adjective *these* or *those*.

> Buy **those** [*not* them] strawberries.

then See *than, then*.

till, until Both are acceptable; except in expressive writing, avoid the contracted form *'til*.

to, too, two *To* is a preposition. *Too* is an adverb meaning "also; more than enough." *Two* is the number.

When you go **to** Chicago, visit the Art Institute. Go **to** Harry Caray's for dinner, **too**. It won't be **too** expensive because **two** people can share an entrée.

try and, sure and See *sure and, try and.*

type *Type* is nonstandard when used to mean *type of.*

Use that **type of** [*not* type] glue on plastic.

unique *Unique* is an absolute adjective; do not combine it with *more, most,* or other qualifiers.

Solar heating is **uncommon** [*not* somewhat unique] in the Northeast. A **unique** [*not* very unique] heating system in one Vermont home uses hydrogen for fuel.

used to See *supposed to, used to.*

utilize Academic writers prefer *use* to *utilize.*

The team **used** [*not* utilized] all its players to win the game.

way, ways When referring to distance, use *way* rather than *ways.*

He is a long **way** [*not* ways] from home.

well See *good, well.*

where *Where* is nonstandard when used for *that* as a subordinating conjunction.

I read **that** [*not* where] Bill Gates is the richest man alive.

Where is your house? [*not* Where is your house at?]

whether See *if, whether.*

which See *that, which.*

who, whom Use *who* as a subject or a subject complement. Use *whom* as an object (see 28M).

who's, whose *Who's* is a contraction of *who is. Whose* is a possessive pronoun.

Who's willing to drive? **Whose** truck should we take?

would of *Would of* is nonstandard. Use *would have* instead.

your, you're *Your* is a possessive. *You're* is the contraction of *you are.*

You're generous to volunteer **your** time at the elementary school.

TERMS GLOSSARY

Words printed in SMALL CAPITAL LETTERS in your *Simon & Schuster Handbook for Writers* indicate important terms that are defined in this glossary. The parenthetical references with each definition tell you the handbook sections where each term is most fully discussed. If you can't find a term's definition in this glossary, look for the term in the Index.

absolute phrase A phrase containing a subject and a participle that modifies an entire sentence: *The semester* [subject] *being* [present participle of *be*] *over, the campus looks deserted.* (28O)

abstract A very short summary that presents all the important ideas of a longer piece of writing. Sometimes appears before the main writing, as in APA style. (26F)

abstract noun A noun that names something not knowable through the five senses: *idea, respect.* (28B)

academic writing The writing people do for college courses and as scholarship published in print and online journals. (6D)

action verb A verb that describes an action or occurrence done by or to the subject. (40E)

active reading Annotating reading to make connections between your prior knowledge and the author's ideas. (3D)

active voice When a verb shows that its action or the condition expressed is done *by* the subject. The *active voice* stands in contrast with the *passive voice,* which conveys that the verb's action or condition is done *to* the subject. (29N)

adjective A word that describes or limits (modifies) a noun, a pronoun, or a word group functioning as a noun: *silly* joke, *three* trumpets. (28F, Ch. 32)

adjective clause A dependent clause, also known as a *relative clause,* that modifies a noun or pronoun that comes before it. An adjective clause begins with a relative word (such as *who, which, that,* or *where*). Also see *clause.* (28P)

advanced searches Also called *guided searches.* Allow you to search by entering information in a form online. (22D)

adverb A word that describes or limits (modifies) verbs, adjectives, other adverbs, phrases, or clauses: *loudly, very, nevertheless, there.* (28G, Ch. 32)

adverb clause A dependent clause beginning with a subordinating conjunction that establishes the relationship in meaning between itself and its independent clause. An adverb clause can modify an independent clause's verb or an entire independent clause. (28P)

agreement The concept of matching number and person of a subject and verb and of a pronoun and its antecedent. See also *antecedent.* (Ch. 31)

analogy An explanation of the unfamiliar in terms of the familiar, often comparing things not usually associated with each other. Analogy is a rhetorical strategy useful for developing a paragraph (6H). Unlike a simile, which uses *like* or *as* in making a comparison, an analogy does not use such words. (37H)

analysis A process of critical thinking, sometimes called *division,* that divides a whole into its component parts that shows how the parts interrelate. Analysis is a rhetorical strategy useful for developing paragraphs. (6H, Ch. 14)

analytical frameworks Systematic ways of investigating a work. (59B)

annotated bibliography Bibliography in which listed sources are accompanied by summaries of, or comments about, each source. (21O)

annotating Brief summaries or comments about a reading, perhaps in the margins, on a separate page, or in a computer file. (3D)

antecedent The noun or pronoun to which a pronoun refers. (30L)

APA style *APA* is the abbreviation for the American Psychological Association. APA style specifies the format and the form of citation and documentation used in source-based papers in many academic disciplines, especially psychology and most other social sciences. (Ch. 26)

appositive A word or group of words that renames the noun or noun phrase coming immediately before or after it: *my favorite month,* ***October***. (28N)

argumentative writing Using rhetorical strategies to convince one's readers to agree with the writer's position about a topic open to debate. (Ch. 15)

articles Also called *determiners* or *noun markers*, the words *a, an*, and *the*. *A* and *an* are indefinite articles; *the* is a definite article. Also see *determiner*. (28F, Ch. 53)

assertion A statement that expresses a point of view about a topic. Often used by writers to develop a thesis statement. (5E)

assumption An idea or value that a writer takes for granted without proof. (3E)

audience The readers to whom a written document is primarily directed. (TIP 4, 5D)

auxiliary verb Also known as a *helping verb*, a form of *be, do, have*, or one of the modal verbs. Auxiliary verbs combine with main verbs to express tense, mood, and voice. Also see *modal auxiliary verbs*. (29E)

balanced sentences Sentences consisting of two short independent clauses that serve to compare or contrast. (39A)

bias Material that is slanted toward beliefs or attitudes and away from facts or evidence. (Ch. 43)

bibliographic note system Documentation system used by the *Chicago Manual of Style*. (27A)

bibliography A list of sources with their authorial and publication facts. (22H)

block style Style used in writing business letters. Block style uses no indents, single spacing within paragraphs and double spacing between paragraphs. All lines start flush left, which means at the left margin. (64E)

blog Shortened form of "Web log," an online journal usually updated on a fairly regular basis. (63B)

body paragraphs Paragraphs in an essay or other document that come between the introductory and concluding paragraphs. (6D)

book catalog Database that lists all books and bound volumes owned by a particular library. (Ch. 22)

Boolean expressions Words such as *AND, OR*, and *NOT* that researchers can use in a search engine to create keyword combinations that narrow and refine their searches. (22D)

brainstorming Listing all ideas that come to mind on a topic, and then grouping the ideas by whatever patterns emerge. (5E)

browser Software that allows people to connect to the Internet. Common examples are Microsoft Internet Explorer and Mozilla Firefox. (22C)

bureaucratic language Sometimes called *bureaucratese;* language that is overblown or overly complex. (37J)

call number Identification number, usually according to the Dewey Decimal System, used to store and retrieve an individual book or other library material. (22F)

case The form of a noun or pronoun that shows whether it's functioning as a subject, an object, or a possessive in a particular context. Nouns change form in the possessive case only (*city* can be a subject or object; *city's* is the possessive form). Also see *pronoun case*. (30A–30K, 45B)

case study Research that relies on the careful, detailed observation and analysis of one person or a small group of people. (60B)

catalog Also called a *card catalog*, often in digitized form an extensive and methodically organized list of all books and other bound volumes in a library. (22F)

cause and effect The relationship between outcomes (effects) and the reasons for them (causes), which is a rhetorical strategy for developing paragraphs. (6H, Ch. 13)

chronological order Also called *time order*, an arrangement of information according to time sequence; an organizing strategy for sentences, paragraphs, and longer pieces of writing. (6H)

citation Information that identifies a source referred to in a piece of writing. Also see *documentation*. (Chs. 25 and 26)

claim States an issue and then takes a position on a debatable topic related to the issue, supported with evidence and reasons. (5E)

classical argument An argument with a structure consisting of introduction, thesis statement, background, evidence and reasoning, response to opposing views, and conclusion. (15A)

classification A rhetorical strategy that organizes information by grouping items according to their underlying shared characteristics. (6H)

clause A group of words containing a subject and a predicate. A clause that delivers full meaning is called an *independent* (or *main*) *clause*. A clause that lacks full meaning by itself is called a *dependent* (or *subordinate*) *clause*. Also see *adjective clause, adverb clause, nonrestrictive element, noun clause, restrictive element*. (28P)

cliché An overused, worn-out phrase that has lost its capacity to communicate effectively: *soft as a kitten, lived to a ripe old age*. (37J)

close reading The practice of reading carefully, analytically, and critically. (3D)

clustering Also called *mapping*, it is an invention technique based on thinking visually about a topic and drawing attached balloons for its increasingly specific subdivisions. (5E)

CM style *CM*, the abbreviation for *Chicago Manual* style, is a form of citation and documentation used in many academic disciplines, including history and the arts. (27A–27B)

coherence The written or spoken progression from one idea to another using transitional expressions, pronouns, selective repetition, and/or parallelism to make connections between ideas explicit. (6G)

collaborative writing Students working together to write a paper. (Ch. 9)

collective noun A noun that names a group of people or things: *family, committee*. (31J)

colloquial language Casual or conversational language. (37J)

comma splice Sometimes called a *comma fault*, the error that occurs when a comma alone connects two independent clauses. (Ch. 34)

common noun A noun that names a general group, place, person, or thing: *dog, house*. (28B)

comparative The form of a descriptive adjective or adverb that expresses a different degree of intensity between two things: *bluer, less blue; more easily, less easily*. Also see *superlative*. (32E)

comparison and contrast A rhetorical strategy for organizing and developing paragraphs by discussing a subject's similarities (by comparing them) and differences (by contrasting them). (6H)

complement A grammatical element after a verb that completes the predicate, such as a direct object after an action verb or a noun or adjective after a linking verb. Also see *object complement* and *subject complement*. (28N, 29A)

complete predicate See *predicate*.

complete subject See *subject*.

complex sentence See *sentence*.

compound-complex sentence See *sentence*.

compound predicate See *predicate*.

compound sentence See *sentence*.

compound subject See *subject*.

compound word Two or more words placed together to express one concept, such as "fuel-efficient" or "proofread." (49G)

conciseness Writing that is direct and to the point. Its opposite, which is undesirable, is *wordiness*. (Ch. 40)

concluding paragraph Final paragraph of an essay, report, or other document. (6J)

concrete noun A noun naming something that can be seen, touched, heard, smelled, or tasted: *smoke, sidewalk*. (28B)

conjunction A word that connects or otherwise establishes a relationship between two or more words, phrases, or clauses. Also see *coordinating conjunction, correlative conjunction, subordinating conjunction*. (28I)

conjunctive adverb An adverb that expresses a relationship between words, such as addition, contrast, comparison, and the like. (28G)

connotation Ideas implied, not directly stated, by a word giving emotional overtones. (37F)

content notes Notes researchers write to record information about what each source they've found says—along with publication information so that the researcher can find the source again if needed. (21P)

context The circumstances that exist when a piece is written. (4F)

contraction A word in which an apostrophe takes the place of one or more omitted letters: *can't, don't, I'm, isn't, it's, let's, they're, we've, won't*, and others. (45D)

coordinate adjectives Two or more adjectives that carry equal weight in modifying a noun (***big, friendly*** *dog*). The order of coordinating adjectives can be changed without changing the meaning. Also see *cumulative adjectives*. (42E)

coordinate sentences Two or more independent clauses joined by either a semicolon or a comma with coordinating conjunction showing their relationship; also called a *compound sentence*. Also see *coordination*. (38F)

coordinating conjunction A conjunction that joins two or more grammatically equivalent structures: *and, or, for, nor, but, so, yet*. (28I, 38G)

coordination The use of grammatically equivalent forms to show a balance in, or sequence of, ideas. (38D)

correlative conjunction A pair of words that joins equivalent grammatical structures: *both . . . and; either . . . or; not only . . . but also*. (28I)

count noun A noun that names items that can be counted: *radio, street, idea, fingernail*. (52A)

critical thinking A form of thinking in which you take control of your conscious thought processes by judging evidence, considering assumptions, making connections, and analyzing implications. (3A)

CSE style *CSE*, the abbreviation for the Council of Science Editors, is a form of citation and documentation used in the natural sciences. (27C–27D)

cue words Words that tell what an assignment suggests that students accomplish in their writing. (58B)

cumulative adjectives Adjectives that build up meaning from word to word as they get closer to the noun (***familiar rock*** *tunes*). The order of cumulative adjectives cannot be changed without destroying the meaning. Also see *coordinating adjectives*. (42E)

cumulative sentence The most common structure for a sentence, with the subject and a verb first, followed by modifiers adding details; also called a *loose sentence*. (38O)

dangling modifier A modifier that illogically attaches its meaning to the rest of its sentence, either because it is closer to another noun or pronoun than to its true subject or because its true subject is not expressed in the sentence. (Ch. 35)

database An electronic collection of citations and, frequently, articles or documents on a particular subject matter or field, or about a specific body of sources. (22C)

declarative sentence A sentence that makes a statement: *Sky diving is exciting.* Also see *exclamatory sentence, imperative sentence, interrogative sentence.* (28L)

deductive reasoning The process of reasoning from general claims to a specific instance. (3H)

definition A rhetorical strategy that defines or gives the meaning of terms or ideas. (6H)

deliberate repetition A writing technique that uses the conscious repetition of a word, phrase, or other element to emphasize a point or to achieve a specific effect on readers. (6G)

demonstrative pronoun A pronoun that points out the antecedent: *this, these; that, those.* (28C)

denotation The dictionary definition of a word. (37F)

dependent clause Also called *subordinate clause,* a subordinate clause can't stand alone as an independent grammatical unit. If it tries to, it is a sentence fragment. Also see *adjective clause, adverb clause, noun clause.* (28P)

description A statement that paints a picture in words. (6H)

descriptive adverb An adverb that describes the condition or properties of whatever it is modifying and has comparative and superlative forms: *happily, more happily, most happily.* (28G)

determiner A word or word group, traditionally identified as an *adjective,* that limits a noun by telling whether a noun is general (**a** noun) or specific (**the** tree). (28F, 52B)

dialect Also called *regional language.* Language that is specific to a particular geographic area. (37B)

diction Word choice. (37F)

digital portfolio A collection of several texts in electronic format to represent the range of your skills and abilities. (8D)

direct address Words naming a person or group being spoken to: *"The solution,* ***my friends****, is in your hands."* (30R)

direct discourse Words that repeat speech or conversation exactly, always enclosed in quotation marks. Also see *indirect discourse.* (36E, 42G)

direct object A noun, pronoun, or group of words functioning as a noun that receives the action (completes the meaning) of a transitive verb. (28M)

direct question A sentence that asks a question and ends with a question mark: *Are you going to the concert?* (41C)

direct quotation See *quotation.*

direct title A title that tells exactly what the essay will be about. (5J)

documentation The acknowledgment of a source's words and ideas being used in any written document by giving full and accurate information about the source of the words used and about where those words can be found. Also see *documentation style.* (Chs. 25–27)

documentation style Any of various systems for providing information about the source of words, information, and ideas that a writer quotes, paraphrases, or summarizes from any source other than the writer. Documentation styles discussed in this handbook are MLA (Ch. 25), APA (Ch. 26), CM (27A–27B), and CSE (27C–27D).

document design The arrangement of words, images, graphics, and space on a page or screen. (Ch. 7)

double negative A nonstandard structure that uses two negative modifiers rather than one. (32C)

drafting The part of the writing process in which writers compose ideas in sentences and paragraphs, thereby creating *drafts*. A *discovery draft* is what some writers call an early, rough draft. (5G)

editing The part of the writing process in which writers check a document for the technical correctness in edited American English of its grammar, sentence structure, punctuation, spelling, and mechanics. (5J)

elliptical construction A sentence structure that deliberately omits words that can be filled in because they repeat words already in the sentence. (36H)

emotional appeal Rhetorical strategy intended to evoke empathy and compassion. Its Greek name is *pathos*. (3B, 15C)

ethical appeal Rhetorical strategy intended to evoke confidence in your credibility, reliability, and trustworthiness. Its Greek name is *ethos*. (3B, 15C)

ethnography A research method that involves careful observation of a group of people or a setting, often over a period of time. Ethnography also refers to the written work that results from this research. (60B)

euphemism Language that attempts to blunt certain realities by speaking of them in "nice" or "tactful" words. (37J)

evaluation Examining new ideas independently and fairly, avoiding biases and prejudices that you might have accepted without question before. (3G)

evidence Facts, data, and examples used to support a writer's assertions and conclusions. (24G)

example Specific incident or instance provided to illustrate a point. (6H)

exclamatory sentence A sentence beginning with *What* or *How* that expresses strong feeling: *What a ridiculous statement!* (28L)

expletive construction The phrase *there is (are), there was (were), it is (was)* at the beginning of a clause, which postpones the subject: *It is Mars that we hope to reach* (a better version would be *We hope to reach Mars*). (40C)

expressive writing Writing that reflects your personal thoughts and feelings. (4B)

fact Information or data widely accepted as true. (3E)

faulty parallelism Grammatically incorrect writing that results from nonmatching grammatical forms linked with coordinating conjunctions. (39D)

faulty predication A grammatically illogical combination of subject and predicate: *The purpose of television was invented to entertain*. (36G)

field research Primary research that involves going into, and taking notes on, real-life situations to observe, survey, interview, or be part of some activity. (21L)

figurative language Words that carry other meanings in addition to their literal meanings, sometimes by making unusual comparisons. Also see *analogy, irony, metaphor, personification, overstatement, simile, understatement*. (37H)

first person See *person*.

focused freewriting Freewriting that starts with a set topic or builds on one sentence taken from earlier freewriting. (5E)

formal outline An outline that lays out the topic levels of generalities or hierarchies and marks them with roman numerals, letters, and numbers indented in a carefully prescribed fashion. (5F)

frame Guides that suggest how to develop or structure an essay or assignment. (Part 2)

freewriting Writing nonstop for a period of time to generate ideas by free association of thoughts. (5E)

future perfect progressive tense The form of the future perfect tense that describes an action or condition ongoing until some specific future time: *I will have been talking when you arrive.* (29G)

future perfect tense The tense indicating that an action will have been completed or a condition will have ended by a specified point in the future: *I will have talked to him by the time you arrive.* (29I)

future progressive tense The form of the future tense showing that a future action will continue for some time: *I will be talking when you arrive.* (29G)

future tense The form of a verb, made with the simple form and either *shall* or *will*, expressing an action yet to be taken or a condition not yet experienced: *I will talk.* (29G)

gender The classification of words as masculine, feminine, or neuter. In English, a few pronouns show changes in gender in third-person singular: *he, him, his; she, her, hers; it, its, its;* also few nouns that define roles change form to show gender difference (*prince, princess*), but most no longer do (*actor, police officer, chairperson*). (37I)

gender-neutral language Nonsexist language. Also see *sexist language.* (37I)

general databases Include sources from a broad range of periodicals and books, both popular and scholarly. (22C)

generalization A broad statement without details. (Ch. 1)

general reference work The starting point for many college researchers that help identify keywords useful in searching for subject headings and catalogs—and for finding examples and verifying facts. (22H)

genre A category of writing characterized by certain features; for example, a short story or a research report. (4E)

gerund A present participle functioning as a noun: ***Walking*** *is good exercise.* Also see *verbal.* (28E, Ch. 56)

gerund phrase A gerund, along with its modifiers and/or object(s), which functions as a subject or an object: ***Walking the dog*** *can be good exercise.* See also *gerund.* (28O)

helping verb See *auxiliary verb.*

homonyms Words spelled differently that sound alike: *to, too, two.* (49F)

home page The opening main page of a Web site that provides access to other pages on the site categories. (63F)

hyperbole See *overstatement.*

hyperlink Connection from one digital document to another online. (63F)

idiom A word, phrase, or other construction that has a different meaning from its usual or literal meaning: *He lost his head. She hit the ceiling.* (Ch. 55)

illustration Provides support for the main idea of a paragraph by giving several examples, often ones that call on the five senses to picture them. (6H)

imperative mood The grammatical form that expresses commands and direct requests, using the simple form of the verb and almost always implying but not expressing the subject: *Watch out.* (29L)

imperative sentence A sentence that gives a command. *Go to the corner to buy me a newspaper.* (28L)

indefinite pronoun A pronoun, such as *all, anyone, each*, and others, that refers to a nonspecific person or thing. (31I, 31R)

independent clause A clause that can stand alone as an independent grammatical unit. (28P)

index List of main terms used in a text and the page(s) on which each term can be found. (22A)

indicative mood The grammatical form of verbs used for statements about real things or highly likely ones: *I think Grace will be arriving today.* (29L)

indirect discourse Reported speech or conversation that does not use the exact structure of the original and so is not enclosed in quotation marks. (36E, 42G)

indirect object A noun, pronoun, or group of words functioning as a noun that tells to whom, or for whom, the action expressed by a transitive verb was done. (28M)

indirect question A sentence that reports a question and ends with a period, not a question mark: *I asked if you are going.* (41C)

indirect quotation A quotation that reports a source's words without quotation marks, unless any words are repeated exactly from the source. It requires documentation of the source to avoid plagiarism. Also see *indirect discourse.* (42H)

indirect title Hints at an essay's topic; tries to catch the reader's interest by presenting a puzzle that can be solved by reading the essay. (5J)

inductive reasoning A form of reasoning that moves from particular facts or instances to general principles. (3H)

inference What is implied, not stated, by words. (3C)

infinitive A verbal made of the simple form of a verb and usually, but not always, preceded by the word *to.* It functions as a noun, an adjective, or an adverb. (Ch. 55)

infinitive phrase An infinitive, with its modifiers and/or object, which functions as a noun, an adjective, or an adverb. (28O)

informal outline Outline that doesn't follow the rules of a *formal outline.* (5F)

informal writing Word choice that creates a tone appropriate for casual writing or speaking. (37D)

intensive pronoun A pronoun that ends in *-self* and that intensifies its antecedent: *Vida **himself** argued against it.* Also see *reflexive pronoun.* (30K)

interjection An emotion-conveying word that is treated as a sentence, starting with a capital letter and ending with an exclamation point or a period: *Oh! Ouch.* (28J)

interrogative pronoun A pronoun, such as *whose* or *what,* that implies a question: *Who called?* (28C)

interrogative sentence A sentence that asks a direct question: *Did you see that?* (28L)

in-text citation Source information placed in parentheses within the body of a research paper. Also see *citation, parenthetical documentation.* (Chs. 25 and 26)

intransitive verb A verb that does not take a direct object. (29F)

introductory paragraph Opening paragraph of document that orients readers and generates interest in the topic or ideas that follow. (6C)

inverted word order In contrast to standard order, the main or auxiliary verb comes before the subject in a sentence: *In **walks*** [verb] *the president* [subject]. Most questions and some exclamations use inverted word order: *Did* [verb] *you* [subject] *see the circus?* (31H, 38B)

irony Using words to imply the opposite of their usual meaning. (37H)

irregular verb A verb that forms the past tense and past participle other than by adding *-ed* or *-d.* (29D)

jargon Specialized vocabulary of a particular field or group that is not familiar to a general reader. (37J)

justify When used as a design term, it refers to aligning text evenly along both the left and right margins. (7C)

keywords Main words in a source's title, or that the author or an editor has identified as central to that source. Sometimes keywords are called *descriptors* or *identifiers.* (22D)

levels of formality The degrees of formality of language, reflected by word choice and sentence structure. A formal level is used for ceremonial and other occasions when stylistic flourishes are appropriate. A semiformal level, which is neither too formal nor too casual, is acceptable for most academic writing. (5J, 37D)

linking verb A main verb that links a subject with a subject complement that renames or describes the subject. Linking verbs convey a state of being, relate to the senses, or indicate a condition. (29A)

literal meaning What is stated "on the line" explicitly by words. (3C)

logical appeal Rhetorical strategy that intends to show readers that the argument depends on formal reasoning, including providing evidence and drawing conclusions from premises. Its Greek name is *logos*. (3B)

logical fallacies Flaws in reasoning that lead to illogical statements that need to be rejected in logical arguments. (3I)

long quotation A direct quotation that in an MLA-style source-based paper occupies, if it is prose, more than four lines of type, and if it is poetry, more than three lines of the poem. In an APA-style source-based paper, if it is more than forty words of prose. Long quotations are block indented on the page. Also see *short quotation*. (46C)

main clause See *independent clause*.

main verb A verb that expresses action, occurrence, or state of being and that shows mood, tense, voice, number, and person. (28D, 29B)

mechanics Conventions governing the use of capital letters, italics, abbreviations, and numbers. (Chs. 48–49)

memo Commonly shortened term for *memorandum*. A brief form of business correspondence with a format that is headed with lines for "To," "From," "Date," and "Subject" (or "Re") and uses the rest of its space for its message. (64D)

metaphor A comparison implying similarity between two things: *a mop of hair*. A metaphor does not use the words *like* or *as*, which are used in a simile to make a comparison explicit: *hair* ***like*** *a mop*. (37H)

misplaced modifier Describing or limiting words that are wrongly positioned in a sentence so that their message either is illogical or relates to the wrong word(s). (Ch. 35)

mixed sentence A sentence that unintentionally changes from one grammatical structure to another incompatible grammatical structure, so that the result is garbled meaning. (36F)

mixed metaphor Inconsistent metaphors in a single expression: *You'll get into hot water skating on thin ice*. (37H)

MLA style *MLA*, the abbreviation for the Modern Language Association, specifies the format and the form of citation and documentation in source-based papers in English and some other humanities courses. (Ch. 25)

modal auxiliary verb A group of auxiliary verbs that communicate possibility, likelihood, obligation, permission, or ability: *can, might, would*. (29E)

modifier A word or group of words functioning as an adjective or adverb to describe or limit (modify) another word or word group. (28N)

mood The attribute of verbs showing a writer's orientation to an action by the way the verbs are used. English has three moods: imperative, indicative, and subjunctive. Also see *imperative mood, indicative mood, subjunctive mood*. (29L)

multimodal The use of a combination of words and images. (3L)

narrative writing Writing that tells a story. (6H)

netiquette Coined from the word *etiquette*, netiquette is good manners when using e-mail, the Internet, and online sites such as bulletin boards, chat rooms, etc. (63G)

noncount noun A noun that names "uncountable" things: *water, time*. (52A)

nonrestrictive clause A clause that is not essential to the sentence's meaning. (30S)

nonrestrictive element A descriptive word, phrase, or dependent clause that provides information not essential to understanding the basic message of the element it modifies; it is therefore set off by commas. Also see *restrictive element.* (42F)

nonsexist language See *sexist language.*

noun A word that names a person, place, thing, or idea. Nouns function as subjects, objects, or complements. (28B)

noun clause A dependent clause that functions as a subject, object, or complement. (28P)

noun phrase A noun along with its modifiers functioning as a subject, object, or complement. (28O)

number The attribute of some words indicating whether they refer to one (singular) or more than one (plural). (31B, 36B)

object A noun, pronoun, or group of words that receives the action of the verb (*direct object;* 28M); tells to whom or for whom something is done (*indirect object;* 28M); or completes the meaning of a preposition (*object of a preposition;* 28H).

object complement A noun or adjective renaming or describing a direct object after certain verbs, including *call, consider, name, elect,* and *think:* Some *call* daily ***joggers*** [object] ***fanatics*** [object complement]. (28N)

objective case The case of a noun or pronoun functioning as a direct object, an indirect object, an object of a preposition, or a verbal. A few pronouns change form to show the objective case (for example, *him, her, whom*). Also see *case.* (30A)

opinion A statement open to debate. (3E)

outline A technique for laying out ideas for writing in an orderly fashion that shows levels of generality. An outline can be formal or informal. (5F)

overstatement Deliberate exaggeration for emphasis; also called *hyperbole.* (37H)

paragraph A group of sentences that work together to develop a unit of thought. (6B)

paragraph development Rhetorical strategies for arranging and organizing paragraphs using specific, concrete details (RENNS) to support a generalization in the paragraph. (6B, 6D, 6F)

parallelism The use of equivalent grammatical forms or matching sentence structures to express equivalent ideas: *singing* and *dancing.* (6G, Ch. 39)

paraphrase A restatement of a source's ideas in language and sentence structure different from that of the original. (18C)

parenthetical documentation Citation of source information enclosed in parentheses that follows quoted, paraphrased, or summarized material from another source. Such citations alert readers that the material comes from a source other than the writer. Parenthetical documentation and a list of bibliographic information at the end of a source-based paper together document the writer's use of sources. (Chs. 25 and 26)

participial phrase A phrase that contains a present participle or a past participle and any modifiers and that functions as an adjective. Also see *verbal.* (28O, 38P)

participle A verb form that indicates the present tense (*-ing* ending) or the past tense (*-ed, -d, -n,* or *-t* ending). A participle can also function as an adjective or an adverb. Also see *present participle, past participle.* (Ch. 29)

parts of speech The names and definitions of types of words that give you a vocabulary for identifying words and understanding how language works to create meaning. (28A–28J)

passive voice The *passive voice* emphasizes the action, in contrast to the *active voice,* which emphasizes the doer of the action. If the subject is mentioned in the sentence, it usually appears as the object of the preposition *by: I was frightened by the thunder* (the active voice form is *The thunder frightened me*). (29N)

past participle The third principal part of a verb, the past participle is formed in regular verbs by adding *-d* or *-ed* to the simple form to create the past tense. In irregular verbs, past and past participle formation varies by adding a letter or two to the simple form: *break, broke, broken*. The past participle functions as a verb only with an auxiliary verb as its partner. (29B)

past perfect progressive tense The past-perfect-tense form that describes an ongoing condition in the past that has been ended by something stated in the sentence: *Before the curtains caught fire,* ***I had been talking***. (29J)

past perfect tense The tense that describes a condition or action that started in the past, continued for a while, and then ended in the past: *I had talked to him before*. (29I)

past progressive tense The past-tense form that shows the continuing nature of a past action: *I was talking when you walked in*. (29J)

past subjunctive The simple past tense in the subjunctive mood. (29M)

past-tense verb The second principal part of a verb. In regular verbs, the past tense is formed by adding *-d* or *-ed* to the simple form. In irregular verbs, the formation of the past tense varies from merely adding a letter or two to the simple form: *break, broke; see, saw*. (29B)

peer-response group Groups of students in your class who gather together to read and constructively react to each other's writing. (9C)

perfect tenses The three tenses—the present perfect (*I have talked*), the past perfect (*I had talked*), and the future perfect (*I will have talked*)—that help to show complex time relationships between two clauses. (29I)

periodic sentence A sentence that begins with modifiers and ends with the independent clause, thus postponing the main idea—and the emphasis—for the end; also called a *climactic sentence*. (38O)

periodicals Magazines, newspapers, and journals published on a regular basis. (22G)

person The attribute of nouns and pronouns showing who or what acts or experiences an action. *First person* is the one speaking (*I, we*); *second person* is the one being spoken to (*you*); and *third person* is the person or thing spoken about (*he, she, it, they*). All nouns are third person. (31B, 36B)

personal pronoun A pronoun that refers to people or things: *I, you, them, it*. (30B)

personality The sense of the writer that comes through his or her writing; for example, friendly, bossy, shy, assertive, concerned, angry, and so on. (37D)

personification Assigning a human trait to something not human. (37H)

persuasive appeal Rhetorical strategies which appeal to the emotions, logic, or ethics of readers. (3B)

persuasive writing Writing that seeks to convince the reader about a matter of opinion. It is also known as *argumentative writing*. (Ch. 15)

phrasal verb A verb that combines with one or more prepositions to deliver its meaning: *ask* ***out***, *look* ***into***. (55C)

phrase A group of related words that does not contain a subject and predicate and thus cannot stand alone as an independent grammatical unit. A phrase can function as a noun, a verb, or a modifier. (28O)

plagiarism A writer's presenting another person's words or ideas without giving credit to that person. Writers use documentation systems to give proper credit to sources in standardized ways recognized by scholarly communities. Plagiarism is a serious offense, a form of intellectual dishonesty that can lead to course failure or expulsion from an institution. (Ch. 19)

planning Early part of the writing process in which writers gather ideas. (5A)

plural See *number*.

podcasts Brief sound files that are shared over the Internet, somewhat like online radio broadcasts. (63E)

point of view The perspective from which a piece is written. (3E)

possessive case The case of a noun or pronoun that shows ownership or possession. Also see *case*. (30A, 45A)

possessive pronoun A pronoun that shows ownership: *his, hers*, and so on. (45C)

predicate The part of a sentence that contains the verb and tells what the subject is doing or experiencing or what is being done to the subject. A *simple predicate* contains only the main verb and any auxiliary verb(s). A *complete predicate* contains the verb, its modifiers, objects, and other related words. A *compound predicate* contains two or more verbs, modifiers, objects, and other related words. (28L)

prediction A major activity of the *reading process*, in which the reader guesses what comes next. (3D)

premises In a deductive argument expressed as a syllogism, statements presenting the conditions of the argument from which the conclusion must follow. (3H)

prefix Letters added at the beginning of a root word to create a new word: ***pre**test*. (47H, 51C)

preposition A word that conveys a relationship, often of space or time, between the noun or pronoun following it and other words in the sentence: *under, over, in, out*. The noun or pronoun following a preposition is called the *object of the preposition*. (28H, Ch. 55)

prepositional phrase A group of words beginning with a preposition and including a noun or pronoun, which is called the *object of the preposition*. (28O)

presentation style The way you deliver what you have to say. Memorization, reading, mapping, and speaking with notes are different types of presentation styles. (62F)

present infinitive Names or describes an activity or occurrence coming together either at the same time or after the time expressed in the main verb. (29G)

present participle A verb's *-ing* form: *talking, singing*. Used with auxiliary verbs, present participles function as main verbs. Used without auxiliary verbs, present participles function as nouns or adjectives. (29B)

present perfect progressive tense The present-perfect-tense form that describes something ongoing in the past that is likely to continue into the future: *I have been talking for a while*. (29J)

present perfect tense The tense indicating that an action or its effects, begun or perhaps completed in the past, continue into the present: *I had talked to her before you arrived*. (29I)

present progressive tense The present-tense form of the verb that indicates something taking place at the time it is written or spoken about: *I am talking right now to her*. (29J)

present subjunctive The simple form of the verb for all persons and numbers in the subjunctive mood. (29M)

present tense The tense that describes what is happening, what is true at the moment, and/or what is consistently true. It uses the simple form (*I talk*) and the *-s* form in the third-person singular (*he talks, she talks, it talks*). (29G)

present-tense participial phrase A verbal phrase that uses the *-ing* form of a verb and functions only as a modifier (whereas a gerund phrase functions only as a noun). (28O)

primary sources Also called *primary evidence*, these sources are "firsthand" work such as written accounts of experiments and observations by the researchers who conducted them; taped accounts, interviews, and newspaper accounts by direct observers; autobiographies, diaries, and journals; and expressive works such as poems, plays, fiction, and essays. They stand in contrast to *secondary sources.* (21B)

process writing Presents instructions, lays out steps in a procedure, explains how objects work, or describes human behaviors. (6H, Ch. 12)

progressive forms Verb forms made, in all tenses, with the present participle and forms of the verb *be* as an auxiliary. Progressive forms show that an action, occurrence, or state of being is ongoing: *I am singing; he was dancing.* (29J)

pronoun A word that takes the place of a noun and functions in the same ways that nouns do. Types of pronouns are demonstrative, indefinite, intensive, interrogative, personal, reciprocal, reflexive, and relative. (28C)

pronoun–antecedent agreement The match required between a pronoun and its antecedent in number and person, including personal pronouns and their gender. (31O)

pronoun case The way a pronoun changes form to reflect its use as the agent of action (*subjective case*), the thing being acted upon (*objective case*), or the thing showing ownership (*possessive case*). (30A–30K)

pronoun reference The relationship between a pronoun and its antecedent. (30L–30S)

proofreading The act of reading a final draft to find and correct any spelling or mechanical mistakes, typing errors, or handwriting illegibility; the final step of the writing process. (5K)

proper noun A noun that names specific people, places, or things; it is always capitalized: *Tom Thumb, Buick.* (48E)

proposal or solution essays A piece of writing intended to persuade readers that a particular problem is best solved by the solution explained in that writing. (16A)

purpose Purposes for writing vary: to narrate, give information, analyze a text, argue or persuade, and evaluate. (4B)

quotation Repeating or reporting another person's words. *Direct quotation* repeats another's words exactly and encloses them in quotation marks. *Indirect quotation* reports another's words without quotation marks except around any words if they are repeated exactly from the source. Both direct and indirect quotation require documentation of the source to avoid plagiarism. (18B)

readers Readers are the audiences for writing; readers process material they read on the literal, inferential, and evaluative levels. (4C)

reciprocal pronoun The pronouns *each other* and *one another* referring to individual parts of a plural antecedent. (28C)

References The title of a list of sources at the end of a research paper or scholarly article or other written work used in many documentation styles, especially that of APA. (Ch. 26)

reflexive pronoun A pronoun that ends in *-self* and that reflects back to its antecedent: *They claim to support* ***themselves.*** (30K)

regular verb A verb that forms its past tense and past participle by adding *-ed* or *-d* to the simple form. Most English verbs are regular. (29D)

relative adverb An adverb that introduces an adjective clause: *The garage* ***where I usually park my car*** *was full.* (28G)

relative clause See *adjective clause.*

relative pronoun A pronoun—such as *who, which, that, whom, whoever,* and a few others—that introduces an adjective clause or sometimes a noun clause. (28P)

RENNS A memory aid for the specific, concrete details used to support a topic sentence in a paragraph: reasons, examples, names, numbers and the five sentences. (6F)

research A systematic process of gathering information to answer a question. (21A)

research log A diary of your research process; useful for keeping yourself organized and on track. (21G)

research or term paper A paper written using the results of research. (21C)

research question A question that provides a clear focus for your research and a goal for your writing process. (21F)

response essay Provides a summary of a source and gives your opinion—supported by reasons—about the source's ideas or quality. (20C)

restrictive clause A dependent clause that gives information necessary to distinguish whatever it modifies from others in the same category. In contrast to a nonrestrictive clause, a restrictive clause is not set off with commas. (30S)

restrictive element A word, phrase, or dependent clause that provides information essential to the understanding of the element it modifies. In contrast to a nonrestrictive element, a restrictive element is not set off with commas. Also see *nonrestrictive clause.* (42F)

revising A part of the writing process in which writers evaluate their rough drafts and, on the basis of their assessments, rewrite by adding, cutting, replacing, moving, and often totally recasting material. (5I)

rhetoric The art and skill of speaking and writing effectively. (6I)

rhetorical patterns Various techniques for presenting ideas to deliver a writer's intended message with clarity and impact, including logical, ethical, and emotional appeals. (3B) Rhetorical strategies involve stylistic techniques such as parallelism and planned repetition as well as patterns for organizing and developing writing such as illustration, description, and definition. (6H)

Rogerian argument An argument technique using principles developed by Carl Rogers in which writers strive to find common ground and thus assure readers who disagree with them that they understand others' perspectives. (15A)

role The position the writer is emphasizing for a given task; for example, student, client, taxpayer, parent, supervisor, helper, critic, or so on.

root The base part of a word; ***use****less.* (47H)

run-on sentence A sentence in which independent clauses run together without the required punctuation that marks them as complete units. Also known as a *fused sentence.* (Ch. 34)

sans serif Font types that do not have little "feet" or finishing lines at the top and bottom of each letter. (7C)

search engine An Internet-specific software program that can look through all files on Internet sites. (22C)

search strategy A systematic way of finding information on a certain topic. (21K)

secondary source A source that reports, analyzes, discusses, reviews, or otherwise deals with the work of someone else. It stands in contrast to a primary source, which is someone's original work or firsthand report. A reliable secondary source must be the work of a person with appropriate credentials, must appear in a respected publication or other medium, must be current or historically authentic, and must reflect logical reasoning. (21B)

second person See *person.*

sentence A group of words, beginning with a capitalized first word and ending with a final punctuation mark, that states, asks, commands, or exclaims something. A sentence must consist of at least one *independent clause.* A *simple sentence* consists of one independent clause. A *complex sentence* contains one independent clause and one or more dependent clauses. A *compound sentence* contains two or more independent clauses joined by a coordinating conjunction. A *compound-complex sentence* contains at least two independent clauses and one or more dependent clauses. (28K–28Q)

sentence fragment A portion of a sentence that is punctuated as though it were a complete sentence. (Ch. 33)

sentence outline A type of outline in which each element is a sentence. (5F)

sentence variety Writing sentences of various lengths and structures; see *coordinate sentence, cumulative sentence, periodic sentence, sentence.* (38B)

serif Font types that are characterized by little "feet" or finishing lines at the top and bottom of each letter. (7C)

server A computer that is always online and available to Internet users. (63F)

sexist language Language that unfairly or unnecessarily assigns roles or characteristics to people on the basis of gender. Language that avoids gender stereotyping is called *gender-neutral* or *nonsexist language.* (37I)

shift An unnecessary change within a sentence in person, number, voice, tense, or other grammatical framework that makes a sentence unclear. (36A–36E)

short quotation A direct quotation that occupies no more than four lines of type in an MLA-style source-based paper (for prose) or no more than three lines of poetry. In an APA-style source-based paper, a short quotation has no more than forty words of prose. Short quotations are enclosed in quotation marks. (46B)

simile A comparison, using *like* or *as*, of otherwise dissimilar things. (37H)

simple form Part of a verb, the simple form shows action, occurrence, or state of being taking place in the present. It is used in the singular for first and second person and in the plural for first, second, and third person. Simple forms divide time into past, present, and future. (29B, 29G)

simple predicate See *predicate.*

simple sentence See *sentence.*

simple subject See *subject.*

simple tenses The present, past, and future tenses, which divide time into present, past, and future. (29G)

singular See *number.*

slang Coined words and new meanings for existing words, which quickly pass in and out of use. Slang is inappropriate for most academic writing except when used intentionally as such. See *colloquial language.*

slanted language Language that tries to manipulate the reader with distorted facts. (37J)

source A print or online book, article, document, CD, other work, or person providing information in words, music, pictures, or other media. (21B)

specialized database A database of sources covering a specific discipline or topic. (22C)

specialized reference work A reference work (such as a dictionary, encyclopedia, biographical compendium) covering a specific discipline or topic. (22H)

specific noun A noun understood to be exactly and specifically referred to; uses the definite article *the.* (53A)

split infinitive One or more words coming between the two words of an infinitive. (35B)

squinting modifier A modifier that is considered misplaced because it isn't clear whether it describes the word that comes before it or the word that follows it. (35A)

standard edited English Written usage of the American English language, expected in academic writing, that conforms to mainstream rules of grammar, sentence structure, punctuation, spelling, and mechanics. Sometimes it is referred to as *standard English,* but given the diversity of dialects in the United States today, the term *standard* is less descriptive than it once was. (37B)

standard word order The most common sentence pattern in English, which places the subject before the verb. (38R, Ch. 54)

stereotype A kind of hasty generalization (a *logical fallacy*) in which a sweeping claim is made about all members of a particular ethnic, racial, religious, gender, age, or political group. (37I)

style The manner in which a writer expresses his or her ideas. (37A)

subject The word or group of words in a sentence that acts, is acted upon, or is described by the verb. A *simple subject* includes only the noun or pronoun. A *complete subject* includes the noun or pronoun and all its modifiers. A *compound subject* includes two or more nouns or pronouns and their modifiers. (28L)

subject complement A noun or adjective that follows a linking verb, renaming or describing the subject of the sentence. (28N)

subject directories Lists of topics or resources and services, with links to sources on those topics and resources. An alternative to keyword searches. (22E)

subjective case The case of the noun or pronoun functioning as a subject. Also see *case*. (30A)

subject–verb agreement The required match in number and person between a subject and a verb. (31B–31N)

subjunctive mood The verb orientation that expresses wishes, recommendations, indirect requests, speculations, and conditional statements: *I wish you were here*. (29L)

subordinate clause See *dependent clause*.

subordinating conjunction A conjunction that introduces a dependent clause and expresses a relationship between the word and the idea in the independent clause. (28I)

subordination The use of grammatical structures to reflect the relative importance of ideas in a sentence. The most important information falls in the independent clause, and less important information falls in the dependent clause or phrases. (38D)

suffix Letters added at the end of a root word to change function or meaning: ***useless***. (47H, 51C)

summary A critical thinking activity to extract the main message or central point of a passage or other discourse. (18D)

superlative The form of an adjective or adverb that expresses the greatest degree of quality among three or more things: *bluest; most easily*. (32E)

syllogism The structure of a deductive argument expressed in two *premises* and a *conclusion*. The first premise is a general assumption or statement of fact. The second premise is a different assumption or statement of fact based on evidence. The conclusion is also a specific instance that follows logically from the premises. (3H)

synonym A word that is close in meaning to another word. (5J)

synthesis A component of critical thinking in which material that has been summarized, analyzed, and interpreted is connected to what one already knows (one's prior knowledge) from reading or experiences. (3F)

tag sentence An inverted verb–pronoun combination added to the end of a sentence that "asks" the audience to agree with the assertion in the first part of the sentence: *You know what a tag question is,* ***don't you?*** A tag is set off from the rest of the sentence with a comma. (42G)

tense The time at which the action of the verb occurs: in the present, the past, or the future. (29G)

tense sequence In sentences that have more than one clause, the sequencing of verb forms to reflect logical time relationships. (29K)

thesis statement A statement of an essay's central theme that makes clear the main idea, the writer's purpose, the focus of the topic, and perhaps the organizational pattern. (5E)

third person See *person*.

title The part of an essay that clarifies the overall point of the piece of writing. It can be *direct* or *indirect*. (5I)

tone The quality, feeling, or attitude that a writer expresses. (37A)

topic The subject of discourse. (5C)

topic outline An outline in which items are listed as words or phrases, not full sentences. (5F)

topic sentence The sentence that expresses the main idea of a paragraph. (6E)

Toulmin model A model that defines the essential parts of an argument as the *claim* (or *main point*), the *support* (or *evidence*), and the *warrants* (or *assumptions behind the main point*). (15B)

transition The word or group of words that connects one idea to another in discourse. Useful strategies for creating transitions include transitional expressions, conjunctive adverbs, parallelism, and planned repetition of key words and phrases. (6G)

transitional expressions Words and phrases that signal connections among ideas and create coherence. (6G)

transitive verb A verb that must be followed by a direct object. (29F)

understatement Figurative language in which the writer uses deliberate restraint for emphasis. (37H)

unity The clear and logical relationship between the main idea of a paragraph and the evidence supporting the main idea. As a design principle, the term refers to whether the elements (color, text, images) work together visually. (7B)

URL *URL* is the abbreviation for *Universal* (or *Uniform*) *Resource Locator*. It is the online address of a site or page on the Web. (22C)

unstated assumptions Premises that are implied but not stated. (3E)

usage A customary way of using language. (37F)

valid Correctly and rationally derived; applied to a deductive argument whose conclusion follows logically from the premises. Validity applies to the structure of an argument, not its truth. (3H)

verb A word that shows action or occurrence, or that describes a state of being. Verbs change form to show time (tense), attitude (mood), and role of the subject (voice). Verbs occur in the predicate of a clause. Verbs can be parts of verb phrases, which consist of a main verb, any auxiliary verbs, and any modifiers. Verbs can be described as transitive or intransitive, depending on whether they take a direct object. (28D, Ch. 29)

verb phrase A main verb, along with any auxiliary verb(s) and any modifiers. (28O)

verbal A verb form that functions as a noun, adjective, or adverb. (28E)

verbal phrase A group of words that contains a verbal (an infinitive, participle, or gerund) and its modifiers. (28O)

voice Attribute of verbs showing whether the subject acts (active voice) or is acted upon (passive voice). (29N)

warrants The writer's underlying assumptions, which are often implied rather than stated, that connect reasons to claims. (15B)

Web site A collection of related files online that may include documents, images, audio, and video. Web sites typically have a *home page* that provides links to this content. (22C, 63F)

wiki A Web site that allows multiple readers to change its content. (63C)

wordiness Writing that is full of words and phrases that don't contribute to meaning. The opposite of *conciseness*. (Ch. 40)

word order The order in which words fall in most English sentences. Usually, the subject comes before the predicate. Inverted word order can bring emphasis to an idea. Multilingual writers are often accustomed to word orders in sentences other than those used in English. (Ch. 54)

working bibliography A preliminary annotated list of useful sources in research writing with a brief summary of each source. (21M)

Works Cited In MLA documentation style, the list of standardized information about all sources drawn upon in a research paper or other scholarly written work. (Ch. 25)

writer's block The desire to start writing, but not being able to do so. (5I)

writing portfolio A collection of written works, often the final project of a writing course. (8A)

writing process Stages of writing in which a writer plans, drafts, revises, edits, and proofreads. The stages often overlap. (5A)

writing situation Elements for writers to consider at the beginning of the writing process: their writing topic, purpose, audience, context, role, and special requirements. (5C)

CREDITS

TEXT

Page 7: From "Harmony and the Dream" by David Brooks from *The New York Times*, August 12, 2008. Copyright © 2008 by The New York Times. www.nytimes.com. All rights reserved. Used by permission and protected by the Copyright Laws of the United States. The printing, copying, redistribution, or retransmission of this Content without express written permission is prohibited; **Figure 3.1:** Screenshot of Doctors Without Borders web page. Reprinted by permission of Doctors Without Borders; **page 49:** From "Diamonds" from *Mammoth Book of Fascinating Information* by Richard B. Manchester, 1980, A&W Visual Books; **pages 50–51:** Excerpt from "Give Students Broad Education, Not Narrow Vocational Tracks." Reprinted by permission of Debra Humphreys; **pages 51–52:** From "Trees Are Living Archives" by James S. Trefil, *Smithsonian*, July 1985, pp 46–54. Copyright © 1985. Reprinted by permission of James S. Trefil; **page 52:** From *The Economics of Attention* by Richard Lanham. Copyright © 2007 by The University of Chicago Press; **page 87:** From *Why Don't Students Like School?: A Cognitive Scientist Answers Questions About How the Mind Works and What It Means for the Classroom* by Daniel T. Willingham, 2009, John Wiley & Sons, Inc.; **page 88:** From "Nothing About These Women Is Real," by Abigail Haworth, *Marie Claire*, July 2005. Copyright © 2005. Reprinted by permission of Abigail Haworth; **page 89, top:** From "Composers and Patrons in the Classical Era" from *Understanding Music*, 3rd Edition, by Jeremy Yudkin. Copyright © 2002. Reprinted by permission of Pearson Education, Upper Saddle River, NJ; **page 89, bottom:** From *Gestures: The Do's and Taboos of Body Language around the World* by Roger E. Axtell, 1998, John Wiley & Sons, Inc.; **page 90:** Excerpt from *Three Uses of the Knife: On the Nature and Purpose of Drama* by David Mamet. Copyright © 1989 by Columbia University Press; **page 93:** Excerpt from *The Relaxation Response* by Herbert Benson, MD, with Miriam Z. Klipper. Copyright © 1975 by William Morrow & Company. Reprinted by permission of HarperCollins Publishers; **page 95:** Excerpt from "Clean House: Getting Laid Off from His Job Gave This Franchisee a Fresh Start" by Sara Wilson from *Entrepreneur*, August 2005; **pages 95–96:** From "The Study of Humanity" from *Cultural Anthropology* by Nancy Bonvillain. Copyright © 2006. Reprinted by permission of Pearson Education, Upper Saddle River, NJ; **page 97:** From "Depth of Field" by Susan Howard from *Newsday*, January 1, 1991. Copyright © 1991 by Newsday, Inc. Reprinted by permission of Newsday, Inc. www.newsday.com; **page 99:** From "Magic by the Numbers" by Daniel Gilbert from *The New York Times*, October 17, 2010. Copyright © 2010 by The New York Times. www.nytimes.com. All rights reserved. Used by permission and protected by the laws of the United States. The printing, copying, redistribution, or retransmission of this Content without express written permission is prohibited; **page 100, top:** From *The Hard Truth about Soft Skills* by Peggy Klaus, © 2007, HarperCollins Publishers; **page 100, mid:** From *Masterworks: A Musical Discovery*, 1st Edition by D. Kern Holoman. Copyright © 1998. Reprinted by permission of Pearson Education, Upper Saddle River, NJ; **page 102:** From *The Language of Clothes* by Alison Lurie, © 1981; **page 103:** From *You Just Don't Understand* by Deborah Tannen. Copyright © 1990 by Deborah Tannen. Reprinted by permission of HarperCollins Publishers; **page 168:** Act Now page from We Won't Fly.com. Reprinted by permission of www.WeWontFly.com; **pages 205 and 206:** From *Alone Together: Why We Expect More from Technology and Less from Each Other* by Sherry Turkle, © 2001, Basic Books; **page 207:** From

"Times of Our Lives" by Karen Wright from *Scientific American*, September 2002; **page 210:** From "Post-Teenage Wasteland?" by Ann Hulbert, © 2005, *The New York Times Magazine;* **pages 217–218:** From "Too Many Choices" from *Consumer Reports on Health* by Ronni Sandoff; **Figure 21.4:** Screenshot from NoodleTools. Copyright © NoodleTools, Inc., http:///www.NoodleTools.com. Permission is given to reproduce this as a handout for teaching or training purposes; **Figure 21.5:** Screenshot from Diigo.com. Reprinted by permission of Diigo.com; **Figure 22.1:** Home Page of Arapahoe Community College Library. Photo courtesy of Lisa Grabowski. Reprinted by permission of Arapahoe Community College; **Figure 22.2:** PsycINFO search, reprinted with permission of the American Psychological Association, publisher of the PsycINFO ® Database. Copyright © 2005. All rights reserved. For more information, contact PsycINFO@apa.org; **Figure 22.3:** EBSCO Research search engine, copyright © 2012 by EBSCO Publishing, Inc. All rights reserved; **Figures 22.6, 22.7, 22.8, and 22.9:** Reprinted by permission of the University of Denver; **Figures 22.10 and 23.1a and b:** Courtesy of Google; **Figures 23.1c and d:** EBSCO Research Engine, Copyright © 2005 by EBSCO Publishing, Inc. All rights reserved; **Figure 25.2:** From "In the Name of Citizenship: The Writing Classroom and the Promise of Citizenship," by Amy J.Wan from *College English*, Volume 74, Number 1, September 2011. Copyright © 2011 by the National Council of Teachers of English. Reprinted by permission of National Council of Teachers of English; **Figure 25.8:** Screenshot of "What Predicts Crime?" by Andrew Sullivan from "The Dish: Biased and Balanced" from *The Daily Beast*, February 21, 2012. Reprinted by permission of The Newsweek/Daily Beast Company LLC. All rights reserved; **page 567:** From "If Only the Pilgrims Had Been Italian" by Thomas J. Craughwell from *The American Spectator*, November 21, 2007. Reprinted by permission of *The American Spectator;* **pages 568–569:** From "Google's Tar Pit" by Joshua Green from *The Atlantic*, December 2007. Reprinted by permission of *The Atlantic*.

PHOTOS

Page 3: © ImageZoo/Alamy; **page 4:** StockbrokerXtra/AGE Fotostock America; **page 7:** © Arco Images GmbH/Alamy; **page 9, top:** © Ian Shaw/Alamy; **page 9, bottom:** Susan Montgomery/Shutterstock; **page 19:** Doctors Without Borders/ Medecins San Frontieres (MSF). South Sudan © Jean-Marc Jacobs; **page 40:** Douglas Hesse; **page 42:** Paul Conklin/Taxi/Getty Images; **page 43, top:** Peter Vadnai; **page 43, bottom:** James McConnachie/Rough Guides/DK Images; **page 44:** Ad Council; **page 45, top:** Ad Council; **page 45, bottom:** Ad Council; **page 48:** Douglas Hesse; **page 108:** Douglas Hesse; **page 112, top:** Douglas Hesse; **page 112, bottom:** Douglas Hesse; **page 113:** Douglas Hesse; **page 116:** Douglas Hesse; **page 120:** Douglas Hesse; **page 330:** MIT Press; **page 763:** AP Images; **page 781:** Douglas Hesse.

INDEX

PROOFREADING MARKS AND RESPONSE SYMBOLS

Your instructor might use response symbols to show where writing should be edited or revised. You can use proofreading marks on hard copy for editing or revision.

PROOFREADING MARKS

- **delete** — take ~~this~~ this out
- ¶ **new paragraph** — This is the end. ¶ This is a new beginning.
- **transpose letters** — transpoes letters
- **transpose words** — words transpose
- ^ **insert** — A ^ signals an addition (caret)
- # **add space** — addspace
- **close up space** — clo se up space
- (SP) **spell out** — They live in (WI.) SP
- rom **use roman type** — That sounds *(silly.)* rom
- ital **use italic type** — Washington Post ital
- (cap) **use capital letters** — anne tyler cap
- (lc) **use lowercase letters** — Drive North and then East. lc

RESPONSE SYMBOLS

ab	abbreviation error	686–690
ad	adjective or adverb error	519–527
ca	pronoun case error	486–495
cap	needs a capital letter	677–683
cl	revise a cliché	578–579
coh	needs coherence	92–97
coord	faulty coordination	585–586, 592–593
cs	comma splice	537–546
dev	needs development	85, 91–104
dm	dangling modifier	550–551
e	needs exact language	573–574
emph	needs emphasis	583, 593–597
frag	sentence fragment	527–537
hyph	hyphen needed	674–676, 693
inc	incomplete sentence	527–537
ital	italics error	683–686
k	awkward	546–551
lc	needs lowercase letter	677–683
mixed	mixed construction	557–561
mm	misplaced modifier	546–550
¶	new paragraph	85–104
no ¶	no new paragraph	85–104
//	faulty parallelism	598–604
pass	passive voice	485–486
pl	faulty plural	694–695
pro agr	pronoun agreement error	514–519
pro ref	pronoun reference error	495–502
p	punctuation error	616–676
,/	comma error	620–639
;/	semicolon error	640–644
:/	colon error	645–649
’/	apostrophe error	649–654
“/”	quotation marks error	655–663
rep	too much repetition	609
shift	sentence shift	552–557
sl	revise slang	572
sp	spelling error	693–703
subord	subordination error	586–593
sxt	sexist language	517, 576–578
t, tense	verb tense error	475–482
trans	needs transition	93–95, 104
u	needs unity	92–97
us	usage error	UG-1–UG-11
v	verb form error	465–475
v agr	verb agreement error	503–514
var	needs sentence variety	582–597
w	wordy	605–613
wc	word choice error	571–574
ww	wrong word	564–582

Detailed Contents